The Parathyroids
Basic and Clinical Concepts

Editor-in-Chief

John P. Bilezikian, M.D.
Professor of Medicine and Pharmacology
Chief, Division of Endocrinology
Director, Metabolic Bone Diseases Program
Departments of Medicine and Pharmacology
College of Physicians and Surgeons
Columbia University
New York, New York

Associate Editors

Robert Marcus, M.D.
Professor of Medicine
Department of Medicine
Stanford University School of Medicine
Stanford, California; and
Director, Aging Study Unit
Veterans Affairs Medical Center
Palo Alto, California

Michael A. Levine, M.D.
Professor of Medicine
Departments of Medicine and Pathology
Johns Hopkins University School of Medicine
Baltimore, Maryland

Raven Press  New York

Raven Press, 1185 Avenue of the Americas, New York, New York 10036

Made in the United States of America

Library of Congress Cataloging-in-Publication Data

The Parathyroids : basic & clinical concepts / editor-in-chief, John
  P. Bilezikian, associate editors, Robert Marcus, Michael A. Levine.
      p.   cm.
    Includes bibliographical references and index.
    ISBN 0-7817-0017-5
    1. Parathyroid glands—Diseases. 2. Parathyroid glands—
Pathophysiology. 3. Parathyroid glands—Physiology.
    4. Parathyroid hormone. 5. Parathyroid hormone-related protein.
    I. Bilezikian, John P. II. Marcus, Robert, 1940–   . III. Levine,
Michael A., 1950–   .
    [DNLM: 1. Parathyroid Diseases—physiopathology. 2. Parathyroid
Diseases—therapy. 3. Parathyroid Glands—physiology.
    4. Parathyroid Hormones—physiology.   WK 300 P2239 1193]
    RC655.P35 1993
    616.4′45—dc20
    DNLM/DLC
    for Library of Congress   93-4126
                                                                 CIP

The material contained in this volume was submitted as previously
unpublished material, except in the instances in which credit has been given
to the source from which some of the illustrative material was derived.

Great care has been taken to maintain the accuracy of the information
contained in the volume. However, neither Raven Press nor the editors can
be held responsible for errors or for any consequences arising from the use of
the information contained herein.

Materials appearing in this book prepared by individuals as part of their
official duties as U.S. Government employees are not covered by the above-
mentioned copyright.

9 8 7 6 5 4 3 2 1

The Parathyroids
Basic and Clinical Concepts

Contents

Section I: Basic Concepts of the Parathyroids

Anatomy and Physiology

Parathyroid Hormone: Structure, Function, Receptors, Mechanisms of Action

Causes and Management of Hypercalcemia Due to Parathyroid Hormone-Related Protein and Other Factors

Section II: Clinical Concepts of the Parathyroids

The Hyperparathyroid States

Contributing Authors

Andrea Amorosi, M.D.
Endocrine Section
Department of Clinical Physiopathology
University of Florence Medical School
Viale Pieraccini 6
50139 Florence, Italy

Andrew Arnold, M.D.
Endocrine Unit
Laboratory of Endocrine Oncology
Harvard Medical School
Massachusetts General Hospital
50 Blossom Street
Boston, Massachusetts 02114

Jane E. Aubin, Ph.D.
M.R.C. Group in Periodontal Physiology
Faculty of Dentistry
University of Toronto
Medical Sciences Building
8 Taddle Creek Road
Toronto, Ontario M5S 1A8, Canada

Allen E. Bale, M.D.
Department of Genetics
Yale University School of Medicine
333 Cedar Street
New Haven, Connecticut 06510

Carlton G. Bellows, Ph.D.
M.R.C. Group in Periodontal Physiology
Faculty of Dentistry
University of Toronto
Medical Sciences Building
8 Taddle Creek Road
Toronto, Ontario M5S 1A8, Canada

John P. Bilezikian, M.D.
Departments of Medicine and
  Pharmacology
College of Physicians and Surgeons
Columbia University
630 West 168th Street, P&S 9-410
New York, New York 10032

Karen Shipp Black, M.D.
Department of Medicine
Division of Endocrinology
University of Texas Health Science Center
7703 Floyd Curl Drive
San Antonio, Texas 78284

Maria-Luisa Brandi, M.D., Ph.D.
Endocrine Section
Department of Clinical Physiopathology
University of Florence Medical School
Viale Pieraccini 6
50139 Florence, Italy

Murray F. Brennan, M.D., F.R.A.C.S.,
  F.A.C.S
Department of Surgery
Memorial Sloan-Kettering Cancer Center
1275 York Avenue
New York, New York 10025

F. Richard Bringhurst, M.D.
Endocrine Unit
Department of Medicine
Harvard Medical School
Masssachusetts General Hospital
Fruit Street
Boston, Massachusetts 02114

Arthur E. Broadus, M.D., Ph.D.
Department of Internal Medicine
Yale University School of Medicine
333 Cedar Street
New Haven, Connecticut 06510

Edward M. Brown, M.D.
Department of Medicine
Endocrine-Hypertension Division
Brigham and Women's Hospital
221 Longwood Avenue
Boston, Massachusetts 02115

Ernesto Canalis, M.D.
Departments of Medicine and Orthopedics
University of Connecticut School of
*   Medicine*
Farmington, Connecticut 06032; and
Department of Research
St. Francis Hospital and Medical Center
114 Woodland Street
Hartford, Connecticut 06105

Robert E. Canfield, M.D.
Department of Medicine
Irving Center for Clinical Research
College of Physicians and Surgeons
Columbia University
622 West 168th Street-PH10
New York, New York 10032

Lewis R. Chase, M.D.
Department of Medicine
Washington University School of Medicine
St. Louis Veterans Affairs Medical Center
St. Louis, Missouri 63106

Michael Chorev, Ph.D.
Department of Pharmaceutical Chemistry
The Hebrew University of Jerusalem
Faculty of Medicine
Jerusalem, 91120, Israel

Jack W. Coburn, M.D.
Departments of Medicine and Pediatrics
UCLA School of Medicine; and
Nephrology Section
West Los Angeles Veterans Affairs
*   Medical Center*
Wilshire and Sawtelle Boulevards
Los Angeles, California 90073

David V. Cohn, Ph.D.
Department of Biological and Biophysical
*   Sciences*
Health Sciences Center
University of Louisville
Louisville, Kentucky 40292

Daniel T. Coleman, Ph.D.
Department of Physiology and Biophysics
Mount Sinai School of Medicine
1 Gustave L. Levy Place
New York, New York 10029

Bess Dawson-Hughes, M.D.
Calcium and Bone Metabolism Laboratory
USDA Human Nutrition Research Center
*   on Aging*
Tufts University
711 Washington Street
Boston, Massachusetts 02111

Leonard J. Deftos, M.D.
Department of Medicine
University of California; and
San Diego Veterans Affairs Medical
*   Center*
3350 La Jolla Village Drive
San Diego, California 92161

David W. Dempster, Ph.D.
Department of Pathology
College of Physicians and Surgeons
Columbia University
630 West 168th Street
New York, New York 10032; and
Regional Bone Center
Helen Hayes Hospital
West Haverstraw, New York 10993

John L. Doppman, M.D.
Department of Radiology
National Institutes of Health
9000 Rockville Pike
Bethesda, Maryland 20892

Robert W. Downs, Jr., M.D.
Department of Medicine
Medical College of Virginia
Virginia Commonwealth University
Richmond, Virginia 23298

Richard C. Eastman, M.D.
Diabetes Branch
National Institute of Diabetes, Digestive,
*   and Kidney Diseases*
National Institutes of Health
9000 Rockville Pike
Bethesda, Maryland 20892

Brigitte H. Fasciotto, Ph.D.
Department of Biological and Biophysical
*   Sciences*
Health Sciences Center
University of Louisville
Louisville, Kentucky 40292

Murray J. Favus, M.D.
Department of Medicine
The University of Chicago
5841 South Maryland Avenue, MC 5100
Chicago, Illinois 60637

Lorraine A. Fitzpatrick, M.D.
Department of Medicine
Mayo Clinic and Mayo Foundation
5-164 West Joseph Building
Rochester, Minnesota 55905

Eitan Friedman, M.D.
Department of Clinical Genetics
Karolinska Hospital
S-10401 Stockholm, Sweden

Robert F. Gagel, M.D.
Section of Endocrinology
M. D. Anderson Cancer Center
1515 Holcombe Boulevard
Houston, Texas 77030

Flore Gartenberg, R.N.
Department of Medicine
Division of Endocrinology
College of Physicians and Surgeons
Columbia University
630 West 168th Street
New York, New York 10032

David Goltzman, M.D.
Departments of Medicine and Physiology
McGill University; and
Calcium Research Laboratory
Royal Victoria Hospital
687 Pine Avenue West
Montreal, Quebec, H3A 1A1, Canada

Sven-Ulrik Gorr, Ph.D.
Department of Biological and Biophysical
  Sciences
Health Sciences Center
University of Louisville
Louisville, Kentucky 40292

Vivian Grill, M.B.B.S., F.R.A.C.P.
Department of Medicine
University of Melbourne
St. Vincent's Hospital
41 Victoria Parade, Fitzroy
Melbourne, Victoria 3065, Australia

David A. Heath, M.B., Ch.B.
Department of Medicine
Selly Oak Hospital
Raddlebarn Road
Birmingham B15 2TH United Kingdom

Johan N. M. Heersche, B.Sc., Drs., Ph.D.
MRC Group in Periodontal Physiology
Faculty of Dentistry
Department of Pharmacology
University of Toronto
Room 4384 Medical Sciences Building
8 Taddle Creek Road
Toronto, Ontario M5S 1A8, Canada

Janet M. Hock, B.D.S., Ph.D.
Skeletal Diseases Research
Eli Lilly and Company
Lilly Research Laboratories, 0403
Indianapolis, Indiana 46285

Thomas P. Jacobs, M.D.
Department of Medicine
Division of Endocrinology
College of Physicians and Surgeons
Columbia University
630 West 168th Street
New York, New York 10032

Robert T. Jensen, M.D.
Digestive Diseases Branch
National Institute of Diabetes, Digestive,
  and Kidney Diseases
National Institutes of Health
9000 Rockville Pike
Bethesda, Maryland 20892

Tae-Sook Kim, R.N.
Department of Medicine
Division of Endocrinology
College of Physicians and Surgeons
Columbia University
630 West 168th Street
New York, New York 10032

Michael Kleerekoper, M.D.
Division of Endocrinology
Wayne State University School of
  Medicine
4201 St. Antoine, UHC-4H
Detroit, Michigan 48201

Vanessa A. Klugman, M.D.
Department of Medicine
The University of Chicago
5841 South Maryland Avenue, MC 5100
Chicago, Illinois 60637

Richard Kremer, M.D., Ph.D.
Department of Medicine
McGill University
Royal Victoria Hospital
687 Pine Avenue West
Montreal, Quebec, H3A 1A1, Canada

Henry M. Kronenberg, M.D.
Endocrine Unit
Department of Medicine
Harvard Medical School
Massachusetts General Hospital
Fruit Street
Boston, Massachusetts 02114

Catharina Larsson, M.D., Ph.D.
Department of Clinical Genetics
Karolinska Hospital
S-10401 Stockholm, Sweden

Michael A. Levine, M.D.
Departments of Medicine and Pathology
The Johns Hopkins University School of
* Medicine*
Ross Research Building
720 Rutland Avenue
Baltimore, Maryland 21205

Virginia A. LiVolsi, M.D.
Department of Pathology
Hospital of the University of Pennsylvania
3400 Spruce Street
Philadelphia, Pennsylvania 19104

Lawrence E. Mallette, M.D., Ph.D.
Division of Endocrinology and Metabolism
Baylor College of Medicine
1 Baylor Plaza
Houston, Texas 77030

Robert Marcus, M.D.
Department of Medicine
Stanford University School of Medicine
Stanford, California 94305; and
Aging Study Unit
Veterans Affairs Medical Center
3801 Miranda Avenue
Palo Alto, California 94304

T. John Martin, M.D., D.Sc., F.R.A.C.P.,
** F.R.C.P.A.**
Department of Medicine
University of Melbourne
St. Vincent's Hospital
41 Victoria Parade, Fitzroy
Melbourne, Victoria 3065, Australia

Kevin J. Martin, M.B., Ch.B.
Division of Nephrology
St. Louis University Medical Center
3635 Vista Avenue
St. Louis, Missouri 63110

Stephen J. Marx, M.D.
Genetics and Endocrinology Section
National Institute of Diabetes, Digestive,
* and Kidney Diseases*
National Institutes of Health
Building 10, Room 9C-101
Bethesda, Maryland 20892

David C. Metz, M.D.
Department of Medicine
Division of Gastroenterology
Hospital of the University of Pennsylvania
University of Pennsylvania
Philadelphia, Pennsylvania 19104

Arnold M. Moses, M.D.
Department of Medicine
University Hospital
State University of New York
750 East Adams Street
Syracuse, New York 13210

Gregory R. Mundy, M.D.
Department of Medicine
Division of Endocrinology
University of Texas Health Science Center
7703 Floyd Curl Drive
San Antonio, Texas 78284

Timothy M. Murray, M.D., F.R.C.P.(C)
Department of Medicine
University of Toronto
St. Michael's Hospital
Suite 212, 38 Shutter Street
Toronto, Ontario, M5B 1A6, Canada

Lynette Nieman, M.D.
Developmental Endocrinology Branch
National Institute of Child Health and
* Human Development*
National Institutes of Health
9000 Rockville Pike
Bethesda, Maryland 20892

Robert A. Nissenson, Ph.D.
Departments of Medicine and Physiology
University of California, San Francisco;
  and
Endocrine Unit
Veterans Affairs Medical Center
4150 Clement Street
San Francisco, California 94121

Jeffrey A. Norton, M.D.
Department of Surgery
Washington University School of Medicine
4960 Audubon Avenue, Box 8109
St. Louis, Missouri 63110

Samuel R. Nussbaum, M.D.
Endocrine Unit
Department of Medicine
Harvard Medical School
Massachusetts General Hospital
Fruit Street
Boston, Massachusetts 02114

J. L. H. O'Riordan, D.M., F.R.C.P.
Department of Metabolic Medicine
University College London
The Middlesex Hospital
Mortimer Street
London, W1N 8AA, United Kingdom

Charles Y. C. Pak, M.D.
Department of Internal Medicine
Division of Mineral Metabolism
University of Texas Southwestern Medical
  Center
5323 Harry Hines Boulevard
Dallas, Texas 75235

A. Michael Parfitt, M.D.
Bone and Mineral Research Laboratory
Henry Ford Hospital
2799 West Grand Boulevard
Detroit, Michigan 48202; and
Department of Medicine
University of Michigan
Ann Arbor, Michigan 48109

May Parisien, M.D.
Department of Pathology
College of Physicians and Surgeons
Columbia University
630 West 168th Street
New York, New York 10032; and
Regional Bone Center
Helen Hayes Hospital
West Haverstraw, New York 10993

John T. Potts, Jr., M.D.
Department of Medicine
Harvard Medical School
Massachusetts General Hospital
Fruit Street
Boston, Massachusetts 02114

Lawrence G. Raisz, M.D.
Department of Medicine
Division of Endocrinology
University of Connecticut Health Center
263 Farmington Avenue
Farmington, Connecticut 06032

Leticia G. Rao, Ph.D.
Department of Medicine
University of Toronto
St. Michael's Hospital
38 Shutter Street
Toronto, Ontario, M5B 1A6, Canada

Rene E. Rizzoli, M.D.
Division of Clinical Pathophysiology
Department of Medicine
University Hospital of Geneva
12211 Geneva 14, Switzerland

Michael Rosenblatt, M.D.
Division of Bone and Mineral Metabolism
Beth Israel Hospital
330 Brookline Avenue
Boston, Massachusetts 02215

Robert K. Rude, M.D.
Department of Medicine
University of Southern California
2025 Zonal Avenue
Los Angeles, California 90033

Kazushige Sakaguchi, M.D., Ph.D.
Bone Research Branch
National Institute of Dental Research
National Institutes of Health
9000 Rockville Pike, Building 30 Room 106
Bethesda, Maryland 20892

Isidro B. Salusky, M.D.
Departments of Medicine and Pediatrics
UCLA School of Medicine; and
Nephrology Section
West Los Angeles Veterans Affairs
  Medical Center
Wilshire and Sawtelle Boulevards
Los Angeles, California 90073

Arthur C. Santora II, M.D., Ph.D.
*Department of Endocrine and Metabolism
    Clinical Research*
Merck Research Laboratories
P.O. Box 2000, WBD-365
Rahway, New Jersey 07065

William F. Schwindinger, M.D., Ph.D.
Department of Medicine
*The Johns Hopkins University School of
    Medicine*
Ross Research Building
720 Rutland Avenue
Baltimore, Maryland 21205

Gino V. Segre, M.D.
Endocrine Unit
Department of Medicine
Harvard Medical School
Massachusetts General Hospital
Fruit Street
Boston, Massachusetts 02114

Elizabeth Shane, M.D.
Department of Medicine
Division of Endocrinology
College of Physicians and Surgeons
Columbia University
630 West 168th Street
New York, New York 10032

Louis M. Sherwood, M.D.
Medical and Scientific Affairs
US Human Health
Merck and Company
P.O. Box 4 Sumneytown Pike
West Point, Pennsylvania 19486; and
Department of Medicine
Albert Einstein College of Medicine
1300 Morris Park Avenue
Bronx, New York 10461

Shonni J. Silverberg, M.D.
Department of Medicine
Division of Endocrinology
College of Physicians and Surgeons
Columbia University
630 West 168th Street
New York, New York 10032

Frederick R. Singer, M.D.
*Osteoporosis and Metabolic Bone
    Diseases Program*
St. John's Hospital and Health Center
1328 22nd Street
Santa Monica, California 90404

Ethel S. Siris, M.D.
Department of Medicine
Division of Endocrinology
College of Physicians and Surgeons
Columbia University
630 West 168th Street
New York, New York 10032

Monica C. Skarulis, M.D.
Division of Intramural Research
*National Institute of Diabetes, Digestive,
    and Kidney Diseases*
National Institutes of Health
9000 Rockville Pike
Bethesda, Maryland 20892

Eduardo Slatopolsky, M.D.
Department of Internal Medicine
Renal Division
*Washington University Medical Center at
    Barnes Hospital*
660 South Euclid Avenue, Box 8129
St. Louis, Missouri 63110

Allen M. Spiegel, M.D.
Molecular Pathophysiology Branch
*National Institute of Diabetes, Digestive,
    and Kidney Diseases*
National Institutes of Health
Building 10, Room 9N-222
9000 Rockville Pike
Bethesda, Maryland 20892

Andrew F. Stewart, M.D.
Division of Endocrinology
Yale University School of Medicine
333 Cedar Street
New Haven, Connecticut 06510; and
*West Haven Veterans Affairs Medical
    Center*
950 Campbell Avenue
West Haven, Connecticut 06516

John L. Stock, M.D.
Endocrinology Division
*The Medical Center of Central
    Massachusetts*
119 Belmont Street
Worcester, Massachusetts 01605

Gordon J. Strewler, M.D.
Department of Medicine
*University of California, San Francisco;
    and*
Endocrine Unit
Veterans Affairs Medical Center
4150 Clement Street
San Francisco, California 94121

Rajesh V. Thakker, M.A., M.R.C.P.
MRC Molecular Medicine Group
Royal Postgraduate Medical School
Hammersmith Hospital
Du Cane Road
London, W12 0NN, United Kingdom

Lee S. Weinstein, M.D.
Molecular Pathophysiology Branch
National Institute of Diabetes, Digestive,
* and Kidney Diseases*
National Institutes of Health
Building 10 Room 8C101
9000 Rockville Pike
Bethesda, Maryland 20892

Samuel A. Wells, Jr., M.D.
Department of Surgery
Washington University School of Medicine
660 South Euclid Avenue, Box 8109
St. Louis, Missouri 63110

G. Donald Whedon, M.D.
880 Mandalay Avenue
Clearwater, Florida 34630

Michael P. Whyte, M.D.
Metabolic Research Unit
Shriners Hospital for Crippled Children
2001 South Lindbergh Avenue;
Division of Bone and Mineral Diseases
The Jewish Hospital of St. Louis; and
Departments of Medicine and Pediatrics,
Division of Endocrinology and Metabolism
Washington University School of Medicine
660 South Euclid Avenue
St. Louis, Missouri 63110

Ji-Xiang Zhang, Ph.D.
Department of Biological and Biophysical
* Sciences*
Health Sciences Center
University of Louisville
Louisville, Kentucky 40292

Preface

One of us (JPB), dreamed of this book about five years ago. It seemed then that advances in our knowledge of the parathyroids represented nothing less than a 30-year revolution of spectacular progress. We gained knowledge over this period at an explosive pace with a concomitant new appreciation of the basic and clinical ramifications of these four tiny endocrine glands. The major secretory product, parathyroid hormone (PTH), was isolated, sequenced, assayed, and cloned. PTH became one of the first hormones to be shown to utilize cAMP as a second messenger. Regulation of PTH synthesis and secretion by calcium and 1,25-dihydroxyvitamin D was appreciated, as well as the cellular effects of PTH on its two major target organs, bone and kidney. The discovery of parathyroid hormone-related protein (PTHrP) as a cause of hypercalcemia of malignancy and a more general appreciation of PTHrP and PTH as polypurpose factors with many diverse biological effects, represent exciting new advances in our field. The recent cloning of a bona fide receptor for both PTH and PTHrP is a tremendous achievement, as is the thinking that both PTH and PTHrP may utilize more than one second messenger pathway, and perhaps interact with more than one receptor. At the clinical level, we have seen a remarkable evolution in the presentation of primary hyperparathyroidism and are beginning to understand molecular features of this disease. Pseudohypoparathyroidism is now appreciated, in its classical form, to be a G protein deficiency disease. Autoimmune and molecular features of hypoparathyroidism have been identified and studied. New knowledge of the pathophysiology of secondary hyperparathyroidism associated with renal failure has had direct impact on management and clinical outcome. PTH is now appreciated to have important anabolic properties on bone that may have implications for its use as a therapeutic agent in osteoporosis. This incomplete summary argues persuasively for how fast and how far this field has advanced.

This is not to say that we were in the dark ages before Aurbach isolated parathyroid hormone. Certainly, it was Fuller Albright who in 1948 correctly pointed out that "back in the dark ages of endocrinology, in the early 1920s, hyperparathyroidism was an unknown fact." It was also Albright who reminded us of the work of Sandstrom, who in 1880, 40 years before the first known cases of hyperparathyroidism wrote, "The existence of a hitherto unknown gland in animals that have so often been a subject of anatomical examination called for a thorough approach to the region around the thyroid gland even in man. Although the probability of finding something hitherto unrecognized seemed so small that it was exclusively with the purpose of completing the investigations rather than with the hope of finding something new that I began a careful examination of this region, so much the greater was my astonishment therefore when in the first individual I examined, I found on both sides at the inferior border of the thyroid gland an organ of the size of a small pea, which judging from its exterior, did not appear to be a lymph gland, or an accessory thyroid gland, and upon histological examination showed a rather peculiar structure."

The first chapters on the parathyroids were indeed written by Albright and a band of spectacular clinical investigators of the 1920s, 30s and 40s. These chapters are recorded in the Albright and Reifenstein classic *The Parathyroid Glands and Metabolic Disease*. We recommend this insightful 45-year-old book as important and provocative reading. *The Parathyroids* is designed to follow the Albright and Reifenstein text. Certainly all endocrinology reference texts routinely include a section on the subject matter of this book. Other texts that are more focused on calcium metabolism provide more information than the standard endocrinology texts on the parathyroids. However, there is no book that is exclusively devoted to a comprehensive examination of basic and clinical concepts of the parathyroids. As indicated by the size and scope of *The Parathyroids*, it is clear that a book devoted to this subject is worthy and long overdue. It is time for such a book to stand on the endocrine shelf near its anatomical partner, the thyroid gland, which in Werner and Ingbar's *The Thyroid* has had its own literary repository since 1955.

This book is intended for students, teachers, practitioners, and investigators of this field. It covers in a current and concise yet complete manner virtually all that we know about the parathyroids. Thus, it is both a basic and a clinical text. The 51 chapters are divided into a presentation of basic knowledge of the parathyroids and the clinical disorders associated with dysfunction of these glands. Section I, Basic Concepts of the Parathyroids, consists of 22 chapters. Chapters 1–7 cover the embryology, anatomy, and pathology of the parathyroid glands; calcium homeostasis; regulation of parathyroid hormone by dietary calcium and vitamin D; anabolic and catabolic effects of parathyroid hormone; cellular actions of parathyroid hormone on osteoblast and osteoclast function; autocrine and paracrine functions of parathyroid tissue; and the chemistry and biology of parathyroid hormone secretory protein. In Chapters 8–16, parathyroid hormone is considered with respect to the discovery by Aurbach of one of its second messengers, cAMP; regulation of its biosynthesis and metabolism; the parathyroid hormone gene; structure-function analysis of parathyroid hormone and parathyroid hormone-related protein; measurement of parathyroid hormone in the circulation; parathyroid hormone and parathyroid hormone-related protein as polyhormones; receptors for parathyroid hormone and parathyroid hormone-related protein; G proteins as transducers of parathyroid hormone action; biochemical mechanisms of parathyroid hormone action. The book proceeds in Chapters 17–20 to a consideration of PTHrP: its structure, physiological processing, and actions; its causative role in hypercalcemia of malignancy; its skeletal and renal actions; and its measurement in the circulation. Other causes of hypercalcemia, besides PTHrP, and the management of PTH and PTHrP-dependent hypercalcemia complete this section (Chapters 21–22).

Section II, Clinical Concepts of the Parathyroids, begins with a 18-chapter section on primary hyperparathyroidism (chapters 23–40). This segment is a full exploration of the hyperparathyroid state from theoretical aspects of parathyroid cell growth to the molecular basis of primary hyperparathyroidism. A discussion of the spectrum of parathyroid tumors leads to a consideration of its modern clinical presentations and the course of primary hyperparathyroidism. The change in clinical presentation of primary hyperparathyroidism from a disease of bones and stones and groans, to a relatively asymptomatic disorder does not lose sight of a major clinical complication, nephrolithiasis, which is still seen in patients on a regular basis. A chapter devoted to newer markers of bone turnover in primary hyperparathyroidism is followed by a discussion of the histomorphometric features of the disease. Medical and surgical management of primary hyperparathyroidism and the role of preoperative localization techniques are covered completely. Unusual manifestations of primary hyperparathyroidism include separate discussions of parathyroid carcinoma and acute primary hyperparathyroidism. The MEN syndromes I and II focus on the parathyroids as does the chapter on familial hypocalciuric hypercalcemia. In Chapters 41 and 42, the parathyroids in renal disease are reviewed with respect to pathophysiology, clinical profile, and management.

Chapters 43–47 cover the hypoparathyroid states with respect to differential diagnosis, autoimmune etiologies, molecular genetics, and a special consideration of the clinical, biochemical, and molecular features of pseudohypoparathyroidism. A separate chapter is devoted to the therapy of hypoparathyroidism.

The last four chapters of the book, Chapters 48–51, cover unusual aspects of the parathyroids: parathyroid function in the pathophysiology of osteoporosis and parathyroid hormone as a potential therapy of osteoporosis. Parathyroid function in Paget's disease of bone and in magnesium deficiency complete the treatise.

We recognize that few readers will read this book from cover to cover, although many of the chapters are closely interrelated. In order to permit virtually all chapters to "stand alone" but also to be connected to the rest of the book, we have liberally included cross-references to other chapters where appropriate. The reader can thus easily refer to other chapters for more information on a given subject. This design also necessarily calls for some interdigitation between chapters so that the reader is not always required to refer to another chapter but, rather, can get a brief summary in the chapter being read of an area that is covered more completely elsewhere.

If it was true that we needed a book on this subject five years ago when the idea was first germinating, why did it take so long to get it done and what was the impetus for finally accomplishing the task? The first of these two questions has a simple answer. Ideas for books are rather easy to develop but it is quite another matter to mobilize an army of over 90 experts to bring that idea to reality. As is true for so many things, this idea was put on the shelf to be admired for its own sake and to be completed later. The mobilizing impetus and the inspiration for this effort eventually did come. Regrettably, it came in the form of a tragic event in our lives, the death of Gerald D. Aurbach.

The death of Jerry on a street in Charlottesville, Virginia, on November 4, 1991, was random, senseless, and violent. At 64 years of age, Jerry was still alive with love for his work, his family, and his friends. In a moment, we suddenly lost a man who guided the very definition of our field for over 30 years. We lost a man who was our teacher and our friend. We lost a brilliant scientist who was involved in most of the major advances in this field over the past three decades. We lost a man who trained an extraordinary number of us for successful careers in basic and clinical investigation of the parathyroids. We lost a gentle man who consistently brought out the best in us. A summary of the many accomplishments that came from Jerry's laboratory and the trainees, collaborators, and associates who worked with him is depicted in the time-line on pages xxvi–xxvii of this book. It is an extraordinary legacy. The two *IN MEMORIA*, by Bilezikian (*Journal of Bone and Mineral Research* 7:ix-x, 1992) and by Potts and Spiegel (*Journal of Clinical Endocrinology and Metabolism* 75:1386–1388, 1992), speak volumes to his career, to his accomplishments, and to his persona.

In a flash, the dream shelved in the recesses of consciousness and relegated to "when I get to it" became an urgent need. *The Parathyroids* had to be written in the memory and honor of Gerald D. Aurbach, and it seemed altogether fitting that it be written by those who were close to Jerry. We who knew him so well and respected him so much would write a volume for the field. Virtually all of the principal authors of this text fit into that category. Maurice Attie who also belongs in this book was tragically killed in a bicycle accident in Philadelphia only a few months after Jerry's death. We remember Maurice and wish that he too were still with us. It is extraordinary that a book designed to be as comprehensive as this could be assembled by a collective authorship whose scientific roots were established by Jerry. His contributions to this field are represented not only by his science but also by his scientific progeny who are the next generation of investigators to study and write about it.

We took up this task with time in mind. *The Parathyroids* had to be published with a short lag time because the book is a timely dedication to Jerry's memory. It had to be published soon because this field is in "fast forward" and if one used the normal publication time for a book of this magnitude, it would run the risk of rapidly becoming outdated. To the credit and thanks to all the authors, virtually all 51 chapters were submitted within a six-month period of time. The dedication of the authors to this task is gratefully acknowledged by us. We also are grateful to Jasna Markovac of Raven Press who helped to ensure that the process ran as efficiently as possible and whose efforts also were instrumental in ensuring a rapid turnaround time to final publication.

John P. Bilezikian
Robert Marcus
Michael A. Levine

Foreword

This new authoritative text on the parathyroid glands is a thoroughly modern and comprehensive assembly of treatises on the diseases of the parathyroids, and on the physiology and biochemistry of parathyroid hormone. Most appropriately, it is dedicated to Gerald D. Aurbach, a warm, humane scientist who contributed as much as any other to our current concepts and understanding of this important area of endocrinology.

Organized into "Basic Concepts" and "Clinical Concepts" sections, the 51 chapters examine in detail nearly every aspect of the relatively tiny glands that are the principal regulators of calcium and bone metabolism. The more than 90 authors have been major contributors to much of the most recent knowledge of bone physiology and calcium metabolism. Many of them trained or worked directly in Dr. Aurbach's laboratory in the NIAMD (later NIADDK, then NIDDK) of NIH or were active collaborators of his in other divisions or institutes of NIH. Many others, in university laboratories in various parts of the United States and in several foreign countries, were influenced by collaborations or contacts with him.

The most significant feature of a sizeable proportion of the chapters in the book is the interrelationship of the so-called basic and clinical research developments, showing the ways in which new knowledge of basic structure and function have led to advances in clinical diagnosis and improved management of diseases. The chapters provide clear supportive evidence for the concept of basic and clinical research as one interwoven fabric, findings in the former being necessary for advances in the latter, and movement of these findings from one to the other being logical and inevitable. This feature of seemingly effortless flow of discovery and understanding is exemplified by the work of Dr. Aurbach and his various collaborators. His studies began with purification and chemical characterization of parathyroid hormone and progressed to the development of assays for its amount in biological fluids, then from discovering cAMP as a second messenger for parathyroid hormone action to its application to clinical diagnosis. Measurement of parathyroid hormone for diagnosis of hyperparathyroidism and in studies to locate the offending tumor followed by subsequent deft surgical removal demonstrates the applicatory nature of imaginative and analytical bioscience. This same use of basic research to explain or account for clinical disease is shown in a number of other descriptions in this book of various familial and genetic forms of hypo- and hyperparathyroidism and of disorders involving hypercalcemia.

No book dedicated to Jerry Aurbach can fail to note the recognition accorded by the scientists of several organizations and countries for his outstanding work over the years. To mention only a few—the William F. Neuman Award of the American Society for Bone and Mineral Research, the Edwin B. Astwood Award of the Endocrine Society, the Andre Lichtwitz Prize from France, the Gairdner Foundation Award from Canada, the Royal Society of Medicine's Burroughs-Wellcome Visiting Professorship and in 1986 election to the National Academy of Sciences. His contributions to scientific organizations were very generous, notably to the Laurentian Hormone Conference, the International Society of Endocrinology (Executive Committee) and the Endocrine Society (Council and later President). He contributed also much time and superb effort as an editor (particularly of *Endocrinology*) and a reviewer for many journals.

My personal memories of Jerry Aurbach began principally in 1965 when I relinquished my position as Chief of the Metabolic Diseases Branch of NIAMD at NIH for administrative responsibilities in the same institute. In so doing I bequeathed to him my secretary, Lillian Perry, for the beginning of a long and very effective and happy association for which he many times expressed his gratitude. My closest continuing contact with Jerry was by attending over many years the weekly rounds of his group. My administrative responsibilities were facilitated, I think, by exposure to the vibrant discussions of both research and clinical management by the many bright members of the group under Jerry's direction. During these years (the 60s to the early 80s) I wrote an occasional paper or editorial on which Jerry was kind enough to give informal critique. I remember him as a tough reviewer, gentle but detailed and specific, for whose comments I was indeed grateful. A related memory is of his comments following oral presentations of the papers of others at national meetings; he nearly always began with a compliment regarding the considerable effort put into the work, but then, to the pleasure of many I think, came the soft, seemingly hesitant, almost apologetic, question or comment which led the presenter (and the audience) to realize how the research could have been done significantly better. Noted by many was his devotion to family, his wife and two daughters, of whom he was both loving and proud; not mentioned, I think, was his care of and for his laboratory family and his affection for the summer ocean beach near Fenwick Island, Delaware.

It is entirely fitting that this book be dedicated to the memory and honor of this modest, gentle, and lovable man.

G. Donald Whedon
Clearwater, Florida

Foreword

A rational approach to understanding the clinical features, diagnosis, and treatment of disorders of calcium and phosphate metabolism requires an integrated understanding of the anatomy and cellular physiology of the parathyroid cell and the biology of parathyroid hormone (PTH) itself. Consisting of 51 chapters contributed by a group of international experts, *The Parathyroids* is a comprehensive review of the rapidly expanding body of knowledge concerning the basic biology of PTH and its cellular actions that regulate mineral ion metabolism and skeletal remodelling. This background provides a logical basis for the interpretation of the pathophysiology of diseases that result from hereditary or acquired perturbations in PTH action and brings reason to the management of these disorders. It is most propitious for *The Parathyroids* to become available at this time considering the rapid and significant advances that have been made in this field over the past few decades.

From a teleological perspective, it is conceivable that the well-developed systems to protect phosphate balance present in terrestrial species—namely, highly efficient conservation of phosphate by the kidney and absorption of phosphate in the intestine—represent adaptations that evolved as ancestral saltwater species acquired mechanisms to prevent phosphate deficiency. By contrast, in the food chain for terrestrial vertebrates, a calorically adequate diet can be deficient in calcium. Despite this potential environmental challenge, renal and intestinal transport mechanisms are less suited to preserve calcium balance than they are to preserve phosphate balance. The teleological explanation here might be that there was less need to develop homeostatic mechanisms for efficient calcium acquisition and retention in the sea. Whatever the validity of the evolutionary speculations, the physiological reality is that regulation of extracellular fluid (ECF) calcium at a constant level during each 24-hour cycle is a major homeostatic challenge in terrestrial vertebrates; calcium losses in urine and intestinal secretions may exceed intake for many hours each day.

This challenge is met by PTH and also by calcitonin and the active forms of vitamin D, the three hormones acting synergistically as the hormonal regulators of calcium homeostasis. PTH is the principal effector of the minute-to-minute regulation of ECF calcium. Vitamin D is vital to maintaining calcium balance and the integrity of bone. (Although readily apparent in many mammalian species, the role of calcitonin in human biology is unclear.)

Phylogenetically, parathyroid glands appear first in amphibians, with the move of vertebrates to land. Parathyroid glands have not been identified in fish, but recent studies in which powerful techniques of molecular biology have been used to scan the fish genome have identified what appears to be a fish PTH. The existence of PTH in a species that lacks a parathyroid gland and that arose in evolution prior to the move of animal life to land raises new questions about possible functions of PTH in earlier evolutionary biology. Further complexity in understanding the evolutionary and biological role of PTH has been introduced through consideration of the role of parathyroid hormone-related protein (PTHrP). PTHrP was discovered through efforts to identify the substance responsible for the hypercalcemia of malignancy. In addition to its causative role in many examples of humoral hypercalcemia of malignancy, PTHrP is now appreciated to be a physiologically important paracrine agent. PTHrP mediates a number of actions in endothelium, skin, uterus, and several other tissues, as well as playing a crucial developmental role in embryogenesis, especially on the skeleton, as outlined in four chapters dealing with this interesting hormone.

Both PTH and PTHrP use the same receptor, now termed the PTH/PTHrP receptor, as revealed by studies with the recently cloned receptor that mediates the actions of PTH on traditional target tissues. It is surprising to find that these two biologically active polypeptides, despite major differences in structure, use the same receptor to mediate their respective endocrine and paracrine functions. The existence of additional receptors for either peptide is an attractive speculation, but remains unproved.

Hypercalcemia may be due to primary hyperparathyroidism, an overactivity of the parathyroid glands. This volume devotes considerable attention to primary hyperparathyroidism and covers virtually all aspects of the disorder. It also covers completely in several chapters the subject of abnormal parathyroid gland growth, a disorder due to a still poorly understood loss of cellular control, which in some cases has definable acquired or hereditary genetic defects of the type seen in other neoplasms. Many clinical features of primary hyperparathyroidism can be logically explained based on information involving normal parathyroid physiology. An accurate diagnosis in patients with hypercalcemia is now greatly facilitated by the recent development of highly reliable immunoassays. Hypoparathyroidism is much less common than primary hyperparathyroidism: specific genetic defects that explain defective PTH production have been identified in some patients. Patients with PTH resistance due to defective target cell response, pseudohypoparathyroidism, have been analyzed in great detail clinically and the molecular pathogenesis has been partly clarified. Although defects in signal transduction mechanisms response, such as G proteins, have been identified, specific defects in receptor structure have not yet been discovered.

The book is dedicated to Dr. Gerald D. Aurbach, a close friend and colleague to many of the authors. His contributions to the parathyroid field and to endocrinology in general are monumental. Several of us have had the privilege of honoring his memory in tributes given at international meetings and written in other volumes. These citations (see Preface) document his scientific accomplishments and his remarkable personal qualities as a wise and gentle mentor to many young physicians and scientists. His early breakthrough in 1957, the isolation and purification of PTH, pioneered the modern era of investigation in PTH. This accomplishment made possible structural analysis and synthesis of the hormone and development of radioimmunoassays. The subsequent application of the techniques of molecular biology to study of the hormone gene and its receptor has further widened our understanding of PTH action. Jerry's interests were broad, and his contributions parallel the breadth of the current volume. He made many seminal contributions to clinical as well as basic investigation of calcium metabolism, as reflected in this volume.

John T. Potts, Jr.
Boston, Massachusetts

To the Memory of
Gerald D. Aurbach
(1927–1991)

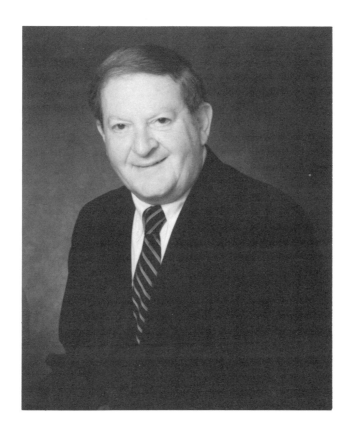

We learned from your wisdom, scientific acumen, investigative skills,
and daring insights.

THE LEGACY OF

Colleagues and Collaborators

Astwood
Whedon / Pastan / Wolff
Anfinsen / Gordon / Rall
Berson / Yalow
Potts
Sherwood
Care / Mayer / O'Riordan
Tashjian / Munson
Gill / Bartter / Melick
Condliffe / Ramberg
Chase / Deftos / Buckle
Keutmann / Niall / Kronfeld
Melson / Fedak
Marcus / White
Winickoff / Dawson
Marx / Desbuquois
Tregear / Sauer
Palmer / Heersche
Wilber / D. Heath
Murray / Habener
Powell / Shimkin
Woodard / Doppman
Wells / Ketcham
Bilezikian / J.D. Gardner
Klaeveman / Mallette
Patten / Monchik
Spiegel / Hauser / Troxler
Broadus / Sode / Beazley
Brown / Rodbard
Hurwitz

Milestones of Basic Research

Cyclic AMP as second messenger for PTH

Calcitonin-stimulated adenylyl cyclase

Guanine nucleotides and hormone action

Regulation of parathyroid hormone secretion

Isolation of human PTH

Catecholamines and cation transport

Beta-adrenergic receptors in turkey erythrocytes

Isolation of bovine PTH

Radioimmunoassay of PTH

Structural basis for biological and immunological activities of PTH

PTH-sensitive adenylyl cyclase in bone and kidney

Iodinated radioligand to detect beta-adrenergic receptors

'60   '61   '62   '63   '64   '65   '66   '67   '68   '69   '70   '71   '72   '73   '74   '75   '76

Milestones of Clinical Research

Defective excretion of cAMP in Pseudohypoparathyroidism

Properative localization of abnormal parathyroid glands

Pseudogout after parathyroidectomy

Neuromuscular disease in primary hyperparathyroidism

GERALD D. AURBACH

Downs
Brennan
Windeck
Koehler / D.G. Gardner
Attie
Levine / Singer
Stock / Reen
Lasker / Krudy
Krawietz / Saxe
Rizzoli / Santora
Moses / Norton
Miller
Brandi
Fitzpatrick
Quarto / Bliziotes
Shawker / Sakeguchi
Santora
Fatterossi / Zimering
Curcio / Streeten
Green / Bale
Friedman
Weinstein / DeGrange
Doi / Coleman

Isolation of guanine nucleotide regulatory unit

Regulation of PTH
secretion by calcium:
G protein dependence

Endothelial cell
line from the
parathyroids

Long-term cultures of
bovine parathyroid cells

PTHrP expressed in rat parathyroid cells

Preparation of viable parathyroid cells; control of PTH secretion by hormones, cations, ionophores, etc.

Endothelin from parathyroid cells

Binding of PTH
to bone cells

Regulation of PTH secretion
via calcium channels

FGF-like factor
in MEN I

| ’76 | ’77 | ’78 | ’79 | ’80 | ’81 | ’82 | ’83 | ’84 | ’85 | ’86 | ’87 | ’88 | ’89 | ’90 | ’91 |

Neonatal primary
hyperparathyroidism

Human parathyroid autografts

Mitogenic activity
for PTH in MEN I

Clonality of PTH
tumors in MEN I

Cryopreservation of
parathyroid tissue

Intraoperative cAMP in parathyroid surgery

Anti-parathyroid cell antibodies in
hypoparathyroidism

Allelic loss
in MEN I

Familial Hypocalciuric
Hypercalcemia

Reoperation for persistent hyperparathyroidism

Ultrasound to detect
PTH adenomas

Rapid assay for cAMP

Multihormone resistance in pseudohypoparathyroidism

Abnormal calcium sensitivity
in hyperparathyroidism

Preoperative localization in primary hyperparathyroidism

Deficient G protein in pseudohypoparathyroidism

The Parathyroids
Basic and Clinical Concepts

The Parathyroids, edited by J.P. Bilezikian, M.A. Levine, and R. Marcus. Raven Press, Ltd., New York © 1994.

CHAPTER 1

Embryology, Anatomy, and Pathology of the Parathyroids

Virginia A. LiVolsi

The morphologic abnormalities seen in the parathyroid glands are predominantly those related to hyperfunction, i.e., primary hyperparathyroidism. This chapter focuses on this aspect of parathyroid pathology, because surgical specimens of parathyroid lesions are virtually all derived from patients with hyperparathyroidism. Since this is an important factor in the surgical treatment of this disease, a review of the embryological development of the parathyroids, their anatomy, and the normal histology is included. A brief discussion of parathyroid pathology in hypoparathyroidism is also given, as is discussion of the pathology of the parathyroid glands in humoral hypercalcemia of malignancy.

DEVELOPMENT OF THE PARATHYROID GLANDS

In the 8–10 mm embryo, the parathyroids begin to develop from the third and fourth branchial pouches. The third branchial pouch gives rise to the thymus and the parathyroid complex. The parathyroids migrate to and remain at the lower poles of the thyroid. Thus, in the usual case, the inferior parathyroids migrating with the thymus come to rest below the parathyroids derived from branchial pouch four (1). The fourth branchial pouch, or the fourth–fifth pharyngeal complex, gives rise to the superior parathyroid glands and, via the ultimobranchial body, to the parafollicular or C cells in the lateral thyroid. The superior parathyroids lie adjacent to the upper poles of the thyroid.

ANATOMY OF PARATHYROID GLANDS

Both the number and the location of the parathyroid glands vary in normal individuals. Variation in location of the parathyroid glands can lead to problems in surgical exploration of the neck. Thus, in searching for abnormal parathyroid tissue in patients with hypercalcemia, there may be difficulty in locating the diseased gland(s). Conversely, the surgeon who is operating on the neck for other reasons, such as thyroid or laryngeal disease, may inadvertently traumatize or remove parathyroid glands because of the vagaries of the parathyroids' anatomic position (1–6).

Although from one to twelve parathyroid glands can be found (1), 84% of normal adults have four parathyroid glands (2). One to seven percent of adults have three glands, and 3–13% have five parathyroids (1–6).

The location of the parathyroid glands also varies, with more marked variability occurring in the lower parathyroid glands. The upper glands may be found close to or actually within the thyroid capsule or located behind the pharynx or the esophagus, lateral to the larynx (4). The lower glands, which usually lie near the lower pole of the thyroid, may be found in the paratracheal area or close to or within the thymus in the superior mediastinum (Fig. 1). The glands tend to be bilaterally symmetrical in location.

The parathyroid glands measure between 2 and 7 mm in length, between 2 and 4 mm in width, and between 0.5 and 2 mm in thickness. They are reniform in shape, of soft consistency, and brown-to-rust in color. However, color varies with fat content, degree of vascular congestion, and number of oxyphil cells present (3,6).

The weight of the parathyroids varies with sex, race, and overall nutritional status (7). The combined weight of all parathyroid tissues in a normal adult male is

V. A. LiVolsi: Department of Pathology, Hospital of the University of Pennsylvania, Philadelphia, Pennsylvania 19104.

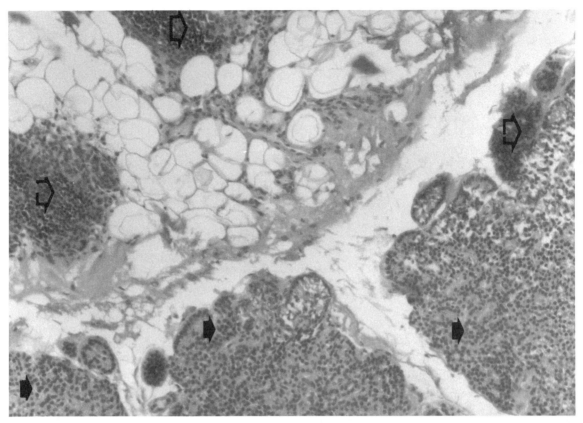

FIG. 1. Parathyroid tissue (*solid arrows*) admixed with thymic tissue (*open arrows*) and fat from mediastinum. Hematoxylin-eosin. ×100.

~120 mg and in adult females ~145 mg (3,6). Weights of individual glands range between 35 and 55 mg (3,6).

HISTOLOGY OF THE PARATHYROIDS

Each parathyroid gland is enveloped by a thin fibrous capsule that extends into the parenchyma as fibrous septa dividing the gland into lobules. A rich capillary network is surrounded by nests and cords of parenchymal cells. Small clusters of cells are interspersed with foci of adipose tissue. The distribution of fat and parenchymal cells in the parathyroid gland is uneven, so that biopsies from a parathyroid may be predominantly fat, or predominantly parenchymal cells, or an equal mixture of the two.

Historically, a ratio of 1:1 parathyroid cells:fat cells has been accepted as normal for adults. However, several studies have indicated that parathyroids from normal individuals show significantly <50% stromal fat (2,3,7–10). Dufour and Wilkerson (7,8) and Dekker et al. (9) have shown that a normal adult parathyroid gland contains only ~17% fat (Fig. 2). Hence the ratio of cells to fat serves little purpose in histological definition of glandular function. Densitometry measure-

ments concur, indicating that parenchymal cell mass accounts for 74% of parathyroid weight (10).

Normal parathyroid cells are chief cells; oxyphil cells and clear cells reflect different morphologic/functional expressions of the same parenchymal cell. The chief cell is polyhedral in shape, measures 6–8 nm in diameter, and contains amphophilic to slightly eosinophilic cytoplasm and a distinct nuclear membrane. Intracellular fat is found in normal chief cells. Clear cells represent chief cells in which there is an excessive amount of glycogen in the cytoplasm (6) (Fig. 3).

Oxyphils initially are found in the glands at puberty, apparently increase with age, and may form small microscopic nodules (Fig. 4). The oxyphil cell is large (~10 nm in diameter), has a well-demarcated cell membrane, and has eosinophilic granular cytoplasm and a pyknotic nucleus (6).

Intracellular fat content may be helpful in defining functional status. Thus in chief cells, the predominant cells in the parathyroid, intracellular fat, i.e., intracytoplasmic fat, is found in the overwhelming majority of cells in the euparathyroid state (~80% of cells) (3,9,10).

Ultrastructurally, the chief cells undergo a cyclic process during synthesis and secretion of parathyroid

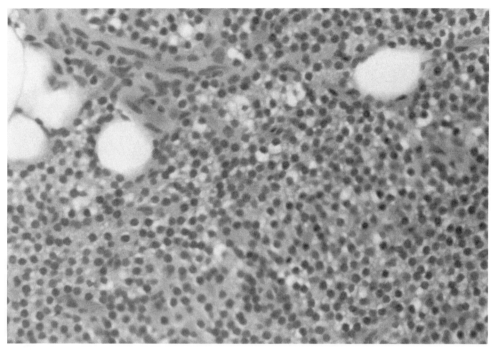

FIG. 2. Normal parathyroid in 36-year-old woman with no calcium abnormalities. This area of the gland contains minimal fat. Hematoxylin-eosin. ×150.

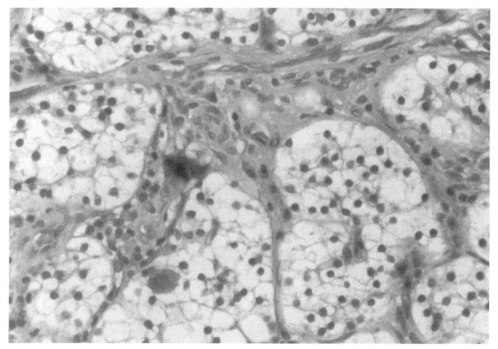

FIG. 3. In some glands, clear cell change can be seen. Hematoxylin-eosin. ×300.

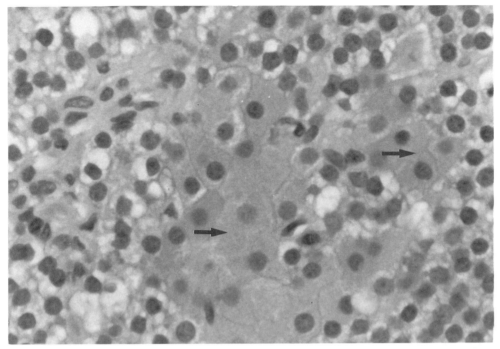

FIG. 4. Oxyphil cells (*arrows*) with normal parathyroid gland from 67-year-old man. Hematoxylin-eosin. ×300.

hormone, with the hormone being synthesized on Golgi apparatus-associated membrane-bound secretory granules. These cells eventually secrete these particles of hormone into the surrounding milieu. Little lipid is present in the actively secreting parathyroid cell (normally ~20% of the parenchymal cell population) (11). In hyperfunctioning parathyroid, a greater percentage of parenchymal cells will show decreased fat content.

DISEASES OF THE PARATHYROIDS

Primary Hyperparathyroidism

The prevalence of primary hyperparathyroidism is estimated as 1–5 cases per 1,000 adults. Most of these patients are asymptomatic and are diagnosed via routine screening test abnormalities (12).

The etiology of primary hyperparathyroidism is unknown. In some families, genetics plays a role [multiple endocrine neoplasia (MEN) syndromes] (13,14). In some individuals, genetic rearrangements have been described (see the chapter by Arnold). In a certain number of individuals with primary hyperparathyroidism, predominantly adenomas, a history of irradiation to the head and neck may be found, although the magnitude and significance of this association are not clear (15,16). Prinz et al. (15) found that 67% of individuals

in their series with combined thyroid and parathyroid tumors gave a history of irradiation.

Pathology of the Parathyroid Glands in Primary Hyperparathyroidism

Parathyroid Adenoma

Reports indicate that a parathyroid adenoma is responsible for 30–90% of cases of primary hyperparathyroidism. This wide range indicates variation in both pathologic and surgical interpretation of the disease. Most authors with great experience believe that ~75–80% of primary hyperparathyroidism is caused by a solitary adenoma (6,17,18).

Recent evidence supports a clonal origin for parathyroid adenomas. Although studies using protein polymorphisms indicated that parathyroid adenomas were nonclonal (19,20), Arnold and colleagues (21–23) using restriction fragment length polymorphism techniques, showed that nonfamilial solitary parathyroid lesions were monoclonal neoplasms.

Grossly, a parathyroid adenoma located more commonly in the lower glands is an oval red-brown nodule that is smooth, circumscribed, or encapsulated. The lesion, which often replaces one parathyroid gland, may show areas of hemorrhage and, if large, cystic degeneration. Occasionally, in small adenomas, a grossly visible rim of normal yellow-brown parathyroid tissue is seen. Weights of adenomas vary from 300 mg to several grams (6).

Microscopically, adenomas are usually encapsulated and comprise parathyroid chief cells arranged in a delicate capillary network. Some lesions appear multinodular. Stromal fat is usually absent (Fig. 5). Approximately 50% of adenomas are associated with a rim of normal parathyroid tissue. Even atrophic parathyroid tissue is sometimes seen outside the adenoma capsule. The cells in the rim tend to be smaller and more uniform, with abundant stromal and cytoplasmic fat. This fat is absent in adenomatous cells. However, the absence of a rim of normal or atrophic tissue does not exclude the diagnosis of adenoma, since large adenomas may have overgrown the preexisting normal gland or, alternatively, the rim may have been lost during the sectioning process.

The cells in the adenoma range from uniform and cytologically bland to severely atypical. Most cells making up the lesion have relatively small, uniform, dark nuclei. Usually, focal, bizarre multinucleated cells with dark, crinkled nuclei can be seen. These nuclei probably represent degenerative changes rather than cells with malignant or premalignant potential. In large tumors, zones of fibrosis may be found in addition to hemorrhage, cholesterol clefts, and hemosiderin as well as occasional areas of calcification (6,24–26). Rarely, lymphocytes are noted within an adenoma (24,27). Thymic tissue may be found in association

with an adenoma, or an adenoma may be found within the thymus.

It has been stated that mitotic activity is never found in a parathyroid adenoma and that the presence of mitoses should lead one to suspect the possibility of parathyroid carcinoma (28,29). This particular area, however, is the subject of debate at this time (see below under Parathyroid Carcinoma).

Nonadenomatous glands in a patient with a parathyroid adenoma may show normal to increased cytoplasmic fat content and normal weight (24–26,30–32). In ~10% of cases, microscopic examination of biopsies from "normal" glands shows areas of hypercellularity, so-called microscopic hyperplasia (24–26,30–32). Although this may represent a true increase in parenchymal cell number, difficulties in defining what is normal along with possible sampling errors may lead to uncertainty. In nonadenomatous glands, cells may be enlarged and may show clear vacuolated cytoplasm; nests of cells may show peripheral nuclear palisading (33) (Fig. 6).

Adenomas can be composed exclusively or almost exclusively of oxyphilic or oncocytic cells (34–38). These tumors, which can function, tend to be larger than chief cell adenomas, but the serum calcium levels tend to be only minimally elevated.

Because of embryologic migration patterns, parathyroid adenomas can occur in ectopic locations. Ectopic locations include the superior mediastinum,

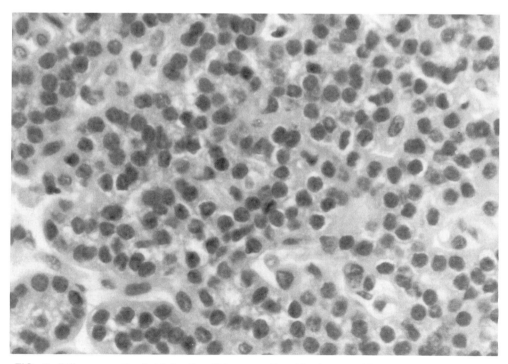

FIG. 5. Diffuse growth of chief cells within a parathyroid adenoma. Hematoxylin-eosin. ×150.

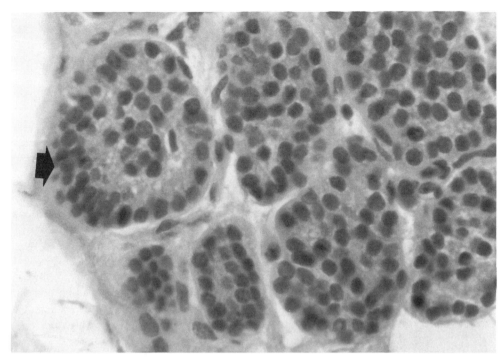

FIG. 6. Biopsy of nontumoral parathyroid gland from patient with adenoma. Note peripheral palisading of cells in aggregate (*arrow*). Hematoxylin-eosin. × 150.

within the thymus, behind the esophagus, and intrathyroidal (39–44) (see chapters by Norton et al. and Doppman).

Double adenomas, if they occur at all, are rare. Most patients who have so-called double adenomas may, over a period of time, return with recurrent hyperparathyroidism and in fact have four-gland hyperplasia. The diagnosis of double adenoma can be made only if two glands are enlarged and histologically abnormal while the remaining glands are normal, there is no family history of parathyroid disease, and permanent cure of hypercalcemia follows excision of only the two enlarged glands (45–52). This subject is covered more completely in the chapters by Mallette, "The Function and Pathologic Spectrum of Parathyroid Abnormalities in Hyperparathyroidism," and Norton et al.

Primary Parathyroid Hyperplasia

Primary parathyroid hyperplasia (32,52–62) is divided into two main types: the more common one, chief cell hyperplasia, and the less common one, water clear cell hyperplasia. Chief cell hyperplasia accounts for 15% of all primary hyperparathyroidism in most series, although a much smaller number of reports indicate that about one-half of primary hyperparathyroidism cases are due to hyperplasia (52–60). The reasons for this discrepancy probably follow from differences in pathologic interpretation. Approximately 30% of patients with chief cell hyperplasia have familial hyperparathyroidism or one of the syndromes of MEN (13,14,63–65).

In chief cell hyperplasia, all four glands are grossly enlarged, but they may be unequal in size. If the glands are unequal in size, the lower glands tend to be larger (6,61,66). Occasionally one gland is much larger than the others, giving the impression of a single gland disease. The weight of all four glands ranges from only minimally enlarged (150 mg) to over 20 g. The usual range is 1–3 g.

Microscopically, diffuse hyperplasia with solid masses of chief cells is seen with minimal, if any, intercellular fat. In some examples, nodular or pseudoadenomatous hyperplasia is present. This lesion consists of circumscribed nodules of chief, transitional, or oxyphil cells, each nodule being devoid of fat, and with little fat in the intervening stroma. In hyperplasia there is usually no rim of normal tissue. Bizarre nuclei are rarely found in primary hyperplasia, but mitoses are identified occasionally. (In the author's experience, ~5% of hyperplastic glands contain mitoses.) Lymphocytic infiltration of some of these glands has been considered an autoimmune disease (24,27).

Clear cell or water clear cell hyperplasia is very rare and represents the only multiglandular condition of the parathyroid in which the superior glands are larger than the lower (6,67–69). Total weights of such parathyroids always exceed 1 g and usually range from 5 to 10 g. The glands are irregular and show pseudopods and cysts; a distinct mahogany color is seen grossly. Histologically, the glands are composed of diffuse sheets of clear cells, without any mixture of other types. No rim is present.

Parathyroid Carcinoma

This condition is responsible for ~1–2% of primary hyperparathyroidism cases (28,70–83), although recent studies suggest that it is even more uncommon (see the chapter by Shane). There is an almost equal sex ratio, which is in contrast to parathyroid adenomas and ordinary hyperplasias, where women predominate. Patients with parathyroid carcinoma tend to be somewhat younger than typical patients with benign disease. They are virtually always symptomatic, with very high levels of serum calcium and parathyroid hormone. Very rarely, parathyroid carcinoma occurs in the setting of familial endocrine disease (84,85) or in a familial setting without antecedent endocrine hyperplasia (86). The development of carcinoma arising in the setting of four-gland hyperplasia (either primary or secondary) is very rare, but this does occur (87–92).

In their classic paper describing the pathology of parathyroid carcinoma, Shantz and Castleman (70) indicate that these parathyroid cancers tend to be large (average weight 12 g) and characteristically show a trabecular arrangement of tumor cells divided by thick fibrous bands. Capsular and blood vessel invasion is seen, and mitotic figures are readily found (28,70).

The presence of capsular invasion is not definitely equated with malignancy, since large parathyroid adenomas may have undergone prior hemorrhage with consequent fibrosis and trapping of tumor cells within the capsule. Vascular invasion may also be difficult to define unless it is seen outside the vicinity of the neoplasm. An important clue to the diagnosis of parathyroid carcinoma is the surgical finding of adherence to and/or invasion of local structures. Metastases at the time of presentation are unusual, but they may be identified in regional lymph nodes. Invasion of nerves, soft tissue, and the esophagus may be noted as well.

Parathyroid carcinoma is an indolent malignancy. Metastases, which may occur in up to one-third of cases, are found in regional lymph nodes, bone, lung, and liver. However, many patients survive for long periods. Multiple recurrences usually develop over time (15–20 years). The severity of the symptoms due to metastatic disease is directly related to tumor burden, because this in turn is related to the amount of parathyroid hormone produced (71,74,77,79–83). Rarely,

nonfunctioning parathyroid carcinomas have been found (93,94). These lesions tend to be large and composed of clear cells.

Since mitotic figures are virtually never found in a benign parathyroid adenoma, their presence in tumor cells should raise the suspicion of malignancy (Fig. 7). However, this principle has been called into question recently, and parathyroid tumors with mitotic activity in fact may be benign (28,29,95,96). However, follow-up in the series that have reported on this point is quite short, so one should still be appropriately very suspicious when mitotic figures are seen. It has been suggested that some of these tumors be called *atypical adenomas*, similar to descriptions of tumors in the thyroid gland, in which similar observations have been made. Many pathologists believe that this term may be useful, although the clinical and biological potential of such lesions remains unknown (29).

Unusual Lesions of the Parathyroid

Parathyroid Cysts

Cysts of the parathyroid glands are unusual. They typically range from 1 to 6 cm in diameter and may be misinterpreted clinically as thyroid nodules (97). Parathyroid cysts occur more frequently among women than among men. Most are found in the lower glands, but occasionally cysts are found in the mediastinum (97–104).

Grossly, parathyroid cysts are almost always unilocular and smooth walled and contain fluid with a high parathyroid hormone content (97–106). The cysts are lined by clear epithelium containing glycogen. The cyst wall is fibrous, with fragments of smooth muscle and nests of normal parathyroid tissue. It is unclear how these cysts arise. Microcysts are found in about one-half of normal parathyroids, and these might possibly enlarge by accumulating secretory products to produce gross cysts. The cysts may arise from embryologic remnants of pharyngeal pouches in the neck undergoing cystic degeneration and entrapping portions of parathyroid tissue. Many authors believe, however, that parathyroid cysts represent degenerated parathyroid adenomas, and in some cases, in fact, the cysts have been associated with hyperparathyroidism (102,103).

Lipoadenoma–Hamartoma of the Parathyroid

These tumors present as masses composed of parathyroid cells arranged in nests similar to normal parathyroid, but they are intimately associated with large areas of adipose tissue (107–110). The lesion may be

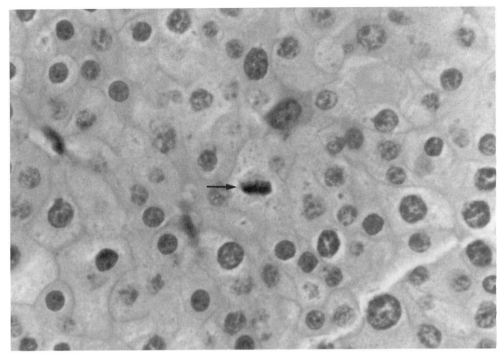

FIG. 7. Prominent mitotic figure (*arrow*) in this field in a large parathyroid tumor. Other features, including invasion of esophagus, were found to confirm diagnosis of carcinoma. Hematoxylin-eosin. ×400.

functional or nonfunctional. It is usually circumscribed, but rarely is it encapsulated. In unusual examples, a rim of normal parathyroid tissue is seen at the periphery. In some instances at least one other histologically normal parathyroid is recognized. In some, there is an unusual myxomatous stroma and other mesenchymal elements, including metaplastic bone. Wolfe and Goodman (107) suggest the term *parathyroid adenomas with stromal component*. Over three-fourths of reported lipoadenomas have been associated with hypercalcemia. When one considers the weight of the lipoadenoma and calculates the weight of parathyroid cells within it, the latter would consist of a rather large parathyroid adenoma.

Parathyromatosis

Rare instances of hyperparathyroidism due to primary hyperplasia show nests of hyperplastic parathyroid cells in the neck outside the confines of the hyperplastic glands (111–114). In some individuals, these cells are discovered at the time of the first neck exploration, so spillage during prior surgery can be excluded. It has been postulated that, during embryologic development, nests of pharyngeal tissue containing parathyroid cells might be scattered throughout the adipose tissue of the neck and medias-

tinum. Normally these nests are inconspicuous. However, in the process of diffuse hyperplasia of the parathyroids, all functioning tissue may become hyperplastic and appear as separate fragments on histologic evaluation. Sometimes a similar lesion occurs following surgery due to spillage and implantation of hyperplastic parathyroid tissue in the neck (112,114). The ability of hyperplastic parathyroid tissue to "take" in soft tissue and skeletal muscle is utilized when treating parathyroid hyperplasia by removal of all parathyroid tissue from the neck and autotransplantation of part of it usually into the forearm (115).

INTRAOPERATIVE ASSESSMENT OF PARATHYROID TISSUE

As is discussed above, in normal parathyroid glands, 80% of the cells are in the nonsecretory phase and contain intracytoplasmic fat (7,9,116,117). Can the assessment of fat content assist in intraoperatively distinguishing adenoma from hyperplasia, since all hyperfunctioning glands should be depleted of fat? Advocates have promoted the use of fat stains (Sudan black or oil red O) on parathyroid tissue removed at surgery (116–123). A sample of an enlarged parathyroid gland is sent for frozen sectioning, and, with hematoxylin and eosin (H&E) staining, it is hypercellular, with little or no stromal fat. Thus, it represents either an adenoma or a hyperplastic gland, but it is not normal. A biopsy of a second parathyroid is frozen and is normocellular or minimally hypercellular. Fat stain shows abundant cytoplasmic fat in the latter biopsy, so this is a normal gland. The enlarged gland, which shows minimal or no fat, represents an adenoma. Many authors have cautioned, however, that the fat stain cannot be the sole procedure on which a diagnosis is based, since, although the fat stain is helpful, accurate results are reported in only ~80% of cases. The fat stain must be considered as an adjunct technique in addition to gross findings and consideration of gland weight and size. It cannot be relied upon in itself (116–125).

Another rapid technique that may prove useful for intraoperative assessment of parathyroid tissue is density gradient measurements (2,126). There is an almost linear relationship between density and parenchymal parathyroid tissue content. The technique utilizes tissue samples from the center and the rim. Their densities are determined in a 25% mannitol solution. Abnormal parathyroid tissue sinks because of decreased fat and higher parenchymal cell mass. Some workers, including Wang and Ryder (126), have found this to be a simple test that can be used by the surgeon in the operating room for distinguishing normal from abnormal glands.

It cannot be overemphasized that, in the intraoperative assessment of parathyroid pathology, close communication between the surgeon and pathologist is essential (127). While being given tissue for analysis, the pathologist must be apprised of the gross findings. The following protocol is recommended: the largest parathyroid gland found is resected in toto and delivered to the pathologist for weighing, measuring, and histological examination. If the gland shows diffuse growth of chief cells, maybe a normal-appearing rim, lack of fat, and bizarre nuclei, a diagnosis of presumed adenoma can be made. It is useful for the surgeon to biopsy and for the pathologist to examine a grossly normal-appearing gland in order to document single-gland disease.

If the histology of the largest gland is that of hypercellularity, but other criteria for adenoma are not seen, biopsy of at least one more gland is needed. In fact, in many centers, pathologists consider that excision of the largest abnormal gland and at least a biopsy of one other gland are essential for adequate diagnostic interpretation of the pathology of hyperparathyroidism. The weight ratio of parenchymal cells to fat and normal or abundant intracytoplasmic fat content in the second gland strongly support that the first is an adenoma.

Some pathologists, especially those with great experience in cytopathology, recommend intraoperative touch imprint smears stained for fat both as an identification method for parathyroid tissue and for assessment of fat-rich vs. fat-poor examples (128).

Preoperative fine needle aspiration (FNA), using ultrasound guidance, of lesions suspected to be parathyroid origin can yield diagnostic material in ~85% of cases (129–132). However, morphologic overlap with thyroid lesions may interfere with accurate diagnosis (130).

OTHER TYPES OF HYPERPARATHYROIDISM

Secondary Hyperparathyroidism

Secondary hyperparathyroidism usually due to renal disease is relatively common in this age of hemodialysis and renal transplantation (133–135). The role of the surgical pathologist in the evaluation of secondary hyperparathyroidism is basically to identify parathyroid tissue at the time of frozen section to allow the surgeon to remove portions of this tissue for autotransplantation. Secondary hyperparathyroidism is really no different histopathologically from multiglandular involvement in primary hyperparathyroidism. Mitotic activity occasionally is found in such glands. Usually all four glands are enlarged, although one or two glands may be of very great size.

Transplanted parathyroid tissue shows a "take" in the majority of cases. When transplantation occurs in the forearm, and if hyperfunction recurs, the tissue can be "shaved" or reduced readily (115,136). Such lesions will show small nests and islands of vascularized parathyroid tissue in the muscle or fat of the forearm.

Tertiary Hyperparathyroidism

Although the existence of this entity has been questioned, most authors believe it represents the autonomous function of one parathyroid gland that develops in the face of longstanding secondary hyperparathyroidism (137). The pathology resembles that of secondary hyperparathyroidism, although one of the four glands is usually disproportionately enlarged.

Familial Hyperparathyroidism

In addition to the multiple endocrine neoplasia (MEN) syndromes, in which hyperparathyroidism is often a prominent clinical problem, familial parathyroid hyperplasia without other endocrine lesions has been reported. The lesions in all these patients resemble those of primary chief cell hyperplasia (13,138–140), although a ribbon pattern of cell growth may be prominent in MEN-I.

Familial Hypocalciuric Hypercalcemia

This condition, inherited as an autosomal dominant, is manifested clinically by familial occurrence, moderate to minimally elevated serum calcium, and reduced urinary calcium excretion (see the chapter by Heath). The parathyroid glands appear normal to mildly hypercellular, and subtotal parathyroidectomy fails to reverse the hypercalcemia. The defect appears not to be in the parathyroid glands themselves (141,142).

FLOW CYTOMETRY AND THE PARATHYROID

Several studies of DNA content have shown that aneuploidy may be found in parathyroid adenomas, and even in hyperplasia, as well as in carcinoma. Approximately 70% of parathyroid carcinomas, 30% of adenomas, and 30–50% of chief cell hyperplasia glands show aneuploid DNA populations (143–146). As in proliferations of other endocrine organs, the finding of aneuploid cell populations does not ensure a diagnosis of malignancy (147–149).

HUMORAL HYPERCALCEMIA OF MALIGNANCY (HHM) OR ECTOPIC PARATHYROIDISM

Hypercalcemia without bone metastasis in nonparathyroid malignancies may be found in association with a malignant tumor. Hypercalcemia is relieved by excision of the tumor and returns with its recurrence. This paraneoplastic endocrine syndrome is due in many cases to a peptide that resembles parathyroid hormone but is distinctly different. The factor responsible for the syndrome of humoral hypercalcemia of malignancy, which is due to parathyroid hormone-related protein (PTHrP), is discussed in other chapters in this volume. PTHrP binds to parathyroid hormone receptors on bone and kidney and mimics the actions of parathyroid hormone itself. The tumors most commonly associated with this syndrome include squamous carcinomas arising in a number of primary sites, including lung, vulva, esophagus, and head and neck, and clear cell cancers, especially of renal and ovarian origin (150–154). The parathyroid glands appear normal or atrophic histologically (33,155).

HYPOPARATHYROIDISM

The most common parathyroid pathology found in patients with hypoparathyroidism is four normal glands. Unfortunately, they have been surgically removed from the patient! Accidental excision of normal parathyroid glands during the course of neck surgery, especially thyroid surgery, is an uncommon but unfortunately not a rare event. In addition to actual excision of the glands, injury to their vascular supply may cause their infarction, or they may be so damaged that they become functionally absent.

Infiltration

Impaired parathyroid function caused by infiltration of parathyroid glands has been described in hemochromatosis, amyloidosis, and metastatic carcinoma to the parathyroids. These are all rare causes of hypoparathyroidism (156).

Radiation

Rarely, patients are reported who have developed hypoparathyroidism after radioactive iodine treatment for hyperthyroidism. The presumed mechanism is radiation damage to and fibrosis of the parathyroids (157).

Autoimmune Parathyroid Destruction

Lymphocytic infiltration of parathyroid tissue, with subsequent autoimmune destruction of the glands, is probably the most common cause of hypoparathyroidism (noniatrogenic cause). It may occur as an isolated event or in association with autoimmune diseases of other endocrine organs, i.e., thyroid, adrenal, or ovary (158–161).

REFERENCES

1. Gilmour JR. The embryology of the parathyroid glands, the thymus and certain associated remnants. *J Pathol Bacteriol* 1937;45:507–522.
2. Grimelius L, Akerstrom G, Johansson H, Bergstrom R. Anatomy and histopathology of human parathyroid glands. *Pathol Annu* 1981;16(Part 1):1–24.
3. Akerstrom G, Malmaeus J, Bergstrom S. Surgical anatomy of human parathyroid glands. *Surgery* 1984;95:14–21.
4. Wang CA. The anatomic basis of parathyroid surgery. *Ann Surg* 1976;183:271–175.
5. Alveryd A. Parathyroid glands in thyroid surgery. *Acta Chir Scand* 1968;389(Suppl):9–36.
6. Castleman B, Roth SI. *Tumors of the parathyroid glands.* Washington, DC: Armed Forces Institute of Pathology, Fascicle 14, Series 2, 1978.

7. Dufour DR, Wilkerson SY. Factors related to parathyroid weight in normal persons. *Arch Pathol Lab Med* 1983; 107:167–172.

8. Dufour DR, Wilkerson SY. The normal parathyroid revisited: percent of stromal fat. *Hum Pathol* 1982;13:717–721.

9. Dekker A, Dunsford HA, Geyer SJ. The normal parathyroid gland at autopsy: the significance of stromal fat in adult patients. *J Pathol* 1979;128:127–132.

10. Akerstrom G, Grimelius L, Johansson H, Pertoft H, Lundquist H. Estimation of parathyroid parenchymal cell mass by density gradients. *Am J Pathol* 1980;99:685–694.

11. Johannessen JV. Parathyroid glands. In: Johannessen JV, ed. *Electron microscopy in human medicine,* Vol 10. New York: McGraw Hill, 1981;111.

12. Heath H, Hodgson SF, Kennedy MA. Primary hyperparathyroidism: incidence morbidity and potential economic impact in a community. *N Engl J Med* 1980;302:189–193.

13. Steiner AL, Goodman AD, Powers SR. Study of a kindred with pheochromocytoma, medullary thyroid carcinoma, hyperparathyroidism and Cushing's diseases: multiple endocrine neoplasia, type 2. *Medicine* 1968;47:371–409.

14. Keiser HR, Beaven MA, Doppmann J, Wells S, Buja LM. Sipple's syndrome: medullary thyroid carcinoma, pheochromocytoma and parathyroid disease. *Ann Intern Med* 1973;78:561–579.

15. Prinz RA, Barbato AL, Braithwaite SS, Brooks MH, Lawrence AM, Paloyan E. Prior irradiation and the development of coexistent differentiated thyroid cancer and hyperparathyroidism. *Cancer* 1982;49:874–877.

16. Russ JE, Scanlon EF, Sener SF. Parathyroid adenoma following irradiation. *Cancer* 1979;43:1078–1083.

17. Palmer JA, Brown WA, Kerr WH, Rosen IB, Walters NA. The surgical aspects of hyperparathyroidism. *Arch Surg* 1975;110:1004–1007.

18. Dolgin C, LoGerfo P, LiVolsi V, Feind C. Twenty-five year experience with primary hyperparathyroidism at Columbia Presbyterian Medical Center. *Head Neck Surg* 1979;2:92–98.

19. Fialkow PJ, Jackson CE, Block MA, Greenwald KA. Multicellular origin of parathyroid "adenomas." *N Engl J Med* 1977;297:695–698.

20. Jackson CE, Cerny JC, Block MA, Fialkow PJ. Probable clonal origin of aldosteronomas versus multicellular origin of parathyroid "adenomas." *Surgery* 1982;92:875–879.

21. Arnold A, Staunton CE, Kim HG, Gaz RD, Kronenberg HM. Monoclonality and abnormal parathyroid hormone genes in parathyroid adenomas. *N Engl J Med* 1988;318:658–662.

22. Arnold A. Kim HG. Clonal loss of one chromosome II in a parathyroid adenoma. *J Clin Endocrinol Metab* 1989;69:496–499.

23. Arnold A, Kim HG, Gaz RD, Eddy RR, Fukushima Y, Beyers MG, Shows TB, Kronenberg HM. Molecular cloning and chromosomal mapping of DNA rearranged with the parathyroid hormone gene in a parathyroid adenoma. *J Clin Invest* 1989;83:2034–2040.

24. Ghandur-Mnaymneh L, Kimura N. The parathyroid adenoma: a histolopathologic definition with a study of 172 cases of primary hyperparathyroidism. *Am J Pathol* 1984;115:70–83.

25. Roth SI. Recent advances in parathyroid gland pathology. *Am J Med* 1972;50:612–622.

26. Williams ED. Pathology of the parathyroid glands. *J Clin Endocrinol Metab* 1974;3:285–303.

27. Bondeson AG, Bondeson L, Ljungberg O. Chronic parathyroiditis associated with parathyroid hyperplasia and hyperparathyroidism. *Am J Surg Pathol* 1984;8:211–215.

28. Evans HL. Criteria for diagnosis of parathyroid carcinoma. *Surg Pathol* 1991;4:244–265.

29. SanJuan J, Fraker D, Norton J, Merino MJ. Significance of mitotic activity and other morphologic parameters in parathyroid adenomas, and their correlation with clinical behavior. *Am J Clin Pathol* 1989;92:523 (abstract).

30. Badder EM, Graham WP, Harrison TS. Functional insignificance of microscopic parathyroid hyperplasia. *Surg Gynecol Obstet* 1977;145:863–868.

31. Block MA, Frame B, Jackson CE, Parfitt ASM, Horn RC. Primary diffuse microscopical hyperplasia of the parathyroid glands. *Arch Surg* 1976;111:348–354.

32. Harrison TS, Duarte B, Reitz RE, et al. Primary hyperparathyroidism: four to eight year postoperative follow-up demonstrating persistent functional insignificance of microscopic parathyroid hyperplasia and decreased autonomy of parathyroid hormone release. *Ann Surg* 1981;194:429–437.

33. Dufour DR, Marx SJ, Spiegel AM. Parathyroid gland morphology in nonparathyroid hormone mediated hypercalcemia. *Am J Surg Pathol* 1985;9:43–51.

34. Jones SH, Dietler P. Oxyphil cell adenoma as a cause of hyperparathyroidism. *Am J Surg* 1981;141:744–745.

35. McGregor DH, Lotuaio LG, Chu LH. Functioning oxyphil adenoma of parathyroid gland. An ultrastructural and biochemical study. *Am J Pathol* 1978;92:691–703.

36. Ordonez NG, Ibanez ML, MacKay B, Samaan NA, Hickey RC. Functional oxyphil cell adenomas of parathyroid gland: evidence of hormonal activity in oxyphil cells. *Am J Clin Pathol* 1982;78:681–689.

37. Rodriquez FH, Sarma DP, Lunseth JH, Guileyardo JM. Primary hyperparathyroidism due to an oxyphil adenoma. *Am J Clin Pathol* 1983;80:878–880.

38. Bedetti CD, Dekker A, Watson CG. Functioning oxyphil cell adenoma of the parathyroid gland: a clinicopathologic study of ten patients with hyperparathyroidism. *Hum Pathol* 1984;15:1121–1126.

39. Nathaniels EK, Nathaniels AM, Wang CA. Mediastinal parathyroid tumors: a clinical and pathological study of 84 cases. *Ann Surg* 1970;171:165–170.

40. Russell CF, Edis AJ, Scholz DA, Sheedy PF, vanHeerden JA. Mediastinal parathyroid tumors: experience with 38 tumors requiring mediastinotomy for removal. *Ann Surg* 1981;193:805–809.

41. Russell CF, Grant CS, vanHeerden JA. Hyperfunctioning supernumerary parathyroid glands: an occasional cause of hyperparathyroidism. *Mayo Clin Proc* 1982;57:121–124.

42. Edis AJ, Purnell DC, vanHeerden JA. The undescended "parathymus": an occasional cause of failed neck exploration for hyperparathyroidism. *Ann Surg* 1979;190:64–68.

43. Sloane JA, Moody HC. Parathyroid adenoma in submucosa of esophagus. *Arch Pathol Lab Med* 1978;102:242–243.

44. Spiegel AM, Marx SJ, Doppmann JL, Beazley RM, Ketcham AS, Kasten B, Aurbach GD. Intrathyroidal parathyroid adenoma or hyperplasia. *JAMA* 1975;234:1029–1033.

45. Harness JK, Ramsbury SR, Nishiyama RH, Thompson NW. Multiple adenomas of the parathyroids; do they exist? *Arch Surg* 1979;114:468–474.

46. Seyfar AE, Sigdestad JB, Hirata RM. Surgical considerations in hyperparathyroidism: reappraisal of the need for multigland biopsy. *Am J Surg* 1976;132:38–340.

47. Schwindt WD. Multiple parathyroid adenomas. *JAMA* 1967;199:945–946.

48. Verdon CA, Edis AJ. Parathyroid "double adenomas." Fact or fiction? *Surgery* 1981;90:523–526.

49. Wang CA. Parathyroid reexploration. *Ann Surg* 1977; 186:140–145.

50. Fulmer DH, Rothschild EO, Myers WPL. Recurrent parathyroid adenoma. *Arch Intern Med* 1969;124:495–501.

51. Balijet L. Recurrent parathyroid adenoma. *JAMA* 1973; 225:1238–1239.

52. Paloyan E, Lawrence AM, Strauss FH. *Hyperparathyroidism.* New York: Grune & Stratton, 1973.

53. Cope OH, Keynes WM, Roth SJ, Castleman B. Primary chief cell hyperplasia of the parathyroid glands: a new entity in the surgery of hyperparathyroidism. *Ann Surg* 1958; 148:375–388.

54. Block MA, Frame B, Jackson CE. The efficacy of subtotal parathyroidectomy for primary hyperparathyroidism due to

multiple gland involvement. *Surg Gynecol Obstet* 1978; 147:1–5.

55. Prinz RA, Gamuros OI, Sellu D, Lynn JA. Subtotal parathyroidectomy for primary chief cell hyperplasia of the multiple endocrine neoplasia type 1 syndrome. *Ann Surg* 1981; 193:26–29.

56. Wang CA, Castleman B, Cope O. Surgical management of hyperparathyroidism due to primary hyperplasia. A clinical and pathologic study of 104 cases. *Ann Surg* 1982;195:384–392.

57. Adams PH, Chalmers TM, Peters N, Rack JH, Truscott BM. Primary chief cell hyperplasia of the parathyroid glands. *Ann Intern Med* 1965;63:454–467.

58. Edis AJ, vanHeerden JA, Scholz DA. Results of subtotal parathyroidectomy for primary chief cell hyperplasia. *Surgery* 1979;86:462–469.

59. Lawrence DAS. A histological comparison of adenomatous and hyperplastic parathyroid glands. *J Clin Pathol* 1978; 31:626–632.

60. Scholz DA, Purnell DC, Edis AJ, vanHeerden JA, Woolner LB. Primary hyperparathyroidism with multiple parathyroid gland involvement. Review of 53 cases. *Mayo Clin Proc* 1978;53:792–797.

61. Black WC, Utley JF. The differential diagnosis of parathyroid adenoma and chief cell hyperplasia. *Am J Clin Pathol* 1968;49:761–775.

62. Haff RC, Ballinger WF. Causes of recurrent hypercalcemia after parathyroidectomy for primary hyperparathyroidism. *Ann Surg* 1971;173:884–889.

63. Wells SA, Farndon JR, Dale JK, Leight GS, Dilley WG. Long term evaluation of patients with primary parathyroid hyperplasia managed by total parathyroidectomy and heterotopic autotransplantation. *Ann Surg* 1980;192:451–458.

64. Marx SJ, Powell D, Shimkin PM, Wells SA, Ketcham AS, McGuigan JE, Bilezikian JP, Aurbach GD. Familial hyperparathyroidism. *Ann Intern Med* 1973;78:371–377.

65. Marx JS, Spiegel AM, Brown EM, Aurbach GD. Familial studies in patients with primary parathyroid hyperplasia. *Am J Med* 1977;62:698–706.

66. Castleman B, Schantz A, Roth SI. Parathyroid hyperplasia in primary hyperparathyroidism. *Cancer* 1976;38:1668–1675.

67. Dorado AE, Hensley G, Castleman B. Water clear hyperplasia of parathyroid. *Cancer* 1976;38:1676–1683.

68. Dawkins RL, Tashjian AH, Castleman B, Moore EW. Hyperparathyroidism due to clear cell hyperplasia. *Am J Med* 1973;54:119–126.

69. Persson S, Hansson G, Hedman I, Tisell LE, Wideehn S. Primary parathyroid hyperplasia of water clear cell type. Transformation of water clear cells into chief cells. *Acta Pathol Microbiol Scand Sect A* 1986;94:391–395.

70. Schantz A, Castleman B. Parathyroid carcinoma: a study of 70 cases. *Cancer* 1973;31:600–605.

71. Shane E, Bilezikian JP. Parathyroid carcinoma: a review of 62 patients. *Endocr Rev* 1982;3:218–226.

72. vanHeerden JA, Weiland LH, ReMine NH, Walls JT, Purnell DC. Cancer of the parathyroid glands. *Arch Surg* 1979;114:475–480.

73. Aldinger KA, Hickey RC, Ibanez ML, Samaan NA. Parathyroid carcinoma. A clinical study of seven cases of functioning and two cases on nonfunctioning parathyroid cancer. *Cancer* 1982;49:388–397.

74. Holmes EC, Morton DL, Ketcham AS. Parathyroid carcinoma: a collective review. *Ann Surg* 1969;169:631–640.

75. Ellis HA, Floyd M, Herbert FK. Recurrent hyperparathyroidism due to parathyroid carcinoma. *J Clin Pathol* 1971;24:596–604.

76. Flye MW, Brennan MF. Surgical resection of metastatic parathyroid carcinoma. *Ann Surg* 1981;193:425–435.

77. Grayzel EF. Hyperparathyroidism in a patient with parathyroid carcinoma: 15 year follow-up. *Arch Intern Med* 1967;120:349–352.

78. O'Bara T, Fujimoto Y, Yamaguchi K, Takanashi R, Kimo I, Sasaki Y. Parathyroid carcinoma of the oxyphil cell type. *Cancer* 1985;55:1482–1498.

79. Zisman E, Buckle RM, Deftos LJ, et al. Production of parathyroid hormone by metastatic parathyroid carcinoma. *Am J Med* 1968;45:619–623.

80. Anderson BJ, Samaan NA, Vassilopoulou-Sellin R, Ordonez NG, Hickey RC. Parathyroid carcinoma: features and difficulties in diagnosis and management. *Surgery* 1983;94:906–915.

81. Wang C, Gaz RD. Natural history of parathyroid carcinoma. *Am J Surg* 11985;149:522–527.

82. Inoue H, Ishihara T, Fukai S, Mikata A, Ito K, Mimura T. Parathyroid carcinoma with tracheal invasion and airway obstruction. *Surgery* 1980;87:113–117.

83. Cohn K, Silverman M, Corrado J, Sedgewick C. Parathyroid carcinoma: the Lahey Clinic experience. *Surgery* 1985; 98:1095–1100.

84. Mallette LE, Bilezikian JP, Ketcham AS, Aurbach GD. Parathyroid carcinoma in familial hyperparathyroidism. *Am J Med* 1974;57:642–648.

85. Dinnen JS, Greenwood RH, Jones JH, Walker DA, Williams ED. Parathyroid carcinoma in familial hyperparathyroidism. *J Clin Pathol* 1977;30:966–975.

86. Streeten EA, Weinstein LS, Norton JA, et al. Studies in a kindred with parathyroid carcinoma. *J Clin Endocrinol Metab* 1992;75:362–366.

87. Haghighi P, Astarita RW, Wepale T, Wolf PL. Concurrent primary parathyroid hyperplasia and parathyroid carcinoma. *Arch Pathol Lab Med* 1983;107:349–350.

88. Desch CE, Arsensis G, Woolf PD, May AG, Amatruda JM. Parathyroid hyperplasia and carcinoma within one gland. *Am J Med* 1984;77:131–134.

89. Berland Y, Olmer M, Lebreuil G, et al. Parathyroid carcinoma, adenoma and hyperplasia in a case of chronic renal insufficiency on dialysis. *Clin Nephrol* 1982;18:154–158.

90. Ireland J, Fleming S, Levison D, et al. Parathyroid carcinoma associated with chronic renal failure and previous radiotherapy to the neck. *J Clin Pathol* 1985;38:1114–1118.

91. Kodama M, Ikegami M, Kmanishi M, et al. Parathyroid carcinoma in a case of chronic renal failure on dialysis. *Urol Int* 1989;44:110–112.

92. Krishna GG, Mendez M, Levy B, Ritchis W, Marks A, Narins RG. Parathyroid carcinoma in a chronic hemodialysis patient. *Nephron* 1989;52:194–195.

93. Merlano M, Conte P, Scarsi P, et al. Nonfunctioning parathyroid carcinoma. A case report. *Tumori* 1985;71:193–196.

94. Yamashita H, Noguchi S, Nakayama I, Togon H, Moriuchi A, Yokoyama S, Mochizuki Y, Nogfuchi A. Light and electron microscopic study of nonfunctioning parathyroid carcinoma. *Acta Pathol Jpn* 1984;34:123–132.

95. Snover DC, Foucar K. Mitotic activity in benign parathyroid disease. *Am J Clin Pathol* 1981;75:345–347.

96. Chaitin BA, Goldman RL. Mitotic activity in benign parathyroid disease (letter). *Am J Clin Pathol* 1981;76:363–364.

97. Wang CA, Vickery AL, Maloof F. Large parathyroid cysts mimicking thyroid nodules. *Ann Surg* 1972;175:448–453.

98. Ginsberg J, Young JEM, Walfish PG. Parathyroid cysts. *JAMA* 1978;240:1506–1507.

99. Thacker WC, Wells VH, Hall ER. Parathyroid cysts of the mediastinum. *Ann Surg* 1971;174:969–975.

100. Hoehn JG, Beahrs OH, Woolner LB. Unusual surgical lesions of the parathyroid gland. *Am J Surg* 1969;118:770–778.

101. Troster M, Chiu HF, McLarty TD. Parathyroid cysts: report of a case with ultrastructural observations. *Surgery* 1978; 83:238–242.

102. Earll JM, Cohen A, Lundberg GD. Functional cystic parathyroid adenoma. *Am J Surg* 1969;118:100–103.

103. Albertson DA, Marshall RB, Jarman WT. Hypercalcemic crisis secondary to a functioning parathyroid cyst. *Am J Surg* 1981;141:175–177.

104. Clark OH. Hyperparathyroidism due to primary cystic parathyroid hyperplasia. *Arch Surg* 1978;113:748–750.

105. Silverman JF, Khazanie PG, Norris T, Fore WW. Parathy-

roid hormone (PTH) assay of parathyroid cysts examined by fine needle aspiration biopsy. *Am J Clin Pathol* 1986;86: 708–776.

106. Marco V, Carrasco MA, Marco C, Bauza A. Cytomorphology of a mediastinal parathyroid cyst. *Acta Cytol* 1983; 27:688–692.

107. Wolff M, Goodman EN. Functioning lipoadenoma of supernumerary parathyroid gland in the mediastinum. *Head Neck Surg* 1980;2:302–307.

108. Grimelius L, Johansson H, Lindquist B. A case of unusual stromal development in a parathyroid adenoma. *Acta Chir Scand* 1972;138:628–629.

109. Ober WB, Kaiser GA. Hamartoma of the parathyroid. *Cancer* 1958;11:601–606.

110. Perosio P, Brooks JJ, LiVolsi VA. Orbital brown tumor as initial manifestation of parathyroid lipoadenoma. *Surg Pathol* 1988;1:77–82.

111. Reddick RL, Costa JC, Marx SJ. Parathyroid hyperplasia and parathyromatosis *Lancet* 1977;1:549.

112. Fitko R, Roth SI, Hines JR, Roxe DM, Cahill E. Parathyromatosis in hyperparathyroidism. *Hum Pathol* 1990;21: 234–237.

113. Rattner DW, Marrone GC, Kasdon E, Silen W. Recurrent hyperparathyroidism due to implantation of parathyroid tissue. *Am J Surg* 1985;149:745–748.

114. Akerstrom G, Rudberg C, Grimelius L, Rastad J. Recurrent hyperparathyroidism due to preoperative seeding of neoplastic or hyperplastic parathyroid tissue. *Acta Chir Scand* 1988;154–219.

115. Jansson S, Tisell LE. Autotransplantation of diseased parathyroid glands into subcutaneous abdominal adipose tissue. *Surgery* 1987;101:549–556.

116. Dekker A, Watson CG, Barnes EL. The pathologic assessment of primary hyperparathyroidism and its impact on therapy: a prospective evaluation of 50 cases with oil-red-O stain. *Ann Surg* 1979;190:671–675.

117. Roth SI, Gallagher MJ. The rapid identification of "normal" parathyroid glands by the presence of intracellular fat. *Am J Pathol* 1976;84:521–528.

118. Black WC. Correlative light and electron microscopy in primary hyperparathyroidism. *Arch Pathol* 1969;88:225–241.

119. Roth SI, Capen CC. Ultrastructural and functional correlations of the parathyroid gland. *Int Rev Exp Pathol* 1974; 13:161–221.

120. Dufour DR, Durkowski C. Sudan IV staining: its limitations in evaluating parathyroid functional status. *Arch Pathol Lab Med* 1982;106:224–227.

121. King DT, Hirose FM. Chief cell intracytoplasmic fat used to evaluate parathyroid disease by frozen section. *Arch Pathol Lab Med* 1979;103:609–612.

122. Kasden EJ, Cohen RB, Rosen S, Silen W. Surgical pathology of hyperparathyroidism: usefulness of fat stains and problems in interpretation. *Am J Surg Pathol* 1981;5:381–384.

123. Ljungberg O, Tibblin S. Perioperative fat staining of frozen sections in primary hyperparathyroidism. *Am J Pathol* 1979;95:633–642.

124. Monchik JM, Farrugia R, Teplitz C, Brown S. Parathyroid surgery: the role of chief cell intracellular fat staining with osmium carmine in the intraoperative management of patients with hyperparathyroidism. *Surgery* 1983;94:877–886.

125. Bondeson AG, Bondeson L, Ljungberg O, Tibblin S. Fat staining in parathyroid disease—diagnostic value and impact on surgical strategy. *Hum Pathol* 1985;16:1255–1263.

126. Wang CA, Reider SV. A density test for the intraoperative differentiation of parathyroid hyperplasia from neoplasia. *Ann Surg* 1978;187:63–67.

127. Roth SI, Wang CA, Potts JT. The team approach to primary hyperparathyroidism. *Hum Pathol* 1975;6:645–648.

128. Silverberg SG. Imprints in the intraoperative evaluation of parathyroid disease. *Arch Pathol* 1975;100:375–378.

129. Guazzi A, Gabrielli M, Guadagni G. Cytologic features of a functioning parathyroid carcinoma. *Acta Cytol* 1982;26:709–713.

130. Halbauer M, Crepinko I, Brzac HT, Simonovic I. Fine needle aspiration cytology in the preoperative diagnosis of ultrasonically enlarged parathyroid glands. *Acta Cytol* 1991;35:728–735.

131. Karstrup S, Glenthoj A, Torp-Pedersen S, Hedegius L, Holm HH. Ultrasonically guided fine needle aspiration in suggested enlarged parathyroid glands. *Acta Radiol* 1988; 29:213–216.

132. Mincione GP, Borrelli D, Cicchi P, Ipponi PL, Fiorini A. Fine needle aspiration sytology of parathyroid adenoma: a review of seven cases. *Acta Cytol* 1986;30:65–69.

133. Roth SI, Marshall RB. Pathology and ultrastructure of human parathyroid glands in chronic renal failure. *Arch Intern Med* 1969;124:397–407.

134. Malmaeus J, Grimelius L, Johansson H, Akerstrom G, Ljunghall S. Parathyroid pathology in hyperparathyroidism secondary to chronic renal failure. *Scand J Urol Nephrol* 1984;18:157–166.

135. Akerstrom G, Malmaeus J, Grimelius L, Ljunghall S, Bergstrom R. Histological changes in parathyroid glands in subclinical and clinical renal disease. *Scand J Urol Nephrol* 1084;18:75–84.

136. Max MH, Flint LM, Richardson JD, Ferris FZ, Nagar D. Total parathyroidectomy and parathyroid autotransplantation in patients with chronic renal failure. *Surg Obstet Gynecol* 1981;153:177–180.

137. Krause MW, Hedinger CE. Pathologic study of parathyroid glands in tertiary hyperparathyroidism. *Human Pathol* 1985;16:772–784.

138. Jackson CE, Norum RA, Boyd SB, et al. Hereditary hyperparathyroidism and multiple ossifying jaw fibromas: a clinically and genetically distinct syndrome. *Surgery* 1990; 108:1006–1013.

139. Mallette LE, Malini S, Rappaport MP, Kirkland JL. Familial cystic parathyroid adenomatosis. *Ann Intern Med* 1987; 107:54–60.

140. Harach HR, Jasane B. Parathyroid hyperplasia in multiple endocrine neoplasia type I. *Histopathology* 1992;20:305–313.

141. Law Wm, Carney JA, Heath H. Parathyroid glands in familial benign hypercalcemia (familial hypocalciuric hypercalcemia). *Am J Med* 1989;76:1021–1026.

142. Thorgeirsson U, Costa J, Marx SJ. The parathyroid glands in familial hypocalciuric hypercalcemia. *Hum Pathol* 1981; 12:229–237.

143. Bengtsson A, Grimelius L, Johansson H, Ponten J. Nuclear DNA content of parathyroid cells in adenomas, neoplastic and normal glands. *Acta Pathol Microbiol Scand* 1977; 85:455–460.

144. Bowlby LS, DeBault LE, Abraham SR. Flow cytometric DNA analysis of parathyroid glands. *Am J Pathol* 1987; 128:338–344.

145. Harlow S, Roth SI, Bauer K, Marshal RB. Flow cytometric DNA analysis of normal and pathologic parathyroid glands. *Mod Pathol* 1991;4:310–315.

146. Mallette LE. DNA quantiation in the study of parathyroid lesions: A review. *Am J Clin Pathol* 1992;98:305–311.

147. Joensuu H, Klemi PJ. DNA aneuploidy in adenomas of endocrine organs. *Am J Pathol* 1988;132:145–151.

148. Obara T, Fujimoto Y, Hirayama A, et al. Flow cytometric DNA analysis of parathyroid tumors with special reference to its diagnostic and prognostic value in parathyroid carcinoma. *Cancer* 1990;65:1789–1793.

149. Levin KE, Chew KL, Ljung BM, Mayali BH, Siperstein AE, Clark OH. Deoxyribonucleic acid cytometry helps identify parathyroid carcinomas. *J Clin Endocrinol Metab* 1988;67:779–784.

150. Rodan SB, Insogna KL, Vignery AM, et al. Factors associated with humoral hypercalcemia of malignancy stimulate adenylate cyclase in osteoblastic cells. *J Clin Invest* 1983;72:1511–1515.

151. Strewler GJ, Stern PH, Jacobs JW, et al. Parathyroid hormone like protein from human renal cell carcinoma cells. *J Clin Invest* 1987;80:1803–1807.
152. Stewart AF, Horst R, Deftos LJ, Cadman EC, Lang R, Broadus AE. Biochemical evaluation of patients with cancer associated hypercalcemia. *N Engl J Med* 1980;303:1377–1383.
153. Burton PBJ, Moniz C, Knight DE. Parathyroid hormone related peptide can function as an autocrine growth factor in human renal cell carcinoma. *Biochem Biophys Res Commun* 1990;167:1134–1138.
154. Mallette LE, Beck P, Vandepol C. Malignancy hypercalcemia. *Am J Med Sci* 1991;302:205–210.
155. Tachimori Y, Watanabe H, Kato H, et al. Hypercalcemia in patients with esophageal carcinoma. *Cancer* 1991;61:2625–2629.
156. Sherman LA, Pfeffernbaum A, Brown EB. Hypoparathyroidism in a patient with longstanding iron storage disease. *Ann Intern Med* 1970;73:259–261.
157. Eipe J, Johnson SA, Kiamko RT, Bronsky D. Hypoparathyroidism following 131 I therapy for hyperthyroidism. *Arch Intern Med* 1968;121:270–272.
158. Kleerekoper M, Basten A, Penny R, Posen S. Idiopathic hypoparathyroidism with primary ovarian failure. *Arch Intern Med* 1974;134:944–947.
159. Marieb NJ, Melby JC, Lyall SS. Isolated hypoaldosteronism associated with idiopathic hypoparathyroidism. *Arch Intern Med* 1974;134:424–429.
160. Van de Casseye M, Gepts W. Primary (autoimmune?) parathyroiditis. *Virchows Arch Pathol Anat* 1973;361:257–261.
161. Neufeld M, Maclaren NK, Blizzard RM. Two types of autoimmune Addison's disease associated with polyglandular autoimmune (PGA) syndromes. *Medicine* 1981;60:335–357.

The Parathyroids, edited by J.P. Bilezikian,
M.A. Levine, and R. Marcus. Raven Press, Ltd.,
New York © 1994.

CHAPTER 2

Homeostatic Mechanisms Regulating Extracellular and Intracellular Calcium Metabolism

Edward M. Brown

Calcium (Ca^{2+}) is an essential element throughout the phylogenetic tree. In mammals, it has a variety of important extracellular as well as intracellular functions (Table 1) (1–5). Its extracellular roles include the provision of a large reservoir of Ca^{2+} within the skeleton that also protects vital soft tissues. The skeletal system likewise acts as a rigid but articulated framework that facilitates bodily movement as well as the intake and digestion of food (e.g., the jaws and teeth). The skeleton represents by far the largest compartment of total body calcium (>99%). Additional extracellular functions of Ca^{2+} include its roles in blood clotting, intercellular adhesion, and maintenance of plasma membrane integrity as well as in providing a source of calcium ions essential for intracellular processes such as hormonal secretion, muscular contraction, and intracellular signalling. Indeed, extracellular Ca^{2+} is ultimately the source of all intracellular calcium. The free extracellular Ca^{2+} concentration is maintained within a narrow range (~1–1.3 mM) by regulating the fluxes of Ca^{2+} into and out of the skeleton as well as across the epithelial cells of the kidneys and intestine (1,2,4,5), thereby ensuring a constant supply of Ca^{2+} for its various extra- and intracellular roles. This tight control of extracellular Ca^{2+} homeostasis is achieved despite fluxes of calcium across these calcium-regulating tissues that can be large relative to the total mass of soluble extracellular Ca^{2+} (~1 g or 0.1% of total body calcium). For example, on the order of 10 g Ca^{2+}

is filtered (and potentially lost) daily by the kidney, but 9.8 g of this (98%) is reabsorbed.

Calcium also serves a variety of intracellular roles (3,6,7). It is a cofactor for certain key intracellular enzymes, such as mitochondrial dehydrogenases and various phospholipases and proteases. Ca^{2+} is also an important intracellular second messenger, regulating multiple cellular functions, such as glycogen metabolism, secretion, motility, and some aspects of cellular proliferation (3). Many of these functions are accomplished through interaction of calcium with intracellular Ca^{2+}-binding proteins or receptors, such as calmodulin or troponins, which then activate enzymes and other effector systems (6,7).

The cytosolic free calcium concentration (Ca_i) in resting cells is on the order of 100 nM, ~10,000-fold lower than the extracellular free Ca^{2+} concentration (6). Thus the total mass of intracellular free Ca^{2+} is minute (on the order of milligrams). Consistent with its role as an intracellular second messenger, Ca_i in activated cells can rise by ten- to 100-fold or more. Such large changes are brought about, in part, by rapid uptake of extracellular Ca^{2+} via plasma membrane calcium channels, with the attendant movement of Ca^{2+} down its electrochemical gradient (the interior of cells is generally electrically negative relative to the outside, providing a further driving force for movement of Ca^{2+} into the cell) (8). In some cells, the efficiency of uptake of extracellular Ca^{2+} is enhanced through specialized invaginations of the plasma membrane (e.g., the T-tubules in striated muscle). Ca^{2+} can also be released from intracellular stores, such as a specialized compartment(s) of the endoplasmic reticulum, in

E. M. Brown: Department of Medicine, Endocrine-Hypertension Division, Brigham and Women's Hospital, Boston, Massachusetts 02115.

TABLE 1. *Selected properties of calcium in humans*[a]

Form	Location	Mass (% of total)	Functions
Intracellular soluble	Cytosol, nucleus	0.2 mg	Action potentials Contraction, motility Metabolic regulation Cytoskeletal function Cell division Secretion
Insoluble (sequestered)	Plasma lemma, ER	9 g (0.9)	Structural integrity Storage
Extracellular soluble	Extracellular fluid	1 g (0.1)	Blood clotting Membrane potential Exocytosis[b] Contraction[b]
Insoluble	Bones, teeth	1–2 kg (99)	Protection Locomotion Ingestion of nutrients Mineral storage

[a]Reprinted from ref. 5 with permission.
[b]Activation of exocytosis and muscle contraction depend, in part, on uptake of extracellular calcium.

which the Ca^{2+} concentration is much higher than in the cytosol (9). Indeed, total cellular calcium is high relative to Ca_i (in the millimolar range and comprising ~9 g or 0.9% of total body calcium). Despite the resting levels of Ca_i being much less than the extracellular calcium concentration, the total fluxes of Ca^{2+} involved in the regulation of Ca_i can be quite large. For example, a liver cell can change its total cellular calcium concentration by some 0.3 mM within a few minutes of stimulation by a hormone such as vasopressin, which mobilizes intracellular Ca^{2+} stores (10).

Thus intra- and extracellular Ca^{2+} homeostasis differs markedly in certain respects (e.g., the dramatic contrast between the near constancy of the extracellular Ca^{2+} concentration and the marked fluctuations that can take place in Ca_i). There are also interesting similarities and analogies, however, between the cellular and molecular mechanisms used to regulate these two systems. In both cases, key components of the regulatory mechanisms are the transport systems that promote either uptake of Ca^{2+} from the outside environment [e.g., movement of Ca^{2+} across the intestinal mucosa into the extracellular fluid (ECF) or across the plasma membrane into and out of the cytosol] or cause release of internal Ca^{2+} stores (i.e., release of skeletal Ca^{2+} or mobilization of that within the endoplasmic reticulum). Extracellular (first) messengers and intracellular (second) messengers, in turn, control these fluxes of calcium in such a way as to maintain extra- or intracellular Ca^{2+} homeostasis, respectively (1–5). Second messengers involved in these processes include cyclic adenosine monophosphate (cAMP), ino-

sitol 1,4,5-trisphosphate, and diacylglycerol, as well as Ca_i itself. Moreover, Ca_i is involved in several aspects of calciotrophic hormone secretion and action. It is not only a key intracellular messenger involved in the control of the synthesis and/or secretion of parathyroid hormone (PTH), calcitonin, (CT) and 1,25-dihydroxy-vitamin D [1,25-$(OH)_2$D], but the mechanisms regulating Ca_i homeostasis have also been adapted in kidney and intestinal cells to effect the vectorial transport of Ca^{2+} across epithelial interfaces, which is a key component of extracellular Ca^{2+} homeostasis in complex organisms.

A major emphasis has traditionally been placed on the role of the calciotropic hormones PTH, 1,25-$(OH)_2$D, and CT in maintaining extracellular Ca^{2+} homeostasis (1,2,4,5). Recent data have suggested, however, that, despite the seeming invariance of the extracellular Ca^{2+} concentration, it, too, like Ca_i, is intimately involved in its own regulation through its role as an extracellular messenger, directly regulating a variety of cell types via cell-surface Ca^{2+} receptors (5,11–13). These include cells involved in the control of extracellular calcium homeostasis, such as parathyroid, bone, and kidney cells, but calcium also has effects on other cell types (e.g., platelets), the significance of which is not at present clear (5). The purpose of this chapter is twofold: first, to describe the mechanisms through which extracellular Ca^{2+} homeostasis is maintained (an area of particular interest to Jerry Aurbach, and one in which he made many outstanding contributions) and, second, to compare and contrast this system with the mechanisms involved in regulating intracellular Ca^{2+} homeostasis.

CALCIUM BALANCE AND OVERALL EXTRACELLULAR CALCIUM HOMEOSTASIS

A complex homeostatic system has evolved in mammalian species that maintains extracellular Ca^{2+} homeostasis through hormone-induced changes in the gastrointestinal, renal, and skeletal handling of calcium ions (1,2,4,5). This end is often accomplished without any change in total body Ca^{2+}. With calcium excess, however, there may be positive Ca^{2+} balance, (i.e., deposition of calcium in bone and/or soft tissues) in order to maintain normal or near normal extracellular Ca^{2+} concentrations. Conversely, under conditions of severe calcium deficiency, skeletal Ca^{2+} may be mobilized to maintain normocalcemia. Thus the calcium homeostatic system exhibits several general properties. Its first priority is to maintain a normal extracellular ionized Ca^{2+} concentration. This component represents approximately 45% of the total circulating calcium concentration. Another 45% of total circulating calcium is bound to proteins (primarily albumin); ~10% is bound to small organic anions. With mild to moderate stresses on the system, intestinal and renal adaptive mechanisms are usually adequate to restore normocalcemia. With severe Ca^{2+} deficiency, however, skeletal calcium is mobilized in the interest of maintaining a normal extracellular Ca^{2+} concentration, potentially compromising the structural integrity of the skeleton and thereby predisposing

to skeletal pain, deformity and/or fractures, as in osteomalacia.

The system has two key components. The first comprises several distinct cell types that sense (i.e., recognize and respond to) physiologically relevant changes in the extracellular ionized calcium concentration, leading to appropriate changes in cellular function (e.g., secretion of calciotropic hormones) designed to normalize extracellular Ca^{2+}. For example, parathyroid cells are key sensors of extracellular Ca^{2+} in mammalian species, responding with changes in PTH secretion that are inversely related to those in Ca^{2+} (5,14–17). In contrast, high Ca^{2+} stimulates hormonal release from the CT-secreting C cells of the thyroid gland (18–20).

The second key component of the homeostatic mechanism is the effector systems, specialized calcium-translocating cells of the kidneys, bones, and intestine, that respond to these calciotropic hormones with changes in the transport of mineral ions so as to restore the extracellular Ca^{2+} concentration to normal (1–5). The average amount of Ca^{2+} translocated across these tissues daily in the process of maintaining skeletal homeostasis is shown in Fig. 1. This must be achieved, however, with minimal perturbation in the extracellular ionized Ca^{2+} concentration, which deviates by only a few percent from its average value during the day. At the same time, the calciotropic hormones of the mineral ion homeostatic system (as well

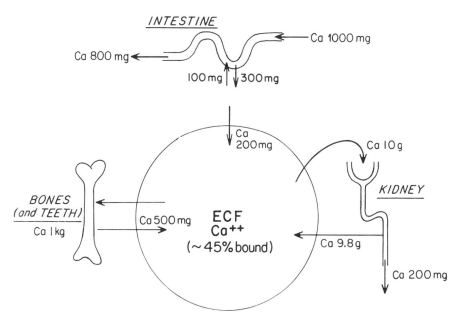

FIG. 1. Example of calcium balance in a hypothetical normal human. Calcium is both absorbed and secreted by the intestine, with a net absorption of ~200 mg/day. This is balanced by the net urinary excretion of 200 mg calcium. Although during young adult life the formation and resorption of bone are equal, during growth there is net bone accretion, and later in life there in net negative skeletal balance. (Reprinted from ref. 5 with permission.)

as a large number of other hormones and neurotransmitters) may employ Ca_i as a messenger that regulates not only their secretion but also their actions, including transcellular, bulk transport of Ca^{2+} in kidney and intestine (3). Therefore, the role of Ca^{2+} as both an extracellular and intracellular messenger as well as the resultant changes in its translocation across Ca^{2+}-regulating tissues must be precisely coordinated in the process of maintaining extra- and intracellular Ca^{2+} homeostasis.

This chapter first discusses the traditional, well-established model of the overall hormonal control of calcium homeostasis. This includes a detailed description of the mechanisms regulating PTH secretion and a brief discussion of the actions of the calciotropic hormones at a cellular level. The discussion that follows then points out certain limitations of this model and discusses newer data and concepts that help to resolve some of these shortcomings. Subsequent sections cover the regulation of intracellular Ca^{2+} homeostasis and its relevance to extracellular Ca^{2+} homeostasis in terms of both hormone action and the interrelationships between intra- and extracellular Ca^{2+} metabolism.

OVERALL HORMONAL CONTROL OF CALCIUM HOMEOSTASIS

Response of the Homeostatic System to Hypocalcemia

Even slight reductions in the extracellular ionized calcium concentration (on the order of 1–2% or less) elicit prompt increases in the rate of PTH secretion (Fig. 2) (14–17). Renal responses to the increased circulating levels of PTH relevant to mineral ion metabolism include phosphaturia (21,22), enhanced distal tubular reabsorption of Ca^{2+} (22), and increased generation of 1,25-$(OH)_2D$ from 25-hydroxyvitamin D [25-(OH)D] (23,24). The increased levels of 1,25-$(OH)_2D$ directly stimulate intestinal absorption of calcium and phosphate. PTH and 1,25-dihydroxyvitamin D also promote net release of calcium and phosphate from bone (25,26). The increased flux of Ca^{2+} into the extracellular fluid, coupled with renal retention of this ion, restores circulating levels of Ca^{2+} toward normal, thereby inhibiting PTH secretion and closing the negative feedback loop. The excess phosphate mobilized from bone and intestine along with calcium is excreted into the urine through the phosphaturic action of PTH.

The magnitude and duration of the hypocalcemic stress impacts significantly on the manner in which the homeostatic system responds. There is a hierarchy of responses by the parathyroid glands as well as by the effector systems that regulate calcium transport in the skeleton, kidney, and intestine. The initial changes in secretory rate for PTH in response to changes in Ca^{2+}

take place within seconds because of the release of preformed hormone (5). Within 15–30 min, there is also an increase in the net rate of synthesis of PTH, without any alteration in the level of its messenger RNA (mRNA), because of reduced intracellular degradation of the hormone (27,28). If the hypocalcemic stimulus persists, modest increases in the levels of PTH mRNA take place within 3–12 hr in the rat in vivo (29) or within 1–2 days in bovine parathyroid cells in vitro (30) that increase the amount of hormone that can be released by each parathyroid cell. Prolonged hypocalcemia promotes parathyroid cellular hypertrophy and proliferation within days to weeks (31,32), which can greatly increase parathyroid cellular mass and PTH secretion in vivo.

The most rapid changes in calcium handling by the target tissues for PTH take place in the kidneys and skeleton. Alterations in renal tubular reabsorption of Ca^{2+} occur within minutes in vitro (33), while release of calcium from the skeleton is observed within 1–2 hr (1,2,4,5). If hypocalcemia persists despite those homeostatic adaptations, continued hypersecretion of PTH causes increased synthesis of 1,25-$(OH)_2D$ within hours to 1 day (34) and promotes the appearance of new osteoclasts within hours to days (4). Only rarely (i.e., with severe vitamin D or dietary Ca^{2+} deficiency) is this full sequence of responses inadequate to restore normocalcemia.

In addition to the calcemic actions of increased circulating levels of 1,25-$(OH)_2D$ (i.e., enhancing intestinal absorption of Ca^{2+} and release of skeletal Ca^{2+}), this sterol hormone also has important actions as a negative feedback regulator of parathyroid function that may limit the response of the gland to hypocalcemia. Elevated levels of 1,25-$(OH)_2D$ inhibit PTH secretion (35) and expression of the PTH gene (29) as well as parathyroid cellular proliferation (36). These inhibitory actions of 1,25-$(OH)_2D$ may modify the overall homeostatic response to calcium or vitamin D deficiency as follows: With pure Ca^{2+} deficiency, 1,25-$(OH)_2D$ levels will be high, and this may limit the magnitude of the parathyroid response by diminishing the extent of cellular hyperplasia and the increase in mRNA for PTH. With renal failure, on the other hand, there is deficient production of 1,25-$(OH)_2D$ that can be accompanied by hypocalcemia, and both factors combined can lead to massive parathyroid cellular hyperplasia.

Parathyroid hormone-related protein (PTHrP) is an additional calcium-elevating factor, which was originally described as a tumor-derived factor responsible for a sizeable proportion of cases of malignancy-associated hypercalcemia (37,38). PTHrP has significant homology to PTH in its amino terminus and exerts its hypercalcemic actions by interacting with PTH receptors, thereby mimicking many of the biochemical features of primary hyperparathyroidism when it is pro-

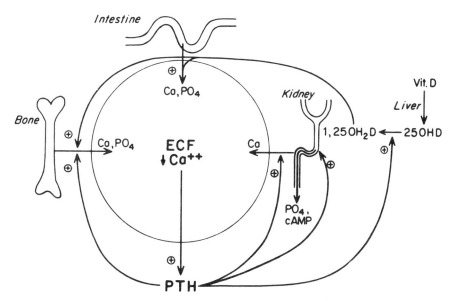

FIG. 2. Overall hormonal control of calcium balance. Decreases in the extracellular ionized calcium concentration stimulate PTH release, which, in concert with 1,25-(OH)₂D, modulates the handling of calcium and phosphate by kidney, intestine, and bone, and restore calcium and phosphate concentrations toward normal. In addition to the effects shown, 1,25-(OH)₂D also feeds back on the parathyroid gland to inhibit expression of the PTH gene, PTH secretion, and parathyroid cellular proliferation. See text for additional details. (Reprinted from ref. 17a with permission.)

duced in excess by tumors (see the chapters by Broadus and Stewart, Grill and Martin, Strewler and Nissenson, and Kremer and Goltzman for details). The normal role of PTHrP, however, remains enigmatic, and it is unlikely that it contributes to normal Ca^{2+} homeostasis during postnatal life in humans. It may be involved in regulating transplacental flow of calcium during pregnancy (39), but much work remains to be carried out in defining its function throughout life.

Response of the Homeostatic System to Hypercalcemia

A calcium load produces responses in the homeostatic system that are largely the opposite of those seen during hypocalcemia. An increase in extracellular ionized Ca^{2+} inhibits PTH secretion, with a resultant renal tubular "leak" of calcium, diminished net release of skeletal calcium, and decreased gastrointestinal absorption of Ca^{2+} because of reduced synthesis of 1,25-(OH)₂D. The remarkable sensitivity of the system to increase in the extracellular Ca^{2+} concentration can be observed with the ingestion of an amount of calcium equivalent to that present in a glass of milk (4). An almost imperceptible increase in serum Ca^{2+} concentration produces an ~30% decrease in circulating PTH levels (as assessed by changes in nephrogenous cAMP excretion), sufficient to promote urinary calcium excretion of much of the absorbed calcium. In response to large loads of calcium, the skeleton can

buffer substantial quantities of the ion, and the kidneys of a normal human are capable of excreting up to ~1 g Ca^{2+} per 24 hr. Hypercalcemia may supervene under these circumstances, however, particularly if renal impairment develops. With a reduction in glomerular filtration rate (GFR), there is a corresponding decrease in the quantity of calcium that can be excreted at a given level of the serum Ca^{2+} concentration, and severe hypercalcemia can supervene over a matter of hours to days (see the chapter, "Acute Management of Hypercalcemia due to Parathyroid Hormone- and Parathyroid Hormone-Related Protein," by Bilezikian and Singer).

In some species, the hypercalcemia-evoked secretion of calcitonin (CT) by the C-cells of the thyroid gland is an important arm of the homeostatic response to hypercalcemia (18). CT directly inhibits osteoclasts, thereby reducing the flux of Ca^{2+} into the extracellular fluid from bone. CT has an additional calciuric action, which contributes to its hypocalcemic actions, as well as an analgesic effect, which may reflect its actions as a neurotransmitter. CT has a substantial hypocalcemic action in certain species, such as the rat, lowering the serum calcium concentration by as much as 50% over a few hours. It has very modest effects in normal humans, however, perhaps because of the relatively low rate of bone turnover in adults. In cases when bone turnover is increased, as in some hypercalcemic individuals and in patients with high-turnover osteoporosis, it can be an effective therapeutic agent.

Control of Phosphate Homeostasis by the Mineral Ion Homeostatic System

An elegant feature of the mineral ion homeostatic system is that it simultaneously contributes to the regulation of the serum phosphate concentration as well. With deficiency of Ca^{2+} leading to secondary hyperparathyroidism, excess phosphate mobilized into the extracellular fluid from bone and intestine is excreted in the urine (mild hypophosphatemia may, in fact, ensue) (1,2,4,5). With oral loading of calcium, on the other hand, the decreases in gastrointestinal and skeletal availability of phosphate are compensated for to some extent by reduced renal phosphate clearance, resulting from a decrease in PTH secretion (Fig. 3).

Primary abnormalities in phosphate metabolism also bring about changes in both serum phosphate and calcium concentrations. Such phosphate-induced changes in the Ca^{2+} homeostatic system can be an important consequence of renal dysfunction and the resultant skeletal disease. Hypophosphatemia, for example, enhances the synthesis of 1,25-$(OH)_2$D (24), thereby increasing intestinal absorption and skeletal release of phosphate as well as calcium. The increased movement of Ca^{2+} into the extracellular fluid from these sources suppresses PTH release, thereby increasing the excretion of the excess calcium as well as retaining phosphate available from intestine and bone. The kidney also reabsorbs phosphate more avidly under these circumstances, although through mechanisms independent of PTH (21). Changes in the extracellular and/or total body phosphate levels have additional effects on phosphate homeostasis, however, that are independent of the classical calciotropic hormones. For example, elevations in ambient phosphate concentration stimulate bone formation, inhibit bone resorption, and reduce the production of 1,25-$(OH)_2$D, while reductions in phosphate have the opposite effects on these processes (21,40,41). It is possible that hyperphosphatemia has direct stimulatory effects on parathyroid function and/or cellular proliferation that are independent of its concomitant actions to reduce the serum Ca^{2+} concentration, 1,25-$(OH)_2$D production, and bone resorption (42).

Does the Mineral Ion Homeostatic System Regulate Magnesium Metabolism?

The serum magnesium concentration is also maintained within a relatively narrow range, but less is known about the mechanisms through which this regulation takes place (1,2,4,5). Magnesium (Mg^{2+}) has direct effects on PTH release, inhibiting PTH release both at low (43) and high Mg^{2+} concentrations (5). The former causes the functional hypoparathyroidism seen in hypomagnesemic individuals, but the mechanism(s) underlying this effect is not known. The latter action appears to result from biochemical mechanisms similar to those through which high Ca^{2+} suppresses PTH release, but its relevance to extracellular Mg^{2+} homeostasis is uncertain, since Mg^{2+} is two- to threefold less potent than Ca^{2+} in suppressing PTH secretion (5). Clear inhibitory effects of Mg^{2+} on PTH secretion in humans can be seen at nonphysiologically high concentrations, such as during the treatment of toxemia of pregnancy by Mg^{2+} infusion (44). The actions of PTH and 1,25-$(OH)_2$D on some of their target tissues affect magnesium as well as calcium transport. For example, PTH stimulates Mg^{2+} reabsorption in the distal renal tubule (45). The overall intestinal absorption of Mg^{2+} is less clearly tied to the action of 1,25-$(OH)_2$D, however, and the skeleton does not serve as a repository for Mg^{2+} as it does for Ca^{2+} (46). The bulk of bodily Mg^{2+} is intracellular, where it plays an important role as a cofactor in the metabolism of compounds containing phosphates linked in high-energy bonds, as in adenosine triphosphate (ATP). It seems likely, therefore, that magnesium homeostasis is maintained by mechanisms in addition to those that regulate calcium homeostasis.

Limitations of Current Models of Mineral Ion Homeostasis

The calciotropic hormones PTH, 1,25-$(OH)_2$D, and CT play critical roles in maintaining mineral ion (i.e.,

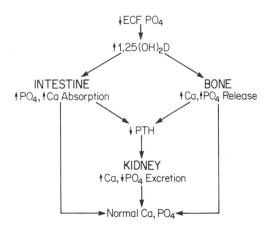

FIG. 3. Response of the mineral ion homeostatic system to hypophosphatemia in a normal individual. Reduced phosphate increases the formation of 1,25-$(OH)_2$D, which increases the efficiency of the absorption of calcium and phosphate from intestine and mobilizes both ions from bone. The resultant increase in the extracellular Ca^{2+} concentration suppresses PTH release, thereby enhancing renal calcium clearance and reducing phosphate clearance to restore the phosphate concentration toward normal while preventing hypercalcemia. (Reprinted from ref. 115 with permission.)

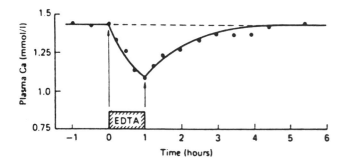

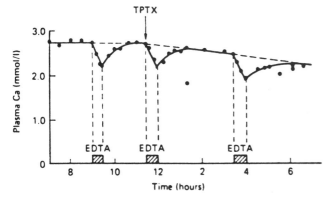

FIG. 4. Effect of the infusion of EDTA on plasma calcium concentration in the euparathyroid (**top**) and hypoparathyroid dog (**bottom**). Even following parathyroidectomy, there is relatively rapid correction of the calcium concentration to the predetermined (albeit slowly decreasing) set point after the infusion of EDTA is stopped. TPTX, thyroparathyroidectomy. (Reprinted from ref. 47, with permission.)

Ca^{2+}, phosphate, and perhaps Mg^{2+}) homeostasis. For magnesium and phosphate homeostasis, however, it is clear that there must be additional, as yet undefined, regulatory mechanisms involved in this process. The same must also be true for extracellular Ca^{2+} homeostasis, as illustrated by the following experiment: Following parathyroidectomy in the dog, the serum Ca^{2+} concentration decreases progressively, dropping by ~20–25% in the first 12 hr (Fig. 4) (47). If the serum Ca^{2+} concentration is reduced further by administering a brief (30 min) infusion of EDTA during this time, however, the Ca^{2+} concentration returns to the slowly decreasing level seen in parathyroidectomized dogs not receiving EDTA within 1–2 hr. Therefore, there must be calcemic mechanisms in addition to the increase in PTH secretion that are capable of some homeostatic regulation of the extracellular Ca^{2+} concentration in response to hypocalcemia, even in the total absence of the parathyroid glands. Recent theoretic discussions of the regulation of calcium homeostasis have emphasized complex and potentially self-regulatory properties of the tissues involved in maintaining mineral ion metabolism (48). Although the cellular and biochemical mechanisms responsible for

these observations in the parathyroidectomized dog are not known, recent studies, described below, on the process of Ca^{2+}-sensing in parathyroid cells and other cell types may provide some clues in this regard. That is, the capacity of ion-translocating as well as hormone-secreting cells of the mineral ion homeostatic system to recognize and respond to changes in their local ionic environment may play a more fundamental role in ion homeostasis than previously recognized (5).

PHYSIOLOGICAL, CELLULAR, AND MOLECULAR MECHANISMS UNDERLYING THE CONTROL OF CALCIUM HOMEOSTASIS BY ION-SENSING AND EFFECTOR CELLS

The Physiology of Ca^{2+}-Regulated Parathyroid Hormone Release and Its Role in Calcium Homeostasis

There is a steep inverse sigmoidal relationship between PTH secretion and the extracellular ionized calcium concentration (Fig. 5), which enables the parathyroid glands to respond to even minute perturbations in extracellular Ca^{2+} (5,15,17). The sigmoidal relationship has been demonstrated both in vivo and in vitro. One way of fitting such curves is by the use of four parameters that include the maximal and minimal secretory rates, the concentration of calcium producing half-maximal inhibition of PTH (termed the "set point"), and the slope of the curve at its midpoint (Fig. 6) (49).

The maximal secretory rate represents the acute secretory reserve of the gland when exposed to a maximally stimulatory, hypocalcemic stimulus. It can increase with an elevated secretory capacity for PTH on a per cell basis, as might occur with increased levels of the mRNA for PTH that occurs in response to hypocalcemia and/or deficiency in 1,25-$(OH)_2D$. An additional cellular mechanism that can modulate maximal rates of parathyroid glandular secretion of PTH has been suggested by the recent studies of Fitzpatrick and coworkers (50) on immunoreactive PTH release from individual parathyroid cells. These studies have shown considerable heterogeneity in the secretion of PTH from single cells: a very significant proportion of individual parathyroid cells studied using the reverse hemolytic plaque assay to quantify PTH release secrete no detectable PTH at high Ca^{2+} concentrations (~80%). The activation of secretion at low Ca^{2+} results from increases in both the fraction of secretory cells as well as the amount of hormone secreted per cell. Even at very low Ca^{2+} concentrations (0.2 mM), however, there is still a substantial percentage of nonsecretory cells (50%). These results are consistent with the previous suggestion of Roth and Raisz (51)

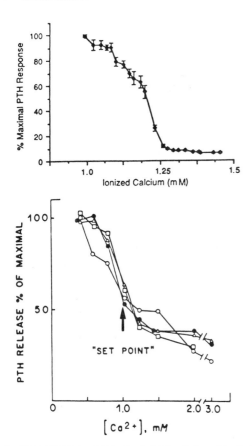

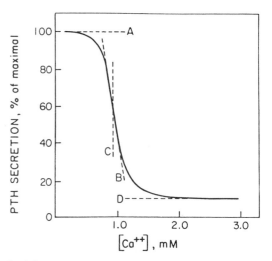

FIG. 6. A four-parameter model of the relationship between extracellular Ca^{2+} and PTH release, based on the relationship $Y = \{(A - D)/[1 + (X/C)^B]\} + D$, where Y is the secretory rate for PTH and X is the free Ca^{2+} concentration. The four parameters are A, maximal secretory rate; B, slope at the midpoint of the curve; C, midpoint or set point of the curve (defined as the Ca^{2+} concentration producing one-half of the maximal inhibition of secretion); and D, minimal secretory rate. (Reprinted from ref. 49 with permission.)

FIG. 5. The steep inverse sigmoidal relationship between PTH release and the extracellular ionized Ca^{2+} concentration in vivo (**top**) and in vitro (**bottom**). The studies in vivo were carried out by infusing EDTA or Ca^{2+} in normal human subjects and measuring the levels of intact PTH as a function of the serum ionized Ca^{2+} concentration, using an immunoradiometric assay specific for intact PTH. The in vitro studies were performed using dispersed cells from normal human parathyroid glands biopsied at the time of thyroidectomy for thyroid cancer. (Reprinted from ref. 5 with permission.)

from ultrastructural studies in the rat that parathyroid cells vary in their secretory state based on morphological criteria, suggesting that they cycle between active and inactive secretory states. Therefore, maximal secretory capacity at the glandular level may be modulated not only by changing the hormonal output of each individual parathyroid cell but also by altering the fraction of parathyroid cells that are in an active secretory state. Even further increases in maximal secretory capacity occur when parathyroid cellular hyperplasia takes place.

The minimal secretory rate has a finite value, even at very high extracellular Ca^{2+} concentrations (i.e., there is a nonsuppressible basal component of PTH secretion) (52). Although there is an increase in the relative proportion of secreted PTH that is inactive fragments with hypercalcemia (predominantly midregion

and carboxyterminal fragments) due to increased intracellular degradation of the hormone, the secretion of intact PTH also persists at high Ca^{2+} (28,52). Therefore, a very large mass of parathyroid tissue would be associated with greater release of intact PTH at high Ca^{2+} even without a change in the inherent suppressibility of individual parathyroid cells. In clinical situations in which there has been a significant increase in parathyroid cellular mass, such as primary or secondary hyperparathyroidism, this residual secretion of PTH at high Ca^{2+} may contribute to the development of hypercalcemia (49).

The set point of normal human parathyroid cells in vitro corresponds to an ionized Ca^{2+} concentration of ~1.0 mM, which is close to the ambient free calcium concentration in normal humans (1–1.3 mM) and plays an important role in determining the level at which the extracellular calcium concentration is set in vivo (49). The set point for the extracellular Ca^{2+} concentration, however, is determined by additional factors in the homeostatic system, including the function of the ion-transporting cells of kidney, intestine, and bone, and their sensitivities to PTH and 1,25-$(OH)_2$D. It should be noted that the extracellular Ca^{2+} concentration is normally ~20% higher than the set point of the parathyroid glands (15), so that the gland is normally functioning at one-third to one-fourth of its maximal, acute secretory capacity. Thus, the gland is particularly well positioned to respond to hypocalcemic stresses, although the capacity of the cell to be suppressed further in response to increases in extracellular Ca^{2+} is a critical part of the defense against hypercalcemia. Interestingly, there is not a universal "normal" serum ionized Ca^{2+} concentration among mammals. Rabbits show serum total and ionized calcium concentrations that can be up to 40% higher than in other mammals, because their parathyroid glands show a corresponding increase in set point that sustains this "hypercalcemia" (53).

In contrast to normal parathyroid cells, cells from parathyroid adenomas show set points of 1.1–1.4 mM, and the serum calcium concentrations in patients with primary hyperparathyroidism are correspondingly set at an elevated level (49). It has recently been shown that enlarged parathyroid glands from patients with uremic hyperparathyroidism may be dominated by cells that have a monoclonal origin (that is, they arose from a single progenitor cell) and have genetic abnormalities, such as deletions on chromosome 11, that are similar to those of parathyroid adenomas (which also have a monoclonal origin) (54). In such cases, uremic hyperparathyroidism may represent true "tertiary" hyperparathyroidism (in the sense that a somatic mutation has generated a clone of cells with inherently abnormal regulation of parathyroid function by Ca^{2+}). These cases may account, in part, for the finding of increased values for set point in cells prepared from some enlarged parathyroid glands from patients with uremic hyperparathyroidism (49).

The fourth parameter describing the sigmoidal relationship between PTH release and the extracellular Ca^{2+} concentration is its slope. The parathyroid function curve has a very steep slope. This ensures large changes in secretory rate with small changes in Ca^{2+} and, in turn, plays a key role in maintaining the extracellular Ca^{2+} concentration within a narrow range. It should be noted that alterations in the "sensitivity" of the parathyroid cell to changes in extracellular Ca^{2+} are reflected not by changes in set point but rather by alterations in the slope of the parathyroid function curve (i.e., the change in PTH that will result from a given alteration in the extracellular Ca^{2+} concentration) (55).

Additional Complexities in the Control of Parathyroid Hormone Secretion by Ca^{2+}

Recent studies have also documented that the regulation of PTH release by the extracellular Ca^{2+} concentration per se cannot explain the changes in PTH levels occurring in vivo during induced hypo- or hypercalcemia. These studies have been greatly facilitated by the development of double antibody assays specific for intact PTH, making it possible to measure changes in the circulating levels of the intact, largely biologically active PTH-(1–84), despite the large excess of inactive fragments of the hormone in the circulation (56).

In normal human subjects, the levels of intact PTH are higher during the induction of hypocalcemia with citrate infusion than they are at the same level of ionized calcium during the normalization of Ca^{2+} following cessation of the infusion (Fig. 7) (57). That is, there is hysteresis in the relationship between Ca^{2+} and PTH following reversal of the direction in which the serum ionized Ca^{2+} concentration is changing. A similar hysteretic relationship between Ca^{2+} and PTH is evident when hypercalcemia induced by calcium infusion is followed by citrate infusion to normalize rapidly the serum Ca^{2+} concentration. Under these circumstances, serum intact PTH levels are also higher when Ca^{2+} is falling than when it is rising. Similar observations have been made in dialysis patients when dialysis against a low-Ca^{2+} bath is followed by dialysis against a high-Ca^{2+} bath, with intact PTH levels being higher at any level of Ca^{2+} when the serum Ca^{2+} concentration is falling (58).

It appears that the hysteresis in the relationship between PTH and Ca^{2+} in vivo results, at least in part, from rate dependence in the control of PTH secretion by Ca^{2+}. When normal human subjects undergo several decremental "steps" in serum ionized Ca^{2+} concentration (brought about by infusion of citrate at progressively greater rates), there is an initial rapid three- to fourfold increase in PTH level with each step that then declines to a lower level despite stable or even declining levels of Ca^{2+} (Fig. 8) (59,60). When the stepwise reductions in Ca^{2+} are made more slowly, on the other hand, the initial, rapid increases in PTH are much smaller (59). The transient nature of the initial increase in PTH cannot result solely from depletion of stored hormone (since it can be elicited repeatedly) and most likely results from a more exuberant PTH response when serum ionized Ca^{2+} decreased more rapidly (i.e., there is rate dependent control of PTH). On the other hand, there is no evidence for rate dependent control of PTH during induced hypercalcemia (59).

The superimposition of rate dependence upon concentration dependent control of PTH during rapid decrements but not increments in Ca^{2+} could produce hysteresis in the relationship between Ca^{2+} and PTH, since PTH levels would be higher at any given Ca^{2+} level during induction of hypocalcemia (either from ambient or frankly hypercalcemic levels). Although the relevance of rate dependent control of PTH dynamics by Ca^{2+} in such studies to PTH dynamics under normal circumstances in vivo is uncertain, it provides a potential mechanism for mobilizing a greater

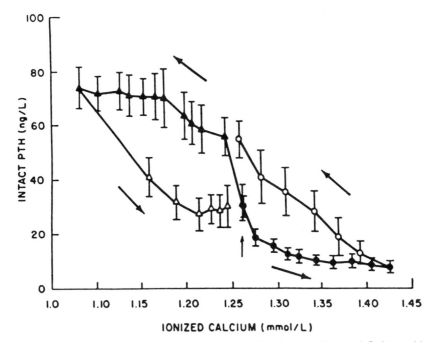

FIG. 7. Hysteresis in the relationship between the circulating levels of ionized Ca²⁺ and intact PTH in normal human subjects when the direction of change of Ca²⁺ is altered. The subjects were initially infused with citrate (*solid triangles*) to lower their ionized calcium, and subsequently Ca²⁺ was allowed to normalize by terminating the citrate infusion (*open triangles*). On a subsequent study day, the same subjects received a calcium infusion (*solid circles*) followed by a citrate infusion (*open circles*). Note that the intact PTH level is higher when the calcium is falling than when it is rising. The *vertical arrow* indicates the basal Ca²⁺ and PTH; the other *arrows* indicate the direction of change of Ca²⁺ during the various phases of the study. (Reprinted from ref. 57 with permission.)

total mass of PTH for a given fall in serum ionized Ca²⁺ concentration when the fall in Ca²⁺ occurs more rapidly.

Mechanisms Underlying Acute and Chronic Ca²⁺-Regulated Parathyroid Hormone Release

The regulation of PTH secretion by Ca²⁺ must involve one or more of the steps regulating the biosynthesis, degradation, and/or secretion of PTH or the control of parathyroid cellular proliferation. The regulation of PTH by Ca²⁺ is unusual in the sense that there is an inverse rather than the usual direct relationship between Ca²⁺ and hormonal secretion (5). Thus the mechanisms regulating acute PTH secretion must ensure the following general features of the secretory mechanism and its control: (a) there must be a substantial rate of PTH secretion even at very low levels of Ca²⁺, to ensure mobilization of Ca²⁺ into the extracellular fluid by the effector cells of the calcium homeostatic system; (b) PTH secretion must be markedly and rapidly inhibited over a very narrow range of physiologically relevant Ca²⁺ concentrations; and (c) the overall magnitude of the curve must be capable of being modulated on a chronic basis when the needs of Ca²⁺ homeostasis dictate it (e.g., the curve must be

scaled upward in the setting of chronic hypocalcemia). The discussion that follows addresses these three properties in turn.

Factors Contributing to Low Ca²⁺-Stimulated Secretion of Parathyroid Hormone

The mechanism(s) that drive PTH secretion at low extracellular Ca²⁺ concentration are not well understood (5). PTH is present in secretory vesicles within the parathyroid cell and is thought to be released by exocytosis. Exocytosis in a variety of cell types is regulated by several different types of mechanisms. Constitutive secretion (61) (e.g., ongoing secretion of proteins such as albumin) shows little minute to minute variation and presumably involves continuous packaging and secretion of secretory vesicles by mechanisms that likely involve an important role for low-molecular-weight guanosine triphosphate (GTP) binding proteins as well as a variety of other proteins that are involved in the biogenesis, targeting, and fusion of various types of vesicles with their cellular membranous destinations (e.g., endosomes, lysosomes, etc.) (62,63). In addition to the basic mechanisms controlling vesicle formation, movement, and fusion with target membranes, regulated secretion of hormones, neu-

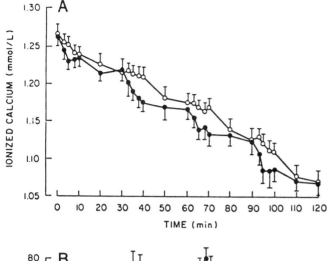

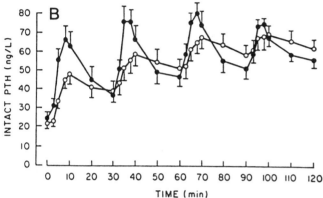

FIG. 8. Rate dependence of the intact PTH response to stepwise decrements in the serum ionized Ca^{2+} concentration in normal human subjects using two different protocols for infusion of citrate. In one protocol (*solid circles*), citrate was given as a bolus followed by a constant infusion rate for each of four 30 min periods, while, in the second protocol (*open circles*), the bolus was omitted. Therefore, the first protocol gives a more rapid approach to the 0.05 mM decrement in Ca^{2+} than the second protocol for each of the 30 min steps (**A**). **B** shows that the more rapid fall in Ca^{2+} in the first protocol elicits a more robust secretory response. (Reprinted from ref. 59 with permission.)

rotransmitters, and other secretory products probably involves additional regulatory mechanism permitting complex control of exocytosis, usually of the dense core secretory vesicles apparent on electron microscopy of secretory cells (64). These additional factors include cAMP, diacylglycerol, and other lipid mediators; Ca^{2+} itself; as well as others; and likely act, in large part, by modulating the activity of cellular kinases, with resultant changes in the phosphorylation of appropriate cellular targets.

The relative contributions of constitutive versus regulated secretion to low Ca^{2+}-stimulated PTH release are not certain. In other cells, constitutive secretion is relatively insensitive to either increase or decreases in Ca$_i$ (65). Therefore, this form of secretion might be able to persist in the parathyroid cell even at low extracellular as well as cytosolic Ca^{2+} concentrations [although, in contrast to previous studies (66,67), Nygren et al. (68) have presented evidence that PTH release decreases if the cytosolic calcium concentration is reduced sufficiently]. It does appear likely that there is also some stimulation of regulated PTH secretion at low extracellular Ca^{2+}. For example, Morrissey et al. (69) found that in response to low Ca^{2+} there was mobilization of the same storage pool of PTH released in response to agents elevating cellular cAMP levels. Moreover, the ultrastructural studies of Habener, Orci, and coworkers (70) showed progressive migration of electron-dense, PTH-containing secretory granules to the plasma membrane with their eventual secretion at low Ca^{2+} concentrations in slices of bovine parathyroid glands. The low Ca^{2+}-induced increase in cellular cAMP in parathyroid cells may contribute to this increase in secretion via the regulated pathway (71). Protein kinase C activity, at least as assessed by its translocation to the plasma membrane, also appears to be increased in parathyroid cells exposed to low ambient Ca^{2+} concentrations (72) and may contribute to stimulation of PTH secretion, in that it is known to enhance secretion of a number of other hormones.

Evidence for a G Protein-Coupled Ca^{2+} Receptor

Accumulating evidence implicates a cell surface, receptor-like mechanism as a key component in the regulation of parathyroid function by extracellular Ca^{2+} (5,12,13). To date, the evidence supporting this concept is largely indirect, based on the effects of the putative Ca^{2+} receptor on intracellular second messengers and PTH secretion. Although Juhlin et al. (73) have raised monoclonal antibodies against parathyroid cells that have been suggested to bind to the Ca^{2+} receptor, the latter has not as yet been isolated in a form that allows detailed characterization of its structure and function.

Largely by analogy with other, more classical receptors for hormones and neurotransmitters, the parathyroid calcium receptor has been suggested to have the following properties (Fig. 9). (a) It is likely to be present on the cell surface and interacts not only with Ca^{2+} but also with a variety of other di- and trivalent cations (13,74,75) as well as with polycations (e.g., neomycin, protamine, and polyarginine) (76,77). The receptor is, therefore, a cell surface polycation receptor, although Ca^{2+} and, to a lesser extent, Mg^{2+} are the only polycations known to circulate in vivo at concentrations capable of modulating its function. (b) The receptor responds over a narrower range of Ca^{2+} concentrations than would be expected if there were a single class of noninteracting binding sites (5,15). This prop-

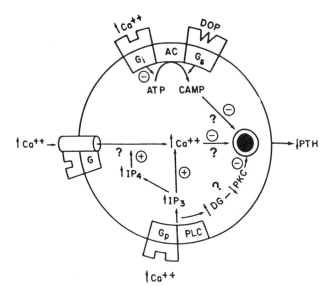

FIG. 9. Model of the possible coupling of cell surface Ca²⁺ receptors to intracellular mediators and PTH secretion in dispersed bovine parathyroid cells. High extracellular Ca²⁺ binds to one or more types of Ca²⁺ receptors, each of which may interact with a separate intracellular effector system. For the adenylate cyclase (AC)–cAMP system, the receptor is coupled to inhibition of AC via the inhibitory G protein Gi. High extracellular Ca²⁺ also activates phospholipase C (PLC), perhaps by a pertussis toxin-insensitive G protein such as Gq. The high level of Ca²⁺-induced, sustained increase in Caᵢ could be due either to the effects of second messengers such as IP₃ or IP₄ or to a separate Ca²⁺ receptor activating Ca²⁺ channels. The links between the resultant changes in intracellular second messengers and PTH secretion remain controversial and are discussed in more detail in the text. (Reprinted from ref. 5 with permission.)

erty most likely results from the receptor having at least two binding sites or possibly several interacting subunits with one or more binding sites for Ca²⁺ (as well as other polycations) that confer positive cooperativity on it. The latter would appear essential to ensure that parathyroid cells respond to Ca²⁺ over a narrow, physiologically relevant range. (c) Carbohydrate moieties likely play a role in the function of the receptor. El-Hajj Fuleihan and coworkers (78) have shown that the lectin concanavalin A renders Ca²⁺ and neomycin twofold less potent in inhibiting PTH release and cAMP accumulation as well as in stimulating the accumulation of inositol phosphates and the transient increase in Caᵢ. A number of cell surface receptors contain consensus glycosylation sites in their extracellular domains, and the Ca²⁺ receptor could also be a glycoprotein. As a practical matter, the use of either lectins or polycations (e.g., polylysine) to attach parathyroid cells to culture dishes or other substrata could directly modulate their function. (d) The putative Ca²⁺ receptor is linked to several intracellular second messenger systems via one or more guanine nucleotide

regulatory (G) proteins (for review, see 5). For example, Ca²⁺ inhibits agonist-stimulated cAMP accumulation in a pertussis toxin-sensitive manner, suggesting that the Ca²⁺ receptor couples to adenylyl cyclase in an inhibitory fashion via Gi (79). Ca²⁺ receptor "agonists" also activate phosphoinositide-specific phospholipase C, resulting in hydrolysis of phosphoinositides with resultant accumulation of the biologically active inositol 1,4,5-trisphosphate (IP₃) and diacylglycerol (12,80,81). IP₃ releases Ca²⁺ from intracellular stores and is most likely the basis for the polycation-induced transient rise in Caᵢ in parathyroid cells. Unlike its effects on cAMP metabolism, pertussis toxin has inconsistent or no effects on inositol phosphate levels and Caᵢ in parathyroid cells (82). While the Ca²⁺ receptor could couple to phospholipase C via a pertussis toxin-insensitive G protein, such as Gq, there is currently no direct evidence for the involvement of a G protein in this process. While it is possible that a single form of Ca²⁺ receptor couples to several second messenger systems in parathyroid cells, it is also possible that there are distinct forms of the receptor that couple to changes in cAMP and phosphoinositide turnover (as for the α-adrenergic receptor, for example). There are also a number of other parameters of parathyroid function that are modulated by extracellular Ca²⁺, including changes in the activity of potassium channels, membrane voltage, cellular respiration, and intracellular pH (for review, see 5). It is not at present clear whether these are regulated by one or more forms of the Ca²⁺ receptor. Another potentially important effect of Ca²⁺ on cellular function is the regulation of cellular stores of PTH. Both in vivo (83) and in vitro (27,28) studies have shown that there is more intracellular degradation of PTH at high than at low extracellular Ca²⁺ concentrations, with a sigmoidal relationship between the extracellular Ca²⁺ concentration and the proportion of secreted PTH that is fragments. The cellular mechanisms and mediators involved in the control of intracellular PTH metabolism, however, are at present unknown.

Efforts are currently underway to use expression cloning strategies with *Xenopus laevis* oocytes to clone Ca²⁺ receptor(s) from parathyroid tissue. Two groups have shown that injection of poly-(A⁺) RNA into such oocytes renders them responsive to extracellular Ca²⁺ presumably because of expression of the Ca²⁺ receptor encoded in the parathyroid-derived RNA on the cell surface of the oocyte and coupling of the receptor to the G proteins and other elements of the signal-transducing and effector mechanisms already present in the oocytes (84,85). A similar strategy has been successfully employed to clone a number of other G protein-coupled cell surface receptors. The availability of a cloned Ca²⁺ receptor would be of great utility in elucidating the regulation of parathyroid cells and other components of the mineral ion homeostatic system.

Coupling of Ca^{2+}-Induced Changes in Intracellular Second Messengers to Alterations in Parathyroid Hormone Secretion

It is currently believed that activation of the parathyroid Ca^{2+} receptor at high extracellular Ca^{2+} concentrations is responsible for the associated inhibition of PTH secretion. There remains considerable uncertainty regarding which, if any, of the high extracellular Ca^{2+}-elicited changes in cellular mediators measured to date are actually coupled to inhibition of PTH secretion (Fig. 9). It is generally agreed that cAMP decreases and Ca$_i$ increases with elevations in extracellular Ca^{2+}, but these changes can be dissociated from the accompanying changes in secretion (5). It is possible that the combined actions of several mediators or even additional mediators that have not yet been characterized in parathyroid cells are essential for Ca^{2+}-regulated PTH secretion. A clue in this regard may be the inhibition of protein kinase C (PKC) activity (72) in parathyroid cells at high extracellular Ca^{2+}, despite the concomitant increases in Ca$_i$ (5,11,86) and diacylglycerol (87) that activate several isoforms of the enzyme (88). Some additional mediator, such as products of the action of phospholipase A$_2$ (89), might be generated at high Ca^{2+} that inhibits PKC and, in turn, PTH release. Moreover, an increasing number of different isoforms of the enzyme have been recognized (88), including those that are Ca^{2+} independent as well as regulated by fatty acids, and a number of different isoforms of PKC could be involved in different aspects of Ca^{2+}-regulated parathyroid function. Future studies should address the regulation of individual isoforms of this enzyme as well as the regulation by extracellular Ca^{2+} and other factors of the various mediators that modulate their activities.

Cellular and Molecular Mechanism Underlying More Chronic Regulation of PTH Secretion by Extracellular Ca^{2+}

Although subsequent chapters address the molecular mechanisms involved in the control of the biosynthesis of PTH, this subject is covered briefly here in the context of the role of these mechanisms in the longer term adaptive processes of the parathyroid gland. As was noted previously, additional ways in which PTH secretion can be increased in response to persistent (hours to days) or chronic (weeks to months) hypocalcemia are through increases in the secretory rate per cell via enhanced expression of the PTH gene or through parathyroid cellular hyperplasia.

Studies carried out both in vivo and in vitro have shown that high extracellular Ca^{2+} concentrations reduce the levels of the mRNA for PTH (29,30). Okazaki et al (90) have recently described a negative calcium-responsive element (nCaRE-PTH) located at -3.5 kilobases (kb) in the upstream flanking region of the PTH gene that confers responsiveness of the gene to extracellular Ca^{2+}. This element is a 15 base palindromic sequence (TGAGACAGGGTCTCA) present in a closely homologous form in certain other genes, such as the rat atrial natriuretic peptide (rANP) gene. The nCaRE may be an important component of a larger gene family regulated in a negative fashion by extracellular Ca^{2+} through interactions of the element with a putative common nuclear protein(s). It is not currently known whether transduction of the extracellular Ca^{2+} signal to the nucleus in such tissues requires an extracellular Ca^{2+} receptor similar to that described above.

A common concomitant of chronic hypocalcemia is vitamin D deficiency, with reduced levels of 1,25-(OH)$_2$D. The latter active metabolite also modulates expression of the PTH gene (91) through the presence in parathyroid cells of a vitamin D receptor (VDR) similar to that present in other target cells for vitamin D. Following binding of 1,25-(OH)$_2$D, the 1,25-(OH)$_2$D–VDR complex binds to specific DNA sequences usually in the upstream region of vitamin D-regulated genes. A sequence motif upstream of the human PTH gene has recently been identified that binds the VDR and likely mediates transcriptional inhibition due to 1,25-(OH)$_2$D (92). In contrast to up-regulatory vitamin D responsive elements, that usually contain a direct, a palindromic, or an inverted palindromic repeat (93), only one copy of the motif is present upstream of the PTH gene. Hypocalcemia accompanied by reductions in 1,25-(OH)$_2$D will produce even further increases in the expression of the PTH gene.

Another essential homeostatic response of the parathyroid gland to chronic hypocalcemia is parathyroid cellular hypertrophy/hyperplasia. The older literature suggested that this was a direct effect of hypocalcemia on the gland (31,32), although many of these studies were carried out in vivo under conditions in which it was difficult to separate out the relative effects of hypocalcemia and attendant changes in vitamin D metabolites. Recent evidence, however, has raised the possibility that hypocalcemia per se, independent of concomitant vitamin D deficiency, promotes parathyroid cellular hypertrophy (including increased levels of the mRNA for PTH as noted) but not hyperplasia (94). In particular, studies carried out in vitro, in which the levels of extracellular Ca^{2+} and 1,25-(OH)$_2$D can be more readily manipulated independently, have more often shown *no* effect of a low ambient Ca^{2+} concentration on parathyroid cellular proliferation (36,95) than they have shown such an effect (96). 1,25 Dihydroxyvitamin D, on the other hand, has been shown in recent studies to have clear inhibitory effects on parathyroid cellular proliferation (36,97). Therefore, a deficiency in this sterol may be an important contributor to parathyroid cellular hyperplasia in hypocalcemic states. The development of a parathyroid cell line in continuous culture that faithfully reproduces the properties of bona fide parathyroid cells in vivo would be of great utility in future studies in this area.

PHYSIOLOGICAL ACTIONS OF PARATHYROID HORMONE AND 1,25-DIHYDROXYVITAMIN D ON TARGET TISSUES

Following a change in the circulating levels of PTH and/or 1,25-$(OH)_2D$, these hormones must modulate the physiological functions of bone, kidney, and intestine in order to restore mineral ion homeostasis (1,2,4,5). The section that follows provides a brief overview of this area as it relates to Ca^{2+} homeostasis, primarily with respect to the physiological actions of these hormones on their target tissues. More detailed discussions of the mechanisms underlying these effects are given in chapters that follow.

Regulation of Bone Cell Function and Ionic Homeostasis

The principal acute actions of PTH and 1,25-$(OH)_2D$ on bone are to increase net release of calcium and phosphate by stimulating breakdown of bone (26,40) and inhibiting its formation (98). Both hormones increase the resorptive activity of preformed osteoclasts in vivo (99). The activated osteoclasts resorb bone more efficiently by forming tight seals with the bone surface and secreting protons and lysosomal enzymes into the space between the osteoclast and bone (100). Several lines of evidence suggest that these hormones stimulate osteoclast function indirectly. Mature osteoclasts are thought to lack receptors for PTH and 1,25-$(OH)_2D$ (101). Moreover, isolated osteoclasts do not respond to these hormones (102). Hormonal responsiveness can be restored by the addition of osteoblast-like cells (103), suggesting that the latter mediate the effects of PTH and active metabolites of vitamin D on the activity of the mature osteoclast through direct cellular contact and/or local humoral mechanisms (100,101).

These calciotropic hormones also increase the numbers of osteoclasts, probably by promoting the differentiation and/or fusion of their mononuclear precursors (99). This action may represent a direct action of the hormones, because receptors for PTH are present on murine mononuclear phagocytes (putative osteoclastic precursors) (104), and 1,25-$(OH)_2D$ promotes maturation and phagocytic activity of mononuclear phagocytes in vitro (105). Characterization of the cellular precursors of osteoclasts and elucidation of the factors regulating their differentiation is the subject of intensive investigation. It is likely that various cytokines, such as interleukin IL-1 and IL-6, play an important role in this process (106) and that some of the beneficial effects of estrogen on osteoporosis, for example, result from inhibition of IL-6 secretion by stromal cells within the bone marrow with an attendant reduction in the activity of osteoclasts (107). In any event, the net effects of increases in the circulating levels of PTH and 1,25-$(OH)_2D$ are to promote a marked activation of bone resorption, and they may act synergistically in this regard. PTH also acutely changes the morphology of osteocytes, and these cells may play some role in the minute-to-minute regulation of the extracellular Ca^{2+} concentration through local release of calcium (4). A postulated role for osteocytes as well as the inactive lining cells covering bone in mineral ion homeostasis (2) remains potentially important but unproved.

In addition to stimulating osteoclastic activity, PTH and 1,25-$(OH)_2D$ both exert direct inhibitory effects on osteoblasts (41,98), thereby further increasing net release of mineral ions from bone. The effect of the former is through interaction with a specific high-affinity cell surface receptor, which has recently been cloned and characterized as a member of the G protein-coupled superfamily of receptors (108). The PTH receptor, which also binds PTHrP with similar affinity, appears to couple to the activation of both adenylyl cyclase and phospholipase C. 1,25 Dihydroxyvitamin D acts predominantly by nuclear actions mediated by the VDR that alter the transcription of specific genes (25). 1,25 Dihydroxyvitamin D also has rapid effects on bone cells, however, as well as other cell types to raise Ca_i that are extranuclear in action (109).

After exposure to PTH, osteoblasts become spindle-shaped rather than cuboidal and show decreases in collagen synthesis and alkaline phosphatase activity (41,98). 1,25 Dihydroxyvitamin D also inhibits osteoblastic collagen synthesis (110). Despite these acute effects, sustained elevations in circulating levels of PTH eventually produce an increase in the rate of bone formation after several weeks (4). This effect most likely results from the coupling of enhanced bone resorption to increased bone formation by the skeletal mechanisms that override the acute inhibitory effects of the hormone on osteoblast function. PTH can also have direct anabolic effects when administered exogenously in an intermittent fashion, which likely result from PTH-induced production of local anabolic factors in bone, such as insulin-like growth factor-I (IGF-I) (111).

The similarity between the actions of 1,25-(OH)$_2$D and PTH on bone may appear paradoxical in view of the well-recognized need for vitamin D in skeletal growth and the consequences of its lack (e.g., rickets or osteomalacia). A major direct action of 1,25-(OH)$_2$D not shared by PTH, however, is to ensure adequate gastrointestinal (GI) absorption of calcium and phosphate in order to promote proper mineralization of bone (1,2,4,5). The skeletal actions of vitamin D presumably contribute indirectly to bone formation by increasing the available supply of calcium and phosphate for mineralization of newly deposited osteoid. 1,25 Dihydroxyvitamin D also directly stimulates the production of the bone-specific protein, osteocalcin, however, so that it may well have direct osteoblastic effects important for optimal bone formation (112).

Renal Handling of Ca^{2+} and Phosphate and Its Regulation by Parathyroid Hormone and 1,25-Dihydroxyvitamin D

A quantity of calcium about ten times that present in all of the ECF is filtered daily by the kidneys (113). Most of this (~65%) is absorbed in the proximal tubule. An additional 20% is reclaimed by Henle's loop, while most of the remainder is reabsorbed in the distal tubule (10%) and collecting duct (5%). Only 1–3% of the filtered Ca^{2+} escapes renal tubular reabsorption and appears in the final urine. Although the amount of calcium reabsorbed in the distal segments of the nephron is relatively small on a quantitative basis, hormonal modulation of this process by PTH plays a major role in mineral ion homeostasis. PTH increases calcium reabsorption by the cortical thick ascending limb, distal convoluted tubule, and connecting tubule in experimental animals (113). The localization of the modulatory effects of PTH on renal reabsorption of calcium in humans is less precise. In effect, PTH resets the renal handling of calcium so that less Ca^{2+} is excreted at a given level of serum Ca^{2+} concentration. Figure 10 illustrates this point by documenting the impact of hyper- and hypoparathyroidism on the calcium excretion as a function of the serum calcium concentration (114).

The effects of vitamin D and its metabolites in modulating renal calcium handling vary depending on the circumstances in which they are administered (115). A vitamin D-dependent Ca^{2+}-binding protein that could be involved in renal Ca^{2+} transport has been localized in the distal convoluted tubule and, to a lesser extent, in the collecting ducts (116). A vitamin D-mediated increase in the level of the Ca^{2+}-binding protein may underlie, in part, the modest vitamin D-induced increase in renal tubular reabsorption of calcium when it is administered to vitamin D-deficient animals. This action may also explain the clinical observation that 1,25-

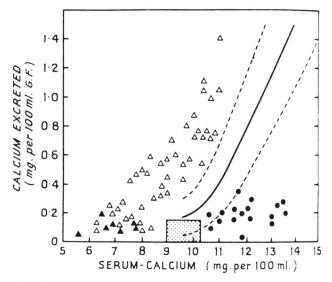

FIG. 10. Urinary excretion of calcium as a function of the total serum calcium concentration in normal subjects (solid line; ± 2 SD, dashed lines), hypoparathyroid individuals (*triangles*), and patients with primary hyperparathyroidism (*circles*). (Reprinted from ref. 114 with permission.)

(OH)$_2$D is required for optimal, PTH-stimulated distal tubular reabsorption of Ca^{2+} (117). In patients with hypoparathyroidism being treated with vitamin D, on the other hand, there is generally an increase in urinary calcium excretion that is primarily an indirect action due to the attendant elevation in the extracellular Ca^{2+} concentration. This then leads to a higher filtered load of calcium that offsets direct, albeit modest, effects of vitamin D metabolites to promote renal tubular reabsorption of Ca^{2+} (115).

The majority of the filtered phosphate load (~80–90%) is reabsorbed proximally. The modulation of this process by PTH represents the major hormonal control of renal phosphate handling relevant to mineral ion homeostasis (21). In contrast to Ca^{2+}, the hormonal control of renal phosphate handling by PTH promotes phosphate excretion by decreasing its proximal tubular reabsorption. The effects of vitamin D and its metabolites on renal phosphate handling are also complex and vary as a function of the metabolic status of the animal (115). As for the effects of vitamin D on renal calcium handling, vitamin D is necessary for optimal PTH-stimulated phosphaturia (21), and this observation could explain the hyperphosphatemia occasionally encountered in patients with severe vitamin D deficiency. More commonly, however, there is phosphate retention following administration of the vitamin to vitamin D-deficient animals or patients (21). Some of this effect likely reflects direct stimulation of the GI absorption of phosphate by vitamin D and indirect inhibition of renal phosphate excretion due to reversal of secondary hyperparathyroidism. However, modest direct stimulatory effects of vitamin D (118), 25-(OH)D (118), and 1,25-(OH)$_2$D (119) on proximal tubular reabsorption of phosphate have also been observed when it is administered to vitamin D-deficient animals. In the hypoparathyroid state, diametrically opposed results can be noted. Administration of vitamin D metabolites to hypoparathyroid humans reduces serum phosphate concentration. In this setting, the vitamin appears to restore the capacity of the proximal renal tubule to excrete phosphate and to adapt to variations in dietary phosphate (more phosphate will be absorbed in this setting and would normally be expected to promote phosphate excretion). The relationships between serum phosphate concentration, body phosphate stores, and the effects of vitamin D on renal phosphate handling are clearly complex and require additional study.

Renal Metabolism of Vitamin D

An important role of the kidney in mineral ion homeostasis is the regulated synthesis of 1,25-(OH)$_2$D from 25-(OH)D (1,2,4,5). PTH-stimulated production of 1,25-(OH)$_2$D in response to hypocalcemia enhances gastrointestinal absorption of both calcium and phosphate as well as skeletal release of these two ions (1,2,4,5). The phosphaturic action of PTH, in turn, clears any excess phosphate mobilized by intestine and bone. Elevated levels of 1,25-(OH)$_2$D enhance the degradation and inhibit the synthesis of 1,25-(OH)$_2$D, thereby acting as a feedback modulator of the net production of 1,25-(OH)$_2$D (1). As was noted above, 1,25-(OH)$_2$D also has an important role as a feedback inhibitor of PTH synthesis and secretion and parathyroid cellular proliferation.

Renal Metabolism of Parathyroid Hormone

In addition to direct parathyroid glandular secretion of fragments of PTH, the liver and to a lesser extent the kidney contribute to the metabolism of PTH and the attendant generation of circulating fragments of PTH (115). The fragments produced by these tissues are largely carboxyterminal, and it has been difficult to detect biologically significant levels of the biologically active N-terminal fragment of PTH under normal circumstances (see the chapter by Kronenberg et al.). Another important role for the kidney is in the metabolic clearance of PTH, which is important in limiting PTH action by assuring a short circulating half time for the hormone. In dogs and in humans, the major route for the clearance of circulating C-terminal fragments of PTH is via glomerular filtration (120). A portion of these fragments is excreted, while some are degraded by renal cells during their passage along the

nephron. In contrast to carboxyterminal fragments, intact PTH and PTH-(1–34) are cleared both by a peritubular (vascular) route [presumably, to a significant degree via interaction with the cell surface receptor(s) through which PTH produces its biological effects] and by glomerular filtration (120).

Renal Magnesium Handling

The proximal tubular concentration of Mg^{2+} rises progressively to levels ~1.5-fold higher than those in the glomerular filtrate, indicating that the reabsorption of this ion lags behind that of other constituents of the tubular fluid in this portion of the nephron (45). Accordingly, in contrast to calcium and phosphate, only 15–30% of the filtered load of Mg^{2+} is reabsorbed proximally. Unlike the case with the former two ions, the major site of reabsorption of Mg^{2+} is Henle's loop, particularly the thick ascending limb (45,121).

In contrast to calcium and phosphate, the importance of hormonal regulation of renal Mg^{2+} handling is uncertain. PTH, calcitonin, glucagon, and vasopressin can all increase Mg^{2+} reabsorption in the kidney, probably acting on the thick ascending limb of Henle's loop. The role of these actions in Mg^{2+} homeostasis is unclear (45), however, particularly since the feedback relationship between Mg^{2+} and PTH secretion may not occur over the range of concentrations present under normal circumstances in vivo. It is also unclear whether the cells secreting calcitonin, glucagon, and ADH can "sense" changes in circulating Mg^{2+} that would then lead to appropriate modulation of renal Mg^{2+} handling by these hormones. As is discussed below, however, Ca^{2+} (and presumably Mg^{2+}) inhibits vasopressin action on the thick ascending limb, which might modify renal Mg^{2+} reabsorption even without a change in vasopressin secretion per se.

THE ROLE OF ION-SENSING IN MINERAL METABOLISM

Figure 4 illustrates that the capacity to maintain extracellular Ca^{2+} homeostasis is not totally lost following parathyroidectomy in the dog. The mechanisms that permit acute correction of induced changes in extracellular Ca^{2+} under these circumstances are not fully understood, but direct effects of extracellular mineral ions on cells other than those secreting PTH and calcitonin represent one possibility.

A growing body of evidence suggests that several cell types in addition to parathyroid cells are capable of sensing changes in the extracellular Ca^{2+} concentration (5). The process of calcium sensing (that is, the capacity to recognize and respond to physiologically meaningful changes in extracellular Ca^{2+}) differs from simple Ca^{2+} dependence. Most, if not all, cells require some extracellular calcium to ensure the maintenance of a variety of calcium-dependent intra- and/or extracellular functions (i.e., muscle contraction, hormonal secretion, and membrane integrity). Most studies addressing the Ca^{2+} dependence of various cellular processes, however, have studied the impact of large reductions in the extracellular Ca^{2+} concentration. It is less clear whether small, physiologically relevant changes in extracellular Ca^{2+} also modulate cellular function and are of some physiological relevance in a variety of cell types. Some cells do respond to relatively small changes in the extracellular Ca^{2+} concentration in a manner that shares one or more features with the parathyroid cell.

Sensing of Extracellular Ca^{2+} by C-Cells

As was noted previously, elevated levels of extracellular Ca^{2+} stimulate hormonal secretion from C-cells rather than inhibiting it as in the parathyroid cell (18,19). Less is known about the process of Ca^{2+}-sensing in the C-cell than in the parathyroid cell, but available data suggest similarities as well as differences in the manner in which the two cell types respond to Ca^{2+} (5). Several studies have investigated the relationship between the extracellular and cytosolic Ca^{2+} concentrations in C-cells (19,20,122,123). These studies have generally employed C-cell lines derived from human or animal medullary thyroid cancers. In several cases, Ca^{2+}-sensing is retained, and these are useful model systems. These could, however, be differences between the ways in which these cells and normal C-cells sense Ca^{2+}. The rat C-cell line rMTC 44-2 shows a transient followed by a sustained rise in Ca_i with even small increases (0.1 mM) in extracellular Ca^{2+} over a physiologically relevant range (20). This response superficially appears very much like that seen in parathyroid cells, but there are several important differences. First, the initial transient increase in Ca_i is essentially abolished by exposure of the cells to a Ca^{2+} channel blocker, unlike the results in parathyroid cells. Thus the Ca_i transient does not appear to arise from intracellular Ca^{2+} stores. Ca^{2+} channel blockers also nearly completely abolish the high Ca^{2+}-evoked increase in Ca_i in C-cells, whereas such blockers have little, if any, effect on the sustained increase in Ca_i in parathyroid cells, even though the latter arises from uptake of extracellular Ca^{2+} (19,20). Thus there are important pharmacological differences between the plasma membrane Ca^{2+} channels activated by elevated extracellular Ca^{2+} concentrations in C-cells and in parathyroid cells. Studies of single C-cells loaded with fura-2 have shown additional differences between Ca_i responses in parathyroid and C-cells. In this case

elevated extracellular Ca^{2+} concentrations evoke repetitive oscillations in Ca_i (122,123), which are not seen in comparable studies of single parathyroid cells.

There are relatively few data available on the role of cAMP, the phosphoinositide–PKC system, and other second messenger systems in Ca^{2+}-regulated CT secretion, although, if anything, high Ca^{2+} elicits increases in cAMP rather than the decreases observed in parathyroid cells (124). Further studies will be necessary to define in more detail the mechanisms underlying Ca^{2+}-sensing in C-cells.

Kidney Cells That Sense Ca^{2+}

Several cell types within the kidney respond directly to changes in the extracellular Ca^{2+} concentration (5). Selected examples have been chosen for discussion here. A number of studies have shown that the synthesis of 1,25-$(OH)_2D$ by the renal proximal tubule is stimulated by decreases and inhibited by increases in the extracellular Ca^{2+} concentration in experimental animals and humans. The first of these responses is accounted for, in part, by the low Ca^{2+}-stimulated increase in circulating PTH levels, which enhances renal 1-hydroxylase activity (23). Studies in parathyroidectomized animals, however, have also shown direct stimulatory and inhibitory effects, respectively, of elevations and reductions in the extracellular Ca^{2+} concentration on the renal 1-hydroxylase (125). This effect takes place over a narrow range of Ca^{2+} concentrations (Fig. 11), similar to that regulating PTH secretion (cf. Fig. 5). The direct inhibitory effect of high Ca^{2+}

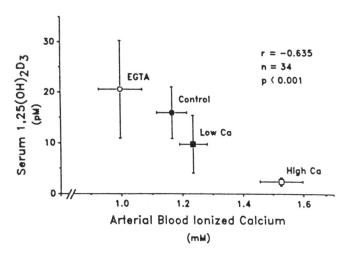

FIG. 11. Relationship between the blood ionized calcium concentration and the levels of 1,25-$(OH)_2D$ in parathyroidectomized rats infused at a constant rate with PTH. The rats received the additional treatments shown next to the symbols to either lower or raise their blood ionized calcium concentration. (Reprinted from ref. 125 with permission.)

on 1,25-$(OH)_2$D synthesis provides an explanation for several observations made previously in vivo. When ruminants (126), dogs (127), or humans (127) receive infusions of PTH, for example, the levels of 1,25-$(OH)_2$D initially rise, owing to the stimulatory effect of PTH on the 1-hydroxylation and perhaps also to the simulation of the same reaction from PTH-induced phosphaturia. As the serum Ca^{2+} concentration becomes frankly elevated, however, the 1,25-$(OH)_2$D levels decline, because of the direct inhibition of the 1-hydroxylation reaction by the hypercalcemia. Patients with severe primary hyperparathyroidism can show a similar response if they have serum Ca^{2+} concentrations sufficiently high to counteract the stimulatory effects of hypophosphatemia and elevated levels of PTH on the formation of 1,25-$(OH)_2$D, thereby resulting in frankly low levels of 1,25-$(OH)_2$D (128).

Additional studies have shown direct effects of extracellular Ca^{2+} and other divalent cations on intracellular second messengers in proximal tubular cells consistent with regulation of tubular function though a mechanism similar to that in parathyroid cells. For instance, elevated extracellular levels of Ca^{2+} (129,130) or Mg^{2+} (131) inhibit PTH-stimulated cAMP production in the proximal tubule both in vivo and in vitro. The concentration dependence of these effects is similar to that for the effects of these ions on parathyroid function. Therefore, 1-hydroxylation of vitamin D in the proximal tubule could be regulated, in part, by Ca^{2+} receptor-mediated modulation of cellular cAMP levels. This possibility has also been suggested by the cross reactivity of monoclonal antibodies thought to bind to the Ca^{2+} receptor in parathyroid cells with proximal tubules (132).

Raising the extracellular Ca^{2+} concentration also increases Ca_i in proximal tubular cells, another effect that could be Ca^{2+} receptor-mediated. Goligorsky and Hruska (133) exposed proximal tubular cells to a single large increase in the extracellular Ca^{2+} concentration from 1.25 to 3.25 mM and observed a transient rise in Ca_i from 20 to 170 nM, which then declined to a level similar to that seen before the addition of the Ca^{2+}. Fujii et al. (134) examined the effects of stepwise increases in extracellular Ca^{2+} on Ca_i in slices of kidney cortex. Raising the extracellular Ca^{2+} concentration produced a dose-dependent increase in Ca_i reminiscent of that observed previously in parathyroid cells loaded with quin-2 (135). This experimental system has several drawbacks in terms of limitations to diffusion of Ca^{2+}, nutrients, and other substances as well as difficulties in resolving the cell types responding with changes in Ca_i. Nevertheless, the results indicate another similarity between the responses of proximal tubular cells and parathyroid cells to increases in extracellular Ca^{2+} that is consistent with the presence of Ca^{2+} receptors in the proximal tubule. Additional studies will be needed to clarify the relative contributions of intra- and extracellular Ca^{2+} to these changes in intracellular calcium dynamics as well as the possible role of phosphoinositide turnover or other second messenger systems in this process.

Several other types of renal cells also respond directly to changes in the extracellular Ca^{2+} concentration in a parathyroid-like manner. In cells of the medullary thick ascending limb of Henle's loop (MTAL) of the mouse, but not in those of the cortical collecting duct, high extracellular concentrations of Ca^{2+} inhibit vasopressin-stimulated cAMP generation (136). The difference between the responses of the two segments of the nephron demonstrates that this response to Ca^{2+} could not be a totally nonspecific response exhibited by all kidney cells. In addition, pretreatment of the tubules of the MTAL with pertussis toxin abrogates the inhibitory effect of high extracellular Ca^{2+} concentrations on cAMP accumulation (136). Thus, in this segment of the nephron, Ca^{2+} may act on adenylyl cyclase through a receptor-like mechanism similar to that thought to be present in the parathyroid cell. Pertussis toxin will also be a useful probe for determining whether high Ca^{2+} acts on cAMP generation in the proximal tubule in a similar or identical fashion.

The effects of high extracellular Ca^{2+} on vasopressin-stimulated cAMP accumulation in the MTAL could well be the basis for the vasopressin-resistant diabetes insipidus observed in some hypercalcemic individuals (1,2,4). Rather than resulting from a nonspecific, direct inhibition of vasopressin-stimulated adenylyl cyclase by an elevated Ca^{2+} concentration, this effect could be due to a more specific Ca^{2+} receptor-mediated process. The role of such a mechanism under normal circumstances is not known.

Quamme (121) has suggested that the MTAL may also represent an important site for the regulation of renal Mg^{2+} (and potentially Ca^{2+}) reabsorption. Elevations in the peritubular but not the luminal concentration of Ca^{2+} or Mg^{2+} inhibit reabsorption of both ions. It is possible that the autoregulation of divalent cation reabsorption in this segment of the nephron contributes to the increased excretion of these two ions that can take place in hypercalcemia and results from a Ca^{2+} receptor-mediated process. Abnormal Ca^{2+} sensing in both parathyroid gland and this portion of the nephron could explain the hypercalcemia, mild hypermagnesemia, and enhanced renal tubular reabsorption of Ca^{2+} and Mg^{2+} in the human disease familial hypocalciuric hypercalcemia (FHH) (137). This defect in renal handling of divalent cations has been suggested to lie in the thick ascending limb, and the location might also explain why these individuals (in contrast to those with primary hyperparathyroidism) concentrate their urine in a normal or near normal fashion despite their hypercalcemia (137).

Renin secretion from the renal juxtaglomerular (JG) cells, similar to PTH secretion, is stimulated by reduced and inhibited by elevated extracellular Ca^{2+} concentrations (138). Many of the studies in this area have investigated the effects of Ca^{2+} on renin release from whole kidneys, tissue slices, or fragments or have employed relatively impure preparations of JG cells. The use of these heterogeneous preparations introduces the risk of confounding effects of extracellular Ca^{2+} mediated indirectly through some other cell type(s). Nevertheless, in more purified preparations of juxtaglomerular cells, a similar inverse relationship between Ca^{2+} and renin secretion has been found. The studies carried out to date also are consistent with Ca$_i$ being an inhibitory mediator in the JG cell as in the parathyroid cell. The atrial natriuretic peptide (ANP)-secreting cells of the cardiac atria, as with JG cells, respond to parameters that are related to the volume of the ECF and have also been reported to respond directly to extracellular Ca^{2+} in an inhibitory fashion. The stretch-activated release of this peptide is reduced by increasing the extracellular Ca^{2+} concentration (139). The mechanism(s) responsible for this effect as well as its physiological significance are uncertain. An additional nephron segment that responds directly to extracellular Ca^{2+} is the distal tubule. Raising the extracellular Ca^{2+} concentration from 0.5 to 2 mM potentiates the 1,25-(OH)$_2$D-mediated increase in the mRNA for calbindin in this region of the kidney (140). It is currently unknown whether the mechanisms responsible for this interaction are related to those through which extracellular Ca^{2+} and 1,25-(OH)$_2$D modulate the mRNA for PTH or whether a Ca^{2+} receptor-like mechanism is involved.

Ca^{2+} Sensing by Osteoclasts

Increasing evidence suggests that osteoclasts recognize and respond to changes in the extracellular Ca^{2+} concentration in a manner similar to that of the parathyroid cell. Cultured chicken and rat osteoclasts exhibit transient followed by sustained increases in Ca$_i$ when the extracellular Ca^{2+} concentration is elevated in the range of 2–6 mM (141,142). Similar to the case with the parathyroid cell, the Ca$_i$ transient is the result of release of Ca^{2+} from intracellular stores. The sustained increase in Ca$_i$, on the other hand, can be blocked by La^{3+} (which inhibits Ca^{2+} channels) suggesting that the latter arises, at least partly, from uptake of extracellular Ca^{2+}. High Ca^{2+} has additional effects on osteoclastic function that may be related to the associated changes in Ca$_i$. Elevating the extracel-

lular Ca^{2+} concentration decreases the expression of podosomes, which mediate the attachment of osteoclasts to bone, and also inhibits bone resorption (142). Therefore, changes in the local extracellular Ca^{2+} concentration accompanying bone resorption could potentially regulate osteoclast activity through a paracrine mechanism. Although the Ca^{2+} concentrations that exert these effects on osteoclasts may appear inordinately high, the Ca^{2+} concentration beneath an active osteoclast may be as high as 26 mM (143). Thus Ca^{2+} within this compartment or that released within the immediate vicinity of an osteoclast could modulate its function or potentially that of nearby osteoclasts. In addition, Ca^{2+} has effects on other bone cells, such as enhancing bone formation in vitro (40,41) and stimulating the release of alkaline phosphatase from osteoblasts, but the mechanisms underlying these effects and their physiological significance are unknown.

Ca^{2+} Sensing in Placental Cells

High extracellular Ca^{2+} concentrations inhibit the secretion of the polypeptide hormone placental lactogen from placental fragments as well as from dispersed or cultured trophoblastic cells, mimicking the effects of high Ca^{2+} on renin and PTH secretion (144). In addition, Juhlin et al. (73) showed that trophoblastic cells exhibit high extracellular Ca^{2+}-induced changes in Ca$_i$ similar to those observed in parathyroid cells and react with the same monoclonal antibody that is thought to interact with the Ca^{2+} receptor in parathyroid cells. Thus Ca^{2+} receptors could play as yet undefined roles in placental function, including modulating the Ca^{2+} concentration in the fetal circulation and/or regulating transplacental Ca^{2+} transport.

Ca^{2+} Sensing and Mineral Ion Homeostasis

These direct effects of extracellular Ca^{2+} on cell types directly involved in mineral ion transport, such as osteoclasts and renal cells, in addition to the cells secreting calciotropic hormones suggest that the mineral ion homeostatic system might be considerably more complex than is suggested in Fig. 1. The latter formulation emphasizes the importance of Ca^{2+}-regulated secretion of PTH, which then acts on distant target tissues to regulate the flux of mineral ions into or out of the extracellular fluid compartment. Systemic and/or local changes in the extracellular Ca^{2+} concentration may, however, also have additional important functions as an extracellular or first messenger in regulating ionic fluxes and skeletal homeostasis. Figure 12 shows a schematic representation of the levels at which Ca^{2+} sensing could modulate the functions of

SYSTEMIC

CONTROL OF
HORMONAL SECRETION

CONTROL OF
HORMONE ACTION

LOCAL

PARACRINE

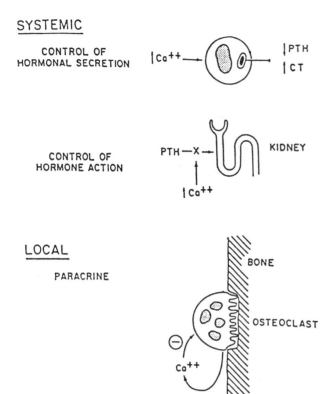

FIG. 12. Schematic diagram of the manner in which changes in the extracellular Ca^{2+} concentration could modulate the function of cells involved in mineral ion homeostasis. Ca^{2+} directly regulates the secretion of calciotropic hormones from parathyroid and C cells. It also inhibits the action of PTH on the proximal tubular synthesis of 1,25-$(OH)_2D$. Finally, Ca^{2+} resorbed from bone by osteoclasts could feed back to inhibit osteoclast activity. Ca^{2+} released during bone resorption also contributes to changes in the systemic Ca^{2+} concentration, thereby regulating PTH and CT secretion in a hormone-like fashion. (Reprinted from ref. 5 with permission.)

cells involved in mineral ion homeostasis. The combination of systemic and local control of these cells by Ca^{2+} could provide a powerful mechanism for maintaining mineral ion homeostasis. Ca^{2+} would thereby not only regulate the secretion of PTH [as well as CT and 1,25-$(OH)_2D$] but could also modulate the action of PTH at the proximal tubule. The direct actions of Ca^{2+} on the reabsorption of Ca^{2+} and Mg^{2+} by the MTAL, on the levels of mRNA for calbindin in the distal tubule, and on osteoclastic function might also locally regulate Ca^{2+} fluxes into the ECF. These local regulatory mechanisms could potentially fine tune the systemic effects of PTH, 1,25-$(OH)_2D$, and CT on Ca^{2+} transport. Moreover, as is discussed in more detail below, these same cells also show responsiveness to changes in the concentrations of phosphate and Mg^{2+} in some cases that could contribute to maintaining homeostasis of these ions.

SENSING OF IONS OTHER THAN Ca^{2+}

Sensing of Phosphate Ions by Cells Involved in Mineral Ion Homeostasis

Changes in the extracellular phosphate concentration also alter cellular function in a physiologically relevant way. Low phosphate concentrations stimulate while high concentrations inhibit 1,25-$(OH)_2D$ production in the proximal tubule (24). Regulation of the synthesis of 1,25-$(OH)_2D$ by phosphate availability can play an important role in mineral ion homeostasis by appropriately modulating the gastrointestinal absorption of phosphate and by enhancing 1,25-$(OH)_2D$-mediated bone resorption. This, in turn, will liberate both phosphate and calcium ions from the skeleton. Body phosphate stores likewise modulate renal tubular reabsorption of phosphate ions, reduced phosphate enhancing and increased phosphate decreasing tubular reabsorption of this ion (21). Phosphate ions can also directly regulate skeletal function (40,41). For instance, elevating the extracellular phosphate concentration reduces bone resorption and stimulates bone formation, while decreasing it has the opposite effects on these parameters. These effects may be partly related to concomitant changes in the synthesis of 1,25-$(OH)_2D$, but similar actions of phosphate have also been seen in vitro (40), suggesting direct effects of variations in extracellular phosphate concentrations on bone cell function.

Thus phosphate-induced changes in the renal, gastrointestinal, and skeletal handling of phosphate ions all contribute to the maintenance of a normal extracellular phosphate concentration, although the mechanisms underlying phosphate-sensing are not understood. It is conceivable that a disorder such as X-linked hypophosphatemia, in which there is abnormal regulation of renal tubular reabsorption of phosphate and the 1-hydroxylation of vitamin D by the extracellular phosphate concentrations, is a disorder in which there is abnormal phosphate-sensing (145).

Possible Role of Mg^{2+} Sensing in Mg^{2+} Homeostasis

Increases in the extracellular Mg^{2+} concentration mimic the actions of elevating the extracellular Ca^{2+} concentration in parathyroid cells (5). These actions are thought to be mediated by the same receptor-like mechanism through which Ca^{2+} acts. Elevated concentrations of Mg^{2+} likewise stimulate CT secretion and inhibit the enhancement of cAMP production by PTH in the renal proximal tubule of the rat both in vivo (131) and in vitro (130). The direct effects of extracellular Mg^{2+} on the secretion of calciotropic hormones could potentially contribute to extracellular Mg^{2+} homeostasis, but it is not clear that this is the case. For instance, Ca^{2+} is 2.5- to threefold more potent on a molar basis than Mg^{2+} in regulating PTH secretion and intracellular second messenger levels, while circulating ionized Mg^{2+} concentrations are comparable to those of Ca^{2+}. Thus it is unlikely that the circulating Mg^{2+} concentrations encountered normally in vivo modulate parathyroid function, at least in the cow. The inhibition of PTH-stimulated cAMP accumulation by Mg^{2+} in the rat proximal renal tubule, on the other hand, takes place at concentrations nearly identical to the Ca^{2+} concentrations that exert the same action (130). As was discussed above, elevated peritubular concentrations of Mg^{2+} directly inhibit the renal tubular reabsorption of Mg^{2+} (as well as Ca^{2+}) in the MTAL (45,121). It is conceivable, therefore, that a significant component of systemic extracellular Mg^{2+} homeostasis could result from the effects on Mg^{2+} on calciotropic hormone action on their target tissues or from other direct actions of Mg^{2+} on the kidney or additional tissues involved in Mg^{2+} handling.

Recognition of Multiple Ions at Cellular Interfaces

The renal proximal tubular and JG cells respond to several different extracellular ions. JG cells are thought to sense K$^+$ (138), Ca^{2+} (138), Cl$^-$ (146), H$^+$ (147), and perhaps Na$^+$ (138). The 1-hydroxylation of vitamin D, on the other hand, is modulated by changes in extracellular Ca^{2+} (125), phosphate (24), and H$^+$ (148), while PTH-stimulated accumulation of cAMP in this nephron segment is also modulated by Mg^{2+} (130,131). Both JG cells and proximal tubular cells have crucial roles in ionic homeostasis. Their capacity to respond to a variety of ionic species may enable them to integrate several different types of ionic input. These two cell types also respond to inputs of a nonionic nature, which include hormonal [e.g., angiotensin II (138) and PTH (1,2,4,5)] and, in the case of the JG cell, nonhormonal (i.e., parameters related to vascular volume) and neural (e.g., sympathetic innervation) modulation (138). Both proximal tubular and JG cells, therefore, may receive several different forms of incoming information that is then integrated to determine the final functional output of the cell.

It may not be surprising that the sensing of multiple ions by individual cell types takes place in the kidney, which acts as a critical interface between the extracellular fluid compartment and the outside environment. This enables it to monitor and modulate the ionic composition of the final urine in response to changes in the extracellular fluid composition. The extracellular concentration of ions also modifies the activity of other cell types residing within the kidney or other cellular interfaces. The cells of the macula densa in the distal tubule may be involved in tubuloglomerular feedback by sensing changes in the ionic composition of the distal tubular fluid (138,149). The gastrointestinal tract also provides examples of cells that have an important impact on the absorption of ions by the organism. Tastebuds sense H$^+$, Na$^+$, and Cl$^-$ (150) and will, therefore, influence the ingestion of substances containing these ions (for a more complete discussion of the sensing of H$^+$, Cl$^-$, and other ions, see 5).

MECHANISMS REGULATING INTRACELLULAR Ca^{2+} HOMEOSTASIS

As was noted above, maintenance of intracellular Ca^{2+} homeostasis involves modulation of the fluxes of calcium across the plasma membrane as well as the regulation of its uptake and release from various intracellular stores (3,6). Unlike the extracellular Ca^{2+} concentration, Ca$_i$ undergoes wide fluctuations, consistent with its role as an intracellular second messenger, due to transient changes in the fluxes of Ca^{2+} into and out of the cytosol. There is considerable variation in the relative importance of the different mechanisms contributing to the regulation of Ca$_i$ in different cell types, which reflect the specialized needs of the wide variety of cells making up complex organisms. This variability, in turn, results from rich diversity in the various molecular forms of uptake, release, and transport mechanisms for Ca^{2+} within these different cell types (Fig. 13). The activity of these transport mechanisms is also regulated by intracellular messengers, such as Ca$_i$ per se, cAMP, and components of the phosphoinositide–PKC system as well as their respective extracellular messengers (3). These regulatory mechanisms again permit great specificity in the control of the basal level of Ca$_i$ as well as its response to extracellular and intracellular signals. The sections that follow provide an overview of the mechanisms through which intracellular Ca^{2+} homeostasis is maintained and provide examples of how these mechanisms are involved in regulating Ca$_i$ in specific cell types. This is followed by a brief outline on how Ca^{2+} is transported across cellular interfaces into the ECF as this relates to maintaining extracellular Ca^{2+} homeostasis.

Extrusion of Ca^{2+} Across the Plasma Membrane

The 10,000-fold lower concentration of Ca$_i$ relative to the extracellular Ca^{2+} concentration requires active transport of calcium ions out of the cytosol. Although the lipid bilayer of the plasma membrane provides some barrier to passive movement of Ca^{2+} down its electrochemical gradient into the cytosol, there is still

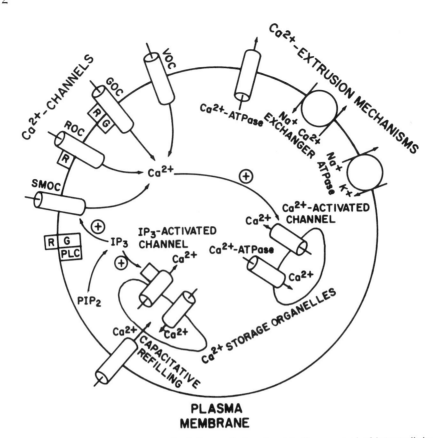

FIG. 13. Schematic diagram of the principal elements involved in the control of intracellular Ca^{2+} homeostasis. Shown are the Ca^{2+} channels, pumps, and exchangers that regulate the movement of calcium ions from the extracellular space into or out of the cytosol or from the latter into or out of the IP_3- and non IP_3-sensitive pools of the endoplasmic reticulum. Abbreviations are as follows: (R) receptor; (G) G-protein; (PLC) phospholipase C; (IP_3) inositol 1,4,5-triphosphate; (PIP_2) phosphatidylinositol 4,5-bisphosphate; (SMOC) second messenger-operated Ca^{2+} channel, (ROC) receptor-operated Ca^{2+} channel; (GOC) G-protein-operated Ca^{2+} channel.

a finite permeability of even a pure lipid bilayer to Ca^{2+} (6). While the uptake of Ca^{2+} into intracellular organelles by the mechanisms described later helps to maintain Ca_i at a low level, the capacity of these uptake systems is limited, and ultimately transport of Ca^{2+} across the plasma membrane is required to maintain Ca_i at its resting level of ~100 nM. There are two main types of Ca^{2+} transport systems involved in active transfer of calcium ions out of the cell: (a) Ca^{2+}–ATPases (151) and (b) the Na^+/Ca^{2+} exchanger (6).

Plasma Membrane Ca^{2+}–ATPases

A family of Ca^{2+}–ATPases has been described whose members are ubiquitous in eukaryotic cells and actively translocate calcium ions out of the cytosol across the plasma membrane by an energy-requiring process that hydrolysis one molecule of ATP for each Ca^{2+} translocated (6,151). The Ca^{2+}–ATPases belong to the family of E1/E2 transport ATPases [also termed P(phosphorylation)-type Ca^{2+} pumps]. These exist in

two conformational states (E1 and E2) during the transport cycle, one of which stores the energy liberated by ATP hydrolysis intramolecularly via a phosphorylated aspartyl residue. Binding of a vanadate ion to this site results in competitive inhibition of the activity of the ATPase by virtue of its stereochemical similarity to PO_4. The plasma membrane Ca^{2+}–ATPases are integral membrane proteins with a molecular mass of ~130–140 kDa. They have an overall topology similar to that of the Na^+/K^+-ATPase and the sarcoplasmic reticulum Ca^{2+}–ATPase, with an even number of transmembrane domains (probably ten) as well as cytoplasmically located amino and carboxyterminal domains. Figure 14 shows a model proposed for the structural organization and topology of the plasma membrane Ca^{2+}–ATPases, illustrating the regions of the molecule thought to be involved in various aspects of the function and regulation of the pump.

Calmodulin (CaM) is a key activator of the plasma membrane Ca^{2+}–ATPases, binding directly to a sequence typical of a calmodulin-binding domain and increasing the affinity of the Ca^{2+}–ATPase for both Ca^{2+}

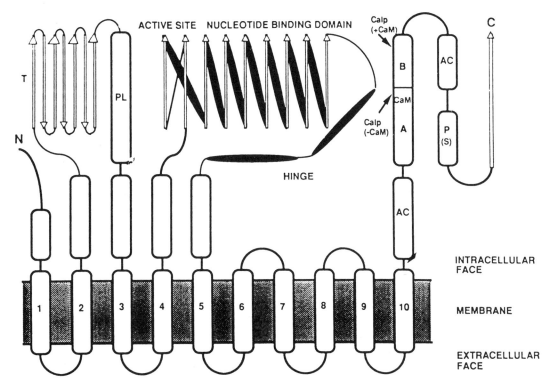

FIG. 14. Model proposed for the overall topology of the plasma membrane Ca²⁺-ATPases. The molecule is shown as a two dimensional representation, with ten transmembrane segments as well as various important intracellular functional domains, including the active (phosphorylation) site and nucleotide-binding regions. From *left* to *right,* abbreviations are as follows: N, amino terminus; T, transduction domain; PL, phospholipid-sensitive region; Calp (±CaM), calpain sensitive sites in the presence and absence of calmodulin; CaM, calmodulin-binding region (with subdomains A and B); AC, acidic regions flanking the CaM binding region; P(S), region containing a serine residue susceptible to phosphorylation by cAMP-dependent protein kinase. *Open rods* and *solid bars* correspond to regions predicted to have α helices, and *arrows* indicate putative β sheet secondary structural elements. (Modified from ref. 151 with permission.)

and ATP, rather than by phosphorylating the enzyme via a CaM-activated kinase (7,152). Therefore, as Ca_i rises during cellular activation, the activity of the Ca²⁺-ATPases increase concurrently through the action of the specifically bound calmodulin and enhance the pumping of calcium ions out of the cell. There is a time lag in the binding of CaM to the enzyme and in its activating effect, permitting an overshoot in the rise in Ca_i before a new steady-state value is reached (153). Several additional activators of the enzyme have been described. These include acidic phospholipids, including polyphosphoinositides, long-chain fatty acids, and PKC (6). Phosphorylation by cAMP-dependent protein kinase is known to activate the Ca²⁺-ATPase from cardiac sarcolemma (6), but not all isoforms of the plasma membrane Ca²⁺-ATPases contain a consensus sequence for phosphorylation by cAMP-dependent protein kinases. The plasma membrane Ca²⁺-ATPases are also activated by limited proteolysis. In the case of the Ca²⁺-activated protease calpain, this could provide an additional level of feedback control of Ca²⁺-ATPase activity by Ca_i (151).

Regulation of Ca_i by the Na⁺/Ca²⁺ Exchanger

The plasma membranes of excitable cells and some nonexcitable cells contain an Na⁺/Ca²⁺ exchanger that is electrogenic and voltage-sensitive because of its coupling ratio of three sodium ions exchanged for each calcium ion (6,154). Although the Na⁺/Ca²⁺ exchanger is not directly driven by ATP, it is thought to be phosphorylated under normal circumstances and is indirectly powered by the transmembrane gradients of monovalent cations maintained by the Na⁺/K⁺-ATPase. Since the phosphorylated exchanger has a high affinity for intracellular Ca²⁺ and extracellular Na⁺, the normally high ratio of extracellular to intracellular Na⁺ favors exchange of inwardly directed sodium ions for outwardly directed calcium ions. If the plasma membrane is depolarized, however, the changes in the electrical driving forces for Na⁺ and Ca²⁺ now favor inward movement of calcium ions. In excitable cells, therefore, the exchanger can contribute to elevation in Ca_i during the action potential and to pumping of calcium out of the cytosol during repolarization (6). While the V_{max} of the exchanger is higher than that of the plasma membrane Ca^{2+}–ATPases, its K_m for Ca^{2+} is considerably higher (~2 μM). Therefore, the importance of the exchanger for the maintenance of resting levels of Ca_i will depend heavily on the absolute level of the cytosolic Ca^{2+} concentration as well as on the relative numbers of Ca^{2+}–ATPases and Na^+/Ca^{2+} exchangers. There appears to be relatively little direct regulation of the exchanger by the intracellular mediators that can modulate the activity of Ca^{2+}–ATPases, but an important forms of indirect regulation takes place with variations in the intracellular sodium concentration. Inhibition of the Na^+/K^+-ATPase by cardiac glycosides, for instance, elevates the intracellular Na^+ concentration, favoring uptake rather than extrusion of Ca^{2+} by the exchanger and resulting in a rise in Ca_i and enhanced cardiac contractility (155).

Uptake of Extracellular Ca^{2+} by Plasma Membrane Ca^{2+} Channels

The opening of plasma membrane Ca^{2+} channels allows rapid, passive movement of Ca^{2+} ions down their electrochemical gradient and represents an important source of Ca^{2+} for intracellular signaling via increases in Ca_i. The plasma membrane Ca^{2+} channels fall into two major groups, depending on whether they are voltage or ligand gated (6).

Voltage-Operated Ca^{2+} Channels

This class of Ca^{2+} channels is present in both excitable and nonexcitable cells. Present nomenclature distinguishes three principal forms of voltage-operated Ca^{2+} channels—the L-type, N-type, and T-type Ca^{2+} channels—that differ in their distribution, kinetic properties, and susceptibility to various pharmacological agents (8). The L-type channels are potently inhibited by the dihydropyridine class of Ca^{2+} channel blockers. They begin to activate at membrane potentials more positive than −30 to −40 mM and inactivate rapidly in cardiac and smooth muscle but more slowly in neurons and particularly in endocrine cells. The purified channel from skeletal muscle comprises a 1:1:1:1 complex of four distinct polypeptide chains, the α_1, α_2, δ, and γ chains (156) [upon reduction of the α_2 chain, a fifth chain (the δ subunit) appears]. Molecular cloning of the individual chains has revealed a considerable degree of homology between one of the predicted membrane spanning domains of the α_1 subunit (the S4 segment) (157) and the corresponding segments of voltage-sensitive K^+ (158) and Na^+ (159) channels. It is thought that the S4 segment contains

structural elements essential for voltage-sensing by all three types of channels.

Cardiac L-type Ca^{2+} channels can be activated by hormones stimulating adenylyl cyclase activity by two distinct mechanisms, one involving cAMP-dependent phosphorylation of the channel and/or an associated protein and the second entailing direct stimulation of channel activity by GS, the G protein that also activates adenylyl cyclase (6). There is considerable heterogeneity in the response of L-type channels to cAMP, however, since Ca^{2+} currents of some neuronal, smooth muscle, and secretory cells are not increased in association with elevations in intracellular cAMP content.

N-type channels are a heterogeneous group of Ca^{2+} channels present predominantly in neurons (8). They are activated over a range of membrane potentials similar to that for L-type channels but have a lower single channel conductance for Ca^{2+}, inactivate more completely at membrane potentials more positive than −20 mV, and are insensitive to dihydropyridines. In further distinction to L-type channels, they are irreversibly blocked by ω-conotoxin. T-type Ca^{2+} channels are found in a much wider range of excitable and nonexcitable cells and activate at membrane potentials ~30–40 mV more negative than L- and T-type channels. They show very substantial voltage-dependent inactivation and are blocked much more potently by Ni^{2+} than are L- or N-type channels but are relatively resistant to both dihydropyridines and ω-conotoxin.

In addition to the regulation of L-type channels by cAMP and G_s, voltage-operated Ca^{2+} channels (most likely the N-type channels) can be inhibited by a pertussis toxin-insensitive G protein, most likely Go (160). Activators or protein kinase C also inhibit voltage-dependent Ca^{2+} currents in many secretory cells, perhaps through actions on L-type channels (161), as noted above, as well as on T-type channels (162).

Receptor- and Second Messenger-Activated Ca^{2+} Channels

Although it has been known for some time that plasma membrane Ca^{2+} channels can be gated by extracellular hormones, neurotransmitters, and other ligands, recent studies have begun to differentiate several distinct mechanisms through which this can take place (6). Three types of channels currently recognized are receptor-operated channels, second messenger-operated channels, and G protein-operated channels. In the first of these, the receptor controls a channel that is either on the same polypeptide chain or is part of the same molecular complex. The clearest example of receptor-operated Ca^{2+} channels are the glutamate-activated channels (NMDA, APMA, and kainate receptors) in the brain (164), which have large extracellular domains thought to contribute to glutamate binding as well as four putative membrane spanning domains that likely make up the Ca^{2+} channel itself.

Regulation of second messenger-operated channels takes place through receptor-mediated generation of a soluble, intracellular second messenger, which then gates a Ca^{2+} channel that is physically distinct from the receptor. The Ca^{2+}-activated Ca^{2+} release channel in the endoplasmic reticulum is an example of this type of channel and is discussed in more detail below, but some studies have suggested that similar channels may exist in the plasma membrane (165). In this formulation, a rise in Ca$_i$ due to release of Ca^{2+} from intracellular stores could then gate Ca^{2+}-activated Ca^{2+} channels in the plasma membrane. Inositol 1,4,5-trisphosphate and perhaps inositol 1,3,4,5-tetrakisphosphate have also been suggested to regulate plasma membrane Ca^{2+} channels (6), but not all investigators have been able to confirm their existence, and further investigation of this mechanism is needed. An alternative or additional explanation for uptake of Ca^{2+} in association with increases in IP$_3$ levels, initially postulated by Putney (166), is that influx of extracellular Ca^{2+} in response to hormones stimulating phosphoinositide turnover is activated in order to refill intracellular Ca^{2+} stores emptied by inositol 1,4,5-trisphosphate (the so-called capacitative model). This model originally suggested that release of Ca^{2+} from intracellular storage organelles in some way promoted a direct, gap junction-like connection between the organelle and the plasma membrane, permitting refilling of the depleted stores. A recent reformulation of this hypothesis has suggested the generation of an as yet unidentified intracellular signal in response to depletion of intracellular Ca^{2+} stores, which then opens plasma membrane Ca^{2+} channels (166). Refilling of the IP$_3$-sensitive stores takes place via the cytosol rather than through a direct connection between these storage organelles and the plasma membrane.

Finally, there is some evidence for receptor-dependent, G protein-mediated gating of plasma membrane Ca^{2+} channels (6) other than the activation of L-type channels by GS described previously. For example, IGF-I and IGF-II activate a nonspecific cation channel, permeable to Ca^{2+} (167). This activation is inhibited by pertussis toxin and can be mimicked in excised membrane patches by addition of GTP or nonhydrolyzable GTP analogs. The activation is not thought to involve the G protein-dependent generation of an intracellular second messenger, however, since, in the cell-attached configuration of the patch clamp (the pipette is attached to an intact cell without disrupting the patch of membrane inside the pipette) extracellular application of the growth factors inside but not outside of the pipette opens channels within the patch (167). In this configuration, the seal between the patch pipette and the plasma membrane is so tight that IGF-I and -II do not have access to their receptors within the membrane patch inside of the patch pipette. If an intracellular second messenger were involved in mediating the effect, it would be able to diffuse through the cytosol from the region of membrane outside the patch pipette to the channels within the patch following application of the hormone to the bath.

In addition to the Ca^{2+} channels and channel-like processes described above, additional mechanisms have been described that could increase the cellular entry of Ca^{2+}. One such mechanism is the purported role of phosphatidic acid (generated directly by the action of phospholipase D or by the sequential actions of phospholipase C and DG kinase) as a Ca^{2+} ionophore (168). The action has been postulated to involve the direct interaction of Ca^{2+} ions with PA, followed by passage of the complex across the plasma membrane by a largely nonspecific, ionophore-like action (113). The relevance of this action to agonist-induced changes in Ca$_i$ is unclear. Moreover, PA appears to be able to exert actions on intracellular second messengers that could be explained by a G protein-coupled cell surface receptor for this or some related lipid (169,170).

Release and Uptake of Cytosolic Ca^{2+} by Intracellular Ca^{2+}-Storage Organelles

Although the extracellular fluid provides an essentially infinite source of Ca^{2+} ions potentially available for intracellular needs, cells have developed an additional source of calcium ions that can be rapidly released into the cytosol in response to appropriate stimuli. In muscle cells, these organelles [the sarcoplasmic reticulum (SR)] are placed into close apposition with myofibrils to improve the efficiency of stimulus–contraction coupling (6). Essentially all cells (with the example of mature erythrocytes) use variations on this theme to provide a rapidly releasable pool(s) of intracellular Ca^{2+} ions. These organelles are likely to be specialized forms of the endoplasmic reticulum, although there is some uncertainty regarding their exact identification, and they vary in their morphological and functional properties between different cell types (171).

Ca^{2+} storage organelles appear to share three basic elements: (a) a Ca^{2+} pump, enabling them to accumulate calcium ions against a concentration gradient, (b) Ca^{2+}-binding proteins within the organelles, and (c) receptor-regulated Ca^{2+}-release channels (6,171). Because of the efficiency of the plasma membrane Ca^{2+}–ATPases, however, some fraction of the Ca^{2+} released from these organelles is generally lost to the extracellular space with each release event. An additional property that is necessary for optimal long-term function of Ca^{2+} storage organelles, therefore, is a mechanism for ensuring proper refilling of these organelles, utilizing Ca^{2+} from the extracellular space when necessary. This was described previously in the context of the capacitative model of refilling of the IP_3-sensitive intracellular Ca^{2+} pool (166).

Ca^{2+} Pumps in Ca^{2+}-Storage Organelles

There is tissue-specific expression of three different intracellular Ca^{2+} pumps: (a) the type I (fast-type) Ca^{2+}–ATPase found in fast-twitch skeletal muscle, (b) the type II (slow-type) Ca^{2+}–ATPase found in slow-twitch skeletal muscle and cardiac muscle, and (c) a nonmuscle form of the slow-type Ca^{2+}–ATPase found in nonmuscle cells (172). All three families are P-type Ca^{2+}–ATPases, but molecular cloning has shown them to be distinct from the plasma membrane Ca^{2+}–ATPases (173). All three have molecular weights of ~100–110 kDa. The fast-type and slow-type Ca^{2+}–ATPases are separate gene products, while the nonmuscle form of slow-type Ca^{2+}–ATPase arises from the same gene as the slow-type Ca^{2+}–ATPase by alternative splicing.

The overall topology of the Ca^{2+}–ATPases of the Ca^{2+}-storage organelles is similar to that of the plasma membrane Ca^{2+} pumps, with ten membrane spanning regions as well as transduction, phosphorylation (active site), and nucleotide-binding domains (6). The smaller molecular size of the intracellular Ca^{2+}–ATPases is accounted for primarily by shortening of the cytoplasmic carboxy terminus of the molecule, which contains important regulatory regions (CaM-binding region and site for cAMP-dependent phosphorylation) in the plasma membrane Ca^{2+}–ATPases. The slow-type Ca^{2+}–ATPase is regulated by an acidic proteolipid, phospholamban, which binds ATP with 1:1 stoichiometry and has phosphorylation sites for both cAMP- and Ca^{2+}–CaM-dependent protein kinases. Phospholamban binds to the Ca^{2+}–ATPase in its dephosphorylated forms and inhibits it; after it is phosphorylated, phospholamban dissociates from the enzyme permitting its activation (174).

Ca^{2+}-Binding Proteins Within Ca^{2+}-Storage Organelles

The most abundant calcium-binding proteins within the Ca^{2+}-storage organelles are calsequestrin within the sarcoplasmic reticulum and calreticulin within nonmuscle endoplasmic reticulum (6). Both are glycoproteins with molecular weights of 40–50 kDa that have multiple (30–50) low-affinity binding sites for Ca^{2+} with values for K_d in the range of 1 mM. Calreticulin also has one high-affinity Ca^{2+}-binding site. The function of these proteins is not known with certainty, but they may provide for buffering of the locally high Ca^{2+} concentrations within the Ca^{2+}-storage organelles or serve to concentrate calcium ions near the sites where Ca^{2+}-release channels are located (175). An additional intriguing possibility that has been put forward is that these or other Ca^{2+}-binding proteins serve as Ca^{2+} sensors that monitor the state of filling of the Ca^{2+}-storage organelles (6). It would not be surprising if the function and Ca^{2+} concentration of this important Ca^{2+}-storage compartment was regulated, in part, by a process of Ca^{2+} sensing analogous to the roles of the extracellular Ca^{2+} receptor(s) and the intracellular Ca^{2+} receptor, CaM, in maintaining extracellular and intracellular (cytosolic) Ca^{2+} homeostasis, respectively.

Ca^{2+}-Release Channels of Ca^{2+}-Storage Organelles

Two principal Ca^{2+} channels have been identified that control the release of Ca^{2+} from its intracellular Ca^{2+}-storage organelles, the ryanodine receptor/channel and the inositol 1,4,5-trisphosphate receptor/channel (6,171). The former releases Ca^{2+} from these stores in response to ryanodine, caffeine, or Ca^{2+} itself and is thought to be the basis for Ca^{2+}-induced release of intracellular Ca^{2+} stores. It was originally defined in muscle cells but has subsequently been found in nonmuscle cells as well. The ryanodine receptor is a very large protein ~5,000 amino acids in length. Only the carboxy terminus contains sequences of amino acids sufficiently hydrophobic to comprise membrane spanning regions, of which there are probably four that make up the Ca^{2+}-release channel. The remainder of the molecule probably represents a huge hydrophilic, cytosolic amino terminus that represents one subunit of the "foot" structures in intact muscle that span the gap between the SR and the T-tubules invaginating from the plasma membrane (6) (Fig. 15). It has been suggested that these "feet" interact with dihydropyridine receptors in the T-tubules that act as voltage sensors to regulate Ca^{2+} release from the sarcoplasmic reticulum (177).

An IP_3-sensitive Ca^{2+} channel has also recently been cloned and is likewise a large protein (predicted molecular weight 313 kDa) with up to six membrane spanning regions, all near the carboxy terminus, as in the ryanodine receptor (178). There is, in fact, significant sequence homology with the ryanodine receptor in specific regions (i.e., 47% identity over 136 residues of the two proteins). There are neuronal and nonneuronal forms of the protein, derived by alternative splicing (171). The N-terminus has been proposed to lie within the cytoplasm, while the C-terminus resides

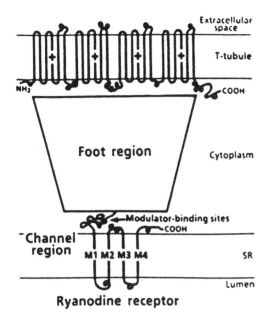

FIG. 15. Structural model proposed for the junctional complex of the sarcoplasmic reticulum. The *looped structures* within the T-tubule represent dihydropyridine receptors, with the *plus signs* representing their voltage sensors within the S4 segment. The ryanodine receptor within the SR, with its large "foot" structure contacting the dihydropyridine receptors, is also shown. (Reprinted from ref. 176 with permission.)

within the lumen of the ER. The protein has a high affinity for inositol 1,4,5-trisphosphate, binds strongly to heparin (which is an inhibitor of IP$_3$ action), and has multiple glycosylation sites and two phosphorylation sites for cAMP-dependent protein kinase.

A wide variety of cell surface receptors, including not only G protein-coupled receptors (e.g., the receptors for PTH and calcitonin as well as the putative Ca^{2+} receptor of the parathyroid cell) but also growth factor receptors, are linked to the action of phosphoinositide-specific PLC (9,88). The ensuing hydrolysis of phosphatidylinositol 4,5-bisphosphate generates both DG and inositol 1,4,5-trisphosphate. The latter releases Ca^{2+} from the IP$_3$-sensitive storage pool(s) in the endoplasmic reticulum by interacting with its specific receptor. As was noted above, IP$_3$-mediated release of Ca^{2+} from these stores is often accompanied by uptake of extracellular Ca^{2+} through several possible mechanisms, including plasma membrane Ca^{2+} channels or other uptake mechanisms activated by IP$_3$ or Ca$_i$ itself (i.e., Ca^{2+}-induced Ca^{2+} uptake or through the capacitative mechanism described previously) (6,166). Recent studies have also shown that increases in Ca$_i$ due to gating of plasma membrane Ca^{2+} channels can enhance release of intracellular Ca^{2+} from intracellular stores not only by Ca^{2+}-induced Ca^{2+} release (6) but also due to direct activation of phospholipase C by increases in Ca$_i$ leading to IP$_3$-mediated release of intracellular Ca^{2+} (179). The effects

of the resultant increases in Ca$_i$ are mediated both through the intracellular Ca^{2+} receptors described in the next section (7,152) as well as through activation of PKC by the combined effects of increases in cellular levels of DG and in Ca$_i$ (9,88).

Additional intracellular mediators have been described that release Ca^{2+} from intracellular stores, but the mechanisms regulating their formation and actions, including the Ca^{2+}-storage organelles upon which they act and the receptors/channels through which they release stored Ca^{2+}, have not yet been fully elucidated. These agents include a metabolite of sphingosine, perhaps sphingosine phosphate (180). The importance of this putative mediator in intracellular Ca^{2+} signaling in a wider variety of cell types has not yet been established.

Other Ca^{2+}-Binding Intracellular Organelles

Secretory vesicles accumulate significant amounts of Ca^{2+} but are not thought to be involved in the regulation of Ca$_i$. Mitochondria also can take up large quantities of Ca^{2+}, but their role in intracellular Ca^{2+} homeostasis is still uncertain (6). It is possible that one function of mitochondria is to act as a low-affinity, high-capacity repository for Ca^{2+} that can buffer pathological increases in Ca$_i$ occurring with cell injury. It is also clear that several important mitochondrial dehydrogenases are Ca^{2+} regulated, and the regulation of mitochondrial Ca^{2+} metabolism is likely to be essential for the proper coordination of their enzymatic activities.

Cytosolic Ca^{2+}-Binding Proteins and Intracellular Ca^{2+} Receptors

There are two broad classes of cytosolic Ca^{2+}-binding proteins: those that are thought to act as intracellular Ca^{2+} buffers and those that act as specific intracellular Ca^{2+} receptors and mediate the effects of changes in Ca$_i$. The parvalbumins are examples of the former class of Ca^{2+}-binding proteins (6). They are small (9–13 kDa) proteins present in many different cell types that, unlike the Ca^{2+}-binding proteins in Ca^{2+}-storage organelles, must be capable of binding Ca^{2+} within the range of concentrations encountered in the cytosol (~0.1–10 μM). Therefore, unlike the low (mM)-affinity Ca^{2+}-binding sites of calsequestrin and calreticulin, these proteins have higher affinity sites, exemplified by those of the so-called EF-hand superfamily of Ca^{2+}-binding proteins (181). The calcium-binding site of this motif comprises an α helix–loop–α helix structure. There is no known function of parvalbumin other than acting as a calcium buffer. It is present in large concentrations in fast-twitch muscle fibers and may facilitate rapid reductions in Ca_i at the end of each contraction by acting as a temporary repository for Ca^{2+} prior to its reuptake into the SR (6).

A number of intracellular Ca^{2+}-binding proteins are now known to act as intracellular Ca^{2+} sensors or receptors and play a key role in transducing changes in Ca_i into alterations in cellular function. Probably the best known of these is the small (16 kDa), ubiquitous Ca^{2+}-binding protein CaM (7,152). It is a dumbbell-shaped molecule with two EF-hand Ca^{2+}-binding sites within each globular end of the molecule. CaM exerts its cellular effects by interacting with and activating target enzymes in a Ca^{2+}-dependent manner. Binding of several (probably three or more) Ca^{2+} ions to CaM greatly increases its affinity for target enzymes. Recently, it has been suggested that CaM exerts its effect on target enzyme activity by derepression rather than direct activation (182). In this formulation, originally suggested for myosin light-chain kinase (MLCK), the CaM-binding domain of MLCK prevents access of the natural substrate to the enzyme in the absence of CaM. Binding of CaM then removes this block and permits the enzyme to phosphorylate myosin (182). Among the enzymatic reactions regulated by CaM are the following: cAMP phosphodiesterase, adenylyl cyclase, phosphorylase kinase, MLCK, plasma membrane Ca^{2+}–ATPase, and phospholipase A_2 (7). This allows this intracellular Ca^{2+} receptor to play a pivotal role in cellular regulation, not only directly mediating the effects of changes in Ca_i on cellular function but also by modulating these changes in Ca_i through its effects on the cellular mechanisms transferring calcium ions into and out of the cytosol (e.g., by the plasma membrane Ca^{2+}–ATPases).

Troponin C is another small, EF-hand-containing protein that plays an important role in the regulation of muscle contraction of striated muscle fibers (6,183). In relaxed muscle fibers, it is an integral part of the thin filament and prevents the interaction of myosin heads with actin. Following a rise in Ca_i, binding of calcium ions to troponin C causes the protein to move away from the thin filament, thereby allowing myosin–actin interactions necessary for muscle contraction to take place (6). It should be pointed out that there are additional intracellular Ca^{2+}-binding proteins that act as Ca^{2+} sensors but do not belong to the EF-hand superfamily of proteins. These include the Ca^{2+}-dependent isoforms of PKC (88), the annexin family involved in mediating Ca^{2+}-dependent interactions with phospholipids, neutral proteases such as calpain, calcineurin (a protein phosphatase), and others (6). These share with troponin C and CaM, however, the capacity to bind calcium ions in the relevant range of Ca_i, with attendant changes in their own function or in the function of proteins they interact with that are relevant to cellular regulation.

THE INTEGRATED CONTROL OF INTRACELLULAR CALCIUM AND ITS ROLE IN REGULATING CELLULAR FUNCTION

The previous sections have pointed out that there are a number of ways in which transient changes in Ca_i can be brought about that utilize varying combinations of alterations in plasma membrane uptake and extrusion of Ca^{2+} into storage organelles. These changes occur most commonly in response to extracellular stimuli that exert their actions through changes in Ca_i and various other intracellular mediators. The development of techniques for directly measuring Ca_i using Ca^{2+}-sensitive intracellular dyes (184,185) as well as for performing high-resolution imaging of Ca_i dynamics at the subcellular level (186) has yielded a host of insights into the regulation and actions of Ca_i in intact cells. The use of these methodologies in combination with techniques for defining the actual mechanisms translocating Ca^{2+} ions into and out of the cytosol are essential for a full understanding of Ca_i and its regulation at the cellular, subcellular, and molecular levels. The regulation of secretion from several cell types and of muscle contraction provides illustrative examples of how these methods have been used in this manner.

Intracellular Calcium Regulation in Adrenal Chromaffin Cells

The studies of Cheek (187) and Burgoyne (64) have utilized digital imaging techniques for measuring Ca_i to show the impact that different patterns of rise in Ca_i have on catecholamine secretion from bovine adrenal chromaffin cells. Direct activation of nicotinic cholinergic receptors (a ligand-gated cation channel) or exposure of the cells to high extracellular K^+ concentrations depolarizes the cell membrane and activates voltage-sensitive Ca^{2+} channels in the plasma membrane (64,187). This results in an increase in Ca_i in the immediate subplasmalemmar space, which is a potent stimulus for exocytosis of secretory vesicles in this region (Fig. 16). There is a subsequent more generalized increase in Ca_i that often becomes polarized toward one side of the cell (Fig. 16). The latter results from diffusion of Ca^{2+} throughout the cytosol, perhaps accompanied by Ca^{2+}-induced Ca^{2+} release, followed by direct activation of PLC by the increase in Ca_i, which then releases Ca^{2+} from the IP_3-sensitive Ca^{2+} stores (which tend to be eccentrically located on one side of the cell).

In contrast, treatment of the cells with a muscarinic agonist or angiotensin II, which activate G protein-coupled receptors linked to PLC, produces little increase in catecholamine secretion, even though the maximal increase in Ca_i is comparable to that seen

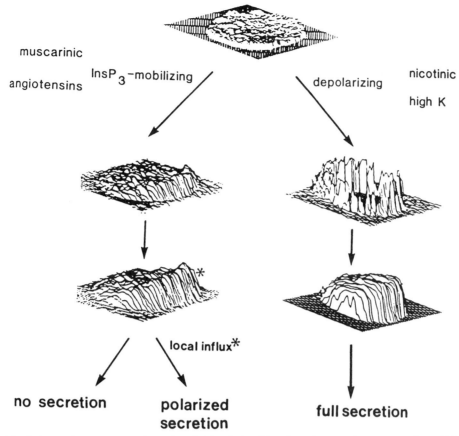

muscarinic

angiotensins   InsP$_3$-mobilizing

nicotinic

high K

depolarizing

local influx*

no secretion

polarized
secretion

full secretion

FIG. 16. Schematic summary of results obtained via video imaging on changes on Ca$_i$ within bovine adrenal chromaffin cells in response to various agonists. Results are depicted as contour plots to illustrate the concentration and distribution of Ca$_i$ within individual chromaffin cells. (Reprinted from ref. 64 with permission and courtesy of Dr. Tim Cheek.)

with nicotinic stimulation (64,187). Digital imaging studies of the changes in Ca$_i$, however, reveal that the changes in Ca$_i$ elicited by agents such as those that increase IP$_3$ show a localized, polarized increase in Ca$_i$ deeper within the cytosol that is compatible with release from the IP$_3$-sensitive stores. This pattern of change in Ca$_i$ is a poor stimulus for secretion, most likely because the accompanying increases in Ca$_i$ immediately under the plasmalemma are not sufficient to activate exocytosis. In some cells stimulated with angiotensin II or muscarinic agonists, however, increases in IP$_3$ result in localized influx of extracellular Ca^{2+} through the mechanisms described previously (6). The resultant increase in Ca$_i$ immediately under the plasma membrane produces localized secretion from the portion of the plasma membrane, where the uptake of extracellular Ca^{2+} takes place. In support of the latter formulation, histamine, which also activates PLC but (for unclear reasons) produces a more generalized increase in uptake of Ca^{2+} by the plasma membrane, is also a considerably more potent secretagogue than muscarinic agonists or angiotensin II (64).

Thus, there is a major impact of the pattern of increase in Ca$_i$ on the resultant enhancement of catecholamine secretion from bovine adrenal chromaffin cells. In other cell types, localized changes in Ca$_i$ are utilized to regulate nonexocytotic secretion. In rat parotid acinar cells (188), there is an IP$_3$-sensitive Ca^{2+}-storage pool near the basolateral plasma membrane. Cholinergic activation of the cells leads to a localized increase in Ca$_i$ in this portion of the cell via the associated rise in IP$_3$, which then activates Ca^{2+}-activated K$^+$ channels in the basolateral plasma membrane. The latter is an important prerequisite for Cl$^-$ uptake and subsequent fluid secretion (189). As is described below, the transcellular transport of Ca^{2+} ions by renal and intestinal epithelial cells represents a further adaptation of the mechanisms regulating intracellular Ca^{2+} dynamics to effect translocation of calcium ions across these epithelial cell interfaces in response to calciotropic hormones.

Elegant studies carried out by Rose and Lowenstein (190) in the 1970s, without the benefit of many of the sophisticated tools used by present day investigators, showed that injection of Ca^{2+} into neurons produced highly localized increases in Ca_i. Spread of the Ca^{2+} did not take place because of the presence of energy-requiring cellular organelles (presumably the ER) that rapidly took up the injected Ca^{2+} and prevented its spread by diffusion. Such precise localization of changes in Ca_i signals is particularly important in neurotransmission, because of the need for accurate targeting of Ca_i signalling to sites of intercellular communication. This can be accomplished in presynaptic neurons by clustering of voltage-sensitive Ca^{2+} channels to "active zones" of the plasma membrane at the specialized sites where synaptic release of neurotransmitters takes place at the nerve terminal (191). In the cases of synapses releasing fast-acting neurotransmitters, such as glutamate, γ-aminobutyric acid (GABA), and acetylcholine, there is also presynaptic localization of several additional components involved in neurotransmission, including synaptic vesicles, cellular elements that recycle vesicular membranes after exocytosis, and Ca^{2+}-binding proteins and Ca^{2+}-sequestering organelles (187,191,192). This permits extremely rapid increases in Ca_i, followed by activation of neurotransmitter release and, in turn, lowering of Ca_i to basal levels and recycling of membrane constituents for subsequent release events.

Stimulus–contraction coupling in cardiac muscle cells provides a further example of the specialized uses of the various mechanisms available for raising and then lowering Ca_i as part of cellular Ca_i signalling (6). Depolarization of the sarcolemma results in activation of voltage-activated Ca^{2+} channels in the plasma membrane as well as in the T-tubules, with attendant uptake of extracellular Ca^{2+}. Cellular depolarization may also enable the Na^+/Ca^{2+} exchanger to operate in the reverse mode to transport Ca^{2+} into the cell as noted previously. Depolarization of the plasma membrane is also coupled in some fashion to activation of the ryanodine-sensitive Ca^{2+} channels in the SR via the T-tubules, resulting in release of Ca^{2+} from these intracellular stores into the immediate vicinity of the myofibrils. Repolarization of the plasma membrane then closes the voltage-activated Ca^{2+} channels and the Ca^{2+}-release channels of the SR and permits removal of Ca^{2+} from the cytosol by the activity of plasma membrane Ca^{2+}–ATPases, exchange of cytosolic Ca^{2+} for extracellular Na^+ by the Na^+/Ca^{2+} exchanger, and reuptake of Ca^{2+} into the SR by its Ca^{2+}–ATPase, all within a time frame of <1 sec.

In addition to the mechanisms described to this point, there are a variety of other forms of regulation of the elements involved in controlling the levels of Ca_i. As was noted above, Ca^{2+} channels can be regulated by membrane voltage, extracellular ligands in a G protein-dependent or -independent fashion, and

phosphorylation by PKC or cAMP-dependent protein kinases (6). Furthermore, the receptor- and G protein-dependent activation of phosphoinositide-specific protein kinase C can also be regulated by the same two protein kinases (193,194), both serving to decrease the activation of PLC in response to a given level of hormonal stimulation. The action of IP_3 on release of Ca^{2+} from intracellular stores, in turn, can be enhanced at low levels of Ca_i and inhibited at higher cytosolic Ca^{2+} concentrations (195). Thus in the appropriate concentration range the Ca_i signal can be amplified both by Ca^{2+} acting as a coagonist for IP_3-mediated Ca^{2+} release as well as by Ca^{2+}-activated Ca^{2+} release from intracellular stores and perhaps also by Ca^{2+}-activated uptake of extracellular Ca^{2+}. Higher levels of Ca_i may feed back in a negative manner by inhibiting IP_3 action (195).

Studies of agonist-stimulated increases in Ca_i in single cells have also revealed complexities not previously appreciated when Ca_i was measured in cell populations (122,123). Single cells frequently exhibit agonist-induced oscillations in Ca_i (122,123,196) that are thought to result from cyclical release of Ca^{2+}, followed by its reuptake into intracellular stores. There can also be intracellular propagation of Ca^{2+} waves (197) as well as communication of such waves between cells by a process that may involve transfer of a soluble second messenger between cells via gap junctions. Boitano et al. (198) recently investigated the mechanisms underlying intracellular Ca_i oscillations and intercellular communication of Ca_i waves in airway epithelial cells. In cells loaded with heparin, which blocks the IP_3 receptor, oscillations persisted, suggesting that they likely arise from cycles of Ca^{2+}-induced Ca^{2+} release. Although the heparin blocked the propagation of Ca_i within that particular cell, it did not prevent the spread of waves into adjacent cells, suggesting that movement of IP_3 rather than Ca_i through gap junctions was the likely mediator of wave propagation. The significance of the more complex Ca_i dynamics seen in single cells in not yet certain, but they may encode information not contained within simple, sustained elevations in Ca_i previously suggested by studies of cell populations.

Not only the mechanisms for influx of Ca^{2+} into the cytosol but also those responsible for its removal are susceptible to specific regulation by Ca_i and other factors. Increase in Ca_i activate the plasma membrane Ca^{2+}–ATPases in a CaM-dependent fashion, while cAMP can accelerate the reuptake of Ca^{2+} into the SR (6). The coordination of these regulatory influences on Ca^{2+} entry and extrusion mechanisms permits the broad range of biological diversity in the regulation of Ca_i observed in complex multicellular organisms.

INTRACELLULAR CALCIUM SIGNALLING AND CALCIOTROPIC HORMONE SECRETION AND ACTION AT TARGET TISSUES

The extracellular Ca^{2+} homeostatic system utilizes Ca_i signalling in a variety of ways. In both parathyroid cells (5,11,12) and C cells (122,123), changes in Ca_i are a prominent component of the extracellular Ca^{2+}-evoked changes in intracellular second messengers. In parathyroid cells the initial increase in Ca_i in this setting is due to release from intracellular Ca^{2+} stores, while in C cells uptake of extracellular Ca^{2+} plays a key role in Ca_i dynamics. It seems possible that the change in Ca_i in the subplasmalemmar region of parathyroid cells with increases in extracellular Ca^{2+} would be less conducive to activating exocytosis than that taking place in C-cells. Perhaps the inhibition of PTH secretion despite the concomitant increases in the extracellular and cytosolic Ca^{2+} concentrations results both from failure to activate secretion as well as concomitant mechanisms that inhibit secretion (such as the decrease in PKC activity). Another difference between the patterns in the extracellular Ca^{2+}-evoked changes in Ca_i between the two cell types is the oscillations that are seen in C cells but not, apparently, in parathyroid cells (122). This difference has not been investigated to any extent in terms of the underlying mechanisms or its impact on secretory control but could potentially also have disparate effects on the exocytotic mechanism. Finally, the PTH-mediated stimulation of the proximal tubular synthesis of 1,25-$(OH)_2D$ is also accompanied by increases in both Ca_i and cAMP and has recently been suggested to be mediated by changes in PKC activity accompanying the former (199).

Calciotropic hormone actions on their target tissues also involve the use of Ca_i as a second messenger. In addition to its actions in regulating proximal tubular 1-hydroxylation, the other proximal tubular actions of the hormone likely utilize not only cAMP but also Ca_i for intracellular signalling (113). The stimulation of distal tubular Ca^{2+} reabsorption is also associated with increases in Ca_i, but, as is described in more detail below, this is a secondary response to increased transcellular Ca^{2+} flux, with cAMP acting as the major intracellular mediator underlying this response (200). PTH also increases phosphatidylinositol (PI) turnover and Ca_i in osteoblasts (201), and these are probably part of the intracellular signalling involved in the inhibitory effects of the hormone on osteoblastic function and, secondarily, on stimulating osteoclasts via osteoblast-derived signals. Both calcitonin and elevated extracellular Ca^{2+} concentrations, on the other hand, inhibit osteoclast function in association with increases in Ca_i (141,142). 1,25 Dihydroxyvitamin D is now known to produce rapid, nongenomic changes in Ca_i that may be involved in intracellular signalling and hormone action (109).

The actions of both PTH and 1,25-$(OH)_2D$ involve stimulation of the transport of calcium ions into the ECF by bone cells, kidney cells, and/or intestinal cells. In some cases this involves extracellular movement of calcium ions out of bone or across the renal tubules by a paracellular (e.g., extracellular) route, but in others there is direct transcellular Ca^{2+} transport by mechanisms similar to those that are involved in regulating Ca_i (Fig. 17) (113,202). The latter form of transport might potentially interfere with intracellular Ca^{2+} signalling within these same cell types. As is pointed

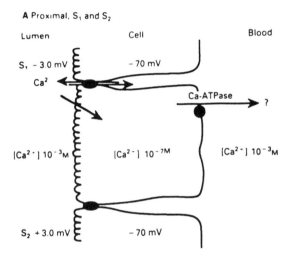

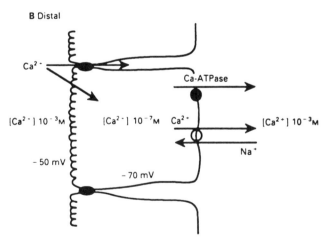

FIG. 17. Cellular mechanisms proposed to be involved in the transport of calcium ions in proximal S1 and S2 tubule (**A**) and distal convoluted tubule (**B**) segments. (Reprinted from ref. 202 with permission.)

out in the discussion that follows, however, the cells acted upon by calciotropic hormones are able to integrate successfully their functions of bulk transfer of Ca^{2+} with their use of Ca^{2+} in intracellular signalling.

In bone, large amounts of Ca^{2+} are mobilized by actively resorbing osteoclasts, but this takes place in an extracellular compartment through the osteoclastic secretion of protons and digestive enzymes (100). Therefore, the mobilized Ca^{2+} should not interfere with intracellular Ca^{2+} regulation of the osteoclast except insofar as it acts on extracellular Ca^{2+} receptors to down regulate resorptive activity through increases in Ca_i (141,142). In the processes of both intestinal absorption of Ca^{2+} and renal tubular reabsorption of Ca^{2+}, on the other hand, there must be actual bulk movement of calcium ions across an epithelial interface to accomplish the functions of these Ca^{2+}-translocating tissues in mineral ion homeostasis. This movement of calcium ions is thought to take place through two distinct mechanisms (113,202,203). In the first, there is paracellular movement of calcium ions. In the kidney, this occurs primarily in the proximal tubule and thick ascending limb, and movement of Ca^{2+} is thought to follow the bulk reabsorption of fluid and monovalent ions, assisted by a luminal Ca^{2+} concentration slightly higher than that in blood (21) and a lumen positive electrical potential in some nephron segments (113,202). This form of transepithelial movement of Ca^{2+} ions, like osteoclastic bone resorption, will not interfere with intracellular Ca^{2+} homeostasis,

since the calcium ions transported do not actually traverse the cytosol.

Although some of these same nephron segments (e.g., the S1 segment of the proximal convoluted tubule) have been postulated to have some degree of active, transcellular Ca^{2+} transport, the bulk of the active, hormonally regulated renal transport of calcium takes place in the distal tubule and collecting duct. Cells in the latter part of the nephron are known to have Ca^{2+}-activated K^+ channels (200) that have been localized to the luminal plasma membrane and may be involved in K^+ secretion in this portion of the nephron (204). If PTH-stimulated tubular reabsorption of Ca^{2+} in this nephron segment were associated with large changes in Ca_i, this might have undesirable consequences in terms of K^+ homeostasis. Bordeau and Lau (200) have recently reviewed their contributions and those of other investigators to our understanding of the mechanisms through which PTH stimulates Ca^{2+} reabsorption in this part of the nephron within the context of understanding how this is accomplished under the constraints imposed by the use of Ca^{2+} as an intracellular messenger.

In the collecting tubule of the rabbit nephron, as in the distal tubule of other species, PTH produces a prominent increase in the reabsorption of calcium ions. This effect persists when the electrochemical forces promoting passive reabsorption of Ca^{2+} are removed, suggesting an active, transcellular mechanism for Ca^{2+} reabsorption. Cell-permeant cAMP analogs

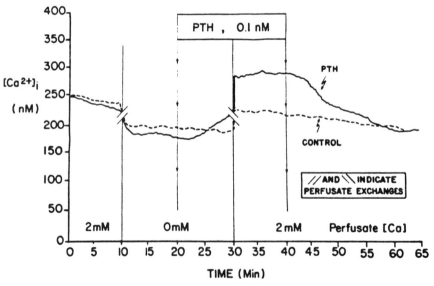

FIG. 18. Effects of PTH in the peritubular fluid on Ca_i in isolated perfused rabbit collecting tubule segments in the presence or absence of luminal calcium. The peritubular calcium concentration of Ca^{2+} was maintained at 2 mM throughout the experiment. The *solid* and *dashed lines* are the mean values for six PTH-treated and five time control tubules, respectively. Note that PTH is able to stimulate an increase in Ca_i only when calcium is present in the luminal fluid, despite the continuous presence of calcium in the peritubular fluid. (Reprinted from ref. 200 with permission.)

quantitatively mimic the actions of PTH, suggesting that cAMP is the predominant intracellular messenger mediating this effect. [The collecting tubule, in fact, is known to contain the highest levels of PTH-stimulated adenylyl cyclase along the rabbit nephron (205).] PTH stimulates a modest (30–40%) increase in Ca$_i$ in collecting tubule cells (200) that is totally dependent on the presence of extracellular Ca^{2+} on the luminal side of the tubule (Fig. 18). Thus PTH appears to have little effect on release of intracellular Ca^{2+} and (by inference) IP$_3$ production in these cells. Instead, the increase in Ca$_i$ arises to a significant extent from uptake of luminal Ca^{2+} through as yet poorly defined pathways, perhaps involving Ca^{2+} channels, in the luminal plasma membrane (200). Bulk movement of Ca^{2+} across the cell would then require transcellular diffusion of calcium ions, followed by pumping of these ions across the basolateral membrane principally by Ca^{2+}–ATPases. The latter would presumably also be stimulated by the associated increase in Ca$_i$ through a Ca^{2+}- and CaM-dependent mechanism. It is also possible that a basolateral Na$^+$/Ca^{2+} exchanger plays some role in this process (200). Although the PTH-induced increases in Ca$_i$ are small and presumably provide only a small driving force for bulk diffusion of Ca^{2+} ions, the presence of high concentrations of the vitamin D-dependent calbindins in this segment of the nephron could potentially facilitate diffusional transport (206–208). This, in turn, could explain the necessity for normal levels of 1,25-(OH)$_2$D for optimal expression of PTH-stimulated renal tubular Ca^{2+} reabsorption (117). Finally, the relatively small magnitude of the increase in Ca$_i$ in these cells in the presence of PTH is apparently not sufficient to activate tubular transport of other ions, such as K$^+$, and to interfere with their homeostatic regulation.

Vitamin D-stimulated absorption of Ca^{2+} by the gastrointestinal tract is also thought to involve active, transcellular movement of calcium ions (203). Again, this must involve (a) movement of Ca^{2+} across the luminal plasma membrane and down its electrochemical gradient into the intestinal cell, (b) translocation across the enterocyte cytosol, and finally (c) active transport of Ca^{2+} across the basolateral plasma membrane. Despite intensive study by a number of investigators, much remains to be learned about the details of these steps in intestinal Ca^{2+} absorption and the manner in which 1,25-(OH)$_2$D stimulates one or more of them. 1,25 Dihydroxyvitamin D does have several clear effects on the intestine. (a) It promotes differentiation of enterocytes in vitamin D-responsive portions of the GI tract (209). (b) It has rapid, nongenomic effects on brush border phospholipid metabolism and uptake of Ca^{2+} that may contribute to the initial steps of vitamin D-stimulated Ca^{2+} absorption (210–212). The rapid increase in Ca$_i$ that has been documented in

a number of cell types could be relevant in this regard (109). (c) It induces increases in the levels or activities of enterocyte proteins that may be involved in Ca^{2+} transport, including Ca^{2+}–ATPase (213) and the vitamin D-dependent calbindins (214). The former, perhaps in concert with Na$^+$/Ca^{2+} exchange (215), likely plays a key role in active transport of Ca^{2+} across the luminal plasma membrane. Despite many years of scrutiny, the calbindins remain enigmas. Some have found that they activate the Ca^{2+}–ATPase, but others have not been able to replicate this observation (203). It has also been postulated that they facilitate diffusion of Ca^{2+} through the cytosol of the enterocyte (208), but this suggestion is far from proved. Nevertheless, vitamin D-stimulated intestinal Ca^{2+} absorption, like renal tubular reabsorption of Ca^{2+}, appears to utilize elements of the Ca$_i$ homeostatic system to achieve net movement of Ca^{2+} across the cell rather than producing regulated changes in Ca$_i$ whose principal function is related to intracellular Ca^{2+} signalling. It would be of interest to apply digital Ca^{2+} imaging techniques as well as molecular biological probes of the various elements of Ca$_i$ homeostasis to probe further the mechanism involved in vectorial Ca^{2+} transport.

COMPARISON BETWEEN THE INTRACELLULAR AND EXTRACELLULAR CA^{2+} HOMEOSTATIC SYSTEMS AND MECHANISMS OF INTERCOMMUNICATION BETWEEN THE EXTRACELLULAR AND CYTOSOLIC CALCIUM CONCENTRATIONS

Table 2 summarizes similarities and differences between various aspects of the regulation of the cytosolic and extracellular Ca^{2+} concentrations that have been alluded to throughout this chapter. The two are linked by a number of features, particularly the messenger functions of Ca^{2+} within both compartments and the presence of receptors for intra- and extracellular Ca^{2+} that contribute importantly (along with other first and second messengers and their respective receptors) to modulation of the effector function of the two homeostatic systems. These effector mechanisms are similar from a broad perspective (i.e., they mobilize internal calcium stores or modulate fluxes of Ca^{2+} into or out of the organism or cell). While they differ in some of their details (i.e., the types of mechanisms used to mobilize calcium ions), there are also shared uses of plasma membrane calcium ion transporters to accomplish different ends. One of the consequences of the transition from unicellular to multicellular organisms, therefore, was the need to develop systems that regulated not only the intracellular Ca^{2+} concentration but also the level of extracellular Ca^{2+}. This apparently involved not only the adaptation of preexisting systems

TABLE 2. *Comparison of properties and regulation of extra- and intracellular Ca²⁺ homeostasis[a]*

Property	Extracellular Ca²⁺ homeostasis	Cytosolic Ca²⁺ homeostasis
Basal Ca²⁺ concentration	1 mM	100 nM
Ca²⁺ buffers	Albumin, other proteins	Parvalbumin, other proteins
Form of Ca²⁺ regulated	Ionized	Ionized
Magnitude of Ca²⁺ excursions	Small ($\pm$ a few %)	Large (ten- to 100-fold)
Rapidity of changes in Ca²⁺	Slow (minutes to hours)	Rapid (milliseconds to seconds)
Ca²⁺ sensors	Extracellular Ca²⁺ receptors	CaM, other intracellular CaBP
Ca²⁺ effectors	Kidney, bone, intestine (via pumps, exchangers, channels)	Membrane pumps, exchangers, and channels
Sources of Ca²⁺	Environment, skeleton	Extracellular Ca²⁺, intracellular Ca²⁺ stores
Direction of Ca²⁺ fluxes that is regulated	Bidirectional (bone) Unidirectional (kidney, intestine)	Bidirectional
Regulators of Ca²⁺ fluxes	Extracellular Ca²⁺, PTH, CT, 1,25-(OH)₂D via second messengers and genomic effects	Ca$_i$, cAMP, cGMP, DAG, etc., via first messengers

[a]Abbreviations: CaM, calmodulin; PTH, parathyroid hormone; CT, calcitonin; 1,25-(OH)₂D, 1,25-dihydroxyvitamin D; Ca$_i$, cytosolic calcium concentration; second messengers, intracellular second messengers; first messengers, hormones, neurotransmitters, and other extracellular stimuli; cAMP, cyclic AMP; cGMP, cyclic GMP; DAG, diacylglycerol.

for regulating Ca$_i$ to effect vectorial Ca²⁺ transport between the organism and the environment but also the development of novel mechanisms (i.e., paracellular Ca²⁺ transport) for this purpose as well as the establishment of extracellular Ca²⁺ stores that could be mobilized in a regulated fashion. These mechanisms for regulating extracellular calcium also required regulatory calciotropic peptides and sterols, but extracellular Ca²⁺ itself may have served as an early calciotropic "hormone" involved in local regulation of Ca²⁺ fluxes by effector tissues of Ca²⁺ homeostasis and continues to subserve this function in mammals.

In addition to the relationships between cellular and subcellular Ca²⁺ homeostasis shown in Table 2, there are additional means of communication between intra- and extracellular Ca²⁺: Extracellular Ca²⁺-induced release of intracellular calcium stores and/or uptake of extracellular Ca²⁺ mediated via cell surface Ca²⁺ receptors plays a key role in regulation of extracellular Ca²⁺ homeostasis both by the ion-sensing and by the effector arms of this system. Changes in Ca$_i$, in turn, may potentially be able to modulate extracellular Ca²⁺ sensing through the effects of changes in protein kinase C on the coupling of the Ca²⁺ receptor to PI turnover in parathyroid cells or other actions on cell function that modulate Ca²⁺ sensing.

There are also interesting interrelationships between the use of intracellular Ca²⁺ stores and extracellular Ca²⁺ in regulating Ca$_i$. Both represent sites with high

(approximately millimolar) Ca²⁺ concentrations that can be made available to promote rapid increases in Ca$_i$. In skeletal muscle, these intra- and extracellular sites of Ca²⁺ "storage" are closely juxtaposed, permitting close temporal and spatial coordination of release and uptake of Ca²⁺ from both. The original formulation of the capacitative model of refilling of the IP₃-sensitive Ca²⁺ stores from the extracellular space addressed intriguing issues concerning the structural and functional interrelationships between the uses of intracellular and extracellular sources of Ca²⁺ in intracellular Ca²⁺ signalling. Secretory vesicles are another element of the intercommunicating system of vesicles and cisternae that concentrate calcium ions and are involved in trafficking of a variety of substances between the intracellular membranous systems and the extracellular space. The inner face of this membranovesicular system (i.e., secretory vesicles, endosomes, ER, etc.) would correspond to the outer face of the plasma membrane. In turn, the systems for translocating, sensing, and regulating Ca²⁺ fluxes across these organelles and the plasma membrane might be homologous (as for the Ca²⁺–ATPases of plasma membrane and ER). Additional studies on the mechanisms involved in the sensing of the Ca²⁺ concentrations and the regulation of Ca²⁺ homeostasis within these organelles may provide further insights into the mechanisms involved in regulating Ca$_i$ and the extracellular calcium concentrations and the evolutionary and functional relationships between these two homeostatic mechanisms.

ACKNOWLEDGMENTS

The time that I spent with Jerry Aurbach in the Metabolic Diseases Branch of the National Institutes of Arthritis, Diabetes and Digestive Diseases at the NIH between 1974 and 1979 had a profound effect on my subsequent life, scientific and otherwise. Jerry was a kind and gentle, but firm, mentor, who had strong opinions about the way scientific research should be conducted, evaluated, and written about. His superb work on the calciotropic hormones made a lasting impression on me and profoundly influenced the way I have thought about my own work in this area ever since. He was, at the same time, a wonderful friend and colleague, who was a peerless example to us all of what it means to exemplify openness, generosity, integrity, and love in all aspects of life. I miss him very much, but welcome the opportunity to be a part of this volume, which is a testament to his impact on his chosen field, his colleagues, his students, and his many friends. We are all fortunate to have had the opportunity to know him. This chapter was made possible through the generous support of the National Institutes of Health (grants DK36796, DE41415, and DE 44588) as well as the St. Giles Foundation. I also appreciate the hard work and creative thinking of my many coworkers, who are coauthors in papers listed in the references.

REFERENCES

1. Aurbach GD, Marx SJ, Spiegel AM. Parathyroid hormone, calcitonin, and the calciferols. In: Wilson J, Foster DW, eds. *Textbook of endocrinology, 7th ed.* Philadelphia: WB Saunders, 1985;1137–1217.
2. Parfitt AM, Kleerekoper M. The divalent ion homeostatic system: physiology and metabolism of calcium, phosphorus, magnesium, and bone. In: Maxwell MH, Kleeman CR, eds. *Clinical disorders of fluid and electrolyte metabolism, 3rd ed.* New York: McGraw-Hill, 1980;269–398.
3. Rasmussen H. Calcium messenger system. *N Engl J Med* 1986;314:1089–1107.
4. Stewart AF, Broadus AE. Mineral metabolism. In: Felig P, Baxter JD, Broadus AE, Frohman LA, eds. *Endocrinology and metabolism, 2nd ed.* New York: McGraw-Hill, 1987; 1317–1453.
5. Brown EM. Extracellular Ca^{2+}-sensing, regulation of parathyroid cell function, and role of Ca^{2+} and other ions as extracellular (first) messengers. *Physiol Rev* 1991;71:371–411.
6. Pietrobon D, Di Virgilio F, Pozzan T. Structural and functional aspects of calcium homeostasis in eukaryotic cells. *Eur J Biochem* 1990;120:599–622.
7. Means AR, Dedman JR. Calmodulin—an intracellular calcium receptor. *Nature* 1980;285:73–77.
8. Nowycky MC, Fox AP, Tsjen RW. Three types of neuronal calcium channels with different calcium agonist sensitivities. *Nature* 1985;316:440–443.
9. Berridge MJ, Irvine RF. Inositol trisphosphate, a novel second messenger in cellular signal transduction. *Nature* 1984; 312:315–321.
10. Blackmore PF, Brumley FT, Marks JL, Exton JH. Studies on α-adrenergic activation of hepatic glucose output. Relationship between α-adrenergic stimulation of calcium efflux and activation of phosphorylase in isolated rat liver parenchymal cells. *J Biol Chem* 1978;253:4851–4858.
11. Nemeth EF, Scarpa A. Rapid mobilization of cellular Ca^{2+} in bovine parathyroid cells by external divalent cations. *J Biol Chem* 1987;262:5188–5196.
12. Shoback DM, Membreno LA, McGhee J. High calcium and other divalent cations increase inositol trisphosphate in bovine parathyroid cells. *Endocrinology* 1988;123:382–389.
13. Nygren P, Gylfe E, Larsson R, et al. Modulation of the Ca^{2+}-sensing function of parathyroid cells in vitro and in hyperparathyroidism. *Biochim Biophys Acta* 1988;253–260.
14. Sherwood LM, Potts JT Jr, Care AD, Mayer GP, Aurbach GD. Evaluation by radioimmunoassay of factors controlling the secretion of parathyroid hormone. *Nature* 1966;209:52–55.
15. Brent GA, LeBoff MS, Seely EW, Conlin PR, Brown EM. Relationship between the concentration and rate of change of calcium and serum intact parathyroid hormone levels in normal humans. *J Clin Endocrinol Metab* 1988;67:944–950.
16. Rudberg C, Akerstrom G, Ljunghall S, Grimelius L, Johansson H, Pertoft H, Wide L. Regulation of parathyroid hormone secretion in primary and secondary hyperparathyroidism: studies in vivo and in vitro. *Acta Endocrinol* 1982; 101:408–413.
17. Mayer GP, Hurst JG. Sigmoidal relationship between parathyroid hormone secretion rate and plasma calcium concentration in calves. *Endocrinology* 1978;102:1036–1042.
18. Austin LA, Heath H. Calcitonin. Physiology and pathophysiology. *N Engl J Med* 1981;304:269–278.
19. Muff R, Nemeth EF, Haller-Brem S, Fischer JA. Regulation of hormone secretion and cytosolic Ca^{2+} by extracellular Ca^{2+} in parathyroid and C-cells: role of voltage-sensitive Ca^{2+} channels. *Arch Biochem Biophys* 1988;265:128–135.
20. Fried RM, Tashjian AH Jr. Unusual sensitivity of cytosolic free Ca^{2+} to changes in extracellular Ca^{2+} in rat C-cells. *J Biol Chem* 1986;261:7669–7674.
21. Dennis VW. Phosphate homeostasis. In: Windhager E, ed. *Handbook of physiology, section 8. Renal physiology.* New York: Oxford University Press, 1992;1785–1816.
22. Agus ZS, Gardner LB, Beck LM, Goldberg M. Effects of parathyroid hormone on renal tubular reabsorption of calcium, sodium, and phosphate. *Am J Physiol* 1973;224:1143–1148.
23. Fraser DR, Kodicek E. Regulation of 25-hydroxy-cholecalciferol-hydroxylase activity in kidney by parathyroid hormone. *Nature* [*New Biol*] 1973;241:163–166.
24. Hughes MR, Brumbaugh PF, Haussler MR, Wergedal JE, Baylink DJ. Regulation of serum 1,25-dihydroxyvitamin D$_3$ by calcium and phosphate in the rat. *Science* 1975;190:578–580.
25. Marx SJ, Liberman UA, Eil CA. Calciferols: actions and deficiencies in actions. *Vitamins Hormones* 1983;40:235–308.
26. Raisz LG, Trummel CL, Holick ME, DeLuca HF. 1,25-Dihydroxyvitamin D: a potent stimulator of bone resorption in tissue culture. *Science* 1972;175:768–769.
27. Morrissey JJ, Hamilton JW, MacGregor RR, Cohn DV. The secretion of parathormone fragments 34–84 and 37–84 by dispersed porcine parathyroid cells. *Endocrinology* 1980;107: 164–171.
28. Hanley DA, Takatsuki K, Sultan JM, Schneider AB, Sherwood LM. Direct release of parathyroid hormone fragments from functioning bovine parathyroid glands in vitro. *J Clin Invest* 1978;62:1247–1254.
29. Naveh-Many T, Silver J. Regulation of parathyroid hormone gene expression by hypocalcemia, hypercalcemia and vitamin D in the rat. *J Clin Invest* 1990;86:1313–1319.
30. Russell J, Lettieri D, Sherwood LM. Direct regulation by calcium of cytoplasmic messenger ribonucleic acid coding for preproparathyroid hormone in isolated bovine parathyroid cells. *J Clin Invest* 1983;72:1851–1855.

31. Riasz LG. Regulation by calcium of parathyroid growth and secretion in vitro. *Nature* 1965;44:103–110.

32. Capen CC, Rowland GN. Ultrastructural evaluation of the parathyroid glands of young cats with experimental hyperparathyroidism. *Z Zellforsch Mikrosk Anat* 1968;90:495–500.

33. Agus ZS, Puschett JG, Senesky D, Goldberg M. Mode of action of parathyroid hormone and cyclic adenosine 3′,5′-monophosphate. *J Clin Invest* 1971;50:617–626.

34. Bilizekian JP, Canfield RE, Jacobs TP, et al. Response of 1,25-dihydroxyvitamin D₃ to hypocalcemia in human subjects. *N Engl J Med* 1978;299:437–441.

35. Cantley LK, Russell J, Lettieri D, Sherwood LM. 1,25-Dihydroxyvitamin D suppresses parathyroid hormone secretion from bovine parathyroid cells in tissue culture. *Endocrinology* 1985;117:2114–2119.

36. Kremer R, Bolivar I, Goltzman D, Hendy GN. Influence of calcium and 1,25-dihydroxycholecalciferol on proliferation and proto-oncogene expression in primary cultures of bovine parathyroid cells. *Endocrinology* 1989;125:935–941.

37. Suva LJ, Winslow GA, Wettenhall EH, et al. A parathyroid hormone-related protein implicated in malignant hypercalcemia: cloning and expression. *Science* 1987;237:893–896.

38. Mangin M, Webb AC, Dreyer BF, et al. Identification of a cDNA clone encoding a parathyroid hormone-like peptide from a human tumor associated with humoral hypercalcemia of malignancy. *Proc Natl Acad Sci USA* 1988;85:597–601.

39. Rodda CP, Caple IW, Martin TJ. Role of PTHrP in fetal and neonatal physiology. In Halloran BP, Nissenson RA, eds. *Parathyroid hormone related protein: normal physiology and its role in cancer.* Boca Raton, FL: CRC Press, 1992; 169–196.

40. Raisz LG. Bone resorption in tissue culture: factors influencing the response to parathyroid hormone. *J Clin Invest* 1965;44:103–110.

41. Raisz LG, Kream BE. Regulation of bone formation. *N Engl J Med* 1983;309:35–39.

42. Slatopolsky E, Berkoben M, Kelber J, Brown A, Delmez J. Effects of calcitriol and non-calcemic vitamin D analogs on secondary hyperparathyroidism. *Kidney Int* 1991;42(Suppl 38):S43–S49.

43. Anast C, Winnacker JL, Forte LR, Burns TW. Impaired release of parathyroid hormone in magnesium deficiency. *J Clin Endocrinol Metab* 1976;42:707–717.

44. Cholst IN, Steinberg SF, Trapper PJ, Fox HE, Segre GV, Bilizekian JP. The influence of hypermagnesemia on serum calcium and parathyroid hormone levels in human subjects. *N Engl J Med* 1984;310:1221–1225.

45. Quamme GA, Dirks JH. The physiology of renal magnesium handling. In: Windhager EE, ed. *Handbook of physiology, section 8. Renal physiology.* New York: Oxford University Press, 1992;1917–1936.

46. Rude RK, Oldham SB. Magnesium metabolism. In Becker KL, ed. *Principles and practice of endocrinology and metabolism.* Philadelphia: JB Lippincott, 1990;531–536.

47. Parfitt AM. Equilibrium and dysequilibrium hypercalcemia: new light on old concepts. *Metab Bone Dis Rel Res* 1979; 1:279–293.

48. Staub JF, Tracquil P, Brezillon P, Milhaud G, Perault-Staub AM. Calcium metabolism in the rat: a temporal self-organized model. *Am J Physiol* 1988;254:R134–R149.

49. Brown EM. Four parameter model of the sigmoidal relationship between PTH release and extracellular calcium concentration in normal and abnormal parathyroid tissue. *J Clin Endocrinol Metab* 1983;56:572–581.

50. Clarke BL, Hassager C, Fitzpatrick LA. Regulation of parathyroid hormone release by protein kinase-C is dependent on extracellular calcium in bovine parathyroid cells. *Endocrinology* 1993;132:1168–1175.

51. Roth SI, Raisz LG. The cause and reversibility of calcium effect on the ultrastructure of the rat parathyroid gland in organ culture. *Lab Invest* 1966;15:1187–1211.

52. Mayer GP, Habener JF, Potts JT Jr. Parathyroid hormone secretion in vivo: demonstration of a calcium-independent, non-suppressible component of secretion. *J Clin Invest* 1976; 57:678–683.

53. Warren HB, Lausen NCC, Segre GV, El-Hajj G, Brown EM. Regulation of calciotropic hormones in vivo in the New Zealand white rabbit. *Endocrinology* 1989;125:2683–2690.

54. Arnold A, Brown M, Urena P, Drueke T, Sarfati E. X-inactivation analysis of clonality in primary and secondary parathyroid hyperplasia. *J Bone Mineral Res* 1992;7(Suppl 1):241A.

55. Felsenfeld AJ, Llach F. Parathyroid gland function in chronic renal failure. *Kidney Int* 1993;43:771–789.

56. Nussbaum SR, Zahradnick RJ, Lavigne JR, et al. A highly sensitive two site immunoradiometric assay of parathyrin (PTH) and its clinical utility in evaluating patient with hypercalcemia. *Clin Chem* 1987;33:1364–1367.

57. Conlin PR, Fajtova VT, Mortensen RM, LeBoff MS, Brown EM. Hysteresis in the relationship between serum ionized calcium and intact parathyroid hormone during recovery from induced hyper- and hypocalcemia in normal humans. *J Clin Endocrinol Metab* 1989;69:593–599.

58. Felsenfeld AJ, Ross D, Rodriguez M. Hysteresis of the parathyroid hormone response to hypocalcemia in hemodialysis patients with low turnover bone disease. *J Am Soc Nephrol* 1991;2:1136–1143.

59. Grant FD, Conlin PR, Brown EM. Rate and concentration dependence of parathyroid hormone dynamics during stepwise changes in serum ionized calcium in normal humans. *J Clin Endocrinol Metab* 1990;71:370–378.

60. Schwarz P, Sorensen HA, Transbol I, McNair P. Regulation of acute parathyroid hormone in normal humans: combined calcium and citrate clamp study. *Am J Physiol* 1992;263 [Endocrinol Metab]:E195–E198.

61. Burgess TL, Kelly R. Constitutive and regulated secretion of proteins. *Annu Rev Cell Biol* 1987;3:243–293.

62. Bennett MK, Scheller RH. The molecular machinery for secretion is conserved from yeast to neurons. *Proc Natl Acad Sci USA* 1993;90:2559–2563.

63. Sollner T, Whiteheart SW, Brunner M, et al. SNAP receptors implicated in vesicle targeting and fusion. *Nature* 1993;362:318–320.

64. Burgoyne RD. Control of exocytosis in adrenal chromaffin cells. *Biochim Biophys Acta* 1991;1071:174–202.

65. Turner MD, Rennison ME, Handel SE, Wilds CJ, Burgoyne RD. Proteins are secreted both by constitutive and regulated secretory pathways in lactating mouse mammary epithelial cells. *J Cell Biol* 1992;117:269–278.

66. Brown EM, Watson EJ, Leombruno R, Underwood RH. Extracellular calcium is not necessary for acute, low calcium- or dopamine-stimulated PTH secretion in dispersed bovine parathyroid cells. *Metabolism* 1983;32:1038–1044.

67. Wallace J, Scarpa A. Parathyroid hormone secretion in the absence of extracellular free Ca²⁺ and transmembrane Ca²⁺ flux. *FEBS Lett* 1983;151:83–88.

68. Nygren P, Larsson R, Lindh F, et al. Bimodal regulation of secretion by cytoplasmic Ca²⁺ as demonstrated by the parathyroid. *FEBS Lett* 1987;213:195–198.

69. Morrissey JJ, Cohn DV. Regulation of secretion of parathyroid hormone and secretory protein-1 from separate intracellular pools by calcium, dibutyryl cAMP and (l)-isoproterenol. *J Cell Biol* 1979;82:93–102.

70. Habener JF, Amherdt M, Ravazzola M, Orci L. Parathyroid hormone biosynthesis. Correlation of conversion of biosynthesis precursors with intracellular protein migration as determined by electron microscopic autoradiography. *J Cell Biol* 1979;80:715–731.

71. Brown EM, Gardner DG, Windeck R, Aurbach GD. Relationship of intracellular 3′,5′ adenosine monophosphate accumulation to parathyroid hormone release from dispersed bovine parathyroid cells. *Endocrinology* 1978;103:2323–2333.

72. Kobayashi N, Russell J, Lettieri D, Sherwood LM. Regulation of protein kinase C by extracellular calcium in bovine parathyroid cells. *Proc Natl Acad Sci USA* 1988;85:4857–4860.

73. Juhlin C, Lundgren S, Johansson H, Rastad J, Akerstrom G, Klareskog L. 500 Kilodalton calcium sensor regulating cytoplasmic Ca²⁺ in cytotrophoblast cells of human placenta. *J Biol Chem* 1990;265:8275–8280.

74. Brown EM, Fuleihan GEH, Chen CJ, Kifor O. A comparison of the effects of divalent and trivalent cations on parathyroid

hormone release, 3',5'-cyclic adenosine monophosphate accumulation, and the levels of inositol phosphates in bovine parathyroid cells. *Endocrinology* 1990;127:1064–1070.

75. Nemeth EF. Regulation of cytosolic calcium by extracellular divalent cations in C-cells and parathyroid cells. *Cell Calcium* 1990;11:323–327.

76. Ridefelt P, Hellman P, Wallfelt C, Akerstrom G, Rastad J, Gylfe E. Neomycin interacts with Ca^{2+} sensing of normal and adenomatous parathyroid cells. *Mol Cell Endocrinol* 1992;83:211–218.

77. Brown EM, Katz C, Butters R, Kifor O. Polyarginine, polylysine, and protamine mimic the effects of high extracellular calcium concentrations on dispersed bovine parathyroid cells. *J Bone Mineral Res* 1991;6:1217–1225.

78. El-Hajj Fuleihan G, Katz C, Kifor O, Gleason R, Brown EM. Effects of the lectin concanavalin-A on the regulation of second messengers and parathyroid hormone release by extracellular Ca^{2+} in bovine parathyroid cells. *Endocrinology* 1991;128:2931–2936.

79. Chen CJ, Barnett J, Brown EM. Divalent cations suppress adenosine monophosphate accumulation by stimulating a pertussis toxin-sensitive guanine nucleotide-binding protein in cultured bovine parathyroid cells. *Endocrinology* 1989;124:233–239.

80. Brown EM, Enyedi P, LeBoff M, Rothberg J, Preston J, Chen C. High extracellular Ca^{2+} and Mg^{2+} stimulate accumulation of inositol phosphates in bovine parathyroid cells. *FEBS Lett* 1987;218:113–118.

81. Kifor O, Kifor I, Brown EM. Effects of high extracellular calcium concentrations on phosphoinositide turnover and inositol phosphate metabolism in dispersed bovine parathyroid cells. *J Bone Mineral Res* 1992;7:1327–1336.

82. Hawkins D, Enyedi P, Brown EM. The effects of high extracellular Ca^{2+} and Mg^{2+} concentrations on the levels of inositol 1,3,4,5-tetrakisphosphate in bovine parathyroid cells. *Endocrinology* 1988;124:838–844.

83. D'Amour P, Palandy J, Bahsali G, Mallette LE, DeLean A, LePage R. The modulation of circulating parathyroid hormone immunoheterogeneity in man by ionized calcium concentration. *J Clin Endocrinol Metab* 1992;74:525–532.

84. Racke FK, Dubyak GR, Nemeth EF. Functional expression of the parathyroid calcium receptor in *Xenopus* oocytes. *J Bone Mineral Res* 1991;6:S118(abstract).

85. Shoback DM, Chen T-H. Injection of poly(A)$^+$ RNA from bovine parathyroid tissue into xenopus oocytes confers sensitivity to extracellular calcium. *J Bone Mineral Res* 1991; 6:S135 (abstract).

86. Shoback DM, Thatcher J, Leombruno R, Brown EM. The relationship between PTH secretion and cytosolic calcium concentration in dispersed bovine parathyroid cells. *Proc Natl Acad Sci USA* 1984;81:3113–3117.

87. Kifor O, Brown EM. Relationship between diacylglycerol levels and extracellular Ca^{++} in dispersed bovine parathyroid cells. *Endocrinology* 1988;123:2723–2729.

88. Nishizuka Y. Intracellular signaling by hydrolysis of phospholipids and activation of protein kinase C. *Science* 1992; 258:607–614.

89. Bourdeau A, Souberbielle J-C, Bonnet P, Herviaux P, Sachs C, Lieberherr M. Phospholipase-A$_2$ action and arachidonic acid metabolism in calcium-mediated parathyroid hormone secretion. *Endocrinology* 1992;130:1339–1344.

90. Okazaki T, Ando K, Igarishi T, Ogata T, Fujita T. Conserved mechanism of negative regulation by extracellular calcium. Parathyroid hormone gene versus atrial natriuretic polypeptide gene. *J Clin Invest* 1992;89:1268–1273.

91. Silver J, Russell J, Sherwood LM. Regulation by vitamin D metabolites of messenger ribonucleic acid for preproparathyroid hormone in isolated bovine parathyroid cells. *Proc Natl Acad Sci USA* 1985;82:4270–4273.

92. DeMay MG, Kiernan MS, DeLuca HF, Kronenberg HM. Sequences in the human parathyroid hormone gene that bind to the 1,25-dihydroxyvitamin D$_3$ receptor and mediate transcriptional repression in response to 1,25-dihydroxyvitamin D$_3$. *Proc Natl Acad Sci USA* 1992;89:8097–8101.

93. Carlberg C, Bondik I, Wyss A, et al. Two nuclear signalling pathways for vitamin D. *Nature* 1993;361:657–660.

94. Wernerson A, Widholm SM, Svensson O, Reinholt FP. Parathyroid cell number and size in hypocalcemic young rats. *APMIS* 1991;99:1096–1102.

95. LeBoff MS, Rennke HG, Brown EM. Abnormal regulation of parathyroid cell secretion and proliferation in primary cultures of bovine parathyroid cells. *Endocrinology* 1983;113: 277–284.

96. Lee MJ, Roth SI. Effect of calcium and magnesium on deoxyribonucleic acid synthesis in rat parathyroid glands in vitro. *Lab Invest* 1975;33:72–79.

97. Nygren P, Larsson R, Johansson H, Ljunghall S, Rastad J, Akerstrom G. 1,25(OH)$_2$D inhibits hormone secretion and proliferation but not functional differentiation of cultured bovine parathyroid cells. *Calcif Tissue Int* 1988;42:213–218.

98. Kream BE, Rowe DW, Gworek SC, Raisz LG. Parathyroid hormone alters collagen synthesis and procollagen mRNA levels in fetal rat calvaria. *Proc Natl Acad Sci USA* 1980; 77:5654–5658.

99. Nijweide PJ, Burger EH, Feyen JHM. Cells of bone: proliferation, differentiation, and hormonal regulation. *Physiol Rev* 1986;66:855–886.

100. Chambers TJ, Hall IJ. Cellular and molecular mechanisms in the regulation and function of osteoclasts. *Vit Hormones* 1991;46:41–86.

101. Rodan GA, Martin TJ. Role of osteoblasts in hormonal control of bone resorption. *Calcif Tissue Int* 1981;33:349–351.

102. Chambers TJ. The effect of parathyroid hormone, 1,25-dihydroxycholecalciferol and prostaglandins on the cytoplasmic activity of isolated osteoclasts. *J Pathol* 1982;137: 193–203.

103. Chambers TJ. Osteoblasts release osteoclasts from calcitonin-induced quiescence. *J Cell Sci* 1982;57:247–260.

104. Minkin CL, Blackman L, Newbrey J, Pokress S, Posek R, Walling M. Effects of parathyroid hormone and calcitonin on adenylate cyclase in murine mononuclear phagocytes. *Biochem Biophys Res Commun* 1977;76:875–881.

105. Roodman GD, Ibbotson KJ, MacDonald BR, Huehl TJ, Mundy GR. 1,25-Dihydroxyvitamin D$_3$ causes formation of multinucleated cells with several osteoclast characteristics in cultures of primate marrow. *Proc Natl Acad Sci USA* 1985;82:8213–8217.

106. Mundy GR. Cytokines and local factors which affect osteoclast function. *Int J Cell Cloning* 1992;10:215–222.

107. Pottratz S, Bellido T, Mocharla H, et al. 17-beta-Estradiol inhibits stimulated transcription from the human IL-6 promoter in transfected Hela and murine bone marrow stromal cells. *J Bone Mineral Res* 1992;7:S126 (abstract).

108. Juppner H, Abou-Samra AB, Freeman M, et al. A G-protein-coupled receptor for parathyroid hormone and parathyroid hormone-related protein. *Science* 1991;254:1024–1126.

109. Baran DT, Milne ML. 1,25-Dihydroxyvitamin D increases hepatocyte cytosolic calcium levels: a potential regulator of vitamin D 25-hydroxylase. *J Clin Invest* 1986;77:1812–1626.

110. Rowe DW, Kream BE. Regulation of collagen synthesis in fetal rat calvaria by 1,25-dihydroxyvitamin D$_3$. *J Biol Chem* 1982;257:8009–8015.

111. Canalis E, McCarthy T, Centrella M. Growth factors and the regulation of bone remodeling. *J Clin Invest* 1988;81:277–281.

112. Hauschka PV, Lian JB, Cole DEC, Gundberg CM. Osteocalcin and matrix gla protein: vitamin K dependent proteins in bone. *Physiol Rev* 1989;69:990–1047.

113. Costanzo LS, Windhager EE. Renal tubular transport of calcium. In Windhager EE, ed. *Handbook of physiology, section 8. Renal physiology*. New York: Oxford University Press, 1992;1759–1783.

114. Peacock M, Robertson WG, Nordin BEC. Relation between serum and urinary calcium with particular reference to parathyroid activity. *Lancet* 1969;1:384–386.

115. Brown EM. Kidney and bone: physiological and pathophysiological relationships. In Windhager EE, ed. *Handbook of physiology, section 8. Renal physiology*. New York: Oxford University Press, 1992;1841–1916.

116. Taylor AN, McIntosh JE, Bourdeau JE. Immunocytochemical localization of vitamin D-dependent calcium-binding

protein in renal tubules of the rabbit, rat, and chick. *Kidney Int* 1982;21:765–773.

117. Yamamoto M, Takuwa Y, Masuko S, Ogata E. Effects of endogenous and exogenous parathyroid hormone on tubular reabsorption of calcium in pseudohypoparathyroidism. *J Clin Endocrinol Metab* 1988;66:618–625.

118. Puschett JB, Maranz J, Kurnick WJ. Evidence for a direct action of cholecalciferol and 25-hydroxycholecalciferol on the renal transport of phosphate, sodium, and calcium. *J Clin Invest* 1972;51:373–385.

119. Puschett JB, Fernandez PC, Boyle IT, Gray RW, Omdahl JL, DeLuca HF. The acute renal tubular effects of 1,25-dihydroxycholecalciferol. *Proc Soc Exp Biol Med* 1972;141:379–384.

120. Martin KJ, Hruska KA, Lewis J, Anderson C, Slatopolsky E. The renal handling of parathyroid hormone: role of peritubular uptake and glomerular filtration. *J Clin Invest* 1977;60:808–814.

121. Quamme G. Control of magnesium transport in the thick ascending limb. *Am J Physiol* 1989;256:F197–F210.

122. Fajtova VT, Quinn ST, Brown EM. Cytosolic calcium responses of single rMTC 44-2 cells to stimulation with external calcium and potassium. *Am J Physiol* 1991;261:E151–E158.

123. Eskert RW, Sherubl H, Petzelt C, Friedhelm R, Ziegler R. Rythmic oscillations of cytosolic calcium in rat C-cells. *Mol Cell Endocrinol* 1989;64:267–270.

124. Zeytin FN, DeLellis R. The neuropeptide-synthesizing rat 44-2C cell line: regulation of peptide synthesis, secretion, 3′5′-cyclic adenosine monophosphate efflux, and adenylate cyclase activation. *Endocrinology* 1987;121:352–360.

125. Weisinger JR, Favus MJ, Langman CB, Bushinsky DA. Regulation of 1,25-dihydroxyvitamin D_3 by calcium in the parathyroidectomized, parathyroid hormone replete rat. *J Bone Mineral Res* 1989;4:929–935.

126. Hove K, Horst RL, Littledike LT, Beitz C. Infusions of parathyroid hormone in ruminants: hypercalcemia and reduced plasma 1,25-dihydroxyvitamin D concentrations. *Endocrinology* 1989;114:897–903.

127. Hulter HN, Halloran BP, Tuto RD, Peterson JC. Long-term control of plasma calcitriol concentration in dogs and humans. Dominant role of plasma calcium concentration in experimental hyperparathyroidism. *J Clin Invest* 1988;76:695–702.

128. Wortsman J, Haddad JG, Posillico JT, Brown EM. Primary hyperparathyroidism with low serum 1,25-dihydroxyvitamin D levels. *J Clin Endocrinol Metab* 1986;62:1305–1308.

129. Beck N, Singh H, Reed SW, Davis RD. Direct inhibitory effect of hypercalcemia on renal actions of parathyroid hormone. *J Clin Invest* 1974;53:717–725.

130. Mathias RS, Brown EM. Divalent cations modulate PTH-dependent 3′,5′-cyclic adenosine monophosphate production in renal proximal tubular cells. *Endocrinology* 1991;128:3005–3012.

131. Slatopolsky E, Mercado A, Morrison A, Yates J, Klahr S. Inhibitory effect of hypermagnesemia on the renal action of parathyroid hormone. *J Clin Invest* 1976;58:1273–1279.

132. Juhlin C, Holmdahl R, Johansson H, Rastad J, Akerstrom G, Klareskog G. Monoclonal antibodies with exclusive reactivity against parathyroid cells and tubule cells of the kidneys. *Proc Natl Acad Sci USA* 1987;84:2990–2994.

133. Goligorsky MS, Hruska HA. Hormonal modulation of cytoplasmic calcium concentration in renal tubular epithelium. *Mineral Electrolyte Metab* 1980;14:58–70.

134. Fujii Y, Fulcase M, Tsutsumi M, Miyauchi A, Tsunenari T, Fujita T. Parathyroid hormone control of cytosolic Ca^{2+} in the kidney. *J Bone Mineral Metab* 1988;3:525–532.

135. Shoback DM, Thatcher J, Leombruno R, Brown EM. Effects of extracellular Ca^{2+} and Mg^{2+} on cytosolic Ca^{2+} in dispersed bovine parathyroid cells. *Endocrinology* 1983;113:424–426.

136. Takaichi K, Kurokawa K. Inhibitory guanosine triphosphate-binding protein-mediated regulation of vasopressin action in isolated single medullary tubules of mouse kidney. *J Clin Invest* 1988;82:1437–1444.

137. Marx SJ, Attie MF, Levine MA, Spiegel AM, Downs RW Jr, Lasker RD. The hypocalciuric or benign variant of familial hypercalcemia: clinical and biochemical features in fifteen kindreds. *Medicine* 1981;60:397–412.

138. Fray JCS, Park CS, Valentine ND. Calcium and the control of renin secretion. *Endocr Rev* 1987;8:53–93.

139. Greenwald E, Apkon M, Hruska K, Needleman P. Stretch-induced atriopeptin secretion in the isolated rat myocyte and its negative modulation by calcium. *J Clin Invest* 1989;83:1061–1065.

140. Clemens TL, McGlade SA, Garrett KP, Craviso GL, Hendy GN. Extracellular calcium modulates vitamin D-dependent calbindin-D_{28K} gene expression in chick kidney cells. *Endocrinology* 1989;124:1582–1584.

141. Malgaroli A, Meldolesi J, Zambone-Zallone A, Teti A. Control of cytosolic free calcium in rat and chicken osteoclasts. The role of extracellular calcium and calcitonin. *J Biol Chem* 1989;264:14342–14349.

142. Zaidi M, Datta HK, Patchell A, Moonga B, MacIntyre I. "Calcium-activated" intracellular calcium elevation: a novel mechanism of osteoclast regulation. *Biochem Biophys Res Commun* 1989;163:1461–1465.

143. Silver IA, Murrils RJ, Etherington DJ. Microelectrode studies in the acid microenvironment beneath adherent macrophages and osteoclasts. *Exp Cell Res* 1988;175:266–276.

144. Handwerger S, Conn PM, Barrett J, Barry S, Golander A. Human placental lactogen release in vitro: paradoxical effects of calcium. *Am J Physiol* 1981;240:E550–E555.

145. Lyles KW, Clark AG, Drezner MK. Serum 1,25-dihydroxyvitamin D levels in subjects with X-linked hypophosphatemic rickets and osteomalacia. *Calcif Tissue Int* 1982;34:125–134.

146. Koletsky RJ, Moore TJ, Dluhy RG, Hollenberg NK, Williams GH. Dietary chloride modifies renin release in normal humans. *Am J Physiol* 1981;241:F361–F363.

147. Quintanella A, Molteni A, Huang Delgreco F. Effect of acid base changes on renin, aldosterone, and cortisol. *Physiologist* 1978;21:95 (abstract).

148. Ro H-K, Tembe V, Krug T, Yang P-Y, Bushinsky DA, Favus MJ. Acidosis inhibits 1,25-$(OH)_2D_3$ but not cAMP production in response to parathyroid hormone in the rat. *J Bone Mineral Res* 1990;5:273–278.

149. Barajas L. The juxtaglomerular apparatus: anatomic considerations in the feedback control of glomerular filtration rate. *Fed Proc* 1981;40:78–86.

150. Biedler LM. Taste receptor stimulation with salts and acids. In Biedler LM, ed, *Handbook of sensory physiology. Taste,* vol 4, part 2. New York: Springer-Verlag, 1971;200–220.

151. Strehler EE. Recent advances in the molecular characterization of plasma membrane Ca^{2+} pumps. *J Membrane Biol* 1991;120:1–15.

152. Cheung WY. Calmodulin plays a pivotal role in cellular regulation. *Science* 1980;207:19–27.

153. Scharf O, Foder B, Skibsted U. Hysteretic activation of the calcium pump revealed by calcium transients in human red cells. *Biochim Biophys Acta* 1983;730:295–305.

154. Blaustein MP. Effects of internal and external cations and of ATP on sodium-calcium and calcium-calcium exchange in squid axons. *Biophys J* 1970;20:79–111.

155. Blaustein MP. Sodium/calcium exchange and the control of contractility in cardiac muscle and vascular smooth muscle. *J Cardiovasc Pharmacol* 1988;12(suppl 5):S56–S68.

156. Catteral WA, Seager MJ, Takahashi M. Molecular properties of dihydropyridine-sensitive Ca^{2+} channels in skeletal muscle. *J Biol Chem* 1988;263:3535–3538.

157. Stuhmer W, Conti F, Suzuki H, et al. Structural parts involved in activation and inactivation of the sodium channels. *Nature* 1989;339:597–603.

158. Papazian DM, Schwartz TL, Tempel BL, Jan Yn, Yan LJ. Cloning of genomic and complementary cDNA from shaker, a putative K^+ channel gene from *Drosophila. Science* 1987;237:749–753.

159. Noda M, Shimuzu S, Tanabe T, et al. Primary structure of Electrophorus electricus sodium channel deduced from cDNA sequence. *Nature* 1984;312:121–127.

160. McFadzean I, Mullaney I, Brown D, Milligan G. Antibodies to GTP binding protein, Go, antagonizes noradrenaline-induced calcium current inhibition in NG10845 hybrid cells. *Neuron* 1989;3:177–182.

161. DiVirgilio F, Pozzan T, Wollheim CB, Vincenti LM, Meldolesi J. Tumor promoter phorbol myristate acetate inhibits Ca^{2+} influx through voltage-gated Ca^{2+} channels in the secretory cell lines PC12 and RINm5F. *J Biol Chem* 1989; 261:32–35.

162. Marchetti C, Brown AM. Protein kinase activator 1-oleoyl-2-acetyl sn-glycerol inhibits two types of calcium currents in GH_3 cells. *Am J Physiol* 1988;254:C206–C210.

163. Plummer MR, Logethetis DE, Hess P. Elementary properties and pharmacological sensitivity of calcium channels in mammalian peripheral neurons. *Neuron* 1989;2:1453–1463.

164. Cotman CW, Iverson LL. Excitatory amino acids in the brain-focus on NMDA receptors. *Trends Neurosci* 1987;10: 263–265.

165. Partridge LD, Swandulla D. Calcium-activated non-specific cation channels. *Trends Neurosci* 1988;11:69–72.

166. Putney JW Jr. Receptor-regulated calcium entry. *Pharmacol Ther* 1990;48:427–434.

167. Matsumaga H, Nishimoto I, Kojima I, Yamashita N, Kurokawa K, Ogata E. Activation of calcium-permeable cation channel by insulin-like growth factor II in Balb/c 3T3 cells. *Am J Physiol* 1988;255:C442–C446.

168. Hruska KA, Mills S, Khalifa S, Hammerman MR. Phosphorylation of renal brushborder membrane vesicles: effect on calcium uptake and membrane content of phosphoinositides. *J Biol Chem* 1983;258:2501–2507.

169. Murayama T, Ui M. Phosphatidic acid may stimulate membrane receptors mediating adenylate cyclase inhibition and phospholipid breakdown in 3T3 fibroblasts. *J Biol Chem* 1990;262:5522–5529.

170. Moolenaar WH, Kruijer W, Tilly BC, Verlaan I, Bierman AJ, de Laat SW. Growth factor-like action of phosphatidic acid. *Nature* 1986;323:171–173.

171. Krause K-H. Ca^{2+}-storage organelles. *FEBS Lett* 1991;285: 225–229.

172. Brandl CJ, Green NM, Korczak B, MacLennan DH. Two Ca^{2+}–ATPase genes: homologies and mechanistic implications of deduced amino acid sequences. *Cell* 1986;44:597–607.

173. Clarke DM, Loo TW, Inesi G, MacLennan DH. Location of high affinity Ca^{2+}-binding sites within the predicted transmembrane domains of sarcoplasmic reticulum Ca^{2+}–ATPase. *Nature* 1989;339:476–478.

174. Inui M, Chamberlain BK, Saito A, Fleischer S. The nature of the modulation of Ca^{2+} transport as studies by reconstitution of cardiac sarcoplasmic reticulum. *J Biol Chem* 1986;261:1794–1800.

175. Jorgensen AO, Shen ACY, Campbell KP, MacLennan DH. Ultrastructural localization of calsequestrin in skeletal muscle by immunoferritin labeling of ultrathin frozen sections. *J Cell Biol* 1983;97:1573–1581.

176. Takashima H, Nishimura S, Matsumoto T, et al. Primary structure and expression from complementary DNA of skeletal muscle ryanodine receptor. *Nature* 1989;339:439–445.

177. Block BA, Imagawa T, Campbell KP, Franzini-Armstrong C. Structural evidence for direct interaction between the molecular components of the transverse tubule/sarcoplasmic reticulum junction in skeletal muscle. *J Cell Biol* 1988;107: 2587–2600.

178. Furuichi T, Yoshikawa S, Miyawaki A, Wada K, Maeda N, Mikoshiba K. Primary structure and functional expression of the inositol 1,4,5-trisphosphate binding protein P_{400}. *Nature* 1989;342:32–38.

179. Eberhard DA, Holz RW. Intracellular Ca^{2+} activates phospholipase C. *Trends Neurosci* 1988;11:517–520.

180. Ghosh TK, Bian J, Gill DL. Intracellular Ca^{2+} release mediated by sphingosine derivative generated in cells. *Science* 1990;248:1653–1656.

181. Persechini A, Moncrief ND, Kretsinger RH. The EF-hand family of calcium-modulated proteins. *Trends Neurosci* 1989; 12:462–467.

182. Kemp BE, Pearson RB, Guerriero V Jr, Means AR. The calmodulin-binding domain of chicken smooth muscle myosin light chain kinase contains a pseudosubstrate sequence. *J Biol Chem* 1987;262:2542–2548.

183. Herzberg O, James MNG. Structure of the calcium regulatory muscle protein troponin C at 2.8 A resolution. *Nature* 1985;313:653–659.

184. Tsien RY, Pozzan T, Rink TJ. Calcium homeostasis in intact lymphocytes: cytoplasmic free calcium monitored with a new intracellularly trapped fluorescent indicator. *J Cell Biol* 1982;94:325–334.

185. Grynkiewicz G, Poenie M, Tsien RY. A new generation of Ca^{2+} indicators with greatly improved fluorescent properties. *J Biol Chem* 1985;266:3440–3450.

186. Poenie M, Alderton J, Tsien RY, Steinhardt RA. Changes in free Ca^{2+} levels with stages of the cell division cycle. *Nature* 1985;315:147–149.

187. Cheek TR. Spatial aspects of calcium signalling. *J Cell Sci* 1989;93:211–216.

188. Foskett JK, Guntu-Smith PJ, Melvin JE, Turner RJ. Physiological localization of an agonist-sensitive pool of Ca^{2+} on parotid acinar cells. *Proc Natl Acad Sci USA* 1989;86:167–171.

189. Peterson OH. Calcium-activated potassium channels and fluid secretion by exocrine glands. *Am J Physiol* 1986;251: G1–G13.

190. Rose B, Loewenstein WR. Calcium ion distribution in cytoplasm visualized by aequorin. Diffusion in cytosol restricted by energized sequestering. *Science* 1975;190:1204–1206.

191. Lipscombe D, Madison DV, Poenie M, Reuter H, Tsien RY, Tsien RW. Spatial distribution of calcium channels and cytosolic calcium transients in growth cones and cell bodies of sympathetic neurons. *Proc Natl Acad Sci USA* 1988;85: 2398–2402.

192. Blaustein MP. Calcium transport and buffering in neurons. *Trends Neurosci* 1988;11:438–443.

193. Kifor O, Congo, Brown EM. Phorbol esters modulate the high Ca^{2+}-stimulated accumulation of inositol phosphates in bovine parathyroid cells. *J Bone Mineral Res* 1990;5:1003–1011.

194. DiMarzo V, Galaderi SHI, Tippins JR, Morris HR. Interactions between second messengers: cAMP and PLA_2 and PLC metabolites. *Life Sci* 1991;49:247–259.

195. Finch EA, Turner TJ, Goldin SM. Ca^{2+} as coagonist of inositol 1,4,5-trisphosphate-induced calcium release. *Science* 1991;252:443–446.

196. Berridge MJ, Cobbold PH, Cuthbertsin KSR. Spatial and temporal aspects of cell signalling. *Phil Trans R Soc London* 1988;320:325–343.

197. Jaffe LF. Sources of Ca^{2+} in egg activation: a review and hypothesis. *Dev Biol* 1983;99:265–276.

198. Boitano S, Dirksen ER, Sanderson MJ. Intercellular propagation of calcium waves mediated by inositol trisphosphate. *Science* 1992;258:292–295.

199. Ro H-K, Tembe V, Favus MJ. Evidence that activation of protein kinase C can stimulate 1,25-dihydroxyvitamin D_3 secretion by rat proximal tubules. *Endocrinology* 1992;131: 1424–1428.

200. Bourdeau JE, Lau K. Regulation of cytosolic free calcium concentration in the rabbit connecting tubule: a calcium-absorbing renal epithelium. *J Lab Clin Med* 1992;119:650–662.

201. Abou-Samra AB, Juppner H, Force T, et al. Expression cloning of a PTH/PTHrP receptor from rat osteoblast-like cells: a single receptor stimulates intracellular accumulation of both cAMP and inositol trisphosphates and increases intracellular free calcium. *Proc Natl Acad Sci USA* 1992;89: 2726–2732.

202. Rouse D, Suki WN. Renal control of extracellular calcium. *Kidney Int* 1990;38:700–708.

203. Gross M, Kumar R. Physiology and biochemistry of vitamin D-dependent calcium binding proteins. *Am J Physiol* 1990; 259:F195–F209.

204. Tam S, Lau K. Regulation of potassium channel in apical

membranes of rabbit connecting tubule by cytoplasmic Ca²⁺ and H⁺. *J Am Soc Nephrol* 1991;2:752 (abstract).

205. Morel F. Sites of hormone action in mammalian nephron. *Am J Physiol* 1981;240:F159–F164.

206. Bronner F, Stein WD. CaBP facilitates intracellular diffusion for Ca pumping in distal convoluted tubule. *Am J Physiol* 1988;255:F558–F562.

207. Kretsinger RH, Mann JE, Simmonds JG. Model of facilitated diffusion of calcium by the intestinal calcium binding protein. In: Norman AW, Schaefer K, von Herrath D, Grigoleit H-G, eds. *Vitamin D: chemical, biochemical, and clinical endocrinology of calcium metabolism.* New York: Walter de Gruyter, 1982;233–248.

208. Feher JJ. Facilitated calcium diffusion by intestinal calcium binding protein. *Am J Physiol* 1983:244:C303–C307.

209. McCarthy JT, Barham SS, Kumar R. 1,25-Dihydroxyvitamin D₃ rapidly alters the morphology of the duodenal mucosa of rachitic chicks: evidence for novel effects of 1,25-dihidroxyvitamin D. *J Steroid Biochem* 1984;21:253–258.

210. Rasmussen H, Fontaine O, Max EE, Goodman DBP. The effect of 1-hydroxyvitamin D₃ administration on calcium transport in chick intestinal brush border membrane vesicles. *J Biol Chem* 1979;254:2993–2999.

211. Norman AW, Putkey JA, Nemere I. Intestinal calcium transport: pleiotropic effects mediated by vitamin D. *Fed Proc* 1982;41:78–83.

212. Rasmussen H, Matsuomto T, Fontaine O, Goodman DBP. Role of changes in membrane lipid structure in the action of 1,25-dihydroxyvitamin D₃. *Fed Proc* 1982;41:72–77.

213. Ghusen WEJM, Van Os OH. 1,25-Dihydroxyvitamin D₃ regulates ATP-dependent calcium transport in basolateral plasma membranes of rat enterocytes. *Biochim Biophys Acta* 1982;689:170–172.

214. Wasserman RH. Intestinal absorption of calcium and phosphorus. *Fed Proc* 1981;40:68–72.

215. Martin DL, DeLuca HF. Influence of sodium on calcium transport by the rat small intestine. *Am J Physiol* 1969; 216:1351–1359.

The Parathyroids, edited by J.P. Bilezikian,
M.A. Levine, and R. Marcus. Raven Press, Ltd.,
New York © 1994.

CHAPTER 3

Regulation of Parathyroid Hormone by Dietary Calcium and Vitamin D

Bess Dawson-Hughes

As the populations of industrialized countries age, focus on prevention and treatment of chronic diseases has increased. Over the past decade, there has been an unprecedented amount of interest and research directed toward preventing and treating osteoporosis. Progress in the field has followed the development of new technologies for indirectly assessing bone mass.

Research in the area of calcium and vitamin D intake, parathyroid hormone (PTH), and bone status draws on advances in densitometry and on important recent developments in assays for PTH. The methodologically weak link is the assessment of calcium and vitamin D intake. Not only do intakes of these nutrients vary widely from day to day in most individuals, but the amounts present in fortified foods (i.e., vitamin D content of milk) can deviate widely from the contents stated on food labels. The vitamin D content of many foods is unknown, and there is the general inclination to underreport food consumption. These and other difficulties with intake assessments limit one's ability to identify associations between intake of these nutrients and bone change in observational studies. Relationships between PTH and calcium and vitamin D intake can be assessed better in controlled-diet (metabolic) studies, and the influence of these nutrients on bone mass can be estimated more effectively with calcium- and vitamin D-intervention studies.

DIETARY CALCIUM, PARATHYROID HORMONE, AND BONE

The amount of calcium available for the skeleton is dependent on the level of dietary intake and on intestinal absorption efficiency. Although the quantity of calcium absorbed varies directly with intake, fractional absorption varies inversely with dietary intake (1) (Fig. 1), providing a partial compensation for dietary calcium insufficiency. This adaptation results from the homeostatic regulation of 1,25-dihydroxyvitamin D [1,25(OH)$_2$D], the metabolite of vitamin D that stimulates active transport of calcium across intestinal mucosal cells. During calcium restriction, the following sequence occurs: the total amount of calcium absorbed decreases, the plasma ionized calcium activity decreases slightly, plasma PTH concentration increases, and this stimulates 1,25(OH)$_2$D production in the kidney. At low to moderate calcium intakes, 1,25(OH)$_2$D-stimulated active transport is the major mechanism by which calcium is absorbed. As intake rises, passive diffusion accounts for a progressively larger proportion of absorption. Regarding the calcium absorbed from an 8 oz glass of milk, the calculations of Ireland and Fordtran (2) indicate that young adults with low usual calcium intakes absorb about 80% by active transport and 20% by passive diffusion.

Early evidence linking PTH to a relationship between calcium intake and bone status was provided by Jowsey and Raisz (3). When fed a low-calcium, high-phosphorus diet, intact adult cats developed osteoporosis, whereas cats with their parathyroid glands removed did not. In man, PTH is the main physiologic activator of bone remodeling, a process that determines the overall bone turnover rate. For 3–6 months following an increase in turnover, whether induced by PTH or by another agent, such as thyroid hormone, resorption will transiently exceed formation and result in a short-term net loss of bone mineral (4). A higher endogenous PTH level is expected to amplify bone loss in those who have an unfavorable resorption/formation ratio. This resorptive characteristic of PTH is

B. Dawson-Hughes: Calcium and Bone Metabolism Laboratory, USDA Human Nutrition Research Center on Aging, Tufts University, Boston, Massachusetts 02111.

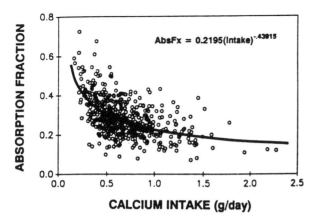

FIG. 1. Relationship of absorption fraction and 24 hr calcium intake in 526 studies in 189 unselected women aged 35–60 years. The curve is the best-fit regression line for the log transforms of the data. (Reprinted from ref. 1 with permission.)

distinct from the anabolic effect that results from pulsatile administration of active PTH fragments (see the chapter by Marcus).

Aging is associated with changes in PTH, calcium absorption, and bone mineral density. Circulating PTH increases with age (5–7). Fractional calcium absorption declines after menopause (1), declines with aging (1,8), and is lower in osteoporotic than in age-matched nonosteoporotic women (8). Bone mineral density declines with aging in men and women. Age-related changes such as these may or may not influence the interrelationships between dietary calcium, serum PTH, and bone. These relationships are examined in the context of aging and of estrogen status.

Mature Young Adults

From the time when peak bone mass is achieved, at about age 30 years, until the approach of menopause, bone mass in healthy women is fairly stable. Young men have a longer period of stability in bone mass. Several metabolic studies allow an evaluation of the dietary calcium–PTH axis in young adults. Adams et al. (9) found that in premenopausal women and young men consuming a mean of 900 mg calcium per day, calcium restriction to 48 mg per day resulted in a significant increase in fasting serum PTH concentration. A 4 g calcium load decreased fasting serum PTH concentrations in this population (9). In several young (and also in older) women, calcium restriction from 2,000 mg to 300 mg per day caused a prompt increase in fasting intact PTH concentration that persisted over a 2 month period of calcium restriction (10). A third recent study supports these findings (11). In contrast,

in a 3 year field study in premenopausal women consuming ~960 mg calcium daily, an additional 600 mg dietary calcium per day did not alter fasting PTH levels measured after 18 and 36 months of supplementation (12). The similar PTH levels with the two calcium intakes may reflect the relatively modest increase in calcium intake during supplementation or the longer dietary intervention. As the authors pointed out, an effect of supplemental calcium on PTH may have been present during the day but undetectable in fasting blood samples. Importantly, the increase in calcium intake did have a beneficial effect on spine bone mineral density (12). These studies indicate that increases in dietary calcium reduce serum PTH concentration, at least transiently, and help stabilize bone mineral density in healthy young adults.

Early Postmenopausal Women

Loss of estrogen at menopause results in very rapid bone loss over about a 5 year period. A small group of normal women in this age range exhibited acute suppression of their PTH levels in response to an oral calcium load of 25 mg/kg (13). Three large prospective studies in early postmenopausal women allow examination of the effect of supplemental calcium on fasting PTH levels and bone mineral density over a several year period. In the largest, involving 295 women consuming a mean of 1,150 mg calcium per day, supplementation with up to 2,000 mg calcium daily had no effect on fasting PTH levels (14). There was a reduction in spinal bone loss in the first but not in the second year in this study (14). In 65 early postmenopausal women with dietary calcium intakes under 650 mg per day, supplementation with 500 mg calcium daily did not alter fasting PTH concentration or significantly influence rates of bone loss from the spine, hip, or radius (15). Nilas et al. (16) found basal PTH levels of early postmenopausal women to be similar across tertiles of calcium intake (mean intakes 403 mg per day, 880 mg per day, and 1,640 mg per day). Neither serum PTH nor bone mineral density changed with calcium supplementation (16).

The rapid bone loss that occurs during this period may provide calcium to the extracellular fluid, suppress PTH secretion, and indirectly also suppress 1,25(OH)$_2$D concentration and calcium absorption. In this circumstance PTH levels would be expected to drop across menopause. Several studies indicate, however, that PTH concentration is not affected by estrogen status. Prince et al. (17) found age-matched pre- and postmenopausal women to have similar PTH levels and similar increases in PTH concentration after calcium restriction. In agreement with this, fasting PTH levels were similar in early and late postmenopausal women recruited for a calcium supplement trial (15).

Another approach has also been used to examine the influence of estrogen on serum PTH and 1,25(OH)₂D concentrations. In several elegant metabolic studies, administration of oral estrogen to women beyond menopause did not alter either fasting (18,19) or day-long (20) PTH levels. Instead, the positive effect of estrogen on calcium balance may result, at least in part, from estrogen-induced increases in 1,25(OH)₂D (18,20,21). Figure 2 (21) illustrates the acute serum calcium, PTH, and 1,25(OH)₂D responses to EDTA-induced hypocalcemia in healthy postmenopausal women, before and after treatment with estrogen for 30 days. After estrogen, free (data not shown) and total 1,25(OH)₂D levels were higher; however, the increases in 1,25(OH)₂D and PTH concentrations following EDTA infusion were similar. From this, estrogen appears to increase the level of 1,25(OH)₂D

acutely but not to alter the 1,25(OH)₂D response to a PTH challenge.

There is some evidence that estrogen also influences calcium balance by a vitamin D-independent action on the gut (22). Fourteen women were studied before and 6 months after bilateral oophorectomy. After the surgery, the women were randomly assigned to treatment with either placebo or estrogen over the 6 month study period. Before and 6 months after surgery, the effect of exogenous 1,25(OH)₂D (1 μg daily for 7 days) on calcium absorption was assessed. As is shown in Fig. 3, basal serum 1,25(OH)₂D levels were similar before and after surgery, and changes in response to 1,25(OH)₂D treatment were also similar (22). In contrast (Fig. 4), fractional calcium absorption was lower after surgery in the placebo-treated women, and their absorption response to treatment with 1,25(OH)₂D was blunted (22). In this study, the loss of estrogen lowered fractional calcium absorption, apparently by a mechanism that is independent of 1,25(OH)₂D concentration. Notably, the acute effect of estrogen on serum 1,25(OH)₂D observed by Cheema et al. (21) was not apparent after 6 months in the above-mentioned study (22).

In conclusion, in early postmenopausal women an inverse relationship between PTH and dietary calcium intake is observed acutely after a change in calcium intake. Supplementation with calcium, however, does not result in a measurable change in fasting PTH level over the long term. Calcium supplementation in this population has, at most, a modest impact on the rate of bone loss. Neither the rapid bone loss that follows menopause nor its prevention with estrogen-replacement therapy appears to involve the PTH concentration directly. This has led to the hypothesis that bone

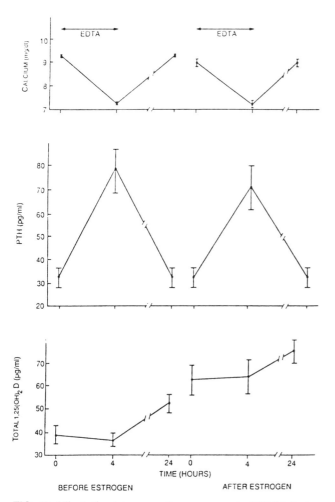

FIG. 2. Effect of estrogen on the response to EDTA infusion in 12 postmenopausal women. **Top:** Serum calcium; **middle:** iPTH; **bottom:** total calcitriol. Arrows at top show duration of EDTA infusion. (Reprinted from ref. 21 with permission.)

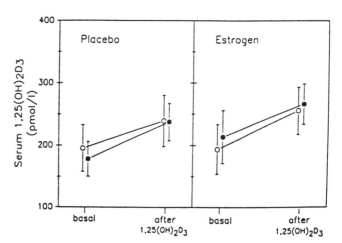

FIG. 3. Changes in serum 1,25(OH)₂D₃ induced by a 7 day course of 1,25(OH)₂D₃ (1 μg/day) in women treated with placebo (**left**) or estrogen (**right**), before (○) and 6 months after (●) oophorectomy. (Reprinted from ref. 22 with permission.)

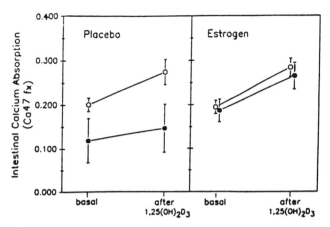

FIG. 4. Changes in intestinal calcium absorption induced by a 7 day course of 1,25(OH)₂D₃ (1 μg/day) in women treated with placebo (**left**) or estrogen (**right**) before (○) and 6 months after (●) oophorectomy. (Reprinted from ref. 22 with permission.)

sensitivity to PTH is altered by estrogen (23,24). The recent development of specific biochemical markers of bone formation and resorption should facilitate further examination of this question.

Late Postmenopausal Women

By this stage, age-related increases in PTH level and decreases in bone mass have been sustained. Throughout a broad range of calcium intakes, dietary calcium influences the fasting serum PTH concentration in elderly men and women. Circulating PTH decreased significantly after dietary calcium was raised from 100 to 1,000 mg per day (25), from 725 to 1,200 mg per day (26), from 750 to 1,750 mg per day (27), and from 950 to 1,950 mg per day (28). In the two studies in which they were measured (25,26), 1,25(OH)₂D concentrations decreased after calcium supplementation.

A role for dietary calcium in reducing bone loss in late postmenopausal women is apparent. In a pilot study of 76 healthy women (29), we observed that those in the lowest quartile of dietary calcium intake (<400 mg/day) had more bone loss from the spine over a 7 month interval than did those in the highest intake quartile (>800 mg/day). We then conducted a large calcium-intervention trial to test the effect of 500 mg supplemental calcium, as either carbonate or citrate malate, on rates of bone loss in healthy postmenopausal women with low (<400 mg/day) and moderate (400–650 mg/day) dietary calcium intakes (15). Changes in bone density in women 6 or more years beyond menopause are shown in Fig. 5. In those with calcium intakes under 400 mg per day, supplementation to a total intake of ~800 mg per day reduced bone loss from the spine, femoral neck, and radius. Those

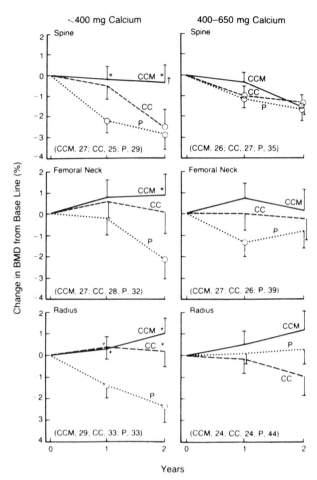

FIG. 5. Effect of calcium on mean adjusted rates of change in bone mineral density (BMD) in late postmenopausal women. The rates were adjusted for baseline bone mineral density and body mass index and for dietary calcium intake during the study for each scan site and calcium-intake category. The panels at **left** show women with calcium intakes of <400 mg per day and the panels at **right** those with intakes of 400–650 mg per day. The sample sizes are shown in parentheses. CCM, calcium citrate malate; CC, calcium carbonate; P, placebo. Within each panel, mean values labeled with asterisks differed significantly from those for the placebo group (*P* < 0.05); the dagger indicates a difference from the calcium carbonate group that is of borderline significance (*P* = 0.081). The open circles indicate values that differed significantly from the baseline values (*P* ≤ 0.05 by repeated-measures analysis of variance). The T bars indicate the SE. (Reprinted from ref. 15 with permission.)

with higher dietary intakes had less bone loss in general and no significant benefit from the supplementation. To examine the overall relationship between calcium intake and rate of bone loss in these women, we computed mean calcium intake from five measurements made over the 2 year study (30). Changes in bone mineral density by quintile of total calcium intake (diet plus supplements) are shown in Fig. 6. These profiles suggest that calcium is a threshold nutrient and that the threshold may differ by skeletal site. More cal-

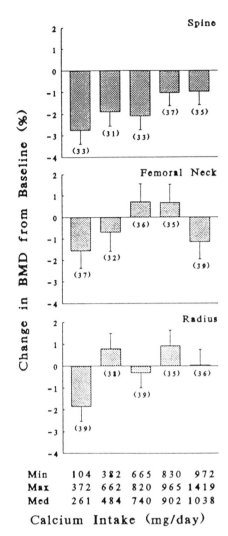

FIG. 6. Bone loss by quintile of total calcium intake in women 6 or more years beyond menopause (15). Rates were adjusted for differences in initial bone mineral density. Minimum, maximum, and median intakes for each quintile are shown. (Reprinted from ref. 30 with permission.)

cium may be needed to minimize bone loss at the spine than at the radius. A threshold at the femoral neck is less certain but may lie between that of the other sites.

Among the late postmenopausal women participating in the 2 year calcium supplement trial described above (15), correlations between hormone levels and bone status were examined (31). Serum PTH and 1,25(OH)$_2$D concentrations decreased after supplementation with calcium. Before treatment, lower serum calcium and higher 1,25(OH)$_2$D concentrations were predictive of a favorable response to added calcium at the femoral neck. During supplementation with calcium, a higher serum calcium concentration was predictive of a positive response at the radius, with similar trends for the spine and hip. Similarly, a lower 1,25(OH)$_2$D level was associated with less bone loss at the spine and radius. Serum intact PTH levels

were not predictive of bone performance at any site, whether measured at baseline or during the intervention.

These studies and the recent work of Lau et al. (32) reveal that a low calcium intake causes bone loss in elderly women and that increasing calcium intake to 800–1,000 mg daily reduces this loss. Reid et al. (27) showed that increasing calcium intake from 750 to 1,750 mg per day reduced whole-body bone loss in the second treatment year. This study is important because it raises the intake level at which a skeletal benefit has been demonstrated in women several years beyond menopause. To date, bone change in this population has been correlated with fasting serum calcium and with 1,25(OH)$_2$D concentrations. PTH concentrations are consistently lowered by increasing calcium intake; however, a more direct relationship between serum PTH and rate of bone change remains to be demonstrated.

VITAMIN D, PTH, AND BONE

Consideration of vitamin D is integral to a discussion of dietary calcium, PTH, and bone, because the active metabolite of this vitamin, 1,25(OH)$_2$D, is the main determinant of calcium absorption at usual levels of intake, it directly suppresses PTH synthesis and secretion, and it exerts concentration-dependent effects on bone. Defining optimal vitamin D nutriture is difficult because of the complex pattern of formation and metabolism of this vitamin.

Vitamin D is derived from diet and is both synthesized and degraded in the skin. Intestinal absorption of vitamin D occurs in the distal ileum and requires the presence of bile salts. Barragry et al. (33) found that vitamin D absorption in healthy women declined by ~40% with aging. Others have not confirmed this observation, possibly because they estimated absorption from supraphysiologic test doses of vitamin D (34,35). Decreased vitamin D absorption also accompanies a variety of gastrointestinal disorders that involve failure of fat emulsification and digestion, decreased gastric transit time, and fat malabsorption. Several commonly used drugs reduce vitamin D availability or enhance 25(OH)D metabolism. Aluminum hydroxide in large amounts precipitates bile acids and thus decreases vitamin D absorption. Cholestyramine binds 25(OH)D during its enterohepatic circulation. Several drugs, including anticonvulsants, rifampin, and primidone, accelerate metabolism of 25(OH)D probably by hepatic microsomal induction.

Vitamin D is synthesized in the skin after exposure to solar ultraviolet B rays. Skin synthesis of vitamin D is reduced in the elderly, apparently because of substrate deficiency. MacLaughlin and Holick (36) have shown that the 7-dehydrocholesterol concentration in the epidermis declines by ~50% from age 20 to age 84 years. Because of age-related decreases in absorption and synthesis, serum 25(OH)D concentrations are reduced in ambulatory elderly individuals and are further reduced among those who are institutionalized.

In the heavily populated temperate zone, skin synthesis of vitamin D varies with time of year. At latitude 42.2°N (Boston), the rays that stimulate vitamin D synthesis (290–315 nm) do not reach the earth's surface over the 5 month period from mid-October through mid-March (37). This interval is longer at higher latitudes, whereas, at the lower latitude of 34°N, skin synthesis apparently occurs year round (37).

Recent in vitro studies reveal that vitamin D is degraded by solar rays of 315–330 nm wavelength (38). Interestingly, at latitude 42.2°N, rays of this wavelength do reach earth's surface year round. Photodegradation of vitamin D in vitro, although more extensive in summer, does occur in the winter (38). The degradation can apparently occur while the vitamin is bound to vitamin D binding protein (38). Ultraviolet rays of wavelength 315–330 nm penetrate the epidermis and dermis (39) and thus have access to bound vitamin D as it circulates through dermal capillaries. From this it seems plausible that vitamin D from both skin and dietary sources may be subject to photodegradation, al-

though there is no clinical evidence presently to support or refute this.

At intakes of vitamin D commonly ingested in the United States, Europe, and Japan, ~75–150 IU per day, sunlight makes a significant contribution to the serum 25(OH)D concentration. At high latitudes, the solar or skin contribution can be estimated from the amplitude of seasonal variation in serum 25(OH)D concentration. As intake increases, the solar contribution becomes relatively less important.

Serum 25(OH)D and PTH concentrations vary inversely (40,41), and both change with season (42,43). Krall et al. (43) examined the influence of vitamin D intake on seasonal changes in serum 25(OH)D and PTH concentrations in 333 healthy postmenopausal women recruited for a 2 year calcium supplement trial. In these ambulatory women with a mean vitamin D intake of 112 IU/day, serum 25(OH)D fell and PTH levels rose in the late winter; however, significant seasonal variation was restricted to the subset of women with vitamin D intakes below 220 IU daily (Fig. 7). Because only one-fourth of the women had intakes above this level, one cannot be certain that an intake somewhat higher than 220 IU is not required to prevent a wintertime rise in serum PTH. In this study, an intake of 220 IU per day corresponded to a 25(OH)D level of 95 nmol/liter (38 ng/ml).

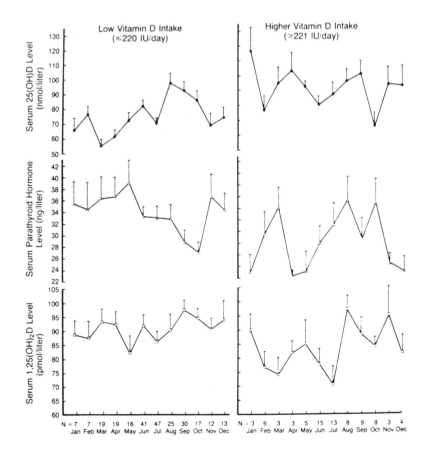

FIG. 7. Month-to-month variations in mean (±SE) serum concentrations of 25(OH)D (●), parathyroid hormone (△), and 1,25(OH)₂D (□) in 333 postmenopausal women grouped according to total vitamin D intake. The number of women studied each month is indicated at the bottom. (Reprinted from ref. 43 with permission.)

Peacock et al. (44) addressed the issue of vitamin D sufficiency by determining what level of 25(OH)D was needed to ensure adequate substrate for 1,25(OH)$_2$D production. Administration of 25(OH)D did not increase the 1,25(OH)$_2$D concentration in subjects with a starting 25(OH)D concentration of 50 nmol/liter or above, whereas it did in those with lower initial 25(OH)D levels (44). The relation between 25(OH)D and vitamin D intake will obviously vary if different methods are used to assess either of these measures. Nonetheless, the different approaches of Peacock and Krall have provided fairly good evidence that the 25(OH)D level needed to minimize perturbation of the calcium-regulating hormones is near the midpoint of what is commonly considered to be the normal range. The observation that supplementation with vitamin D reduces PTH levels in those with low dietary vitamin D intakes (45,46) but not in those who are better nourished (47) illustrates this point.

The relationship between PTH and vitamin D is clinically relevant if it has implications for bone status. Several recent studies have related vitamin D intake to PTH concentration, bone mineral density, rates of bone loss, and fracture rates. Available data for different age groups are reviewed below.

Pre- and Early Postmenopausal Women

Lukert et al. (41) followed 22 healthy women for 5 years as they went through menopause. Their mean calcium intake was 1,000 mg (range 476–3,118) per day, and vitamin D intake was 340 IU (range 48–823) per day. Dietary vitamin D intake was positively correlated with change in bone mineral content of the distal radius (Fig. 8) and accounted for 26% of the variability in this change over the 5 year period. In contrast, calcium intake was not correlated with bone change. Serum PTH concentration was inversely related to change in proximal radius BMC in the year before (Fig. 9) but not during the interval following cessation of menses (41). These associations led to the conclusion that vitamin D insufficiency contributes to bone loss in perimenopausal women, probably by a PTH-induced increase in the bone turnover rate (41). This is consistent with an earlier 1 year study of perimenopausal women, in which rate of change in distal radius BMC was inversely related to serum PTH (48).

Late Postmenopausal Women, Men

In cross-sectional studies, associations of vitamin D status and PTH with bone mineral density have been observed by some (49,50) but not other (5) study groups. In middle-aged women in England, circulating 25(OH)D was positively correlated and PTH nega-

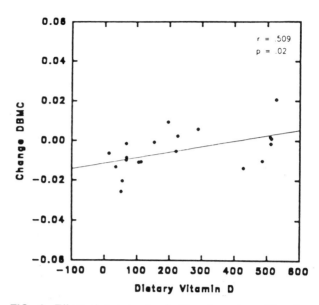

FIG. 8. Effect of dietary vitamin D on bone loss. The slope of the change in distal radius bone mineral content (DBMC) over 5 years was highly correlated with dietary intake of vitamin D. (Reprinted from ref. 41 with permission.)

tively correlated with density of the spine and femur (49). Among women being evaluated for osteoporosis (50), 10% had low serum 25(OH)D levels (>2 SD below the reference mean) but no clinical evidence of osteomalacia. In this subset, spinal bone mineral density was correlated positively with serum 25(OH)D (r =

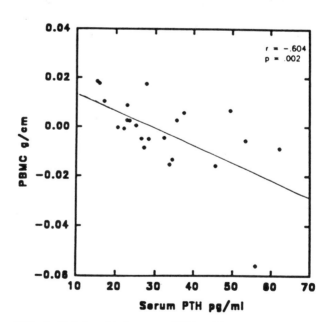

FIG. 9. Relationship between PTH and bone loss premenopausal. The proximal radius bone mineral content (PBMC) slope was negatively correlated with the mean serum PTH during the year before the rise of FSH. (Reprinted from ref. 41 with permission.)

0.41, $P < 0.01$) and inversely with PTH ($r = -0.47$, $P < 0.01$) concentration (Fig. 10). These relationships were not observed in the larger number of women with normal 25(OH)D levels. Collectively, these findings suggest that vitamin D insufficiency contributes to bone loss in many older women residing in the temperate zone.

On the basis of seasonal fluctuation in the serum PTH, we postulated that rates of bone loss may vary during the year. To test this hypothesis, we examined the rates of change in spinal and whole-body bone mineral density in 246 late postmenopausal women over two 6 month intervals (51). The intervals were timed to flank the periods when PTH concentration in a similar population (Fig. 7) was lowest (June and July through December and January) and highest (December and January through June and July). All of the women received supplemental calcium, and equal numbers were randomized to 400 IU vitamin D or placebo. Both groups consumed about 100 IU vitamin D daily in their diets. The placebo-treated group had a significant winter/spring decrease in serum 25(OH)D and increase in serum PTH concentrations, whereas the vitamin D-treated group did not (51). Changes in spinal bone density in the summer/fall (period 1), winter/spring (period 2), and overall are shown in Fig. 11. Both groups demonstrated seasonality in the bone measurements. There was an overall benefit from vitamin D supplementation after 1 year that resulted from decreased bone loss in the winter. Cumulative benefit over a longer period remains to be demonstrated; however, it appears likely based on the studies cited earlier (41,48,52). Because 400 IU supplemental vitamin D eliminated seasonal change in PTH concentrations, one might suspect that this intake is sufficient

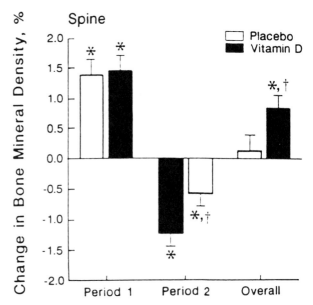

FIG. 11. Effect of vitamin D on annualized rates of change in spinal bone mineral density during the year. Period 1 is June–July through December–January, and period 2 is December–January through the following June–July. Bars labeled with asterisks differed from zero ($P < 0.01$); daggers indicate a difference between treatment groups ($P < 0.05$). Standard errors are also shown. (Reprinted from ref. 51 with permission.)

to minimize bone loss; however, this too remains to be demonstrated. Seasonal change in bone mineral density but no treatment effect was noted for the whole-body site.

Relationships between 25(OH)D concentration and bone mass, when noted, have been at skeletal sites rich in trabecular bone, the most distal radius and spine (41,50,51). This is in contrast to recent observations that cortical bone is affected most in hyperparathyroidism (53). The explanation may be related to the different PTH concentrations in normal vs. hyperparathyroid subjects.

Some information is available on calcium and vitamin D nutritional status and fracture rates. A higher calcium intake has been associated with lower hip fracture rates in several (54,55) but not in other (56) observational studies. Lips et al. (52) noted that elderly hip fracture patients had lower levels of 25(OH)D than elderly controls. Annual injections of vitamin D reduced upper body fractures in elderly subjects in Finland (57). Finally, in a randomized trial in over 3,000 elderly nursing home residents in France (58), supplementation with 1,200 mg calcium and 800 IU vitamin D daily for 18 months reduced hip and other nonvertebral fracture rates (Fig. 12). In the subset measured, treatment caused a sustained increase in serum 25(OH)D (from 16 to 40 ng/ml), decreases in PTH

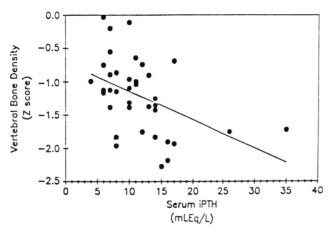

FIG. 10. Correlation between vertebral bone density and serum iPTH in subjects with low 25(OH)D. (Reprinted from ref. 50 with permission.)

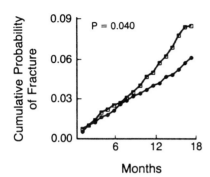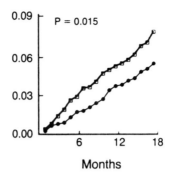

FIG. 12. Cumulative probability of hip fracture (**left**) and other nonvertebral fracture (**right**) in the placebo group (□) and the group treated with vitamin D_3 and calcium (●), estimated by the life-table method and based on the length of time to the first fracture. (Reprinted from ref. 58 with permission.)

(from 54 to 35 pg/ml) and osteocalcin (from 8 to 7 μg/l), and no change in $1,25(OH)_2D$ concentration. This important study provides convincing evidence that calcium and vitamin D supplementation, even when started very late in life, can reduce fracture rates in people whose usual calcium and vitamin D intakes are low.

In conclusion, there is mounting evidence that an inadequate intake of vitamin D as well as calcium contributes to bone loss in adults residing in the temperate zone. The mechanism by which this loss occurs is unknown, but the evidence cited here suggests that secondary increases in PTH concentrations, well within the normal range, may trigger the bone loss. Definition of the vitamin D intake that is optimal and safe for men and women of different ages and residing at different latitudes merits further research.

REFERENCES

1. Heaney RP, Recker RR, Stegman MR, Moy AJ. Calcium absorption in women: relationships to calcium intake, estrogen status, and age. *J Bone Mineral Res* 1989;4:469–475.
2. Ireland P, Fordtran JS. Effect of dietary calcium and age on jejunal calcium absorption in humans studied by intestinal perfusion. *J Clin Invest* 1973;52:2672–2681.
3. Jowsey J, Raisz LG. Experimental osteoporosis and parathyroid activity. *Endocrinology* 1968;82:384–396.
4. Frost HM. Remodeling as a determinant of envelop physiology. In: Frost HM, ed. *Bone remodeling and its relationship to metabolic bone diseases. Orthopaedic Lectures.* Vol III. Springfield, IL: Charles C. Thomas Publishers, 1973;28–53.
5. Sherman SS, Tobin JD, Hollis BW, Gundberg CM, Roy TA, Plato CC. Biochemical parameters associated with low bone density in healthy men and women. *J Bone Mineral Res* 1992;7:1123–1130.
6. Eastell R, Yergey AL, Vieira NE, Cedel SL, Kumar R, Riggs BL. Interrelationships among vitamin D metabolism, true calcium absorption, parathyroid function, and age in women: evidence of an age-related intestinal resistance to 1,25-dihydroxyvitamin D action. *J Bone Mineral Res* 1991;6:125–132.
7. Quesada JM, Coopmans W, Ruiz B, Aljama P, Jans I, Bouillon R. Influence of vitamin D on parathyroid function in the elderly. *J Clin Endocrinol Metab* 1992;75:494–501.
8. Avioli LV, McDonald JE, Lee SW. The influence of age on the intestinal absorption of ^{47}Ca in women and its relation to ^{47}Ca absorption in postmenopausal osteoporosis. *J Clin Invest* 1965;44:1960–1967.
9. Adams ND, Gray RW, Lemann J. The effects of oral $CaCO_3$ loading and dietary calcium deprivation on plasma 1,25-dihydroxyvitamin D concentrations in healthy adults. *J Clin Endocrinol Metab* 1979;48:1008–1016.
10. Dawson-Hughes B, Stern DT, Shipp CC, Rasmussen HM. Effect of lowering dietary calcium intake on fractional whole body calcium retention. *J Clin Endocrinol Metab* 1988;67:62–68.
11. Barger-Lux MJ, Heaney RP. Effects of calcium restriction on metabolic characteristics of premenopausal women. *J Clin Endocrinol Metab* 1993;76:103–107.
12. Baran D, Sorensen A, Grimes J, et al. Dietary modification with dairy products for preventing vertebral bone loss in premenopausal women: a three-year prospective study. *J Clin Endocrinol Metab* 1990;70:264–270.
13. Tohme JF, Bilezikian JP, Clemens TL, Silverberg SJ, Shane E, Lindsay R. Suppression of parathyroid hormone secretion with oral calcium in normal subjects and patients with primary hyperparathyroidism. *J Clin Endocrinol Metab* 1990; 70:951–956.
14. Elders PJ, Netelenbos JC, Lips P, et al. Calcium supplementation reduces vertebral bone loss in perimenopausal women: a controlled trial in 248 women between 46 and 55 years of age. *J Clin Endocrinol Metab* 1991;73:533–540.
15. Dawson-Hughes B, Dallal GE, Krall EA, Sadowski L, Sahyoun N, Tannenbaum S. A controlled trial of the effect of calcium supplementation on bone density in postmenopausal women. *N Engl J Med* 1990;323:878–883.
16. Nilas L, Christiansen C, Rodbro P. Calcium supplementation and postmenopausal bone loss. *Br Med J* 1985;289:1103–1106.
17. Prince RL, Dick I, Garcia-Webb P, Retallack RW. The effects of the menopause on calcitriol and parathyroid function: responses to a low dietary calcium stress test. *J Clin Endocrinol Metab* 1990;70:1119–1123.
18. Civitelli R, Agnusdei D, Nardi P, Zacchei F, Avioli LV, Gennari C. Effects of one-year treatment with estrogens on bone mass, intestinal calcium absorption, and 25-hydroxyvitamin D-1α-hydroxylase reserve in postmenopausal osteoporosis. *Calcif Tissue Int* 1988;42:77–86.
19. Marcus R, Villa ML, Cheema M, Cheema C, Newhall K, Holloway L. Effects of conjugated estrogen on the calcitriol response to parathyroid hormone in postmenopausal women. *J Clin Endocrinol Metab* 1992;74:413–418.
20. Packer E, Holloway L, Newhall K, Kanwar G, Butterfield G, Marcus R. Effects of estrogen on daylong circulating calcium, phosphorus, 1,25-dihydroxyvitamin D, and parathyroid hormone in postmenopausal women. *J Bone Mineral Res* 1990;5:877–884.
21. Cheema C, Grant BF, Marcus R. Effects of estrogen on circulating "free" and total 1,25-dihydroxyvitamin D and on the parathyroid-vitamin D axis in postmenopausal women. *J Clin Invest* 1989;83:537–542.
22. Gennari C, Agnusdei D, Nardi P, Civitelli R. Estrogen preserves a normal intestinal responsiveness to 1,25-dihydroxyvitamin D_3 in oophorectomized women. *J Clin Endocrinol Metab* 1990;71:1288–1293.

23. Heaney RP. A unified concept of osteoporosis. *Am J Med* 1965;39:877–880.
24. Kotowicz MA, Klee GG, Kao PC, et al. Relationship between serum intact parathyroid hormone concentrations and bone remodeling in type 1 osteoporosis: evidence that skeletal sensitivity is increased. *Osteoporosis Int* 1990;1:14–22.
25. Bikle DD, Herman RH, Hull S, Hagler L, Harris D, Halloran B. Adaptive response of humans to changes in dietary calcium: relationship between vitamin D regulated intestinal function and serum 1,25-dihydroxyvitamin D levels. *Gastroenterology* 1983;84:314–323.
26. Kochersberger G, Westlund R, Lyles KW. The metabolic effects of calcium supplementation in the elderly. *J Am Geriatr Soc* 1991;39:192–196.
27. Reid IR, Ames RW, Evans MC, Gamble GD, Sharpe SJ. Effect of calcium supplementation on bone loss in postmenopausal women. *N Engl J Med* 1993;328:460–464.
28. Kochersberger G, Bales C, Lobaugh B, Lyles KW. Calcium supplementation lowers serum parathyroid hormone levels in elderly subjects. *J Gerontol* 1990;45:M159–M162.
29. Dawson-Hughes B, Jacques P, Shipp C. Dietary calcium intake and bone loss from the spine in healthy postmenopausal women. *Am J Clin Nutr* 1987;46:685–687.
30. Dawson-Hughes B. Effects of calcium intake on calcium retention and bone density in postmenopausal women. In: Burckhardt P, Heaney R, eds. *Nutritional aspects of osteoporosis.* Serono Symposia Publications, Vol 85. New York: Raven Press, 1991;331–345.
31. Dawson-Hughes B, Harris S, Dallal G. Serum predictors of a favorable bone response of postmenopausal women to supplementation with calcium (abstract). *Third International Symposium on Osteoporosis, Cophenhagen*, 1990;398.
32. Lau EMC, Woo J, Leung PC, Swaminathan R, Leung D. The effects of calcium supplementation and exercise on bone density in elderly Chinese women. *Osteoporosis Int* 1992;2:168–173.
33. Barragry JM, France MW, Corless D, et al. Intestinal cholecalciferol absorption in the elderly and in younger adults. *Clin Sci Mol Sci* 1978;55:213–220.
34. Lo CW, Paris PW, Clemens TL, Nolan J, Holick MF. Vitamin D absorption in healthy subjects and in patients with intestinal malabsorption syndromes. *Am J Clin Nutr* 1985;42:644–649.
35. Clemens TL, Zhou XY, Myles M, Endres D, Lindsay R. Serum vitamin D_2 and vitamin D_3 metabolite concentrations and absorption of vitamin D_2 in elderly subjects. *J Clin Endocrinol Metab* 1986;63:656–660.
36. MacLaughlin J, Holick MF. Aging decreases the capacity of human skin to produce vitamin D_3. *J Clin Invest* 1985;76:1536–1538.
37. Webb AR, Kline L, Holick MF. Influence of season and latitude on the cutaneous synthesis of vitamin D_3: exposure to winter sunlight in Boston and Edmonton will not promote vitamin D_3 synthesis in human skin. *J Clin Endocrinol Metab* 1988;67:373–378.
38. Webb AR, DeCosta BR, Holick MF. Sunlight regulates the cutaneous production of vitamin D_3 by causing its photodegradation. *J Clin Endocrinol Metab* 1989;68:882–887.
39. Everett MA, Yeargers E, Sayer RM, Olson RL. Penetration of the epidermis by ultraviolet rays. *Photochem Photobiol* 1966;5:533–542.
40. Lukert BP, Carey M, McCarty B, et al. Influence of nutritional factors on calcium regulating hormones and bone loss. *Calcif Tissue Int* 1987;40:119–125.
41. Lukert B, Higgins J, Stoskopf M. Menopausal bone loss is partially regulated by dietary intake of vitamin D. *Calcif Tissue Int* 1992;51:173–179.
42. Lips P, Hackeng WHL, Jongen MJM, van Ginkel FC, Netelenbos JC. Seasonal variation in serum concentrations of parathyroid hormone in elderly people. *J Clin Endocrinol Metab* 1983;57:204–206.
43. Krall EA, Sahyoun N, Tannenbaum S, Dallal GE, Dawson-Hughes B. Effect of vitamin D on seasonal variations in parathyroid hormone secretion in postmenopausal women. *N Engl J Med* 1989;321:1777–1783.
44. Peacock M, Selby PL, Francis RM, Brown WB, Hordon L, Vitamin D deficiency, insufficiency, sufficiency and intoxication: what do they mean? In: Norman AW, Schaefer K, Grigoleit H-G, von Herrath D, eds. *Vitamin D: chemical, biochemical, and clinical update: sixth workshop on vitamin D.* New York: Walter de Gruyter, 1985;569–570.
45. Chapuy M-C, Chapuy P, Meunier PJ. Calcium and vitamin D supplements: effects on calcium metabolism in elderly people. *Am J Clin Nutr* 1987;46:324–328.
46. Lips P, Wiersinga A, van Ginkel FC, et al. The effect of vitamin D supplementation on vitamin D status and parathyroid function in elderly subjects. *J Clin Endocrinol Metab* 1988;67:644–650.
47. Orwoll ES, Oviatt SK, McClung MR, Deftos LJ, Sexton G. The rate of bone mineral loss in normal men and the effects of calcium and cholecalciferol supplementation. *Ann Intern Med* 1990;112:29–34.
48. Aloia JF, Vaswani AN, Yeh JK, Ross P, Ellis K, Cohn SH. Determinants of bone mass in postmenopausal women. *Arch Intern Med* 1983;143:1700–1704.
49. Khaw K-T, Sneyd M-J, Compston J. Bone density parathyroid hormone and 25-hydroxyvitamin D concentrations in middle aged women. *Br Med J* 1992;305:273–277.
50. Villareal DT, Civitelli R, Chines A, Avioli LV. Subclinical vitamin D deficiency in postmenopausal women with low vertebral bone mass. *J Clin Endocrinol Metab* 1991;72:628–634.
51. Dawson-Hughes B, Dallal GE, Krall EA, Harris S, Sokoll LJ, Falconer G. Effect of vitamin D supplementation on wintertime and overall bone loss in healthy postmenopausal women. *Ann Intern Med* 1991;115:505–512.
52. Lips P, van Ginkel FC, Jongen MJM, Rubertus F, van der Vijgh WJF, Netelenbos JC. Determinants of vitamin D status in patients with hip fracture and in elderly control subjects. *Am J Clin Nutr* 1987;46:1005–1010.
53. Parisien M, Silverberg SJ, Shane E, et al. The histomorphometry of bone in primary hyperparathyroidism: preservation of cancellous bone structure. *J Clin Endocrinol Metab* 1990;70:930–938.
54. Matkovic V, Kostial K, Simonovic I, Buzina R, Brodarec A, Nordin BEC. Bone status and fracture rates in two regions of Yugoslavia. *Am J Clin Nutr* 1979;32:540–549.
55. Holbrook TL, Barrett-Connor E, Wingard DL. Dietary calcium and risk of hip fracture: 14-year prospective population study. *Lancet* 1988;2:1046–1049.
56. Pagnini-Hill A, Chao A, Ross RK, Henderson BE. Exercise and other factors in the prevention of hip fracture: the leisure world study. *Epidemiology* 1991;2:16–25.
57. Heikinheimo RJ, Inkovaara JA, Harju EJ, et al. Annual injection of vitamin D and fractures of aged bones. *Calcif Tissue Int* 1992;51:105–110.
58. Chapuy MC, Arlot ME, Duboeuf F, et al. Prevention of hip fractures in elderly women with vitamin D_3 and calcium. *N Engl J Med* 1992;327:1637–1642.

The Parathyroids, edited by J.P. Bilezikian, M.A. Levine, and R. Marcus. Raven Press, Ltd., New York © 1994.

CHAPTER 4

Anabolic and Catabolic Effects of Parathyroid Hormone on Bone and Interactions with Growth Factors

Ernesto Canalis, Janet M. Hock, and Lawrence G. Raisz

The concept that parathyroid hormone (PTH) has both anabolic and catabolic effects on the skeleton was first proposed about half a century ago (1). This paradox was confirmed in subsequent studies on the anabolic effect of PTH in experimental animals and in patients. The major mechanism for the catabolic action is a stimulation of bone resorption, and this is discussed elsewhere in this volume. Interest in the anabolic effect of PTH has been greatly heightened by clinical studies showing that intermittent administration of this hormone can increase trabecular bone mass. This work has received recent attention after in vitro and animal studies suggested that the anabolic effect of PTH is dependent on a complex interaction between PTH and the growth factors for bone.

Growth factors are polypeptides that modify the replication and differentiated function of cells (2). Frequently, growth factors are mitogens, and as such they stimulate cell replication. However, under certain experimental conditions, specific factors fail to display a mitogenic effect or may even inhibit mitogenesis. The effects of growth factors on cell replication and differentiation vary with diverse target cells and experimental conditions. For the most part, during an active phase of replication, cells do not express their differentiated function, and growth factors with marked mitogenic activity have a tendency to inhibit differentiation. Growth factors are present in the systemic circulation and are synthesized by a variety of cells in different tissues throughout the organism. As such, they can act as systemic or as local regulators of cell metabolism. When present in serum, growth factors may be found either free or bound to specific binding proteins, or they may be present in platelet granules from which they are released during platelet aggregation. At a local level, the target cell for a growth factor may be a cell of the same class or a cell different from that synthesizing the factor so that the factor can act as an autocrine or paracrine regulator of cell function. Cells synthesizing growth factors frequently synthesize specific growth factor binding proteins, which modify either the activity or the half-life of the factor.

Growth factors are regulated by hormones, such as PTH, which modify their synthesis or activate factors secreted in an inactive form (3,4). Hormones also alter the activity of growth factors by modulating their binding to cell surface receptors or to binding proteins. This is achieved by changes in binding affinity, number of receptors, or amounts of binding protein (5). It is important to note that, in addition to systemic hormones, growth factors may have positive feedback and enhance their own synthesis or may regulate the synthesis of their binding proteins or other locally produced growth factors (6). Although there are no specific growth factors secreted by skeletal or nonskeletal

E. Canalis: Departments of Medicine and Orthopedics, University of Connecticut School of Medicine, Farmington, Connecticut 06032; and Department of Research, St. Francis Hospital and Medical Center, Hartford, Connecticut 06105.

J. M. Hock: Skeletal Diseases Research, Eli Lilly and Company, Lilly Research Laboratories, Indianapolis, Indiana 46285.

L. G. Raisz: Department of Medicine, Division of Endocrinology, University of Connecticut Health Center, Farmington, Connecticut 06032.

tissues, hormones may target a growth factor to cells expressing specific hormonal receptors. For instance, PTH enhances the production of growth factors, specifically in bone tissue, because osteoblasts express PTH receptors, while other growth factor producing cells do not (3). This chapter provides a review of 1) data on the effects of PTH on bone formation and growth factor production in cell and organ culture models, 2) recent studies using animal models to elucidate further the anabolic effect of PTH, and 3) human studies related to the anabolic and catabolic effects of PTH, which emphasize some of the important unanswered questions.

EFFECTS OF PTH ON BONE REMODELING IN VITRO

The stimulatory effects of PTH on bone resorption and calcium metabolism are well established. However, its effects on bone formation are more complex, and PTH has been shown to have both stimulatory and inhibitory actions on this phase of bone remodeling. This dual anabolic and inhibitory effect of PTH was first reported in 1932 by Selye, who showed that, in vivo, continuous treatment with PTH resulted in an inhibition of bone formation, whereas intermittent administration of the hormone resulted in a stimulatory effect. Although the definition of intermittent PTH treatment has varied among investigators, it is known that continuous exposure of bone cells to PTH results in a dose-dependent inhibition of collagen synthesis (7,8). PTH at concentrations of 1 pM to 10 nM

for 24 hr decreases collagen synthesis in cultured fetal rat calvariae by ~50% (Fig. 1). PTH does not modify the synthesis of noncollagen protein, so the inhibitory effect on collagen synthesis is specific. This inhibition of collagen synthesis is observed as early as 6 hr after treatment, and it is sustained for periods of 96 hr (Fig. 2). The effect is dose and time dependent, and it is more pronounced after longer exposure to the hormone (7,8). The decrease in collagen synthesis occurs at least in part at the transcriptional level, since PTH was shown to decrease type I collagen promoter activity in calvarial cells from neonatal transgenic mice (9). The inhibitory effect of PTH of collagen synthesis appears to be due to a direct action on the osteoblast. It is likely to be mediated by cyclic adenosine monophosphate (cAMP), since dibutyryl cAMP and other cAMP inducers in bone cells, such as forskolin, mimic the inhibitory effects of PTH on collagen synthesis and type I collagen promoter activity. Furthermore, continuous treatment with parathyroid hormone-related protein (PTHrP), which acts by way of the PTH receptor to increase cAMP, also results in an inhibition of collagen synthesis in cultured calvariae (10).

In contrast, when cultures of intact calvariae are exposed to PTH at 0.1–10 nM for 24 hr and are transferred to control medium for the subsequent 24 or 48 hr, an increase in collagen and noncollagen protein synthesis is observed (Fig. 3). This stimulatory effect is noted only after bone cultures are transiently exposed to PTH and is detected in the nonperiosteal central calvarial bone, which is rich in osteoblasts (8). Intermittent PTH enhances type I collagen synthesis, indicating a direct action on the differentiated function

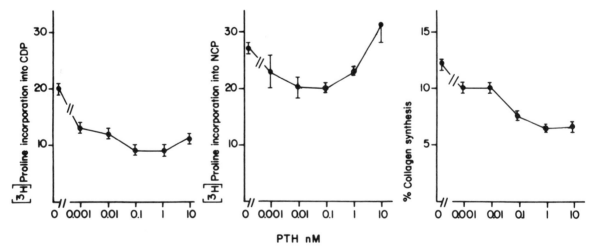

FIG. 1. Effect of continuous treatment with PTH on [³H]proline incorporation into collagenase digestible protein (collagen; CDP); and noncollagen protein (NCP), and on percentage of collagen synthesized in calvariae cultured for 24 hr in the continuous presence of PTH. (Reproduced from ref. 8 with permission.)

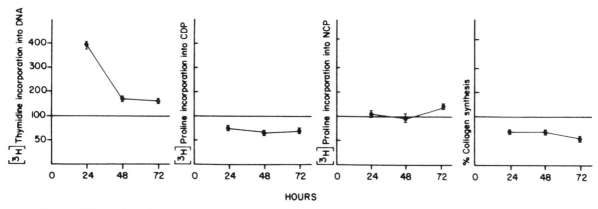

FIG. 2. Effect of continuous treatment with 1 nM PTH for 24–72 hr on [³H]thymidine incorporation into DNA, on [³H]proline incorporation into collagenase-digestible protein (collagen; CDP) and noncollagen protein (NCP), and on the percentage of collagen synthesized in calvariae. (Reproduced from ref. 8 with permission.)

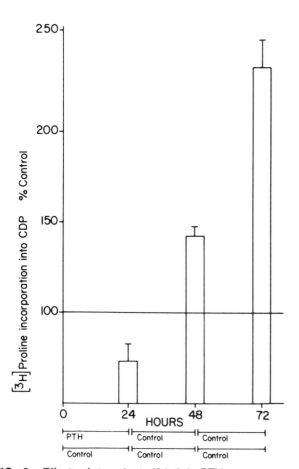

FIG. 3. Effect of transient (24 hr) PTH treatment on [³H]proline incorporation into collagenase digestible protein (collagen; CDP) in calvariae treated only for the first 24 hr of culture and transferred to control medium for the remainder of the incubation as indicated. Values are expressed as percentage of control. (Reproduced from ref. 8 with permission.)

of the osteoblast. Analogous to this effect, transient exposure of calvarial cultures to PTHrP results in an increase in collagen and noncollagen synthesis of a magnitude similar to that of PTH (10).

In addition to its regulatory actions on collagen synthesis, PTH stimulates DNA synthesis and cell replication in intact rat calvariae and in cells derived from human bone (Fig. 2) (8,11). The exact target cell for the mitogenic effect of PTH is not known. However, increments in collagen and noncollagen protein synthesis are independent of changes in cell number and are not modified by DNA synthesis inhibitors such as hydroxyurea. The physiological relevance of the increased cell replication induced by PTH should be determined. The regulation of collagen by PTH is complex not only because of its dual stimulatory and inhibitory effect on synthesis but also because PTH increases the degradation of collagen. In calvarial cultures, treatment with PTH for 48 hr enhances the degradation of newly synthesized collagen by about twofold after 48 hr, an effect that is likely due to a direct increase in collagenase production by the osteoblast (12,13). The mechanism of action of PTH on the production of collagenase by osteoblastic cells was examined in osteosarcoma cell lines and was shown to be cAMP dependent. The calcium ionophore ionomycin was ineffective, and phorbol esters, known to activate the protein kinase C pathway, had only marginal effects on collagenase production (13). This suggests that, for this purpose, the main signal transduction pathway used by PTH is cAMP.

SKELETAL GROWTH FACTORS

Although PTH undoubtedly has direct effects on bone cells, recent investigations have shown that some of its actions are mediated by locally produced growth factors. Studies performed in the late 1970s demonstrated that bone cells secrete growth factors, and some of these factors might mediate the coupling of bone resorption to bone formation observed after treatment with PTH (14). Over the past decade, a number of growth factors synthesized by bone cells have been characterized. We now know that bone cells synthesize insulin-like growth factors (IGF)-I and -II; transforming growth factor-β (TGFβ), -β₂, and β₃; platelet-derived growth factor AA; heparin-binding growth factors (HBGF)-1 and -2; and several bone morphogenetic proteins (BMP) or osteoinductive factors (15). Skeletal cells also synthesize and respond to cytokines known to have primary effects on immune and hematological cells. These cytokines include interleukins 1 and 6, tumor necrosis factor-α and selected colony-stimulating factors. A detailed description of the growth factors synthesized by skeletal cells is beyond the scope of this chapter and our discussion is limited to a selected group of factors.

Insulin-Like Growth Factors-I and -II

IGF-I and -II are polypeptides with a molecular mass (Mr) of 7,600. IGF-I and -II have 66% amino acid sequence homology and have similar biological activities. IGFs are present in the systemic circulation and are synthesized by skeletal and a variety of nonskeletal cells. The role of IGFs as systemic regulators of bone metabolism has not been demonstrated fully, and significant abnormalities in serum levels of IGF-I or -II have not been shown in patients with various metabolic bone disorders. It is believed that IGF-I and -II act as local regulators of musculoskeletal cell function. IGFs stimulate bone formation in vitro (16,17). They increase the replication of cells, primarily of preosteoblasts, and independently stimulate osteoblastic collagen synthesis and matrix apposition rates (Figs. 4, 5). IGF-I and -II have similar effects, although IGF-I is somewhat more potent than IGF-II. In addition to their effects of enhancing collagen synthesis, IGFs decrease collagen degradation. Because of their important effects on bone cell replication and differentiation, it is believed that these polypeptides are major regulators of bone formation and are important in the maintenance of bone mass.

Skeletal cells also secrete a variety of IGF binding proteins (IGFBPs). So far, six structurally related IGFBPs have been described, and it is known that five of them, IGFBP-2, -3, -4, -5, and -6, are synthesized by skeletal cells (18–23). The exact role of IGFBPs in bone cell metabolism is not entirely known. It is postulated that IGFBPs are important for the storage of IGF and to prolong its half-life. They also may be relevant in the regulation of IGF activity by competing with cell surface receptors for IGF binding. Studies testing continuous exposure of high doses of IGFBP-2 and -3 to bone cells have shown that they cause an inhibition of DNA and protein synthesis (24,25). However, much remains to be learned about the physiological role of IGFBPs in skeletal tissue and their temporal expression in relationship to IGF-I and -II. This knowledge is essential in that, under different experimental conditions, IGFBPs enhance or decrease the activity of IGF-I or -II (26,27).

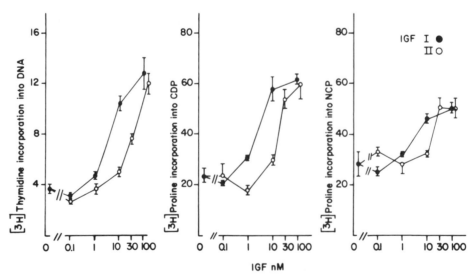

FIG. 4. Effect of IGF I (●) and IGF II (○) on [³H]thymidine incorporation into DNA and [³H]proline incorporation into collagenase-digestible protein (collagen; CDP) and noncollagen protein (NCP) in calvariae cultured for 24 hr. (Reproduced from ref. 17 with permission.)

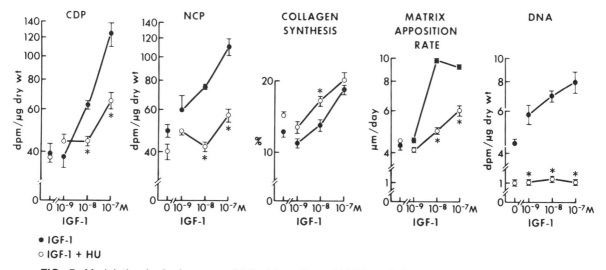

• IGF-1
○ IGF-1 + HU

FIG. 5. Modulation by hydroxyurea (HU) of the effect of IGF-I on [³H]proline incorporation into collagenase-digestible protein (collagen; CDP) and noncollagen protein (NCP), percentage collagen synthesis, matrix apposition rate, and [³H]thymidine incorporation in calvariae cultured for 24 hr. (Reproduced from ref. 16 with permission.)

Transforming Growth Factor-β and Related Polypeptides

TGFβ is a dimer polypeptide with an Mr of 25,000. In general TGFβ is secreted as a homodimer. Five TGFβ isoforms have been described and are termed TGFβ₁, -β₂, -β₃, -β₄, and -β₅ (28). Heterodimers of TGFβ also have been isolated from various tissues. Skeletal cells synthesize TGFβ₁, -β₂, and -β₃, and bovine bone has been shown to contain TGFβ₁,₂ and TGFβ₂,₃ heterodimers (29–31). The reason for the presence of various TGFβ isoforms in bone tissue is not clear, particularly in that the various forms tested have virtually the same effects on bone cell function, with modest differences of potency (32). For the most part, studies using cultures of normal osteoblasts and intact calvariae have demonstrated that TGFβ stimulates cell replication as well as collagen and noncollagen protein synthesis (33). TGFβ enhances biochemical parameters of bone formation as well as matrix apposition rates (34). TGFβ is secreted as a high-molecular-weight complex consisting of the polypeptide, a precursor, and a binding protein. TGFβ is present in the tissue matrix in an inactive form, and it is activated by various mechanisms, including lowering of the pH, which could occur in the bone environment during the process of bone resorption (3). Thus TGFβ may be important in the coupling of bone resorption to bone formation.

In addition to the five TGFβ isoforms described above, other related polypeptides share up to 30% amino acid sequence homology with TGFβ and possibly have similar biological activities. These polypeptides include inhibins, activin, Muellerian inhibiting substance, the gene products of *Drosophila decapentaplegic*, and six of the seven known bone morphogenetic proteins (BMPs) or osteoinductive substances (35). Initially, the primary function of BMPs was considered to be the induction of new bone formation occurring after the implantation of demineralized bone matrix in soft tissues. Recent studies have indicated that the BMPs not only induce growth and differentiation of cells but also stimulate bone cell replication and protein synthesis in a manner analogous to that shown for TGFβ (36,37).

Platelet-Derived Growth Factor

Platelet-derived growth factor is a dimer with an Mr of 30,000. PDGF is the product of two genes, PDGF A and B, which give rise to two distinct PDGF chains with 60% homology (38). PDGF exists as a homodimer or heterodimer of these two chains, which can combine to form PDGF AA, BB, and AB. PDGF is stored in platelet granules, and thus it can act as a systemic regulator of cell function. In humans, the circulating forms of PDGF are, for the most part, PDGF BB and AB (39), whereas normal human and rat bone cells express only the PDGF A gene. This is in contrast to osteosarcoma cells, which also express the PDGF B gene (40,41). The three PDGF isoforms stimulate cell replication in intact calvariae and in osteoblast cultures (42,43). PDGF BB is more potent than PDGF AA, and PDGF AB has an intermediate effect. As a consequence of its effects on cell replication, PDGF causes a small increase in bone protein synthesis. However, PDGF does not seem to stimulate the differentiated function of the osteoblast, and it is, to some extent, inhibitory. At present, the production of specific PDGF binding proteins by bone cells is uncertain, and it is believed that skeletal PDGF is secreted in a biologically active form.

Heparin-Binding Growth Factors-1 and -2

HBGFs are a group of polypeptides with mitogenic activity. HBGF-1, or acidic fibroblast growth factor, and HBGF-2, or basic fibroblast growth factor, are secreted by bovine osteoblastic cells (44,45). HBGFs have a M_r of ~17,000, and HBGF-1 and -2 have ~55% amino acid sequence homology. HBGFs are not secreted proteins and are likely to be bound to the bone matrix, where they probably act as local regulators of skeletal cell function. HBGFs are bone cell mitogens and do not appear to have potent direct stimulatory effects on osteoblastic differentiated function (46,47). Currently, it is unknown if bone cells also secrete specific binding proteins for these factors, and the presence of HBGFs in the circulation has been debated.

INTERACTIONS OF PTH AND SKELETAL GROWTH FACTORS IN VITRO

PTH stimulates IGF-I synthesis by osteoblastic cells (2). This effect is observed at PTH concentrations of 0.1–10 nM and possibly involves the transcriptional regulation of IGF-I synthesis. PTH increases both IGF-I mRNA and polypeptide levels about threefold (Figs. 6,7). The effect of PTH appears to be mediated, at least in part, by an increase in cAMP, since other agents known to enhance cAMP production by osteoblastic cells, such as prostaglandin E_2 (PGE_2) and forskolin, also increase skeletal IGF-I synthesis (48,49) (Fig. 8). In contrast, the calcium ionophore ionomycin and phorbol esters do not alter IGF-I synthesis by osteoblastic cells. The effect of PTH on IGF-I production is mimicked by PTHrP in bone cells (50).

The fact that PTH and PGE_2 both increase IGF-I production and that PTH can increase PGE_2 production in bone could suggest a possible mechanism for the anabolic effect of PTH. However, in cell culture, indomethacin, which inhibits PGE_2 synthesis, has little effect on the ability of PTH to increase IGF-I production. Nevertheless, it is possible that under some circumstances, for example, in estrogen deficiency, when PGE_2 production is enhanced, this amplification of the anabolic effect of PTH could play a relevant clinical role.

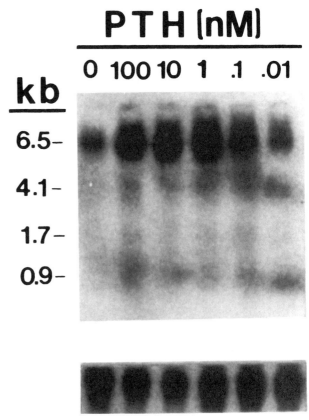

FIG. 6. Northern blot analysis of prepro-IGF-I (**upper panel**) and β-actin (**lower panel**) transcripts in osteoblast-enriched cultures from rat calvariae treated with PTH for 6 hr. RNA standards were used to determine the length (in kilobases) of prepro-IGF-I transcripts shown on the left. (Reproduced from ref. 3 with permission.)

Although PTH stimulates IGF-I synthesis and IGF-I increases bone collagen synthesis, continuous exposure of bone cells to PTH results in a decrease in bone collagen production (8). This inhibitory effect seems to be the result of PTH overriding the stimulatory actions of IGF-I, and, when calvarial explants are concomitantly exposed to PTH and IGF-I, only the inhibitory effect of PTH on collagen synthesis is observed. In contrast, transient exposure to PTH, which results in an induction of skeletal IGF-I, causes a stimulation of collagen synthesis (8). The stimulatory effect of PTH on collagen synthesis is blocked by IGF-I neutralizing antibodies, suggesting that IGF-I is at least in part responsible for the increase in bone collagen.

In addition to changes in IGF-I synthesis, PTH also modifies the synthesis of IGFBPs. However it does not alter IGF-II synthesis or the binding of IGFs to specific cell surface receptors (50). The synthesis of IGFBP-3, -4, and -5 in bone cells is cAMP dependent, and transcripts for IGFBP-4 have been shown to be elevated by PTH in human bone cells (21). It is apparent that the induction of cAMP in bone cells results in

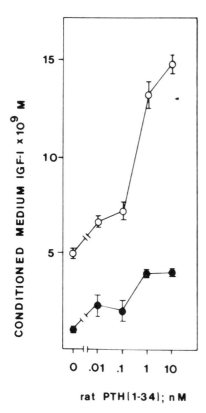

FIG. 7. Effect of PTH on IGF-I levels in medium of osteoblast-enriched cultures from rat calvariae treated for 6 hr (●) or 24 hr (○) with rat PTH (1–34) at the concentrations shown. (Reproduced from ref. 3 with permission.)

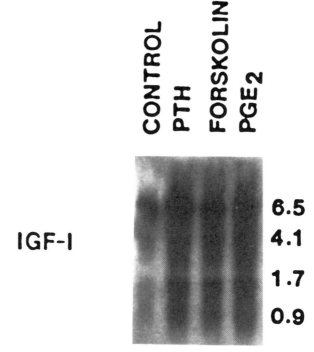

FIG. 8. Comparison of the effect of PTH (10 nM) forskolin (1 μM) and prostaglandin E_2 (PGE$_2$; 1 μM) on prepro-IGF-I transcript levels in osteoblast-enriched cultures from rat calvariae treated for 6 hr. RNA standards are used to determine the length (in kilobases) of prepro-IGF-I transcripts shown on the right. (Reproduced from ref. 49 with permission.)

an increased production not only of IGF-I but also of selected IGFBPs (19). Although the role of the binding proteins is not entirely known, it is possible that they are important in mechanisms regulating the exposure of bone cells to endogenous IGF-I.

PTH and other agents that stimulate bone resorption increase the secretion of TGFβ activity in bone cultures during this process (4). It has been suggested that this phenomenon is due to the activation of TGFβ in the osteoclastic microenvironment, possibly the result of lowering the pH. PTH does not increase TGFβ mRNA levels in osteoblastic cells, and it is likely to activate previously synthesized TGFβ. TGFβ may play an important role in the local control of bone resorption, since it has been shown to inhibit this process as a result of a decrease in the formation of osteoclast-like cells (51,52). In addition to its effects on TGFβ activation, PTH regulates the binding and activity of TGFβ in osteoblast cultures (53). PTH increases the number of apparent TGFβ receptors, but, for reasons not entirely understood, it opposes the activity of TGFβ on bone DNA and collagen synthesis.

Preliminary investigations have revealed that PTH does not modify the concentrations of PDGF AA in bone cell cultures or the binding of PDGF to its bone cell receptors, suggesting that PDGF is not an important mediator of PTH function in bone. At present no information is available regarding the effects of PTH on the synthesis or binding of HBGF or the activity of various BMPs.

ANABOLIC RESPONSE OF PTH IN VIVO IN ANIMAL MODELS

The in vitro actions of PTH to stimulate osteoclastic resorption and to inhibit osteoblastic formation represent the action of high doses of PTH. In vivo, as in vitro, PTH can produce an anabolic effect. The finding that low doses of crude preparations of parathyroid extract (PTE) increased trabecular bone density was first reported in the 1930s by Selye, Pugsley, and Burrows (1,54,55) but was largely ignored. When the synthetic fragment hPTH 1–34 became available in the early 1970s, there was renewed interest in the anabolic effect of PTH. Synthetic hPTH 1–34 increased bone in rats (56–74), retired greyhounds (75–80), and osteoporotic humans (77,81–84). A recent study showed no difference in the anabolic bone response to full-length PTH or the 1–34 human fragment (85).

The anabolic effect of PTH in vivo may be best defined as a net increase in bone mass or bone mineral. Measures of only the rate of bone formation may be misleading in that PTH, under certain experimental conditions and in hyperparathyroidism, may increase the rate of formation as a consequence of the activation of an increased number of resorption sites. This results in an increased rate of bone turnover but with no net gain in bone mass.

PHENOMENOLOGY OF THE ANABOLIC RESPONSE TO PTH IN BONE IN VIVO

Universal Effect of PTH in Healthy and Osteopenic Animal Models

The increase in bone mass induced by PTH has been demonstrated in a wide variety of animal models and confirmed in humans (81,82,86). Extensive work has been done on male and female rats (56–74,87–92) and retired racing greyhounds with assumed disuse osteopenia (75–79). These studies demonstrated that the anabolic effect of PTH does not depend on whether the animals are young; it can be induced in adult and aged rats with closed epiphyses (67,70,87,88,93). The anabolic response to PTH in bone may be induced rapidly and in a shorter time frame than the remodeling cycle, even in adult and aged animals (67,69,70,89–91). Continued treatment with PTH for up to 15 weeks leads to a steady accumulation of bone in rats (Mitlak and Neer, personal communication) and humans (81,82,86). The anabolic effect of PTH is independent of gender and sexual maturity; it occurs in middle-aged and osteoporotic men and women (81–84,94) and in intact and castrated osteopenic male and female rats (60,69,70,87–89,91). PTH also increases bone mass in animals with osteopenia induced by denervation (92,95), immobilization (96), or discontinuation of exercise (75–77).

Dose-response experiments have shown that, in trabecular bone, a statistically significant increase in bone mass of 20–30% could be detected in young male rats given 8 μg or 16 μg hPTH 1–34/100 g by once daily subcutaneous injection for 12 days (Fig. 9). A similar increase in bone mineral was present in proximal tibia (Fig. 10) and in the trabecular bone volume of lumbar vertebrae (Fig. 11). The increase in distal femur mass amounted to an increase of 3–10 mg of both calcium and dry weight, due to a two- to threefold increase in trabecular bone forming surfaces (Fig. 11) and osteoblast number, with no appreciable stimulation of resorption in trabecular bone (59,61,65,70,87,88). Matrix apposition rate (MAR) was comparable to that in controls (61,65). In thyroparathyroidectomized (TPTX) rats and aged rats, there is a small but signifi-

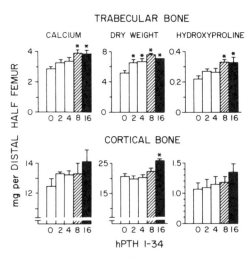

FIG. 9. Anabolic effects of PTH on calcium content and dry weight of cortical and trabecular bone of distal femurs of young male rats treated with vehicle or hPTH 1–34 once daily for 12 days. (Reproduced from ref. 56 with permission.)

cant stimulation of MAR by PTH (65,67,71–73). Thus, the striking effect of PTH on bone surfaces appears to be due to a stimulation of osteoblast differentiation rather than to a stimulation of osteoblast function in intact rats.

Anabolic Effect of PTH on Trabecular and Cortical Bone

In earlier studies, the fact that cortical bone density could be decreased by PTH at the same time that trabecular bone volume was increased led to the hypothesis that the anabolic effect of PTH on trabecular bone might be secondary to loss of cortical bone (81,97). Cortical bone mass is decreased while trabecular mass is maintained or increased in mild primary hyperparathyroidism (86,98,99).

We developed a method to separate mechanically trabecular and cortical bone in the distal one-half of the femur to determine if PTH had differential effects on cortical and trabecular bone (56). For young rats, we found that cortical bone mass is consistently and significantly increased if PTH treatment is continued for >24 days (59). In aged rats with age-related trabecular bone loss, the increase in cortical bone on metaphyseal endosteal surfaces necessarily predominates (67). Histomorphometry has shown that the anabolic effect of PTH on cortical bone was to stimulate endosteal and periosteal bone formation. This resulted in an expansion of the cross-sectional area of bone and marrow, with some resorption within the cortical bone matrix as the cortical bone width increased (87). However, this combined effect on cortical periosteal and endosteal bone resulted in increased mechanical strength (85).

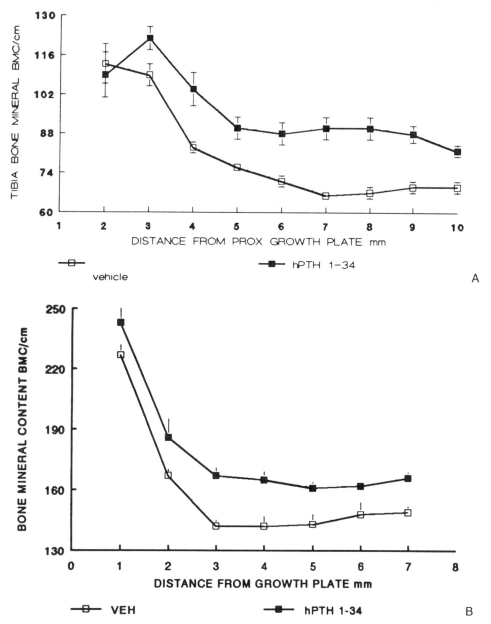

FIG. 10. Single photon absorptiometry scans of the bone mineral content of proximal tibia of rats. **A:** Young 4-week-old male rats given PTH for 12 days. **B:** Aged 24-month-old female rats given PTH for 32 days.

Differential effects on cortical and trabecular bone were observed when TPTX rats were infused continuously with PTH and were given intermittent PTH concurrently by once daily injections (64). Metaphyseal trabecular bone in the proximal tibia was increased, while bone resorption and enhanced vascularization were observed on the endosteal surface of the diaphysis (64).

The rate of administration of PTH appears to be critical in determining its effect on bone. The anabolic effect of PTH requires intermittent administration (65,72,78). Increasing the number of injections of PTH from once to twice per day did not augment its anabolic effect on total body calcium in female rats (100). PTH, given by continuous infusion at a daily dose comparable to doses that were anabolic when given by once daily injection, induced hypercalcemia and death in rats and dogs (65,78,79). At sublethal doses, continuous infusion of PTH for 12 days did not increase trabecular bone mass in intact rats (65). In TPTX rats, intermittent PTH increased trabecular bone volume by stimulating formation, while continuous PTH stimulated both formation and resorption, with no net change in bone volume (64,65,71–73). These differen-

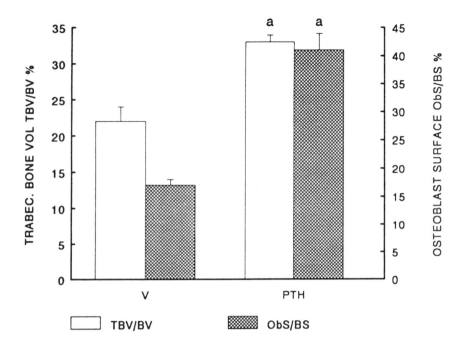

FIG. 11. Histomorphometry of lumbar vertebrae, showing the percentage trabecular volume and percentage osteoblastic surface of trabecular bone of young male rats treated with PTH for 12 days.

tial responses may be regulated by effects on the PTH receptor. Following a single PTH pulse, PTH cell surface receptors in the kidney rapidly reappeared after being down-regulated. In contrast, down-regulation of PTH receptors was prolonged and was only slowly reversed when PTH was given by infusion (101,102).

Interaction With Endogenous PTH

It has been hypothesized that changes in endogenous PTH secretion are important to the anabolic action of exogenous PTH. Exogenous PTH in humans causes a sharp drop in endogenous PTH, which rebounds above normal values during recovery, before stabilization (94,103–105). It was speculated that this change in endogenous PTH was required for the anabolic effect of PTH. However, variations in endogenous PTH do not appear to be critical for the anabolic effect of PTH on bone in experimental models. For example, an anabolic effect can be induced by exogenous PTH in the absence of endogenous PTH in TPTX rats (64,71–73). Moreover, a combination of continuous infusion of low doses of PTH with intermittent PTH increased bone mass in TPTX rats to a greater extent than intermittent PTH alone (64). This suggests that steady levels of endogenous PTH, while not required for the anabolic effect of exogenous PTH, may enhance the bone response.

Reversal of the Anabolic Effect Upon Withdrawal of PTH

The anabolic effect of PTH on bone mass was lost 24–48 hr after the last PTH injection in young rats (59).

This reversal can be attributed to inactivation of forming surfaces. There are marked decreases in percentage calcein-labeled bone surface (DLS/BS) and percent osteoblast surface (ObS/BS) but little change in the number of osteoclasts and osteoclast surface (59). Loss of bone forming surface can be detected within 48 hr in young rats after PTH treatment has been stopped. On the other hand, whole-body calcium measurements by neutron activation showed that PTH-treated, mature, lactating female rats retained calcium after treatment was discontinued for 6 months (100).

POTENTIAL MEDIATORS OF THE ANABOLIC EFFECT OF PTH ON BONE IN VIVO

Interaction With Calcium

The target organs for PTH are bone, kidney, and, by an interaction with 1,25-dihydroxyvitamin D [1,25(OH)₂D₃], intestines. Hence it is possible that the anabolic effect of PTH on bone is indirect, associated with changes in another target organ, which then modify skeletal homeostasis. Although there is a transient increase in serum calcium within 1 hr of PTH injection (62,76,78), variations in serum calcium do not seem to be critical for the anabolic effect of PTH on bone. PTH-related protein 1–34 (PTHrP 1–34) induced an anabolic response in bone in the presence of sustained increased serum calcium in intact rats (62). PTH increased bone in the presence of hypocalcemia, induced either in ovariectomized rats fed a low-calcium diet (68–70,87,88) or in TPTX rats (64). In general, serum calcium, phosphate, alkaline phosphatase, urea nitrogen, and creatinine and kidney calcium content in intact young rats treated with hPTH 1–34 remain within physiologic range (60–67).

Interaction With 1,25-Dihydroxyvitamin D

The interdependence of PTH and $1,25(OH)_2D_3$ suggested the hypothesis that the anabolic effect of PTH might be mediated by its stimulation of $1,25(OH)_2D_3$ synthesis (83,84). However, we have found that $1,25(OH)_2D_3$ neither enhanced nor mimicked the anabolic effect of PTH (58,77). At doses of $1,25(OH)_2D_3$ that do not increase serum calcium, bone mass was unchanged; at doses that induced hypercalcemia, matrix formation was increased, but mineralization was impaired (58,77).

Serum $1,25(OH)_2D_3$ (106–108) vitamin D receptors (109), intestinal calcium binding protein (106), and $1,25(OH)_2D_3$-dependent intestinal calcium absorption (106–110) are all known to decline with age. In senile male rats with reduced serum $1,25(OH)_2D_3$, PTH increased serum $1,25(OH)_2D_3$ to levels comparable to those induced in young male rats (111). Aged female rats (67) and osteopenic greyhounds (75), given intermittent PTH, showed both increased serum $1,25(OH)_2D_3$ and increased calcium absorption (67). Despite these consistent stimulatory effects, no clear correlation has been found between the magnitude of the increases in serum $1,25(OH)_2D_3$ and calcium absorption and the presence of an anabolic response in bone in aged rats (67). It remains to be determined if $1,25(OH)_2D_3$ has a permissive role in the anabolic effect of PTH.

Coupling of Formation to Initiation of Resorption

A popular hypothesis has been that the initial stimulation of resorption by PTH, which has been demonstrated repeatedly in vitro, results in the release of a coupling factor(s) that stimulates bone formation (14,112). The early histologic studies of the bone effects of intermittent parathyroid extract (PTE) in young rats (1,54,55) reported a resorptive phase in the first few days that was followed later by a significant gain in bone density. In vitro studies of avian bones treated by transient exposure to PTH (14,112) showed increases in resorption and the rate of hydroxyproline incorporation. However, in vivo, blocking resorption with calcitonin or bisphosphonates did not modify the anabolic effect of PTH (61,65). Even in the presence of a loss of body weight and inhibition of resorption associated with 12 days of calcitonin treatment, PTH continued to increase bone mass (61). When PTH was given by continuous infusion and bone resorption was blocked with a bisphosphonate, the inhibition of bone

formation associated with bisphosphonate was reversed by PTH to control levels, suggesting that the formation and resorption effects of PTH were not coupled (65).

Interactions With Prostaglandins

PTH increases prostaglandin synthesis in bone organ cultures (113,114), and we hypothesized that the anabolic effect of PTH might be mediated by prostaglandins. In cultured fetal rat calvaria, prostaglandins have been shown to have dose-dependent, biphasic effects on bone formation (113,115). In vivo, indomethacin given in a range of doses, either by twice daily injection or by continuous infusion, did not modify the increase in bone mass induced by PTH in young intact rats (116). While it is possible that indomethacin, despite the range of doses tested, did not totally block local prostaglandin synthesis in bone, these experiments suggest that prostaglandins do not mediate the anabolic action of PTH in vivo.

Interactions With Growth Hormone

Early studies in which calvariae from hypophysectomized (HX) rats were treated with high doses of PTE in vivo and then cultured showed less hydroxyproline incorporation than calvariae from intact rats treated with PTE (116). This suggested the hypothesis that a pituitary hormone, most likely growth hormone (GH), might be required for the anabolic effect of PTH on bone (65). We found that HX rats, supplemented with corticosterone and thyroxine and treated with intermittent PTH, showed a 50–70% inhibition of the PTH anabolic effect. GH not only reversed this inhibition but also enhanced the anabolic effect of PTH on bone (65). To determine if this was due to GH stimulation of systemic growth, young intact rats were given PTH and either pair-fed to the dietary intake of age- and weight-matched HX rats or fed a 50% calorie-restricted diet to prevent the increase in body weight associated with growth. In that the increase in bone mass of distal femurs of the restricted rats was equivalent to that of age-matched, treated, intact rats fed ad libitum (65), and in that the anabolic effect of PTH has been induced in adult (86,87) and aged ovariectomized female rats (117) or senile male rats (111), it is unlikely that the requirement for GH is based on stimulation of longitudinal bone growth.

GH secretion declines with age (118–120). If GH is required for the anabolic action of PTH, aged animals should show a loss of responsiveness to PTH in bones. In a study of aged, intact females rats, neither PTH nor GH alone increased bone mass, but the combination of PTH and GH increased femoral trabecular bone mass and vertebral trabecular bone volume (67).

Interactions With Skeletal Growth Factors

Because GH does not stimulate bone matrix formation in bone organ culture (121), it may be that GH-dependent factors such as IGF-I mediate the anabolic effect of PTH. In vitro, a single pulse of PTH increased mRNA and polypeptide synthesis of IGF-I in fetal bone organ culture (3,8,122). As with PTH, the anabolic effect of IGF-I in vivo appears to be dependent on the route of administration. When given by twice daily injections, IGF-I augmented the effect of PTH on the femur and tibia of HX rats, but the magnitude of its anabolic effect was significantly less than that of GH given alone or in combination with PTH (J. Hock, unpublished data). When given by continuous infusion, IGF-I reduced cortical bone mass in distal femurs of young HX rats (J. Hock, unpublished data) and stimulated tunneling resorption of the diaphyseal cortex in aged female rats (117). Most recently, IGF-I was shown to stimulate osteoclastic bone resorption in vitro by regulating osteoclast differentiation (123). In that PTH has been shown to regulate not only IGF-I but also its binding proteins in vitro (3,23), it may be that, in vivo, intermittent PTH transiently modifies the IGFBPs to activate IGF-I and initiate its anabolic action in bone.

Circulating IGF-I also could play a role in regulating the anabolic effects of PTH. Preliminary data, obtained from young HX rats and aged female rats, showed that, while PTH did not alter serum IGF-I levels, GH increased IGF-I, and PTH given with GH partially inhibited this stimulatory effect of GH on serum IGF-I (63). Because long-term energy restriction of rats results in a 50% decrease in circulating IGF-I (124), we tested the response to PTH and GH in aged rats from the same colony that had been energy restricted in their dietary intake by 60% since weaning. These rats showed an attenuated response in their femur bone mass and tibia bone mineral when treated with PTH alone or in combination with GH (J. Hock, unpublished data).

It remains to be determined if skeletally derived IGF-I or its binding proteins play a critical role in mediating the anabolic effect of PTH. Although bone organ culture studies showed that corticosterone inhibited IGF-I induced by pulsed PTH in vitro, in vivo corticosterone, given in the morning or in the evening to HX rats treated with PTH alone or in combination with GH, did not modify the anabolic effect of PTH and GH (66). These results suggest that other growth factors, such as TGFβ, which is known to alter PTH receptors in vitro (4,29,33,125), may also play a contributing role.

ANABOLIC AND CATABOLIC EFFECTS OF PTH IN HUMANS

The earliest cases of primary hyperparathyroidism showed severe bone disease (126). In 1925, Mandel carried out the first successful parathyroidectomy on a streetcar conductor with multiple fractures, who promptly recovered. Captain Martel, a famous American case, had multiple appendicular and vertebral crush fractures but did not recover after surgery because he also had nephrocalcinosis and renal failure. However, Albright and Reifenstein (127) pointed out in their classic monograph that "it is a mistake to think of bone disease as an essential part of hyperparathyroidism." They also described a patient in whom osteosclerosis developed in hyperparathyroidism apparently as a consequence of giving a high-calcium diet. Jowsey measured formation and resorption surfaces by microradiography and concluded that hyperparathyroidism led to increases in both forming and resorbing surfaces (128). The first effort to quantitate bone formation in patients with hyperparathyroidism by dynamic histomorphometry using tetracycline labeling showed a decrease in the mineral apposition rate but a remarkably wide range in the extent of bone forming surface, with some samples showing bone formation rates at the tissue level that were ten times normal (129). Subsequent studies of histomorphometry in hyperparathyroidism have confirmed this wide variation (130,131). Bone resorption, as evidenced by the extent of resorbing surface as well as the number of osteoclasts, is almost invariably increased, and this is usually associated with a coupled increase in bone forming surfaces. The net effect on bone mass appears to vary with skeletal site and with severity of the disease. A decrease in mean wall thickness has been reported, consistent with a decrease in osteoblast renewal or in the function of individual osteoblasts (132), but trabecular bone volume is maintained or even increased in mild to moderate cases (86,97,98), although it may be decreased in severe hyperparathyroidism (132). In contrast, cortical bone volume is generally decreased. These changes are discussed in detail elsewhere in this volume. There is a marked decrease in bone turnover following successful parathyroid surgery (99), but treatment with estrogen, which presumably inhibits the resorptive response to PTH, produces little change in bone formation (133).

Results of studies on the role of PTH in osteoporosis are conflicting. Kotowicz et al. (134) reported that higher PTH values were associated with lower trabecular bone volume in patients with vertebral crush fractures, while Silverberg et al. (135) found that vertebral crush fracture patients had a diminished PTH response to phosphate loading compared to age-matched controls. Increased PTH levels have been associated with senile osteoporosis and hip fractures, presumably secondary to calcium deficiency and decreased renal function, which leads to decreased 1,25-dihydroxyvitamin D synthesis (136). Thus, in elderly women with fractures and hyperparathyroidism, low creatinine clearance and serum 1,25-dihydroxyvitamin D levels have been reported, and the skeletal changes may not be due to effects of PTH (137).

Many studies have shown decreased bone mineral density at various skeletal sites in primary hyperparathyroidism and an effect of surgical cure on the recovery of bone mineral density. However, these studies did not yield consistent findings. In mild to moderate primary hyperparathyroidism, radial bone mineral density is decreased more than lumbar bone density, and this is consistent with the findings of decreased cortical and maintained or increased trabecular bone volume on biopsies (86,99,138). On the other hand, the trabecular deficit in the distal radius appears to be greater than the cortical deficit in the midradius in patients with parathyroid adenomas (139). The decrease in bone mass appears to be proportional to the severity of hyperparathyroidism (140).

There are two observations that might be explained by the existence of an anabolic effect of PTH in mild primary hyperparathyroidism. The first is that decreases in bone mineral density are not completely reversed after parathyroidectomy, although there was an early transient increase in bone mass in some studies (141–146). The second is that patients with low bone mass and mild primary hyperparathyroidism followed over time do not show biochemical progression or accelerated bone loss (147). This could be explained if both the initial loss phase and the recovery phase were due to changes in bone resorption and if the anabolic effect of PTH was sufficient to maintain bone mass through stimulating bone formation during a steady state of increased PTH production. Thus the initial loss would be due to an increased number of resorption cavities, and, if these were being filled in at an accelerated overall formation rate, no further bone loss would occur.

If trabecular bone is maintained and cortical bone is decreased in hyperparathyroidism, then one might expect a relatively low rate of vertebral in Colles' fractures and an increase in fractures of the femoral neck and other appendicular cortical sites. However, this would require that trabecular bone mass be maintained in the distal radius as it appears to be in the iliac crest and vertebrae, as was noted above (139), and there are data contradicting this possibility. Unfortunately, clinical data on these points are quite limited. Increased risk for Colles' fracture and a possible increased risk of vertebral fractures have been reported (148–150). However, in other studies the incidence of peripheral fractures was relatively high, but that for vertebral fractures was actually lower than predicted (151–153).

Since intermittent PTH administration is more effective than continuous administration in increasing bone mass in animal models, studies of intermittent administration of exogenous PTH or intermittent stimulation of endogenous PTH secretion would provide the most important validation of the hypothesis that PTH is anabolic in humans. Here, again, the data are not consistent. The most striking study was that reported in 1986 by Slovik et al. (84). These authors showed a substantial increase in vertebral trabecular bone mass in a small group of osteoporotic men as measured by computerized tomography during 1 year of treatment with daily injections of hPTH 1–34 and low doses of oral calcitriol. Studies using cyclic therapy for osteoporosis with neutral phosphate suggest that an increase in bone density may be in part dependent on the ability of phosphate to stimulate PTH secretion (154). Initial human studies using PTH alone regularly demonstrated an increase in markers of bone formation and in osteoblastic surfaces, as were previously described in primary hyperparathyroidism, but did not always show an increase in bone mass (77,81,83). Many studies have been difficult to interpret because multiple agents were used in treatment. For example, Reeve et al. combined intermittent PTH therapy with hormone replacement therapy to provide an antiresorptive agent and showed substantial increases in cancellous bone volume in osteoporotic patients (82). Hesch et al. (105,155,156) carried out similar studies using pulsatile HPTH 1–38 together with either calcitonin or bisphosphonate. The patients treated with calcitonin appeared to show a better response than those treated with the bisphosphonate.

Clearly, more extensive controlled trials of intermittent PTH therapy are needed to determine whether this approach might be effective in the treatment of osteoporosis. However, the possibility that cortical bone will be lost during PTH treatment makes it difficult to justify long-term, large-scale studies unless an additional agent that inhibits bone resorption is added to the regimen. There remains the concern that an increase in trabecular bone mass will not be associated with an increase in bone strength, because the new bone formed may not be in continuity with existing trabeculae. This possibility has already been suggested for sodium fluoride, which has effects on trabecular bone similar to those of PTH (157). PTH does resemble fluoride in being a bone cell mitogen (158). However, recent comparisons of the trabecular architecture in patients with hyperparathyroidism and osteoporosis suggest that cancellous bone architecture is preserved in hyperparathyroid patients (159,160).

UNANSWERED QUESTIONS AND NEW APPROACHES

While there is ample evidence that PTH can stimulate bone formation under certain circumstances, we know remarkably little about the conditions that favor this anabolic response. The fact that trabecular bone mass can be increased both in primary hyperparathyroidism and in patients with osteoporosis given intermittent PTH makes it critical to resolve some of the unanswered questions. Probably the most important of these is the reason for the difference in the response of cortical and trabecular bone and perhaps also the difference in the response of trabecular bone in the spine and ilium compared with the distal radius. If we accept the hypothesis that the anabolic effect of PTH is mediated by local growth factors and that the direct effect of PTH is to inhibit osteoblastic collagen synthesis at high concentrations, then variations in the production of or response to these growth factors could be responsible for the local differences. It has been reported that PTH stimulates the proliferation of cells derived from human trabecular bone, and a comparison of cells derived from different skeletal sites might help resolve these questions. Current methods of molecular and cellular biology, such as in situ hybridization and immunocytochemical identification of local regulatory factors, might be successful if these differences are due to differences in growth factor production. However, it will first be necessary to identify precisely which growth factors are involved. The data summarized in this chapter point to IGF-I as a potential mediator, but the mitogenic effect of PTH may not be mediated by this growth factor. Activation of TGFβ during resorption could be important in the increased bone turnover seen in hyperparathyroidism. TGFβ is a potent mitogen and can inhibit resorption, so it is possible to ascribe a net anabolic effect to this mediator. On the other hand, there are few data concerning the effects of PTH on growth factors other than IGF-I and TGFβ. This information will be important not only because it will help define the mechanism of the anabolic effect but also because it may provide an alternative approach to therapy that might circumvent some of the undesirable effects of intermittent PTH administration.

ACKNOWLEDGMENTS

Portions of this work were supported by National Institutes of Health grants AR 21707, DK 42424, DK 45227, AR 18063, and AR 38933. The authors thank Miss Beverly Faulds for valuable secretarial assistance.

REFERENCES

1. Selye H. On the stimulation of new bone formation with parathyroid extract and irradiated ergosterol. *Endocrinology* 1932;16:547–588.
2. Canalis E, McCarthy TL, Centrella M. The role of growth factors in skeletal remodeling. *Endocrinol Metab Clin North Am* 1989;18:903–918.
3. McCarthy TL, Centrella M, Canalis E. Parathyroid hormone enhances the transcript and polypeptide levels of insulin-like growth factor I in osteoblast-enriched cultures from fetal rat bone. *Endocrinology* 1989;124:1247–1253.
4. Pfeilschifter J, Mundy GR. Modulation of type B transforming growth factor activity in bone cultures by osteotropic hormones. *Proc Natl Acad Sci USA* 1987;84:2024–2028.
5. Centrella M, McCarthy TL, Kusmik WF, Canalis E. Isoform-specific regulation of platelet-derived growth factor activity and binding in osteoblast-enriched cultures from fetal rat bone. *J Clin Invest* 1992;89:1076–1084.
6. Canalis E, Varghese S, McCarthy TL, Centrella M. Role of platelet derived growth factor in bone cell function. *Growth Regul* 1992;2:151–155.
7. Dietrich JW, Canalis EM, Maina DM, Raisz LG. Hormonal control of bone collagen synthesis in vitro: effects of parathyroid hormone and calcitonin. *Endocrinology* 1976;98:943–949.
8. Canalis E, Centrella M, Burch W, McCarthy TL. Insulin-like growth factor I mediates selective anabolic effects of parathyroid hormone in bone cultures. *J Clin Invest* 1989;83:60–65.
9. Kream BE, LaFrancis D, Petersen DN, et al. Parathyroid hormone represses α1(1) collagen promoter activity in calvariae from neonatal transgenic mice. *J Bone Mineral Res* 1991;6(Suppl 1):S135.
10. Canalis E, McCarthy TL, Centrella M. Differential effects of continuous and transient treatment with parathyroid hormone related peptide (PTHrP) on bone collagen synthesis. *Endocrinology* 1990;126:1806–1812.
11. MacDonald BR, Gallagher JA, Russell RGG. Parathyroid hormone stimulates the proliferation of cells derived from human bone. *Endocrinology* 1986;118:2445–2449.
12. Rydziel S, Canalis E. Analysis of hydroxyproline by high performance liquid chromatography and its application to collagen turnover studies in bone cultures. *Calcif Tissue Int* 1989;44:421–424.
13. Civitelli R, Hruska KA, Jeffrey JJ, Kahn AJ, Avioli LV, Partridge NC. Second messenger signaling in the regulation of collagenase production by osteogenic sarcoma cells. *Endocrinology* 1989;124:2928–2934.
14. Howard GA, Bottemiller BL, Turner RT, Rader JI, Baylink DJ. Parathyroid hormone stimulates bone formation and resorption in organ culture: evidence for a coupling mechanism. *Natl Acad Sci USA* 1981;5:3204–3208.
15. Canalis E, McCarthy TL, Centrella M. Growth factors and cytokines in bone cell metabolism. *Annu Rev Med* 1991;42:17–24.
16. Hock JM, Centrella M, Canalis E. Insulin-like growth factor I has independent effects on bone matrix formation and cell replication. *Endocrinology* 1988;122:254–260.
17. McCarthy TL, Centrella M, Canalis E. Regulatory effects of insulin-like growth factors I and II on bone collagen synthesis in rat calvarial cultures. *Endocrinology* 1989;124:301–309.
18. Shimasaki S, Gao L, Shimonaka M, Ling N. Isolation and molecular cloning of insulin-like growth factor-binding protein-6. *Mol Endocrinol* 1991;5:938–948.
19. Canalis E, Centrella M, McCarthy TL. The role of insulin-like growth factors in bone remodelling. In: Cohn DV, Gennari C, Tashjian AH, eds. *Calcium regulating hormones and bone metabolism: basic and clinical aspects*. Amsterdam: Excerpta Medica, 1992;258–265.
20. Schmid C, Ernst M, Zapf J, Froesch ER. Release of insulin-like growth factor carrier proteins by osteoblasts: stimulation by estradiol and growth hormone. *Biochem Biophys Res Commun* 1989;160:788–794.
21. LaTour D, Mohan S, Linkhart TA, Baylink DJ, Strong DD. Inhibitory insulin-like growth factor-binding protein: cloning, complete sequence, and physiological regulation. *Mol Endocrinol* 1990;4:1806–1814.

22. Moriwake T, Tanaka H, Kanzaki S, Higuchi J, Seino Y. 1,25-Dihydroxyvitamin D3 stimulates the secretion of insulin-like growth factor binding protein 3 (IGFBP-3) by cultured human osteosarcoma cells. *Endocrinology* 1992;130:1071–1073.

23. McCarthy TL, Centrella M, Canalis E. Regulation of insulin-like growth factor (IGF) binding protein (IGF-BP) expression in primary rat osteoblast (Ob) enriched cultures. *J Bone Mineral Res* 1991;6(Suppl 1):S204.

24. Schmid CH, Rutishauser J, Schlapfer I, Froesch ER, Zapf J. Intact but not truncated insulin-like growth factor binding protein-3 (IGFBP-3) blocks IGF I-induced stimulation of osteoblasts: control of IGF signalling to bone cells by IGFBP-3-specific proteolysis? *Biochem Biophys Res Commun* 1991; 179:579–585.

25. Feyen JH, Evans DB, Blinkert C, Heinrich GF, Geisse S, Kocher HP. Recombinant human (Cys281) insulin-like growth factor-binding protein 2 inhibits both basal and insulin-like growth factor I-stimulated proliferation and collagen synthesis in fetal rat calvariae. *J Biol Chem* 1991; 266:19469–19474.

26. DeMellow JSM, Baxter RC. Growth hormone-dependent insulin-like growth factor (IGF) binding protein both inhibits and potentiates IGF-I-stimulated DNA synthesis in human skin fibroblasts. *Biochem Biophys Res Commun* 1988; 156:199–204.

27. Conover CA. Glycosylation of insulin-like growth factor binding protein-3 (IGFBP-3) is not required for potentiation of IGF-I action: evidence for processing of cell-bound IGFBP-3. *Endocrinology* 1991;129:3259–3268.

28. Barnard JA, Lyons RM, Moses HL. The cell biology of transforming growth factor β. *Biochim Biophys Acta* 1990; 1032:79–87.

29. Centrella M, McCarthy TL, Canalis E. Transforming growth factor-beta and remodeling of bone. *J Bone Joint Surg* 1991;73A:1418–1428.

30. Pelton RW, Dickinson ME, Moses HL, Hogan BLM. In situ hybridization analysis of TGF β3 RNA expression during mouse development: comparative studies with TGF β1 and β2. *Development* 1990;110:609–620.

31. Ogawa Y, Schmidt DK, Dasch JR, Chang R-J, Glaser CB. Purification and characterization of transforming growth factor β2.3 and β1.2 heterodimers from bovine bone. *J Biol Chem* 1991;267:2325–2328.

32. Ten Dijke P, Iwata KK, Goddard C, Pieler C, Canalis E, McCarthy TL, Centrella M. Recombinant transforming growth factor type β3: biological activities and receptor binding properties in isolated bone cells. *Mol Cell Biol* 1990; 10:4473–4479.

33. Centrella M, McCarthy TL, Canalis E. Transforming growth factor beta is a bifunctional regulator of replication and collagen synthesis in osteoblast-enriched cell cultures from fetal rat bone. *J Biol Chem* 1987;262:2869–2874.

34. Hock JM, Canalis E, Centrella M. Transforming growth factor beta (TGF-beta-1) stimulates bone matrix apposition and bone cell replication in cultured fetal rat calvariae. *Endocrinology* 1990;126:421–426.

35. Wozney JM, Rosen V, Celeste AJ, et al. Novel regulators of bone formation: molecular clones and activities. *Science* 1988;242:1528–1534.

36. Hiraki Y, Inoue H, Shigeno C, et al. Bone morphogenetic proteins (BMP-2 and BMP-3) promote growth and expression of the differentiated phenotype of rabbit chondrocytes and osteoblastic MC3T3-E1 cells in vitro. *J Bone Mineral Res* 1991;6:1373–1385.

37. Chen TL, Bates RL, Dudley A, Hammonds RG, Amento EP. Bone morphogenetic protein-2b stimulation of growth and osteogenic phenotypes in rat osteoblast-like cells: comparison with TGFβ1. *J Bone Mineral Res* 1991;6:1387–1393.

38. Heldin CH, Westermark B. PDGF-like growth factors in autocrine stimulation of growth. *J Cell Physiol* 1987;5:31–34.

39. Bowen-Pope DF, Hart CE, Seifert RA. Sera and conditioned media contain different isoforms of platelet-derived growth factor (PDGF) which bind to different classes of PDGF receptor. *J Biol Chem* 1989;264:2502–2508.

40. Rydziel S, Ladd C, McCarthy TL, Centrella M, Canalis E. Determination and expression of platelet-derived growth factor-AA in bone cell cultures. *Endocrinology* 1992; 130:1916–1922.

41. Graves DT, Owen AJ, Barth RK, et al. Detection of c-sis transcripts and synthesis of PDGF-like proteins by human osteosarcoma cells. *Science* 1984;226:972–974.

42. Canalis E, McCarthy TL, Centrella M. Effects of platelet-derived growth factor on bone formation in vitro. *J Cell Physiol* 1989;140:530–537.

43. Centrella M, McCarthy TL, Canalis E. Platelet-derived growth factor enhances deoxyribonucleic acid and collagen synthesis in osteoblast-enriched cultures from fetal rat parietal bone. *Endocrinology* 1989;125:13–19.

44. Burgess WH, Maciag T. The heparin-binding (fibroblast) growth factor family of proteins. *Annu Rev Biochem* 1989;58:575–606.

45. Globus RK, Plouet J, Gospodarowicz D. Cultured bovine bone cells synthesize basic fibroblast growth factor and store it in their extracellular matrix. *Endocrinology* 1989; 124:1539–1547.

46. Canalis E, Centrella M, McCarthy T. Effects of basic fibroblast growth factor on bone formation in vitro. *J Clin Invest* 1988;81:1572–1577.

47. McCarthy TL, Centrella M, Canalis E. Effects of fibroblast growth factors on deoxyribonucleic acid and collagen synthesis in rat parietal bone cells. *Endocrinology* 1989; 125:2118–2126.

48. McCarthy TL, Centrella M, Canalis E. Cyclic AMP induces insulin-like growth factor I synthesis in osteoblast-enriched cultures. *J Biol Chem* 1990;265:15353–15356.

49. McCarthy TL, Centrella M, Raisz LG, Canalis E. Prostaglandin E2 stimulates insulin-like growth factor I synthesis in osteoblast-enriched cultures from fetal rat bone. *Endocrinology* 1991;128:2895–2900.

50. Canalis E, Centrella M, McCarthy TL. Regulation of insulin-like growth factor II production in bone cultures. *Endocrinology* 1991;129:2457–2462.

51. Pfeilschifter J, Seyedin SM, Mundy GR. Transforming growth factor beta inhibits bone resorption in fetal rat long bone cultures. *J Clin Invest* 1988;82:680–685.

52. Chenu C, Pfeilschifter J, Mundy GF, Roodman GD. Transforming growth factor β inhibits formation of osteoclast-like cells in long-term human marrow cultures. *Proc Natl Acad Sci USA* 1988;85:5683–5687.

53. Centrella M, McCarthy TL, Canalis E. Parathyroid hormone modulates transforming growth factor β activity and binding in osteoblast-enriched cell cultures from fetal rat parietal bone. *Proc Natl Acad Sci USA* 1988;85:5889–5893.

54. Pugsley L, Selye H. The histological changes in bone responsible for the action of parathyroid hormone on the calcium metabolism of the rat. *J Physiol (London)* 1933;79:113–117.

55. Burrows R. Variations produced in bones of growing rats by parathyroid extracts. *Am J Anat* 1938;62:237–290.

56. Gunness-Hey M, Hock JM. Increased trabecular bone mass in rats treated with synthetic parathyroid hormone. *Metab Bone Rel Dis* 1984;5:177–181.

57. Gunness-Hey M, Hock JM, Gera I, et al. Human parathyroid hormone (1–34) and salmon calcitonin do not reverse impaired mineralization produced by high doses of 1,25 dihydroxyvitamin D3. *Calcif Tissue Int* 1986;38:234–238.

58. Gunness-Hey M, Gera I, Fonseca J, Raisz LG, Hock JM. 1,25 Dihydroxyvitamin D3 alone or in combination with parathyroid hormone does not increase bone mass in young rats. *Calcif Tissue Int* 1988;43:284–288.

59. Gunness-Hey M, Hock JM. Loss of anabolic effect of parathyroid hormone on bone after discontinuation of hormone in rats. *Bone* 1990;10:447–452.

60. Hock JM, Gera I, Fonseca J, Raisz LG. Human parathyroid hormone (1–34) increases bone mass in ovariectomized and orchidectomized rats. *Endocrinology* 1988;122:2899–2904.

61. Hock JM, Hummert JR, Boyce R, Fonseca J, Raisz LG. Resorption is not essential for the stimulation of bone growth

by human parathyroid hormone 1–34 in rats in vivo. *J Bone Mineral Res* 1989;4:449–458.

62. Hock JM, Fonseca J, Gunness-Hey M, Kemp BE, Martin TJ. Comparison of the anabolic effects of synthetic parathyroid hormone-related protein (PTHrP) 1–34 and PTH 1–34 on bone in rats. *Endocrinology* 1989;125:2022–2027.

63. Hock JM, Fonseca J. Anabolic effect of human synthetic parathyroid hormone (1–34) depends on growth hormone. *Endocrinology* 1990;127:1804–1810.

64. Hock JM, McOsker J. The anabolic effect of parathyroid hormone on bone does not depend on suppression of endogenous PTH (abstract). *Endocrine Society 73rd Annual Meeting, Washington, DC*, 1991.

65. Hock JM, Gera I. Effects of continuous and intermittent administration and inhibition of resorption on the anabolic response of bone to parathyroid hormone. *J Bone Mineral Res* 1992;7:65–72.

66. Hock JM, Berrol. Synthetic parathyroid hormone (hPTH 1–34) does not require corticosterone for its anabolic effect on bone in growth-hormone-and-thyroxine-supplemented hypophysectomized rats (abstract). *J Bone Mineral Res* 1991;6(Suppl 1):382.

67. Hock JM, Wood R. Bone response to parathyroid hormone in aged rats. *Cells Materials* 1991;Suppl 1:53–58.

68. Kalu DN, Pennock J, Doyle FH, Foster GV. Parathyroid hormone and experimental osteosclerosis. *Lancet* 1970;1:1363–1366.

69. Kalu DN, Hardin RH, Cockerham R, Yu P. Aging and dietary modulation of rat skeleton and parathyroid hormone. *Endocrinology* 1984;115:1239–1247.

70. Kalu DN, Echon R, Hollis BW. Modulation of ovariectomy-related bone loss by parathyroid hormone in rats. *Mech Ageing Dev* 1990;56:49–62.

71. Tam C, Cruikshank B, Swinson D, Anderson W, Little H. The response of the bone apposition rate to some non-physiologic conditions. *Metabolism* 1979;28:751–755.

72. Tam C, Heersche J, Murray T, Parsons JA. Parathyroid hormone stimulates the bone apposition rate independently of its resorptive action: differential effects of intermittent and continuous administration. *Endocrinology* 1982;110:506–512.

73. Turnbull RS, Heersche JN, Tam CS, Howley TP. Parathyroid hormone stimulates dentin and bone apposition in the thyroparathyroidectomized rat in a dose-dependent fashion. *Calcif Tissue Int* 1983;35:586–590.

74. Walker D. The induction of osteopetrotic changes in hypophysectomized thyroparathyroidectomized and intact rats of various ages. *Endocrinology* 1971;89:1389–1406.

75. Parsons JA, Reit B. Chronic response of dogs to parathyroid hormone infusion. *Nature* 1974;250:254–255.

76. Parsons JA. Parathyroid physiology and the skeleton. In: Bourne GJ, ed. *Biochemistry and Physiology of Bone,* Vol 4. New York: Academic Press, 1976;271–298.

77. Parsons JA, Bernat M, Bijvoet OL, et al. Low doses of a synthetic fragment of human parathyroid hormone (hPTH 1–34) as a stimulus to bone formation. In: US Barzel, ed. *Osteoporosis II.* New York: Grune & Stratton, 1979;151–159.

78. Podbesek RD, Eduoard C, Meunier PJ, et al. Effects of two treatment regimens with synthetic human parathyroid hormone fragment on bone formation and the tissue balance of trabecular bone in greyhounds. *Endocrinology* 1983;113:1000–1006.

79. Podbesek RD, Mawer EB, Zanelli GD, Parsons JA, Reeve J. Intestinal absorption of calcium in greyhounds: the response to intermittent and continuous administration of human synthetic parathyroid hormone fragment 1–34 (hPTH 1–34). *Clin Sci* 1984;67:591–599.

80. Malluche HH, Sherman D, Meyer W, Ritz E, Norman AW, Massry SG. Effects of long-term infusion of physiologic doses of 1–34 PTH on bone. *Am J Physiol* 1982;242:F197–F201.

81. Reeve J, Meunier PJ, Parsons JA, et al. Anabolic effect of parathyroid hormone fragment on trabecular bone in invo-

82. Reeve J, Bradbeer JN, Arlot M, et al. hPTH 1–34 treatment of osteoporosis with added hormone replacement therapy: biochemical, kinetic and histological responses. *Osteoporosis Int* 1991;1:162–170.

83. Slovik DM, Neer RM, Potts JT. Short-term effects of synthetic human parathyroid hormone (1–34) administration on bone mineral metabolism in osteoporotic patients. *J Clin Invest* 1981;68:1261–1271.

84. Slovik DM, Rosenthal DI, Doppelt SH, Potts JT, Daly MA, Neer RM. Restoration of spinal bone in osteoporotic men by treatment with human parathyroid hormone (1–34) and 1,25-dihydroxyvitamin D. *J Bone Mineral Res* 1986;1:377–381.

85. Mosekilde L, Sogard CH, Danielsen CC, Torring O. The anabolic effects of human parathyroid hormone (hPTH) on rat vertebral body mass are also reflected in the quality of bone, assessed by biomechanical testing: a comparison study between hPTH 1–34 and hPTH 1–84. *Endocrinology* 1991;129:421–428.

86. Silverberg JS, Shane E, de la Cruz L, et al. Skeletal disease in primary hyperparathyroidism. *J Bone Mineral Res* 1989;4:283–291.

87. Liu CC, Kalu DN. Human parathyroid hormone (1–34) prevents bone loss and augments bone formation in sexually mature ovariectomized rats. *J Bone Mineral Res* 1990;5:973–981.

88. Liu CC, Kalu DN, Salerno E, Echon R, Hollis BW, Ray M. Preexisting bone loss associated with ovariectomy is reversed by parathyroid hormone. *J Bone Mineral Res* 1991;6:1071–1080.

89. Takahashi HE, Tanizawa T, Hori M, Uzawa T. Effect of intermittent administration of human parathyroid hormone (1–34) on experimental osteopenia of rats induced by ovariectomy. *Cells Materials* 1991;S1:105–112.

90. Shen V, Dempster DW, Mellish RW, Birchman R, Horbert W, Lindsay R. Effects of combined and separate intermittent administration of low-dose human parathyroid hormone fragment (1–34) and 17-beta estradiol on bone histomorphometry in ovariectomized rats with established osteopenia. *Calcif Tissue Int* 1992;50:214–230.

91. Wronski TJ, Yen CF, Oi H, Dann LM. Parathyroid hormone is more effective than estrogen or diphosphonates for reversal of osteopenia in ovariectomized rats (abstract). *J Bone Mineral Res* 1992;7(Suppl 1):95.

92. Hori M, Uzawa T, Morita K, Noda T, Takahashi H, Inoue J. Effect of human parathyroid hormone (PTH 1–34) on experimental osteopenia of rats induced by ovariectomy. *Bone Mineral* 1988;3:193–199.

93. Johnston CC, Deiss WP. Some effects of hypophysectomy and parathyroid extract on bone matrix biosynthesis. *Endocrinology* 1965;76:198–202.

94. Hodsman AB, Steer BM, Fraher LJ, Drost DJ. Bone densitometric and histomorphometric responses to sequential human parathyroid hormone (1–38) and salmon calcitonin in osteoporotic patients. *Bone Mineral* 1991;14:67–83.

95. Steen-Hackett L, Gera I, Fonseca J, Raisz LG, Hock JM. Human parathyroid hormone 1–34 increases bone mass in denervated legs of rats. *J Bone Mineral Res* 1987;1(Suppl):57A.

96. Tada K, Younamura T, Okamura R, Kasai R, Takahashi H. Restoration of axial and appendicular bone volumes by hPTH (1–34) in parathyroidectomized and osteopenic rats. *Bone* 1990;11:163–169.

97. Seeman E, Wahner HW, Offord KP, Kumar R, Johnson WJ, Riggs BL. Differential effects of endocrine dysfunction on the axial and appendicular skeleton. *J Clin Invest* 1982;69:1302–1309.

98. Parisien M, Silverberg SJ, Shane E, et al. The histomorphometry of bone in primary hyperparathyroidism: preservation of cancellous bone structure. *J Clin Endocrinol Metab* 1990;70:930–938.

99. Christiansen P, Steiniche T, Vesterby A, Mosekilde L, Hes-

sov I, Melsen F. Primary hyperparathyroidism: iliac crest trabecular bone volume, structure, remodeling and balance evaluated by histomorphometric methods. *Bone* 1992;13:41–49.

100. Hefti E, Trechsel U, Bonjour J-P, Fleisch H, Schenk R. Increase of whole body calcium and skeletal mass in normal and osteoporotic adult rats treated with parathyroid hormone. *Clin Sci* 1982;62:389–396.

101. Mahoney CA, Nissenson RA. Canine renal receptors for parathyroid hormone. Down-regulation in vivo by exogenous parathyroid hormone. *J Clin Invest* 1983;72:411–421.

102. Pun KK, Ho PWM, Nissenson RA, Arnaud CD. Desensitization of parathyroid hormone receptors on cultured bone cells. *J Bone Mineral Res* 1990;5:1193–1200.

103. Harms HM, Kaptaina U, Kulpmann WR, Brabant G, Hesch RD. Pulse amplitude and frequency modulation of parathyroid hormone in plasma. *J Clin Endocrinol Metab* 1989;69:843–851.

104. Harms HM, Prank K, Brosa U, et al. Classification of dynamical diseases by new mathematical tools: application of multidimensional phase space analysis to the pulsatile secretion of parathyroid hormone. *Eur J Clin Invest* 1992;22:371–377.

105. Hesch RD, Rittinghaus EF, Harms HM, Delling G. Die fruhtherapie der osteoporose mit (1–38) parathormon und calcitonin-nasalspray [Early treatment of osteoporosis with parathyroid hormone 1–38 and calcitonin nasal spray]. *Med Klin* 1989;84:488–498.

106. Armbrecht HJ, Wongsurawat N, Paschal RE. Effect of age on renal responsiveness to parathyroid hormone and calcitonin in rats. *J Endocrinol* 1987;114:173–178.

107. Armbrecht HJ, Bolz M, Strong R, Richardson A, Bruns ME, Cristakos S. Expression of calbindin-D decreases with age in intestine and kidney. *Endocrinology* 125:2950–2956, 1989.

108. Armbrecht HJ. Effect of age on calcium and phosphate absorption. Role of 1,25-dihydroxyvitamin D. *Mineral Electrolyte Metab* 16:159–166, 1990.

109. Horst RL, Goff JP, Reinhardt TA. Advancing age results in reduction of intestinal and bone 1,25-dihydroxyvitamin D receptor. *Endocrinology* 1990;126:1053–1057.

110. Wood RJ, Theall C, Contois JH, Rosenberg IH. Intestinal and organ resistance to 1,25-dihydroxyvitamin D stimulation of calcium absorption in the senescent rat. In: Norman AW, ed. *Vitamin D Molecular, cellular and clinical endocrinology.* New York: Walter De Gruyter, 1988;907–908.

111. Mitlak BH, Williams DC, Bryant HU, Paul DC, Neer RM. Intermittent administration of bovine PTH (1–34) increases serum dihydroxyvitamin D concentration and spinal bone density in senile (23 month) rats. *J Bone Mineral Res* 1992;7:479–484.

112. Howard GA, Bottemiller BL, Baylink D. Evidence for the coupling of bone formation to bone resorption in vitro. *Metab Bone Dis* 1980;2:131–135.

113. Chyun YS, Raisz LG. Stimulation of bone formation by prostaglandin E2. *Prostaglandins* 1984;27:97–103.

114. Klein-Nulend J, Pilbeam CC, Harrison JR, Fall PM, Raisz LG. Mechanism of regulation of prostaglandin production by parathyroid hormone, interleukin 1 and cortisol in cultured mouse parietal bones. *Endocrinology* 1991;128:2503–2510.

115. Raisz LG, Fall PM. Biphasic effects of prostaglandin E2 on bone formation in cultured fetal rat calvariae: interaction with cortisol. *Endocrinology* 1990;126:1654–1659.

116. Gera I, Hock JM, Raisz LG, Gunness-Hey M, Fonseca J. Indomethacin does not inhibit the anabolic effect of parathyroid hormone in rats. *Calcif Tissue Int* 1988;40:206–211.

117. Ibbotson KJ, Orcutt CM, D'Souza SM, et al. Contrasting effects of parathyroid hormone and insulin-like growth factor I in an aged ovariectomized rat model of postmenopausal osteoporosis. *J Bone Mineral Res* 1992;7:425–432.

118. Deslauriers N, Gadreau P, Abribat T, Renier G, Petitclerc D, Brazeau P. Dynamics of growth hormone responsiveness to growth hormone releasing factor in aging rats: peripheral and central influences. *Neuroendocrinology* 1991;53:439–446.

119. Goya RG, Quigley KL, Takahashi S, Reichhart R, Meites J. Effect of homeostatic thymus hormone on plasma thyrotropin and growth hormone in young and old rats. *Mech Ageing Dev* 1989;49:119–128.

120. Takahashi S, Gottshall PE, Quigley KL, Goya RG, Meites J. Growth hormone secretory patterns in young, middle-aged and old female rats. *Neuroendocrinology* 1987;46:137–142.

121. Canalis E, Hintz RL, Dietrich JW, Maina DM, Raisz LG. Effect of somatomedin and growth hormone on bone collagen synthesis in vitro. *Metabolism* 1977;25:1079–1087.

122. Linkhardt TA, Mohan S. Parathyroid hormone stimulates release of insulin-like growth factor-I (IGF-I) and IGF-II from neonatal mouse calvaria in organ culture. *Endocrinology* 1989;125:1484–1491.

123. Mochizuki H, Hakeda Y, Wakatsuki N, et al. Insulin-like growth factor I supports formation and activation of osteoclasts. *Endocrinology* 1992;131:1075–1080.

124. Breese CR, Ingram RL, Sonntag WE. Influence of age and longterm dietary restriction on plasma insulin-like growth factor-I, IGF-I gene expression and IGF-binding proteins. *J Gerontol* 1991;46:B180–B187.

125. Oursler MJ, Cortese C, Keeting F, Anderson MA, Bonde SK, Riggs BL, Spelsberg TC. Modulation of transforming growth factor-beta in normal human osteoblast-like cells by 17-beta estradiol and parathyroid hormone. *Endocrinology* 1991;129:3313–3320.

126. Albright F. In: Loriaux L, ed. *Uncharted seas.* Portland, OR: JBK Publishing, 1990.

127. Albright F, Reifenstein EC. *The parathyroid glands and metabolic bone disease.* Baltimore: Williams & Wilkins, 1948.

128. Jowsey J. Indirect measurement of bone resorption. *J Clin Endocrinol Metab* 1965;25:1408–1416.

129. Wilde CD, Jawarski ZF, Villanueva AR, Frost HM. Quantitative histological measurements of bone turnover in primary hyperparathyroidism. *Calcif Tissue Int* 1973;12:137–142.

130. Charhon SA, Edouard CM, Arlot ME, Meunier PJ. Effects of parathyroid hormone on remodeling of iliac trabecular bone packets in patients with primary hyperparathyroidism. *Clin Orthop* 1982;162:255–263.

131. Eriksen EF, Mosekilde L, Melson F. Trabecular bone remodeling and balance in primary hyperparathyroidism. *Bone* 1986;7:213–221.

132. Cundy T, Darby AJ, Barry HE, Parsons V. Bone metabolism in acute parathyroid crisis. *Clin Endocrinol* 1985;22:787–793.

133. Marcus R, Madvig P, Crim M, Pont A, Kosek J. Conjugated estrogens in the treatment of postmenopausal women with hyperparathyroidism. *Ann Intern Med* 1984;100:633–640.

134. Kotowicz MA, Klee GG, Kao PC, et al. Relationship between serum intact parathyroid hormone concentrations and bone remodeling in type I osteoporosis: evidence that skeletal sensitivity is increased. *Osteoporosis Int* 1992;1:14–22.

135. Silverberg SJ, Shane E, de la Cruz L, Segre GV, Clemens TL, Bilezikian JP. Abnormalities in parathyroid hormone secretion and 1,25 dihydroxyvitamin D_3 in women with osteoporosis. *N Engl J Med* 1989;320:277–281.

136. Marcus R, Madvig P, Young G. Age-related changes in parathyroid hormone and parathyroid hormone action in normal humans. *J Clin Endocrin Metab* 1984;58:223–230.

137. Mori S, Shiraki M, Fujimaki H, Ito H. Bone fracture in elderly female with primary hyperparathyroidism: relationship among renal function, vitamin D status and fracture risk. *Horm Metab Res* 1987;19:183–189.

138. Silverberg SJ, Gartenberg F, Bilezikian JP. Primary hyperparathyroidism protects cancellous bone density in postmenopausal women (abstract). *J Bone Miner Res* 1992;7:S296.

139. Hesp R, Tellez M, Davidson L, Elton A, Reeve J. Trabecular and cortical bone in the radii of women with parathyroid ad-

enomata: a greater trabecular deficit, with a preliminary assessment of recovery after parathyroidectomy. *Bone Mineral* 1987;2:301–310.

140. de Deuxchaisnes CN, Derogelaer JP, Huaux JP. Long-term follow up of untreated primary hyperparathyroidism. *Br Med J* 1985;290:64–65.

141. Martin P, Bergmann P, Gillet C, et al. Partially reversible osteopenia after surgery for primary hyperparathyroidism. *Arch Intern Med* 1986;146:689–691.

142. Martin P, Bergmann P, Gillet C, Fuss M, Corvilain S, Vangeertruden J. Long-term irreversibility of bone loss after surgery for primary hyperparathyroidism. *Arch Intern Med* 1990;150:1495–1500.

143. Eastell R, Kennedy NSJ, Smith MA, Tothill P, Edwards CRW. Changes in total body calcium following surgery for primary hyperparathyroidism. *Bone* 1986;7:269–272.

144. Block MA, Dailey GE, Muchmore DE. Bone demineralization, a factor of increasing significance in the management of primary hyperparathyroidism. *Surgery* 1990;106:1063–1069.

145. Aburgassa S, Nordenstrom J, Eriksson S, Mollerstrom G, Alveryd A. Skeletal remineralization after surgery for primary and secondary hyperparathyroidism. *Surgery* 1990;107:128–133.

146. Mautalen C, Reyes HR, Ghiringhelli G, Fromm G. Cortical bone mineral content in primary hyperparathyroidism—changes after parathyroidectomy. *Acta Endocrinol* 1986;111:494–497.

147. Rao DS, Wilson RJ, Kleerekoper M, Parfitt AM. Lack of biochemical progression or continuation of accelerated bone loss in mild asymptomatic primary hyperparathyroidism: Evidence for biphasic disease course. *J Clin Endocrinol Metab* 1988;67:1294–1298.

148. Larsson K, Lindh E. Increased fracture risk in hypercalcemia: bone mineral content measured in hyperparathyroidism. *Acta Orthop Scand* 1989;60:268–270.

149. Kochersberger G, Buckley NJ, Leight GS, et al. What is the clinical significance of bone loss in primary hyperparathyroidism. *Arch Intern Med* 1987;147:1951–1953.

150. Chalmers J, Irvine GR. Fractures of the femoral neck in elderly patients with hyperparathyroidism. *Clin Orthop Rel Res* 1988;229:125–130.

151. Wilson RJ, Rao DS, Ellis B, Kleerekoper M, Parfitt AM. Mild asymptomatic primary hyperparathyroidism is not a risk factor for vertebral fractures. *Ann Intern Med* 1988;109:959–962.

152. Peacock M. Interpretation of bone mass determinations as they relate to fracture: implications for asymptomatic primary hyperparathyroidism. *J Bone Mineral Res* 1991;6(Suppl 2):S77–S82.

153. Wishart J, Horowitz M, Need A, Nordin BEC. Relationship between forearm and vertebral mineral density in postmenopausal women with primary hyperparathyroidism. *Arch Intern Med* 1990;150:1329–1331.

154. Mallette LE, LeBlanc AD, Pool JL. Cyclic therapy of osteoporosis with neutral phosphate and brief, high-dose pulses of etidronate. *J Bone Mineral Res* 1989;4:143–148.

155. Hesch R-D, Busch U, Prokop M. Increase of vertebral density by combination therapy with pulsatile (1–38)hPTH and sequential addition of calcitonin nasal spray in osteoporotic patients. *Calcif Tissue Int* 1989;44:176–180.

156. Hesch R-D, Heck J, Delling G, et al. Results of a stimulatory therapy of low bone metabolism in osteoporosis with (1–38)hPTH and disphosphonate EHDP. *Klin Wochenschr* 1988;66:976–984.

157. Reeve J, Davies UM, Hesp R, McNally E, Katz D. Treatment of osteoporosis with human parathyroid peptide and observation on effect of sodium fluoride. *Br Med J* 1990;301:314–317.

158. MacDonald BR, Gallagher JA, Russell RGG. Parathyroid hormone stimulates the proliferation of cells derived from human bone. *Endocrinology* 1986;118:2445–2549.

159. Parisien M, Mellish RW, Schnitzer M, et al. Cancellous bone structure in post-menopausal women: comparison among osteoporosis or primary hyperparathyroidism and normals (abstract). *J Bone Mineral Res* 1992;7:S114.

160. Parisien M, Mellish RWE, Silverberg SJ, et al. Maintenance of cancellous bone connectivity in primary hyperparathyroidism—trabecular strut analysis. *J Bone Mineral Res* 1992;7:913–920.

The Parathyroids, edited by J.P. Bilezikian,
M.A. Levine, and R. Marcus. Raven Press, Ltd.,
New York © 1994.

CHAPTER 5

Cellular Actions of Parathyroid Hormone on Osteoblast and Osteoclast Differentiation

Johan N. M. Heersche, Carlton G. Bellows, and Jane E. Aubin

Bone is a highly organized tissue, the structure of which reflects its primary functions to provide support and protection and the environment for hematopoiesis. To maintain the structural integrity of bone, large numbers of new cells must be recruited continuously: osteoblasts responsible for bone formation and osteoclasts responsible for bone resorption. These two cell types belong to two different lineages; the osteoblasts derive from mesenchymal cells, the osteoclasts from hematopoietic cells.

This chapter considers the direct and indirect effects of parathyroid hormone (PTH) on the differentiation of osteoblasts and osteoclasts and discusses observations made in vivo; in organ cultures of bone in vitro; in mixed primary cultures of osteoblast-like cells, osteoclast-like cells, or bone marrow; and in clonal populations of osteoblast-like cells. Despite advances in this field, much greater knowledge is required of the characteristics of bone cells and their progenitors at various stages of differentiation to resolve the multiplicity of pathways through which PTH regulates osteoblast and osteoclast number and activity.

EFFECTS OF PARATHYROID HORMONE ON OSTEOCLAST AND OSTEOBLAST DIFFERENTIATION IN VIVO: STUDIES IN HUMAN SUBJECTS AND RATS

A prolonged increase in circulating concentrations of PTH is associated with increased bone turnover,

i.e., increased osteoclastic bone resorption and increased osteoblastic activity (1–3). In severe hyperparathyroidism, this results in loss of both cortical and cancellous bone (4,5). However, mild hyperparathyroidism is associated with normal or increased bone mineral density and increased bone volume in areas that are primarily cancellous, such as vertebrae (6–9), but bone is still lost in cortical areas (6). Daily injections of human PTH-1–34 for 6–12 months also increases the cancellous bone area in iliac crest biopsies (10) and decreases femoral cortical bone density of osteoporotic patients (11). Thus, under certain conditions, PTH can affect cancellous bone and cortical bone differently, with a net increase in bone mass occurring in cancellous bone concomitant with a net loss of cortical bone. Of particular interest is the observation that the adverse effects of treatment with PTH on cortical bone density might be ameliorated by simultaneous treatment with estrogen (12) or calcitriol (13).

In agreement with these results, intermittent injection of PTH-1–34 increased cancellous bone in the secondary spongiosa of thyroparathyroidectomized rats (14,15), an effect that was independent of resorptive activity (14,16). It is also of interest to note that the anabolic effects of PTH on bone apposition were abolished in vitamin D-deficient rats and were restored by vitamin D supplementation (17). This interaction seemed to be dependent on the presence of growth hormone (18).

The mechanism whereby excess PTH is thought to affect bone metabolism in humans is an increase in remodeling resulting from a 50% increase in activation frequency (19). Why this should maintain or increase cancellous bone volume and decrease cortical bone volume remains to be determined. One explanation, suggested by results of Parfitt and colleagues (20,21) is that the depth of osteoclastic resorption lacunae on the endocortical surface is greater than the depth of

J. N. M. Heersche: M.R.C. Group in Periodontal Physiology, Faculty of Dentistry, Department of Pharmacology, University of Toronto, Toronto, Ontario M5S 1A8 Canada.

C. G. Bellows, and J. E. Aubin: M.R.C. Group in Periodontal Physiology, Faculty of Dentistry, University of Toronto, Toronto, Ontario M5S 1A8 Canada.

the lacunae on cancellous bone surfaces. The reasons for this difference, however, are not known.

EFFECTS OF PARATHYROID HORMONE ON OSTEOBLAST AND OSTEOCLAST DIFFERENTIATION IN BONE ORGAN CULTURE SYSTEMS

Early studies with mouse long bone rudiments showed conclusively that PTH affected both osteoblast and osteoclast numbers and activity in a dose- and time-dependent fashion (22). With culture in the presence of low concentrations of PTH (0.01–0.001 U/ml), decreased activity of osteoblasts was seen after 12–24 hours, whereas multinucleated osteoclasts increased in numbers and became active after 24–48 hr. The three types of tissue represented in such bone rudiments, that is, bone, cartilage, and marrow stroma, all responded to PTH, but timing and dose responsiveness differed. Low concentrations of PTH (0.01–0.001 U/ml) had no effect on cartilage or marrow stroma. Higher concentrations of PTH, however, induced increased proliferation of cartilage and of connective tissue and more pronounced effects on osteoblasts and osteoclasts.

These early experiments point out three aspects of PTH action on bone-related tissues that have been of major interest over the past 30 years: (a) the time delay between PTH effects on osteoblasts and osteoclasts (compatible with a cause and effect relationship); (b) reduction of osteoprogenitor differentiation into osteoblasts and enhanced proliferation of a fibroblast-like cell type; and (c) the effects of PTH on cartilage differentiation and proliferation. Numerous authors have since confirmed and extended these early investigations using a variety of experimental systems. The resulting consensus is that culture of bone tissue in the continuous presence of PTH causes extensive osteoclastic resorption, stimulates proliferation and differentiation of osteoclast progenitors if they are present in the cultured tissues (23), increases the activity of osteoclasts already present in the tissue (24–26), and decreases osteoblastic activity and differentiation of functioning osteoblasts (27,28). Further experimentation suggested that, although continuous culture in PTH-containing media results in inhibition of collagen synthesis during the first 24–72 hr of culture, stimulation of collagen synthesis may occur after longer incubation (29). These latter results thus raise the possibility that under certain culture conditions the anabolic effect of PTH observed in vivo can also be detected in vitro. This view was confirmed by the studies of Canalis et al. (30), who showed that treatment with PTH for the first 24 hr of culture followed by 48–72 hr of incubation in control medium stimulated rather than inhibited collagen synthesis in rat calvaria (see the previous chapter by Canalis et al.) This stimulation was shown to be mediated by tissue production of insulin-like growth factor type I (IGF-I). In agreement with these results, Kream et al. (31) showed that PTH blocked the effects of IGF-I on collagen synthesis in cultured 21 day fetal rat calvariae. However, Spencer et al. (32) found that PTH potentiated the mitogenic effects of IGF-I in embryonic chick osteoblast-like cells. Thus, although effects in different systems may vary, these results illustrate that the effects of PTH on bone tissue may be modulated or mediated by locally produced factors, a mechanism that has recently become the central issue in elucidating the effects of PTH (and of PTHrP) on osteoblast and osteoclast differentiation.

PARATHYROID HORMONE EFFECTS ON DIFFERENTIATION AND PROLIFERATION OF OSTEOGENIC PROGENITORS AND ON OSTEOBLAST ACTIVITY IN ISOLATED CELL SYSTEMS

By analogy with the hematopoietic lineages, it is thought that the stromal cell compartment of bone contains pluripotential stem cells with the ability to generate committed progenitors, which then give rise to the different cells formed in or near bone, such as the osteogenic, chondrogenic, and various other mesenchymal cell lineages (for reviews, see 33–35). Detailed knowledge of osteoblast lineage, including identification of transitional steps from stem cell to committed osteoprogenitor to osteoblast, interactions of cells within the lineage, and identification and regulation of stem cells and other progenitors, is limited. However, several features have been useful in partial characterization of osteoblasts and their immediate progenitors. Of these, high alkaline phosphatase (AP) activity, PTH binding, a PTH-stimulated adenylyl cyclase, and ability to synthesize a number of noncollagenous bone matrix proteins have been most frequently used.

It is not clear at which stage of differentiation osteoprogenitor cells first acquire PTH receptors. We attempted to answer this question by analyzing the effects of PTH on osteoprogenitor differentiation in long-term cultures of isolated fetal rat calvaria cell populations (36). Such cultures, when continuously maintained in media containing 15% fetal calf serum, ascorbic acid, and β-glycerophosphate, form discrete, three-dimensional, mineralized, nodular areas with the histological, immunohistological (37,38), and ultrastructural (39) appearance of woven bone. Limiting dilution analysis indicates that ~0.4% of these cells are osteoprogenitors and that one osteoprogenitor cell gives rise to a single bone nodule under standard culture conditions without added hormones or growth factors (40). Thus, by counting the number of nodules formed at a given cell density, the effects of hormones and growth factors on proliferation and differentiation of a particular cell type and its progeny can be evaluated. In our experiments studying the effects of PTH on osteoprogenitor differentiation, PTH was present continuously or for different intervals during the culture period (36). Continuous presence of PTH for the entire culture period (21 days) prevented bone nodule formation independently of a change in cell proliferation or saturation density of the total cell population. When PTH was removed 6–8 days before the end of the culture period, the number of nodules approached the number formed under control conditions, and clusters of differentiated osteoblasts could be observed within 3 days after removing PTH from the medium. The rate at which such clusters developed after PTH removal suggested to us that PTH acts late in the progression from osteoprogenitor cell to osteoblast, most likely at the stage just before differentiation of preosteoblasts into osteoblasts. Such an effect may synchronize the appearance of mature osteoblasts after a temporary increase in the concentration of PTH in vivo and in vitro.

Other data support the concept that the number of progenitor cells with the ability to proliferate and differentiate is not affected by PTH during the proliferative phase of the population. A single 48 hr treatment with PTH at any time during the 17 day culture period, or removal of PTH earlier than 6–8 days before the end of the culture period, did not significantly affect the number of nodules ultimately formed. Thus it appears that PTH has no effect on early osteoblast progenitors, which could imply that receptors for PTH appear only during the later stages of differentiation. Consequently, the PTH-induced increases in IGF-I production (41), interleukin-6 (IL-6) production (42), or interleukin-1 (IL-1) binding (43) in cultures of osteoblast-like cells are likely to represent regulatory mechanisms involving late-stage osteoprogenitors.

PTH receptors were demonstrated on the osteoblast and its immediate precursors in early studies by Silve et al., and Rao et al. (44,45). More recent studies suggest, however, that the highest number of receptors may be on a cell type distinct from the mature osteoblast, possibly an immediate osteoblast progenitor or preosteoblast (46,47). On the other hand, higher levels of PTH receptor mRNA have been localized in bone tissue via in situ hybridization in mature osteoblasts than in the less differentiated precursor cells (48,49). The latter observation agrees with observations of Bernier et al. (50), whose studies with UMR 106 cells suggest that the cells binding the highest levels of PTH are relatively quiescent and possibly more mature.

The mechanism of the PTH-induced suppression of bone nodule formation requires further examination with respect to which second messengers may be involved. It is now well established that cellular responses to PTH are mediated through multiple second messenger signals, such as increased intracellular free Ca^{2+}, cyclic adenosine monophosphate (cAMP), and inositol-1,4,5-trisphosphate levels (see the chapter by Coleman et al.). These pathways are likely to play a role in differentiation as has been found to occur with several other cell types. In the bone nodule system described above, the concentration of PTH required to inhibit osteoprogenitor differentiation is lower than that required to elicit a detectable cAMP response (36). To evaluate further the involvement of cAMP-mediated events in the regulation of osteoprogenitor differentiation in this system, we analyzed the effects of forskolin (51). Forskolin stimulates the formation of cAMP by mechanisms that bypass hormone receptors. Low concentrations of forskolin (1 nM), which did not affect cAMP levels, were stimulatory, while higher concentrations (1 and 10 μM), which caused significant increases in cAMP levels, were inhibitory. Short 1 hr pulses with 10 μM forskolin at each medium change were also inhibitory (51), similar to the effects of short-term pulses with PTH (Bellows et al., unpublished observations). Thus it seems likely that the inhibition of bone nodule formation by PTH is mediated by both cAMP and other messenger systems.

THE COMPLEXITY OF INTERACTIONS THAT DETERMINE THE RESPONSIVENESS OF OSTEOBLAST-LIKE CELLS TO PARATHYROID HORMONE

We and others have previously reviewed and summarized the effects of hormones and cytokines in a variety of bone cell systems (52–54) and discussed possible reasons for the disparate effects in the different model systems. Part of the problem is the wide variety of conditions under which such effects have been assayed. For example, in some cases, a serum supplement [10–15% fetal calf serum (FCS)] was present; in other cases, reduced serum (0.2–2%) was used; in other cases, no serum was present. Also of importance is the possibility that the different model systems comprised mixtures of osteoblastic cells at different stages of differentiation. The presence of bone matrix as a repository of growth factors that may be released during resorption in tissue culture systems is an additional factor that could radically alter the environment in which osteoblast differentiation takes place. Finally, establishment of cell lines to immortal growth (MC3T3-E1) or transformation (ROS 17/2.8, UMR 106) may alter the nature of the responses. All these points should be addressed more definitively in the models currently under investigation. Newer methods to identify cell types will facilitate meeting this need.

In an attempt to find model systems in which the properties of osteoblast-lineage cells at distinct stages of differentiation could be analyzed, clonal cell lines have been isolated. Osteoblast-like osteosarcoma lines from rat tissue [e.g., ROS 17/2.8 (55) and UMR 106 (56)] or human tissue [e.g., SaOS-2 (57), MG-63 (58), and TE-85 (59)] as well as clonal lines derived from normal bone cell populations [e.g., mouse (MC3T3-E1) (60), rat calvariae (61,62)] and mouse bone marrow stroma (63) have helped to establish the correlation of particular features with osteoblast and/or other cell types. Interestingly, most of these cell lines have been characterized as osteoblastic based on the presence of PTH responsiveness (i.e., PTH-stimulatable adenylyl cyclase activity.

To illustrate the complexity of the interactions involved in regulating the responsiveness of osteoblast-like cells to PTH, this chapter next reviews some of the results obtained using cloned osteoblast-like cells, in particular UMR 106 cells. This cell line and other clonal cell lines are more homogeneous than primary populations derived from bone tissue in that all cells are from the same lineage, but they are still heterogeneous in that they comprise a majority of proliferating cells at early stages of culture and mostly nonproliferating and possibly more differentiated cells at postconfluent stages of culture.

In UMR 106.01 cells, PTH at concentrations of 0.1 nM or greater inhibits both cell replication and DNA synthesis in both the presence and the absence of serum (64). This inhibition was directly linked by Kano et al. (65) to activation of a cAMP-dependent protein kinase. Furthermore, by using a mutant cAMP-resistant osteoblastic clone (UMR 4-7), it was confirmed that growth inhibition of UMR cells is dependent on activation of cAMP-dependent protein kinase A (66). By contrast, in other cell lines, PTH has been found to stimulate proliferation [TE 85 cells (67), human osteoblast-like cells (68)]. Moreover, in TE-85 cells, PTH-induced stimulation of proliferation did not appear to involve increases in intracellular cAMP, nor increases in IGF-I, IGF-II, or transforming growth factor-β (TGFβ) production (67).

Effects of parathyroid hormone-related protein (PTHrP) on osteoblast-like cell populations are generally the same or similar to those of PTH (for review, see 69; see also 70,71), presumably because both activate common receptors (48). As a consequence, endogenous production of PTHrP by osteoblast-like cells, in particular those derived from osteosarcomas, may affect the number of receptors for PTH and thus modulate the effects of exogenously added PTH. This was shown to occur in the clonal human osteosarcoma-derived cell line SAOS-2/B-10, in which lack of PTH-stimulatable adenylyl cyclase activity correlated with production of PTHrP (72). Interestingly, epider-

mal growth factor (EGF) stimulated PTHrP production in this cell line, suggesting that the EGF-induced decrease in the number of cells displaying high binding of ^{125}I-PTH when UMR 106 cells are cultured with EGF (50) may not be related to the proliferative stage or the degree of maturity of the cells but rather to endogenous PTHrP production.

The effects of PTH, PTHrP, and EGF may also be affected by PTH-induced down-regulation of EGF receptors. This was shown to occur in the PTH- and EGF-responsive osteoblastic cell line MC3T3-E1 (73) and also in UMR 106 cells (74). TGFα similarly attenuated PTH- and PTHrP-induced cAMP responses in UMR 106 cells (75).

An additional factor influencing the PTH-PTHrP–EGF interaction in osteoblastic cells is 1,25-dihydroxyvitamin D_3 [1,25-$(OH)_2D_3$] receptor levels. In UMR 106 cells, PTH up-regulates 1,25-$(OH)_2D_3$ receptors, and this up-regulation is inhibited by EGF (76). Since circulating levels of 1,25-$(OH)_2D_3$ increase when levels of circulating PTH increase, it is evident that PTH-induced effects on osteoblast proliferation are affected by 1,25-$(OH)_2D_3$.

The complexity of interactions between PTH, PTHrP, 1,25-$(OH)_2D_3$, EGF, and TGFα is further underscored by the involvement of additional factors present in the osteoblast environment, such as TGFβ, IL-1, tumour necrosis factor-α (TNFα) and prostaglandins of the E series (PGEs). Incubation of UMR cells with TGFβ for 48–72 hr, for example, has been shown to increase both the cAMP response to PTH and the PTH receptor numbers in the total population (77,78). Schneider et al. (78) concluded that TGFβ induced a shift of the population to a more mature osteoblastic phenotype, an explanation consistent with the observation of Bernier et al. (50) that nonproliferative UMR 106 cells bind PTH to a greater degree than proliferative cells. Interleukin-1 and TNFα also modulate the effects of PTH. Both have been shown to inhibit PTH-responsive adenylyl cyclase in UMR 106 cells after culture with IL-1 or TNFα for 48 hr (79). Conversely, PTH has also been shown to increase IL-6 production in UMR 106 cells (42), and IL-1 and IL-6 production in MC3T3-E1 cells (80). How the observation that IL-1 and TNFα synergistically interact with PTH in stimulating resorption (81), and also potentiate PTHrP effects (82), fits in with some of the results mentioned above is unclear at present.

The presence of a growth factor is obviously important, but the form it is in is also a crucial feature of the ultimate response. This is true for TGFβ and IL-1β (active vs. latent) and for fibroblast growth factors (FGFs) and IGFs (release from matrix and cell surfaces). The major enzyme identified to be involved in activation and/or release of these growth factors is plasmin, which in turn is stored in latent form as plasminogen and is activated by plasminogen activators (PAs), a process inhibited by plasminogen activator inhibitors (PAIs). Both PAs and PAIs are produced by osteoblast-like cells, and their production and release are regulated not only by PTH but also by prostaglandins, IL-1, and TGFβ. One example of such regulation is the observation that PTH and PGE$_1$ increased PA activity (83–85) and decreased PAI activity in osteoblast-like cells (84,85). It seems abundantly clear that effects of PTH on PA and PAI secretion could either directly or indirectly (for example, through PTH-induced increases in IL-1 production) affect the concentration of cytokines in the osteoblastic environment and thus have a major effect on osteoblast differentiation.

The results obtained with cloned osteoblast-like osteosarcoma cell lines are generally comparable to those obtained with isolated mixed bone cell populations derived from fetal or adult bone tissue; with cloned, nontransformed, but immortal populations; and with intact embryonic bone tissue. However, major discrepancies between results obtained with different systems have been observed, particularly with regard to the regulation of proliferation. It is beyond the scope of this chapter to analyze the possible causes of the differences observed, and the reader is referred to other reviews of bone cell heterogeneity to obtain further information on this topic (33,52). As a general conclusion, however, it seems that an approach in which single cell characteristics, responses, and differentiation potential are analyzed would be likely to generate the next wave of insight into regulation of osteoblast proliferation and differentiation. Such analyses are now in progress in several laboratories (see, e.g., 35,86).

EFFECTS OF PARATHYROID HORMONE ON OSTEOCLAST DIFFERENTIATION

When embryonic long bone rudiments or calvariae are explanted and maintained in culture for several days, osteoclast progenitors located in either marrow spaces or periosteum proliferate and differentiate to form osteoclasts (87,88). Osteoclast-like cells also develop in bone marrow cultures. Hematopoietic progenitor cells derived from mouse bone marrow form colonies of osteoclast-like cells, but generally 1,25-(OH)$_2$D$_3$ is required to obtain significant numbers of such colonies (89). Progenitors present in mouse spleen can also differentiate into osteoclasts, but only in the presence of bone marrow-derived stroma and not in the presence of spleen-derived stromal cells (90,91). This suggests that osteoclast differentiation from hematopoietic progenitors is controlled, at least in part, by specific stromal cells present in the marrow

cultures. Similar interactions have been proposed between the stromal layer and progenitors of other hematopoietic cells (92).

In the experiments referred to above, osteoclast formation and tartrate-resistant acid phosphatase (TRAP)-positive colony formation were always closely associated with AP-positive stromal cells. However, as was mentioned in an extensive review of the literature on osteoclast differentiation (93), the characteristics of this stromal cell type, beyond its AP positivity, are largely unknown. An interesting observation with regard to the effects of PTH on osteoclast differentiation in cocultures of spleen cells and stromal cell lines is that PTH-induced osteoclast-like cell formation was observed only in cocultures with a cell line that responded to PTH with an increase in cAMP [KS-4 cells (94)] and not with cell lines not responsive to PTH. However, the observation that stromal cell lines not responsive to PTH, but responsive to PGE$_2$ or 1,25-(OH)$_2$D$_3$ (95), mediated PGE$_2$- or 1,25-(OH)$_2$D$_3$-induced osteoclast formation in spleen cell coculture systems indicates that several types of stromal osteoblast-like or nonosteoblast-like cells that differ in hormone responsiveness may be involved in the regulation of osteoclast formation. Furthermore, we observed that stimulation of the development of TRAP-positive osteoclast-containing colonies was clearly associated with formation of AP-positive stromal cell colonies in cocultures of mouse bone marrow with a chondrogenic cell line (RCJ 3.1.C5.18) (96), suggesting that proliferation of this type of AP-positive stromal cell was stimulated by factors elaborated by or associated with the chondrogenic cells. The fact that the C5.18 cell line responds to PTH with an increase in cAMP levels (97) supports the view that a PTH-induced increase in osteoclast development could also be mediated by a cascade of events involving more than one cell type.

Other factors whose concentration is, at least in part, regulated by PTH, such as macrophage colony-stimulating factor (MCSF), IL-1, IL-6, and granulocyte–macrophage colony-stimulating factor (GMCSF) (42,80,98–100) have also been found to alter osteoclast differentiation. For example, production of MCSF by stromal or other cells is necessary for proliferation and differentiation of osteoclast progenitors in most systems studied (101–104), although other reports indicate that MCSF can also inhibit osteoclast formation (105–107). With regard to the role of other cytokines, the evidence is also somewhat conflicting. For example, IL-6 is strongly implicated in stimulating osteoclastogenesis in vivo in ovariectomized rats (108) and has been shown to stimulate osteoclast-like cell formation in long-term human marrow cultures by inducing IL-1 release (109). However, Shinar et al. (105) found no effect of IL-6 on osteoclast formation in mouse marrow cultures. Shinar et al. (105) also found no effects of GMCSF, while others observed either inhibition (107) or stimulation (101) of osteoclast development in marrow cultures maintained in the continuous presence of added GMCSF.

Whether osteoclasts or osteoclast progenitors can also directly respond to PTH or PTHrP would seem to depend on whether these cells possess receptors for this hormone. Results to date are inconclusive. Specific binding of PTH has been found in hematopoietic blast cells (110), and specific binding of iodinated or biotinylated bovine PTH-1–84 to chicken osteoclasts was reported by Teti et al. (111), Agarwala and Gay (112), and Duong et al. (113). However, others have been unable to demonstrate specific binding of PTH-1–34 to osteoclasts or osteoclast precursors in chicken long bones (44) or long bones of rats infused with iodinated PTH-1–34 (114). Until this issue is resolved, the question of whether PTH has direct effects on osteoclasts or their progenitors will remain unresolved.

In summary, it seems clear that PTH stimulates osteoclast differentiation in vivo and in vitro and that stromal AP-positive cells are involved. However, the specific interactions between "osteoblast-lineage" cells and the "osteoclast-lineage" cells and the mechanisms whereby PTH affects these interactions are still for the most part obscure. Further delineation and characterization of the hormone and growth factor responsiveness of cells at various stages in these pathways will be necessary to clarify these issues.

REFERENCES

1. Meunier P, Vignon G, Bernard J, Edouard C, Courpron P. Quantitative bone histology as applied to the diagnosis of hyperparathyroid states. In: Frame B, Parfitt AM, Duncan H, eds. *Clinical aspects of metabolic bone disease*. Amsterdam: Exerpta Medica, 1973;215.
2. Parfitt AM. The actions of parathyroid on bone: Relation to bone remodeling and turnover, calcium homeostasis and metabolic bone disease. Part III. *Metabolism* 1976;25:1033–1069.
3. Eriksen EF, Mosekilde L, Melsen F. Trabecular bone remodelling and balance in primary hyperparathyroidism. *Bone* 1986;7:213.
4. Seeman E, Wahner HW, Offord KP, et al. Differential effects of endocrine dysfunction on the axial and the appendicular skeleton. *J Clin Invest* 1982;69:1302–1309.
5. Richardson ML, Pozzi-Mucelli RS, et al. Bone mineral changes in primary hyperparathyroidism. *Skel Radiol* 1986; 15:85–95.
6. Silverberg SJ, Shane E, de la Cruz L, et al. Skeletal disease in primary hyperparathyroidism. *J Bone Mineral Res* 1989;4:283–291.
7. Delling G. Bone morphology in primary hyperparathyroidism—a quantitative and qualitative study of 391 cases. *Appl Pathol* 1987;5:147–159.
8. Parisien M, Silverberg SJ, Shane E, et al. The histomorphometry of bone in primary hyperparathyroidism: preservation of cancellous bone structure. *J Clin Endocrinol Metab* 1990;70:930–938.
9. Parisien M, Mellish RWE, Silverberg SJ, et al. Maintenance of cancellous bone connectivity in primary hyperparathy-
roidism: trabecular strut analysis. *J Bone Mineral Res* 1992;7:913–919.
10. Reeve J, Meunier PJ, Parsons JA, et al. Anabolic effect of human parathyroid hormone fragment on trabecular bone in involutional osteoporosis: a multicentre trial. *Br Med J* 1980;280:1340–1344.
11. Hesp R, Hulme P, Williams D, Reeve J. The relationship between changes in femoral bone density and calcium balance in patients with involutional osteoporosis treated with human parathyroid hormone fragment (hPTH 1–34). *Metab Bone Dis Rel Res* 1981;2:331–334.
12. Reeve J, Bradbeer JN, Arlot M, et al. hPTH 1–34 treatment of osteoporosis with added hormone replacement therapy: biochemical, kinetic and histological responses. *Osteoporosis Int* 1991;1:162–170.
13. Slovik DM, Rosenthal DI, Doppelt SH, et al. Restoration of spinal bone in osteoporostic men by treatment with human parathyroid hormone (1–34) and 1,25 dihydroxyvitamin D. *J Bone Mineral Res* 1986;1:377–381.
14. Tam C, Heersche JNM, Murray TM, Parsons JA. Parathyroid hormone stimulates the bond apposition rate independently of its resorptive action: differential effects of intermittent and continuous administration. *Endocrinology* 1982;110:506–512.
15. Tada K, Yamamuro T, Okumura H, Kasai R, Takahashi H. Restoration of axial and appendicular bone volumes by hPTH (1–34) in parathyroidectomized and osteopenic rats. *Bone* 1990;11:163–169.
16. Hock JM, Hummert JR, Boyce R, Fonseca J, Raisz LG. Resorption is not essential for the stimulation of bone growth by hPTH-(1–34) in rats in vivo. *J Bone Mineral Res* 1989;4:449–458.
17. Tam CS, Jones G, Heersche JNM. The effect of vitamin D restriction and repletion on bone apposition in the rat and its dependence on parathyroid hormone. *Endocrinology* 1981; 109:1448.
18. Hock JM, Fonseca J. Anabolic effect of human synthetic parathyroid hormone (1–34) depends on growth hormone. *Endocrinology* 1990;127:1804–1810.
19. Christiansen P, Steiniche T, Vesterby A, Mosekilde L, Hessov I, Melsen F. Primary hyperparathyroidism: iliac crest trabecular bone volume, structure, remodeling, and balance evaluated by histomorphometric methods. *Bone* 1992;13:41–49.
20. Parfitt AM, Kleerekoper M, Rao D, Stanciu J, Villanueva AR. Cellular mechanisms of cortical thinning in primary hyperparathyroidism (PHPT). *J Bone Mineral Res* 1987; 2(Suppl 1):384.
21. Parfitt AM. Surface specific bone remodeling in health and disease. In: Kleerekoper M, Krane SM, eds. *Clinical disorders of bone and mineral metabolism*. New York: Mary Ann Ciebgott, 1989;7–13.
22. Gaillard PJ. The influence of parathormone on the explanted radius of albino mouse embryos. *Proc Kon Ned Akad Wet* 1960;C64:25.
23. Liskova-Kiar M. Mode of action of cortisol on bone resorption in fetal rat fibrilae cultured in vitro. *Am J Anat* 1979;156:63.
24. Holtrop ME, Raisz LG. Comparison of the effects of 1,25 dihydroxycholecalciferol, Prostaglandin E$_2$ and osteoclast activating factor with parathyroid hormone on the ultrastructure of osteoclasts in cultural long bone of fetal rats. *Calcif Tissue Int* 1979;29:201.
25. King GJ, Holtrop ME, Raisz LG. The relation of ultrastructural changes in osteoclasts to resorption in bone cultures stimulated with parathyroid hormone. *Metab Bone Dis Rel Res* 1978;1:67.
26. Feldman RS, Krieger NS, Tashjian AH Jr. Effects of parathyroid hormone and calcitonin on osteoclast formation in vitro. *Endocrinology* 1980;107:1137–1143.
27. Kream BE, Rowe DW, Gworek S, Raisz LG. Parathyroid hormone alters collagen synthesis and procollagen mRNA levels in fetal rat calvaria. *Proc Natl Acad Sci USA* 1980;77:5654.

28. Heersche JNM, de Voogd van der Straaten WA. A radioautographic and radiometric analysis of the influence of parathyroid extract on the proline binding capacity of cultivated mouse radius rudiments. *Proc Kon Ned Akad Wet* 1965; C68:277.

29. Howard GA, Bottemiller BL, Turner RT, Rader JI, Baylink DJ. Parathyroid hormone stimulates bone formation and resorption in organ culture: evidence for a coupling mechanism. *Proc Natl Acad Sci USA* 1981;78:3204–3208.

30. Canalis E, Centrella M, Burch W, McCarthy TL. Insulin-like growth factor-1 mediates selective anabolic effects of parathyroid hormone in bone cultures. *J Clin Invest* 1989;83:60–65.

31. Kream BE, Petersen DN, Raisz LG. Parathyroid hormone blocks the stimulatory effect on insulin-like growth factor-I on collagen synthesis in cultured 21-day fetal rat calvariae. *Bone* 1990;11:411–415.

32. Spencer EM, Si EC, Liu CC, Howard GA. Parathyroid hormone potentiates the effect of insulin-like growth factor-I on bone formation. *Acta Endocrinol* 1989;121:435–442.

33. Aubin JE, Turksen K, Heersche JNM. Osteoblastic cell lineage. In: Noda M, ed. *Cellular and molecular biology of the bone.* In press.

34. Nijweide PJ, Van der Plas A, Olthof AA. Osteoblastic differentiation. In: *Cell and molecular biology of vertebrate hard tissues.* Evered D, Harnett S, eds. New York: John Wiley & Sons, 1988;61–72.

35. Aubin JE, Bellows CG, Turksen K, Liu F, Heersche JNM. Analysis of the osteoblast lineage and regulation of differentiation. In: *Chemistry and biology of mineralized tissues.* Slavkin H, Price P, eds. Amsterdam: Elsevier, 1992;267–276.

36. Bellows CG, Ishida H, Aubin JE, Heersche JNM. Parathyroid hormone reversibly suppresses the differentiation of osteoprogenitor cells into functional osteoblasts. *Endocrinology* 1990;127:3111–3116.

37. Nefussi J-R, Boy-Lefevre ML, Boulekbache H, Forest N. Mineralization in vitro of matrix formed by osteoblasts isolated by collagenase digestion. *Differentiation* 1985;29:160–168.

38. Bellows CG, Aubin JE, Heersche JNM, Antosz ME. Mineralized bone nodules formed in vitro from enzymatically released rat calvaria cell populations. *Calcif Tissue Int.* 1986;38:143–154.

39. Bhargava U, Bar-Lev M, Bellows CG, Aubin JE. Ultrastructural analysis of bone nodules formed in vitro by isolated fetal rat calvaria cells. *Bone* 1988;9:155–163.

40. Bellows CG, Aubin JE. Determination of numbers of osteoprogenitors present in isolated fetal rat calvaria cells in vitro. *Dev Biol* 1989;133:8–13.

41. McCarthy TL, Centrella M, Canalis E. Parathyroid hormone enhances the transcript and polypeptide levels of insulin-like growth factor I in osteoblast-enriched cultures from fetal rat bone. *Endocrinology* 1989;124:1247–1253.

42. Lowik CW, van der Pluijm G, Bloys H, et al. Parathyroid hormone (PTH) and PTH-like protein (PLP) stimulate interleukin-6 production by osteogenic cells: a possible role of interleukin-6 in osteoclastogenesis. *Biochem Biophys Res Commun* 1989;162:1546–1552.

43. Shen V, Cheng SL, Kohler NG, Peck WA. Characterization and hormonal modulation of IL-1 binding in neonatal mouse osteoblastlike cells. *J Bone Mineral Res* 1990;5:507–515.

44. Silve CM, Hradek GT, Jones AL, Arnaud CD. Parathyroid hormone receptor in intact embryonic chicken bone: characterization and cellular localization. *J Cell Biol* 1982; 94:379–386.

45. Rao LG, Murray TM, Heersche JNM. Immunohistochemical demonstration of parathyroid hormone binding to specific cell types in fixed rat bone tissues. *Endocrinology* 1983;113:805–810.

46. Rouleau MF, Mitchell J, Goltzman D. In vivo distribution of parathyroid hormone receptors in bone: evidence that a predominant osseous target cell is not the mature osteoblasts. *Endocrinology* 1988;123:187–191.

47. Rouleau MF, Mitchell J, Goltzman D. Characterization of the major parathyroid hormone target cell in the endosteal

metaphysis of rat long bones. *J Bone Mineral Res* 1990; 5:1043–1053.

48. Abou-Samra A-B, Juppner H, Force T, et al. Expression cloning of a common receptor for parathyroid hormone-related peptide from rat osteoblast-like cells: A single receptor stimulates intracellular accumulation of both cAMP and inositol trisphosphates and increases intracellular free calcium. *Proc Natl Acad Sci USA* 1992;89:2732–2736.

49. Urena P, Lee K, Weaver D, et al. PTH/PTHrP receptor mRNA expression as assessed by Northern blot and in situ hybridization. *J Bone Mineral Res* 1992;7:S119.

50. Bernier SM, Rouleau MF, Goltzman D. Biochemical and morphological analysis of the interaction of epidermal growth factor and parathyroid hormone with UMR 106 osteosarcome cells. *Endocrinology* 1991;128:2752–2760.

51. Turksen K, Grigoriadis AE, Heersche JNM, Aubin JE. Forskolin has biphasic effects on osteoprogenitor cell differentiation in vitro. *J Cell Physiol* 1990;142:61–69.

52. Heersche JNM, Aubin JE. Regulation of cellular activity of osteoblasts. In: Hall BK, ed. *The osteoblast and osteocyte.* Caldwell: The Telford Press, 1990;327–349.

53. Canalis E, McCarthy TL, Centrella M. The regulation of bone formation by local growth factors. *Bone Mineral Res* 1989;6:27–56.

54. Nijweide PJ, Burger EH, Feyen JHM. Cells of bone: proliferation, differentiation and hormonal regulation. *Physiol Rev* 1986;66:855–886.

55. Majeska RJ, Rodan SB, Rodan GA. Maintenance of parathyroid hormone response in clonal rat osteosarcoma lines. *Exp Cell Res* 1978;111:465–468.

56. Partridge NC, Alcorn D, Michelangeli VP, Ryan G, Martin TJ. Morphological and biochemical characterization of four clonal osteogenic sarcoma cells of rat origin. *Cancer Res* 1983;43:4308–4314.

57. Rodan SB, Imai Y, Thiede MA, et al. Characterization of a human osteosarcoma cell. 1987.

58. Franceschi RT, Romano PR, Park KY. Regulation of type I collagen synthesis by 1,25-dihydroxyvitamin D_3 in human osteosarcoma cells. *J Biol Chem* 1988;263:18938–18945.

59. McAllister RM, Gardner MB, Greene AE, Bradt C, Nichols WW, Landing BH. Cultivation in vitro of cells derived from a human osteosarcoma. *Cancer* 1971;27:397–402.

60. Kodama H, Amagai Y, Sudo H, Kasai S, Yamamoto S. Establishment of a clonal osteogenic cell line from newborn mouse calvaria. *Jpn J Oral Biol* 1982;23:899–904.

61. Aubin JE, Heersche JNM, Merrilees MJ, Sodek J. Isolation of bone cell clones with differences in growth hormone responses and extracellular matrix production. *J Cell Biol* 1982;92:452–462.

62. Guenther HL, Cecchini MG, Elford PR, Fleisch H. Effects of transforming growth factor type beta upon bone cell populations grown either in monolayer of semisolid medium. *J Bone Mineral Res* 1988;3:269–278.

63. Benayahu D, Fried A, Zipori D, Weintroub S. Subpopulations of marrow stromal cells share a variety of osteoblastic markers. *Calcif Tissue Int* 1991;49:202–207.

64. Partridge NC, Opie AL, Opie RT, Martin TJ. Inhibitory effects of parathyroid hormone on growth of osteogenic sarcoma cells. *Calcif Tissue Int* 1985;37:519–525.

65. Kano J, Sugimoto T, Fukase M, Fujita T. The activation of cAMP-dependent protein kinase is directly linked to the inhibition of osteoblast proliferation (UMR-106) by parathyroid hormone-related protein. *Biochem Biophys Res Commun* 1991;179:97–101.

66. Zajac JD, Kearns AK, Skurat RM, Kronenberg HM, Bringhurst FR. Regulation of gene transcription and proliferation by parathyroid hormone is blocked in mutant osteoblastic cells resistant to cyclic AMP. *Mol Cell Endocrinol* 1992; 87:69–77.

67. Finkelman RD, Mohan S, Linkhart TA, et al. PTH stimulates the proliferation of TE-85 human osteosarcoma cells by a mechanism not involving either increased cAMP or increased secretion of IGF-I, IGF-II or TGF beta. *Bone Mineral* 1992;16:89–100.

68. MacDonald BR, Gallagher JA, Russell RGG. Parathyroid

hormone stimulates the proliferation of cells derived from human bone. *Endocrinology* 1986;118;2445–2449.

69. Moseley JM, Suva LJ. Isolation, biochemistry and molecular biology of the PTH-related protein of malignant hypercalcaemia. In: Heersche JNM, Kanis JA, eds. *Bone and mineral research 7*. Amsterdam: Elsevier, 1990;175–208.

70. Murrills RJ, Stein LS, Fey CP, Dempster DW. The effects of parathyroid hormone (PTH) and PTH-related peptide on osteoclast resorption of bone slices in vitro: an analysis of pet size and the resorption focus. *Endocrinology* 1990;127: 2648–2653.

71. Lopez-Hilker S, Martin KJ, Sugimoto T, Slatopolsky E. Biologic activities of parathyroid hormone (1–34) and parathyroid hormone-related peptide (1–34) in isolated perfused rat femur. *J Lab Clin Med* 1992;119:738–743.

72. Rodan SB, Wesolowski G, Ianacone J, Thiede MA, Rodan GA. Production of parathyroid hormone-like peptide in a human osteosarcoma cell line: stimulation by phorbol esters and epidermal growth factor. *J Endocrinol* 1989;122:219–227.

73. Ohta S, Shigeno C, Yamamoto I, et al. Parathyroid hormone down-regulates the epidermal growth factor receptors in clonal osteoblastic mouse calvarial cells, MC3T3-E1: possible mediation by adenosine 3'5'-cyclic monophosphate. *Endocrinology* 1989;124:2419–2426.

74. Borst SE, Catherwood BD. Regulation of osteosarcoma EGF receptor affinity by phorbol ester and cyclic AMP. *J Bone Mineral Res* 1989;4:185–191.

75. Pizurki L, Rizzoli R, Caverzasio J, Bonjour JP. Stimulation by parathyroid hormone-related protein and transforming growth factor-alpha of phosphate transport in osteoblast-like cells. *J Bone Mineral Res* 1991;6:1235–1241.

76. van Leeuwen JP, Pols HA, Schilte JP, Visser TJ, Birkenhager JC. Modulation by epidermal growth factor of the basa 1,25(OH)₂D₃ receptor level and the heterologous up-regulation of the 1,25(OH)₂D₃ receptor in clonal osteoblast-like cells. *Calcif Tissue Int* 1991;49:35–42.

77. Gutierrez GE, Mundy GR, Manning DR, Hewlett EL, Katz MS. Transforming growth factor beta enhances parathyroid hormone stimulation of adenylate cyclase in clonal osteoblast-like cells. *J Cell Physiol* 1990;144:438–447.

78. Schneider HG, Michelangeli VP, Frampton RJ, et al. Transforming growth factor-beta modulates receptor binding of calciotropic hormones and G protein-mediated adenylate cyclase responses in osteoblast-like cells. *Endocrinology* 1992;131:1383–1389.

79. Katz MS, Gutierrez GE, Mundy GR, et al. Tumor necrosis factor and interleukin 1 inhibit parathyroid hormone-responsive adenylate cyclase in clonal osteoblast-like cells by down-regulating parathyroid hormone receptors. *J Cell Physiol* 1992;153:206–213.

80. Li NH, Ouchi Y, Okamoto Y, et al. Effect of parathyroid hormone on release of interleukin 1 and interleukin 6 from cultured mouse osteoblastic cells. *Biochem Biophys Res Commun* 1991;179:236–242.

81. Dewhirst FE, Ago JM, Peros WJ, Stashenko P. Synergism between parathyroid hormone and interleukin 1 in stimulating bone resorption in organ culture. *J Bone Mineral Res* 1987;2:127.

82. Sato K, Fujii Y, Kasono K, et al. Parathyroid hormone-related protein and interleukin-1 alpha synergistically stimulate bone resorption in vitro and increase the serum calcium concentration in mice in vivo. *Endocrinology* 1989;124: 2172–2178.

83. Hamilton JA, Lingelbach SR, Partridge NC, Martin TJ. Stimulation of plasminogen activator in osteoblast-like cells of bone resorbing hormones. *Biochem Biophys Res Commun* 1985;131:774.

84. Pfeilschifter J, Erdmann J, Schmidt W, et al. Differential regulation of plasminogen activator and plasminogen activator inhibitor by osteotropic factors in primary cultures of mature osteoblasts and osteoblast precursors. *Endocrinology* 1990; 126:703–711.

85. Fukumoto S, Allan EH, Yee JA, Gelehrter TD, Martin TJ. Plasminogen activator regulation in osteoblasts—parathy-

roid hormone inhibition of type-1 plasminogen activator inhibitor and its messenger RNA. *J Cell Physiol* 1992;152:346–355.

86. Liu F, Gupta AK, Aubin JE. Molecular analysis of osteoblast heterogeneity at the single cell level. *Bone Mineral* 1992;17(Suppl 1):198.

87. Scheven BAA, Kawilaragn-De Haas EWM, Wasserman EM, Nyweide PJ. Differentiation kinetics of osteoclasts in the periosteum of embryonic bones in vivo and in vitro. *Anat Rec* 1986;214:418.

88. Burger E, van der Meer J, van der Gevel J, et al. In vitro formation of osteoclasts from long term cultures of bone marrow mononuclear phagocytes. *J Exp Med* 1982;156:1604–1614.

89. Takahashi N, Yamana H, Yoshiki S, et al. Osteoclast-like cell formation and its regulation by osteotropic hormones in mouse narrow cultures. *Endocrinology* 1988;122:1373–1377.

90. Takashashi N, Akatsu T, Udagawa N, et al. Osteoblastic cells are involved in osteoclast formation. *Endocrinology* 1988;123:2600–2603.

91. Udagawa N, Nakahashi N, Akatsu T, et al. The bone marrow-derived stromal cell lines MC3T3-G2/PA6 and ST2 support osteoclast-like cell differentiation in cocultures with mouse spleen cells. *Endocrinology* 1989;125:1805–1813.

92. Avraham H, Scadden DT, Chi S, et al. Interaction of human bone marrow fibroblasts with megakaryocytes: Role of c-kit ligand. *Blood* 1992;80:1679–1684.

93. Suda T, Takahashi N, Martin TJ. Modulation of osteoclast differentiation. *Endocrinology* 1992;13:66–80.

94. Yamashita T, Asano K, Takahashi N, et al. Cloning of an osteoblastic cell line involved in the formation of osteoclast-like cells. *J Cell Physiol* 1990;145:587.

95. Akatsu T, Takahashi N, Udagawa N, et al. Role of prostaglandins in interleukin-1-induced bone resorption in mice in vitro. *J Bone Mineral Res* 1991;6:183–190.

96. Taylor L, Turksen K, Aubin JE, Heersche JNM. Osteoclast differentiation in co-cultures of a clonal chondrogenic cell line and mouse bone marrow cells. *Endocrinology* (in press).

97. Grigoriadis AE, Aubin JE, Heersche JNM. Effects of dexamethasone and vitamin D₃ on cartilage differentiation in a clonal chondrogenic cell population. *Endocrinology* 1989;125:2103–2110.

98. Greenfield EM, Horowitz MC, Gornik SA, Shaw SM, Khoury MA. The role of interleukin-6 production and cAMP signaling in stimulation of bone resorption by parathyroid hormone. In: *Proc 39th Ann Meeting Orthopaed Res Soc*, 1993;170.

99. Weir EC, Insogna KL, Horowitz MC. Osteoblast-like cells secrete granulocyte-macrophage colony-stimulating factor in response to parathyroid hormone and lipopolysaccharide. *Endocrinology* 1989;124:899–904.

100. Horowitz MC, Coleman DL, Ryaby JT, Einhorn TA. Osteotropic agents induce the differential secretion of granulocyte-macrophage colony-stimulating factor by the osteoblast cell line MC3T3-E1. *J Bone Mineral Res* 1989;4:911–921.

101. Takahashi N, Udagawa N, Akatsu T, et al. Deficiency of osteoclasts in osteopetrotic mice is due to a defect in the local microenvironment provided by osteoblastic cells. *Endocrinology* 1991;128:1792.

102. Felix R, Cecchini MG, Fleisch H. Macrophage colony stimulating factor restores in vivo bone resorption in the op/op osteopetrotic mouse. *Endocrinology* 1990;127:2592.

103. Yoshida H, Hayashi S, Kunisada T, et al. The murine mutation osteopetrosis is in the coding region of the macrophage colony stimulating factor gene. *Nature* 1990;345:442.

104. Kodama H, Yamasaki A, Nose M, et al. Congenital osteoclast deficiency in osteopetrotic (op/op) mice is cured by injections of macrophage colony-stimulating factor. *J Exp Med* 1991;173:269.

105. Shinar DM, Sato M, Rodan GA. The effect of hemopoietic growth factors on the generation of osteoclast-like cells in mouse bone marrow cultures. *Endocrinology* 1990;126:1728–1735.

106. Van de Wijngaert EP, Tas MC, van der Meer JWM, Burger

EH. Growth of osteoclast precursor-like cells from whole mouse bone marrow: inhibitory effect of CSF-1. *Bone Mineral* 1987;3:97.

107. Hattersley G, Chambers TJ. Effects of interleukin 3 and of granulocyte-macrophage and macrophage colony stimulating factors on osteoclast differentiation from mouse hemopoietic tissue. *J Cell Physiol* 1990;142:201–211.

108. Jilka RL, Hangoc G, Girasole G, et al. Increased osteoclast development after estrogen loss—mediation by interleukin-6. *Science* 1992;257:88–91.

109. Kurihara N, Bertolini D, Suda T, Akiyama Y, Roodman GD. IL-6 stimulates osteoclast-like multinucleated cell formation in long term human marrow cultures by inducing IL-1 release. *J Immunol* 1990;144:4226–4230.

110. Hakeda Y, Hiura K, Sato T, et al. Existence of parathyroid hormone binding sites on murine hemopoietic blast cells. *Biochem Biophys Res Commun* 1989;163:1481.

111. Teti A, Rizzoli R, Zambonin-Zallone A. Parathyroid hormone binding to cultured avian osteoclasts. *Biochem Biophys Res Commun* 1991;174:1217–1222.

112. Agarwala N, Gay CV. Specific binding of parathyroid hormone to living osteoclasts. *J Bone Mineral Res* 1992;7:531–539.

113. Duong LT, Grasser W, DeHaven PA, Sato M. Parathyroid hormone receptors identified on avian and rat osteoclasts. *J Bone Mineral Res* 1990;5:S203.

114. Rouleau MF, Warshawsky H, Goltzman D. Parathyroid hormone binding in vivo to renal, hepatic, and skeletal tissues of the rat using a radioautographic approach. *Endocrinology* 1986;118:919–931.

The Parathyroids, edited by J.P. Bilezikian, M.A. Levine, and R. Marcus. Raven Press, Ltd., New York © 1994.

CHAPTER 6

Autocrine and Paracrine Functions of Parathyroid Tissue

Kazushige Sakaguchi

THE CONCEPTS OF AUTOCRINE AND PARACRINE CONTROL

Sporn and Todaro (1) defined *autocrine secretion* as a mechanism by which a cell secretes a hormone-like substance for which the cell itself has functional external receptors. The autocrine concept originated from the observation that cancer cells are less dependent on exogenous hormones or growth factors for growth than normal cells. However, secretion of autocrine growth factors may occur as a normal, transient physiological process during repair of tissue injury, during normal embryological development, or under circumstances when particularly rapid growth of cells is needed (2). The autocrine mechanism in normal cell physiology is a transient, regulated system as compared to the persistent, unregulated autocrine system observed in cancer cells.

Excess secretion of growth factors is only one means of autocrine stimulation of cell growth. Other autocrine mechanisms to account for unregulated growth of malignant cells are increases in receptor number or affinity, alteration in receptor structure or function, amplification of postreceptor signal transduction mechanisms, or failure of ligand binding to reduce the number of cell surface receptors (2). Each of these autocrine mechanisms has been described in cancer cells or transformed cells, but their roles in normal cell physiology have not yet been studied extensively.

The concept of paracrine regulation involves the secretion by one cell type of factors, which include hormones, growth factors, and cytokines that diffuse through the extracellular space to their ultimate cellular targets (3). Usually the type of cell that produces a factor is different from the cell that responds to the factor. However, for cells with similar or perhaps identical characteristics and in confined space (e.g., endocrine organs), both autocrine and paracrine mechanisms can be operative simultaneously. The paracrine function is well illustrated in endocrine organs, with their rich network of capillaries into which hormone is secreted. Endothelial cells that line the capillaries were once regarded as simple diffusion barriers, but they have been proved to have important paracrine functions (4–6). The synthesis of growth factor by the endothelial cell, for example, is believed to affect in a paracrine fashion the neighboring hormone-producing parenchymal cells.

There is reason to believe that the parathyroids are likely to be regulated by autocrine and paracrine mechanisms more significantly than other endocrine organs because the parathyroids are not controlled by the higher order hypothalamic–pituitary axis of the other endocrine glands (7). Extracellular calcium concentration is the principal physiological regulator of parathyroid cell function (8).

Modulation of this ionic regulation and independent influence are potential key areas of autocrine and paracrine control. Until recently, hypotheses based on these concepts were difficult to test because clonal lines of functional parathyroid cells were unavailable. Establishment of clonal lines of rat parathyroid epithelial cells that are functional and bovine parathyroid endothelial cells (5,9) has moved this area of investigation forward in the past 5 years. This chapter summarizes what is currently known about the several autocrine and paracrine systems in parathyroid tissue

K. Sakaguchi: Bone Research Branch, National Institute of Dental Research, National Institutes of Health, Bethesda, Maryland 20892.

that have been discovered to have important roles in cell growth and hormone secretion.

CLONAL RAT PARATHYROID EPITHELIAL CELLS (PT-r) AND BOVINE PARATHYROID ENDOTHELIAL CELLS (BPE-1)

The clonal rat parathyroid cell line (PT-r cells) was established by serial cloning of parathyroid cells from young adult rats that had been maintained on a low-calcium, high-phosphorus diet. The PT-r cell line retains several characteristics of differentiated parathyroid chief cells; however, it does not secrete parathyroid hormone (PTH). Rather, the calciotropic peptide released by this cell line is parathyroid hormone-related protein (PTHrP). The observation that PTHrP may be the principal calciotropic peptide secreted from fetal parathyroid glands (10) suggests that this cell line represents an early stage in parathyroid gland development. Release of PTHrP is inversely regulated by extracellular calcium concentrations, similar to the mechanism for release of PTH in mature parathyroid cells. Other mature, differentiated characteristics of this cell line are regulation of intracellular calcium concentration by physiological concentrations of extracellular calcium (K. Sakaguchi et al., unpublished data), increased production of cAMP in response to secretin, and regulation of cell growth by calcium (9).

Cloning of the bovine parathyroid endothelial cell line (BPE-1 cells) was accomplished by use of a culture medium that favors endothelial cell growth and by methods that provide a selective advantage for growth of endothelial cells in primary culture (5). The BPE-1 cell line retains differentiated endothelial cell characteristics, including production of factor VIII-related antigen and the ability to take up exogenous acetylated low-density lipoproteins and PTH. It also shows morphological features that are characteristic of endothelial cells. BPE-1 cells have been maintained in culture by serial passage for >40 months without showing signs of senescence. Cell growth is not suppressed by high concentrations of extracellular calcium.

AUTOCRINE AND PARACRINE FUNCTIONS AFFECTING PARATHYROID CELL GROWTH

Controversies About Parathyroid Cell Growth
Calcium Regulation

There is little controversy about the principal, controlling role for calcium in PTH synthesis and secretion (8) (see the chapter by Brown). The importance of calcium as a regulator of parathyroid cell growth, however, is much more uncertain. In part, the uncertainty is due to differences in the experimental systems used

for the studies. In an in vivo study, chickens fed a low-, normal-, or high-calcium diet, constant in phosphorus, for 2 weeks showed significantly different parathyroid weights (11). Parathyroid weight was inversely related to the dietary calcium concent. Serum levels of 1,25-dihydroxyvitamin D [1,25-$(OH)_2$D] were not measured but were assumed to be high in the low-calcium group. In a second in vivo study, in which both calcium and vitamin D in the diet were varied, workers did not assess parathyroid weight but instead used a unique technique to determine parathyroid cell number (12). Thyroparathyroid tissue from rats was digested by collagenase and the dispersed cells were separated by size using flow cytometry. The smaller cells in the first peak were parathyroid cells; the larger cells in the second peak were thyroid cells. The number of parathyroid cells was 1.7-fold greater in the animals kept on a vitamin D- and calcium-deficient diet for 3 weeks [serum calcium 4.4 mg/dl; serum 1,25-$(OH)_2$D 90.7 ± 13 pg/ml] than in those on normal diet [serum calcium 10.4 mg/dl; serum 1,25-$(OH)_2$D 154 ± 20 pg/ml; $P < 0.05$ for differences in both calcium and 1,25-$(OH)_2$D]. Since 1,25-$(OH)_2$D is regarded to be a potent independent regulator of parathyroid cell growth (13,14), the data do not substantiate a direct role for serum calcium in the regulation of parathyroid cell proliferation. In another study, the effects of hypercalcemia induced by a low-phosphorus diet and the effects of hypocalcemia induced by a low-calcium diet were analyzed morphologically in weanling rats. Hypercalcemic rats showed a reduction in parathyroid cell number and cell volume that was proportional to the reduction in body weight; hypocalcemic rats showed an increase in parathyroid size that was due to parathyroid cell hypertrophy rather than hyperplasia (15,16). Serum 1,25-$(OH)_2$D levels, although not measured, could well have affected the results in these studies. In a different study (14), parathyroid hyperplasia, rather than hypertrophy, was observed to develop in a uremic rat model in which both serum calcium and 1,25-$(OH)_2$D levels were significantly reduced. The hyperplastic parathyroid cells were unchanged in protein/DNA ratio in size of nuclei or in overall size.

Organ cultures permitted a distinction between the effects of vitamin D and those of calcium on parathyroid growth. In 1963, Raisz (17) reported that parathyroid cells both from chick embryos and from adult rats respond to *low* calcium with an increase in the ratio of cytoplasmic-to-nuclear volume, indicating cytoplasmic growth. Parathyroid cells from chick embryos also increased their mitotic rate (17). Lee and Roth (18) also demonstrated a direct effect of calcium on rat parathyroid cell proliferation in organ cultures. Thymidine incorporation was stimulated maximally by total calcium concentrations between 0.9 and 1.3 mM and was suppressed by higher calcium concentrations.

Autoradioagraphs of sections of parathyroid glands after labeling with ^{3}H-thymidine also showed more than a doubling of the thymidine index in chief cells that had been maintained in a low-calcium medium.

Primary cultures of parathyroid cells established from various animals have also been used to study questions related to calcium regulation of growth (19–26). There is agreement among several studies that parathyroid cells in primary culture quickly dedifferentiate over a few days and lose calcium responsiveness. Cells different from hormone-secreting epithelial cells (e.g., endothelial cells) overgrow these epithelial cells and predominate thereafter. These parathyroid-derived endothelial cells take up PTH (5) and stain positively by immunocytochemistry using an anti-PTH antibody, a potentially confusing observation with regard to using this technique to identify hormone-producing cells. Several groups have examined the effect of extracellular calcium on parathyroid cell proliferation in primary culture (19,21–24). Only one study, by Brandi et al. (19), has succeeded in maintaining differentiated characteristics of bovine parathyroid cells (>140 population doublings) using serum-free medium and shown negative mitogenic effect of calcium. All other reports have failed to show an effect of ambient calcium on parathyroid cell growth. Four groups (21,22,27,28) tested the effect of 1,25-$(OH)_2$D on parathyroid cell proliferation and found an inhibitory effect of the steroid. The inhibitory effect of 1,25-$(OH)_2$D, however, does not seem to be specific to parathyroid parathyroid cells (14,29).

In summary, the effect of extracellular calcium on parathyroid cell growth has been examined by several groups using three different systems: in vivo systems, organ cultures, and primary cell cultures. Each system has its own strengths and weaknesses. Because 1,25-$(OH)_2$D and calcium influence each other in in vivo systems, it is impossible to distinguish their unique effects. Parathyroid cells in primary culture have a general tendency toward dedifferentiation over a few days, so this system may not be appropriate for evaluation of cell growth. Organ culture may be a good system in which to evaluate growth regulation of an entire parathyroid gland. However, it is difficult to examine regulatory mechanisms, in that the whole gland contains several different cell types. Therefore, no consensus has been reached on the effect of calcium on parathyroid cell growth, nor has a putative mechanism for growth regulation by calcium been clarified.

Autocrine and Paracrine Regulation of Parathyroid Cell Growth: Fibroblast Growth Factors

FGFs and Their Receptors (Review)

Fibroblast growth factors (FGFs) may be part of an autocrine and paracrine system in the parathyroids that is responsible, at least in part, for the regulation of parathyroid cell growth by calcium. Before describing the relationship of FGF to the autocrine and paracrine system in parathyroid tissue, FGF biology and molecular biology are reviewed briefly.

The family of FGFs currently comprises seven polypeptides, which vary in size from 155 to 268 amino acids and share 33–65% amino acid sequence homology. Because they all bind to heparin tightly, the FGFs are also called heparin-binding growth factors (30). Acidic FGF (aFGF) and basic FGF (bFGF) were the first FGFs to be purified, cloned, and sequenced (31,32). Both aFGF and bFGF are predicted to have 155 amino acids in their complete forms, but purified preparations exhibit microheterogeneity due to post-translational processing and to extraction artifacts. The gene for human aFGF is located between 5q31.3 and 5q33.2 (32); the gene for human bFGF is located on chromosome 4 (33). The proteins encoded by the two genes share 55% amino acid identity. Both aFGF and bFGF lack classical consensus signal peptide sequences that, if present, could account for their secretion (32,34). In addition to release of these growth factors following cell lysis, an alternative release mechanism is suspected (35,36).

The other members of the FGF family are *int-2*, *K-fgf/hst-1*, FGF-5, FGF-6, and keratinocyte growth factor (KGF). Readers are referred to recent reviews for more complete discussion of these FGFs (30,37–39). Unlike aFGF and bFGF, these other FGFs do have signal peptide sequences. In adult mice, expression of the product of the *int-2* protooncogene (40) is limited to the brain. During embryogenesis, there is tight developmental control over its expression in different tissues. Virus activation of *int-2* gene expression has been implicated in the formation of mouse mammary tumors. The *int-2* gene product seems to be a poor mitogen for cells that respond to aFGF and bFGF. The *K-fgf/hst-1* protooncogene was discovered in Kaposi's sarcoma (41) and in human stomach cancers (42). Its expression in normal mice is detectable only during very early embryonal development (43). Inappropriate levels of gene expression, rather than gene mutation, lead to transformation. The transforming capacity of *K-fgf/hst-1* appears to require the presence of the signal peptide (44). Human FGF-5 was originally identified as an oncogene product (45). FGF-5 expression seems to be regulated spatially and temporally in the developing mouse embryo (43). Low levels of expression have been detected in adult mouse brain. The FGF-6 gene was originally isolated using the *hst* gene as a probe (46). FGF-6 is expressed in heart and skeletal muscle during embryogenesis and in the adult. Transformation of NIH3T3 cells transfected by the FGF-6 gene is dependent on the presence of the signal peptide. The newest member of the FGF family is KGF, which was purified from dermal fibroblasts.

Unlike all other FGFs, KGF lacks mitogenic activity on NIH3T3 cells and is specifically mitogenic to epithelial cells (47).

Receptors for fibroblast growth factors appear to belong to two distinct families: high-affinity glycoproteins with tyrosine kinase activity, and low-affinity heparan sulfate proteoglycans. Four genes have been identified for the high-affinity receptors. They constitute a unique class of membrane-anchored tyrosine kinases. Based on analysis of the coding sequences of four cloned human FGF receptors, their genes encode highly homologous FGF receptors that share 56–92% amino acid sequence identity and similar predicted structures (Fig. 1). All of the fundamental structural features are conserved among the other species. The FGF receptor genes encode proteins of 800–822 amino acids. The proteins are predicted to have an 18–24-amino-acid signal peptide, an extracellular domain of 346–356 amino acids, a transmembrane domain of 21 amino acids, and a cytoplasmic domain of 410–425 amino acids. The extracellular domain of all FGF receptor tyrosine kinases contains three immunoglobu-

lin-like domains. An "acidic box" consisting of four to eight adjacent acidic amino acids is located between the first and second immunoglobulin-like domains. The cytoplasmic domain consists of a 74–81 residue juxtamembrane region; the kinase domain, which contains a hydrophilic 14 amino acid insertion, and a C-terminal tail of 59–69 residues. The diversity of FGF receptors is further increased as a result of alternative splicing or alternative cleavage of their primary transcripts (48).

A clone for FGF receptor 1 (FGFR1) was originally isolated from a human endothelial cell cDNA library by low-stringency screening using the kinase domain of v-fms as a probe (49). FGFR1 was initially identified as a novel tyrosine kinase, an fms-like gene (flg). Its identity as an FGF receptor was not recognized until the chicken bFGF receptor was purified and its gene was cloned (50). Among the numerous variants of FGFR1 receptors, it is notable that the first immunoglobulin-like domain is dispensable and that variation in the third immunoglobulin-like domain determines specificity of FGF binding (51,52). The first one-half of the third immunoglobulin-like domain of FGFR1 may be followed by either of two alternative exons, IIIb and IIIc (Fig. 1) or by eight amino acids and a termination codon. L6 skeletal muscle myoblasts that have been transfected with mouse FGFR1 cDNA containing exon IIIb express receptors that display ~50-fold less affinity for bFGF than for aFGF. By contrast, receptors expressed by cells transfected with FGFR1 containing exon IIIc show equivalent affinity for aFGF and bFGF. Some cells co-express all of the three forms of the FGFR1 mRNA.

FGFR2 was cloned as a novel receptor tyrosine kinase by screening a mouse liver expression cDNA library in λgt11 with antiphosphotyrosine antibodies. This screening strategy resulted in the isolation of a partial cDNA clone encoding a *bacterial expressed kinase (bek)* (53). The identification of human and chicken flg as an FGF receptor and its homology to the mouse bek sequence suggested that bek was likely to be a receptor for an FGF receptor. A number of FGFR2 variants were found that were similar to those for FGFR1. The first immunoglobulin-like domain is dispensable. As is the case for FGFR1, variants are produced by alternative splicing of exons IIIb and IIIc encoding the second one-half of the third immunoglobulin-like domain (Fig. 1). FGFR2 forms containing exon IIIb, which were recognized as KGF receptors (54,55), display high affinity for both aFGF and KGF but not for bFGF. By contrast, FGFR2 forms with exon IIIc show high affinity for aFGF and bFGF but not for KGF. Use of exon IIIb or exon IIIc is tissue specific, and a given cell will express only one of the two forms of the FGFR2 mRNA. Exon IIIb seems to be used in epithelial-derived cells and chicken embryo fibroblasts (56).

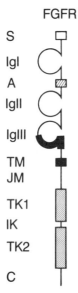

FIG. 1. Schematic presentation of fibroblast growth factor receptor (FGFR) protein structure for the four distinct FGFRs reported thus far. For FGFR1 and FGFR2, many variations generated by alternative splicing have been reported. Among these, the second one-half of the third immunoglobulin-like domain (shown as a *bold line*), which is encoded by either exon IIIb or IIIc, is important in determining the ligand specificity (described in the text). Exon IIIa at this position in FGFR1 produces a secreted form of the FGFR. Exon IIIa is not known in FGFR2. The following structural features are identified in the figure: S, signal peptide (*open box*); IgI, II and III, immunoglobulin-like domains; A, acidic box (*hatched box*); TM, transmembrane domain (*solid box*); JM, juxtamembrane domain; TK1 and 2, tyrosine kinase domains (*stippled boxes*); IK, interkinase domain; C, carboxyl terminal domain.

FGFR3 was cloned by screening a chicken embryo fibroblast expression cDNA library with antiphosphotyrosine antibodies and was originally named *chicken embryo kinase 2 (cek2)* (57,58). A human homolog of cek2 has also been cloned (59,60). No splicing variants of FGFR3 have been reported. When expressed in *Xenopus* oocytes by microinjection, FGFR3 is activated by both aFGF and bFGF as measured by $^{45}Ca^{2+}$ efflux assay (59). FGFR4 was cloned from human K-562 erythroleukemia cells (60,61) and lung (62). No splicing variants have been found. FGFR4 binds to aFGF but not to bFGF.

Heparin is well known to bind tightly to aFGF and bFGF (63,64) and to potentiate the biological activity of aFGF (65,66). This interaction between heparin and FGFs is the basis for an efficient affinity chromatography method for the purification of these growth factors (63,64). Heparin protects the growth factors from degradation (67–71), stabilizes the tertiary structure of aFGF (72,73), and increases the apparent affinity of the aFGF receptor for the ligands (73). Heparan sulfate (HS) glycosaminoglycan, a homolog of heparin that is located on the cell surface or in the extracellular matrix, binds FGFs with low affinity (74–77), protects FGFs from proteolytic degradation (9,69,70,78), and is regarded as an extracellular reservoir for FGFs (76,78–82). Recently, several groups have demonstrated that heparin or HS glycosaminoglycan is required for high-affinity binding of bFGF to FGF receptors encoded by flg and bek (83–85). The mechanism for these observations is unknown. In one proposed mechanism, interaction of bFGF with cell-surface HS glycosaminoglycan changes the conformation of bFGF so that it can interact with the high-affinity receptor. Alternatively, it is possible that cell-surface HS glycosaminoglycan modulates the structure of the high-affinity receptor, allowing it to bind bFGF. This might suggest a dual receptor system, composed of a classical protein-type receptor and a lower affinity glycosaminoglycan-type receptor, is necessary for bFGF binding (86). It is not currently known if this concept can be generalized for all FGF members and all FGF receptors.

Fibroblast Growth Factors

The development of clonal parathyroid epithelial cells and endothelial cells gave us an opportunity to develop model systems for cell–cell interaction in parathyroid tissue. We used whole parathyroid tissue as a control to ensure that clones represent the characteristics of the original cells. In a morphological examination, rat parathyroid epithelial cells (PT-r cells), originally polygonal cells, change their appearance to elongated, fibroblast-like cells after many passages or after keeping cells in confluency for a long period without trypsinization (87). This resembles the shape change of the cells bearing bFGF receptors after pro-

longed exposure to exogenously added bFGF (37). Northern blot hybridization with cDNA probes specific to aFGF, bFGF, and KGF revealed that epithelial cells (PT-r cells) express only aFGF and that capillary endothelial cells express bFGF and a small amount of KGF (88) (KGF data unpublished). The amount of aFGF mRNA in PT-r cells is regulated by calcium, as is the amount of aFGF peptide, with more mRNA and peptide at lower calcium concentrations. Cells produce aFGF and retain the peptide by intracellular or extracellular attachment; aFGF is not detectable in the culture medium by a Western blot analysis using a specific anti-aFGF antibody. This is true for almost all cells synthesizing aFGF or bFGF (30).

The receptors expressed by PT-r cells bear have at least 20-fold higher affinity for aFGF than for bFGF (89). Affinity-labeling experiments show that the receptors can be divided into two subgroups of 130 kDa and 150 kDa. A subset of the 150 kDa receptor seems to carry HS glycosaminoglycan chains. Digestion with heparitinase, an enzyme that digests HS glycosaminoglycans, shifts a part of the 150 kDa receptor mass to 130 kDa. aFGF receptors cross-linked with ^{125}I-aFGF bind to an anion-exchange column and are eluted with 0.5 M sodium chloride, which is a typical elution concentration for HS proteoglycans, but the receptor is different from the major HS proteoglycans that PT-r cells bear on their cell surface (89,90). Scatchard analysis shows that there are two binding sites, of K_d 4 pM and 110 pM, for aFGF. Both these are high-affinity receptors based on the K_d values reported for other cells (75,76). Interestingly, cells lose the higher affinity binding site (K_d 4 pM) after treatment with heparitinase. Therefore, we speculate that the receptor with HS glycosaminoglycan is responsible for the higher affinity binding and that the receptor has two requirements for high affinity binding: (a) a peptide region that promotes receptor specificity and affinity and (b) an HS glycosaminoglycan, that stabilizes ligand tertiary structure, reduces proteolytic attack, and enhances affinity as described above. Betaglycan or a transforming growth factor-β (TGFβ) type III receptor (91,92) is another growth factor receptor/proteoglycan containing chondroitin and HS glycosaminoglycans. However, betaglycan does not require any glycosaminoglycans for ligand binding (93). In this sense, the aFGF receptor in PT-r cells is unique.

We found that the aFGF receptors apparently translocate as a function of changing extracellular calcium concentrations, with more receptors in a cell surface ligand-accessible compartment at low calcium concentrations (88). They translocated with a half-time ($t_{1/2}$) of 15–20 min when cells were washed with a buffer containing EGTA. The translocation is temperature dependent (no apparent translocation occurs at 4°C) and is independent of *de novo* protein synthesis (no effect of cycloheximide on the translocation). The nature of the apparent translocation is unknown. Mechanisms other than a simple translocation, such as chemical modification of aFGF receptor or change in cell surface structure, might be involved. Scatchard analysis of ^{125}I-aFGF binding to PT-r cells in monolayer culture shows that the receptor with K_d 110 pM increases its number of binding sites without changing affinity after decreasing extracellular calcium concentrations. The receptor with K_d 4 pM does not change its affinity or number of binding sites for aFGF. In accordance with these results, thymidine incorporation and cell growth are stimulated under low calcium conditions and are suppressed by anti-aFGF neutralizing antibody at low calcium concentrations. From these observations, an aFGF autocrine system including the apparent translocation of aFGF receptors and the regulation of aFGF production may explain, at least in part, the mechanism by which calcium regulates parathyroid cell growth (Fig. 2).

We have also characterized two major cell surface HS proteoglycans, HSPG-I and HSPG-II, which are believed to act as low-affinity binding sites for FGF in PT-r cells (90) (Fig. 3). HSPG-I has a mass of ~160 kDa, with a single HS chain (~12 kDa) and a core protein of ~150 kDa, including oligosaccharides. HSPG-II has a mass of ~170 kDa, with three or four HS chains (~30 kDa each) and a core protein of 70–80 kDa, including oligosaccharides. The distribution of proteoglycans, examined by digesting the molecules with trypsin, which cleaves core proteins, after metabolic labeling with ^{35}S-sulfate and counting ^{35}S radioactivity incorporated into the proteoglycans, was dramatically influenced by extracellular calcium concentration (94); at low calcium levels, 50–60% of the HS proteoglycans are trypsin-accessible, while ~20% are accessible at high calcium levels. Similar results were obtained by treatment with heparitinase. Since HSPG-II contains >90% of the radioactivity incorporated into proteoglycans in all cell compartments when ^{35}S-sulfate is used as a metabolic precursor, these data reflect primarily, if not exclusively, the metabolism of the HSPG-II molecules.

Cell-associated HS proteoglycans are redistributed in response to changing extracellular calcium concentrations, with a $t_{1/2}$ <4 min; more HS proteoglycans appear on the cell surface as extracellular calcium concentration decreases (94). Furthermore, HS proteoglycans on the cell surface recycle in low-calcium environments, with an average cycling time of 9.2 min, to and from an intracellular compartment approximately ten times before their degradation. They are not recycled under high calcium conditions. The distribution but not the biosynthesis of HS proteoglycans is regulated by extracellular calcium concentrations. We have partially categorized three subpopulations of the HS proteoglycans by use of pulse-chase and trypsin-treatment experiments. The 10 min pulse-chase

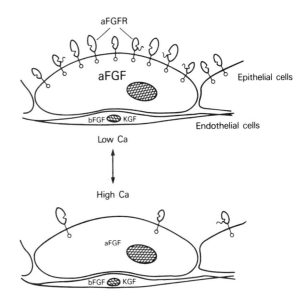

FIG. 2. Schematic representation of FGF biology in parathyroid tissue. In parathyroid epithelial cells, more aFGF receptors are expressed on the cell surface and more aFGF is synthesized under low rather than high ambient calcium conditions. The change of receptor number occurs with a half time of 15–20 min. Contents of cytosolic mRNA for aFGF do not change until 6–8 hr after the change in ambient calcium concentration. aFGF, acidic fibroblast growth factor; bFGF, basic fibroblast growth factor; KGF, keratinocyte growth factor; aFGFR, acidic fibroblast growth factor receptor.

experiments define the following three kinetically distinct proteoglycan subpopulations (94) (Fig. 4). Subpopulation 1 has a long half-life (>4 hr) on the cell surface or in a pericellular matrix and makes up 10–15% of the total HS proteoglycans. Subpopulation 2, accounting for at least 50% of the total HS proteoglycans, is most apparent in cultures maintained in low calcium. Molecules in this subpopulation cycle between the cell surface and an intracellular compartment. Subpopulation 2 has a functional life of at least 90 min before depolymerization in lysosomes, a process that occurs sometime between 120 and 240 min of chase. Under high calcium conditions, the cycling between the cell surface and an intracellular compartment does not occur. When extracellular calcium concentration is changed, however, a proportion of HS proteoglycans similar to that of subpopulation 2 rapidly ($t_{1/2}$ ~4 min) changes its distribution to reflect the final calcium concentration. Subpopulation 3, ~25% of the total newly synthesized HS proteoglycans, is secreted into the medium with kinetics that distinguish it from subpopulations 1 and 2. The proportion of this subpopulation secreted in a high-calcium medium (2.1 mM Ca^{2+}) is about one-half that secreted in a low-calcium medium (0.05 mM Ca^{2+}). When the extracellular calcium concentration is decreased, however, there is a rapid secretion of the remaining HS proteoglycans from this subpopulation.

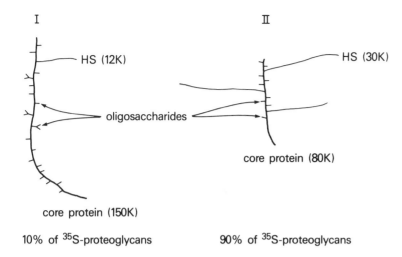

FIG. 3. Proteoglycans in PT-r cells. PT-r cells bear two major proteoglycans, both of which are heparan sulfate (HS) proteoglycans. They are termed *HSPG-I* and *HSPG-II*. These HS proteoglycans were isolated by two consecutive ion-exchange chromatography steps and analyzed by gel filtration, SDS-PAGE, and specific enzyme and chemical reactions after metabolic labeling with ^{35}S-sulfate and ^{3}H-glucosamine as precursors. For more details, see Yanagishita et al. (90). HSPG-I and HSPG-II make up 10% and 90% of all the ^{35}S-labeled proteoglycans, respectively. HS, heparan sulfate glycosaminoglycan chain. Molecular sizes of the core proteins and those of the glycosaminoglycan chains are expressed in daltons in parentheses.

Summary and Speculation on Fibroblast Growth Factor Biology in the Parathyroids

Three members of an FGF family, aFGF, bFGF, and KGF, are expressed by parathyroid tissue; aFGF is synthesized by epithelial cells, bFGF and KGF by endothelial cells. The amount of KGF mRNA appears to be low compared to that of aFGF or bFGF. Since the receptors borne by epithelial hormone-producing cells have high affinity for aFGF but low affinity for bFGF (affinity for KGF not tested), an aFGF autocrine system is likely to play an important role in the physiology of parathyroid tissue.

The production of aFGF increases under low calcium conditions. High-affinity aFGF receptors and HS proteoglycans, low-affinity FGF receptors, are translocated or redistributed in response to a change in extracellular calcium concentration, with more receptors in a cell-surface ligand-accessible compartment at lower calcium conditions. These responses to calcium shifts by the epithelial cells accentuate the prominence of the aFGF autocrine system in the normal parathyroid physiology, especially in the growth regulation by calcium. This seems to be the first example of autocrine stimulation by increased receptor number as a transient, normal physiological mechanism.

The kinetics and the metabolism of major HS proteoglycans have been well studied. They can be divided into three subpopulations as shown in Fig. 4. The mechanism and physiological significance of the subpopulation 2 proteoglycan recycling and redistribution are unknown, but the recycling may help to move aFGFs from the inside to the outside of parathyroid cells, or *vice versa*, and to facilitate their binding to high-affinity receptors. The redistribution following a change in extracellular calcium concentration may function to redistribute aFGF between the cell surface and an intracellular compartment to regulate the availability of aFGF to high-affinity receptors. Calcium seems to be a specific stimulator of the proteoglycan

movement among other divalent cations in PT-r cells (94,95). The mechanism of the apparent translocation of the high-affinity receptors remains to be elucidated, but it appears to be different from that of the redistribution of proteoglycans, since the rate of change for the high-affinity receptors is much slower than that for proteoglycans in both directions. Furthermore, the ap-

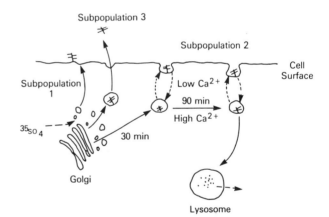

FIG. 4. Schematic model for HS proteoglycans of PT-r cells in each of the subpopulations. HS proteoglycans in subpopulation 2 have a "programmed" metabolism. Approximately 30 min after completion of the sulfation in a trans-Golgi compartment, they appear in the sequestered (high Ca^{2+}) or cycling (low Ca^{2+}) compartment, where they reside for at least 90 min. Subsequently, sometime between 120 and 240 min of chase, they are completely degraded in lysosomes. Thus these HS proteoglycans follow membrane flow from trans-Golgi to lysosomes. HS proteoglycans in subpopulation 3 are secreted into the medium, with more secretion at lower extracellular Ca^{2+}. Whether some of the HS proteoglycans in this population are ultimately degraded in lysosomes if they are not secreted is at present unknown. Likewise, it is not known to what extent their protein and complex carbohydrate constituents differ from HS proteoglycans in the other subpopulations. Less is known about subpopulation 1. It appears on the cell surface or in a closely associated extracellular matrix with similar kinetics to the entry of subpopulation 2 HS proteoglycans into the cycling compartment at low extracellular Ca^{2+}. (Modified from ref. 127 with permission.)

parent translocation of high-affinity receptors is temperature dependent (88), but the redistribution of proteoglycans does not seem to be inhibited completely by low temperature (96).

One mechanism to be considered is the redistribution of proteoglycans as a possible means of influencing the binding of aFGF to its high-affinity aFGF receptors. For FGFR1–bFGF interaction, HS glycosaminoglycan or heparin appears to be essential for the binding, as was described above (84,85). In PT-r cells, a smaller number of HS glycosaminoglycans/proteoglycans on the cell surface at high calcium (90,94) may influence the binding of aFGF to the high-affinity receptors, if the same mechanism as for the FGFR1–bFGF interaction is applicable to the interaction between aFGF and the high-affinity receptors. However, addition of heparin, which can substitute for HS glycosaminoglycan, does not affect the binding of aFGF to the high-affinity receptors at high calcium concentrations (88), indicating that the apparent translocation of high-affinity receptors is not explainable by the mere redistribution of the proteoglycans. The dependence of aFGF–aFGF receptor interaction on heparin or HS glycosaminoglycan remains to be examined further.

The high-affinity aFGF receptor with HS glycosaminoglycan(s) is a unique receptor in that the carbohydrate component gives higher affinity to the peptide component of the receptor. However, HS glycosaminoglycan appears not to be on all of the aFGF receptors/core proteins, based on the observations that heparitinase does not shift all the affinity-labeled 150 kDa receptor mass to 130 kDa and that Scatchard analysis shows two high-affinity binding sites for aFGF, heparitinase-sensitive and -insensitive sites. The aFGF receptors with HS glycosaminoglycan(s), which are responsible for the higher affinity binding sites ($K_d = 4$ pM), do not appear to be translocated after changing the extracellular calcium concentrations (88). These receptors may be related to the basal growth of the cells.

Other Autocrine and Paracrine Growth Factors

Epidermal growth factor (EGF) receptors have been analyzed by studying the binding of radioiodinated EGF to crude membrane fractions from parathyroid tumors (97). It was found that seven of ten solitary parathyroid adenomas showed no EGF binding and three showed only low-affinity EGF binding. In two patients with multiple adenomas and one patient with hyperplastic parathyroid glands secondary to renal failure, high-affinity EGF binding sites were found. In one patient with persistent hyperparathyroidism following a successful renal transplant, only a low-affinity EGF binding site was found. The production of

EGF from the parathyroid tumors was not described in that paper (97).

We have examined the expression of mRNA for growth factors and their receptors in PT-r cells by Northern blot hybridization (98). Transforming growth factor-α (TGFα), TGFβ, platelet-derived growth factor (PDGF) β-chain, and the EGF receptor are expressed in PT-r cells. Their functions remain to be examined.

AUTOCRINE AND PARACRINE FUNCTIONS AFFECTING PARATHYROID HORMONE SECRETION

Endothelin in the Parathyroids

Endothelin 1 (ET-1) is a potent vasoconstrictor originally purified from the conditioned medium of cultured porcine aortic endothelial cells (99). Initially, ET-1 was believed to act as a voltage-sensitive calcium channel agonist. Later, it became apparent that ET-1 binds to a specific cell surface receptor linked to phospholipase C rather than binding to a dihydropyridine-sensitive calcium channel complex (100). However, since ET-1 activates dihydropyridine-sensitive, voltage-dependent L-type calcium channels without depolarization of the membrane potential (101), the mechanism of activation remains to be elucidated. Four distinct endothelin isoforms have been identified; ET-1, ET-2, ET-3, and vasoactive intestinal contractor or endothelin-β (81,99,102–104). Endothelin displays a panoply of biological functions. It causes contraction of smooth muscles in blood vessels, trachea, intestine, and uterus (105–110); it also affects the release of many hormones, including gonadotropin, prolactin, substance P, oxytocin, vasopressin, aldosterone, atrial natriuretic peptide (ANP), renin, and norepinephrine (111–121). Among these, the inhibition of renin secretion by ET-1 from juxtaglomerular cells, ET-1-induced stimulation of catecholamine release from adrenomedullary cells, and ET-1-mediated substance P release in isolated spinal cord have also been reported to be dependent on extracellular calcium concentrations and sensitive to calcium channel antagonists derived from dihydropyridine (100).

Two distinct but homologous (about 63% amino acid identity) cDNAs for ET receptors have been cloned (122) and designated as ET_A and ET_B receptors. They consist of seven domains of hydrophobic amino acid residues, which are likely to represent transmembrane regions. The proteins exhibit significant sequence and topographical similarity to G protein-coupled receptors. The order of affinity of ETs for ET_A receptor is ET-1 > ET-2 >> ET-3. Affinity for ET-1 is ~100 times higher than that for ET-3. The ET_B receptor shows equal affinity for all three ETs and for sarafo-toxins.

The parathyroid glands are highly vascularized endocrine organs, and their function is regulated physiologically by calcium. Voltage-dependent calcium channels have been implicated as one of the mechanisms whereby parathyroid hormone secretion from epithelial cells is regulated (123,124). In view of these anatomical and functional characteristics, we were interested in examining endothelins and their receptors in parathyroid cells (125).

We examined preproendothelin mRNA expression in different bovine tissues and found that the parathyroid glands and the lung are the two organs expressing the largest amounts of preproendothelin mRNA (Fig. 5A). Furthermore, we found evidence from mRNA content and immunoreactivity that this peptide is synthesized by rat parathyroid epithelial cells (PT-r cells) and bovine parathyroid chief cells but not by bovine parathyroid endothelial cells (BPE-1 cells) (Fig. 5B). The ET synthesized in the parathyroid cells is identified as ET-1 by high-performance liquid chromatography (HPLC) analysis and by radioimmunoassay. Prepro-ET-1 mRNA expression by PT-r cells and ET-1 peptide production are regulated by calcium. Shifts in extracellular calcium, either from high to low concentrations or *vice versa,* elicit a similar evanescent increase in expression of mRNA with a peak at 1 hr.

Currently, no physiological explanation is apparent for this biphasic effect of calcium. Synthesis of the peptide seems to be controlled by mRNA expression, and peptide in the medium appears to be continuously degraded or taken up by the cells, because its concentration in the medium shows a time course similar to that of mRNA expression. PT-r cells also bear a single class of receptors highly specific for ET-1, with >100-fold lower affinity for ET-3 and sarafotoxin. The receptor is probably an ET_A receptor based on these binding inhibition data. The facile regulation of ET concentrations in the medium by shifts in extracellular calcium concentration and possible autocrine regulation by ET-1 suggest that this peptide may mediate, at least in part, effects of calcium on the parathyroid system. BPE-1 cells do not express ETs but express receptors for ET.

Eguchi et al. (126) reported expression of ET_A and ET_B receptor mRNAs and ET-1 mRNA in human parathyroid adenomas. They also reported suppression of basal PTH release from dispersed parathyroid adenoma cells by ET-1, although the effect of ET on normal parathyroid cells remains to be examined. Much work remains to be done to understand the function of the ET autocrine system in the parathyroids, to uncover possible regulation of ET receptors by calcium, and to find any modification of signal transduction by calcium.

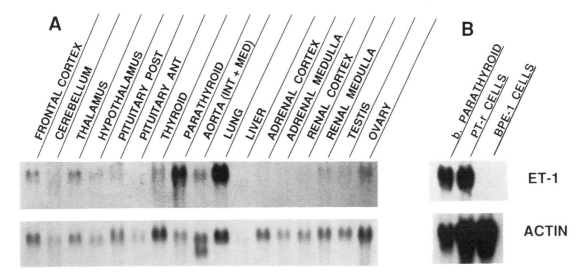

FIG. 5. A: RNA was extracted form the bovine tissues indicated. Total RNA (20 μg) from each tissue was fractionated in a 1% agarose/formaldehyde gel, blotted onto a nylon membrane, and hybridized with an antisense ET-1 RNA probe or with an actin cDNA probe. B: Total RNA was extracted from bovine parathyroid glands, PT-r cells, or BPE-1 cells, and poly(A)⁺ RNA was selected with an oligo-d(T) column. Poly(A)⁺ RNA (15 μg) was fractionated, blotted onto a nylon membrane, and hybridized with probes (125). The parathyroid glands and the lung are the two organs expressing the largest amounts of prepro-ET-1 mRNA. The differentiated endothelial cells cloned from bovine parathyroid cells (BPE-1 cells) did not express the mRNA, whereas rat parathyroid epithelial cells (PT-r cells) or chief cells from bovine glands are replete with prepro-ET-1 mRNA and the peptide itself [from immunohistochemical studies (125) not shown here].

ACKNOWLEDGMENT

The author is grateful to Dr. S.J. Marx for critical reading of the manuscript.

REFERENCES

1. Sporn MB, Todaro GJ. Autocrine secretion and malignant transformation of cells. *N Engl J Med* 1980;303:878–880.
2. Sporn MB, Roberts AB. Introduction: autocrine, paracrine and endocrine mechanisms of growth control. *Cancer Surv* 1985;4:627–632.
3. Dockray GJ. Evolutionary relationships of the gut hormones. *Fed Proc* 1979;38:2295–2301.
4. Banerjee DK, Ornberg RL, Youdim MBH, Heldman E, Pollard HB. Endothelial cells from bovine adrenal medulla develop capillary-like growth patterns in culture. *Proc Natl Acad Sci USA* 1985;82:4702–4706.
5. Brandi ML, Ornberg RL, Sakaguchi K, et al. Establishment and characterization of a clonal line of parathyroid endothelial cells. *FASEB J* 1990;4:3152–3158.
6. Mizrachi Y, Lelkes PI, Ornberg RL, Goping G, Pollard HB. Specific adhesion between pheochromocytoma (PC12) cells and adrenal medullary endothelial cells in co-culture. *Cell Tissue Res* 1989;256:356–372.
7. Wison JD, Foster DW. Hormones and hormone action. In: Wison JD, Foster DW, eds. *Williams textbook of endocrinology, 8th ed.* Philadelphia: W.B. Saunders, 1992;1–8.
8. Aurbach GD, Marx SJ, Spiegel AM. Parathyroid hormone, calcitonin, and the calciferols. In: Wison JD, Foster DW, eds. *Williams textbook of endocrinology, 8th ed.* Philadelphia: W.B. Saunders, 1992;1397–1476.
9. Sakaguchi K, Santora A, Zimering M, Curcio F, Aurbach GD, Brandi ML. Functional epithelial cell line cloned from rat parathyroid glands. *Proc Natl Acad Sci USA* 1987;84:3269–3273.
10. MacIsaac RJ, Caple IW, Danks JA, et al. Ontogeny of parathyroid hormone-related protein in the ovine parathyroid gland. *Endocrinology* 1991;129:757–764.
11. Mueller GL, Anast CS, Breitenbach RP. Dietary calcium and ultimobrachial body and parathyroid gland in the chicken. *Am J Physiol* 1970;218:1718–1722.
12. Naveh-Many T, Silver J. Regulation of parathyroid hormone gene expression by hypocalcemia, hypercalcemia, and vitamin D in the rat. *J Clin Invest* 1990;86:1313–1319.
13. Slatopolsky E, Weerts C, Thielan J, Horst R, Harter H, Martin KJ. Marked suppression of secondary hyperparathyroidism by intravenous administration of 1,25-dihydroxycholecalciferol in uremic patients. *J Clin Invest* 1984;74:2136–2143.
14. Szabo A, Merke J, Beier E, Mall G, Ritz E. 1,25(OH)₂ vitamin D₃ inhibits parathyroid cell proliferation in experimental uremia. *Kidney Int* 1989;35:1049–1056.
15. Wernerson A, Svensson O, Reinholt F. Parathyroid cell number and size in hypercalcemic rats: a stereologic study employing modern unbiased estimators. *J Bone Miner Res* 1989;4:705–713.
16. Wernerson A, Widholm SM, Svensson O, Reinholt FP. Parathyroid cell number and size in hypocalcemic young rats. *APMIS* 1991;99:1096–1102.
17. Raisz LG. Regulation by calcium of parathyroid growth and secretion in vitro. *Nature* 1963;197:1115–1116.
18. Lee M, Roth SI. Effect of calcium and magnesium on deoxyribonucleic acid synthesis in rat parathyroid glands in vitro. *Lab Invest* 1975;33:72–79.
19. Brandi ML, Fitzpatrick LA, Coon HG, Aurbach GD. Bovine parathyroid cells: cultures maintained for more than 140 population doublings. *Proc Natl Acad Sci USA* 1986;83:1709–1713.
20. Hornicek FJ, Reiss E, Malinin TI, Malinin GI. Establishment of primary cell cultures from human and canine parathyroid gland explants. *Bone Mineral* 1988;4:157–165.
21. Ishimi Y, Russel J, Sherwood LM. Regulation by calcium and 1,25-(OH)₂D₃ of cell proliferation and function of bovine parathyroid cells in culture. *J Bone Mineral Res* 1990;5:755–760.
22. Kremer R, Bolivar I, Goltzman D, Hendy GN. Influence of calcium and 1,25-dihydroxycholecalciferol on proliferation and proto-oncogene expression in primary cultures of bovine parathyroid cells. *Endocrinology* 1989;125:935–941.
23. LeBoff MS, Rennke HG, Brown EM. Abnormal regulation of parathyroid cell secretion and proliferation in primary cultures of bovine parathyroid cells. *Endocrinology* 1983;113:277–284.
24. MacGregor RR, Sarras MP Jr., Houle A, Cohn DV. Primary monolayer cell culture of bovine parathyroids: effect of calcium, isoproterenol and growth factors. *Mol Cell Endocrinol* 1983;30:313–328.
25. Matalanis G, Clunie GJ, Whitehead RH. A technique for the in vitro culture of human parathyroid gland tissue. *Aust NZ J Surg* 1988;58:407–411.
26. Nygren P, Larsson R, Gylfe E, et al. Development of abnormal parathyroid cell function during monolayer culture and its relation to cellular hypertrophy and proliferation. *Acta Path Microbiol Immunol Scand [A]* 1987;95:207–214.
27. Brandi ML, Carter AD, Fitzpatrick LA, Sakaguchi K, Marx SJ, Aurbach GD. Vitamin D₃ regulation of growth and differentiation of bovine parathyroid cells in culture. In: Cohn DV, Martin TJ, Meunier PJ, eds. *Calcium regulation and bone metabolism: basic and clinical aspects,* Vol 9. Amsterdam: Elsevier Science Publishers, 1987;238–242.
28. Nygren P, Larsson R, Johansson H, Ljunghall S, Rastad J, Akerstrom G. 1,25(OH)₂D₃ inhibits hormone secretion and proliferation but not functional dedifferentiation of cultured bovine parathyroid cells. *Calcif Tissue Int* 1988;43:213–218.
29. Bikle DD. Clinical counterpoint: vitamin D: new actions, new analogs, new therapeutic potential. *Endocr Rev* 1992;13:765–784.
30. Burgess WH, Maciag T. The heparin-binding (fibroblast) growth factor family of proteins. *Annu Rev Biochem* 1989;58:575–606.
31. Abraham JA, Mergia A, Whang JL, et al. Nucleotide sequence of a bovine clone encoding the angiogenic protein, basic fibroblast growth factor. *Science* 1986;233:545–548.
32. Jaye M, Howk R, Burgess W, et al. Human endothelial cell growth factor: cloning, nucleotide sequence, and chromosomal localization. *Science* 1986;233:541–545.
33. Mergia A, Eddy R, Abraham JA, Fiddes JC, Shows TB. The genes for basic and acidic fibroblast growth factors are on different human chromosomes. *Biochem Biophys Res Commun* 1986;138:644–651.
34. Abraham JA, Whang JL, Tumolo A, et al. Human basic fibroblast growth factor: nucleotide sequence and genomic organization. *EMBO J* 1986;5:2523–2528.
35. Mignatti P, Morimoto T, Rifkin DB. Basic fibroblast growth factor released by single, isolated cells stimulates their migration in an autocrine manner. *Proc Natl Acad Sci USA* 1991;88:11007–11011.
36. Mignatti P, Morimoto T, Rifkin DB. Basic fibroblast growth factor, a protein devoid of secretory signal sequence, is released by cells via a pathway independent of the endoplasmic reticulum–Golgi complex. *J Cell Physiol* 1992;151:81–93.
37. Gospodarowicz D, Ferrara N, Schweigerer L, Neufeld G. Structural characterization and biological functions of fibroblast growth factor. *Endocr Rev* 1987;8:96–113.
38. Korhonen J, Partanen J, Eerola E, et al. Five FGF receptors with distinct expression patterns. *EXS* 1992;61:91–100.
39. Robinson CJ. Multiple receptors found for the growing FGF family. *Trends Pharmacol Sci* 1991;12:123–124.
40. Dickson C, Peters G. Potential oncogene product related to growth factors. *Nature* 1987;326:833.
41. Delli Bovi P, Curatora AM, Kern FG, Greco A, Ittmann M, Basilico C. An oncogene isolated by transfection of Kaposi's

sarcoma DNA encodes a growth factor that is a member of the FGF family. *Cell* 1987;50:729–737.

42. Taira M, Yoshida T, Miyagawa K, Sakamoto H, Terada M, Sugimura T. cDNA sequence of human transforming gene hst and identification of the coding sequence required for transforming activity. *Proc Natl Acad Sci USA* 1987;84: 2980–2984.

43. Hebert JM, Basilico C, Goldfarb M, Haub O, Martin GR. Isolation of cDNA encoding four mouse FGF family members and characterization of their expression pattern during embryogenesis. *Dev Biol* 1990;138:454–463.

44. Talarico D, Basilico C. The K-*fgf*/*hst* oncogene induces transformation through an autocrine mechanism that requires extracellular stimulation of the mitogenic pathway. *Mol Cell Biol* 1991;11:1138–1145.

45. Zhan X, Bates B, Hu X, Goldfarb M. The human FGF-5 oncogene encodes a novel protein related to fibroblast growth factors. *Mol Cell Biol* 1988;8:3487–3495.

46. Marics I, Adelaide J, Raybaud F, et al. Characterization of the *HST*-related *FGF.6* gene, a new member of the fibroblast growth factor gene family. *Oncogene* 1989;4:335–340.

47. Finch PW, Rubin JS, Miki T, Ron D, Aaronson SA. Human KGF is FGF-related with properties of a paracrine effector of epithelial cell growth. *Science* 1989;245:752–755.

48. Jaye M, Schlessinger J, Dionne CA. Fibroblast growth factor receptor tyrosine kinase: molecular analysis and signal transduction. *Biochim Biophys Acta* 1992;1135:185–199.

49. Ruta M, Howk R, Ricca G, et al. A novel protein tyrosine kinase gene whose expression is modulated during endothelial cell differentiation. *Oncogene* 1988;3:9–15.

50. Lee PL, Johnson DE, Cousens LS, Fried VA, Williams LT. Purification and complementary DNA cloning of a receptor for basic fibroblast growth factor. *Science* 1989;245:57–60.

51. Johnson DE, Lee PL, Lu J, Williams LT. Diverse forms of a receptor for acidic and basic fibroblast growth factors. *Mol Cell Biol* 1990;10:4728–4736.

52. Werner S, Duan D-SR, de Vries C, Peters KG, Johnson DE, Williams LT. Differential splicing in the extracellular region of fibroblast growth factor receptor 1 generates receptor variants with different ligand-binding specificities. *Mol Cell Biol* 1992;12:82–88.

53. Kornbluth S, Paulson KS, Hanafusa H. Novel tyrosine kinase identified by phosphotyrosine antibody screening of cDNA libraries. *Mol Cell Biol* 1988;8:5541–5544.

54. Miki T, Bottaro DP, Fleming TP, et al. Determination of ligand-binding specificity by alternative splicing: two distinct growth factor receptors encoded by a single gene. *Proc Natl Acad Sci USA* 1992;89:246–250.

55. Miki T, Fleming TP, Bottaro DP, Rubin JS, Ron D, Aaronson SA. Expression cDNA cloning of the KGF receptor by creation of a transforming autocrine loop. *Science* 1991;251:72–75.

56. Sato M, Kitazawa T, Iwai T, et al. Isolation of chicken-*bek* and a related gene: identification of structural variation in the ligand-binding domains of the FGF-receptor family. *Oncogene* 1991;6:1279–1283.

57. Pasquale EB. A distinctive family of embryonic protein-tyrosine kinase receptors. *Proc Natl Acad Sci USA* 1990; 87:5812–5816.

58. Pasquale EB, Singer SJ. Identification of a developmentally regulated protein-tyrosine kinase by using anti-phosphotyrosine antibodies to screen cDNA expression library. *Proc Natl Acad Sci USA* 1989;86:5449–5453.

59. Keegan K, Johnson DE, Williams LT, Hayman MJ. Isolation of an additional member of the fibroblast growth factor receptor family, FGFR-3. *Proc Natl Acad Sci USA* 1991; 88:1095–1099.

60. Partanen J, Makela TP, Alitalo R, Lehvaslaiho H, Alitalo K. Putative tyrosine kinases expressed in K-562 human leukemia cells. *Proc Natl Acad Sci USA* 1990;87:8913–8917.

61. Partanen J, Makela TP, Eerola E, et al. FGFR-4, a novel acidic fibroblast growth factor receptor with a distinct expression pattern. *EMBO J* 1991;10:1347–1354.

62. Holtrich U, Brauninger A, Strebhardt K, Rubsamen-Waig-

mann H. Two additional protein-tyrosine kinases expressed in human lung: fourth member of the fibroblast growth factor receptor family and an intracellular protein-tyrosine kinase. *Proc Natl Acad Sci USA* 1991;88:10411–10415.

63. Maciag T, Mehlman T, Friesel R, Schreiber AB. Heparin binds endothelial cell growth factor, the principal endothelial cell mitogen in bovine brain. *Science* 1984;225:932–935.

64. Shing Y, Folkman J, Sullivan R, Butterfield C, Murray J, Klagsbrun M. Heparin affinity: purification of a tumor-derived capillary endothelial cell growth factor. *Science* 1984; 223:1296–1299.

65. Lobb R, Sasse J, Sullivan R, et al. Purification and characterization of heparin-binding endothelial cell growth factors. *J Biol Chem* 1986;261:1924–1928.

66. Thornton SC, Mueller SN, Levine EM. Human endothelial cells: use of heparin in cloning and long-term serial cultivation. *Science* 1983;222:623–625.

67. Damon DH, Lobb RR, D'Amore PA, Wagner JA. Heparin potentiates the action of acidic fibroblast growth factor by prolonging its biological half-life. *J Cell Physiol* 1989;138: 221–226.

68. Gospodarowicz D, Cheng J. Heparin protects basic and acidic FGF from inactivation. *J Cell Physiol* 1986;128:475–484.

69. Lobb RR. Thrombin inactivates acidic fibroblast growth factor but not basic fibroblast growth factor. *Biochemistry* 1988;27:2572–2578.

70. Rosengart TK, Johnson WV, Friesel R, Clark R, Maciag T. Heparin protects heparin-binding growth factor-1 from proteolytic inactivation in vitro. *Biochem Biophys Res Commun* 1988;152:432–440.

71. Sommer A, Rifkin DB. Interaction of heparin with human basic fibroblast growth factor: protection of the angiogenic protein from proteolytic degradation by a glycosaminoglycan. *J Cell Physiol* 1989;138:215–220.

72. Jaye M, Burgess WH, Shaw AB, Drohan WN. Biological equivalence of natural bovine and recombinant human alpha-endothelial cell growth factors. *J Biol Chem* 1987;262: 16612–16617.

73. Schreiber AB, Kenney J, Kowalski WJ, Friesel R, Mehlman T, Maciag T. Interaction of endothelial cell growth factor with heparin: characterization by receptor and antibody recognition. *Proc Natl Acad Sci USA* 1985;82:6138–6142.

74. Bashkin P, Doctrow S, Klagsbrun M, Svahn CM, Folkman J, Vlodavsky I. Basic fibroblast growth factor binds to subendothelial extracellular matrix and is released by heparitinase and heparin-like molecules. *Biochemistry* 1989;28: 1737–1743.

75. Kan M, DiSorbo D, Hou J, Hoshi H, Mansson PE, McKeehan WL. High and low affinity binding of heparin-binding growth factor to a 130-kDa receptor correlates with stimulation and inhibition of growth of a differentiated human hepatoma cell. *J Biol Chem* 1988;263:11306–11313.

76. Moscatelli D. High and low affinity binding sites for basic fibroblast growth factor on cultured cells: absence of a role for low affinity binding in the stimulation of plasminogen activator production by bovine capillary endothelial cells. *J Cell Physiol* 1987;131:123–130.

77. Vigny M, Ollier-Hartmann MP, Lavigne M, et al. Specific binding of basic fibroblast growth factor to basement membrane-like structures and to purified heparan sulfate proteoglycan of the EHS tumor. *J Cell Physiol* 1988;137:321–328.

78. Saksela O, Moscatelli D, Sommer A, Rifkin DB. Endothelial cell-derived heparan sulfate binds basic fibroblast growth factor and protects it from proteolytic degradation. *J Cell Biol* 1988;107:743–751.

79. Folkman J and Klagsbrun M. Angiogenic factors. *Science* 1987;235:442–447.

80. Moscatelli D. Metabolism of receptor-bound and matrix-bound basic fibroblast growth factor by bovine capillary endothelial cells. *J Cell Biol* 1988;107:753–759.

81. Saida K, Mitsui Y, Ishida N. A novel peptide, vasoactive intestinal constrictor, of a new (endothelin) peptide family. *J Biol Chem* 1989;264:14613–14616.

82. Vlodavsky I, Folkman J, Sullivan R, et al. Endothelial cell-derived basic fibroblast growth factor: Synthesis and deposition into subendothelial extracellular matrix. *Proc Natl Acad Sci USA* 1987;84:2292–2296.

83. Mansukhani A, Dell'Era P, Moscatelli D, Kornbluth S, Hanafusa H, Basilico C. Characterization of the murine BEK fibroblast growth factor (FGF) receptor: activation by three members of the FGF family and requirement for heparin. *Proc Natl Acad Sci USA* 1992;89:3305–3309.

84. Rapraeger AC, Krufka A, Olwin BB. Requirement of heparan sulfate for bFGF-mediated fibroblast growth and myoblast differentiation. *Science* 1991;252:1705–1708.

85. Yayon A, Klagsbrun M, Esko JD, Leder P, Ornitz DM. Cell surface, heparin-like molecules are required for binding of basic fibroblast growth factor to its high affinity receptor. *Cell* 1991;64:841–848.

86. Klagsbrun M, Baird A. A dual receptor system is required for basic fibroblast growth factor activity. *Cell* 1991;67:229–231.

87. Sakaguchi K, Ikeda K, Curcio F, Aurbach GD, Brandi ML. Subclones of a rat parathyroid cell line (PT-r): regulation of growth and production of parathyroid hormone-related peptide (PTHRP). *J Bone Mineral Res* 1990;5:863–869.

88. Sakaguchi K. Acidic fibroblast growth factor autocrine system as a mediator of calcium-regulated parathyroid cell growth. *J Biol Chem* 1992;267:24554–24562.

89. Sakaguchi K, Yanagishita M, Takeuchi Y, Aurbach GD. Identification of heparan sulfate proteoglycan as a high affinity receptor for acidic fibroblast growth factor (aFGF) in a parathyroid cell line. *J Biol Chem* 1991;266:7270–7278.

90. Yanagishita M, Brandi ML, Sakaguchi K. Characterization of proteoglycans synthesized by a rat parathyroid cell line. *J Biol Chem* 1989;264:15714–15720.

91. Cheifetz S, Andres JL, Massague J. The transforming growth factor-β receptor type III is a membrane proteoglycan domain structure of the receptor. *J Biol Chem* 1988;263:16984–16991.

92. Segarini PR, Seyedin SM. The high molecular weight receptor to transforming growth factor-β contains glycosaminoglycan chains. *J Biol Chem* 1988;263:8366–8370.

93. Cheifetz S, Massague J. Transforming growth factor-β (TGF-β) receptor proteoglycan. Cell surface expression and ligand binding in the absence of glycosaminoglycan chain. *J Biol Chem* 1989;264:12025–12028.

94. Takeuchi Y, Sakaguchi K, Yanagishita M, Aurbach GD, Hascall VC. Extracellular calcium regulates distribution and transport of heparan sulfate proteoglycans in a rat parathyroid cell line. *J Biol Chem* 1990;265:13661–13668.

95. Takeuchi Y, Yanagishita M, Hascall VC. Effects of MgCl$_2$ on the release and recycling of heparan sulfate proteoglycans in a rat parathyroid cell line. *Arch Biochem Biophys* 1992;298:371–379.

96. Takeuchi Y, Yanagishita M, Hascall VC. Recycling of transferrin receptors and heparan sulfate proteoglycans in a rat parathyroid cell line. *J Biol Chem* 1992;267:14685–14690.

97. Duh QY, Gum ET, Sancho JJ, Levine KE, Raper SE, Clark OH. Epidermal growth factor receptors in parathyroid tumors. *J Surg Res* 1986;46:569–573.

98. Sakaguchi K, Brandi ML, Aurbach GD. Expression of mRNAs for growth factors and their receptors in parathyroid epithelial and capillary endothelial cells. In: *The Endocrine Society 71st Annual Meeting Program & Abstracts.* 1989;471.

99. Yanagisawa M, Kurihara H, Kimura S, et al. A novel potent vasoconstrictor peptide produced by vascular endothelial cells. *Nature* 1988;332:411–415.

100. Yanagisawa M, Masaki T. Molecular biology and biochemistry of the endothelins. *Trends Pharmacol Sci* 1989;10:374–378.

101. Goto K, Kasuya Y, Matsuki N, et al. Endothelin activates the dihydropyridine-sensitive, voltage-dependent Ca^{2+} channel in vascular smooth muscle. *Proc Natl Acad Sci USA* 1989;86:3915–3918.

102. Inoue A, Yanagisawa M, Kimura S, et al. The human endothelin family: Three structurally and pharmacologically distinct isopeptides predicted by three separate genes. *Proc Natl Acad Sci USA* 1989;86:2863–2867.

103. Itoh Y, Yanagisawa M, Ohkubo S, et al. Cloning and sequence analysis of cDNA encoding the precursor of a human endothelium-derived vasoconstrictor peptide, endothelin: identity of human and porcine endothelin. *FEBS Lett* 1988;231:440–444.

104. Yanagisawa M, Inoue A, Ishikawa T, et al. Primary structure, synthesis, and biological activity of rat endothelin, an endothelium-derived vasoconstrictor peptide. *Proc Natl Acad Sci USA* 1988;85:6964–6967.

105. Auguet N, Delaflotte S, Chabrier PE, Pirotzky E, Clostre R, Braquet P. Endothelin and Ca^{++} agonist Bay K8644: different vasoconstrictive properties. *Biochem Biophys Res Commun* 1988;156:186–192.

106. Eglen RM, Michel AD, Sharif NA, Swank SR, Whiting RL. The pharmacological properties of the peptide, endothelin. *Br J Pharmacol* 1989;97:1297–1307.

107. Marsden PA, Dansuluri NR, Brenner BM, Ballermann BJ, Brock TA. Endothelin action on vascular smooth muscle involves inositol triphosphate and calcium mobilization. *Biochem Biophys Res Commun* 1989;158:86–93.

108. Tomobe Y, Miyauchi T, Saito A, et al. Effects of endothelin on the renal artery from spontaneously hypertensive and Wistar Kyoto rays. *Eur J Pharmacol* 1988;152:373–374.

109. Uchida Y, Ninomiya H, Saotome H, et al. Endothelin, a novel vasoconstrictor peptide, as potent bronchoconstrictor. *Eur J Pharmacol* 1988;154:227–228.

110. Withrington PG, deNucci G, Vane JRJ. Endothelin-1 causes vasoconstriction and vasodilation in the blood perfused liver of the dog. *J Cardiovasc Pharmacol* 1989;13:S209–S210.

111. Boarder M, Marriott DB. Characterization of endothelin-1 stimulation of catecholamine release from adrenal chromaffin cells. *J Cardiovasc Pharmacol* 1989;13:S223–S224.

112. Calvo JJ, Gonzalez R, DeCarvalho LF, et al. Release of substance P from rat hypothalamus and pituitary by endothelin. *Endocrinology* 1990;126:2288–2295.

113. Cozza EN, Gomez-Sanchez CE, Foecking MF, Chiou S. Endothelin binding to cultured calf adrenal zona glomerulosa cells and stimulation of aldosterone secretion. *J Clin Invest* 1989;84:1032–1035.

114. Fukuda Y, Hirata Y, Yoshimi H, et al. Endothelin is a potent secretagogue for atrial natriuretic peptide in cultured rat atrial myocytes. *Biochem Biophys Res Commun* 1988;155:167–172.

115. Hu JR, Berninger UG, Lang RE. Endothelin stimulates atrial natriuretic peptide (ANP) release from rat atria. *Eur J Pharmacol* 1988;158:177–178.

116. Morishita R, Higaki J, Ogihara T. Endothelin stimulates aldosterone biosynthesis by dispersed rabbit adreno-capsular cells. *Biochem Biophys Res Commun* 1989;160:628–632.

117. Rakugi H, Nakamaru N, Saito J, Higaki J, Ogihara T. Endothelin inhibits renin release from isolated rat glomeruli. *Biochem Biophys Res Commun* 1988;155:1244–1247.

118. Samson WK, Skala KD, Alexander BD, Huang F-LS. Pituitary site of action of endothelin: selective inhibition of prolactin release in vitro. *Biochem Biophys Res Commun* 1990;169:737–743.

119. Stojilkovic SS, Merelli F, Iida T, Krsmanovic LZ, Catt KJ. Endothelin stimulation of cytosolic calcium and gonadotropin secretion in anterior pituitary cells. *Science* 1990;248:1663–1666.

120. Takagi N, Matsuoka K, Atarashi K, Yagi S. Endothelin: a new inhibitor of renin release. *Biochem Biophys Res Commun* 1988;157:1164–1168.

121. Yoshizawa T, Shinmi O, Giaid A, et al. Endothelin: a novel peptide in the posterior pituitary system. *Science* 1990;247:462–464.

122. Sakurai T, Yanagisawa M, Masaki T. Molecular characterization of endothelin receptors. *Trends Pharmacol Sci* 1992;13:103–108.

123. Fitzpatrick LA, Brandi ML, Aurbach GD. Control of PTH secretion is mediated through calcium channels and is

blocked by pertussis toxin treatment of parathyroid cells. *Biochem Biophys Res Commun* 1986;138:960–965.

124. Fitzpatrick LA, Chin H, Nirenberg M, Aurbach GD. Antibodies to an α subunit of skeletal muscle calcium channels regulate parathyroid cell secretion. *Proc Natl Acad Sci USA* 1988;85:2115–2119.

125. Fuji Y, Moreira JE, Orlando C, et al. Endothelin as an autocrine factor in the regulation of parathyroid cells. *Proc Natl Acad Sci USA* 1991;88:4235–4239.

126. Eguchi S, Hirata Y, Imai T, et al. Endothelin receptors in human parathyroid gland. *Biochem Biophys Res Commun* 1992;184:1448–1455.

127. Takeuchi Y, Sakaguchi K, Yanagishita M, Hascall VC. Heparan sulfate proteoglycans on rat parathyroid cells recycle in low Ca^{2+} medium. *Biochem Soc Trans* 1990;18:816–818.

The Parathyroids, edited by J.P. Bilezikian,
M.A. Levine, and R. Marcus. Raven Press, Ltd.,
New York © 1994.

CHAPTER 7

Chemistry and Biology of Chromogranin A (Secretory Protein-I) of the Parathyroid and Other Endocrine Glands

David V. Cohn, Brigitte H. Fasciotto, Ji-Xiang Zhang, and Sven-Ulrik Gorr

For most of the history of the study of the parathyroid gland, the focus has been on the chemistry, regulation of synthesis, and secretion of parathyroid hormone (PTH) (1). Recently, there has been a growing awareness and interest in a second major calcium-regulated secretory protein of the gland, referred to as *chromogranin A (CgA)* or *secretory protein-I (SP-I)*. Interest in CgA and the other members of the granin class—chromogranin B and secretogranin-II—is heightened because these proteins may play important physiological roles in structural and functional aspects of endocrine gland secretion and intercommunication.

Although this review highlights parathyroid CgA, we refer often to studies of CgA from other tissues since this protein is widespread in the endocrine/neuroendocrine system (2) and is the product of one gene (3). On the other hand, we dwell only briefly on the other granins, since these are present in only limited amounts, if at all, in the parathyroid. The interested reader is referred to recent reviews (4–7), for details on these latter proteins as well as additional information on CgA itself.

DISCOVERY OF PARATHYROID CHROMOGRANIN A

Kemper et al. (8) were the first to describe the secretion of a new protein, referred to as *parathyroid secretory protein (PSP)*, by parathyroid tissue in culture. As is the case with PTH, the secretion of this protein was inhibited at physiologically high concentrations of calcium in the medium. Shortly thereafter, secretion of this protein (now termed *SP-I*) was described by Morrissey and coworkers (9), who subsequently isolated and characterized the SP-I protein, including determination of the partial amino acid sequence and generation of specific antiserum (10,11). On a relative basis, Ca^{2+} more effectively decreased SP-I secretion than it did that of PTH (Fig. 1).

Independent of studies on SP-I, other investigators interested in adrenal physiology were characterizing soluble proteins of the adrenal medullary chromaffin granule. One of these, chromogranin A (CgA), was of particular interest in that it represented almost 50% of the soluble protein of the granule (12). Comparison of SP-I and CgA showed that they were alike in charge, amino acid and carbohydrate compositions, and partial amino acid sequence. Antisera raised to either protein cross reacted with the other (13). Subsequent studies confirmed that parathyroid SP-I and adrenal CgA are the same protein (14), although differences may exist as a result of posttranslational modification.

CgA was soon recognized to be widely distributed in endocrine and neuroendocrine cells, including the pancreas and the pituitary gland (2,15,16). CgA has enjoyed a long evolutionary history; it has been detected

D. V. Cohn, B. H. Fasciotto, J.-X. Zhang, S.-U. Gorr: Department of Biological and Biophysical Sciences, Health Sciences Center, University of Louisville, Louisville, Kentucky 40292.

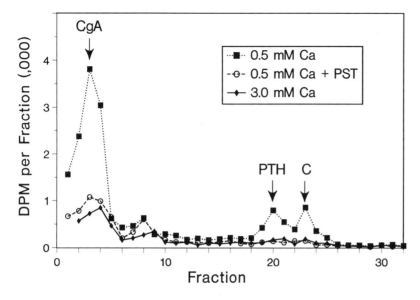

FIG. 1. Inhibition of secretion of chromogranin A (CgA) and parathyroid hormone (PTH) by calcium and pancreastatin (PST). Porcine parathyroid cells were incubated with ^{3}H-lysine at 0.5, 3.0 mM Ca or 0.5 mM Ca + PST (1 μM) for 2.5 hr. Radioactive secreted proteins were separated by electrophoresis on an acid/urea gel. The *arrows* indicate the migration positions of CgA, PTH, and the PTH-C-terminal fragment (C). (Adapted from ref. 53 with permission.)

```
            -18               -1   1
Bovine    MRSAAVLALLLCAGQVIA    LPVNSPMNKGDTEVMKCIVEVISDTLSKPSPM    32
Human     MRSAAVLALLLCAGQVTA    LPVNSPMNKGDTEVMKCIVEVISDTLSKPSPM    32
Pig       XXSAAALALLLCAGQVIA    LPVMSPMNKGDTEVMKCIVEVISDTLSKPSPM    32
Rat       MRSSAALALLLCAGQVFA    LPVNSPMTKGDTKVMKCVLEVISDSLSKPSPM    32
Mouse     MRSTAVLALLLCAGQVFA    LPVNSPMTKGDTKVMKCVLEVISDSLSKPSPM    32
          .. *  * *********** *    ***.*** **** ****  ***** *******


Bovine    PVSKECFETLRGDERILSILRHQNLLKELQDLALQGAKERTHQ-------    75
Human     PVSKECFETLRGDERILSILRHQNLLKELQDLALQGRKERAHQ-------    75
Pig       PVSQECFETLRGDERILSILRHQNLLKELQDLALQGAKERSHQ-------    75
Rat       PVSPECLETLQGDERVLSILRHQNLLKELQDLALQGAKERAQQ-----QQ    77
Mouse     PVSPECLETLQGDERILSILRHQHLLKELQDLALQGAKEREQQPLKQQQP    82
          *** ** *** **** .******* .*************** ** *


Bovine    -------------QKKHSSYEDELSEVLEKPNDQAEPKEVTEEVSSKDAA    112
Human     -------------QKKHSGFEDELSEVLENQSSQAELKQAVEEPSSKDVM    112
Pig       -------------QKKQSSYEDELSEVLEKQNDQAELKEGTEEASSKEAA    112
Rat       QQQQQQQQQQQQQQQHSSFEDELSEVFENQSPAAKHGDAASEAPSKDTV    127
Mouse     PKQQQQQQQQQQQQEQQHSSFEDELSEVFENQSPDAKHRDAAAEVPSRQTM    132
                       . *. ******* * .     *      * *.


Bovine    EKRDDFKEVEKSD--EDSDGDRPQASPGLGPGPKVEEDNQAPGEEEEA--    158
Human     EKREDSKEAEKSG--EATDGARPQALPEPMQESKAEGNKQAPGEEEEEEE    160
Pig       EKRGDSKEVEKND--EDADGAKPQA--SLEPPXXXEAEDQTPGEE-----    153
Rat       EKREDSDKGQQDAFEGTTEGPRPQAFPEPKQESSMMGNSQSPGEDT----    173
Mouse     EKRKDSDKGQQDGFEATTEGPRPQAFPEPNQESPMMGDSESPQEDT----    178
          *** *.          * .***  .               . *.*


Bovine    -PSNAHPLASLPSPKYPGPQAKEDSE-GPS-QGPASREKGLSAEQGRQTE    205
Human     EATNTHPPASLPSQKYPGPQAKGDSE-GLS-QGLVDREKGLSVEPGWQAK    208
Pig       EAASTHPLASLPSKKRPGAQAEEDHE-GPS-QGPVDREKGPSAEQGPQA    201
Rat       -ANNTQSPTSLPSQEHGIPQTTEGSERGPSAQQQARKAKQEEKEEEEEEK    222
Mouse     -ATNTQSPTSLPSQEHVDPQATGDSERGLSAQQQARKAKQEEKEEEE---    224
          .  .. ****     *. ..* * * *        * *  *
```

FIG. 2. Deduced amino acid sequences of bovine, human, pig, rat, and mouse CgAs. The sequences are aligned and gaps are added to provide the best homology among the sequences. Perfect conservation of a sequence is indicated by an asterisk, good conservation by a point. Sequences used are as follows: bovine (3), human (21), porcine (23a), rat (25), and mouse (24). Potential basic amino acid cleavage sites are shown in boldface.

immunologically with antisera to mammalian CgA in fish (17,18) and paramecium (19).

CHEMISTRY AND PHYSICAL PROPERTIES OF CHROMOGRANIN A

Primary Structure

The amino acid sequences of pre-CgA of human (20,21), bovine (3,22,23), pig (23a), mouse (24), and rat (25) origin have been deduced from the cloned mRNAs (Fig. 2). The homology of the various species of CgA ranges between 67% and 91%.

Each CgA is translated as a preprotein containing an 18-amino-acid hydrophobic NH_2-terminal sequence, the hallmark of proteins destined for secretion, and ~450 amino acid residues making up the mature chain. Of these, ~25% are Glu and Asp that account for an

acidic pI of ~4.5, and ~9% are Pro residues. In all species a single internal disulfide link exists between cysteine residues 18 and 37 (26). CgA is modified substantially after translation.

The mature molecule contains ~5% carbohydrate consisting of O-linked tri- and tetrasaccharides that include sialic acid, galactose, and N-acetylgalactosamine (13,27–29). Sulfate (1,30) and phosphate residues (31) are present, covalently joined through undefined serine and/or threonine but not tyrosine residues (32).

Estimates of molecular mass based on sodium dodecyl sulfate (SDS)-polyacrylamide gel electrophoresis yield values of ~70 kDa, considerably above the value of 48–50 kDa derived from the amino acid composition alone. Posttranslational additions account for perhaps 5 kDa more as judged from equilibrium sedimentation study in the presence of guanidinium chloride (33). In the parathyroid, CgA exhibits a molecular

```
Bovine   REEEEEKWEEAEAREKAVPEEESPPTAAFKPPPSLGNKETQRAAP----G      251
Human    REEEEEEEEEAEAGEEAVPEEEGP-TVVLNPHPSLGYKEIRKGES-RSEA    256
Pig      REEEEE----AEAGEKAVPEEEGPRSEAFDSHPSLGYKEMQRG---WPQA    244
Rat      EEEEEEKEEEKAIAREKAGPKE--VPTAASSSHFYSGYKKIQKDDDGQSES   270
Mouse    ------EEEAVAREKAGPEE--VPTAASSSHFHAGYKAIQKDD-GQSDS     264
         .....  . * * * .* * *.*       ..   . *.*   .

Bovine   WPEDGAGKMGAEEAKPPEGKGEWAHSRQ--EEEE-MARAPQVLFRGGKSG       298
Human    LAVDGAGKPGAEEAQDPEGKGEQEHSQQKEEEEE-MAVVPQGLFRGGKSG       305
Pig      PAMDGAGKTGAEEAQPPEGKGAREHSRQ-EEEEE-TAGAPQGLFRGGKRG       292
Rat      QAVNG--KTGASEAVPSEGKGELEHSQQEEDGEEAMAGPPQGLFP-GGKG       317
Mouse    QAVDGDGKTEASEALPSEGKGELEHSQQEEDGEEAMVGTPQGLFPQGGKG       314
         .  .* .* .* ** . **** . ** * .  ** .. **.** * *

Bovine   -------EPEQEEQ--LSKEWEDAKRWSKMDQLAKELTAEKRLEGEEEE        339
Human    -------ELEQEEE-RLSKEWEDTNRWSKMDQLAKELTAEKRLEGQEEEE       347
Pig      -------EPAQEEEERLSEEWENAKRWSKMDRLAKELTAEKRLQGEEEEE       335
Rat      QELERKQQEEEEEEERLSREWED-KRWSRMDQLAKELTAEKRLEGED---       363
Mouse    RELEHKQEEEEEEEERLSREWED-KRWSRMDQLAKELTAEKRLEGED---       360
                .. **  .** ***  .*** **.**********  *.

Bovine   E---DPDRSMRLSFRARGYGFRGPGLQLRRGWRPNSREDSVEAGLPLQVR      386
Human    D---NRDRSMRLSFRARGYGFRGPGPQLRRGSRPNSWEDSLEAGLPLQVR      394
Pig      EEEEDPDRSMKLSFRAPAYGFRGPGLQLRRGWRPSSREDSVEAGLPLQVR      385
Rat      ----DPDRSMKLSFRARAYGFRDPGPQLRRGWRPSSREDSVEA------R      403
Mouse    ----DPDRSMKLSFRTRAYGFRDPGPQLRRGWRPSSREDSVEA------R      400
             ..**** ****.. **** ** ***** .** *.***.**        *

Bovine   GYPEEKKEEEGSANRRPEDQELESLSAIEAELEKVAHQLEELRRG           431
Human    GYPQEKKEEEGSANRRPEDQELESLSAIEAELEKVAHQLQALRRG           439
Pig      XYLEEKKEEEGSANRRPEDQELESLSAIEAELEKVAPQLQSLRRG           430
Rat      GDFEEKKEEEGSANRRAEDQELESLSAIEAELEKVAHQLQALRRG           448
Mouse    SDFEEKKEEEGSANRRAEQQELESLSAIEAELEKVAHQLQALRRG           445
         . ********** *.***************** .**..****
```

FIG. 2. *Continued.*

mass of 52 kDa by sedimentation equilibrium analysis (34). The large discrepancy between measured migration and theory could result from a low affinity of SDS to the acidic protein in gel electrophoresis and to a high axial ratio of the protein in aqueous solution (10). In nondenaturing solutions, moreover, CgA migrates as a tetramer, evidence of electrostatic interactions between the monomeric protein chains (10).

CgA contains six perfectly conserved pairs of basic residues (Lys-Lys, Lys-Arg, Arg-Arg) and 22 single basic residues that are either Lys or Arg. Basic residues, and particularly dibasic regions, are often favored cleavage sites for posttranslational proteolytic processing. Some examples are pro-PTH (35), pre-provasoactive intestinal peptide (VIP) (36), and pro-opiomelanocortin (37) among many others. The presence of basic pairs distributed throughout the sequence was the initial clue that CgA was a precursor of smaller peptides.

Calcium-Binding and Aggregation

The calcium binding activity of CgA was established by Gratzl and coworkers (38–40). Calcium-binding has also been reported for chromogranin B (41) and secretogranin-II (42–44).

CgA binds calcium with low affinity but high capacity: 150–1,150 nmol Ca^{2+}/mg protein, with a dissociation constant of 31 μM to 4 mM (34,38,39,45–48). These differences in experimental results are partly due to the effect of pH and salt concentration on calcium binding (39,47). For example, CgA exhibits a decreased affinity for calcium at lower pH values. The decreased affinity for calcium may allow calcium exchange at the high calcium concentrations and low pH found in secretory granules.

The binding of calcium is accompanied by conformational changes that may play a role in the affinity of the ion to the protein (47a). At pH 5.5, for example, the α-helix content of CgA decreased from 40% to 30% upon calcium binding, whereas at pH 7.5 an increase in α-helicity was noted.

THE CHROMOGRANIN A GENE

The gene for CgA has been isolated from bovine (49) and mouse (24) genomic libraries. It exists as a single copy (3) and resides on chromosome 14 (50,51), separate from that of PTH and other hormones (50). The bovine gene contains eight exons and seven introns that span 13.6 kbp. The CgA transcript contains 1,943 bases. In general, the exons encode distinct functional domains in the CgA protein: exon 1 encodes the entire 5′-untranslated region and 15 residues of the 18 residue amino acid signal peptide; exon 2 encodes the remain-

der of the signal peptide and 13 residues of the NH_2-terminal sequence; exon 3 encodes a 33-amino-acid segment containing the two cysteine residues that presumably exist as an internal disulfide (26); exons 4 and 5 encode highly conserved regions of the NH_2-terminal domain; exon 6 encodes a variable domain that differs most among the animal species examined and codes for a central region of the protein that contains chromostatin; exon 7 encodes most of the COOH terminus of CgA that includes the region coding for pancreastatin and parastatin; and exon 8 encodes the remaining portion of CgA and all of the 3′-untranslated region. For the most part the structure of the mouse gene is similar to that of the bovine gene. The first three and the last two exons of the CgA and CgB genes, corresponding to the signal peptide, NH_2 terminus, disulfide loop, and COOH terminus, are similar in these two genes. These structural similarities suggest that these genes (and their respective proteins) may have evolved from a common ancestral gene and may constitute a gene family (6).

Chromogranin A Promoter Region

The promoter region in the bovine and mouse CgA genes contains a TATA box as well as consensus sequences for a cyclic adenosine monophosphate (cAMP)-response element, SP1-binding site, and possible glucocorticoid-, estrogen-, and phorbol ester-response elements (49). As was pointed out by Iacangelo et al. (49), these several potential transcriptional elements provide the opportunity for multiple hormones and second messengers to interact in the regulation of gene expression.

REGULATION OF CHROMOGRANIN A AND PARATHYROID HORMONE SECRETION AND GENE TRANSCRIPTION

Calcium

Parathyroid secretion of CgA, as well as PTH (1), is exquisitely sensitive to Ca^{2+}, responding within seconds to changes in the extracellular concentration of this ion (1,52,53) (Fig. 1). The concordant secretion of CgA and PTH results from both substances residing in the same secretory granules (54).

In experiments conducted over several minutes to a few hours, changes in secretion of PTH and CgA appear to be independent of changes in cellular levels of the respective mRNAs (55-57). Rather, in acute experiments with PTH, the cells modify the degree of proteolytic degradation of the hormone (58). Definitive data of this type do not exist for CgA.

Upon chronic exposure to elevated calcium levels, PTH mRNA (57,59–61) and CgA mRNA levels (57) decrease. In earlier studies, Russell et al. (61) and Mouland and Hendy (60) did not observe an effect of Ca^{2+} on CgA mRNA. This apparent discrepancy may relate to differences in parathyroid cell preparation employed by the latter workers compared to the study of Zhang et al. (57).

Vitamin D Metabolites

1,25-Dihydroxyvitamin D_3 [$1,25(OH)_2D_3$] is a potent modulator of parathyroid gland function. Chronic exposure of parathyroid cells to this agent gradually decreases PTH secretion and PTH mRNA levels while increasing CgA secretion and CgA mRNA (60–65). The action of $1,25(OH)_2D_3$ on PTH mRNA levels results from decreased transcription of the PTH gene. In the case of CgA, Mouland and Hendy (60) have reported that $1,25(OH)_2D_3$ has a post-transcriptional effect on CgA synthesis by decreasing peptide chain elongation and hence CgA translatability.

Glucocorticoids

The effect of dexamethasone has been tested on several CgA-secreting cell types. Dexamethasone increases CgA secretion and/or CgA mRNA in the pituitary (66,67), in primary adrenal chromaffin cells (49), and in rat insulinoma (49) and AtT-20 mouse corticotropic cell lines (68). Hypophysectomy has been correlated with selective decreases in CgA in the adrenal (69). The action of glucocorticoid on CgA mRNA is consistent with the presence of glucocorticoid-response elements in the CgA gene (49), as was mentioned above.

In the parathyroid, the effect of dexamethasone on CgA secretion and cellular mRNA levels, unlike that on PTH secretion and PTH mRNA, is uniquely dependent on the concentration of extracellular Ca^{2+}. Dexamethasone increased CgA secretion and CgA mRNA at 3.0 mM Ca^{2+} but decreased secretion at 0.5 mM Ca^{2+} (57). In contrast, dexamethasone enhanced PTH secretion and PTH mRNA cellular level irrespective of calcium concentration (57,70–72). This result emphasizes that the parathyroid uses independent mechanisms to regulate the cellular levels of PTH and CgA mRNAs.

Other Agents Affecting Chromogranin A Secretion and Synthesis

There are several agents that operate through "second messengers" that have been shown to affect CgA

synthesis and secretion. Among these, phorbol ester and forskolin stimulate CgA secretion and CgA mRNA levels in human calcitonin-producing cell lines of thyroid (MTC) and lung (BEN) carcinomas (73,74). On the other hand, phorbol ester decreased CgA mRNA in bovine chromaffin cells, had no effect in a rat insuloma cell line (RIN), and blocked stimulation by dexamethasone in both cell types (49). Forskolin increased CgA mRNA in chromaffin cells but was inactive in the RIN cells. This suggests that inhibition of CgA gene expression by phorbol ester in the chromaffin and RIN cells is mediated via the glucocorticoid receptor.

The calcium ionophore A23187, which enhances entry of extracellular Ca^{2+} into cells, increased secretion of CgA and calcitonin in the BEN cell line but did not affect secretion of these substances in the MTC cell line. On the other hand, A23187 did not alter CgA mRNA levels in either cell line (74). These results show significant cell specificity and imply that development of an encompassing hypothesis relating to CgA gene regulation will be difficult.

CHROMOGRANIN A AS A PEPTIDE PRECURSOR

Single and paired basic amino acids often represent specific processing sites for the generation of hormones from prohormone molecules (75). Well known examples of prohormones containing pairs of basic processing sites are proinsulin, progonadotropin, prosomatostatin, pro-PTH, and proopiomelanocortin. Examples of prohormones containing single basic processing sites include human atrial natriuretic factor (ANF), gastrin, and insulin-like growth factors-I and -II (IGF-I and -II) (see 75). The existence of eight pairs of basic amino acids in bovine CgA, the first sequence to be deduced, was immediately suggestive that CgA serves as a peptide precursor (76,77). Furthermore, as the CgA sequences of other species became known, conservation of dibasic and monobasic putative processing sites was apparent (Fig. 2).

The Discovery and Actions of Pancreastatin

Definitive evidence that CgA serves as a peptide precursor arose from independent studies by Tatemoto et al. (78). These workers isolated from porcine pancreatic tissue a 49-amino-acid, C-terminally amidated peptide termed *pancreastatin* that was found to be a potent inhibitor of glucose-stimulated insulin release by the perfused pancreas (78,79). The authors determined the amino acid sequence of pancreastatin and showed that its activity resided in the latter one-third of the molecule (78). Shortly after this information became known, Eiden (76) and Huttner and Benedum

(77) pointed out that the sequence of porcine pancreastatin was >70% homologous to a central region of bovine CgA. When the deduced sequence of pCgA became available (23), it was noted that the sequence of pancreastatin and pCgA$_{240-288}$ matched exactly (Figs. 2 and 3). Because the pancreastatin region of CgA is highly conserved across different animal species, it is likely that this region is functionally important.

The action of pancreastatin on secretion is not confined to the pancreas. It is a powerful inhibitor of parathyroid secretion (Fig. 1) (53), cholecystokinin-stimulated release by the exocrine pancreas (80), and acid secretion by parietal cells (81). In some secreting systems, pancreastatin is stimulatory, enhancing glucagon- and L-arginine-stimulated insulin release from the isolated perfused rat pancreas (82).

Processing of Chromogranin A

Although intact CgA has been reported to inhibit insulin secretion by the perfused pancreas (83) and PTH secretion by parathyroid cells in culture (84), these actions appear to require extracellular proteolytic processing of the CgA (85). Fasciotto et al. (84) reported that addition of CgA antibodies to parathyroid cells incubated in hypocalcemic medium enhanced PTH secretion above what had been believed to be a maximum level. This finding represents primary evidence that CgA and its derived peptides play a physiological role in down-regulating parathyroid secretion.

Chromostatin and Adrenal Chromaffin Secretion

Simon et al. (86) tested the effect of CgA on the secretion of catecholamines by nicotine-stimulated chromaffin cells in culture. They noted that, for CgA to be effective, it required incubation for a time in the medium or had to be proteolytically degraded by exposure to trypsin. Galindo et al. (87) treated CgA with endoproteinase Lys-C in order to prepare peptides that were derived by cleaving at the carboxyl side of Lys residues. They determined that inhibition of catecholamine secretion was due to a fragment of CgA representing at the minimum CgA$_{124-143}$ (Figs. 2 and 3), a region apart from that comprising pancreastatin. Galindo et al. (87) synthesized CgA$_{124-143}$, which they termed *chromostatin*, and showed that it was active. Subsequently, Galindo et al. (88) detected a receptor to chromostatin on the chromaffin cell. Of particular interest, pancreastatin did not affect chromaffin cell secretion.

β-Granin [CgA$_{(1-114)}$] and Subfragments

β-Granin is formed in the rat pancreatic islet cells, from which it is cosecreted with insulin (89). Drees et al. (90) have recently determined that β-granin inhibits parathyroid cell secretion; CgA$_{1-40}$, generated in vitro by proteolysis of CgA, stimulated release of calcitonin (CT) gene-related peptide but inhibited CT and parathyroid hormone-related protein (PTHrP) release by the BEN human lung tumor cell line (91,92). Vasostatin (CgA$_{1-76}$) has been reported to lower vascular tension (93).

Parastatin and Parathyroid Secretion

Despite the great potency of pancreastatin in inhibiting parathyroid secretion, Drees and Hamilton (94) question whether pancreastatin plays a biologically

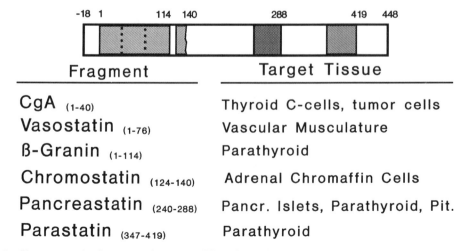

Fragment	Target Tissue
CgA (1-40)	Thyroid C-cells, tumor cells
Vasostatin (1-76)	Vascular Musculature
β-Granin (1-114)	Parathyroid
Chromostatin (124-140)	Adrenal Chromaffin Cells
Pancreastatin (240-288)	Pancr. Islets, Parathyroid, Pit.
Parastatin (347-419)	Parathyroid

FIG. 3. Chromogranin A as a prohormone. The *shaded areas* show the regions of active peptides derived from CgA. Residues −18 to 1 represent the signal peptide of the CgA proprotein. Since the lengths of the CgA from different species differ somewhat, so will the residue numbers of the derived peptides. The reader should refer to Fig. 2 for exact start and stop residues for each fragment.

relevant role in this gland. They found little if any pancreastatin immunoactivity in bovine parathyroid tissue and have been unable to demonstrate that it is formed under physiological conditions. To test whether hitherto undescribed portions of the CgA molecule were active on parathyroid gland secretion, Fasciotto et al. (95) tested several CgA fragments derived by endoproteinase Lys-C digestion. Only one fragment, CgA$_{347-419}$, termed *parastatin,* inhibited parathyroid secretion. This fragment is distinct from other regions of the CgA chain that comprise β-granin, chromostatin, and pancreastatin (see Fig. 3).

PUTATIVE PHYSIOLOGICAL ROLE(S) OF CHROMOGRANIN A

At the outset, we should note that no role for CgA or the other members of the granin family has been confirmed. Rather, speculation continues based on unique properties of CgA that have already been mentioned in this chapter. These include coresidency with hormones and neurotransmitters in endocrine cells, conservation within the molecule of basic amino acid residues that represent potential cleavage sites, the actions on secretory processes of the intact molecule and derived fragments, and the binding of large amounts of calcium to the protein that can lead to molecular aggregation.

Two hypotheses currently being tested are particularly noteworthy: first, that CgA and/or its derived peptides are autocrine or paracrine inhibitors of endocrine secretion; second, that calcium-binding allows the molecule to target it and other hormones into secretory vesicles, leading to condensation and maturation of the granule's contents.

CgA as an Autocrine/Paracrine Regulator

CgA and its derived peptides such as pancreastatin and chromostatin most often inhibit secretion of those cells in which it resides (Fig. 4). The studies of Fasciotto et al. (84), for example, showed that CgA or pancreastatin inhibited low-calcium-stimulated secretion of PTH by parathyroid cells in culture and that CgA or pancreastatin antibodies added to the culture medium potentiated stimulated secretion. Thus, at what had been long considered to be maximal, physiologic secretory activity of those cells appeared to be held below a true maximum by secreted CgA peptides. Wand et al. (68) noted similar results for corticotropin-releasing hormone-stimulated proopiomelanocortin secretion by a corticotropic cell line (AtT20 cells) treated with CgA or CgA antiserum.

What advantage would accrue to a cell that upon stimulation secreted a substance that immediately antagonized further stimulation? One possibility is that the rapid down-regulation of secretion in the continued presence of the stimulus would lead to a sharper secretory pulse and hence more precise control of cell secretion. This hypothetical concept is illustrated in Fig. 5.

In accordance with CgA's role as a physiological regulator of PTH secretion, one would anticipate that under certain defined conditions an inverse relationship would exist between PTH and CgA synthesis and secretion. Specific examples of this inverse relationship have been recognized. 1,25-Dihydroxyvitamin D$_3$, whose synthesis from 25-(OH)$_2$D$_3$ in the kidney is enhanced by PTH (96), feeds back on the parathyroid to lower PTH cellular mRNA levels and the amount of PTH secreted by the gland (56,59,60) while increasing CgA secretion and mRNA levels (60).

Dexamethasone treatment of parathyroid tissue pro-

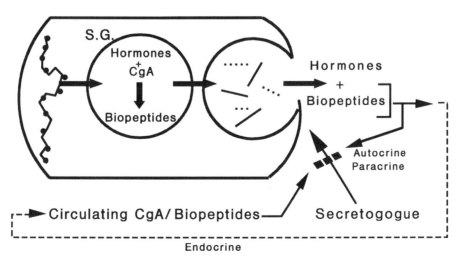

FIG. 4. Proposed autocrine/paracrine and endocrine nature of CgA-derived peptides. See text for details. S.G., secretory granules.

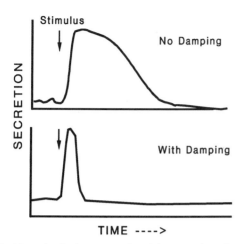

FIG. 5. Hypothetical concept involving a pulse-sharpening role of CgA-derived peptides in endocrine cell secretion. See text for details.

vides another example of this inverse relationship between PTH and CgA synthesis and secretion (57). Dexamethasone substantially increases PTH secretion and PTH mRNA levels at all Ca^{2+} concentrations. In the presence of the glucocorticoid, there is a decrease in CgA mRNA levels at low Ca^{2+}, but an increase occurs at high Ca^{2+} levels. These results have been interpreted to mean that, when the gland senses the "inappropriately high" secretion of PTH at high Ca^{2+}, it synthesizes and secretes more CgA in an attempt to reduce PTH secretion (57).

To determine whether CgA released by a parathyroid cell suppresses subsequent secretion by the same cell (direct autocrine regulation; Fig. 4), Ritchie et al. (97) employed a unique sequential reverse hemolytical plaque assay. Although they found that cells "cycled" between secretory and nonsecretory phases, they did not obtain evidence that CgA plays a role in this cycling.

It is possible that circulating forms of CgA act as endocrine agents on distal peripheral tissues and glands. In this regard, it would be important to learn if tissue-specific processing, which appears to exist (89,90,98,99), generates CgA peptides that have unique activities on targets.

Seidah et al. (100) noted that processing of adrenocorticotropic hormone (ACTH) and proenkephalin by a serine protease was inhibited by addition of CgA to the assay system. Conversely, CgA processing was inhibited by addition of ACTH to the assay system, suggesting that CgA is a substrate for the protease rather than a specific inhibitor. The subsequent identification of the serine protease as plasma kallikrein (101) raises the possibility that an extracellular processing pathway exists for the circulating form of CgA. This pathway might support an endocrine role for CgA or

merely represent a mechanism to clear the protein from the circulation.

CgA and Secretory Vesicle Formation, Maturation, and Stability

The Ca^{2+}-binding properties of CgA are consistent with CgA serving as an intragranular calcium storage protein (Fig. 6). The total calcium concentration in secretory granules has been estimated at between 8 and 40 mM (40,102), while the free Ca^{2+} concentration is in the micromolar range (40). Calcium is not released by chromaffin granules treated with calcium ionophore alone, whereas it is readily released from granule ghosts, suggesting that calcium is primarily bound to the granule contents rather than to granule membranes (103–105). Such a role would be similar to that played by calsequestrin (106). The secretory granule can then be thought of as a "calcium sink" that expels excess calcium upon exocytosis (107). Such a mechanism may act in concert with membrane calcium-adenosine triphosphatases (Ca-ATPases) to regulate intracellular calcium.

At the high calcium concentration and low pH present in secretory granules, CgA forms high-molecular-weight aggregates (34,41,45,47a,48). The size of the aggregates and the extent of aggregation depend on the total calcium concentration, with the most complete aggregation detected at 10–30 mM calcium (34,41,47a). The efficiency of aggregation is significantly enhanced at low pH. Chromogranin A precipitates in the absence of calcium at a pH <6.0, where the protein exists as tetramers (10,41,47). The conditions required for efficient aggregation of chromogranins are found in endocrine secretory granules and are approximated in the trans-Golgi network, suggesting that CgA may aggregate in these compartments.

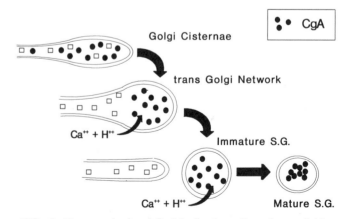

FIG. 6. Proposed role of CgA in the targeting of exportable peptides into secretory granules (S.G.) of the regulated pathway and maturation of these granules via calcium aggregation. See text for details.

These observations have led to a model for the packaging of chromogranins into secretory granules in endocrine cells (6,45,108). As the proteins are transported through the Golgi apparatus, they encounter an increasing calcium concentration and an acidic pH. Under these conditions the chromogranins aggregate. The aggregates could trigger the formation of secretory granules from the membrane of the trans-Golgi network (TGN) granules and would thus exclude non-aggregated proteins. Further condensation might occur in the maturing granule, in agreement with the apparent darkening of maturing granules observed by electron microscopy.

The evidence supporting this model includes the aggregation of chromogranins and the coprecipitation of chromogranins with other peptide hormones, including PTH (41) and luteinizing hormone (6). Proatrial natriuretic factor also exhibits calcium-induced aggregation (109), while proinsulin and prolactin precipitate at acidic pH in the absence of calcium (44,110,111). Constitutive secretory proteins, on the other hand, do not precipitate with chromogranins under these conditions (41,43). Trans-Golgi network-derived membrane vesicles that have been permeabilized and incubated at low pH in the presence of calcium release sulfated glycosaminoglycans, a marker for the constitutive secretory pathway, but not chromogranins. The latter are released at pH 7.4 in the absence of calcium (112), indicating that the calcium complexes are formed in the TGN.

There is evidence that calcium is involved in stabilization of the mature secretory granules as well. Isolated chromaffin granules lyse after removal of calcium from the granules, and this lysis can be prevented by increasing the osmolality of the incubating medium (103). Insulin storage granules appear translucent in cells deprived of calcium, indicating that the protein contents are less tightly packed in these granules (113).

CHROMOGRANIN A AND SOME CLINICAL CORRELATIONS

Chromogranin A as a Neuroendocrine Tumor Marker

CgA in tissue and serum was first determined to be elevated in a case of human pheochromocytoma by O'Connor and Bernstein (114). Subsequently, it was reported that CgA is elevated in a variety of tumors of peptide-secreting cells not normally thought to secrete CgA. These include medullary (C-cell) thyroid carcinoma, prostatic tumor, pancreatic islet cell tumor, and pituitary tumor (115–118) but not primary hyperparathyroidism (119,120). The circulating level of CgA in human serum is ~60 ng/ml. Patients with carcinoid tumors and pheochromocytomas may exhibit up to 500-fold higher levels of serum CgA (121).

Schürmann et al. (122) investigated 33 patients with neuroendocrine tumors and found that serum CgA was elevated in 92% of the subjects. The mean CgA levels varied with tumor location but did not differ between functioning and nonfunctioning tumors. The cell line QGP-1 derived from human nonfunctioning pancreatic islet cell tumor has been found to produce pancreastatin and CgA, which is helpful in the diagnosis of this tumor (98).

Immunohistochemical detection of CgA is also useful in detecting tumors. Immunoactive CgA was found to be present in practically all 122 cases of medullary thyroid carcinoma reported by Harach et al. (123). The serum level of CgA did not correlate well with the stage of medullary thyroid carcinoma, because the levels were elevated in most patients only when the disease was advanced (124).

Abrahamsson et al. (125) used iCgA and the Grimelius silver staining technique in a search for neuroendocrine cells. They reported a correlation between the progression of the prostatic carcinoma in 25 cases and the number of neuroendocrine cells and suggested that CgA may be a sensitive marker for this type of carcinoma. The investigation of the relative distribution of CgA in prospectively sampled prostatectomy specimens indicated that all prostatic adenocarcinomas exhibited CgA immunoreactivity (126).

Eriksson et al. (127) reported that all of their 84 patients with endocrine pancreatic tumors had significantly elevated levels of plasma CgA. Schmid et al. (128) studied 42 pituitary adenomas using immunohistochemical methods. Thirteen of 16 null cell adenomas contained CgA, whereas CgA was not found in prolactinomas.

CgA is a more widely distributed marker for neuroendocrine tumors than either CgB or secretogranin-II. CgA can be detected in serum or tumors from patients with some rare neuroendocrine tumors, e.g., Merkel cell tumor of skin and carotid body tumors. CgA is also currently used in diagnosis of neuroendocrine tumors of respiratory and gastrointestinal tracts, such as small-cell lung cancer and gastrointestinal carcinoid.

Does Chromogranin A Play a Role in Hypertension?

Aardal and Helle (93) demonstrated that vasostatin (CgA_{1-76}) inhibits endothelin-induced vasoconstriction in isolated saphenous vein, providing the first direct evidence that CgA can affect blood pressure. Intriguing indirect evidence exists. Pheochromocytoma is typified by hypertension and is accompanied by elevated circulating levels of intracellular CgA (114,129). The adrenal glands of spontaneously hypertensive and stroke-prone rats exhibit increased amounts of chromaffin granule contents, including CgA (130,131).

Recently it was noted that CgA is costored with Atrial natriuretic factor (ANF) in the heart (132). ANF is released from atrial myocytes upon atrial distension and acts upon vasculature and kidney to lower blood pressure. The issue to be determined is whether CgA-derived peptides can block ANF release as they do for other secreting cells. If so, the high circulating levels of CgA in pheochromocytoma patients and in genetic hypertensive rats might act to limit ANF release and contribute to elevated blood pressure.

Injection of plasma from spontaneously hypertensive rats into normotensive rats led to increased blood pressure and vascular calcium uptake in the latter (133). This effect has been linked to the presence of a hypertensive factor of parathyroid origin in the hypertensive rat model (134). This heat-stable factor exhibited a molecular weight of ~3 kDa and was inactivated by trypsin. We may wonder if this hypertensive factor from the parathyroid is not a CgA-derived peptide.

CONCLUSIONS

This chapter points out that CgA, initially linked to the parathyroids and adrenals by chance of discovery, should be looked upon in a broader light. The possibility grows stronger that CgA is a paracrine agent that regulates secretion of the cells in which it is generated and secreted. We should also keep in mind the possibility that this protein is one member of a family of granins that integrates function and secretion of related glands in the endocrine system.

REFERENCES

1. Cohn DV, Elting J. Biosynthesis, processing and secretion of parathormone and secretory protein-I. *Rec Progr Horm Res* 1983;39:181–209.
2. Cohn DV, Elting JJ, Frick M, Elde R. Selective localization of the parathyroid secretory protein-I/adrenal medulla chromogranin A protein family in a wide variety of endocrine cells of the rat. *Endocrinology* 1984;114:1963–1974.
3. Ahn TG, Cohn DV, Gorr S-U, Ornstein DL, Kashdan MA, Levine MA. Primary structure of bovine pituitary secretory protein I (chromogranin A) deduced from the cDNA sequence. *Proc Natl Acad Sci USA* 1987;84:5043–5047.
4. Winkler H, Apps DK, Fischer-Colbrie R. The molecular function of adrenal chromaffin granules: established facts and unresolved topics. *Neuroscience* 1986;18:261–290.
5. Simon J-P, Aunis D. Biochemistry of the chromogranin A protein family. *Biochem J* 1989;262:1–13.
6. Huttner WB, Gerdes H-H, Rosa P. The granin (chromogranin/secretogranin) family. *Trends Biochem Sci* 1991;16:27–30.
7. Winkler H, Fischer-Colbrie R. The chromogranins A and B: the first 25 years and future perspectives. *Neuroscience* 1992;49:497–528.
8. Kemper B, Habener JF, Rich A, Potts JT Jr. Parathyroid secretion: discovery of a major calcium-dependent protein. *Science* 1974;184:167–169.
9. Morrissey JJ, Hamilton JW, Cohn DV. The secretion of par-athormone and glycosylated proteins by parathyroid cells in culture. *Biochem Biophys Res Commun* 1978;82:1279–1286.
10. Cohn DV, Morrissey JJ, Hamilton JW, Shofstall RE, Smardo FL, Chu LLH. Isolation and partial characterization of secretory protein-I from bovine parathyroid glands. *Biochemistry* 1981;20:4135–4140.
11. Cohn DV, Morrissey JJ, Shofstall RE, Chu LLH. Cosecretion of secretory protein-I and parathormone by dispersed bovine parathyroid cells. *Endocrinology* 1982;110:625–630.
12. Winkler H, Carmichael SW. The chromaffin granule. In: Poisner AM, Trifaro JM, eds. *The secretory granule.* Amsterdam: Elsevier, 1982;3–79.
13. Cohn DV, Zangerle R, Fischer-Colbrie R, Chu LLH, Elting JJ, Hamilton JW, Winkler H. Similarity of secretory protein-I from parathyroid gland to chromogranin A from adrenal medulla. *Proc Natl Acad Sci USA* 1982;79:6056–6059.
14. Kruggel W, O'Connor DT, Lewis RV. The amino terminal sequences of bovine and human chromogranin A and secretory protein. *Biochem Biophys Res Commun* 1985;127:380–383.
15. O'Connor DT. Chromogranin: widespread immunoreactivity in polypeptide hormone producing tissues and in serum. *Regul Pept* 1983;6:263–280.
16. Eiden LE, Huttner WB, Mallet J, O'Connor DT, Winkler H, Zanini A. A nomenclature proposal for the chromogranin/secretogranin proteins. *Neuroscience* 1987;21:1019–1021.
17. Deftos LJ, Bjornsson BT, Burton DW, O'Connor DT, Copp DH. Chromogranin A is present in and released by fish endocrine tissue. *Life Sci* 1987;40:2133–2136.
18. Tisserand-Jochem EM, Lopez E, Milet C, et al. Co-localization and secretion of parathyrin of stannius corpuscles (immunoreactive parathyroid hormone) and of secretory glycoproteins including secretory protein-I in the European eel (*Anguilla angilla* L.). *Bone Mineral* 1987;2:163–174.
19. Peterson JB, Nelson DL, Ling E, Hogue-Angeletti R. Chromogranin A-like proteins in the secretory granules of a protozoan, Paramecium tetraurelia. *J Biol Chem* 1987;262:17264–17267.
20. Konecki DS, Benedum UM, Gerdes H-H, Huttner WB. The primary structure of human chromogranin A and pancreastatin. *J Biol Chem* 1987;262:17026–17030.
21. Helman LJ, Ahn TG, Levine MA, et al. Molecular cloning and primary structure of human chromogranin A (secretory protein-I) cDNA. *J Biol Chem* 1988;263:11559–11563.
22. Benedum UM, Baeuerle PA, Konecki DS, et al. The primary structure of bovine chromogranin A: a representative of a class of acidic secretory proteins common to a variety of peptidergic cells. *Eur Mol Biol Org J* 1986;5:1495–1502.
23. Iacangelo A, Affolter HU, Eiden LE, Herbert E, Grimes M. Bovine chromogranin A sequence and distribution of its messenger RNA in endocrine tissues. *Nature* 1986;323:82–86.
23a. Iacangelo AL, Fischer-Colbrie R, Koller KJ, Brownstein MJ, Eiden LE. The sequence of porcine chromogranin A messenger RNA demonstrates chromogranin A can serve as the precursor for the biologically active hormone, pancreastatin. *Endocrinology* 1988;122:2339–2341.
24. Wu H-J, Rozansky DJ, Parmer RJ, Gill BM, O'Connor DT. Structure and function of the chromogranin A gene. Clues to evolution and tissue-specific expression. *J Biol Chem* 1991;266:13130–13134.
25. Iacangelo A, Okayama H, Eiden LE. Primary structure of rat chromogranin A and distribution of its mRNA. *FEBS Lett* 1988;227:115–121.
26. Benedum UM, Lamouroux A, Konecki DS, et al. The primary structure of human secretogranin I (chromogranin B): comparison with chromogranin A reveals homologous terminal domains and a large intervening variable region. *EMBO J* 1987;6:1203–1211.
27. Smith AD, Winkler H. Purification and properties of an acidic protein from chromaffin granules of bovine adrenal medulla. *Biochem J* 1967;103:483–492.
28. Kiang WL, Krusius T, Finne J, Margolis RU, Margolis RK. Glycoproteins and proteoglycans of the chromaffin granule matrix. *J Biol Chem* 1982;257:1651–1659.

29. Majzoub JA, Dee PC, Habener JF. Cellular and cell-free processing of parathyroid secretory proteins. *J Biol Chem* 1982;257:3581–3588.

30. Kumarasamy R, Cohn DV. Sulfation of porcine parathyroid secretory protein-I. *J Biol Chem* 1986;261:16473–16477.

31. Bhargava G, Russel J, Sherwood LM. Phosphorylation of parathyroid secretory protein-I. *Proc Natl Acad Sci USA* 1983;80:878–881.

32. Gorr S-U, Hamilton JW, Cohn DV. Sulfated secreted forms of bovine and porcine parathyroid chromogranin A (secretory protein-I). *J Biol Chem* 1991;266:5780–5784.

33. Kirshner N. Molecular organization of the chromaffin vesicles of the adrenal medulla. In: Ceccarelli B, Medlolesi J, Clementi F, eds. *Cytopharmacology of secretion.* New York: Raven Press, 1974;265–272.

34. Gorr S-U, Dean WL, Radley TL, Cohn DV. Calcium-binding and aggregation properties of parathyroid secretory protein-I (chromogranin A). *Bone Mineral* 1988;4:17–25.

35. Cohn DV, MacGregor RR, Chu LLH, Kimmel JR, Hamilton JW. Calcemic fraction-A: Biosynthetic peptide precursor of parathyroid hormone. *Proc Natl Acad Sci USA* 1972;69:1521.

36. Tsukada T, Horovitch SJ, Montminy MR, Mandel G, Goodman RH. Structure of the human vasoactive intestinal polypeptide gene. *DNA* 1985;4:293–300.

37. Eipper BA, Mains RE. Structure and biosynthesis of proadrenocorticotropin/endorphin and related peptides. *Endocrine Rev* 1980;1:1–17.

38. Reiffen FU, Gratzl M. Ca^{2+} binding to chromaffin vesicle matrix proteins: effects of pH, Mg^{2+}, and ionic strength. *Biochemistry* 1986;25:4402–4406.

39. Reiffen FU, Gratzl M. Chromogranins, widespread in endocrine and nervous tissue, bind Ca^{2+}. *FEBS Lett* 1986;195:327–330.

40. Bulenda D, Gratzl M. Matrix free Ca^{2+} in isolated chromaffin vesicles. *Biochemistry* 1985;24:7760–7765.

41. Gorr S-U, Shioi J, Cohn DV. Interaction of calcium with porcine adrenal chromogranin A (secretory protein-I) and chromogranin B (secretogranin I). *Am J Physiol* 1989;257:E247–E254.

42. Cozzi MG, Zanini A. Secretogranin II is a Ca^{2+}-binding protein. *Cell Biol Int Rep* 1988;12:493.

43. Gerdes H-H, Rosa P, Phillips E, Baeuerle PA, Frank R, Argos P, Huttner WB. The primary structure of human secretogranin II, a widespread tyrosine-sulfated secretory granule protein that exhibits low pH- and calcium-induced aggregation. *J Biol Chem* 1989;264:12009–12015.

44. Thompson ME, Zimmer WE, Haynes AL, Valentine DL, Forss-Petter S, Scammell JG. Prolactin granulogenesis is associated with increased secretogranin expression and aggregation in the golgi apparatus of GH$_4$C$_1$ cells. *Endocrinology* 1992;131:318–326.

45. Gorr S-U, Dean WL, Kumarasamy R, Cohn DV. Calcium binding properties of parathyroid secretory protein-I. In: Cohn DV, Martin TJ, Meunier PJ, eds. *Calcium regulation and bone metabolism: basic and clinical aspects, Vol 9.* Amsterdam: Elsevier, 1987;49–55.

46. Leiser M, Sherwood LM. Calcium-binding proteins in the parathyroid gland. *J Biol Chem* 1989;264:2792–2800.

47. Yoo SH, Albanesi JP. High capacity, low affinity Ca^{2+} binding of chromogranin A. Relationship between the pH-induced conformational change and Ca^{2+} binding property. *J Biol Chem* 1991;266:7740–7745.

47a. Yoo SH, Albanesi JP. Ca^{2+}-induced conformational change and aggregation of chromogranin A. *J Biol Chem* 1990;265:14414–14421.

48. Videen JS, Mezger MS, Chang Y-M, O'Connor DT. Calcium and catecholamine interaction with adrenal chromogranins. *J Biol Chem* 1992;267:3066–3073.

49. Iacangelo A, Grimes M, Eiden LE. The bovine chromogranin A gene: structural basis for hormone regulation and generation of biologically active peptides. *Mol Endocrinol* 1991;5:1651–1660.

50. Murray SS, Deaven LL, Burton DW, O'Connor DT, Mellon PL, Deftos LJ. The gene for human chromogranin A (CgA)

51. is located on chromosome 14. *Biochem Biophys Res Commun* 1986;142:141–146.

52. Modi WS, Levine MA, Seuanez HN, Dean M, O'Brien SJ. The human chromogranin A gene: chromosome assignment and RFLP analysis. *Am J Hum Genet* 1989;45:814–818.

52. Morrissey JJ, Cohn DV. The effects of calcium and magnesium on the secretion of parathormone and parathyroid secretory protein by isolated porcine parathyroid cells. *Endocrinology* 1978;103:2081–2090.

53. Fasciotto BH, Gorr S-U, DeFranco DJ, Levine MA, Cohn DV. Pancreastatin, a presumed product of chromogranin-A (secretory protein-I) processing, inhibits secretion from porcine parathyroid cells in culture. *Endocrinology* 1989;125:1617–1622.

54. Arps H, Dietel M, Lauritzen B, Elting JJ, Niendorf A, Cohn DV. Co-localization of parathyroid hormone and secretory protein-I in bovine parathyroid glands: a double immunocytochemical study at the electron microscopical level. *Bone Mineral* 1987;2:175–183.

55. Heinrich G, Kronenberg HM, Potts JT Jr, Habener JF. Parathyroid hormone messenger ribonucleic acid: effect of calcium on cellular regulation in vitro. *Endocrinology* 1983;112:449–457.

56. Russell J, Lettieri D, Sherwood LM. Direct regulation by calcium of cytoplasmic messenger ribonucleic acid coding for preproparathyroid hormone in isolated bovine parathyroid cells. *J Clin Invest* 1983;72:1851–1855.

57. Zhang JX, Fasciotto BH, Cohn DV. Dexamethasone and calcium interact in the regulation of parathormone and chromogranin A secretion and mRNA levels in parathyroid cells. *Endocrinology* (in press).

58. Morrissey JJ, Cohn DV. Secretion and degradation of parathormone as a function of intracellular maturation of hormone pools. *J Cell Biol* 1979;83:521–528.

59. Brookman JJ, Farrow SM, Nicholson L, O'Riordan JLH, Hendy GN. Regulation by calcium of parathyroid hormone mRNA in cultured parathyroid tissue. *J Bone Mineral Res* 1986;1:529–537.

60. Mouland AJ, Hendy GN. Regulation of synthesis and secretion of chromogranin-A by calcium and 1,25-dihydroxycholecalciferol in cultured bovine parathyroid cells. *Endocrinology* 1991;128:441–449.

61. Russell J, Lettieri D, Adler J, Sherwood LM. 1,25-Dihydroxyvitamin D3 has opposite effects on the expression of parathyroid hormone genes. *Mol Endocrinol* 1990;4:505–509.

62. Silver J, Russell J, Sherwood LM. Regulation by vitamin D metabolites of messenger ribonucleic acid for preproparathyroid hormone in isolated bovine parathyroid cells. *Proc Natl Acad Sci USA* 1985;82:4270–4273.

63. Russell J, Lettieri D, Sherwood LM. Suppression by 1,25-(OH)2 D3 of transcription of the preproparathyroid hormone gene. *Endocrinology* 1986;119:2865–2866.

64. Silver J, Naveh-Many T, Mayer H, Schemelzer H, Popovtzer MM. Regulation by vitamin D metabolites of parathyroid hormone mRNA gene transcription in vivo in the rat. *J Clin Invest* 1986;78:1297–1301.

65. Ridgeway RD, MacGregor RR. Opposite effects of 1,25-(OH)2D3 on synthesis and release of PTH compared with secretory protein I. *Am J Physiol* 1988;254:E279–E286.

66. Fischer-Colbrie R, Wohlfarter T, Schmid KW, Grino M, Winkler H. Dexamethasone induces an increased biosynthesis of chromogranin A in rat pituitary gland. *J Endocrinol* 1989;121:487–494.

67. Grino M, Wohlfarter T, Fischer-Colbrie R, Eiden LE. Chromogranin A messenger RNA expression in the rat anterior pituitary is permissively regulated by the adrenal gland. *Neuroendocrinology* 1989;49:107–110.

68. Wand GS, Takiyuddin M, O'Connor DT, Levine MA. A proposed role for chromogranin A as a glucocorticoid-responsive autocrine inhibitor of proopiomelanocortin secretion. *Endocrinology* 1991;128:1345–1351.

69. Sietzen M, Schober M, Fischer-Colbrie R, Scherman D, Sperk G, Winkler H. Rat adrenal medulla: levels of chromogranins, enkephalins, dopamine β-hydroxylase and of the

amine transporter are changed by nervous activity and hypophysectomy. *Neuroscience* 1987;22:131–139.

70. Fucik RF, Kukreja SC, Hargis GK, Bowser EN, Henderson WJ, Williams GA. Effect of glucocorticoids on function of the parathyroid glands in man. *J Clin Endocrinol Metab* 1975;40:152–155.

71. Sugimoto T, Brown AJ, Ritter C, Morrissey J, Slatopolsky E, Martin KJ. Combined effects of dexamethasone and 1,25-dihydroxyvitamin D3 on parathyroid hormone secretion in cultured bovine parathyroid cells. *Endocrinology* 1989;125:638–641.

72. Peraldi MN, Rondeau E, Jousset V, et al. Dexamethasone increases preproparathyroid hormone messenger RNA in human hyperplastic parathyroid cells in vitro. *Eur J Clin Invest* 1990;20:392–397.

73. Murray SS, Burton DW, Deftos LJ. The coregulation of secretion and cytoplasmic ribonucleic acid of chromogranin A and calcitonin by phorbol ester in cells that produce both substances. *Endocrinology* 1988;122:495–499.

74. Murray SS, Burton DW, Deftos LJ. The effects of forskolin and calcium ionophore A23187 on secretion and cytoplasmatic RNA levels of chromogranin-A and calcitonin. *J Bone Mineral Res* 1988;3:447–452.

75. Loh YP, Beinfeld MC, Birch NP. Proteolytic processing of prohormone and proneuropeptides. In: Loh YP, ed. *Mechanisms of intracellular trafficking and processing of proproteins.* Boca Raton, FL: CRC Press, 1993:180–224.

76. Eiden LE. Is chromogranin a prohormone? *Nature* 1987;325:301.

77. Huttner WB, Benedum UM. Chromogranin A and pancreastatin. *Nature* 1987;325:305.

78. Tatemoto K, Efendic S, Mutt V, Makk G, Feistner GJ, Barchas JD. Pancreastatin, a novel pancreatic peptide that inhibits insulin secretion. *Nature* 1986;324:476–478.

79. Efendic S, Tatemoto K, Mutt V, Quan C, Chang D, Östenson C-G. Pancreastatin and islet hormone release. *Proc Natl Acad Sci USA* 1987;84:7257–7260.

80. Funakoshi A, Miyasaka K, Nakamura R, et al. Bioactivity of synthetic human pancreastatin on exocrine pancreas. *Biochem Biophys Res Commun* 1988;156:1237–1242.

81. Lewis JJ, Zdon MJ, Adrian TE, Modlin IM. Pancreastatin: a novel peptide inhibitor of parietal cell secretion. *Surgery* 1988;104:1031–1036.

82. Ishizuka J, Tatemoto K, Cohn DV, Thompson JC, Greeley GH Jr. Effects of pancreastatin and chromogranin A on insulin release stimulated by various insulinotropic agents. *Regul Pept* 1991;34:25–32.

83. Greeley GH Jr, Thompson JC, Ishizuka J, et al. Inhibition of glucose-stimulated insulin release in the perfused rat pancreas by parathyroid secretory protein-I (chromogranin-A). *Endocrinology* 1989;124:1235–1238.

84. Fasciotto BH, Gorr S-U, Bourdeau AM, Cohn DV. Autocrine regulation of parathyroid secretion: inhibition of secretion by chromogranin-A (secretory protein-I) and potentiation of secretion by chromogranin-A and pancreastatin antibodies. *Endocrinology* 1990;127:1329–1335.

85. Fasciotto BH, Gorr S-U, Cohn DV. Autocrine inhibition of parathyroid cell secretion requires proteolytic processing of chromogranin A. *Bone Mineral* 1992;17:323–333.

86. Simon J-P, Bader M-F, Aunis D. Secretion from chromaffin cells is controlled by chromogranin A-derived peptides. *Proc Natl Acad Sci USA* 1988;85:1712–1716.

87. Galindo E, Rill A, Bader M-F, Aunis D. Chromostatin, a 20-amino acid peptide derived from chromogranin A, inhibits chromaffin cell secretion. *Proc Natl Acad Sci USA* 1991;88:1426–1430.

88. Galindo E, Mendez M, Calvo S, et al. Chromostatin receptors control calcium channel activity in adrenal chromaffin cells. *J Biol Chem* 1992;267:407–412.

89. Hutton JC, Davidson HW, Peshavaria M. Proteolytic processing of chromogranin A in purified insulin granules. Formation of a 20 kDa N-terminal fragment (betagranin) by the concerted action of a Ca^{2+}-dependent endopeptidase and carboxypeptidase H (EC 3.4.17.10). *Biochem J* 1987;244:457–464.

90. Drees BM, Rouse J, Johnson J, Hamilton JW. Bovine parathyroid glands secrete a 26-kDa N-terminal fragment of chromagranin-A which inhibits parathyroid cell secretion. *Endocrinology* 1991;129:3381–3387.

91. Deftos LJ, Hogue-Angeletti R, Chalberg C, Tu S. A chromogranin A-derived peptide differentially regulates the secretion of calcitonin gene products. *J Bone Mineral Res* 1990;5:989–991.

92. Deftos LJ, Hogue-Angeletti R, Chalberg C, Tu S. PTHrP secretion is stimulated by CT and inhibited by CgA peptides. *Endocrinology* 1989;125:563–565.

93. Aardal S, Helle KB. The vasoinhibitory activity of bovine chromogranin A fragment (vasostatin) and its independence of extracellular calcium in isolated segments of human blood vessels. *Regul Pept* 1992;41:9–18.

94. Drees BA, Hamilton JW. Pancreastatin and bovine parathyroid cell secretion. *Bone Mineral* 1992;17:335–346.

95. Fasciotto BH, Trauss CA, Greeley GH, Cohn DV. Parastatin (porcine chromogranin $A_{347-419}$, a novel chromogranin A-derived peptide, inhibits parathyroid cell secretion. *Endocrinology* (in press).

96. DeLuca HF. Metabolism and mechanisms of action of vitamin D—1982. In: Peck WA, ed. *Bone and mineral research annual I.* Amsterdam: Excerpta Medica, 1983;7.

97. Ritchie CK, Cohn DV, Maercklein PB, Fitzpatrick LA. Individual parathyroid cells exhibit cyclic secretion of parathyroid hormone and chromogranin-A (as measured by a novel sequential hemolytic plaque assay). *Endocrinology* 1992;131:2638–2642.

98. Funakoshi A, Tateishi K, Tsuru M, Jimi A, Wakasugi H, Ikeda Y, Kono A. Pancreastatin producing cell line from human pancreatic islet cell tumor. *Biochem Biophys Res Commun* 1990;168:741–746.

99. Deftos LJ, Gazdar AF, Hogue-Angeletti R, Mullen PS, Burton DW. Distinct patterns of chromogranin-A-related species can be demonstrated in endocrine cells. *Bone Mineral* 1990;9:169–178.

100. Seidah NG, Hendy GN, Hamelin J, et al. Chromogranin A can act as a reversible processing enzyme inhibitor. Evidence from the inhibition of the IRCM-serine protease I cleavage of pro-enkephalin and ACTH at pairs of basic amino acids. *FEBS Lett* 1987;211:144–150.

101. Seidah NG, Paquin J, Hamelin J, Benjannet S, Chretien M. Structural and immunological homology of human and porcine pituitary and plasma IRCH-serine protease I to plasma kallikrein: marked selectivity for pro-enzyme processing. *Biochimie* 1988;70:33–46.

102. Ornberg RL, Kuipers GAJ, Leapman RD. Electron probe microanalysis of subcellular compartments of bovine adrenal chomaffin cells. *J Biol Chem* 1988;263:1488–1493.

103. Südhof TC. Evidence for a divalent cation dependent catecholamine storage complex in chromaffin granules. *Biochem Biophys Res Commun* 1983;116:663–668.

104. Krieger-Brauer HI, Gratzl M. Effects of monovalent and divalent cations on Ca^{2+} fluxes across chromaffin secretory membrane vesicles. *J Neurochem* 1983;41:1269–1276.

105. Shioi J, Gorr S-U, Cohn DV. Stability of intragranular proteins in chromaffin granules after removal of calcium. *J Cell Biol* 1988;107:117a.

106. MacLennan DH, Wong PTS. Isolation of a calcium-sequestering protein from sarcoplasmic reticulum. *Proc Natl Acad Sci USA* 1971;68:1231–1235.

107. Phillips JH. Dynamic aspects of chromaffin granule structure. *Neuroscience* 1982;7:1595–1609.

108. Cohn DV, Gorr S-U. Physiological and biochemical roles of the chromogranin family of proteins. In: Bronner F, Peterlik M, eds. *Extra- and intracellular calcium and phosphate regulation.* Boca Raton, FL: CRC Press Inc., 1991.

109. Thibault G, Doubell AF. Binding and aggregation of proatrial natriuretic factor by calcium. *Am J Physiol* 1992;262:C907–C915.

110. Frank BH, Veros AJ. Physical studies on proinsulin–association behavior and conformation in solution. *Biochem Biophys Res Commun* 1968;32:155–160.

111. Gorr S-U. Calcium-induced aggregation of proteins that are

sorted to the regulated secretory pathway in endocrine cell. *Mol Biol Cell* 1992;3:56a.

112. Chanat E, Huttner WB. Milieu-induced, selective aggregation of regulated secretory proteins in the trans-golgi network. *J Cell Biol* 1991;115:1505–1519.

113. Howell SL, Tyhurst M, Duvefelt H, Andersson A, Hellerstrom C. Role of zinc and calcium in the formation and storage of insulin in the pancreatic β-cell. *Cell Tissue Res* 1978;188:107–118.

114. O'Connor DT, Bernstein KN. Radioimmunoassay of chromogranin A in plasma as a measure of exocytotic sympathoadrenal activity in normal subjects and patients with pheochromocytoma. *N Engl J Med* 1984;311:764–770.

115. Deftos LJ, Woloszczuk W, Krisch L, et al. Medullary thyroid carcinomas express chromogranin A and a novel neuroendocrine protein recognized by monoclonal antibody HISL-19. *Am J Med* 1988;85:780–784.

116. Sobol RE, Memoli V, Deftos LJ. Hormone-negative, chromogranin A-positive endocrine tumors. *N Engl J Med* 1989; 320:444–447.

117. Deftos LJ, O'Connor DT, Wilson CB, Fitzgerald PA. Human pituitary tumors secrete chromogranin-A. *J Clin Endocrinol Metab* 1989;68:869–872.

118. Deftos LJ. Chromogranin A: its role in endocrine function and as an endocrine and neuroendocrine tumor marker. *Endocrine Rev* 1991;12:181–187.

119. Nanes MS, O'Connor DT, Marx SJ. Plasma chromogranin-A in primary hyperparathyroidism. *J Clin Endocrinol Metab* 1989;69:950–955.

120. Levine MA, Dempsey MA, Helman LJ, Ahn TG. Expression of chromogranin-A messenger ribonucleic acid in parathyroid tissue from patients with primary hyperparathyroidism. *J Clin Endocrinol Metab* 1990;70:1668–1673.

121. O'Connor DT, Deftos LJ. Secretion of chromogranin A by peptide-producing endocrine neoplasms. *N Engl J Med* 1986;314:1145–1151.

122. Schürmann G, Raeth U, Wildenmann B, Buhr H, Herfarth C. Serum chromogranin A in the diagnosis and follow-up of neuroendocrine tumors of the gastroenteropancreatic tract. *World Surg* 1992;16:697–702.

123. Harach HR, Wilander E, Grimelius L, Bergholm U, Westermark P, Falkmer S. Chromogranin A immunoreactivity compared with argyrophilia, calcitonin immunoreactivity, and amyloid as tumor markers in the histopathological diagnosis of medullary (C-cell) thyroid carcinoma. *Pathol Res Pract* 1992;188:123–130.

124. Blind E, Schmidt-Gayk H, Sinn HP, O'Connor DT, Raue F. Chromogranin A as tumor marker in medullary thyroid carcinoma. *Thyroid* 1992;2:5–10.

125. Abrahamsson PA, Falkmer S, Falt K, Grimelius L. The course of neuroendocrine differentiation in prostatic carcinomas. An immunohistochemical study testing chromogranin A as an "endocrine marker." *Pathol Res Pract* 1989;185:373–380.

126. Bonkhoff H, Wernert N, Dhom G, Remberger K. Relation of endocrine-paracrine cells to cell proliferation in normal, hyperplastic, and neoplastic human prostate. *Prostate* 1991;19:91–98.

127. Eriksson B, Arnberg H, Lindgren PG, et al. Neuroendocrine pancreatic tumors: clinical presentation, biochemical and histopathological findings in 84 patients. *J Intern Med* 1990;228:103–113.

128. Schmid KW, Kroll M, Hittmair A, et al. Chromogranin A and B in adenomas of the pituitary. An immunohistochemical study of 42 cases. *Am J Surg Pathol* 1991;15:1072–1077.

129. Hsiao RJ, Parmer RJ, Takiyyuddin MA, O'Connor DT. Chromogranin A storage and secretion: sensitivity and specificity for the diagnosis of pheochromocytoma. *Am J Med* 1991;88:607–613.

130. Schober M, Howe PRC, Sperk G, Fischer-Colbrie R, Winkler H. An increased pool of secretory hormones and peptides in adrenal medulla of stroke-prone spontaneously hypertensive rats. *Hypertension* 1989;13:469–474.

131. Takiyyuddin MA, Cervenka JH, Hsiao RJ, Barbosa JA, Parmer RJ, O'Connor DT. Chromogranin A. Storage and release in hypertension. *Hypertension* 1990;15:237–246.

132. Steiner H-J, Weiler R, Ludescher C, Schmid KW, Winkler H. Chromogranins A and B are co-localized with atrial natriuretic peptides in secretory granules of rat heart. *J Histochem Cytochem* 1990;38:845–850.

133. Lewanczuk RZ, Wang J, Zhang ZR, Pang PKT. Effects of spontaneously hypertensive rat plasma on blood pressure and tail artery calcium uptake in normotensive rats. *Am J Hypertens* 1989;2:26–31.

134. Benishin CG, Lewanczuk RZ, Pang PKT. Purification of parathyroid hypertensive factor from plasma of spontaneously hypertensive rats. *Proc Natl Acad Sci USA* 1991;88:6372–6376.

The Parathyroids, edited by J.P. Bilezikian,
M.A. Levine, and R. Marcus. Raven Press, Ltd.,
New York © 1994.

CHAPTER 8

Parathyroid Hormone and Cyclic Adenosine Monophosphate

The Early Days

Lewis R. Chase

In 1957 T.W. Rall, Earl W. Sutherland, and colleagues working at Western Reserve University were studying the mechanism of activation of hepatic phosphorylase by glucagon and epinephrine. They discovered that incubation of particulate fractions from liver with these hormones in the presence of adenosine triphosphate (ATP) and magnesium resulted in formation of a heat-stable factor (1). This factor in turn stimulated formation of active hepatic phosphorylase in supernatant fractions of homogenates in which the hormones themselves were inactive. An identical heat-stable factor was isolated from particulate fractions of heart, skeletal muscle, and brain (2) and was found to be an adenine ribonucleotide that was identical to a compound produced chemically by digestion of adenosine triphosphate with barium hydroxide and identified by Cook, Lipkin, and Markam (3) as cyclic adenosine-3',5'-monophosphate (cAMP). Rall and Sutherland (4) developed the first quantitative assay for this cyclic nucleotide based on stimulation of phosphorylase in liver homogenates. The finding of an intracellular mediator of hormone action formed the basis of the "second messenger" hypothesis. This hypothesis, based on data involving glucagon, epinephrine, and cAMP, postulated that hormones and biogenic amines interact with specific receptors located on the cell surface and do not have to enter the cell in order to act. Interaction

with the receptor results in activation of the enzyme adenylyl cyclase and subsequent generation of intracellular cAMP. The increased intracellular concentration of cAMP in turn activates other intracellular events, which constitute the physiological action(s) of the hormone. This hypothesis formed the basis for our current understanding of hormone receptors, the adenylyl cyclase complex, and the structure and actions of protein kinases as well as the discovery of numerous other intracellular second messengers that are coupled to cell surface receptors.

In 1965, Dr. Sutherland was invited to be an outside lecturer in a seminar series that had been organized by Dr. Gerald Aurbach and several of his colleagues at the National Institutes of Health. During this lecture, Dr. Sutherland cited data indicating that large amounts of cAMP were excreted by the kidney into the urine (5). The excretion of cAMP was not affected by hypophysectomy. Based on the earlier observation of Beutner and Munson (6) that administration of parathyroid hormone, intravenously, to the rat resulted in a prompt increase in urinary phosphate excretion and the new information from Sutherland that cAMP was a mediator of peptide hormone action and was excreted into the urine, Aurbach reasoned that cAMP may be a mediator of the phosphaturic action of parathyroid hormone (PTH) and that its concentration in urine may be responsive to PTH.

To test this hypothesis, Aurbach and Houston (7) developed a more sensitive and specific assay for cAMP. The bioassay methodology based on activation of phosphorylase b kinase by cAMP was cumbersome,

L. R. Chase: Department of Medicine, Washington University School of Medicine, and St. Louis Veterans Affairs Medical Center, St. Louis, Missouri 63106.

nonlinear, and insensitive. Improved methods based on conversion of cAMP to ATP and subsequent measurement of ATP by amplification reactions were insensitive at low concentration of cAMP due to interfering substances. Aurbach solved the contamination problem by removing nucleotides, phosphate, and other interfering substances using a zinc sulfate-barium hydroxide precipitation method he learned from a colleague at the NIH, Dr. Gopal Krishna, and removing contaminating ions by anion-exchange chromatography. The purified cAMP was converted to adenosine 5'-monophosphate by cyclic nucleotide phosphodiesterase and then to ATP by myokinase and pyruvate kinase in the presence of phosphoenolpyruvate. The ATP was then measured using a radioactive phosphate/ATP exchange reaction with the coupled enzymes phosphoglycerate kinase–glyceraldehyde phosphate dehydrogenase. The assay was sensitive to as little as 6×10^{-12} moles of cAMP, which allowed for measurement of physiological concentrations of the cyclic nucleotide in both urine and tissues. Although not as sensitive and simple as the radioimmunoassay or the competitive binding assay for cAMP that were described subsequently, this highly imaginative application of basic biochemistry allowed Aurbach to test his hypothesis.

During the development of the assay for cAMP in Aurbach's laboratory, a Clinical Associate, who had been struggling rather unsuccessfully to improve the radioimmunoassay for parathyroid hormone, volunteered to test whether PTH increased urinary excretion of cAMP in the rat. The bovine hormone was now in plentiful supply; it had been purified, sequenced, and partially synthesized as the result of a long-standing collaborative effort between Aurbach and Dr. John Potts. The Clinical Associate injected parathyroid hormone into hydrated, parathyroidectomized rats and noted a rapid (within minutes) increase in urinary excretion of cAMP that preceded the increased excretion of urinary phosphate (8). Additional experiments demonstrated that calcium suppressed cAMP excretion in rats with intact parathyroid glands. Clearance studies suggested that the cAMP responsive to PTH came directly from the kidney and could not be attributed to increased renal clearance. The subsequent, elegant studies of Broadus, Sutherland, and colleagues (9) assaying both urine and plasma cAMP confirmed these findings and firmly established the concept of "nephrogenous cAMP." These studies provided the basis for using urinary cAMP as a diagnostic test for hyperparathyroidism (10), as an index of successful parathyroidectomy in patients undergoing reoperations for primary hyperparathyroidism (11), and as an early "clue" to the existence of PTH-related protein (PTHrP) as causative factor in the humoral hypercalcemia of malignancy (12).

Sutherland had suggested that three criteria must be met in order to establish that cAMP mediated the physiological response to a given hormone. The hormone should increase the concentration of cAMP in target tissues, the hormone should increase the activity of adenylyl cyclase in plasma membrane preparations from target tissues, and cAMP or its more stable analog dibutyryl cAMP should mimic the physiological actions of the hormone. The initial observations of the effects of PTH on cAMP in urine generated considerable activity at the NIH and elsewhere to test the criteria for the actions of PTH in renal and skeletal tissue. Many different laboratories at the NIH were working concurrently on different cAMP systems, and new discoveries were being made almost daily. Gopal Krishna's laboratory was improving methodology for assaying cAMP and adenylyl cyclase. Martin Rodbell's laboratory was studying the effects of multiple hormones on cAMP metabolism in fat cells and liver, which provided early evidence for the presence of a guanosine triphosphate (GTP)-binding site in the adenylyl cyclase complex. Jesse Roth's laboratory was investigating the effects of thyroid-stimulating hormone (TSH) and adrenocorticotropin (ACTH) on cAMP in thyroid and adrenal tissues. Ira Pastan learned at Sutherland's lecture that there was a high concentration of cAMP in *Escherichia coli*. This finding stimulated his laboratory to initiate innovative studies on the role of cAMP in control of protein synthesis and enzyme induction. Each of these investigators provided useful information and constructive criticism, which greatly facilitated studies that were carried out by Aurbach and his associates.

Demonstration that PTH activated adenylyl cyclase in renal plasma membranes was greatly facilitated by Krishna's new methodology (13), which was based on conversion of $\alpha^{32}P$-ATP to cAM^{32}P and separation of the cAMP formed from substrate and other labeled metabolites. Chase and Aurbach (14) used this methodology to show that PTH activated adenylyl cyclase specifically in plasma membrane fractions from renal cortex, whereas vasopressin activated the enzyme preferentially in renal medulla. These experiments contributed to the emerging concept that specificity for hormone action was conferred at the level of the receptor in the plasma membrane. These findings were rapidly confirmed (15) and extended in Aurbach's laboratory in purified renal tubules (16) and in enriched renal plasma membrane fractions (17).

Marcus and Aurbach (18) adapted the technique into a sensitive bioassay for the hormone, which was utilized to great advantage in Potts's laboratory in developing analogs and inhibitors of PTH. Studies in Rodbell's laboratory (19) demonstrating a GTP requirement for glucagon activation of hepatic adenylyl cyclase stimulated extensive research in Aurbach's laboratory (20) directed toward characterizing the guanine nucleotide binding protein in the adenylyl cyclase complex in turkey erythrocytes and then in renal plasma membranes.

Sutherland's two other criteria were demonstrated concurrently with the adenylyl cyclase data. Parathyroid hormone was shown to cause a rapid increase in the concentration of endogenous cAMP in vivo (21), in renal cortical tubules (22), and in renal slices (23). Infusion of cAMP or its analog dibutyryl cAMP mimicked the phosphaturic action of PTH in rats (24), dogs (25), and man (26).

Attention was next focused on the effect of PTH on the adenylyl cyclase–cAMP system in skeletal tissue. Wells and Lloyd (27) carried out a series of infusion experiments in parathyroidectomized rats in which they showed that dibutyryl cAMP or theophylline, an inhibitor of cyclic nucleotide phosphodiesterase, caused significant hypercalcemia and hypophosphatemia. The results were confirmed and extended by Rasmussen (24), who also demonstrated a significant increase in hydroxyproline excretion. Raisz's laboratory had developed a technique for studying the actions of PTH in organ cultures of fetal rat calvaria labeled with radioactive calcium. Dibutyryl cAMP was shown to mimic the effects of PTH in this system both histologically and biochemically (28). The fetal rat calvaria model provided the opportunity for Aurbach's laboratory to apply the adenylyl cyclase and cAMP assays to skeletal tissue. Chase, Aurbach, and colleagues showed that PTH caused a rapid and concentration-dependent increase in adenylyl cyclase in broken cell preparations (29) and an increase in the concentration of cAMP (30) in whole tissue from fetal rat calvaria. Thus Sutherland's criteria were also satisfied for the effects of PTH on bone. An interesting incidental finding from these studies was that prostaglandin E_1 (PGE_1) was added to the organ culture system, fortuitously, as an "on-the-shelf" control and was found to increase cAMP formation. Raisz was notified of these results and quickly showed that PGE_1 also caused significant bone resorption. These findings stimulated others to test the hypothesis (still without conclusive support) that prostaglandins were a mediator of the hypercalcemia of malignancy.

The late 1960s at the NIH was a period of intense and exciting clinical activity in addition to the basic science that was being carried out concurrently. G. Donald Whedon had been promoted to Director of the (then) National Institute of Arthritis and Metabolic Diseases, and Aurbach had assumed Whedon's position as Chief of the Metabolic Diseases Branch of this Institute. The clinical focus of the branch shifted from Whedon's classic balance studies on patients with osteoporosis to Aurbach's major interest in disorders of the parathyroid glands. Aurbach was a skilled clinician

and endocrinologist as well as a scientist, and he immediately realized the clinical implications of his cAMP studies in disorders of the parathyroids. Early studies were facilitated by the availability of purified PTH that had been prepared in Potts's laboratory. With this preparation, the potential effects of contaminating factors in commercially available crude parathyroid extract did not require consideration. It was quickly demonstrated that PTH caused a marked increase in urinary cAMP in normal human volunteers and that this effect preceded, temporally, the phosphaturic effect of the hormone and exceeded it, significantly, in magnitude.

It had been postulated in the 1940s by Fuller Albright that the X-linked dominant disorder pseudohypoparathyroidism was characterized by peripheral resistance to PTH. In the classic diagnostic test described by Ellsworth and Howard, patients with pseudohypoparathyroidism did not develop the expected phosphaturic response to an injection of parathyroid extract; the test was inconsistent and insensitive. A mother with pseudopseudohypoparathyroidism and her daughter with pseudohypoparathyroidism were admitted to the Clinical Center at the NIH, and Chase, Melson, and Aurbach (31) demonstrated the first case of a deficient urinary cAMP response to PTH in the affected daughter. In a subsequent flurry of activity, Aurbach contacted colleagues around the country to locate patients with pseudohypoparathyroidism and other causes of PTH deficiency. The findings in the original case were confirmed. In additional studies, elevated concentrations of PTH in serum of patients with pseudohypoparathyroidism were demonstrated and suppressed with calcium. The cAMP response to exogenous PTH was not restored after suppression of endogenous PTH, indicating that a biologically inactive form of the hormone could not account for the peripheral resistance. Thus, the resistance to PTH in pseudohypoparathyroidism was localized to an abnormality in the receptor–adenylyl cyclase complex. Direct studies of adenylyl cyclase activation in renal tissue from two patients with pseudohypoparathyroidism were not consistent with an abnormal receptor or adenylyl cyclase catalytic activity and suggested an abnormality in the "G" protein (32,33). Aurbach's uncanny ability to link seemingly unrelated areas of investigation further extended and defined this hypothesis. Studies from his and Bourne's laboratories to define the β-adrenergic receptor/adenylyl cyclase/ cAMP complex in avian erythrocytes provided the basis for localizing the abnormality in pseudohypoparathyroidism to defective activation of the guanine nucleotide-regulatory protein (34,35). These studies anticipated subsequent definition of the molecular basis of the G protein abnormality (36,37). These early studies on the role of cAMP in the mechanism of action of PTH and its extension to clinical disorders of the parathyroids established the legacy through which Gerald Aurbach influenced and inspired a generation of investigators.

REFERENCES

1. Rall TW, Sutherland EW, Berthet J. The relationship of epinephrine and glucagon to liver phosphorylase. *J Biol Chem* 1957;224:463–475.
2. Sutherland EW, Rall TW. Fractionation and characterization of a cyclic adenine ribonucleotide formed by tissue particles. *J Biol Chem* 1957;232:1077–1091.
3. Cook WH, Lipkin D, Markham R. The formation of a cyclic dianhydrodiadenylic acid (I) by the alkaline degradation of adenosine-5′-triphosphoric acid (II). *J Am Chem Soc* 1957; 79:3607–3608.
4. Rall TW, Sutherland EW. Formation of a cyclic adenine ribonucleotide by tissue particles. *J Biol Chem* 1957;232:1065–1076.
5. Hardman JG, Davis JW, Sutherland EW. Measurement of guanosine 3′,5′-monophosphate and other cyclic nucleotides. Variations in urinary excretion with hormonal state of the rat. *J Biol Chem* 1966;241:4812–4815.
6. Beutner EH, Munson PL. Time course of urinary excretion of inorganic phosphate by rats after parathyroidectomy and injection of parathyroid extract. *Endocrinology* 1960;66:610.
7. Aurbach GD, Houston BA. Determination of 3′,5′-adenosine monophosphate with a method based on a radioactive phosphate exchange reaction. *J Biol Chem* 1968;243:5935–5940.
8. Chase LR, Aurbach GD. Parathyroid function and the renal excretion of 3′,5′-adenylic acid. *Proc Natl Acad Sci USA* 1967;58:518–525.
9. Broadus AE, Kaminsky NI, Hardman JG, Sutherland EW, Liddle GW. Kinetic parameters and renal clearances of plasma adenosine 3′,5′cyclic monophosphate and guanosine 3′,5′-monophosphate in man. *J Clin Invest* 1970;49:2222–2236.
10. Broadus AE, Mahaffey JE, Bartter FC, Neer RM. Nephrogenous cyclic adenosine monophosphate as a parathyroid function test. *J Clin Invest* 1977;60:771–783.
11. Darling GE, Marx SJ, Spiegel AM, Aurbach GD, Norton JA. Prospective analysis of intraoperative and postoperative urinary cyclic adenosine 3′,5′-monophosphate levels to predict outcome of patients undergoing reoperations for primary hyperparathyroidism. *Surgery* 1988;104:1128–1136.
12. Stewart AF, Horst R, Deftos LJ, Cadman EC, Lang R, Broadus AE. Biochemical evaluation of patients with cancer-associated hypercalcemia: evidence for humoral and nonhumoral groups. *N Engl J Med* 1980;30:1377–1383.
13. Krishna G, Weiss B, Brodie BB. A simple sensitive method for the assay of adenylyl cyclase. *J Pharmacol Exp Ther* 1968;163:379–385.
14. Chase LR, Aurbach GD. Renal adenyl cyclase: anatomical separation of sites sensitive to parathyroid hormone and vasopressin. *Science* 1968;159:545–547.
15. Dousa T, Rychlik I. The effect of parathyroid hormone on adenyl cyclase in rat kidney. *Biochim Biophys Acta* 1968; 158:484–486.
16. Melson GL, Chase LR, Aurbach GD. Parathyroid hormone-sensitive adenylyl cyclase in isolated renal tubules. *Endocrinology* 1970;86:511–518.
17. Marx SJ, Fedak SA, Aurbach GD. Preparation and characterization of a hormone-responsive renal plasma membrane fraction. *J Biol Chem* 1972;247:6913–6918.
18. Marcus R, Aurbach GD. Bioassay of parathyroid hormone in vitro with a stable preparation of adenyl cyclase from rat kidney. *Endocrinology* 1969;85:801–810.
19. Rodbell M, Krans HM, Pohl SL, Birnbaumer L. The glucagon-sensitive adenyl cyclase system in plasma membranes of rat liver. *J Biol Chem* 1971;246:1872–1876.
20. Spiegel AM, Downs RW, Levine MA, et al. The role of guanine nucleotides in regulation of adenylate cyclase activity. *Rec Progr Horm Res* 1981;37:635–665.
21. Aurbach GD, Potts JT, Chase LR, Melson GL. Polypeptide hormones and calcium metabolism. *Ann Intern Med* 1969; 70:1243–1265.
22. Rasmussen H, Tenenhouse A. Cyclic adenosine monophosphate, calcium and membranes. *Proc Natl Acad Sci USA* 1968;59:1364–1370.
23. Steiner AL, Pagliara AS, Chase LR, Kipnis DM. Radioimmunoassay for cyclic nucleotides. *J Biol Chem* 1972; 247:1114–1120.
24. Rasmussen H, Pechet M, Fast D. Effect of dibutyryl cyclic adenosine 3′,5′-monophosphate, theophylline, and other nucleotides upon calcium and phosphate metabolism. *J Clin Invest* 1968;47:1843–1850.
25. Gill JR, Casper AG. Renal effects of adenosine 3′,5′-cyclic monophosphate and dibutyryl adenosine 3′,5′-cyclic monophosphate. *J Clin Invest* 1971;50:1231–1240.
26. Bell NH, Avery S, Sinha T, Clark CM, Allen DO, Johnston C. Effects of dibutyryl cyclic adenosine 3′,5′-monophosphate and parathyroid extract on calcium and phosphorus metabolism in hypoparathyroidism and pseudohypoparathyroidism. *J Clin Invest* 1972;51:816–823.
27. Wells J, Lloyd W. Hypercalcemic and hypophosphatemic effects of dibutyryl cyclic AMP in rats after parathyroidectomy. *Endocrinology* 1969;84:861–867.
28. Raisz LG, Brand JS, Klein DC, Au WY. Hormonal regulation of bone resorption. In: Gual C, ed. *Progress in endocrinology*. Amsterdam: Excerpta Medica Foundation, 1969;696–703.
29. Chase LR, Fedak SA, Aurbach GD. Activation of skeletal adenyl cyclase by parathyroid hormone in vitro. *Endocrinology* 1969;84:761–768.
30. Chase LR, Aurbach GD. The effect of parathyroid hormone on the concentration of adenosine 3′,5′-monophosphate in skeletal tissue in vitro. *J Biol Chem* 1970;245:1520–1526.
31. Chase LR, Melson GL, Aurbach GD. Pseudohypoparathyroidism: defective excretion of 3′,5′-AMP in response to parathyroid hormone. *J Clin Invest* 1969;48:1832–1844.
32. Marcus R, Wilber JF, Aurbach GD. Parathyroid hormone-sensitive adenylyl cyclase from the renal cortex of a patient with pseudohypoparathyroidism. *J Clin Endocrinol Metab* 1971;33:537–541.
33. Drezner MK, Burch WM. Altered activity of the nucleotide regulating site in the parathyroid hormone sensitive adenylate cyclase from the renal cortex of a patient with pseudohypoparathyroidism. *J Clin Invest* 1978;62:1222–1227.
34. Levine MA, Downs RW, Singer M, Marx SJ, Aurbach GD, Spiegel AM. Deficient activity of guanine nucleotide regulatory protein in erythrocytes in patients with pseudohypoparathyroidism. *Biochem Biophys Res Commun* 1980;94:1319–1324.
35. Farfel Z, Brickman AS, Kaslow HR, Brothers VM, Bourne HR. Defect of receptor-cyclase coupling protein in pseudohypoparathyroidism. *N Engl J Med* 1980;31:237–242.
36. Weinstein LS, Gejman PV, Friedman E, et al. Mutations of the G_S alpha-subunit gene in Albright hereditary osteodystrophy detected by denaturing gradient gel electrophoresis. *Proc Natl Acad Sci USA* 1990;87:8287–8290.
37. Patten JL, Johns DR, Valle D, et al. Mutation of the gene encoding the stimulatory G protein of adenylate cyclase in Albright's hereditary osteodystrophy. *N Engl J Med* 1990; 322:1412–1419.

The Parathyroids, edited by J.P. Bilezikian,
M.A. Levine, and R. Marcus. Raven Press, Ltd.,
New York © 1994.

CHAPTER 9

Parathyroid Hormone Biosynthesis and Metabolism

Henry M. Kronenberg, F. Richard Bringhurst, Gino V. Segre, and John T. Potts, Jr.

The parathyroid hormone (PTH) gene has many jobs. It must encode a peptide that can bind to and activate receptors on target tissues. Equally importantly, the amount of hormone produced must be carefully controlled to maintain the blood level of calcium within a narrow range. Nature's solution to these problems has involved the specific synthesis of PTH primarily in the parathyroid chief cell, a cell designed to sense the blood level of calcium. In the chief cell, synthesis and secretion of the hormone can be carefully regulated. Furthermore, the structure of the hormone is designed for rapid metabolic degradation, even in the absence of receptor binding. In this way, the rapid turnover of the hormone can ensure that circulating blood concentrations of hormone change quickly in response to changes in hormone secretory rate. This rapid metabolism of hormone is required of a system designed to respond quickly to sudden changes in the amounts of calcium entering and leaving the bloodstream. Studies over the last 2 decades have shown that the sequences of PTH and its precursors are designed to steer the hormone through the chief cell's secretory pathway, to direct the hormone's binding to receptors, and to ensure rapid metabolism of the hormone. More recent studies have begun to unravel the mechanisms whereby synthesis of PTH is regulated in the chief cell. This chapter describes the structure of the PTH gene and summarizes the current understanding of

how this structure allows the gene to accomplish its multiple functions.

BIOSYNTHESIS OF PARATHYROID HORMONE

Parathyroid hormone is synthesized as part of the larger precursor molecule, preproPTH. Only trace amounts of this full-length precursor are found in parathyroid chief cells, because the "pre" or signal sequence is cleaved from the amino terminus while the protein is being synthesized (see Fig. 1). As the signal sequence emerges from the ribosome, it binds to a signal recognition particle, an RNA–protein complex that recognizes signal sequences on most secreted proteins. The signal recognition particle then binds to a receptor on the rough endoplasmic reticulum and directs the nascent preproPTH molecule to a protein-lined channel, through which the preproPTH molecule is transported. A signal peptidase located on the inner surface of the membrane of the endoplasmic reticulum then cleaves off the signal sequence, leaving the intermediate precursor, proPTH, in the cisternae of the endoplasmic reticulum. ProPTH then travels via a series of vesicles to and through the Golgi apparatus (see Fig. 2). In the Golgi, the short, amino-terminal "pro" sequence is removed, leaving the mature PTH molecule. Parathyroid hormone is then concentrated in dense core secretory vesicles; these vesicles fuse with the plasma membrane and release PTH in response to a fall in extracellular calcium. The hormone secreted is predominantly the intact 84-residue PTH molecule, although a variable fraction made up of carboxy-terminal PTH fragments is secreted as well.

H. M. Kronenberg, G. V. Segre, F. R. Bringhurst, and J. T. Potts, Jr.: Endocrine Unit, Department of Medicine, Massachusetts General Hospital, and Harvard Medical School, Boston, Massachusetts 02114.

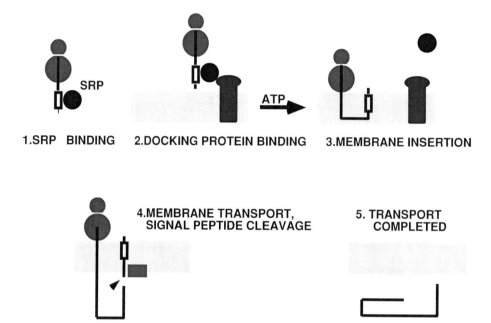

FIG. 1. The signal or "pre" sequence directs the nascent polypeptide to the apparatus for transport across the membrane of the endoplasmic reticulum.

Function of the Signal or "Pre" Sequence

The specific sequences of each of the three portions of the preproPTH molecule are responsible for directing the hormone through this complicated pathway of transport and cleavage. The known preproPTH sequences from human (1), bovine (2), rat (3), pig (4), and chicken (5,6) share a 25-residue "pre" sequence and a six-residue "pro" sequence (see Fig. 3). Each "pre" sequence contains a hydrophobic stretch of amino acids preceded by a positively charged residue. The signal sequence ends with a small amino acid at the last and third-to-last positions. These characteristics are typical of most signal sequences. PreproPTH's signal sequence was first discovered (7) when parathyroid gland mRNA was translated in a cell-free

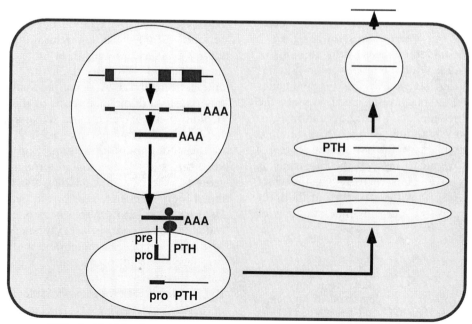

FIG. 2. Multiple cleavages occur during the intracellular transport of PTH.

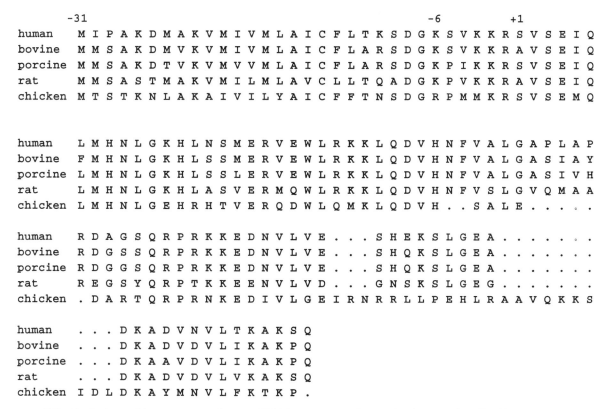

FIG. 3. Amino acid sequences of preproPTH from mammalian and avian species. Residues −31 to −7 constitute the "pre" sequences; residues −6 to −1 constitute the "pro" sequences. *Dots* represent residues found in chicken PTH without corresponding residues in the mammalian sequences. Amino acid residues are indicated by the single letter code: ala A, arg R, asn N, asp D, cys C, gln Q, glu E, gly G, his H, ile I, leu L, lys K, met M, phe F, pro P ser S, thr T, trp W, tyr Y, val V.

extract devoid of endoplasmic reticulum. Directed mutations have demonstrated the importance of each of the regions of the preproPTH's signal sequence for normal signal function (8–10). Furthermore, when a synthetic "prepro" peptide was added to a cell-free extract, it blocked the transport and cleavage of proPTH by microsomal membranes (11). Most strikingly, a point mutation was found in the signal sequence of a preproPTH gene in a family with inherited hypoparathyroidism (12). A point mutation at residue 18 changed the cysteine to arginine and thereby inserted a charged residue into the hydrophobic core of the signal sequence. When this mutant preproPTH was expressed in cell-free extracts or in cultured cells, the precursor was inefficiently transported and cleaved.

Function of the "Pro" Sequence

The signal sequence of proPTH thus resembles the signal sequences of other secreted proteins and performs the important role of directing the protein across the membrane of the endoplasmic reticulum and into the secretory pathway. The function of the "pro" sequence is less well established. In all known preproPTH sequences, the "pro" sequence is six residues long. The first is always positively charged, the third is hydrophobic, and the last two residues are lys-arg. This pattern closely resembles that found in rat proalbumin (arg-gly-val-phe-arg-arg) and that predicted to be present in the "pro" sequence of preproparathyroid hormone-related protein (PTHrP) (arg-arg-leu-lys-arg) (see the chapter by Broadus and Stewart). ProPTH was first discovered as a large PTH-related molecule that was the predominant form of the hormone found in parathyroid cells after pulse labeling with radioactive amino acids (13,14). Subsequent chase incubations demonstrated that the proPTH was converted to PTH in ~15 min; this correlated in time with transport to the Golgi (15). After this time, no trace of the "pro" peptide or possible fragments could be found in the cell or medium (16). These data strongly suggest that the "pro" sequence serves an exclusively intracellular function, probably involved in movement through the secretory pathway. Wiren et al. (17) tested this hypothesis by deleting the DNA sequences encoding the "pro" hexapeptide from cloned cDNA encoding human preproPTH and by subsequently expressing the cDNA in cell-free protein-synthesizing extracts and in intact rat pituitary GH4 cells. The mutant precursor functioned abnormally in both expression systems. The precursor crossed the membrane of the endoplasmic reticulum inefficiently, and, consequently, the subsequent cleavage of the signal sequence was inefficient. Cells secreted PTH but also secreted a molecule slightly bigger than PTH. Sequence analysis showed that the abnormal protein included the last two residues of the signal sequence. Thus the removal of the "pro" sequence resulted in imprecise and inefficient function of the signal sequence. The "pro" sequence of preproPTH should be considered part of the functional unit responsible for transport and cleavage of the precursor upon its entry into the secretory pathway. This result is not surprising. In other precursor proteins, the sequences immediately distal to the signal sequence can affect signal sequence function. One can speculate that the constraints on this region conflict with the constraints on the amino terminus of the mature PTH molecule. The PTH receptor, for example, requires very specific residues at the amino terminus of PTH for subsequent activation of adenylyl cyclase (see chapter by Chorev and Rosenblatt). The experiments of Wiren et al. (17) show that these residues cannot be placed immediately distal to the signal sequence. The "pro" sequence can be considered a linker region that allows efficient signal sequence function and physically separates the signal sequence from the mature hormone sequence, which has its own and separate evolutionary constraints. The possibility that the "pro" sequence has additional functions, such as the promotion of proper folding of the PTH molecule in the endoplasmic reticulum, has not been rigorously examined.

The enzyme responsible for cleavage of the "pro" sequence of proPTH has not yet been characterized, but a number of arguments suggest that the recently characterized protein furin (or a close relative) is the cleavage enzyme (18). Furin is a subtilisin-like enzyme that is located in the Golgi cisternae of probably all mammalian cells. The enzyme cleaves sequences like the "pro" sequence of rat proalbumin that end in dibasic residues and are preceded by other basic residues. Unlike the related PC2 and PC1 proteases, which are found in cells with secretory granules, furin cleaves precursors in cells such as hepatocytes, which have no secretory granules. Cleavage by furin probably explains why proPTH, in contrast to proinsulin, for example, is cleaved normally when the hormone is synthesized in all sorts of cells, from parathyroid chief cells to fibroblasts and kidney cells (19,20). One can only speculate on why proPTH, which is normally synthesized virtually exclusively in specialized parathyroid chief cells, uses an enzyme designed for cleav-

age of proteins secreted from nonendocrine cells. One plausible explanation is an evolutionary argument. The PTH gene may well be derived from the gene encoding PTHrP. The PTHrP gene is widely expressed, both in cells with secretory granules, such as parathyroid chief cells and neurons, and in cells without secretory granules, such as smooth muscle cells (see the chapter by Broadus and Stewart). Therefore, it would be expected that the "pro" sequence of proPTHrP would be designed for cleavage by an enzyme expressed in most cells. The "pro" sequence of proPTH may well share this property because of its evolutionary heritage, even though proPTH is normally expressed only in cells with a secretory granule apparatus.

Intracellular Roles of the Mature Parathyroid Hormone Sequence

Like the "prepro" sequence, portions of the mature PTH molecule serve to facilitate intracellular handling of PTH (21). Shortened versions of preproPTH are not stable in transfected cells. When the human preproPTH cDNA was modified to encode preproPTH (1–40) (where the numbers refer to the mature PTH sequence), the signal sequence functioned, and proPTH (1–40) was produced in transfected cells. The proPTH-(1–40) was not further cleaved to PTH-(1–40), however. Instead, it was degraded intracellularly; no PTH peptides were secreted from the cells. A similar, though less dramatic, defect in secretion was exhibited by preproPTH-(1–52). These short precursors were long enough for the signal sequence to direct them into the secretory pathway, but they were unstable and were not transported through the entire pathway. These results may partly explain the role of the carboxy-terminal portion of the PTH molecule. One function of the full 84-residue protein may be to allow stable and efficient transport through the secretory apparatus. Since all secreted peptides are synthesized as rather large precursors, this need for a minimal length of translation product may be a general one for secreted proteins.

Even the 84-residue PTH molecule is not completely stable in the parathyroid chief cell. Though the major secretory product of the cell is normally the 84-residue peptide, the hormone secreted by calves in vivo under conditions of hypercalcemia consists largely of carboxy-terminal fragments of PTH (22). Secretion of fragments of PTH was studied in detail by Habener et al. (23) and by Chu et al. (24). These workers noted that the degradation of newly synthesized PTH is influenced by the level of extracellular calcium. Few fragments were secreted when the gland was stimulated in vitro by medium containing low levels of calcium. In contrast, most of the hormone secreted under conditions of hypercalcemic suppression consisted of fragments. Thus calcium regulated the amount of available intact PTH by causing the intracellular degradation of hormone. This effect could have been caused by the activation of a PTH-degrading pathway. Alternatively, the intracellular degradation rate might have been constant; the decrease in total degradation of PTH associated with low calcium levels might simply have resulted from rapid secretion of hormone and the concomitant shorter time of exposure to the intracellular degradation mechanism.

Phorbol ester treatment of parathyroid cells in vitro has also been shown to result in the secretion of an increased fraction of PTH fragments, in both high- and low-calcium conditions (25). Phorbols are either activating a proteolytic mechanism or may be selectively stimulating secretion from secretory granules containing a high proportion of PTH fragments. The physiologic correlate in vivo of this action of phorbol esters has not yet been established. In any case, the parathyroid gland has the capability of varying the fraction of PTH secreted as the biologically active, intact molecule. This seemingly wasteful capability makes it possible for the gland to vary quickly and dramatically the amount of biologically active hormone secreted. This regulatory capability provides a rationale for the intracellular instability of the hormone. (The secretion of hormonal fragments is addressed below under Peripheral Metabolism of Parathyroid Hormone.)

To sum up, it can be seen that all portions of the preproPTH molecule have intracellular functions. The "prepro" region is required for efficient introduction of the hormone to the secretory pathway. The carboxy-terminal region of the mature hormone is required for efficient and stable transport of PTH through the secretory pathway. Inherent instability of even the full-length hormone provides a regulatory mechanism that allows extracellular calcium to alter rapidly the amount of active hormone available for secretion.

THE PARATHYROID HORMONE GENE

The genomic DNAs encoding human (26), bovine (27), rat (28), and chicken (29) preproPTH have been cloned; the complete sequences of the human (30) and bovine (27) genes have been determined. Each gene contains three exons separated by two introns (see Fig. 4). The introns vary in size from species to species, though the first intron is invariably large, and the second intron in the human, bovine, and rat genes is ~100 base pairs (bp) in length. This length is close to

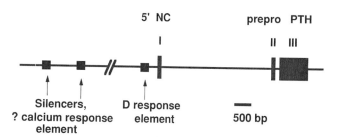

FIG. 4. The parathyroid hormone gene.

the minimum length that can be recognized by the splicing machinery. The introns interrupt the sequences encoding mRNA at precisely the same locations in each species. The first exon contains most of the 5' noncoding sequence. The second exon encodes most of the "prepro" sequence; the second intron comes in the middle of the triplet encoding the lysine residue that precedes the dibasic cleavage sequence lys-arg found at the end of the known "pro" sequences. The third exon encodes the lys-arg sequence, the mature PTH sequence, and the 3' noncoding region of the gene.

The human and bovine genes are preceded by two functional TATA boxes that determine the two closely spaced start sites of the human are bovine transcripts. The rat and chicken genes are preceded by only one TATA box, found in a position equivalent to the second TATA box in the human and bovine genes. Though both start sites of transcription are used in the human and bovine genes, no conditions have been found that favor the use of one start site over the other. No data suggest that the two transcripts have importantly different stabilities or translatability, but such questions have not been exhaustively studied.

The 5' noncoding regions of each gene extend ~120 base pairs. The 3' noncoding regions of each gene vary substantially in length, from the bovine at 227 base pairs to the chicken at >1,600 base pairs. Possible functional properties of these sequences have not been systematically examined.

The human, rat, and bovine PTH genes are represented only once in the haploid genomes of each species. The human PTH gene is located on the short arm of chromosome 11 at band 11p15 (31–33). A series of restriction fragment length polymorphisms (34,35) have made it possible to show that the human PTH gene is linked to the genes encoding catalase, calcitonin, *H-ras,* insulin, and β-globin (36). Two other polymorphisms have been identified through the use of denaturing gel electrophoresis (37). All of these polymorphisms have been useful in defining the inheritance of specific alleles of the PTH gene in families with calcium disorders (38).

Several features of the PTH gene suggest that the gene is related to that encoding PTHrP (39–41). Most importantly, the major coding exon of both genes starts precisely at the same nucleotide, one base before the codons encoding the lys-arg residues of the "pro" sequences of each hormone. After the lys-arg sequences, the PTH and PTHrP amino acid sequences are identical in eight of the next 13 residues. Further, the PTHrP gene is located on chromosome 12, a chromosome known to encode many genes that resemble genes on chromosome 11; for this reason, the chromosomes are thought to have arisen by an ancient duplication event (42). One can speculate that the PTH gene may represent a variation of the PTHrP gene; the PTH hormone takes advantage of the PTHrP receptor to regulate calcium metabolism. If this hypothesis is correct, then the gene had to change in order to ensure expression primarily in the parathyroid chief cell and to ensure appropriate regulation by modulators such as extracellular calcium and 1,25-dihydroxyvitamin D_3 [1,25-$(OH)_2D_3$].

REGULATION OF PARATHYROID HORMONE BIOSYNTHESIS

The minute-to-minute stability of the level of blood calcium depends on the regulation of PTH secretion by calcium. Longer term homeostasis depends on several other levels of control (see Fig. 5). The number of parathyroid chief cells is carefully regulated; when appropriately stimulated, the parathyroid glands can increase in size dramatically. The parathyroid chief cell is uniquely designed to express the PTH gene; the state of differentiation of the chief cell can, therefore, influence the rate of PTH biosynthesis. Specific blood-borne signals, most notably calcium and 1,25-$(OH)_2D_3$, regulate the activity of the PTH gene as well. In this section, these several levels of regulation of PTH biosynthesis are discussed.

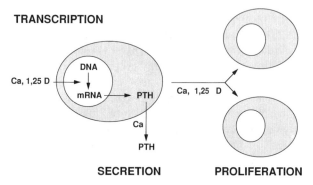

FIG. 5. Levels of parathyroid cell regulation.

Regulation of Parathyroid Cell Number

Little is known about the regulation of parathyroid cell number. The relatively uniform morphology of chief cells suggests that all chief cells have the potential to divide, if appropriately stimulated, but the alternative hypothesis that a subset of chief cells has the unique, stem cell-like capability to proliferate has not been evaluated. Furthermore, there is the general impression that parathyroid cells are long-lived, since mitoses are seldom seen in normal glands of mature animals and because hyperplastic glands only slowly decrease in size after stimulation. Nevertheless, specific studies to define potential modulators of chief cell longevity have not been performed. Despite this paucity of information, the dramatic hyperplasia of parathyroid cells in patients and animals with renal failure demonstrates the likely roles of calcium and 1,25-$(OH)_2D_3$ in regulating parathyroid cell proliferation. Dietary manipulation alone can similarly lead to chief cell hyperplasia. Naveh-Many and Silver (43), for example, used flow cytometry to count parathyroid cells and showed that 3 weeks of a calcium- and vitamin D-deficient diet fed to weanling rats led to a 1.7-fold increase in parathyroid cell number. Other issues related to parathyroid cell growth are covered in the chapter by Parfitt.

The possibly independent roles of calcium and 1,25-$(OH)_2D_3$ in the regulation of parathyroid cell proliferation have not been studied extensively. In vivo, these variables are difficult to manipulate independently in the intact animal. In studies of cultured parathyroid chief cells, it has been possible to vary the levels of calcium and 1,25-$(OH)_2D_3$ separately. Several groups have shown that 1,25-$(OH)_2D_3$ can regulate parathyroid cell proliferation in vitro. Whether the cells were grown in the presence of serum (44,45) or serum-free growth factors (46), administration of 1,25-$(OH)_2D_3$ decreased their rate of proliferation. Studies of the effects of calcium on parathyroid cell proliferation in vitro have yielded differing results. Several studies have shown that lowering of calcium leads to increased cellular proliferation (47–49). Other studies of dispersed, early-passage chief cells have demonstrated no effect of calcium on the rate of cell proliferation, however (45,46,50).

Although extracellular levels of calcium and 1,25-$(OH)_2D_3$ can be independently regulated in vitro, it is hard to be sure that parathyroid cells in culture respond to modulators of proliferation in this setting in the same way that they do in vivo. Thus, while the combined effects of low calcium and low levels of 1,25-$(OH)_2D_3$ to stimulate parathyroid cell proliferation are well established, the individual roles of calcium and 1,25-$(OH)_2D_3$ remain uncertain. The direct effects of 1,25-(OH)$_2$D$_3$ have been demonstrated consistently in vitro; the possible direct effects of calcium have been less uniformly demonstrated.

Cell-Specific Parathyroid Hormone Gene Expression

Expression of the PTH gene occurs almost exclusively in the parathyroid chief cell. [Expression has been noted in the rat hypothalamus as well (98).] When the chief cell is disrupted by neoplastic transformation, the regulation of PTH gene expression can be altered. For example, parathyroid cancers may stop synthesizing PTH completely, although this is rare (51). Presumably, specific DNA sequences associated with the PTH gene respond to the environment of the chief cell to activate gene expression. Because no well-differentiated cell line expressing the PTH gene has been established, it has been difficult to determine the sequences responsible for chief cell-specific PTH gene expression. Occasional "experiments of nature" have provided important clues, however. Very rarely, human nonparathyroid tumors have been found to produce PTH ectopically, for example. In one case studied carefully (52), the PTH regulatory region upstream from the gene was disrupted in tumor cells. Presumably, this gene rearrangement allowed the gene to be expressed in nonparathyroid cells by providing new regulatory signals or abolishing normal silencing mechanisms found upstream of the gene. Furthermore, in a subset of parathyroid adenomas, the entire upstream portion of the PTH gene and the first, noncoding exon are separated from the rest of the gene and rearranged adjacent to the PRAD1 gene (see the chapter by Arnold) (53). As a consequence of this rearrangement, the PRAD1 gene, a regulator of the cell cycle, is dramatically overexpressed. These observations suggest that the PTH gene upstream region contain sequences that stimulate gene transcription in parathyroid chief cells. Further analysis of the sequences that determine chief cell expression of the PTH gene must await studies of transgenic animals or the establishment of well-differentiated parathyroid chief cell lines.

Modulators of Parathyroid Hormone Gene Expression

The effects of calcium on PTH gene expression were first demonstrated in experiments using primary parathyroid cells in culture. Russell et al. (54) found that high levels of calcium resulted in a fall in PTH mRNA levels over a period of several days. In those studies, no difference was noted between the effects of low and normal levels of extracellular calcium. The fall in PTH mRNA levels in response to high calcium could be re-

versed by lowering the calcium level; thus the suppressive effect of calcium was not an irreversible, toxic effect. These in vitro observations have been confirmed by Brookman et al. (55), who noted a slight increase in PTH mRNA under low-calcium conditions at one time point. Subsequent studies by Russell and Sherwood (56) showed that the rate of transcription of the PTH gene in nuclei of dispersed bovine parathyroid cells fell within 6 hr in response to high levels of extracellular calcium. The rate of transcription of the actin gene was unchanged; therefore, the effect of calcium was shown to be specific.

Two groups have studied the acute effects of changes in blood calcium on PTH mRNA levels in the intact rat. Both showed that acute lowering of blood calcium (with phosphate, calcitonin, or EDTA) led to a prompt increase in PTH mRNA levels (57,58). Elevations in blood calcium, in contrast, led to no change in PTH mRNA levels after 6 hr (57) and to a slight decrease in PTH mRNA levels after 48 hr (58). The parathyroid gland apparently, then, in the normal state rests near the bottom of the calcium dose–response curve. The gland is well equipped to increase PTH production but poorly prepared to decrease production in the face of hypercalcemia.

The results of studies in intact animals resemble those in vitro, but they differ in two respects. The time course of the in vivo response is extremely rapid, with maximal responses occurring in a few hours. In contrast, the in vitro responses take days. Furthemore, the in vitro studies show little difference between the effects of low and normal extracellular calcium levels. Only high calcium levels lead to a fall in PTH mRNA levels. Thus the in vitro mRNA response to calcium is shifted to the right in comparison to the response in vivo. These differences cannot be clearly explained at present but may well represent some damage to the calcium response machinery when parathyroid cells are placed in culture. Alternatively, but less likely, the effects of calcium in vivo could be a consequence of the alteration of some other blood constituent in response to hypocalcemia or could reflect effects of calcium on organs other than the parathyroid.

The lack of parathyroid cell lines that produce PTH has hampered the search for DNA sequences responsible for the transcriptional effects of calcium. Okazaki et al. (59) have identified short sequences several thousand base pair upstream from the start site of PTH gene transcription that may well be important for calcium regulation, however. These investigators identified the region by showing that several short sequences in the region could decrease gene transcription from many different promoters, including the PTH gene promoter (60). Furthermore, when the level of extracellular calcium was varied, after transfection of fusion genes containing a short oligonucleotide from this region, high calcium further suppressed transcription from genes containing the sequence but had no effect on control plasmids. Intriguingly, almost identical sequences were found in the gene encoding rat atrial natriuretic polypeptide, another gene negatively regulated by calcium. This DNA sequence could also confer calcium sensitivity to a fusion gene in fibroblast transfection experiments. While these experiments are very suggestive, further studies will be necessary to show that the regulatory region can confer calcium sensitivity in its normal location far upstream from the PTH gene transcription start site. Ultimately, studies using well-differentiated parathyroid cells will be required as well.

1,25-Dihydroxyvitamin D_3 has been shown to be an important regulator of PTH gene transcription in studies both in vitro and in vivo. Silver et al. (61) used primary parathyroid cells in culture to show that exposure to 1,25-$(OH)_2D_3$ led to a fall in PTH mRNA levels. This work has been confirmed by studies of Karmali et al. (62) and Brown et al. (63). Russell et al. (64) then showed that 1,25-$(OH)_2D_3$ lowers the PTH gene transcription rate as early as 2 hr after exposure of cells to 1,25-$(OH)_2D_3$. Similarly, in intact rats, intraperitoneal injections of 1,25-$(OH)_2D_3$ rapidly led to decreased transcription of the PTH gene and decreased PTH mRNA levels (65). The doses of 1,25-$(OH)_2D_3$ were so low that blood calcium did not change; the precise blood levels of 1,25-$(OH)_2D_3$ required to suppress PTH gene transcription acutely in vivo have not been established, however.

The effects of low levels of 1,25-$(OH)_2D_3$ have not been studied extensively in intact animals. Such studies are difficult to interpret, because of confounding effects of vitamin D deficiency on blood calcium and parathyroid cell number. Weanling rats fed a vitamin D-deficient diet for 3 weeks had a modest increase in their PTH mRNA levels (43). This increase occurred with no apparent decrease in blood calcium.

In the intact organism, calcium and 1,25-$(OH)_2D_3$ seldom vary independently; consequently, the effects of changes in both parameters simultaneously have important physiologic relevance. When rats were made acutely hypocalcemic with phosphate and were at the same time given 1,25-$(OH)_2D_3$ intraperitoneally, the suppressive effect of 1,25-$(OH)_2D_3$ reversed the effect of hypocalcemia and led to a fall in PTH mRNA (57). In contrast, when rats were fed a low-calcium diet for 3 weeks, blood calcium fell and blood levels of 1,25-$(OH)_2D_3$ increased dramatically. In this setting, PTH mRNA levels rose severalfold; thus the effects of low calcium were more influential than the effects of high 1,25-$(OH)_2D_3$ levels. The differing results of the acute and chronic studies suggest that the net effect of changes in calcium and 1,25-$(OH)_2D_3$ will depend on the chronicity of the manipulation and the degree of the changes in each variable.

In experimental uremia, the double stimulus of hypocalcemia and low levels of 1,25-$(OH)_2D_3$ has consistently led to increases in PTH mRNA (66,67). Administration of 1,25-$(OH)_2D_3$ could reverse this increase. This effect of 1,25-$(OH)_2D_3$ is likely to contribute importantly to the fall in PTH blood levels seen in dogs with experimental uremia (68) and in dialysis patients (69).

A series of transfection studies and DNA binding assays have been used to identify DNA sequences in the PTH gene responsible for modulating transcription of the PTH gene. When a fusion gene containing 684 bp of DNA upstream of the human PTH gene was introduced stably into rat pituitary GH4 cells, expression of the gene was specifically suppressed by 1,25-$(OH)_2D_3$ (70). Two groups have identified DNA sequences upstream of the PTH gene that bind to 1,25-$(OH)_2D_3$ receptors in vitro. Filter binding assays showed that 1,25-$(OH)_2D_3$ receptors can bind to bovine PTH gene sequences between -485 and -100 base pairs upstream from the transcription start site (71). Subsequently, gel mobility shift assays were used to identify a specific 26-base-pair sequence, located 125 base pairs upstream from the start site of transcription of the human PTH gene, that bind 1,25-$(OH)_2D_3$ receptors (72). When this short sequence was linked to a reporter gene and expressed in pituitary GH4 cells, 1,25-$(OH)_2D_3$ decreased expression of the reporter gene. This suppression of transcription was even greater when the number of 1,25-$(OH)_2D_3$ receptors in the GH4 cells was increased by cotransfection of a 1,25-$(OH)_2D_3$ receptor expression vector. The negative 1,25-$(OH)_2D_3$ response element contains one copy of a motif found in two copies in the mouse osteopontin gene, a gene up-regulated by 1,25-$(OH)_2D_3$. The role of this sequence in down-regulation of the PTH gene and the identification of other sequences that may be involved in this down regulation are under active investigation.

Though calcium and 1,25-$(OH)_2D_3$ are certainly the most important physiological regulators of PTH gene transcription, other circulating factors are likely to modulate PTH gene transcription as well. The PTH gene contains a consensus cyclic adenosine monophosphate (cAMP) response element that can function in the context of a fusion gene in transfection experiments (73). Thus hormones that stimulate adenylyl cyclase may increase PTH gene transcription. Glucocorticoids have been shown to increase PTH mRNA in dispersed, hyperplastic human parathyroid cells (74) and to abolish the decrease in PTH mRNA in response to 1,25-$(OH)_2D_3$ in dispersed bovine parathyroid cells (62). These cell culture studies should be confirmed by studies in vivo to determine their physiologic significance. In ovariectomized rats, estradiol administration led within 24 hr to a fourfold increase in PTH mRNA (75). Estrogen receptors were identified in rat parathyroids. These observations may have important implications for an understanding of postmenopausal osteoporosis and hyperparathyroidism. The possibility that the effect of estrogen on PTH mRNA levels is a direct effect on the parathyroid gland should be tested by studies using cultured parathyroid cells.

PERIPHERAL METABOLISM OF PARATHYROID HORMONE

Intact PTH is rapidly cleared from the circulation, with a disappearance half-time of ~2 min (76–79). Removal of PTH from the blood occurs mainly (60–70%) in the liver but also in the kidneys (20–30%) and, to a much lesser extent, in other organs (76,78,79). Clearance of PTH by the liver is mediated mainly by a high-capacity, nonsaturable uptake by Kupffer cells and is followed by rapid and extensive proteolysis (80). Renal clearance occurs almost entirely by glomerular filtration. The hormone is also reabsorbed by the renal tubules and then extensively degraded, so that little or no intact PTH appears in the final urine (78). In both the liver and kidney, as in bone, some PTH is removed by high-affinity binding to cell-surface receptors, but this constitutes only a small fraction (<1%) of overall PTH clearance (78,81,82). Thus it appears that the main role of the liver and kidney in PTH metabolism is rapidly to remove and degrade circulating biologically active hormone. This rapid metabolism ensures that the concentration of hormone available to receptors in target tissues is dictated exclusively by the rate at which PTH is secreted by the parathyroid glands.

This simple, first-order model, in which secreted intact PTH not bound to specific high-affinity cellular receptors is rapidly cleared by peripheral organs, was found to be inadequate when it was recognized that multiple species of immunoreactive PTH molecules are present in the circulation (83,84). Early observations with region-specific immunoassays in vivo and in medium from perfused organs in vitro, followed later by direct analysis of the peripheral metabolism of intravenously administered radioactive PTH, confirmed that intact PTH not only is rapidly cleared from the blood but also is rapidly cleaved by endoproteases to a series of carboxyl-terminal (C-) fragments, some of which reenter the circulation (76,78,79,83,85,86). The chemical identities of these fragments have not been established definitively. Microradiosequencing of radioactive fragments recovered from blood of rats following intravenous administration of [^{125}I-Tyr^{43}]bPTH or [^{3}H-Tyr^{43}]bPTH has shown that PTH peptides produced by cleavages between residues 33–34, 36–37,

40–41, and 42–43 are the predominate large "signature" C fragments (79,80,82,85). These fragments exhibit apparent molecular weights of 4,000–7,000, and it is not certain that they all extend entirely to the original C terminus (i.e., to residue 84) of the intact hormone. Also, because fragments shorter than PTH-(43–84) would have been invisible to these radiosequencing analyses, it is possible that such shorter fragments also exist in blood. Other evidence, derived from detailed analysis by region-specific immunoassays of circulating forms of PTH, points to the presence in blood of shorter "midmolecule" fragments, presumably derived from proteolysis within both the amino (N-) and C-terminal portions of the intact hormone (83,87, 88).

In vitro, isolated hepatic Kupffer cells, but not hepatocytes, generate C fragments that are chemically identical to the major circulating forms (80,89). Also, liver ablation, but not nephrectomy, blocks the production of circulating C fragments that otherwise are produced by proteolysis of administered radiolabeled intact PTH (79). These findings suggest that hepatic Kupffer cells are responsible for both the rapid clearance and the extensive proteolysis of PTH that occur in the liver. Moreover, Kupffer cells appear also to be the source of the major circulating C fragments identified so far that result from postsecretory metabolism of PTH. In the kidney, extensive proteolysis of PTH occurs also, but the kidney does not contribute significantly to the circulating pool of PTH C fragments (76,79,85). Studies of the cellular enzymes responsible for these cleavages are most consistent with a role for lysosomal enzymes of the cathepsin B/D family (82,90).

Quantitatively, <10–20% of secreted intact PTH is converted to circulating C fragments by peripheral metabolism (76,79,85). On the other hand, C fragments make up between 50% and 90% of total circulating PTH immunoreactivity (78,82,83,87,88,91). This disparity results from at least two factors. First, the clearance of C fragments, which does not occur in the liver but rather proceeds mainly via glomerular filtration in the kidney, is significantly slower than that of intact PTH (78,92). Second, it is now clear that C fragments are secreted along with intact PTH by the parathyroid glands, which thus constitute an independent source of these fragments (90,91,93–95). Remarkably, the major C fragments secreted by the parathyroids are chemically identical (at their N termini) with the principal circulating products of peripheral metabolism of PTH (90,94). The impact of these factors is especially obvious in renal insufficiency, where delayed renal clearance (up to 100-fold) of C fragments, combined with their accelerated generation, both within the hyperplastic parathyroid glands and during peripheral metabolism of overproduced intact hormone, leads to massive accumulation of C fragments vs. intact hormone in the circulation.

Metabolism of PTH, both peripherally and within the parathyroid glands, involves cleavages within the region PTH-(33–43). Cleavage within this region, at least potentially, could generate biologically active N-terminal fragments. Accordingly, considerable interest has focused upon the possibility that such circulating N fragments might result from PTH metabolism and, further, that the overall rate or pattern of PTH proteolysis might be regulated physiologically to modulate the production of such fragments. Circulating N-terminal PTH fragments have been demonstrated occasionally, almost exclusively in the setting of renal failure or hyperparathyroidism, or both, but it has been difficult to exclude postcollection proteolysis as the explanation in these circumstances (82,83,96). Moreover, immunochemical analyses of normal plasma have not provided convincing evidence of circulating N-terminal PTH fragments. More recently, direct analysis of the fate of the N terminus of PTH has been possible using biologically active hormone radiolabeled with ^{35}S-methionine to high specific activity within the N-terminal region of the molecule. These studies in normal rats have shown that N-terminal PTH fragments produced by isolated Kupffer cells in vitro or by the liver or kidney in vivo are rapidly degraded in situ and do not reenter the circulation, at least at concentrations above 50 fm (76). Similar investigations have provided no evidence that peripheral metabolism of PTH is regulated physiologically in response to alterations in serum or dietary calcium, vitamin D intoxication, or parathyroid status (77,97). In contrast, secretion of C fragments by the parathyroid glands is strikingly influenced by extracellular calcium, in that hypercalcemia increases the ratio of secreted C fragments to intact hormone whereas the opposite occurs in hypocalcemia (83,91,93,94). These alterations in the intracellular proteolysis of PTH are reflected by corresponding changes in the predominant immunoreactive forms of PTH in the circulation observed during hypercalcemia and hypocalcemia (83,87).

In summary, the extremely rapid peripheral clearance and proteolysis of intact PTH plays an important role in limiting the duration of hormone action and in ensuring that the secretory activity of the parathyroid glands is the overriding determinant of the circulating concentration of biologically active PTH. Whereas a small percentage of degraded PTH molecules reappears in the blood, these are exclusively composed of large carboxyl and midregion fragments that are devoid of classical PTH bioactivity. Additional fragments are released directly by the parathyroid glands, reflecting an intraglandular mechanism involved in calcium regulation of hormone secretion, but these, too, are biologically inactive. It remains possible that such carboxyl and midregion PTH fragments exert novel biological actions in some tissues via receptors other than those known to be activated by intact PTH or N-terminal PTH fragments, but there is little evidence at present in support of a critical physiologic role for such fragments.

CONCLUSIONS

The blood level of PTH is regulated at several levels, each designed to respond to different challenges to calcium homeostasis. Over short times, the regulation of secretion of PTH by calcium, coupled to the rapid metabolism of the hormone, ensures that the blood level of PTH can adjust to sudden changes in calcium flux. Turnover of PTH within the parathyroid gland decreases under hypocalcemic conditions; this adjustment provides rapid increases in available hormone. Over longer times, both calcium and 1,25-$(OH)_2D_3$ regulate PTH biosynthesis. It is, of course, reasonable that 1,25-$(OH)_2D_3$ should regulate PTH biosynthesis, because the need for PTH can be expected to be great in face of vitamin D deficiency, no matter what the instantaneous level of blood calcium. Although the physiological studies are not extensive, the synthetic machinery seems designed particularly to respond dramatically to falls in blood calcium and 1,25-$(OH)_2D_3$ levels. Over longer times, calcium and, perhaps even more so, 1,25-$(OH)_2D_3$ regulate the number of parathyroid cells. This is a relatively crude and slow process. The slow turnover of parathyroid chief cells suggests that the parathyroid gland is not meant to rely on frequent changes in parathyroid cell number but uses this method of amplifying its signal only when other alternatives are insufficient. This perspective on parathyroid control, with its emphasis on multiple levels of regulation, provides a framework for understanding the alterations caused by disease and may suggest therapeutic strategies as well.

REFERENCES

1. Hendy GN, Kronenberg HM, Potts JT Jr, Rich A. Nucleotide sequence of cloned cDNAs encoding human preproparathyroid hormone. *Proc Natl Acad Sci USA* 1981;78:7365–7369.
2. Kronenberg HM, McDevitt BE, Majzoub JA, et al. Cloning and nucleotide sequence of DNA coding for bovine preproparathyroid hormone. *Proc Natl Acad Sci USA* 1979;76:4981–4985.
3. Heinrich G, Kronenberg HM, Potts JT Jr, Habener JF. Gene encoding parathyroid hormone: nucleotide sequence of the rat gene and deduced amino acid sequence of rat preproparathyroid hormone. *J Biol Chem* 1984;259:3320–3329.
4. Schmelzer H-J, Gross G, Widera G, Mayer H. Nucleotide sequence of a full-length cDNA clone encoding preproparathyroid hormone from pig and rat. *Nucleic Acids Res* 1987;15:6740.

5. Khosla S, Demay M, Pines M, Hurwitz S, Potts JT Jr, Kronenberg HM. Nucleotide sequence of cloned cDNAs encoding chicken preproparathyroid hormone. *J Bone Mineral Res* 1988;3;689–698.

6. Russell J, Sherwood LM. Nucleotide sequence of the DNA complementary to avian (chicken) preproparathyroid hormone mRNA and the deduced sequence of the hormone precursor. *Mol Endocrinol* 1989;3:325–331.

7. Kemper B, Habener JF, Mulligan RC, et al. Preproparathyroid hormone: a direct translation product of parathyroid messenger RNA. *Proc Natl Acad Sci USA* 1974;71:3731–3735.

8. Freeman M, Wiren K, Rapoport A, et al. Consequences of amino-terminal deletions of preproparathyroid hormone signal sequence. *Mol Endocrinol* 1987;1:628–638.

9. Cioffi JA, Allen KL, Lively MO, Kemper B. Parallel effects of signal peptide hydrophobic core modifications on co-translational translocation and post-translational cleavage by purified signal peptidase. *J Biol Chem* 1989;264:15052–15058.

10. Wiren KM, Potts JT Jr, Kronenberg HM. Importance of the propeptide sequence of human preproparathyroid hormone for signal sequence function. *J Biol Chem* 1988;263:19771–19777.

11. Majzoub JA, Rosenblatt M, Fennick, et al. Synthetic preproparathyroid hormone leader sequence inhbits cell-free processing of placental, parathyroid, and pituitary prehormones. *J Biol Chem* 1980;255:11478–11483.

12. Arnold A, Horst SA, Gardella TJ, Baba H, Levine MA, Kronenberg HM. Mutation of the signal peptide-encoding region of the preproparathyroid hormone gene in familial isolated hypoparathyroidism. *J Clin Invest* 1990;86:1084–1087.

13. Cohn DV, MacGregor RR, Chu LL, et al. Calcemic fraction-A: biosynthetic peptide precursor of parathyroid hormone. *Proc Natl Acad Sci USA* 1972;69:1521–1525.

14. Kemper B, Habener JF, Potts JT Jr, Rich A. Proparathyroid hormone: identification of a biosynthetic precursor to parathyroid hormone. *Proc Natl Acad Sci USA* 1972;69:643–647.

15. Habener JF, Amherdt M, Ravazzola M, Orci L. Parathyroid hormone biosynthesis: Correlation of conversion of biosynthetic precursors with intracellular protein migration as determined by electron microscope autoradiography. *J Cell Biol* 1979;80:715–731.

16. Habener JF, Stevens TD, Tregear GW, Potts JT Jr. Radioimmunoassay of human proparathyroid hormone: analysis of hormone content in tissue extracts and in plasma. *J Clin Endocrinol Metab* 1976;42:520–530.

17. Wiren KM, Ivashkiv L, Ma P, Freeman MW, Potts JT Jr, Kronenberg HM. Mutations in signal sequence cleavage domain of preproparathyroid hormone alter protein translocation, signal sequence cleavage, and membrane-binding properties. *Mol Endocrinol* 1989;3:240–250.

18. Lindberg I. The new eukaryotic precursor processing proteinases. *Mol Endocrinol* 1991;5:1361–1365.

19. Hellerman JC, Cone RC, Potts JT Jr, et al. Secretion of human parathyroid hormone from rat pituitary cells infected with a recombinant retrovirus encoding preproparathyroid hormone. *Proc Natl Acad Sci USA* 1984;81:5340–5344.

20. Gardella TJ, Axelrod D, Rubin D, et al. Mutational analysis of the receptor-activating region of human parathyroid hormone. *J Biol Chem* 1991;266:13141–13146.

21. Lim SK, Gardella TJ, Thompson A, et al. Full-length chicken parathyroid hormone: biosynthesis of *Escherichia coli* and analysis of biological activity. *J Biol Chem* 1991;266:3709–3714.

22. Mayer GP, Keaton JA, Hurst JG, Habener JF. Effects of plasma calcium concentration on the relative proportion of hormone and carboxyl fragments in parathyroid venous blood. *Endocrinology* 1979;104:1778–1784.

23. Habener JF, Kemper B, Potts JT Jr. Calcium-dependent intracellular degradation of parathyroid hormone: a possible mechanism for the regulation of hormone stores. *Endocrinology* 1975;97:431–441.

24. Chu LLH, MacGregor RR, Anast CS, et al. Studies on the biosynthesis of rat parathyroid hormone and proparathyroid

hormone: adaptation of the parathyroid gland to dietary restriction of calcium. *Endocrinology* 1973;93:915–924.

25. Tanguay KE, Mortimer ST, Wood PH, Hanley DA. The effects of phorbol myristate acetate on the intracellular degradation of bovine parathyroid hormone. *Endocrinology* 1991;128:1863–1868.

26. Vasicek T, McDevitt BE, Freeman MW, et al. Nucleotide sequence of the human parathyroid hormone gene. *Proc Natl Acad Sci USA* 1983;80:2127.

27. Weaver CA, Gordon DF, Kissil MS, et al. Isolation and complete nucleotide sequence of the gene for bovine parathyroid hormone. *Gene* 1984;28:319–329.

28. Heinrich G, Kronenberg HM, Pott JT Jr, Habener JF. Gene encoding parathyroid hormone: nucleotide sequence of the rat gene and deduced amino acid sequence of rat preproparathyroid hormone. *J Biol Chem* 1984;259:3320.

29. Russell J, Olivera A, Liu S, Sherwood LM. Isolation and complete nucleotide sequence of the avian parathyroid hormone gene. *Endocrine Society Program and Abstracts, 73rd Annual Meeting, June 19–22, 1991.*

30. Reis A, Hecht W, Gröger R, et al. Cloning and sequence analysis of the human parathyroid hormone gene region. *Hum Genet* 1990;84:119–124.

31. Naylor SL, Sakaguchi AY, Szoka P, et al. Human parathyroid hormone gene (PTH) is on short arm of chromosome 11. *Somat Cell Genet* 1983;9:609–616.

32. Mayer H, Breyel E, Bostock C, Schmidtke J. Assignment of the human parathyroid hormone gene to chromosome 11. *Hum Genet* 1983;64:283–285.

33. Zabel BU, Kronenberg HM, Bell GI, Shows TB. Chromosome mapping of genes on the short arm of human chromosome 11: parathyroid hormone gene is at 11p15 together with the genes for insulin, c-Harvey-*ras* 1, and b-hemoglobin. *Cytogenet Cell Genet* 1985;39:200–205.

34. Antonarakis SE, Phillips JA III, Mallonee RL, et al. b-globin locus is linked to the parathyroid hormone (PTH) locus and lies between the insulin and PTH loci in man. *Proc Natl Acad Sci USA* 1983;80:6615–6619.

35. Schmidtke J, Pape B, Krengel U, et al. Restriction fragment length polymorphisms at the human parathyroid hormone gene locus. *Hum Genet* 1984;67:428–431.

36. Kittur SD, Hoppener JWM, Antonarakis SE, et al. Linkage map of the short arm of human chromosome 11: location of the genes for catalase, calcitonin, and insulin-like growth factor II. *Proc Natl Acad Sci USA* 1985;82:5064–5067.

37. Miric A, Levine MA. Analysis of the preproPTH gene by denaturing gradient gel electrophoresis in familial isolated hypoparathyroidism. *J Clin Endocrinol Metab* 1991;74:509–516.

38. Ahn TG, Antonarakis SE, Kronenberg HM, et al. Familial isolated hypoparathyroidism: a molecular genetic analysis of 8 families with 23 affected persons. *Medicine* 1986;65:73–81.

39. Suva LJ, Winslow GA, Wettenhall REH, et al. A parathyroid hormone-related protein implicated in malignant hypercalcemia: cloning and expression. *Science* 1987;237:893–896.

40. Mangin M, Ikeda K, Dreyer BE, Broadus AE. Isolation and characterization of the human parathyroid hormone-like peptide gene. *Proc Natl Acad Sci USA* 1989;86:2408–2412.

41. Yasuda T, Banville D, Hendy GN, Goltzman D. Characterization of the human parathyroid hormone-like peptide gene: functional and evolutionary aspects. *J Biol Chem* 1989;264:7720–7725.

42. Comings DE. Evidence for ancient tetraploidy and conservation of linkage groups in mammalian chromosomes. *Nature* 1972;238:455–457.

43. Naveh-Many T, Silver J. Regulation of parathyroid hormone gene expression by hypocalcemia, hypercalcemia, and vitamin D in the rat. *J Clin Invest* 1990;86:1313–1319.

44. Nygren P, Larsson R, Johansson H, Ljunghall S, Rastad J, Akerström G. 1,25(OH)$_2$D$_3$ inhibits hormone secretion and proliferation but not functional dedifferentiation of cultured bovine parathyroid cells. *Calcif Tissue Int* 1988;43:213–218.

45. Kremer R, Bolivar I, Goltzman D, Hendy GN. Influence of calcium and 1,25-dihydroxycholecalciferol on proliferation

and proto-oncogene expression in primary cultures of bovine parathyroid cells. *Endocrinology* 1989;125:935–941.

46. Ishimi Y, Russell J, Sherwood LM. Regulation by calcium and 1,25-(OH)$_2$D$_3$ of cell proliferation and function of bovine parathyroid cells in culture. *J Bone Mineral Res* 1990;5:755–760.

47. Lee MJ, Roth SI. Effect of calcium and magnesium on deoxyribonucleic acid synthesis in rat parathyroid glands in vitro. *Lab Invest* 1975;33:72–79.

48. Raisz LG. Regulation by calcium of parathyroid growth and secretion in vitro. *Nature* 1963;197:1115–1117.

49. Brandi ML, Fitzpatrick LA, Coon HG, Aurbach GD. Bovine parathyroid cells maintained for more than 140 population doublings. *Proc Natl Acad Sci USA* 1986;83:1707–1713.

50. Leboff MS, Rennke HG, Brown EM. Abnormal regulation of parathyroid cell secretion and proliferation in primary cultures of bovine parathyroid cells. *Endocrinology* 1983;113:227–284.

51. Baba H, Kishihara M, Tohmon M, et al. Identification of parathyroid hormone messenger ribonucleic acid in an apparently nonfunctioning parathyroid carcinoma transformed from a parathyroid carcinoma with hyperparathyroidism. *J Clin Endocrinol Metab* 1986;62:247–252.

52. Nussbaum SR, Gaz RD, Arnold A. Hypercalcemia and ectopic secretion of parathyroid hormone by an ovarian carcinoma with rearrangement of the gene for parathyroid hormone. *N Engl J Med* 1990;323:1324–1328.

53. Motokura T, Bloom T, Kim HG, et al. A BCL1-linked candidate oncogene which is rearranged in parathyroid tumors encodes a novel cyclin. *Nature* 1991;350:512–515.

54. Russell J, Lettieri D, Sherwood LM. Direct regulation of calcium of cytoplasmic messenger ribonucleic acid coding for pre-preparathyroid hormone in isolated bovine parathyroid cells. *J Clin Invest* 1983;72:1851–1855.

55. Brookman JJ, Farrow SM, Nicholson L, O'Riordan JLH, Hendy GN. Regulation by calcium of parathyroid hormone mRNA in cultured parathyroid tissue. *J Bone Mineral Res* 1986;1:529–537.

56. Russell J, Sherwood LM. The effects of 1,25-dihydroxyvitamin D$_3$ and high calcium on transcription of the preproparathyroid hormone gene are direct. *Trans Assoc Am Physicians* 1987;100:256–262.

57. Naveh-Many T, Friedlander MM, Mayer H, Silver J. Calcium regulates parathyroid hormone messenger ribonucleic acid (mRNA), but not calcitonin mRNA in vivo in the rat. Dominant role of 1,25-dihydroxyvitamin D. *Endocrinology* 1989;125:275–280.

58. Yamamoto M, Igarishi T, Muramatsu M, Fukagawa M, Motokura T, Ogata E. Hypocalcemia increases and hypercalcemia decreases the steady state level of parathyroid hormone messenger ribonucleic acid in the rat. *J Clin Invest* 1989;83:1053–1058.

59. Okazaki T, Zajac JD, Igarashi T, Ogata E, Kronenberg HM. Negative regulatory elements in the human parathyroid hormone gene. *J Biol Chem* 1991;266:21903–21910.

60. Okazaki T, Ando K, Igarashi T, Ogata E, Fujita T. Conserved mechanism of negative gene regulation by extracellular calcium. *J Clin Invest* 1992;89:1268–1273.

61. Silver J, Russell J, Sherwood LM. Regulation by vitamin D metabolites of messenger ribonucleic acid for preproparathyroid hormone in isolated bovine parathyroid cells. *Proc Natl Acad Sci USA* 1985;82:4270–4273.

62. Karmali R, Farrow S, Hewison M, Barker S, O'Riordan JLH. Effects of 1,25-dihydroxyvitamin D$_3$ and cortisol on bovine and human parathyroid cells. *J Endocrinol* 1989;123:137–142.

63. Brown AJ, Ritter CR, Finch JL, et al. The noncalcemic analogue of vitamin D, 22-oxacalcitriol, suppresses parathyroid hormone synthesis and secretion. *J Clin Invest* 1989;84:728–732.

64. Russell J, Lettieri D, Sherwood LM. Direct suppression by 1,25-(OH)$_2$D$_3$ of transcription of the parathyroid hormone gene. *Clin Res* 1986;34:726A.

65. Silver J, Naveh-Many T, Mayer H, Schmelzer HJ, Popovtzer MM. Regulation by vitamin D metabolites of parathyroid hormone gene transcription in vivo in the rat. *J Clin Invest* 1986;78:1296–1301.

66. Shvil Y, Naveh-Many T, Barach P, Silver J. Regulation of parathyroid cell gene expression in experimental uremia. *J Am Soc Nephrol* 1990;1:99–104.

67. Fukagawa M, Kaname S, Igarashi T, Ogata E, Kurokawa K. Regulation of parathyroid hormone synthesis in chronic renal failure in rats. *Kidney Int* 1991;39:874–881.

68. Lopez-Hilker S, Galceran T, Chan YL, Rapp N, Martin KJ, Slatopolsky E. Hypocalcemia may not be essential for the development of secondary hyperparathyroidism in chronic renal failure. *J Clin Invest* 1986;78:1097–1102.

69. Delmez JA, Tindira C, Grooms P, Dusso A, Windus DW, Slatopolsky E. Parathyroid hormone suppression by intravenous 1,25-dihydroxyvitamin D: a role for increased sensitivity to calcium. *J Clin Invest* 1989;83:1349–1355.

70. Okazaki T, Igarashi T, Kronenberg HM. 5'-Flanking region of the parathyroid hormone gene mediates negative regulation by 1,25(OH)$_2$ vitamin D$_3$. *J Biol Chem* 1988;263:2203–2208.

71. Farrow SM, Hawa NS, Karmali R, Hewison M, Walters JC, O'Riordan JLH. Binding of the receptor for 1,25-dihydroxyvitamin D$_3$ to the 5'-flanking region of the bovine parathyroid hormone gene. *J Endocrinol* 1990;126:355–359.

72. Demay MB, Kiernan MS, DeLuca HF, Kronenberg HM. Sequences in the human parathyroid hormone gene that bind the 1,25-dihydroxyvitamin D$_3$ receptor and mediate transcriptional repression in response to 1,25-dihydroxyvitamin D$_3$. *Proc Natl Acad Sci USA* 1992;89:8097–8101.

73. Rupp E, Mayer H, Wingender E. The promoter of the human parathyroid hormone gene contains a functional cyclic AMP-response element. *Nucleic Acids Res* 1990;18:5677–5683.

74. Peraldi MN, Rondeau E, Jousset V, et al. Dexamethasone increases preproparathyroid hormone messenger RNA in human hyperplastic parathyroid cell in vitro. *Eur J Clin Invest* 1990;20:392–397.

75. Naveh-Many T, Almogi G, Livni N, Silver J. Estrogen receptors and biologic response in rat parathyroid tissue and C cells. *J Clin Invest* 1992;90:2434–2438.

76. Bringhurst FR, Stern AM, Yotts M, Mizrahi N, Segre GV, Potts JT Jr. Peripheral metabolism of PTH: fate of biologically active amino terminus in vivo. *Am J Physiol* 1988;255:E886–E893.

77. Fox J, Scott M, Nissenson RA, Heath H. Effects of plasma calcium concentration on the metabolic clearance rates of parathyroid hormone in the dog. *J Lab Clin Medicine* 1983;102:70–77.

78. Martin KJ, Hruska KA, Freitag JJ, Klahr S, Slatopolsky E. The peripheral metabolism of parathyroid hormone. *N Engl J Med* 1979;302:1092–1098.

79. Segre GV, D'Amour P, Hultman A, Potts JT Jr. Effects of hepatectomy, nephrectomy, and nephrectomy/uremia on the metabolism of parathyroid hormone in the rat. *J Clin Invest* 1981;67:439–448.

80. Bringhurst FR, Segre GV, Lampman GW, Potts JT Jr. Metabolism of parathyroid hormone by Kupffer cells: analysis by reverse-phase high-performance liquid chromatography. *Biochemistry* 1982;21:4252–4258.

81. Rouleau MF, Warshawsky H, Goltzman D. Parathyroid hormone binding in vivo to renal, hepatic and skeletal tissues of the rat using a radioautographic approach. *Endocrinology* 1986;118:919–931.

82. Rosenblatt M, Kronenberg HM, Potts JT Jr. Parathyroid hormone. Physiology, chemistry, biosynthesis, secretion, metabolism and mode of action. In: DeGroot LJ, ed. *Endocrinology*, vol II. Philadelphia: W.B. Saunders, 1989;848–891.

83. Dambacher MA, Fischer JA, Hunziker WH, et al. Distribution of circulating immunoreactive components of parathyroid hormone in normal subjects and in patients with primary and secondary hyperparathyroidism: the role of the kidney and of serum calcium concentration. *Clin Sci* 1979;57:435–443.

84. Berson SA, Yalow RS. Immunochemical heterogeneity of parathyroid hormone in plasma. *J Clin Endocrinol Metab* 1968;28:1037–1047.

85. Segre GV, D'Amour P, Potts JT Jr. Metabolism of radioiodinated bovine parathyroid hormone in the rat. *Endocrinology* 1976;99:1645–1652.

86. Daugaard H, Egfjord M, Olgaard K. Metabolism of intact parathyroid hormone in isolated perfused rat liver and kidney. *Am J Physiol* 1988;254:E740–E748.

87. D'Amour P, Palardy J, Bahsali G, Mallette LE, DeLean A, Lepage R. The modulation of circulating parathyroid hormone immunoheterogeneity in man by ionized calcium concentration. *J Clin Endocrinol Metab* 1992;74:525–532.

88. Roos BA, Lindall AW, Aron DC, et al. Detection and characterization of small midregion parathyroid hormone fragment(s) in normal and hyperparathyroid glands and sera by immunoextraction and region-specific radioimmunoassays. *J Clin Endocrinol Metab* 1981;53:709–721.

89. Segre GV, Perkins AS, Witters LA, Potts JT Jr. Metabolism of parathyroid hormone by isolated rat Kupffer cells and hepatocytes. *J Clin Invest* 1981;67:449–457.

90. MacGregor RR, Jilka RL, Hamilton JW. Formation and secretion of fragments of parathormone. Identification of cleavage sites. *J Biol Chem* 1986;261:1929–1934.

91. D'Amour P, LaBelle F, LeCavalier L, Plourde V, Harvey D. Influence of serum Ca concentration on circulating molecular forms of PTH in three species. *Am J Physiol* 1986;251:E680–E687.

92. D'Amour P, Lazure C, LaBelle F. Metabolism of radioiodinated carobxy-terminal fragments of bovine parathyroid hormone in normal and anephric rats. *Endocrinology* 1985;117:127–134.

93. Flueck JA, DiBella FP, Edis AJ, Kehrwald JM, Arnaud CD. Immunoheterogeneity of parathyroid hormone in venous effluent serum of hyperfunctioning parathyroid glands. *J Clin Invest* 1977;69:1367–1375.

94. Hanley DA, Ayer LM. Calcium-dependent release of carboxyl-terminal fragments of parathyroid hormone by hyperplastic human parathyroid tissue in vitro. *J Clin Endocrinol Metab* 1986;63:1075–1079.

95. Tanguay KE, Mortimer ST, Wood PH, Hanley DA. The effects of phorbol myristate acetate on the intracellular degradation of bovine parathyroid hormone. *Endocrinology* 1991;128:1863–1868.

96. Goltzman D, Henderson B, Loveridge M. Cytochemical bioassay of parathyroid hormone. Characteristics of the assay and analysis of circulating hormonal forms. *J Clin Invest* 1980;65:1309–1317.

97. Bringhurst FR, Stern AM, Yotts M, Mizrahi N, Segre GV, Potts JT Jr. Peripheral metabolism of [35S]parathyroid hormone in vivo: influence of alterations in calcium availability and parathyroid status. *J Endocrinol* 1989;122:237–245.

98. Fraser RA, Kronenberg HM, Pang PK, Harvey S. Parathyroid hormone messenger ribonucleic acid in the rat hypothalamus. *Endocrinology* 1990;127:2517–2522.

The Parathyroids, edited by J.P. Bilezikian,
M.A. Levine, and R. Marcus. Raven Press, Ltd.,
New York © 1994.

CHAPTER 10

Structure–Function Analysis of Parathyroid Hormone and Parathyroid Hormone-Related Protein

Michael Chorev and Michael Rosenblatt

GENERAL GOALS AND USES OF ANALOGS

Remarkably, both parathyroid hormone (PTH) and parathyroid hormone-related protein (PTHrP) are able to bind to and activate the same membranous receptor (apparently a single subtype) present on the surface of cells in target tissues such as bone and kidney. This binding occurs despite major differences between the two hormones in their amino acid sequence, their distribution in tissues in which they are synthesized, their role in normal physiology, and their contribution to various disorders of calcium metabolism.

Considerable insight regarding the structural determinants essential for productive hormone–receptor interactions has been obtained in the PTH/PTHrP system, as well as in other peptide hormone–receptor systems, through the synthesis and biological evaluation of native-sequence hormone and hormone fragments and analogs (1–4). Since the first synthesis of a peptide hormone, oxytocin, by du Vigneaud and coworkers in 1953 (5), selective modification of hormonal structure has become a powerful research tool in endocrinology. By studying the relation between the structure and the activity of various peptide hormones, investigators very often generate fragments or analogs of hormones that have advantageous properties, such as increased potency, prolonged duration of action, increased stability, greater selectivity within

the spectrum of biologic activity of a given hormone, or antagonism of hormonal action.

Hormone analogs have also been designed and synthesized to serve specialized applications. Synthetic fragments of PTH and PTHrP have been used in immunization programs to generate region-specific antisera, which have been very useful in the development of clinically applied immunoassays (see the chapter by Nussbaum and Potts). Similarly, hormonal fragments have been covalently tethered to solid supports in order to generate affinity columns for the purification of antisera or solubilized receptors (6). For this purpose, hormone analogs were modified by affinity tags such as biotin to allow purification of hormone–receptor complexes based on biotin–avidin interaction (7,8). Other fragments have been used as alternate substrates for native hormone in order to inhibit the metabolic processes that degrade and clear hormone (see the chapter by Kronenberg et al.) and in research efforts to determine the role of hormonal cleavage in normal physiology. Hormone analogs containing a radiolabel at specific sites have been useful in studying the metabolism of hormone and identifying the precise location within the hormone molecule where cleavage occurs both in vitro and in vivo (see the chapter by Kronenberg et al.). Analogs incorporating photoreactive moieties have been critically important in photoaffinity labeling and subsequent physicochemical characterization of receptor (9–13). The design and synthesis of radiolabeled analogs that retain bioactivity have allowed the development of radioreceptor assays (14–16). In turn, these assays have permitted investigators to study directly hormone–receptor interactions, facilitating the design of potent hormone agonists and antagonists (17–19).

M. Chorev: Department of Pharmaceutical Chemistry, The Hebrew University of Jerusalem, Faculty of Medicine, Jerusalem 91120, Israel.

M. Rosenblatt: Division of Bone and Mineral Metabolism, Beth Israel Hospital, Boston, Massachusetts 02215.

The full spectrum of utilities and design directions for analogs of PTH and PTHrP, discussed above, although important to a number of avenues of research, are not discussed further here. Rather, this chapter focuses on analysis of the nature of the interaction of PTH and PTHrP with receptors.

PARATHYROID HORMONE/PARATHYROID HORMONE-RELATED PROTEIN–RECEPTOR INTERACTIONS IN GENERAL

In the PTH/PTHrP system, extensive structure–activity studies have defined the essential structural features responsible for hormonal binding to receptor and subsequent activation of receptor leading to generation of intracellular second messengers (1,20) (Fig. 1). Some analogs can bind to the PTH/PTHrP receptor without causing increasing cyclic adenosine monophosphate (cAMP) levels or other events in the biochemical cascade of hormonal action (19,21). These analogs can serve as effective antagonists of PTH both in vitro and in vivo (17,18).

This review describes some general approaches and principles for the design of peptide hormone antagonists and shows how they have been applied to the design and evaluation of parathyroid hormone analogs and subsequent development of antagonists effective in vivo. In addition, we discuss the potential clinical utility of these antagonists.

Peptide hormone antagonists that are effective *in vivo* are uniquely precise tools for biomedical research. They can be used to determine a hormone's mechanism of action, to define its role in normal physiologic processes, and to delineate its contribution to pathophysiologic conditions. In addition, antagonists have potential clinical utility in the diagnosis and treatment of syndromes of hormone excess (1).

Antagonists

PTH or PTHrP antagonists have potential therapeutic application in a variety of clinical disorders. Since the hypercalcemia that accompanies malignancy is mediated in many, if not most, cases by PTHrP, administration of antagonists that competitively occupy PTH/PTHrP receptors is a conceptually appealing approach to therapy as it is mechanism based. Similarly, there are several other clinical situations in which excess PTH secretion occurs and in which a PTH or PTHrP antagonist might be useful (Table 1). These include treatment of "parathyroid storm" and medical therapy of high-risk surgical candidates with hyperparathyroidism, parathyroid carcinoma, chronic renal failure, or persistent hyperparathyroidism after renal transplantation.

Despite intensive research on many hormone systems over the past 30 years, peptide analogs that are effective as antagonists in animals or humans have been generated for only a few peptide hormones: vasopressin (22,23), glucagon (24,25), luteinizing hormone-releasing hormone (26–29), angiotensin II (30), and PTH. The issues and challenges that arose during the design and evaluation of PTH/PTHrP antagonists have important implications for the development of other peptide hormone antagonists, since similar problems have been encountered in other hormonal systems.

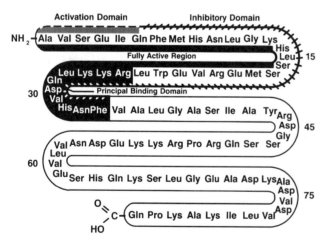

FIG. 1. Amino acid sequence of bovine parathyroid hormone. The region of full biological activity (sequence 1–34), indicated by the solid stripe, is subdivided into a short activation domain (sequence 1–6?) (*stippled area*) followed by a longer inhibitory or binding domain (sequence 7–34) (*crossed lines*). White-on-black lettering indicates the principal binding domain (sequence 25–34), representing the minimal structural requirements for detectable receptor occupancy.

TABLE 1. *Potential uses of parathyroid hormone antagonists*

1. Short-term treatment of hypercalcemic crisis ("parathyroid storm") due to parathyroid adenoma, hyperplasia, or carcinoma; for preoperative optimization of blood calcium levels
2. Long-term treatment of hyperparathyroidism
   In high-risk surgical candidates
   In patients who have undergone unsuccessful surgery
   In parathyroid carcinoma (inoperable)
   For general medical management of hyperparathyroidism(?)
3. Adjunct treatment
   After renal transplantation, when there is persistent "secondary" hyperparathyroidism

Limited Sequence Homology

Comparison of the sequences for PTH and PTHrP of human and rat origins reveals striking sequence homology between the isohormones (Fig. 2). However, the homology between PTH and PTHrP sequences is limited to a small region at the amino terminus. Eight of the first 13 amino acids are identical [PTH-(1–13) and PTHrP-(1–13)]. In the region 14–34, only four of 21 residues are identical. The "homology" is also limited because even many of the nonidentical residues lack structural similarity; for example, Ile^5, Asn^{10}, Leu^{11}, His^{14}, and Ser^{17} in PTH vs. His^5, Asp^{10}, Lys^{11}, Ser^{14}, and Asp^{17} in PTHrP. Furthermore, the distribution of charges, polar, and hydrophobic groups are different between the two hormones in the 14–34 region, and entire structural motifs are "displaced." The basic triad in PTH, Arg^{25}-Lys-Lys^{27}, also appears in PTHrP, but it is shifted closer to the N-terminus (Arg^{19}-Arg-Arg^{21}). The motif of two glutamic acid residues in positions 19 and 22 in PTH does not have a counterpart in PTHrP. This theme of a short region of similarity followed by prominent structural divergence is even more pronounced in analogs truncated from the N-terminus. Such modification in both hormones produces fully effective antagonists, which inhibit the action of both hormones with comparable potency, despite the marked structural dissimilarities between the hormones and the shorter antagonists. Assuming that

there is only one PTH/PTHrP receptor, it is an intellectual challenge to understand the presumed structural or conformational compatibility of both hormones with the same receptor in what is an unusual "structure–function experiment" of nature.

Similarities in Secondary Structure

Different primary structures that assume closely related bioactive conformations may interact with and activate the same receptor, producing similar intracellular signals. In spite of differences in primary structure, the 1–34 sequences of PTH and PTHrP adopt similar basic elements of secondary structure (Fig. 3) (31). Employing the Chou-Fasman algorithm (32a) to both sequences, α-helices are predicted to be present at the N-termini (1–28 and 1–18 for PTH and PTHrP, respectively), interrupted by β-turns (12–15 and 9–12 for PTH and PTHrP, respectively). The probability for the presence of a β-turn is higher in PTHrP than in PTH. The N-terminal α-helical domain is followed by a stretch of β-sheet in both hormones (29–34 and 23–28 for PTH and PTHrP, respectively). For PTHrP, a second β-turn (residues 19–22) and an additional α-helical structure for the C-terminus (residues 29–34) are predicted. Very similar conformations were recently predicted by Cohen and coworkers employing both Chou-Fasman-Robson (33) and helical-wheel (34)

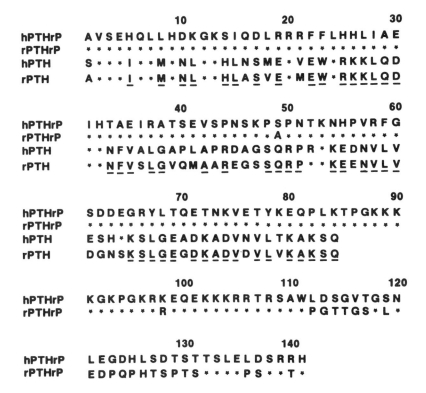

FIG. 2. Alignment of sequences of PTH and PTHrP from human and rat species. The homology within the PTHrP sequences and between PTHrP and PTH is indicated by *asterisks*. Identity between the PTH sequences is indicated by the *underscored residues*. The most significant homology between PTH and PTHrP is confined to the amino-terminal 13 amino acids.

A.

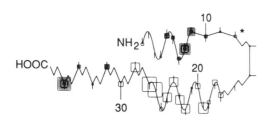

B.

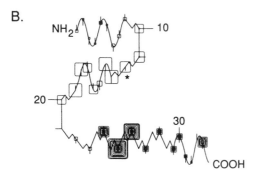

FIG. 3. Secondary structure prediction of the N-terminal 1–34 sequences of human PTH (**A**) and human PTHrP (**B**) predicted by Chou and Fasman (32) analysis. The different structural elements are depicted as follows: sine wave, α-helix; zigzag, β-sheet; and reversed direction, β-turn. Hydrophobic and hydrophilic residues are indicated by *open* and *solid circles,* respectively. The diameter of the circle is proportional to the magnitude of the hydrophobicity calculated by the method of Kyte and Doolittle. (Reprinted from ref. 31 with permission.)

PTH-(1–34) is mostly nonstructured, except for a short nonrandomly structured region localized around Trp[23] (42–44). However, the titration profile of the histidine residues in either bPTH-(1–34) or bPTH-(1–84), as monitored by the pH dependence of some aromatic chemical shifts and accompanying nuclear Overhauser effect (NOE) correlations, suggests that a nonrandom structure may be present (45,46). Recently ^{1}H-NMR studies of hPTH-(1–34) in TFE/water (~11% v/v) identified medium-range NOEs, that were then used in a constrained molecular modeling simulation (47). A family of structures was generated in which two helical domains (residues 3–9 and 17–28) are linked via a flexible nonstructured sequence (residues 10–16). By extrapolation from previous studies (47,48), more recent comparative CD studies, and secondary structure predictions, Cohen and coworkers (35) were able to propose a common three-dimensional model for both sequences. In this model, the amino- and carboxy-α-helical domains are lined up side by side, in an antiparallel fashion, with hydrophobic residues facing inward. The hydrophilic residues make up the loop, connecting the helices, and their outward faces (Fig. 4).

A more detailed, experimentally based structure for hPTHrP-(1–34) emerged from an extensive two-dimensional ^{1}H-NMR and CD study carried out by Barden and Kemp (49). Their model depicts a compact structure in which an α-helical portion (residues 3–6) is followed by two type I β-turns (Gly[12]-Lys[13]-Ser[14]-Ile[15] and Gln[16]-Asp[17]-Leu[18]-Arg[19]) and a coiled stretch (residues

analyses, which are pattern-based semiempirical approaches (35).

Folding PTH-(1–34) into an α-helical conformation generates a hydrophobic domain twisted along the helix. This structure is characteristic of an amphiphatic helix (36). Folding PTHrP-(1–34) in an identical manner also produces an amphiphatic helix, which closely resembles that of PTH.

Actual determinations of secondary structure or content (based on experimental data) for PTH-(1–34) and, more recently, PTHrP-(1–34) are inconclusive. The helical content of PTH in aqueous solution as determined by circular dichroism (CD) is minimal: the peptide resides in an unordered structure (37–40). In the presence of 45% trifluoroethanol (TFE) (a solvent that promotes secondary structure), the total helical content in bovine PTH (bPTH) and human PTHrP (hPTHrP)-(1–34) is 73%. In the absence of TFE, only 20–30% of residues are involved in helical structure (35). Similarly, in the presence of lipids, there is an increase in the α-helical content of PTH-(1–34) (36,41). Early [1]H-nuclear magnetic resonance (NMR) studies conducted in water (D₂O) led to the conclusion that

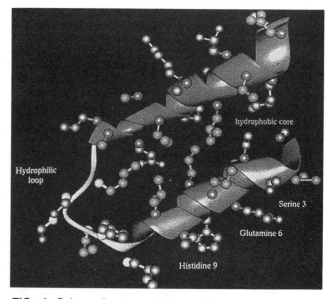

FIG. 4. Schematic representation of the paired helix model for bPTH-(1–34) and hPTHrP-(1–34). The amino and carboxy α-helical regions are connected by a hydrophilic loop. The hydrophobic residues in the α-helical regions are facing inward, while the hydrophilic residues are outwardly oriented. (Reprinted from ref. 35 with permission.)

23–34). Medium to strong interresidue NOEs indicate close proximity between N-terminal and C-terminal residues. Based on this analysis, a space-filling model was constructed, which reveals clustering of hydrophobic and hydrophilic residues on opposite surfaces of the structure. This model also suggests that salt bridges exist between proximal residues Asp[10]···Lys[13], Asp[10]---Lys[13] and Asp[17]···Arg[19], Asp[17]---Arg[19], which may play a role in stabilizing the β-turns (49). Additional considerations regarding salt bridge formation in this region of the molecule are addressed later in this chapter.

Linear Functional Architecture

It has been demonstrated that a tumor-secreted factor from malignancies associated with the paraneoplastic syndrome of humoral hypercalcemia was able to stimulate PTH-like action in vitro and in vivo (50–56). Similar to observations for bPTH-(1–34), a preparation containing endogenous PTHrP can inhibit sodium-dependent phosphate transport in renal epithelial cells (54,56,60). More recently, the same observations were reported for PTHrP produced by recombinant DNA biosynthetic technology (57–59). Recombinant PTHrP stimulates adenylyl cyclase in osteoblast-like cells (57,59) and in renal cortical membranes (59). Moreover, PTHrP stimulation of adenylyl cyclase in renal tissue and osteoblast-like cells is inhibited by a PTH antagonist (50–53,56,57). PTH and PTHrP compete with radiolabeled PTHrP for binding to canine renal cortical membranes (54). The hormone causes release of $^{45}Ca^{2+}$ from fetal rat bone and induces hypercalcemia in rats following a 3-day infusion (59). Like PTH, PTHrP inhibits Ca^{2+} release from intracellular stores in cells derived from an osteogenic sarcoma line (58).

The pronounced homology between PTH and PTHrP at the N-terminus led to the assumption that the established linear sequential organization of functional domains in PTH (61) (Fig. 1) is also present in PTHrP (2,3,62,63). Similar to observations made on the N-terminal one-third of PTH, peptides corresponding to the amino-terminal region of PTHrP, namely, PTHrP-(1–34) (2,3,63) and PTHrP-(1–36) (62), demonstrated the full range and potency of PTH-like in vitro and in vivo activities (Fig. 5). PTHrP-(1–34)NH₂ competes for renal receptor binding with a PTH-radioligand analog, [Nle[8,18], 3-^{125}I-Tyr[34]]bPTH-(1–34)NH₂ (2). Binding of [125]I-[Tyr[40]]PTHrP-(1–40)NH₂ and [Nle[8,18],3-^{125}I-Tyr[34]]bPTH-(1–34)NH₂ to osteoblast-like cells was inhibited by synthetic PTHrP peptides (16). Both radiolabeled PTHrP-(1–34)NH₂ and [Tyr[34]]bPTH-(1–34)NH₂ photoaffinity analogs cross link to the same components of renal membranes; this

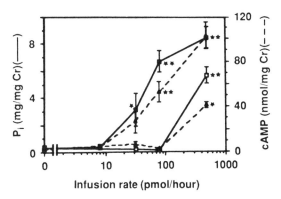

FIG. 5. Effects of bPTH-(1–84) and PTHrP-(1–34)NH₂ on urinary excretion of phosphate and cAMP in a thyroparathyroidectomized rat. Peptides were continuously infused (8–480 pmol/hr) for 4 hr beginning 4 hr after surgery. The ordinates indicate average of urinary excretion of phosphate (*solid lines*) or cAMP (*dashed lines*) per 30 min interval following treatment with either bPTH-(1–84) (*open symbols*) or PTHrP-(1–34)NH₂ (*solid symbols*). (Reprinted from ref. 2 with permission.)

cross linking is inhibited by an excess of the nonradiolabeled peptides (64). In a similar manner, radioiodinated [Nle[8,18],Tyr[34]]bPTH-(1–34)NH₂ and [Tyr[40]] PTHrP-(1–40)NH₂ cross link to an identical membrane protein in osteoblast-like cells (16).

In both PTH and PTHrP, truncation from the C-terminus to produce peptides shorter than 30 residues markedly *reduces* adenylyl cyclase activity (3,65) (Fig. 1). Peptides such as PTHrP-(1–25) and PTHrP-(1–29) do not stimulate isolated osteoclasts (in the presence of osteoblasts) to resorb bone at concentrations up to 24 nM (66). The shortest sequence that still binds to the receptor with measurable affinity is PTH-(1–26) (3). These studies suggest that the sequence 1–34 in both PTH and PTHrP makes up, quite closely, the fully active region of these hormones (for activities relevant to PTH-like effects on mineral metabolism) and that the principal binding domain of PTH resides in the sequence 25–34 (21,67) (Fig. 1).

Recently, Kronenberg and coworkers (68) elegantly demonstrated that carboxy-terminal sequence beyond the fully active region (1–34) of PTH is essential for correct hormone processing and efficient secretion. A series of carboxy-terminal deleted mutants of human prepro-PTH were expressed in a cell-free system and in transfected COS 7 cells. Prepro-PTH-(1–40) and prepro-PTH-(1–34), respectively, are either poorly or not at all translocated across the membrane of the endoplasmic reticulum. Prepro-PTH-(1–40) and prepro-PTH-(1–52) were converted inefficiently to the corresponding pro-PTH sequences. Only full-length prepro-PTH-(1–84) was processed to pro-PTH-(1–84), allowing for the efficient secretion of mature PTH (68).

Analogous to effects observed in PTH by truncation of two amino acid residues from the amino terminus, amino-terminal truncation of PTHrP yields peptides that inhibit both PTH- and PTHrP-mediated stimulation of adenylyl cyclase (16,69). For many years [Nle^{8,18},Tyr^{34}]bPTH(3–34)NH$_2$ was the inhibitor of choice for blocking PTH action in vitro in renal- and bone-derived assays (1,20, and references therein). The analog's avidity for the PTH receptor is comparable to that of native PTH and the inhibitory potency is high [K$_i$ = 9.0 × 10^{-8}M, 200-fold higher than that of bPTH-(3–34) and similar to the binding constant (K$_b$) of PTH] (20,21). Nevertheless, weak PTH-like agonist activity for the analog, e.g., producing elevation of urinary P$_i$, urinary cAMP, and plasma Ca^{2+} levels, was observed in several in vivo studies (18,70,71). We have not found any report of comparable studies for the 3–34 fragment of PTHrP.

The emergence of a second generation of PTH antagonists followed from the finding that the activation domain for PTH extends beyond Ser^3 (Fig. 1): PTH-(3–34) possesses some agonist properties. This finding provided impetus for undertaking further truncation from the amino-terminus and led to synthesis of [Tyr^{34}]bPTH-(7–34)NH$_2$, a weakly potent antagonist in vitro but one devoid of any measurable PTH-like agonist activity in vivo (19). The potency of this antago-

nist was considerably lower than the related, but longer, analog [Nle^{8,18},Tyr^{34}]PTH-(3–34)NH$_2$ (binding affinity ratio ≈15; inhibition of PTH-stimulated cAMP ≈25 in bovine renal cortical membranes) (15,67). Using [Tyr^{34}]bPTH-(7–34)NH$_2$, Horiuchi and coworkers (19) were able to demonstrate inhibition of PTH-stimulated urinary P$_i$ and cAMP excretion in vivo (PTH/PTH antagonist molar ratio of 200:1) (Fig. 6). The same antagonist blocked PTH-stimulated calcium elevations in thyroparathyroidectomized rats (1).

In summary, these studies identified the amino-terminal sequence 1–6 in PTH as the hormone's "activation" domain, thus bringing to completion the mapping of functional domains in the fully active 1–34 region of PTH. Nevertheless, as is discussed later, studies on amino-terminal peptides derived from PTHrP suggest possible extension of the "activation" domain further toward the C-terminus from the 1–6 sequence.

Based on these structure–activity studies for PTH, the peptide PTHrP-(7–34)NH$_2$ was prepared (72). The homology between PTH and PTHrP is markedly reduced after truncation of six amino acid residues from the amino terminus (five of eight identical amino acid residues within the sequences 1–13 are deleted) (Fig. 7). Nevertheless, PTHrP-(7–34)NH$_2$ is a potent inhibitor of PTH action in vitro in both renal- and bone-based assays (72,73). PTHrP-(7–34)NH$_2$ also has a sevenfold higher binding affinity, and it is eight- to 12-fold more potent an antagonist of either PTH- or PTHrP-stimu-

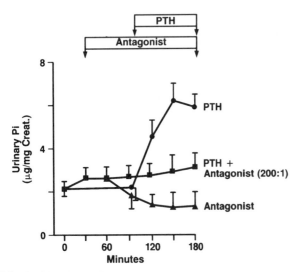

FIG. 6. Inhibition of PTH-stimulated urinary phosphate excretion in rats by PTH antagonist [Tyr^{34}]bPTH-(7–34)NH$_2$. Nine animals received native PTH alone (0.27 nmol/h) (●), 11 animals received both the antagonist and native PTH at a molar dose ratio of 200:1 (■), and four animals received the antagonist alone (54 nmol/hr) (▲). Infusion of antagonist began 1 hr prior to the beginning of the infusion of native PTH. Antagonist and native PTH were infused intravenously through separate cannulas. (Reprinted from ref. 19 with permission.)

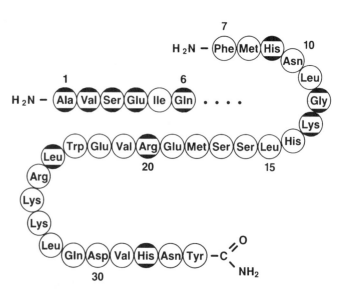

FIG. 7. Deletion of the first six amino acid residues from the aminoterminus of [Tyr^{34}]bPTH-(1–34)NH$_2$ eliminates a considerable portion of homology shared by the hormones. The homologous residues are indicated by the partially darkened circles.

lated adenylyl cyclase in rat osteosarcoma cells than is the PTH-(7–34)NH$_2$-derived antagonist (72).

However, PTHrP-(7–34)NH$_2$ differs from [Tyr^{34}] PTH-(7–34)NH$_2$ in one important way: it is a weak, but definite, partial agonist. When added (8 μM) to media bathing rat osteosarcoma cells, it elicits a 2.4-fold increase in cAMP, similar to that with [Nle^{8,18},Tyr^{34}]bPTH-(3–34)NH$_2$ (72). This observation suggests that the activation domain in PTHrP extends beyond the 1–6 region found for PTH. Interestingly, both [Nle^{8,18},Tyr^{34}]bPTH-(3–34)NH$_2$ and PTHrP-(7–34)NH$_2$, despite possessing partial agonist activity, are able to inhibit PTH actions either in vitro (52,53) or in vivo (73) (Fig. 8).

The PTH-derived antagonist inhibits cAMP production in renal membranes stimulated by either extracts (52) or conditioned media (53) obtained from tumors removed from patients suffering with humoral hypercalcemia of malignancy. PTHrP-(7–34)NH$_2$ antagonizes PTHrP-(1–34)-induced rises in blood calcium in nude mice when administered by infusion (73). These studies provide great impetus to efforts directed at designing clinically relevant PTH/PTHrP antagonists for use as drugs in treatment of the hypercalcemia of malignancy. Furthermore, it is not without precedent that mixed agonist/antagonist compounds may be of greater therapeutic potential in certain clinical disorders than either pure agonists or antagonists.

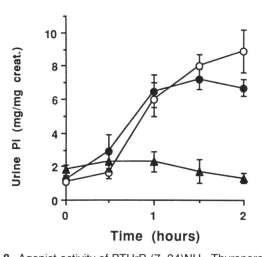

FIG. 8. Agonist activity of PTHrP-(7–34)NH$_2$. Thyroparathyroidectomized rats received PTHrP-(7–34)NH$_2$ alone at a dose of 8 nmol/hr. Urine phosphate was measured in 30 min fractions for a 2 hr period (○). The increases observed in urine phosphate excretion were comparable to those achieved in rats receiving PTHrP-(1–34)NH$_2$ at 0.16 nmol/hr (●). Infusion of [Tyr^{34}]bPTH-(7–34)NH$_2$ alone at a dose of 32 nmol/hr (▲) resulted in no appreciable phosphaturia. Values are mean ± SEM from three to five rats. (Reprinted from ref. 117 with permission.)

NONHOMOLOGOUS SEQUENCES OF PARATHYROID HORMONE AND PARATHYROID HORMONE-RELATED PROTEIN

Progressive stepwise truncation of amino acid residues from the amino terminus of PTH and PTHrP 1–34 fragments further reduces sequence homology (Fig. 2). Amino acid residues common to both hormones and carboxy-terminal to position 6 are: Leu^7, His^9, Gly^{12}, and Lys^{13} (67,73). The peptides [Tyr^{34}]PTH-(14–34)NH$_2$, PTHrP-(14–34)NH$_2$, and [Tyr^{34},Cys^{38}]PTHrP-(14–38) have been synthesized and biologically evaluated (74,75). Both [Tyr^{34}]bPTH-(14–34)NH$_2$ and [Tyr^{34}, Cys^{38}]PTHrP-(14–38) compete for binding to intact rat osteosarcoma cells with the radiolabeled ligands of either PTH or PTHrP with similar avidity (K$_d$ = 50 and 10 μM for radioiodinated [Nle^{8,18},Tyr^{34}] bPTH-(1–34)NH$_2$, K$_d$ = 10 and 30 μM for radioiodinated [Tyr^{36}]PTHrP-(1–36)NH$_2$, respectively) (74). Whereas the PTH and PTHrP analogs were equipotent in inhibiting PTH-stimulated adenylyl cyclase and binding in bovine renal membranes, PTHrP-(14–34)NH$_2$ was at least tenfold more potent than PTH-(14–34)NH$_2$ in other bone- or renal-based assays (75).

Caulfield and coworkers (75) studied two hybrid analogs of PTH and PTHrP. These hybrids were constructed by exchanging the C-terminal portions of PTH- and PTHrP-derived antagonists starting at position 19. The hybrids, [Nle^{8,18},D-Trp^{12}]bPTH-(7–18)–PTHrP-(19–34)NH$_2$ and [D-Trp^{12}]PTHrP-(7–18)–[Tyr^{34}]bPTH-(19–34)NH$_2$, maintained high affinity for PTH/PTHrP receptors and potently inhibited PTH-stimulated adenylyl cyclase in bovine renal membranes and rat osteosarcoma cells. These observations further support the localization of the principal receptor binding domain in both PTH and PTHrP to a site carboxy-terminal to position 14 and outside the sequence displaying the highest degree of sequence homology between the two hormones (Fig. 1).

The binding affinity and inhibition of PTH-stimulated adenylyl cyclase activity of [Nle^{18},Tyr^{34}]bPTH-(10–34)NH$_2$ in renal membranes was ~50% weaker than that of [Nle^{8,18},Tyr^{34}]bPTH-(7–34)NH$_2$ (21,67). The inhibition of PTH-stimulated adenylyl cyclase activity by PTHrP-(10–34)NH$_2$ in rat osteosarcoma cells was threefold lower than that of PTHrP-(7–34)NH$_2$ (73).

The lack of PTH-like agonist activity and the significant inhibitory potency of the similar sequence regions reinforces previous observations that indicate the binding domain is contained within the 14–34 sequences of both hormones. Furthermore, assuming that these nonhomologous peptides interact with a single type of PTH receptor, they must also share similar bioactive conformations.

RATIONAL DESIGN OF HIGHLY POTENT ANTAGONISTS: ROLE OF HYDROPHOBICITY

Very little is known about the interaction of a peptide agonist compared to an antagonist with receptors. Therefore, there are no established rules for converting an agonist into an antagonist with comparable affinity for the receptor. Also, there is no reliable information regarding the relationship between the so-called bioactive conformations of agonists and corresponding antagonists.

Elimination of residues 1–6 (the "activation" domain) in PTH led to the analog [Nle^{8,18},Tyr^{34}]bPTH-(7–34)NH$_2$, a pure antagonist devoid of PTH-like agonist activity. However, this modification was accompanied by an ~240-fold reduction in binding affinity compared to [Nle^{8,18},Tyr^{34}]bPTH-(1–34)NH$_2$ (K$_b$ = 145 nM vs. K$_b$ = 0.6 nM in bovine renal membranes).

Substituting either N-MePhe or desamino-Phe for Phe^7 in [Tyr^{34}]bPTH-(7–34)NH$_2$ and N-MeMet for Met^8 yielded antagonists that were equipotent to the parent compound [Tyr^{34}]bPTH-(7–34)NH$_2$ in receptor avidity (15). This finding greatly diminishes the likelihood that the reduced affinity of the antagonists stemmed from greater susceptibility to aminopeptidases than occurs with the corresponding agonist.

Our two-phase strategy for recovering the lost receptor affinity of antagonists consists of (a) stabilizing the hypothetical bioactive conformation and (b) identification of sites within the PTH molecule that are tolerant of hydrophobic substitutions and therefore can be made to serve as auxiliary receptor binding elements. This approach is based on two assumptions. The first assumption is that recognition and binding of agonist and antagonist to the same receptor imply that both share closely related bioactive conformations. The second assumption is that the reduced binding affinity of [Nle^{8,18},Tyr^{34}]bPTH-(7–34)NH$_2$ results principally from the elimination of interactions between the "activation" domain and the receptor. In β-adrenergic receptors, ligand interactions that stimulate signal transduction cause a reduction in enthalpy. This reduction is probably brought about by concomitant conformational change in either receptor or ligand or both. Comparable interactions are missing in the antagonist; compensation for these lost interactions can occur by increasing entropy through provision of extra hydrophobic interactions in the receptor–antagonist complex (76).

Several conformational studies of PTH- and PTHrP-derived peptides suggest that Gly^{12} is part of either an α-helix or a β-turn. Position 12 is occupied exclusively by a glycine residue throughout the isohormone series of PTH and PTHrP sequences (Fig. 2). Therefore, we probed for the conformational latitude permitted at this position by substituting amino acid residues that can be used as conformational reporters (31). We tried sarcosine and proline, both of which are N-alkylated amino acids known as helix breakers. Other substitutions included L- and D-alanine, α-aminoisobutyric acid, and β-alanine. Only the helix breakers failed to maintain binding affinity comparable to the Gly^{12}-containing parent agonist and antagonist (31). Position 12 was therefore designated a substitution-tolerant site and was targeted for incorporation of a highly hydrophobic aromatic residue. Introduction of D-Trp in position 12 yielded, the first time, an antagonist with binding affinity in the low nanomolar range (77). A ten- to 20-fold enhancement in bind affinity and inhibition of PTH-stimulated adenylyl cyclase was observed: K$_b$ = 7 and 15 nM in renal membranes and 60 and 182 nM in osteosarcoma cells, and K$_i$ = 69 and 125 nM in renal membranes and 211 and 69 nM in osteosarcoma cells for [D-Trp^{12},Tyr^{34}]- and [Nle^{8,18},D-Trp^{12},Tyr^{34}]bPTH-(7–34)NH$_2$, respectively (77). When closely related highly hydrophobic aromatic residues such as D-α- and β-naphthylalanine were substituted in position 12, potencies similar to that of [Nle^{8,18},D-Trp^{12},Tyr^{34}]bPTH-(7–34)NH$_2$ were displayed (31). A similar modification in PTHrP-(7–34)NH$_2$ resulted in [D-Trp^{12}]PTHrP-(7–34)NH$_2$, which was about six-fold more potent than the nonsubstituted parent peptide (31). Again, parallel effects are observed for the two hormones following introduction of D-Trp^{12}, suggesting a similar role for Gly^{12} in both sequences.

Position 13 in PTH and PTHrP and position 18 in PTH were also identified as sites tolerant of hydrophobic substitution, allowing for substitutions designed to promote either PTH-like agonist activity in 1–34 fragments or binding affinity in the corresponding antagonists (7,9,78–85). Replacement of Met^{18} with Trp led to a three- to fourfold enhancement in receptor binding and inhibition of PTH-stimulated activation of adenylyl cyclase in renal membranes (K$_b$ = 45 vs. 145 nM and K$_i$ = 420 vs. 1600 nM for [Nle^8, Trp^{18},Tyr^{34}]- and [Nle^{8,18},Tyr^{34}]bPTH-(7–34)NH$_2$, respectively) (78). A similar potentiation has been observed using a more hydrophobic modification, as evidenced by the properties of [Nle^8,D-Trp^{12,18},Tyr^{34}]bPTH-(7–34)NH$_2$ compared to [Nle^{8,18},D-Trp^{12},Tyr^{34}]bPTH-(7–34)NH$_2$ (78). Introduction of either Lys(N-ε-biotinyl) (7,80–82) or Lys(N-ε-p-azido-2-nitrophenyl) (9,83,84) in position 13 in PTH-derived agonists resulted in maintenance of biological potency. Replacement of the endogenous residue at position 13 by Lys(N-ε-dihydrocinnamoyl) in PTH analogs (85) or by Lys(N-ε-biotinyl) in PTHrP analogs (7) produced slight enhancement of antagonistic properties.

RESOLVING THE PARTIAL AGONIST/ANTAGONIST PUZZLE: THE "TRANSPLANTED CASSETTE"

The first divergence of PTHrP from the established PTH structure–function pattern emerged when we found that PTHrP-(7–34)NH$_2$, unlike [Tyr^{34}]PTH-(7–34)NH$_2$, possesses partial agonist activity (86). In untreated ROS 17/2.8 cells, PTHrP-(7–34)NH$_2$ stimulated adenylyl cyclase activity sixfold above basal at a dose of 5 μM. In contrast, [Tyr^{34}]PTH-(7–34)NH$_2$ had no stimulatory effect on cyclase activity. An assay was devised to facilitate detection of weak PTH-like agonist properties. The presence of pertussis toxin eliminates the inhibitory activity of the G$_i$ protein on adenylyl cyclase. Addition of dexamethasone increases the number of PTH receptors. Together, the modifi-

cations increase responsiveness to PTH. In the modified assay, both [Tyr^{34}]PTH-(7–34)NH$_2$ and PTHrP-(7–34)NH$_2$ displayed weak agonist activity. The PTH-derived peptide stimulated cAMP production 2.6-fold and the PTHrP-derived peptide 14-fold above the basal level at concentrations of 10 and 1.25 μM, respectively (86).

Nutt and coworkers (87) further dissected the structural source of agonism in these peptides. They demonstrated that removal of the residual agonist activity from PTHrP-(7–34)NH$_2$ and introduction of partial agonist activity into [Tyr^{34}]PTH-(7–34)NH$_2$ could be accomplished by swapping one or two amino acid residues between the two peptides (Fig. 9A) (87). Substituting Asp^{10} and Lys^{11} in PTHrP-(7–34)NH$_2$ with the corresponding amino acids taken from the native PTH sequence, namely, Asn^{10} and Leu^{11}, eliminated

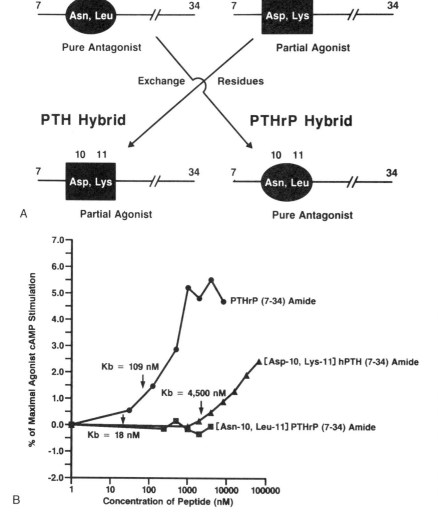

FIG. 9. Exchanging amino acid residues between PTHrP-(7–34)NH$_2$ and [Tyr^{34}]bPTH-(7–34)NH$_2$ removes partial agonist properties from the former and introduces partial agonist properties into the latter. **A:** The "PTH hybrid" containing Asp^{10}-Lys^{11} (originating from the PTHrP sequence) becomes a partial agonist, while the "PTHrP hybrid" containing Asn^{10}-Leu^{11} (originating from the PTH sequence) becomes a pure agonist. **B:** Effect of modification in positions 10 and 11 in PTH and PTHrP analogs on cAMP accumulation in ROS 17/2.8 cells, which were grown in the presence of 30 nM dexamethasone for 3 days and 40 ng/ml pertusis toxin for 1 day prior to assay. (Reprinted from ref. 87 with permission.)

the PTH-like agonist activity. Conversely, substituting Asn[10] and Leu[11] in [Tyr[34]]PTH-(7–34)NH$_2$ with the corresponding amino acid residues taken from the native PTHrP sequence, namely, Asp[10] and Lys[11], resulted in a sixfold reduction in antagonist potency and introduced weak agonist properties into the previously "pure" antagonist (Fig. 9B).

Moreover, unlike the case with [Tyr[34]]PTH-(7–34)NH$_2$ in which substitution of Gly[12] by D-Trp led to 13-fold potentiation of antagonist activity (K$_i$ = 210 nM in ROS 17/2.8 cells) (86), the same substitution in PTHrP yielded [D-Trp[12]]PTHrP-(7–34)NH$_2$, an analog that possesses sixfold enhancement in antagonist potency yet retains weak agonist activity (87), i.e., a partial agonist. Introduction of Leu in position 11, as is found in native PTH, led to [Leu[11],D-Trp[12]]PTHrP-(7–34)NH$_2$, which not only is over 100-fold more potent than PTHrP-(7–34)NH$_2$ in inhibiting PTH-stimulated adenylyl cyclase in ROS 17/2.8 cells but also is devoid of agonist activity (even in cells pretreated to enhance PTH responsiveness) (86,87).

The trisubstituted [Asn[10],Leu[11],D-Trp[12]]- and the disubstituted [Leu[11],D-Trp[12]]PTHrP-(7–34)NH$_2$ are highly potent antagonists (at inhibiting PTH-stimulated production of cAMP in ROS 17/2.8 cells) compared to the sixfold less potent [Asn[10],Leu[11]]PTHrP-(7–34)NH$_2$. In addition, these analogs are devoid of PTH-like agonist activity, emphasizing the role of Lys[11] in PTHrP as an integral part of the "activation" domain of the hormone. Introduction of Leu[11] in [D-Trp[12]]PTHrP-(7–34)NH$_2$ also removes agonist activity and augments the potency enhancement of D-Trp[12], leading to a tenfold increase in antagonist activity (K$_i$ = 7 vs. 70 nM at inhibiting PTH-stimulated adenylyl cyclase activity in ROS 17/2.8 cells, respectively) (87).

The finding that PTH-like agonist activity can be inserted or deleted in "cassette" fashion is a new concept in structure–function relations. These observations also indicate that the activation domain in both PTH and PTHrP involves residues 1–11, extending the activation domain further from the N-terminus than was appreciated earlier (67).

GLOBAL CONFORMATIONAL CONSTRAINT: THE ALTERNATIVE APPROACH

A generally held hypothesis in analog design is that stabilization of biologically relevant conformations results in enhancement of biological activity. Stabilizing a receptor-favored conformation for PTH or PTHrP may be an especially promising approach to analog design, since these linear peptides have a great degree of conformational freedom in solution. The so-called bioactive conformations, conformations that interact

with receptor, may represent only a minor fraction of the total array of energetically allowed conformations. Hence adaptation of a "bioactive" conformation may be the rate-limiting factor in hormonal expression of bioactivity for a linear peptide in solution. Introduction of a structural modification that conformationally constrains a peptide may stabilize the bioactive conformation during receptor interaction and/or prevent an extensive departure from it while the peptide is free in solution. For example, replacement of a reversible salt bridge (which stabilizes an α-helical domain) by i-to-(i + 4) side chain–to–side chain lactamization can globally constrain this domain and lock it into the same conformation (Fig. 10).

The amino-terminal portion of PTH and PTHrP was suggested in several studies to remain predominantly in an α-helical structure (31,35,36,41,47,49). If this structural feature is an important element in the bioactive conformation of PTHrP-(7–34)NH$_2$, it can be transiently stabilized by a salt bridge such as the one formed between side chains of Lys[13] and Asp[17] (which are juxtaposed in an α-helical pitch; see Fig. 11A). This hypothesis was tested by replacement of the salt bridge electrostatic interaction with a covalent bond. A lactam linkage was formed between the ε-NH$_2$ of Lys[13] and β-carboxy group of Asp[17], locking in a cyclic structure. Enhanced potency accompanied the increase in α-helical nature of this analog (see Fig. 11B) (79).

As anticipated, [Lys[13],Asp[17]]PTHrP-(7–34)NH$_2$ has tenfold higher affinity for the PTH receptor and is fivefold more potent in inhibiting PTH-stimulated adenylyl cyclase in human osteosarcoma (B-10) cells than the linear parent analog PTHrP-(7–34)NH$_2$ (79). The conformational effect is specific: closely related analogs that cannot form a salt bridge, such as [Lys[13](ε-Ac),Asn[17]]PTHrP-(7–34)NH$_2$ (a linear analog), or lactam analogs in which D-isomers of Lys[13] and/or Asp[17] were introduced (79) are markedly reduced in potency. Moreover, the introduction of lactam linkage conformational constraint, as in [Lys[13],Asp[17]]PTHrP-(7–34)NH$_2$, not only enhanced antagonist potency but also eliminated partial agonist activity as an accompaniment of the increased α-helical content (88). CD measurement of [Lys[13],Asp[17]]PTHrP-(7–34)NH$_2$ in the presence or absence of dimyristoylphosphatidylglycerol (an anionic lipid mimicking the membrane environment), revealed initial high helicity, which was further enhanced by the lipid (from 30% to 45%) as compared to lower helical content in the parent linear analog, PTHrP-(7–34)NH$_2$ (from 20% to 30%).

This CD study provided additional insights regarding possible different mechanisms for potentiating PTH-antagonist activity. Merging the structural modifications in the hydrophobically substituted analog (Leu[11],D-

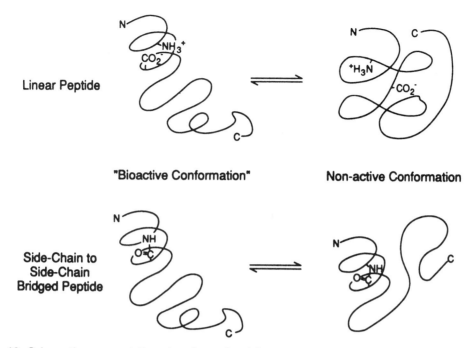

Linear Peptide

"Bioactive Conformation"   **Non-active Conformation**

Side-Chain to Side-Chain Bridged Peptide

FIG. 10. Schematic representation of conformational dynamic equilibrium of a linear peptide containing a transient salt bridge or side chain–to–side chain lactam-linked peptide. In the latter case, "locking in" the α-helical motif of the "bioactive" conformation prevents spontaneous and complete randomization of the cyclic structure. (Reprinted from ref. 79 with permission.)

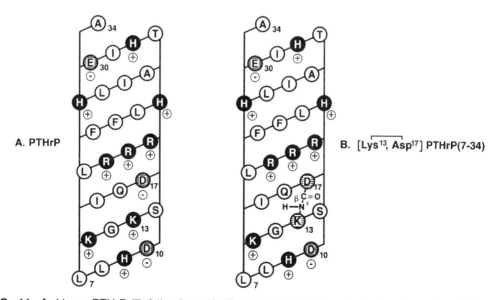

A. PTHrP   **B. [Lys¹³, Asp¹⁷] PTHrP(7-34)**

FIG. 11. A: Linear PTHrP-(7–34) schematically represented in an α-helical conformation. **B:** A cyclic lactam formed between Lys¹³ and Asp¹⁷ stabilizes an α-helical conformation. Key amino acids are highlighted: positively charged residues (*heavily shaded*), negatively charged residues (*lightly shaded*), and residues participating in the cyclization (*striped*). (Reprinted from ref. 79 with permission.)

Trp^{12}]PTHrP-(7–34)NH$_2$ and the globally constrained lactam [Lys^{13},Asp^{17}]PTHrP-(7–34)NH$_2$ yielded Ac[Leu^{11}, D-Trp^{12},Lys^{13},Asp^{17}]PTHrP-(7–34) NH$_2$. However, the affinity of the latter analog for the PTH receptor in renal membrane was less than anticipated had the combined substitutions been synergistic (K$_b$ = 4, 15, and 45 nM, respectively). The helical content of this analog was low (20%) in the absence of lipid and did not change with addition of lipid (88). It appears that additional hydrophobicity in the linear antagonist may create auxiliary interactions with the receptor and thus enhance binding affinity.

Structural rigidification via lactam formation theoretically could enhance potency by an unrelated mechanism, namely, stabilization of a biologically relevant conformation. Unfortunately, in the PTHrP analogs, these two modifications are mutually exclusive in terms of both effects on biological activity and α-helical content (88). Perhaps the hydrophobic interactions of Leu^{11} and D-Trp^{12} with the PTH receptor compromise the potential to form an α-helix, or at the same time the presence of the lactam linkage between Lys^{13} and Asp^{17} compromises optimal hydrophobic interactions with the receptor.

PARATHYROID HORMONE AND PARATHYROID HORMONE-RELATED PROTEIN ANALOGS AS SPECIALIZED MOLECULAR TOOLS FOR PROBING RECEPTOR INTERACTION

Analogs specialized for studying hormone–receptor interactions include radioligands, photoaffinity ligands, and affinity cross-linking ligands. To be used most effectively, such analogs must be fully characterized physiochemically and biologically. In our laboratory, we have "custom designed" and synthesized specialized analogs of rigorously defined structure for use in several PTH/PTHrP studies (7,15,80) (Fig. 12). The nonradioactive version **I** of the widely used radioligand monoiodinated ^{125}I-[Nle^{8,18},Tyr^{34}(3-^{125}I)]bPTH-(1–34)NH$_2$ was prepared, for the first time, by *de novo* synthesis rather than postsynthetic iodination, using Boc-Tyr(O-Bzl,3-I)-OH as a building block (15). The availability of **I** allowed us to demonstrate that its binding affinity for PTH receptors in renal membranes is very similar to [Nle^{8,18},Tyr^{34}]bPTH-(1–34)NH$_2$ (IC$_{50}$ = 1.3 and 1.1 nM, respectively). This nonradioactive iodinated agonist was used as a standard to develop a reliable and reproducible reversed-phase (RP)-high-performance liquid chromatography (HPLC) purification method for the radioiodinated compound (15).

Difficulties encountered in the radiolabeling of a PTH-derived antagonist and a PTHrP-derived agonist

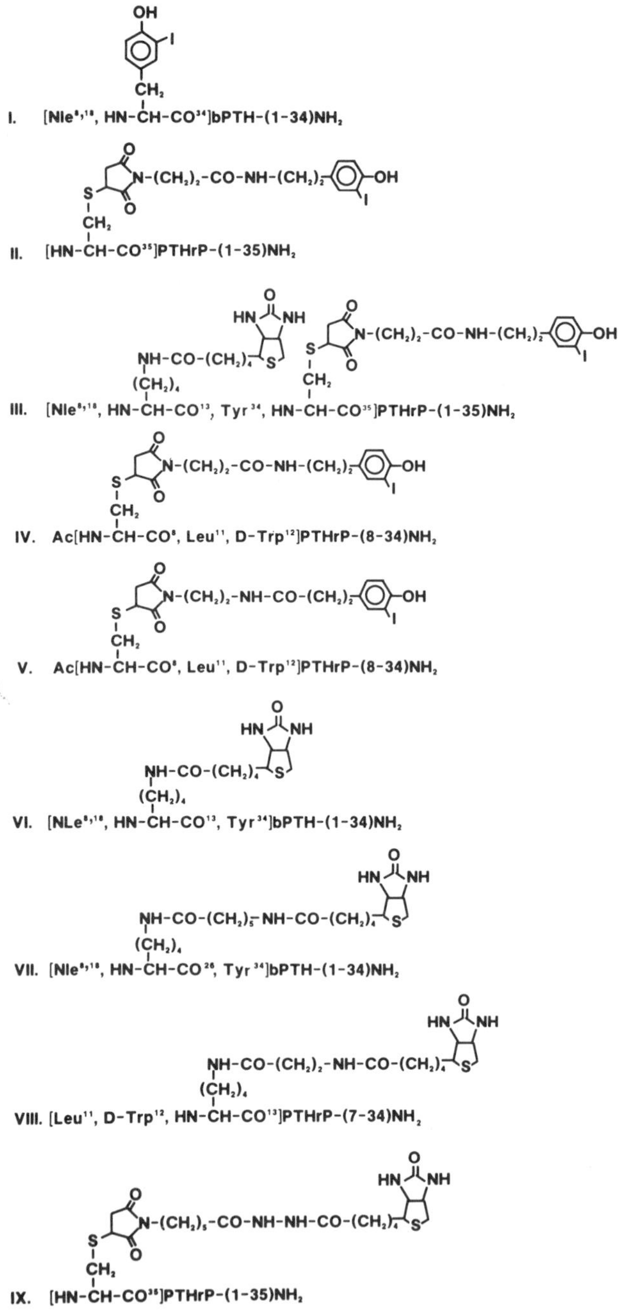

FIG. 12. Structures of analogs of PTH and PTHrP containing specialized additions.

were overcome by the development of a novel, mild, specific, indirect, and nonoxidative method for radioiodination (80). Based on thiol-maleimido chemistry, we synthesized cysteine-containing analogs of PTH and PTHrP, which were then modified postsynthetically by reaction with newly developed iodine-substituted maleimido agents (radioactive and nonradioactive). In this manner, we were able to prepare not only highly potent nonradioactive iodinated agonists of PTHrP and PTH, **II** and **III,** respectively, but also for the first time nonradioactive iodinated PTHrP antagonists **IV** and **V.** Analogs **II–V** were also prepared as radioiodinated analogs; the corresponding nonradioactive analogs were used as standards in RP-HPLC purification (80).

De novo synthesis of PTH agonists biotinylated on either Lys^{13} or Lys^{26} (e.g., **VI** and **VII**) and a PTHrP antagonist biotinylated on Lys^{13} (**VIII**) produced highly potent compounds (K_b = 1.52, 1.89 and 37.3 nM, for **VI–VIII** respectively, K_m = 0.33 and 2.91 nM for **VI** and **VII,** respectively, and K_i = 2.6 nM for **VIII** in human osteosarcoma B-10 cells) (7). We were able to obtain a highly potent biotinylated PTHrP antagonist, **IX,** by postsynthetic modification of [Cys^{35}]PTHrP-(7–35)NH$_2$ using maleimido-substitution biotin. These analogs maintain high affinity for the PTH receptor (porcine renal cortical membranes), even in the presence of large accompanying molecules such as avidin, strepavidin, and antibiotin antibodies. Radioiodination yielded highly potent radioligands, that effectively cross linked to a single (receptor) component in renal membranes ($M_r \approx 75,000$). Unlike the case with previously reported postsynthetic biotinylation procedures (81,82), our *de novo* synthesis provided sufficient quantities of material for full chemical and biological characterization. Taken together, these biotinylated analogs serve as important tools for the identification and isolation of PTH receptors (7).

THE MISSING DIMENSION: PARATHYROID HORMONE/PARATHYROID HORMONE-RELATED PROTEIN RECEPTOR

Classical in vitro studies of PTH and its fragments and analogs were conducted on membranes and cells derived from bone and kidney of several species. The accumulated data reflect either true species-specific differences in PTH/PTHrP receptors or a possible divergence of intracellular signaling mechanisms across target tissues (89–91). On the other hand, comparisons of PTH responses in bone- and kidney-derived systems within a single species suggest identity of bone and renal PTH receptors (64,90,92,93).

An example of the complexity derived when target tissue is obtained from more than one species is exemplified in a recent study by Gaedella et al. (94), which utilized opossum kidney and rat osteosarcoma (bone) cell lines. The analog [Arg^2,Tyr^{34}]hPTH-(1–34)NH$_2$ binds to ROS 17/2.8 with affinity similar to that of [Tyr^{34}]hPTH-(3–34)NH$_2$ (K_d = 31 and 89 nM, respectively) and is nearly as effective in inhibiting PTH-stimulated increases in cAMP (<10% of maximal cAMP response at an analog concentration of 1 μM).

Nevertheless, the Arg^2 analog is a weak partial agonist in this bone system. With the opossum kidney cell line, this same analog had slightly lower affinity than the PTH-(3–34) analog but surprisingly was a full agonist (maximal stimulation of cAMP at a concentration of 1 μM). The disparity between the properties of the Arg^2 analog in the two target tissue cell lines led to the suggestion that this analog should be used as a probe to distinguish between different PTH receptors (94).

Complementary DNA (cDNA) clones encoding the PTH/PTHrP receptor have been isolated and sequenced from opossum kidney (95), rat osteosarcoma ROS 17/2.8 cells (96), and human kidney and bone (SaOS-2) phage libraries (97). Transient expression has been achieved in African green monkey kidney (COS 7) cells. The rat bone PTH/PTHrP receptor was stably transfected into the murine corticotroph cell line AtT-20, where it binds [Nle^{8,18},Tyr^{34}]bPTH-(1–34)NH$_2$ with high affinity and potently stimulates cAMP increases (K_d = 0.5 and ED$_{50}$ = 0.6 nM, respectively) (98).

Structure–function analysis of PTH/PTHrP receptors cloned from different species and target tissues (based on transfection into identical expressing cells for study of ligand binding and intracellular signaling) may provide a more controlled setting for comparative studies than use of harvested tissue or cell lines. Mutated PTH/PTHrP receptors may represent novel receptor phenotypes and reveal functional domains within the receptor or may provide an explanation for the heterogeneity displayed in coupling to multiple G proteins (99,100).

Until the recent cloning of the PTH/PTHrP receptor (96,97,101), the process of designing antagonists has differed in several important ways from that of designing enzyme inhibitors. First, for several enzymes, the critical structural features of the substrate that interact with the active site of the enzyme are known, as are, in many cases, the crystalline structure of the enzyme and the spatial relation of the enzyme to the substrate in the transition state. In general, this information has been obtained because substantial quantities of pure enzyme have been isolated and the substrate is relatively small, containing only a few structural determinants. Such detailed structural information about the interaction between a peptide hormone and its receptor has only recently begun to be assembled. The example of cocrystallization of growth hormone with the soluble form of its receptor is a spectacular example of the power of such information (102). The insights obtained from a detailed picture of growth hormone–growth hormone receptor interaction led directly to the design of effective growth hormone antagonists (103), an accomplishment not thought to be possible by many just a few years ago.

Despite advances in PTH antagonist design, none of

the antagonists prepared to date has had sufficient potency or duration of action in vivo to permit its practical use as a therapeutic agent in the treatment of hypercalcemic disorders due to excess PTH or PTHrP secretion (Table 1). It is hoped that further insights into hormone–receptor interactions will permit reduction of the size of analogs to only a few essential structural elements, allowing the design of small molecule (and perhaps nonpeptide) mimetics or antagonists of PTH and PTHrP.

Already, important observations concerning the role of certain regions of the PTH/PTHrP receptor in hormone binding and intracellular signalling have been made. Much of this information has been gathered by comparing the sequences and biological properties of the rat and opossum isoforms of the PTH/PTHrP receptor (see the chapter by Segre et al.). Site-directed mutagenesis, in which portions of one receptor have been deleted, altered, or transferred and incorporated into the counterpart receptor from another species, has identified critical regions involved in expression of hormonal bioactivity (see the chapter by Segre et al.). This approach will be facilitated by the wide array of PTH and PTHrP analogs already available.

FUTURE DIRECTIONS

We anticipate that the most powerful insights into the nature of hormone–receptor interactions are yet to come. Manipulating hormonal structure for purposes of structure–function studies was undertaken previously in a manner that was "blind" to structural information about the receptor (out of necessity) until the recent cloning of the PTH/PTHrP receptor. Similarly, recent structure–activity studies based on alteration of receptor structure using site-directed mutagenesis techniques follow a similar pattern of focus on only one component of the hormone–receptor complex, the receptor.

Knowledge of the nature of the bimolecular interaction between hormone and receptor will allow analog design in a manner not previously possible. The design and synthesis of cross-linking moieties that can be strategically placed along the hormone sequence will permit the elucidation of amino acid-to-amino acid point-to-point interactions between hormone and receptor (Fig. 13). A hormone–receptor conjugate thus generated can be fragmented using enzymatic or chemical cleavage methods. The radiolabeled complex of hormone fragment covalently linked to a segment of the receptor binding domain then can be isolated and sequenced, thereby identifying small regions of hormone and receptor that are in contact with or in proximity to each other. Furthermore, as a result of the photoreaction, there are modified amino acids within

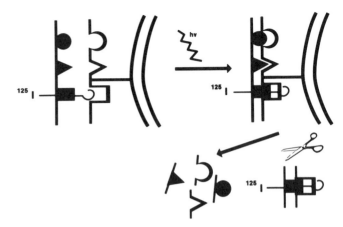

FIG. 13. Schematic approach to photoaffinity labeling of PTH/PTHrP receptors, followed by fragmentation of the resulting conjugate. The site of adduct formation is radiolabeled. After purification, a covalently linked fragment of the hormone–receptor complex can be microsequenced, identifying the cross-linked residue in the receptor.

the receptor (at the site of cross linking), which are radiolabeled and are definitely known to be in contact with hormone. By moving the photoreactive cross-linking moiety along the peptide sequence to certain discrete positions in PTH or PTHrP where bioactivity can be maintained, it will be possible to map precisely the true binding domain of the receptor and to identify at a highly localized level the structural elements critical for hormone–receptor interaction.

Once identified, the role of a given amino acid in hormone-receptor contact can be confirmed or disproven by chemical synthesis of an amino acid-substituted hormone analog (based on the cross-linking insight) and evaluation of its biological properties. In an analogous fashion, site-directed mutagenesis can be employed to produce a substituted form of the receptor that can be used to test the validity of the putative hormone–receptor contact point. By pursuing such an approach systematically, the nature of receptor interaction with hormone agonists, antagonists, and partial agonists can be studied and the mechanisms responsible for differences in biological profile of these categories can be elucidated. Coupled with computer-based molecular modeling, these insights should facilitate greatly the design of therapeutically advantageous analogs of PTH and PTHrP.

One area of investigation that has grown steadily in interest over the last decade is the potential utility of PTH or PTHrP agonists for the treatment of osteoporosis. Low-dose intermittent administration of several forms of PTH has been demonstrated to stimulate bone formation and to have an overall anabolic effect on bone (104,105). Further observations have been made in vivo in animal and in human studies conducted for periods as long as 1 year (106–113). This beneficial effect on bone occurs despite the well-documented action of PTH of stimulating bone resorption via increased osteoclast number and activity.

The precise cellular mechanism by which PTH action produces a gain in bone mass, as opposed to the more commonly observed bone loss that characterizes hyperparathyroidism, may derive from the central role occupied by the osteoblast in overall regulation of cellular bone metabolism (114–116). The osteoblast possesses functional PTH/PTHrP receptors. The osteoblast is thought to release cytokines (interleukin-1, interleukin-6, tumor necrosis factor-α, etc.) that act either directly or indirectly through intermediary cells on osteoclasts. Osteoclasts themselves, although quite prominent in the histological picture of hyperparathyroidism, possess few, if any, PTH/PTHrP receptors. It may be possible to stimulate the PTH/PTHrP receptors on osteoblasts sufficiently through administration of PTH by special regimens and thereby instigate osteoblastic bone formation without concomitant activation of osteoclasts and resultant bone resorption.

Whether PTHrP or its analogs also have the same potential as PTH to be used for treatment of osteoporosis remains to be determined. Although the data indicate that both PTH and PTHrP interact with the same receptor, an interesting and potentially important clinical observation suggests a different biological profile for the two hormones. In the syndrome of primary hyperparathyroidism, osteoblast activity and bone formation are increased; however, osteoclast-mediated bone resorption outstrips any net gain in bone mass. In hypercalcemia of malignancy due to secretion of PTHrP, bone formation does not appear to increase. Hence excess bone resorption is relatively unopposed. How these contradictory phenomena can be explained when the expression of hormonal bioactivity for both PTH and PTHrP is through the same receptor remains to be clarified.

In any case, even if one hormone or both hormones prove promising for treatment of osteoporosis, issues of safety and drug delivery will have to be addressed. Thus far, these peptides can be administered only parenterally. It is anticipated that, in addition to the available agents such as estrogens, calcitonin, and vitamin D analogs, orally active bisphosphonates will be available in the next several years. To be attractive as therapeutic agents, PTH or PTHrP agonists will have to be very effective at restoring lost bone and even forming new bone and/or these peptides will have to be administered conveniently by a regimen acceptable more widely than once-daily injection.

For PTH and PTHrP antagonists as well as agonists, development of improved drug delivery systems would greatly enhance therapeutic potential. Improved delivery may be accomplished through specialized formulations such as that used for a gonadotropin-releasing hormone analog, in which injection once per month has favorably transformed patient and physician acceptance of a peptide therapeutic agent (118–120). Given the probability of substantial progress in analog design and in peptide delivery systems, PTH or PTHrP agonists or antagonists are likely to find clinical utility in treatment of disorders of calcium and bone metabolism.

ACKNOWLEDGMENT

The authors gratefully acknowledge the expert secretarial assistance of Ms. Dawn Griffiths.

REFERENCES

1. Rosenblatt M. Peptide hormone antagonists that are effective in vivo. *N Engl J Med* 1986;315:1004–1013.
2. Horiuchi N, Caulfield MP, Fisher JE, et al. Similarity of synthetic peptide from human tumor to parathyroid hormone in vivo and in vitro. *Science* 1987;238:1566–1588.
3. Kemp BE, Moseley JM, Rodda CP, et al. Parathyroid hormone-related protein of malignancy: active synthetic fragments. *Science* 1987;238:1568–1570.
4. Habener JF, Rosenblatt M, Potts JT Jr. Parathyroid hormone: biochemical aspects of biosynthesis, secretion, action, and metabolism. *Physiol Rev* 1984;64:985–1053.
5. du Vigneaud V, Ressler C, Swan JM, Roberts CW, Katsoyannis PG, Gordon S. The synthesis of an octapeptide amide with the hormonal activity of oxytocin. *J Am Chem Soc* 1953;75:4879–4880.
6. Wright BS, Tyler GA, O'Brien R, Caporale LH, Rosenblatt M. Immunoprecipitation of the parathyroid hormone receptor. *Proc Natl Acad Sci USA* 1987;84:26–30.
7. Roubini E, Doung LT, Gibbons SW, et al. Synthesis of fully active biotinylated analogs of parathyroid hormone and parathyroid hormone-related peptide as tools for the characterization of PTH receptors. *Biochemistry* 1992;31:4026–4033.
8. Brennan DP, Levine MA. Characterization of soluble and particulate parathyroid hormone receptors using a biotinylated bioactive hormone analog. *J Biol Chem* 1987;262:14795–14800.
9. Coltrera MD, Potts JT Jr, Rosenblatt M. Identification of a renal receptor for parathyroid hormone by photoaffinity radiolabeling using a synthetic analogue. *J Biol Chem* 1981;256:10555–10559.
10. Goldring SR, Tyler GA, Krane SM, Potts JT Jr, Rosenblatt M. Photoaffinity labeling of parathyroid hormone receptors: comparison of receptors across species and target tissues and after desensitization to hormone. *Biochemistry* 1984;23:498–502.
11. Nissenson RA, Karpf D, Bambino T. Covalent labeling of a high-affinity, guanyl nucleotide sensitive parathyroid hormone receptor in canine renal cortex. *Biochemistry* 1987;26:1874–1878.
12. Karpf DB, Arnaud CD, King K, et al. The canine renal parathyroid hormone receptor is a glycoprotein: Characterization and partial purification. *Biochemistry* 1987;26:7825–7833.
13. Shigeno C, Hiraki Y, Westerberg DP, Potts JT Jr, Segre GB. Parathyroid hormone receptors are plasma membrane glycoproteins with asparagine-linked oligosaccharides. *J Biol Chem* 1988;263:3872–3878.
14. Rosenblatt M, Goltzman D, Keutmann TH, Tregear GW, Potts JT Jr. Chemical and biological properties of synthetic, sulfur-free analogues of parathyroid hormone. *J Biol Chem* 1976;251:159–164.

15. Goldman ME, Chorev M, Reagan JE, Nutt RF, Levy JJ, Rosenblatt M. Evaluation of novel parathyroid hormone analogs using a bovine renal membrane receptor binding assay. *Endocrinology* 1988;123:1468–1475.

16. Shigeno C, Yamamoto I, Kitamura N, et al. Interaction of human parathyroid hormone-related peptide with parathyroid hormone receptors in clonal rat osteosarcoma cells. *J Biol Chem* 1988;263:18369–18377.

17. Doppelt SH, Neer RM, Nussbaum SR, Federico P, Potts JT Jr, Rosenblatt M. Inhibition of the in vivo parathyroid hormone-mediated calcemic response in rats by a synthetic hormone antagonist. *Proc Natl Acad Sci USA* 1986;83:7557–7560.

18. Segre GV, Rosenblatt M, Tully GL III, Laughran J, Reit B, Potts JT Jr. Evaluation of in vitro parathyroid antagonist in vivo in dogs. *Endocrinology* 1985;116:1024–1029.

19. Horiuchi N, Holick MF, Potts JT Jr, Rosenblatt M. A parathyroid hormone inhibitor in vivo: design and biological evaluation of a hormone analog. *Science* 1983;220:1053–1055.

20. Rosenblatt M, Callahan EN, Mahaffey JE, Pont A, Potts JT Jr. Parathyroid hormone inhibitors, design synthesis and biological evaluation of hormone analogues. *J Biol Chem* 1977;252:5847–5851.

21. Nussbaum SR, Rosenblatt M, Potts JT Jr. Parathyroid hormone-renal receptor interactions. *J Biol Chem* 1980;255:10183–10187.

22. Sawyer WH, Manning M. The development of vasopressin antagonists. *Fed Proc* 1984;43:87–90.

23. Manning M, Sawyer WH. Design of potent and selective in vivo antagonists of the neurohypophysial peptides. In: Cross BA, Leng G, eds. *The neurohypophysis: structure, function, and control.* New York: Elsevier, 1983;367–382.

24. Hruby VJ. Structure-conformation-activity studies of glucagon and semisynthetic glucagon analogs. *Mol Cell Biochem* 1982;44:49–64.

25. Johnson DG, Goebel CU, Hruby VJ, Bregman MD, Trivedi D. Hyperglycemia of diabetic rats decreased by a glucagon receptor antagonist. *Science* 1982;215:1115–1116.

26. Coy DH, Horvath A, Nekola MV, Coy EJ, Erchegyi J, Schally AV. Peptide antagonists of LH-RH: large increases in antiovulatory activities produced by basic D-amino acids in the six position. *Endocrinology* 1982;110:1445–1447.

27. Folkers K, Bowers CY, Kubiak T, Stepinski J. Antagonists of luteinizing hormone-releasing hormone with pyridyl-alanines which completely inhibit ovulation at nanogram dosage. *Biochem Biophys Res Commun* 1983;111:1089–1095.

28. Rivier C, Vale W, Rivier J. Effects of gonadotropin-releasing hormone agonists and antagonists on reproductive functions. *J Med Chem* 1983;26:1545–1550.

29. Karten MJ, Rivier JE. Gonadotropin-releasing hormone analog design. Structure-function studies toward the development of agonists and antagonists: Rationale and perspective. *Endocr Rev* 1986;7:44–66.

30. Bravo EL, Khosla MC, Bumpus FM. Vascular and adrenocortical responses to a specific antagonist of angiotensin II. *Am J Physiol* 1975;228:110–114.

31. Chorev M, Goldman ME, McKee RL, et al. Modifications of position 12 in parathyroid hormone and parathyroid hormone-related protein: toward the design of highly potent antagonists. *Biochemistry* 1990;29:1580–1586.

32. Chou PY, Fasman GD. Conformational parameters for amino acids in helical, beta-sheet, and random coil regions calculated from proteins. *Biochemistry* 1974;13:211–222.

32a. Chou PY, Fasman GD. Prediction of protein conformation. *Biochemistry* 1974;13:222–245.

33. Garnier J, Osguthorpe DJ, Robson B. Analysis of accuracy and implications of simple methods for predicting the secondary structure of globular proteins. *J Mol Biol* 1978;120:97–120.

34. Schiffer M, Edmundson AB. Use of helical wheels to represent the structures of proteins and to identify with helical potential. *Biophys J* 1967;7:121–135.

35. Cohen FE, Strewler GJ, Bradley MS, et al. Analogues of

36. Epand RM, Epand RF, Hui SW, He NB, Rosenblatt M. Formation of water-soluble complex between the 1–34 fragment of parathyroid hormone and dimyristoylphosphatidylcholine. *Int J Peptide Protein Res* 1985;25:594–600.

37. Aloj S, Edelhoch H. Structural studies on polypeptide hormones. II. Parathyroid hormone. *Arch Biochem Biophys* 1972;150:782–785.

38. Brewer HB Jr, Fairwell T, Rittel W, Littledike T, Arnaud CD. Recent studies on the human, bovine and porcine parathyroid hormones. *Am J Med* 1974;56:759–766.

39. Zull JE, Smith SK, Wiltshire R. Effect of methionine oxidation and deletion of amino-terminal residues on the conformation of parathyroid hormone. *J Biol Chem* 1990;265:5671–5676.

40. Hong B-S, Yang MCM, Liang JN, Pang PKT. Correlation of structural changes in parathyroid hormone with its vascular action. *Peptides* 1986;7:1131–1135.

41. Willis KJ, Szabo AG. Conformation of parathyroid hormones: time-resolved fluorescence studies. *Biochemistry* 1992;31:8924–8931.

42. Lee SC, Russell AF. Two-dimensional ^{1}H-NMR study of the 1–34 fragment of human parathyroid hormone. *Biopolymers* 1989;28:1115–1127.

43. Bundi A, Andreatta RH, Wutrich K. Characterization of a local structure in the synthetic parathyroid hormone fragment 1–34 by ^{1}H nuclear-magnetic-resonance techniques. *Eur J Biochem* 1978;91:201–208.

44. Bundi A, Andreatta RH, Rittel W, Wutrich K. Conformational studies of the synthetic fragment 1–34 of human parathyroid hormone by NMR techniques. *FEBS Lett* 1976;64:126–129.

45. Smith LM, Jentoft J, Zull JE. Proton NMR studies of the biologically active 1–34 fragment of bovine parathyroid hormone: examination of a structural model. *Arch Biochem Biophys* 1987;253:81–86.

46. Coddington JM, Barling PM. Proton nuclear magnetic resonance studies of intact native bovine parathyroid hormone. *Mol Endocrinol* 1989;3:749–753.

47. Klaus W, Dieckmann T, Wray V, Schaumburg D. Investigations of the solution structure of the human parathyroid hormone fragment (1–34) by ^{1}H NMR spectroscopy, distance geometry, and molecular dynamic calculations. *Biochemistry* 1991;30:6936–6942.

48. Zull JE, Lev NB. A theoretical study of the structure of parathyroid hormone. *Proc Natl Acad Sci USA* 1980;77:3791–3795.

49. Barden JA, Kemp BE. ^{1}H-NMR study of a 34-residue N-terminal fragment of the parathyroid-hormone-related protein secreted during hormonal hypercalcemia of malignancy. *Eur J Biochem* 1989;184:379–394.

50. Moseley JM, Kubota M, Diefenbach-Jagger HD, et al. Parathyroid hormone-related protein purified from human lung cancer cell line. *Proc Natl Acad Sci USA* 1987;84:5048–5052.

51. Rodan SB, Insogna KL, Vignery AM-C, et al. Factors associated with humoral hypercalcemia of malignancy stimulate adenylate cyclase in osteoblastic cells. *J Clin Invest* 1983;72:1511–1515.

52. Stewart AF, Insogna KL, Goltzman D, Broadus AE. Identification of adenylate cyclase-stimulating activity and cytochemical bioactivity in extracts of tumors from patients with humoral hypercalcemia of malignancy. *Proc Natl Acad Sci USA* 1983;80:1454–1458.

53. Strewler GJ, Williams RD, Nissenson RA. Human renal carcinoma cells produce hypercalcemia in nude mouse and a novel protein recognized by parathyroid hormone receptors. *J Clin Invest* 1983;71:769–774.

54. Strewler GJ, Stern PH, Jacobs JW, et al. Parathyroid hormone-like protein from human renal carcinoma cells. Structural and functional homology with parathyroid hormone. *J Clin Invest* 1987;80:1803–1807.

55. Pizurki L, Rizzoli R, Moseley J, Martin TJ, Caverzasio J, Bonjour J-P. Effect of synthetic tumoral PTH-related pep-

tide on cAMP production and Na-dependent P, transport. *Am J Physiol* 1988;255:F957–F961.

56. Sartori L, Weir EC, Stewart AF, et al. Synthetic and partially-purified adenylate cyclase-stimulating proteins from tumors associated with humoral hypercalcemia of malignancy inhibit phosphate transport in a PTH-responsive renal cell line. *J Clin Endocrinol Metab* 1988;66:459–461.

57. Suva LJ, Winslow GA, Wettenhall REH, et al. A parathyroid hormone-related protein implicated in malignant hypercalcemia: cloning and expression. *Science* 1987;237:893–896.

58. Civitelli R, Martin TJ, Fausto A, Gunsten SL, Hruska KA, Avioli LV. Parathyroid hormone-related peptide transiently increases cytosolic calcium in osteoclast-like cell. Comparison with parathyroid hormone. *Endocrinology* 1989;125:1204–1210.

59. Thorikay M, Kramer S, Reynold FH, et al. Synthesis of a gene encoding parathyroid hormone-like protein-(1–141): purification and biological characterization of the expressed protein. *Endocrinology* 1989;124:111–118.

60. Pizurki L, Rizzoli R, Caverzasio J, Mundy G, Bonjour J-P. Factors derived from human lung carcinoma associated with hypercalcemia mimics the effects of parathyroid hormone on phosphate transport in cultured renal epithelia. *J Bone Mineral Res* 1988;3:233–239.

61. Potts JT Jr, Tregear GW, Keutmann HT, et al. Synthesis of biologically active N-terminal tetratriacontapeptide of parathyroid hormone. *Proc Natl Acad Sci USA* 1971;68:63–67.

62. Stewart AF, Mangin M, Wu T, et al. Synthetic human parathyroid hormone-like protein stimulates bone resorption and causes hypercalcemia in rats. *J Clin Invest* 1988;81:596–600.

63. Yates AJP, Gutierrez GE, Smolens P, et al. Effects of a synthetic peptide of parathyroid hormone-related protein on calcium homeostasis, renal tubular calcium reabsorption, and bone metabolism in vivo and in vitro in rodents. *J Clin Invest* 1988;81:932–938.

64. Nissenson RA, Diep D, Strewler GJ. Synthetic peptides comprising the amino-terminal sequences of parathyroid hormone-like protein from human malignancies. *J Biol Chem* 1988;263:12866–12871.

65. Tregear GW, van Rietschoten J, Greene E, et al. Bovine parathyroid hormone: minimum chain length of synthetic peptide required for biological activity. *Endocrinology* 1973;93:1349–1353.

66. Evely RS, Bonomo A, Schneider H-G, Moseley JM, Gallagher J, Martin TJ. Structural requirements for the action of parathyroid hormone-related protein (PTHrP) on bone resorption by isolated osteoclasts. *J Bone Mineral Res* 1991;6:85–93.

67. Mahaffey JE, Rosenblatt M, Shepard GL, Potts JT Jr. Parathyroid hormone inhibitors. *J Biol Chem* 1979;254:6496–6498.

68. Lim SK, Gardella TJ, Baba H, Nussbaum SR, Kronenberg HM. The carboxy-terminus of parathyroid hormone is essential for hormone processing and secretion. *Endocrinology* 1992;131:2325–2330.

69. Goltzmann D, Peytremann A, Callahan E, Tregear GW, Potts JT Jr. Analysis of the requirements for parathyroid hormone action in renal membranes with the use of inhibiting analogues. *J Biol Chem* 1975;250:3199–3203.

70. Horiuchi N, Rosenblatt M, Keutmann HT, Potts JT Jr, Holick MF. A multiresponse parathyroid hormone assay: an inhibitor has agonist properties in vivo. *Am J Physiol* 1983;244:E589–E595.

71. Martin KJ, Bellorin-Font E, Freitag J, Rosenblatt M, Slatopolski E. The arterio-venous difference for immunoreactive parathyroid hormone and the production of adenosine 3',5'-monophosphate by isolated perfused bone: studies with analogs of parathyroid hormone. *Endocrinology* 1981;109:956–959.

72. McKee RL, Goldman ME, Caulfield MP, et al. The 7–34-fragment of human hypercalcemia factor is a partial agonist/antagonist for parathyroid hormone-stimulated cAMP production. *Endocrinology* 1988;122:3008–3010.

73. Nagasaki K, Yamaguchi K, Miake Y, et al. In vitro and in vivo antagonists against parathyroid hormone-related protein. *Biochem Biophys Res Commun* 1989;158:1036–1042.

74. Abou-Samra A-B, Ueno S, Jueppner H, et al. Non-homologous sequences of parathyroid hormone and the parathyroid hormone related peptide bind to a common receptor on ROS 17/2.8 cells. *Endocrinology* 1989;125:2215–2217.

75. Caulfield MP, McKee RP, Goldman ME, et al. The bovine renal parathyroid hormone (PTH) receptor has equal affinity for two different amino acid sequences: the receptor binding domains of PTH and PTH-related protein are located within the 14–34 region. *Endocrinology* 1990;127:83–87.

76. Abramson SN, Molinoff PB. In vitro interactions of agonists and antagonists with β-adrenergic receptors. *Biochem Pharmacol* 1984;33:869–875.

77. Goldman ME, McKee RL, Caulfield MP, et al. A new highly potent parathyroid hormone antagonist [D-Trp^{12},Tyr^{34}]bPTH-(7–34)NH$_2$. *Endocrinology* 1988;123:2597–2599.

78. Chorev M, Roubini E, Goldman ME, et al. Effects of hydrophobic substitutions at position 18 on the potency of parathyroid hormone antagonists. *Int J Peptide Protein Res* 1990;36:465–470.

79. Chorev M, Roubini E, McKee RL, et al. Cyclic parathyroid hormone related antagonists: lysine 13 to aspartic acid 17 [i to (i + 4)] side chain to side chain lactamization. *Biochemistry* 1991;30:5968–5974.

80. Chorev M, Caulfield MP, Roubini E, et al. A novel, mild specific and indirect thiol-maleimido based radioiodolabeling method: radiolabeling of analogs derived from parathyroid hormone (PTH) and PTH-related protein. *Int J Peptide Protein Res* 1992;40:445–455.

81. Abu-Samra A-B, Freeman M, Juppner H, Uneno S, Segre GV. Characterization of fully active biotinylated parathyroid hormone analogs. *J Biol Chem* 1990;265:58–62.

82. Newman W, Beall LD, Levine MA, Cone JL, Randhawa ZI, Bertolini DR. Biotinylated parathyroid hormone as a probe for the parathyroid hormone receptor. *J Biol Chem* 1989;264:16359–16366.

83. Shigeno C, Hiraki Y, Westerberg DP, Potts JT Jr, Segre GV. Photoaffinity labeling of parathyroid hormone receptors in clonal rat osteosarcoma cells. *J Biol Chem* 1988;263:3864–3871.

84. Shigeno C, Hiraki Y, Keutmann HT, Stern AM, Potts JT Jr, Segre GV. Preparation of photoreactive analog of parathyroid hormone [Nle^8,Lys(N-ε-azido-2-nitrophenyl)^{13}, Nle^{18},Tyr^{34}] bovine parathyroid hormone (1–34) NH$_2$, a selective, high-affinity ligand for characterization of parathyroid hormone receptors. *Anal Biochem* 1989;179:268–273.

85. Chorev M, Roubini E, McKee RL, et al. Biological activity of parathyroid hormone antagonists substituted at position 13. *Peptides* 1991;12:57–62.

86. McKee RL, Caulfield MP, Rosenblatt M. Treatment of bone-derived ROS 17/2.8 cells with dexamethasone and pertussis toxin enables detection of partial agonist activity for parathyroid hormone antagonists. *Endocrinology* 1990;127:76–82.

87. Nutt RF, Caulfield MP, Levy JJ, Gibbons SW, Rosenblatt M, McKee RL. Removal of partial agonist from parathyroid hormone (PTH)-related protein-(7–34)NH$_2$ by substitution of PTH amino acids at positions 10 and 11. *Endocrinology* 1990;127:491–493.

88. Chorev M, Epand RF, Rosenblatt M, Caulfield MP, Epand RM. Circular dichroism (CD) studies of antagonists derived from parathyroid hormone-related protein. *Int J Peptide Protein Res* (in press).

89. McKee RL, Caulfield MP, Fisher JE, Duong LT, Rosenblatt M. Differences in human and rat parathyroid (PTH) receptors: agonists and antagonists are 3- to 130-fold more potent in human derived systems (abstract). *J Bone Mineral Res* 1989;4:S341.

90. Orloff JJ, Goumas D, Wu TL, Stewart AF. Interspecies comparison of renal cortical receptors for parathyroid hormone and parathyroid hormone-related protein. *J Bone Mineral Res* 1991;6:279–287.

91. Takano T, Takatsuki K, Yoneda M, Tomita A, Ogawa K, Matsui N. Studies of structure-function relationship of hu-

man parathyroid hormone using rat and human renal cortical cells in culture. *Acta Endocrinol* 1988;118:551–558.

92. Juppner H, Abou-Samra A-B, Uneno S, Gu WX, Potts JT Jr, Segre GV. The PTH-like peptide associated with humoral hypercalcemia of malignancy and parathyroid hormone bind to the same receptor on the plasma membranes of ROS 17/2.8 cells. *J Biol Chem* 1988;263:1071–1078.

93. Orloff JJ, Ribaudo AE, McKee RL, Rosenblatt M. A pharmacological comparison of parathyroid hormone receptors in human bone and kidney. *Endocrinology* 1992;131:1603–1611.

94. Gaedella TJ, Axelrod D, Rubin D, et al. Mutational analysis of the receptor-activating region of human parathyroid hormone. *J Biol Chem* 1991;266:13141–13146.

95. Juppner H, Abou-Samra A-B, Freeman M, et al. A G protein linked receptor for parathyroid hormone and parathyroid hormone-related peptide. *Science* 1991;254:1024–1026.

96. Abou-Samra A-B, Juppner H, Force T, et al. Expression cloning of a common receptor for parathyroid hormone and parathyroid hormone-related peptide from rat osteoblast-like cells: a single receptor stimulates intracellular accumulation of both cAMP and inositol triphosphates and increases intracellular free calcium. *Proc Natl Acad Sci USA* 1992;89:2732–2736.

97. Schipani E, Karga H, Karaplis AC, et al. Characterization of the cDNA encoding the human PTH/PTHrP receptor (abstract). *J Bone Mineral Res* 1992;7:S246.

98. Abou-Samra A-B, Juppner H, Khalifa A, et al. Parathyroid hormone (PTH) stimulates adrenocorticotropin release in AtT-20 cells stably expressing a common receptor for PTH and PTH-related peptide. *Endocrinology* 1993;132:801–805.

99. Juppner H, Gardella T, Lee CW, et al. Mapping of a ligand binding domain by using mutant PTH/PTHrP receptors (abstract). *J Bone Mineral Res* 1992;7:S93.

100. Abou-Samra A-B, Juppner H, Force T, et al. The PTH/PTHrP receptor activates adenylate cyclase and phospholipase C through two distinct molecular domains (abstract). *Seventy-Fourth Annual Meeting of the Endocrine Society, San Antonio, Texas*, Bethesda, Maryland: The Endocrine Society Press, 1992;260.

101. Juppner H, Abou-Samra AB, Freeman M, et al. A G protein-linked receptor for parathyroid hormone and parathyroid hormone-related peptide. *Science* 1991;254:1024–1026.

102. de Vos AM, Ultsch M, Kossiakoff AA. Human growth hormone and extracellular domain of its receptor: crystal structure of the complex. *Science* 1992;255:306–312.

103. Fuh G, Cunningham BC, Fukunaga R, Nagata S, Goeddel DV, Wells JA. Rational design of potent antagonists to the human growth hormone receptor. *Science* 1992;256:1677–1680.

104. Howard GA, Bottemiller BL, Turner RT, Rader JI, Baylink DJ. Parathyroid hormone stimulates bone formation and resorption in organ culture: evidence for a coupling mechanism. *Proc Natl Acad Sci USA* 1981;78:3204–3208.

105. Tam CS, Heersche JNM, Murray TM, Parsons JA. Parathyroid horone stimulates the bone apposition rate independently of its resorptive action: differential effects of inter-

mittent and continual administration. *Endocrinology* 1982;110:506–512.

106. Reeve J, Davies UM, Hesp R, McNally E, Katz D. Treatment of osteoporosis with human parathyroid peptide and observations on effect of sodium fluoride. *Br Med J* 1990;301:3140–3144.

107. Reeve J, Williams D, Hesp R, et al. Anabolic effect of low doses of a fragment of human parathyroid hormone on the skeleton in postmenopausal osteoporosis. *Lancet* 1976;1:1035–1038.

108. Tada K, Yamamuro T, Okumura H, Kasai R, Takahashi H. Restoration of axial and appendicular bone volumes by h-PTH(1–34) in parathyroidectomized and osteopenic rats. *Bone* 1990;11:163–169.

109. Hock JM, Gera I, Fonseca J, Raisz LG. Human parathyroid hormone-(1–34) increases bone mass in ovariectomized and orchidectomized rats. *Endocrinology* 1988;122:2899–2904.

110. Hodsman AB, Fraher LJ. Biochemical responses to sequential human parathyroid hormone (1–38) and calcitonin in osteoporotic patients. *Bone Mineral* 1990;9:137–152.

111. Tsai K-S, Ebeling PR, Riggs BL. Bone responsiveness to parathyroid hormone in normal and osteoporotic postmenopausal women. *J Clin Endocrinol Metab* 1989;69:1024–1027.

112. Slovik DM, Rosenthal DI, Doppelt SH, et al. Restoration of spinal bone in osteoporotic men by treatment with human parathyroid hormone (1–34) and 1,25-dihydroxyvitamin D. *J Bone Mineral Res* 1986;1:377–381.

113. Wronski TJ, Yen C-F, Qi H, Dann LM. Parathyroid hormone is more effective than estrogen or bisphosphonates for restoration of lost bone mass in ovariectomized rats. *Endocrinology* 1993;132:823–831.

114. Rodan GA, Martin TJ. Role of osteoblasts in hormonal control of bone resorption—a hypothesis. *Calcif Tissue Int* 1982;33:349–351.

115. McSheehy PM, Chambers TJ. Osteoblastic cells mediate osteoclastic responsiveness to parathyroid hormone. *Endocrinology* 1986;118:824–828.

116. Rodan GA. Introduction to bone biology. *Bone* 1992;13(Suppl 1):S3–S6.

117. Horiuchi N, Hongo T, Clemens TL. A 7–34 analog of parathyroid hormone-related protein has potent antagonist and partial agonist activity in vivo. *Bone Mineral* 1991;12:181–188.

118. Parmar H, Rustin G, Lightman SL, Phillips RH, Hanham IW, Schally AV. Response to D-Trp-6-luteinising hormone releasing hormone (Decapeptyl) microcapsules in advanced ovarian cancer. *Br Med J* 1988;296:1229.

119. Zorn JR, Mathieson J, Risquez F, Comaru-Schally AM, Schally AV. Treatment of endometriosis with a delayed release preparation of the agonist D-Trp6-luteinizing hormone-releasing hormone: long-term follow-up in a series of 50 patients. *Fertil Steril* 1990;53:401–406.

120. Korkut E, Bokser L, Comaru-Schally AM, Groot K, Schally AV. Inhibition of growth of experimental prostate cancer with sustained delivery systems (microcapsules and microgranules) of the luteinizing hormone-releasing hormone antagonist SB-75. *Proc Natl Acad Sci USA* 1991;88:844–848.

The Parathyroids, edited by J.P. Bilezikian,
M.A. Levine, and R. Marcus. Raven Press, Ltd.,
New York © 1994.

CHAPTER 11

Advances in Immunoassays for Parathyroid Hormone

Clinical Applications to Skeletal Disorders of Bone and Mineral Metabolism

Samuel R. Nussbaum and John T. Potts, Jr.

Advances in our understanding of parathyroid hormone (PTH) secretion in clinical disorders of mineral ion homeostasis and metabolic bone diseases have resulted from more sensitive and precise measurement of PTH, especially the biologically active intact hormone PTH-(1–84). This chapter reviews the advantages of double antibody techniques that measure exclusively the intact hormone over earlier techniques that used a single antiserum in displacement assays that were sensitive to circulating fragments. In addition, we will examine the role of PTH immunoassays in the diagnosis and management of patients with hypercalcemia and secondary hyperparathyroidism.

PARATHYROID HORMONE SECRETION AND METABOLISM: AN OVERVIEW

Although PTH was one of the first hormones to be measured by the technique of radioimmunoassay (RIA) 30 years ago (1), determination of circulating levels of PTH in man has been fraught with challenges. The difficulties involved in the measurement of PTH are related to the extremely low (picomolar) circulat-

ing levels of the hormone in normal physiology and to the heterogeneity of PTH that results from the presence of circulating fragments of the hormone secreted from the parathyroid glands (2–10) and/or derived from peripheral metabolism (11–21).

Parathyroid hormone, like other peptide hormones (as reviewed in the chapter by Kronenberg et al.), is synthesized as a larger precursor, preproparathyroid hormone: a 115-amino-acid peptide. The 25-amino-acid amino-terminal leader sequence, a hydrophobic precursor essential for transport of PTH across the endoplasmic reticulum to secretory granules, and the six-amino-acid *pro* sequence are removed and destroyed within the gland; only the polypeptide of 84 amino acids PTH-(1–84) survives (Fig. 1) (22).

Parathyroid hormone-(1–84) is stored in secretory granules awaiting two fates: secretion in response to hypocalcemic stimuli or intracellular degradation. Surprisingly, degradation via proteolytic cleavage of the stored hormone provides a dynamic mechanism for regulation of PTH stores. Evidence in vitro indicates that rates of intracellular degradation of hormone *increase* in states of hypercalcemia, when hormone secretion rates from the parathyroid glands are lower. By contrast, the absolute rate of hormone degradation decreases in hypocalcemic conditions when tissue release of hormone PTH-(1–84) is greatest (5,6,8,23). These in vitro studies have been confirmed in vivo by analysis of immunoreactive PTH peptides in parathyroid gland effluent blood of cows subjected to experimentally induced changes in extracellular fluid (ECF)

S. R. Nussbaum: Endocrine Unit, Department of Medicine, Harvard Medical School, Massachusetts General Hospital, Boston, Massachusetts 02114

J. T. Potts, Jr.: Department of Medicine, Harvard Medical School, Massachusetts General Hospital, Boston, Massachusetts 02114.

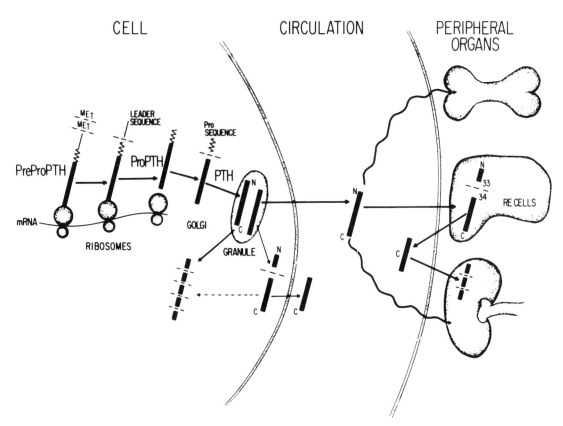

FIG. 1. Biosynthesis, secretion, and metabolism of parathyroid hormone. The predominant species of PTH in the circulation is represented by C-terminal fragments derived largely from hepatic metabolism of the intact 1–84 molecule. These C terminal fragments are derived from cleavage of PTH-(1–84) at positions 33–34 (and other midmolecule sites) and from glandular secretion.

calcium concentration that suppress (hypercalcemia) or stimulate (hypocalcemia) hormone production. Secretion of PTH-(1–84) hormone is suppressed greatly but still persists at a low level in hypercalcemia; under these conditions the ratio of middle and carboxyl-terminal fragments to intact hormone is much higher than during normocalcemic or hypocalcemic conditions (3,6,24). Hence variable amounts of fragments accompany the release of intact hormone PTH-(1–84) from the gland (9). Amino-terminal fragments are generally not detected in parathyroid gland effluent (6,10,25–27).

Intact PTH is efficiently cleared from the circulation within several minutes (28). Hepatic, renal, and skeletal cells extract PTH from blood, with the liver playing the dominant quantitative role in PTH metabolism (13–15,19,20,29). Fragments similar to those detected in parathyroid gland effluent result from peripheral metabolism of the hormone, as reviewed in Chapter 9. As with metabolism of PTH-(1–84) within the gland, the potentially biologically active amino-terminal fragment does not survive to reenter the circulation after peripheral metabolism of hormone (11,13,15,20, 29,30).

Overall, in normal physiology, ~10–20% of circulating PTH immunoactivity represents the intact hormone, the remainder being a heterogeneous collection of fragments corresponding to the middle and carboxyl regions of the molecule but not, apparently, amino-terminal fragments. In advanced renal disease, biologically inactive fragments may make up >95% of immunologically detectable PTH; this problem in assessing concentrations of biologically active PTH has been largely circumvented (see below) by assays that detect only intact hormone. It is the presence of circulating PTH fragments that, in part, is responsible for the confusion regarding serum PTH levels in pathophysiologic states.

HISTORICAL PERSPECTIVE: PARATHYROID HORMONE RADIOIMMUNOASSAY

Gerald Aurbach, to whom this volume is dedicated, working with Berson and Yalow, developed the first RIA for bovine and human PTH 30 years ago (1). RIA refers to a displacement assay technique in which a radiolabeled ligand (usually the antigen) is bound to a high-affinity polyclonal antibody raised in a heterologous species. The addition of unlabeled standards or an unknown amount of hormone present in a serum or plasma sample results in a competition between labeled and unlabeled hormone for antibody binding, with the displacement of labeled hormone. As increasing quantities of unlabeled ("cold") hormone (or ligand) are added to the radiolabeled ligand-antibody reaction, there is a progressive reduction of the amount of radioactivity bound, and a standard curve plotting concentration of hormone ligand versus bound radiolabeled ligand can be generated.

Many technical issues must be considered to optimize performance of displacement type RIAs. These include the affinity of the antibody, efficient labeling of the antigen (often with ^{125}I for tyrosine-containing peptide ligands) without loss of immunoreactivity (31,32), stability of labeled and unknown hormone (33), presence of potential interfering substances, and reaction conditions including time and temperature for incubation (34). Overall, despite the large number of displacement assays developed for PTH, most have lacked the sensitivity required to detect circulating levels of PTH in normal physiology and have lacked specificity for the biologically active intact hormone, PTH-(1–84). Moreover, most RIAs require several days of incubation, delaying the availability of the result. Also, many have failed to achieve the absolutely essential clinical criterion for a reliable PTH assay, namely, complete separation of those individuals with primary hyperparathyroidism from those with other causes of hypercalcemia not mediated by PTH, such as hypercalcemia associated with malignancy. Despite the overall clinical utility of displacement-type assays, there have been serious problems in application and interpretation, especially with the occurrence of false-positive results in patients with nonparathyroid malignancy. These issues have been reviewed and their causes analyzed extensively elsewhere (25,35,36).

Many of the reasons for the suboptimal clinical performance of these assays are known (37); others, such as false-positive results in patients with cancer (38–42), remain speculative. Initially, PTH used as an immunogen was prepared from bovine parathyroid glands. Bovine hormone was used for labeling because of its availability, and only the bovine hormone contains tyrosine (22). This resulted in displacement assays in which the bovine or human standards and human samples produced nonparallel dose-response curves (32). To deal with this problem of nonparallelism, standards for human hormone were developed from pools of sera of patients with hyperparathyroidism. The epitopes that were recognized were variable, and sometimes several epitopes were detected by polyclonal antisera. The sensitivity was sufficiently low that it was ambiguous at best whether normal levels of PTH were detectable. Results were reported in terms of microliter equivalents of an arbitrary pooled standard (33,39,41,42).

Some of these limitations were overcome when synthetic human PTH peptides became available for use as immunogens and standards. The availability of synthetic PTH fragments allowed the mapping of the epitopic recognition sites of polyclonal antibodies directed against the intact molecule. Anti-PTH antibodies appear to recognize linear sequences of amino acids rather than conformational features of the molecule. Despite the use of synthetic peptides, the heterogeneity of circulating forms of PTH continued to cause confusion in the interpretation of PTH assays. The synthetic peptides PTH-(1–34), PTH-(28–48), PTH-(44–68), and PTH-(53–84) were used to develop assays that recognized amino-, middle-, and carboxyl-terminal portions of PTH (7,26,27,31,32,43–49). Although each antiserum recognizes to varying degrees the intact molecule, assays based on the middle and carboxyl-terminal region predominantly detect the inactive mid and carboxyl fragments that circulate often at tenfold higher concentrations than with intact hormone (10,14,22,27,31,32,43,45–48).

Ideally, clinicians and clinical investigators would derive the greatest benefit from a PTH assay that is sufficiently sensitive to measure the secreted hormone in normal physiologic states and can (a) identify all individuals with primary hyperparathyroidism and distinguish these patients from patients with other causes of hypercalcemia, (b) assess parathyroid gland responses to changes in renal function or vitamin D status, and (c) be used to analyze PTH secretion in other clinical disease states such as nephrolithiasis (50) and metabolic bone diseases (51). In addition, the optimal assay would be easy to perform, provide results rapidly, and have satisfactory technical characteristics, including reproducibility and an extended standard range. An extended standard range would allow measurement of circulating levels of PTH in patients with significant oversecretion (renal failure, hypocalcemia) and those with decreased secretion of PTH (hypoparathyroidism, hypomagnesemia) in the same assay without multiple dilutions. Overall, displacement RIAs do not satisfy all these criteria for an ideal assay. While they identify hypercalcemic patients with hyperparathyroidism in 90–95% of circumstances, the 10–25% rate of false-positive results in malignancy-associated hypercalcemia in most assays limits their utility (Fig. 2). Furthermore, in many of these assays, PTH is undetectable in blood from many normal people and subjects with hypoparathyroidism. Marked elevations of PTH are reported in renal insufficiency with assays that detect middle and carboxyl-terminal PTH regions; the elevations are not reliably proportional to the secretion of PTH-(1–84) because of pro-

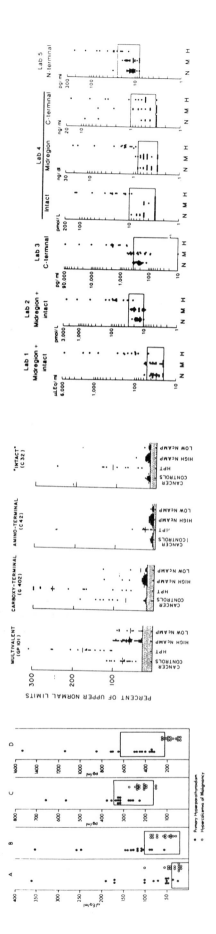

FIG. 2. Comparison of region-specific radioimmunoassays in the diagnosis of hypercalcemic patients with hyperparathyroidism and those with hypercalcemia associated with malignancy. Note the overlap of values. (Reprinted from refs. 39, 41, and 42 with permission.)

longed clearance of carboxyl fragments in renal failure. RIAs based on amino-terminal regions of PTH are clinically useful in renal failure but are less useful in the diagnosis of primary hyperparathyroidism because of low sensitivity.

In summary, although various region-specific displacement assays have been developed, they are generally insufficiently sensitive or specific to measure normal circulating levels of PTH and therefore cannot determine short-term responses to physiologic stimuli for PTH release. While many of these assays can distinguish most patients with primary hyperparathyroidism from normal individuals, many of these assays yield falsely elevated PTH values in malignancy-associated hypercalcemia.

IMMUNOMETRIC ASSAYS

Immunometric assays (52,53), also called *sandwich assays, two-site assays,* and *labelled antibody assays,* have been developed to measure PTH (28,36,54–66) and have been widely applied in clinical research and practice. They have greatly improved our knowledge of PTH secretion in physiologic and pathophysiologic conditions. These noncompetitive immunometric assays take advantage of saturation kinetics rather than competitive binding (52,53) of radiolabeled PTH with PTH in the serum sample. Immunometric assays for PTH-(1–84) employ two antibodies directed against different epitopic determinants within PTH-(1–84) (Fig. 3). Binding of these two antibodies to antigenic recognition sites on the PTH molecule requires that each antibody must not sterically interfere with the other. One antibody is present in relative excess and is immobilized on a plastic bead or support. This antibody serves as a "capture" antibody that "extracts" PTH-(1–84) and other fragments that contain the epitopic determinant from the serum sample (54,56,57, 59,64,66). A second antibody, generally of higher affinity, is labeled with either radioactive iodine (termed an *immunoradiometric assay;* IRMA) or with a chemiluminescent molecule (termed an *immunochemiluminometric assay;* ICMA) (57,61) in order to facilitate detection and quantitation of intact PTH bound to the capture antibody (Fig. 3).

Most of the immunometric assays for PTH apply similar formats for construction of the assay. Antibodies are developed against amino- and carboxyl-regions of PTH either by an immunization program involving synthetic fragments corresponding to these regions or by using affinity chromatography to purify a class of region-specific antibodies generated with PTH-(1–84) as the immunogen. These antibodies may be monoclonal antibodies, raised and expanded in mice, or polyclonal antibodies, which have been affinity-purified to

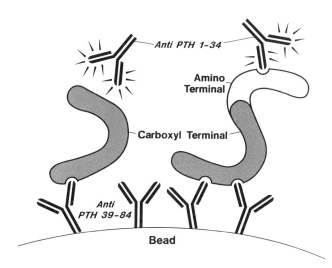

FIG. 3. Schematic representation of an immunometric (double antibody or "sandwich") assay for PTH. An antibody recognizing PTH-(39–84) binds middle and carboxyl fragments and the intact molecule. A high-affinity antibody recognizing the amino-terminal region of PTH is either iodinated or complexed to a chemiluminescent compound.

select a high-affinity class that is specific for a region of PTH. Often the monoclonal antibody serves the role of the more abundant capture antibody with lower affinity, whereas the polyclonal antibody is of higher affinity and is labeled (56,57). Binding cooperativeness between these two antibodies provides a higher avidity of binding and can greatly increase the sensitivity of the assay. The apparent affinity of the immunometric assay can be much greater than the affinity of either antibody used alone in a displacement, solution-phase RIA because of their cooperative effect (52,53).

One general scheme for the commercially available immunometric assays involves immobilization onto a solid support of an antibody that recognizes the middle and carboxyl-terminal regions of PTH. This antibody captures intact PTH-(1–84) and the more abundant midcarboxyl fragments that are present in plasma or serum (36). The second "signal," or reporter, antibody recognizes and binds to the intact hormone only and not to the carboxyl-terminal fragments. The second, labeled, antibody is added in excess, but antibody that does not bind is washed away. Signal antibodies have been labeled with radioactive ^{125}I or a chemiluminescent aryl acridinium ester. The amount of labeled antibody that binds to PTH that has been immobilized to the solid support via binding to the capture antibody (in a sandwich fashion) increases as a function of intact PTH. The amount of intact PTH in a serum sample is directly proportional to the amount of detector "activity" that is quantified with a gamma counter (radioactivity) or with a luminometer (chemiluminescence). The concentration of PTH can be accurately determined by comparison with standard curves generated using synthetic PTH-(1–84) standards. High concentrations of midregion and carboxyl fragments that accumulate in renal failure with severe secondary hyperparathyroidism do not interfere with assay performance. Although these middle and carboxyl fragments are found by the capture antibody, they are not detected by the reporter antibody for which they lack epitopic recognition. Under unusual circumstances in which the concentrations of middle and carboxyl-terminal fragments vastly exceed the concentration of intact PTH, the capture antibody may be "overwhelmed," and few antibody binding sites may be available to immobilize intact hormone molecules. These conditions may lead to an underestimation of the level of intact hormonepresent in a sample. Although these considerations may be more theoretical than practical, these conditions occasionally occur in measuring intact PTH present in samples obtained by aspiration of parathyroid adenomas.

Immunometric assays have several advantages compared to displacement RIAs. They have enhanced sensitivity that allows PTH measurements within and below the normal range (useful for physiological studies and for detection of hypoparathyroid patients) (55,57,64,66); specificity for the circulating biologically active PTH-(1–84) peptide; higher precision; improved tracer stability that results from chemiluminescent tags or iodination of antibodies rather than PTH; freedom from nonspecific serum effects; technical simplicity because of the addition of serum or plasma and reporter antibody to a solid support; speed of performance, with a turnaround time of minutes to hours (65) (although most assays give optimal performance at ~24 hr); and the practical advantage of a dose-response curve which extends over three orders of PTH-(1–84), making reassay of diluted samples, as often occurred in renal failure with earlier assays, unnecessary.

Theoretical considerations suggest that immunochemiluminometric assays should have greater sensitivity than immunoradiometric assays (52,53), but data are insufficient to support this prediction for PTH at present (57,61,64,67). There remains a strong interest, however, in using assays that do not involve radioactivity because of issues associated with disposal of radioactivity.

BIOASSAYS FOR PARATHYROID HORMONE

Several bioassays based on measurement of cAMP in urine or serum or on the accumulation of cAMP in rat osteosarcoma cells have been developed to measure PTH (68–71). None of these assays are more sensitive than immunometric assays for PTH. The discovery of parathyroid hormone-related protein (PTHrP)

as a frequent cause for hypercalcemia associated with malignancy has provided an important breakthrough in understanding the pathophysiologic basis for the hypercalcemia of cancer. More recently, the cloning of a common receptor for PTH and PTHrP has provided evidence that both peptides bind to this receptor with equal affinities and stimulate adenylyl cyclase and cAMP to comparable degrees, thus explaining the similarities in renal calcium and phosphate handling in hyperparathyroidism and malignancy-associated hypercalcemia. Because PTH or PTHrP binding to a common PTH/PTHrP receptor on kidney and bone results in an increase in adenylyl cyclase and cAMP, the classic signal transduction pathway for PTH action, bioassays based on these biologic responses lack the ability to discriminate between malignancy associated with PTHrP and primary hyperparathyroidism. An extremely sensitive cytobiochemical assay (72,73) that measures the ability of PTH to increase glucose-6-phosphate dehydrogenase activity in guinea pig renal distal convoluted tubules is also not specific for PTH; it detects PTHrP in patients with hypercalcemia associated with malignancy (40). Therefore, this technically demanding and time-consuming assay, despite its sensitivity of <1 pg/ml, has limited practical or clinical utility.

CLINICAL APPLICATIONS OF PARATHYROID HORMONE ASSAYS: DIFFERENTIAL DIAGNOSIS OF HYPERCALCEMIC DISORDERS, DISTINCTION BETWEEN PRIMARY HYPERPARATHYROIDISM, AND OTHER CAUSES OF HYPERCALCEMIA

The two most frequent causes for hypercalcemia are primary hyperparathyroidism and hypercalcemia associated with malignancy. Together, these two diagnoses account for at least 90% of all cases of hypercalcemia. The majority of asymptomatic ambulatory patients with hypercalcemia have hyperparathyroidism, whereas hypercalcemia associated with malignancy is more often associated with symptoms and generally occurs in hospitalized patients. However, hypercalcemia is only rarely the presenting manifestation of malignancy.

In the past, many individuals with primary hyperparathyroidism would undergo extensive diagnostic evaluation for other causes of hypercalcemia, particularly cancer, because earlier displacement type RIAs could not reliably distinguish individuals with primary hyperparathyroidism from those with cancer. Analysis of the large number of reports of PTH measurements in hypercalcemic disorders reveals that normal rather than suppressed values are present in 25–50% of patients with malignancy associated hypercalcemia and, on occasion, elevated values may be found (Fig. 2) (25,36,39,41,42,59,61,67). In one widely applied clinical assay that shows excellent separation of normal individuals from those with primary hyperparathyroidism, apparent elevations of PTH are present in 27% of serum samples from patients with malignancy and hypercalcemia (74).

Several recently reported displacement assays compare favorably with assays of PTH-(1–84) in the diagnosis of hyperparathyroidism (25). When patients with primary hyperparathyroidism are compared with normal subjects who have normal renal function, immunoreactive PTH levels are found to be elevated in at least 90% of hyperparathyroid patients (Fig. 2), and some assays claim complete separation (67) (Fig. 4). From a theoretical perspective, high rates of secretion and slower clearance of middle and carboxyl fragments in hyperparathyroidism should provide for a higher integrated value as an index of PTH secretion than intact PTH per se, essentially minimizing the effects of pulsatile secretion of intact hormone (75,76).

In general, it appears that the overlap of PTH values is greatest in cancer and hyperparathyroid patients who have mildly elevated serum calcium concentrations. In those patients with severe hypercalcemia

from hyperparathyroidism (termed *parathyroid storm* or *parathyroid crisis*), often there are marked elevations of PTH values in contrast to severe hypercalcemia of malignancy, in which the apparent PTH serum values may be only minimally elevated.

Why do most carboxyl- and midmolecule assays give false-positive results in patients with hypercalcemia of malignancy? Even though there is strong structural homology between the amino terminal regions of PTH and PTHrP (nine of 13 amino acids are identical, and synthetic peptides based on the sequence of the amino terminal 34 residues of either peptide bind to and activate the PTH receptor equivalently), no antisera generated against PTH have been reported to recognize PTHrP or its fragments in displacement assays. Furthermore, approaches such as charcoal stripping of serum have been shown to reduce the false-positive signals for PTH in hypercalcemia of malignancy seen in displacement assays (Segre, unpublished). Taken together, this information suggests that there are substances in the serum of some patients with cancer that interfere nonspecifically with displacement-type PTH assays (65,77–79). It is also clear that, at least in the short term, PTH secretion (both a small amount of intact hormone and

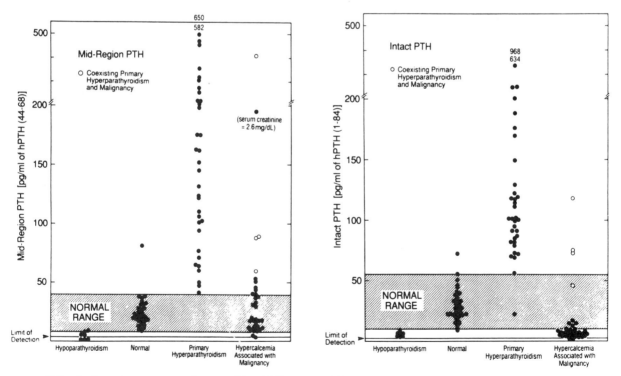

FIG. 4. A contemporary region-specific middle region PTH assay continues to identify apparent PTH in the serum of patients with hypercalcemia associated with malignancy, although four patients (represented by *open circles*) had coexisting hyperparathyroidism and cancer. This can be contrasted with results from the same patients measured in an immunochemiluminometric assay. (Reprinted from ref. 25 with permission.)

a larger quantity of fragments) continues despite hypercalcemia. Such persistent secretion could account for detection of hormone, especially in fragment-based assays, although the levels detected should be less than in normal subjects. However, absolutely increased levels are reported in some patients in some region-specific displacement assays (Fig. 2).

Based on studies of PTH messenger RNA extracted from tumors producing the clinical syndrome of humoral hypercalcemia of malignancy and from results with immunometric assays, production of authentic PTH by nonparathyroid tumors is extremely rare. In fact, there are only three well documented examples of PTH production by nonparathyroid tumors (80–82). With one case of a woman with hypercalcemia due to an ovarian cancer (80), our group demonstrated PTH production by the tumor by measuring gradients in hormone concentration across the arterial and venous circulation of tumor, disappearance of PTH from the serum after tumor resection, and the production of authentic PTH-(1–84) and not PTHrP by this tumor in tissue culture. The other reports of PTH secretion involve a lung cancer and a small cell carcinoma that secreted both PTH and PTHrP-(81,82).

How well do immunometric assays distinguish patients with primary hyperparathyroidism from normal individuals and those with other causes for hypercalcemia? A compilation of several large assay validation studies indicates that, overall, approximately 90% of patients with clinically suspected or surgically proven primary hyperparathyroidism have PTH values above the upper range of normal in the IRMA or ICMA assays, and the remaining patients have serum PTH values that are inappropriately elevated for the degree of hypercalcemia (Fig. 5) (25,36,38,55,57,61,63,64,66, 67,83–88).

A critical feature of the IRMA assay for PTH is its effectiveness in discriminating between primary hyperparathyroidism and malignancy-associated hypercalcemia. In contrast to the small to moderate overlap seen when PTH is measured by displacement-type RIAs, the IRMA assay will virtually always give below normal or undetectable serum levels of PTH in subjects with hypercalcemia of malignancy (Fig. 5) (25,36,38,55,57,61,63,64,66,67).

The pulsatile secretion of intact PTH may account for the failure to detect an absolute increase in measured immunoreactive PTH levels in all patients with hyperparathyroidism in the immunometric assays. This is only a theoretical issue at present, as repeated assays in the same patient to confirm this premise have not been reported. Also, displacement assays, which have, as a group, their greatest difficulty in false-positive results in malignancy also, with many of the reported mid region and carboxyl terminal assays, report false-negative results in hyperparathyroidism. As

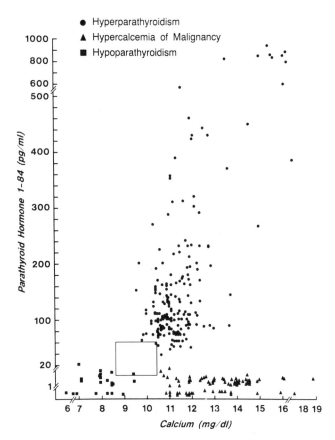

FIG. 5. Immunometric assay for PTH-(1–84) consistently demonstrates complete separation of 177 consecutive hyperparathyroid patients from 79 with malignancy-associated hypercalcemia at the Massachusetts General Hospital. The area within the box represents normal serum calcium and serum intact PTH concentrations.

with other endocrine disorders, there is some overlap in hormone levels between normal subjects and those with hormone excess syndromes; multiple explanations are offered, including a variable host response or an abnormal new "steady state."

A more problematic issue is the performance of both conventional displacement radioimmunoassays and immunometric assays in distinguishing individuals with familial hypocalciuric hypercalcemia (FHH; also termed *familial benign hypercalcemia*) from patients with primary hyperparathyroidism. The pathophysiologic defect in FHH is uncertain but appears to involve an abnormality in sensing or responding to ECF calcium that is shared by the parathyroids and the kidney, accounting for persistent PTH secretion and abnormally high urinary calcium reabsorption, respectively. In FHH, PTH serum levels measured by immunometric assay are often normal and not suppressed. Most clinicians find family screening for hypercalcemia and urinary calcium excretion, particularly in young children, to be of greater value than PTH assays in establishing the diagnosis of FHH.

PARATHYROID HORMONE ASSAYS TO ASSESS RECOVERY OF PARATHYROID GLAND SECRETION

The ability of immunometric assays to measure PTH within and below the normal circulating concentration of the hormone has permitted studies of the clearance of the hormone following surgery for primary hyperparathyroidism (28,62), the rate of recovery of PTH secretion following surgical care of hyperparathyroidism (28,62,65), or correction of hypercalcemia associated with malignancy (77–79). In studies of PTH secretion following removal of a parathyroid adenoma, serum concentrations of PTH became undetectable within 1 hr following surgery, with a half-life of the intact hormone calculated to be in minutes (28,66). Recovery of parathyroid gland function by remaining parathyroid tissue occurred within 2 days (Fig. 6) (28), although PTH secretion in response to hypocalcemia remains impaired for a longer interval (62).

Shortened incubation times and speed of performance of immunometric assays make them ideal tools in the perioperative management of selected patients with primary hyperparathyroidism. Taking advantage of the shortened incubation times of immunoradiometric assays, coupled with the rapid clearance of PTH-(1–84) from the circulation, these assays can be used intraoperatively to assess surgical cure of hyperparathyroidism in patients with parathyroid adenoma or parathyroid hyperplasia and can be of value in intraoperative venous sampling for localization of abnormal parathyroid tissue (65).

By altering incubation conditions, a standard curve with a detection limit of ~25 ng/liter (nl sensitivity 1 ng/liter) can be generated within 15 min (65). The accelerated performance of this assay can be used to replace selective venous catheterization should the surgeon be unsuccessful in the initial neck exploration. The results obtained from such an assay can show a marked "step-up" in PTH levels from the thyroid vein draining the abnormal parathyroid adenoma that has defied surgical identification. At times, this approach to intraoperative sampling, with results obtained within 30 min, can direct the surgeon to the mediastinum or to a high cervical location for the elusive parathyroid adenomas.

Recent experience suggests another application. Intraoperative measurement of PTH can help in distinguishing parathyroid hyperplasia from adenoma (or two "adenomas" from one) at the time of surgery. Samples, obtained intraoperatively before and 15 min after the vascular pedicle to what proved to be the single enlarged parathyroid gland was tied off, show a >50% decline from baseline values. In 40 patients with parathyroid adenoma who we have studied, no patient with a decline of 50% or greater of baseline PTH values had persistent hyperparathyroidism after removal of a single abnormal gland (Nussbaum, unpublished observations). Those with hyperplasia had a gradual, stepwise drop in PTH values over the course of resection of several parathyroid glands. Such intraoperative PTH determination might find special use in patients with asymmetric hyperplasia or double adenoma in whom all parathyroid glands are not identified at the first operation or in certain reoperations in which scarring makes bilateral neck exploration more problematic and increases the risk for nerve injury or hypoparathyroidism.

An extension of the usefulness of rapid determination of serum levels of PTH-(1–84) can be in the evaluation of patients with hypercalcemic crisis. Severe hypercalcemia is most often associated with malignancy, but, at times, it may herald the presentation of acute primary hyperparathyroidism. The finding of markedly elevated serum PTH levels may lead to recognition of acute primary hyperparathyroidism and expedite prompt surgical intervention (see the chapter by Fitzpatrick).

Patients with hypercalcemia associated with malignancy studied via IRMA or ICMA assays have undetectable or below normal values for PTH 95% of the time; the remaining 5% have values in the low normal range (25,36,38,55,57,61,63,64,66,67). Measurement of

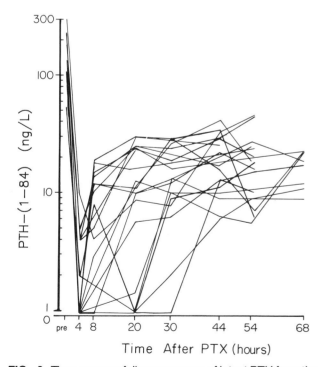

FIG. 6. Time course of disappearance of intact PTH from the serum of 19 patients following the removal of a single parathyroid adenoma and recovery of secretion from "suppressed" remaining glands within 20–30 hours following parathyroidectomy. (Reprinted from ref. 28 with permission.)

serum levels of PTH after therapy for hypercalcemia of malignancy with bisphosphonates, which inhibit osteoclastic bone resorption and result in a normalization of serum calcium, has led to recovery of PTH secretion within days after normocalcemia has been achieved (77–79,89). Preliminary studies of PTH secretion in malignancy-associated hypercalcemia suggest that patients with osteolytic skeletal metastases have greater degrees of elevation of PTH with the return of normocalcemia than do patients who have the clinical syndrome of humoral hypercalcemia of malignancy (79,89,90). It is possible that PTHrP may have a direct action on PTH secretion or that patients with humoral hypercalcemia of malignancy have greater chronicity to their hypercalcemia; therefore, a longer time is required for recovery of parathyroid gland secretory activity.

PARATHYROID HORMONE MEASUREMENTS IN HYPOPARATHYROIDISM

Displacement-type RIAs are not sufficiently sensitive to measure PTH serum levels reliably in patients with hypoparathyroidism. ICMA and IRMA assays have generally revealed undetectable or low serum PTH values in hypocalcemia patients with hypoparathyroidism (Fig. 5) in contrast to the elevated serum levels of PTH seen in hypocalcemia caused by renal insufficiency or from vitamin D deficiency. In our experience, autoimmune destruction of the parathyroids produces lower levels of serum PTH than operative removal of parathyroid tissue: patients with idiopathic hypoparathyroidism as a component of the syndrome of polyglandular failure type I have undetectable levels of PTH, whereas patients with postsurgical hypoparathyroidism may have detectable although low levels of PTH (64).

PARATHYROID HORMONE MEASUREMENT IN RENAL INSUFFICIENCY

The biologically inactive middle and carboxyl fragments of PTH accumulate markedly in the blood of patients with renal disease (17,25,27,91–94). Measurement of these fragments in renal insufficiency, therefore, provides an overestimation of the concentration of biologically active hormone. A more accurate measure of parathyroid gland secretory activity in renal insufficiency is reflected by the level of intact PTH-(1–84) determined by immunometric assay (93,94). In recent years there has been an enhanced understanding of the role of hyperphosphatemia and hypocalcemia, and of impaired 1,25-dihydroxyvitamin D [1,25(OH)$_2$D] synthesis by the kidney, in the development of the secondary hyperparathyroidism that ac-

companies advancing renal disease. In addition, our understanding of the spectrum of bone diseases that accompanies renal insufficiency (renal osteodystrophy) has been clarified by study of the role of increased aluminum in bone and its relationship to aplastic bone disease as well as the contribution of elevated PTH to osteitis fibrosa cystica (95,96 and the chapter by Coburn and Salusky). Correlation of circulating intact PTH concentrations and osseous indices of hyperparathyroidism determined by quantitative bone histomorphometric analysis of iliac crest bone biopsies has shown that PTH levels correlated linearly with bone formation and marrow fibrosis (92).

Early intervention with calcium acetate to control hyperphosphatemia and provide calcium supplementation, and with 1,25(OH)$_2$D to decrease PTH gene transcription, as well as use of dialysates with supraphysiologic concentrations of calcium, may control secondary hyperparathyroidism and limit the development of hyperparathyroid bone disease. An elevation of intact PTH-(1–84) along with a decrease in 1,25(OH)$_2$D, is the earliest indication of altered mineral ion homeostasis, earlier than hyperphosphatemia and hypocalcemia. Recent unpublished studies (Segre, personal communication) of therapy with 1,25(OH)$_2$D have shown decreases in serum intact PTH by 60% (to approximately three times the upper limit of normal) contrasted with more modest decreases of 27% (to 100 times the upper limit of normal) in a mid region assay. Regression of parathyroid gland secretory activity may be associated with improvement in osteitis fibrosa cystica and can thus be more effectively monitored by measuring the intact PTH molecule.

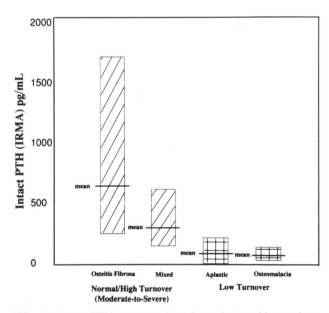

FIG. 7. Intact PTH serum values in patients with renal osteodystrophy. In general, values >300 pg/ml correlate with osteitis fibrosa cystica. (Modified from refs. 95 and 96.)

In one important recent study (96), 259 patients were analyzed to identify laboratory parameters that were predictive indices for the different types of renal osteodystrophy (determined by bone histomorphometry); PTH assay results seemed especially useful. Intact PTH levels were excellent predictors of osteitis fibrosa cystica vs. aplastic bone disease or osteomalacia, with the highest values seen in osteitis fibrosa cystica, 586 ± 51 pg/ml (mean $\pm$ SE), vs. aplastic lesions 87 ± 7 pg/ml, and osteomalacia, 83 ± 10 pg/ml (Fig. 7). The data indicate that, when intact PTH values are >500 pg/ml, osteitis fibrosa cystica is likely; values <200 pg/ml suggest aplastic bone disease or osteomalacia. This information may be useful for directing therapy with 1,25-$(OH)_2D$ or newer vitamin D analogs and may also define a group of patients for whom parathyroidectomy will not likely be of benefit.

SUMMARY

Improvements in measurement of PTH by immunoassay over the last 3 decades have paralleled basic advances in PTH chemistry, physiology, and metabolism. More recently, the development of immunometric or double antibody "sandwich" assays with improved sensitivity and specificity has led to significant advances in the accurate diagnosis of patients with hypercalcemia, especially in distinguishing patients with primary hyperparathyroidism from those with hypercalcemia of malignancy. These immunometric assays have become the diagnostic test of choice in the differential diagnosis of hypercalcemia. The capacity to measure PTH within and below the normal range should permit the standard suppression and stimulation tests (e.g., hypercalcemia and hypocalcemia) to be used to study normal and abnormal parathyroid secretion patterns and thereby improve our understanding of the contribution of PTH to disorders of calcium metabolism and skeletal homeostasis. Further technical refinements, including the increased use of chemiluminescent detection methods, may enhance assay sensitivity further. Two-site assays with these refinements will likely provide even greater assistance in the operative management of hyperparathyroidism and enhance our understanding of the etiologic role of PTH in renal osteodystrophy.

REFERENCES

1. Berson SA, Yalow RS, Aurbach GD, Potts JT Jr. Immunoassay of bovine and human parathyroid hormone. *Proc Natl Acad Sci USA* 1963;49:613–617.
2. Berson SA, Yalow RS. Immunochemical heterogeneity of parathyroid hormone in plasma. *J Clin Endocrinol Metab* 1968;28:1037–1047.
3. D'Amour P, Labelle F, LeCavalier L, Plourde V, Harvey D. Influence of serum Ca concentration on circulating molecular forms of PTH in three species. *Am J Physiol* 1986;251:E680–E687.
4. D'Amour P, Labelle F, Wolde-Giorghis R, Hamel L. Immunological evidences for the presence of small late carboxyl-terminal fragment(s) of human parathyroid hormone (PTH) in circulation in man. *J Immunoassay* 1989;10:191–205.
5. Flueck JA, DiBella FP, Edis AJ, et al. Immunoheterogeneity of parathyroid hormone in venous effluent serum from hyperfunctioning parathyroid glands. *J Clin Invest* 1977;60:1367–1375.
6. Kubler N, Krause U, Wagner PK, Beyer J, Rothmund M. The secretion of parathyroid hormone and its fragments from dispersed cells of adenomatous parathyroid tissue at different calcium concentrations. *Exp Clin Endocrinol* 1986;88:101–108.
7. Kubler N, Krause U, Wagner PK, Beyer J, Rothmund M. The influence of parathyroid hormone and its fragments on results from midregion and C-terminal specific radioimmunoassays. *Exp Clin Endocrinol* 1987;89:61–69.
8. Mayer GP, Keaton JA, Hurst JG, Habener JF. Effects of plasma calcium concentration on the relative proportion of hormones and carboxyl fragments in parathyroid venous blood. *Endocrinology* 1979;104:1778–1784.
9. Morissey JJ, Hamilton JW, MacGregor R, Cohn DV. The secretion of parathormone fragments 34–84 and 37–84 by dispersed porcine parathyroid cells. *Endocrinology* 1980;107:164–171.
10. Schachter PP, Christy MD, Shabtay M, Ayalon A, Leight GS Jr. The role of circulating N-terminal parathyroid hormone fragments in the early postparathyroid adenomectomy period. *Surgery* 1991;110:1048–1052.
11. Bringhurst FR, Stern AM, Yotts M, Mizrahi N, Segre GV, Potts JT Jr. Peripheral metabolism of PTH: Fate of biologically active amino terminus in vivo. *Am J Physiol* 1988;255:E886–E893.
12. Bringhurst FR, Stern AM, Yotts M, Mizrahi N, Segre GV, Potts JT Jr. Peripheral metabolism of [^{35}S]parathyroid hormone in vivo: influence of alterations in calcium availability and parathyroid status. *J Endocrinol* 1989;122:237–245.
13. Hruska KA, Korkor A, Martin K, Slatopolsky E. Peripheral metabolism of intact parathyroid hormone: Role of liver and kidney and the effect of chronic renal failure. *J Clin Invest* 1981;67:885–892.
14. Martin KJ, Freitag JJ, Conrades MB, et al. Selected uptake of the synthetic amino-terminal fragment of bovine parathyroid hormone by isolated perfused bone. *J Clin Invest* 1978;62:256–261.
15. Martin KJ, Hruska KA, Freitag JJ, et al. The peripheral metabolism of parathyroid hormone. *N Engl J Med* 1979;301:1092–1098.
16. Segre GV, Haberner JF, Powell D, et al. Parathyroid hormone in human plasma: Immunochemical characterization and biological implications. *J Clin Invest* 1972;5:3163–3172.
17. Segre GV, Tregear GW, Potts JT Jr. Development and application of sequence-specific radioimmunoassays for analysis of the metabolism of parathyroid hormone. *Methods Enzymol* 1975;37:38–66.
18. Segre GV, D'Amour P, Potts JT Jr. Metabolism of parathyroid radioiodinated hormone in the rat. *Endocrinology* 1976;99:1645–1652.
19. Segre GV, D'Amour P, Hultman A, Potts JT Jr. Effects of hepatectomy, nephrectomy, and nephrectomy/uremia on the metabolism of parathyroid hormone in the rat. *J Clin Invest* 1981;67:439–448.
20. Segre GV, Perkins AS, Witters LA, Potts JT Jr. Metabolism of parathyroid hormone by isolate rat Kupffer cells and hepatocytes. *J Clin Invest* 1981;67:449–457.
21. Silverman R, Yalow RS. Heterogeneity of parathyroid hormone: Clinical and physiologic implications. *J Clin Invest* 1973;52:1958–1971.
22. Rosenblatt M, Kronenberg HK, Potts JT Jr. Parathyroid hormone: Physiology, chemistry, biosynthesis, secretion metabolism and mode of action. In: DeGroot LJ, ed. *Endocrinology, 2nd ed.* Philadelphia: W.B. Saunders, 1989;848.
23. MacGregor RR, Hamilton JW, Kent GN, et al. The degrada-

tion of proparathormone and parathormone by parathyroid and liver cathepsin B. *J Biol Chem* 1979;254:4428.

24. D'Amour P, Palardy J, Bahsali G, Mallette LE, DeLean A, Lepage R. The modulation of circulating parathyroid hormone immunoheterogeneity in man by ionized calcium concentration. *J Clin Endocrinol Metab* 1992;74:525–532.
25. Endres DB, Villanueva R, Sharp CF Jr, Singer FR. Measurement of parathyroid hormone. *Endocrinol Metab Clin North Am* 1989;18:611–629.
26. Papapoulos SE, Manning RM, Hendy GN, et al. Studies of circulating parathyroid hormone in man using a homologous amino-terminal specific immunoradiometric assay. *Clin Endocrinol* 1980;13:57–67.
27. Segre GV. Amino-terminal radioimmunoassays for human parathyroid hormone. In: Frame B, Potts JT Jr, eds. *Clinical Disorders of Bone and Mineral Metabolism*. Amsterdam: Excerpta Medica, 1983;14–17.
28. Brasier AR, Wang CA, Nussbaum SR. Recovery of parathyroid hormone secretion after parathyroid adenomectomy. *J Clin Endocrinol Metab* 1988;66:495–500.
29. MacGregor RR, Jilka RL, Hamilton JW. Formation and secretion of fragments of parathormone: Identification of cleavage sites. *J Biol Chem* 1986;261:1929.
30. Martin KJ, Hruska KA, Lewis J, et al. The renal handling of parathyroid hormone: Role of peritubular uptake and glomerular filtration. *J Clin Invest* 1977;60:808.
31. D'Amour P, Labelle F, Lazure C. Comparison of four different carboxyl-terminal tracers in a radioimmunoassay specific to the 68–84 region of human parathyroid hormone. *J Immunoassay* 1984;5:183–204.
32. Mallette LE, Tuma SN, Berger RE, Kirkland JL. Radioimmunoassay for the middle region of human parathyroid hormone using an homologous antiserum with a carboxyl-terminal fragment of bovine parathyroid hormone as radio-ligand. *J Clin Endocrinol Metab* 1982;54:1017–1024.
33. Zanelli JM, Gaines Das RE. The first international reference preparation of human parathyroid hormone for immunoassay: Characterization and calibration by international collaborative study. *J Clin Endocrinol Metab* 1983;57:462–469.
34. Minne HW. Quality control in parathyroid hormone radioimmunoassays: A multicenter study performed by the European Parathyroid Hormone Study Group. *Eur J Clin Invest* 1984;14:16–23.
35. Measuring the PTH level. *Lancet* 1988;1:94–95.
36. Nussbaum SR, Potts JT Jr. Immunoassays for parathyroid hormone 1–84 in the diagnosis of hyperparathyroidism. *J Bone Mineral Res* 1991;6:S43–S50.
37. Kasono K, Sato K, Suzuki T, et al. Falsely elevated serum parathyroid hormone levels due to immunoglobulin G in a patient with idiopathic hypoparathyroidism. *J Clin Endocrinol Metab* 1991;72:217–222.
38. Birkeland KI, Gallefoss F, Olsson S, Haug E. Primary hyperparathyroidism or hypercalcaemia of malignancy? *Scand J Clin Lab Invest* 1992;52:347–349.
39. Lufkin EG, Kao PC, Heath H III. Parathyroid hormone radioimmunoassays in the differential diagnosis of hypercalcemia due to primary hyperparathyroidism or malignancy. *Ann Intern Med* 1987;106:559–560.
40. Orloff JJ, Wu TL, Stewart AF. Parathyroid hormone-like proteins: biochemical responses and receptor interactions. *Endocrine Rev* 1989;10:476–495.
41. Raisz LG, Yajnik CH, Bockman RS, Bower BF. Comparison of commercially available parathyroid hormone immunoassays in the differential diagnosis of hypercalcemia due to primary hyperparathyroidism or malignancy. *Ann Intern Med* 1979;91:739–740.
42. Stewart AF, Horst R, Deftos LJ, Cadman EC, Land R, Broadus AE. Biochemical evaluation of patients with cancer associated hypercalcemia: Evidence for humoral and nonhumoral groups. *N Engl J Med* 1980;303:1377–1383.
43. Fischer JA, Binswanger U, Dietrich FM. Human parathyroid hormone: Immunological characterization of antibodies against a glandular extract and the synthetic amino-terminal fragments 1–22 and 1–34 and their use in the determination of immunoreactive hormone in human sera. *J Clin Invest* 1974; 54:1382–1394.

44. Ingle AR, Bailey JE, Matthews HL, Harrop JS. Performance and clinical utility of a commercially available 'C-terminal' PTH assay. *Ann Clin Biochem* 1986;23:434–439.
45. Jüppner H, Rosenblatt M, Segre GV, Hesch RD. Discrimination between intact and mid-C-region PTH using selective radioimmunoassay systems. *Acta Endocrinol* 1983;102:543–548.
46. Lindall AW, Elting J, Ellis J, Roos BA. Estimation of biologically active intact parathyroid hormone in normal and hyperparathyroid sera by sequential N-terminal immunoextraction and mid-region radioimmunoassay. *J Clin Endocrinol Metab* 1983;57:1007–1014.
47. Marx SJ, Sharp ME, Krudy A, Rosenblatt M. Radioimmunoassay for the middle region of human parathyroid hormone: Studies with a radioiodinated synthetic peptide. *J Clin Endocrinol Metab* 1981;53:76–84.
48. Segre GV, Potts JT Jr. Differential diagnosis of hypercalcemia: Methods and clinical application of parathyroid hormone assays. In: DeGroot LJ, ed. *Endocrinology, 2nd ed.* Philadelphia: W.B. Saunders, 1989;984.
49. Wood PJ. The measurement of parathyroid hormone. *Ann Clin Biochem* 1992;29:11–21.
50. Ashby JP, Loveridge N, Brown RC, Zanelli JM, Rinsler MG, Watts RW. Anomalies in the assay of parathyroid hormone in normocalcaemic patients with renal stone disease. *Clin Endocrinol* 1988;29:131–140.
51. Stock JL, Coderre JA, Posillico JT. Effects of estrogen on mineral metabolism in postmenopausal women as evaluated by multiple assays measuring parathyrin bioactivity. *Clin Chem* 1989;35:18–22.
52. Ekins R. Towards immunoassays of greater sensitivity, specificity and speed: An overview. In: Albertini A, Ekins R, eds. *Monoclonal Antibodies and Developments in Immunoassay.* Amsterdam: Elsevier/North Holland, 1981;3–21.
53. Hales CN, Woodhead JS. Labelled antibodies and their use in the immunoradiometric assay. *Methods Enzymol* 1980; 70:334.
54. Blind E, Schmidt-Gayk H, Armbruster FP, Stadler A. Measurement of intact human parathyrin by an extracting two-site immunoradiometric assay. *Clin Chem* 1987;33:1376–1381.
55. Blind E, Schmidt-Gayk H, Scharla S, et al. Two-site assay of intact parathyroid hormone in the investigation of primary hyperparathyroidism and other disorders of calcium metabolism compared with a midregion assay. *J Clin Endocrinol Metab* 1988;67:353–360.
56. Bouillon R, Coopmans W, Degrotte DEH, Radoux D, Ellard PH. Immunoradiometric assay of parathyrin with polyclonal and monoclonal region-specific antibodies. *Clin Chem* 1990; 36:271–276.
57. Brown RC, Aston JP, Weeks I, Woodhead S. Circulating intact parathyroid hormone measured by a two-site immunochemiluminometric assay. *J Clin Endocrinol Metab* 1987;65: 407–414.
58. Flentje D, Schmidt-Gayk H, Fischer S, et al. Intact parathyroid hormone in primary hyperparathyroidism. *Br J Surg* 1990;77:168–172.
59. Frolich M, Walma ST, Paulson C, Pappapoulos SE. Immunoradiometric assay for intact human parathyroid hormone: characteristics, clinical application and comparison with a radio-immunoassay. *Ann Clin Biochem* 1990;27:69–72.
60. Hackeng WHL, Lips P, Netenlenbos JC, Lipps CJM. Clinical implications of estimation of intact parathyroid hormone (PTH) versus total immunoreactive PTH in normal subjects and hyperparathyroid patients. *J Clin Endocrinol Metab* 1986;63:447–453.
61. Kao PC, van Heerden JA, Grant CS, Klee GG, Khosla S. Clinical performance of parathyroid hormone immunometric assays. *Mayo Clin Proc* 1992;67:637–645.
62. Mazzuoli G, Minisola S, Scarnecchia L, et al. Two-site assay of intact parathyroid hormone in primary hyperparathyroidism: studies in basal condition, following adenoma removal and during calcium and EDTA infusion. *Clin Chim Acta* 1990;190:239–248.

63. Minisola S, Scarnecchia L, Romagnoli E, et al. Conventional and new diagnostic applications of a two-site immunoche-miluminometric assay for parathyroid hormone. *J Endocrinol Invest* 1992;15:483–489.
64. Nussbaum SR, Zahradnik RJ, Lavigne JR, et al. Highly sensitive two-site immunoradiometric assay of parathyrin, and its clinical utility in evaluating patients with hypercalcemia. *Clin Chem* 1987;33:1364–1367.
65. Nussbaum SR, Thompson AR, Hutcheson KA, Gaz RD, Wang CA. Intraoperative measurement of PTH 1–84: A potential use of the clearance of PTH to assess surgical cure of hyperparathyroidism. *Surgery* 1988;104:1121–1127.
66. Ratcliffe WA, Heath DA, Ryan M, Jones SR. Performance and diagnostic application of a two-site immunoradiometric assay for parathyrin in serum. *Clin Chem* 1989;35:1957–1961.
67. Endres DB, Villanueva R, Sharp CF Jr, Singer FR. Immuno-chemiluminometric and immunoradiometric determinations of intact and total immunoreactive parathyrin: performance in the differential diagnosis of hypercalcemia and hypopara-thyroidism. *Clin Chem* 1991;37:162–168.
68. Broadus AE, Mahaffey JE, Bartter FC, Neer RM. Nephro-genous cyclic adenosine monophosphate as a parathyroid function tests. *J Clin Invest* 1977;60:771–783.
69. Broadus AE. Nephrogenous cyclic AMP. *Rec Progr Hormone Res* 1981;37:667–701.
70. Nissenson RA, Abbott SR, Teitelbaum AP, et al. Endogenous biologically active human parathyroid hormone: Measure-ment by a guanyl nucleotide amplified renal adenylate cyclase assay. *J Clin Endocrinol Metab* 1981;52:840.
71. Klee G, Preissner CM, Schloegel IW, Kao PC. Bioassay of parathyrin: Analytical characteristics and clinical perfor-mance in patients with hypercalcemia. *Clin Chem* 1988;34:482.
72. Fenton S, Somers S, Heath DA. Preliminary studies with the sensitive cytochemical bioassay for parathyroid hormone. *Clin Endocrinol* 1978;9:381–384.
73. Goltzman D, Henderson B, Loveridge N. Cytochemical bioassay of parathyroid hormone: Characteristics of the as-say and analysis of circulating hormonal forms. *J Clin Invest* 1980;65:1309–1317.
74. Slatopolsky E, Hruska K, Martin K, Freitag J. Physiological and metabolic effects of parathyroid hormone. In: Brenner B, Stein J, eds. *Contemporary Issues in Nephrology, Vol. 4.* New York: Churchill-Livingstone, 1979;169–193.
75. Harms HM, Kaptaina U, Kulpmann WR, Brabant G, Hesch RD. Pulse amplitude and frequency modulation of parathy-roid hormone in plasma. *J Clin Endocrinol Metab* 1989;69:843–851.
76. Kitamura N, Shigeno C, Shiomi K, et al. Episodic fluctuation in serum intact parathyroid hormone concentration in men. *J Clin Endocrinol Metab* 1990;70:252–263.
77. Mallette LE, Beck P, Vandepol C. Malignancy hypercal-cemia: evaluation of parathyroid function and response to treatment. *Am J Med Sci* 1991;302:205–210.
78. Body JJ, Dumon JC, Seraj F, Cleeren A. Recovery of para-thyroid hormone secretion during correction of tumor-asso-ciated hypercalcemia. *J Clin Endocrinol Metab* 1992;74:1385–1388.
79. Body JJ, Dumon JC, Thirion M, Cleeren A. Circulating PTHrP concentrations in tumor-induced hypercalcemia: In-fluence on the response to bisphosphonate and changes after therapy. *J Bone Mineral Res* 1993;8:701–706.
80. Nussbaum S, Gaz R, Arnold A. Hypercalcemia and ectopic secretion of parathyroid hormone by an ovarian carcinoma with rearrangement of the gene for parathyroid hormone. *N Engl J Med* 1990;323:1324–1326.
81. Yoshimoto K, Yamasaki R, Hideki S, et al. Ectopic production of parathyroid hormone by small cell lung cancer in a patient with hypercalcemia. *J Clin Endocrinol Metab* 1989;68:976–981.
82. Strewler GJ, Budayr AA, Clark OH, Nissenson RA. Produc-tion of parathyroid hormone by a malignant nonparathyroid tumor in a hypercalcemia patient. *J Clin Endocrinol Metab* 1993;76:1373–1375.
83. Hollenberg AN, Arnold A. Hypercalcemia with low-normal serum intact PTH: a novel presentation of primary hyper-parathyroidism. *Am J Med* 1991;91:547.
84. Endres DB, Morgan CH, Garry PJ, Omdahl JL. Age-related changes in serum immunoreactive parathyroid hormone and its biological action in healthy men and women. *J Clin En-docrinol Metab* 1987;65:724–731.
85. Gallagher JC, Riggs BL, Jerpbak CM, Arnaud CD. The effect of age on serum immunoreactive parathyroid hormone in nor-mal and osteoporotic women. *J Lab Clin Med* 1980;95:373–385.
86. Insogna KL, Lewis AN, Lipinski BA, et al. Effect of age on serum immunoreactive parathyroid hormone and its biologi-cal effects. *J Clin Endocrinol Metab* 1981;53:1072–1075.
87. Marcus R, Madvig P, Young G. Age-related changes in para-thyroid hormone action in normal humans. *J Clin Endocrinol Metab* 1984;58:223–230.
88. Wiske PS, Epstein S, Bell NH, et al. Increases in immuno-reactive parathyroid hormone with age. *N Engl J Med* 1979;300:1419–1421.
89. Nussbaum SR, Younger J, VandePol CJ, et al. Single-dose intravenous therapy with pamidronate for the treatment of hy-percalcemia of malignancy: comparison of 30-, 60-, and 90-mg dosages. *Am J Med* 1993;95:297–304.
90. Dodwell DJ, Abbas SK, Morton AR, et al. Parathyroid hor-mone-related protein[50–69] and response to pamidronate therapy for tumour-induced hypercalcaemia. *Eur J Cancer* 1991;27:1629–1633.
91. Andress DL, Endres DB, Maloney NA, Kopp JB, Coburn JW, Sherrard DJ. Comparison of parathyroid hormone assays with bone histomorphometry in renal osteodystrophy. *J Clin Endocrinol Metab* 1986;63:1163–1169.
92. Quarles LD, Lobaugh B, Murphy G. Intact parathyroid hor-mone overestimates the presence and severity of parathyroid-mediated osseous in uremia. *J Clin Endocrinol Metab* 1992;75:145–150.
93. St John A, Thomas MB, Davies CP, et al. Determinants of intact parathyroid hormone and free 1,25-dihydroxyvitamin D levels in mild and moderate renal failure. *Nephron* 1992;61:422–427.
94. Togashi K, Takahashi N, Ando K, Tsukamoto Y, Marumo F. Comparison of different parathyroid hormone radioimmu-noassays in uremic patients with secondary hyperparathy-roidism. *Int J Artif Organs* 1990;13:77–82.
95. Sherrard DJ, Hercz G, Pei Y, et al. The spectrum of bone disease in end-stage renal failure—An evolving disorder. *Kid-ney Int* 1993;43:436–442.
96. Pei Y, Hercz G, Greenwood C, et al. Non-invasive prediction of aluminum bone disease in hemo- and peritoneal dialysis patients. *Kidney Int* 1992;41:1374–1382.

The Parathyroids, edited by J.P. Bilezikian, M.A. Levine, and R. Marcus. Raven Press, Ltd., New York © 1994.

CHAPTER 12

Parathyroid Hormone and Parathyroid Hormone-Related Protein as Polyhormones

Evolutionary Aspects and Nonclassical Actions

Lawrence E. Mallette

With the explosion of biological and genetic information in the past quarter century has come the discovery of previously unknown hormones and growth factors, of unexpected genetic relatedness among receptors and among hormones, and of unanticipated additional actions of classical hormones. This chapter reviews current knowledge concerning parathyroid hormone (PTH) and its sister molecule, parathyroid hormone-related protein (PTHrP), and then discusses the probable evolutionary derivation of PTH, its relationship to PTHrP, and its possible relationship to the melanocyte-stimulating hormone (MSH) family of peptides. This chapter concludes with a discussion of the multiple nonclassical actions of PTH and PTHrP.

EVOLUTION OF PREPROPARATHYROID HORMONE: REPLICATION OF A PRIMITIVE GENE

The preproparathyroid hormone (prepro-PTH) molecule contains a fourfold internal homology that probably represents four copies of a primitive gene. The first evidence for this internal homology was given by Cohn and coworkers (1), who found a significant twofold homology within the amino acid sequence of bovine prepro-PTH, specifically between the −27 to +22 and the +26 to +74 regions (Fig. 1). In addition to significant amino acid sequence homology, these two regions were calculated to show significant structural homology, based on their estimated degree of helical, β-sheet, and β-turn structure. These authors proposed that the mammalian prepro-PTH gene arose by reduplication of at least a portion of a primitive gene. The original gene would have encoded both a "prepro-" region and at least enough of a secretory peptide to impart biological activity, i.e., from the current initiating methionine at −31 to approximately amino acid +22 or beyond. After the reduplication step, the carboxyl-terminal segment of the new gene doublet was presumably subject to less evolutionary constraint and evolved separately to lose its hypercalcemic activity (1).

The author has readdressed the question of homology within prepro-PTH (2). Dr. H.T. Pretorius and I were examining the structure of the PTH molecule to estimate the location of probable antigenic epitopes. He noted that a rare tripeptide, RKK (arg-lys-lys), is contained twice within the PTH molecule (positions +25 and +52; Fig. 1) and referred me to a published uniqueness analysis[1] of the tripeptide sequences of prepro-PTH (3). The analysis revealed that the RKK tripeptide seemed unique to PTH at the time; it was not found anywhere else in the available databank of human protein sequences, then containing over 32,500 amino acids.

---

[1]Peptides can be described in terms of their multiple overlapping tripeptide sequences: peptides of N amino acids contain $N - 2$ tripeptide sequences. Certain tripeptides occur commonly in mammalian proteins, and others occur rarely. The frequency with which each tripeptide occurs can be catalogued and the data used to analyze the uniqueness of structure of individual peptides (3).

L. E. Mallette: Division of Endocrinology and Metabolism, Baylor College of Medicine, Houston, Texas 77030.

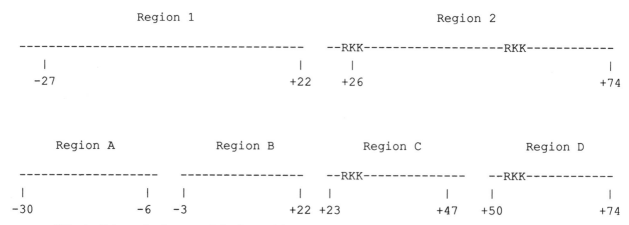

FIG. 1. Schematic diagram of the internal homologies in prepro-PTH. The top structure shows the homology of amino acid sequence between regions 1 and 2 as found by Cohn et al. (1). The RKK tripeptide occurs twice, at the boundary of and within region 2. The rarity of this tripeptide suggested an additional homology, between regions C and D of the lower structure, as detailed in Fig. 2. Accommodating both the Cohn and RKK homologies suggested that there might be four contiguous regions of homology. A full alignment of the codon sequences of these four regions is given in Fig. 3.

Such a rare sequence would be unlikely to arise twice by chance within the same peptide. Genetic reduplication would be a more likely explanation. I therefore aligned the two RKK motifs and their flanking amino acid sequences and found further homology nearby (Fig. 2). In a span of nine amino acid positions, there were four identical amino acids and two amino acid pairs whose codons differ by only one base. The homology was different from the homology described by Cohn et al.: both RKK sequences were contained within Cohn et al.'s second region (Fig. 1).

To accommodate both the Cohn et al. homology and the RKK homology in the same scheme, I postulated a fourfold replication (2) (Fig. 3). This scheme uses the published nucleotide sequences of human prepro-PTH messenger RNA and the human PTH gene (4–6). It aligns four regions of the PTH gene containing 25 codons each. There are two codons left over at the carboxyl-terminal end of regions A and C. The RKK mo-

tifs are in regions C and D, but possible homolog remnants of this motif are seen in regions A and B as well (—K— in region A and R— — in region B).

Is there statistical evidence for homology among the four 25 codon regions? Each sequence represents 75 DNA base positions, among which are 33 consensus positions, i.e., positions that carry the same base in at least three of the four sequences. With a computer, Dr. John Thornby and I showed that random assembly of the 104 codons in this overall span of prepro-PTH would produce 33 or more "matches" with a frequency of <0.0001. The known ability of DNA sequences to replicate provides the most likely explanation for such strong homology.

The exact boundaries of the actual replications can only be surmised. If, however, one were to begin the alignment with a nearby codon instead of codon −30, the number of consensus base positions would be reduced. The array in Fig. 3 places the breakpoint with codon −30. I chose this specific location because of the observation of Südhof and colleagues (7) that intervening sequences (introns) often mark the boundaries of regions that have undergone reduplication. These investigators found in the low-density lipoprotein (LDL) receptor seven contiguous repeats of a cysteine-rich region. Introns were located before and after the codon sequence for each repeat except two: introns were missing after regions 3 and 4. The missing introns were proposed to have been lost during evolution. By analogy, I propose that the single intron of the mammalian prepro-PTH gene within codon −2 is likely to mark the boundary of the replicated region.

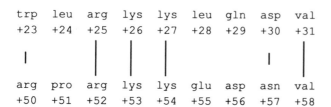

FIG. 2. Amino acid sequence of the regions flanking the two RKK tripeptides in PTH, aligned to display the homology. In a span of nine amino acid positions, four are identical, and the codons for two others differ by only one base (+23/ +50 Trp/Arg TGG/AGG; +30/+57 Asp/Asn GAT/AAT).

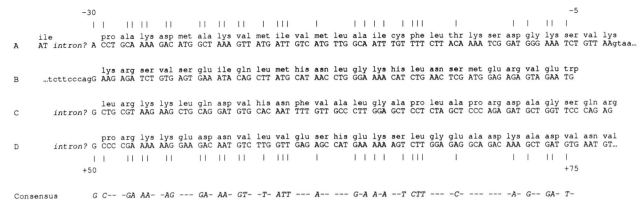

FIG. 3. Codon structure of human preproPTH from −31 to +77, aligned to show the fourfold homology. Positions where at least three of the four copies contain an identical base (consensus positions) are marked with vertical lines, and the consensus base is given in italics below. The four copies are aligned to give the maximum number (33) of consensus positions. The specific breakpoint was chosen as the location of the single intron of the prepro-PTH gene (see text). Part of the intron sequence is shown in lowercase letters. Three putative copies of the intron, which may have been deleted during evolution, are indicated as *intron?*. To determine how frequently 33 consensus position would arise from a chance assembly of these codons, Dr. Thornby placed the 104 codons in random order 300 times, and determined the number of consensus positions for each randomization. The observed number of consensus positions in the 300 individual randomizations ranged from 12 to 28, with a mean of 18.88, standard deviation 3.48, and an approximately normal distribution. Given this population sample, 33 or more matches would be predicted to occur with a frequency of <0.0001.

By analogy with the LDL receptor, one might hypothesize that three other introns have been lost during evolution after the reduplication events (Fig. 3). Alternately, two other introns might have been lost, with the third now represented by the intron that is found in the prepro-PTH gene five bases upstream from the codon for methionine −31 (6).

Figure 4 illustrates the evolutionary steps that I have postulated to explain the fourfold internal homology and the two dipeptide "tags" at the ends of regions A

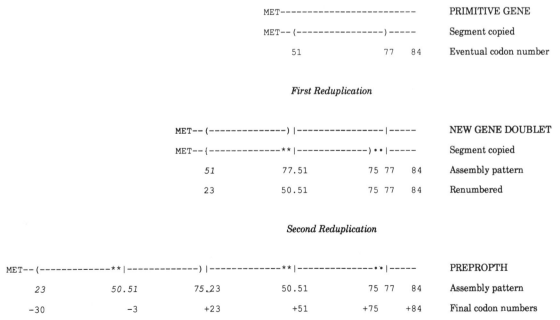

FIG. 4. Diagram of the putative reduplications giving rise to the present prepro-PTH gene. *Dots* indicate the two codons that were not included in the second reduplication. *Asterisks* indicate two homologous codons that were included and code for the extra dipeptide at the ends of regions A and C in Fig. 3.

preproPTH	+16 to +22	Asn	**Ser**	**Met**	**Glu**	*Arg*	*Val*	*Glu*	**Trp**
POMC α–MSH	+2 to +9	**Tyr**	Ser	**Met**	**Glu**	His	Phe	Arg	Trp
POMC β–MSH	+88 to +95	**Tyr**	*Lys*	**Met**	**Glu**	His	Phe	Arg	Trp
POMC γ–MSH	−55 to −48	**Tyr**	*Val*	**Met**	*Gly*	His	Phe	Arg	Trp
POMC "δ–MSH"	−111 to −105		**Ser**	**Met**	**Glu**	*Val*	*Arg*	*Gly*	**Trp**

FIG. 5. Homology of amino acid structure between human PTH and the four MSH copies in bovine POMC. The fourth MSH copy, unnamed and less complete, is labeled "δ*MSH*." Four of the eight amino acids in PTH match the MSH consensus amino acid, while Asn/Tyr forms a close match (TAC/AAC).

and C. First, a 27 codon portion of a primitive gene replicated to lengthen the original gene by 27 codons. Of these 54 codons, 52 then participated in a second duplication event, to lengthen the gene again, this time by 52 codons. Alternately, one would have to postulate a series of three precise replications of a 27 codon sequence, followed by a two codon deletion from the end of the B sequence. The relationship of the proposed reduplication scheme to the biologically active regions of the PTH molecule is discussed below.

PARATHYROID HORMONE–MELANOCYTE-STIMULATING HORMONE HOMOLOGY

Several years ago it was recognized that PTH-(15–25) and ACTH-(1–11) contain small domains that are homologous (8). These regions contain much of the information that directs PTH receptor binding (9) and most of the α-MSH sequence (10), respectively. In fact the homology imparts enough similarity of structure that each peptide can interact, albeit weakly, with the other's cell membrane receptor (11). The homologies of amino acid structure between human PTH and each of the four copies of MSH in the mammalian proopiomelanocortin (POMC) molecule are shown in Fig. 5.

The similarity of structure has generally been regarded as a coincidence. We should consider the pos-

sibility, however, that prepro-PTH and POMC had a common origin. Might the precursor gene for prepro-PTH also have been the precursor for the MSH family? To test this hypothesis, we can reconstruct our best estimate of the prepro-PTH precursor gene for comparison with MSH. The reconstructed prepro-PTH precursor would consist of one copy of the replicating 25 codon segment plus the nonreplicating "tail" (Fig. 6). For the replicating segment, I chose the current structure of the calcemic region of PTH (region B in Fig. 3), since it is probably the region under the most evolutionary constraint. The tail is juxtaposed to the calcemic region—codons 23 and 76 abut. For the "tail," I used the consensus codon sequence among three mammalian 76–84 regions (bovine, porcine, and human).

Figure 6 aligns the reconstructed proto-PTH gene with mammalian and salmon MSH. For the mammalian MSH structure, I first determined a consensus mammalian sequence for each of the four MSH copies within POMC, using the published sequences for human, murine, bovine, and porcine POMC (10,12–14). I then used the consensus sequence among the four MSH versions as the best estimate of the proto-MSH sequence. The salmon POMC gene contains only two MSH copies. Since no consensus sequence could be derived, I arbitrarily chose the α-MSH copy for comparison (15).

```
consensus mammalian MSH    AAG AAG GAC TCG GGG TCT TAC TCC ATG GAA CAC TTC CGC TGG GGC AGC CCG GTG AAG GGC AAG CGG CGG CGC
                            ||   | |           || || ||| ||     |     ||| |         |  ||  |  || | |   |

protoPTH +10 to 23^76 to 84 AAC CTG GGA AAA CAT CTG AAC TCG ATG GAG AGA GTA GAA TGG GAT GTA TTA ATT AAA GCT AAA CCC CAG
                            ||           ||      || || ||| |||     |     ||| |    |     |||           ||| | | |

salmon alpha-MSH -2 to +40  AAG AGA         CAC TCC TAC TCC ATG GAG CAC TTC CGC TGG GGC AAA CCC ATT GGG CAC AAA CGC CCC ATC
```

FIG. 6. Codon sequence of the putative proto-PTH aligned with the sequence of the consensus mammalian MSH and with salmon α-MSH. Computerized randomization analyses (Dr. John Thornby) showed that the observed degree of homology for the entire 23 codons would be highly unlikely to arise by a chance arrangement of the specific codons ($P = 0.00021$ for mammalian MSH and $P = 0.00001$ for salmon α-MSH). A similar analysis limited to the 76–84 "tail" of PTH and the corresponding MSH region showed that the observed number of base matches with the MSH sequences would also be unlikely to have occurred by chance ($P = 0.040$ for mammalian MSH and $P = 0.056$ for salmon α-MSH).

For the region of recognized amino acid homology, this alignment reveals the expected strong homology of base structure. There is also significant homology between the PTH "tail" and the corresponding portion of MSH, confirmed by computerized randomization analyses (see legend to Fig. 6). The homology between the PTH "tail" and the MSH sequence is compatible with the hypothesis that prepro-PTH and POMC arose from a common precursor. This leads me to wonder what evolutionary constraints might have been operating on the PTH-(76–84) region to have preserved its apparent homology with MSH.

PARATHYROID HORMONE AND PARATHYROID HORMONE-RELATED PROTEIN: GENETIC RELATEDNESS

PTHrP was isolated as a peptide with PTH-like adenylyl cyclase-stimulating ability, a property of the PTH amino-terminal region. The structure of the two peptides showed identity of eight of the first 13 amino acids as well as of the last two amino acids of their prohormone segments (16–18). Otherwise, the amino acid structures diverge markedly. Since the genes for PTH and PTHrP are located in similar positions on sibling chromosomes 11 and 12, it is likely that they arose from a common precursor by chromosomal duplication.

At the time of chromosomal duplication, how was the ancestral PTH/PTHrP gene configured? Had the fourfold homology found in prepro-PTH evolved yet? If so, two predictions can be made: (a) there should be residual homology of codon base structure (if not of amino acid sequence) beyond the calcemic regions of the two sequences and (b) prepro-PTHrP might retain evidence of a fourfold internal homology.

Figure 7 aligns the prepro-PTHrP and prepro-PTH codons in parallel, with each gene divided into the four regions used for prepro-PTH in Fig. 3. The homology of base sequence does appear to extend beyond their calcemic regions. For the B region, with the strong amino acid homology between PTH and PTHrP, there is a 50% homology of base sequence for codon positions 1 and 2 (the more strongly preserved codon positions). For both the C and the D regions, the homology of base sequence is still 40% at codon positions 1 and 2, probably more than would be expected by chance. For the A region the extent of homology is only the 25% predicted by random events, but prohormone sequences are known to be subject to less evolutionary constraint.

There is, however, no evidence that prepro-PTHrP preserves the fourfold homology found within prepro-PTH (Fig. 7). Alignment of the prepro-PTHrP gene into the four regions produces only 14 consensus base positions, far fewer than the 33 consensus bases for the prepro-PTH array and easily explainable by chance.

These observations suggest that the chromosomal duplication that gave rise to PTH and PTHrP as separate entities occurred relatively soon after at least three of the four homologous regions in prepro-PTH had been formed but that the internal homology originally present within prepro-PTHrP was subsequently lost by virtue of regions C and D being subject to less evolutionary constraint than the corresponding regions of prepro-PTH. The fact that prepro-PTH did

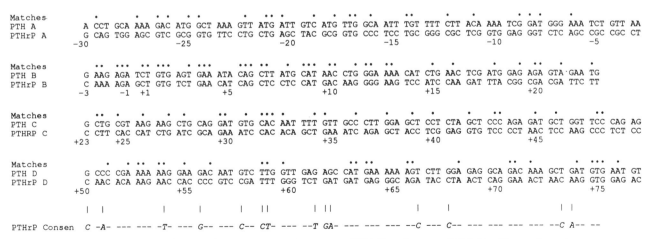

FIG. 7. Alignment of the codon sequences for prepro-PTHrP and prepro-PTH. Positions where base matches occur between the two sequences are indicated with dots. The sequences are divided into four regions according to the prepro-PTH internal homology scheme of Fig. 3. The 14 consensus base positions in prepro-PTHrP are marked with *vertical lines,* and the consensus bases are given in italics below.

conserve the evidence of internal homology leads us to ask what forces applied the necessary constraint. Did the individual regions retain their own biological activities after the reduplication step?

PARATHYROID HORMONE AND PARATHYROID HORMONE-RELATED PROTEIN AS POLYHORMONES

According to the classical concept of a hormonally active polypeptide, a given hormone gene encodes a peptide that contains a single active region, which can interact with a unique receptor on the target cell membrane to initiate hormone action. Tissue specificity is governed by the location of cells that express the hormone's receptor. Over the years, several revisions have been made to this traditional scheme. More than one gene can exist for a given hormone (usually only one being functional). A single gene may encode messenger RNAs for more than one hormone, usually through alternative splicing (calcitonin and calcitonin gene-related peptide, for example). A hormone may interact with more than one receptor, and some receptors can recognize more than one hormone (insulin and insulin-like growth factors and their receptors, for example).

PRESENTATION AND EXPANSION OF THE POLYHORMONE CONCEPT

Another revision is the concept of the polyactive hormone, or polyhormone: a single secretory polypeptide that contains more than one potentially biologically active region (19). Each active region has a different structure and presumably interacts with its own unique receptor in a different target tissue. PTH and PTHrP have each been found to contain at least three active regions and are therefore good examples of polyhormones. This section summarizes the evidence for the multiple actions of these peptides and points out areas where further information is needed.

As a prelude to this discussion, I will begin by amplifying our original concept of the polyhormone in several ways. Receptors for each active region need not necessarily lie in different tissues. Theoretically they might all reside in the same tissue or even on the same cell type (although it would not be clear to what purpose this would be so), nor do the receptors for each region have to be in a tissue remote from the cell secreting the peptide. Endocrine activity might coexist in the same molecule with paracrine or autocrine activities.

For the actions of a polyactive peptide that are endocrine in nature, the classical characteristics of a hormone (generation in one tissue and action in a remote

tissue) should be demonstrable, and negative feedback control of secretion can be expected in most cases. There might also be feedback control of autocrine and paracrine activities.

A polyhormone might be regarded as a prohormone, since it is the parent molecule for one or more active hormones. The polyhormone is likely to bear a "pre-" or "prepro-" sequence to facilitate entry into the secretory apparatus. However, since the polyhormone contains more than one active region, it is more than simply a prohormone.

If the organism is to take advantage of the different potential activities in the polyhormone molecule, a mechanism must exist to allow each active region to be presented with some selectivity to its receptor. Conceptually it is possible that the actions of two different regions on two different tissues might be required exactly in parallel, so that it would suffice for them to arrive at their respective target cells traveling in the same polyhormone molecule. This would, however, present a remarkable redundancy; a single peptide region interacting with the same receptor in the two target cell types would have sufficed.

More flexibility would be provided, however, if the different regions could be mobilized separately and selectively, depending on physiologic need, tissue of origin, or stage of ontogeny. Cleavage to select the needed region might occur in the cell of origin before secretion, perhaps by selection of alternative cleavage sites in the parent polyhormone molecule. We know that multiple potential cleavage sites do exist within many polypeptides. Differing proteolytic processing might occur instead at a remote site after secretion, either in the target tissue or in a tissue traversed on the way there (liver or lung, for example). Differential splicing of mRNA can be viewed as an alternative means of providing the same service (the selection of a specific subset of the total information stored in a sequence) but is more efficient in that it avoids the necessity of synthesizing a complete polyhormone sequence, part of which would be discarded.

An alternative means to select the activity of one or the other region of a polyhormone would be to vary the expression of its receptors in the target tissues. A given region cannot have activity when its receptor is not expressed. This area of research is only beginning to be explored.

PARATHYROID HORMONE: MULTIPLE ACTIONS

The secretory form of PTH is a straight-chain 84-amino-acid peptide, with the classical biological function of increasing plasma calcium concentration. Other important effects include stimulation of renal tubular phosphate excretion, calcium reabsorption, and 1α-hydroxylation of 25-hydroxyvitamin D. Activities different from these classical ones have been discovered for PTH, some of which reside outside the amino-terminal region classically thought to mediate PTH action (Fig. 8).

Parathyroid Hormone-(1–34) Region: One or Two Receptors?

The discovery that PTH stimulates cyclic adenosine 3',5'-monophosphate (cAMP) synthesis in kidney (20) and bone (21) provided a tool for the study of structure–activity relationships. Stimulation of cAMP formation was found to reside in the amino-terminal 1–34 region and to require as a minimum the 2–27 sequence (9,22). Among the responses currently thought to result from a stimulation of the cAMP pathway are renal 1α-hydroxylation of 25-hydroxyvitamin D and keratinocyte differentiation (Fig. 8). PTH-(3–34) competitively inhibits cAMP formation in response to PTH-(1–34) or PTH-(1–84), suggesting that the binding domain of PTH for the receptor is in the 3–34 region but that the first two amino acids are required in order to signal the adenylyl cyclase-coupled Gs protein that the receptor is occupied.

Studies in the whole animal showed unexpectedly that PTH-(3–34) was hypercalcemic (23), one of the first indications that signaling pathways not involving cAMP might be involved in PTH action. It is now recognized that PTH-(1–34) can also activate the response pathway that uses protein kinase C and intracellular calcium. Two examples are kidney and cartilage.

Urinary phosphate excretion is increased by picomolar concentrations of PTH that do not increase urinary cAMP excretion (24). This was originally interpreted to mean that a rise had occurred in a critical intracellular cAMP pool, none of which spilled over for urinary excretion. It has now been shown convincingly, however, that the protein kinase C pathway mediates the change in renal phosphate transport. Certain analogs of PTH-(1–34) that do not increase cAMP production will nevertheless inhibit phosphate transport by opossum kidney cells (25). Both the inhibition of phosphate transport and the activation of the protein kinase C pathway in these cells are half-maximal at ~10 pM, whereas a much higher concentration is required to activate protein kinase A (26). Direct activation of protein kinase C by phorbol myristate will alter phosphate transport with no change in cellular cAMP values (27). Exactly which part of the PTH-(3–34) region is needed for protein kinase C activation has not been determined.

PTH-(1–34) widens the epiphyseal growth plate and increases the number of chondrocytes along the zone of ossification (28). In rat epiphyseal cartilage cell cul-

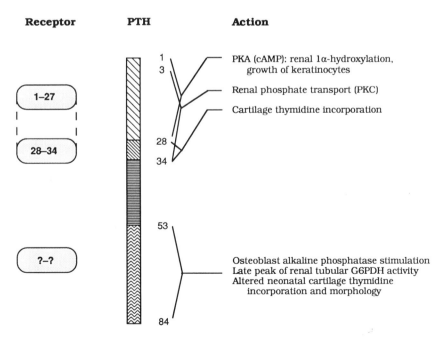

FIG. 8. Schematic diagram of the biologically active regions in PTH and their putative receptors. PKA and PKC represent protein kinases A and C, respectively. The 1–27 and 28–34 receptors are connected by dotted lines because the relationship between these two binding activities is not fully understood. The classic PTH-(1–34) receptor coupled to cAMP generation may also be coupled to the PKC pathway, but there may be a separate receptor mediating some or all of the effects of the 3–34 region on PKC (see text).

tures, PTH-(1–34) increases creatine kinase levels and thymidine incorporation, effects that are reproduced by PTH-(28–48) and occur with no change in cAMP (29). Thymidine incorporation by chick chondrocytes can be stimulated by a peptide containing the 30–34 region of PTH, as long as a few amino acids are included on either side of the 30–34 region. PTH-(13–34) and PTH-(30–47) were equally effective, but PTH-(31–47) was inactive (30). These observations may explain why the structure of PTH is highly conserved among species as far as amino acid 37. A change in cellular cAMP was not required for the increase in thymidine incorporation, but extracellular calcium was required. It was postulated that the protein kinase C pathway might be involved in opening a membrane calcium channel in these cells.

Different models could be proposed to explain these observations: *model 1:* separate receptors for the cAMP-mediated effects of the 2–27 region and for the protein kinase C-mediated effects of the 28–34 region; *model 2:* separate receptors, one for the 1–34 region able to stimulate both cAMP formation and the protein C pathway, and a second mediating only the effects of the 30–34 region on the protein C pathway, perhaps with a different affinity; *model 3:* a single receptor that can interact with different G proteins to couple it to either the cAMP or the protein kinase C pathway, the choice of G proteins being influenced by the precise length and configuration of the bound PTH ligand. For either model 1 or 2, the receptors might be genetically separate or might arise via alternative RNA splicing or by differing posttranslational modifications.

In support of model 2, rat osteosarcoma cells can be induced to increase their membrane-bound protein kinase C by a physiologically low concentration of PTH-(1–34) (5 pM), an effect not accompanied by an increase in cAMP and one that is reproduced by similar levels of PTH-(3–34) or PTH-(13–34) (31). This increase is down-regulated rapidly at higher concentrations, but, as the concentration of PTH-(1–34) is increased even further, a second increase in membrane-bound protein kinase C activity occurs at ~15 nM, accompanied by a parallel increase in cAMP. PTH-(3–34) and PTH-(13–34) also produce the secondary increase in membrane-bound protein kinase C but do not increase cAMP. The suggested model is a high-affinity receptor for the 3–34 region coupled to protein kinase C plus a low-affinity receptor for 1–34 coupled to both kinases. Perhaps the high-affinity receptor might also recognize the 30–47 peptide, as does the chick chondrocyte. The recent cloning of a PTH-(1–34) receptor (32) may facilitate the search for the putative 30–34 receptor, but, if the latter receptor exists as a separate entity, it may or may not be homologous with the receptor already cloned.

Parathyroid Hormone-(53–84) Region

When the sequence of PTH was first determined, it was recognized that the RKK motif at 52–54 represented a potential proteolytic cleavage site, but there seemed to be no obvious reason for cleavage here, since the amino-terminal portion of PTH was found to be responsible for the classical biological activities. Studies with biologically active radiolabeled PTH-(1–84) and synthetic fragments of PTH showed that the 53–84 region accounts for 30–70% of the binding of PTH-(1–84) to renal or bone cell membranes (33–35). The 53–84 binding is saturable and reversible. The calculated K_d of 53–84 binding is higher than the K_d for binding of the 1–34 region, but fragments of PTH that contain at least a portion of the 53–84 region are known to circulate at concentrations more than tenfold higher than that of PTH-(1–84). This suggests that a 53–84 receptor could potentially receive significant occupancy *in vivo.*

Is there any evidence for a biological effect of PTH-(53–84)? The peptide is not hypercalcemic (22), but at least three biological effects have been identified. (a) It increases glucose-6-phosphate dehydrogenase (G6PDH) activity in renal tubular cells (36). This effect was discovered during work examining the specificity of a PTH bioassay using renal cortical slices. PTH-(1–84) produces a rise in G6PDH activity at 8 min that is specific for the PTH-(1–34) region. PTH-(53–84) also increases G6PDH but at a later time point. (b) PTH-(53–84) increases alkaline phosphatase activity in glucocorticoid-primed osteoblast-like cells (37). (c) PTH-(53–84) abolishes the mitogenic effect of PTH-(1–34) in neonatal mouse condylar cartilage explants and produces distinctive structural changes in the mineralized hypertrophic zone of the explant (38).

The physiologic importance and consequences of these clear biological effects of PTH-(53–84) in vivo are not known. The author has proposed that the osteosclerosis that occasionally complicates intense primary or secondary hyperparathyroidism might be mediated by the midregion fragments of PTH (2) that are known to be secreted by many parathyroid adenomas (39) and to accumulate in renal failure (40). Might some of the growth retardation of secondary hyperparathyroidism be mediated by the effects of the 53–84 region of PTH on epiphyseal cartilage?

Relationship of the Active Regions of Parathyroid Hormone to Evolutionary Reduplications

Figure 9 illustrates the relationship of the three active regions of PTH to the proposed genetic reduplication scheme for the prepro-PTH gene. Starting at the

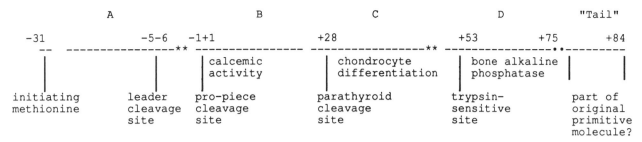

FIG. 9. Correlation of biologically active regions of PTH and sites of proteolytic cleavage with the fourfold reduplication scheme.

left of the figure, the codon for the initiating methionine of the prepro-PTH gene and the next codon (ATC AT) were probably present in the original gene but were not part of the reduplication process.

Three of the replications of the RKK motif seem to represent sites of significant proteolytic cleavage. In the B region, the remnant of the RKK site forms the site of cleavage of the "pro-" piece at $-1/+1$. In the C region, the RKK tripeptide marks a site of natural cleavage ($+27/+28$) in the parathyroid gland. MacGregor and coworkers (41) have shown that a PTH fragment that begins at $+28$ is secreted by human and bovine parathyroid glands. The RKK motif of the D region is a known trypsin sensitive cleavage site, but whether this is utilized in vivo is not known.

Regions B, C, and D correspond to the three different biologically active regions in PTH. Region B represents the heart of the region responsible for cAMP-mediated activities and perhaps for some protein kinase C-mediated actions as well. Region C represents the 30–34 region capable of altering chondrocyte replication and probably other effects on skeletal tissue. Region D represents the 53–84 region, with several activities. The fact that three of the four reduplicated regions seem to have unique biological activity suggests that after reduplication each region and its receptor were free to evolve their own set of unique activities. In return, these activities provided evolutionary constraints to help maintain evidence of the fourfold internal homology in prepro-PTH. The three active regions may originally have interacted with the same receptor. It will be of interest to learn whether the putative 30–34 and 53–84 receptors are members of the same receptor family as the 1–29 receptor or whether the new replicated regions adopted their own, unrelated receptors.

PARATHYROID HORMONE-RELATED PROTEIN

PTHrP was isolated based on its ability to stimulate cAMP formation in PTH-like fashion (16,42). Knowledge about normal biological roles of PTHrP is being acquired rapidly. Many tissues synthesize PTHrP, including most epidermal derivatives, smooth muscle under stretch, breast under prolactin stimulation, fetal parathyroid gland, and placenta. The gene for PTHrP can encode peptides of 139, 141, and 173 amino acids, depending on which alternative splice occurs in its mRNA (43). The molecule is known to contain several basic amino acid pairs that represent potential cleavage sites (43) and is now known to contain several biologically active regions (Fig. 10).

Parathyroid Hormone-Related Protein-(1–34) Region

In the process of mimicking the cAMP stimulatory effect of PTH, synthetic PTHrP-(1–34) binds to the PTH-(2–27) receptor (44). This was demonstrated by competition experiments using membranes from cells that showed a cAMP response to either peptide: unlabeled aminoterminal fragments of PTH or PTHrP would inhibit binding of the other labeled peptide, and each could be affinity linked to an apparently identical 80,000 Dalton membrane macromolecule (45). That these two peptides can use a common receptor has now been proved conclusively: expression of the cloned PTH receptor in cells that were originally receptor negative induced cAMP responsiveness to the aminoterminal fragments of both PTH and PTHrP (32,46). The biological reasons for this redundancy of effect are not fully understood, but the peptides are presumably presented to the PTH-(2–27) receptor in different tissues at different times and for different reasons.

Potential physiological roles for interaction of PTHrP with the 2–27 receptor may include keratinocyte differentiation (47), smooth muscle relaxation (48), and fetal skeletal modeling. Fetal parathyroidectomy arrests fetal skeletal development by slowing bone remodeling (49), and PTHrP-(1–34) can restore this remodeling. Cord blood contains little or no immunoreactive PTH (50–53) but is rich in PTH-like biological activity (53) that is attributable to PTHrP (54).

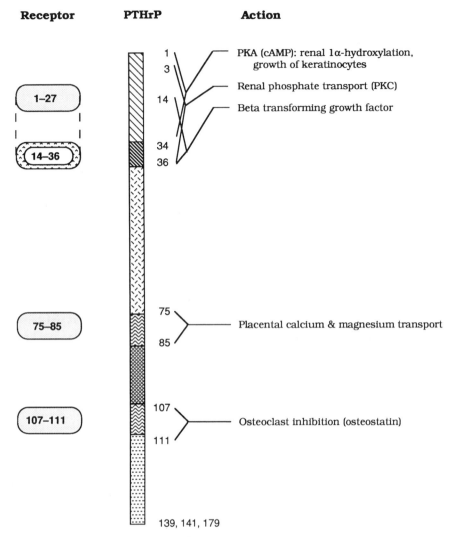

FIG. 10. Schematic diagram of the biologically active regions in PTHrP and their putative receptors. The two receptors for the amino-terminal region are connected by dotted lines because their relationship is not well understood. The exact extent of the 1–34 region needed for the transforming growth factor-β activity is not known.

Thus the interaction of PTHrP with a 2–27 receptor is probably essential for normal fetal skeletal maturation.

Parathyroid Hormone-Related Protein-(14–35) Region

PTHrP-(1–141) and ³⁶Tyr-PTHrP-(1–36) both possess transforming growth factor-β (TGFβ) activity not found in PTH-(1–34). Specifically, these peptides induce large colony formation by NRK cells in soft agar and stimulate fibronectin biosynthesis by human dermal fibroblasts (55). Assuming that the full-length PTH-(1–84) molecule does not show TGFβ activity [not tested by Insogna et al. (55)], we must conclude that PTHrP interacts with a receptor not available to PTH itself. The interaction would presumably involve the region of the molecule where the primary structures of PTH and PTHrP differ, i.e., the 14–35 regions

(Fig. 10). Further work is needed to discover the biologic importance of this activity and to characterize the receptor mediating the effect.

Parathyroid Hormone-Related Protein-(75–85) Region

Placental transport of divalent cations normally generates a 10–40% higher concentration of calcium and magnesium in the fetus than in the mother (56). The transplacental gradients for both ions are abolished by parathyroidectomy of the fetus but not of the mother (57,58). The activity of the placental divalent cation pump in sheep was studied by perfusing placentas *in situ* in the absence of the fetus. Fetuses were parathyroidectomized a few days before the study to allow placental divalent cation transport to diminish. The placentas were perfused with hypoparathyroid fetal lamb blood to which various substances could be added for testing.

An extract of the fetal parathyroid glands stimulated placental calcium and magnesium transport. PTH, however, was not the agent responsible, since neither PTH-(1–34) nor PTH-(1–84) added directly would stimulate the cation pump. Fetal parathyroid extracts were rich in immunoreactive PTHrP but contained little PTH (59,60). PTHrP-(1–141) was therefore tested in the perfusate and was found to stimulate the divalent cation pump. Cord blood has subsequently been shown to contain significant PTHrP, which could be the factor mediating the fetal parathyroid's effect on the placenta (54).

Synthetic fragments of PTHrP were used to determine which region of the PTHrP molecule is responsible for stimulating the placental pump. Since PTH-(1–34) was inactive, it was not surprising that PTHrP-(1–34) was also inactive. The pump-stimulating activity was found to reside in the 75–85 region of PTHrP, requiring at least the 75–84 segment (61).

The current hypothesis is that a peptide containing the 75–85 region of PTHrP is the fetal calcemic hormone, with the placenta as one of its target tissues. Since the 1–34 region of PTHrP is important for fetal bone remodeling, the secreted PTHrP peptide would be expected to span at least the 1–84 region. The immunoassay used to demonstrate the presence of PTHrP in cord blood may have been reading such a peptide, since it was a biterminal assay that used antibodies against the 1–40 and 60–72 regions of PTHrP (54). Experiments are still needed, however, to show specifically that the fetal parathyroid gland does secrete a PTHrP peptide, to determine the structure of the secreted species, and to show that its secretion is responsive to ambient calcium values.

The actual source of the PTHrP in fetal serum has not been established, and nonparathyroid sources are possible. The placenta itself is the most likely alternative or additional source of fetal serum PTHrP. The placenta is known to synthesize and secrete PTHrP (60,62,63). More exciting are the observations that the cytotrophoblast (a) stains with an antibody thought to be specific for the parathyroid cell membrane calcium receptor, (b) is able to sense the ambient calcium ion concentration, and (c) will adjust its secretion of PTHrP downward in the presence of high calcium concentrations in parathyroid-like fashion (63). These observations suggest that the placenta might be able to control the divalent cation pump in paracrine fashion.

If so, then why is the parathyroid gland necessary? How can we reconcile these two models (parathyroid vs. placental origin of the PTHrP that controls the placental pump)? *Hypothesis 1:* PTHrP from both the fetal parathyroid and placenta is important, with the dual source providing a protective degree of redundancy.

Hypothesis 2: one tissue provides a bone-active peptide (containing the 1–34 region of PTHrP but not an intact 75–85 region), while the other provides a placental-active peptide (containing the 75–85 region of PTHrP but perhaps without a complete 1–34 region). *Hypothesis 3:* the fetal parathyroid gland secretes little PTHrP but produces another factor that increases placental PTHrP production. Other parathyroid secretory products that might be tested for such an action include the 26 kD betagranin-like peptide derived from chromogranin A and recently shown to be secreted by normal bovine parathyroid cells (64) and the tissue plasminogen activator or urokinase activity secreted by human and bovine parathyroid cells, respectively (65).

Might the biologically active site at 75–85 in PTHrP have arisen as a fifth replicant of the primitive gene that gave rise to prepro-PTH? If so, then one might expect homology between the PTHrP-(75–85) active core and the other four regions, especially with the calcemic 1–34 regions of PTH and PTHrP (which may have been subject to the most evolutionary constraint). Aligning the codons for PTHrP-(75–85) and PTHrP-(1–11) reveals homology at 11 of the 22 first and second base positions, statistically more than the 7.6 ± 1.9 SD matches that would occur by a random assembly of either codon sequence ($P = 0.037$). A similar alignment of PTHrP-(75–85) with PTH-(1–11) gives agreement at nine of the 22 first and second base positions vs. the 6.6 ± 1.9 SD matches that would occur by chance ($P < 0.10$). This modest evidence for residual homology is most easily explained by supposing that the 75–85 region of PTHrP does represent a fifth replicant of the primitive gene. If so, we can hypothesize that the placental receptor for PTH-(75–85) will be found to be a member of the same receptor family as the 2–27 receptor already cloned.

Parathyroid Hormone-Related Protein-(107–111) Region

Studies of the bone resorbing activities of PTHrP-(1–141) vs. PTHrP-(1–34) unexpectedly showed a reduced activity of the longer peptide. This led to the discovery that the 107–111 region of PTHrP can directly inhibit activity of the osteoclast (66,67) and may decrease osteoclast recruitment (68), actions that tend to counteract the stimulation of osteoclast activity produced by the 1–34 region. The fact that the 107–111 region is highly conserved in evolution suggested that this region would have an important function, and a proteolytic cleavage site exists at 106–107. Rat and chick osteoclasts both show this response to the 107–111 region (66,69). The postulated physiological peptide containing this activity has been called *osteo-*

statin. A peptide as short as the five amino acids of PTHrP-(107–111) retains this biological activity. The physiologic significance of this inhibitory action, the sources of the peptide that might act *in vivo* on the osteoclast or its precursors, the structure of this peptide, and the biology of its putative receptor are not yet understood. The author could discover no homology of base sequence between PTHrP-(107–111) and the 1–34 regions of PTH or PTHrP.

SUMMARY

The sister peptides PTH and PTHrP have multiple active regions and could be regarded as the prototypical polyhormones. The presence of multiple biologically active sites in a single polypeptide provides additional versatility. It also expands the number of potential loci of endocrine control to include the peptide regions rich in basic amino acids (likely sites of proteolytic cleavage) that often lie adjacent to the biologically active regions. Most of the recognized functions of the active regions of PTH and PTHrP affect some facet of bone and mineral metabolism, suggesting that the evolutionary precursors of these peptides may have been involved in regulating divalent cation fluxes for many eons. At least for PTH, the three activities may have arisen by divergent evolution after reduplication produced four copies of a primitive gene. For each of the actions of PTH and PTHrP, as for other polyhormones, the factors that function at the pre- or postsecretory level to control the structure and concentration of the circulating (or paracrine-acting) molecules must be identified.

ACKNOWLEDGMENTS

This work was supported by the U.S. Department of Veterans Affairs.

REFERENCES

1. Cohn DV, Smardo FJ, Morissey JJ. Evidence for internal homology in bovine preproparathyroid hormone. *Proc Natl Acad Sci USA* 1979;76:1469–1471.
2. Mallette L, Thornby J, Pretorius HT. Internal homology in preproparathyroid hormone. Four copies of a primitive gene. *J Bone Mineral Res* 1986;1:58.
3. Saroff HA, Pretorius HT. The uniqueness of protein sequences. *o*-uniqueness and infrequent peptides. *Bull Math Biol* 1983;45:117–139.
4. Kronenberg HM, McDevitt BE, Majzoub JA, et al. Cloning and nucleotide sequence of DNA coding for bovine preproparathyroid hormone. *Proc Natl Acad Sci USA* 1979;76:4981–4985.
5. Hendy GN, Kronenberg HM, Potts JT Jr, Rich A. Nucleotide sequence of cloned cDNAs encoding human preproparathyroid hormone. *Proc Natl Acad Sci USA* 1981;78:7365–7369.
6. Vasicek TJ, McDevitt BE, Freeman MW, et al. Nucleotide sequence of the human parathyroid hormone gene. *Proc Natl Acad Sci USA* 1983;80:2127–2131.
7. Südhof TC, Goldstein JL, Brown MS, Russell DW. The LDL receptor gene: a mosaic of exons shared with different proteins. *Science* 1985;228:815–822.
8. Parsons JA. Parathyroid physiology and the skeleton. In: Bourne GH, eds. *Biochemistry and physiology of bone.* New York: Academic Press, 1976;159–225.
9. Potts JT Jr, Kronenberg HM, Rosenblatt M. Parathyroid hormone: chemistry, biosynthesis, and mode of action. *Adv Protein Chem* 1982;35:323–396.
10. Nakanishi S, Inoue A, Kita T, et al. Nucleotide sequence of cloned cDNA for bovine corticotropin-β-lipotropin precursor. *Nature* 1979;278:423–427.
11. Rafferty B, Zanelli JM, Rosenblatt M, Schulster D. Corticosteroidogenesis and adenosine 3′,5′-monophosphate production by the amino-terminal (1–34) fragment of human parathyroid hormone in rat adrenocortical cells. *Endocrinology* 1983;113:1036–1042.
12. Takahashi H, Hakamata Y, Watanabe Y, Kikuno R, Miyata T, Numa S. Complete nucleotide sequence of the human corticotropin-beta-lipotropin precursor gene. *Nucleic Acids Res* 1983;11:6847–6858.
13. Uhler M, Herbert E. Complete amino acid sequence of mouse pro-opiomelanocortin derived from the nucleotide sequence of pro-opiomelanocortin cDNA. *J Biol Chem* 1983;258:257–261.
14. Boileau G, Barbeau C, Jeannotte L, Chrétien M, Drouin J. Complete structure of the porcine pro-opiomelanocortin mRNA derived from the nucleotide sequence of cloned cDNA. *Nucleic Acids Res* 1983;11:8063–8071.
15. Soma G, Kitahara N, Nishizawa T, et al. Nucleotide sequence of a cloned cDNA for proopiomelanocortin precursor of chum salmon, *Onchorynchus keta. Nucleic Acids Res* 1984;12:8029–8041.
16. Suva LJ, Winslow GA, Wettenhall REH, et al. A parathyroid hormone-related protein implicated in malignant hypercalcemia: cloning and expression. *Science* 1987;237:893–896.
17. Stewart AF, Wu T, Goumas D, Burtis WJ, Broadus AE. N-terminal amino acid sequence of two novel tumor-derived adenylate cyclase-stimulating proteins: Identification of parathyroid hormone-like and parathyroid hormone-unlike domains. *Biochem Biophys Res Commun* 1987;146:572–578.
18. Mangin M, Webb AC, Dreyer BE, et al. Identification of a cDNA encoding a parathyroid hormone-like peptide from a human tumor associated with humoral hypercalcemia of malignancy. *Proc Natl Acad Sci USA* 1988;85:597–601.
19. Mallette LE. The parathyroid polyhormones: new concepts in the spectrum of peptide hormone action. *Endocr Rev* 1991;12:110–117.
20. Chase LR, Aurbach GD. Parathyroid function and the renal excretion of 3′,5′-adenylic acid. *Proc Natl Acad Sci USA* 1967;58:518–525.
21. Chase LR, Fedak SA, Aurbach GD. Activation of skeletal adenyl cyclase by parathyroid hormone in vitro. *Endocrinology* 1969;84:761–768.
22. Rosenblatt M. Parathyroid hormone: chemistry and structure-activity relations. In: Ioachim HL, eds. *Pathobiology Annual, Vol 11.* New York: Raven Press, 1981;53–86.
23. Segre GV, Rosenblatt M, Tully GL III, Gaugharn J, Reit B, Potts JT Jr. Evaluation of an *in vitro* parathyroid hormone antagonist *in vivo* in dogs. *Endocrinology* 1985;116:1024–1029.
24. Puschett JB, Winaver J, Chen T, Fragula J, Syck DB, Robertson JS. Study of the renal tubular sites and mechanisms of action of parathyroid hormone. *Mineral Electrolyte Metab* 1981;6:190–209.
25. Cole JA, Carnes DL, Forte LR, Eber S, Poelling RE, Thorne PK. Structure-activity relationships of parathyroid hormone analogs in the opossum kidney cell line. *J Bone Mineral Res* 1989;4:723–730.
26. Muff R, Fischer JA, Biber J, Murer H. Parathyroid hormone receptors in control of proximal tubular function. *Annu Rev Physiol* 1992;54:67–79.

27. Kaufman M, Muff R, Fischer JA. Effect of dexamethasone on parathyroid hormone and parathyroid hormone related protein regulated phosphate uptake in opossum kidney cells. *Endocrinology* 1991;128:1819–1824.

28. Havelka S, Babicky A, Musilova J, Rohozkove D, Tesavek B. Effect of osteotropic hormones on cartilage metabolism. *Hormone Metab Res* 1979;11:83–84.

29. Sömjen D, Binderman I, Schlüter K, Wingender E, Mayer H, Kaye AM. Stimulation by defined parathyroid hormone fragments of cell proliferation in skeletal-derived cell cultures. *Biochem J* 1990;272:781–785.

30. Schlüter K, Hellstern H, Wingender D, Mayer H. The central part of parathyroid hormone stimulates thymidine incorporation of chondrocytes. *J Biol Chem* 1989;294:11087–11092.

31. Jouishomme H, Whitfield JF, Chakravarthy B, et al. The protein kinase-C activation domain of the parathyroid hormone. *Endocrinology* 1992;130:53–60.

32. Abou-Samra A, Juppner H, Force T, et al. Expression cloning of a common receptor for parathyroid hormone and parathyroid hormone-related peptide from rat osteoblast-like cells: a single receptor stimulates intracellular accumulation of both cAMP and inositol trisphosphates and increases intracellular free calcium. *Proc Natl Acad Sci USA* 1992;89:2732–2736.

33. Rizzoli RE, Murray TM, Marx SJ, D. AG. Binding of radio-iodinated bovine parathyroid hormone (1–84) to canine renal cortical membranes. *Endocrinology* 1983;112:1303–1312.

34. Rao LG, Murray TM. Binding of intact parathyroid hormone to rat osteosarcoma cells: major contribution of binding sites for the carboxyl-terminal region of the hormone. *Endocrinology* 1985;117:1632–1638.

35. McKee MD, Murray TM. Binding of intact parathyroid hormone to chicken renal plasma membranes: evidence for a second binding site with carboxyl-terminal specificity. *Endocrinology* 1985;117:1930–1939.

36. Arber CE, Zanelli JM, Parsons JA, Bitensky L, Chapman J. Comparison of the bioactivity of highly purified human parathyroid hormone and of synthetic amino- and carboxy-region fragments. *J Endocrinol* 1980;85:55–56.

37. Murray TM, Rao IG, Muzaffar SA, Ly H. Human parathyroid hormone carboxylterminal peptide (53–84) stimulates alkaline phosphatase activity in dexamethasone-treated rat osteosarcoma cells in vitro. *Endocrinology* 1989;124:1097–1099.

38. Silbermann M, Shurtz-Swirski R, Lewinson D, Shenzer P, Mayer H. In vitro response of neonatal condylar cartilage to simultaneous exposure to the parathyroid hormone fragments 1–34, 28–48, and 53–84 hPTH. *Calcif Tissue Int* 1991;48:250–266.

39. Marx SJ, Sharp ME, Krudy A, Rosenblatt M, Mallette LE. Radioimmunoassay for the middle region of human parathyroid hormone: studies with a radioiodinated synthetic peptide. *J Clin Endocrinol Metab* 1981;53:76–84.

40. Mallette LE, Tuma SN, Berger RE, Kirkland J. Radioimmunoassay for the middle region of human parathyroid hormone using an homologous antiserum with a carboxy-terminal fragment of bovine PTH as radioligand. *J Clin Endocrinol Metab* 1982;54:1017–1024.

41. MacGregor RR, McGregor DH, Lee SH, Hamilton JW. Structural analysis of parathormone fragments elaborated by cells cultured from a hyperplastic human parathyroid gland. *Bone Mineral* 1986;1:41–50.

42. Mangin M, Ikeda K, Dreyer BE, Broadus AE. Isolation and characterization of the human parathyroid hormone-like peptide gene. *Proc Natl Acad Sci USA* 1989;86:2408–2412.

43. Burtis WJ, Brady TG, Orloff JJ, et al. Immunochemical characterization of circulating parathyroid hormone-related protein in patients with humoral hypercalcemia of cancer. *N Engl J Med* 1990;322:1106–1112.

44. Juppner H, Abou-Samra AB, Uneno S, Gu WX, Potts JT Jr, Segre GV. The parathyroid hormone-like peptide associated with humoral hypercalcemia of malignancy and parathyroid hormone bind to the same receptor on the plasma membrane of ROS 17/2.8 cells. *J Biol Chem* 1988;263:8557–8560.

45. Shigeno C, Yamamoto I, Kitamura N, et al. Interaction of human parathyroid hormone-related peptide with parathyroid hormone receptors in clonal rat osteosarcoma cells. *J Biol Chem* 1988;263:18369–18377.

46. Schipani E, Karga H, Karaplis AC, et al. Characterization of the cDNA encoding the human PTH/PTHrP receptor. *J Bone Mineral Res* 1992;7:S246.

47. Henderson JE, Kremer R, Rhim JS, Goltzman D. Identification and functional characterization of adenylate cyclase-linked receptors for parathyroid hormone-like peptides on immortalized human keratinocytes. *Endocrinology* 1992;130:449–457.

48. Thiede MA, Harm SC, McKee RL, Grasser WA, Duong LT, Leach RMJ. Expression of the parathyroid hormone-related protein gene in the avian oviduct: potential role as a local modulator of vascular smooth muscle tension and shell gland motility during the egg-laying cycle. *Endocrinology* 1991;129:1958–1966.

49. Aaron JE, Abbas SK, Colwell A, et al. Parathyroid gland hormones in the skeletal development of the ovine foetus: the effect of parathyroidectomy with calcium and phosphate infusion. *Bone Mineral* 1992;16:121–129.

50. Root A, Gruskin A, Reber RM, Stopa A, Duckett G. Serum concentrations of parathyroid hormone in infants, children and adolescents. *J Pediatr* 1974;8:329–336.

51. Hillman OS, Slatopolsky E, Haddad JG. Perinatal vitamin D metabolism in maternal and cord serum. 24,25-Dihydroxyvitamin D concentration. *J Clin Endocrinol Metab* 1978;47:1073–1077.

52. Wieland P, Fisher JA, Trechsel U, et al. Perinatal parathyroid hormone, vitamin D metabolites, and calcitonin in man. *Am J Physiol* 1980;239:E385–E390.

53. Allgrove J, Adami S, Manning RM, O'Riordan JL. Cytochemical bioassay of parathyroid hormone in mternal and cord blood. *Arch Dis Child* 1985;60:110–115.

54. Thiébaud D, Pecherstorfer M, Janisch S, Jacquet AF, Burchhardt P. Direct evidence of a parathyroid related protein gradient between the mother and the newborn in humans. *J Bone Mineral Res* 1992;7:S228.

55. Insogna KL, Stewart AF, Morris CA, Hough LM, Milstone LM, Centrella M. Native and a synthetic analogue of the malignancy-associated parathyroid hormone-like protein have in vitro transforming growth factor-like properties. *J Clin Invest* 1989;83:1057–1060.

56. Pitkin RM. Calcium metabolism in pregnancy and the perinatal period. *Am J Obstet Gynecol* 1985;151:99–109.

57. Care AD, Caple IW, Abbas SK, Pickard DW. The effect of fetal thyroparathyroidectomy on the transport of calcium across the ovine placenta of the fetus. *Placenta* 1986;7:417–424.

58. Care AD. The placental transfer of calcium. *J Dev Physiol* 1991;15:253–257.

59. Rodda DP, Kubota M, Heath JA, et al. Evidence for a novel parathyroid hormone-related protein in fetal lamb parathyroid glands and sheep placenta: comparisons with a similar protein implicated in humoral hypercalcemia of malignancy. *J Endocrinol* 1988;117:261–271.

60. Abbas SK, Pickard DW, Illingworth D, et al. Measurement of parathyroid hormone-related protein in extracts of fetal parathyroid glands and placental membranes. *J Endocrinol* 1990;124:319–325.

61. Care AD, Abbas SK, Pickard DW, et al. Stimulation of ovine placental transport of calcium and magnesium by mid-molecule fragments of human parathyroid hormone-related protein. *Exp Physiol* 1990;75:605–608.

62. Ng KW, Martin TJ. Humoral hypercalcemia of malignancy. *Clin Biochem* 1990;23:11–16.

63. Hellman P, Ridefelt P, Juhlin C, Akerstrom G, Rastad J, Gylfe E. Parathyroid-like regulation of parathyroid-hormone-related protein release and cytoplasmic calcium in cytotrophoblast cells of human placenta. *Arch Biochem Biophys* 1992;293:174–180.

64. Drees BM, Rouse J, Johnson J, Hamilton JW. Bovine parathyroid glands secrete a 26-kDa N-terminal fragment of chromogranin-A which inhibits parathyroid cell secretion. *Endocrinology* 1991;129:3381–3387.

65. Bansal DD, MacGregor RR. Calcium-regulated secretion of tissue plasminogen activator and parathyroid hormone from human parathyroid cells. *J Clin Endocrinol Metab* 1992;74: 266–271.

66. Fenton AJ, Kemp BE, Kent GN, et al. A carboxyl-terminal peptide from the parathyroid hormone-related protein inhibits bone resorption by osteoclasts. *Endocrinology* 1991;129: 1762–1768.

67. Fenton AJ, Kemp BE, Hammonds RGJ, et al. A potent inhibitor of osteoclastic bone resorption within a highly conserved pentapeptide region of parathyroid hormone-related protein; PTHrP [107–111]. *Endocrinology* 1991;129:3424–3426.

68. Dudley A, King K, Mathias J, et al. Effect of human parathyroid hormone related peptide 107–139 on osteoclast formation and bone resorption in vitro. *J Bone Mineral Res* 1992;7: S309.

69. Fenton AJ, Martin TJ, Nicholson GC. Carboxyl-terminal parathyroid hormone-related protein inhibits basal and stimulated resorption in populations of isolated chicken osteoclasts. *J Bone Mineral Res* 1992;7:S314.

The Parathyroids, edited by J.P. Bilezikian,
M.A. Levine, and R. Marcus. Raven Press, Ltd.,
New York © 1994.

CHAPTER 13

Interactions of Parathyroid Hormone, Parathyroid Hormone-Related Protein, and their Fragments with Conventional and Nonconventional Receptor Sites

Timothy M. Murray, Leticia G. Rao, and Rene E. Rizzoli

The major physiological roles of parathyroid hormone (PTH) in the regulation of calcium and bone metabolism are now well established and have been recently reviewed (1,2). Parathyroid hormone homeostatically regulates plasma and extracellular fluid (ECF) calcium concentrations in a negative feedback mechanism via actions on kidney and bone (and indirectly on the intestine) such that plasma calcium is maintained within narrow physiological limits. Parathyroid hormone is secreted by the parathyroid gland in response to hypocalcemia and, in turn, elevates the serum calcium concentration in an effort to restore homeostasis; it does this by increasing bone resorption, increasing calcium reabsorption in the renal tubule, and increasing the intestinal absorption of calcium indirectly by increasing renal synthesis of the vitamin D-derived hormone 1,25-dihydroxyvitamin D_3 [1,25-$(OH)_2D_3$]. In addition to regulating plasma and ECF calcium concentration, PTH is a regulator of bone turnover (3). PTH accomplishes these actions in its primary target tissues, kidney and bone, via interaction with guanine nucleotide-linked cell surface receptors, in a manner analogous to other peptide hormones.

The amino acid sequence of the PTH molecule is shown in Figure 1. The major actions of PTH on bone and kidney can be expressed by amino-terminal (N-terminal) fragments of the hormone, principally the fragment comprising amino acid residues 1–34 (4–6). As examples, the skeletal actions of PTH on bone formation and resorption and the renal actions on ion transport and vitamin D metabolism have been reproduced in vitro and in vivo by the PTH-(1–34) fragment. The discovery in the early 1970s that the amino-terminal 1–34 fragment retained full biological activity (4,5) gave rise to the hypothesis that the secreted 84-residue peptide might be cleaved in the circulation prior to exerting its hormonal effects in target tissues. However, subsequent experiments demonstrated that intact hormone was able to exert its full effect in kidney (7) and bone (8), both in vitro (8) and in vivo (9), under conditions in which cleavage to fragments did not occur and that radioiodinated intact PTH-(1–84) could bind to receptors and activate adenylyl cyclase in kidney membranes (10) and bone cells (11,12) without cleavage of the hormone in the amino-terminal region prior to the tyrosine at position 43. Furthermore, experiments that employed the sensitive cytochemical bioassay coupled with plasma fractionation by high-performance liquid chromatography (HPLC) have shown that the principal circulating form of the hormone possessing bioactivity related to calcium and phosphorus metabolism is the intact 84-residue hormone; biologically active amino-terminal fragments are not detected (13). Thus, while a number of hormonal fragments have been detected in vivo, the prevailing view is that most of the circulating fragments of PTH are biologically inactive and that the parathy-

R.E. Rizzoli: Division of Clinical Pathophysiology, Department of Medicine, University Hospital of Geneva, 1211 Geneva, 14, Switzerland.

T.M. Murray and L.G. Rao: Department of Medicine, University of Toronto, St. Michael's Hospital, Toronto, Ontario, M5B 1A6 Canada.

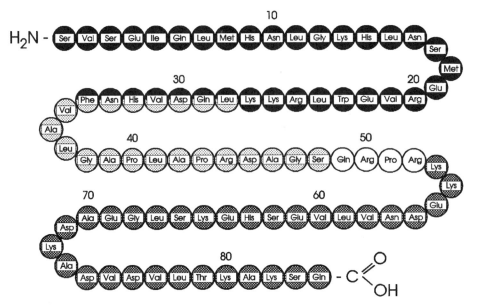

FIG. 1. Amino-acid sequence of human parathyroid hormone. The *solid area* represents the 1–34 region, responsible for the classical calcium and bone-regulating activities of the hormone now known to be mediated by a common amino-terminal PTH/PTHrP receptor that activates adenylyl cyclase, phospholipase C, and PKC, and for which the cDNA has recently been cloned (see text). The *lightly hatched area* represents the midregion fragment hPTH-(28–48), shown to stimulate mitogenesis without an effect on adenylyl cyclase. The *more darkly hatched area* represents the carboxyl-terminal 53–84 fragment, shown to stimulate alkaline phosphatase and osteocalcin expression in differentiated osteoblastic cells. The activities of these three epitopes of PTH are also summarized in Table 1.

roid hormone molecule involved in the regulation of calcium and phosphorus metabolism is the native 84-residue peptide. This classical view of PTH physiology incorporates the concept that the native 1–84 hormone exerts its calciotropic and bone-regulating effects via a receptor that is activated by the region encompassing the amino-terminal one-third of the hormone molecule (see Fig. 1).

The structure–function relationships of the PTH molecule have been extensively studied (see the chapter by Chorev and Rosenblatt). Early reviews (14,15) point out the major features discussed above. On the other hand, the subject continues to undergo active investigation and refinement, particularly through the techniques of peptide synthesis (16) and site-directed mutagenesis (17–19). While recent studies have extended our view of PTH action, they have, at the same time, introduced interesting new complexities. Thus, PTH and its amino-terminal fragments and analogs have been shown to interact with a G protein-coupled receptor for which the cDNA has recently been cloned and sequenced (20,21) (see below and the following chapter by Segre). Expression of the cloned receptor indicates that it clearly represents the conventional PTH receptor, which, at least on the basis of currently available evidence, is linked to the physiological actions of PTH. On the other hand, there is now some evidence that PTH may also interact with other unconventional or nonclassical sites in various tissues and exerts a variety of nonclassical effects, presumably receptor-mediated, both in vitro and in vivo (see the preceding chapter by Mallette). Included among these nonconventional sites are receptors for regions of the hormone other than the classically recognized region for biological activity. Thus, in addition to receptors for the amino-terminal 1–34 region of the hormone, there are now suggestions that distinct receptors may exist for midregion (28–48) epitopes and for the carboxyl-terminal 53–84 region. Figure 1 summarizes these major structural concepts. This chapter reviews these effects critically and attempts to place these various putative actions of the hormone in a useful conceptual framework.

A parathyroid hormone-related protein (PTHrP) has been isolated, initially from tumor cells associated with the syndrome of hypercalcemia of malignancy (22–24), its cDNA cloned, and its amino acid sequence deduced (24–29). The gene encoding PTH is on human chromosome 11 (30,31), while the gene for PTHrP is on human chromosome 12 (27); the genes encoding these two peptides are thought to be derived from a common ancestral gene (32). PTHrP is thought to be a major mediator of the hypercalcemia associated with malignant disease (see the chapter by Grill and Martin). A large body of evidence, both in vitro and in vivo, suggests that PTH and PTHrP share a common receptor in various tissues (33–45). This is particularly interesting in view of the limited homology between the amino acid and sequences of the two peptides. While there is strong homology in the first half of the active amino-terminal core, with eight of the first 13 amino acid residues being identical, the remainder of the 1–34 portions of the two peptides differ. It is now evident that nonhomologous sequences within the 14–34 regions of the two peptides share sufficient three-dimensional structure to explain their ability to bind to the same receptor (37,41). On the other hand, some observations of differential effects of various inhibitory analogs of PTH and PTHrP suggest that some distinct receptors for either peptide may exist in rat osteosarcoma cells (46). In addition, some activities have been attributed to PTHrP that are not shared by PTH. While PTHrP was suggested to have a unique transforming growth factor-β (TGFβ)-like activity in one study (47), the results of another study (48) did not support these findings. On the other hand, PTHrP was also shown to augment fibronectin synthesis in dermal fibroblasts, while PTH does not (47). Some reports have suggested that PTH and PTHrP are not equipotent in all systems. For example, PTHrP was found to be less potent than PTH in canine renal membranes but more potent than PTH in UMR cells (34). Also, in vivo infusion to human volunteers of hPTH-(1–34) and hPTHrP-(1–34) suggested that PTHrP may be three- to tenfold less potent than PTH (49). These observations notwithstanding, the major concept that arises from a review of the recent literature is that amino-terminal regions of PTH and PTHrP bind to the same receptor and exert similar effects in all systems, and usually with equimolar potency. As an example, a comparison of the two peptides in stimulating cyclic adenosine monophosphate (cAMP) accumulation in OK cells is illustrated in Fig. 2. Most differences may result from the difficulty in standardizing different batches of various peptides, in addition to some differences between species, particularly in receptor coupling (50), and perhaps also as a result of pharmacokinetic differences (49). It is of interest that recent direct comparisons between transfected cloned opossum and rat PTH/PTHrP receptors do reveal some minor but distinct species differences (51), and minor differences have also been shown between the properties of transfected cloned rat and human PTH/PTHrP receptors (52). There is 91% identity, however, between the deduced amino acid sequences of rat and human PTH/PTHrP receptors (52).

The discovery that PTH and PTHrP share a common receptor requires that any discussion of PTH receptor(s) reflect this special relationship. We therefore include interactions of PTHrP with its receptor in this review, but concentrate primarily on interactions of PTH with its receptor. It is currently thought that PTHrP, expressed in many tissues in humans (53,54), acts mainly in a paracrine rather than in an endocrine mode (see the chapter by Broadus and Stewart). In addition, it is recognized that receptors for PTH/PTHrP are widely distributed in mammalian tissues (55,56). To what extent these receptors, located in various tissues, may subserve physiological actions of circulating PTH and to what extent they subserve physiological paracrine or even autocrine actions of PTHrP are not known, but this distinction is important, and where possible available data are discussed with this question in mind. We therefore approach the topic by considering data relating to binding of chemically defined PTH radioligands to various cells and tissues and

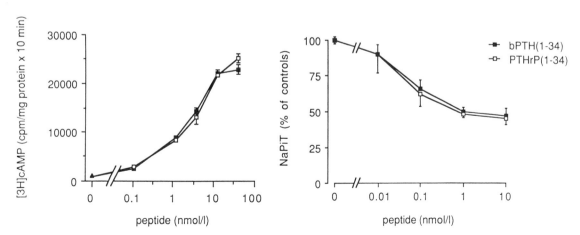

FIG. 2. Effect of synthetic PTHrP-(1–34) or bPTH-(1–34) on cAMP production (**left panel**) and P$_i$ transport in OK epithelial cells (**right panel**). Seven days after plating, cAMP response to either agent was determined in confluent OK cells during a 10 min period at 37°C, and sodium-dependent phosphate transport was measured. Values are means of four to seven determinations. The effects of PTHrP-(1–34) and PTH-(1–34) are indistinguishable. From Pizurki et al. (313).

then discuss the physiologic and pathophysiologic implications associated with the various receptors and/or binding sites.

"CONVENTIONAL" PARATHYROID HORMONE RECEPTORS

Historical Aspects

The study of PTH responses in target tissues began even before the precise structure of PTH was known, with the discovery by Chase and Aurbach (57) in 1968 that PTH action in renal tissue was concomitant with the ability of PTH to activate adenylyl cyclase. A similar relationship was subsequently shown in bone (58). Almost simultaneously, Aurbach's group determined that infusion of PTH failed to activate renal adenylyl cyclase activity in patients with pseudohypoparathyroidism (59), the syndrome of PTH unresponsiveness initially described by Albright et al. in 1941 (60). These observations formed the basis for the realization that the calciotropic actions of PTH were associated with activation of adenylyl cyclase in target tissues, probably via a receptor linked to adenylyl cyclase. Marcus and Aurbach (61) utilized this activity of PTH to design the first in vitro bioassay for PTH, the well-known rat renal membrane adenylyl cyclase bioassay. Thus the elucidation of PTH action began in the laboratory of Gerry Aurbach. These early events in the study of PTH action are reviewed in the chapter by Chase.

Development of Labeled Probes for Parathyroid Hormone Receptors

Throughout the 1970s, receptors for various peptide hormones were analyzed to determine their binding activity and their regulation. However, characterization of PTH receptors lagged behind the study of other receptors, principally because of the difficulty of obtaining a biologically active PTH radioligand. Conventional iodination methods with chloramine-T resulted in loss of biological activity because they resulted in the oxidation of labile methionine residues in the N-terminal one-third of the hormone molecule, at residues 8 and 18 of bovine PTH (62). In the late 1970s, however, two groups developed methods for the production of biologically active bPTH-(1–34) fragment radioligands. The Boston group substituted isoleucine for the methionine residues to produce oxidation-resistant analogs (63), and the San Francisco group utilized a milder electrolytic method for radioiodination of bPTH-(1–34) followed by an affinity purification step using chicken renal membranes (64). Other groups had attempted to radiolabel the intact 84-residue native PTH molecule. Zull and colleagues (65,66) initially developed a method to produce a biologically active tritiated PTH-(1–84) preparation using an acetamidation technique, while Nielsen et al. (67) and Rosenberg et al. (68) used electrochemical approaches to radioiodinate intact PTH. Kremer et al. (69) employed a gentle lactoperoxidase iodination, which, when followed by HPLC purification, yielded a biologically active intact PTH preparation. While radiolabeling of bovine or human peptide has been used in most experiments, it has been shown that, for rat tissues, a rat PTH radioligand is not only preferable but indeed necessary (70). Recently it has been possible to develop biologically active biotinylated derivatives of both PTH-(1–34) and PTH-(1–84) that allow tagging of PTH-responsive bone cells. These biologically active ligands permit analysis of PTH binding by fluorescence-activated flow cytometry (71,72) and localization of PTH binding sites (73).

PTH Structure–Function Relations

Initial studies of PTH receptor binding and activation of adenylyl cyclase provided significant insights regarding the structure–function relationships of the PTH molecule. Occupancy of the amino-terminal PTH receptor correlates closely with activation of adenylyl cyclase in target tissues (10,64,74). Shortening of the PTH-(1–34) fragment from the amino-terminal end reduces the ability of the peptide to activate adenylyl cyclase, but fragments thus shortened retain their ability to bind to the receptor and thus act as competitive inhibitors of PTH activity. The minimum length of peptide that is capable of binding to the PTH receptor corresponds to residues 25–34 of bPTH (75,76).

Intracellular Mediators in Parathyroid Hormone

Some early observations suggested that not all actions of PTH could be explained by the activation of adenylyl cyclase. For example, Hermann-Erlee et al. (77) observed that fragments of PTH-(1–34) truncated at the amino-terminal end stimulated bone resorption without activating adenylyl cyclase. Recently it has been increasingly appreciated that other mediators, including cytosolic free Ca^{2+}, inositol trisphosphate (IP_3), and diacylglycerol (DAG), not only are involved in PTH action but may be separately regulated under some circumstances, particularly by PTH fragments lacking the first few amino-terminal residues (see below for further details).

Studies of Parathyroid Hormone Receptors Using Amino-Terminal Parathyroid Hormone Radioligands

Studies in Kidney

Initial studies of PTH receptor binding were performed in renal membranes. Studies by Nissenson and Arnaud (64) of chick renal plasma membranes demonstrated a single high-affinity binding site for electrolytically radioiodinated membrane-purified bPTH-(1–34) with a K_d of 7–10 nM. Binding activity correlated closely with activation of adenylyl cyclase in the membranes. Other studies carried out at virtually the same time by Segre et al. (74) used radioiodinated 8,18 Nle-substituted bPTH-(1–34) as radioligand to study PTH receptors in dog renal cortical membranes and produced similar results, with a K_d also in the low nanomolar range. These studies also showed parallel activities of synthetic hormone analogs in receptor binding and adenylyl cyclase assays, indicating a linkage between hormone binding and subsequent adenylyl cyclase activation. Receptor-mediated endocytosis and degradation of the [Nle^{8,18}, ^{125}I-Tyr^{34}]bPTH-(1–34)NH$_2$ radioligand have been demonstrated following hormone binding to the opossum renal (OK) cell line (78). Down-regulation of PTH receptors by PTH (homologous desensitization) was observed in vitro (79) and in vivo (80). The mechanism of homologous desensitization may be mediated by protein kinase (PKC) (79).

Studies of the association of hormone binding to the renal PTH receptor with subsequent activities of the hormone in kidney have revealed the existence of multiple cellular mediators of PTH action. Although it has been firmly established that binding of PTH to renal tissue correlates closely with activation of adenylyl cyclase (10,64,70,80–82), it is now also evident that PTH is coupled to other signal transduction mechanisms, including stimulation of membrane-bound phospholipase C with consequent production of the intracellular messengers DAG and IP$_3$ (21,83,84). Thus the second messengers cAMP (10,64,70,80–82), DAG (83), IP$_3$ (83,84), and cytosolic Ca^{2+} [Ca]$_i$ [released by IP$_3$ from intracellular stores (85,86)], may also be regarded as mediators of the biological actions of PTH in kidney. The cellular mediators of two important renal actions of the hormone have been studied in detail; the effects of PTH on vitamin D metabolism (see 87, for review) and on Na/phosphate cotransport (88–90). In vitro studies in cultured chicken kidney cells in the OK cell line have contributed greatly to the elucidation of these and other aspects of the renal actions of PTH. The stimulatory effect of PTH on 1,25-(OH)$_2$D$_3$ production and the inhibitory effect of PTH on 24,25-(OH)$_2$D$_3$ production in cultured chicken kidney cells have been shown to be mediated by cAMP (87,91,92). Recently, however, it has also been shown that PKC,

possibly via DAG, also mediates PTH effects on production of vitamin D metabolites; PKC inhibits PTH-stimulated cAMP production and 1,25-(OH)$_2$D$_3$ synthesis and stimulates 24,25-(OH)$_2$D$_3$ production in cultured chick kidney cells (87). Although these studies did not include an analysis of PTH receptor binding, these data suggest that PKC down-regulates the PTH receptor and agree with the data of Pernalete et al. (79), who showed that PKC modulates desensitization of PTH receptor–adenylyl cyclase in OK cells. Recent evidence also indicates that the inhibitory effect of PTH on phosphate transport is exerted via two apparently independent pathways: first, through cAMP production and, second, through activation of phospholipase C. Although the effect of PTH on sodium-dependent phosphate transport can be mimicked by cAMP, or agents that stimulate the production of cAMP (88), the half-maximal concentration of PTH required for inhibition of Na/phosphate cotransport is $\sim 10^{-11}$ M (93), a concentration commensurate with that required for DAG and IP$_3$ production and much lower than the concentration required for cAMP stimulation (10^{-9}–10^{-8} M). These findings were taken to suggest that phospholipase C might be a more physiologically relevant mediator than cAMP at normal levels of PTH (93), but additional evidence will be necessary to establish this.

Studies in Bone

Early studies of the major effects of PTH on skeletal tissue were reviewed in 1982 by Wong (94). The initial studies of bPTH-(1–34) binding suggested very similar characteristics of bPTH-(1–34) binding to kidney and bone (95,96), and current evidence based on nucleotide sequences of cloned receptor cDNAs of skeletal and renal origin also indicates that the amino-terminal PTH/PTHrP receptors in bone and kidney are the same at the molecular level (52).

Homologous desensitization of PTH binding was shown to occur after treatment of rat ROS 17/2 (97) and ROS 17/2.8 cells (97,98), rat UMR-106 cells (99,100), and human SaOS-2 cells (101) by PTH agonists. In UMR-106 cells, it was observed that part of this desensitization was associated with receptor events and part with postreceptor events; maximal loss of adenylyl cyclase-stimulating ability was observed after 2 hr, while maximal loss of receptor binding was not reached until 14 hr (99). In ROS 17/2.8 cells, the agonist-induced receptor down-regulation was reversed by inactivation of G$_i$ with pertussis toxin (98). By contrast, in SaOS-2 cells, agonist-induced receptor desensitization requires the activation of PKA and possibly PKC, but does not involve G$_i$ (101). While Pun et al. (100) did not observe heterologous desensitization by isoprenaline, prostaglandin (PG) E$_1$, or PGE$_2$, Mitchell and Goltzman (99) observed that heterologous desensitization by PGE$_2$ was associated with a reversible modification of the amino-terminal PTH receptor. A number of investigators have found that 1,25-(OH)$_2$D$_3$ can reduce the cAMP response to PTH in osteoblastic cells (97,102–104). Down-regulation of PTH receptors in osteoblastic osteosarcoma cells and embryonic chick bone cells is associated with receptor-mediated internalization of the hormone (105,106). While acute exposure (2 hr) to PTH results in down-regulation of the hormone response (106), it has recently been shown that chronic exposure to PTH (48 hr) results in potentiation of PTH responsiveness in osteoblasts derived from human bone, at least at the level of cAMP production, and this potentiation occurs at hormone concentrations at or below the physiological range (10^{-14} M) (107). PTH receptor density is also regulated by agents that regulate cell differentiation, including glucocorticoids, 1,25-(OH)$_2$D$_3$, retinoic acid, and various growth factors (see below).

As with renal tissue, current data indicate that multiple intracellular second messengers are generated by PTH receptor binding and are responsible for the subsequent actions of the hormone in bone. However, structure–function analyses in bone provide clearer evidence for distinct postreceptor regulatory pathways. Thus very early studies demonstrated that amino-terminally truncated analogs that have little or no adenylyl cyclase-stimulating potential still have calcemic properties in vivo (5), findings that were confirmed in later studies (108). Early observations in vitro on bone resorption indicated that amino-terminally truncated PTH analogs, while lacking the ability to stimulate adenylyl cyclase in rat calvarial bone, did possess biological activity in bone resorption assays (77,109). Furthermore, potent inhibitors of adenylyl cyclase do not block PTH-stimulated bone resorption in vitro (110). These data indicate that a mediator(s) other than cAMP/PKA must be associated with PTH-induced bone resorption. Later experiments revealed that DAG (111) and IP$_3$ (112,113), generated via activation of phospholipase C (114), as well as [Ca^{2+}]$_i$ released from intracellular stores by IP$_3$ (115–118), are mediators of the skeletal actions of PTH. Cross-talk between the adenylyl cyclase and phospholipase C pathways occurs at multiple levels, involving postreceptor modulation of adenylyl cyclase (119–121) and down-regulation of PTH receptors (98,101,122). The latter interactions have been ascribed to PKC and the former also to calmodulin (120). Furthermore, different domains of the PTH-(1–34) fragment have been shown to be responsible for the activation of PKA, PKC, PLC, and the cytosolic [Ca^{2+}]$_i$ responses in bone. Jouishomme et al. (123) demonstrated in ROS 17/2.8 cells that both hPTH-(1–84) and hPTH-(1–34) stimulated PKC in two distinct peaks of activity, one at PTH concentrations of 1–50 pM and another at 5–

50 nM, while PTH stimulated cAMP production only in the nanomolar range. The authors have shown further that the PKC activation is associated with PTH peptides as short as the 28–34 fragment. At the same time, Fujimori et al. showed in UMR-106-01 cells that bPTH-(1–34), bPTH-(2–34), propionyl-bPTH-(2–34), and bPTH-(3–34) elicited a transient spike of [Ca^{2+}]$_i$ (124), activation of PKC, and stimulation of IP$_3$ production (125), while bPTH-(7–34)-amide and bPTH-(30–34) were ineffective. On the other hand, only bPTH-(1–34) and bPTH-(2–34) stimulated PKA activity. The results from these two laboratories, although studies were performed in two different cell types and at different hormone concentrations, demonstrate that PTH signal transduction through these two pathways can be dissociated; the activation of PKA requires the first two amino-terminal residues, while activation of PKC and PLC does not. In this respect there may be a difference between the transduction mechanisms in kidney and bone; hPTH-(3–34), an analog that does not activate adenylyl cyclase, is able to stimulate PKC activity in osteoblastic cells (123,126) but is unable to do so in the OK renal cell line (127). The PKA and PKC pathways have now been implicated in the action of PTH on collagenase production (128), mitogenic activity (129), and ornithine decarboxylation (130) as well as others. A strategy that is proving most useful in sorting out the various interrelated signal transduction pathways involved in PTH action is the use of transfected cultured bone cell lines (e.g., transfected UMR-106 and SaOS-2 cells) that express an inactive form of PKA (131–133). As an example, these studies reveal that PTH-induced inhibition of alkaline phosphatase release by SaOS-2 cells is dependent on PKA; cAMP-resistant mutant cell lines release <10% of the alkaline phosphatase activity of wild-type cells (133). Additional new mediators of hormone action are also likely to be found in osteoblasts. In this regard, it has been recently noted that nitric oxide is produced in UMR-106 cells and rat osteoblasts in primary culture (134).

Further complexities in the skeletal actions of PTH remain to be unraveled, particularly concerning which PTH target cells in bone exert which actions. The osteoblast lineage consists of several cell types that are still relatively uncharacterized, and it is likely that these different cell types will have unique patterns of PTH responsiveness, perhaps both qualitatively and quantitatively. The main source of heterogeneity is the variety of cell types representing different stages of differentiation. It is now becoming more evident that hormonal responses of cells of the osteoblastic lineage are modified by the stage of differentiation; moreover, this dependence has been documented in the case of PTH binding and PTH responsiveness. Thus Rouleau et al. (135,136) demonstrated that the major target cells for PTH in bone are not mature osteoblasts but instead are less differentiated cells that have long cytoplasmic extensions and that are located near the endosteal surface. The same group showed that heterogeneity of PTH binding to osteoblastic cells could also be demonstrated in UMR 106 cell cultures, which contained three morphologically distinct subtypes (106). The subtype with the most abundant [^{125}I]rPTH-(1–34) binding was found to have long cytoplasmic extensions (106); these cells exhibited more frequent cytosolic calcium [Ca^{2+}]$_i$ spikes in response to PTH (137). The dependence of PTH binding and responsiveness on cell differentiation has also been documented using dexamethasone and/or 1,25-(OH)$_2$D$_3$ in rat osteoblast-like cells (138), the rat osteosarcoma cell line ROS 17/2.8 (103,104,139–142), the human osteosarcoma cell line SaOS-2 (143), normal osteoblast cells derived from human trabecular explants (144–146), and cultured mouse osteoblastic cells (147). Thus it has been shown that glucocorticoid stimulates (103,104,138–141) and 1,25-(OH)$_2$D$_3$ inhibits (102–104,142) adenylyl cyclase activity and cAMP production in a manner that may also involve postreceptor events, including inhibition of phosphodiesterase (138), enhanced G protein–adenylyl cyclase expression and coupling efficiency (139), and the interaction between adenylyl cyclase and PKC (104) as well as an effect on PTH/PTHrP receptor density (103,142). The PTH/PTHrP receptor density on rat osteosarcoma cells is increased two- to tenfold by glucocorticoids (103,142). Suarez and Silve (147) have suggested that the permissive action of dexamethasone on PTH regulation of free arachidonic acid levels in mouse osteoblast cells implicates the involvement of the phospholipase C transduction pathway. The findings that dexamethasone augments the PTH-(1–34)-induced inhibition of alkaline phosphatase (ALP) activity, a marker of osteoblast differentiation, in ROS 17/2.8 cells (148) and has a permissive effect on estrogen-induced potentiation of PTH-stimulated ALP activity in SaOS-2 cells (143) both strongly support the hypothesis that the PTH response is differentiation stage dependent. Other differentiating agents that have been shown to affect PTH responsiveness and PTH receptor density include tumor necrosis factor-α (149), retinoic acid (149), epidermal growth factor (EGF) (150), TGFα (151), and TGFβ (152,153). Interestingly, chronic exposure to PTH-(1–84) itself suppresses the differentiation of rat calvarial preosteoblasts into mature osteoblasts in bone nodule formation assays (154). Although this effect was tested only with intact PTH-(1–84), it is likely that the effect occurs via the amino-terminal PTH/PTHrP receptor, in view of the many other observations that PTH suppresses bone formation in vitro (155,156). The subject of the effects of PTH on bone cell differentiation is reviewed in the chapter by Heersche et al.

An additional complexity requiring further investi-

gation and clarification is that there are differences in vitro in hormonal responses of osteoblastic cells derived from different areas of the skeleton. This has been explored and reviewed by Heersche et al. (157). An example relevant to PTH receptors is that PTH receptor mRNA levels were suppressed by estrogen in human osteoblastic cells derived from femoral head but not in iliac crest (158), indicating that PTH acts differently at different sites in the skeleton.

The long-standing question of why PTH stimulates bone resorption preferentially at subperiosteal sites may have been at least partially resolved by recent in situ hybridization studies of whole rat tibiae using a cDNA probe for the amino-terminal PTH receptor. These studies revealed striking localization of high densities of amino-terminal PTH/PTHrP receptors in the subperiosteal region (159).

The question of why PTH-stimulated bone formation occurs primarily in trabecular as opposed to cortical bone (160,161) has yet to be clarified. The stimulation of bone formation by PTH (162–166) and PTHrP (165,166) is favored by intermittent hormone treatment and is suppressed by continuous treatment, both in vivo (162,165,168) and in vitro (166). The similar actions of PTH and PTHrP in this respect suggest that the two hormones act via the common amino-terminal PTH/PTHrP receptor. However, the basis for the positive effect of intermittent receptor signaling is not currently understood. The formation-inducing effects of both PTH and PTHrP appear to be dependent on human growth hormone (HGH) and/or insulin-like growth factor type I (IGF-I) (166,169).

Studies Using Intact Parathyroid Hormone Radioligands

Studies by Zull and colleagues (65,66,170) in which tritiated PTH-(1–84) was used as a radioligand first characterized the binding of the intact PTH molecule to target tissues. These tritiated radioligands were of relatively low specific activity, and it was generally thought that higher specific activities were necessary to probe physiologically relevant receptors. The subsequent development of radiodinated intact hormone radioligands (68,69) confirmed and extended these findings, however. Using an intact PTH-(1–84) radioligand, Rizzoli et al. (10) observed that specific hormone binding to dog renal membranes generated a two-site Scatchard plot; binding of intact hormone to the high-affinity renal site (K$_d$ 2–5 nM) correlated with activation of adenylyl cyclase. McKee and Murray (81) demonstrated two-site Scatchard plots for intact PTH binding to chick kidney membranes; the high-affinity (K$_d$ 1.21 nM) amino-terminal site was linked to activation of adenylyl cyclase, while the low-affinity (K$_d$ 333 nM) site was not. The low-affinity site corresponded kinetically to sites probed by competition with the carboxyl-terminal hPTH-(53–84) fragment (see Fig. 3). These authors also presented evidence for separate regulation of the two binding sites in chick kidney; the low-affinity renal binding site was differentially regulated by Mg^{2+} (10,81). Other laboratories also observed differences between binding of intact and amino-terminal radioligands (69,170–172). In particular, it was observed in bovine (170) and canine (172) renal membranes that PTH-(1–34) was incapable of completely inhibiting the binding of radiolabeled PTH (1–84). The inability of these other investigators to observe two-site Scatchard plots probably reflected methodological differences, in that the low-affinity carboxyl-terminal PTH site in renal membranes is labile during storage at $-20°C$, and its demonstration requires longer incubation times (81). Kinetic analysis of intact PTH-(1–84) binding to OK cells also gave rise to a biphasic Scatchard plot (173).

Experiments in skeletal tissue using intact PTH radioligands also showed differences from studies employing amino-terminal tracers. Studies by Rao and Murray (12) in ROS 17/2.8 cells suggested two distinct binding sites, one for the 1–34 amino-terminal region linked to adenylyl cyclase and the other for the carboxyl-terminal 53–84 region. These findings are illustrated in Fig. 4. While the affinities of these two binding sites were too similar to provide a two-component Scatchard plot, the existence of two separate binding sites was strongly suggested both by direct comparison of binding of radioiodinated bPTH-(1–34) and bPTH-(1–84) and by competition studies with various

hormonal fragments using radiolabeled bPTH-(1–84) as radioligand (12). Demay et al. (171) also found evidence in UMR-106 cells for a significant contribution to hormone binding by residues beyond position 34 of intact PTH and observed that this interaction was greater in the UMR-106 osteosarcoma cells than in canine renal membranes. However, the demonstration of distinct binding sites was less clear in those studies than in those of Rao and Murray (12) using ROS 17/2.8 cells. This may be due to the differences in target tissues employed, as Murray et al. (174) also observed fewer carboxyl-terminal binding sites on UMR-106 cells than on ROS cells, consistent with the less differentiated phenotype of these cells in comparison to that of ROS 17/2.8 cells.

The results of the PTH receptor studies that have utilized intact hormone radioligands suggest (a) that intact hormone binds to the same receptor to which amino-terminal radioligands bind and (b) that there is at least one other site to which intact hormone binds in target tissues. It is likely that the major additional binding site for intact PTH is specific for the region of PTH encompassing the residues 53–84 (see below).

Cloning of the cDNA for the Amino-Terminal Parathyroid Hormone/Parathyroid Hormone-Related Protein Receptor

Recently the cDNA for the amino-terminal PTH/PTHrP receptor was cloned by COS-7 cell expression

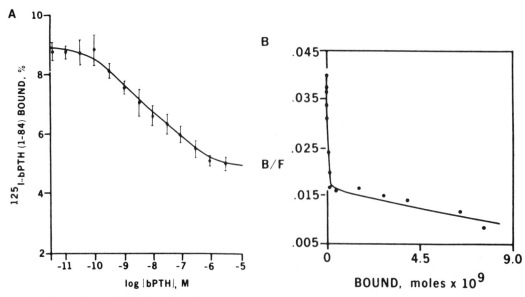

FIG. 3. **A:** Binding of [^{125}I]bPTH-(1–84) to chicken renal plasma membranes in the presence of varying amounts of unlabeled bPTH-(1–84). Pooled data from eight experiments in quadruplicate. **B:** The Scatchard plot of the data from A is distinctly biphasic. From McKee and Murray (81).

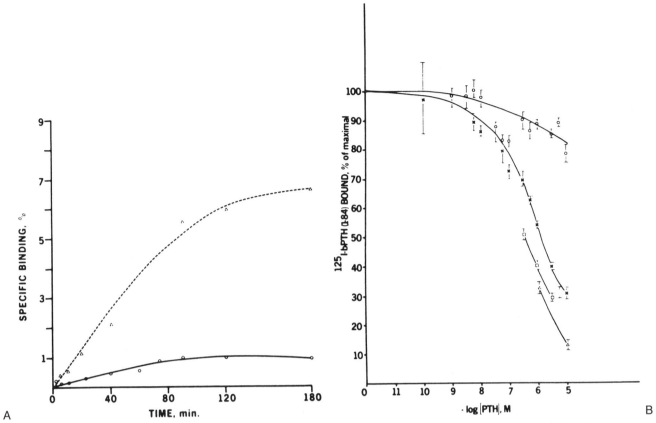

FIG. 4. A: Time course of PTH binding to ROS 17/2.8 cells. [^{125}I]bPTH-(1–84) (△) or [^{125}I]bPTH-(1–34) (○) was added to confluent cultures of ROS 17/2.8 cells and binding studies carried out with or without added unlabelled bPTH-(1–84) (1 × 10^{-5} M). Each point is the mean of duplicate determinations. Nonspecific binding is ~1–2% of total added radiolabel. There is a much higher binding capacity for [^{125}I]bPTH-(1–84) than for [^{125}I]-bPTH-(1–34) in these rat osteoblastic cells. B: Competitive inhibition of [^{125}I]bPTH-(1–84) binding to ROS 17/2.8 cells by unlabeled bPTH-(1–84) (△), hPTH-(53–84) (×), bPTH-(1–34) (○), and hPTH-(53–84) + bPTH-(1–34) (□). The major competing PTH peptide in this system is hPTH-(53–84), which accounts for >70% of the binding of intact PTH to ROS 17/2.8 cells. From Rao and Murray (12).

from an OK cell cDNA library (20) and from a rat ROS 17/2.8 osteosarcoma cell library (see the chapter by Segre; 21). The deduced amino acid sequence of the rat bone receptor had 78% identity to the opossum kidney receptor, indicating striking conservation across distant mammalian species. The same receptor not only binds both ligands, PTH and PTHrP, but is linked to at least two intracellular transduction pathways, adenylyl cyclase and phospholipase C (21,51). The knowledge gained through expression studies of these receptor cDNAs and studies utilizing cDNA probes for this amino-terminal PTH/PTHrP receptor indicate that the cloned receptor is indeed the signal detector protein that mediates the effects of both amino-terminal fragments and intact forms of PTH and PTHrP (see the chapter by Segre). It also appears that this amino-terminal PTH/PTHrP receptor mediates the anabolic effects of the hormone; the 1–34 fragment appears to be equipotent with native PTH in stimulating apposi-

tional bone growth (162) and also in increasing bone mass (163,164).

PUTATIVE OR "UNCONVENTIONAL" PARATHYROID HORMONE RECEPTORS

Amino-Terminal 1–34 Region

The consensus regarding the available information suggests that there is only one binding site for the PTH-(1–34) molecule. However, some studies have suggested that there may be more than one receptor for the amino-terminal portion of the molecule. While the recently cloned amino-terminal receptor cDNA appears to code for the physiologically important amino-terminal PTH receptor, there continues to be some question about whether additional receptors for this region exist. For example, in addition to the major 2.3–

2.5 kb PTH/PTHrP receptor transcripts noted in classical PTH target tissues, and many other tissues, additional transcripts of different sizes have been found in kidney, liver, skin, and testis (56). Some of these transcripts could represent cross-hybridizing PTH/PTHrP receptors with different functional properties, different splicing forms of the cloned PTH receptor, or methodological artefacts. Further investigation will be required to clarify their significance.

Putative Parathyroid Hormone Receptors Possibly Related to Calcium and Phosphorus Metabolism

In kidney, PTH and PTHrP have been shown to play a major role in the regulation of apical sodium–proton exchange, and sodium–phosphate cotransport in proximal tubular cells. This effect occurs via the aminoterminal domain of these hormones and appears to be mediated largely by cAMP (88,151). Other intracellular mediators are likely to play a role as well (175). Experiments performed on PTH-responsive kidney cells grown on permeant filters have provided the opportunity to differentially assess hormonal responses on the apical and/or basolateral cell surfaces. By adding the amino-terminal fragment of PTH to either side of the polarized cell system, a higher affinity for PTH-induced inhibition of P_i uptake was demonstrated when the hormone was added to the apical surface. The opposite was found, however, for cAMP generation (176,177). These results indicate the presence of PTH receptors on both the apical and basolateral surfaces of cultured renal cells, each capable of stimulating sodium–proton exchange and sodium–phosphate cotransport but with differing sensitivities to the hormone. Whether these findings reflect intrinsic differences in PTH receptors or in postreceptor events has not yet been established.

With regard to skeletal tissue, studies of the binding of rat PTH-(1–34) to rat ROS 17/2.8 osteosarcoma cells was shown to fit a two-site kinetic model (178), suggesting two distinct binding sites within the 1–34 region. It is not known whether this observation, not made in other studies, is explained by methodological factors or whether it is species-specific. Perhaps the most persuasive argument for two amino-terminal PTH receptors in bone is provided by the work of Jouishomme et al. (123) with ROS 17/2.8 cells, in which a two-component dose–response curve was seen for PTH stimulation of PKC. PKC was stimulated at doses of 1–50 pM (in the same order of magnitude as circulating PTH concentrations) and 5–50 nM, but not at intermediate concentrations, suggesting that, in addition to the "classical" receptor for PTH/PTHrP, which has an affinity in the nanomolar range, there is a PTH receptor that is 100-fold more sensitive that preferentially activates PKC. The existence of a separate PTH receptor in bone not linked to adenylyl cyclase was first proposed by Herrmann-Erlee et al. (109).

Parathyroid Hormone Receptors on Osteoclasts

Rao et al. (179) first demonstrated binding of PTH to osteoclasts. They utilized intact, unlabeled bPTH-(1–84), visualized immunohistochemically in sections of neonatal rat radii by an anti-PTH antibody with specificity towards the midregion of the PTH molecule (179). Bovine PTH bound specifically to mature multinucleated osteoclasts (as well as osteoblasts and osteocytes). Autoradiographic studies by others (180,181) have failed to demonstrate specific binding of radiolabeled aminoterminal or intact PTH ligands to osteoclasts in intact embryonic chick bone in vitro (180) or in mature rat skeletal tissue in vivo (181). In a more recent study (182), radioiodinated PTHrP-(1–34) and PTHrP-(1–84) did not bind to isolated osteoclasts, whereas these ligands labeled cultured osteoblasts. In the last few years, however, three other groups have provided additional evidence for specific binding of PTH to osteoclasts or preosteoclasts (73,183,184). Teti et al. (184) reported specific binding of electrolytically labeled intact bPTH-(1–84) to cultured avian marrow-derived tartrate-resistant acid phosphatase (TRAP)-positive cells with a K_d of 3×10^{-7} M. Agarwala and Gay (73) demonstrated PTH binding to isolated chicken osteoclasts using a biotinylated intact bPTH-(1–84) derivative and fluorescein isothiocyanate (FITC)–avidin. PTH binding was specifically displaced by unlabeled PTH-(1–84) and was saturable, with a K_d of 10^{-7} M, in the same order of magnitude as that observed by Teti et al. (184). Duong et al. (183) demonstrated specific binding of radioiodinated [Nle^{8,18},^{125}I-Tyr^{34}]bPTH-(1–34)NH$_2$ to isolated avian and rat osteoclasts. Additionally, studies of PTH binding to murine hematopoietic blast cells revealed a binding site for the aminoterminal ligand [Ne^{8,18},^{125}I-Tyr^{34}]bPTH-(1–34)NH$_2$ with a K_d of 5×10^{-9} M (185). This suggests that PTH receptors are expressed by osteoclast precursors, and the observation that treatment of these cells with PTH-(1–34) stimulated the formation of multinucleated cells suggests that the receptors are physiologically important (185). The aggregate results of five separate studies (73,179,183–185) strongly support the hypothesis that there are specific receptors for PTH on osteoclasts. On the other hand, the failures to demonstrate direct effects of PTH on stimulation of cAMP production in relatively pure preparations of isolated osteoclasts (186) or resorption of bone in a devitalized bone resorption assay (187) have cast doubts on whether PTH exerts any direct actions on cells of the osteoclast lineage. Stimulation of bone resorption was observed in such systems only when osteoclasts were cocultured with or in the presence of contaminating osteoblasts (187,188). These latter studies support the hypothesis of Rodan and Martin (189) and others (182,187), that PTH binds to osteoblasts, which then trigger osteoclasts secondarily, but does not interact directly with osteoclasts (182,187,188). Methodological differences between the various studies may explain the apparent discrepancies. It is also possible that PTH might activate osteoclasts via an intracellular mediator other than cAMP. Other actions of PTH on osteoclasts, such as changes in cellular pH (190) and activation of carbonic anhydrase (191), have also been proposed as evidence for direct effects of PTH on osteoclasts. Further studies will be necessary to establish the physiological relevance of PTH binding sites on osteoclasts.

Parathyroid Hormone Receptors on Chondrocytes

Studies with $[Nle^{8,18}, {}^{125}I\text{-}Tyr^{34}]bPTH\text{-}(1–34)NH_2$ revealed binding sites on cultured rabbit costal chondrocytes with a binding affinity in the nanomolar range (192). Receptor density was significantly higher in growth cartilage than in resting cartilage. These receptors can be linked to expression of the differentiated chrondrocyte phenotype, since PTH increases ornithine decarboxylase and glycosaminoglycan (GAG) synthesis in chondrocytes in vitro, in a cAMP-dependent manner (193), although other mediators appear to be involved as well (194). DAG, IP_3, the subsequent release of Ca^{2+} from intracellular pools, and the activation of PKC have all been shown to be involved in this response (195). At the same time, PTH appears to inhibit the expression of cellular activity related to cartilage mineralization; i.e., PTH inhibits ALP and the incorporation of ^{45}Ca into the insoluble fraction of cultures of growth plate chondrocytes (196). The association between PTH receptor binding and GAG synthesis seems strong; both binding and GAG synthesis were coordinately increased by IGF-I and TGFβ and decreased by retinoic acid, epidermal growth factor (EGF), and fibroblast growth factor (FGF) (197). Presumably the chondrocyte receptors are linked to the effects of PTH on cartilage in growing bone. In the developing mouse mandibular condyle, a model for endochondral bone formation, PTH stimulates proliferation of chondroprogenitor cells (198). In addition, PTH promotes chondrocyte differentiation in costal chondrocyte cultures (288).

Intestinal Receptors for Parathyroid Hormone

Increased intestinal calcium absorption is a prominent feature of hyperparathyroidism, and stimulation of calcium absorption by the gut is recognized as an important in vivo effect of PTH. It is generally thought that the stimulatory effect of the hormone on intestinal calcium transport is indirect, via enhanced renal synthesis of $1,25\text{-}(OH)_2D$, but evidence has been presented supporting a direct effect of PTH on the intestine (199). By contrast, other work fails to confirm a direct effect of PTH on intestinal calcium transport; with the bisphosphonate etidronate to block 25-hydroxyvitamin D 1α-hydroxylase activity in thyroparathyroidectomized rats, even large doses of native PTH were unable to correct the low levels of calcium absorption, although hormonal changes in renal tubular transport could still be detected (200,201).

Placental Parathyroid Hormone Receptors

Lafond et al. (202) detected binding sites for amino-terminal PTH-(1–34) in human placental tissue and proposed that these sites are physiologically relevant PTH receptors. The K_d for these binding sites (2.0 nM) was similar to that found for PTH receptors in other classical PTH target tissues. PTH was shown to stimulate cAMP production (202) and to increase placental brush border phosphate transport (203). Also, PTH-(1–34) has been shown to stimulate placental calcium transport in ewes in vivo (204). Data from Care's laboratory (205,206) demonstrated that this activity could be subserved by PTHrP derived from the fetus. The observations that PTH does not cross the placenta (207,208) and that PTH is not secreted in significant amounts during fetal life (208,209), have further supported a role for PTHrP as the fetal calciotropic hormone. Thus the majority of evidence now suggests that placental PTH/PTHrP receptors regulate placental calcium transport in response to PTHrP derived from the fetal parathyroid (205,206).

Parathyroid Cell Receptors for PTH

Parathyroid cells may express amino-terminal receptors for PTH, in view of recent observations that low (10^{-12} M) concentrations of PTH-(1–34) can inhibit PTH secretion from cultured bovine parathyroid cells (210).

Putative Parathyroid Hormone Receptors Not Related to Calcium and Phosphorus Metabolism

Amino-terminal PTH and/or PTH fragments have been shown to have biological activity in several cells and tissues that are not considered classical PTH targets. While the physiological role of these nonclassical activities is for the most part unclear, their existence confirms the widespread distribution of PTHrP and its receptors.

Vasodilation and Relaxation of Smooth Muscle

A hypotensive effect of PTH was noted in the first analysis of a biologically active parathyroid gland extract by Collip and Clark (212) and subsequently confirmed by several other investigators (reviewed in 213,214). The vascular effects of the hormone were called to modern attention by the work of Charbon (211), who demonstrated potent and rapid effects of the hormone on celiac and renal artery blood flow. The hypotensive effect has been demonstrated in many species and with the synthetic 1–34 fragment as well as the native hormone. Hypotension occurs as the result of vasodilatation, a direct effect on arterial resistance vessels (215,216), and is consistent with the ability of PTH to relax smooth muscle (214). The vasorelaxant effect of bPTH-(1–34) is associated with stimulation of adenylyl cyclase activity (214,217) and the subsequent cAMP-dependent inhibition of an L-type calcium channel (218). The effect does not require interaction with endothelial cells (217). The endocrine effects of PTH on vascular smooth muscle may be of less important physiological relevance than the local paracrine or autocrine interactions of PTHrP on this tissue, as PTHrP is abundantly expressed in blood vessel walls, and its expression is induced by angiotensin II and other vasoconstrictors such as serotonin and bradykinin (219).

PTH can induce relaxation of smooth muscle in sites other than blood vessels. Thus PTH has a direct relaxant effect on smooth muscle from uterus and vas deferens, trachea, and gastrointestinal (GI) tract smooth muscle (214). Myorelaxant effects of PTHrP have been noted in uterus in bladder. Finally, PTHrP stimulates cAMP production in a cell model recently described by Ferrari et al. (220) that may represent a model for mammary myoepithelial cells.

Lymphocyte Receptors for Parathyroid Hormone

MacManus et al. (221) presented the earliest suggestion that PTH receptors might be present on lymphocytes. These workers described the dose-related stimulation by PTH of cAMP accumulation in thymic lymphocytes (221). Early studies had analyzed binding of intact PTH to cultured B lymphocytes using a labeled antibody assay for amino-terminal PTH binding and showed a K_d in the 10^{-11}–10^{-10} M range (222). In other studies, Yamamoto et al. (223) demonstrated specific binding of [Nle^{8,18},^{125}I-Tyr^{34}]bPTH-(1–34)NH$_2$ to heterogeneous populations of circulating bovine lymphocytes and presented evidence suggesting that such cells possess a PTH-stimulated adenylyl cyclase activity. Using radioiodinated [Nle^{8,18},^{125}I-Tyr^{34}]bPTH-(1–34)NH$_2$ as radioligand, Yamamoto et al. (224) found that PTH receptors on circulating bovine lymphocytes had a ($\sim 10^{-9}$M K_d) binding affinity for amino-terminal

PTH similar to that of receptors in renal membranes, on intact rat osteosarcoma cells, and on OK cells. They further observed that PTH peptides activated adenylyl cyclase in lymphocytes in a manner similar to that which occurs in cells from classical PTH target tissues. On the other hand, studies in T lymphocytes ndicate that PTH causes an increase in [Ca^{2+}]$_i$ without stimulating an increase in cAMP (225). Thus there are at least two different types of responses in cells of the lymphocyte series, one that involves adenylyl cyclase and one that does not. Recently it was shown that PTH-(1–84) stimulated phytohemagglutinin (PHA)-induced proliferation of T cells in a dose-dependent manner (226). The physiological significance of PTH binding sites on lymphocytes is not clear, but it has been shown that T lymphocytes can synthesize PTHrP (227), and it has been suggested that PTHrP may serve as an autocrine growth factor for T lymphocytes (225,228).

Parathyroid Hormone Receptors in Skin

Goldring et al. (229) were the first to suggest that dermal fibroblasts expressed PTH receptors, when they demonstrated that PTH stimulated adenylyl cyclase in fibroblasts from human skin. Pun and colleagues (40,230) have provided direct evidence for the presence of binding sites for human and bovine PTH-(1–34) in human dermal fibroblasts. The K_d for these sites is similar to that in classical PTH target tissues, ~ 1 nM (230). In the CRL 1564 human dermal fibroblast cell line, a second, lower affinity site (Kd 1.5 μM) was also found, not linked to adenylyl cyclase and of unknown significance (230). It is currently thought that the high-affinity binding sites represent targets for PTHrP that is released in a paracrine fashion from nearby keratinocytes (231). On the other hand, an autocrine role for PTHrP produced by keratinocytes is suggested by experiments showing that PTH-(1–34) stimulates PKC in these cells. Surprisingly, PTH does not stimulate adenylyl cyclase in mouse epidermal keratinocytes (232). This latter observation cannot be explained on the basis of current information regarding the cloned amino-terminal PTH/PTHrP receptor and raises the question of whether different receptors are expressed in keratinocytes or whether the differences in signaling pathways reflect cell (or species)-specific postreceptor differences. Immunohistological studies have demonstrated PTHrP in normal human skin, in cells of the prickle cell layer of skin, and in the cells of hair follicles (233).

Parathyroid Hormone Receptors on Adipocytes

Sinha et al. (235) observed dose-dependent stimulation of lipolysis by PTH in isolated human fat cells.

Dose–response curves for PTH-stimulated adenylyl cyclase activity in fat tissue suggest that the fat cell expresses a PTH receptor with binding affinity similar to that of amino-terminal PTH/PTHrP receptors in classical target tissues (234). PTH produces significant increases in glycerol production in human adipocytes at hormone concentrations as low as 10^{-9} M. Moreover, glycerol production is accompanied by a dose-related increase in cAMP content; effects are seen with both PTH-(1–84) and PTH-(1–34) (235). In vivo infusions of parathyroid extract to normal volunteers consistently produced transient increases in plasma free fatty acids (235). PTH may also affect lipid removal from plasma (236) and may also impair oxidation of fatty acids in target tissues (237). It is difficult to be definitive about the physiological significance of the PTH response in fat tissue, but the role of PTH in lipid metabolism is an anabolic one and has been linked to the general anabolic effects of PTH (238) and may play a role in the hyperlipidemia associated with chronic renal failure (236).

Pancreatic Parathyroid Hormone Receptors

Parathyroid hormone augments glucose-stimulated insulin release from normal rat pancreatic islets (239). It has also been shown that PTHrP is expressed in normal human and rat pancreatic islets (240,241). PTHrP binds specifically to rat insulinoma cells with a K_d in the 100 nM range. As in keratinocytes, PTH does not activate adenylyl cyclase (241) but does activate PKC (242).

Parathyroid Hormone Receptors in Brain

When bovine PTH-(1–34) was administered to rats in vivo, it induced calcium transport in brain synaptosomes independently of adenylyl cyclase (243). Also, it has been shown that PTHrP is expressed in mammalian brain. Brain adenylyl cyclase-stimulating activity could be detected in brain extracts that was inhibitable by anti-PTHrP but not anti-PTH antibodies, suggesting the production of PTHrP by brain (244). The data suggest the possibility of PTHrP paracrine or autocrine loops in brain. PTHrP transcripts could be localized to neurons of the hippocampus and cerebral cortex (244).

Liver Receptors for Parathyroid Hormone

The first demonstrated role for the liver in PTH action was that of hepatic uptake and metabolism of intact PTH (254–247). Uptake of PTH is selective for intact PTH rather than its fragments (246), and this uptake has been shown to occur specifically in Kuppfer cells (see the chapter by Kronenberg et al.) (181). Kuppfer cells metabolize intact PTH to C-terminal fragments by endopeptidase cleavage; hepatocytes do not metabolize the hormone (248). Hepatic uptake and/or enzymatic cleavage of PTH is blocked by bPTH-(28–48) (249). The subject of hepatic metabolism of PTH has been reviewed by Martin et al. (250).

The earliest indication that PTH could generate a biological response in liver was suggested by the finding that PTH-(1–84), but not PTH-(1–34), stimulates hepatic glucose release in dogs in vivo (251). The significance of this finding is not clear, because the specific uptake mechanism for intact PTH is in Kuppfer cells rather than hepatocytes. It seems likely that this observation reflected a nonphysiological effect. Nonetheless, amino-terminal and intact PTH can interact with liver tissue to activate adenylyl cyclase (245). In 1980, Neuman and Schneider (252) showed that both intact PTH and its amino-terminal 1–34 fragment stimulated adenylyl cyclase in rat liver. Intact PTH exhibited greater ability to activate adenylyl cyclase than PTH-(1–34), but direct binding studies of intact PTH to liver membranes showed binding of very low affinity ($K_d \sim 10^{-5}$ M) (252). Subsequent studies by Bergeron et al. (253) demonstrated that PTH was less effective than glucagon in stimulating hepatic adenylyl cyclase activity. Much later studies have demonstrated that PTH is capable of binding with low affinity to glucagon receptors in rat liver membranes (254), and the aggregate data suggest that some of the binding and adenylyl-cyclase-stimulating activity of PTH in rat liver may be mediated by the glucagon receptor rather than the PTH receptor.

In vivo binding of PTH-(1–34) and PTH-(1–84) to liver tissue was demonstrated autoradiographically by Goltzman and coworkers (181,253). Whereas binding of both PTH ligands occurred on hepatocytes and sinusoidal cells, only PTH-(1–84) bound to Kuppfer cells. Thus there are also specific receptors for amino-terminal PTH on hepatocytes. The binding sites on Kuppfer cells are clearly linked to degradation of circulating PTH. The biological actions associated with the amino-terminal PTH/PTHrP receptors on hepatocytes remain to be elucidated but appear to be linked to adenylyl cyclase. Further investigation of these questions is necessary, but at present no physiological role for PTH in the liver has been identified.

Parathyroid Hormone Actions That May Be Mediated by Amino-Terminal Ligand Receptors

Both PTH-(1–34) and PTH-(1–84), but not the 53–84 fragment, have chronotropic effects on cultured rat heart cells (255) and increase erythrocyte osmotic fragility in vitro (256).

Receptors Specific for the Midmolecular Region (28–48) of Parathyroid Hormone

Recent studies by Mayer and coworkers (257) have focused attention on the middle portion of the PTH molecule as a potentially bioactive region of PTH. Initially it was demonstrated that midregion fragments possessed mitogenic activity in chondrocytes and in a kidney cell line and that this activity was independent of cAMP (257). Detailed studies using a series of smaller fragments showed that PTH residues 30–34 defined a core region for mitogenic activity. Later studies demonstrated that bPTH-(28–48) and other midregion fragments are capable of stimulating creatine kinase activity and cell proliferation in rat calvarial cells and ROS 17/2.8 cells in vitro (129,258). Human PTH-(28–48) does not bind to the amino-terminal receptor for PTH-(1–34) (76). On the other hand, Mayer (259) has recently studied the binding of ^{27}Tyr-hPTH-(28–48) to ROS 17/2.8 cells and found specific competition for binding by hPTH-(28–48); hPTH-(1–34) was tenfold less potent than hPTH-(28–48) in competing for binding (259). At the same time, hPTH-(28–48) does not activate adenylyl cyclase at any dose but does activate PKC (123). The data suggest the possibility of a separate receptor for the midregion 28–48 portion of the PTH molecule. Another potentially significant function of the midregion of PTH was suggested by earlier in vivo studies, which demonstrated that hepatic extraction of intact PTH from blood and its subsequent degradation depended on the 28–48 region (260).

Receptors Specific for the Carboxyl-Terminal 53–84 Region

Studies in the 1970s of bovine (4) or human (261) PTH-(53–84) fragments showed that these molecules lacked either hypercalcemic activity or renal adenylyl cyclase activity. From these early observations it has generally been concluded that the carboxyl-terminal region of the PTH molecule is biologically inactive. In 1980, Arber et al. (271) first suggested that carboxyl-terminal PTH fragments might have biological activity. Using a cytochemical assay to detect PTH activity, they showed that guinea pig kidney slices contained two peaks of activity, one associated with PTH-(1–34) and a later peak associated with hPTH-(53–84) stimulation; PTH-(1–84) produced activity in both peaks (271). This early study of the effects of carboxyl-terminal PTH, published in abstract form only, went largely unnoticed. However, many later PTH receptor binding studies in which intact PTH radioligands were used to analyze receptors in kidney and bone disclosed that binding to the amino-terminal receptor for PTH-(1–34) could not account for all the binding of intact hormone to target tissue, strongly suggesting the ex-

istence of additional hormone binding sites for epitopes distal to residue 35 (10,12,81,170–172). Two of these studies from Murray's laboratory have demonstrated that hPTH-(53–84) is capable of competitively inhibiting the binding of intact radiolabeled bPTH-(1–84) to target tissues (12,81). It was also shown that competition isotherms of intact PTH binding to dog (10) or chick (81) renal membranes generated biphasic Scatchard plots, indicating the presence of two binding sites for intact PTH. The affinity and capacity of the high-affinity site were similar to the high-affinity binding observed when amino-terminal fragments were used as radioligands (64,74) (see above). In addition, a lower affinity site was also observed that matched closely in affinity and capacity the parameters observed when the binding of intact hormone tracer was competitively inhibited by hPTH-(53–84) (81). This study also showed differences between the amino-terminal and carboxyl-terminal binding sites in chicken kidney membranes in stability of receptors during storage at $-20°C$ and in regulation of their binding activity by guanyl nucleotides and magnesium (81). Also, while the amino-terminal site was linked to stimulation of adenylyl cyclase, the carboxyl-terminal site was not. In another study, 72% of the binding of radiolabeled intact hormone to ROS 17/2.8 rat osteosarcoma cells could be competitively inhibited by hPTH-(53–84) compared to only ~20% by PTH-(1–34) or [Nle^{8,18},Tyr^{34}]b PTH-(1–34)NH$_2$ (12) (see Fig. 4). At the same time, hPTH-(53–84) did not activate adenylyl cyclase in these osteoblastic cells. All these observations suggested the existence of distinct carboxyl-terminal receptors for PTH in classical target tissues that were not linked to adenylyl cyclase and were of unknown physiological function. To date it has not been possible, however, to show specific binding of a radiolabeled carboxyl-terminal PTH fragment radioligand to PTH target tissues. For example, unpublished information from several laboratories, including our own, indicates that radioiodinated [^{52}Tyr]hPTH-(53–84) does not bind to PTH target tissues. This may be due to a combination of methodological problems. First, there is the possibility that radioiodination induces conformational changes in carboxyl-terminal PTH fragments that alter their binding properties. Second, in bone, carboxyl-terminal binding sites may be expressed only during specific stages of osteoblast differentiation. This would make it difficult to demonstrate specific binding in mixed cell populations, especially if the proportion of cells with carboxyl-terminal PTH receptors is small.

For some time little significance was attributed to these observations of carboxyl-terminal PTH binding. Recently, however, Murray et al. (262,263) have shown that hPTH-(53–84) is capable of stimulating alkaline phosphatase (ALP) activity in dexamethasone-treated ROS 17/2.8 cells in a dose- and time-dependent

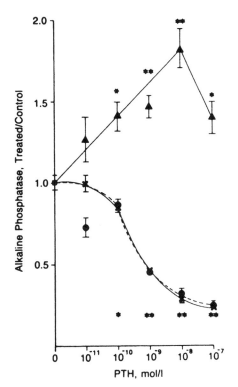

FIG. 5. Stimulation by hPTH-(53–84) (▲) and inhibition by bPTH-(1–84) (●) and bPTH-(1–34) (×) of alkaline phosphatase activity in dexamethasone-treated ROS 17/2.8 cells. $P < 0.01$, $**P < 0.001$, significantly different from zero added hormone. Pooled data from three experiments. There is significant dose-related stimulation of enzyme activity by the carboxyl-terminal hPTH-(53–84) fragment, the opposite of the inhibitory effect of either the amino-terminal bPTH-(1–34) or the intact bPTH-(1–84) hormone. From Murray et al. (262).

fashion (see Fig. 5). These findings have now been confirmed and extended by Nakamoto et al. (264), who also used this system to study the effects of a series of truncated C-terminal fragments. The major ALP-stimulatory activity appears to reside within the residues 53–68; the 69–84 fragment was inhibitory in this system, as was the 1–34 fragment (264). Murray et al. (265) have also observed that hPTH-(53–84) can regulate expression of several genes in SaOS-2 human osteosarcoma cells, including ALP, osteocalcin, and

the vitamin D receptor. Table 1 compares the distinctive pattern of gene regulation in these osteoblastic cells by hPTH-(53–84) and by either intact hormone or PTH-(1–34). These latter observations were made in the absence of added corticosteroid. Thus corticosteroids are not an absolute requirement for this effect. A likely explanation for the observation that physiological doses of dexamethasone are required for stimulation of ALP in ROS 17/2.8 cells is that the physiological concentrations of corticosteroid used in the ROS cell experiments promote cell differentiation in vitro, as discussed above. It is also notable that, for both ALP-stimulating activity and gene regulation, the activity of hPTH-(53–84) was clearly distinguishable from that of either bPTH-(1–34) or bPTH-(1–84) (262–265). Thus hPTH-(53–84) stimulated ALP activity in ROS 17/2.8 cells, while in concurrent experiments bPTH-(1–34) inhibited ALP activity (262–264). In the SaOS-2 experiments, hPTH-(53–84) stimulated the expression of ALP and osteocalcin mRNAs without any effect on type 1 procollagen expression, whereas hPTH-(1–34) had a strong stimulatory effect on type I procollagen expression without any significant effect on the expression of either ALP or osteocalcin mRNA (265). Silbermann et al. (266) also showed that hPTH-(53–84) has specific effects in a model of mouse endochondral bone formation; the addition of the carboxyl-terminal PTH peptide produced resorptive changes. In this study, PTH-(1–34), hPTH-(28–48), and hPTH-(53–84) each had distinct effects.

All these recent studies contradict earlier findings that hPTH-(53–84) is biologically inactive and suggest that the carboxyl-terminal region of PTH has significant and distinct regulatory effects in bone. The signaling pathway for the action of this region of PTH is not known. It does not stimulate adenylyl cyclase (12) or PKC (123) in ROS 17/2.8 cells.

Other recent studies have shown that the carboxyl-terminal portion of PTH is essential for normal processing and secretion of the intact hormone (267). Thus there appear to be at least two separate roles for the carboxyl-terminal region of the hormone in PTH physiology. Additional evidence in support of an important biological activity for the late carboxyl-terminal region

TABLE 1. *Effects of PTH peptides on gene expression in SaOS-2 cells[a]*

Peptide	ALP	Osteocalcin	Type 1 collagen	Vitamin D receptor
hPTH-(53–84)	1.53 (0.22)*	1.33 (0.12)*	1.11 (0.17)	1.31 (0.17)*
bPTH-(1–84)	1.08 (0.13)	1.09 (0.08)	1.56 (0.25)*	1.76 (0.19)*
bPTH-(1–34)	1.04 (0.11)	1.32 (0.26)	1.87 (0.24)*	1.55 (0.14)*

[a]SaOS-2 cells were grown to confluence, then treated with PTH peptides at a concentration of 10 nM. Total RNA was then extracted and subjected to slot blot hybridization analysis. Values are expressed as treated/control ratios. The pattern of gene regulation after treatment with hPTH-(53–84) is quite different from that of PTH-(1–34) or PTH-(1–84). Data are from Murray et al. (265).

*Different from 1.0 at $P < .05$.

has been provided by experiments in which deamidation of residue 76 of human PTH resulted in considerable reduction of potency of the hormone (268). Also, the carboxyl-terminal region contributes significant inhibitor potency, in that hPTH-(3–84) was found to be 100 times more potent as an inhibitor in the renal cytochemical bioassay than hPTH-(3–34) (269). Recently Massry et al. (270) found that the carboxyl-terminal fragment bPTH-(19–84), but not bPTH-(1–34), stimulates elastase release from human polymorphonuclear leukocytes.

IMPLICATIONS FOR PATHOPHYSIOLOGICAL RELEVANCE OF UNCONVENTIONAL PARATHYROID HORMONE RECEPTORS

It appears that the amino-terminal PTH-PTHrP receptor mediates a variety of nonclassical biological effects of PTH in diverse tissues. Furthermore, different biological activities may be ascribed to different amino-terminal, midmolecular, and carboxyl-terminal domains of the hormone, as summarized in Table 2.

Because the secretion of PTH (and probably its fragments) is regulated by changes in the serum calcium concentration, overall concepts of the significance of unconventional PTH–PTHrP receptor interactions must take into consideration whether the interaction is modulated by serum calcium levels in vivo. Moreover, it is unknown whether bioactive PTH fragments are generated within the parathyroid gland, locally in target tissues, or, in both sites, in response to other signals. At present there is no coherent evidence for physiological roles of most of these interactions with unconventional PTH receptors. However, the diversity of the observations we have summarized here should encourage some speculation, and this section discusses some possible implications.

Interaction of Parathyroid Hormone with Local Tissue Parathyroid Hormone-Related Protein Response Systems

For bone and kidney, native PTH-(1–84) is likely to be the ligand of major physiological significance, particularly in view of the major classical interactions of PTH with these tissues. Specifically, parathyroidectomy results in major alterations in renal handling of calcium and phosphorus and in bone turnover. In spite of these obvious major interactions, it is quite possible that PTHrP, produced locally, also interacts with these same receptors under physiological conditions in which the local tissue concentration of PTHrP might exceed the local concentration of PTH. Further in vivo studies will be necessary to explore these possibilities.

There are several cells and tissues that have not

TABLE 2. *Effects of PTH peptides from three hormonal domains*

	1–34	28–48	53–84
Ca^{2+} metabolism	+	– [a]	–
Adenylyl cyclase	↑	–	–
DNA synthesis	↑	↑	–
Protein kinase C	↑	↑	–
Alkaline phosphatase in dexamethasone-treated ROS 17/2.8 cells	↓	n.t.[b]	↑

[a] –, No effect.
[b] n.t., Not tested.

been considered classical PTH targets in which amino-terminal PTH and/or PTH fragments have been shown to have biological activity. For some of these sites, it is possible that experimental responses to PTH may result from nonphysiological interaction of PTH with receptors that under normal physiological circumstances are activated by locally produced PTHrP in a paracrine or autocrine fashion. The indirect evidence for PTHrP receptors in nonclassical target tissues has been recently reviewed by Orloff et al. (55). More recent in situ hybridization studies have demonstrated expression of mRNA encoding PTH/PTHrP receptors in aorta, adrenal gland, bladder, brain, breast, heart, liver, lung, skeletal muscle, ovary, placenta, skin, spleen, stomach, and testis, in addition to bone and kidney, of normal rats (56). For a particular biological effect to be attributed to a PTHrP autocrine/paracrine loop, several criteria should be met: (a) PTHrP should be shown to be produced locally in the area, either in cells neighboring the target cells or in the target cells themselves; (b) a PTH/PTHrP receptor should be demonstrable, preferably by in situ hybridization, in the target cells; and (c) the hormonal action should not be regulated by changes in serum calcium in animals with intact parathyroids. Although such studies have only begun, the colocalization of expression of PTHrP and the PTH/PTHrP receptor to the same tissue may ultimately be a difficult criterion to satisfy. For example, the respective mRNAs for PTHrP and its receptor are expressed in various tissues in the developing rat fetus, but, while they are often expressed in the same tissue, they are not necessarily expressed together at the same time of development, suggesting that such local paracrine loops may function only for limited periods during fetal development (272). Despite the widespread tissue distribution of both PTHrP (53,54) and PTH/PTHrP receptors (56), there are few if any examples that fulfill the criteria defined above for local tissue autocrine or paracrine PTHrP systems. However, blood vessels, lymphocytes, brain, and pancreatic islets are examples of sites in which paracrine/autocrine effects of PTHrP/PTH are likely to be documented. The relaxant effect of PTH on arterial smooth muscle may be an example of the interation of PTH with a local PTHrP system in that (a) PTHrP is produced locally in vascular smooth muscle (273); this relaxant effect can be elicited by the amino-terminal 1–34 region of PTHrP (274); and (b) PTHrP receptors are expressed in arterial walls (56). On the other hand, the response of blood pressure to changes in serum calcium implies that PTH rather than PTHrP may be the active hormone in some cases. Perhaps the outstanding feature that would differentiate PTH (and PTH fragments) from PTHrP physiologically in vivo is that PTH and C-terminal PTH fragments are produced by the parathyroid gland and may be secreted in response to changes in serum Ca^{2+} concentration. This property should be utilized in experiments designed to delineate further the physiological relevance of the various PTH and PTHrP peptides in a way that putative physiological effects may be correlated with change in PTH.

Parathyroid Hormone as a Polyhormone

With new and diverse information implicating biological activities in various structural domains of the hormone, it is difficult to summarize this information within a simple context of hormonal activity that fits a single physicochemical or biological concept. It seems that, in particular, some of the observations concerning active midregion and carboxyl-terminal epitopes may be explained more readily by a concept involving separately active PTH fragments. Such a concept has recently been advanced by Mallette (275) (see also the chapter "Parathyroid Hormone and Parathyroid Hormone-Related Protein as Polyhormones," by Mallette). He suggests that both PTH and PTHrP are polyhormones, proteins that contain several different functional epitopes that may each be separately regulated under unique different circumstances. Thus PTHrP has been shown to have a PTH-like amino-terminal domain that can regulate mineral homeostasis through skeletal and renal receptors (see above), a midmolecular domain (residues 67–86) that is capable of regulating placental calcium transport (206), and a carboxyl-terminal domain that can regulate the function of isolated osteoclasts (276). Similarly, PTH may have three separate domains, the amino-terminal domain subserving the regulation of calcium and phosphorus metabolism, a midmolecular domain regulating cell replication and osteogenesis, and a carboxyl-terminal domain regulating osteoblast function or differentiation. Currently available data related to activities of these various epitopes are summarized in Table 2. This polyhormone hypothesis remains undeveloped at present and requires much further investigation.

Receptors for the Carboxyl-Terminal 53–84 Region

At present the physiological significance of the binding sites for this region of the hormone and their related biological activities are unknown. However, several specific bone responses, including augmentation of ALP activity (262,263), ALP mRNA levels, and osteocalcin mRNA levels (265) in the absence of a concomitant mitogenic effect (277), suggest either a stimulatory effect on the function of differentiated osteoblasts or an effect on osteoblast differentiation.

It is important to point out that under physiological circumstances significant concentrations of carboxyl-terminal PTH fragments are present in the blood. Thus it has been shown in three different species, bovine, canine, and human, that, when blood calcium is normal, the serum concentration of carboxyl-terminal PTH fragments is three- to tenfold greater than that of intact PTH (278). Furthermore, the relative concentrations of at least some carboxyl-terminal PTH fragments are regulated by changes in plasma calcium, such that in hypocalcemia the relative concentration of intact hormone is greater, whereas in hypercalcemia the relative proportion of carboxyl-terminal PTH fragments increases in the circulation (278–281). The same effects have been observed in vitro: incubation of cultured bovine parathyroid cells in high-calcium medium leads to release of a higher proportion of carboxyl-terminal fragments than incubation in low-calcium medium (282,283). It is possible that there is some physiological importance to calcium-regulated changes in the ratio of carboxyl-terminal/intact PTH released from parathyroid tissue and also that these changes play some role in the syndrome of malignancy-associated hypercalcemia. A recent study has demonstrated that the increase in carboxyl-terminal fragments that normally occurs with hypercalcemia does not seem to occur in primary hyperparathyroidism (284), although even in hyperparathyroidism there is a preponderance of carboxyl-terminal PTH fragments in the circulation (284,285).

Activities of Various Parathyroid Hormone Epitopes in Endochondral Bone Formation

Studies by Silbermann et al. (266) in the developing mouse mandibular condyle suggest that epitopes in the mid- and carboxyl-terminal regions of the hormone may have distinctive actions in normal endochondral bone formation. This process takes place in an orderly sequence, involving replication of chondroprogenitors, hypertrophy of chondrocytes, mineralization of the cartilage, and resorption (198). In the Silbermann et al. studies, hPTH-(1–34) stimulated cell proliferation in the layer of proliferating chondrocyte precursors, whereas the addition of hPTH-(28–48) to hPTH-(1–34) augmented the layer of hypertrophic chondrocytes and their mineralization. The further addition of hPTH-(53–84) to the other two fragments induced a separate later phase, perhaps involving resorption (266). On the other hand, hPTH-(53–84) had no effects on either mitogenicity or morphology when added alone to these cultures (286). The effect of PTH on chondrocytes depends on their anatomical location; while the hormone has strong specificity for growth plate chondrocytes, it has no effects on articular chondrocytes (287). PTH is also capable of promoting differentiation in costal chondrocyte cultures (288).

Psychiatric Symptoms Associated With Hyperparathyroidism

Mental and psychological symptoms are observed not infrequently in hyperparathyroidism (289), especially when they are sought by specialized testing (290). These symptoms are believed by some to be alleviated after successful parathyroidectomy (see the chapter by Kleerekoper) (290). Elevated levels of intracellular calcium have been demonstrated in normal rats treated with PTH-(1–84) and PTH (1–34) (291), and also in brain synaptosomes of hyperparathyroid rats with chronic renal failure (292). Although some of these symptoms in subjects with primary hyperparathyroidism may be due to elevated serum levels of calcium, it is possible that some (or all) of the psychiatric symptoms are mediated via activation of PTH/PTHrP receptors in brain.

Genetic Hypertension in Rats

Studies in spontaneously hypertensive (SHR) rats show subtle abnormalities in responsiveness to both PTH and PTHrP in comparison to normotensive Wistar controls (293). It was suggested that these abnormalities (fourfold higher PTH levels without differences in serum calcium concentration, reduced numbers of renal PTH/PTHrP receptors, and decreased chronotropic responses to PTH) implicate the amino-terminal PTH/PTHrP receptor in regulation of blood pressure. In these studies, the relative hypotensive effects of PTH and PTHrP did not differ between SHR rats and Wistar controls. However, the difference in circulating PTH levels implicates PTH in this syndrome and points to the importance of PTH/PTHrP receptors in the modulation of blood pressure. In further support of this hypothesis are the findings that serum PTH is also elevated in the Dahl salt-sensitive (DS) rat and the John Rapp DS strain rat (294). In humans, hypertension occurs in 22–56% of subjects with primary hyperparathyroidism (295); moreover, hyperparathyroidism was diagnosed in seven of 900 patients with

hypertension (296). However, there is no direct evidence that hypertension is abolished or reduced by surgical correction of hyperparathyroidism (see the chapters by Bilezikian et al. and Kleerekoper). While modest decreases in blood pressure have been noted after parathyroid surgery in some reports (297), other reports have not confirmed such reductions (298). In a recent prospective study of 56 patients with primary hyperparathyroidism who were followed for a period of 60 months postparathyroidectomy, none of the 21.8% of patients with preoperative hypertension became normotensive, while 32% of the normotensive patients became hypertensive during follow-up (298). In the patients who were hypertensive preoperatively, midregion PTH levels were more than threefold higher than in normotensive patients ($P = .018$), while preoperative creatinine levels were lower ($P < .002$) (298).

Carbohydrate Intolerance: Possible Role of Pancreatic Parathyroid Hormone/Parathroid Hormone-Related Protein Receptors

Carbohydrate intolerance is common in patients with chronic renal failure (299). Massry and coworkers (300) have studied glucose tolerance in uremic dogs using intravenous glucose tolerance tests and both euglycemic and hyperglycemic clamps. These workers found a strong association between abnormal carbohydrate tolerance and parathyroid hyperfunction; there was a clear relationship between elevated PTH and decreased insulin secretion and no evidence for increased metabolic clearance of insulin (300). Furthermore, in perifused pancreas from rats with chronic renal failure, dynamic insulin secretion was reduced, an abnormality that was reversed by parathyroidectomy (307). Abnormalities in carbohydrate tolerance have also been observed in primary hyperparathyroidism (302–304). In view of the evidence cited above suggesting the presence of PTHrP receptors and PTHrP expression in pancreas, it is conceivable that these situations represent the interaction of pathologically high concentrations of PTH with tissue-specific paracrine or autocrine mechanism(s) involving PTHrP. In one of these reports, six of nine patients showed an improvement in carbohydrate tolerance following surgical correction of the hyperparathyroidism (303). On the other hand, a large clinical study in 441 patients with primary hyperparathyroidism (305) showed that, although there was enhanced insulin response to glucose in patients with primary hyperparathyroidism, the effect was relatively mild. In 26 of these patients studied prospectively, surgical correction of the hyperparathyroidism did not alter fasting blood glucose, hemoglobin A_{1c} values, or insulin requirements (294). Thus, while pancreatic PTH receptors may be involved in the glucose intolerance associated with either primary or secondary hyperparathyroidism, no evidence has yet been provided that establishes this directly.

Treatment of Osteoporosis

Synthetic amino-terminal fragments of PTH have been proposed as a treatment for osteoporosis for well over a decade on the basis of animal experiments (167,168,306) and clinical trials (see the chapter by Marcus) (307–309). Recent structure–function studies have suggested that the anabolic effects of PTH may be exerted preferentially by peptides that activate PKC and include domain(s) of the hormone encompassing the 28–34 region (123,124). It has been proposed that PTH analogs that take advantage of this property may be clinically useful in the treatment of osteoporosis (123). This suggestion is especially interesting in that some recent therapeutic trials of PTH-(1–34) have shown a plateau in the anabolic response associated with cortical bone loss; it has been postulated that agents that do not activate adenylyl cyclase may be anabolic in vivo but have relatively less bone resorption activity. Further in vivo studies of this issue are necessary.

Liver Regeneration

Experiments reported in 1971 by Rixon and Whitfield (310), in which liver regeneration after partial hepatectomy was blocked by parathyroidectomy, have implicated PTH in the process of liver regeneration. These initial experiments left open the question of whether the effect of parathyroidectomy was due to the induced hypocalcemia or was the effect of the removal of PTH. Subsequent experiments and reanalysis suggested that some of the acute effects of TPTX also may be related to calcitonin deficiency and concluded that the major effect of PTH in liver regeneration is probably indirect and is a result of its effects on serum calcium and phosphorus concentrations (311). On the other hand, more recent data indicate that PTH can have a significant effect on hepatic IGF-I production (312). Thus the mechanism of liver regeneration following partial hepatectomy should be re-evaluated with regard to the interaction of IGF-I, and other growth factors, either produced locally or liberated from bone in response to PTH (see the chapter by Canalis et al.).

SUMMARY

The cloning of the cDNA for the common amino-terminal receptor for PTH/PTHrP present in bone and kidney has greatly advanced our understanding of the major interactions of PTH with its target tissues in the regulation of calcium and phosphorus metabolism. On the other hand, this single hormone–receptor interaction does not explain many observations regarding the interaction between PTH and nonclassical target tissues or the observations of interactions between PTH fragments comprising residues beyond the 1–34 region with target tissues. It is entirely possible that there is more than one type of amino-terminal receptor for PTH and/or PTHrP. While PTH/PTHrP receptors may be expressed in a variety of tissues, and may mediate a number of nonclassical activities of PTH, none of these activities can be assigned a definite physiological role at present. The many discoveries that have emerged recently have opened up this field and will no doubt spark further interest. It is likely that the field of nonclassical activities of PTH will continue to expand.

Of particular interest is the possibility of a distinct physiological role for carboxyl-terminal PTH fragments, since, in addition to having distinct biological activities in vitro, these fragments circulate in high enough concentrations to activate some of these responses, and their concentrations may be regulated by the serum calcium concentration. This area should also be an important one for further study.

ACKNOWLEDGMENT

The authors are grateful to Dr. Robert Josse for his critical review of the manuscript.

REFERENCES

1. Murray TM. Parathyroid hormone and hyperparathyroidism. In: *Metabolic bone disease: cellular and tissue mechanisms.* CS Tam, JNM Heersche, TM Murray, eds. Boca Raton, FL: CRC Press, 1989;106–113.
2. Aurbach GD, Marx SJ, Spiegel AM. Parathyroid hormone, calcitonin, and the calciferols. In: *Williams textbook of endocrinology,* 8th ed. JD Wilson, DW Foster, eds. Philadelphia: WB Saunders, 1992;1406–1415.
3. Parfitt AM. The actions of parathyroid hormone on bone: relation to bone remodeling and turnover, calcium homeostasis, and metabolic bone disease (review). *Metabolism* 1976;25:809–844, 904–955ff.
4. Potts JT Jr, Murray TM, Peacock M, et al. Parathyroid hormone: sequence, synthesis, and immunoassay studies. *Am J Med* 1971;50:639–649.
5. Tregear GW, van Reitschoten J, Saver R, et al. Bovine parathyroid hormone: minimum chain length for biological activity. *Biochemistry* 1977;16:2817–2823.
6. Habener JF, Rosenblatt M, Potts JT Jr. Parathyroid hormone: biochemical aspects of biosynthesis, secretion, action, and metabolism. *Physiol Rev* 1984;64:985–1053.
7. Goltzman D, Peytremann A, Callahan EN, Segre GV, Potts JT Jr. Metabolism and biological activity of parathyroid hormone in renal cortical membranes. *J Clin Invest* 1976;57:8.
8. Goltzman D. Examination of the requirement for metabolism of parathyroid hormone in skeletal tissue before biological action. *Endocrinology* 1978;102:1555.
9. Calvo MS, Fryer MJ, Laakso KJ, et al. Structural requirements for parathyroid hormone action in mature bone: effects on release of cyclic adenosine monophosphate and

bone gamma-carboxyglutamic acid-containing protein from perfused rat hindquarters. *J Clin Invest* 1985;76:2348–2354.

10. Rizzoli RE, Murray TM, Marx SJ, Aurbach GD. Binding of radioiodinated bone parathyroid hormone-(1–84) to canine renal cortical membranes. *Endocrinology* 1983;112:1303–1312.

11. Rizzoli RE, Somerman M, Murray TM, Aurbach GD. Binding of radioiodinated parathyroid hormone to cloned bone cells. *Endocrinology* 1983;113:1832.

12. Rao LG, Murray TM. Binding of intact parathyroid hormone to rat osteosarcoma cells: major contribution of binding sites for the carboxyl-terminal region of the hormone. *Endocrinology* 1985;117:1632–1638.

13. Goltzman D, Henderson B, Loveridge N. Cytochemical bioassay of parathyroid hormone: characteristics of the assay and analysis of circulating hormonal forms. *J Clin Invest* 1980;65:1309.

14. Draper MW. The structure of parathyroid hormone; its effects on biological action. *Mineral Electrolyte Metab* 1982;8:159–172.

15. Rosenblatt M. Pre-proparathyroid hormone, proparathyroid hormone, and parathyroid hormone: the biologic role of hormone structure. *Clin Orthop Rel Res* 1982;170:260–276.

16. Cohen FE, Strewler GJ, Bradley S, et al. Analogs of parathyroid hormone modified at positions 3 and 6: effective receptor binding and activation of adenylyl cyclase in kidney and bone. *J Biol Chem* 1991;266:1997–2004.

17. Gardella TJ, Axelrod D, Rubin D, et al. Mutational analysis of the receptor-activating region of human parathyroid hormone. *J Biol Chem* 1991;266:13141–13146.

18. Gardella TJ, Wilson AK, Keutmann HT, et al. Analysis of parathyroid hormone's principal receptor-binding region by site-directed mutagenesis and analog design. *Endocrinology* 1993;132:2024–2030.

19. Reppe S, Gabrielsen OS, Olstad OK, et al. Characterization of a K26Q site-directed mutant of human parathyroid hormone expressed in yeast. *J Biol Chem* 1991;266:14198–14201.

20. Juppner H, Abou-Samra A-B, Freeman M, et al. A G-protein-linked receptor for parathyroid hormone and parathyroid hormone-related peptide. *Science* 1991;254:1024–1026.

21. Abou-Samra A-B, Juppner H, Force T, et al. Expression cloning of a common receptor for parathyroid hormone and parathyroid hormone-related peptide from rat osteoblast-like cells: a single receptor stimulates intracellular accumulation of both cAMP and inositol trisphosphates and increases intracellular free calcium. *Proc Natl Acad Sci USA* 1992;89:2732–2736.

22. Burtis WJ, Wu T, Bunch C, et al. Identification of a novel 17,000-dalton parathyroid hormone-like adenylate cyclase-stimulating protein from a tumour associated with humoral hypercalcemia of malignancy. *J Biol Chem* 1987;262:7151–7156.

23. Moseley JM, Kubota M, Diefenbach-Jagger H, et al. Parathyroid hormone-related protein purified from a human lung cancer cell line. *Proc Natl Acad Sci USA* 1987;84:5048–5052.

24. Strewler GJ, Stern PH, Jacobs JW, et al. Parathyroid hormone-like protein from human renal carcinoma cells: structural and functional homology with parathyroid hormone. *J Clin Invest* 1987;80:1803–1807.

25. Stewart AF, Wu T, Goumas D, Burtis WJ, Broadus AE. N-terminal amino acid sequence of two novel tumor-derived ac1-stimulating proteins: identification of parathyroid hormone-like and parathyroid hormone-unlike domains. *Biochem Biophys Res Commun* 1987;146:672–678.

26. Suva LJ, Winslow GA, Wettenhall RE. A parathyroid hormone-related protein implicated in malignant hypercalcemia: cloning and expression. *Science* 1987;237:893–896.

27. Mangin M, Webb AC, Dreyer BE, et al. Identification of a cDNA encoding a parathyroid hormone-like peptide from a human tumor associated with hypercalcemia of malignancy. *Proc Natl Acad Sci USA* 1988;85:597–601.

28. Mangin M, Ikeda K, Dreyer BE, Broadus AE. Isolation and characterization of the human parathyroid hormone-like peptide gene. *Proc Natl Acad Sci USA* 1989;86:2408–2412.

29. Broadus AE, Mangin M, Isogna KL, Weir EC, Burtis WJ, Stewart AF. Humoral hypercalcemia of cancer: identification of a novel parathyroid hormone-like peptide. *N Engl J Med* 1988;319:556–563.

30. Lebo RV, Cheung M-C, Bruce BD, Riccardi VM, Kao F-T, Kau YW. Mapping parathyroid hormone, beta-globin, insulin and LDH-A genes within the human chromosome 11 short arm by spot blotting sorted chromosomes. *Hum Genet* 1985;69:316.

31. Chaganti RSK, Jhanwar SC, Antonarakis SE, Hayward WS. Germ-line chromosomal localization of genes in chromosome 11p linkage: parathyroid hormone, beta-globin, c-Ha-ras-1, and insulin. *Somat Cell Mol Genet* 1985;11:197.

32. Yasuda T, Banville D, Hendy GN, Goltzman D. Characterization of the human parathyroid hormone-like peptide gene: functional and evolutionary aspects. *J Biol Chem* 1989;264:7720–7725.

33. Juppner H, Abou-Samra A-B, Uneno S, Gu W-X, Potts JT Jr, Segre GV. The parathyroid hormone-like peptide associated with humoral hypercalcemia of malignancy and parathyroid hormone bind to the same receptor on the plasma membrane of ROS 17/2.8 cells. *J Biol Chem* 1988;263:8557–8560.

34. Nissenson RA, Diep D, Strewler GJ. Synthetic peptides comprising the amino-terminal sequence of a parathyroid hormone-like protein from human malignancies: binding to parathyroid hormone receptors and activation of adenylate cyclase in bone cells and kidney. *J Biol Chem* 1988;263:12866–12871.

35. Thompson DD, Seedor JG, Fisher JE, Rosenblatt M, Rodan GA. Direct action of the parathyroid hormone-like human hypercalcemic factor on bone. *Proc Natl Acad Sci USA* 1988;85:5673–5677.

36. Akatsu T, Takahashi N, Udagawa N, et al. Parathyroid hormone (PTH)-related protein is a potent stimulator of osteoclast-like multinucleated cell formation to the same extent as PTH in mouse marrow cultures. *Endocrinology* 1989;125:20–27.

37. Abou-Samra A-B, Uneno S, Jueppner H, et al. Non-homologous sequences of parathyroid hormone and the parathyroid hormone related peptide bind to a common receptor on ROS 17/2.8 cells. *Endocrinology* 1989;125:2215–2217.

38. Civitelli R, Martin TJ, Fausto A, Gunsten SL, Hruska KA, Avioli LV. Parathyroid hormone-related peptide transiently increases cytosolic calcium in osteoblast-like cells: comparison with parathyroid hormone. *Endocrinology* 1989;125:1204–1210.

39. Hock JM, Fonseca J, Gunness-Hey M, Kemp BE, Martin TJ. Comparison of the anabolic effects of synthetic parathyroid hormone-related protein (PTHrP) 1–34 and PTH 1–34 on bone in rats. *Endocrinology* 1989;125:2022–2027.

40. Pun K-K, Ho PWM. Identification and characterization of parathyroid hormone receptors on dog kidney, human kidney, chick bone and human dermal fibroblast: a comparative study of functional and structural properties. *Biochem J* 1989;259:785–789.

41. Caulfield MP, McKee RL, Goldman ME, et al. The bovine renal parathyroid hormone (PTH) receptor has equal affinity for two different amino acid sequences: the receptor binding domains of PTH and PTH-related protein are located within the 14–34 region. *Endocrinology* 1990;127:83–87.

42. Caulfield MP, McKee RL, Goldman ME, et al. Parathyroid hormone-related protein (PTHrP): studies with synthetic peptides indicate that parathyroid hormone and PTHrP interact with the same receptor. *Int J Radiat Appl Instrument Part B Nucl Med Biol* 1990;17:633–637.

43. Raisz LG, Simmons HA, Vargas SJ, Kemp BE, Martin TJ. A comparison of the effects of amino-terminal synthetic parathyroid hormone-related peptide of malignancy and parathyroid hormone on resorption of cultured fetal rat long bones. *Calcif Tissue Int* 1990;46:233–238.

44. Karpf DB, Bambino T, Alford G, Nissenson RA. Features of the renal parathyroid hormone-related protein receptor derived from structural studies of receptor fragments. *J Bone Mineral Res* 1991;6:173–182.

45. Loveridge N, Dean V, Goltzman D, Hendy GN. Bioactivity

of parathyroid hormone and parathyroid hormone-like peptide: agonist and antagonist activities of amino-terminal fragments as assessed by the cytochemical bioassay and in situ biochemistry. *Endocrinology* 1991;128:1938–1946.

46. Donahue HJ, Fryer MJ, Heath H III. Structure-function relationships for full-length recombinant parathyroid hormone-related peptide and its amino-terminal fragments: effects on cytosolic calcium ion mobilization and adenylate cyclase activation in rat osteoblast-like cells. *Endocrinology* 1990;126:1471–1477.

47. Isogna KL, Stewart AF, Morris CA, Hough LM, Milstone LM, Centrella M. Native and a synthetic analogue of the malignancy-associated parathyroid hormone-like protein have in vitro transforming growth factor-like properties. *J Clin Invest* 1989;83:1057–1060.

48. Kikuchi H, Shigeno C, Lee K, et al. On the transforming growth factor beta-like activity of synthetic polypeptides comprising the aminoterminal sequence of the human parathyroid hormone-related peptide. *Endocrinology* 1991;128:1229–1237.

49. Fraher LJ, Hodsman AB, Jonas K, et al. A comparison of the in vivo biochemical responses to exogenous parathyroid hormone (PTH)-(1–34) and PTH-related peptide-(1–34) in man. *J Clin Endocr Metab* 1992;75:417–423.

50. Orloff JJ, Goumas D, Wu TL, Stewart AE. Interspecies comparison of renal cortical receptors for parathyroid hormone and parathyroid hormone-related protein. *J Bone Mineral Res* 1991;6:279–287.

51. Bringhurst FR, Juppner H, Giro G, et al. Cloned stably-expressed parathyroid hormone (PTH)/PTH-related peptide receptors activate multiple messenger signals and biological responses in LLC-PK$_1$ kidney cells. *Endocrinology* 1993;132:2090–2098.

52. Schipani E, Karga H, Karaplis AC, et al. Identical complementary deoxyribonucleic acids encode a human renal and bone parathyroid hormone (PTH)/PTH-related peptide receptor. *Endocrinology* 1993;132:2157–2165.

53. Ikeda K, Weir EC, Mangin M, et al. Expression of messenger ribonucleic acids encoding a parathyroid hormone-like peptide in normal human and animal tissues with abnormal expression in human parathyroid adenomas. *Mol Endocrinol* 1988;2:1230–1236.

54. Campos RV, Asa SL, Drucker DJ. Immunocytochemical localization of parathyroid hormone-like peptide in rat fetus. *Cancer Res* 1991;51:6351–6357.

55. Orloff JJ, Wu TL, Stewart AF. Parathyroid hormone-like proteins: biochemical responses and receptor interactions. *Endocr Rev* 1989;10:476–495.

56. Urena P, Kong X-F, Abou-Samra A-B, et al. PTH and PTHrP related peptide receptor mRNAs are widely distributed in rat tissues. *Endocrinology* 1993;133:617–623.

57. Chase LR, Aurbach GD. Renal adenyl cyclase: anatomical separation of sites sensitive to parathyroid hormone and vasopressin. *Science* 1968;159:545–547.

58. Chase LR, Fedak SA, Aurbach GD. Activation of skeletal adenyl cyclase by parathyroid hormone in vitro. *Endocrinology* 1969;84:761–768.

59. Chase LR, Melson GL, Aurbach GD. Pseudohypoparathyroidism: defective excretion of 3'5'-AMP in response to parathyroid hormone. *J Clin Invest* 1969;48:1832.

60. Albright F, Burnett CH, Smith PH, Parson W. Pseudohypoparathyroidism—an example of "Seabright-Bantam syndrome." *Endocrinology* 1941;30:922–932.

61. Marcus R, Aurbach GD. Bioassay of parathyroid hormone in vitro with a stable preparation of adenyl cyclase from rat kidney. *Endocrinology* 1969;85:801–810.

62. Tashjian AH Jr, Ontjes DA, Munson PL. Alkylation and oxidation of methionine in bovine parathyroid hormone: effects on hormonal activity and antigenicity. *Biochemistry* 1964;3:1175–1182.

63. Rosenblatt M, Goltzman D, Keutmann H, Tregear GW, Potts JT Jr. Chemical and biological properties of synthetic, sulfur-free analogues of parathyroid hormone. *J Biol Chem* 1976;251:159.

64. Nissenson RA, Arnaud CD. Properties of the parathyroid hormone receptor-adenylate cyclase system in chicken renal plasma membranes. *J Biol Chem* 1976;254:1469–1475.

65. Zull JE, Repke DW. Studies with tritiated polypeptide hormones. I The preparation and properties of an active, highly tritiated derivative of parathyroid hormone: acetamidino-PTH. *J Biol Chem* 1972;247:2183.

66. Zull JE, Chuang J. Further studies on acetamidination as a technique for preparation of a biologically valid ^{3}H-labeled tracer for PTH. *J Biol Chem* 1975;250:1668–1675.

67. Nielsen ST, Barrett PQ, Neuman MW, Neuman WE. The electrolytic preparation of bioactive radioiodinated parathyroid hormone of high specific activity. *Anal Biochem* 1979;92:67–73.

68. Rosenberg RA, Muzaffar SA, Heersche JNM, Jez D, Murray TM. Preparation and properties of biologically active radioiodinated parathyroid hormone. *Anal Biochem* 1983;128:331–341.

69. Kremer R, Bennett HPJ, Mitchell J, Goltzman D. Characterization of the rabbit renal receptor for native parathyroid hormone employing a radioligand purified by reverse phase liquid chromatography. *J Biol Chem* 1982;257:14048–14054.

70. Nickols GA, Metz-Nickols MA, Pang PKT, Roberts MS, Cooper CW. Identification and characterization of parathyroid hormone receptors in rat renal cortical plasma membranes using radioligand binding. *J Bone Mineral Res* 1989;4:615–623.

71. Newman W, Beall LD, Levine MA, Cone JL, Randhawa ZI, Bertolini DR. Biotinylated parathyroid hormone as a probe for the parathyroid hormone receptor. *J Biol Chem* 1989;264:16359–16366.

72. Roubini E, Duong LT, Gibbons SW, Leu CT, Caulfield MP, Chorev M, Rosenblatt M. Synthesis of fully active biotinylated analogues of parathyroid hormone (PTH) and PTH-related protein as tools for the characterization of PTH receptors. *Biochemistry* 1982;31:4026–4033.

73. Agarwala N, Gay CV. Specific binding of parathyroid hormone to living osteoclasts. *J Bone Mineral Res* 1992;7:531–539.

74. Segre GV, Rosenblatt M, Reiner BL, Mahaffey JE, Potts JT Jr. Characterization of parathyroid hormone receptors in canine renal cortical plasma membranes using a radioiodinated sulfur-free hormone analogue: correlation of binding with adenylate cyclase activity. *J Biol Chem* 1979;254:6980–6986.

75. Nussbaum SR, Rosenblatt M, Potts JT Jr. Parathyroid hormone renal interactions: demonstration of two binding domains. *J Biol Chem* 1980;255:10183–10187.

76. Rosenblatt M, Segre GV, Tyler GA, Shepard GA, Nussbaum SR, Potts JT Jr. Identification of a receptor-binding region in parathyroid hormone. *Endocrinology* 1980;106:545–550.

77. Herrmann-Erlee M, Heersche J, Hekkelman J, et al. Effects on bone in vitro of bovine PTH and synthetic fragments representing residues 1–34, 2–34, and 3–34. *Endocrinol Res Commun* 1976;3:21.

78. Brown RC, Silver AC, Woodhead JS. Binding and degradation of NH$_2$-terminal parathyroid hormone by opossum kidney cells. *Am J Physiol* 1991;260 [Endocrinol Metab 23]:E544–E552.

79. Pernalete L, Garcia JC, Betts CR, Martin KJ. Inhibitors of protein kinase-C modulate desensitization of the parathyroid hormone receptor–adenylate cyclase system in opossum kidney cells. *Endocrinology* 1990;126:407–413.

80. Mahoney CA, Nissenson RA, Sarnacki P, Kong P. Canine renal receptors for parathyroid hormone: down-regulation in vivo by exogenous parathyroid hormone. *J Clin Invest* 1983;72:411–421.

81. McKee MD, Murray TM. Binding of intact parathyroid hormone to chicken renal plasma membranes: evidence for a second binding site with carboxyl-terminal specificity. *Endocrinology* 1985;117:1930–1939.

82. Keutmann HT, Griscom AW, Nussbaum SR, et al. Rat parathyroid hormone (1–34) fragment: renal adenylate cyclase activity and receptor binding properties in vitro. *Endocrinology* 1985;117:1230.

83. Hruska KA, Moskowitz D, Esbrit P, Civitelli R, Westbrook S, Huskey M. Stimulation of inositol triphosphate and dia-

cylglycerol production in renal tubular cells by parathyroid hormone. *J Clin Invest* 1987;79:230–239.

84. Coleman DT, Bilezikian JP. Parathyroid hormone stimulates formation of inositol phosphates in a membrane preparation of canine renal tubular cells. *J Bone Mineral Res* 1990;5:299–306.

85. Hruska KA, Goligorsky M, Scoble J, Tsusumi M, Westbrook S, Moskowitz D. Effect of parathyroid hormone on cytosolic calcium in renal proximal tubular primary cultures. *Am J Physiol* 1986;251:F188.

86. Goligorsky MS, Loftus DJ, Hruska KA. Cytoplasmic calcium in individual proximal tubular cells in culture. *Am J Physiol* 1986;251:F938

87. Henry HL, Dutta C, Noreen C, et al. The cellular and molecular regulation of 1,25(OH)$_2$D$_3$ production. *J Steroid Biochem Mol Biol* 1992;41:401–407.

88. Caverzasio J, Rizzoli R, Bonjour J-P. Sodium-dependent phosphate transport inhibited by parathyroid hormone and cyclic AMP stimulation in an opossum kidney cell line. *J Biol Chem* 1986;261:3233–3237.

89. Nakai M, Kinoshita Y, Fukase M, Kujita T. Phorbol esters inhibit phosphate uptake in opossum kidney cells: a model of proximal renal tubular cells. *Biochem Biophys Res Commun* 1987;145:303–308.

90. Cole JA, Forte LR, Eber S, Throne K, Poelling RE. Regulation of sodium-dependent phosphate transport by parathyroid hormone in opossum kidney cells: adenosine 3'5'-monophosphate-dependent and -independent mechanisms. *Endocrinology* 1986;122:2981–2989.

91. Henry HL. The role of parathyroid hormone in the regulation of the metabolism of 25-hydroxyvitamin D$_3$. *Mineral Electrolyte Metab* 1982;8:179–187.

92. Armbrecht HJ, Wongsurawat N, Zenser TV, Davis BB. Effects of PTH and 1,25(OH)$_2$D$_3$ on renal 25(OH)D$_3$ metabolism, adenylate cyclase, and protein kinase. *Am J Physiol* 1984;246:E102–E107.

93. Quamme G, Pfeilschifter J, Murer H. PTH inhibition of Na$^+$/phosphate cotransport in OK cells: generation of second messengers in the regulatory cascade. *Biochem Biophys Res Commun* 1989;158:951–957.

94. Wong G. Skeletal actions of parathyroid hormone (review). *Mineral Electrolyte Metab* 1982;8:188–198.

95. Nissenson RA. Functional properties of parathyroid hormone receptors. *Mineral Electrolyte Metab* 1982;8:151–158.

96. Teitelbaum AP, Pliam NB, Silve C, Abbott SR, Nissenson RA, Arnaud CD. Functional properties of parathyroid hormone receptors in kidney and bone. *Adv Exp Med Biol* 1982;151:535–548.

97. Yamamoto I, Shigeno C, Potts JT Jr, Segre GV. Characterization and agonist-induced down-regulation of parathyroid hormone receptors in clonal rat osteosarcoma cells. *Endocrinology* 1988;122:1208–1217.

98. Abou-Samra A-B, Jueppner H, Potts JT Jr, Segre GV. Inactivation of pertussis toxin-sensitive guanyl nucleotide-binding proteins increased parathyroid receptors and reverse agonist-induced receptors down regulation in ROS 17/2.8 cells. *Endocrinology* 1989;125:2594–2599.

99. Mitchell J, Goltzman D. Mechanisms of homologous and heterologous regulation of parathyroid hormone receptors in the rat osteosarcoma cell line UMR-106. *Endocrinology* 1990;126:2650–2660.

100. Pun KK, Ho PWM, Nissenson RA, Arnaud CD. Desensitization of parathyroid hormone receptors on cultured bone cells. *J Bone Mineral Res* 1990;5:1193–1200.

101. Fukayama S, Tashjian AH Jr, Bringhurst FR. Mechanism of desensitization to parathyroid hormone in human osteoblast-like SaOS-2 cells. *Endocrinology* 1992;131:1757–1769.

102. Rizzoli R, Fleisch H. Heterologous desensitization by 1,25-dihydroxyvitamin D3 of cyclic AMP response to parathyroid hormone in osteoblast-like cells and the role of the stimulatory guanine nucleotide. *Biochim Biophys Acta* 1986;887:214–221.

103. Titus L, Jackson E, Nanes MS, Rubin JE, Catherwood BD. 1,25-dihydroxyvitamin D reduces parathyroid hormone receptor number in ROS 17/2.8 cells and prevents the gluco-

corticoid-induced increase in these receptors: relationship to adenylate cyclase activation. *J Bone Mineral Res* 1991;6:631–637.

104. Rao LG, Wylie JN. The effects of dexamethasone and 1,25-dihydroxyvitamin D3 on protein kinase C modulation of parathyroid hormone-stimulated adenylate cyclase in ROS 17/2.8 cells. *Bone Mineral* (in press).

105. Teitelbaum AP, Silve CM, Nyiredy KO, Arnaud CD. Down-regulation of parathyroid hormone receptors in cultured bone cells is associated with agonist-specific intracellular processing of PTH-receptor complexes. *Endocrinology* 1986;118:595–602.

106. Mitchell J, Rouleau MF, Goltzman D. Biochemical and morphological characterization of parathyroid hormone receptor binding to the rat osteosarcoma cell line UMR-106. *Endocrinology* 1990;126:2327–2335.

107. Avioli LV, Halstead LR, Scott MJ, Roberts ML, Rifas L. Parathyroid hormone positively regulates its own cAMP response in cultured human osteoblasts. *J Endocrinol Invest* 1991;15(Suppl 6):19–26.

108. Segre GV, Rosenblatt M, Tully GL, Laugharn J, Reit B, Potts JT Jr. Evaluation of an in vitro parathyroid hormone antagonist in vivo in dogs. *Endocrinology* 1985;116:1024–1029.

109. Herrmann-Erlee MPM, Nijweide PJ, van der Meer JM, Ooms MAC. Action of bPTH and bPTH fragments on embryonic bone in vitro; dissociation of the cyclic AMP and bone-forming response. *Calcif Tissue Int* 1983;35:70–77.

110. Reid IR, Lowe C, Cornish J, Gray DH, Skinner SJM. Adenylate cyclase blockers dissociate PTH-stimulated bone resorption from cAMP production. *Am J Physiol* 1990;256:E708–E714.

111. Civitelli R, Reid IR, Westbrook S, Avioli LV, Hruska KA. Parathyroid hormone elevates inositol polyphosphate and diacylglycerol in a rat osteoblast-like cell line. *Am J Physiol* 1988;252:E45–E51.

112. Farndale RW, Sandy JR, Atkinson SJ, Pennington SR, Meghji S, Meikle MC. Parathyroid hormone and prostaglandin E2 stimulate both inositol phosphates and cyclic AMP accumulation in mouse osteoblast cultures. *Biochem J* 1988;252:263–268.

113. Cosman F, Morrow B, Kopal M, Bilezikian JP. Stimulation of inositol phosphate formation in ROS 17/2.8 cell membranes by guanine nucleotide, calcium, and parathyroid hormone. *J Bone Mineral Res* 1989;4:413–420.

114. Babich M, King KL, Nissenson RA. G protein-dependent activation of a phosphoinositide-specific phospholipase C in UMR-106 osteosarcoma cell membranes. *J Bone Mineral Res* 1989;4:549–556.

115. Lowik CWGM, van Leeuwen JPTM, ven der Meer JM, van Zeeland JK, Scheven BAA, Herrmann-Erlee MPM. A two-receptor model for the action of parathyroid hormone on osteoblasts: a role for intracellular free calcium and cAMP. *Cell Calcium* 1985;6:311–326.

116. Yamaguchi DT, Hahn TJ, Iida-Klein A, Kleeman CR, Muallem S. Parathyroid hormone-activated calcium channels in an osteoblast-like clonal osteosarcoma cell line. *J Biol Chem* 1987;262:7711–7718.

117. Reid IR, Civitelli R, Halstead LR, Avioli LV, Hruska KA. Parathyroid hormone acutely elevates intracellular calcium in osteoblast-like cells. *Am J Physiol* 1987;252:E45–E51.

118. Donahue HJ, Fryer MJ, Eriksen EF, Heath H III. Differential effects of parathyroid hormone and its analogues on cytosolic calcium ion and cAMP levels in cultured rat osteoblast-like cells. *J Biol Chem* 1988;263:13522–13527.

119. Rao LG, March M, Murray TM. Calcium and protein kinase C enhance parathyroid hormone- and forskolin-stimulated adenylate cyclase in ROS 17/2.8 cells. *Calcif Tissue Int* 1989;45:354–359.

120. Rao LG, March M, Murray TM. Calcium modulation of the parathyroid hormone-sensitive adenylate cyclase in ROS 17/2.8 cells: effects of N-(6-aminohexyl-5-Cl-napthalene sulfonamide) (W-7) and trifluoperazine (TFP). *Bone Mineral* 1989;7:191–204.

121. Koch HM, Muir H, Gelderblom D, Hough S. Protein kinase

C modulates parathyroid hormone- but not prostaglandin E₂-mediated stimulation of cyclic AMP production via the inhibitory guanine nucleotide binding protein in UMR-106 osteosarcoma cells. *J Bone Mineral Res* 1992;7:1353–1362.

122. Ikeda K, Sugimoto T, Fukase M, Fujita T. Protein kinase C is involved in PTH-induced homologous desensitization by directly affecting PTH receptor in the osteoblastic osteosarcoma cells. *Endocrinology* 1991;128:2901–2906.

123. Jouishomme H, Whitfield JF, Chakravarthy B, et al. The protein kinase-C activation domain of parathyroid hormone. *Endocrinology* 1992;130:53–60.

124. Fujimori A, Cheng S-L, Avioli LV, Civitelli R. Dissociation of second messenger activation by PTH fragments in osteosarcoma cells. *Endocrinology* 1991;128:3032–3039.

125. Fujimori A, Cheng S-L, Avioli LV, Civitelli R. Structure-function relationship of parathyroid hormone: activation of phospholipase-C, protein kinase-A and -C in osteosarcoma cells. *Endocrinology* 1992;130:29–36.

126. Chakravarthy BR, Durkin JP, Rixon RH, Whitfield JF. Parathyroid hormone fragment (3–34) stimulates protein kinase C activity in rat osteosarcoma and murine T-lymphoma cells. *Biochem Biophys Res Commun* 1990;171:1105–1110.

127. Tamura T, Sakamoto H, Filburn CR. Parathyroid hormone 1–34, but not 3–34 or 7–34, transiently translocates protein kinase C in cultured renal OK cells. *Biochem Biophys Res Commun* 1989;159:1352–1358.

128. Civitelli R, Hruska KA, Jeffrey JJ, Kahn AJ, Avioli LV, Partridge NC. Second messenger signaling in the regulation of collagenase production by osteogenic sarcoma cells. *Endocrinology* 1989;124:2928–2934.

129. Somjen D, Schluter KD, Wingender Z, Mayer H, Kaye AM. Stimulation of cell proliferation in skeletal tissues of the rat by defined parathyroid hormone fragments. *Biochem J* 1991;277:863–868.

130. van Leeuwen JPTM, Bos MP, Herrmann-Erlee MPM. Modulatory function of protein kinase C in the activation of ornithine decarboxylase and in cAMP production in rat osteoblasts. *J Cell Physiol* 1989;138:548–554.

131. Bringhurst FR, Zajac JD, Daggett AS, Skurat RN, Kronenberg HM. Inhibition of parathyroid hormone responsiveness in clonal osteoblastic cells expressing a mutant of 3′5′-cyclic adenosine monosphosphate-dependent protein kinase. *Mol Endocrinol* 1989;3:60–67.

132. Abou-Samra A-B, Zajac JD, Schiffer-Alberts D, et al. Cyclic adenosine 3′5′-monophosphate (cAMP)-dependent and cAMP-independent regulation of parathyroid hormone receptors on UMR-106-01 osteoblastic osteosarcoma cells. *Endocrinology* 1991;129:2547–2554.

133. Fukayama S, Kearns AK, Skurat RM, Tashjian AH Jr, Bringhurst FR. Protein kinase A-dependent inhibition of alkaline phosphatase release by SaOS-2 human osteoblastic cells: studies in new mutant cell lines that express a cyclic AMP-resistant phenotype. *Cell Regul* 1991;2:889–896.

134. Lowik CWGM, van der Ruit M, Nibbering PH. Cytokine-induced nitric oxide production in osteoblast-like cells and bone explants is involved in the inhibition of osteoclastic bone resorption. *Calcif Tissue Int* 1993;53(Suppl 1):S13 (abstract).

135. Rouleau MF, Mitchell J, Goltzman D. In vivo distribution of parathyroid hormone receptors in bone: evidence that a predominant osseous target cell is not the mature osteoblast. *Endocrinology* 1988;123:187–191.

136. Rouleau MF, Mitchell J, Goltzman D. Characterization of the major parathyroid hormone target cell in the endosteal metaphysis of rat long bones. *J Bone Mineral Res* 1990;5:1043–1053.

137. Civitelli R, Fujimori A, Bernier SM, et al. Heterogeneous intracellular free calcium responses to parathyroid hormone correlate with morphology and receptor distribution in osteogenic sarcoma cells. *Endocrinology* 1992;130:2392–2400.

138. Chen TL, Feldman D. Glucocorticoid potentiation of the adenosine 3′,5′-monophosphate response to parathyroid hormone in cultured rat bone cells. *Endocrinology* 1978;102:589–596.

139. Rodan SB, Rodan GA. Dexamethasone effects on β-adren-

ergic receptors and adenylate cyclase regulatory proteins G_s and G_i in ROS 17/2.8 cells. *Endocrinology* 1986;118:2510–2518.

140. Catherwood BD. 1,25-Dihydroxycholecalciferol and glucocorticoid regulation of adenylate cyclase in an osteoblast-like cell line. *J Biol Chem* 1985;260:736–745.

141. Rizzoli R, von Tscharner V, Fleisch H. Increase of adenylate cyclase catalytic-unit activity by dexamethasone in rat osteoblast-like cells. *Biochem J* 1986;237:447–454.

142. Yamamoto I, Potts JT, Segre GV. Glucocorticoids increase parathyroid hormone receptors in rat osteoblastic osteosarcoma cells (ROS 17/2). *J Bone Mineral Res* 1988;3:707–712.

143. Rao LG, Wylie J, Sutherland M, Murray TM. The potentiation by estrogen of parathyroid hormone-stimulated alkaline phosphatase activity and mRNA in human osteosarcoma cells is differentiation stage-dependent. *Calcif Tissue Int* 1993;52(Suppl 1):44.

144. Wong MM, Rao LG, Hao L, et al. Long-term effects of physiologic concentrations of dexamethasone on human bone-derived cells. *J Bone Mineral Res* 5:803–813.

145. Silve C, Fritsch J, Grosse B, Tau C, Edelman A, Delmas P, Balsan S, Garabedian M. Corticosteroid-induced changes in the responsiveness of human osteoblast-like cells to parathyroid hormone. *Bone Mineral* 1989;6:65–75.

146. Subramaniam M, Colvard D, Keeting PE, Rasmussen K, Riggs BL, Spelsberg TC. Glucocorticoid regulation of alkaline phosphatase, osteocalcin, and proto-oncogenes in normal human osteoblast-like cells. *J Cell Biochem* 1992;50:411–424.

147. Suarez F, Silve C. Effect of parathyroid hormone on arachidonic acid metabolism in mouse osteoblasts: permissive action of dexamethasone. *Endocrinology* 1992;130:592–598.

148. Majeska RJ, Nair BC, Rodan GA. Glucocorticoid regulation of alkaline phosphatase in the osteoclastic osteosarcoma cell line ROS 17/2.8. *Endocrinology* 1985;116:170–179.

149. Schneider H-G, Allan EH, Moseley JM, Martin TJ, Findlay DM. Specific down-regulation of parathyroid hormone receptors and responses to PTH by tumor necrosis factor α and retinoic acid in UMR 106-06 osteoblastic osteosarcoma cells. *Biochem J* 1991;280:451–457.

150. Bernier SM, Rouleau MF, Goltzman D. Biochemical and morphological analysis of the interaction of epidermal growth factor and parathyroid hormone with UMR 106 osteosarcoma cells. *Endocrinology* 1991;128:2752–2760.

151. Pizurki L, Rizzoli R, Caverzasio J, Bonjour J-P. Stimulation by parathyroid hormone-related protein and transforming growth factor-alpha of phosphate transport in osteoblast-like cells. *J Bone Mineral Res* 1991;6:1235–1241.

152. Schneider H-G, Michelangeli VP, Frampton RJ, et al. Transforming growth factor-β modulates receptor binding of calciotropic hormones and G protein-mediated adenylate cyclase responses in osteoblast-like cells. *Endocrinology* 1992;131:1383–1389.

153. Seitz PK, Zhu B-T, Cooper CW. Effect of transforming growth factor β on parathyroid hormone receptor binding and cAMP formation in rat osteosarcoma cells. *J Bone Mineral Res* 1992;7:541–546.

154. Bellows CG, Ishida H, Aubin JE, Heersche JNM. Parathyroid hormone reversibly suppresses the differentiation of osteoprogenitor cells into functional osteoblasts. *Endocrinology* 1990;127:3111–3116.

155. Raisz LG, Dietrich JW, Canalis EM. Factors affecting bone formation. *Israel J Med Sci* 1976;12:108–114.

156. Dietrich JW, Canalis EM, Maina DM, Raisz LG. Hormonal control of bone collagen synthesis in vivo: effects of parathyroid hormone and calcitonin. *Endocrinology* 1976;98:943–949.

157. Heersche JNM, Reimers S, Denkovski P, Bellows CG, Aubin JE. Heterogeneity of osteoblasts in vivo and in vitro. Proc. Fourth International Symposium on Osteoporosis, Hong Kong, March, 1993;11 (abstract).

158. Rao LG, Sutherland M, Muzaffar S, et al. Estrogen affects osteoblastic marker mRNA levels in normal human osteoblasts from femoral but not iliac crest trabecular bone. *J Bone Mineral Res* 1993;8(Suppl 1):S300.

159. Fermot B, Mason DJ, Lee K, et al. Differences in periosteal and trabecular gene expression in growing bone. *J Bone Min Res* 1993;8(Suppl 1):S198.
160. Reeve J, Davies UM, Hesp R, McNally E, Katz D. Treatment of osteoporosis with human parathyroid peptide and observations on effect of sodium fluoride. *Br Med J* 1990; 301:314–318.
161. Mueller KR, Cortesi R, Jeker H. The PTH-induced increase of trabecular bone in the rat: a pharmacological study. *Calcif Tissue Intl* 1993;52(Suppl 1):55.
162. Tam CS, Heersche JN, Murray TM, Parsons JA. Parathyroid hormone stimulates the bone apposition rate independently of its resorptive action: differential effects of intermittent and continuous administration. *Endocrinology* 1982; 110:506–512.
163. Gunness-Hey M, Hock JM. Increased trabecular bone mass in rats treated with human synthetic parathyroid hormone. *Metab Bone Dis Rel Res* 1984;5:177–181.
164. Tada K, Yamamuro T, Okumura H, Kasai R, Takahashi H. Restoration of axial and appendicular bone volumes by hPTH (1–34) in parathyroidectomized and osteopenic rats. *Bone* 1990;11:163–169.
165. Gera I, Dorbrolet N, Hock JM. Intermittent but not continuous parathyroid hormone [hPTH (1–34)] increases bone mass independently of resorption. *J Bone Mineral Res* 1989;4:S303.
166. Canalis E, McCarthy TL, Centrella M. Differential effects of continuous and transient treatment with parathyroid hormone-related peptide on bone collagen synthesis. *Endocrinology* 1990;126:1806–1812.
167. Parsons JA, Reit B. Chronic response of dogs to parathyroid hormone infusion. *Nature* 1974;250:254.
168. Hefti E, Trechsel U, Bonjour J-P, Fleisch H, Schenk R. Increase of whole body calcium and skeletal mass in normal and osteoporotic adult rats treated with parathyroid hormone. *Clin Sci* 1982;63:389–396.
169. Hock JM, Fonseca J. Anabolic effect of human synthetic parathyroid hormone-(1–34) depends on growth hormone. *Endocrinology* 1990;127:1804–1810.
170. Zull JE, Chuang J. Kidney membrane binding of native parathyroid hormone compared to binding of its synthetic 1–34 fragment. *J Receptor Res* 1980;1:69–89.
171. Demay M, Mitchell J, Goltzman D. Comparison of renal and osseous binding of parathyroid hormone and hormonal fragments. *Am J Physiol* 1985;249:E437–E446.
172. Garcia JC, McConkey CC, Martin KJ. Separate binding sites for intact parathyroid hormone (1–84) and synthetic PTH (1–34) in canine kidney. *Calcif Tissue Int* 1989;44:214–219.
173. Ruth JD. *Parathyroid hormone action in a renal cell line.* MS Thesis, University of Toronto, 1988.
174. Murray TM, Ruth JD, MacLellan WR, Rao LG. Binding of intact PTH and its amino and carboxylterminal fragments to cells of renal and skeletal origin: further evidence for C-terminal binding site. Paper presented at the IXth Meeting of ICCRH, Nice, France, Abstract 762, 1986.
175. Murer H, Werner A, Reshkin S, Wuarin F, Biber J. Cellular mechanisms in proximal tubular reabsorption of inorganic phosphate. *Am J Physiol* 1991;260:C885–C898.
176. Reshkin SJ, Forgo J, Murer H. Functional assymetry in phosphate transport and its regulation in opossum kidney cells—parathyroid hormone inhibition. *Pflugers Arch* 1990; 416:624–631.
177. Reshkin SJ, Forgo J, Murer H. Apical and basolateral effects of PTH in OK cells. Transport inhibition, messenger production, effects of pertussis toxin, and interaction with a PTH analog. *J Membrane Biol* 1991;124:227–237.
178. Seitz PK, Nickols GA, Nickols MA, McPherson MB, Cooper CW. Radioiodinated rat parathyroid hormone-(1–34) binds to its receptor on rat osteosarcoma cells in a manner consistent with two classes of binding sites. *J Bone Mineral Res* 1990;5:353–359.
179. Rao LG, Murray TM, Heersche JNM. Immunohistochemical demonstration of parathyroid hormone binding to specific cell types in fixed rat bone tissue. *Endocrinology* 1990;113:805–810.
180. Silve CM, Hredek GT, Jones AL, Arnaud CD. Parathyroid hormone receptor in intact embryonic chicken bone: characterization and cellular localization. *J Cell Biol* 1982;94: 379.
181. Rouleau MF, Warshawsky H, Goltzman D. Parathyroid hormone binding in vivo to renal, hepatic, and skeletal tissues of the rat using a radioautographic approach. *Endocrinology* 1986;118:919–931.
182. Evely RS, Bonomo A, Schreider H-G, Mosely JM, Gallagher J, Martin TJ. Structural requirements for the action of parathyroid hormone-related protein on bone resorption by isolated osteoclasts. *J Bone Mineral Res* 1991;6:85–93.
183. Duong LT, Grasser W, DeHaven PA, Sato M. Parathyroid hormone receptors identified on avian and rat osteoclasts. *J Bone Mineral Res* 1990;5:S203.
184. Teti A, Rizzoli R, Zambonin Zallone A. Parathyroid hormone binding to cultured avian osteoclasts. *Biochem Biophys Res Commun* 1991;174:1217–1222.
185. Hakeda Y, Hiura K, Sato T, et al. Existence of parathyroid hormone binding sites on murine hemopoietic blast cells. *Biochem Biophys Res Commun* 1989;163:1481–1486.
186. Ito MB, Schraer H, Gay CV. The effects of calcitonin, parathyroid hormone, and prostaglandin E_2 on cyclic AMP levels of isolated osteoclasts. *Comp Biochem Physiol* 1985;81A: 653–657.
187. McSheehy PM, Chambers TJ. Osteoblast-like cells in the presence of parathyroid hormone release soluble factor that stimulates osteoclastic bone resorption. *Endocrinology* 1986; 119:1654–1659.
188. Murrills RJ, Stein LS, Fey CP, Dempster DW. The effects of parathyroid hormone (PTH) and PTH-related peptide on osteoclast resorption of bone slices in vitro: an analysis of pit size and the resorption focus. *Endocrinology* 1990;127: 2648–2653.
189. Rodan GA, Martin TJ. Role of osteoblasts in hormonal control of bone resorption: a hypothesis. *Calcif Tissue Int* 1981;33:349–351.
190. Hunter SJ, Schraer H, Gay CV. Characterization of isolated and cultured chick osteoclasts: the effects of acetazolamide, calcitonin, and parathyroid hormone on acid production. *J Bone Mineral Res* 1988;3:287–303.
191. Anderson RE, Jee WSS, Woodbury DM. Stimulation of carbonic anhydrase in osteoclasts by parathyroid hormone. *Calcif Tissue Int* 1985;37:646–650.
192. Enomoto M, Kinoshita A, Pan H-O, Suzuki F, Yamamoto I, Takigawa M. Demonstration of receptors for parathyroid hormone on cultured rabbit costal chondrocytes. *Biochem Biophys Res Commun* 1989;162:1222–1229.
193. Takano T, Takigawa M, Shirai E, Suzuki F, Rosenblatt M. Effects of synthetic analogs and fragments of bovine parathyroid hormone on adenosine 3'5'-monophosphate level, ornithine decarboxylase activity, and glycosaminoglycan synthesis in rabbit costal chondrocytes in culture: structure-activity relations. *Endocrinology* 1985;116:2536–2542.
194. Kato Y, Koike T, Iwamoto M, et al. Effects of limited exposure of rabbit chondrocyte cultures to parathyroid hormone and dibutyryl adenosine 3'5'-monophosphate on cartilage-characteristic prostaglandin synthesis. *Endocrinology* 1988;122:1991–1997.
195. Iannotti JP, Brighton CT, Iannotti V, Ohisi T. Mechanism of action of parathyroid hormone-induced proteoglycan synthesis in the growth plate chondrocyte. *J Orthop Res* 1990;8:136–145.
196. Kato Y, Shimazu A, Nakashima K, Suzuki F, Jikko A, Iwamoto M. Effects of parathyroid hormone and calcitonin on alkaline phosphatase activity and matrix calcification in rabbit growth-plate cultures. *Endocrinology* 1990;127:114–118.
197. Takigawa M, Kinoshita A, Enomoto M, Asada A, Suzuki F. Effects of various growth and differentiation factors on expression of parathyroid hormone receptors on rabbit costal chondrocytes in culture. *Endocrinology* 1991;129:868–876.
198. Lewinson D, Silbermann M. Parathyroid hormone stimulates proliferation of chondroprogenitor cells in vitro. *Calcif Tissue Int* 1986;38:155–162.

199. Nemere I, Norman AW. Parathyroid hormone stimulates calcium transport in perfused duodenum from normal chicks: comparison with the rapid (transcaltachic) effect of 1,25-dihydroxyvitamin D₃. *Endocrinology* 1986;119:1406.

200. Bonjour JP, Fleisch H, Trechsel J. Calcium absorption in diphosphonate-treated rats: effect of parathyroid function, dietary calcium and phosphorus. *J Physiol* 1977;264:125–139.

201. Rizzoli R, Fleisch H, Bonjour J-P. Role of 1,25-dihydroxyvitamin D₃ on intestinal phosphate absorption in rats with a normal vitamin D supply. *J Clin Invest* 1977;60:639–647.

202. Lafond J, Auger D, Fortier J, Brunette MG. Parathyroid hormone receptor in human placental syncytiotrophoblast brush border and basal renal plasma membranes. *Endocrinology* 1988;123:2834–2840.

203. Brunette MG, Auger D, Lafond J. Effect of parathyroid hormone on PO₄ transport through the human placenta microvilli. *Pediatr Res* 1989;25:15–18.

204. Barlet JP, Davicco M-J, Coxam V. Synthetic parathyroid hormone-related peptide (1–34) fragment stimulates placental calcium transfer in ewes. *J Endocrinol* 1990;127:33–37.

205. Rodda CP, Kubota M, Heath JA, et al. Evidence for a novel parathyroid hormone-related protein in fetal lamb parathyroid glands and sheep placenta: comparisons with a similar protein implicated in human hypercalcemia of malignancy. *J Endocrinol* 1988;117:261–271.

206. Care AD, Abbas SK, Pickard DW, et al. Stimulation of ovine placental transport of calcium and magnesium by mid-molecule fragments of human parathyroid hormone-related protein. *Exp Physiol* 1990;75:605–608.

207. Pitkin RM. Calcium metabolism in pregnancy: a review. *Am J Obstet Gynecol* 1975;121:724–737.

208. Reitz RE, Daane TA, Woods JR, Weinstein RL. Calcium, magnesium, phosphorus, and parathyroid hormone interrelationships in pregnancy and newborn infants. *Obstet Gynecol* 1977;50:701–705.

209. Fleischman AR, Lerman S, Oakes GK, Epstein MF, Chez RA, Mintz DH. Perinatal primate parathyroid hormone metabolism. *Biol Neonate* 1975;27:40–49.

210. Fujimi T, Baba H, Fukase M, Fujita T. Direct inhibitory effect of aminoterminal parathyroid hormone fragment PTH (1–34) on parathyroid hormone secretion from bovine parathyroid primary cultured cells in vitro. *Biochem Biophys Res Commun* 1991;178:953–958.

211. Charbon GA, Hulstaert PF. Augmentation of arterial hepatic and renal blood flow by extracted and synthetic parathyroid hormone. *Endocrinology* 1974;95:621.

212. Collip JB, Clark EP. Further studies on the physiological action of a parathyroid hormone. *J Biol Chem* 1925;64:485.

213. Nickols GA. Actions of parathyroid hormone in the cardiovascular system. *Blood Vessels* 1987;24:120.

214. Mok LLS, Nickols GA, Thompson JC, Cooper CW. Parathyroid hormone as a smooth muscle relaxant. *Endocrine Rev* 1989;10:420–436.

215. Pang PKT, Tenner TE Jr, Yee JA, Janssen HF. Hypotensive action of parathyroid hormone preparations on rats and dogs. *Proc Natl Acad Sci USA* 1980;77:675–678.

216. Pang PKT, Yang MCM, Shew R, Tenner TE Jr. The vasorelaxant action of parathyroid hormone fragments on isolated rat tail artery. *Blood Vessels* 1985;22:57–64.

217. Nickols GA, Metz MA, Cline WH Jr. Endothelium-independent linkage of parathyroid hormone receptors of rat vascular tissue with increased adenosine 3′5′-monophosphate and relaxation of vascular smooth muscle. *Endocrinology* 1986; 119:349–356.

218. Wang R, Wir L, Karpinski E, Pang PKT. The effects of parathyroid hormone on L-type voltage-dependent calcium channel currents in vascular smooth muscle cells and ventricular nyocytes are mediated by a cyclic AMP-dependent mechanism. *FEBS Lett* 1991;282:331–334.

219. Pirola CJ, Wang H-M, Kamyar A, et al. Angiotensin II regulates parathyroid hormone–related protein expression in cultured rat aortic smooth muscle cells through transcriptional and post-transcriptional mechanisms. *J Biol Chem* 1993;268:1987–1994.

220. Ferrari S, Rizzoli R, Chaponnier C, Gabbiani G, Bonjour J-P. Parathyroid hormone-related protein increased cAMP production in mammary epithelial cells. *Am J Physiol* 1993;264:E471–E475.

221. MacManus JP, Youdale T, Whitfield JF, Franks DJ. The mediations by calcium and cyclic AMP of the stimulatory action of parathyroid hormone on thymic lymphocyte proliferation. In: *Calcium, parathyroid hormone, and the calcitonins.* Talmage RV, Munson PL, eds. International Congress Series 243, Amsterdam: Exerpta Medica, 1972;338–350.

222. Bialasiewicz AA, Juppner H, Diehl V, Hesch R-D. Binding of bovine parathyroid hormone to surface receptors of cultured lymphocytes. *Biochim Biophys Acta* 1979;584:467–478.

223. Yamamoto I, Potts JT Jr, Segre GV. Circulating bovine lymphocytes contain receptors for parathyroid hormone. *J Clin Invest* 1983;71:404–407.

224. Yamamoto I, Bringhurst FR, Potts JT Jr, Segre GV. Properties of parathyroid hormone receptors on circulating bovine lymphocytes. *J Bone Mineral Res* 1988;3:289–295.

225. McCauley LK, Rosol TJ, Merryman JI, Capen CC. Parathyroid hormone-related protein binding to human T-cell lymphotropic virus type 1-infected lymphocytes. *Endocrinology* 1992;130:300–306.

226. Klinger M, Alexiewicz JM, Linkenisraeli M, et al. Effect of parathyroid hormone on human T-cell activation. *Kidney Int* 1990;37:1543–1551.

227. Fukumoto S, Matsumoto T, Watanabe T, Takashashi H, Miyoshi I, Ogata E. Secretion of parathyroid hormone-like activity from human T-cell lymphotropic virus type I-infected lymphocytes. *Cancer Res* 1989;49:3849–3852.

228. Adachi N, Yamaguchi K, Miyake Y, et al. Parathyroid hormone-related protein is a possible autocrine growth factor for lymphocytes. *Biochem Biophys Res Commun* 1990;166:1088–1094.

229. Goldring SR, Mahaffey JE, Rosenblatt M, Dayer J-M, Potts JT Jr, Krane SM. Parathyroid hormone inhibitors; comparison of biological activity in bone- and skin-derived tissue. *J Clin Endocrinol Metab* 1979;48:655.

230. Pun K-K, Arnaud CD, Nissenson RA. Parathyroid hormone receptors in human dermal fibroblasts: structural and functional characterization. *J Bone Mineral Res* 1988;3:453–460.

231. Kaiser SM, Laneuville P, Bernier SM, Rhim JS, Kremer R, Goltzman D. Enhanced growth of a human keratinocyte cell line induced by antisense RNA for parathyroid hormone-related peptide. *J Biol Chem* 1992;267:13623–13628.

232. Whitfield JF, Chakravarthy BR, Durkin JP, et al. Parathyroid hormone stimulates protein kinase C but not adenylate cyclase in mouse epidermal keratinocytes. *J Cell Physiol* 1992;150:299–303.

233. Hayman JA, Danks JA, Ebeling PR, Moseley JM, Kemp BE, Martin TJ. Expression of parathyroid hormone related protein in normal skin and in tumours of skin and skin appendages. *J Pathol* 1989;158:293–296.

234. Kather H, Simon B. Adenylate cyclase of human fat cell ghosts. Stimulation of enzyme activity by parathyroid hormone. *J Clin Invest* 1977;59:730–733.

235. Sinha TK, Thajchayapong P, Queener S, Allen DO, Bell NH. On the lipolytic action of parathyroid hormone in man. *Metabolism* 1976;25:251–260.

236. Akmal M, Kasim SE, Soliman AR, Massry SG. Excess parathyroid hormone adversely affects lipid metabolism in chronic renal failure. *Kidney Int* 1990;37:854–858.

237. Smogorewski M, Perna AF, Borum PR, Massry SG. Fatty acid oxidation in the myocardium: effects of parathyroid hormone and CRF. *Kidney Int* 1988;34:797–803.

238. Hueck CC, Ritz E. Does parathyroid hormone play a role in lipid metabolism? *Contrib Nephrol* 1980;20:118–128.

239. Fadda GZ, Akmal M, Lipson LG, Massry SG. Direct effect of parathyroid hormone on insulin secretion from pancreatic islets. *Am J Physiol* 1990;258:E975–E984.

240. Drucker DJ, Asa SL, Henderson J, Goltzman D. The parathyroid hormone-like peptide (PLP) gene is expressed in the normal and neoplastic human endocrine pancreas. *Mol Endocrinol* 1989;3:1589–1595.

241. Gaich G, Orloff JJ, Attillasoy EJ, Burtis WJ, Ganz MB, Stewart AF. Amino-terminal parathyroid hormone-related protein: specific binding and cytosolic calcium responses in rat insulinoma cells. *Endocrinology* 1993;132:1402–1409.

242. Sahai A, Fadda GZ, Massry S. Parathyroid hormone activates protein kinase C of pancreatic islets. *Endocrinology* 1992;131:1889–1894.

243. Fraser CL, Sarnacki P, Budayr A. Evidence that parathyroid hormone-mediated calcium transport in rat brain synaptosomes is independent of cyclic adenosine monophosphate. *J Clin Invest* 1988;81:982–988.

244. Weir EC, Brines ML, Ikeda K, Burtis WJ, Broadus AE, Robbins RJ. Parathyroid hormone-related peptide gene is expressed in the mammalian nervous system. *Proc Natl Acad Sci USA* 1990;87:108–112.

245. Canterbury JM, Levy G, Ruiz E, Reiss E. Parathyroid hormone activation of adenylate cyclase in liver. *Proc Soc Exp Biol Med* 1974;147:366–370.

246. Martin K, Hruska K, Greenwalt A, Klahr S, Slatopolsky E. Selective uptake of intact parathyroid hormone by the liver: differences between hepatic and renal uptake. *J Clin Invest* 1976;58:781–788.

247. Barrett PQ, Teitelbaum AP, Neuman WF, Neuman MW. The role of the liver in the peripheral metabolism of parathyroid hormone. In: *Endocrinology of calcium metabolism.* Copp DH, Talmage RV, eds. Amsterdam: Excerpta Medica, 1978;324–328.

248. Segre GV, Perkins AS, Witters LA, Potts JT Jr. Metabolism of parathyroid hormone by isolated rat Kuppfer cells and hepatocytes. *J Clin Invest* 1981;67:449–457.

249. Rosenblatt M, Segre GV, Potts JT Jr. Synthesis of a fragment of parathyroid hormone, bPTH-(28-48): an inhibitor of hormone cleavage in vivo. *Biochemistry* 1977;16:2811–2816.

250. Martin KJ, Hruska K, Tamayo J, Arbelaez M, Slatopolsky E. Hepatic metabolism of parathyroid hormone. *Mineral Electrolyte Metab* 1982;8:173–178.

251. Hruska KA, Blondin J, Bass R, et al. Effect of intact parathyroid hormone on hepatic glucose release in the dog. *J Clin Invest* 1974;64:1016–1023.

252. Neuman WF, Schneider N. The parathyroid hormone-sensitive adenylate cyclase system in plasma membranes of rat liver. *Endocrinology* 1980;107:2082–2087.

253. Bergeron JJM, Tchervenkov S, Rouleau MF, Rosenblatt M, Goltzman D. In vivo demonstration of receptors in rat liver to the amino-terminal region of parathyroid hormone. *Endocrinology* 1981;109:1552–1559.

254. Shah GV, Epand RM, Orlowski RC. Conformational determinants in receptor recognition of peptide hormones: interaction of parathyroid hormone with the glucagon receptor. *Mol Cell Endocrinol* 1987;49:203–210.

255. Bogin E, Massry SG, Harary I. Effect of parathyroid hormone on rat heart cells. *J Clin Invest* 1981;67:1215–1227.

256. Bogin E, Massry SG, Levi J, Djaldeti M, Bristol G, Smith J. Effect of parathyroid hormone on osmotic fragility of human erythrocytes. *J Clin Invest* 1982;69:1017–1025.

257. Schluter K-D, Hellstern H, Wingender E, Mayer H. The central part of parathyroid hormone stimulates thymidine incorporation of chondrocytes. *J Biol Chem* 1989;264:11087–11092.

258. Somjen D, Binderman I, Schluter K-D, Wingender E, Mayer H, Kaye A. Stimulation by defined parathyroid hormone fragments of cell proliferation in skeletal-derived cell cultures. *Biochem J* 1990;272:781–785.

259. Mayer H. The mid-region (28–48) of parathyroid hormone exerts its effects via a mechanism that is distinct from the classical cAMP-dependent pathway; structure/function relationship of PTH-fragments on bone-forming cells. Proceedings of the First International Forum on Calcified Tissue and Bone Metabolism, Yokohama, 1992, Tokyo: Chugai Pharmaceuticals, 1992;44–47.

260. D'Amour P, Huet P, Segre GV, Rosenblatt M. Characteristics of bovine parathyroid hormone extraction by dog liver in vivo. *Am J Physiol* 1981;241:E208–E214.

261. Rosenblatt M, Segre GV, Tregear GW, Shepard GL, Tyler GA, Potts JT Jr. Human parathyroid hormone: synthesis and chemical, biological, and immunological evaluation of the carboxylterminal region. *Endocrinology* 1978;103:978–984.

262. Murray TM, Rao LG, Muzaffar SA, Ly H. Human parathyroid hormone carboxy–terminal peptide (53–84) stimulates alkaline phosphatase activity in dexamethasone-treated rat osteosarcoma cells in vitro. *Endocrinology* 1989;124:1097–1099.

263. Murray TM, Rao LG, Muzaffar SA. Dexamethasone-treated ROS 17/2.8 rat osteosarcoma cells are responsive to human carboxylterminal parathyroid hormone peptide hPTH (53–84): stimulation of alkaline phosphatase. *Calcif Tissue Int* 1991;49:120–123.

264. Nakamoto C, Baba H, Fukase M, et al. Individual and combined effects of intact PTH, amino-terminal, and a series of truncated carboxyl-terminal PTH fragments on alkaline phosphatase activity in dexamethasone-treated rat osteoblastic osteosarcoma cells ROS 17/2.8. *Acta Endocrinol* 1993;128:367–372.

265. Murray TM, Sutherland M, Ly H, Wylie J, Haussler M, Rao LG. Gene regulation in osteoblastic cells by the carboxyterminal (53–84) fragment of parathyroid hormone: Effects of hPTH (53–84) in human osteoblastic SaOS-2 cells. In: *Calcium regulating hormones and bone metabolism: basic and clinical aspects.* Vol II. DV Cohn, C Gennari, AH Tashjian Jr eds. Amsterdam: Excerpta Medica, 1992;105–109.

266. Silbermann M, Shurtz-Swirski R, Lewinson D, Shenzer P, Mayer H. In vitro response of neonatal condylar cartilage to simultaneous exposure to the parathyroid hormone fragments 1–34, 28–48, and 53–84 hPTH. *Calcif Tissue Int* 1991;48:260–266.

267. Lim SK, Gardella TJ, Baba H, Nussbaum SR, Kronenberg HM. The carboxy-terminus of parathyroid hormone is essential for hormone processing and secretion. *Endocrinology* 1992;131:2325–2330.

268. Zaman G, Saphieri PW, Loveridge N, et al. Biological properties of synthetic human parathyroid hormone: effects of deamidation at position 76 on agonist and antagonist activity. *Endocrinology* 1991;128:2583–2590.

269. Born W, Loveridge N, Petermann JB, Kronenberg HM, Potts JT Jr, Fischer JA. Inhibition of parathyroid hormone bioactivity by human parathyroid hormone (PTH)-(3–84) and PTH-(8–84) synthesized in Escherichia coli. *Endocrinology* 1988;123:1848–1853.

270. Massry SG, Schaefer RM, Teschner M, Roeda M, Zull JF, Heidland A. Effect of parathyroid hormone on elastase release from human polymorphonuclear leucocytes. *Kidney Int* 1989;36:883–890.

271. Arber CE, Zanelli JM, Parsons JA, Bitensky L, Chayen J. Comparison of the bioactivity of highly purified human PTH and of synthetic amino- and carboxy-region fragments. *J Endocrinol* 1980;85:55.

272. Lee K, Karaplis A, Bond AT, Segre GV. Expression of PTHrP and PTH/PTHrP receptor transcripts is not spatially or temporally correlated in rat fetal development. *J Bone Min Res* 1992;7(Suppl 1):S134.

273. Hongo T, Kupfer J, Enomoto H, et al. Abundant expression of parathyroid hormone-related protein in primary rat aortic smooth muscle cells accompanies serum-induced proliferation. *J Clin Invest* 1991;88:1841–1847.

274. Winquist RJ, Baskin EP, Vlasuk GP. Synthetic tumor-derived human hypercalcemic factor exhibits parathyroid hormone-like relaxation in renal arteries. *Biochem Biophys Res Commun* 1987;149:227.

275. Mallette LE. The parathyroid polyhormones: new concepts in the spectrum of peptide hormone action. *Endocrine Rev* 1991;12:110–117.

276. Fenton AJ, Kemp BE, Kent GN, et al. A carboxyl-terminal peptide from the parathyroid hormone-related protein inhibits bone resorption by osteoclasts. *Endocrinology* 1991;129:1762–1768.

277. Murray TM, Rao LG, Muzaffar SA. Studies of the interactions between parathyroid hormone, its N- and C-terminal fragments, insulin-like growth factor-1, and dexamethasone in the regulation of mitogenesis in osteoblastic ROS 17/2.8 cells. *J Bone Mineral Res* 6(Suppl 1):S115.

278. D'Amour P, Labelle F, Lecavalier L, Plourde V, Harvey D. Influence of serum Ca concentration on circulating molecular forms of PTH in three species. *Am J Physiol* 1986; 251:E680–E687.

279. Mayer GP, Keaton JA, Hurst JG, Habener JF. Effects of plasma calcium concentration on the relative proportion of hormone and carboxyl fragments in parathyroid venous blood. *Endocrinology* 1979;104:1778–1784.

280. D'Amour P, Labelle F, Wolde-Giorghis R, Hamel L. Immunological evidences for the presence of small late carboxyl-terminal fragments of human parathyroid hormone in circulation in man. *J Immunoassay* 1989;10:191–205.

281. D'Amour P, Palardy J, Bahsali G, Mallette LE, DeLean A, Lepage R. The modulation of circulating parathyroid hormone immunoheterogeneity in man by ionized calcium concentration. *J Clin Endocrinol Metab* 1992;74:525–532.

282. Hanley DA, Ayer LM. Calcium-dependent release of carboxyl-terminal fragments of parathyroid hormone by hyperplastic human parathyroid tissue in vitro. *J Clin Endocrinol Metab* 1986;63:1075.

283. Watson PH, Mortimer ST, Tanguay KE, Hanley DA. Activation and inhibition of protein kinase C in cultured bovine parathyroid cells: effect on the release of C-terminal fragments of parathyroid hormone. *J Bone Mineral Res* 1992; 7:667–674.

284. Brossard J-H, Whittom S, Lepage R, D'Amour P. Carboxylterminal fragments of parathyroid hormone are not preferentially secreted in primary hyperparathyroidism as they are in other hypercalcemic conditions. *J Clin Endocrinol Metab* 1993;77:413–419.

285. Habener JF, Segre GV, Powell D, Murray TM, GP, Potts JT Jr. Immunoreactive parathyroid hormone in circulation of man. *Nature* 1971;238:152–154.

286. Shurtz-Swirski R, Lewinson D, Shenzer P, Mayer H, Silbermann M. Effects of parathyroid hormone fragments on the growth of murine mandibular condylar cartilage in vitro. *Acta Endocrinol* 1990;122:217–226.

287. Crabb ID, O'Keefe RJ, Puzas JE, Rosier R. Differential effects of parathyroid hormone on chick growth plate and articular chondrocytes. *Calcif Tissue Int* 1992;50:61–66.

288. Takigawa M, Fukuo K, Takano T, Suzuki F. Restoration by parathyroid hormone and dibutyryl cyclic AMP of expression of the differentiated phenotype of chondrocytes inhibited by a tumor promoter, 12-O-tetradecanoylphorbol-13-acetate. *Cell Differ* 1983;13:283–291.

289. Petersen P. Psychiatric disorders in primary hyperparathyroidism. *J Clin Endocrinol Metab* 1968;28:1491–1495.

290. Rastad J, Joborn C, Akerstrom G, Ljunghall S. Incidence, type, and severity of psychic symptoms in patients with sporadic primary hyperparathyroidism. *J Endocrinol Invest* 1991;15(Suppl 6):149–162.

291. Fraser CL, Sarnacki P, Budayr A. Evidence that parathyroid hormone-mediated calcium transport in rat brain synaptosomes is independent of cyclic adenosine monophosphate. *J Clin Invest* 1988;81:982–988.

292. Smogorzewski M, Fadda GZ, Massry SG. Mechanisms underlying elevated $[Ca^{2+}]_i$ in brain synaptosomes in states with chronic excess of PTH. *J Endocrinol Invest* 1991; 15(Suppl 6):97–104.

293. DiPette DJ, Christenson W, Nickols MA, Nickols GA. Cardiovascular responsiveness to parathyroid hormone (PTH) and PTH-related protein in genetic hypertension. *Endocrinology* 1992;130:2045–2051.

294. Schleiffer R. Involvement of parathyroid hormone in genetic models of hypertension. *J Endocrinol Invest* 1991;15(Suppl 6):87–95.

295. Scholtz DA. Hypertension and hyperparathyroidism. *Arch Intern Med* 1977;137:1123.

296. Rosenthal FD, Roy S. Hypertension and hyperparathyroidism. *Br Med J* 1972;4:396–397.

297. Diamond TW, Botha JR, Wing J, Meyers AM, Kalk WJ. Parathyroid hypertension: a reversible disorder. *Arch Intern Med* 1986;146:1709.

298. Sancho JJ, Rouco J, Riera-Vidal R, Sitges-Serra A. Long-term effects of parathyroidectomy for primary hyperparathyroidism on arterial hypertension. *World J Surg* 1992; 16:732–736.

299. De Fronzo RA, Andres R, Edgar P, Walker WG. Carbohydrate metabolism in uremia: a review. *Medicine* 1977;52: 469–481.

300. Akmal M, Massry SG, Goldstein DA, Fanti P, Weisz A, DeFronzo RA. Role of parathyroid hormone in the glucose intolerance of chronic renal failure. *J Clin Invest* 1985;75: 1037–1044.

301. Fadda GZ, Smogorzewski M, Massry SG. Abnormalities in pancreatic islet function and metabolism in presence and absence of excess PTH: role of high Ca^{2+}. *J Endocrinol Invest* 1992;15(Suppl 6–9):163–169.

302. Yasuda K, Hurukawa Y, Okuyama M, Kikuchi M, Yoshinaga K. Glucose tolerance and insulin secretion in patients with parathyroid disorders: effects of serum calcium on insulin release. *N Engl J Med* 1975;292:501–504.

303. Hamilton DV, Pryor JS. Endocrine abnormalities in primary hyperparathyroidism. *Postgrad Med J* 1981;57:167–161.

304. Prager R, Schernthaner G, Kovarik J, Cichini G, Klaushofer K, Willvonseder R. Primary hyperparathyroidism is associated with decreased insulin receptor binding and glucose intolerance. *Calcif Tissue Int* 1984;36:253–258.

305. Ljunghall S, Palmer M, Akerstrom G, Wide L. Diabetes mellitus, glucose intolerance and insulin response to glucose in patients with primary hyperparathyroidism before and after parathyroidectomy. *Eur J Clin Invest* 1983;13:373–377.

306. Podbesek R, Edouard C, Meunier PJ, Parsons JA, Reeve J. Treatment with human parathyroid hormone fragment (hPTH 1–34) stimulates bone formation and intestinal calcium absorption in the greyhound: comparison with data from the osteoporosis trial. In: *Hormonal control of calcium metabolism*. DV Cohn, RV Talmage, JL Matthews, eds. Amsterdam: Excerpta Medica, 1981;118–123.

307. Reeve J, Hesp R, Wooton R. Clinical trial of hPTH (1–34) in "idiopathic" osteoporosis. In: *Endocrinology of calcium metabolism*. DH Kopp, RV Talmage, eds. ICS Congress Series 421. Amsterdam: Exerpta Medica, 1978;71–74.

308. Slovik DM, Rosenthal DC, Coppelt SH, et al. Restoration of spinal bone in osteoporotic men by treatment with human parathyroid hormone (1–34) and 1,25-dihydroxyvitamin D. *J Bone Mineral Res* 1986;1:377–382.

309. Reeve J, Meunier PS, Parsons JA, et al. Anabolic effect of human parathyroid hormone fragment on trabecular bone in involutional osteoporosis: a multicenter trial. *Br Med J* 1980;280:1340–1344.

310. Rixon RH, Whitfield JF. Parathyroid hormone: a possible initiator of liver regeneration. *Proc Soc Exp Biol Med* 1971;141:93–97.

311. Rixon RH, MacManus JP, Whitfield JF. The control of liver regeneration by calcitonin, parathyroid hormone and 1,25-dihydroxycholecalciferol. *Mol Cell Endocrinol* 1979;15: 79–89.

312. Coxam V, Davicco M-J, Durand D, Bauchart D, Lefaivre J, Barlet J-P. The influence of parathyroid hormone-related protein on hepatic IGF-1 production. *Acta Endocrinol* 1992;126:430–433.

313. Pizurki LR, Rizzoli R, Moseley J, Martin TJ, Caverzasio J, Bonjour J-P. Effect of synthetic tumoral parathyroid hormone related peptide on cAMP production and sodium-dependent phosphate transport in cultured renal epithelial cells. *Am J Physiol* 1988;255:F957–F961.

The Parathyroids, edited by J.P. Bilezikian,
M.A. Levine, and R. Marcus. Raven Press, Ltd.,
New York © 1994.

CHAPTER 14

Receptors for Parathyroid Hormone and Parathyroid Hormone-Related Protein

Gino V. Segre

Parathyroid hormone (PTH) is well-recognized to be the most critical homeostatic regulator of extracellular calcium and phosphorus, through actions that begin with its binding to cell surface receptors, particularly on renal tubule cells and on osteoblasts (1). Chase and Aurbach's (2) report that PTH increased urinary cAMP immediately before it elicited its classic phosphaturic response was a seminal observation indicating that this hormone acts by stimulating adenylyl cyclase. These observations were soon confirmed and extended by evidence that PTH activated adenylyl cyclase in vitro in both renal and bone cell preparations (3,4). The mechanism by which agonist-occupied receptors, such as the PTH receptor, function was subsequently complicated by the discovery of heterotrimeric guanyl nucleotide-binding proteins (G proteins) that transduce signals from these cell-surface receptors to intracellular effectors, including adenylyl cyclase, and amplify them.

The agonist-occupied receptor must have two general properties; it must modulate events that alter the biological actions of the cell, while also initiating processes to terminate these events and restore the cell's capacity to respond to subsequent stimulation. The following cascade of events is thought to occur when all G protein-coupled receptors, including the PTH receptor, are occupied by agonists: the agonist-occupied receptor activates a G protein, a process during which guanosine diphosphate (GDP) bound to the G protein's α-subunit is exchanged for guanosine triphosphate (GTP). This, in turn, results in the dissociation of the α-subunit from the $\beta\gamma$-subunits that remain bound to each other, and the subsequent activation or

inhibition of an effector system by the GTP-occupied Gα-subunit. Most of PTH's distal actions, if not all, were thought to be the consequence of PTH's capacity to activate the stimulatory G protein (Gs), and the subsequent stimulation of adenylyl cyclase by the dissociated, active α-subunit. More recently, however, hormonal stimulation of PTH receptors also has been shown to activate phospholipase C, as evidenced by hormone-stimulated increases of intracellular free calcium ($[Ca^{++}]_i$) and acceleration of inositol phosphate hydrolysis rates (5–11). PTH also promotes Ca^{2+} entry through the cell's plasma membrane (10) and may have direct effects on phospholipase A$_2$ (12,13). The physiological relevance of these complex cellular responses to PTH are discussed elsewhere in this volume, as is the issue of whether these responses are all primary, or are secondary consequences of postreceptor "crosstalk" between effector-activated pathways.

Direct analysis of PTH/receptor interactions lagged because developing high specific-activity PTH ligands was a formidable problem. PTH receptor properties have been characterized primarily using ^{125}I-labeled amino-terminal PTH fragments and analogs as radioligands rather than intact hormone. Although this limitation must be recognized, it is acceptable because the properties of these shortened molecules are, for the most part, closely similar to, or indistinguishable from those of the full-length, 84-amino-acid hormone (1). Studies of endogenous receptors by radioreceptor assay and by affinity cross-linking of the ligand to its receptor have defined many of its pharmacological and physicochemical properties. Mostly kidney and bone, traditional PTH targets, have been studied, although it is now quite clear that PTH also binds to a variety of other cells or preparations of their plasma membranes. These include fibroblasts (14), circulating lymphocytes (15), chondrocytes (16), vascular smooth muscle

G. V. Segre: Endocrine Unit, Department of Medicine, Harvard Medical School, Massachusetts General Hospital, Boston, Massachusetts 02114.

(17), fat cells (18), and placental trophoblasts (19). Receptors in these nonclassical locations appear to be authentic; their activation by PTH is associated with increased cAMP production, and ligand-receptor cross-linking does not distinguish these receptors from those present in bone and kidney, when such studies have been performed (14). The issue of whether osteoclasts directly respond to PTH is still controversial, although several lines of evidence suggest that mature osteoclasts do not have PTH receptors and respond to PTH only indirectly (20,21). Additional binding sites that are specific for portions of the PTH sequence carboxyl-terminal to position 53 have been reported. However, based on competitive radioreceptor assays that used biologically active PTH-(1–84) as the radioligand, the biological significance of these so-called carboxyl-terminal PTH receptors has been elusive (22,23).

Details of parathyroid hormone-related protein's (PTHrP) structure and function are provided elsewhere in this volume (see the chapters by Broadus and Stewart, Grill and Martin, Strewler and Nissenson, and Kremer and Goltzman). The following short summary, however, will facilitate discussions of the PTH/PTHrP receptor's biological properties. PTHrP was originally identified in extracts of tumors from cancer patients with elevated blood calcium levels (24–26). It appears to be the causal factor responsible for most instances of hypercalcemia associated with malignancies, perhaps the most common paraneoplastic syndrome in human beings. In this capacity, PTHrP functions principally as a circulating hormone. It also may circulate in the blood of patients without malignancies, although its functions in normal human adult physiology are unknown (27,28). PTH and PTHrP share identical amino acids at eight of their 13 most amino-terminal positions, although the remainder of their sequences are completely different. Northern blot analyses of PTHrP mRNA, prepared from human cancers, reveal multiple transcripts that are likely due to alternative mRNA splicing, and perhaps result from other mechanisms, such as transcription initiated from more than one promoter. If all these mRNAs are translated, they would encode peptides that are about 50–90 amino acids longer than PTH (29). The capacity of both PTH and PTHrP peptides to bind to the same receptor (see below) and for PTHrP to mimic PTH's capacity to induce hypercalcemia undoubtedly relates to this limited amino-terminal sequence homology (30). PTHrP is also synthesized in multiple adult and fetal tissues, where it is thought to mediate several paracrine/autocrine functions.

Parathyroid hormone-related protein activation of its receptors certainly plays an important role in embryogenesis. Homologous recombination has been used to remove the major coding exon from one copy of the mouse PTHrP gene (31). Homozygous mutants, the products of matings between heterozygotic animals that transmit the mutant allele through their germlines, die soon after birth and have a multitude of skeletal anomalies (see below). As discussed elsewhere in this volume, the importance of activated PTH/PTHrP receptors in early fetal development also can be inferred from the wide distribution of PTHrP in all three germ layers and from PTHrP's expression in trophectoderm cells in the morula stage in mice embryos, where it has been proposed to serve a paracrine/autocrine role in parietal endoderm development (32). Although PTHrP's roles in fetal and adult physiology are under intensive study, they remain somewhat elusive (30,33). Perhaps, its best defined and most unique physiological property is to actively transport calcium across the placenta against a gradient from the ewe to the lamb. In carrying out this function, PTHrP most probably acts as a hormone rather than through paracrine/autocrine mechanisms (33).

Although PTHrP has been implicated in the control of fetal blood calcium levels, it apparently does not regulate blood calcium levels in animals after birth. Obviously, the profound hypocalcemia that accompanies total parathyroidectomy demonstrates that PTHrP cannot serve as a surrogate for PTH. PTHrP's distribution in many tissues has fueled speculation that receptors in these unorthodox targets might serve, physiologically, to mediate PTHrP's actions, rather than actions of PTH. Evidence in support of these hypotheses is only currently becoming available.

The properties of PTH receptors were first characterized using renal cortical plasma membranes and radioligands of the amino-terminal portion of the PTH molecule. For example, all earlier studies and most recent experiments from this laboratory have used [Nle⁸, Nle¹⁸, Tyr³⁴]bovine PTH-(1–34) amide, a ¹²⁵I-labeled sulfur-free PTH analog, as the radioligand (34,35). PTH receptors were shown to be of high affinity (K_ds between 0.8 and 5 nM) and linked to adenylyl cyclase activation, as evidenced by direct measurements of hormonally-stimulated enzyme activity or increased intracellular cAMP in plasma cell membrane preparations and in intact cells, respectively (34–36). Furthermore, addition of nonhydrolyzable GTP analogs to membrane preparations accelerated dissociation of the ligand, a characteristic of G protein-coupled receptors (37).

Responses to PTH are determined in large part, of course, by its circulating blood level. The agonist-occupied receptor's second major role, to set in motion mechanisms that regulate the cell's response to further exposure to the ligand, also is thought to play a key role. Cells regulate their responsiveness by many mechanisms that include modulating the number of functional receptors and influencing postreceptor events important to their mechanism of action. In intact animals with induced primary and secondary hyperparathyroidism, functional PTH receptors are diminished in number, when expressed per milligram of renal membrane protein, but have unaltered affinity (38,39). Resistance to PTH action is well recognized, especially in patients with chronic renal failure, who also have elevated PTH levels (40). This decreased responsiveness may be due, at least in part, to agonist-induced down-regulation of their PTH receptors (40a).

Decreased PTH binding and desensitization of adenylyl cyclase responsiveness to a subsequent PTH challenge occur in vitro in a dose- and time-dependent manner, when cells expressing endogenous PTH receptors are continuously treated with PTH agonists (34,41–45). Interestingly, homologous down-regulation of PTH receptors in ROS 17/2.8 cells occurs with hormonal concentrations too low to be measured by competitive radioreceptor assays (34). This has at least two implications; certain cellular responses to PTH occur with receptor occupancy too low to measure and, its corollary, PTH-responsive cells have many "spare" receptors. The mechanisms that underlie these regulatory phenomena are under investigation. Preliminary analyses suggest that homologous down-regulation in clonal ROS 17/.28 and OK cells is primarily determined at the posttranscriptional level, because functional PTH receptors are markedly diminished by several days of hormonal treatment, but steady-state levels of receptor mRNA are not altered (46). These data confirm and extend the earlier report by Teitelbaum et al. (47) of marked reduction of PTH binding by pretreatment of primary avian bone cells with compounds that interfere with receptor recycling and the lack of effect on PTH binding by inhibitors of protein synthesis. Acutely, homologous PTH receptor down-regulation in primary bone cells appeared to be dependent largely on internalization and intracellular processing of ligand-receptor complexes, and subsequent catabolism or reinsertion of PTH receptors into the plasma membrane, rather than to rely on new receptor synthesis. Teitelbaum and her colleagues (47) also showed that internalization of PTH-receptor complexes was agonist-induced and energy-dependent.

Heterologous regulation of the PTH receptor, that is, regulation by factors other than PTH and PTHrP, also occurs in a dose- and time-dependent manner. Glucocorticoids dramatically increase the number of PTH receptors in osteoblast-like ROS 17/2.8 osteosarcoma cells (48), and they have been reported to decrease PTH receptor number in OK cells (49). Both retinoic acid (50) and 1,25-dihydroxyvitamin D [1,25(OH)$_2$D] (51) down-regulate PTH receptors in ROS 17/2.8 cells. In the few examples thus far studied, heterologous regulation is associated with parallel changes in the steady-state levels of receptor mRNA, in contrast to homologous down-regulation of PTH receptors (G.V. Segre, unpublished data).

The physicochemical properties of PTH receptors have been partially characterized by affinity cross-linking radioiodinated PTH ligands to them, solubilizing the ligand-receptor complex, and identifying the receptor as a radioactively-labeled band after sodium dodecyl sulfate (SDS)-polyacrylamide gel electrophoresis. These receptors are glycoproteins with a molecular size of ~80,000 daltons; the peptide backbone accounts for ~59,000 daltons, and the remainder is due to asparagine-linked oligosaccharides (52–54). Essentially, two principal methods have been used. (a) N-hydroxysuccinimidyl-4-azido-benzoate, a heterobifunctional reagent has been used to crosslink ^{125}I-PTH (1–34) bound to its receptor. This method also demonstrated the extraordinary susceptibility of the receptor to proteolysis (55). (b) Binding of photoreactive derivatives of amino-terminal analogs of both PTH and PTHrP that were first covalently modified by addition of 4-fluoro-3-nitrophenylazide to the α-amino group of the first amino acid or to ε-amino functions of lysine residues, then radioiodinated, and finally incubated with intact cells before crosslinking them to receptors with ultraviolet (UV) light. The biological properties of the family of derivatived PTH and PTHrP analogs have been characterized in detail, after their separation via high-performance liquid chromatography (HPLC). These studies have contributed to understanding functionally important residues in the ligand, by distinguishing analogs that retained activity from those where modifications of the molecule impaired the hormone's activity (56–58).

Amino-terminal analogs of PTHrP, which subsequently became available and could also be made photoreactive, allowed comparisons between the binding properties of PTH-(1–34) and PTHrP-(1–36) or -(1–40). Receptors bound the two peptides with the same affinity. The receptors that bound either ligand were of same apparent molecular size, and both PTH and PTHrP down-regulated receptors that bound either ligand (59,60) (Figs. 1, 2). These studies provided strong evidence that the same receptor binds both ligands, an issue that was definitively resolved when cloned opossum renal and rat receptors were shown to bind amino-terminal PTH and PTHrP analogs with equal affinity (5,61). The cloned human receptor also binds both peptides, although it prefers PTH (62). All the actions of PTH and PTHrP, however, may not be mediated through PTH/PTHrP receptors that have been cloned. Receptor mRNAs with differing lengths have been identified in several tissues and organs (63) (Fig. 3),

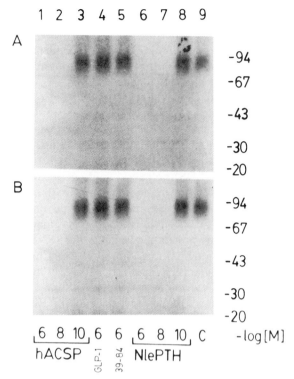

1 2 3 4 5 6 7 8 9

A

-94
-67
-43
-30
-20

B

-94
-67
-43
-30
-20

6 8 10 6 6 6 8 10 C -log[M]
hACSP GLP-1 39-84 NlePTH

FIG. 1. Photoaffinity labeling of ROS 17/2.8 cell PTH receptors. ROS 17/2.8 cells were incubated in the dark (4 hr, 15°C) with either ^{125}I-photoreactive [Nle^{8,18},Tyr^{34}]bovine PTH-(1–34) amide or (**A**) ^{125}I-photoreactive [Tyr^{36}] human PTHrP-(1–36) amide (labeled hASCP) (**B**). Competing unlabeled ligands are [Tyr^{36}] human PTHrP-(1–36) amide (range from 10^{-6} to 10^{-10} M; *lanes 1–3*), GLP-1 (10^{-6} M; *lane 4*), human PTH-(53–84) (10^{-6} M, *lane 5*), or [Nle^{8,18},Tyr^{34}]bovine PTH-(1–34) amide (range 10^{-6}–10^{-10} M, *lanes 6–8*). Incubation of the cells in the presence of either photoligand alone is shown in lane 9 (C, control). After rinsing, photolysis, and solubilization, the samples were analyzed by SDS-PAGE with subsequent autoradiography. (Reprinted from ref. 58 with permission.)

and, as was mentioned above, there may be receptors that specifically bind carboxyl-terminal portions of the PTH molecule. Additional PTHrP receptors that do not share binding with PTH or preferentially bind PTHrP may well exist (30,33).

The recent cloning of cDNAs encoding PTH receptors has made it possible to study its ligand-binding and signal-transduction properties in much greater detail through experiments in which receptors are expressed, transiently or stably, in "neutral" cells that do not express PTH receptors endogenously. The availability of cloned receptor cDNAs also has permitted detection of PTH receptor mRNA by both Northern blotting and in situ nucleotide hybridization. These studies have characterized the size and distribution of receptor mRNA. The cellular locations of receptor transcripts have raised many provocative questions concerning potential functions of these receptors

in signal transduction, embryogenesis, cell proliferation, and cell differentiation.

The cDNAs encoding opossum renal and rat bone PTH/PTHrP receptors were independently cloned by minor modifications of the mammalian expression methods described by Gearing et al. (64) in their successful cloning of the granulocyte-macrophage colony-stimulating factor (GM-CSF) receptor. This technique relies on identifying COS-7 cells that transiently express the receptor of interest by their capacity to bind the relevant radiolabeled ligand, which is then detected by emulsion autoradiography. This approach, which has now been used to clone a large number of cell-surface receptors, has three essential requirements: (a) an appropriate plasmid vector, (b) a high-efficiency expression system, and (c) a highly selective screening system. Additionally, the method's efficiency is enhanced through the use of non-self annealing adapters and a high-quality, size-selected cDNA library. The plasmid vector, CDM-8 (65), which is commercially available as pcDNA1, was used to express and clone the cDNAs encoding several PTH/PTHrP receptors (5,61). This plasmid features a tyrosine tRNA amber suppressor gene, a polylinker for insertion of the DNAs, a bacterial origin of replication for efficient cloning of the plasmid, a simian virus 40 (SV40) viral origin of replication that permits rapid multiplication of plasmids in mammalian cells, a strong promoter derived from cytomegalovirus (CMV) to drive transcription of DNA inserted in the polylinker, and an M13 origin of replication that permits rapid single-strand DNA sequencing.

To isolate cDNAs that encode PTH/PTHrP receptors, cDNA libraries were prepared from poly-A$^+$ RNAs, which were independently extracted from clonal opossum kidney (OK) and clonal rat osteosarcoma (ROS 17/2.8) cells. After second-stranding the DNAs, the libraries were independently ligated to Bst-X1 non-self-annealing adapters. (Use of these adapters avoids adapter-adapter and cDNA-cDNA polymers and improves yield because dephosphorylation is not required.) These libraries were then size-selected for cDNAs >700 bp in length and were used to transform *Escherichia coli,* which contain the amber mutation encoding resistance to ampicillin and tetracycline. Plasmid cDNA pools from ~10,000 independent bacterial colonies were transfected into subconfluent COS-7 cells, which were grown in "slideflasks." After a 48 hr incubation to permit maximal expression of the cDNAs, cells were incubated with ^{125}I-[Tyr^{36}]PTHrP-(1–36) amide. The slides then were washed with appropriate buffer, the cells were fixed with glutaraldehyde, and the slides then were dipped in photoemulsion for autoradiography. Slides were developed after 2–4 days and examined by microscopy (darkfield is more effi-

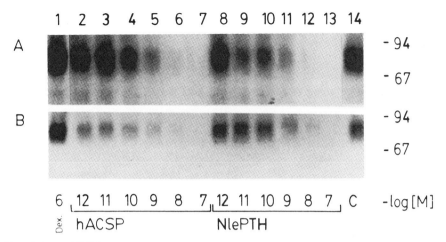

FIG. 2. Regulation of ROS 17/2.8 cell receptors by NlePTH, [Tyr36]human PTHrP-(1–36) amide, and dexamethasone. ROS 17/2.8 cells were initially treated for 3 days with either [Tyr36]human PTHrP-(1–36) amide (labeled hACSP), 10^{-12}–10^{-7} M, *lanes 2–7*). NlePTH (10^{-12}–10^{-7}, *lanes 8–13*), dexamethasone (10^{-6} M, *lane 1*), or vehicle alone (lane 14). The cells were then incubated in the dark (4 hr, 15°C), with either ^{125}I-photoreactive [Nle^{8,18},Tyr^{34}] bovine PTH-(1–34) amide (NlePTH) (**A**) or ^{125}I-photoreactive [Tyr36]human PTHrP-(1–36) amide (**B**). After rinsing, photolysis, and solubilization, the samples were analyzed by SDS-PAGE with subsequent autoradiography. (Reprinted from ref. 59 with permission.)

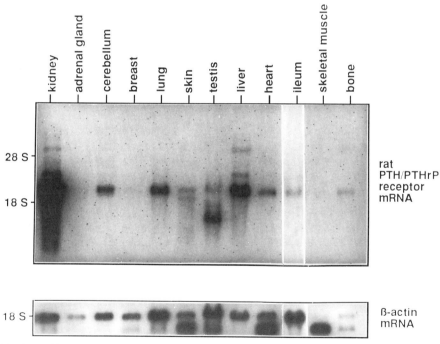

FIG. 3. Northern blot analysis of poly-A$^+$ RNA prepared from different rat tissues. Approximately 5 μg of poly-A$^+$ RNA was loaded in each lane, hybridized with the cDNA probe and washed at high stringency conditions; 30 min at 42°C with 300 ml of 1 × SSC and 0.1% SDS, and 30 min at 65°C with the same solution. The autoradiograph was developed after 7 days of exposure at −80°C. After hybridization with the PTH/PTHrP receptor probe, and exposure, the filter was washed and rehybridized with the β-actin probe, and then exposed for 20 hours at −80°C. (Reprinted from ref. 62 with permission.)

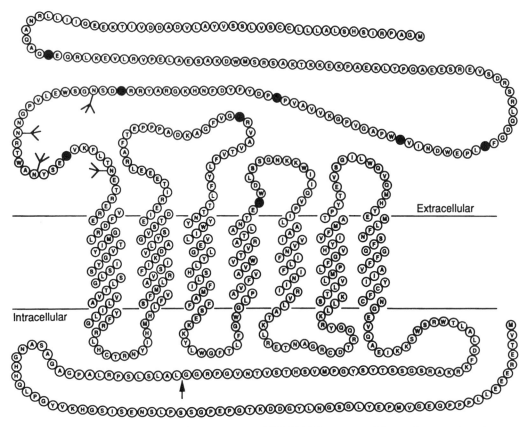

FIG. 4. Schematic representation of the opossum PTH/PTHrP receptor. The amino-terminus is extra-cellular; potential glycosylation sites (Υ) and conserved cysteines (•) are indicated. In OK-H, a carboxyl-terminally truncated receptor, residues 508–515 (to the left of the arrow) are WPCPSALD. This mutant receptor ends eight residues after the arrow. (Reprinted from ref. 61 with permission.)

cient than brightfield). The bacterial pools responsible for generating the positive autoradiographic signals were then sequentially subdivided and screened until clones that expressed PTH/PTHrP receptors were isolated (5,61). Complementary DNAs encoding rat renal and human renal and bone PTH/PTHrP receptors were subsequently cloned by standard nucleotide hybridization techniques in which phage cDNA libraries that

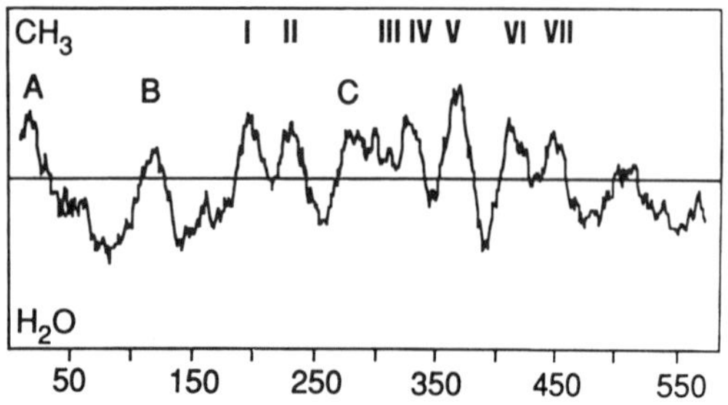

FIG. 5. Hydrophobicity plot of the deduced opossum PTH/PTHrP receptor sequence with a 20-residue window. The seven membrane-spanning helices are indicated as are additional hydrophobic regions A, B, and C. (Reprinted from ref. 61 with permission.)

had been synthesized from poly-A⁺ RNA isolated from the respective organs were screened initially with portions of the rat receptor sequence (62).

The cDNAs encoding these PTH/PTHrP receptors predicted them to have general topographic features common to other members of the G protein-linked receptor superfamily; amino-terminal extracellular sequences (although not all G protein-linked receptors have a signal sequence), three extracellular loops, three intracellular loops, and a carboxyl-terminal cytoplasmic region. These relatively hydrophilic regions are linked by seven relatively hydrophobic membrane-spanning helices (Figs. 4, 5).

The PTH/PTHrP receptor's amino acid sequences are highly homologous, and their lengths vary from 585 to 594 amino acids (5,61,62). Rat and mouse PTH/PTHrP receptors are 99% identical at the amino acid level, and the human and rat PTH/PTHrP receptors are 91% identical; opossum and rat receptors, whose amino acids are 78% identical, are the most widely divergent of the sequences thus far reported. This phylogenetic conservation across such distantly related mammals is striking. The greatest amino acid differences among these receptors are limited to discrete

```
                  **                                      *
H  MGTARIAPGL ALLLCCPVLS SAYALVDADD VMTKEEQIFL LHRAQAQCEK  50
R  ..A.....S. .......... .......... ...F....... ........D.  50
O  ..AP..SHS. ......S.... .V........ ...I......I. .RN......Q  50

H  RLKEVLQRPA SIMESDKGWT SASTSGKPRK DKASGKLYPE SEEDKEAPTG 100
R  L......HTA. N......... P.......... E.....F... .K.N.DV... 100
O  ......RV. ELA..A.D. M.R.A.TK. E.PAE....SQ A..SR.VSDR  97

            '*          *                *            *
H  SRYRGRPCLP EWDHILCWPL GAPGEVVAVP CPDYIYDFNH KGHAYRRCDR 150
R  ..R....... ...N.V.... .......... .......... .......... 150
O  ..LQDGF... ...N.V...A .V..K..... .......... ..R......S 147

      $       $    $   *      $                   I
H  NGSWELVPGH NRTWANYSEC VKFLTNETRE REVFDRLGMI YTVGYSVSLA 200
R  .....V.... .......... L..M...... .......... .......M... 200
O  .........N .......... .......... .......... ....I..G 197

                            II
H  SLTVAVLILA YFRRLHCTRN YIHMHLFLSF MLRAVSIFVK DAVLYSGATL 250
R  .......... .......... ....M..... ...A...... .......F.. 250
O  .........G .......... ....V.. ........I. .......VST 247

                     *
H  DEAERLTEEE LRAIAQAPPP PATAAAGYAG CRVAVTFFLY FLATNYYWLL 300
R  .......... .HI...V.. ..A..V.... .......... .......... 300
O  ..I..I.... ...FTE ... DK..FV. ......V.... ..T...... 294

   III          FMAFFSEKKY IV
H  VEGLYLHSLI FMAFFSEKKY LWGFTVFGWG LPAVFVAVWV SVRATLANTG 350
R  .......... .......... ....I..... .......... G........ 350
O  .......... .......... ....L.. .......... T........E 344

      *                     V
H  CWDLSSGNKK WIIQVPILAS IVLNFILFIN IVRVLATKLR ETNAGRCDTR 400
R  .......H.. .......... .....V.... ...I...... .......... 400
O  .......... .......... ....A..V... ...I...... .... ... 394

              VI
H  QQYRKLLKST LVLMPLFGVH YIVFMATPYT EVSGTLWQVQ MHYEMLFNSF 450
R  ......R... ...V...... .T....L... .......... ...I...... 450
O  .......... .......... .......... ...I...... .......... 444

   VII
H  QGFFVAIIYC FCNGEVQAEI KKSWSRWTLA LDFKRKARSG SSSYSYGPMV 500
R  .......... .......... .R........ .......... .......... 500
O  .......... .......... .......... .......... ..T...... 494

H  SHTSVTNVGP RVGLGLPLSP RLLPTAT T NGHPQLPGHA KPGTPALETL 548
R  .......... .A..S..... ..P. .. ....S...... ..A..T.. 546
O  .......... .G..A.S.... ..A.G.GASA ...H.....YV .H.SISENS. 544

H  ETTPPAMAAP KDDGFLNGSC SGLDEEASGP ERPPALLQEE WETVM      593
R  ..L.VT..V. .......... .......... A...P..... .....      591
O  PSSG.E PGT ....Y.... ..Y.PMV. .Q..P..E.. R....       585
```

FIG. 6. Alignment of the human (H), rat (R), and opossum (O) PTH/PTHrP receptors. Identical amino acids between the human and rat, or human and opossum receptors (·), conserved extracellular cysteines (*), conserved extracellular potential glycosylation sites ($), and putative membrane-spanning regions (*underscored, I–VII*) are indicated. (Reprinted from ref. 62 with permission.)

portions of their amino-terminal extracellular region and first extracellular loop and to their carboxyl-terminal intracellular sequences. Other portions of their amino-terminal extracellular region and the sequences that putatively span the membrane are especially highly conserved (Fig. 6). All PTH receptors have three additional hydrophobic regions; the location and sequence of the first suggest that it is a signal peptide, although whether it is retained in the mature peptide or cleaved during processing is unknown; the second lies within the amino-terminal extracellular region, and third within the first putative extracellular loop

(Fig. 5). Ten cysteine residues (including two in the putative signal sequence, six in the amino-terminal extension, and one in each of the first two extracellular loops), several charged amino acids and prolines within the receptor's membrane-spanning portions, and four potential glycosylation sites in the amino-terminal extension all are positioned identically (Fig. 6). Although the nucleotide sequences encoding human and rat PTH/PTHrP receptors differ, renal and bone receptors are identical within each species, indicating that the same receptor transcript is present in these two traditional PTH targets. Of course, other receptors that might bind PTH or PTHrP exclusively or preferentially are not excluded. These may not have been detected by the methods employed (62).

Parathyroid hormone/parathyroid hormone-related protein receptors are now appreciated to belong to a newly discovered and growing family within the very large superfamily of G protein-linked receptors. Other members of this family, all of which have been cloned over the last 2 years, include receptors for secretin (66), calcitonin (67), vasoactive intestinal peptide (68), glucagon-like peptide-1 (69), glucagon (70) and growth hormone-releasing hormone (71). Classifying these receptors as members of a distinct G protein-coupled receptor family is warranted because they have no significant sequence identity (<12%) with the other G protein-linked receptors presently in data banks (72,73). Sequence alignment of members of this receptor family shows them to be highly homologous with many identical or highly conserved amino acids (Fig. 7). All members have relatively long amino-terminal, extracellular extensions; a highly conserved pattern of cysteine residues in the amino-terminal extension and in each of the first two putative extracellular loops, and multiple potential asparagine-linked glycosylation sites. Their last three membrane-spanning domains and the initial portion of their carboxyl-terminal intracellular region are especially highly conserved; 16 of 18 and 17 of 18 amino acids in this region are identical between secretin and PTH/PTHrP receptors and between calcitonin and PTH/PTHrP receptors, respectively.

Interesting implications and speculations arise from the unexpectedly close relationships among these receptors and their respective ligands. For example, when animals moved from an oceanic environment, which contains abundant calcium, to terrestrial habitats, where calcium is in short supply, a hormonal system for preventing hypocalcemia would have provided a clear evolutionary advantage. The similarities between the genes encoding PTH and PTHrP suggest that they evolved from a common ancestral molecule by a translocation event and that PTHrP is likely to be the older gene. Chromosomal translocations also are thought to explain the evolutionary relationship among

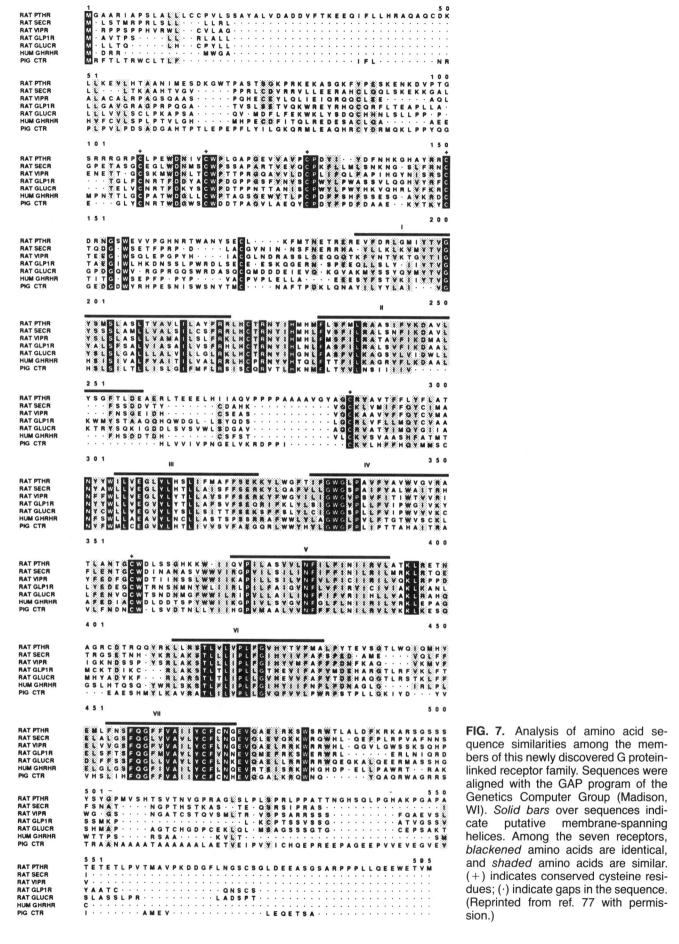

FIG. 7. Analysis of amino acid sequence similarities among the members of this newly discovered G protein-linked receptor family. Sequences were aligned with the GAP program of the Genetics Computer Group (Madison, WI). *Solid bars* over sequences indicate putative membrane-spanning helices. Among the seven receptors, *blackened* amino acids are identical, and *shaded* amino acids are similar. (+) indicates conserved cysteine residues; (·) indicate gaps in the sequence. (Reprinted from ref. 77 with permission.)

ligands that belong to the secretin/glucagon family of peptides. The existence of a remote common ancestor for the superfamily of G protein-coupled receptors is quite plausible, and the interrelationships among members of this newly discovered family, based on their relative homologies, is consistent with the G protein-coupled seven membrane-spanning receptor phylogenetic-tree presented in Fig. 8. Other receptors belonging to this family certainly will be identified, and their properties will further clarify the evolutionary and functional relationships among its members.

The enormous array of critical roles served by the G protein-linked receptor superfamily is especially noteworthy. Receptors that share this common motif of seven membrane-spanning helices are found both in invertebrates and vertebrates, including mammalian as well as submammalian species. Their versatility is exemplified by their capacity to be activated by such diverse stimuli as photons, odors, opioids, catecholamines, prostaglandins, compounds important for cellular metabolism (such as glutamate and adenosine), thrombin, cAMP (in *Dictyostelium discoideum*), mating factor (in yeast), large glycopeptide hormones [such as thyroid-stimulating hormone (TSH), luteinizing hormone/human chorionic gonadotropin (LH/hCG), and follicle-stimulating hormone (FSH)], and small peptide hormones, including somatostatin, va-

sopressin, oxytocin, and a rapidly growing number of others (for review, see 74–77).

The specific molecular determinants required for PTH/PTHrP-receptor and receptor-G protein interactions are under intense investigation. These must involve the three-dimensional organization of each of these moieties, and the modifications that occur when they bind each other. Interactions between PTH (and PTHrP) and its receptor(s) are undoubtedly complex, as they occur between ligands that are at least 84 amino acids in length and highly ordered seven membrane-spanning receptors consisting of about 590 amino acids. Receptor-transducer interactions also are likely to be very complex, because of the myriad of potential interaction sites between these large molecules. Additionally, the cloned activated PTH/PTHrP receptors all stimulate multiple effectors, including both adenylyl cyclase and phospholipase C, almost certainly through their interactions with multiple G proteins (5) (Fig. 9). This property is shared with at least some other members of this newly discovered receptor family (78–80) and may be common to all of them. It also is a property of activated LH (81) and TSH (82) receptors.

Some domains of the PTH/PTHrP receptor involved in ligand-binding have been deduced by characterizing

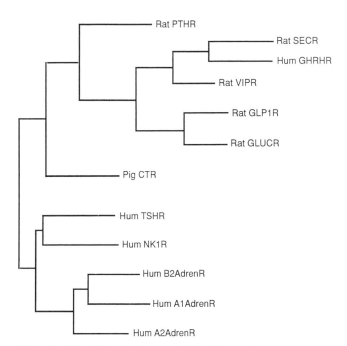

FIG. 8. Plausible phylogeny of the G protein-receptor superfamily. The *upper portion* depicts the seven receptors members of this newly-discovered receptor family. Hum TSHR, Hum NK1R, Hum B2AdrenR, HumA1AdrenR, and Hum A2AdrenR refer to the human homologs of receptors for thyroid-stimulating hormone; neurokinen 1; and β_2-, α_1-, and α_2-adrenergic compounds. (Reprinted from ref. 109 with permission.)

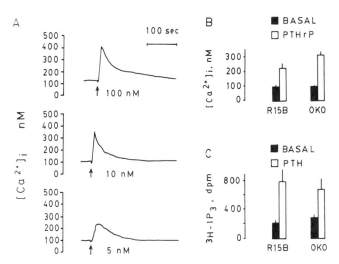

FIG. 9. PTH- and PTHrP-stimulated increases of intracellular free [Ca²⁺] transients and total inositol phosphate production in COS-7 cells transiently expressing either the rat or opossum PTH/PTHrP receptors. Increases in intracellular free [Ca²⁺] or the rate of inositol phosphate hydrolysis stimulated by either PTH-(1–34) amide or PTHrP-(1–36) amide were measured in COS-7 cells expressing either the rat or opossum PTH/PTHrP receptor. **A:** Effects of PTH-(1–34) amide (5, 10, 100 nM) on intracellular free [Ca²⁺] in COS-7 cells expressing the rat receptor. **B:** Effects of PTHrP-(1–36) (100 nM) on intracellular free [Ca²⁺] in COS-7 cells expressing either the rat or opossum receptor. **C:** Stimulation of total inositol phosphate production (60 sec, 37°C, 5 mM LiCl) by PTH-(1–34) amide in COS-7 cells expressing either rat or opossum receptors. (Reprinted from ref. 5 with permission.)

the interactions among several synthetic PTH and PTHrP fragments and analogs with receptors having authentic sequences and those that have been mutated by truncations, deletions, and single- and clustered-substitutions and through binding of ligands with chimeric receptors (83). To distinguish between mutant receptors that are poorly expressed, or are not expressed at all, and those that are expressed and have altered binding characteristics, an epitope, such as a short DNA sequence encoding a portion of the MYC protein, has been incorporated into the receptor's extracellular regions. Also, epitope-tagged PTH/PTHrP receptors have been used to define the PTH/PTHrP receptor's general topographical features. Many of the extracellular and intracellular assignments that had been predicted from computer algorithms of hydrophobic and hydrophilic amino acids have been confirmed experimentally by inserting the epitope into stretches of DNA encoding the many putative extracellular and intracellular regions, expressing these modified sequences, and then reacting the cells with labeled second antiserum with or without permeabilizing the cells with detergent.

Some of the extracellular regions are required for ligand binding, but not all of them. Receptors with deletions of many segments of the amino-terminal extracellular extension either fail to be expressed and/or fail to bind. Receptors in which 45 amino acids of the amino-terminal region (the portion encoded by the E-2 exon; see below) have been deleted have unimpaired capacity to be expressed, to bind, and to activate adenylyl cyclase, however. Through use of discrepancies in binding of amino-terminal fragments to PTH/PTHrP receptors from different species and to chimeric receptors between these different PTH receptors, the receptor's amino-terminal, extracellular domain has been shown to largely determine binding specificity and affinity for amino-terminally truncated forms of PTH-(1–34), such as PTH-(7–34) and PTH-(15–34). Receptors in which any of the PTH/PTHrP receptor's six cysteine residues in the amino-terminal extension are mutated, excluding the two cysteines in the signal peptide and with exception of the first in the amino-terminal region, are not expressed. However, mutating the first cysteine residue markedly reduces expression. Mutating either cysteine residue in the putative first or second extracellular loop similarly impairs expression, but to a lesser degree. Thus proper processing, folding, and membrane insertion of the receptor rely on the integrity of these cyteine residues (84,85). These data complement and extend the previous report showing complete loss of ligand binding with treatment of renal plasma membranes with reducing agents, suggesting that the PTH receptor's functional integrity requires intact cysteine bonds (37).

The PTH/PTHrP receptor's membrane-spanning helices, which are strongly conserved across species, are clearly vital for signal transduction across the cell's plasma membrane. Analyses of mutant and chimeric PTH/PTHrP receptors has generated a partial map of the receptor's ligand-binding domains and has partially distinguished them from determinants required to induce an "active" receptor conformation, one that allows the receptor to couple productively with G proteins. Preliminary data indicate that portions of the membrane-spanning helices may be critical for PTH binding and receptor activation, as has now been shown for other hormones and their G protein-linked receptors (74), although this has not yet been demonstrated with certainty with PTH/PTHrP receptors. From these initial structure-function studies, it is clear that multiple receptor regions are involved in both ligand binding and receptor activation; the former requires at least portions of the amino-terminal extracellular region and the third extracellular loop and/or adjacent membrane-spanning regions, while the latter appears to require regions of the receptor that lie between its third and sixth membrane-spanning helices (84,85).

The activated PTH/PTHrP receptor's capacity to stimulate multiple second messenger pathways, which was initially reported with COS-7 cells transiently expressing them, has recently been confirmed and extended by studies with stably transfected LLC-PK$_1$ cells. These porcine cells lack endogenous PTH/PTHrP receptors, but express abundant calcitonin receptors and many features of a proximal renal tubular epithelial cell. Subclones of LLC-PK$_1$ cells expressing either the rat or opossum receptor exhibited high-affinity PTH binding and dose-dependent activation by PTH of both cAMP accumulation and increased release of cytosolic $[Ca^{2+}]$ from intracellular stores. The EC_{50} of the cAMP response was 20–50-fold lower, however, than the intracellular $[Ca^{2+}]$ response. Like calcitonin, PTH reduced the rate of cell proliferation and augmented the rate of inorganic phosphate transport. This effect on cell growth was mimicked by cAMP analogs, forskolin, phorbol esters, and calcium ionophores. Regulation of phosphate transport, however, was mimicked only by phorbol esters. Thus cloned PTH/PTHrP receptors stably expressed at near-physiological levels mediate more than one second messenger response, as they did when transiently expressed at high receptor copy-number. Modulation of phosphate transport by agonist-occupancy of the same receptor also provides strong evidence that activation of pathways, in addition to those dependent on cAMP, is relevant to cellular physiology (86).

Scanning mutagenesis of the receptor's putative intracellular regions, which is in its preliminary stages, has defined a few intracellular regions critical for both receptor expression and G protein-coupling. Alanine scanning, that is, individually substituting alanine for amino acids in the highly conserved, putative first intracellular loop, reduced receptor binding, presumably because these modifications interfere with receptor processing, folding, or membrane insertion (83). Earlier studies, suggesting that OK-H, a mutant receptor with a 70-amino-acid deletion of its carboxyl-terminal tail, had unimpaired capacity to stimulate adenylyl cyclase have been confirmed, but the interpretation that this truncated receptor had reduced capacity to stimulate phospholipase C was probably erroneous (84,85). At least two confounding factors had not been adequately considered. First, expression of truncated receptors containing as much as one-half of the putative carboxyl-terminal receptor tail, is impaired even in transient expression systems, and, second, it is now appreciated that 20–50-fold more ligand is required for stimulating phospholipase C than for adenylyl cyclase. Thus failure to detect activation of phospholipase C by stimulating OK-H probably reflected its reduced expression and not the deletion of structural features required for signaling this alternative pathway.

Other data from studies of authentic and mutant receptors that are equally well expressed do not indicate that the tail region is required for activation of phospholipase C. They do suggest, however, that one putative intracellular loop or more is required to stimulate phospholipase C, that different portions of the receptor intracellular regions are involved in activation of these two effectors, and that regions critical for PTH/PTHrP receptor coupling to transducer molecules are quite likely to differ from those of the adrenergic and muscarinic receptors, the most thoroughly explored models (G.V. Segre, unpublished data). Clearly, much more work is needed before structural determinants that are responsible for the PTH/PTHrP receptor's ligand-binding and G-protein activation are understood. Unraveling the specific intermolecular events that occur between the activated PTH/PTHrP receptors and transducer molecules and between activated G proteins and effectors will be a difficult task. These studies must consider the involvement of the PTH/PTHrP receptors with more than one G protein and must take the complexities among the G protein subunits and multiple effector molecules into consideration. The number of G protein α, β, and γ subunits is growing (74,87), and there now appear to be at least four different adenylyl cyclases (88–90), at least 12 phospholipase-C (PLC) enzymes that have been classified into four groups (91), and evidence that G-protein α-β complexes act catalytically in certain circumstances (92,93).

Parathyroid hormone/parathyroid hormone-related protein receptors with other sequences also may exist, although the renal and osseous receptors thus far

cloned in humans and rats are identical within each species. Northern blot analyses show considerable receptor mRNA heterogeneity that appears to be tissue-specific (Fig. 3). Although a common 2.3 kb transcript is expressed in many tissues, larger transcripts are present in the kidney and liver and smaller transcripts in kidney, skin, and testes (63). These alternatively sized mRNAs could be processed from multiple genes and/or alternatively processed mRNAs from one or more genes. Whether any of these alternative transcripts are translated remains to be determined.

Most G protein-coupled receptors, however, exist in several receptor subtypes, either as products of different genes or from alternative splicing of their mRNAs. Multiple adrenergic (94), dopaminergic (95–97), muscarinic (98), serotoninergic (99,100), vasopressin (101,102), and angiotensin II (103–106) receptor subtypes are encoded by more than one gene, and alternatively spliced receptors have been reported for LH/hCG (107,108) and dopamine (109) receptors. Receptor subtypes often can provide functional and tissue specificity in complex hormonal systems. Current data are

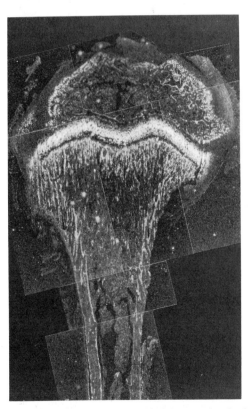

FIG. 10. PTH/PTHrP receptor mRNA expression in the tibia of a 4-week-old rat. Paraffin sections of tibias from 4-week-old rats were hybridized with ^{35}S-labeled antisense PTH/PTHrP receptor cRNA, and hybridization signals were detected via emulsion autoradiography. Overlapping darkfield images of the proximal portion of the tibia are shown. Bar = 1 mm. (Reprinted from ref. 21 with permission.)

consistent, however, with only a single receptor: cDNAs cloned from both bone and kidney are the same in both rats and humans. Homology is close among rat, human, opossum, and mouse receptors and there is only one copy of the PTH/PTHrP receptor gene, which has been mapped to the short arm of chromosome 3 (H. Heath, personal communication). Nonetheless, the diversity of PTH- and PTHrP-me-

diated effects mandates a careful search for multiple PTH/PTHrP receptor subtypes that might mediate these many biological actions.

Localizing PTH/PTHrP receptor transcripts by in situ hybridization complement studies of PTHrP gene and protein expression, which are discussed in detail elsewhere in this volume. Rat long bones show high levels of PTH/PTHrP receptor mRNA in a highly dis-

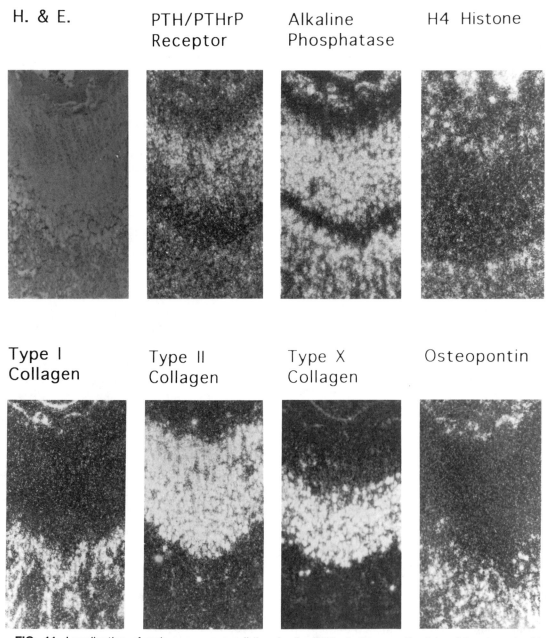

FIG. 11. Localization of various osseous cell "marker" mRNAs in the growth plate of the 4-week-old rat tibia. Sequential paraffin-embedded sections of a 4-week-old rat tibia were hybridized with ^{35}S-labeled antisense cRNAs for the various proteins. Darkfield views of hybridized sections are shown with a hematoxylin and eosin staining of the section hybridized with PTH/PTHrP receptor cRNA. Hematoxylin and eosin staining. Bar = 250 μm. (Reprinted from ref. 21 with permission.)

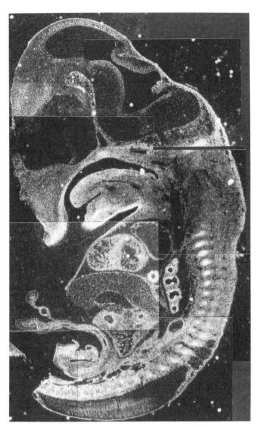

FIG. 12. Expression of PTH/PTHrP receptor mRNA in 15-day-old rat fetus. Midline paraffin sections of a 15-day-old rat fetus were hybridized with ^{35}S-labeled antisense PTH/PTHrP receptor cRNA, and hybridization signals were detected via emulsion autoradiography. Note extensive expression in many organs and tissues, which is most intense in vertebrae, skin, bronchi, heart, and tooth bud. Overlapping darkfield images of the whole fetus are shown.

crete portion of the growth plate that includes the lower proliferative and the upper hypertrophic chondrocyte layers, in mononuclear cells that line bony trabeculae, in cortical endosteal and periosteal cells, and in some marrow stromal cells (21) (Figs. 10,11). Histological examinations of "PTHrP-less" mice, who die immediately after birth from yet to be determined causes, show that PTHrP is critical for regulating endochondral bone formation. Homozygous mutants have many skeletal abnormalities, including widespread, premature skeletal mineralization, and an abnormal chondrocyte development that is most evident in endochondral bone. The mutant animal's deformed long bones are shorter in length and wider than those of normal littermates and show short, disorganized columns of proliferative growth-plate chondrocytes and distorted remnants of calcified cartilage. In situ hybridization with cRNAs for the PTH/PTHrP receptor, and several chondrocyte and bone-cell marker cRNAs reveal the layer of less well differentiated, receptor-negative chondrocytes in the growth plate that express type II collagen to be dramatically reduced, but show the thickness of the hypertrophic chondrocyte layer containing cells that express both type II and type X collagen to be normal. Since cells that do not express PTH/PTHrP receptor mRNA show the most obvious abnormalities, these morphological data suggest that the development of these receptor-negative cells may be regulated directly or indirectly by adjacent chondrocytes that express receptors and thus can respond to PTHrP (110,111). Additionally, the wide distribution of PTH/PTHrP receptor mRNA in many organs, other than bone and cartilage (Fig. 12), suggests that activated PTH/PTHrP receptors have more general and perhaps critical roles in embryogenesis.

The rat, mouse, and human receptor genes are organized similarly, but are quite distinct from the genes of most other members of the G protein-linked receptor superfamily. Adrenergic receptors and many other related receptors are intronless. In contrast, the receptors for the glycoprotein hormones TSH, FSH, and LH have multiple introns in portions of their genes that encode their amino-terminal extracellular extensions, but have only a single exon that encodes their membrane-spanning helices (74). The PTH/PTHrP receptor gene contains at least 14 exons encoding the receptor, many of which are quite short. Also, at least two additional exons lie in the 5′ upstream region (Fig. 13). The introns range considerably in size, and some are shorter than 100 bp. This novel and complex gene organization will require considerable effort to understand (112). The presence of relatively short intronic/exonic sequences obviously complicates analysis of the receptor mRNAs because alternative splicing may yield multiple transcripts of similar lengths, but containing different sequences, which must be investigated by hybridization with exon-specific probes and by use of the polymerase chain reaction with appropriately constructed primers.

Future experiments will define the functional characteristics that are determined by the many novel structural features of this PTH/PTHrP receptor as well as the properties that are associated with its complex gene organization. These studies will both broaden our understanding of this particular receptor and its roles in calcium homeostasis and embryogenesis and in the physiology and development of tissue and organs in which receptor transcripts are widely distributed after birth. Additionally, defining the properties of PTH/PTHrP receptors will contribute to knowledge concerning this newly discovered G protein-linked receptor family and the evolutionary and functional relationships among its members.

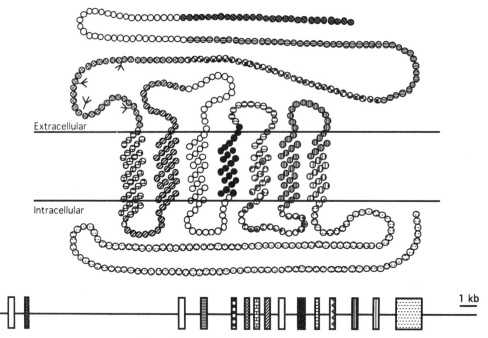

FIG. 13. Schematic representation of the rat PTH/PTHrP receptor gene. The rat PTH/PTHrP receptor gene is highly complex, with 14 exons encoding the receptor protein and an additional two exons in the 5' upstream portion of the gene.

ACKNOWLEDGMENTS

The author is grateful to A-B. Abou-Samra, T. Gardella, A. Iida-Klein, H. Jüppner, L.F. Kolakowski, Jr., H. Kronenberg, C. W. Lee, and K. Lee for sharing unpublished data and their figures. Also, the author thanks J. T. Potts, Jr., and H. Kronenberg for helpful comments in review of the manuscript. This work was supported in part by NIH grants DK-11794 and DK-47034.

REFERENCES

1. Rosenblatt M, Kronenberg HM, Potts JT Jr. Parathyroid hormone physiology, chemistry, biosynthesis, secretion, metabolism and mode of action. In: DeGroot LJ, ed. *Endocrinology, Vol. II.* Philadelphia: W.B. Saunders Co, 1989; 848–891.
2. Chase LR, Aurbach GD. Parathyroid function and the renal secretion of 3',5'-adenylic acid. *Proc Natl Acad Sci USA* 1967;58:518–525.
3. Marcus R, Aurbach GD. Bioassay of parathyroid hormone in vitro in a stable preparation of adenyl cyclase from rat kidney. *Endocrinology* 1969;85:801–810.
4. Rodan SB, Rodan GA. The effect of parathyroid hormone and thyrocalcitonin on the accumulation of cyclic 3'-5'-monophosphate in freshly isolated bone cells. *J Biol Chem* 1974;249:3068–3074.
5. Abou-Samra AB, Jüppner H, Force T, et al. Expression cloning of a common receptor for parathyroid hormone and parathyroid hormone-related peptide from rat osteoblast-like cells: a single receptor stimulates intracellular accumulation of both cAMP and inositol trisphosphates and in-creases intracellular free calcium. *Proc Natl Acad Sci USA* 1992;89:2732–2736.
6. Civitelli R, Fujimori A, Bernier SM, et al. Heterogeneous intracellular free calcium responses to parathyroid hormone correlate with morphology and receptor distribution in osteogenic sarcoma cells. *Endocrinology* 1992;130:2392–2400.
7. Dunlay R, Hruska K. PTH receptor coupling to phospholipase C is an alternate pathway of signal transduction in bone and kidney. *Am J Physiol* 1990;258:F223–F231.
8. Rappaport MS, Stern PH. Parathyroid hormone and calcitonin modify phospholipid metabolism in fetal rat limb bones. *J Bone Mineral Res* 1986;2:173–179.
9. Cosman F, Morrow B, Kopal M, Bilezikian JP. Stimulation of inositol phosphate formation in ROS 17/2.8 cell membranes by guanine nucleotide, calcium and parathyroid hormone. *J Bone Mineral Res* 1989;4:413–420.
10. Yamaguchi TD, Hhan TJ, Iida-Klein A, Kleeman CR, Muallem S. Parathyroid hormone-activated calcium channels in an osteoblast-like clonal osteosarcoma cell line. cAMP independent calcium channels. *J Biol Chem* 1987;262:7711–7718.
11. Donahue HJ, Fryer MJ, Eriksen EF, Heath H. Differential effects of parathyroid hormone and its analogues on cytosolic calcium ion and cAMP levels in cultured osteoblast-like cells. *J Biol Chem* 1988;263:13522–13527.
12. Feyen JHM, van der Wilt G, Moonen P, DiBon A, Nijweide PJ. Stimulation of arachidonic acid metabolism in primary cultures of osteoblast-like cells by hormones and drugs. *Prostaglandins* 1984;28:769–781.
13. MacDonald BR, Gallagher JA, Ahnfelt-Ronne I, Beresford JN, Gowen M, Russell RGG. Effects of bovine parathyroid hormone and 1,25-dihydroxyvitamin D on the production of prostaglandins by cells derived from human bone. *FEBS Lett* 1984;169:49–52.
14. Goldring SR, Tyler GA, Krane SM, Potts JT Jr, Rosenblatt M. Photoaffinity labeling of parathyroid hormone receptors: comparison of receptors across species and target tissues and after desensitization to hormone. *Biochemistry* 1984;23:498–502.

15. Yamamoto I, Potts JT Jr., Segre GV. Circulating bovine lymphocytes contain receptors for parathyroid hormone. *J Clin Invest* 1983;71:404–407.

16. Enomoto M, Kinashita A, Pan HO, Suzuki F, Yamamoto I, Takigawa M. Demonstration of receptors for parathyroid hormone on cultured rabbit costal chondrocytes. *Biochem Biophys Res Commun* 1989;162:1222–1229.

17. Mok LL, Nickols GA, Thompson JC, Cooper CW. Parathyroid hormone as a smooth muscle relaxer. *Endocr Rev* 1989;10:420–436.

18. Taniguchi A, Kataoka K, Kono T, et al. Parathyroid hormone-induced lipolysis in human adipose tissue. *J Lipid Res* 1987;28:490–494.

19. Lafond J, Auger D, Fortier J, Brunetta MG. Parathyroid hormone receptor in human syncytotrophoblast brush border and basal plasma membranes. *Endocrinology* 1988;123:2834–2840.

20. McSheehy PMJ, Chambers TJ. Osteoblastic cells mediate osteoclastic responsiveness to parathyroid hormone. *Endocrinology* 1986;118:824–828.

21. Lee K, Deeds JD, Chiba S, Unno M, Bond AT, Segre GV. Parathyroid hormone induces sequential c-*fos* expression in bone cells in vivo: in situ localization of its receptor and c-*fos* mRNAs. *Endocrinology* (in press).

22. Rao LG, Murray TM. Binding of intact parathyroid hormone to rat osteosarcoma cells: major contribution of binding sites for the carboxyl-terminal region of the hormone. *Endocrinology* 1985;117:1632–1638.

23. McKee MD, Murray TM. Binding of intact parathyroid hormone to chicken renal membranes: evidence for a second binding site with carboxyl-terminal specificity. *Endocrinology* 1985;117:1930–1939.

24. Suva LJ, Winslow GA, Wettenhall RE, et al. A parathyroid hormone-related protein implicated in malignant hypercalcemia: cloning and expression. *Science* 1987;237:893–896.

25. Strewler GJ, Stern PH, Jacobs JW, et al. Parathyroid hormone-like protein from human renal carcinoma cells. Structural and functional homology with parathyroid hormone. *J Clin Invest* 1987;80:1803–1807.

26. Mangin M, Webb AC, Dreyer BE, et al. Identification of a cDNA encoding a parathyroid hormone-like peptide from a human tumor associated with humoral hypercalcemia of malignancy. *Proc Natl Acad Sci USA* 1988;85:597–601.

27. Burtis WJ, Brady TG, Orloff JJ, et al. Immunochemical characterization of circulating PTHrP in patients with humeral hypercalcemia of malignancy. *N Engl J Med* 1990; 322:1106–1112.

28. Pandian MR, Morgan CH, Carlton E, Segre GV. Modified immunoradiometric assay of PTHrP: clinical application in the differential diagnosis of hypercalcemia. *Clin Chem* 1992;28:282–288.

29. Mangin M, Ikeda K, Dreyer B, Broadus AE. Isolation and characterization of the human PTH-like peptide gene. *Proc Natl Acad Sci USA* 1989;86:2408–2412.

30. Orloff JJ, Wu TL, Stewart AF. Parathyroid hormone-like protein: biochemical responses and receptor interactions. *Endocr Rev* 1989;10:476–495.

31. Karaplis AC, Tybulewicz V, Mulligan RC, Kronenberg HM. Disruption of parathyroid hormone-related peptide gene leads to multiple skeletal abnormalities and perinatal mortality. *J Bone Mineral Res* 1992;7(Suppl 1):S93.

32. van de Stolpe A, Karperien M, Lowik CWGM, et al. Parathyroid hormone-related peptide as an endogenous inducer of parietal endoderm differentiation. *J Cell Biol* 1993;120: 235–242.

33. Martin TJ, Moseley JM, Gillespie MT. Parathyroid hormone-related protein, biochemistry and molecular biology. *Crit Rev Biochem Mol Biol* 1991;26:377–395.

34. Yamamoto I, Shigeno C, Potts JT Jr, Segre GV. Characterization and agonist-induced down-regulation of parathyroid hormone receptors in clonal rat osteosarcoma cells. *Endocrinology* 1988;122:1208–1217.

35. Segre GV, Rosenblatt M, Reiner BL, Mahaffey JE, Potts JT Jr. Characterization of parathyroid hormone receptors in canine renal critical plasma membranes using a radioiodinated sulfin-free hormone analogue: correlation of binding with adenylate cyclase activity. *J Biol Chem* 1979;254:6980–6986.

36. Nissenson RA, Arnaud CD, Properties of the parathyroid hormone receptor-adenylate cyclase system in chicken renal plasma membranes. *J Biol Chem* 1979;254:1469–1475.

37. Teitelbaum AP, Nissenson RA, Arnaud CD. Coupling of the canine renal parathyroid hormone receptor to adenylate cyclase: modulation by guanyl nucleotides and N-ethylmaleimide. *Endocrinology* 1982;111:1524–1533.

38. Mahoney CA, Nissenson RA. Canine renal receptors for parathyroid hormone. Down-regulation in vivo by exogenous parathyroid hormone. *J Clin Invest* 1983;72:411–421.

39. Forte LR, Langeluttig SG, Foelling RE, Thomas ML. Renal parathyroid hormone receptors in the chick: downregulation in secondary hyperparathyroid animal models. *Am J Physiol* 1982;243:E154–E163.

40. Quarles LD, Lobaugh B, Murphy G. Intact parathyroid hormone overestimates the presence and severity of parathyroid-mediated osseous abnormalities in uremia. *J Clin Endocrinol Metab* 1992;75:145–150.

40a. Ureña P, Kubrusly M, Mannstadt M, et al. The renal PTH/PTHrP receptor is down-regulated in rats with chronic renal failure. *Kidney Int* (in press).

41. Pun KK, Ho PWM, Nissenson RA, Arnaud CD. Desensitization of parathyroid hormone receptors on cultured bone cells. *J Bone Mineral Res* 1990;5:1193–1200.

42. Mitchell J, Goltzman D. Mechanisms of homologous and heterologous regulation of parathyroid hormone receptors in the rat osteosarcoma cell line UMR-106. *Endocrinology* 1990;126:2650–2660.

43. Hanai H, Brennan DP, Cheng L, et al. Downregulation of parathyroid hormone receptors in renal membranes from aged rats. *Am J Physiol* 1990;259:F444–F450.

44. Ikeda K, Sugimoto T, Fukase M, Fujita T. Protein kinase C is involved in PTH-induced homologous desensitization by directly affecting PTH receptor in the osteoblastic osteosarcoma cell. *Endocrinology* 1991;128:2901–2906.

45. Abou-Samra AB, Zajac JD, Schiffer AD, et al. Cyclic adenosine 3′,5′-monophosphate (cAMP)-dependent and cAMP-independent regulation of parathyroid hormone receptors on UMR 106-01 osteoblastic osteosarcoma cells. *Endocrinology* 1991;129:2547–2554.

46. Urena P, Iida-Klein A, Kong XF, et al. Regulation of parathyroid hormone (PTH)/PTH-related peptide receptor mRNA by glucocorticoids and PTH in ROS 17/2.8 and OK cells. *Endocrinology* (in press).

47. Teitelbaum AP, Silve CM, Nyiredy KO, Arnaud CD. Down-regulation of parathyroid hormone (PTH) receptors in cultured bone cells is associated with agonist-specific intracellular processing of PTH-receptor complexes. *Endocrinology* 1986;118:595–602.

48. Yamamoto I, Potts JT Jr, Segre GV. Glucocorticoids increase parathyroid hormone receptors in osteoblastic osteosarcoma cells (ROS 17/2). *J Bone Mineral Res* 1988;3:707–712.

49. Teitelbaum AP, Strewler GJ. Parathyroid hormone receptors couple to cyclic adenosine monophosphate in an established renal cell line. *Endocrinology* 1984;114:980–985.

50. Schneider HG, Allan EH, Moseley JM, Martin TJ, Findlay DM. Specific down regulation of parathyroid hormone (PTH) receptors and responses to PTH by tumour necrosis factor alpha and retinoic acid in UMR 106-06 osteoblast-like osteosarcoma cells. *Biochem J* 1991;280:451–457.

51. Titus L, Jackson E, Nanes MS, Rubin JE, Catherwood BD. 1,25-Dihydroxyvitamin D reduces parathyroid hormone receptor number in ROS 17/2.8 cells and prevents the glucocorticoid-induced increase in these receptors: relationship to adenylate cyclase activation. *J Bone Mineral Res* 1991;6: 631–637.

52. Karpf DB, Arnaud CD, King K, et al. The canine renal parathyroid hormone receptor is a glycoprotein: characterization and partial purification. *Biochemistry* 1987;26:7825–7833.

53. Shigeno C, Hiraki Y, Westerberg DP, Potts JT Jr., Segre GV. Parathyroid hormone receptors are plasma membrane glycoproteins with asparagine-linked oligosaccharides. *J Biol Chem* 1988;263:3872–3878.

54. Shigeno C, Hiraki Y, Westerberg DP, Potts JT Jr., Segre GV. Photoaffinity labeling of parathyroid hormone receptors in clonal rat osteosarcoma cells. *J Biol Chem* 1988;263:3864–3871.

55. Karpf DB, Arnaud CD, Bambino T, et al. Structure properties of the renal parathyroid hormone receptor: hydrodynamic analysis and protease sensitivity. *Endocrinology* 1988;123:2611–2619.

56. Shigeno C, Hiraki Y, Stern AM, Potts JT Jr., Keutmann HT, Segre GV. Preparation of a photoactive analog of parathyroid hormone, [Nle⁸,Lys(N-ε-4-azido-2-nitrophenyl)¹³Nle¹⁸, Tyr³⁴] bovine parathyroid hormone-(1–34)NH₂, a selective, high-affinity ligand for characterization of parathyroid hormone receptors. *Anal Biochem* 1989;179:268–273.

57. Jüppner H, Abou-Samra AB, Uneno S, Keutmann HT, Potts JT Jr., Segre GV. Preparation and characterization of [Nα-(4-azido-2 nitrophenyl)Ala¹Tyr³⁶] parathyroid hormone-related peptide (1–36) amide: a high affinity, partial agonist having high cross-linking efficiency with its receptors on ROS 17/2.8 cells. *Biochemistry* 1990;29:6941–6946.

58. Jüppner H, Abou-Samra AB, Uneno S, et al. Properties of amino-terminal parathyroid hormone-related peptides modified at positions 11–13. *Peptides* 1990;11:1139–1142.

59. Nissenson RA, Diep D, Strewler GJ. Synthetic peptides comprising the amino-terminal sequence of a parathyroid hormone-like protein from human malignancies. Binding to parathyroid hormone receptors and activation of adenylate cyclase in bone cells and kidney. *J Biol Chem* 1988;263:12866–12871.

60. Jüppner H, Abou-Samra AB, Uneno S, Gu WX, Potts JT Jr., Segre GV. The parathyroid hormone-like peptide associated with humoral hypercalcemia of malignancy and parathyroid hormone bind to the same receptor on the plasma membrane of ROS 17/2.8 cells. *J Biol Chem* 1988;263:8557–8560.

61. Jüppner H, Abou-Samra AB, Freeman M, et al. A G protein-linked receptor for parathyroid hormone and parathyroid hormone-related peptide. *Science* 1991;254:1024–1026.

62. Schipani E, Karga H, Karaplis AC, et al. Identical cDNAs encode a human renal and bone parathyroid hormone/parathyroid hormone-related peptide receptor. *Endocrinology* 1993;132:2157–2165.

63. Urena P, Kong XF, Abou-Samra AB, et al. Parathyroid hormone (PTH)/PTH-related peptide (PTHrP) receptor mRNA is widely distributed in rat tissues. *Endocrinology* 1993;133:617–623.

64. Gearing DP, King JA, Gough NM, Nicola NA. Expression cloning of the receptor for human granulocyte-macrophage colony-stimulating factor. *EMBO J* 1989;8:3667–3676.

65. Seed B, Aruffo A. Molecular cloning of the CD2 antigen, the T-cell erythrocyte receptor by a rapid immunoselection procedure. *Proc Natl Acad Sci USA* 1987;84:3365–3369.

66. Ishihara T, Nakamura S, Kaziro Y, Takahashi T, Takahashi K, Nagata S. Molecular cloning and expression of a cDNA encoding the secretin receptor. *Embo J* 1991;7:1635–1641.

67. Lin HY, Harris TL, Flannery MS, et al. Expression cloning of an adenylate cyclase-coupled calcitonin receptor. *Science* 1991;254:1022–1024.

68. Ishihara T, Shigemoto R, Mori K, Takahashi K, Hagata S. Functional expression and tissue distribution of a novel receptor for vasoactive intestinal polypeptide. *Neuron* 1992; 8:811–819.

69. Thorens B. Expression cloning of a pancreatic β cell receptor for the gluco-incretin hormone, glucagon-like peptide 1. *Proc Natl Acad Sci USA* 1992;89:8641–8645.

70. Jelinek LJ, Lok S, Rosenberg GB, et al. Expression cloning and signalling properties of the rat glucagon receptor. *Science* 1993;259:1614–1616.

71. Mayo KE. Molecular cloning and expression of a pituitary-specific receptor for growth hormone-releasing hormone. *Mol Endocrinol* 1992;6:1734–1744.

72. Attwood TK, Eliopoulos EE, Findlay JB. Multiple sequence alignment of protein families showing low sequence homology: a methodological approach using database pattern-matching discriminators of G-protein-linked receptors. *Gene* 1991;98:153–159.

73. Probst WC, Snyder LA, Schuster DI, Brosius J, Sealfon SC. Sequence alignment of the G-protein coupled receptor superfamily. *DNA Cell Biol* 1992;11:1–20.

74. Dohlman HG, Thorner J, Caron MG, Lefkowitz RJ. Model systems for the study of seven-transmembrane-segment receptors. *Annu Rev Biochem* 1991;60:653–688.

75. Reed RR. Signaling pathways in odorant detection. *Neuron* 1992;8:205–209.

76. O'Dowd BF, Lefkowitz RJ, Caron MG. Structure of the adrenergic and related receptors. *Annu Rev Neurosci* 1989; 12:67–83.

77. Segre GV, Goldring SR. Receptors for secretin, calcitonin, parathyroid hormone (PTH)/PTH-related peptide, vasoactive intestinal peptide, glucagon-like peptide 1, growth hormone-releasing hormone, and glucagon belong to a newly discovered G protein-linked receptor family. *Trends Endocrinol Metab* (in press).

78. Chabre O, Conklin BR, Lin HY, et al. A recombinant calcitonin receptor independently stimulates cAMP and calcium/inositol phosphate signalling pathways. *Mol Endocrinol* 1992;6:551–556.

79. Force T, Bonventre JV, Flannery MR, Gorn AH, Yamin M, Goldring SR. A cloned porcine renal calcitonin receptor couples to adenyl cyclase and phospholipase C. *Am J Physiol* 1992;262:F1110–F1115.

80. Wheeler MB, Lu M, Dillon JS, Leng XH, Chen C, Boyd AE III. Functional expression of the rat glucagon-like peptide-I receptor, evidence for coupling to both adenylyl cyclase and phospholipase-C. *Endocrinology* 1993;133:57–62.

81. Gudermann T, Nichols C, Levy FO, Birnbaumer M, Brinbaumer L. Calcium mobilization by the LH receptor expressed in xenopus oocytes independent of cAMP formation: evidence for parallel activation of two signalling pathways. *Mol Endocrinol* 1992;6:272–278.

82. Sande JV, Raspe E, Lejeune PC, Mainhaut C, Vassart G, Dumont JE. Thyrotropin activates both the cyclic AMP and the PIP2 cascades in CHO cells expressing the human cDNA of TSH receptor. *Mol Cell Endocrinol* 1990;74:R1–R6.

83. Drake M, Gardella T, Abou-Samra AB, Segre GV. Mutational analysis of the rat PTH/PTHrP receptor: structural determinants for activation of the stimulatory G protein. *J Bone Mineral Res* 1993;8(Suppl 1):S128.

84. Kronenberg HM, Abou-Samra AB, Jüppner H, Potts JT Jr., Segre GV. Characterization of a receptor that binds both PTH and PTHrP. In: Cohn DV, Gennari C, Tashjian AH Jr., eds. *Proceedings of the XIth International Conference on Calcium Regulating Hormones, Florence, Italy.* Amsterdam: Elsevier Science Publishers BV, 1992;79–82.

85. Segre GV, Abou-Samra AB, Gardella TJ, et al. Structural analysis of the PTH/PTHrp receptor's functional domains. In: Cohn DV, Gennari C, Tashjian AH Jr., eds. *Proceedings of the XIth International Conference on Calcium Regulating Hormones, Florence, Italy.* Amsterdam: Elsevier Science Publishers BV, 1992;92–96.

86. Bringhurst FR, Jüppner H, Guo J, et al. Cloned, stably expressed parathyroid hormone (PTH)/PTH-related peptide receptors activate multiple messenger signals and biologic responses in LLC-PK1 kidney cells. *Endocrinology* 1993; 132:2090–2098.

87. Simon MI, Strathmann MP, Gautam N. Diversity of G proteins in signal transduction. *Science* 1991;252:802–808.

88. Tang WJ, Gilman AG. Type-specific regulation of adenylyl cyclase by G protein beta gamma subunits. *Science* 1991; 254:1500–1503.

89. Tang WJ, Krupinski J, Gilman AG. Expression and characterization of calmodulin-activated (type I) adenylyl cyclase. *J Biol Chem* 1991;266:8595–8603.

90. Tang WJ, Gilman AG. Adenylyl cyclases. *Cell* 1992;70:869–872.

91. Rhee SG, Ryu SH, Lee KY, Cho KS. Assays of phosphoino-

sitide-specific phospholipase C and different modes of activation. *Methods Enzymol* 1991;197:502–511.

92. Birmbaumer L. Receptor-to-effector signalling through G proteins: roles for beta-gamma dimers as well as alpha subunits. *Cell* 1992;71:1069–1072.

93. Federman AD, Conklin BR, Schrader KA, Reed RR, Bourne HR. Hormonal stimulation of adenylyl cyclase through Gi-protein beta gamma subunits. *Nature* 1992;356:159–161.

94. Bylund DB. Subtypes of alpha 1- and alpha 2-adrenergic receptors. *FASEB J* 1992;6:832–839.

95. Monsma FJ Jr, Mahan LC, McVittie LD, Gerfen CR, Sibley DR. Molecular cloning and expression of a Dl dopamine receptor linked to adenylyl cyclase activation. *Proc Natl Acad Sci USA* 1990;87:6723–6727.

96. Van THH, Bunzow R, Guan HC, et al. Cloning of the gene for a human dopamine D4 receptor with high affinity for the antipsychotic clozapine. *Nature* 1991;350:610–614.

97. Weinshank RL, Adham N, Macchi M, Olsen MA, Branchek TA, Hartig PR. Molecular cloning and characterization of a high affinity dopamine receptor (D1 beta) and its pseudogene. *J Biol Chem* 1991;266:22427–22435.

98. Bonner TI, Buckley NJ, Young AC, Brann MR. Identification of a family of muscarinic acetylcholine receptor genes. *Science* 1987;237:527–532.

99. Levy FO, Gudermann T, Birnbaumer M, Kaumann AJ, Birnbaumer L. Molecular cloning of a human gene (S31) encoding a novel serotonin receptor mediating inhibition of adenylyl cyclase. *FEBS Lett* 1992;296:201–206.

100. Saudou F, Boschert U, Amlaiky N, Plassat JL, Hen R. A family of Drosophila serotonin receptors with distinct intracellular signalling properties and expression patterns. *EMBO J* 1992;11:7–17.

101. Lolait SJ, O'Caroll AM, McBride OW, Konig M, Morel A, Brownstein MJ. Cloning and characterization of a vasopressin V2 receptor and possible link to nephrogenic diabetes insipidus. *Nature* 1992;357:336–339.

102. Birnbaumer M, Seibold A, Gilbert S, et al. Molecular cloning of the receptor for human antidiuretic hormone. *Nature* 1992;357:333–335.

103. Takayanagi R, Ohnaka K, Sakai Y, et al. Molecular cloning, sequence analysis and expression of a cDNA encoding human type-1 angiotensin II receptor. *Biochem Biophys Res Commun* 1992;183:910–916.

104. Sasaki K, Yamano Y, Bardhan S, et al. Cloning and expression of a complementary DNA encoding a bovine adrenal angiotensin II type-1 receptor. *Nature* 1991;351:230–233.

105. Murphy TJ, Alexander RW, Griendling KK, Runge MS, Bernstein KE. Isolation of a cDNA encoding the vascular type-1 angiotensin II receptor. *Nature* 1991;351:233–236.

106. Iwai N, Yamano Y, Chaki S, et al. Rat angiotensin II receptor: cDNA sequence and regulation of the gene expression. *Biochem Biophys Res Commun* 1991;177:299–304.

107. Ji I, Ji TH. Exons 1–10 of the rat LH receptor encode a high affinity hormone binding site and exon 11 encodes G-protein modulation and a potential second hormone binding site. *Endocrinology* 1991;128:2648–2650.

108. Loosfelt H, Misrahi M, Atger M, et al. Cloning and sequencing of porcine LH-hCG receptor cDNA: variants lacking transmembrane domain. *Science* 1989;245:525–528.

109. Monsma FJ Jr, McVittie LD, Gerfen CR, Mahan LC, Sibley DR. Multiple D2 dopamine receptors produced by alternative RNA splicing. *Nature* 1989;342:926–929.

110. Amizuka N, Warshawsky H, Goltzman D, Karaplis AC. Morphological analysis of endochondral bone formation in normal and PTHrP-deficient fetal mice. *J Bone Mineral Res* 1993;8(Suppl 1):S148.

111. Kong XF, Joun H, Jüppner H, Segre GV, Kronenberg H, Abou-Samra AB. Characterization of the rat gene encoding the receptor for parathyroid hormone (PTH) and PTH-related peptide (PTHrP). *J Bone Mineral Res* 1993;8(Suppl 1):S183.

The Parathyroids, edited by J.P. Bilezikian,
M.A. Levine, and R. Marcus. Raven Press, Ltd.,
New York © 1994.

CHAPTER 15

G Proteins as Transducers of Parathyroid Hormone Action

Allen M. Spiegel and Lee S. Weinstein

The classic studies of Chase and Aurbach showed that cyclic adenosine monophosphate (cAMP) acts as a second messenger for parathyroid hormone (PTH), that urinary cAMP excretion could be used as an index of PTH action in humans, and that in pseudohypoparathyroidism (PHP), an inherited disorder in which affected individuals are resistant to PTH action, the defect resides proximal to cAMP generation (1). More recent studies have shown that, in both kidney (2) and bone (3), PTH may also act via stimulation of phosphoinositide breakdown with resultant generation of the dual second messengers diacylglycerol (DAG) and inositol trisphosphate (IP3).

It is now clear that not only PTH, but many other hormones, as well as neurotransmitters, growth factors, chemotactic agents, and sensory signals, act via stimulation of second messengers such as cAMP, DAG, and IP3. The general mechanism of action of each of these first messengers involves binding to a specific receptor that in turn interacts with a particular G protein; the G protein regulates the activity of specific effector proteins such as enzymes of second messenger metabolism. The past few years have seen a dramatic advance in our understanding of each of the components: receptors, G proteins, and effectors. PTH receptor cDNAs have been cloned from opposum kidney (OK) cells (4) and from rat osteoblast-like (ROS) cells (5). A family of adenylyl cyclase (AC) cDNAs (6) and a family of phospholipase C (PLC) cDNAs (7) have also been cloned. The PTH receptor

(see the chapter by Segre) and the second messenger pathways involved in PTH action (see the chapter by Coleman et al.) are discussed in depth elsewhere in this volume. This chapter focuses on the structure and function of the G proteins, particularly those that act as transducers of PTH action. We have recently reviewed in detail the general subject of receptor–effector coupling by G proteins (8). Here we highlight more recent developments in the G protein field.

GENERAL FEATURES OF RECEPTOR–EFFECTOR COUPLING BY G PROTEINS

The heterotrimeric G proteins are members of a superfamily that includes other proteins, including ras and the ras-like proteins and initiation and elongation factors in protein synthesis, that bind guanine nucleotides with high affinity and specificity. All members of this superfamily also possess intrinsic guanosine triphosphatase (GTPase) activity and function as molecular switches; they are "on" in the GTP-bound conformation, and hydrolysis of GTP to guanosine diphosphate (GDP) leads to the "off," GDP-bound conformation (9). Members of the superfamily are typically regulated by "exchange factors" that catalyze release of bound GDP, and may also be regulated by GTPase-activating proteins (GAPs) that stimulate the intrinsic GTPase activity of the GTP-binding protein (9).

The G proteins are composed of alpha (α), beta (β), and gamma (γ) subunits, each the product of a separate gene. The α subunit is the GTP-binding homolog of other members of the superfamily. The β and γ subunits are tightly but noncovalently associated to form

A. M. Spiegel and L. S. Weinstein: Molecular Pathophysiology Branch, National Institute of Diabetes and Digestive and Kidney Diseases, National Institutes of Health, Bethesda, Maryland 20892.

TABLE 1. *Mammalian α subunit diversity*

α Subunit	Toxin substrate	Expression	Effector
Gs	CTX	Ubiquitous	↑ Adenylyl cyclase, Ca^{2+} channel
Golf	CTX	Olfactory	↑ Adenylyl cyclase
Gt1	PTX/CTX	Rod photoreceptors	↑ cGMP-phosphodiesterase
Gt2	PTX/CTX	Cone photoreceptors	↑ cGMP-phosphodiesterase
Ggust	PTX/CTX?	Taste cells	?
Gi1	PTX	Neural > other tissues	
Gi2	PTX	Ubiquitous	↓ Adenylyl cyclase,
Gi3	PTX	Other tissues > neural	↑ K^+ channel
Go	PTX	Neural, endocrine	↓ Ca^{2+} channel
GZ	—	Neural, platelets	?
Gq	—	Ubiquitous	
G11	—	Ubiquitous	
G14	—	Liver, lung, kidney	↑ Phospholipase C-β1
G15/16	—	Blood cells	
G12	—	Ubiquitous	?
G13	—	Ubiquitous	?

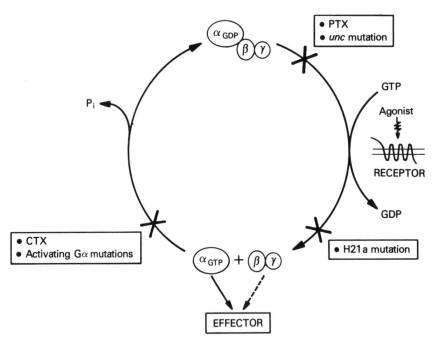

FIG. 1. The G protein GTPase cycle. In their basal, inactive state, α subunits contain tightly bound GDP and are associated as a heterotrimer with the βγ complex. Interaction with the intracellular portion of an agonist-bound, activated, receptor (shown in the schematic with seven putative transmembrane-spanning domains) leads to release of bound GDP and binding of ambient GTP. Binding of GTP leads to dissociation of G protein from receptor and of α subunit from βγ. GTP-bound α interacts with and regulates effector. The dashed line indicates that in some cases (see text) the βγ complex may also regulate effector activity. Intrinsic GTPase activity of the α subunit leads to hydrolysis of bound GTP to GDP, with liberation of inorganic phosphate. This causes dissociation of α subunit from effector and reassociation with βγ. Bacterial toxins covalently modify α subunits and thereby alter signal transduction. Pertussis toxin (PTX) blocks signal transduction by several G proteins by uncoupling them from receptors. Cholera toxin (CTX) constitutively activates its substrate $α_s$, causing agonist-independent cAMP formation. Mutations identified in $α_s$ block signal transduction by uncoupling it from receptors (unc) or preventing GTP activation (H21a). Certain α subunit mutations (see text) can also lead to constitutive activation of the α subunit and effector pathway by inhibiting GTPase activity. (Reproduced from ref. 8 with permission.)

a heterodimer that dissociates from the α subunit when the latter is activated. There is substantial diversity in the G protein subset of the superfamily (10). Sixteen distinct mammalian genes encoding α subunits have been identified in Table 1. Additional diversity is created by alternative splicing of mRNAs encoding Gs- and Go-α subunits (11,12). More recently, substantial diversity among the β and γ subunits has also been recognized (10). Thus, in contrast to what has been believed earlier, specificity of receptor–effector coupling by G proteins may not be determined solely by the α subunit within the heterotrimer.

The most clearly defined function for G proteins is in transduction of information from extracellular "first messengers" (peptides, amines, prostaglandins, sensory signals) into intracellular "second messengers." This function correlates with the location of most G proteins on the inner surface of the plasma membrane, juxtaposed to the transmembrane receptors for first messengers and to the various effector molecules. Posttranslational lipid modifications of α and γ subunits appear to be critical in anchoring G proteins to the inner surface of the plasma membrane (13). The rod photoreceptor G protein transducin is associated with the cytoplasmic surface of the specialized outer segment disk membrane. Recent evidence indicates that other G proteins may also be localized to specialized intracellular compartments such as the Golgi complex and the apical surface of polarized epithelial cells (8). This may indicate a broader role for the G proteins in transmembrane signalling.

A GTPase cycle (Fig. 1) is a critical feature of the function of each G protein. G proteins must be in the inactive, heterotrimeric form to associate with activated (agonist-bound) receptors. The latter act catalytically to release GDP from inactive heterotrimers and permit binding of ambient GTP. The α subunit is thought to undergo a conformational change upon binding of GTP that leads to its activation and dissociation from the βγ dimer. Activated G protein α subunits bind to and regulate the activity of specific effector molecules. It is now clear that βγ dimers can also modulate the activity of certain effectors (6,14). Ordinarily, α subunit activation is transient, terminated by the intrinsic GTPase activity that hydrolyzes bound GTP to GDP. After GTP hydrolysis, the GDP-bound α subunit reassociates with the βγ dimer to reform the inactive heterotrimer. Under artificial conditions, binding of nonhydrolyzable GTP analogs leads to persistent activation. Fluoride anions (complexed with aluminum) activate GDP-bound α subunits by mimicking the γ phosphate of GTP. Covalent modification by cholera toxin of the α subunit of the G protein (Gs) mediating stimulation of cAMP formation inhibits its GTPase activity and thereby leads to persistent activation.

G PROTEIN α SUBUNIT STRUCTURE AND FUNCTION

Mammalian α subunits can be divided into four classes based on their degree of primary sequence conservation (Table 1). Each is between 40% and 90% identical in amino acid sequence, and their overall length varies between 350 and 395 residues. The most conserved regions are those thought to be involved in guanine nucleotide binding, and these show varying degrees of identity to similar domains within more distantly related members of the GTP-binding protein superfamily (9). As of this writing, the three-dimensional structure of an α subunit has not been determined, but extrapolations based on the crystal structure of ras p21 have been performed (15). These show that five noncontiguous regions (designated G1–G5 in ref. 9) come together in the tertiary structure to form the guanine nucleotide-binding pocket.

An arginine residue (Arg 201 in the 394 residue form of Gs-α) within the G2 region is the site of cholera toxin-catalyzed ADP-ribosylation that leads to inhibition of GTPase activity. Mutations of this residue or of a glutamine residue (Gln 227 in Gs-α, which is the equivalent of Gln 61 in ras p21, a known oncogenic "hot spot") in the G3 region lead to constitutive G protein activation by inhibition of GTPase activity (16). Mutation of a glycine residue (226 in Gs-α) to alanine (H21A mutation) prevents activation by GTP (17,18).

The amino terminal region ~(1–2 kDa) of the α subunit appears necessary for interaction with the βγ complex. Certain α subunits (Gi, Go, Gz) undergo cotranslational myristoylation on the amino terminal glycine (19,20). This modification is required both for membrane attachment and for high-affinity interaction with the βγ complex (21).

A number of lines of evidence suggest that the carboxy terminal portion of the α subunit is critical for specific receptor interaction. The Gi-α and Go-α subunits have a cysteine in the fourth position from the carboxyl terminus which is ADP-ribosylated in a reaction catalyzed by pertussis toxin. This modification leads to uncoupling of the G protein from receptor (Fig. 1). Certain mutations near the carboxy terminus (22), as well as binding of specific peptide antibodies to this region (23,24), prevent receptor coupling to G protein.

Effector interaction regions have also been localized within the carboxy terminal portion of the α subunit (15,25). These regions are postulated to be exposed on the surface of the native protein on the side opposite the membrane interaction domain. By analogy with ras p21, activation of the G protein should lead to conformational changes exposing the effector interaction domains to promote protein–protein interaction (15). The divergent regions of α subunit primary sequence are thought to be those that confer specificity in receptor and effector interactions. The specific function of a large, divergent region within the amino terminal one-half of G protein α subunits has, however, not been defined.

The earliest G proteins identified were discovered through functional assays, e.g., Gs as the stimulator of adenylyl cyclase (AC). More recently, G proteins have been identified by homology cloning (10). As a result, at present, the functions of several G proteins (e.g., α-12, α-13, α-z) are unknown. The cAMP pathway is one of the best studied G protein-regulated systems. Even in this pathway, however, the mechanism of AC inhibition remains unclear. Inhibition involves pertussis toxin-sensitive Gi proteins, but the relative importance of α vs. βγ subunits in inhibition is controversial.

Stimulation of PLC to generate the dual second messengers DAG and IP3 involves pertussis toxin-sensitive G proteins in certain cells (neutrophils and monocytes) but is pertussis toxin-insensitive in most cells. Recently, the Gq family of α subunits, including Gq, G11, G14, and G16 (Table 1), has been identified as the mediators of pertussis toxin-insensitive PLC stimulation (26,27). Agonist-stimulated PLC activity can be reconstituted with three components: an appropriate receptor such as the M1 muscarinic, either Gq or G11, and PLC β1 (28). Assays utilizing transient expression of defined α subunits have shown that all members of the Gq family can stimulate PLC of the β subtype but that there may be quantitative differences depending on the G protein and PLC β subtype. For PLC β1 stimulation, Gq = G11 > G16 > G14 (29), whereas, for the PLC β2 subtype, G16 appears to be most effective (29,30). In *Xenopus* oocytes microinjected with Gq or G11, Gq was found to be less effective than G11 in opening of a chloride channel that is thought to depend on PLC stimulation (31).

G PROTEIN β AND γ SUBUNIT STRUCTURE AND FUNCTION

There are at least four distinct mammalian genes encoding β subunits of ~ 340 amino acids. They are highly conserved, with the β4 subtype 80–90% identical to the three previously cloned subtypes (32). They are composed of an amino terminal domain of ~35 amino acids predicted to form a coiled-coil structure (33) followed by eight repetitive segments each ~40 amino acids long. The latter have been termed "WD-40" repeats because of a characteristic tryptophan-aspartate pair and are found not only in the G protein β subunits but also in a diverse group of proteins not known to be involved in signal transduction (34). The

structural and functional significance of the WD-40 motif is unknown at present.

The diversity of γ subunits is greater than that of the β subunits, with at present seven distinct mammalian γ genes identified. There is evidence for tissue-specific patterns of expression of both types of subunit (35–37). Certain forms may be highly localized in expression, e.g., γ1 only in rod photoreceptors. In the retinas β3 is expressed only in cones and β1 is expressed only in rods (38,39). The γ subunits are ~70 amino acids in length and are more divergent in primary sequence (27–75% conserved) than are the β subunits. Each terminates with a "CAAX" motif, which has been shown to undergo three sequential posttranslational modifications (40). These involve isoprenylation of the cysteine, proteolytic cleavage of the "AAX" tripeptide, and methylation of the cysteine carboxyl group. These modifications are not critical for γ subunit association with the β subunit, but they are required for membrane association of the heterodimer (41).

Combining each form of β subunit with each form of γ could in theory lead to a tremendous diversity of heterodimers, but there is evidence that the number of heterodimers that can be formed is more limited due to selectivity in the interactions of specific subtypes (42,43). The structural basis for this selectivity and the domains involved in the tight association between β and γ subunits have not yet been defined. Diversity of native heterodimers purified from brain can be shown with sensitive analytic methods (44,45). There is also evidence for selectivity of association of α subunits with different βγ heterodimers (45,46).

What is the functional significance, if any, of βγ heterodimer diversity? Using antisense methods, it has been shown that not only α subunits (47) but also specific β subunits may be critical in defining the interaction of muscarinic vs. somatostatin receptors with Go heterotrimers in pituitary GH3 cells (48). Recent evidence (discussed below) indicates that βγ heterodimers are also involved in effector modulation and in desensitization. It is likely that diversity contributes to functional specificity in these aspects as well.

RECEPTOR–G PROTEIN COUPLING

Rhodopsin and the β-adrenergic receptor were the first G protein-coupled receptors defined at the molecular level (49). Their structure has been extrapolated to the dozens (hundreds if one includes putative odorant receptors) of G protein-coupled receptors whose primary sequences have since been defined (50,51). Hydrophobicity plots of the primary sequence of members of this family predict seven membrane-spanning domains composed largely of hydrophobic residues. Each receptor comprises a single polypeptide chain, with the amino terminus external and the carboxy terminus internal to the cell membrane. In addition, there are three predicted extracellular and three intracellular loops connecting the membrane-spanning domains. This basic structure is embellished with varying degrees of glycosylation of the amino terminus and occasionally of the extracellular loops and palmitoylation of one or more cysteines in the proximal portion of the carboxy terminal tail.

The tremendous diversity in the ligands binding to this class of receptors is reflected in the diversity of the primary sequences as well as important variations on the basic architectural theme (49,51). For small (e.g., monoamine) ligands, the binding site may be within a pocket comprising the membrane-spanning domains. Larger ligands such as the glycoprotein hormones bind to exterior sites as well; members of the glycoprotein hormone receptor subclass have a dramatically longer (>300 residue) extracellular amino terminus involved in ligand binding. There is also substantial diversity in the length of the third intracellular loop and of the carboxy terminus, which may relate to the specificity of G protein coupling (see below).

The molecular mechanism of G protein-coupled receptor action is undefined and, minimally, awaits definition of the three-dimensional structure of the receptor and G protein. A speculative model suggests that binding of an agonist ligand (or, in the case of the opsins, photoisomerization of covalently bound retinal, which converts an "antagonist" to an "agonist") leads to a conformational change in the receptor that is transmitted to the intracellular loops and carboxy terminus. A change in conformation of the latter promotes high-affinity binding to heterotrimeric G protein(s) and initiates the signal transduction cascade by catalyzing release of GDP from the G protein α subunit.

A variety of techniques, including site-directed mutagenesis, formation of chimeric receptors, and study of peptides corresponding to discrete portions of the intracellular loops of receptors, has been used in an effort to define the critical residues involved in G protein coupling and in defining the specificity of receptor coupling to a particular G protein subtype (49). Most of these studies have focussed attention on the third intracellular loop and, in particular, its proximal and distal portions. A synthetic peptide corresponding to the distal portion of the β-adrenergic receptor was shown to be capable of activating the Gs protein equivalently to the intact receptor (52). Exchanging portions of the third intracellular loops of M2 and M3 muscarinic receptors switched the G protein-coupling properties of the mutant receptor to those of the donor subtype (53). Detailed studies of the β-adrenergic receptor, however, indicate that not only the third intracellular loop but also the proximal portion of the carboxy terminus is critical in defining G protein-coupling specificity (54).

There are many more G protein-coupled receptors than there are G proteins. It is possible that more G proteins remain to be identified, but it is already clear that multiple distinct receptors may couple to the same G protein subtype. The receptors coupled to Gz, G12, and G13 (Table 1) are undefined, but other receptors fall into one of several major groups that couple to (a) Gs, [e.g., the mammalian β-adrenergic receptor and the vasopressin V2 receptor (55)], (b) the Gi/Go family (e.g., M2 muscarinic and somatostatin), (c) the Gq family (e.g., M3 muscarinic and V1 vasopressin), and (d) transducins (photoreceptor opsins). Recent evidence suggests that certain receptors may couple to more than one G protein subtype. In particular, the PTH receptor (4,5), the calcitonin receptor (56), and the glucagon-like peptide 1 receptor (57) may all be coupled to both Gs and Gq. Each of these receptors has been shown to stimulate both cAMP formation and phosphoinositide breakdown, the latter generally with an EC_{50} one order of magnitude higher than that for AC stimulation. Definitive evidence that these receptors couple to both G protein subtypes and elucidation of the structural basis for this unique specificity are still lacking.

G protein-coupled pathways often display marked desensitization, i.e., reduced response despite continued presence of agonist. The mechanism of homologous (agonist-specific) desensitization has been extensively studied (58,59) and involves, in addition to receptor and G protein, a specific kinase termed β-adrenergic receptor kinase (β-ARK), and a protein termed β-arrestin (the photoreceptor homologs are rhodopsin kinase and arrestin, respectively). The change in receptor conformation presumed to occur upon agonist binding leads not only to G protein activation but also to susceptibility of the receptor to phosphorylation by β-ARK. Phosphorylation is generally, but not exclusively, in a serine/threonine-rich portion of the receptor carboxy terminus. Such agonist-dependent phosphorylation by β-ARK appears to occur both in receptors coupled to Gs (e.g., β-adrenergic, from which the kinase originally derived its name) and those coupled to Gi (e.g., M2 muscarinic). Reconstitution studies indicate that receptor phosphorylation *per se* is insufficient to inhibit receptor–G protein coupling (59). An additional protein, β-arrestin, was discovered to be necessary to block receptor–G protein coupling. β-Arrestin appears to act by competing with G protein for receptor binding. Receptor phosphorylation dramatically enhances β-arrestin affinity for receptor. cDNA cloning indicates the existence of multiple forms of both β-arrestin and β-ARK (58). It remains to be seen if this diversity corresponds to specificity in receptor interactions.

Both β-ARK and β-arrestin appear to be cytosolic proteins. Each presumably translocates to the plasma membrane in the course of receptor interaction. This has been demonstrated for β-ARK but not yet for β-arrestin. For β-ARK, targeting to membrane-bound receptors appears to involve the G protein βγ complex (42). As was discussed above, prenylation of the γ subunit leads to membrane association of the βγ hetero-dimer (41). β-ARK in turn binds specifically to the βγ complex when the latter is dissociated from the G protein α subunit. This mechanism serves to link receptor activation (with ensuing G protein activation and dissociation of component subunits) to receptor desensitization (with β-ARK binding to the βγ subunit).

G PROTEIN–EFFECTOR COUPLING

Effectors regulated by G proteins are diverse in structure and function. They include peripheral membrane proteins (cGMP phosphodiesterase and PLC) and integral membrane proteins (AC and various ion channels). For AC (6) and for PLC (7) substantial diversity exists at the molecular level. The functional significance of this diversity is not yet fully understood, but certain interesting points have emerged with respect to G protein regulation. The multiple subtypes of AC are each stimulated by Gs-α, but only a subset are sensitive to calmodulin stimulation. Interestingly, the subtypes vary in terms of the effects of βγ subunits. For example type I (calmodulin-sensitive) AC is inhibited whereas type II is stimulated by βγ subunits (60). Stimulation by βγ subunits can be demonstrated in intact cells transfected with appropriate cDNAs (61), but the physiologic significance of these effects is not yet clear.

Of the PLC subtypes, the γ variety are regulated by tyrosine kinase-type receptors rather than G proteins (7). The β variety are regulated by G proteins. As was discussed above, α subunits of the Gq family are known to stimulate PLC β. It now appears that βγ subunits can also stimulate certain PLC subtypes, particularly the β2 variety (14,62). This may explain the pertussis toxin-sensitive PLC stimulation seen in certain cells such as neutrophils. In this instance, activation of a pertussis-sensitive G protein (perhaps Gi2) by receptors such as the chemotactic peptide f-Met-Leu-Phe receptor could lead to dissociation of a βγ subunit capable of stimulating PLC.

There is also recent evidence that certain effectors may actually stimulate the intrinsic GTPase activity of the G protein α subunits to which they bind. This has been shown in kinetic studies involving Gq and PLC-β1 (63) and for transducin and cGMP phosphodiesterase (64). Low-molecular-weight GTP-binding proteins of the ras family generally display little intrinsic GTPase activity and have specific GAPs that regulate their GTPase activity. Although heterotrimeric G proteins display significant intrinsic GTPase activity, physiologic considerations suggest that stimulation of GTPase activity by effector may be critical in "turning off" effector activity rapidly. Thus, for example, the kinetics of ion channel closure following receptor-stimulated opening are too rapid to be explained by the intrinsic GTPase activity of the responsible G protein. By acting as a GAP, the ion channel may speed the G protein GTPase sufficiently to explain the observed kinetics (63). Further work is needed to establish the generality of this phenomenon as well as to define the domains involved in the GAP effect.

CLINICAL CONSIDERATIONS

It is already clear that defects at the G protein level can lead to clinical disease. Inherited deficiency of Gs-α appears to be responsible for pseudohypoparathyroidism type Ia (65–67). The generalized resistance to hormone action characteristic of pseudohypoparathyroidism Ia conforms to the ubiquitous role of Gs in mediating hormonal stimulation of cAMP formation. Pseudohypoparathyroidism is discussed in detail in the chapter by Levine et al.

Constitutive activation of Gs occurs secondary to somatic mutations encoding substitutions of either arginine 201 or glutamine 227 (16). Such mutations are found in, and may explain the development of, pituitary somatotroph tumors. The McCune-Albright syndrome (MAS) is a sporadic disease characterized by café-au-lait skin pigmentation, polyostotic fibrous dysplasia, and hyperfunction of multiple endocrine glands. Patients with this syndrome harbor a mutation of arginine 201 of Gs-α in a mosaic pattern. This suggests a somatic mutational event that apparently occurs in early embryonic life (68). The resultant constitutive activation of cAMP formation explains the pleiotropic autonomous endocrine hyperfunction observed in this disease. Recent discovery of the same mutation in fibrous dysplasia bone lesions (Shenker A, Weinstein LS, Spiegel AM, unpublished observations) suggests that activation of Gs may be responsible for this bone lesion characterized by proliferation and abnormal differentiation of mesenchymal bone cells. Occasional patients with MAS show hypophosphatemia (and resultant rickets or osteomalacia). It had previously been suggested that this metabolic disturbance may be secondary to either secretion of a phosphaturic substance from dysplastic bone lesions or to hypersensitivity of the renal proximal tubules to PTH (69–71). The finding of activating Gs-α mutations in these patients makes the latter hypothesis a more likely explanation for the observed hypophosphatemia.

To date, Gi2 is the only α subunit other than Gs in which mutations have been found in association with human disease. Constitutively activating mutations of Gi2-α have been identified in certain ovarian and adrenal cortical tumors (72). It seems likely that additional G protein defects remain to be discovered in other human diseases.

REFERENCES

1. Chase LR, Melson GL, Aurbach GD. Pseudohypoparathyroidism: defective excretion of 3′,5′-AMP in response to parathyroid hormone. *J Clin Invest* 1969;48:1832–1844.
2. Hruska KA, Moskowitz D, Esbrit P, Civitelli R, Westbrook S, Huskey M. Stimulation of inositol triphosphate and diacylglycerol production in renal tubular cells by parathyroid hormone. *J Clin Invest* 1987;79:230–239.
3. Cosman F, Morrow B, Kopal M, Bilezikian JP. Stimulation of inositol phosphate formation in ROS 17/2.8 cell membranes by guanine nucleotide, calcium, and parathyroid hormone. *J Bone Mineral Res* 1989;4:413–420.
4. Jüppner H, Abou-Samra A-B, Freeman M, et al. A G protein-linked receptor for parathyroid hormone and parathyroid hormone-related peptide. *Science* 1991;254:1024–1026.
5. Abou-Samra A-B, Jüppner H, Force T, et al. Expression cloning of a common receptor for parathyroid hormone and parathyroid hormone-related peptide from rat osteoblast-like cells: a single receptor stimulates intracellular accumulation of both cAMP and inositol trisphosphates and increases intracellular free calcium. *Proc Natl Acad Sci USA* 1992;89:2732–2736.
6. Tang W-J, Gilman AG. Adenylyl cyclases. *Cell* 1992;70:869–872.
7. Rhee SG, Choi KD. Regulation of inositol phospholipid-specific phospholipase C isozymes. *J Biol Chem* 1992;267:12393–12396.
8. Spiegel AM, Shenker A, Weinstein LS. Receptor–effector coupling by G proteins: implications for normal and abnormal signal transduction. *Endocr Rev* 1992;13:536–565.
9. Bourne HR, Sanders DA, McCormick F. The GTPase superfamily: conserved structure and molecular mechanism. *Nature* 1991;349:117–127.
10. Simon MI, Strathmann MP, Gautam N. Diversity of G proteins in signal transduction. *Science* 1991;252:802–808.
11. Bray P, Carter A, Simons C, et al. Human cDNA clones for four species of $G_{\alpha s}$ signal transduction protein. *Proc Natl Acad Sci USA* 1986;83:8893–8897.
12. Kaziro Y, Itoh H, Kozasa T, Nakafuku M, Satoh T. Structure and function of signal-transducing GTP-binding proteins. *Annu Rev Biochem* 1991;60:349–400.
13. Spiegel AM, Backlund PS Jr, Butrynski JE, Jones TLZ, Simonds WF. The G protein connection: molecular basis of membrane association. *Trends Biochem Sci* 1991;16:338–341.
14. Camps M, Hou C, Sidiropoulos D, Stock JB, Jakobs KH, Gierschik P. Stimulation of phospholipase C by guanine-nucleotide-binding protein βγ subunits. *Eur J Biochem* 1992;206:821–831.
15. Berlot CH, Bourne HR. Identification of effector-activating residues of $G_{s\alpha}$. *Cell* 1992;68:911–922.
16. Landis CA, Masters SB, Spada A, Pace AM, Bourne HR, Vallar L. GTPase inhibiting mutations activate the alpha chain of Gs and stimulate adenylyl cyclase in human pituitary tumours. *Nature* 1989;340:692–696.
17. Miller RT, Masters SB, Sullivan KA, Beiderman B, Bourne HR. A mutation that prevents GTP-dependent activation of the α chain of G_s. *Nature* 1988;334:712–715.
18. Lee E, Taussig R, Gilman AG. The G226A mutant of $G_{s}\alpha$ highlights the requirement for dissociation of G protein subunits. *J Biol Chem* 1992;267:1212–1218.
19. Jones TLZ, Simonds WF, Merendino JJ Jr, Brann MR, Spiegel AM. Myristoylation of an inhibitory GTP-binding protein α subunit is essential for its membrane attachment. *Proc Natl Acad Sci USA* 1990;87:568–572.
20. Mumby SM, Heukeroth RO, Gordon JI, Gilman AG. G-protein α-subunit expression, myristoylation, and membrane association in COS cells. *Proc Natl Acad Sci USA* 1990;87:728–732.
21. Linder ME, Pang I-H, Duronio RJ, Gordon JI, Sternweis PC, Gilman AG. Lipid modifications of G protein subunits. Myristoylation of $G_o\alpha$ increases its affinity for βγ. *J Biol Chem* 1991;266:4654–4659.
22. Sullivan KA, Miller RT, Masters SB, Beiderman B, Heideman W, Bourne HR. Identification of receptor contact site involved in receptor-G protein coupling. *Nature* 1987;330:758–760.
23. Simonds WF, Goldsmith PK, Codina J, Unson CG, Spiegel AM. G_{i2} mediates α_2-adrenergic inhibition of adenylyl cyclase in platelet membranes: *in situ* identification with Gα C-terminal antibodies. *Proc Natl Acad Sci USA* 1989;86:7809–7813.
24. Shenker A, Goldsmith P, Unson CG, Spiegel AM. The G protein coupled to the thromboxane A_2 receptor in human platelets is a member of the novel G_q family. *J Biol Chem* 1991;266:9309–9313.
25. Rarick HM, Artemyev NO, Hamm HE. A site on rod G protein α subunit that mediates effector activation. *Science* 1992;256:1031–1033.
26. Smrcka AV, Hepler JR, Brown KO, Sternweis PC. Regulation of polyphosphoinositide-phospholipase C activity by purified G_q. *Science* 1991;251:804–807.
27. Taylor SJ, Chae HZ, Rhee SG, Exton JH. Activation of the β1 isozyme of phospholipase C by α subunits of the G_q class of G proteins. *Nature* 1991;350:516–518.
28. Berstein G, Blank JL, Smrcka AV, et al. Reconstitution of agonist-stimulated phosphatidylinositol 4,5-bisphosphate hydrolysis using purified m1 muscarinic receptor, $G_{q/11}$, and phospholipase C-β1. *J Biol Chem* 1992;267:8081–8088.
29. Lee CH, Park D, Wu D, Rhee SG, Simon MI. Members of the $G_q\alpha$ subunit gene family activate phospholipase C β isozymes. *J Biol Chem* 1992;267:16044–16047.
30. Schnabel P, Schreck R, Schiller DL, Camps M, Gierschik P. Stimulation of phospholipase C by a mutationally activated G protein α_{16} subunit. *Biochem Biophys Res Commun* 1992;188:1018–1023.
31. Lipinsky D, Gershengorn MC, Oron Y, $G\alpha_{11}$ and $G\alpha_q$ guanine nucleotide regulatory proteins differentially modulate the response to thyrotropin-releasing hormone in *Xenopus* oocytes. *FEBS Lett* 1992;307:237–240.
32. von Weizsäcker E, Strathmann MP, Simon MI. Diversity among the beta subunits of heterotrimeric GTP-binding proteins: characterization of a novel β-subunit cDNA. *Biochem Biophys Res Commun* 1992;183:350–356.
33. Lupas A, Van Dyke M, Stock J. Predicting coiled coils from protein sequences. *Science* 1991;252:1162–1164.
34. Van der Voorn L, Ploegh HL. The WD-40 repeat. *FEBS Lett* 1992;307:131–134.
35. Gautam N, Northrup J, Tamir H. Simon MI. G protein diversity is increased by associations with a variety of γ subunits. *Proc Natl Acad Sci USA* 1990;87:7973–7977.
36. Fisher KJ, Aronson NN Jr. Characterization of the cDNA and genomic sequence of a G protein γ subunit (γ5). *Mol Cell Biol* 1992;12:1585–1591.
37. Cali JJ, Balcueva EA, Rybalkin I, Robishaw JD. Selective tissue distribution of G protein γ subunits, including a new form of the γ subunits identified by cDNA cloning. *J Biol Chem* 1992;267:24023–24027.
38. Peng Y-W, Robishaw JD, Levine MA, Yau K-W. Retinal rods and cones have distinct G protein β and γ subunits. *Proc Natl Acad Sci USA* 1992;89:10882–10886.
39. Lee RH, Lieberman BS, Yamane HK, Bok D, Fung BK-K. A third form of the G protein β subunit: 1. Immunochemical identification and localization to cone photoreceptors. *J Biol Chem* 1992;267:24776–24781.

40. Backlund PS Jr., Simonds WF, Spiegel AM. Carboxyl-methylation and terminal processing of the brain G-protein gamma subunit. *J Biol Chem* 1990;265:15572–15577.

41. Simonds WF, Butrynski JE, Gautam N, Unson CG, Spiegel AM. G-protein βγ dimers: membrane targeting requires subunit coexpression and intact gamma CAAX domain. *J Biol Chem* 1991;266:1–2.

42. Pitcher JA, Inglese J, Higgins JB, et al. Role of βγ subunits of G proteins in targeting the β-adrenergic receptor kinase to membrane-bound receptors. *Science* 1992;257:1264–1267.

43. Pronin AN, Gautam N. Interaction between G-protein β and γ subunit types is selective. *Proc Natl Acad Sci USA* 1992;89:6220–6224.

44. Sohma H, Hashimoto H, Ohguro H, Akino T. Two γ-subunits, γ-I and γ-II, complex with the same β-subunits in bovine brain G-proteins (Gi/o). *Biochem Biophys Res Commun* 1992;184:175–182.

45. Kontani K, Takahashi K, Inanobe A, Ui M, Katada T. Molecular heterogeneity of the βγ-subunits of GTP-binding proteins in bovine brain membranes. *Arch Biochem Biophys* 1992;294:527–533.

46. Cerione RA, Gierschik P, Staniszewski C, et al. Functional differences in the βγ complexes of transducin and the inhibitory guanine nucleotide regulatory protein. *Biochemistry* 1987;26:1485–1491.

47. Kleuss C, Hescheler J, Ewel C, Rosenthal W, Schultz G, Wittig B. Assignment of G-protein subtypes to specific receptors inducing inhibition of calcium currents. *Nature* 1991;353:43–48.

48. Kleuss C, Scherübl H, Hescheler J, Schultz G, Wittig B. Different beta-subunits determine G-protein interaction with transmembrane receptors. *Nature* 1992;358:424–426.

49. Dohlman HG, Thorner J, Caron MG, Lefkowitz RJ. Model systems for the study of seven-transmembrane-segment receptors. *Annu Rev Biochem* 1991;60:653–688.

50. Buck L, Axel R. A novel multigene family may encode odorant receptors: a molecular basis for odor recognition. *Cell* 1991;65:175–187.

51. Probst WC, Snyder LA, Schuster DI, Brosius J, Sealfon SC. Sequence alignment of the G-protein coupled receptor superfamily. *DNA Cell Biol* 1992;11:1–20.

52. Okamoto T, Murayama Y, Hayashi Y, Inagaki M, Ogata E, Nishimoto I. Identification of a Gs activator region of the β₂-adrenergic receptor that is autoregulated via protein kinase A-dependent phosphorylation. *Cell* 1991;67:723–730.

53. Lechleiter J, Hellmiss R, Duerson K, et al. Distinct sequence elements control the specificity of G protein activation by muscarinic acetylcholine receptor subtypes. *EMBO J* 1990; 9:4381–4390.

54. Liggett SB, Caron MG, Lefkowitz RJ, Hnatowich M. Coupling of a mutated form of the human β₂-adrenergic receptor to Gi and Gs. Requirement for multiple cytoplasmic domains in the coupling process. *J Biol Chem* 1991;266:4816–4821.

55. Gudermann T, Birnbaumer M, Birnbaumer L. Evidence for dual coupling of the murine luteinizing hormone receptor to adenylyl cyclase and phosphoinositide breakdown and Ca²⁺ mobilization. Studies with the cloned murine luteinizing hormone receptor expressed in L cells. *J Biol Chem* 1992; 267:4479–4488.

56. Chabre O, Conklin BR, Lin HY, et al. A recombinant calcitonin receptor independently stimulates 3′,5′-cyclic adenosine monophosphate and Ca²⁺/inositol phosphate signaling pathways. *Mol Endocrinol* 1992;6:551–556.

57. Thorens B. Expression cloning of the pancreatic β cell receptor for the gluco-incretin hormone glucagon-like peptide 1. *Proc Natl Acad Sci USA* 1992;89:8641–8645.

58. Attramadal H, Arriza JL, Aoki C, et al. β-Arrestin2, a novel member of the arrestin/β-arrestin gene family. *J Biol Chem* 1992;267:17882–17890.

59. Lohse MJ, Andexinger S, Pitcher J, et al. Receptor-specific desensitization with purified proteins. Kinase dependence and receptor specificity of β-arrestin and arrestin in the β₂-adrenergic receptor and rhodopsin systems. *J Biol Chem* 1992;267:8558–8564.

60. Iñiguez-Lluhi JA, Simon MI, Robishaw JD, Gilman AG. G protein βγ subunits synthesized in Sf9 cells. Functional characterization and the significance of prenylation of gamma. *J Biol Chem* 1992;267:23409–23417.

61. Federman AD, Conklin BR, Schrader KA, Reed RR, Bourne HR. Hormonal stimulation of adenylyl cyclase through Gi-protein βγ subunits. *Nature* 1992;356:159–161.

62. Blank JL, Brattain KA, Exton JH. Activation of cytosolic phosphoinositide phospholipase C by G-protein βγ subunits. *J Biol Chem* 1992;267:23069–23075.

63. Berstein G, Blank JL, Jhon D-Y, Exton JH, Rhee SG, Ross EM. Phospholipase C-β1 is a GTPase-activating protein for Gq/11, its physiologic regulator. *Cell* 1992;70:411–418.

64. Pagès F, Deterre P, Pfister C. Enhanced GTPase activity of transducin when bound to cGMP phosphodiesterase in bovine retinal rods. *J Biol Chem* 1992;267:22018–22021.

65. Patten JL, Johns DR, Valle D, et al. Mutation in the gene encoding the stimulatory G protein of adenylyl cyclase in Albright's hereditary osteodystrophy. *N Engl J Med* 1990; 322:1412–1419.

66. Weinstein LS, Gejman PV, Friedman E, et al. Mutations of the Gs α-subunit gene in Albright hereditary osteodystrophy detected by denaturing gradient gel electrophoresis. *Proc Natl Acad Sci USA* 1990;87:8287–8290.

67. Weinstein LS, Gejman PV, De Mazancourt P, American N, Spiegel AM. A heterozygous 4-bp deletion mutation in the Gsα gene (GNAS1) in a patient with Albright hereditary osteodystrophy. *Genomics* 1992;13:1319–1321.

68. Weinstein LS, Shenker A, Gejman PV, Merino MJ, Friedman E, Spiegel AM. Activating mutations of the stimulatory G protein in the McCune-Albright syndrome. *N Engl J Med* 1991;325:1688–1695.

69. McArthur RG, Hayles AB, Lambert PW. Albright's syndrome with rickets. *Mayo Clin Proc* 1979;54:313–320.

70. Ryan WG, Nibbe AF, Schwartz TB, Ray RD. Fibrous dysplasia of bone with vitamin D resistant rickets: a case study. *Metabolism* 1968;17:988–998.

71. Tanaka T, Suwa S. A case of McCune-Albright syndrome with hyperthyroidism and vitamin D-resistant rickets. *Helv Paediatr Acta* 1977;32:263–273.

72. Lyons J, Landis CA, Harsh G, et al. Two G protein oncogenes in human endocrine tumors. *Science* 1990;249:655–659.

The Parathyroids, edited by J.P. Bilezikian,
M.A. Levine, and R. Marcus. Raven Press, Ltd.,
New York © 1994.

CHAPTER 16

Biochemical Mechanisms of Parathyroid Hormone Action

Daniel T. Coleman, Lorraine A. Fitzpatrick, and John P. Bilezikian

Parathyroid hormone (PTH) is a principal hormone responsible for calcium homeostasis in mammals. Through its action on target cells in bone and kidney, a positive net calcium balance results under physiological conditions (1–5) (see the chapter by Brown). It is generally accepted that many cellular responses induced by PTH are due to receptor-mediated activation of adenylyl cyclase, which leads to increases in intracellular concentrations of 3',5'-cyclic adenosine monophosphate (cAMP). The fundamental contribution in this area was made by Chase and Aurbach and helped to establish not only a key biochemical messenger of PTH but also cAMP as a key messenger system for a great number of other polypeptide hormones. This exciting chapter in the history of the study of hormone action is reviewed elsewhere in this volume (see the chapter by Chase). Knowledge that PTH stimulates cAMP production has helped to account for many of the actions of PTH on its major target organs, bone and kidney. For many years, it was believed that cAMP was utilized exclusively by PTH for all its cellular actions. Evidence has accumulated over the past 10 years that PTH also utilizes another major biochemical pathway for hormone action, namely, phosphatidylinositol hydrolysis. Actions of PTH on this pathway lead to the generation of the inositol phosphates and diacylglycerol, a set of key messengers that are responsible for many cellular events. The recent cloning of the PTH/PTH-related protein (PTHrP) receptor from bone and kidney cells has led to important insights into how these two distinct second messenger systems are activated by PTH. This chapter reviews the effects of PTH in initiating cellular events through actions on these two pathways.

TARGET TISSUES FOR PARATHYROID HORMONE ACTION

The physiologic actions of PTH provide a framework for a discussion of the biochemical effects of PTH. Plasma calcium concentration is maintained within an extremely narrow range in human beings ($\sim$ 8.5–10.5 mg/dl). By releasing PTH in response to a reduction in extracellular calcium, the parathyroid glands very rapidly initiate a series of responses in several tissues that lead to restoration of circulating calcium levels (4,5).

Physiological Effects in Bone

The work of Neuman et al. (6) and Talmage and Meyer (7) indicates that the maintenance of calcium homeostasis in response to PTH involves transport of calcium to the extracellular environment by osteocytes and/or lining cells on bone surfaces. Cells lining the endosteal surfaces of bone release radiolabeled calcium in < 1 hr after administration of PTH (8). This initial rapid response to PTH involves structural changes of endosteal surface cells and is an important regulatory mechanism for maintenance of calcium homeostasis.

PTH causes a release of calcium from bone by stimulating osteoclast-mediated resorption (9,10). PTH

D. T. Coleman: Department of Physiology and Biophysics, Mount Sinai School of Medicine, New York, New York 10029.

L. A. Fitzpatrick: Department of Medicine, Mayo Clinic and Mayo Foundation, Rochester, Minnesota 55905.

J. P. Bilezikian: Departments of Medicine and Pharmacology, College of Physicians and Surgeons, Columbia University, New York, New York 10032.

rapidly mobilizes calcium in vivo as early as 3 h after administration, a process that does not require new protein synthesis. This first phase of PTH action is associated with increased metabolic activity of osteoclasts. A second phase, which depends on new protein synthesis, occurs within 24 hr of PTH administration. This second phase is characterized by an increase in both the number and the metabolic activity of osteoclasts. Despite these actions on the osteoclast, it is often stated that PTH does not appear to have a direct effect on the osteoclast (11). Recent studies, however, have described the binding of ^{125}I-bovine PTH-(1–84) to cultured avian osteoclasts (12), and other investigators have indicated direct activation of and resorption by the osteoclast in response to PTH (13–15). Although the use of mixed cell populations in many of these studies has resulted in difficulty in interpretation of the osteoclast response, many investigators now propose a direct effect of PTH on osteoclast action.

In contrast to its actions on osteoclasts, PTH has well-known direct effects on the osteoblast (16–20). Key actions of PTH on the osteoblast, the cell responsible for bone formation, are inhibition of type I collagen synthesis, stimulation of collagenase synthesis, and reduction of alkaline phosphatase activity (21–23). Increases in osteoclast number and alterations in function could occur through intercellular signals generated by direct effects of PTH on the osteoblast (24). The observation that osteoclasts become responsive to PTH when they are incubated with osteoblasts supports this idea. Osteoclast activation could also occur via an effect of PTH on early cells in the osteoblast lineage, such as bone marrow-derived mononuclear cells (25).

The biochemical mechanisms by which PTH stimulates osteoclast-mediated bone resorption are incompletely understood. Enzymes and other factors released or activated via metabolic events stimulated by PTH include collagenase, lysosomal hydroxylases, acid phosphatases, carbonic anhydrase, H^+,K^+-adenosine triphosphatases (ATPases), Na^+/Ca^{2+} exchange systems, cathepsin B, and cysteine protease. An acidic extracellular environment is necessary during bone resorption for protonation of hydroxyapatite. Ultrastructural studies of the osteoclast show that this acidic microenvironment is created by "podosomes," specialized structures in the osteoclast membrane that help to seal off the space between the osteoclast and the mineralized surface. Several enzymes have been identified that contribute to creation of this acidic microenvironment. An H^+,K^+-ATPase, similar to the proton pump in renal intercalated cells (26), may be involved, because inhibition of this proton pump by omeprazole blocks PTH-mediated bone resorption (27). This ATPase activity, localized by immunocytochemistry to the cell–bone attachment site, is found at

the resorptive site in the osteoclast, the ruffled border (28). Carbonic anhydrase, another enzyme activated by PTH, may generate hydrogen ion and provide the H^+,K^+-ATPase proton pump with substrate. In osteopetrosis, a disease characterized by inadequate bone resorption, type II carbonic anhydrase is absent in skeletal tissue, supporting a role for this enzyme in bone resorption. PTH stimulates carbonic anhydrase II activity, and, when this enzyme is inhibited, PTH-mediated bone resorption is attenuated (29).

Several investigators have proposed that Na^+/Ca^{2+} exchange also plays an important role in bone resorption. Inhibition of the Na^+/Ca^{2+}-exchanger with amiloride or an analog, 3′4′-dichlorobenzamil (DCB), prevents PTH-induced bone resorption in neonatal mouse calvaria (30). DCB also affects other calcium transport systems such as ATP-dependent calcium pumps, which may also play a role in bone resorption. Other studies indicate that PTH is not required for proton buffering in neonatal mouse calvaria and that PTH may instead inhibit this process by bone (31).

Physiological Effects in the Kidney

When PTH secretion is stimulated by a reduction in the ionized calcium concentration, the net effect on the kidney is to conserve calcium by increasing fractional reabsorption of calcium from the glomerular fluid (see the chapter by Brown). The sites of this effect appear to be the thick ascending limb of the loop of Henle, the distal convoluted tubule, and the early portion of the cortical collecting tubule (32). PTH also inhibits proximal tubular reabsorption of sodium, bicarbonate, and phosphate (33,34). In fact, PTH is recognized classically as a phosphaturic agent. The ability of PTH to induce phosphaturia is the basis for the Ellsworth-Howard test, the first clinically useful test to monitor renal PTH responsiveness (35). Recent studies have localized the site of this phosphaturic action of PTH to the proximal convoluted tubule and to the pars recta (36). Phosphate reabsorption is also inhibited, but less importantly, by PTH in the distal tubule. The phosphaturic actions of PTH are of interest in view of PTH's action of mobilizing calcium and phosphate from the skeleton. When PTH secretion is stimulated by hypocalcemia, the net effects on circulating calcium and phosphate concentrations are to restore the serum calcium level, without any substantial change in serum phosphate concentration. As part of the pathophysiology of primary hyperparathyroidism, in contrast, the excessive secretion of PTH leads to phosphaturia, presumably not compensated adequately by skeletal phosphate mobilization. Hence serum phosphate levels are in the low to low-normal range in primary hyperparathyroidism.

In primary hyperparathyroidism, excess PTH leads to a negative calcium balance despite its action to conserve renal tubular calcium. Many patients with primary hyperparathyroidism in fact are hypercalciuric. The apparent explanation for this observation is that the amount of calcium filtered at the glomerulus exceeds even the enhanced capacity for renal tubular calcium conservation. However, for any serum calcium level, urinary calcium excretion will be less in the presence of PTH than in the absence of PTH.

Another key action of PTH in the kidney that works to restore the serum calcium in response to hypocalcemia is stimulation of 1,25-dihydroxyvitamin D [1,25-$(OH)_2$D] formation. Renal 1α-hydroxylase, the enzyme responsible for the conversion of 25-hydroxyvitamin D to 1,25-$(OH)_2$D, is found in the proximal tubule (37). PTH is one of several regulators of this enzyme (38,39) (Fig. 1). Reduction in serum phosphate concentration is another major stimulus to 1,25-$(OH)_2$D formation. High levels of calcium also appear to directly inhibit the renal 1α-hydroxylase (40). The action of PTH of enhancing 1,25-$(OH)_2$D formation accounts for its indirect actions of stimulating gastrointestinal absorption of calcium.

PTH receptors are found on glomerular podocytes and on the antiluminal surface of the proximal and distal tubules and the thick ascending limb of the loop of Henle (18). PTH-sensitive adenylyl cyclase activity is found in renal proximal and distal tubules (41,42) but has also been noted in renal blood vessels (41).

Other Target Tissues of Parathyroid Hormone

The literature has been dominated over the past 50 years by studies of PTH action in its classic targets, bone and kidney. While there can be no disputing the prominent roles for these organs in PTH action, more recent studies have pointed out that non-conventional target systems may also be a focus of PTH action (see the chapter "Parathyroid Hormone and Parathyroid Hormone-Related Protein as Polyhormones" by Mallette). These other tissues and apparent actions include chondrocytes and the development of cartilage (43); uterine (44), vascular (45–49), and gastrointestinal tract smooth muscle relaxation (50); inotropy in the heart (51,52); chronotropy in the heart; and hypotension (53–56). Moreover, effects of PTH to stimulate a transient increase in cellular calcium in dermal fibroblasts are noteworthy (57). A discussion of the biochemical actions of PTH will have to account ultimately for effects in these other organ systems. In fact, clues can sometimes be obtained from cells that do not possess both signalling pathways for PTH, such as mouse epidermal keratinocytes (58) and rat brain synaptosomes (59), in which the adenylyl cyclase response to PTH appears to be attenuated.

ACTIVATION OF THE CYCLIC ADENOSINE MONOPHOSPHATE SECOND-MESSENGER SYSTEM BY PARATHYROID HORMONE

As was noted above, PTH was one of the first hormones to be shown to utilize the cAMP second messenger system (60–62). In the kidney, cAMP is involved in PTH-mediated effects to reduce calcium excretion, to enhance phosphate excretion, and to stimulate 1,25-$(OH)_2$D formation (1–3,5,60,63,64). cAMP is also believed to be a mediator for many of the actions of PTH in bone (20,65,66). Increases in urinary cAMP, a classic marker of PTH action, are associated with known physiological responses to PTH, such as a rise in serum calcium and phosphaturia (60). Dibutyryl cAMP, a cAMP analog that gains cellular entry, mimics the effects of PTH in renal tissue (34,67). Clinical evidence is also available indicating a pivotal role for cAMP in mediating the effects of PTH. Patients suffering from a genetic disorder of PTH resistance, pseudohypoparathyroidism type 1, do not show increases in urinary cAMP after PTH administration (see the chapter by Levine et al.). The expected

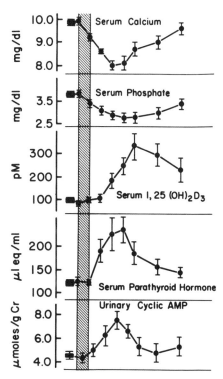

FIG. 1. Response of 1,25$(OH)_2D_3$, PTH, and urinary cAMP to hypocalcemia. Eight patients with Paget's disease received plicamycin (25 μg/kg) by intravenous infusion. The rapid decline in serum calcium is followed by increases in PTH and 1,25$(OH)_2D_3$. (Modified from ref. 39 with permission.)

phosphaturia and increase in serum calcium after PTH administration also do not occur (68–71). Hence patients with pseudohypoparathyroidism type 1 have reduced serum calcium and elevated serum phosphate levels. Chase et al. (72) discovered that pseudohypoparathyroidism type 1 is associated with impaired production of cAMP. The precise biochemical defects in the cAMP pathway and its molecular basis are reviewed in the chapter by Levine et al.

STRUCTURE–ACTIVITY RELATIONSHIP OF PARATHYROID HORMONE ACTIVATION OF ADENYLYL CYCLASE

Detailed structure–function studies of the PTH molecule (Fig. 2) have helped to determine regions required for activation of adenylyl cyclase. A detailed exposition of this subject is found in the chapter by Chorev and Rosenblatt; a brief summary is provided here. A fundamental observation is that the full-length, 84-amino-acid polypeptide is not required for complete expression of the adenylyl cyclase-stimulating properties of the hormone. A shorter amino-terminal fragment, PTH-(1–34), is as potent as the intact molecule (73–77). Carboxy-terminal fragments of PTH

such as PTH-(53–84) are completely inactive. PTH is metabolized in the liver, where several smaller peptides are generated, one of which is PTH-(1–34) or an analog closely related to it. This peptide, however, is not released into the circulation but is subjected to further proteolytic digestion. Nevertheless, production of a fully active but shorter form of PTH in vivo has led to speculation that an active fragment might be produced at target tissues and act locally. In view of the fact that PTH-(1–34) does not gain entrance from the liver into the circulation, an important physiological role for the amino-terminal fragment would require production of this fragment at target sites. In the chapter by Kronenberg et al. a further discussion of the peripheral metabolism of PTH is provided.

Progressive loss in adenylyl cyclase-stimulating properties occurs with stepwise deletion of amino acids from the C-terminal end of PTH-(1–34) (74). Amino-terminal fragments of PTH that are shorter than PTH-(1–25) in length are inactive. These observations have led to the notion that the region defined by positions 25–34 are important for binding of PTH to its receptor (17,78–80). At the other end of the molecule, stepwise removal of amino-terminal amino acids from position 1 leads to a dramatic loss in adenylyl cyclase-stimulating properties, in contrast to the gradual loss of adenylyl-cyclase-stimulating properties when carboxy-terminal amino acids are sequentially removed from PTH-(1–34). PTH-(2–34), for example, is a much weaker stimulator of adenylyl cyclase PTH-(1–34).

Effective PTH antagonists have been designed based on these structure–function considerations. PTH-(3–34), which lacks the first two amino-terminal amino acids, is an effective competitive antagonist in vitro. However, in vivo this analog has weak agonist properties. Further shortening of the amino-terminal region, along with amidation of the carboxy terminus, leads to more effective antagonists, such as PTH-(7–34) amide, a potent antagonist possessing neither in vitro nor in vivo agonist properties. These observations and others detailed in the chapter by Chorev and Rosenblatt have led to a model of the 1–34 fragment of PTH in which domains of activation, inhibition, and binding have been defined (73).

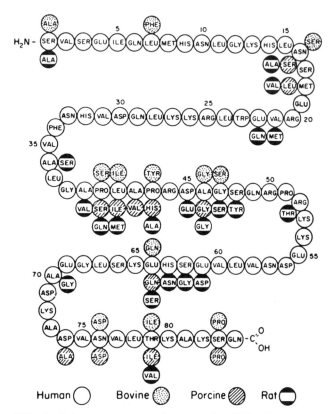

FIG. 2. Primary structure of mammalian PTH. The amino acid sequence of mammalian PTH-(1–84) is shown comparing human (backbone sequence) with bovine, porcine, and rat hormones as indicated.

DISCREPANCIES IN THE STRUCTURE–ACTIVITY RELATIONSHIPS OF PARATHYROID HORMONE FOR ADENYLYL CYCLASE ACTIVITY AND FOR PHYSIOLOGICAL ACTIONS

The relative stimulatory or inhibitory potencies of PTH fragments in bioassays have correlated well in general with their relative potencies in in vitro assays of adenylyl cyclase activity (76,81). However, the conventional adenylyl cyclase assay may not be sensitive enough to detect latent agonism of some of these analogs (73). For example, Rosenblatt and colleagues (82) have observed that responsiveness of adenylyl cyclase to PTH in osteoblast-like ROS 17/2.8 cells is markedly amplified by dexamethasone and/or pertussis toxin. Discrepancies between in vivo and in vitro assay systems thus may be based on experimental conditions (83).

Discrepancies between agonist properties of PTH in assays conducted in vitro and in vivo may also be due to the possibility that PTH utilizes second messengers other than cAMP. PTH-(2–34) is virtually inactive in the conventional adenylyl cyclase assay but can induce substantial hypercalcemia and phosphaturia in several in vivo models (74,84). Another analog generally inactive as a stimulator of adenylyl cyclase is the antagonist [Nle^{8,18}Tyr^{34}]bPTH-(3–34) amide, which induces hypercalcemia, phosphaturia, and increased plasma 1,25-(OH)$_2$D$_3$ concentrations in dogs and rats (85,86). In fact, this peptide produces effects on urinary phosphate and plasma 1,25-(OH)$_2$D$_3$ levels similar to bPTH-(1–34) if sufficiently high concentrations of [Nle^{8,18}Tyr^{34}]bPTH-(3–34) amide are used. This PTH analogue decreases Na$^+$/H$^+$ exchange and Na$^+$, K$^+$-ATPase activity in rat proximal tubules (87). These observations could be explained by the ability of PTH-(3–34) amide to act as an agonist for adenylyl cyclase under very special conditions. However, the special circumstances required to demonstrate agonism in the adenylyl cyclase assay do not necessarily suggest that this signal transduction pathway is stimulated by PTH-(3–34) amide in vivo.

ACTIVATION OF A CALCIUM SECOND-MESSENGER SYSTEM BY PARATHYROID HORMONE

An important response to PTH that cannot be easily ascribed to mechanisms involving the generation of cAMP is that related to changes in intracellular free calcium. The transient hypocalcemia that occurs prior to the better known hypercalcemic effects of PTH was an important observation (Fig. 3) (88,89). Now, years later, it is apparent that the initial hypocalcemia is due to the action of PTH to induce cellular uptake of calcium (90–94). That this response does not appear to be mediated by cAMP is supported by five lines of evidence. (a) cAMP does not reproduce the actions of PTH to raise intracellular concentrations of free calcium in renal tubular cells (95). (b) The ability of PTH to raise intracellular free calcium levels is not altered by continued exposure to PTH (96–98). Repeated stimulation of these cells by PTH, however, leads to loss of the cAMP response. (c) Forskolin, an agent that increases cellular cAMP in virtually all cells, can-

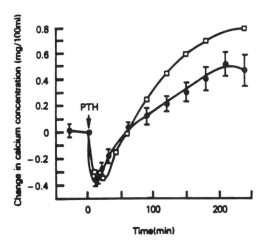

FIG. 3. Initial hypocalcemic action of PTH; bPTH-(1–34) induces a brief, transient hypocalcemia before causing hypercalcemia. Observations shown are from administration of bPTH-(1–34) to dogs in vivo (*open squares*) and to mouse calvaria in vitro (*solid circles*). (From refs. 88 and 89, as modified by ref. 2.)

not mimic actions of PTH to elevate free calcium in osteoblast-like UMR-106 cells (99,100). (d) Rat brain synaptosomes respond to PTH with an increase in calcium uptake, but without any increase in cAMP (59). (e) [Nle^{8,18}Tyr^{34}]PTH-(3–34) amide can elevate intracellular free calcium, although it is an antagonist of PTH-mediated adenylyl cyclase activation (101,102). In addition to the effects of PTH on intracellular calcium, recent observations indicate that the effect of PTH on the renal phosphate transport system may be, in part, independent of cAMP (67,103,104).

The ability of PTH to increase intracellular calcium without perturbing levels of cAMP produced evidence for PTH activation of messenger systems that alter cytosolic calcium concentrations. The pathway of hydrolysis of phosphatidylinositides (PIs), which results in the generation of calcium-mobilizing inositol polyphosphates (IPs), was a likely target of PTH action. The observation that many hormones initially shown to utilize the cAMP pathway also utilize the PI pathway strengthened the idea that PTH also has multiple biochemical mechanisms of action. Moreover, over the past 20 years, the importance of the PI system as a major biochemical pathway for many hormones has been shown clearly to rival that of cAMP (105–108).

TRANSDUCTION OF HORMONE SIGNALS BY POLYPHOSPHOINOSITIDE HYDROLYSIS: FEATURES OF PHOSPHATIDYLINOSITOL HYDROLYSIS

Phosphatidylinositols are present in minute quantities in the plasma membrane of the cell. The three most important compounds are phosphatidylinositol

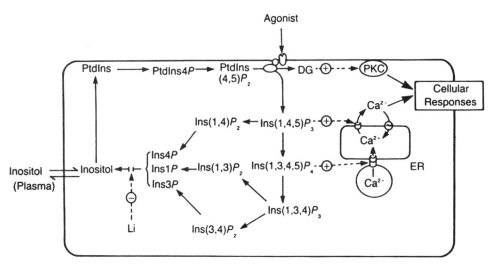

FIG. 4. Scheme of the phospholipase C-dependent second-messenger system. Agonist-mediated receptor activation results in G protein-mediated activation of phospholipase C. Hydrolysis of PIP$_2$ results in formation of Ins(1,4,5)P$_3$ and diacylglycerol (DG). Ins(1,4,5)P$_3$ is metabolized to inositol primarily via the routes shown. Ins(1,4,5)P$_3$ and Ins(1,3,4,5)P$_4$ increase intracellular free Ca^{2+} by actions on the endoplasmic reticulum and plasma membrane calcium channels, respectively. DG and its metabolite arachidonic acid stimulate protein kinase C (PKC). Arachidonic acid may also affect intracellular Ca^{2+} and may be further metabolized to other potential second messengers. DG is also a precursor of phosphatidic acid (PA), which is further metabolized to cytosine diphosphate-DG (CDP-DG). CDP-DG and inositol are recombined by PI synthetase to yield PI and CMP. (Reprinted from ref. 171 with permission.)

(PI), phosphatidylinositol 4-phosphate (PIP), and phosphatidylinositol 4,5-bisphosphate (PIP$_2$) (Fig. 4). PI kinases phosphorylate PI to PIP and then to PIP$_2$. The dynamic state in which these PIs are interconvertible also depends on a dephosphorylation mechanism by phosphatases. Under basal conditions PIP$_2$ can be dephosphorylated to PIP and then to PI. These PIs are substrates for a family of enzymes known as *phospholipase C*, which hydrolyze PIs yielding a series of products known as the "inositol phosphates" (IPs) (109–115). PI is hydrolyzed to inositol 1-monophosphate [Ins(1)P$_1$]; PIP is hydrolyzed to inositol 1,4-bisphosphate [Ins(1,4)P$_2$]; PIP$_2$ is hydrolyzed to inositol 1,4,5-trisphosphate [Ins(1,4,5)P$_3$]. For each IP formed, diacylglycerol is a concomitant product of the hydrolysis. Diacylglycerol and its metabolites have their own important actions as second messengers (116–119) but are not discussed further in this chapter. The IPs can be subjected to cyclization in which the phosphate in position 1 is linked to the 2 position leading to Ins(1,2cyclic)P$_1$, Ins(1,2cyclic,4)P$_2$, or Ins(1,2cyclic, 4,5)P$_3$ compounds (120–123). A key IP$_3$, Ins(1,4,5)P$_3$, can be phosphorylated to inositol 1,3,4,5-tetrakisphosphate [Ins(1,3,4,5)P$_4$] by Ins(1,4,5)P$_3$ 3-kinase (124–132); and Ins(1,3,4,5)P$_4$ can also be formed by direct hydrolysis of another substrate for phospholipase C, phosphatidylinositol 3,4,5-trisphosphate (PIP$_3$) (133).

The metabolism of Ins(1,3,4,5)P$_4$ involves a series of dephosphorylation steps leading initially to an inactive

and isometrically distinct IP$_3$, inositol 1,3,4-trisphosphate [Ins(1,3,4)P$_3$]. This product is formed much more slowly than the active triphosphate isomer Ins(1,4,5)P$_3$. If the inactive and active isomers of IP$_3$ are not separated biochemically, the major product measured is the inactive compound Ins(1,3,4)P$_3$. Many protocols assume that the amount of total IP$_3$ reflects the amount of generation of Ins(1,4,5)P$_3$ by agonist (125,127,130,134,135). However, direct assay of the active product, Ins(1,4,5)P$_3$, is a much more reliable indicator of agonist action. The inactive isomer Ins(1,3,4)P$_3$ undergoes a series of subsequent dephosphorylation steps to 1,3-IP$_2$ and 3,4-IP$_2$ and then to the monophosphates Ins(1)P$_1$ and Ins(3)P$_1$, respectively (132,136). The inactivation of Ins(1,4,5)P$_3$ leads to a different set of dephosphorylated IPs, namely, Ins(1,4)P$_2$ and Ins(4)P$_1$. Ins(1)P$_1$ [formed by the direct action of phospholipase C on PI (113)] and Ins(4)P$_1$ [the product of Ins(1,4)P$_2$ hydrolysis] are then metabolized ultimately to inositol. The formation of inositol serves as a reentrant substrate for PI formation.

Although PIP$_2$ is present at the lowest concentration among the PIs, it is preferentially hydrolyzed to Ins(1,4,5)P$_3$ by phospholipase C in response to agonists such as PTH. Ins(1,4,5)P$_3$ binds to specific receptors and thereby mediates release of calcium directly from intracellular, nonmitochondrial stores (137–140). Ins(1,4,5)P$_3$ is formed rapidly, with peak levels of IP$_3$ and changes in intracellular calcium occurring seconds after exposure to agonist. Only a small fraction of phosphoinositides serve as substrates for receptor-stimulated phospholipase C activity (141,142). Larger, hormone-insensitive pools of PIs have been identified (141,143–149). The relative sizes of hormone-sensitive vs. hormone-insensitive pools of PIs differ according to the tissue. Distinct pools of PIs with different turnover rates may be located in different structures within the cell or may exist as functionally distinct compartments within the plasma membrane (141).

The activation pathway of polyphosphoinositide hydrolysis is exceedingly complex. Some of this complexity is due to the fact that activation appears to be an intrinsic aspect of inactivation. Moreover, the number of IPs that could be produced theoretically as a result of hydrolysis, metabolism, and interconversions is an astounding array of compounds exceeding 50. Many have already been isolated (124,150–155). It is possible that some of these compounds are not mere metabolic products but are active second messengers themselves.

INTERACTION BETWEEN THE CALCIUM AND INOSITOL PHOSPHATE PATHWAYS OF CELLULAR ACTIVATION

Changes in the concentrations of intracellular free Ca^{2+} are responsible for the regulation of a large number of enzyme activities, such as those of adenylyl cyclase, phosphodiesterase, phospholipase A_2, and protein kinases (138,139,156–159). The cellular Ca^{2+} signal is generated by three major mechanisms: (a) release from intracellular Ca^{2+} stores, (b) effects on calcium channels in the plasma membrane, and (c) direct or G protein-mediated effects on calcium channels. Release of Ca^{2+} from intracellular stores is thought to be responsible for rapid, transient Ca^{2+} signals that are independent of extracellular Ca^{2+} (105,106,137–140,160). However, continued release of Ca^{2+} from intracellular stores is ultimately dependent on extracellular Ca^{2+} for replenishment. Thus intracellular changes in Ca^{2+} may show the same dependence on extracellular Ca^{2+} that is usually attributed to simple transmembrane fluxes of Ca^{2+} (161,162). However, this is not the case in the early phase, when changes in intracellular Ca^{2+} can be demonstrated in the absence of extracellular Ca^{2+}. After the initial rapid change in intracellular calcium, a subsequent stimulation of calcium influx across the plasma membrane usually occurs. Influx of Ca^{2+} across the plasma membrane may occur through direct or G protein-mediated, receptor-activated channel openings (157,163–166). Ca^{2+} influx may also be triggered by $Ins(1,3,4,5)P_4$ and possibly also by $Ins(1,4,5)P_3$ or by the combined action of $Ins(1,3,4,5)P_4$ and $Ins(1,4,5)P_3$ (115,167–170). There is also evidence for calcium-activated calcium chan-

nels that open in direct response to an elevation in intracellular calcium (158).

Ca^{2+} signals generated in response to many hormones have been found to result from the formation of IPs through activation of phospholipase C by those hormones (136,156,157,171). Another possibility, namely, activation of phospholipase C by calcium itself, is not believed to be the mechanism underlying phospholipase C activation in response to most hormones (108,172–175). Rather, it is believed that the hormone directly stimulates phospholipase C activity. The resulting Ca^{2+} signal could provide a positive feedback loop, amplifying the initial activation of phospholipase C by the hormone.

EFFECTS OF PARATHYROID HORMONE ON MOBILIZATION OF INOSITOL PHOSPHATES

In renal tissue, PTH stimulates the metabolism of membrane PIs in a manner that reflects increased turnover of these substrates (176–181). Our present understanding of PI metabolism indicates a general rise in PI turnover when one step in the pathway, namely, phospholipase C, is activated. The mechanism by which PTH activates this pathway is independent of cAMP (179,181), as has been shown in bone (182) and in renal cells (183,184). PTH increases levels of IPs and turnover of PIs, suggesting that PTH may stimulate phospholipase C directly. PTH raises levels of IPs in intact bone cell preparations as well as in the kidney (183–185). Hruska et al. (184) have demonstrated a rapid increase in IP_3 release after exposure to PTH in the opossum kidney (OK) cell line. A concomitant reduction in the amount of PIP_2 was also observed. Similar data were obtained when PTH was exposed to primary cultures of canine proximal tubule cells. In ROS 17/2.8 cells, both full-length (1–84) and N-terminal (1–34) PTH are associated with significant stimulation of IP_3 formation (186).

Although the data suggest that PTH stimulates phospholipase C activity, direct assessment of enzyme activity requires the addition of known amounts of substrate and accurate determination of the amount of product formed. Such studies also require that the product formed not be subject to further metabolism. With few exceptions (187), studies of the IP intracellular signaling system have not focused on the direct measurement of phospholipase C activity. Substrates are typically prepared by prelabeling cells with ^3H-inositol. Over time, the ^3H-inositol becomes incorporated into the phosphoinositides, PI, PIP, and PIP_2. Cells containing labeled PIs of unknown specific activity are then stimulated with the agonist in question. Results from studies conducted using this methodology are usually confined to observations of increases in radioactivity in chromatographic fractions containing various IPs. One might consider in this context the distinction between measuring cellular cAMP and adenylyl cyclase activities. Measurement of cAMP does not always reflect the activity of the enzyme; similarly, measurement of IP does not necessarily reflect the activity of phospholipase C.

A variation of this protocol is to utilize membranes prepared from cells previously labeled with ^{3}H-inositol. This approach tends to lower background levels of IPs and permits the study of ions and other modulators of the enzymes involved in the formation and hydrolysis of IPs. Use of membrane preparations labeled previously by incubating the cells from which they were obtained permits a closer approximation of enzyme activity, but it is still indirect. For example, an increase in Ins(1,4,5)P$_3$ with this broken-cell method could result from increased PI(4)P$_1$-5-kinase activity, from decreased Ins(1,4,5)P$_3$ metabolism, or from direct stimulation of phospholipase C activity.

The most direct approach to measure phospholipase C activity is to introduce labeled substrate, PIP$_2$, of known specific activity to membrane preparations much in the way that labeled ATP, of known specific activity, is utilized to study adenylyl cyclase activity. Use of such protocols has been attempted (187), but this is difficult because of the challenge of incorporating an exogenous substrate such as PIP$_2$ in effective proximity to the enzyme machinery that hydrolyzes this substrate.

In canine renal cortical tubular membranes, PTH increases IPs in a concentration-dependent fashion between 1 and 100 nM, similar to published reports of the concentration dependence of PTH stimulation of adenylyl cyclase activity in other membrane preparations. Our own observations of adenylyl cyclase activity in this preparation confirm the same concentration–response relationship for bPTH-stimulated generation of cAMP as for bPTH-stimulated increases in IPs (Fig. 5) (185). This correlates well with concentration responses for PTH-mediated increases in IP$_3$

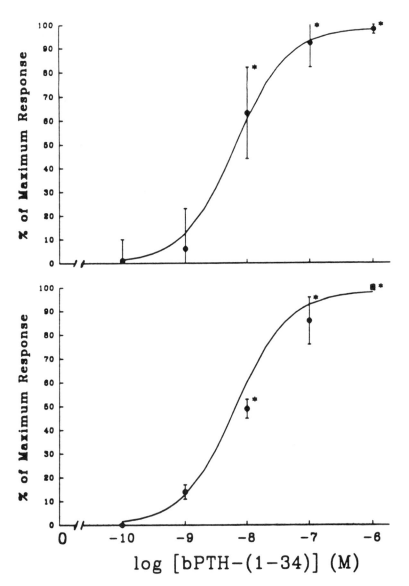

FIG. 5. Relationship of bPTH-(1–34) concentration to ^{3}H-IP$_1$ and cAMP formation in canine renal cortex. Half-maximal stimulation of ^{3}H-IP$_1$ is ~6 nM (**top**). Half-maximal stimulation of cAMP (**bottom**) is ~7 nM. (Reprinted from ref. 185 with permission.)

production in OK cells (184) and the Ca^{2+} response in UMR-106 cells (188). While these similar dose–response relationships do not have any à priori significance, the findings do support the hypothesis that PTH acts on both second messenger systems through receptors with similar affinities for PTH.

The concentrations of bPTH-(1–34) required to increase cAMP and IPs in membranes (EC_{50} ~5 nM) are slightly higher than the concentrations of PTH required to stimulate production of cAMP or to elevate intracellular Ca^{2+} in whole cells and are considerably higher than those required to have effects on physiologic responses such as inhibition of phosphate transport, stimulation of calcium reuptake, and stimulation of 1α-hydroxylase activity of 25-hydroxyvitamin D_3. The half-maximal concentration for PTH-mediated increases in intracellular cAMP in renal cells is 1 nM, while renal phosphate transport is inhibited by PTH with a half-maximal concentration of 50 pM (67,104). Decreased sensitivity in cell-free assay systems is typically due to the loss of activity associated with disruption of cell integrity. The greater sensitivity of the physiological responses compared to the sensitivity of cellular biochemical responses could be a result of the signal amplification that results from the cascade of biochemical reactions following generation of second messengers. These differences in sensitivity to PTH do not argue against an important biological role for PTH as an activator of either phospholipase C or adenylyl cyclase.

CHANGES IN INTRACELLULAR CALCIUM INDUCED BY PARATHYROID HORMONE

The data implicating PTH in the perturbation of cellular calcium are reviewed in this section. In the osteosarcoma cell line UMR-106, PTH perturbs cytosolic calcium in three distinct phases: a rapid increase in the first few seconds, followed by a rapid decrease to basal levels within the first minute, and finally by a slower increment in cellular calcium (189). The initial rise in intracellular calcium is inhibited by lanthanum and verapamil, calcium-channel blockers. The slower, subsequent increase in intracellular calcium may be mediated by intracellular cAMP and is relatively insensitive to calcium-channel antagonists. It seems likely that the initial change in cellular calcium after exposure to PTH is due to activation of a cAMP-independent calcium channel. Further classification led to a description of calcium release from intracellular pools after activation of protein kinase C by phorbol esters (189). Reid et al. (190) also demonstrated that changes in intracellular calcium after stimulation of UMR-106 cells by PTH were independent of cAMP.

Exposure of cells to pertussis toxin reduces PTH-stimulated elevations in intracellular calcium, suggest-

ing a role for a guanine regulatory protein(s) in this system. Analogs of cAMP also reduced intracellular levels of calcium, indicating that the adenylyl cyclase pathway may dampen the effects of the PI pathway. Using the photoprotein aequorin, Donahue et al. (191) demonstrate agonist properties of rat PTH-(1–34), bovine PTH-(3–34), and bovine PTH-(7–34) on cellular calcium in ROS 17/2.8 cells. Desensitization of ROS 17/2.8 cells after PTH exposure has underscored further the importance of calcium as a physiological effector of PTH-stimulated PI hydrolysis. Exposure of cells to rat PTH-(1–34) reduced the cAMP response to PTH but did not attenuate the PTH-induced rise in intracellular calcium (192).

The effects of PTH to regulate renal tubular handling of calcium, as reviewed in an earlier section, are likely to be related directly to actions of PTH on cellular calcium. In opossum kidney cells, human PTH-(1–34) raised intracellular calcium concentration (193). Although hPTH-(1–34) also increased cAMP levels in these cells, forskolin and dibutyryl cAMP failed to elicit an increase in cytosolic calcium concentrations. These data suggest stimulation of intracellular calcium release by PTH.

THE EFFECT OF PARATHYROID HORMONE TO INCREASE INTRACELLULAR CALCIUM MAY BE DUE TO INCREASES IN INOSITOL PHOSPHATES

Demonstration that PTH can stimulate the IP pathway places earlier demonstrations of its ability to perturb cellular Ca^{2+} in a mechanistic context. PTH does not increase intracellular Ca^{2+} through its actions to stimulate cellular cAMP (59,90,91,95,96,99,101). Thus it is reasonable to consider the distinct possibility that PTH stimulates an increase in intracellular Ca^{2+} via its actions to stimulate $Ins(1,4,5)P_3$ formation. The well-established observation that $Ins(1,4,5)P_3$ can cause an increase in cellular Ca^{2+} via its ability to release Ca^{2+} from intracellular stores in a wide variety of tissues (138,139) suggests that the PTH-related increase in intracellular Ca^{2+} is secondary to stimulation of phospholipase C and associated generation of $Ins(1,4,5)P_3$.

$Ins(1,4,5)P_3$ is phosphorylated to form $Ins(1,3,4,5)P_4$, under appropriate conditions. $Ins(1,3,4,5)P_3$ has been shown to open membrane channels, allowing the influx of extracellular Ca^{2+} (115,167–170). This action would explain the transient hypocalcemia in response to PTH that precedes its hypercalcemic action. The hypocalcemic effect of PTH could also be the result of an influx of extracellular Ca^{2+} directly into intracellular storage pools. Such a mechanism has been hypothesized as an explanation for the dependence of IP-mediated release of Ca^{2+} from intracellular pools on extracellular Ca^{2+} (161,162,194).

SPECIFICITY OF THE BIOCHEMICAL PATHWAY OF PARATHYROID HORMONE ACTION

Parathyroid hormone shares the ability to activate two major pathways of hormone action with a growing number of polypeptide hormones. Questions of the specificity of these responses thus arise. One might expect that PTH could produce specific actions on one or another pathway as a function of the tissue itself. However, both pathways are stimulated by PTH in renal and skeletal tissue so that, at least for the major target cells, specificity must be achieved by other means. Newly recognized target cells for PTH (rat brain synaptosomes and dermal keratinocytes) appear to contain the machinery only for the PI response to PTH, but most other cells have the potential to activate both pathways. The following discussion covers several of the more likely possibilities for achieving specificity of the PTH response.

The Cellular Environment

The cellular milieu could dictate the predominant pathway in a given physiological situation. Three observations support this hypothesis. (a) When ROS 17/2.8 cells are grown in the presence of retinoic acid, the distribution of IP products is shifted in favor of the active metabolite IP_3. (b) When the pH of the incubating buffer is lowered, there is a marked increase in phospholipase C activity of ROS 17/2.8 cells (186). (c) Glucocorticoids enhance adenylyl cyclase stimulation by PTH (195) and reduce phospholipase C activity. These observations suggest that experimental conditions could be a factor leading to the preferential activation of one pathway over another. The mechanism of this "switch" to one or another pathway is under active investigation (196). Of course, one does not have to require that only one pathway is stimulated at a given time in the cell. It is possible that each messenger system is regulating a different set of cellular responses and that both sets of responses are important to achieving the end result of PTH action.

THE CELL CYCLE

Baron and colleagues (197) have established elegantly that the cell cycle can be a determining factor in directing the specificity of the calcitonin response in LLCPK cells. A similar mechanism could also direct the specificity of the actions of PTH. Baron et al. have revealed that calcitonin activates both the adenylyl cyclase and the protein kinase C pathways in LLCPK cells. When cells are synchronized in their cell cycle, calcitonin had marked and opposite effects on the activity of the sodium pump depending on the phase of the cell cycle. In the G2 phase, calcitonin increased sodium pump activity; in the S phase, calcitonin markedly reduced sodium pump activity. In the latter phase, the actions of calcitonin are independent of cAMP but mimicked by protein kinase C activation. In G2 phase, calcitonin effects are mimicked by cAMP analogs. To date, these types of studies have not been conducted with PTH, but this is an avenue for new investigation.

Structure–Activity Relationship of Parathyroid Hormone for Activation of Phospholipase C vs. Adenylyl Cyclase

Both bPTH-(1–34) and bPTH-(1–84) are fully active in assays of adenylyl cyclase activity. Although bPTH-(1–84) may be slightly more potent than bPTH-(1–34) in some bioassays, this is attributed to its longer half-life and not to a direct effect of the carboxy-terminal 35–84 portion of the molecule on receptors. Similarly, bPTH-(1–34) and bPTH-(1–84) have almost indistinguishable effects on levels of IPs in assays of phospholipase C activity. These results indicate that the carboxy-terminal portion of the molecule is not required for activation of PI hydrolysis. It should be pointed out, however, that carboxy-terminal fragments of PTH and PTHrP have not been carefully studied in this regard. Recent data on the effects of the pentapeptide fragment of PTH-related protein (PTHrP)-(107–111) to regulate osteoclast activity (198), although controversial (199), suggest that portions of PTH and PTHrP previously unrecognized to have biological activity may prove to be important. Mallette in the chapter "Parathyroid Hormone and Parathyroid Hormone-Related Protein as Polyhormones" has reviewed the concept of PTH as a polyhormone, a notion that fits well in this discussion.

The strongest evidence that the structure–function relationship for PTH stimulated PI hydrolysis diverges from the structure–function relationship for PTH stimulated adenylyl cyclase activation comes from work with PTH analogs that inhibit adenylyl cyclase activation. [Nle^{8,18}Tyr^{34}]bPTH-(3–34)NH$_2$ inhibits PTH-stimulated adenylyl cyclase, but it stimulates increases in IPs in canine renal cortical tubular membranes (200) and in UMR-106 cells (201). In UMR-106 cells, this analog also increases protein kinase C but not protein kinase A activity and causes rapid transient increases in intracellular calcium (101,102). bPTH-(3–34) stimulates bone to produce IP_3 (202) and diacylglycerol (203).

The responsiveness of the PI pathway to stimulation by PTH-(3–34) suggests that the amino terminal adenylyl cyclase "activation domain" of PTH is not a key structural feature in stimulation of the PI pathway. As a result, the minimum sequence necessary for activation of the phospholipase C response is different from the minimum sequence needed for activation of adenylyl cyclase. The weak, but definite, agonist activity of [Nle[8,18]Tyr[34]]bPTH-(3–34)NH$_2$ in vivo in rats and dogs (85,86,204) may be due to its activation of the IP second-messenger system.

To determine the minimum sequence necessary for activation of the IP response, several groups have tested [Tyr[34]]bPTH-(7–34)NH$_2$, which has been shown to be devoid of virtually all agonist properties in vivo (204). This fragment is equally devoid of agonist properties in assays for phospholipase C, protein kinase C or Ca^{2+} responses. PTHrP shares many features of PTH activity in several in vivo and in vitro assays despite its lack of sequence homology with PTH (205–209). Thus, the 1–34 fragment of PTHrP increases levels of ^{3}H-IP$_1$ in canine renal tubular membranes, and, like [Tyr[34]]bPTH-(7–34)NH$_2$, PTHrP-(7–34)NH$_2$ is inactive (200).

There are two other major areas that are important in conferring the PTH response insofar as these dual messenger systems are concerned. These areas are the two other macromolecular components of the PTH receptor complex, the transducing guanine nucleotide binding proteins and the PTH receptor per se. Discussions of these two areas make up the last two sections of this chapter.

COUPLING OF THE PARATHYROID HORMONE RESPONSE TO ADENYLYL CYCLASE AND TO PHOSPHOLIPASE C: GUANINE NUCLEOTIDE-BINDING PROTEINS

The chapter by Spiegel and Weinstein covers the subject of the transducing guanine nucleotide binding proteins. Material is reviewed here only as it contributes to a consideration of G proteins that may couple the PTH receptor(s) to one or another messenger pathway.

G proteins are membrane-associated proteins that facilitate activation or inhibition of second-messenger effector systems in response to receptor activation (Fig. 6) (210–215). These proteins are heterotrimers

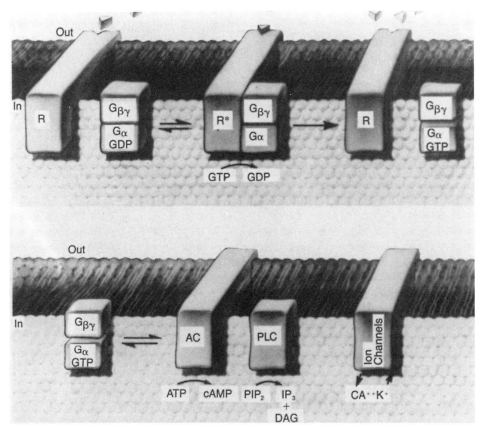

FIG. 6. Scheme of G protein-mediated activation of adenylyl cyclase, phospholipase C, and other effector systems. Receptor activation induces exchange of GTP for GDP and dissociation of the activated G protein from its receptor. GTPγS or AlF$_4$ can induce subunit dissociation in the absence of receptor activation, while GDPβS can inhibit G-protein activation (not shown). Activated G protein α subunits then activate their appropriate target enzymes. (Reprinted from ref. 250 with permission.)

composed of α, β and γ subunits. The α-subunit of each G protein is distinct, defining in part its linkage to and identification with receptor and effector targets. Occupation of a receptor by hormone or drug agonist induces an exchange of active GTP for inactive GDP, and dissociation of the α-GTP from βγ subunits. The activated α subunit is then free to activate or to inhibit its effector enzyme. Intrinsic GTPase activity of α subunits of G proteins leads to hydrolysis of GTP to GDP and dissociation of the resulting α-GDP from the effector. Dissociated βγ subunits have also been implicated in regulation of signal-transducing effector enzymes (216), including adenylyl cyclase (217–219) and phospholipase C (220–222), although the means by which this occurs remains controversial (223).

GTP and its nonhydrolyzable analogs guanosine 5'-O-(3-thiotriphosphate) (GTPγS) and 5'-guanylimidodiphosphate [Gpp(NH)p] can directly activate G proteins in the absence of receptor activation (224). Conversely, activated G·protein-coupled receptors require GTP or GTP analogs to activate their effector enzymes through their respective G proteins. GDP, or its nonhydrolyzable analog guanosine 5'-O-(2-thiodiphosphate) (GDPβS), can stoichiometrically inhibit G protein-mediated effector activation by the activated hormone–receptor complex.

α Subunits of many G proteins are substrates for ADP-ribosylation by bacterial toxins. The α subunit of the stimulatory G protein of the hormone-sensitive adenylyl cyclase system (Gs) is a substrate for this action of cholera toxin. By stabilizing the α subunit of Gs in the active GTP-bound state indirectly by inhibiting its GTPase activity, cholera toxin persistently activates adenylyl cyclase. The α subunit of the inhibitory G protein of the hormone-sensitive adenylyl cyclase system (Gi) is a substrate for ADP-ribosylation by pertussis toxin. This toxin blocks the inhibitory action of the activated α subunit of Gi on adenylyl cyclase (225,226). The net effect of this action is to leave Gs "unopposed" and for the effector systems mediated by Gs to be stimulated further. When a pertussis toxin substrate is a positive transducer, in contrast to the adenylyl cyclase pathway, exposure to pertussis toxin will result in inhibition of the agonist-mediated effect.

Knowledge of other G proteins and the effectors to which they are linked is increasing rapidly (215,223,227). There are now known to be three Gi proteins coupled negatively to adenylyl cyclase, a Gk protein coupled to ion channel gating, and a Gz protein, whose function is unknown. Recently five new Gs-like G proteins have been cloned. A total of 17 distinctly identifiable mammalian genes encoding α subunits have already been identified, and it is likely that additional ones will be forthcoming (see chapter by Weinstein and Spiegel).

The relationships between G proteins and PI turnover are not as well understood. For a number of hormones, receptor-mediated stimulation of phospholipase C has been shown to be mediated by a pertussis toxin-insensitive G protein. There are also pertussis toxin-sensitive G proteins that activate phospholipase C. At least five members of the G protein family have been implicated in this pathway (Gq, Gi, G11, G14, G15) (228,229). For the purpose of this discussion, this family is referred to as Gq because the specific identity of individual G proteins that couple most receptors to phospholipase C is not known (Fig. 6) (107,108,230–234). Six lines of evidence obtained from a variety of systems implicate a G protein in the activation of phospholipase C: (a) GTP or GTPγS alone can activate phospholipase C or responses known to be linked to the generation of IPS (235,236). (b) Calcium-mobilizing hormones that utilize the PI pathway (212,230,231), including PTH (182,185,186), are enhanced by GTP or GTPγS. (c) In membrane preparations, hormonal stimulation of phospholipase C can be greatly enhanced by GTP or GTPγS. (d) Stimulation of phospholipase C by hormones or by GTP (or GTPγS) is inhibited by the GDP analog GDPβS, which favors the uncoupled, inactivated state of G proteins (235). (e) Aluminum fluoride, a known activator of G proteins, stimulates phospholipase C activity as well as adenylyl cyclase activity (231,235–240). (f) Pertussis toxin inhibits phospholipase C activation in some systems (231–233,241); in other systems, it does not (231,242). Although this Gq family of G proteins must bear considerable structural similarity to Gi for some of its members to be substrates for pertussis toxin, it is immunochemically distinguishable from the Gi of neutrophils (243). Diversity among the Gq-type G proteins is also evidenced by variable sensitivity to pertussis toxin. In addition, cholera toxin inhibits basal and stimulated metabolism of (poly)phosphoinositides in liver membrane and T-cell preparations, respectively (244,245). Thus there may be several different G proteins responsible for coupling of PTH to PI hydrolysis.

G PROTEINS AND PARATHYROID HORMONE ACTION

Similar to all other polypeptide hormones that stimulate adenylyl cyclase activity, PTH is dependent on guanine nucleotides. Many of the general properties of G proteins, insofar as their interactions with hormone receptors are concerned, appear to be valid for PTH. These features include alteration by GTP of agonist binding properties and amplification of agonist properties of PTH for adenylyl cyclase activity. Similar to the case in other systems, the presence of the nonhydrolyzable guanine nucleotide Gpp(NH)p leads to a much greater adenylyl cyclase activation by PTH than can be seen in its absence. Amplification of PTH responsiveness by guanine nucleotides has been utilized to develop a very sensitive in vitro assay for PTH. This assay covers a range of PTH concentrations that is much closer to the range in which PTH induces physiological effects (246). Thus the in vitro assay shows agonist effects more easily.

The effects of guanine nucleotides on the other major effector system stimulated by PTH, namely, phospholipase C, has been more difficult to establish. In ROS cells, GTP stimulates basal phospholipase C activity (186). When GTP is present with PTH, the resultant activity is additive, with individual stimulation afforded by GTP and PTH independently. In UMR-106 cells, the stimulation of phospholipase by PTH is more clearly dependent on GTP (182).

Interrelationships between PTH and GTP have also been studied in canine renal tubular membranes. Increases in all three IPs are induced by GTP analogs with a time course that is somewhat slower to develop than with PTH alone but that is maintained for a longer period of time. The changes are greater than the increases observed for PTH alone. PTH-(1–34) and GTP together resulted in higher maximal levels for all IPs. The time course of formation of these IPs was accelerated (185).

The additive effect of GTP and PTH on IP accumulation suggests an effect on the phospholipase C enzyme. An alternative hypothesis is possible. The GTP-associated increase in IP_3 could result from inhibition of the phosphatase responsible for the metabolism of IP_3. Coleman et al. (200) have shown that, under unstimulated conditions, $Ins(1,4,5)P_3$ is rapidly hydrolyzed, with over 80% lost within the first 1 min. GTP slows the rate of hydrolysis of $Ins(1,4,5)P_3$ by >70%. Neither PTH-(1–34) nor PTH-(3–34) had any effects on the metabolism of $Ins(1,4,5)P_3$. The cooperative actions of GTP and PTH on phospholipase C activity therefore could reflect independent actions at two different sites, with PTH acting rather exclusively at the phospholipase C site and GTP acting both at the site of IP_3 hydrolysis and possibly also at the phospholipase C site. Complete understanding of G protein effects on this pathway will require more investigation, and even more work will be required to appreciate how this system relates to the actions of PTH to activate PI hydrolysis.

THE PARATHYROID HORMONE RECEPTOR: RELATIONSHIP TO STIMULATION OF ADENYLYL CYCLASE ACTIVITY AND PHOSPHATIDYLINOSITIDE HYDROLYSIS

The recent cloning of the PTH receptor by Segre and his colleagues is an exciting development that had

eluded many laboratories for a number of years. The characteristics of this receptor, which may belong to a new family of G protein-linked receptors, are covered in the chapter by Segre et al. Reviewed here are those features of the PTH receptor that contribute to our understanding of the specificity of actions of PTH to link via the receptor to these two biochemical pathways.

The PTH receptor was initially cloned from opossum kidney cells and subsequently from rat osteosarcoma cells using an expression cloning screening strategy (247). The receptors from rat bone and opossum kidney are strikingly homologous to each other. Both PTH and PTHrP bind to this receptor with equivalent affinity; it has thus been termed the *PTH/PTHrP receptor*. When rat bone receptor or opossum receptor is expressed in COS-7 cells, which do not contain a native gene for the PTH receptor, PTH acquires the capacities to stimulate adenylyl cyclase activity, to increase cellular calcium, and to stimulate the accumulation of inositol phosphates (Fig. 7). The expressed receptor stimulates adenylyl cyclase activity in a GTP-dependent manner. cDNAs cloned from bone and kidney cells from three species (rat, human, and opossum) and from a murine embryonic carcinoma cell line (P19EC) are identical within species and are highly conserved across species (248). These results suggest

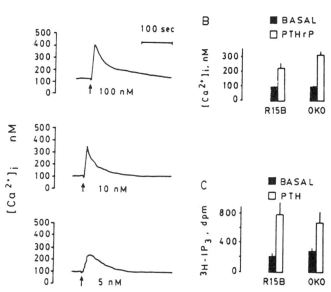

FIG. 7. $[Ca^{2+}]$ and IP_3 responses to PTH and PTHrP in COS-7 cells expressing PTH receptors cloned from rat bone (R15B) or opossum kidney (OK). **A:** Rapid transient increases in intracellular calcium (measured by fura-2 fluorescence) in response to 5, 10, and 100 nM PTH-(1–34) in COS-7 cells expressing R15B. **B:** Mean peak $[Ca^{2+}]$ responses to PTHrP in R15B and OK receptor expressing COS-7 cells. **C:** Mean IP_3 responses to PTH-(1–34) in R15B- and OK-expressing COS-7 cells. (Reprinted from ref. 248 with permission.)

that (a) a single PTH/PTHrP receptor is sufficient to bind two key calcium regulating hormones, PTH and PTHrP; (b) a single receptor is found in cells from the two major target organs of PTH, namely, bone and kidney; and (c) a single receptor can couple to the two biochemical pathways of PTH action. Further studies by the Segre group have shown that this single receptor can be altered by molecular biological techniques to a truncated analog missing the C-terminal region. This truncated receptor R480 has a 111-amino-acid deletion (there is a stop codon at position 481). When the truncated receptor is expressed in COS-7 cells, it maintains its ability to stimulate adenylyl cyclase activity but no longer is capable of stimulating cellular calcium or linking to the PI pathway. Thus there clearly is support for the idea that a single receptor is sufficient to account for the actions of PTH and PTHrP in its many different target cells (especially bone and kidney) and that it can be linked to both biochemical pathways. However, much more work is needed in this area before one concludes that there is only one PTH receptor. In fact, recent studies have revealed via Northern blot analysis transcripts in tissues that are heterogeneous, suggesting multiple PTH receptors or alternative splicing mechanisms (249).

SUMMARY

Parathyroid hormone appears to activate at least two messenger pathways in target cells (Fig. 8). Both messenger systems appear to play pivotal roles in mediating the actions of PTH. They may both be mediated by G proteins. It is unlikely that these two pathways are specific to the two major target organs for PTH, because PTH stimulates both pathways in both bone and kidney (182,184,202) as well as in many other more newly recognized sites of PTH action. These two pathways can be activated by PTHrP as well as by PTH. The single receptor cloned for PTH/PTHrP appears to be able to initiate the signal generated by PTH or PTHrP to lead to the generation of the products of the two pathways. However, it is still possible that other PTH and/or PTHrP receptors will be identified and shown to have preferential action in stimulating one or another pathway. In this regard, the PTH/PTHrP receptor is known to have regions of specificity for transducing the adenylyl cyclase or the PI signal. Work over the next 5 years should clarify this area and should lead to a greater understanding of the biochemical pathways of PTH action.

REFERENCES

1. Aurbach GD, Phang JM. Vitamin D, parathyroid hormone, and calcitonin. In: Mountcastle VB, ed. *Medical physiology*. St. Louis: CV Mosby, 1980;1519–1557.
2. Aurbach GD, Marx SJ, Spiegel AM. Parathyroid hormone, calcitonin, and the calciferols. In: Wilson JD, Foster DW, eds. *Williams textbook of endocrinology*. Philadelphia: WB Saunders, 1981;1137–1217.
3. Arnaud CD, Kolb FO. The calciotropic hormones & metabolic bone disease. In: Greenspan FS, Forsham PH, eds. *Basic & clinical endocrinology*. Los Altos, CA: Lange Medical Publications, 1986;202–271.
4. Cohn DV, MacGregor RR. The biosynthesis, intracellular processing and secretion of parathormone. *Endocr Rev* 1981; 2:1–26.
5. Habener JF, Rosenblatt M, Potts JT Jr. Parathyroid hor-

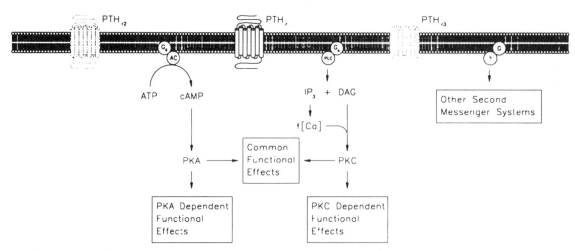

FIG. 8. Scheme of PTH-mediated activation of second messenger systems. Cloned PTH receptors (PTH$_{r1}$) couple PTH and PTHrP to both adenylyl cyclase and phospholipase C in target cells. Additional receptors for PTH are likely to exist. These putative receptors (PTH$_{r2}$ and PTH$_{r3}$) may couple more specifically to either second messenger system or may be present only in certain tissues.

mone: Biochemical aspects of biosynthesis, secretion, action, and metabolism. *Physiol Rev* 1984;64:985–1053.

6. Neuman WF, Neuman MW, Myers CR. Blood:bone disequilibrium III. Linkage between cell energetics and calcium fluxes. *Am J Physiol* 1979;236:C244-C248.

7. Talmage RV, Meyer RA. Physiological role of parathyroid hormone. In: Grup RO, Astwood EB, eds. *Handbook of physiology.* Washington, DC: American Physiological Society, 1967;343–351.

8. Talmage RV. The demand for bone calcium in maintenance of plasma calcium concentration. In: Horton JE, Tarplay TM, Davis WF, eds. *Mechanisms of localized bone loss.* Washington, DC: Info Retrieval, 1978;73–92.

9. Stern PH, Stewart PJ. Vertebral bone resorption in vitro: effects of parathyroid hormone, calcitonin, 1-25 dihydroxyvitamin D_3, epidermal growth factor, prostaglandin E_2, and estrogen. *Calcif Tissue Int* 1987;40:21–26.

10. McSheehy PMJ, Chambers TJ. Osteoblastic cells mediate osteoclastic responsiveness to parathyroid hormone. *Endocrinology* 1986;118:824–828.

11. Chambers TJ, McSheehy PM, Thomson BM, Fuller K. The effect of calcium-regulating hormones and prostaglandins on bone resorption by osteoclasts disaggregated from neonatal rabbit bones. *Endocrinology* 1985;116:234–239.

12. Teti A, Rizzoli R, Zambonin Zallone A. Parathyroid hormone binding to cultured avian osteoclasts. *Biochem Biophys Res Commun* 1991;174:1217–1222.

13. Murrills RJ, Stein LS, Fey CP, Dempster DW. The effects of parathyroid hormone (PTH) and PTH-related peptide on osteoclast resorption of bone slices in vitro: an analysis of pit size and the resorption focus. *Endocrinology* 1990;127:2648–2653.

14. Miller SC and Kenny AD. Activation of avian medullary bone osteoclasts by oxidized synthetic parathyroid hormone (1–34). *Proc Soc Exp Biol Med* 1985;179:38–43.

15. Mears DC. Effects of parathyroid hormone and thyrocalcitonin on the membrane potential of osteoclasts. *Endocrinology* 1971;88:1021.

16. Demay M, Mitchell J, Goltzman D. Comparison of renal and osseous binding of parathyroid hormone and hormonal fragments. *Am J Physiol* 1985;249:E437–E446.

17. Rizzoli RE, Somerman M, Murray TM, Aurbach D. Binding of radioiodinated parathyroid hormone to cloned bone cells. *Endocrinology* 1983;113:1832–1838.

18. Roleau MF, Warshawsky H, Goltzman D. Parathyroid hormone binding in vivo to renal, hepatic, and skeletal tissues of the rat using a radioautographic approach. *Endocrinology* 1986;118:919–931.

19. Peck WA, Carpenter J, Messinger K, DeBra D. Cyclic 3'5' adenosine monophosphate in isolated bone cells: response to low concentrations of parathyroid hormone. *Endocrinology* 1973;92:692–697.

20. Majesca RJ, Rodan SB, Rodan GA. Parathyroid hormone-responsive clonal cell lines from rat osteosarcoma. *Endocrinology* 1980;107:1494–1503.

21. Heath JK, Atkinson SJ, Meikle MC, Reynolds JJ. Mouse osteoblasts synthesize collagenase in response to bone resorbing agents. *Biochim Biophys Acta* 802:151–154.

22. Simon LS, Slovik DM, Neer RM, Krane SM. Changes in serum levels of type I and III procollagen extension peptides during infusion of human parathyroid hormone fragment (1–34). *J Bone Mineral Res* 1988;3:241–246.

23. Hall AK, Dickson IR. The effects of parathyroid hormone on osteoblast-like cells from embryonic chick calvaria. *Acta Endocrinol* 1985;108:217–223.

24. Rodan GA, Martin TJ. Role of osteoblasts in hormonal control of bone resorption—a hypothesis. *Calcif Tissue Int* 1981;33:349.

25. Rouleau MF, Mitchell J, Goltzman D. In vivo distribution of parathyroid hormone receptors in bone: evidence that a predominant osseous target cell is not the mature osteoblast. *Endocrinology* 1988;123:187–191.

26. Baron R, Neff L, Roy C, Boisvert A, Caplan M. Evidence for a high and specific concentration of (Na^+,K^+)ATPase in

the plasma membrane of the osteoclast. *Cell* 1986;46:311–320.

27. Tuukkanen J, Vaananen HK. Omeprazole, a specific inhibitor of H^+-K^+-ATPase, inhibits bone resorption in vitro. *Calcif Tissue Int* 1986;38:123–125.

28. Blair HC, Teitelbaum SL, Ghiselli R, Gluck S. Osteoclastic bone resorption by a polarized vacuolar proton pump. *Science* 1989;245:855–857.

29. Hall GE, Kenny AD. Bone resorption induced by parathyroid hormone and dibutyryl cyclic AMP: role of carbonic anhydrase. *J Pharmacol Exp Ther* 1986;238:778–782.

30. Krieger NS, Kim SG. Dichlorobenzamil inhibits stimulated bone resorption in vitro. *Endocrinology* 1988;122:415–420.

31. Bushinsky DA. Effects of parathyroid hormone on net proton flux from neonatal mouse calvariae. *Am J Physiol* 1987;252:F585–F589.

32. Bourdeau JE. Renal handling of calcium. In: Brenner BM, Stein JH, eds. *Contemporary issues in nephrology. Vol. 2. Divalent ion homeostasis.* New York: Churchill Livingstone, 1983.

33. Pollock AS, Warnock DG, Strewler GJ. Parathyroid hormone inhibition of Na^+-H^+ antiporter activity in a cultured renal cell line. *Am J Physiol* 1986;250:f217–f225.

34. Agus ZS, Puschett JB, Senesky D, Goldberg M. Mode of action of parathyroid hormone and cyclic adenosine 3',5'-monophosphate on renal tubular phosphate reabsorption in the dog. *J Clin Invest* 1971;50:617–626.

35. Ellsworth R, Howard JE. Studies on physiology of parathyroid glands: some responses of normal human kidneys and blood to intravenous parathyroid extract. *Bull Johns Hopkins Hosp* 1934;55:296.

36. Agus ZS, Wasserstein A, Goldfarb S. PTH, calcitonin, cyclic nucleotides and the kidney. *Annu Rev Physiol* 1981;43:583.

37. Kawashima H, Jorika S, Kurokawa K. Localization of 25-hydroxyvitamin D_3-1-alpha-hydroxylase and 24-hydroxylase along the rat nephron. *Proc Natl Acad Sci USA* 1981;78:1199.

38. Slovik DM, Daly MA, Potts JT Jr, Neer RM. Renal 1,25-dihydroxyvitamin D, phosphaturic, and cyclic-AMP responses to intravenous synthetic human parathyroid hormone-(1–34) administration in normal subjects. *Clin Endocrinol* 1984;20:369–375.

39. Bilezikian JP, Canfield RE, Jacobs TP, et al. The response of 1-alpha,25-dihydroxyvitamin D_3 to hypocalcemia in human subjects. *N Engl J Med* 1978;299:437–441.

40. Bushinsky DA, Riera GS, Favus MJ, and Coe FL. Evidence that blood ionized calcium can regulate serum $1,25(OH)_2D_3$ independently of parathyroid hormone and phosphorus in the rat. *J Clin Invest* 1985;76:1599–1604.

41. Helwig JJ, Yang MC, Bollack C, Judes C, Pang PK. Structure-activity relationship of parathyroid hormone: relative sensitivity of rabbit renal microvessel and tubule adenylate cyclases to oxidized PTH and PTH inhibitors. *Eur J Pharmacol* 1987;140:247–257.

42. Morel F, Chabardes D, Imbert-Teboul M, Le Bouffant F, Hus-Citharel A, Montegut M. Multiple hormonal control of adenylate cyclase in distal segments of the rat kidney. *Kidney Int* 1982;21(Suppl. 2)S55–S62.

43. Chin JE, Shalk EM, Kemick ML, Wurthier RE. Effects of synthetic human parathyroid hormone on levels of alkaline phosphatase activity and formation of alkaline phosphatase-rich matrix vessicles by primary cultures of chicken epiphyseal growth plate chondrocytes. *Bone Mineral* 1986;1:421–436.

44. Barri ME, Abbas SK, Care AD. The effects in the rat of two fragments of parathyroid hormone-related protein on uterine contractions in situ. *Exp Physiol* 1992;77:481–490.

45. Nickols GA, Metz MA, Cline WH Jr. Endothelium-independent linkage of parathyroid hormone receptors of rat vascular tissue with increased adenosine 3',5'-monophosphate and relaxation of vascular smooth muscle. *Endocrinology* 1986;119:349–356.

46. Wang R, Karpinski E, Pang PK. Parathyroid hormone selec-

tively inhibits L-type calcium channels in single vascular smooth muscle cells of the rat. *J Physiol* 1991;441:325–346.

47. Trizna W, Edwards RM. Relaxation of renal arterioles by parathyroid hormone and parathyroid hormone-related protein. *Pharmacology* 1991;42:91–96.

48. Pang PK, Wang R, Shan J, Karpinski E, Benishin CG. Specific inhibition of long-lasting, L-type calcium channels by synthetic parathyroid hormone. *Proc Natl Acad Sci USA* 1990;87:623–627.

49. Thiede MA, Nickols GA. *Local expression and action of parathyroid hormone related peptide in the cardiovascular system.* Boca Raton, FL: CRC Press, 1993.

50. Cooper CW, Seitz PK, McPherson MB, Selvanayagam P, Rajaraman S. Effects of parathyroid hormonal peptides on the gut. *Contrib Nephrol* 1991;91:26–31.

51. Rampe D, Lacerda AE, Dage RC, Brown AM. Parathyroid hormone: an endogenous modulator of cardiac calcium channels. *Am J Physiol* 1991;261:H1945–H1950.

52. Wang R, Karpinski E, Pang PK. Two types of voltage-dependent calcium channel currents and their modulation by parathyroid hormone in neonatal rat ventricular cells. *J Cardiovasc Pharmacol* 1991;17:990–998.

53. Jordan LR, Dallemagne CR, Cross RB. Cardiovascular effects of parathyroid hormone in conscious sheep. *Exp Physiol* 1991;76:251–257.

54. Roca Cusachs A, DiPette DJ, Nickols GA. Regional and systemic hemodynamic effects of parathyroid hormone-related protein: preservation of cardiac function and coronary and renal flow with reduced blood pressure. *J Pharmacol Exp Ther* 1991;256:110–118.

55. Kishimoto H, Tsumura K, Fujioka S, et al. Effects of parathyroid hormone-related protein on systemic and regional hemodynamics in conscious rats. A comparison with human parathyroid hormone. *Contrib Nephrol* 1991;90:72–78.

56. Mok LLS, Nickols GA, Thompson JC, Cooper CW. Parathyroid hormone as a smooth muscle relaxant. *Endocr Rev* 1989;10:420–436.

57. Gupta A, Martin KJ, Miyauchi A, Hruska KA. Regulation of cytosolic calcium by parathyroid hormone and oscillations of cytosolic calcium in fibroblasts from normal and pseudohypoparathyroid patients. *Endocrinology* 1991;128: 2825–2836.

58. Whitfield JF, Chakravarthy BR, Durkin JP, et al. Parathyroid hormone stimulates protein kinase C but not adenylate cyclase in mouse epidermal keratinocytes. *J Cell Physiol* 1992;150:299–303.

59. Fraser CL, Sarnacki P, Budayr A. Evidence that parathyroid hormone-mediated calcium transport in rat brain synaptosomes is independent of cyclic adenosine monophosphate. *J Clin Invest* 1988;81:982–988.

60. Chase LR, Aurbach GD. Parathyroid function and the renal excretion of 3'5'-adenylic acid. *Proc Natl Acad Sci USA* 1967;58:518–525.

61. Chase LR, Fedack SA, Aurbach GD. Activation of skeletal adenyl cyclase by parathyroid hormone in vitro. *Endocrinology* 1969;84:761–768.

62. Chase LR, Aurbach GD. Renal adenyl cyclase: Anatomically separate sites for parathyroid hormone and vasopressin. *Science* 1968;159:545–547.

63. Dolson GL, Hise MK, Weinman EJ. Relationship among parathyroid hormone, cAMP, and calcium on proximal tubule sodium transport. *Am J Physiol* 1989;249:F409–F416.

64. Walker DA, Davies SJ, Siddle K, Woodhead JS. Control of renal tubular resorption by parathyroid hormone in man. *Clin Sci Mol Med* 1977;53:431–438.

65. Chase LR, Aurbach GD. The effect of parathyroid hormone on the concentration of adenosine 3',5'-monophosphate in skeletal tissue in vitro. *J Biol Chem* 1970;245:1520–1526.

66. Rodan GA, Rodan SB. Hormone-adenylate cyclase coupling in osteosarcoma clonal cell lines. *Adv Cyclic Nucleotide Protein Phosphorylation Res* 1984;17:127–134.

67. Cole JA, Forte LR, Eber SL, Thorne PK, Poelling RE. Regulation of sodium-dependent phosphate transport by parathyroid hormone in opossum kidney cells: cAMP dependent

68. and independent mechanisms. *Endocrinology* 1988;122: 2981–2989.

69. Spiegel AM, Levine MA, Aurbach GD, et al. Deficiency of hormone receptor-adenylate cyclase coupling protein: basis for hormone resistance in psudohypoparathyroidism. *Am J Physiol* 1982;243:E37–E42.

69. Farfel Z, Brickman AS, Kaslow HR, Brothers VM, Bourne HR. Defect of receptor-cyclase coupling protein in pseudohypoparathyroidism. *N Engl J Med* 1980;303:237–242.

70. Levine MA, Downs RW Jr, Singer M, Marx SJ, Aurbach GD, Spiegel AM. Deficient activity of guanine nucleotide regulatory protein in erythrocytes from patients with pseudohypoparathyroidism. *Biochem Biophys Res Commun* 1980;94:1319–1324.

71. Van Dop C, Bourne HR. Pseudohypoparathyroidism. *Annu Rev Med* 1983;34:259–266.

72. Chase LR, Melson GL, Aurbach GD. Pseudohypoparathyroidism: defective excretion of 3',5'-AMP in response to parathyroid hormone. *J Clin Invest* 1969;48:1832–1844.

73. Rosenblatt M. Peptide hormone antagonists that are effective in vivo. *N Engl J Med* 1986;315:1004–1013.

74. Tregear GW, Van Rietschoten J, Greene E, et al. Bovine parathyroid hormone: Minimum chain length of synthetic peptide required for biological activity. *Endocrinology* 1973;93:1349–1353.

75. Sabatini S, Yang W-C, Kurtzman NA. Effect of parathyroid hormone fragments on calcium transport in toad bladder. *J Pharmacol Exp Ther* 1987;241:448–452.

76. Calvo MS, Fryer MJ, Laakso KJ, et al. Structural requirements for parathyroid action in mature bone. *J Clin Invest* 1981;76:2348–2354.

77. Pliam NB, Nyiredy KO, Arnaud CD. Parathyroid hormone receptors in avian bone cells. *Proc Natl Acad Sci USA* 1982;79:2061–2063.

78. Kremer R, Bennett HPJ, Mitchell J, Goltzman D. Characterization of the rabbit renal receptor for native parathyroid hormone employing a radioligand purified by reversed-phase liquid chromatography. *J Biol Chem* 1982;257:14048–14054.

79. Nussbaum SR, Rosenblatt M, Potts JT Jr. Parathyroid hormone–renal receptor interactions. *J Biol Chem* 1980;255:10183–10187.

80. Segre GV, Rosenblatt M, Reiner BL, Mahaffey JE, Potts JT Jr. Characterization of the parathyroid hormone receptors in canine renal cortical plasma membranes using a radioiodinated sulfur-free hormone analogue. *J Biol Chem* 1979;254:6980–6986.

81. Silver J, Naveh-Many T, Mayer H, Schmelzer HJ, Popovetzer MM. Regulation by vitamin D metabolites of parathyroid hormone gene transcription in vivo in the rat. *J Clin Invest* 1986;78:1296–1301.

82. McKee RL, Caulfield MP, Rosenblatt M. Treatment of bone-derived ROS 17/2.8 cells with dexamethasone and pertussis toxin enables detection of partial agonist activity for parathyroid hormone antagonists. *Endocrinology* 1990;127: 76–82.

83. Nutt RF, Caulfield MP, Levy JJ, Gibbons SW, Rosenblatt M, McKee RL. Removal of partial agonism from parathyroid hormone (PTH)-related protein-(7–34)NH$_2$ by substitution of PTH amino acids at positions 10 and 11. *Endocrinology* 1990;127:491–493.

84. Parsons JA, Rafferty B, Grat D, et al. Pharmacology of parathyroid hormone and some of its fragments and analogues. In: Talmage RV, Owen M, Parsons JA, eds. *Calcium regulating hormones.* Amsterdam: Excerpta Medica, 1975;33–39.

85. Segre GV, Rosenblatt M, Tully GL III, Laugharn J, Reit B, Potts JT Jr. Evaluation of an in vitro parathyroid hormone antagonist in vivo in dogs. *Endocrinology* 1985;116:1024–1029.

86. Horiuchi N, Rosenblatt M, Keutmann HT, Potts JT Jr, Holick MF. A multiresponse parathyroid hormone assay: an inhibitor has agonist properties in vivo. *Am J Physiol* 1983;244:E589–E595.

87. Ribeiro CP, Mandel LJ. Parathyroid hormone inhibits prox-

imal tubule Na(+)-K(+)-ATPase activity. *Am J Physiol* 1992;262:F209–F216.

88. Parsons JA, Neer RM, Potts JT Jr. Initial fall of plasma calcium after intravenous injection of parathyroid hormone. *Endocrinology* 1971;89:735–740.

89. Robertson WG, Peakock M, Atkins D, Webster LA. The effect of parathyroid hormone on the uptake and release of calcium by bone in tissue culture. *Clin Sci* 1972;43:715–718.

90. Scoble JE, Hruska KA. Calcium transport in canine renal basolateral membrane vesicles: effects of parathyroid hormone. *J Clin Invest* 1985;75:1096–1105.

91. Khalifa S, Mills S, Hruska KA. Stimulation of calcium uptake by parathyroid hormone in renal brush-border membrane vesicles. *J Biol Chem* 1983;258:14400–14406.

92. Boland CJ, Fried RM, Tashjian AH Jr. Measurement of cytosolic free Ca^{++} concentrations in human and rat osteosarcoma cells: actions of bone resorption-stimulating hormones. *Endocrinology* 1986;118:980–989.

93. Schofl C, Cuthbertson KS, Gallagher JA, et al. Measurement of intracellular Ca^{2+} in single aequorin-injected and suspensions of fura-2-loaded ROS 17/2.8 cells and normal human osteoblasts. Effect of parathyroid hormone. *Biochem J* 1991;274:15–20.

88. Parsons JA, Neer RM, Potts JT Jr. Initial fall of plasma calcium after intravenous injection of parathyroid hormone. *Endocrinology* 1971;89:735–740.

89. Robertson WG, Peakock M, Atkins D, Webster LA. The effect of parathyroid hormone on the uptake and release of calcium by bone in tissue culture. *Clin Sci* 1972;43:715–718.

90. Scoble JE, Mills S, Hruska KA. Calcium transport in canine renal basolateral membrane vesicles: effects of parathyroid hormone. *J Clin Invest* 1985;75:1096–1105.

91. Khalifa S, Mills S, Hruska KA. Stimulation of calcium uptake by parathyroid hormone in renal brush-border membrane vesicles. *J Biol Chem* 1983;258:14400–14406.

92. Boland CJ, Fried RM, Tashjian AH Jr. Measurement of cytosolic free Ca^{++} concentrations in human and rat osteosarcoma cells: actions of bone resorption-stimulating hormones. *Endocrinology* 1986:118:980–989.

93. Schofl C, Cuthbertson KS, Gallagher JA, et al. Measurement of intracellular Ca^{2+} in single aequorin-injected and suspensions of fura-2-loaded ROS 17/2.8 cells and normal human osteoblasts. Effect of parathyroid hormone. *Biochem J* 1991;274:15–20.

94. Babich M, Choi H, Johnson RM, et al. Thrombin and parathyroid hormone mobilize intracellular calcium in rat osteosarcoma cells by distinct pathways. *Endocrinology* 1991;129:1463–1470.

95. Hruska KA, Goligorsky M, Scoble J, Tsutsumi M, Westbrook S, Moskowitz D. Effects of parathyroid hormone on cytosolic calcium in renal proximal tubular primary cultures. *Am J Physiol* 1986;251:F188–F198.

96. Goligorsky MS, Loftus DJ, Hruska KA. Cytoplasmic calcium in individual proximal tubular cells in culture. *Am J Physiol* 1986;251:F938–F944.

97. Bidwell JP, Carter WB, Fryer MJ, Heath H. Parathyroid hormone (PTH)-induced intracellular Ca^{2+} signalling in naive and PTH-desensitized osteoblast-like cells (ROS 17/2.8): pharmacological characterization and evidence for synchronous oscillation of intracellular Ca^{2+}. *Endocrinology* 1991; 129:2993–3000.

98. Bidwell JP, Fryer MJ, Firek AF, Donahue HJ, Heath H. Desensitization of rat osteoblast-like cells (ROS 17/2.8) to parathyroid hormone uncouples the adenosine 3',5'-monophosphate and cytosolic ionized calcium response limbs. *Endocrinology* 1991;128:1021–1028.

99. Reid IR, Civitelli R, Halstead LR, Avioli LV, Hruska KA. Parathyroid hormone acutely elevates intracellular calcium in osteoblastlike cells. *Am J Physiol* 1987;252:E45–E51.

100. Short AD, Brown BL, Dobson PR. The effect of retinoic acid on parathyroid hormone- and parathyroid hormone-related peptide-induced intracellular calcium in a rat osteosarcoma cell line, UMR106. *J Endocrinol* 1991;129:75–81.

101. Lowik CWGM, van Leeuwen JPTM, van der Meer JM, van

Zeeland JK, Scheven BAA, Herrmann-Erlee MPM. A two-receptor model for the action of parathyroid hormone on osteoblasts: a role for intracellular free calcium and cAMP. *Cell Calcium* 1985;6:311–326.

102. Fujimori A, Cheng SL, Avioli LV, Civitelli R. Dissociation of second messenger activation by parathyroid hormone fragments in osteosarcoma cells. *Endocrinology* 1991;128: 3032–3039.

103. Murer H, Malmstrom K. Intracellular regulatory cascades: examples from parathyroid hormone regulation of renal phosphate transport. *Klin Wochenschr* 1986;64:824–828.

104. Cole JA, Eber SL, Poelling RE, Thorne PK, Forte LR. A dual mechanism for regulation of kidney phosphate transport by parathyroid hormone. *Am J Physiol* 1987;253:E221–E227.

105. Michell RH. Inositol phospholipids and cell surface receptor function. *Biochim Biophys Acta* 1975;415:81–147.

106. Berridge MJ. Inositol trisphosphate and diacylglycerol as second messengers. *Biochem J* 1984;220:345–360.

107. Berridge MJ, Irvine RF. Inositol trisphosphate, a novel second messenger in cellular signal transduction. *Nature* 1984;312:315–321.

108. Abdel-Latif AA. Calcium-mobilizing receptors, polyphosphoinositides, and the generation of second messengers. *Pharmacol Rev* 1986;38:227–272.

109. Rhee SG, Suh PG, Ryu SH, Lee SY. Studies of inositol phospholipid-specific phospholipase C. *Science* 1989;244:546–550.

110. Suh PG, Ryu SH, Moon KH, Suh HW, Rhee SG. Cloning and sequence of multiple forms of phospholipase C. *Cell* 1988;54:161–169.

111. Ryu SH, Suh PG, Cho KS, Lee KY, Rhee SG. Bovine brain cytosol contains three immunologically distinct forms of inositolphospholipid-specific phospholipase C. *Proc Natl Acad Sci USA* 1987;84:6649–6653.

112. Carter HR, Bird IM, Smith AD. Two species of phospholipase C isolated from lymphocytes produce specific ratios of inositol phosphate products. *FEBS Lett* 1986;204:23–27.

113. Ackermann KE, Gish BG, Honchar MP, Sherman WR. Evidence that inositol 1-phosphate in brain of lithium-treated rats results mainly from phosphatidylinositol metabolism. *Biochem J* 1987;242:517–524.

114. Nakanishi H, Nomura H, Kikkawa U, Kishimoto A, Nishizuka Y. Rat brain and liver soluble phospholipase C: resolution of two forms with different requirements for calcium. *Biochem Biophys Res Commun* 1985;132:582–590.

115. Slack BE, Bell JE, Benos DJ. Inositol-1,4,5-trisphosphate injection mimics fertilization potentials in sea urchin eggs. *Am J Physiol* 1986;250:C340–C344.

116. Berridge MJ. Inositol trisphosphate and diacylglycerol: two interacting second messengers. *Annu Rev Biochem* 1987;56: 159–193.

117. Naor Z. Signal transduction mechanisms of Ca2+ mobilizing hormones: the case of gonadotropin-releasing hormone. *Endocr Rev* 1990;11:326–353.

118. Nishizuka Y. The molecular heterogeneity of protein kinase C and its implications for cellular regulation. *Nature* 1988;334:661–665.

119. Housey GM, O'Brian CA, Johnson MD, Kirschmeier P, Weinstein IB. Isolation of cDNA clones encoding protein kinase C: evidence for a protein kinase C-related gene family. *Proc Natl Acad Sci USA* 1987;84:1065–1069.

120. Wilson DB, Connolly TM, Ross TS, et al. Phosphoinositide metabolism in human platelets. *Adv Prostaglandin Thromboxane Leukotriene Res* 1987;17:558–562.

121. Wilson DB, Connolly TM, Bross TE, et al. Isolation and characterization of the inositol cyclic phosphate products of polyphosphoinositide cleavage by phospholipase C. Physiological effects in permeabilized platelets and Limulus photoreceptor cells. *J Biol Chem* 1985;260:13496–13501.

122. Connolly TM, Wilson DB, Bross TE, Majerus PW. Isolation and characterization of the inositol cyclic phosphate products of phosphoinositide cleavage by phospholipase C. Metabolism in cell-free extracts. *J Biol Chem* 1986;261:122–126.

123. Ishii H, Connolly TM, Bross TE, Majerus PW. Inositol cyclic triphosphate [inositol 1,2-(cyclic)-4,5-triphosphate] is formed upon thrombin stimulation of human platelets. *Proc Natl Acad Sci USA* 1986;83:6397–6401.

124. Nahorski SR, Batty I. Inositol tetrakisphosphate: recent developments in phosphoinositide metabolism and receptor function. *TIPS* 1986;2:83–85.

125. Irvine RF, Letcher AJ, Heslop JP, Berridge MJ. The inositol tris/tetrakisphosphate pathway—demonstration of Ins(1,4,5)-P3 3-kinase activity in animal tissues. *Nature* 1986;320: 631–634.

126. Stewart SJ, Prpic V, Powers FS, Bocckino SB, Isaacks RE, Exton JH. Perturbation of the human T-cell antigen receptor–T3 complex leads to the production of inositol tetrakisphosphate: evidence for conversion from inositol trisphosphate. *Proc Natl Acad Sci USA* 1986;83:6098–6102.

127. Balla T, Guillemette G, Baukal AJ, Catt KJ. Metabolism of inositol 1,3,4-trisphosphate to a new tetrakisphosphate isomer in angiotensin stimulated adrenal glomerulosa cells. *J Biol Chem* 1987;262:9952–9955.

128. Biden TJ, Comte M, Cox JA, Wollheim CB. Calcium-calmodulin stimulates inositol 1,4,5-trisphosphate kinase activity from insulin-secreting RINm5F cells. *J Biol Chem* 1987;262:9437–9440.

129. Osborn JE. The AIDS epidemic: an overview of the science. *Issues Technol* 1986;1986:40–55.

130. Tennes KA, McKinney JS, Putney JW Jr. Metabolism of inositol 1,4,5-trisphosphate in guinea-pig hepatocytes. *Biochem J* 1987;242:797–802.

131. Rossier MF, Capponi AM, Vallotton MB. Metabolism of inositol 1,4,5-trisphosphate in permeabilized rat aortic smooth-muscle cells. Dependence on calcium concentration. *Biochem J* 1987;245:305–307.

132. Shears SB, Storey DJ, Morris AJ, et al. Dephosphorylation of myo-inositol 1,4,5-trisphosphate and myo-inositol 1,3,4-triphosphate. *Biochem J* 1987;242:393–402.

133. Traynor-Kaplan AE, Harris AL, Thompson BL, Taylor P, Sklar LA. An inositol tetrakisphosphate-containing phospholipid in activated neutrophils. *Nature* 1988;334:353–356.

134. Homcy CJ, Rockson SG, Haber E. An antiidiotypic antibody that recognizes the β-adrenergic receptor. *J Clin Invest* 1982;69:1147–1154.

135. Hansen CA, Mah S, Williamson JR. Formation and metabolism of inositol 1,3,4,5-tetrakisphosphate in liver. *J Biol Chem* 1986;61:8100–8103.

136. Berridge MJ, Irvine RF. Inositol phosphates and cell signalling. *Nature* 1989;341:197–205.

137. Streb H, Irvine RF, Berridge MJ, Schulz I. Release of Ca²⁺ from a nonmitochondrial intracellular store in pancreatic acinar cells by inositol-1,4,5-trisphosphate. *Nature* 1983;306:67–68.

138. Rasmussen H. The calcium messenger system (first of two parts). *N Engl J Med* 1986;314:1094–1101.

139. Rasmussen H. The calcium messenger system (second of two parts). *N Engl J Med* 1986;314:1164–1170.

140. Rasmussen H, Barrett PQ. Calcium messenger system: An integrated view. *Physiol Rev* 1984;64:938–984.

141. Michell RH, King CE, Guy GR, Hawkins PT, Stephens L. Metabolic pooling of inositol lipids in mature erythrocytes and in hormone-stimulated mammalian cells. *Progr Clin Biol Res* 1987;249:159–167.

142. Monaco ME, Gershengorn MC. Subcellular organization of receptor-mediated phosphoinositide turnover. *Endocr Rev* 1992;13:707–718.

143. Rana RS, Mertz RJ, Kowluru A, Dixon JF, Hokin LE, MacDonald MJ. Evidence for glucose-responsive and -unresponsive pools of phospholipid in pancreatic islets. *J Biol Chem* 1985;260:7861–7867.

144. Monaco ME, Woods D. Characterization of the hormone-sensitive phosphatidylinositol pool in WRK-1 cells. *J Biol Chem* 1983;258:15125–15129.

145. Monaco ME. The phosphatidylinositol cycle in WRK-1 cells: evidence for a separate, hormone-sensitive phosphatidylinositol pool. *J Biol Chem* 1982;257:2137–2139.

146. Monaco ME. Inositol metabolism in WRK-1 cells. Relationship of hormone-sensitive to -insensitive pools of phosphoinositides. *J Biol Chem* 1987;262:13001–13006.

147. Koreh K, Monaco ME. The relationship of hormone-sensitive and hormone-insensitive phosphatidylinositol to phosphatidylinositol 4,5-bisphosphate in the WRK-1 cell. *J Biol Chem* 1986;261:88–91.

148. Rana RS, Kowluru A, MacDonald MJ. Secretagogue-responsive and -unresponsive pools of phosphatidylinositol in pancreatic islets. *Arch Biochem Biophys* 1986;245:411–416.

149. Imai A, Gershengorn MC. Independent phosphatidylinositol synthesis in pituitary plasma membrane and endoplasmic reticulum. *Nature* 1987;325:726–728.

150. Higashijima T, Ferguson KM, Sternweis PC, Smigel MD, Gilman AG. Effects of Mg²⁺ and the beta gamma-subunit complex on the interactions of guanine nucleotides with G proteins. *J Biol Chem* 1987;262:762–766.

151. Dean NM, Moyer JD. Separation of multiple isomers of inositol phosphates formed in GH3 cells. *Biochem J* 1987;242:361–366.

152. Woodcock EA, Smith IA, Wallace CA, White BL. Evidence for a lack of inositol-(1,4,5)trisphosphate kinase activity in norepinephrine perfused rat hearts. *Biochem Biophys Res Commun* 1987;148:68–77.

153. Renard D, Poggioli J. Does the inositol Tris/tetrakisphosphate pathway exist in the rat heart? *FEBS Lett* 1987;217:117–123.

154. Majerus PW, Connolly TM, Deckmyn H, et al. The metabolism of phosphoinositide-derived messenger molecules. *Science* 1986;234:1519–1526.

155. Heslop JP, Irvine RF, Tashjian AH Jr, Berridge MJ. Inositol tetrakis- and pentakisphosphates in GH4 cells. *J Exp Biol* 1985;119:395–401.

156. Berridge MJ. Calcium: a universal second messenger. *Triangle* 1985;24:79–90.

157. Exton JH. Mechanisms involved in calcium-mobilizing agonist responses. *Adv Cyclic Nucleotide Protein Phosphorylation Res* 1986;20:211–262.

158. von-Tscharner V, Prod'hom B, Baggiolini M, Reuter H. Ion channels in human neutrophils activated by a rise in free cytosolic calcium concentration. *Nature* 1986;324:369–372.

159. Steinheardt RA, Epel D. Activation of sea-urchin eggs by a calcium ionophore. *Proc Natl Acad Sci USA* 1974;71:1915–1919.

160. Williamson JR, Cooper RH, Joseph SK, Thomas AP. Inositol trisphosphate and diacylglycerol as intracellular second messengers in the liver. *Am J Physiol* 1985;248:C203–C216.

161. Putney JW Jr, Aub DL, Taylor CW, Merritt JE. Formation and biological action of inositol 1,4,5-trisphosphate. *Fed Proc* 1986;45:2634–2638.

162. Putney JW Jr. Formation and actions of calcium-mobilizing messenger, inositol 1,4,5-trisphosphate. *Am J Physiol* 1987;252:G149–G157.

163. Benham CD, Tsien RW. A novel receptor-operated Ca⁺⁺ permeable channel activated by ATP in smooth muscle. *Nature* 1987;328:275–278.

164. Gomperts BD. Involvement of guanine nucleotide-binding protein in the gating of Ca⁺⁺ by receptors. *Nature* 1983;306:64–66.

165. Holz GG, Rane SG, Dunlap K. GTP-binding proteins mediate transmitter inhibition of voltage-dependent calcium channels. *Nature* 1986;670–672.

166. Hescheler JW, Rosenthal W, Trautwein W, Schultz G. The GTP-binding protein, Go, regulates neuronal calcium channels. *Nature* 1987;325:445–447.

167. Irvine RF, Moor RM. Micro-injection of inositol 1,3,4,5-tetrakisphosphate activates sea urchin eggs by a mechanism dependent on external Ca²⁺. *Biochem J* 1986;240:917–920.

168. Michell B. A second messenger function for inositol tetrakisphosphate. *Nature* 1986;324:613.

169. Kuno M, Gardner P. Ion channels activated by inositol 1,4,5-trisphosphate in plasma membrane of human T-lymphocytes. *Nature* 1987;326:301–304.

170. Whitaker M, Irvine RF. Inositol 1,4,5-trisphosphate mi-

croinjection activates sea urchin eggs. *Nature* 1984;312:636–639.

171. Berridge MJ. The Albert Lasker Medical Awards. Inositol trisphosphate, calcium, lithium, and cell signaling. *JAMA* 1989;262:1834–1841.

172. Rogers SA, Hammerman MA. Calcium activated phospholipase C associated with canine renal basolateral membranes. *Am J Physiol* 1987;252:F74–F82.

173. Knepper SM, Rutledge CO. Effects of calcium depletion on norepinephrine- and A23187-induced stimulation of inositol phosphate formation. *Biochem Pharmacol* 1987;36:3043–3050.

174. Taylor CW, Merritt JE, Putney JW Jr, Rubin RP. Effects of Ca^{2+} on phosphoinositide breakdown in exocrine pancreas. *Biochem J* 1986;238:765–772.

175. Lew PD, Monod A, Krause KH, Waldvogel FA, Biden TJ, Schlegel W. The role of cytosolic free calcium in the generation of inositol 1,4,5-trisphosphate and inositol 1,3,4-trisphosphate in HL-60 cells. Differential effects of chemotactic peptide receptor stimulation at distinct Ca^{2+} levels. *J Biol Chem* 1986;261:13121–13127.

176. Bidot-Lopez P, Farese RV, Sabin MA. Parathyroid hormone and adenosine-3',5'-monophosphate acutely increase phospholipids of the phosphatidate-polyphosphoinositide pathway in rabbit kidney cortex tubules in vitro by a cycloheximide-sensitive process. *Endocrinology* 1981;108:2078–2081.

177. Wirthensohn G, Lefrank S, Guder WG. Phospholipid metabolism in rat kidney cortical tubules: 1. Effect of renal substrates. *Biochim Biophys Acta* 1984;795:392–400.

178. Wirthensohn G, Lefrank S, Guder WG. Phospholipid metabolism in rat kidney cortical tubules: 2. Effects of hormones on ^{32}P incorporation. *Biochim Biophys Acta* 1984;795:401–410.

179. Lo H, Lehotay DC, Katz D, Levey GS. Parathyroid hormone-mediated incorporation of ^{32}P-orthophosphate into phosphatidic acid and phosphatidylinositol in renal cortical slices. *Endocrine Res Commun* 1976;3:377–385.

180. Esbrit P, Navarro E, Manzano F. A possible mechanism whereby parathyroid hormone stimulates phospholipid synthesis in canine renal tubules. *Bone Mineral* 1988;4:7–16.

181. Meltzer V, Weinreb S, Bellorin-Font E, Hruska KA. Parathyroid hormone stimulation of renal phosphoinositide metabolism is a cyclic nucleotide independent effect. *Biochim Biophys Acta* 1982;712:258–267.

182. Babich M, King KL, Nissenson RA. G Protein-dependent activation of a phosphoinositide-specific phospholipase C in UMR-106 osteosarcoma cell membranes. *J Bone Mineral Res* 1989;4:549–556.

183. Ruth JD, Murray TM. PTH binding and PTH stimulated inositol triphosphate production in a clonal line of opossum kidney cells. *J Bone Mineral Res* 1986;1:451s (abstract).

184. Hruska KA, Moskowitz D, Esbrit P, Civitelli R, Westbrook S, Huskey M. Stimulation of inositol trisphosphate and diacylglycerol production in renal tubular cells by parathyroid hormone. *J Clin Invest* 1987;79:230–239.

185. Coleman DT, Bilezikian JP. Parathyroid hormone stimulates formation of inositol phosphates in a membrane preparation of canine renal cortical tubular cells. *J Bone Mineral Res* 1990;5:299–306.

186. Cosman F, Morrow B, Kopal M, Bilezikian JP. Stimulation of inositol phosphate formation in ROS 17/2.8 cell membranes by guanine nucleotide, calcium and parathyroid hormone. *J Bone Mineral Res* 1989;4:413–420.

187. Litosch I, Fain JN. 5-Methyltryptamine stimulates phospholipase C-mediated breakdown of exogenous phosphoinositides by blowfly salivary gland membranes. *J Biol Chem* 1985;260:16052–16055.

188. Civitelli R, Reid IR, Westbrook S, Avioli LV, Hruska KA. PTH elevates inositol phosphates and diacylglycerol in a rat osteoblast-like cell line. *Am J Physiol* 1988;255:E660–E667.

189. Yamaguchi DT, Hahn TJ, Iida Klein A, Kleeman CR, Muallem S. Parathyroid hormone-activated calcium channels in an osteoblast-like clonal osteosarcoma cell line. cAMP-dependent and cAMP-independent calcium channels. *J Biol Chem* 1987;262:7711–7718.

190. Reid IR, Civitelli R, Halstead LR, Avioli LV, Hruska KA. Parathyroid hormone acutely elevates intracellular calcium in osteoblastlike cells [published erratum appears in *Am J Physiol* 1988;255(2 Pt 1):preceding E99]. *Am J Physiol* 1987;253:E45–E51.

191. Donahue HJ, Fryer MJ, Eriksen EF, Heath H. Differential effects of parathyroid hormone and its analogues on cytosolic calcium ion and cAMP levels in cultured rat osteoblast-like cells. *J Biol Chem* 1988;263:13522–13527.

192. Bidwell JP, Fryer MJ, Firek AF, Donahue HJ, Heath H III. Desensitization of rat osteoblast-like cells (ROS 17/2.8) to parathyroid hormone uncouples the adenosine 3',5'-monophosphate and cytosolic ionized calcium response limbs. *Endocrinology* 1991;128:1021–1028.

193. Yamada H, Tsutsumi M, Fukase M, et al. Effects of human PTH-related peptide and human PTH on cyclic AMP production and cytosolic free calcium in an osteoblastic cell clone. *Bone Mineral* 1989;6:45–54.

194. Daniel JL, Dangelmaier CA, Selak M, Smith JB. ADP stimulates IP_3 formation in human platelets. *FEBS Lett* 1986;206:299–303.

195. Rodan SB, Rodan GA. Dexamethasone effects on β-adrenergic receptors and adenylate cyclase regulatory proteins G_s and G_i in ROS 17/2.8 cells. *Endocrinology* 1986;118:2510–2518.

196. Glusman J, Morris SA, Rohde S, Chen G, Camacho JA, Bilezikian JP. Opposing influences of dexamethasone and retinoic acid on adenylate cyclase activity in ROS 17/2.8 cells. *Endocrinology* 1993;132:261–268.

197. Chakraborty M, Chatterjee D, Kellokumpu S, Rasmussen H, Baron R. Cell cycle-dependent coupling of the calcitonin receptor to different G proteins. *Science* 1991;251:1078–1082.

198. Fenton AJ, Kemp BE, Hammonds RG Jr, et al. A potent inhibitor of osteoclastic bone resorption within a highly conserved pentapeptide region of parathyroid hormone-related protein; PTHrP [107–111]. *Endocrinology* 1991;129:3424–3426.

199. Sone T, Kohno H, Kikuchi H, et al. Human parathyroid hormone-related peptide (107–111) does not inhibit bone resorption in neonatal mouse calvariae. *Endocrinology* 1992;131:2742–2746.

200. Coleman DT, Morrow BS, Bilezikian JP. Effects of guanine nucleotides and parathyroid hormone on inositol 1,4,5-trisphosphate metabolism in canine renal cortical tubular cell membranes. *J Bone Mineral Res* 1991;6:599–607.

201. Fujimori A, Cheng SL, Avioli LV, Civitelli R. Structure-function relationship of parathyroid hormone: activation of phospholipase-C, protein kinase-A and -C in osteosarcoma cells. *Endocrinology* 1992;130:29–36.

202. Stathopoulos VM, Rosenblatt M, Stern PH. Actions of nleu^{8,18}tyr^{34}-bPTH-(3–34)amide on resorption and inositol phosphate production in fetal rat limb bones. *J Bone Mineral Res* 1988;3:S110.

203. Stewart PJ, Stathopoulos VM, Stern PH. Parathyroid hormone (1–34) and Nleu8,18Tyr34-parathyroid hormone (3–34) amide increase diacylglycerol in neonatal mouse calvaria. *Hormone Metab Res* 1991;23:535–538.

204. Horiuchi N, Rosenblatt M. Evaluation of a parathyroid hormone antagonist in an in vivo multiparameter bioassay. *Am J Physiol* 1987;253:E187–E192.

205. Horiuchi N, Caulfield MP, Fisher JE, et al. Similarity of synthetic peptide from human tumor to parathyroid hormone in vivo and in vitro. *Science* 1987;238:1566–1568.

206. Stewart AF, Elliot J, Burtis WJ, Wu T, Insogna KL. Synthetic parathyroid hormone-like protein-(1–74): biochemical and physiological characterization. *Endocrinology* 1989;124:642–648.

207. Rodan SB, Noda M, Wesolowski G, Rosenblatt M, Rodan GA. Comparison of postreceptor effects of 1–34 human hypercalcemia factor and 1–34 human parathyroid hormone in rat osteosarcoma cells. *J Clin Invest* 1988;81:924–927.

208. Yates AJ, Gutierrez GE, Smolens P, et al. Effects of a synthetic peptide of a parathyroid hormone-related protein on calcium homeostasis, renal tubular calcium reabsorption,

and bone metabolism in vivo and in vitro in rodents. *J Clin Invest* 1988;81:932–938.

209. Rabbani SA, Mitchell J, Roy DR, Hendy GN, Goltzman D. Influence of the amino-terminus on in vitro and in vivo biological activity of synthetic parathyroid hormone-like peptides of malignancy. *Endocrinology* 1988;123:2709–2716.

210. Gilman AG. G proteins: transducers of receptor-generated signals. *Annu Rev Biochem* 1987;56:615–649.

211. Johnson GL, Dhanasekaran N. The G-protein family and their interaction with receptors. *Endocr Rev* 1989;10:317–331.

212. Spiegel AM. G proteins in clinical medicine. *Hosp Pract* 1988;88:71–88.

213. Rodbell M. The role of hormone receptors and GTP-regulatory proteins in membrane transduction. *Nature* 1980;284:17–22.

214. Gilman AG. G proteins and dual control of adenylate cyclase. *Cell* 1984;36:577–579.

215. Spiegel AM, Shenker A, Weinstein LS. Receptor–effector coupling by G proteins: implications for normal and abnormal signal transduction. *Endocr Rev* 1992;13:536–565.

216. Logothetis DE, Kurachi Y, Galper J, Neer EJ, Clapham DE. The beta gamma subunits of GTP-binding proteins activate the muscarinic K$^+$ channel in heart. *Nature* 1987;325:321–326.

217. Federman AD, Conklin BR, Schrader KA, Reed RR, Bourne HR. Hormonal stimulation of adenylyl cyclase through Gi-protein beta gamma subunits. *Nature* 1992;356:159–161.

218. Tang WJ, Gilman AG. Type-specific regulation of adenylyl cyclase by G protein beta gamma subunits. *Science* 1991;254:1500–1503.

219. Tang WJ, Krupinski J, Gilman AG. Expression and characterization of calmodulin-activated (type I) adenylylcyclase. *J Biol Chem* 1991;266:8595–8603.

220. Katz A, Wu D, Simon MI. Subunits βγ of the heterotrimeric G protein activate β$_2$ isoform of phospholipase C. *Nature* 1992;360:686–689.

221. Camps M, Carozzi A, Schnabel P, Scheer A, Parker PJ, Gierschik P. Isozyme-selective stimulation of phospholipase C-β2 and Cβ3 through protein βγ-subunits. *Nature* 1992;360:684–686.

222. Camps M, Hou C, Sidiropoulos D, Stock JB, Jakobs KH, Gierschik P. Stimulation of phospholipase C by guanine-nucleotide-binding protein beta gamma subunits. *Eur J Biochem* 1992;206:821–831.

223. Birnbaumer L. Receptor-to-effector signaling through G proteins: roles for βγ dimers as well as α subunits. *Cell* 1992;71:1069–1072.

224. Litosch I. Guanine nucleotide and NaF stimulation of phospholipase C activity in rat cerebral-cortical membranes. Studies on substrate specificity. *Biochem J* 1987;244:35–40.

225. Katada T, Ui M. Direct modification of the membrane adenylate cyclase system by islet-activating protein due to ADP-ribosylation of a membrane protein. *Proc Natl Acad Sci USA* 1982;79:3129–3133.

226. Katada T, Ui M. ADP-ribosylation of the specific membrane protein of C6 cells by islet-activating protein associated with modification of adenylate cyclase activity. *J Biol Chem* 1982;257:7210–7216.

227. Harris BA, Robishaw JD, Mumby SM, Gilman AG. Molecular cloning of complimentary DNA for the alpha subunit of the G protein that stimulates adenylate cyclase. *Science* 1985;229:1274–1277.

228. Wu D, Katz A, Lee CH, Simon MI. Activation of phospholipase C by α1-adrenergic receptors is mediated by the α subunits of the Gq family. *J Biol Chem* 1992;267:25798–25802.

229. Wu DQ, Lee CH, Rhee SG, Simon MI. Activation of phospholipase C by the alpha subunits of the Gq and G11 proteins in transfected Cos-7 cells. *J Biol Chem* 1992;267:1811–1817.

230. Fain JN, Wallace MA, Wojcikiewicz RJH. Evidence for involvement of guanine nucleotide-binding regulatory proteins in the activation of phospholipases by hormones. *FASEB J* 1988;2:2569–2574.

231. Cockcroft S. Polyphosphoinositide phosphodiesterase: regulation by a novel guanine nucleotide binding protein, Gp. *TIBS* 1987;12:75–78.

232. Steinberg SF, Chow YK, Robinson RB, Bilezikian JP. A pertussis toxin substrate regulates alpha1-adrenergic dependent phosphatidylinositol hydrolysis in cultured rat myocytes. *Endocrinology* 1987;120:1889–1895.

233. Nakamura T, Ui M. Simultaneous inhibition of inositol phospholipid breakdown, arachidonic acid release, and histamine secretion in mast cells by islet-activating protein, pertussis toxin. *J Biol Chem* 1985;260:3584–3593.

234. Cockcroft S, Gomperts BD. Role of guanine nucleotide binding protein in the activation of polyphosphoinositide phosphodiesterase. *Nature* 1985;314:534–536.

235. Harden TK, Stephens L, Hawkins PT, Downes CP. Turkey erythrocyte membranes as a model for regulation of phospholipase C by guanine nucleotides. *J Biol Chem* 1987;262:9057–9061.

236. Guillion G, Mouillac B, Balestre M-N. Activation of polyphosphoinositide phospholipase C by fluoride in WRK1 cell membranes. *FEBS Lett* 1986;204:183–188.

237. Shoback DM, McGhee JM. Fluoride stimulates the accumulation of inositol phosphates, increases intracellular free calcium, and inhibits parathyroid hormone release in dispersed bovine parathyroid cells. *Endocrinology* 1988;122:2833–2839.

238. Kienast J, Arnout J, Pfliegler G, Deckmyn H, Hoet B, Vermylen J. Sodium fluoride mimics effects of both agonists and antagonists on intact human platelets by simultaneous modulation of phospholipase C and adenylate cyclase activity. *Blood* 1987;69:859–866.

239. Blackmore PF, Bocckino SB, Waynick LE, Exton JH. Role of a guanine nucleotide-binding protein in the hydrolysis of hepatocyte phosphatidylinositol 4,5-bisphosphate by calcium-mobilizing hormones and the control of cell calcium. *J Biol Chem* 1985;260:14477–14483.

240. Graff I, Mockel J, Laurent E, Erneux C, Dumont JE. Carbachol and sodium fluoride, but not TSH, stimulate the generation of inositol phosphates in the dog thyroid. *FEBS Lett* 1987;210:204–210.

241. Ohta H, Okajima F, Ui M. Inhibition by islet-activating protein of a chemotactic peptide-induced early breakdown of inositol phospholipids and Ca^{2+} mobilization in guinea pig neutrophils. *J Biol Chem* 1985;260:15771–15780.

242. Williamson JR. Role of inositol lipid breakdown in the generation of intracellular signals. State of the art lecture. *Hypertension* 1986;8:II140–II156.

243. Milligan G, Gierschik P, Spiegel AM, Klee WA. The GTP-binding regulatory proteins of neuroblastoma x glioma, NG108-15, and glioma, c6, cells. *FEBS Lett* 1986;195:225–230.

244. Biffen M, Martin RB. Polyphosphoinositide labeling in rat liver plasma membrane is reduced by preincubation with cholera toxin. *J Biol Chem* 1987;262:7744–7750.

245. Imboden JB, Shoback DM, Pattison G, Stobo JD. Cholera toxin inhibits the T-cell antigen receptor-mediated increases in inositol trisphosphate and cytoplasmic free calcium. *Proc Natl Acad Sci USA* 1986;83:5673–5677.

246. Nissenson RA, Abbott SR, Teitelbaum AP. Endogenous biologically active human parathyroid hormone: measurement by a guanyl nucleotide-amplified renal adenylate cyclase assay. *J Clin Endocrinol Metab* 1981;52:840.

247. Juppner H, Abou Samra AB, Freeman M, et al. A G protein-linked receptor for parathyroid hormone and parathyroid hormone-related peptide. *Science* 1991;254:1024–1026.

248. Abou Samra AB, Juppner H, Force T, et al. Expression cloning of a common receptor for parathyroid hormone and parathyroid hormone-related peptide from rat osteoblast-like cells: a single receptor stimulates intracellular accumulation of both cAMP and inositol trisphosphates and increases intracellular free calcium. *Proc Natl Acad Sci USA* 1992;89:2732–2736.

249. Orloff JJ, Viena P, Schipani E. Human carcinoma cells and normal human keratinocytes express mRNAs related to but distinct from human PTH receptor mRNA. *J Bone Mineral Res* 1992;7(Suppl.):5230a.

250. Graziano MP, Gilman AG. Guanine nucleotide-binding regulatory proteins: mediators of transmembrane signaling. *TIPS* 1987;8:478–481.

The Parathyroids, edited by J.P. Bilezikian,
M.A. Levine, and R. Marcus. Raven Press, Ltd.,
New York © 1994.

CHAPTER 17

Parathyroid Hormone-Related Protein

Structure, Processing, and Physiological Actions

Arthur E. Broadus and Andrew F. Stewart

Parathyroid hormone-related protein (PTHrP) was initially identified by virtue of its production by tumors associated with the syndrome of humoral hypercalcemia of malignancy (HHM) (1–3) (see also the chapter by Grill and Martin). In this circumstance, the peptide enters the circulation in sufficient quantity to stimulate prototypical parathyroid hormone (PTH) receptors in bone and kidney. These "endocrine" effects, as defined classically, appear to account for the clinical and biochemical features that typify HHM but probably have little or nothing to do with PTHrP biology.

It is now known that the PTH and PTHrP genes arose by duplication and represent two members of a small gene family. What remains from this common origin is a similar organization of the three exons of the PTH gene and the middle portion of the PTHrP gene together with a short stretch of homologous amino-terminal sequence. Otherwise, the two genes clearly have evolved separately. The PTH gene has a simple organization and is expressed predominantly by the parathyroid chief cell, and its product functions as a classical systemic peptide hormone. The PTHrP gene (particularly the human gene) has a complex structure and is expressed in a remarkable variety of normal cell types and tissues, and its product(s) seems to function primarily in an autocrine and/or paracrine fashion. The two genes also appear to be subject to very different types of control. Thus the PTH/PTHrP gene family

consists of two regulatory molecules whose functions seem to be remarkably different.

The structure of the PTHrP gene is more informative than is that of most genes and serves as a useful bridge between the story of the discovery of PTHrP as a product of HHM-associated tumors (see the chapter by Grill and Martin) and the more recent and ever-enlarging literature concerning the biological role(s) of the peptide. Correspondingly, this chapter begins with a description of the organization of the PTHrP gene. Subsequent sections review the sites and control of PTHrP gene expression, the steps in PTHrP processing and secretion, and the case for and against the existence of a single PTH/PTHrP receptor. The final sections of the chapter describe the systems and tissues from which sufficient data have been developed to lead to hypotheses regarding PTHrP function.

Chase and Aurbach initially described the effects of PTH on cyclic adenosine monophosphate (cAMP) excretion in 1967 (4). That the tumor-derived product responsible for HHM might have similar effects was recognized 13 years later (5–7), and this proved to be the key marker that ultimately led to the isolation of the peptide (1–3). Gerald Aurbach followed the "PTHrP problem" with great interest as it developed during the 1980s and provided encouragement to the authors at several points when it was sorely needed. We are particularly honored to be sharing in this tribute to his memory.

A. E. Broadus: Department of Internal Medicine, Yale University School of Medicine, New Haven, Connecticut 06510.
A. F. Stewart: Division of Endocrinology, Yale University School of Medicine, New Haven, Connecticut 06510; and West Haven Veterans Affairs Medical Center, West Haven, Connecticut 06516.

PARATHYROID HORMONE-RELATED PROTEIN GENE STRUCTURE

The human PTHrP gene comprises eight exons spanning more than 15 kb of genomic DNA (Fig. 1) (8–

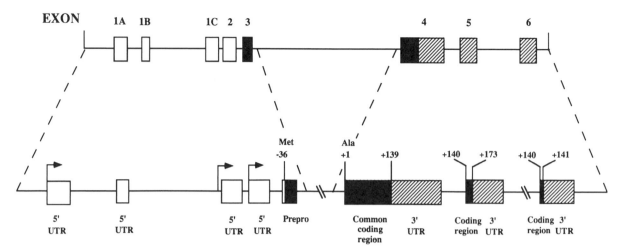

FIG. 1. Organization of the human PTHrP gene. The exons are numbered according to the numbering system given by Mangin et al. (8,13). The *open boxes* represent 5'-untranslated (5' UTR) sequences, the *solid boxes* coding sequences, and the *hatched boxes* 3'-untranslated (3' UTR) sequences. The arrows define the start sites used by the three promoter elements. The initiating methionine (Met), the first amino acid of the mature peptide (Ala), and the C termini of the three PTHrP isoforms are indicated.

10). It is sometimes referred to as a *complex transcriptional unit* because it gives rise to multiple PTHrP mRNA species, and these, in turn, encode more than one product. Four of the exons (1A, 1B, 1C, and 2) are noncoding exons, which can be fused together in various ways as a function of promoter usage and/or different splicing patterns to generate 5' untranslated regions (UTRs) that differ among PTHrP mRNA species (11–13); the designation of three different exons as 1A, 1B, and 1C is a bit awkward and is based on the fact that the two most 5' exons (1A and 1B) were not identified until several years after the main body of the gene was isolated.[1] Exon 3 encodes the prepro- region of the peptide, except for the dibasic endoproteolytic cleavage site, which is carried on exon 4 (see Fig. 2). Exon 4 encodes the bulk of the PTHrP coding region that is common to all PTHrP isoforms; it also contains a common stop codon-splice donor sequence and a 3' UTR. Exons 5 and 6 contain the sequences that encode the carboxy-terminal regions of the 173- and 141-amino-acid PTHrP isoforms, respectively; each of these exons also contains a stop codon and a unique 3' UTR. The structure of the PTHrP gene is highly informative with respect to the gene's heritage, its products, and the complexity of its control. These three features are treated separately below.

First, the organization of the PTHrP gene confirms, in structural terms, its relatedness to the PTH gene. Figure 2 compares the middle portion of the PTHrP gene, comprising exons 2–4, to the simple 3-exon PTH gene and reveals that the intron–exon organization of the two genes is identical in these regions. This similarity of structure includes the positioning of the second intron of both genes such that nucleotides -7 to $+1$, which encode the Lys-Arg dibasic cleavage site, are partitioned to the exon that encodes the bulk of the coding region of both peptides. Since this dibasic cleavage is absolutely essential to generate a functional amino terminus, there would necessarily be strong evolutionary pressure to maintain this organizational feature during the subsequent evolutionary divergence of the two genes. The relatedness of the PTH and PTHrP genes was initially suspected from the amino-terminal sequence similarity of the two peptides and also from chromosomal mapping studies, in which the PTH and PTHrP loci were assigned to the short arms of human chromosomes 11 and 12, respec-

---

[1]Unfortunately, each of the groups that initially isolated parts or all of the human PTHrP gene used a different numbering system for exons (8–10,13). We have maintained the numbering system employed by our own group but would readily agree that a logical alternative would be simply to refer to the exons as 1–8 (14).

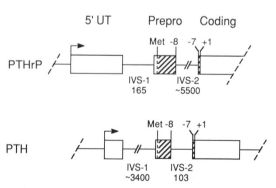

FIG. 2. Comparison of exons 2, 3, and 4 of the human PTHrP gene with the three exons of the PTH gene. Intron (IVS) 2 interrupts the precursor sequence in both genes at nucleotide -7, so that the dibasic residues required for endoproteolytic cleave are a part of the exons encoding the mature peptides. (Reprinted from ref. 8 with permission.)

tively (10,12). The short arms of these two chromosomes bear a number of related genes (e.g., the A isoform of LDH on chromosome 11 and the B isoform on chromosome 12) and are thought to have arisen by an ancient tetraploidization event from a single ancestral chromosome (10,12). The gene clusters in question have also been maintained on paired chromosomes in the rat and mouse genomes, even though the chromosome pairs differ in these species (15). Thus there is abundant evidence that the PTH and PTHrP genes are two members of a small gene family. This evidence, however, does not speak to the "chicken-and-egg" question of which gene might be the oldest, in that what antedated both genes was a common ancestral gene. Given the mounting evidence for a fundamental regulatory role for PTHrP in various tissues, many in the field would argue that PTHrP is perhaps the more ancient of the two molecules.

Second, the human PTHrP gene contains three alternatively spliced 3′ exons (4, 5, and 6) that give rise to three mRNA classes encoding three PTHrP isoforms, each with a unique carboxy terminus (Fig. 3) (11,12,16,17). The splicing pattern here is unusual in that exon 4 can either remain unspliced to generate the mRNA encoding one of the PTHrP isoforms or be alternatively spliced to exons 5 or 6 to generate the other two; the common coding region for 139 amino acids from exon 4 is included in all three products (Fig. 3). The key "hinge" sequence in this regard occurs at the end of the coding region in exon 4. This four-base sequence, GTAA, plays the dual role of splice donor site (GT consensus) or a stop codon (TAA). Although there is Northern blotting evidence for apparent tumor-specific preferential splicing (8,18), virtually nothing is known with respect to possible cell-specific preferential splicing patterns or the regulation of splice choices in normal human tissues. All three mRNA species seem to exist in similar abundance in normal keratinocytes (17), but the mRNA encoding the 139-amino-acid product appears to be relatively enriched in amnion (19).

Although the three PTHrP mRNA classes encode different isoforms, examination of their 3′ UTRs reveals an important common feature, in that each is AU-rich and contains multiple copies of an AUUUA "instability" motif (indicated by the Y symbols in Fig. 3) or AU-rich element (ARE) that has been shown previously to confer rapid turnover on a number of cyto-

kine and protooncogene mRNAs (20,21). Several aspects of the presence of these AREs in the 3′ ends of PTHrP mRNAs are noteworthy from an evolutionary perspective. First, this AU-rich, multiple AUUUA motif sequence is highly conserved in all PTHrP mRNAs from chicken to man (11,12,16,17,22–28) but is not present in PTH mRNA from any species (29,30). Second, the chicken, mouse, and rat PTHrP genes have a somewhat simpler organization than the human gene (see below), so that the unspliced 3′ end of human exon 4 or its equivalent seems to have evolved separately, and it is clear that human exon 5 has evolved quite recently. Nevertheless, all of these 3′ ends are AU rich and bear multiple copies of the AU motif (22–28). Finally, comparison of the three human 3′ ends with each other as well as across species reveals no significant sequence similarity apart from the AREs. These findings would be anticipated only if rapid mRNA turnover is critical for proper regulation of PTHrP mRNA expression and PTHrP biological function.

Third, the 5′-flanking region of the human PTHrP gene has a highly complex organization, consisting of four alternatively spliced, noncoding exons that are transcribed from at least three independent promoter elements (Fig. 4). These elements are referred to as the *upstream* and *downstream TATA promoters* and the *midregion GC promoter* (Fig. 4; see legend for alternative terminology) (8–10,13,14,31). The downstream TATA promoter was the first element to be recognized and is an interesting, short (45-base) structure, the size of which is delimited precisely by its location between exons 1C and 2 (Fig. 4). This seems to be the dominant element in the rodent PTHrP genes, which have a simpler 5′-flanking region than the human gene (26,27). The upstream TATA promoter lies 2.7 kb 5′ of the downstream TATA element. Apart from the TATA consensus, these two promoters bear no resemblance to one another, nor does either resemble the PTH gene promoter (8–10,13,29,30,32). The midregion GC promoter lies just 5′ of exon 1C in a GC-rich region that lacks canonical TATA or CAAT sequences but is enriched in SP1 binding sites (31). The use of both TATA- and GC-rich promoters by the PTHrP gene is very unusual, there being few other reported examples of genes that are transcribed from both classes of promoter elements (31). Many housekeeping genes and some cytokine/growth factor genes operate from GC-

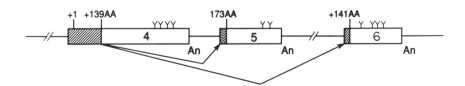

FIG. 3. Schematic representation of the alternatively spliced 3′ exons of the human PTHrP gene. Coding regions are *hatched,* and the locations of the ATTTA motifs are designated by the *Ys.*

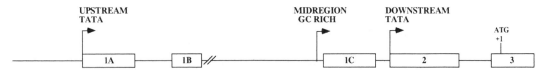

FIG. 4. Schematic representation of the 5′-flanking region of the human PTHrP gene. The exons are numbered according to Mangin et al. (13); the transcription initiation sites used by the three promoters are indicated by *arrows,* and the translocation start site (ATG) is defined as nucleotide +1. The upstream and downstream TATA promoters were designated P_1 and P_2, respectively, in the literature that appeared before the identification of the GC-rich midregion promoter (8–10,13,14). The midregion promoter does not correspond to the putative element reported by Yasuda et al. (9). It is unknown whether promoter usage and/or 5′-splice choices has any influence on 3′-splicing events.

rich promoters (15,31), so that it is tempting to infer that the GC-rich PTHrP gene promoter might have something to do with its widespread expression, at least in human tissues. To date, preferential or cell-specific promoter usage has been examined in only a limited number of studies, and there is evidence for both multiple and preferential promoter use in certain malignant and normal tissues, without a clear pattern having emerged (13,14,19,31).

A computer search of 4.8 kb of DNA upstream of exon 2 of the human PTHrP gene reveals a number of putative binding sites for transcription factors such as SP1, AP1, and AP2, two regions that resemble a cAMP consensus element, and six sequences that are identical to a steroid hormone response element half-site; no 15-base consensus sequences corresponding to a complete hormone response element are present, even allowing for three base mismatches. However, it is clear that steroid hormones are among the host of influences that seem to regulate PTHrP mRNA expression; these controls are summarized in detail below under Control of PTHrP Gene Expression. Possibly because of the complexity of the 5′-flanking region of the PTHrP gene, only a limited number of functional studies of basal promoter activity and/or regulated transcription have been performed (14,31,33–36). An important aspect of control that has been recognized only recently is that of negative regulation or inhibition of basal PTHrP gene transcription. For example, there appear to be multiple negative regulatory or "silencer" sequences located upstream of the midregion GC promoter (14,36). In essence, the general picture beginning to emerge is that the complex structure of the human PTHrP gene 5′-flanking region correlates with an equivalent complexity in terms of control and that the transcription of the gene is subject to finely tuned checks and balances in the form of both positive and negative controls.

PTHrP cDNAs and/or the gene have been isolated from three additional species, rat, mouse, and chicken (22–28). These structures are informative in several ways. First, the PTHrP coding region is highly conserved (98%) through amino acid residue 111, whereas distal to residue 112 there is significant divergence (only 25% sequence similarity). However, if this carboxy-terminal region is realigned with gaps, there is 60% amino acid conservation, and the region remains serine and threonine rich (25). Overall, the PTHrP coding region is more highly conserved than is the case for the PTH coding region across species (29,30,32). Second, the chicken, mouse, and rat genes all have a simpler organization than the human gene. The mouse and rat genes seem to use predominantly the downstream TATA promoter element (25,26); exon 1-like sequences are present upstream of the mouse gene but are represented in mouse PTHrP mRNA in such low abundance that it has been impossible to map a putative upstream promoter (26). With respect to available 3′ splice choices, the mouse and rat genes seem to use exclusively the equivalent of the human exon 4 to 6 splicing pattern (Fig. 3) to generate a single major PTHrP mRNA species; these genes do not contain the equivalents of human exon 5 or the 3′ UTR of exon 4 (25,26). In contrast, while the chicken gene appears to use predominantly the exon 4–6 splicing pattern, it also contains sequences equivalent to the 3′ UTR of human exon 4 (27,28). These findings have been taken as evidence that the avian and rodent genes probably evolved in parallel rather than in a linear sequence.

SITES OF PARATHYROID HORMONE-RELATED PROTEIN GENE EXPRESSION

Secretory PTH-like bioactivity was identified in conditioned medium from normal human keratinocytes in primary culture in 1986 (37). The lead that resulted in this observation was the striking frequency of squamous cell neoplasms among HHM-associated tumors and the implication that PTHrP might be a normal product of nonmalignant epidermal cells. Although most investigators working in the field in the mid-1980s considered it likely that the tumor-derived factor responsible for HHM would prove to be a normal gene product, the actual demonstration that this was the case was of some importance. That this would be the tip of the iceberg in terms of an extraordinarily widespread distribution of expression could not have been foreseen in 1986 and is somewhat difficult to fathom even today.

The sites of PTHrP gene expression in adult and fetal tissues are summarized in Tables 1 and 2, respectively, and a sampling of PTHrP mRNA expression in selected rat tissues is shown in Fig. 5. In general, there is reasonable agreement between laboratories and across techniques for scoring either mRNA or protein, although there is disagreement with respect to some individual findings. Certainly, there is general agreement on two points: 1) widespread expression is observed irrespective of technique and 2) PTHrP mRNA and peptide are present in low abundance and require sensitive methods for detection. The distribution of PTHrP gene expression is covered in the following paragraphs in some brevity, in that there is no functionally harmonious way in which to weave all this information together, unless it be the obvious implication that PTHrP must be playing a predominantly autocrine and/or paracrine role in these many sites. Five areas (skin, placenta, breast, bone, and smooth muscle) have been sufficiently well studied that they have produced reasonable working hypotheses regard-

ing function; these are summarized in some detail at the end of this chapter.

The PTHrP gene is expressed in a wide variety of endocrine tissues and cell types. With the exception of the proposal that PTHrP derived from the fetal parathyroids may be involved in regulating placental calcium transport (38), however, the PTHrP produced in these various endocrine cells is not envisioned as playing a traditional endocrine role in distant target tissues. Indeed, the presence of PTHrP in so many typical endocrine secretory cells with such a diversity of hormonal products is enigmatic. These sites include the pituitary, thyroid, adrenal cortex and medulla, pancreatic islet, ovary, testes, placenta, and parathyroids (26,39–41). In the human pituitary, PTHrP antisera stain growth hormone- and prolactin-producing cells most strongly (40); estrogen-regulated PTHrP gene expression has also been reported in prolactin-producing cultured rat GH_4C_1 pituitary cells (42). In the thyroid, PTHrP is present in follicular cells (40) and in the adrenal the zona reticularis has the strongest immu-

TABLE 1. *PTHrP gene expression in adult mammalian tissues*

Adrenal cortex
Adrenal medulla
Amnion
Bone
Brain
Endothelium
Epidermis and other epithelia
Heart
Kidney
Lung
Mammary gland
Ovary
Pancreatic islets
Parathyroid
Pituitary
Placenta
Prostate
Skeletal muscle
Small intestine
Smooth muscle
   Vascular
   Uterine
   Bladder
   Gastric
Spleen
Stomach mucosa
Testis
Thyroid
Thymus
Urothelium
Uterus (endometrium)

TABLE 2. *PTHrP gene expression during embryogenesis*

Chicken	Human and rat
Day 3–10 embryo	Nervous system
Body and head	Brain
Allantois	Spinal cord
Yolk sac	Dorsal root ganglion
Chorioallantoic membrane	Developing eye
Day 15 embryo	Epithelia
Brain	Epidermis and hair follicles
Gizzard	Pharynx and larynx
Intestine	Bronchial epithelium
Liver	Stomach and intestine
Lung	Pancreatic acini
Skeletal muscle	Liver
Chorioallantoic membrane	Salivary ducts
and yolk sac	Endocrine glands
	Parathyroid
	Thyroid
	Adrenal
	Gonad
	Muscle
	Cardiac muscle
	Striated muscle
	Smooth muscle
	Urogenital tract (human)
	8–10 weeks: glomeruli,
	mesonephros, and
	metanephros
	20 weeks and beyond:
	proximal tubule, distal
	tubule, collecting duct,
	urothelium
	Bone and teeth
	Dental lamina
	Immature chondrocytes
	Mature chondrocytes
	Osteoblast-like cells

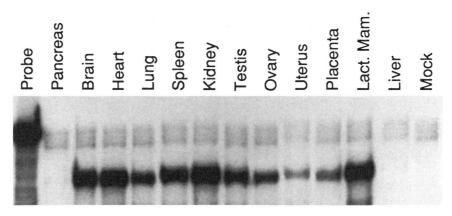

FIG. 5. PTHrP mRNA expression in selected adult rat tissues as determined by RNase protection analysis. Each specimen was assayed at 100 μg total RNA. The probe contains polylinker sequences from the vector and is larger than the protected PTHrP mRNA fragment. The control (Mock) digestion contained 10 μg yeast (RNA). (Reproduced from ref. 26 with permission.)

nostaining (40). All four principal endocrine cell types in the islets stain with PTHrP antisera (Fig. 6) (41). In the ovary, both granulosa and theca cells stain positively, and testicular Leydig cells are intensively positive (40). As was noted, PTHrP is produced in the parathyroids of fetal sheep and is thought to maintain the placental calcium gradient during gestation (38); PTHrP is also present in the parathyroids of newborn sheep but has been reported to be absent in maternal parathyroids (43). This area is reviewed in more detail

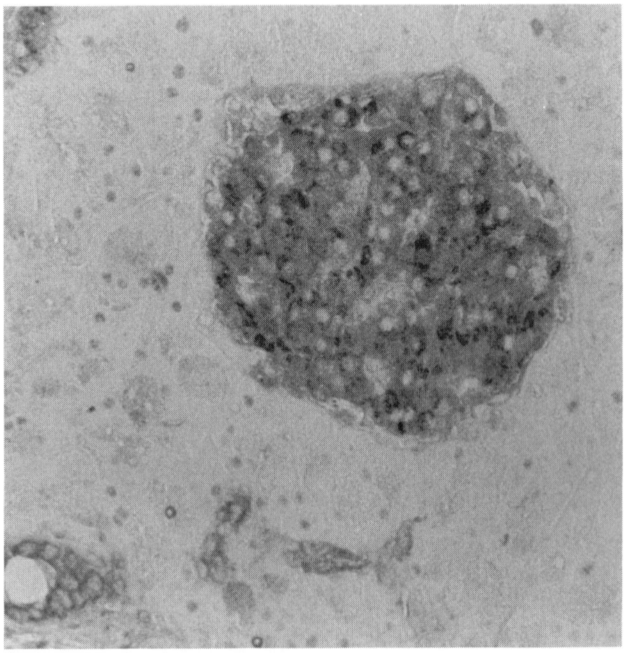

FIG. 6. Normal rat pancreatic islet stained by the peroxidase-antiperoxidase method using an affinity-purified rabbit anti-PTHrP-(1–36) antibody. Note that all cell types within the islet are PTHrP-positive. × 250. (Reprinted from ref. 176 with permission.)

below. The PTHrP gene is also variably expressed in human parathyroid lesions. It is overexpressed, to the extent seen in HHM-associated neoplasms, in about two-thirds of parathyroid adenomas but is expressed at very low levels in primary and secondary parathyroid hyperplasia and in parathyroid carcinoma (Fig. 7) (18,39,44). Curiously, the PTHrP gene is also expressed in a cultured rat parathyroid cell line (PT-r) that has lost the capacity to express the PTH gene (45). The variable PTHrP gene expression seen in abnormal human parathyroid glands is of some interest in that it implies some fundamental abnormality associated with disordered regulation of both the PTH and PTHrP genes but is not of apparent pathophysiological consequence; PTHrP is undetectable in the peripheral circulation of patients with primary hyperparathyroidism and is even absent in the venous drainage of parathyroid adenomas (46).

The PTHrP gene is also expressed in a remarkable variety of nonendocrine tissues (Table 1, Fig. 5). PTHrP is present throughout the epidermis (Fig. 8) and in hair follicles (47,48). The peptide is also present in many other epithelial cells, including the urothelium, stomach mucosa, and lining of the cervix, pharynx, and bronchioles (39,49,50). In the kidney, PTHrP staining is seen in the proximal and distal tubules and in the collecting duct (49). The three principal types of muscle (cardiac, skeletal, and smooth) all contain PTHrP (Fig. 5) (26,49). The gene is particularly widely expressed in different smooth muscle beds, including vascular and gastric smooth muscle and the muscular layers of the uterus and bladder (49,51–53). PTHrP mRNA is present in specific neuronal populations in the brain, being particularly enriched in regions of the cerebral cortex, hippocampus, and cerebellum (Fig. 9) (54). These neuronal populations share a high degree of electrical activity and bear a large number of calcium channels of the L type and excitatory amino acid

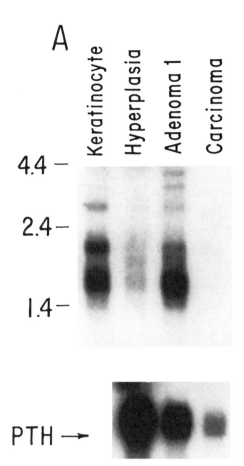

FIG. 7. Northern analysis of poly(A)⁺ RNA prepared from normal human keratinocytes and from single examples of a secondarily hyperplastic parathyroid gland, a parathyroid adenoma, and a parathyroid carcinoma. The filter was hybridized to both PTHrP (*upper panel*) and PTH (*lower panel*) probes. Note the multiple PTHrP mRNA species. (Reprinted from ref. 39 with permission.)

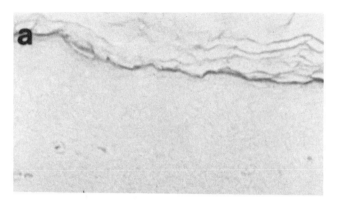

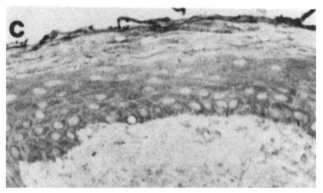

FIG. 8. Immunoperoxidase staining of human skin in the absence (**a**) or presence (**c**) of an affinity-purified anti-PTHrP-(1–36) antibody. Note staining of all layers of keratinocytes. (Reprinted from ref. 47 with permission.)

receptors (54). PTHrP is also present in the hypothalamus (55).

PTHrP gene expression has been studied during embryogenesis in the chicken, rat, and human. In general, the findings mirror those summarized above, namely, very widespread expression involving all three germ layers. In some instances, the level of expression has been found to change as a function of development.

In chick embryos aged 3–10 days, PTHrP mRNA is expressed in the body and head of the embryos and in the extraembryonic membranes (Table 2) (28). In day 15 embryos, PTHrP mRNA is widely expressed, being present in brain, cardiac and skeletal muscle, lung, solid and hollow viscera, and extraembryonic membranes (Table 2). The chorioallantoic membrane is involved in calcium transport during embryogenesis, so that the identification of PTHrP mRNA in this structure is consistent with the proposed role of the peptide

in mediating placental calcium transport in mammals (38).

Fetal rat and human tissues have been examined at various stages of gestation using both in situ hybridization histochemistry and immunohistochemistry (56–60). PTHrP is found not only in the developing brain but also in the spinal cord, dorsal root ganglion, and developing eye (Table 2) (56). PTHrP mRNA and/ or immunoreactivity is present in a wide variety of epithelia, including the epidermis and hair follicles; the lining of the oropharynx, larynx, lungs, and intestine; the pancreatic acini; and the salivary ducts (56,57,59,60). PTHrP immunostaining is seen in the parathyroids and a number of other endocrine glands and also in the three principal types of developing muscle (Table 2) (56,59,60). In the human urogenital tract, PTHrP is present in the glomeruli and developing mesonephros and metanephros at 8–10 weeks; at 20 weeks and beyond, the peptide is detected in the proximal and distal renal tubules, in the collecting duct, and throughout the urothelium (58). The dental lamina are strongly positive for PTHrP mRNA in the rat (57). PTHrP immunostaining is also seen in areas of both endochondral and intramembranous bone formation in the rat and human (56,57,59,60). Here, the pattern seems to change as a function of chondroge-

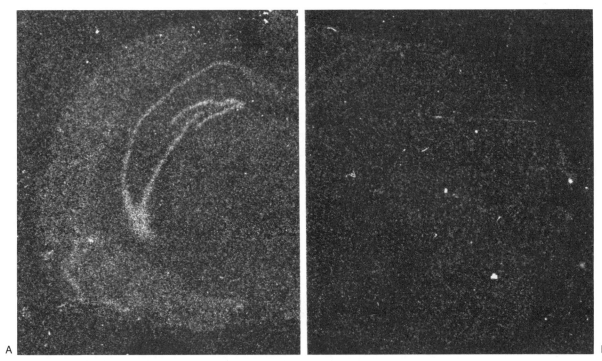

FIG. 9. In situ hybridization histochemistry of PTHrP mRNA in rat brain. The antisense (**A**) oligonucleotide probe hybridized most intensely to regions of the hippocampal formation and cerebral cortex, while only a low level of background hybridization was seen with the sense (**B**) probe. (Reprinted from ref. 54 with permission.)

nesis and bone formation; PTHrP is present early in immature mesenchymal cells and later in "mature" chondrocytes and osteoblast-like cells (56,57,59,60).

Although PTHrP gene expression has not been carefully studied in a large number of tissues in a longitudinal fashion during embryogenesis, both spatial and temporal differences in expression have been seen in the few tissues so studied. These include changing patterns of PTHrP expression in the early mouse embryo (61), dental lamina (57), epidermis and hair follicles (56), and perichondrium and periosteum (56,57,59,60). PTHrP mRNA is also expressed in fetal rat liver, while it is absent in adult liver (39). In addition, PTHrP and the PTH/PTHrP receptor have been found to be induced during differentiation of mouse F9 embryonal carcinoma cells to parietal endoderm (61,62). PTHrP has also been detected in developing trophoectoderm cells in the late morula stage and has been proposed to play a paracrine or autocrine role in the control of parietal endoderm differentiation in the early mouse embryo (61,62).

There has been no shortage of interpretations offered to explain the various findings summarized above, and three of these merit mention. The first and most obvious is that PTHrP may have something to do with embryogenesis, growth, and/or differentiation. The second is that the peptide may be regulating calcium transport, not only in the placenta but also in lo-

cal sites such as the chorioallantoic membrane and distal nephron. The third, based on the localization of PTHrP in the dental lamina and developing cartilage and bone, is that the peptide may play a role in chondrogenesis and/or ossification. Each of these three areas is discussed in more detail in subsequent sections. The most compelling functional data reported to date are those derived from targeted overexpression of the PTHrP gene in the basal keratinocytes of transgenic mice (see below under Parathyroid Hormone-Related Protein as an Autocrine/Paracrine Factor in Skin) (63) and inactivation of the mouse PTHrP gene by homologous recombination (see below under Bone) (64).

CONTROL OF PARATHYROID HORMONE-RELATED PROTEIN GENE EXPRESSION

A fundamental aspect of the evolutionary divergence of the PTH and PTHrP genes has been the development of very different mechanisms of control. The PTH gene is expressed predominantly by the parathyroid chief cell and is subject to a very limited repertoire of transcriptional controls [calcium and $1,25(OH)_2D$] (65). The critical regulatory step in terms of PTH physiology is not transcriptional control of PTH mRNA expression but rather regulation of PTH secretion from storage granules by the extracellular calcium concentration. In contrast, the PTHrP gene is widely expressed, is subject to a large number of transcriptional controls, and is also subject to posttranscriptional regulation; the dual operation of both transcriptional and posttranscriptional mechanisms provides for very tight control of PTHrP mRNA expression. Although there is evidence that PTHrP secretion is regulated, it is not clear that the classical processing–storage–regulated secretion pathway traversed by PTH applies to PTHrP in any cell type, nor is it known whether PTHrP is ever stored in appreciable quantities, even in cells that have this pathway [e.g., it has been reported that the content of PTHrP in bovine parathyroid tissue is 1/400 that of PTH (66)].

The organizational features of the PTHrP gene that relate to the complexity of its control vis-à-vis the PTH gene were summarized above. The complex 5'-flanking region of the PTHrP gene is responsible for at least three aspects of its control: 1) its widespread expression, 2) the large variety of influences that appear to regulate its expression, and 3) the fact that it is subject to negative control in terms of both its basal expression and its regulated expression. The posttranscriptional control of PTHrP mRNA expression appears to reside in the ARE "instability" sequences present in the 3' UTRs of PTHrP mRNAs. Certain basic aspects of the control of PTHrP mRNA expression are discussed below. This discussion is followed by separate sections describing (a) the mechanisms of PTHrP gene expression in HHM-associated tumors and (b) the physiological and pharmacological regulation of PTHrP gene expression and peptide secretion.

In all tissues and cells examined carefully to date, PTHrP mRNA seems to be expressed at a low constitutive level and to be modulated by exogenous influences over a relatively narrow range, in many cases with a rapid peak followed by a rapid decay in mRNA expression. This low constitutive level of PTHrP mRNA is not the result of a low rate of transcription, for in a number of systems runoff analysis has revealed that the gene is transcribed at a rate approximating that of the actin or cyclophilin genes, which encode abundant mRNAs (67–69). Rather, the low level of steady-state PTHrP mRNA seems to reflect predominantly rapid turnover, with estimated half-times both in vivo (22,51) and in vitro (42,67,69,70) of from 30 min to several hours. These kinetics are reminiscent of those of a number of cytokine, lymphokine, and protooncogene mRNAs (20,21,71), and the ARE instability motifs that were initially identified in these mRNAs are also present in PTHrP mRNAs (see above). A short mRNA $T_{1/2}$ reduces the level of mRNA associated with a given rate of transcription and produces a corresponding reduction in "translational yield" of protein (20). In addition, rapid induction-deinduction

kinetics (which require also an element of transcriptional inhibition; see below) limit the duration of response. These limitations in terms of both magnitude and duration of response are thought to be very important in controlling the effects of the powerful regulatory cytokine molecules noted above (20,21,71) and are presumably just as important in limiting PTHrP biological effects. Parenthetically, this "low-abundance" issue presented a major problem in isolating PTHrP as well as PTHrP cDNAs and continues to represent an analytical problem, in that the detection of PTHrP mRNA and peptide requires sensitive techniques. Indeed, the widespread expression of PTHrP mRNA went largely unappreciated by laboratories that employed Northern analysis of total RNA in carrying out their initial tissue surveys.

The essential picture that emerges is one of "tight" control of PTHrP mRNA expression by a finely balanced combination of transcriptional and posttranscriptional mechanisms. These features are given some emphasis herein because they are highly relevant to the production of PTHrP by cells that process and secrete the peptide by the constitutive secretory pathway; these would appear to include most cells that produce PTHrP normally and virtually all malignant cells associated with HHM. In constitutive secretory cells, the rate of PTHrP production/secretion is a direct, linear function of the steady-state level of PTHrP mRNA, so that understanding the production of the peptide by such cells reduces fundamentally to a study of the controls of PTHrP mRNA expression. As was noted above, it is not clear how the "tight" control of PTHrP mRNA expression would bear on PTHrP secretion by a classical regulated secretory pathway.

Parathyroid Hormone Gene Expression in Humoral Hypercalcemia of Malignancy-Associated Tumor Cells

The questions here are basically two: 1) why the PTHrP rather than the PTH gene is so commonly expressed by HHM-associated tumors and 2) why the PTHrP gene is expressed by certain tumor cells of a given cell type and not others. One cannot avoid the terms *ectopic* and *eutopic* in discussing these questions, yet the semantics are rather unimportant as compared to an actual understanding of mechanism. The problem of hormone production by tumors has become in most instances a question of gene regulation, and there are growing numbers of reports on the mechanisms involved. For instance, selective stabilization of the normally labile transcripts for basic fibroblast growth factor and granulocyte-macrophage colony-stimulating factor (GM-CSF) has recently been shown to cause their overexpression in astrocytoma and lymphoid tumor lines, respectively (72,73). The ectopic expression of adrenocorticotropin (ACTH) by several tumors has been shown to involve a shift in proopiomelanocortin (POMC) promoter usage to one mimicking the pattern normally restricted to the pituitary (74). The shift has been correlated with changes in the methylation status of specific regions of the POMC promoter (75). Finally, the excessive activity of transacting factors and the lack of a specific trans-repressing factor have been shown to be responsible for the overexpression of the granulocyte colony-stimulating factor (G-CSF) and α-fetoprotein genes, respectively, in carcinoma cells (76,77). As can be seen from these examples, there appears to be a great deal of heterogeneity in the mechanisms responsible for "ectopic" hormone production, and it is likely that most of the normal regulatory mechanisms that control expression of a given peptide hormone gene may be targets for dysregulation in malignancy.

Only a limited amount of information is available concerning the relative infrequency/frequency of PTH and PTHrP gene expression by "HHM"-associated tumors. The most fundamental general point bearing on this question is the extreme cell specificity of the expression of the PTH gene as compared to the widespread expression of the PTHrP gene. That is, in nonparathyroid tissues, the PTH gene is "off" (presumably because of methylation and other modifications that make the gene inaccessible to the transcriptional apparatus), whereas the PTHrP gene may be "on" (and thus subject to malignancy-associated dysregulation of gene expression of the types discussed in the preceding paragraph). It would follow from this rather simplistic line of reasoning that activation of the PTH gene in a nonparathyroid tumor might require a rather drastic lesion in molecular terms, and in the best-studied example (78) of the three cases reported to date (78–80) this was, in fact, the case. This example involved rearrangement and amplification of the upstream regulatory region of the PTH gene in an ovarian carcinoma (78). This is an unusual mechanism, which has not been described thus far for any PTHrP-producing tumor.

The mechanisms underlying PTHrP gene expression by HHM-associated tumor cells are only beginning to be carefully examined, but use of three tumor systems has begun to shed some light on this process. Given the preceding comments regarding the precedent for multiple molecular mechanisms for hormone production by tumors, it comes as no particular surprise that a different mechanism appears to apply in each of these three systems.

The first involves PTHrP production by human T-cell lymphoma virus type 1 (HTLV-1)-infected T cells in patients with the adult T-cell leukemia syndrome. This is a common neoplasm in Japan, and some 70% of affected patients develop HHM during their course.

PTHrP appears to be responsible for all instances of HHM (81–83), and there is evidence that the PTHrP gene is expressed by virtually 100% of HTLV-1-infected T cells (83). It has been proposed on the basis of transfection studies that the PTHrP gene is being overexpressed because it is being activated or stimulated in trans by Tax, a viral product that is a known transactivator of other cellular genes (83). This is an appealing mechanism, but the initial report did not include appropriate controls (83), and a subsequent preliminary report could not reproduce these findings (84). Nevertheless, given the specificity of HTLV-1 infection to the pathogenesis of this syndrome, it is likely that some viral protein is directly or indirectly responsible for stimulating PTHrP gene expression in infected T cells.

The second tumor system to be studied involves PTHrP gene expression in human renal carcinomas. Renal carcinoma is second only to squamous carcinoma as a cause of HHM, and ~25% of cultured renal carcinoma cells appear to be capable of producing PTHrP (85). Working with six examples each of PTHrP-producing (PTHrP+) and non-producing (PTHrP−) renal carcinoma cell lines as defined by RNase protection analysis, Holt et al. (86) found that the status of PTHrP gene expression in these cells correlated absolutely with the methylation status of four CpG dinucleotides in a 550-bp region located upstream of the midregion GC promoter (Fig. 10). The promoter itself is contained in a 900 bp CpG island, which was found to be unmethylated in all cells (Fig. 10). This analysis was carried out using a series of methylation-sensitive and -insensitive isoschizomers, which either fail to cleave or cleave DNA as a function of methylation of CpG residues in their recognition sequences. Holt et al. (86) further demonstrated that demethylation of PTHrP− cells by 5-azacytidine converted them to a PTHrP+ phenotype, although the level of PTHrP mRNA expression achieved was less than that seen in the native PTHrP+ cells. Methylation is an important means of silencing gene expression, and the results in this system clearly indicate that this cis modification is the functional equivalent of an "off–on" switch in terms of PTHrP gene expression. This phenotypic characterization is directly relevant to the clinical syndrome, in that these same cell lines have been previously shown to be capable (PTHrP+ cells) or incapable (PTHrP− cells) of inducing HHM in nude mice on the basis of their PTHrP phenotype (85). It is unclear how these data might bear on the "eutopic–ectopic" question, and there are two possibilities. One is that the methylation status of the PTHrP gene in renal carcinoma cells reflects the status of the gene in the untransformed cell of origin and that PTHrP+ cells are basically expressing the gene in a eutopic fashion. The other is that methylation of the gene changes as a func-

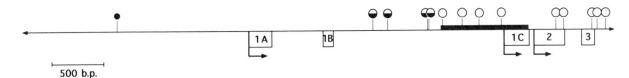

500 b.p.

FIG. 10. Methylation pattern of the PTHrP gene in human renal carcinoma cell lines. The exons and start sites are as designated in Fig. 4. The *half-filled* circles correspond to CpG dinucleotides that were found to be unmethylated in renal carcinoma cells that express the PTHrP gene and methylated in cells that do not express the gene; these are located just upstream of a CpG island (*bold horizontal bar*). Other CpG dinucleotides were found to be methylated (*solid circle*) or unmethylated (*open circles*) in all cells examined and did not correlate with PTHrP gene expression. (Reprinted from ref. 86 with permission.)

tion of transformation and that this is a dysregulated mechanism that is actually responsible for PTHrP gene expression.

The third system involves PTHrP gene expression in human squamous carcinoma cells, the most common cause of HHM. The data here are preliminary (87), but it is clear that the findings in this system are very different from those in the renal carcinoma system just described. Whereas renal carcinoma cells seem to fall into two clear phenotypic subpopulations with respect to PTHrP gene expression, squamous carcinoma cells display a continuum of PTHrP mRNA expression covering an ~20-fold range, from barely detectable expression to abundant expression. Initial transfection studies indicate that the activity of introduced PTHrP-CAT constructs correlates with endogenous gene activity, suggesting that dysregulation of PTHrP gene expression in squamous carcinoma cells resides in one or another trans-acting mechanism (87). The working hypothesis here is that the potential of a given malignant squamous cell for producing HHM may reside in the quantitative capacity of that cell to express the PTHrP gene.

Factors Affecting Parathyroid Hormone-Related Protein Gene Expression In Vivo and In Vitro

There is now a substantial literature on the regulation of PTHrP mRNA expression and protein production both in vivo and in vitro, as indicated by the extensive listing in Table 3. This listing is intended to be reasonably comprehensive, and it is acknowledged that the citations include work that is uneven in terms of mechanistic detail and also include a number of preliminary reports. It is the purpose of this section not to catalog all this information but rather to summarize it in as cohesive a fashion as possible, viewed from a biological perspective. This summary in general follows the vertical organization of Table 3, beginning with physiological stimuli, and ends with a brief discussion of regulated PTHrP secretion.

The physiological stimuli are presented only briefly in this section because they are covered in detail in later sections on potential biological functions of PTHrP in skin, breast, and smooth muscle (see separate sections below under Physiological Functions of PTHrP). Suckling has been found to elicit a rapid and transient increase in PTHrP gene expression in lactating mammary tissue in the rat (22). This response can be reproduced by prolactin administration early in lactation (88), but the more sustained increase in PTHrP mRNA levels seen late in lactation seems to require some additional stimulus (89). A large peak in PTHrP mRNA and peptide content has been observed in rat myometrium in the 48 hr immediately preceding parturition, and this was found to be dependent on uterine occupancy by the fetoplacental unit (i.e., it was not seen in an unoccupied uterine horn at the same stage of gestation) (51). It has subsequently become clear that this response can be reproduced quite exactly by balloon-induced stretch of the uterus (90). As is shown in Fig. 11, stretch has also been found to increase PTHrP mRNA expression in the urinary bladder (52). Similar phenomena may be occurring in the human amnion late in pregnancy (91) and in the chicken oviduct during the egg-laying cycle (92). In the amnion, PTHrP mRNA declines severalfold after membrane rupture (i.e., with decreasing stretch), and in the isthmus and shell gland of the chicken oviduct PTHrP localizes to the smooth muscle of the oviduct and its vascular supply (i.e., perhaps reflecting stretch or increased blood flow, respectively). Differentiation, either spontaneous or induced (see Table 3), has been found to be associated with a modest but sustained increase in PTHrP mRNA in cultured mouse embryonal carcinoma cells (62), rat insulinoma cells (93), and human keratinocytes (34). A similar increase has been seen in the developing trophoectoderm cells in embryogenesis in the mouse (61).

Both glucocorticoids and $1,25(OH)_2D$ have been found to produce a sustained inhibition of basal PTHrP gene transcription in a number of cell types (Fig. 12) (34,45,67,69,70,93). One or the other steroid has also

TABLE 3. *Regulation of PTHrP gene expression*

Agent	Tissue or cell type	PTHrP mRNA[a]	PTHrP content[a]	PTHrP secretion[a]	Mechanism[b]	References
Physiological stimuli						
Suckling	Lactating breast (rat)	↑	↑			22
Uterine occupancy	Myometrium (rat)	↑	↑			51
Stretch	Myometrium (rat)	↑	↑			90
Stretch	Urinary bladder (rat)	↑				52
?Stretch	Amnion (human)	↑	↑			91
Egg-laying cycle	Oviduct (chicken)	↑	↑			92
Differentiation	Embryonal carcinoma (mouse)	↑				61,62
Differentiation	Insulinoma (rat)	↑			?Tx	93
Differentiation	Keratinocyte (human)	↑				34
Differentiation	Trophoectoderm (mouse)		↑			61
Pharmacological stimuli						
Glucocorticoids	Medullary carcinoma (human)	↓			Tx	67
Glucocorticoids	Carcinoid (human)	↓			Tx	69
Glucocorticoids	Insulinoma (rat)	↓				93
Glucocorticoids	Aortic smooth muscle (rat)	↓				53
Glucocorticoids	Keratinocyte (rat)	↓				70
$1,25\text{-}(OH)_2D$	Medullary carcinoma (human)	↓			Tx	67
$1,25\text{-}(OH)_2D$	Keratinocyte (human)	↓			Tx (transfection)	34
$1,25\text{-}(OH)_2D$	Fetal long bones (rat)			↑		96
$1,25\text{-}(OH)_2D$	Keratinocyte (rat)	↓				70
$22\text{-oxa-}1,25\text{-}(OH)_2D$	T cell (MT-2) (human)	↓		↓	Tx	94
EB-1089	Leydig cell tumor (rat)	↓		↓		95
Estrogen	Uterus (rat)	↑			Tx	97
Estrogen	Pituitary, hypothalmus (rat)	↑				55
Estrogen	Myometrial cell (rat)	↑				98
Estrogen	Pituitary GH_4C_1 (rat)	↑			Tx	42
Estrogen	Kidney (monkey)	↑			Tx (cotransfection)	35
Serum	Insulinoma (rat)	↑				93
Serum	Keratinocyte (human)	↑		↑	Tx (transfection)	34
Serum	Keratinocyte (human)			↑		99
Serum	Keratinocyte (rat)	↑		↑		70
Serum	Aortic smooth muscle (rat)	↑	↑	↑		53
Growth factors	Keratinocyte (human)	↑		↑	Tx (transfection)	34
EGF	Osteosarcoma (human)	↑		↑		100
EGF	Keratinocyte (rat)	↑				70
EGF	Mammary epithelial (human)	↑		↑		101
IGF-I	Mammary epithelium (human)	↑		↑		101
TGFβ	Renal carcinoma (human)	↑			post-Tx	102
TGFβ	Myometrial (human)	↑	↑			103
TGFβ	Endometrial (human)	↑	↑			103
TGFβ	Keratinocyte (rat)	↑				70
Prolactin	Mammary gland (rat)	↑				88
Cycloheximide	Multiple (rat and human)	↑			Tx and post-Tx	68
Cycloheximide	Osteosarcoma (human)	↑				100
Cycloheximide	Insulinoma (rat)	↑				93
Cycloheximide	Keratinocyte (rat)	↑				70
Tax	T cells (human)	↑			Tx (transfection)	83
Tax	T cells (human)	—			Tx (transfection)	84
Forskolin	Neuroendocrine (human)	—		↑		106
Forskolin	T cell (MT-2) (human)	↑		↑	Tx (transfection)	107
Calcitonin	Squamous carcinoma (human)			↑		104
Calcitonin	Squamous carcinoma (human)	↑			Tx (transfection)	33
Calcitonin	Unspecified	↑			Tx (transfection)	105
Phorbol ester	Neuroendocrine (human)	—		↑		106
Phorbol ester	Osteosarcoma (human)	↑		↑		100
Phorbol ester	T cells (human)	↑			Tx (transfection)	84
Phorbol ester	Carcinoid (human)			↑		108
Endothelin-I	Aortic smooth muscle (rat)	↑				53
Thrombin	Aortic smooth muscle (rat)	↑				53
Angiotensin II	Aortic smooth muscle (rat)	↑			?Tx and post-Tx	109,232
Ionomycin	Carcinoid (human)			↑		108
$Chromogranin_{1-40}$	Squamous carcinoma (human)			↓		104
Calcium	Leydig cell tumor (rat)			↑		110
Calcium	Parathyroid (PTr) (rat)			↓		45,111
Calcium	Parathyroid (bovine)			—		66

[a]Designations: ↑, increased; ↓, decreased; —, no change.

[b]Abbreviations: Tx, transcriptional; post-Tx, posttranscriptional; transfection, studied by transient transfection; ?, mechanism not studied.

Filling

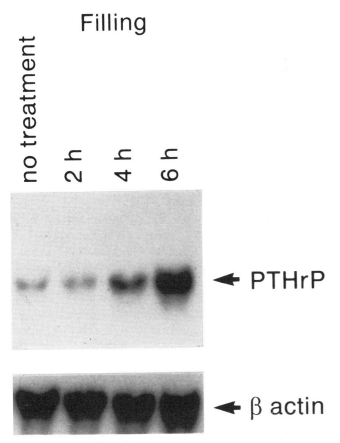

FIG. 11. PTHrP mRNA expression in rat urinary bladder as a function of increasing distention. RNA was prepared from bladder of control rats or rats following urethral ligation for 2, 4, and 6 hr. (Reprinted from ref. 52 with permission. Photograph courtesy of M. Thiede.)

been reported to blunt or block the effects of various agonists (e.g., serum in rat aortic smooth muscle cells) (34,45,93), although this is not a uniform observation (70). An interesting twist on the vitamin D response has been use of "noncalcemic" analogs of vitamin D in attempt to decrease PTHrP mRNA and PTHrP secretion in HTLV-1-infected MT-2 cells and the rat HMM-associated Leydig cell tumor (94,95); these findings hold therapeutic promise but are preliminary. In contrast, 1,25(OH)$_2$D has been reported to increase PTHrP content in medium conditioned by fetal rat long bones in culture, but nothing is known concerning the cell of origin in this system (96). Estrogens have been found to produce a rapid and transient increase in PTHrP mRNA in rat uterus, pituitary, and hypothalamus in vivo (55,97) and in rat GH$_4$C$_1$ pituitary cells in vitro (42); this effect seems to be transcriptional (35,42). In contrast, the estrogen-induced increase in PTHrP mRNA seen in cultured rat myometrial cells appears to be of slower onset and is sustained for at least 5 days (98). As was summarized above, the 5'-flanking region of the PTHrP gene bears a number of hormone response element half-sites, but it does not contain any consensus 15-base response elements. At the same time, it should be noted that "minus" glucocorticoid and vitamin D response elements are much less well defined than the classical "positive" response elements.

Serum, epidermal growth factor (EGF), and insulin-like growth factor type I (IGF-I) have been reported to increase PTHrP mRNA and/or peptide secretion in a variety of cell types, including keratinocytes, rat insulinoma cells, human osteosarcoma cells, and rat aortic smooth muscle cells (34,70,83,99–101). All these examples share a common pattern of PTHrP mRNA response, namely, rapid induction–deinduction kinet-

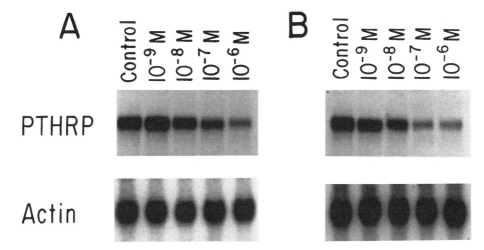

FIG. 12. Dose-dependent regulation of PTHrP mRNA expression in a human C-cell line by dexamethasone (**A**) and 1,25-dihydroxyvitamin D (**B**). PTHrP mRNA was assayed by RNase protection analysis and actin mRNA by Northern analysis. (Reprinted from ref. 67 with permission.)

ics, with a peak within minutes to several hours and a rapid decline thereafter (Fig. 13) (34,45,70,100,101). When it has been studied, this response seems to be transcriptional, but the PTHrP gene does not contain a serum response element of the *c-fos*/β-actin type (34). Transforming growth factor-β (TGFβ), on the other hand, has been found to produce an entirely different kinetic response. In human renal carcinoma cells and in human myometrial and endometrial cells in primary culture, this agent has been shown to elicit a slower PTHrP mRNA response that peaks at 12–24 hr and seems to be sustained (102,103). In the renal carcinoma cell system, this sustained increase in PTHrP mRNA appears to be due, at least in part, to a posttranscriptional effect (i.e., a stabilization of PTHrP mRNA) (102). Cycloheximide (and other protein synthesis inhibitors) increase or "superinduce" PTHrP mRNA in a number of cell types (68,70, 93,100). This response is in large part posttranscriptional and reflects the effect of protein synthesis inhibition on the ARE-mediated instability pathway (68); the exact mechanism of this effect is unknown. The cycloheximide response also has a transcriptional component, and this is presumed to be due to inhibition of the synthesis of a labile repressor of PTHrP gene transcription (68). This is in keeping with the negative regulation of basal PTHrP gene transcriptional summarized above.

Calcitonin and forskolin have been found to increase PTHrP mRNA and PTHrP secretion in several cell types (33,104–107). These effects appear to be transcriptional on the basis of both nuclear runoff analysis and transient transfection experiments and are presumed to be mediated by the cAMP response elements in the 5'-flanking region of the PTHrP gene (see above) (33,107). Phorbol esters also have been reported to increase PTHrP mRNA and/or secretion in several cell types (84,100,106,108), and one preliminary study suggests that this response may be transcriptional (84). As a group, agonists for smooth muscle contraction appear to increase PTHrP mRNA expression (53,109), an interesting finding that is discussed below.

It is clear from the information summarized above that there exist two quite characteristic patterns of PTHrP mRNA response, one having rapid induction–deinduction kinetics and the second representing a more prolonged, plateau response. The rapid response characterizes the effects of (a) estrogen on the uterus, pituitary, and hypothalamus in vivo (55,97) and also on GH$_4$C$_1$ cells in vitro (42); (b) suckling and prolactin on mammary tissue in vivo (22,88); (c) serum, EGF, and IGF-I on a variety of cells in vitro (34,70,100,101); and (d) a putative labile repressor protein in a number of cell types in vitro (68). The plateau pattern is seen (a) in the rat myometrium at term (51); (b) in the rat uterus (90) and bladder (52) following mechanical stretch or distension; (c) in response to estrogen in rat myometrial cells in primary culture (98); (d) following differentiation of keratinocytes, islet cells, and F9 mouse embryonal carcinoma stem cells (34,62,93); and (e) in response to TGFβ treatment of human renal carcinoma cells and of human endometrial and myometrial cells in primary culture (102,103). The different mechanisms responsible for these two patterns of response are only beginning to be understood (see below).

A number of investigators have commented on the similarity of the rapid PTHrP gene response to classical protooncogene and growth factor early gene responses (42,53,70,93,97), but the mechanisms and criteria for distinguishing between a primary and a secondary response gene have not in general been carefully examined. The characteristics of a primary response or immediate early gene (112,113) include the following: (a) expression is low or undetectable in unstimulated cells; (b) expression is rapidly induced at a transcriptional level by mechanisms that are independent of new protein synthesis; (c) this induction is transient; (d) the subsequent cessation or shut-off of transcription requires new protein synthesis; and (e) the transcribed mRNA typically has a very short half-life (113). All five of these criteria have been met experimentally only in the case of estrogen stimulation of PTHrP mRNA expression in rat GH$_4$C$_1$ cells (42), but it is likely that they would also be met, if examined, in most of the other rapid-response systems described in the previous paragraph. One of the more interesting of these criteria in a mechanistic sense is criterion d, involving the induction of a repressor that

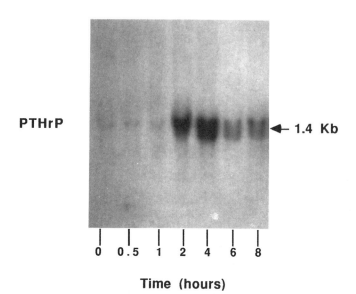

PTHrP ← **1.4 Kb**

0   0.5   1   2   4   6   8

Time (hours)

FIG. 13. Time course of PTHrP mRNA expression in rat aortic smooth muscle cells following exposure to serum. (Reprinted from ref. 53 with permission. Photograph courtesy of T. Clemens.)

mediates the rapid poststimulation inhibition of transcription and that is specific for the stimulus and gene in question (113). At a given new rate of transcription, a short mRNA half-life decreases the time required to reach a new steady-state concentration of mRNA and also reduces this concentration (20) but cannot account in itself for a transient response; this requires an additional mechanism, namely, transcriptional inhibition (113). The details of this phenomenon are not well understood with the exception of the *c-fos* gene, in which case it is the Fos protein that inhibits *c-fos* gene transcription, in a form of autoregulation (114). Clearly, this type of transcriptional control combined with the rapid dissipation of the mRNA provides mechanisms for very fine regulation of gene expression.

The above discussion is intended to establish the credentials of the PTHrP gene as a primary response gene in selected circumstances and also to introduce feedback transcriptional inhibition as an important mechanism that might explain, in part, the two kinetic patterns of PTHrP mRNA response. In fact, given the information summarized in the previous paragraph, a sustained or plateau PTHrP mRNA response would be anticipated in two circumstances: (a) when feedback transcriptional inhibition does not come into play after a given stimulus and/or (b) when there is an induced stabilization of PTHrP mRNA. These mechanisms represent a very important area for future work. The physiological implications of viewing the PTHrP gene as a primary response gene are not entirely clear, although this characterization is certainly compatible with growing evidence that the peptide acts in a predominantly paracrine and/or autocrine fashion.

The question of whether PTHrP is processed, stored, and subsequently subject to regulated secretion as is the case for PTH was touched on in the early portions of this section. Although PTHrP secretion was measured in a number of the studies summarized in Table 3, in many instances early time points were not examined, and clear criteria for separating regulated secretion from other potential effects were not established (34,45,70,99–101,103,104,106,107). The most convincing single example of regulated secretion is the stimulation of PTHrP secretion by ionomycin and/or phorbol esters in human carcinoid cells; here, an increase in PTHrP secretion was seen within minutes of stimulation, and this effect was uninhibited by actinomycin D or cycloheximide (108). Additional supporting examples are the stimulation of PTHrP secretion by calcium in rat Leydig tumor cells (110) and the inhibition of phorbol-induced PTHrP secretion in human squamous carcinoma (BEN) cells by chromogranin A_{1-40} (104). Calcium has only a modest effect on PTHrP secretion by PT-r cells (45,111) and no effect in cultured bovine parathyroid cells (66). On bal-

ance, it seems clear that PTHrP in some vesicular compartment can be mobilized to the cell surface by selected secretagogues, at least in certain cell types. It is not clear, however, how one is to envision regulated secretion in the context of the elaborate checks and balances that have been put in place to regulate PTHrP mRNA expression, that is, why such elaborate mechanisms would exist for a molecule that is destined to be stored in any quantity. Perhaps the seeming contradictions here are more apparent than real, and both constitutive and regulated secretion will be found to be physiologically important in specific cell populations. This is an area that requires much more critical work.

POSTTRANSLATIONAL PROCESSING OF PARATHYROID HORMONE-RELATED PROTEIN

As soon as the three cDNA-predicted PTHrP amino acid sequences became available, it was clear that PTHrP was likely to undergo extensive posttranslational processing and might serve as a prohormone or polyprotein from which a family of peptide hormones could be derived. Work in progress in a number of laboratories has shown that this is indeed the case. This section reviews both documented as well as speculative steps in the posttranslational processing of PTHrP. The reader is referred to Fig. 14 throughout this section.

Signal Peptide Cleavage

The mature PTHrP sequence is preceded by a 36-amino-acid putative "leader" or "prepro-" sequence. The amino-terminal region of this sequence has the features of a classic signal peptide in that it begins with methionine, has a short, charged amino acid domain, and is followed by a strikingly hydrophobic 10–15-amino-acid domain consisting of leucine, valine, phenylalanine, alanine, and tyrosine (115). While this has yet to be documented by pulse-chase metabolic labeling studies, it would appear that the first 20–30 amino acids of PTHrP represent a signal peptide that is important in guiding the nascent peptide from the cytosolic compartment through the rough endoplasmic reticulum lipid bilayer into the interior of the rough endoplasmic reticulum cistern (115). As occurs with other secretory peptides, it is presumed that cleavage of the signal peptide is a cotranslational event, accomplished in the endoplasmic reticulum by the endoproteolytic enzyme complex signal peptidase (115). The exact site of the cleavage within the peptide is unknown, but is likely to be somewhere in the -15 to -5 region (Fig. 14).

A.

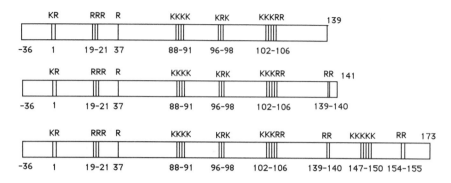

B.

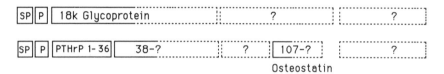

C.

FIG. 14. Posttranslational processing of PTHrP. **A:** The three cDNA-predicted PTHrP initial translation products, each containing a "signal" or "prepro-" peptide (from amino acid −36 to amino acid −1) and, thereafter, mature PTHrPs of 139, 141, or 173 amino acids. These isoforms are identical through amino acid 139 but have different carboxy termini. The regions that are rich in basic amino acids and that are believed to represent posttranslational endoproteolytic processing sites are indicated by *K* (for lysine) and *R* (for arginine). The prolines that are candidate sites for carboxy-terminal amidation are in positions 86 and 94. **B:** Functional domains of PTHrP. These include a signal peptide (*SP*) and a "pro-peptide" (*P*) domain, as described in the text. The "PTH-like" region, "conserved," and "unique" regions are also described in the text. **C:** Secretory forms of PTHrP that have been postulated or actually shown to exist (see text).

Propeptide Cleavage

No direct experimental evidence documents the existence of a PTHrP propeptide segment. On the other hand, the circumstantial evidence that such a peptide exists is overwhelming. As was discussed above, one must assume, by analogy to a wide variety of other secretory peptides, that signal peptidase releases a nascent pro-PTHrP by cleavage in the −15 to −5 region of the peptide following the hydrophobic leader sequence. However, the mature PTHrP peptide, as purified in three independent laboratories (116–118), begins with alanine at position +1. Moreover, as has also been shown in the case of PTH (reviewed in 119), amino acid substitutions and deletions in the 1 and 2 positions of PTHrP markedly diminish bioactivity (120). Thus direct sequencing data from three independent laboratories as well as functional data indicate that the mature peptide begins with alanine in position 1.

Further evidence for the existence of a propeptide is the finding from the PTHrP cDNA sequence that amino acids −2 and −1 are lysine and arginine, a dibasic motif used in a number of peptides, including insulin, albumin, PTH, and POMC, as a site of propeptide cleavage (115,121). As is shown in Fig. 2 and discussed above, this dibasic cleavage site is carried on the exon that encodes the bulk of the coding region, as is the case for the PTH gene. The cellular location in which propeptide cleavage occurs may be the Golgi apparatus or it may be secretory granules, depending on the peptide and cell in question. The cellular function of the propeptide in the case of PTHrP is unknown.

Parathyroid Hormone-Related Protein-(1–36)

With the availability of the cDNA-predicted amino acid sequences for PTHrP, a number of groups proceeded to synthesize amino-terminal PTHrP fragments for use in bioassays, in receptor binding studies, and in immunoassay development (122,123). Generally, peptides including the 1–34, 1–36, and 1–40 sequence were synthesized, although both shorter and longer peptides were synthesized or expressed in bacteria by some investigators (122–125). The selection of the short amino-terminal PTHrPs described above was based not on biochemical evidence of their existence in nature but on the presumption that bioactive PTHrP would be similar to bioactive PTH (1–34) in structure. Alanine was selected as amino acid 1 in synthetic PTHrPs for the reasons outlined in the preceding section. The 1–13 region was included because of the striking homology of this region with PTH, also described above. The 14–34 region was included for two reasons. First, it includes the 19–21 tribasic region that appears to be analogous to tribasic amino acids 25–27 in the PTH sequence, which are believed to be important in the binding of PTH to its receptor (126). Second, based on the extensive structure–function work previously carried out with the PTH molecule (119,126), one would assume that a PTHrP peptide comparable in length to PTH-(1–34) would be biologically active.

Recently, Soifer et al. (12) have shown that the single arginine at position 37 is a cleavage site and that PTHrP-(1–36) is in fact a mature form of the peptide (Fig. 14). This was shown through purification techniques using anti-PTHrP-(37–74) affinity columns, which identified a midregion PTHrP species that begins at alanine 38 of the cDNA-predicted sequence. Interestingly, cleavage of proneuroendocrine peptides and growth factors at single arginine residues is very common. Approximately 90 such sites have been demonstrated to date and exist in peptides such as somatostatin, atrial natriuretic peptide, dynorphin, IGF-I, IGF-II, pancreatic polypeptide, cholecystokinin, vasopressin, growth hormone-releasing hormone, EGF, the molluscan egg-laying hormone, and others (128, 129). Most often, as is the case for PTHrP, the single arginine is followed either by alanine or by a serine. In most cases, the cleavage is carboxy-terminal to arginine, and, in many and probably most instances, the carboxy-terminal arginine is subsequently cleaved by a carboxypeptidase E-like enzyme (reviewed in 130). This would yield, in the case of PTHrP, a mature 1–36 form of the peptide.

The monobasic prohormone cleaving enzyme (or enzymes) that accomplishes these cleavages has not been identified. A number of candidate enzymes have been partially purified from anglerfish islets (for somatostatin) (131), intestinal mucosa (also for somatostatin) (132,133), and cardiac atria (for atrial natriuretic peptide) (134). These enzymes appear to bear no relationship to the subtilisin family of prohormone converting enzymes (121,129,135,136), which cleave precursor peptides at dibasic and tetrabasic residues.

Midregion Parathyroid Hormone-Related Protein Species

The studies of Soifer et al. (127) described above confirm the existence of a midregion species of PTHrP that begins at alanine 38 (Fig. 14). This peptide was found in extracts of PTHrP-producing cell lines as well

as in protease-protected conditioned medium. That is, the midregion peptide was found both within cells during processing and storage and outside of cells following secretion. The complete structure of the midregion peptide is unknown at present, but, by sodium dodecyl sulfate-polyacrylamide electrophoresis (SDS-PAGE), it appears to have a molecular mass of ~7,000 Daltons. This suggests that the midregion peptide would contain ~50–70 amino acids and this would place its carboxy terminus in the 80–108 region of the predicted sequence. This region is rich in tetrabasic putative processing sites (Fig. 14), which would be ideal substrates for members of the subtilisin/KEX-2 family of dibasic and tetrabasic processing enzymes, such as furin, PC-2, and PC-1/3 (121,129,135,136). Work in progress is aimed at determining the precise carboxy terminus of the midregion peptide.

The midregion peptide appears to be packaged into secretory granules both in rat insulinoma cells and in renal carcinoma cells (127). This is in contrast to amino-terminal PTHrP peptides, as assessed by histochemical techniques, which appear predominantly in the Golgi apparatus (127). These findings suggest that midregion and amino-terminal PTHrP fragments are packaged and secreted separately. This is unusual; only one other example exists (molluscan egg-laying hormone) in which distinct regions of a single peptide are sorted into both the regulated and the constitutive secretory pathways (115). Furthermore, these findings imply that the cleavage at arginine 37 occurs in the Golgi apparatus or the trans-Golgi network, prior to the budding of secretory granules.

Several lines of evidence suggest that the midregion peptide will prove to be an important product in functional or physiological terms, rather than simply a biosynthetic intermediate. Perhaps the most important piece of evidence in this regard is the striking interspecies evolutionary conservation of this region. For example, a putative human 38–108 peptide would differ in only two amino acids from its rat and mouse counterparts (22,26) and in only 11 amino acids from the corresponding chicken sequence (28). At present, however, the function of the midregion PTHrP species is unknown. The work of Care et al. (137), using a pregnant ewe model, indicates that a midregion fragment may play a role in the placental transport of calcium from the maternal to fetal circulation (137,138) (see discussion below under Placental Calcium Transport).

Carboxy-Terminal Parathyroid Hormone-Related Protein Species

Examination of the carboxy-terminal sequences of PTHrP-(1–139), -(1–141), and -(1–173) suggests that an additional carboxy-terminal PTHrP species may exist

(Fig. 14). This possibility is supported by three observations. First, the data described above suggest that the midregion PTHrP secretory species likely ends at one of the three multibasic amino acid clusters at amino acids 88–91, 96–98, or 102–106. A cleavage at any of these sites would mandate that a carboxy-terminal PTHrP fragment be created. Second, the sequences of human, mouse, rat, and chicken PTHrP through residue 111 are extremely well conserved, as is discussed in some detail below. This degree of conservation would imply that conserved carboxy-terminal determinants may have functional importance. Third, based on these considerations, Fenton and collaborators (139,140) from Australia have synthesized PTHrP-(107–111) and -(107–139) peptides. These particular peptides were selected for synthesis with the presumed subtilisin processing protease cleavage site at amino acids 102–106 in mind, together with the evolutionary conservation of the 107–111 region mentioned above. Interestingly, these peptides, but not control peptides with similar sequences, have proven to be potent inhibitors of osteoclastic bone resorption in isolated osteoclast assays and in rat long bone organ culture. Fenton et al. (139,140) propose that a carboxy-terminal region of PTHrP that includes PTHrP-(107–111) be named *osteostatin* to reflect its potent resorption-inhibiting capability. If the "osteostatin" idea is confirmed, a scenario arises in which a PTH-like bone resorption-enhancing peptide is encoded by the 1–36 region of the parent peptide and a separate bone resorption-inhibiting peptide is encoded by the 107–111 region. These studies suggest that PTHrP biological activity may be regulated at the posttranslational level by the degree to which the precursor peptide is processed to yield functional and counterbalancing amino- and carboxy-terminal peptides. Whether opposing or counterbalancing amino- and carboxy-terminal peptides will be found to exist in tissues other than bone remains largely unexplored. It is possible, as was suggested by the studies of Kaiser et al. (142), that amino-terminal PTHrP species stimulate proliferation of keratinocytes, while carboxy-terminal species inhibit this process. Clarification of this issue must await further study.

In closing this section, two cautionary notes are in order. First, Sone and collaborators (141) have been unable to reproduce the antiresorptive effects of "osteostatin." The reason for this discrepancy is at present unclear but may relate to the fact that Sone et al. studied osteostatin in a neonatal mouse calvarial system, whereas Fenton et al. employed different systems. Second, it is important to emphasize that the studies of Fenton et al. were based on a synthetic peptide that has yet to be shown to exist in nature. One report by Imamura et al. (143) suggests that a PTHrP peptide with 127–141 immunoreactivity is excreted in the urine of humans and mice with HHM, but the precise sequence of this peptide is unknown. Similarly, preliminary work by dePapp et al. (144) suggests that a separate carboxy-terminal PTHrP fragment is secreted by a variety of human and animal cell lines.

Extreme Carboxy-Terminal "Tail-Region" Parathyroid Hormone-Related Protein Peptide

The possible existence of an extreme carboxy-terminal PTHrP species derived from the 173–amino-acid isoform of the peptide is suggested by three observations. First, in humans, three distinct PTHrP primary translation products, or isoforms, have evolved, the longest of which contains this "tail region." The 1–140 region of the 1–173 peptide is redundant with PTHrP-(1–139) and -(1–141). Thus the only unique portion of this peptide is the 141–173 region encoded by exon 5 of the human gene (Fig. 1). This region does not exist in rodent or avian species (see above) and might therefore have unique physiological effects in primates. Second, the dibasic arginine site at 139–140 of the 1–173 product would appear to be a typical subtilisin-type protease cleavage site such as exists, for example, in insulin and POMC, both of which are cleaved at arginine–arginine dibasic sites (115,121). Such a cleavage would generate a PTHrP species beginning at amino acid 141. Third, two investigators have found evidence for PTHrP-(141–173) peptides in human tissues. Burtis et al. (145), using a sensitive radioimmunoassay for the 141–173 region of PTHrP, have shown that a peptide that contains epitopes in this domain is present in human milk as well as in the supernatants of cultured human keratinocytes and human renal, squamous, and prostate carcinomas. This peptide has not yet been further characterized. Along similar lines, Brandt and colleagues (19) have shown that a PTHrP species recognized by a monoclonal antibody directed to the PTHrP-(140–173) region is present in human amniotic membranes. Again, a note of caution should be included here. While this circumstantial evidence suggests the existence of an extreme carboxy-terminal PTHrP species, the actual existence of such a fragment has yet to be documented. The functional role of such a peptide is at present entirely speculative.

Posttranslational O-Linked Glycosylation

The first nonmalignant human cell type demonstrated to produce and secrete PTHrP was the epidermal keratinocyte (37). With the advent of immunoaffinity purification techniques for PTHrP, it was therefore natural to examine the secretory forms of PTHrP produced by normal human epidermal keratinocytes. When keratinocyte-conditioned medium was harvested under protease-protected conditions and subjected to affinity purification on an anti-PTHrP-(1–36) antibody column, the purified amino-terminal

PTHrP species was shown by SDS-PAGE to migrate with a molecular weight of 18,000 Daltons (146). This affinity-purified PTHrP migrated not as a discrete sharp band but rather as a broad protein band characteristic of a glycoprotein. The glycoprotein nature of this product was confirmed by treating the purified peptide with the peptide deglycosylating agent trifluoromethanesulfonic acid (TFMS), which deglycosylated the aminoterminal keratinocyte-derived PTHrP species to yield a core or backbone peptide with a molecular weight of $\sim$10,000 (Fig. 14) (146). Since the keratinocyte-derived glycoprotein was bioactive in an adenylyl cyclase bioassay, it is apparent that the amino terminus of the peptide is intact; that is, it begins with alanine as amino acid 1. The Mr of 10,000 for the core protein would predict a peptide of 85–100 amino acids, which would put the carboxy terminus of this peptide in the multibasic region described earlier.

Examination of the cDNA-predicted PTHrP sequence reveals an absence of consensus sequences for N-glycosylation. Thus it is presumed that the glycosylation of PTHrP is based on O-glycosylation. The precise amino acids that are glycosylated are currently unknown. However, since each of the three research groups that sequenced the N terminus of purified PTHrPs correctly identified the serine and threonine residues in the first 20–30 amino acids, it is unlikely that the glycosylation occurs in the amino-terminal region (glycosylated residues are not detected by routine sequencing techniques). It is therefore likely that glycosylation occurs in one of the clusters of serine and threonines in the midregion of the cDNA-predicted sequence.

O-linked glycosylation of peptide hormones typically occurs in the Golgi apparatus. The functional significance of O-glycosylation in the case of PTHrP is uncertain. It may be that O-glycosylation plays a role in the intracellular sorting or targeting of PTHrP (115,121). For example, in the case of POMC, the extent of glycosylation in a given tissue may regulate the site at which subsequent proteolytic cleavages occur (115,121), or, as in the case of human chorionic gonadotropin (hCG) and erythropoietin, O-glycosylation may play a role in prolonging peptide half-life in plasma and may thereby enhance the bioactivity of glycosylated forms of the peptide (147,150). It is at present uncertain whether the ability to O-glycosylate PTHrP is unique to keratinocytes or whether other cells that secrete PTHrP may also secrete glycosylated forms of the peptide.

Carboxy-Terminal Amidation of Parathyroid Hormone-Related Protein Fragments

The carboxy-terminus of PTHrP may consist of either a free carboxyl group or an amide group. Car-

boxy-terminal amidation of neuroendocrine peptides has been proved to be extremely common. Examples include POMC-derived peptides, oxytocin, vasopressin, chromogranin A-derived peptides, gastrin, cholecystokinin, corticotropin-releasing hormone, calcitonin gene-related peptide, thyrotrophin-releasing hormone, secretin, and many others (115,121,151). In fact, more than one-half of neuroendocrine peptides are amidated at their carboxy termini (115,121,151). In the past several years, major advances in the understanding of carboxy-terminal amidation have been made. The consensus sequence for carboxy-terminal amidation is X-gly-dibasic, where X indicates any amino acid. This "X" amino acid will ultimately become the amidated amino acid in the completely processed peptide. The dibasic amino acids are usually lysine–arginine or arginine–arginine and, as was mentioned above, are presumed, or in some cases documented, cleavage sites for members of the subtilisin-like family of endoproteolytic processing enzymes. The enzymes that lead to carboxy-terminal amidation have been identified through the work of Bradbury et al. (152), Eipper and Mains (151), and other investigators (153–155). It is now clear that amidation occurs via the actions of the enzyme peptidyl-α-amidating-monooxygenase (PAM). This enzyme contains two separate catalytic domains, which act in sequence. The first is peptidyl-glycine-amino-hydroxylating-monooxygenase (PHM), and the second is peptidyl-α-hydroxyglycine-alpha amidating lyase (PAL). PAM is the only peptide-processing enzyme known to include two distinct enzymatic activities. PAM acts on peptides that have previously been cleaved at dibasic sites by members of the subtilisin-like/KEX-2 protease family discussed above that have had their carboxy-terminal basic residues trimmed by carboxypeptidase. PAM is then free, in essence, to cleave all but the amino group of the carboxy-terminal glycine and leave the new carboxy-terminal amino acid, the "X" amino acid, with a carboxy-terminal amide derived from the α-amino group of glycine. The deaminated glycine becomes glyoxalate.

PAM is expressed in a broad range of tissues (115,121,152–155). Initially, it was presumed that its expression was limited to the central nervous system (CNS) and to classical neuroendocrine tissues such as the pituitary, thyroid parafollicular cells, adrenal medulla, testis, parathyroid, and pancreatic islet. More recently, it has become apparent that cells not classically regarded as neuroendocrine cell types, including renal medullary cells, salivary gland cells, intestinal epithelial cells, osteoblasts, and Chinese hamster ovarian (CHO) fibroblasts, and even plasma, also contain PAM protein and enzymatic activity.

Carboxy-terminal amidation is required for full potency of most amidated peptides. For example, non-amidated forms of corticotropin-releasing hormone

(CRH), cholecystokinin (CCK), and gastrin are orders of magnitude less potent than their amidated counterparts (115,121,152,156). Synthetic carboxy-terminal amidation of PTH-(1–34), a peptide that is not normally amidated, yields a peptide that is approximately ten times more potent than the nonamidated natural form of the peptide (157). In some cases, carboxy-terminal amidation is tissue-specific. For example, gastrin synthesized in the gastric antrum is amidated, whereas the same peptide is not amidated in the pituitary, where it is also normally produced (158).

In the case of PTHrP, there are two potential carboxy-terminal amidation signals. The first is Pro^{86}, Gly^{87}, Lys^{88}, Lys^{89}, Lys^{90}, Lys^{91} and the second is Pro^{94}, Gly^{95}, Lys^{96}, Arg^{97}, Lys^{98} (Fig. 14). These sites are slightly atypical in that the glycine is followed not by a dibasic pair of amino acids but by tetrabasic and tribasic motifs. No evidence yet exists to indicate that either of the two proline sites is, in fact, amidated. Indeed, there is no evidence that either of the two basic clusters at 88–92 or 96–98 is actually an endoproteolytic processing site. On the other hand, given the frequency with which neuroendocrine peptides are amidated, the two consensus signals for carboxy-terminal amidation, and the widespread tissue distribution of both PTHrP and PAM, it would perhaps be surprising if at least one of the two potential prolines was not amidated by one of the many tissues that produce PTHrP. At present, one can only guess at the functional consequences of carboxy-terminal amidation of a midregion fragment of PTHrP. That is an important area for future exploration.

Summary of Posttranslational Processing Parathyroid Hormone-Related Protein

As can be gleaned from the above sections, the regulation of PTHrP gene expression and peptide secretion is extraordinarily complex. Complexity exists at the level of tissue-specific transcriptional control, at the level of mRNA stability, and clearly at the level of posttranslational processing. Posttranslational processing can be viewed as yet another level of functional regulation of expression, which in this case results in multiple peptide species. To date, three secretory forms of PTHrP and two cleavage sites have been clearly documented. O-glycosylation in at least one cell type has also been documented. Counterbalancing or opposing functions of carboxy-terminal and amino-terminal fragments may also be operative. Furthermore, given the widespread tissue distribution of PTHrP, it would seem likely that tissue-specific processing of PTHrP, as occurs in a number of other neuroendocrine peptides, is likely. Studies aimed at clearly delineating the secretory forms of PTHrP are critical; one cannot carefully address its physiological

functions without having a clear idea of the actual secretory forms of this peptide.

UNIQUE RECEPTORS FOR PARATHYROID HORMONE-RELATED PROTEIN

There appears to be little question that the PTH-like effects of PTHrP on the kidney and on bone cells in patients with HHM are mediated through the PTH/PTHrP receptor, which has recently been characterized in molecular terms (see the chapter by Segre et al.) On the other hand, there is a mounting body of evidence suggesting that PTHrP may employ, in addition to the classical PTH receptor, its own unique receptors. Evidence for the existence of unique PTHrP receptors is both direct and circumstantial, and is discussed in this section.

Precedent

By simple precedent alone, it seems likely that PTHrP will prove to act through unique PTHrP receptors. With only two exceptions, this has been proved to be the case for every peptide hormone studied to date. These exceptions are hCG and luteinizing hormone (LH), which share a common receptor (159), and EGF and TGFα which also share a common receptor (160). By contrast, even closely related families of peptides (such as the enkephalins, insulin and the insulin-like growth factors, MSH and ACTH, prolactin and growth hormone, vasopressin, and oxytocin) employ distinct receptors for every member of the family (161–163). Often, as is the case for vasopressin, a single peptide employs not a single receptor but multiple receptor subtypes (163,164).

Differences Between the Clinical Syndromes of Primary Hyperparathyroidism and Humoral Hypercalcemia of Malignancy

These two clinical syndromes differ in three important ways. In HHM (a) the activity of renal 1-α-hydroxylase seems to be decreased, (b) bone formation is uncoupled from resorption, and (c) distal tubular calcium reabsorption is relatively diminished (5,123,165). These three discrepancies between the two clinical syndromes have yet to be explained in clear pathophysiological terms. While a number of explanations for these differences are possible (see full discussion in the chapter by Strewler and Nissenson) it is conceivable that they reflect in part the existence of PTH/PTHrP receptor subclasses. For example, it is possible that the actions of PTH and PTHrP in the proximal tubule to stimulate adenylyl cyclase and to inhibit phosphate reabsorption are mediated by a sub-class of PTH/PTHrP receptor that recognizes both PTH and PTHrP with equal affinity. By this scenario, the relative inability of PTHrP to stimulate renal 1-α-hydroxylase activity or to stimulate maximally distal tubular calcium reabsorption could be due to the existence of a subclass of PTH/PTHrP receptor that has a higher affinity for PTH than for PTHrP. Similar formulations can be constructed to explain the uncoupling of osteoblastic activity from osteoclastic activity in patients with HHM.

Parathyroid Hormone and Parathyroid Hormone-Related Protein Actions in "Nonclassical" Parathyroid Hormone Target Tissues

It is important to bear in mind that the "endocrine" or "systemic" actions of PTHrP on distant target tissues differ in the syndrome of HHM from the normal physiological circumstance, in which PTHrP appears to be produced by and to act on cells in an autocrine or paracrine fashion. Many of the cells now known to produce PTHrP (Tables 1 and 2) have been shown to have PTH-like ligand binding or to display physiological responses to PTH. For example, PTH-(1–34) has been known for some time (a) to stimulate mitogenesis in lymphocytes; (b) to stimulate adenylyl cyclase and cytosolic calcium uptake in islet cells, keratinocytes, and fibroblasts; (c) to relax vascular and uterine smooth muscle; and (d) to induce calcium fluxes across CNS synaptosomes (166–171). Before the identification of PTHrP in 1987, it was difficult to visualize a physiological scheme in which circulating PTH might serve as a regulator, for example, of lymphocyte proliferation or keratinocyte differentiation. With the identification of PTHrP as a product in a broad array of these same "nonclassical" PTH-responsive tissues, it seems very likely that PTHrP, not PTH, is the actual agonist for the receptors present on "nonclassical" PTH-responsive tissues. Logically, the receptors on these tissues would best be considered PTHrP, and not PTH, receptors.

Unique Actions of Parathyroid Hormone-Related Protein

The most direct evidence for the existence of a unique subclass of PTHrP receptors comes from studies in tissues or cell lines that display responses to PTHrP but are less responsive to PTH. For example, Insogna and collaborators (172,173) have shown that PTHrP has the ability to mimic the actions of transforming growth factor-β in fibroblasts (stimulation of large colony formation and of fibronectin synthesis) and that these actions are not shared by PTH. Rodda

and colleagues (138) have shown that PTHrP and not PTH stimulates calcium transport across the placenta.

More recently, using affinity crosslinking techniques, Orloff et al. (174) have shown that PTH and PTHrP bind to a cell membrane protein that is larger than the PTH receptor in human squamous carcinoma cell lines. Further, in benign keratinocytes and in malignant squamous carcinoma cell lines, PTHrP produces an increase in cytosolic calcium but not in cyclic AMP (174). Since other agonists, such as isoproterenol, stimulate adenylyl cyclase in these cell lines, it is apparent that these cells contain receptors that, like the PTH receptor, are coupled to protein kinase C but, unlike the PTH receptor, do not couple to adenylyl cyclase. McCauley et al. (175) and Gaich et al. (176) have recently reported very similar results in lymphocytes and in a pancreatic islet β cell line. These results argue for the existence of a unique receptor, at least in these three cell types, which both produce and respond to PTHrP.

Molecular Evidence for the Existence of Unique Parathyroid Hormone/Parathyroid Hormone-Related Protein Receptors or Receptor Isoforms

With the availability of the rat and human PTH/PTHrP receptor cDNAs, Urena et al. (177) have shown that certain tissues, such as rat testis, contain mRNA species that hybridize to PTH receptor DNA probes but that differ substantially in size from the PTH receptor mRNA seen in bone and kidney. Moreover, multiple hybridizing mRNA species are seen even in rat kidney, suggesting the possible existence of multiple renal PTH receptor subtypes or isoforms. Along similar lines, Orloff et al. (178) have shown that human PTH receptor probes hybridize to mRNA species in human squamous carcinomas and keratinocytes that are both larger and smaller than the prototypical PTH receptor transcript. Studies are in progress in both laboratories to determine whether these novel mRNA species are derived from the classical PTH/PTHrP receptor gene (e.g., by alternative splicing) or whether they represent novel PTHrP receptor mRNAs that are the product of a separate gene.

Receptors for Nonamino-Terminal Parathyroid Hormone-Related Protein Secretory Forms

Since PTHrP seems to undergo extensive posttranslational processing to yield a family of peptides that share no homology with other known peptides, it is likely that each of these products will be found to have its own unique receptor. That is, the midregion, carboxy-terminal, and extreme carboxy-terminal PTHrP species may well each prove to have its own cognate receptor. While no direct evidence for the existence of such receptors has yet been developed, it is implicit in the studies of Rodda et al. and Care et al. (137) on the effects of PTHrP(67–86)amide on placental calcium transport and the studies of Fenton et al. (140) on the effects of PTHrP-(107–111) or "osteostatin" on isolated osteoclasts that placental cells of some type have receptors for midregion PTHrP and that osteoclasts have receptors for "osteostatin." Given the unique sequences in question, there is no reason to suppose that these receptors would have any relationship to the classical bone/kidney PTH/PTHrP receptor. This area is explored more completely in the chapter by Murray et al.

PHYSIOLOGICAL FUNCTIONS OF PARATHYROID HORMONE-RELATED PROTEIN

Parathyroid Hormone-Related Protein as an Autocrine/Paracrine Factor in Skin

Squamous carcinomas are the prototypical PTHrP-producing tumor, and normal human keratinocytes were the first nonmalignant cells shown to secrete PTHrP (37). Human and rodent keratinocytes have been shown to produce PTHrP bioactivity and immunoreactivity in tissue culture (34,37,99,146,179), and the mRNA species encoding all three PTHrP isoforms have been detected in RNA prepared from human keratinocytes (12,17,180). More recently, PTHrP has been directly visualized in epidermal keratinocytes using immunohistochemical techniques (47,48,181). Although PTHrP immunoreactivity can be detected throughout the epidermis, some data suggest that there may be relatively greater quantities in the outer, more differentiated layers of the epidermis (47,48,181). PTHrP has been demonstrated in keratinocytes from human skin biopsies (47,48,181), in both adult and fetal keratinocytes (59), and, interestingly, in the fetal amniotic membrane (91), which, through the umbilical cord, is contiguous with the fetal epidermal keratinocyte layer.

With respect to posttranslational processing of PTHrP, at least three distinct PTHrP species have been shown to be produced by keratinocytes. As was noted above, a 10,000 Da amino-terminal O-glycosylated form of the peptide (5), a midregion species beginning at amino acid 38 (127), and a short, 36-amino-acid, amino-terminal form of the peptide (127) have been demonstrated to exist in cultured keratinocytes (Fig. 14). Immunohistochemical studies have shown that PTHrP species with amino-terminal and midregion epitopes are present in keratinocytes in vivo as well as in vitro (47). It is likely that carboxy-terminal PTHrP species with either or both of (109–141) and (141–173) immunoreactivities will be identified in keratinocytes as the posttranslational processing of PTHrP is studied further.

The levels of PTHrP mRNA expression and/or peptide secretion by cultured human keratinocytes have been shown to be subject to regulation by a number of factors. As with the histochemistry described above, this is a rapidly unfolding field, and in some cases results in these initial studies appear to conflict. Data from several studies indicate that PTHrP expression is inhibited by 1,25-(OH)$_2$D in normal cultured human keratinocytes (34). This is of interest in that 1,25-(OH)$_2$D (a) is produced by keratinocytes, (b) is itself subject to regulation in keratinocytes by PTH and presumably by PTHrP, and (c) is itself a regulator of keratinocyte differentiation (168,182). Fetal bovine serum (FBS) dramatically up-regulates PTHrP production in keratinocytes, although the specific component or components in FBS that account for this up-regulation remain undefined (34,99). Medium calcium concentration, insulin, and epidermal growth factor (EGF) have no effect on PTHrP expression (34,99, 179). Hydrocortisone had no effect on normal keratinocyte production of PTHrP in one study but diminished expression by malignant keratinocytes in another (34). Hoekman et al. (183) and Lowik et al. (184) have suggested that dermal fibroblasts may produce factors that enhance PTHrP production. Clearly, the list of candidate factors that might influence PTHrP expression in keratinocytes is long, and only a few have been examined.

One presumes that the effects of PTHrP on keratinocytes are autocrine or paracrine in nature. One might also presume, for the reasons described above, that the actions of PTHrP on keratinocytes will prove to be mediated through a unique class of PTHrP receptors distinct from the PTH receptor. In support of this presumption, Orloff et al. (174) have shown, using affinity cross-linking studies, that radiolabeled PTHrP is bound to a cell surface protein in squamous cells that is larger than the PTH receptor in bone or kidney. Further, the signal transduction pathways employed by PTHrP in keratinocytes appear to differ from those activated by the PTH receptor in bone and kidney (174). Finally, molecular evidence is beginning to emerge that may indicate the presence of unique PTHrP receptors in keratinocytes (178).

The most pressing questions concerning keratinocyte–PTHrP interactions involve the normal physiological role of PTHrP in the keratinocyte as well as how PTHrP gene expression relates to the malignant transformation of keratinocytes into squamous carcinomas. As was discussed in earlier sections, the PTHrP gene is expressed in a variety of tissues during embryogenesis, and there is evidence that the peptide may play a role in growth and/or differentiation (61,172,175,185–187). There is considerable evidence for this in keratinocytes. Several investigators have reported that amino-terminal PTHrP species stimulate proliferation of keratinocytes in vitro. In the most thorough of these studies, Henderson and colleagues (99) in Montreal demonstrated that virally transformed human neonatal keratinocytes display adenylyl cyclase and weak proliferative responses to PTHrP-(1–34). Similar results have been reported in preliminary form from other laboratories (188). In one report, EGF induced proliferation in keratinocytes, and this proliferation appeared to be mediated by PTHrP, in that antibodies directed against PTHrP blocked EGF-induced mitogenesis (189). In a subsequent study by the Montreal group, antisense RNA technology was employed to neutralize PTHrP mRNA and to prevent PTHrP production in a virally transformed keratinocyte line (142). In these studies, perhaps surprisingly, elimination of the PTHrP production led to increased, not decreased, proliferation. One interpretation of the two seemingly conflicting studies from the Montreal group is that, while the amino terminus of PTHrP may stimulate keratinocyte proliferation, mid- or carboxy-terminal regions might inhibit proliferation, in a fashion analogous to the "osteostatin" story described above (139). In addition to the effects of PTHrP on proliferation, it has been suggested that PTHrP may enhance differentiation of keratinocytes, as evidenced by the increased expression of markers of keratinocyte differentiation in cells exposed to PTHrP (188). Recently, Wysolmerski et al. (63) have developed a transgenic murine model of PTHrP overexpression targeted to the epidermis. While analysis of this model is as yet incomplete, it appears that a five- to tenfold overexpression of PTHrP in the skin of transgenic mice leads to epidermal hyperkeratosis and to interference with normal hair follicle development (63).

Based on the information described above, two tentative models of PTHrP actions in skin can be proposed. In the first, PTHrP made by differentiated cells in the outer layers of the epidermis is seen as acting to inhibit proliferation and stimulate differentiation of basal, inner-layer keratinocytes. When the outer layer of the epidermis is damaged or removed, the basal layers are free to proliferate in order to repair the epidermis. This growth and repair are halted when a mature outer layer of epidermis has been regenerated and can once again secrete PTHrP. In this model, PTHrP overproduction in squamous carcinomas is seen as the result of dysregulated expression of the PTHrP gene. In this setting, PTHrP gene expression is clearly not tied to differentiation, and the peptide is also clearly incapable of controlling cell proliferation.

In the second model, PTHrP is seen as a factor that coordinates the normal interaction of epidermal keratinocytes and dermal fibroblasts. For example, Wu et al. (190) have reported that PTHrP stimulates adenylyl cyclase activity in dermal fibroblasts, and Insogna et al. (172) found that PTHrP stimulates proliferation and fibronectin production in human dermal fibro-

blasts. Conversely, the group in The Netherlands has shown that as yet undefined soluble factors produced by rat fibroblasts and by human dermal fibroblasts stimulate PTHrP production in squamous cells (183,184). Thus, it would appear that the epidermis makes factors (including PTHrP) that modulate dermal fibroblast function and that dermal fibroblasts, in turn, make as yet unidentified factors that modulate epidermal function.

Both these models should be viewed as preliminary but useful exercises in developing testable hypotheses. Complete understanding of the role of PTHrP in keratinocyte and dermal fibroblast biology will have to take into account the complex regulation of PTHrP production by keratinocytes, the complexities of PTHrP posttranslational processing, and the possible opposing effects of different PTHrP secretory species on keratinocyte and dermal fibroblast function.

Placental Calcium Transport

A fetoplacental calcium gradient is established early in pregnancy and is maintained throughout gestation in most mammals. This gradient subserves fetal mineral demands and also results in a fetal serum calcium concentration that exceeds that in the maternal circulation by a factor of about 1.4 to 1. There is a growing body of evidence suggesting that PTHrP, principally derived from the fetal parathyroids, is responsible for maintaining this gradient (38). In this circumstance, PTHrP would act as a fetal hormone in a conventional endocrine sense; to date, this is the only proposed normal PTHrP effect involving actions in distant target tissues.

Pieces of this puzzle were already being put in place in the mid-1980s. Using a sensitive cytochemical bioassay, Allgrove et al. (191) reported in 1985 that PTH-like bioactivity in human cord blood was elevated compared to maternal levels, while immunoreactive PTH was low or undetectable in cord blood. Further, it was found that fetal parathyroidectomy in the lamb resulted in a reversal of the fetomaternal calcium gradient and a fall in the fetal serum calcium concentration and that these changes could not be reversed by administering PTH to the fetus in vivo or to the placenta directly via placental perfusion (192,193). Together, these observations suggested that a factor with PTH-like actions derived from the fetal parathyroids was responsible for maintaining the calcium gradient and relative fetal hypercalcemia.

In 1988, it was reported that biological activity resembling that of PTHrP was present in extracts of fetal lamb parathyroid glands and that perfusion of sheep placenta with these extracts or with PTHrP partially purified from HHM-associated tumor cell-conditioned medium stimulated calcium transport (138). Extracts of maternal parathyroid glands were without effect, as were PTH-(1–34) and PTH-(1–84) (138). The sheep placenta is a useful system for such studies in that it exhibits essentially unidirectional calcium transport, and twin fetuses can be used to obtain paired placentas from control and parathyroidectomized fetuses (38). PTHrP was subsequently identified by radioimmunoassay in extracts of fetal lamb and calf parathyroids and also in extracts of human amnion and chorion (194), and it was also reported that PTHrP could be identified by immunohistochemistry in the parathyroids of fetal and newborn lambs but was not present in the maternal parathyroid (43). Using the perfused sheep placenta system, it was next found that recombinant PTHrP-(1–84), PTHrP-(1–108), and PTHrP-(1–141) were capable of stimulating calcium transport, while synthetic PTHrP-(1–34) was inactive (195). It was then reported that amidated midregion fragments of PTHrP, such as PTHrP-(67–86) amide, were fully active and that this activity could be seen in placentas derived from both normal and parathyroidectomized fetuses (137). Shorter peptides and/or elimination of the carboxy-terminal amide group decreased activity substantially (137). These results imply not that such midregion fragments actually exist and are solely responsible for mediating the placental response (although this is possible) but rather that the midregion of the PTHrP molecule seems to be the biologically active domain in the placenta and that carboxy-terminal cleavage and amidation may be important processing steps in this regard. On the surface, these results would appear to require the presence of a unique PTHrP receptor in the placenta, but additional evidence (e.g., binding studies) for the existence of such a receptor has not been reported thus far. The classical PTH/PTHrP receptor does seem to be expressed at an RNA level in rat placenta (137).

The identification of PTHrP in the chorioallantoic membrane in the chick embryo (38) is consistent with a proposed role in calcium transport, but the patterns of PTHrP gene expression seen in the preterm rat myometrium and in the chicken oviduct during the egg-laying cycle are seen as more likely to be related to smooth muscle function than to calcium transport (see below under Smooth Muscle). It is also unclear what role PTHrP derived from the placental or fetal membranes might play in placental calcium transport (138,194).

In essence, based on the data summarized above, it has been proposed that PTHrP plays a PTH-like systemic role in the fetus, with the key target tissue being the placenta (38). It is also possible that the kidney participates in a systemic response to PTHrP in the fetus, but bone is an unlikely target, since bone mineralization is the intended end result of the entire pro-

cess. This is an attractive proposal, but there remain a number of unresolved questions. First, there is disagreement concerning whether immunoreactive PTHrP concentrations in cord blood are elevated vis-à-vis the concentration in the maternal circulation (38). Second, PTHrP-(75–86) amide has been reported not to stimulate calcium transport in the perfused rat placenta (196). The placenta is structurally dissimilar in the sheep and the rat, so the unresponsiveness of the rat placenta to the midregion peptide might reflect a species difference (196).

Lactating Breast

It is useful to keep in mind several salient features of mammary gland physiology by way of introduction to the findings concerning PTHrP gene expression in lactating mammary tissue (for additional details, see 38,89,197, and references therein). First, extensive developmental changes (referred to collectively as *mammogenesis*) take place in the mammary glands during pregnancy (38,197); lactation itself is triggered by the fall in circulating estrogen and progesterone and the release of prolactin that occur at birth. Second, a large number of biologically active peptides are present in milk, and some of these have been proposed to play one or another role in the neonate, one example being the possible effects of EGF derived from milk on eyelid opening in the newborn (197,198). These proposals are based on the ability of the neonatal intestine to absorb macromolecules such as immunoglobulins by a process of pinocytosis for a variable period after birth (197–199). In the rat, this process diminishes after the second week of nursing and is completely lost by days 21–22, the time of weaning (197–199). Third, there appears to be a "missing link" in the control of maternal systemic mineral metabolism and calcium mobilization into milk during lactation, in that neither PTH nor 1,25-$(OH)_2D$ seems to be necessary or sufficient to account for the mineral fluxes that take place during this period (38,200,201). The available data indicate that this is the case in both rats and humans, although the physiological details differ for these two species (38,200,201). In both species, a substantial quantity of the calcium deposited into milk appears to be derived from bone (38,200,201).

In 1988, Thiede and Rodan (22) reported that suckling induced a rapid and transient increase in PTHrP mRNA and protein content in lactating mammary tissue in the rat. When the pups were removed, a precipitous decline in PTHrP mRNA was seen, reaching basal levels in ~4 hr (22). In subsequent studies, it was found that this phenomenon could be reproduced by prolactin injection in unsuckled puerperal animals and also that the PTHrP mRNA response to suckling could be blocked by bromocriptine administration (88). A year later, Budayr et al. (202) reported that enormous quantities of PTHrP were present in fresh human, bovine, and rat milk and also in commercial milk products and formulas. This observation has been repeatedly confirmed in multiple species, and the average PTHrP concentration in milk has been found to be some 1,000-fold higher than the concentration of the peptide measured in the circulation of patients with HHM (46,202–210). A substantial portion of the PTHrP in milk appears to be biologically active based on the rat osteosarcoma cell bioassay or equivalent assays (199,202,207), but there is some disagreement regarding the form or forms of the peptide present in milk (203–206). In human, bovine, and ovine milk, there is evidence that large peptides corresponding to either full-length PTHrP-(1–141) or PTHrP-(1–108) represent the major PTHrP species present (203,206), but there is evidence that smaller peptides are also present (204,205). It is unclear whether the smaller forms represent differentially processed or degraded products (203–206).

Additional studies have focused on the cells that express the PTHrP gene in mammary tissue and also on the control of PTHrP gene expression during lactation, which appears to be somewhat more complex than was initially thought. By immunohistochemistry and in situ hybridization histochemistry, PTHrP and PTHrP mRNA have been localized to mammary epithelial cells during both mammogenesis and lactation in the rat (209). Cultured rat and human epithelial cells in primary culture have also been shown to contain PTHrP mRNA and/or to secrete the peptide (101,211). PTHrP immunostaining has been reported in one unusual example of massive myoepithelial cell hyperplasia associated with hypercalcemia (212), but it is unknown whether normal myoepithelial cells produce PTHrP (209). Thus PTHrP appears to be produced by the principal alveolar epithelial cells during lactation, as might have been anticipated from the extraordinary content of the peptide in milk, but it has not been established that the expression of the PTHrP gene is confined to these cells, since myoepithelial cells and vascular smooth muscle were not resolved in the histochemical studies in the rat (209).

With respect to control of PTHrP production, careful longitudinal studies have revealed a very substantial increase in PTHrP content in milk and PTHrP mRNA in lactating mammary tissue as a function of the duration of lactation (199,206,209,210). For example, the concentration of PTHrP in rat milk is eightfold higher at day 21 than at day 7 of lactation (Fig. 15) (209,210), and the same trend is also seen in cow's milk over a longer time frame (199,206). In addition, in the rat, the kinetics of PTHrP mRNA expression differ in early and late lactation, in that PTHrP mRNA does not

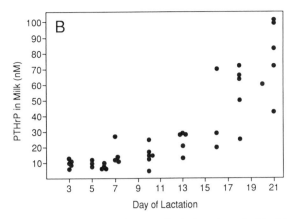

FIG. 15. PTHrP content in rat milk during days 3–21 of lactation. The results are from individual animals. (Reprinted from ref. 52 with permission. Photograph courtesy of M. Yamamoto.)

decline precipitously after cessation of suckling late in lactation (89,210). Although suckling and prolactin appear to be important stimuli to PTHrP production throughout lactation, it is unlikely that the gradual, sustained increase in PTHrP production that occurs later in lactation is mediated by prolactin, since circulating prolactin levels decrease rather than increase at that time (210). It has been pointed out that there is a strong positive correlation between PTHrP content and the volume of milk production in the rat (210), but this correlation does not seem to hold in the cow (199). In essence, it appears that some factor(s) in addition to prolactin contributes to PTHrP production in mid- to late lactation, but it is unclear what the stimulus might be. It is presumably systemic and not local, since the intensity of the suckling stimulus does not correlate with PTHrP content in milk, and PTHrP concentrations are not different in milk samples obtained from suckled and nonsuckled nipples (210,213).

There have been a half-dozen proposals for what function PTHrP has in maternal and/or neonatal physiology. Three of these proposals have been examined with some care, and the data for and against them are considered in the following paragraphs. The other three represent ideas based on very limited data, and these are considered together here. First, the identification of PTHrP in developing nests of epithelial cells in rat mammary tissue as early as day 14 of pregnancy has led to the suggestion that the peptide might have some effect on mammary epithelial growth and development (209). Studies of mammary epithelial cells in vitro have attempted to correlate PTHrP production with growth conditions and various stimuli, but there is no evidence for an actual effect of PTHrP on cell proliferation and/or differentiation (101,211). Second, in a preliminary study it was found that PTHrP was able to block the calcium transient induced by oxytocin in cultured myoepithelial cells, leading to the suggestion that PTHrP might regulate the tone of myoepithelial cells during lactation (214). Third, based on the pronounced increase in blood flow to the breast during lactation and the precedent for PTHrP-induced relaxation of smooth muscle in other systems (see below under Smooth Muscle), it has been proposed that PTHrP might regulate vascular tone and blood flow during lactation (208). This proposal has not been formally examined, and, as was noted above, it is not known whether the PTHrP gene is expressed in the smooth muscle of the vessels feeding the breast, although this seems likely.

Based on PTHrP effects in bone and kidney (see the chapter by Strewler and Nissenson) and the evidence that the peptide is involved in calcium transport across the placenta (see above under Placental Calcium Transport), it has been widely supposed that PTHrP might be involved in the active transfer of calcium from blood to milk during lactation. Few data actually bear directly on this question. In one report, a weak correlation was found between PTHrP and calcium concentrations in bovine milk (206), but this positive correlation was not seen in a longitudinal study of bovine milk (199) or in two longitudinal studies of rat milk (209,210). In the longitudinal studies, milk calcium content was found to be relatively constant throughout lactation, whereas PTHrP concentrations increased progressively, by as much as eightfold late in lactation in the rat (Fig. 15) (199,209,210). While these findings do not support the calcium transport proposal, they do not represent very powerful evidence in this regard. By Northern analysis, PTH/PTHrP receptor mRNA has been reported to be expressed in RNA prepared from the adult rat breast (177), but cellular localization studies have not yet been performed. This remains an intuitively attractive hypothesis, which has yet to be carefully tested in physiological experiments.

It also has been widely supposed that PTHrP might be the "missing link" referred to in the opening paragraph of this section. According to this proposal, PTHrP derived from lactating breast would enter the systemic maternal circulation and be responsible for mobilizing calcium from the skeleton and possibly also for stimulating calcium conservation in the distal nephron. There is evidence for a suckling-induced increase in phosphaturia and cyclic AMP excretion in the rat (201), and a small PTHrP arteriovenous gradient across lactating breast has been found in the goat (208). However, there is disagreement whether circulating concentrations of PTHrP are increased in lactating women compared to either normal subjects or pregnant (nonlactating) women (202,207, 215). In addition, passive immunization with anti-PTHrP antisera in lactating mice has been found to have no influ-

ence on the calcium and phosphorus content in milk, the serum calcium concentration, or the calcium content in the femur (216). Thus, the "missing link" hypothesis is also attractive but is unproven. Methods for measuring PTHrP concentrations in the subpicomolar range will be very useful in evaluating this hypothesis further.

The capacity of the neonatal intestine to absorb proteins by pinocytosis was touched on in the opening paragraph of this section. An additional factor that allows this process to occur is the relative absence of proteolytic enzymes in the intestine of the newborn. Since other proteins seem to be absorbed by this process, it seemed quite logical to propose that this might also be the case for PTHrP, particularly given the high concentrations of the peptide in milk. PTHrP absorption has been demonstrated in calves fed colostrum (199). In these animals, plasma immunoreactive PTHrP rises rapidly after feeding and is maintained at a relatively high level for up to 60 hr thereafter (199). However, this immunoreactive material is devoid of PTH-like bioactivity in the osteosarcoma cell assay (199). In 1-day-old neonatal mice, passive immunization with an anti-PTHrP antiserum targeted at the amino terminus of the peptide has been reported to be without effect on the serum calcium concentration or whole-body calcium content (217). Similarly, the oral administration of PTHrP-(1–34) in the newborn mouse has been found not to influence the serum calcium concentration (217). On balance, these various findings speak against a conventional PTH-like biological effect from milk-derived PTHrP in the newborn, but it seems clear that some PTHrP species do enter the neonatal circulation, at least in calves. The nature of these species and/or what nonconventional effects they might have is unknown. It is also unknown whether PTHrP derived from milk might have a local physiological effect on the neonatal intestine.

In summary, in spite of the clear evidence of physiological regulation of PTHrP gene expression in lactating breast and the several intriguing hints concerning PTHrP function that have been pursued, no specific PTHrP function has been established in the breast or in the neonate. This is but one of several physiological areas in which a null approach would be very powerful experimentally, and it is unfortunate that the "knockout" mouse does not survive and cannot be used for this purpose (64).

Bone

The skeletal effects of PTHrP in the setting of the syndrome of HHM are summarized in detail in the chapter by Strewler and Nissenson, so the discussion in this section is confined to evidence that the peptide(s) has a physiological function in bone. Several of the points summarized in the chapter by Strewler and Nissenson are germane to this discussion and are briefly restated here. First, PTHrP has different effects on bone cells depending on whether the cells are exposed to the peptide continuously or transiently; when the exposure is transient, the effects of PTHrP are anabolic (218). The same is true for PTH (218). Second, there is evidence that portions of the PTHrP molecule including its amino terminus may have growth factor-like actions (172,219). Third, it has been reported that a portion of the PTHrP molecule towards its carboxy terminus is capable of inhibiting osteoclastic bone resorption in purified osteoclasts, osteoblast–osteoclast cocultures, and fetal long bone assays (139,140) but not in a neonatal mouse calvarial assay (141). This sequence was initially defined as the region PTHrP-(107–139) and subsequently as the pentapeptide PTHrP-(107–111), which was referred to as *osteostatin* (139,140). These findings were interpreted as additional evidence that PTHrP might function as a polyprotein, with an amino-terminal sequence stimulating osteoclastic bone resorption via indirect effects involving osteoblasts and a carboxy-terminal sequence inhibiting osteoclastic bone resorption by direct effects on these cells (139,140). The growth factor and osteostatin hypotheses are active areas of research and debate (139–141,172,219) (see also the chapter by Strewler and Nissenson).

There is abundant evidence that the PTHrP gene is expressed in bone cells and chondrocytes and that there is a temporal sequence of expression in these cells during different stages of endochondral and intramembranous bone formation (56,57,59,60,96,100,220). PTHrP-like bioactivity is present in medium conditioned by 19-day-old fetal rat long bones and increases in amount when bone resorption is stimulated by PTH or 1,25-$(OH)_2$D (96). It was subsequently found that PTHrP-like activity could be extracted from bone matrix, and it was proposed that the peptide might be taken up and stored in the matrix and subsequently liberated during the resorptive process (220), as is the case for some growth factors (185). The source of the PTHrP was not defined in these studies but is presumably local (96,220). PTHrP production has been reported in a subclone (Saos-2/B-10) of a human osteosarcoma cell line (100), but the gene is not expressed in basal rat osteosarcoma cells (ROS 17/2.8) (68). PTHrP mRNA and protein production have been studied in both rat and human fetuses using a combination of immunohistochemistry and in situ hybridization histochemistry, and there is generally good agreement among the findings (56,57,59,60). Early in development (e.g., day 13 in the rat), PTHrP immunostaining is seen in immature chondrocytes in the mesenchyme of the developing limbs and the sclerotome of the vertebral column (56,60). This staining is lost as cartilage develops (56,57,60), but PTHrP immunostaining reap-

pears at the time of ossification in both endochondral and intramembranous locations (56,57,59,60). In these sites, PTHrP immunostaining is seen in the "mature" chondrocytes of cartilage and in cells in the perichondrium and periosteum (56,57,59,60). Thus both temporal and spatial variations in PTHrP gene expression have been observed in developing cartilage and bone, involving three different cell types, immature chondrocytes, prechondroblast-like cells in the perichondrium, and possibly osteoblasts (56,57,59,60). PTHrP mRNA expression is also seen in the dental lamina in the rat (57). Very limited information is available concerning the site(s) of expression of the PTH/PTHrP receptor in bone, but the receptor appears to be present in the prehypertrophic chondrocytes in epiphyseal cartilage (a zone between proliferative chondrocytes and hypertrophic chondrocytes) and in mononuclear cells on the periosteal, endosteal, and trabecular bone surfaces, presumed to be osteoblasts (Fig. 16) (177,221).

The findings described above assume greater significance in light of the phenotypic abnormalities ob-

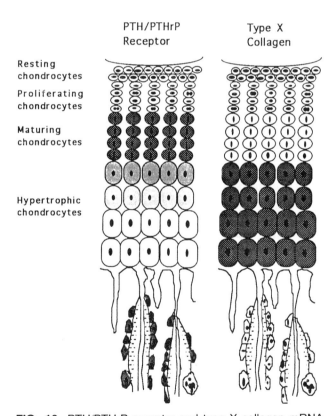

FIG. 16. PTH/PTHrP receptor and type X collagen mRNA expression in the femur of a 4-week-old rat as determined by in situ hybridization histochemistry. The relative levels of mRNA expression are depicted by the shading, from absent (*white*) to highly expressed (*black*). As shown, PTH/PTHrP receptor mRNA is highly expressed in the maturing (prehypertrophic) chondrocytes and trabecular osteoblasts, and type X collagen mRNA is highly expressed in hypertrophic chondrocytes. (Reprinted from ref. 221 with permission. Photograph courtesy of K. Lee.)

served in mice following targeted disruption of the PTHrP gene (64). These mice display a form of chondrodysplasia and die at birth because of acute respiratory distress and/or the impingement of craniofacial abnormalities on the brainstem. The animals appear to lack other obvious abnormalities, although the window of observation is very limited because the mice do not survive. Grossly, the mice have a foreshortened and domed cranium, greatly foreshortened long bones, and a fixed chest wall. Histologically, two abnormalities are seen. The first is disruption of the normal architecture of the epiphyseal growth plate. This abnormality is manifest early (before the onset of ossification in endochondral bone) and consists of a decrease in the numbers of resting and proliferative chondrocytes; the numbers of prehypertrophic and hypertrophic chondrocytes appear to be normal. This finding accounts for the dwarfing. The second abnormality is abnormal endochondral/perichondral ossification in a number of locations, including the costal cartilages (resulting in a fixed thorax) and the base of the skull (resulting in premature closure of the synchondroses of the endochondral bones in this location). It is these two abnormalities that seem to account for the perinatal mortality.

These findings clearly implicate PTHrP in the developmental program that controls the orderly sequence of events associated with epiphyseal growth and cartilaginous mineralization. Although the exact signaling pathways in this regard are not known, it is possible to synthesize what is known into a coherent explanation for both of the key abnormalities seen in the gene-targeted mice. The elements in the synthesis are basically three. First, the PTH/PTHrP receptor gene is expressed in the zone of maturing (prehypertrophic) chondrocytes but is not expressed in other chondrocyte populations (221). Second, PTH (presumably in this setting PTHrP) has been shown to be mitogenic to embryonic chick and rabbit chondrocytes; this response is delayed and is therefore thought to reflect PTH (PTHrP) induction of cytokines (222). Third, PTH (PTHrP) has been shown to inhibit the mineralization of cartilage mediated by hypertrophic chondrocytes in both organ culture (223) and a chondrocyte culture system (224). In essence, PTHrP effects on PTH/PTHrP receptors in prehypertrophic chondrocytes are envisioned as leading to linear growth of the zone of proliferating chondrocytes that lies just above the prehypertropic zone and inhibition of mineralization by the hypertrophic chondrocytes that lie just beneath this zone; both effects are presumably mediated by paracrine signals downstream of the PTHrP–PTH/PTHrP receptor interaction. The absence of these effects in the gene-targeted mice would be predicted to result in exactly the abnormalities that have been observed. In this synthesis of information, neither the source nor the timing of PTHrP production is entirely clear; potential sources would include immature mesenchymal cells (56,60) or cells in the perichondrium in proximity to prehypertrophic chondrocytes (57). PTH itself derived from the systemic circulation is not a serious candidate in this regard, because the growth plate is avascular. The interpretation of the findings described in this paragraph should be regarded as provisional, pending a detailed analysis of these animals.

It is curious that these mice do not appear to display abnormalities other than those described, although many functional abnormalities might well escape histological detection and/or might become apparent later if the mice survived. One potentially contributing feature is the fact that cartilage is avascular and therefore beyond the reach of circulating factors that might "salvage" function (e.g., PTH itself); this point is purely speculative. Another is that the phenotype reflects essentially developmental abnormalities and does not provide a window on putative function(s) beyond birth [e.g., the epidermal abnormalities seen in transgenic mice with keratin promoter-driven PTHrP overexpression in basal keratinocytes are not apparent at birth (63)]. Irrespective of the explanation for the circumscribed nature of the phenotype in the gene-targeted mice, the findings of this experiment provide compelling evidence for a developmental role for PTHrP in cartilaginous growth and endochondral mineralization in vivo.

Smooth Muscle

PTH was first reported to have hypotensive effects in the mid-1920s (reviewed in 170). Over the next 60 years, it was learned that PTH was capable of relaxing not only vascular smooth muscle but also nonvascular smooth muscle in tissues such as the stomach and intestine, trachea, vas deferens, and uterus (170). In the vasculature, the most potent vasorelaxant actions were found to be in the small-resistance vessels. PTH was also reported to have chronotropic and inotropic effects on the heart. All these effects were taken to be direct, in that they could be demonstrated in a variety of systems in vitro as well as in vivo (170). Vasoactivity was found to require an intact amino terminus, but there has been considerable disagreement with respect to mediation via the cAMP and calcium signaling pathways (170). Since PTH is present in the systemic circulation in concentrations that are a direct function of calcium sensing in the parathyroid chief cell, it was never clear that PTH itself was a viable candidate for physiological regulation in any smooth muscle bed.

PTHrP clearly is a viable candidate for such a regulatory role. The lines of evidence in this regard are basically four. First, PTHrP peptides comprising its amino terminus have been found to relax a number of smooth muscle systems (225–230). These include PTHrP-induced hypotensive effects in vivo and the relaxation of aortic strips, renal artery segments, gastric strips, and acetylcholine-stimulated rat uterine horns in vitro (225–230). By the microsphere technique, it has been shown that PTHrP effects in the rat in vivo result from a decrease in total peripheral resistance, with a redistribution of flow that favors some vascular beds such as the coronaries and the vessels of the skin (229). PTHrP has also been found to have both chronotropic and inotropic effects in the perfused rat heart (225). Details of mechanism are unclear; the relaxation of aortic strips was reported to be endothelium independent (225), but the use of arginine analogs has implicated nitric oxide in PTHrP-induced relaxation in the uterus (230). Second, by immunohistochemistry, in situ hybridization histochemistry, or Northern/RNAse protection analysis, the PTHrP gene has been found to be almost uniformly expressed in smooth muscle tissues throughout the organism. These sites include aorta; myometrium; bladder; chicken oviduct; stomach; colon; vessels of the lung, liver, and skin; and the heart (26,49,51–53,90,92,103). Third, although published information is limited, the 2.5 kb PTH/PTHrP receptor mRNA seems to be expressed in many of these same locations (109,177,231). Finally, in cultured rat aortic smooth muscle cells, vasoconstrictive agents such as norepinephrine, endothelin, thrombin, and angiotensin II have been reported to increase PTHrP mRNA expression, implying the existence of a direct autocrine feedback loop (53,232).

Perhaps the most intriguing results implicating PTHrP in the regulation of smooth muscle function have been those concerning physiological control of PTHrP gene expression in expandable tissues such as the uterus, bladder, and chicken oviduct shell gland (19,51,52,90–92,232). The first of these tissues to be studied was the rat uterus. Here, a peak in PTHrP mRNA expression was found in the myometrium during the 48 hr immediately proceeding parturition, with

a rapid decline thereafter (51). This peak was dependent on uterine occupancy by the fetoplacental unit and was not seen in nongravid uterine horns at the same stage of gestation (51). This finding implied that a local signal, either humoral or mechanical, was responsible for regulating PTHrP gene expression in the preterm myometrium. It was subsequently shown that this signal was mechanical stretch and that the peak in PTHrP mRNA expression could be reproduced experimentally by inflating a balloon in the unoccupied uterine horn of the postpartum, unilaterally pregnant (tubal), or virgin animals (Fig. 17) (90). Virtually identical observations have been made in the rat bladder, in which the degree of stretch imposed was a function of distension by urine accumulation following urethral ligation (see Fig. 11) (52). In this system, when distension was limited to one-half of the bladder, the increase in PTHrP mRNA was confined to that one-half (52). Somewhat similar findings have also been reported in the chicken oviduct shell gland during the egg-laying cycle (92). In the shell gland, however, the increase in PTHrP mRNA was found to anticipate the actual arrival of the egg by several hours and to be most pronounced in the serosal vessels overlying the gland (92). These observations suggest that PTHrP-induced relaxation of smooth muscle in the shell gland might serve to accommodate egg movement through the oviduct and/or that a principal effect might be on blood flow to the gland (92). In the human uteroplacental unit, the most abundant source of PTHrP seems to be the amnion, specifically that portion of the amnion directly overlying the placenta (19,91,233). Here, too, mechanical stretch may be the critical signal, in that the level of PTHrP mRNA expression in the amnion was found to fall dramatically following rupture of the fetal membranes (91).

On the basis of the findings reviewed above, it seems clear that mechanotransduction (the means by which physical forces are converted into cellular signals) is a major stimulus controlling PTHrP gene expression in smooth muscle. This is an area of con-

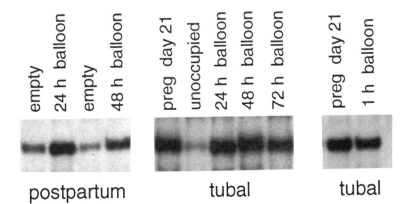

FIG. 17. Balloon-induced PTHrP mRNA expression rat uterus. Experiments were performed in postpartum or unilaterally pregnant ("tubal") animals. Empty or unoccupied uterine horns served as negative controls, and the level of PTHrP mRNA expression in gravid uterine horns at 21 days of gestation served as positive control. The duration of balloon inflation is shown at top. (Reprinted from ref. 90 with permission.)

siderable recent interest in cardiac muscle and smooth muscle physiology and appears to involve membrane-associated signal transduction pathways such as stretch-activated/inactivated channels and adenylyl cyclase (234). In the case of the PTHrP gene, stretch induction would result in the local production of a molecule capable of counterbalancing or accommodating the mechanical force being applied. The specific PTH/PTHrP receptor targets and the resultant physiological effects may well differ depending on the tissue in question. For example, in the vasculature in general, and in the serosal vessels overlying the chicken oviduct and the chorionic and villous vessels underlying the human placental amnion in particular, the principal effect may be an increase in blood flow. In the bladder and smooth muscle of the chicken oviduct, the principal effect may be a gradual relaxation to accommodate volume. In the rat myometrium, PTHrP may function in the complex control of the force and rhythmicity of myometrial contractility that ultimately leads to parturition.

ACKNOWLEDGMENTS

The authors are grateful to T. Clemens, A. Karaplis, K. Lee, L. Milstone, M. Thiede, R. Vasavada, E. Weir, J. Wysolmerski, and M. Yamamoto for sharing artwork, ideas, and unpublished information and to N. Canetti for preparing the manuscript. The authors are supported by grants from the NIH (AR 30102), the American Cancer Society (BE-152B), and the Department of Veterans Affairs.

REFERENCES

1. Broadus AE. Identification of the parathyroid hormone-related peptide. In: Halloran BP, Nissenson RA, eds. *Parathyroid hormone-related protein: normal physiology and its role in cancer.* Boca Raton, FL: CRC Press, 1992;1–23.
2. Martin TJ. Properties of parathyroid hormone-related protein and its role in malignant hypercalcemia. *Q J Med* 1990;76:771–786.
3. Strewler GJ, Nissenson RA. Hypercalcemia in malignancy. *West J Med* 1990;153:635–640.
4. Chase LR, Aurbach GD. Parathyroid function and the renal excretion of 3′,5′-adenylic acid. *Proc Natl Acad Sci USA* 1967;58:518–522.
5. Stewart AF, Horst R, Deftos LJ, Cadman EC, Lang R, Broadus AE. Biochemical evaluation of patients with cancer-associated hypercalcemia: evidence for humoral and nonhumoral groups. *N Engl J Med* 1980;303:1377–1383.
6. Kukreja SC, Shemerdiak WP, Lad TE, Johnson PA. Elevated nephrogenous cyclic AMP with normal parathyroid hormone levels in patients with lung cancer. *J Clin Endocrinol Metab* 51:167–169, 1980.
7. Rude RK, Sharp CF, Fredericks RS, et al. Urinary and nephrogenous adenosine 3′5′-monophosphate in the hypercalcemia of malignancy. *J Clin Endocrinol* 1981;52:765–771.
8. Mangin M, Ikeda K, Dreyer BE, Broadus AE. Isolation and characterization of the human parathyroid hormone-like peptide gene. *Proc Natl Acad Sci USA* 1989;86:2408–2412.
9. Yasuda T, Banville D, Hendry GN, Goltzman D. Characterization of the human parathyroid hormone-like peptide gene. *J Biol Chem* 1989;264:7720–7725.
10. Suva LJ, Mather KA, Gillespie MT, et al. Structure of the 5′ flanking region of the gene encoding human parathyroid hormone-related protein (PTHrP). *Gene* 1989;77:95–105.
11. Suva LJ, Winslow GA, Wettenhall EH, et al. A parathyroid hormone-related protein implicated in malignant hypercalcemia: cloning and expression. *Science* 1987;237:893–896.
12. Mangin M, Webb AC, Dreyer BE, et al. Identification of a cDNA encoding a parathyroid hormone-like peptide from a human tumor associated with humoral hypercalcemia of malignancy. *Proc Natl Acad Sci USA* 1988;85:597–601.
13. Mangin M, Ikeda K, Dreyer BE, Broadus AE. Identification of an upstream promoter of the human parathyroid hormone-related peptide gene. *Mol Endocrinol* 1990;4:851–858.
14. Campos RV, Wang C, Drucker DJ. Regulation of parathyroid hormone-related peptide (PTHrP) gene transcription: cell- and tissue-specific promoter utilization mediated by multiple positive and negative cis-acting DNA elements. *Mol Endocrinol* 1992;6:1642–1652.
15. Hendy GN, Goltzman D. Molecular biology of parathyroid hormone-like peptide. In: Halloran BP, Nissenson RA, eds. *Parathyroid hormone-related protein: normal physiology and its role in cancer.* Boca Raton, FL: CRC Press, 1992;25–55.
16. Thiede MA, Strewler GH, Nissenson RA, Rosenblatt M, Rodan GA. Human renal carcinoma expresses two messages encoding a parathyroid hormone-like peptide: evidence for the alternative splicing of a single-copy gene. *Proc Natl Acad Sci USA* 1988;85:4605–4609.
17. Mangin M, Ikeda K, Dreyer BE, Milstone L, Broadus AE. Two distinct tumor-derived parathyroid hormone-like peptides result from alternative ribonucleic acid splicing. *Mol Endocrinol* 1988;2:1049–1055.
18. Ikeda K, Arnold A, Mangin M, et al. Expression of transcripts encoding a parathyroid hormone-related peptide in abnormal human parathyroid tissues. *J Clin Endocrin Metab* 1989;69:1240–1248.
19. Brandt DW, Bruns ME, Bruns DW, Ferguson JE, Burton DW, Deftos LJ. The parathyroid hormone-related protein (PTHrP) gene preferentially utilizes a GC-rich promoter and the PTHrP 1-139 coding pathway in normal human amnion. *Biochem Biophys Res Commun* 1992;189:938–943.
20. Hargrove JL, Schmidt FH. The role of mRNA and protein stability in gene expression. *FASEB J* 1989;3:2360–2370.
21. Shaw G, Kamen R. A conserved AU sequence from the 3′ untranslated region of GM-CSF mRNA mediates selective mRNA degradation. *Cell* 1986;46:659–667.
22. Thiede MA, Rodan GA. Expression of a calcium-mobilizing parathyroid hormone-like peptide in lactating mammary tissue. *Science* 1988;242:278–280.
23. Yasuda T, Banville D, Rabbani SA, Hendy GN, Goltzman D. Rat parathyroid hormone-like peptide: comparison with the human homologue and expression in malignant and normal tissue. *Mol Endocrinol* 1989;3:518–525.
24. Thiede MA, Rutledge SU. Nucleotide sequence of a parathyroid hormone-related peptide expressed by the 10 day chicken embryo. *Nucleic Acid Res* 1990;18:3062.
25. Karaplis AC, Yasuda T, Hendy GN, Goltzman D, Banville D. Gene encoding parathyroid hormone-like peptide: nucleotide sequences of the rat gene and comparison with the human homologue. *Mol Endocrinol* 1990;4:441–446.
26. Mangin M, Ikeda K, Broadus AE. Structure of the mouse gene encoding the parathyroid hormone-related peptide. *Gene* 1990;95:195–202.
27. Haddad JG, Rutledge SJ, Thiede MA. Structure and expression of the parathyroid hormone-related peptide gene in the chicken. *J Bone Mineral Res* 1990;5(Suppl 1):S257 (abstract).
28. Schermer PT, Chan SDH, Bruce R, Nissenson RA, Wood WI, Strewler GJ. Chicken parathyroid hormone-related protein and its expression during embryologic development. *J Bone Mineral Res* 1991;6:149–155.

29. Heinrich G, Kronenberg HM, Potts JT Jr, Habener JF. Gene encoding parathyroid hormone. Nucleotide sequence of the rat gene and deduced amino acid sequence of rat preproparathyroid hormone. *J Biol Chem* 1984;259:3320–3329.

30. Khosla S, Demay M, Pines M, Hurwitz S, Potts JT, Kronenberg HM. Nucleotide sequence of cloned cDNAs encoding chicken preparathyroid hormone. *J Bone Mineral Res* 1988;3:689–698.

31. Vasavada R, Wysolmerski JJ, Broadus AE, Philbrick WM. Identification and characterization of a GC-rich promoter of the human parathyroid hormone-related peptide gene. *Mol Endocrinol* 1993;7:273–282.

32. Vasicek TJ, McDevitt BE, Freeman MW, et al. Nucleotide sequence of the human parathyroid hormone gene. *Proc Natl Acad Sci USA* 1983;80:2127–2131.

33. Chilco PJ, Gerardi SM, Kaczmarzyk SJ, Chu S, Leopold V, Zajac JD. Calcitonin increases transcription of parathyroid hormone-related protein via cyclic AMP. *Mol Endocrinol* (in press).

34. Kremer R, Karaplis AC, Henderson J, et al. Regulation of parathyroid hormone-like peptide in cultured normal human keratinocytes. *J Clin Invest* 1991;87:884–893.

35. Suva LJ, Gillespie MT, Center RJ, et al. A sequence in the human PTHrP gene promoter responsive to estrogen. *J Bone Mineral Res* 1991;6(Suppl 1):S196 (abstract).

36. Vasavada R, Wysolmerski JJ, Philbrick WM, Broadus AE. A negative regulatory element in th PTHrP gene promoter. *J Bone Mineral Res* 1992;7(Suppl 1):S118 (abstract).

37. Merendino JJ, Insogna KL, Milstone LM, Broadus AE, Stewart AF. Cultured human keratinocytes produce a parathyroid hormone-like protein. *Science* 1986;231:388–390.

38. Rodda CP, Caple IW, Martin TJ. Role of PTHrP in fetal and neonatal physiology. In: Halloran BP, Nissenson RA, eds. *Parathyroid hormone-related protein: normal physiology and its role in cancer.* Boca Raton, FL: CRC Press, 1992; 169–196.

39. Ikeda K, Weir EC, Mangin M, et al. Expression of messenger ribonucleic acids encoding a parathyroid hormone-like peptide in normal human and animal tissues with abnormal expression in human parathyroid adenomas. *Mol Endocrinol* 1988;2:1230–1236.

40. Asa SL, Henderson J, Goltzman D, Drucker DJ. Parathyroid hormone-like peptide in normal and neoplastic human endocrine tissues. *J Clin Endocrinol Metab* 1990;71:1112–1118.

41. Drucker DJ, Asa SL, Henderson J, Goltzman D. The parathyroid hormone-like peptide gene is expressed in the normal and neoplastic human endocrine pancreas. *Mol Endocrinol* 1989;3:1589–1595.

42. Holt EH, Lu C, Dreyer BE, Dannies PS, Broadus AE. Regulation of parathyroid hormone-related peptide gene expression by estrogen in GH$_4$C$_1$ rat pituitary cells has the pattern of a primary response gene. (Submitted).

43. MacIsaac RJ, Caple IW, Danks PA, et al. Ontogeny of parathyroid hormone-related protein in the ovine parathyroid gland. *Endocrinology* 1991;129:757–764.

44. Docherty HM, Ratcliffe WA, Heath DA, Docherty K. Expression of parathyroid hormone-related protein in abnormal human parathyroids. *J Endocrinol* 1991;129:431–438.

45. Ikeda K, Weir EC, Sakaguchi K, et al. Clonal rat parathyroid cell line expresses a parathyroid hormone-related peptide but not parathyroid hormone itself. *Biochem Biophys Res Commun* 1989;162:108–112.

46. Burtis WJ, Brady TG, Orloff JJ, et al. Immunochemical characterization of circulating parathyroid hormone-related protein in patients with humoral hypercalcemia of cancer. *N Engl J Med* 1990;322:1106–1112.

47. Atillasoy EJ, Burtis WJ, Milstone LM. Immunochemical localization of parathyroid hormone-related protein in normal human skin. *J Invest Dermatol* 1991;96:277–280.

48. Hayman JA, Danks JA, Ebeling PR, Moseley JM, Kemp BE, Martin TJ. Expression of parathyroid hormone-related protein in normal skin and in tumors of skin and skin appendages. *J Pathol* 1989;158:293–296.

49. Kramer S, Reynolds FH, Castillo M, Valenzuela DM, Thorikay M, Sorvillo JM. Immunological identification and distribution of parathyroid hormone-like protein polypeptide in normal and malignant tissues. *Endocrinology* 1991;128:1927–1937.

50. Kitazawa S, Kitazawa R, Fukase M, Fujimori T, Maeda S. Immunohistochemical evaluation of parathyroid hormone-related protein (PTHrP) in the uterine cervix. *Int J Cancer* 1992;50:731–735.

51. Thiede MA, Daifotis AG, Weir EC, et al. Intrauterine occupancy controls expression of the parathyroid hormone-related peptide gene in pre-term rat myometrium. *Proc Natl Acad Sci USA* 1990;87:6969–6973.

52. Yamamoto M, Harm SC, Grasser WA, Thiede MA. Parathyroid hormone-related protein in rat urinary bladder: a smooth muscle relaxant produced locally in response to mechanical stretch. *Proc Natl Acad Sci USA* 1992;89:5326–5330.

53. Hongo T, Kupfer J, Enomoto H, et al. Abundant expression of parathyroid hormone-related protein in primary rat aortic smooth muscle cells accompanies serum-induced proliferation. *J Clin Invest* 1991;88:1841–1847.

54. Weir EC, Brines ML, Ikeda K, Burtis WJ, Broadus AE, Robbins RJ. Parathyroid hormone-related peptide gene is expressed in the mammalian central nervous system. *Proc Natl Acad Sci USA* 1990;87:108–112.

55. Grasser WA, Peterson DN, Smoch SL, Thiede MA. Estrogen regulation of PTHrP gene expression in the rat nervous system is tissue-specific. *J Bone Mineral Res* 1992;7(Suppl 1):S240 (abstract).

56. Burton PBJ, Moniz C, Quirke P, et al. Parathyroid hormone-related peptide: expression in fetal and neonatal development. *J Pathol* 1992;167:291–296.

57. Senior PV, Heath DA, Beck F. Expression of parathyroid hormone-related protein mRNA in the rat before birth: demonstration by hybridization histochemistry. *J Mol Endocrinol* 1991;6:281–290.

58. Burton PBJ, Moniz C, Quirke P, et al. Parathyroid hormone-related peptide in the human urogenital tract. *Mol Cell Endocrinol* 1990;69:R13–R17.

59. Moseley MJ, Hayman JA, Danks JA, et al. Immunochemical detection of parathyroid hormone-related protein in human fetal epithelia. *J Clin Endocrinol Metab* 1991;73:478–484.

60. Moniz C, Burton PBJ, Malik AN, et al. Parathyroid hormone-related peptide in normal human fetal development. *J Mol Endocrinol* 1990;5:259–266.

61. de Stolpe A, Karperian M, Lowik CWGM, et al. Parathyroid hormone-related peptide as an endogenous inducer of parietal endoderm differentiation. *J Cell Biol* 1993;120:235–243.

62. Chan SDH, Strewler GS, King KL, Nissenson RA. Expression of a parathyroid hormone-like protein and its receptor during differentiation of embryonal carcinoma cells. *Mol Endocrinol* 1990;4:638–646.

63. Wysolmerski J, Philbrick W, Zhou J, Broadus A, Milstone L. Overexpression of parathyroid hormone-related peptide in skin causes abnormal hair growth, hyperkeratosis, and abnormal pigmentation. *Proc 75th Ann Mtg Endo Soc.* Las Vegas, Nevada, June, 1993; 544 (abstract).

64. Karaplis AC, Tybulewicz V, Mulligan RC, Kronenberg HM. Disruption of parathyroid hormone-related peptide gene leads to multitude of skeletal abnormalities and perinatal mortality. *J Bone Mineral Res* 1992;7(Suppl 1):S93 (abstract).

65. Okazaki T, Ando K, Igarashi T, Ogata E, Fujita T. Conserved mechanism of negative gene regulation by extracellular calcium. *J Clin Invest* 1992;89:1268–1273.

66. Connor CS, Drees BM, Thurston A, Forte L, Hermreck AS, Hamilton JW. Bovine parathyroid tissue: a model to compare the biosynthesis and secretion of parathyroid hormone and parathyroid hormone-related peptide. *Surgery* 1989;106:1057–1062.

67. Ikeda K, Lu C, Weir EC, Mangin M, Broadus AE. Transcriptional regulation of the parathyroid hormone-related

peptide gene by glucocorticoids and vitamin D in a human C-cell line. *J Biol Chem* 1989;264:15743–15746.

68. Ikeda K, Lu C, Weir EC, Mangin M, Broadus AE. Regulation of parathyroid hormone-related peptide gene expression by cycloheximide. *J Biol Chem* 1990;265:5398–5402.

69. Lu C, Ikeda K, Deftos LJ, Gazdar AF, Mangin M, Broadus AE. Glucocorticoid regulation of parathyroid hormone-related peptide gene transcription in a human neuroendocrine cell line. *Mol Endocrinol* 1989;3:2034–2040.

70. Allinson ET, Drucker DJ. Parathyroid hormone-like peptide shares features with members of the early response gene family: rapid induction by serum, growth factors, and cycloheximide. *Cancer Res* 1992;52:3103–3109.

71. Caput D, Beutler B, Hartog K, Thayer R, Brown-Shimer S, Cerami A. Identification of a common nucleotide sequence in the 3'-untranslated region of mRNA molecules specifying inflammatory mediators. *Proc Natl Acad Sci USA* 1986; 85:1670–1674.

72. Schuler GD, Cole MD. GM-CSF and oncogene mRNA stabilities are independently regulated in trans in a mouse monocytic tumor. *Cell* 1988;55:1115–1122.

73. Murphy PR, Guo JZ, Friesen HG. Messenger RNA stabilization accounts for elevated basic fibroblast growth factor transcript levels in a human astrocytoma cell line. *Mol Endocrinol* 1990;4:196–200.

74. Texier PL, de Keyzer Y, Lacave R, et al. Proopiomelanocortin gene expression in normal and tumoral human lung. *J Clin Endocrinol Metab* 1991;73:414–420.

75. Lavender P, Clark A, Besser G, Rees L. Variable methylation of the 5'-flanking DNA of the human pro-opiomelanocortin gene. *J Mol Endocrinol* 1991;6:53–61.

76. Nishizawa M, Tsuchiya M, Watanabe-Fukunaga R, Nagata S. Multiple elements in the promoter of granulocyte colony-stimulating factor gene regulate its constitutive expression in human carcinoma cells. *J Biol Chem* 1990;265:5897–5902.

77. Nakabayashi H, Hashimoto T, Miyao Y, Tjong K, Chan J, Tamaoki T. A position-dependent silencer plays a major role in repressing α-fetoprotein expression in human hepatoma. *Mol Cell Biol* 1991;11:5885–5893.

78. Nussbaum S, Gaz R, Arnold A. Hypercalcemia and ectopic secretion of parathyroid hormone by an ovarian carcinoma with rearrangement of the gene for parathyroid hormone. *N Engl J Med* 1990;323:1324–1328.

79. Yoshimoto K, Yamasaki R, Sakai H, et al. Ectopic production of parathyroid hormone by small cell lung cancer in a patient with hypercalcemia. *J Clin Endocrinol Metab* 1989; 68:976–981.

80. Strewler GJ, Budayr AA, Bruce RJ, Clark OH, Nissenson RA. Secretion of authentic parathyroid hormone by a malignant tumor. *Clin Res* 1990;38:462A (abstract).

81. Fukumoto S, Matsumoto T, Ikeda K, et al. Clinical evaluation of calcium metabolism in adult T-cell leukemia/lymphoma. *Arch Intern Med* 1988;148:921–925.

82. Motokura T, Fukumoto S, Matsumoto T, et al. Parathyroid hormone-related protein in adult T-cell leukemia-lymphoma. *Ann Intern Med* 1989;111:484–488.

83. Watanabe T, Yamaguchi K, Takatsuki K, Osama M, Yoshika M. Constitutive expression of parathyroid hormone-related protein gene in human T cell leukemia virus type I (HTLV-1) carriers and adult T cell leukemia patients that can be trans-activated by HTLV-1 tax gene. *J Exp Med* 1990; 172:759–765.

84. Prager D, Massari M, Gebremedhin S, Yamasaki H, Hendy GN, Clemens TL. Transcriptional activation of the human parathyroid hormone-related protein gene in T lymphocytes. *J Bone Mineral Res* 1991;6(Suppl):S225 (abstract).

85. Weir EC, Insogna KL, Brownstein DG, Bander NH, Broadus AE. In vitro adenylate cyclase-stimulating activity predicts the occurrence of humoral hypercalcemia of malignancy in nude mice. *J Clin Invest* 1988;81:818–821.

86. Holt EH, Vasavada R, Broadus AE, Philbrick WM. Region-specific methylation of the PTH-related peptide gene determines its expression in human renal carcinoma cell lines. *J Biol Chem* (in press).

87 Wysolmerski JJ, Vasavada R, Burtis WJ, Broadus AE, Phil-

brick WM. PTHrP gene expression in human squamous carcinoma cells. *J Bone Mineral Res* 1992;7(Suppl 1):S231 (abstract).

88. Thiede MA. The mRNA encoding a parathyroid hormone-like peptide is produced in mammary tissue in response to elevations in serum prolactin. *Mol Endocrinol* 1989;3:1443–1447.

89. Thiede MA. Expression and regulation of the parathyroid hormone-related protein gene in tumors and normal tissues. In: Halloran BP, Nissenson RA, eds. *Parathyroid hormone-related protein: normal physiology and its role in cancer.* Boca Raton, FL: CRC Press, 1992;57–91.

90. Daifotis AG, Weir EC, Dreyer BE, Broadus AE. Stretch-induced parathyroid hormone-related peptide gene expression in the rat uterus. *J Biol Chem* 1992;267:23455–23458.

91. Ferguson JE, Gorman JV, Bruns DE, et al. Abundant expression of parathyroid hormone-related protein in human amnion and its association with labor. *Proc Natl Acad Sci USA* 1992;89:8384–8388.

92. Thiede WA, Harm SC, McKee RL, Grasser WH, Duong MT, Leach RM. Expression of the parathyroid hormone-related protein gene in the avian oviduct: potential role as a local modulator of vascular smooth muscle tension and shell gland motility during the egg-laying cycle. *Endocrinology* 1991; 129:1958–1966.

93. Streuker C, Drucker DJ. Rapid induction of parathyroid hormone-like peptide gene expression by sodium butyrate in a rat islet cell line. *Mol Endocrinol* 1991;5:703–708.

94. Inuoe D, Ikeda K, Matsumoto T. 22-oxa-calcitriol, a noncalcemic analog of calcitriol, suppresses cell proliferation as well as production and secretion of PTH-related peptide by HTLV-1-infected T cells. *J Bone Mineral Res* 1992;7(Suppl 1):S173 (abstract).

95. Haq M, Goltzman D, Kremer R, Rabbani SA. A vitamin D analogue (EB-1089) prevents the development of malignancy-associated hypercalcemia in vivo. *J Bone Mineral Res* 1992;7(Suppl 1):S119 (abstract).

96. Bergmann P, Nijs-DeWolf N, Pepersack T, Corvilain J. Release of parathyroid hormone-like peptides by fetal long bones in culture. *J Bone Mineral Res* 1990;5:741–753.

97. Thiede MA, Harm SC, Hasson DM, Gardner RM. In vivo regulation of parathyroid hormone-related peptide messenger ribonucleic acid in the rat uterus by 17β-estradiol. *Endocrinology* 1991;128:2317–2323.

98. Weir E, Daifotis A, Dreyer B, Burtis W, Broadus A. Estrogen-responsive expression of the parathyroid hormone-related peptide gene by cultured primary myometrial cells. *J Bone Mineral Res* 1991;6(Suppl 1):S233 (abstract).

99. Insogna KL, Stewart AF, Ikeda K, Centrella M, Milstone LM. Characterization of a parathyroid hormone-like peptide secreted by human keratinocytes. *Ann NY Acad Sci* 1988;548:146–159.

100. Rodan SB, Wesolowski G, Ianacone J, Thiede MA, Rodan GA. Production of parathyroid hormone-like peptide in a human osteosarcoma cell line: stimulation by phorbol esters and epidermal growth factor. *J Endocrinol* 1989;122:219–227.

101. Sebag M, Henderson J, Papavasiliou V, Goltzman D, Kremer R. Regulation of parathyroid hormone-related peptide expression in normal human mammary epithelial cells. *J Bone Mineral Res* 1992;7(Suppl 1):S244 (abstract).

102. Zakalik D, Diep D, Hooks MA, Nissenson RA, Strewler GJ. Transforming growth factor beta increases stability of parathyroid hormone-related protein messenger RNA. *J Bone Mineral Res* 7(Suppl 1):S118 (abstract).

103. Casey ML, Mike M, Erk A, MacDonald PC. Transforming growth factor-β₁ stimulation of parathyroid hormone-related protein expression in human uterine cells in culture: mRNA levels and protein secretion. *J Clin Endocrinol Metab* 1992; 74:950–952.

104. Deftos LJ, Hogue-Angeletti R, Chalberg C, Su T. PTHrP secretion is stimulated by CT and inhibited by CgA peptides. *Endocrinology* 1989;125:563–565.

105. Deftos LJ, Burton DW, Brown TF, Fieck A, Brandt DW. Calcitonin-responsive elements are present in the CT and

PTH-like protein genes. *J Bone Mineral Res* 1992;7(Suppl 1):S235.

106. Deftos LJ, Gazdar AF, Ikeda K, Broadus AE. The parathyroid hormone-related protein associated with malignancy is secreted by neuroendocrine tumors. *Mol Endocrinol* 1984; 3:503–508.

107. Ikeda K, Okazaki R, Inoue D, Ogata E, Matsumoto T. Transcription of the gene for parathyroid hormone-related peptide from the human is activated through a cAMP-dependent pathway by prostaglandin E₁ in HLTV-1-infected T cells. *J Biol Chem* 1993;268:1174–1179.

108. Brandt DN, Pandol SJ, Deftos LJ. Calcium-stimulated parathyroid hormone-like protein secretion: potentiation through a protein kinase C pathway. *Endocrinology* 1991;128:2999–3004.

109. Pirola CJ, Wang HM, Wu S, et al. Regulated expression of parathyroid hormone-related protein and its receptor mRNA in rat aortic smooth muscle cells suggests an autocrine vasoactive role. *J Bone Mineral Res* 1992;7(Suppl 1):S144 (abstract).

110. Rizzoli R, Bonjour J-P. High extracellular calcium increases the production of a parathyroid hormone-like activity by cultured Leydig tumor cells associated with humoral hypercalcemia. *J Bone Mineral Res* 1989;4:839–844.

111. Zajac JD, Callaghan J, Eldridge C, et al. Production of parathyroid hormone-related protein by a rat parathyroid cell line. *Mol Cell Endocrinol* 1989;67:107–112.

112. Heschman HR. Primary response genes induced by growth factors and tumor promoters. *Annu Rev Biochem* 1991; 60:281–319.

113. Sheng M, Greenberg ME. The regulation and function of c-fos and other immediate early genes in the nervous system. *Neuron* 1990;4:477–485.

114. Ofir R, Dwarki VJ, Rashid D, Verma IM. Phosphorylation of the C terminus of Fos protein is required for transcriptional transrepression of the c-fos promoter. *Nature* 1990; 348:80–82.

115. Loh YP. *Mechanisms of intracellular trafficking and processing of proproteins.* Boca Raton, FL: CRC Press, 1993.

116. Moseley JM, Kubota M, Diefenbach-Jagger H, et al. Parathyroid hormone-related protein purified from a human lung cancer line. *Proc Natl Acad Sci USA* 1987;84:5048–5052.

117. Strewler GJ, Stern PH, Jacobs JW, et al. Parathyroid hormone-like protein from human renal carcinoma cells. *J Clin Invest* 1987;80:1803–1807.

118. Stewart AF, Wu T, Goumas D, Burtis WJ, Broadus AE. N-terminal amino acid sequence of two novel tumor-derived adenylate cyclase-stimulating proteins. *Biochem Biophys Res Commun* 1987;146:672–678.

119. Gardella TJ, Axelrod D, Rubin D, et al. Mutational analysis of the receptor activating region of human parathyroid hormone. *J Biol Chem* 1991;266:13141–13146.

120. Rabbani SA, Mitchell J, Roy DR, Hendy GN, Goltzman D. Influence of the aminoterminus on in vitro and in vivo biological activity of synthetic PTH-like peptides of malignancy. *Endocrinology* 1988;123:2709–2716.

121. Fricker LD. *Peptide biosynthesis and processing.* Boca Raton, FL: CRC Press, 1991.

122. Orloff JJ, Stewart AF. Parathyroid hormone-like proteins: biochemical responses and receptor interactions. *Endocrine Rev* 1989;10:476–495.

123. Soifer NE, Stewart AF. Measurement of PTH-related protein and the role of PTH-related protein in malignancy-associated hypercalcemia. In: Nissenson RA, Halloran B, eds. *Parathyroid hormone-related protein: normal physiology and its role in cancer.* Boca Raton, FL: CRC Press, 1992;93–143.

124. Hammonds RG, McKay P, Winslow GA, et al. Purification and characterization of recombinant human parathyroid hormone-related protein. *J Biol Chem* 1989;264:14806–14811.

125. Thorikay M, Kramer S, Reynolds F, et al. Synthesis of a gene encoding parathyroid hormone-like protein (1–141): purification and biological characterization of the expressed protein. *Endocrinology* 1989;124:111–118.

126. Nussbaum SR, Rosenblatt M, Potts JT. Parathyroid hor-

mone/renal receptor interactions: demonstration of two receptor binding domains. *J Biol Chem* 1980;255:10183–10187.

127. Soifer NE, Dee KE, Insogna KL, et al. Secretion of a novel mid-region fragment of parathyroid hormone-related protein by three different cell lines in culture. *J Biol Chem* 1992; 267:18236–18243.

128. Devi L. Peptide processing at monobasic sites. In: Fricker L, ed. *Peptide biosynthesis and processing.* Boca Raton, FL: CRC Press, 1991;175–198.

129. Loh P, Beinfeld MC, Birch NP. Proteolytic processing of prohormones and proneuropeptides. In: Loh YP, ed. *Mechanisms of intracellular trafficking and processing of proproteins.* Boca Raton, FL: CRC Press, 1993;179–224.

130. Fiedorek FT, Parkinson D. Carboxypeptidase H processing and secretion in rat clonal β cell lines. *Endocrinology* 1992;131:1054–1062.

131. Mackin RB, Noe BD, Speiss J. The anglerfish somatostatin-28-generating propeptide converting enzyme in an aspartyl-protease. *Endocrinology* 1991;129:1951–1957.

132. Beinfeld MC, Bourdais J, Kuks P, Morel P, Cohen P. Characterization of an endoprotease from rat small intestinal mucosal secretory granules which generates somatostatin-28 from prosomatostatin by cleavage after a single arginine residue. *J Biol Chem* 1989;264:4460–4465.

133. Bourdais J, Pierotti AR, Boussetta H, Barre N, Devilliers G, Cohen P. Isolation and functional properties of an arginine-selective endoprotease from rat intestinal mucosa. *J Biol Chem* 1991;266:23386–23391.

134. Imada T, Takayaranagi R, Inagami T. Atrioactivase, a specific peptidase in bovine atria for the processing of proANF. *J Biol Chem* 1988;263:9515–9519.

135. Barr PJ. Mammalian subtilisins: the long sought dibasic processing endoproteases. *Cell* 1991;66:1–3.

136. Watanbe T, Nakagawa T, Ikemizu J, Nagahama M, Murakami K, Nakayama K. Sequence requirements for precursor cleavage within the constitutive secretory pathway. *J Biol Chem* 1992;267:8270–8274.

137. Care AD, Abbas SK, Pickard DW, et al. Stimulation of ovine placental transport of calcium and magnesium by mid-molecular fragments of human PTHRP. *Exp Physiol* 1990; 75:605–608.

138. Rodda CP, Kubota M, Heath JA, et al. Evidence for a novel parathyroid hormone-related protein in fetal lamb parathyroid gland and sheep placenta. *J Endocrinol* 1988;117:261–271.

139. Fenton AJ, Kemp BE, Kent GN, et al. A carboxyterminal peptide from the parathyroid hormone-related peptide inhibits bone resorption by osteoclasts. *Endocrinology* 1991; 129:1762–1768.

140. Fenton AJ, Kemp BE, Hammonds RG, et al. A potent inhibitor of osteoclastic bone resorption within a highly conserved pentapeptide region of PTHrP; PTHrP[107–111]. *Endocrinology* 1991;129:3424–3426.

141. Sone T, Kohno H, Kikuchi H, et al. Human PTHrP(107–111) does not inhibit bone resorption in neonatal mouse calvarie. *Endocrinology* 1992;131:2742–2746.

142. Kaiser SM, Laneuville P, Bernier SM, Rhims JS, Kremer R, Goltzman D. Enhanced growth of a human keratinocyte line by antisense RNA for PTHrP. *J Biol Chem* 1992;267:13623–13628.

143. Imamura H, Sato K, Shizume K, et al. Urinary excretion of parathyroid hormone-related protein fragments in patients with humoral hypercalcemia of malignancy and hypercalcemic tumor-bearing nude mice. *J Bone Mineral Res* 1991; 6:77–84.

144. dePapp A, Yang KH, Soifer NE, et al. Post-translational processing and secretion of a novel carboxyterminal PTHrP species. *Proc 75th Ann Mtg Endo Soc.* Las Vegas, Nevada, June 1993; 545 (abstract).

145. Burtis WJ, Debeyssey M, Philbrick WM, et al. Evidence for the presence of an extreme carboxyterminal PTHrP in biological specimens. *J Bone Mineral Res* 1992;7(Suppl 1):S225 (abstract).

146. Wu TL, Soifer NE, Burtis WJ, Milstone LM, Stewart AF. Glycosylation of parathyroid hormone-related peptide se-

creted by human epidermal keratinocytes. *J Clin Endocrinol Metab* 1991;73:1002–1007.

147. Sairam MR. Role of carbohydrates in glycoprotein hormone signal transduction. *FASEB J* 1989;3:1915–1926.

148. Rao-Thotakura N, Desai RK, Bates LG, Cole EX, Pratt BM, Weintraub BD. Biological activity and metabolic clearance of a recombinant human TSH produced in CHO cells. *Endocrinology* 1991;128:341–348.

149. Narki LO, Arakawa T, Aoki KH, et al. Effect of carbohydrate on the structure and stability of erythropoitin. *J Biol Chem* 1991;266:23077–23086.

150. Kaetzel DM, Browne JK, Wondisford F, Nett TM, Thomason AR, Nilson JH. Expression of biologically active bovine LH in CHO cells. *Proc Natl Acad Sci USA* 1985;82:7280–7283.

151. Eipper BA, Mains RE. Peptide alpha-amidation. *Annu Rev Physiol* 1988;50:333–344.

152. Bradbury AF, Finnie MDA, Smyth DG. Mechanism of C-terminal amide formation by pituitary enzymes. *Nature* 1982;298:686–688.

153. Eipper BA, Green CB-R, Campbell TA, et al. Alternative splicing and endoproteolytic processing generate tissue-specific forms of pituitary PAM. *J Biol Chem* 1992;267:4008–4015.

154. Braas KM, Harakall SA, Ouafik L'H, Eipper BA, May V. Expression of PAM: an *in situ* hybridization and immunocytochemical study. *Endocrinology* 1992;130:2778–2788.

155. Mains RE, Bloomquist BT, Eipper BA. Manipulation of neuropeptide biosynthesis through the expression of antisense RNA to PAM. *Mol Endocrinol* 1991;5:187–193.

156. Vale W, Speiss J, Rivier C, Rivier J. Characterization of a 41 residue ovine hypothalamic peptide that stimulates secretion of corticotrophin and β endorphins. *Science* 1981;213:1394–1397.

157. Rosenblatt M, Potts JT. Design and synthesis of parathyroid hormone analogues of enhanced biological activity. *Endocrinol Res Commun* 1977;4:115–133.

158. Dickinson CJ, Yamada T. Gastrin amidating enzyme in the porcine pituitary and antrum. *J Biol Chem* 1991;266:334–338.

159. McFarland KC, Sprengel R, Phillips HS, et al. Lutrophin-choriogonadotropin receptor: an unusual member of the G-protein-coupled receptor family. *Science* 1989;245:494–499.

160. Moroni MC, Willingham MC, Bequinot L. EGF-R antisense RNA blocks expression of the EGF receptor and suppresses transforming phenotype of a human carcinoma line. *J Biol Chem* 1992;267:2714–2722.

161. Abbott AM, Bueno R, Pedrinin MT, Murray JM, Smith RJ. Insulin-like growth factor gene structure. *J Biol Chem* 1992;267:10759–10763.

162. Cunningham BC, Ultsch M, deVos AM, Mulkerrin MB, Clauser KR, Wells JA. Derivitization of the extracellular domain of the human growth hormone receptor by a single molecule. *Science* 1991;254:821–825.

163. Mountjoy KG, Robbins LS, Mortud MT, Cone RD. The cloning of a family of genes that includes the melanocortin receptors. *Science* 1992;257:1248–1251.

164. Marchingo AJ, Abrahams JM, Woodcock EA, Smith AI, Mendelsohn FAO, Johnston CI. Properties of ³H-1-desamino-8-D-arginine vasopressin as a radioligand for vasopressin V₂ receptors in rat kidney. *Endocrinology* 1988;122:1328–1336.

165. Stewart AF, Vignery A, Silvergate A, et al. Quantitative bone histomorphometry in humoral hypercalcemia of malignancy: uncoupling of bone cell activity. *J Clin Endocrinol Metab* 1982;55:219–227.

166. Atkinson MJ, Hesch R-D, Cade C, Wadwah M, Perris AD. Parathyroid hormone stimulation of mitosis in rat thymic lymphocytes is independent of cyclic AMP. *J Bone Mineral Res* 1987;2:303–309.

167. Fadda GZ, Akmal M, Lipson LG, Massry S. Direct effects of parathyroid hormone on insulin secretion from pancreatic islets. *Am J Physiol* 1990;258:E975–E984.

168. Bikle DD, Nemanic MK, Gee E, Elias P. 1,25(OH)₂D pro-

duction by human keratinocytes. *J Clin Invest* 1986;78:557–566.

169. Goldring SR, Mahaffey JE, Krane SM, Potts JT, Dayer JM, Rosenblatt M. Parathyroid hormone inhibitors, comparison of biological activity in bone- and skin-derived tissues. *J Clin Endocrinol Metab* 1979;48:655–662.

170. Mok LLS, Nickols GA, Thompson JC, Cooper CW. Parathyroid hormone as a smooth muscle relaxant. *Endocrine Rev* 1989;10:420–436.

171. Fraser CL, Sarnacki P, Arieff AI. Calcium transport abnormality in uremic rat brain synaptosomes. *J Clin Invest* 1985;76:1789–1795.

172. Insogna KL, Stewart AF, Morris CA, Hough LM, Milstone LM, Centrella M. Native and synthetic analogue of the malignancy-associated parathyroid hormone-like protein have in vitro transforming growth factor-like properties. *J Clin Invest* 1989;83:1057–1060.

173. Mitnick MA, Isales C, Paliwal I, Insogna KL. Parathyroid hormone-related protein stimulates prostaglandin E₂ release from human osteoblast-like cells. *J Bone Mineral Res* 1992;7:887–896.

174. Orloff JJ, Ganz MB, Ribaudo AE, et al. Analysis of parathyroid hormone-related protein binding and signal transduction mechanisms in benign and malignant squamous cells. *Am J Physiol* 1992;262:E599–E607.

175. McCauley LK, Rosol TJ, Merryman JI, Capen CC. PTHrP binding to HTLV-1-infected lymphocytes. *Endocrinology* 1992;130:300–306.

176. Gaich G, Orloff J, Atillasoy EJ, Burtis WJ, Ganz MB, Stewart AF. Amino-terminal parathyroid hormone-related protein: specific binding and cytosolic calcium responses in rat insulinoma cells. *Endocrinology* 1993;132:1402–1409.

177. Urena P, Lee K, Weaver D, et al. PTH/PTHrP receptor mRNA expression as assessed by Northern blot and *in situ* hybridization. *J Bone Mineral Res* 1992;7(Suppl 1):S118 (abstract).

178. Orloff JJ, Urena P, Schipani E, et al. Human squamous carcinoma cells and normal human keratinocytes express mRNAs related to but distinct from human PTH receptor mRNA. *J Bone Mineral Res* 1992;7(Suppl 1):S230 (abstract).

179. Henderson JE, Kremer R, Rhim JS, Goltzman D. Identification and functional characterization of adenylate cyclase-linked receptors for parathyroid hormone-like peptides on immortalized human keratinocytes. *Endocrinology* 1992;130:449–457.

180. Ikeda K, Mangin M, Dreyer BE, et al. Identification of transcripts encoding a parathyroid hormone-like peptide in messenger RNAs from a variety of human and animal tumors associated with humoral hypercalcemia of malignancy. *J Clin Invest* 1988;81:2010–2014.

181. Danks JA, Ebeling PR, Hayman R, et al. PTH-related protein: immunohistochemical localization in cancers and in normal skin. *J Bone Mineral Res* 1989;4:273–278.

182. Pillai S, Bikle DD, Elias PM. 1,25-Dihydroxyvitamin D production and receptor binding in human keratinocytes varies with differentiation. *J Biol Chem* 1988;263:5390–5395.

183. Hoekman K, Lowik CWGM, Ruit M, Kempenaar J, Bijvoet OLM, Ponce M. Modulation of the production of a parathyroid hormone-like protein in human squamous cell lines by interaction with fibroblasts. *Cancer Res* 1990;50:3589–3594.

184. Lowik CWGM, Hoekman K, Offringa R, et al. Regulation of parathyroid hormone-like protein production in cultured normal and malignant keratinocytes. *J Invest Dermatol* 1992;98:198–203.

185. Centrella M, Canalis E, McCarthy TL, Stewart AF, Orloff JJ, Insogna KL. Regulation of DNA and collagen synthesis in fetal rat bone through changes in TGF-β action by parathyroid hormone-related protein. *Endocrinology* 1989;125:199–208.

186. Burton PBJ, Moniz C, Knight DE. Parathyroid hormone related peptide can function as an autocrine growth factor in human renal cell carcinoma. *Biochem Biophys Res Commun* 1990;167:1134–1138.

187. deMiguel F, Garcia-Canero R, Esbrit P. Co-purification of

calcium transport-stimulating and DNA synthesis-stimulating agents with parathyroid hormone-like activity from the hypercalcemic strain of the Walker 256 tumor. *Eur J Cancer* 1991;27:1022–1026.

188. Holick MF, Nussbaum S, Persons KS. PTH-like humoral hypercalcemia factor of malignancy may be an epidermal differentiation factor. *J Bone Mineral Res* 1988;3(Suppl 1):S214 (abstract).

189. Ernst M, Rodan GA, Thiede MA. Rapid induction of parathyroid hormone-like peptide in keratinocytes. *J Bone Mineral Res* 1989;4(Suppl 1):S195 (abstract).

190. Wu TL, Insogna KL, Milstone LM, Stewart AF. Skin-derived fibroblasts respond to human PTH-like adenylate cyclase-stimulating proteins. *J Clin Endocrinol Metab* 1987; 65:105–109.

191. Allgrove J, Adami S, Manning RM, O'Riordan JLH. Cytochemical bioassay of parathyroid hormone in maternal and cord blood. *Arch Dis Child* 1985;60:110–115.

192. Care AD, Caple IW, Pickard DW. The roles of the parathyroid and thyroid glands on calcium homeostasis in the ovine fetus. In: Jones CT, Nathaniels PW, eds. *The physiological development of the fetus and newborn.* London: Academic Press, 1985;135–140.

193. Care AD, Caple IW, Abbas SK, Pickard DW. The effect of fetal thyroparathyroidectomy on the transport of calcium across the ovine placenta in the fetus. *Placenta* 1986;7:417–424.

194. Abbas SK, Pickard DW, Illingworth D, et al. Measurement of parathyroid hormone-related protein in extracts of fetal parathyroid glands and placental membranes. *J Endocrinol* 1990;124:319–325.

195. Abbas SK, Pickard DW, Rodda CP, et al. Stimulation of ovine placental calcium transport by purified natural and recombinant parathyroid hormone-related protein (PTHrP) preparations. *Q J Exp Physiol* 1989;74:549–552.

196. Shaw AJ, Mughal MZ, Maresh MJA, Sibley CA. Effects of two synthetic parathyroid hormone-related protein fragments on maternofetal transfer of calcium and magnesium and release of cyclic AMP by the in situ perfused rat placenta. *J Endocrinol* 1991;129:399–404.

197. Hazum E. Neuroendocrine peptides in milk. *Trends Endocrinol Metab* 1991; Jan-Feb, pp 25–28.

198. Shaw GV, Kacsoh B, Seshadri R, Grosvenor CE, Crowley WR. Presence of calcitonin-like peptide in rat milk: possible physiological role in regulation of neonatal prolactin secretion. *Endocrinology* 1989;125:61–67.

199. Goff JP, Reinhardt TA, Lee S, Hollis BW. Parathyroid hormone-related peptide content of bovine milk and calf blood assessed by radioimmunoassay and bioassay. *Endocrinology* 1991;129:2815–2819.

200. Garner SC, Boass A, Toverud SU. Parathyroid hormone is not required for normal milk composition or secretion or lactation-associated bone loss in normocalcemic rats. *J Bone Mineral Res* 1990;5:69–75.

201. Yamamoto M, Doung LT, Fisher JE, Thiede MA, Caulfield MP, Rosenblatt M. Suckling-mediated increases in urinary phosphate and 3′-5′-cyclic adenosine monophosphate excretion in lactating rats: possible systemic effects of parathyroid hormone-related protein. *Endocrinology* 1991;129:2614–2622.

202. Budayr AA, Halloran BR, King JC, Diep D, Nissenson RA, Strewler GJ. High levels of a parathyroid hormone-like protein in milk. *Proc Natl Acad Sci USA* 1989;86:7183–7185.

203. Thurston AW, Cole JA, Hillman LS, et al. Purification and properties of parathyroid hormone-related peptide isolated from milk. *Endocrinology* 1990;126:1183–1190.

204. Stewart AF, Wu TL, Insogna KL, Milstone LM, Burtis WJ. Immunoaffinity purification of parathyroid hormone-related protein from bovine milk and human keratinocyte-conditioned medium. *J Bone Mineral Res* 1991;6:305–311.

205. Ratcliffe WA, Green E, Emly J, et al. Identification and partial characterization of parathyroid hormone-related protein in human and bovine milk. *J Endocrinol* 1990;127:167–176.

206. Law FML, Moate PJ, Leaver DD, et al. Parathyroid hor-

mone-related protein in milk and its correlation with bovine milk calcium. *J Endocrinol* 1991;128:21–26.

207. Khosla S, Johansen KL, Ory SJ, O'Brien PC, Kao PC. Parathyroid hormone-related peptide in lactation and in umbilical cord blood. *Mayo Clin Proc* 1990;65:1408–1414.

208. Ratcliffe WA, Thompson GE, Care AD, Peaker M. Production of parathyroid hormone-related protein by the mammary gland of the goat. *J Endocrinol* 1992;133:87–93.

209. Rakopoulos M, Vargas SJ, Gillespie MT, et al. Production of parathyroid hormone-related protein by the rat mammary gland in pregnancy and lactation. *Am J Physiol* 1992; 263:E1077–E1085.

210. Yamamoto M, Fisher JE, Thiede A, Caulfield MP, Rosenblatt M, Duong LT. Concentrations of parathyroid hormone-related protein in rat milk change with duration of lactation and interval from previous suckling, but not with milk calcium. *Endocrinology* 1992;130:741–747.

211. Ferrari SL, Rizzoli R, Bonjour JP. Parathyroid hormone-related protein production by primary cultures of mammary epithelial cells. *J Cell Physiol* 1992;150:304–411.

212. Khosla S, van Heerden JA, Gharib H, et al. Parathyroid hormone-related protein and hypercalcemia secondary to massive mammary hyperplasia. *N Engl J Med* 1990;322:1157.

213. Yamamoto M, Duong LT, Caulfield MP. Parathyroid hormone related protein concentrations in rat milk: relationships with the intensity of suckling, food intake, and prolactin. *J Bone Mineral Res* 1992;7(Suppl 1):S237 (abstract).

214. Cooper KM, Ives KL, Seitz PK, Ishizuka J, Townsend CM Jr, Cooper CW. Parathyroid hormone-related peptide 1-34 blocks the oxytocin-induced increase in intracellular Ca²⁺ in cultured human breast myoepithelial cells. *J Bone Mineral Res* 1992;7(Suppl 1):S234 (abstract).

215. Grill V, Hillary J, Ho PMW, et al. Parathyroid hormone-related protein: a possible endocrine function in lactation. *Clin Endocrinol* 1992;37:405–410.

216. Melton ME, D'Anza JJ, Wimbiscus SA, Grill V, Martin TJ, Kukreja SC. Parathyroid hormone-related protein and calcium homeostasis in lactating mice. *Am J Physiol* 1990; 259:E792–E796.

217. Kukreja SC, D'Anza JJ, Melton ME, Wimbiscus SA, Grill V, Martin TJ. Lack of effects of neutralization of parathyroid hormone-related protein on calcium homeostasis in neonatal mice. *J Bone Mineral Res* 1991;6:1197–1201.

218. Canalis E, McCarthy TL, Centrella M. Differential effects of continuous and transient treatment with parathyroid hormone related peptide on bone collagen synthesis. *Endocrinology* 1990;126:1806–1812.

219. Kikuchi H, Shigeno C, Lee K, et al. On the transforming growth factor β-like activity of synthetic polypeptides comprising amino-terminal sequence of human parathyroid hormone-related peptide. *Endocrinology* 1991;128:1229–1237.

220. Nijs-DeWolf N, Pepersack T, Corvilain J, Karmali R, Bergmann P. Adenylate cyclase-stimulating activity immunologically similar to parathyroid hormone-related peptide can be extracted from fetal rat long bones. *J Bone Mineral Res* 1991;6:921–927.

221. Lee K, Deeds JD, Bond AT, Jüppner H, Abou-Samra A-B, Segre GV. In situ localization of PTH/PTHrP receptor mRNA in the bone of fetal and young rats. *Bone* 1993;14:341–345.

222. Koike T, Iwamoto M, Shimazu A, Nakashima K, Suzuki F. Kato Y. Potent mitogenic effects of parathyroid hormone (PTH) on embryonic chick and rabbit chondrocytes. *J Clin Invest* 1990;85:626–631.

223. Burger EN, Gaillard PJ. Structural and ultrastructural responses of calcifying cartilage to parathyroid hormone in vitro. *Calcif Tissue Res* 1976;21:75–80.

224. Kato Y, Shimazu A, Nakashima K, Suzuki F, Jikko A, Iwamoto M. Effects of parathyroid hormone and calcitonin on alkaline phosphatase activity and matrix calcification in rabbit growth plate chondrocyte cultures. *Endocrinology* 1990; 127:114–118.

225. Nichols GA, Nana AD, Nichols MA, DiPette DJ, Asimakis GK. Hypotension and cardiac stimulation due to the para-

thyroid hormone-related protein, humoral hypercalcemia of malignancy factor. *Endocrinology* 1989;125:834–841.

226. Winquist RJ, Baskin EP, Vlasuk GP. Synthetic tumor-derived human hypercalcemic factor exhibits parathyroid hormone-like vasorelaxation in renal arteries. *Biochem Biophys Res Commun* 1987;149:227–232.

227. Mok LLS, Ajiwe E, Martin TJ, Thompson JC, Cooper CW. Parathyroid hormone-related protein relaxes rat gastric smooth muscle and shows cross desensitization with parathyroid hormone. *J Bone Mineral Res* 1989;4:433–439.

228. Shew RL, Yee JA, Kliewer DB, Ketlemariam YJ, McNeill DL. Parathyroid hormone-related protein inhibits stimulated uterine contraction in vitro. *J Bone Mineral Res* 1991;6:955–959.

229. Roca-Cusachs A, DiPette DJ, Nichols GA. Regional and systemic hemodynamic effects of parathyroid hormone-related protein: preservation of cardiac function and coronary blood flow and renal flow with reduced blood pressure. *J Pharmacol Exp Ther* 1991;256:110–118.

230. Shew RL, Yee JA. Inhibition of uterine contraction by parathyroid hormone-related peptide is dependent on nitric oxide formation. *J Bone Mineral Res* 1992;7(Suppl 1):S237 (abstract).

231. Thiede MA, Peterson DN, Grasser WA, Jüppner H, Abou-Samra AB, Segre GV. Coexpression of PTHrP and PTH/PTHrP receptor mRNA in vasculature supports a local mechanism of action in cardiovascular tissues. *J Bone Mineral Res* 1992;7(Suppl 1):S240 (abstract).

232. Pirola CJ, Wang H, Kamyar A, et al. Angiotensin II regulates parathyroid hormone-related protein expression in cultured rat aortic smooth muscle cells through transcriptional and post-transcriptional mechanisms. *J Biol Chem* 1993;268:1987–1994.

233. Germain AM, Attaroglu H, MacDonald PC, Casey ML. Parathyroid hormone-related protein mRNA in avascular human amnion. *J Clin Endocrinol Metab* 1992;75:1173–1175.

234. Watson P. Function follows form: generation of intracellular signals by cell deformation. *FASEB J* 1991;5:2013–2019.

The Parathyroids, edited by J.P. Bilezikian, M.A. Levine, and R. Marcus. Raven Press, Ltd., New York © 1994.

CHAPTER 18

Parathyroid Hormone-Related Protein as a Cause of Hypercalcemia in Malignancy

Vivian Grill and T. John Martin

The discovery of parathyroid hormone-related protein (PTHrP) as a likely cause of hypercalcemia in many patients with cancer has provided new insights into the pathogenesis of the skeletal complications of malignancy. It reveals PTHrP to be a previously unrecognized hormone, important in fetal development and in the pathogenesis of hypercalcemia when produced in excess in certain cancers, but otherwise exerting paracrine actions in a number of fetal and adult tissues.

HYPERCALCEMIA IN CANCER

Hypercalcemia is a very common complication of several cancers, especially squamous cell carcinoma of the lung, breast cancer, renal cortical carcinoma, and a number of hematological malignancies. Indeed malignancy is the most frequent cause of hypercalcemia in a general hospital inpatient population, whereas primary hyperparathyroidism is a more common cause of elevated blood calcium in the community at large. Because the pathophysiology of hypercalcemia is heterogeneous, it has been traditionally considered as three separate syndromes in cancer: (a) humoral hypercalcemia of malignancy, (b) hypercalcemia associated with localized osteolysis due to bone metastases, and (c) hypercalcemia associated with myeloma and other hematological malignancies.

Our understanding of the ways in which various tumors induce hypercalcemia has increased rapidly in the last few years with the identification of several tumor-derived factors that elevate the plasma calcium concentration. The discovery of PTHrP, followed by the establishment of assays that allow its detection in the circulation, has provided new insights into the mechanisms for the hypercalcemia in these three syndrome classes. As a consequence, the division into these classes is now less clear cut than it was, and the reasons for this are expanded in the following discussion.

Humoral Hypercalcemia of Malignancy

The term *humoral hypercalcemia of malignancy* (HHM) was introduced to describe patients with certain cancers in whom the blood calcium is elevated in the absence of skeletal metastases (1). The most common cause of this is squamous cell carcinoma of the lung. Squamous cell cancers at other sites, including skin, esophagus, and head and neck, and also renal cortical carcinoma, primary liver cancer, breast cancer, pancreatic cancer, bladder and prostatic carcinoma, as well as melanoma may all be associated with humoral hypercalcemia. In the absence of secondary lesions, removal of the primary tumor leads to resolution of the hypercalcemia (2). Tumor factors are secreted that act on the skeleton generally to increase bone resorption, and on the kidney to reduce calcium excretion and increase phosphorus excretion (1). Nephrogenous cyclic adenosine monophosphate (cAMP) excretion is also increased (3–5), and there is often a mild hypokalemic, hypochloremic alkalosis.

In squamous cell carcinoma of the bronchus, as an example, mild hypercalcemia occurs in as many as 40% of patients. The degree of hypercalcemia can remain constant for many months; sometimes it progresses steadily and is associated with a mild hypokalemic hypochloremic alkalosis, and sometimes apparently stable hypercalcemia progresses rapidly to severe, and even life-threatening, forms. This may occur without any obvious explanation or may be asso-

V. Grill, T. J. Martin: Department of Medicine, University of Melbourne, and St. Vincent's Hospital, Melbourne, Victoria, 3065 Australia.

TABLE 1. *Clinical and biochemical features of primary hyperparathyroidism and humoral hypercalcemia of malignancy*

	HHM	Primary hyperpara-thyroidism
History	Rapid onset (<6 months)	Slow progression (>12 months)
	Marked weight loss	No weight loss
	No renal calculi	Renal calculi
Serum calcium	High	High
Serum phosphorus	Low	Low
Nephrogenous cAMP	High	High
Serum chloride	Low	High
Serum bicarbonate	High	Low
Serum calcitriol	Low	High

ciated with rapid progression of tumor. Alternatively, it may be a consequence of dehydration in the patient in association with treatment or coexistent infection. It is clear that patients with HHM resemble those with primary hyperparathyroidism in their main biochemical features (Table 1), a similarity that has been recognized for many years. Exceptions to this similarity are the serum concentrations of bicarbonate, which are low in many patients with primary hyperparathyroidism and high in many patients with HHM, and the serum concentration of 1,25-dihydroxyvitamin D [1,25-(OH)$_2$D], which is elevated in many patients with primary hyperparathyroidism but is depressed in many patients with HHM (4).

Hypercalcemia Associated With Bone Metastases

Despite many improvements in early cancer detection and more effective treatment, metastatic disease remains the leading cause of cancer-related deaths. Bone is the most common site of metastasis in breast cancer, and 25% of early stage patients will develop this complication. This figure increases to 75% in patients with advanced disease (6). Currently there is no single, accurate predictor to identify which patients will develop this complication. In the clinical follow-up of patients with breast cancer especially, bone scanning at regular intervals is important in the detection of bone metastases. Recognition of the symptoms of early hypercalcemia is of the utmost importance, since progression to severe hypercalcemia can be prevented by appropriate measures, including increased fluid intake and antitumor therapy. A "flare up" of hypercalcemia can accompany the use of antiestrogen therapy in some patients with breast cancer (7).

Although for many years it was considered that the main mechanism of hypercalcemia in patients with breast cancer was the release of calcium from bone by osteolytic deposits (8), there is increasing evidence for a humoral contribution in these patients also. The extent of metastatic bone disease correlates poorly with both the occurrence and the degree of hypercalcemia in malignancy (9). In 80–90% of cases of unselected solid tumor patients with hypercalcemia, irrespective of whether bone metastases are present, there is evidence of an underlying humoral mechanism (9). The putative humoral mediator produces hypercalcemia both by stimulating generalized osteolysis and, in most cases, by impairing the renal excretion of the resultant increase in filtered calcium load. Reduced renal phosphate threshold and increased tubular calcium reabsorption were observed in hypercalcemic patients compared with their normocalcemic counterparts, emphasizing the importance of renal mechanisms in mediating the hypercalcemia.

Hypercalcemia in Hematological Malignancy

Hematological malignancies may be associated with osteolytic bone destruction and with hypercalcemia. Lymphoproliferative disorders such as malignant lymphomas can be associated with hypercalcemia. Occasional patients with chronic myeloid (10) and acute lymphoblastic leukemia (11) develop hypercalcemia. Hypercalcemia occurs in approximately one-third of all patients with multiple myeloma (8,12), a disease resulting from uncontrolled clonal proliferation of plasma cells. In multiple myeloma, hypercalcemia is almost invariably associated with widespread bone involvement, as well as with some irreversible impairment of renal function, which reduces the ability of the kidney to clear the excess calcium load due to increased bone resorption. Bone involvement in myeloma is characterized by extensive bone destruction accompanied by pain and susceptibility to fracture. Skeletal X-rays reveal abnormalities in 79% of patients (12); these consist of osteoporosis, lytic lesions, and fractures, with over one-half of patients having a combination of all three. Bone resorption leading to hypercalcemia in myeloma is due to the secretion by myeloma cells of bone resorbing cytokines. A number of cytokines previously described by the generic name *osteoclast-activating factor* (13,14) have now been identified in activated leukocyte cultures: interleukin-1, tumor necrosis factor-α (TNFα; cachectin), and tumor necrosis factor-β (TNFβ; lymphotoxin). It is not yet known whether one of these cytokines or more is responsible for the stimulation of osteoclastic bone resorption in multiple myeloma (see the chapter by Black and Mundy). A study found that most, but not all, of the bone-resorbing activity from a human myeloma cell line could be suppressed by neutralizing antibodies to TNFβ (15). Although production of this bone-resorbing cytokine may be related to osteoclastic bone destruction and hypercalcemia in patients with myeloma, other cytokines may also be involved.

The overall incidence of hypercalcemia in patients with lymphoma in the Western world is relatively low compared to that in patients with solid tumors or with multiple myeloma (16) and accounts for ~5% of cases of hypercalcemia in malignancy. Hypercalcemia is uncommon in both non-Hodgkin's and Hodgkin's lymphomas, as shown by a series in which only one of 190 cases of Hodgkin's disease and only three of 104 cases of non-Hodgkin's lymphoma (17) were associated with hypercalcemia. A number of case reports have documented hypercalcemia without lytic bone lesions in both Hodgkin's and non-Hodgkin's lymphoma, which was associated with elevated 1,25-(OH)$_2$D levels and low parathyroid hormone (PTH) levels in plasma (18–24). Involvement of the lymphoma in the extrarenal synthesis of 1,25-(OH)$_2$D was suggested by demonstration of in vitro conversion of 25-(OH)D to 1,25-(OH)$_2$D by lymphoma tissue (21), as was shown to occur with lymph node tissue in sarcoidosis (25). Support for such a humoral mechanism of hypercalcemia was provided by the report that excision of an isolated splenic lymphoma resulted in resolution of the hypercalcemia (19) and by the demonstration that effective chemotherapy regimens produced a substantial decrease in the level of 1,25-(OH)$_2$D and calcium in patients with lymphoma (20,22). Although hypercalcemia is an infrequent complication of lymphoma, a particular diagnostic subgroup of patients with adult T-cell lymphoma/leukemia has a very high incidence of hypercalcemia, varying from 26% to 100% in different reports (26–28); 1,25-(OH)$_2$D levels in this group of patients are uniformly suppressed (29). This disease, with predominant geographic distribution in Japan and a small cluster in the West Indies, is strongly associated with a retrovirus, human T-cell lymphotrophic virus type 1 (HTLV-1) (30–32). Hypercalcemia is the most important prognostic determinant in this disease and also is a frequent cause of death. Hypercalcemia in these patients is associated with elevated nephrogenous cAMP (NcAMP) levels, low to normal immunoreactive PTH levels, and reduced serum 1,25-(OH)$_2$D concentrations (33) in the absence of lytic lesions in bone. These features are similar to those seen in HHM.

DISCOVERY OF PARATHYROID HORMONE-RELATED PROTEIN

Hypercalcemia as a complication of malignancy has been recognized since the 1920s (34). In 1941, Fuller Albright (35) discussed a patient in whom hypercalcemia and hypophosphatemia resolved after the radiation of a single bone metastasis from a renal carcinoma. Albright proposed that the hypercalcemia might be due to production by the cancer of PTH. In later years, this idea gained acceptance, and the term *ectopic PTH syndrome* was widely used to apply to patients with cancer who had a high plasma calcium, low phosphorus, and minimal or no bony metastases (36). Support for this came in 1966, when Berson and Yalow (37) published results from the first radioimmunoassay for PTH; they found significant elevations of the PTH level in a number of unselected patients with lung cancer. Over the next several years, until the early 1970s, several reports were published of measurable PTH (by radioimmunoassay) in extracts of cancer from such patients (reviewed in 1,8). There was one report of an arteriovenous gradient across a tumor bed, indicating release of PTH from tumor (38), and production of immunoreactive PTH was shown by a cell culture established from a renal cortical carcinoma of a hypercalcemic patient (39). Throughout this period, however, it was evident that the radioimmunoassay of PTH presented technical problems, and in none of the abovementioned instances were circulating levels of PTH convincingly very high, certainly not at the levels frequently found with corresponding degrees of elevation of plasma calcium in patients with primary hyperparathyroidism. Two groups of workers in the early 1970s published results indicating that the circulating immunoreactive PTH in the cancer patients differed from "authentic" PTH (40–42). The levels in plasma were in these cases lower than in primary hyperparathyroidism. In one series, measurements of plasma samples in serial dilution were not parallel to PTH standards in the radioimmunoassay (41) and, in the other, the tumor product was of higher molecular weight than PTH (42).

Thus the early 1970s saw some doubt arising that PTH itself was a major contributor to the clinical and biochemical features of this cancer syndrome. This doubt became more firmly based when Powell and colleagues (2) showed in studies of several patients with humoral hypercalcemia that PTH could not be detected in plasma or in tumor extracts, despite the use of a wide range of PTH antisera directed against different parts of the molecule.

The more comprehensive clinical and biochemical investigations that followed (3–5) indicated that the manifestations of HHM were mediated via PTH receptors in kidney and bone (8), and the development of sensitive bioassays for PTH led to exciting developments in understanding of the syndrome. The bioassays revealed that these tumor extracts could stimulate adenylyl cyclase in PTH-responsive renal cortical membranes (43,44). A sensitive cytochemical assay for PTH in kidney cells could detect PTH-like bioactivity in the serum of patients in whom immunoreactive PTH was undetectable (45). Studies in PTH-responsive osteogenic sarcoma cells showed that tumor extracts of rat and human origin could also stimulate adenylyl cyclase in this system (46). Peptide antagonists of PTH blocked biological activity, but preincu-

```
PTHrP    A V S E H Q L L H D K G K S I Q D L R R R F F L H H L I A E I H T A
PTH      S V S E I Q L M H F L G K H L N S M E R V E W L R K K L Q D V H N F
```

FIG. 1. Amino acid sequences of PTH-(1–34) and PTHrP-(1–34).

bation with PTH antisera was ineffective in blocking biological activity (46), indicating that the active material acted on PTH receptors but was immunologically distinct from PTH. Messenger RNA for PTH could not be detected in any of a series of tumors associated with the HHM syndrome (47).

These observations led to the identification and isolation of the factor responsible for the syndrome of HHM. Experimental animal models were developed and cell cultures established from them and from human tumors (48–51). Purification of the active factor to homogeneity on gels was reported (52,53), and PTHrP was finally purified, sequenced, and cloned from a cultured human lung cancer cell line (BEN) (52,54) and from other sources (55,56). The amino-acid sequence of PTHrP bears 60% homology with that of PTH over the first 13 amino acids (Fig. 1). The gene codes for a protein of 141, 139, or 173 amino acids determined by alternate 3' splicing of mRNA. A prepro sequence of 36 amino acids contains potential cleavage points at residues −8 or −6, leaving a short prosequence. The PTH-like biological activity of PTHrP is contained within the first 34 amino acids. Beyond this region, the two molecules have unique sequences.

The limited homology at the amino-terminal region of the mature protein between PTHrP and PTH seemed to be sufficient to account for the similar actions of PTHrP and PTH. PTHrP mimics the actions of PTH in vitro and in vivo (57–63). Immunohistochemical analyses of tumor sections using specific antibodies raised predominantly to PTHrP-(1–34), but also to unique mid-(50–69) and C-terminal-(106–141) epitopes, have shown that PTHrP is present in the cells of all squamous cell cancers investigated (64), indicating the potential of these tumors to produce HHM. In a nude mouse model of HHM, both the hypercalcemia (Fig. 2) and the bone abnormalities are effectively attenuated by treatment with neutralizing antisera against PTHrP (65,66). These passive immunization experiments established that PTHrP was at least a major, if not the sole, mediator of hypercalcemia in these models of HHM, even if they did not exclude the possibility that there could be other contributing factors. There are some discrepancies between the features of HHM and hyperparathyroidism (8), which may relate either to interactions with other tumor factors that may be cosecreted with PTHrP, or possibly to actions mediated via regions of the PTHrP molecule beyond the first 34 amino acids. An example

is the hypokalemic alkalosis seen in hypercalcemia of cancer, whereas mild hyperchloremic acidosis is more commonly noted in primary hyperparathyroidism (Table 1). As a possible explanation for this difference, altered renal handling of bicarbonate by the rat kidney perfused with PTHrP-(1–141) has been found compared to that in PTHrP-(1–34) (67). Prolonged infusion with PTHrP-(1–141) resulted in restricted bicarbonate excretion, after the initial increased excretion noted in response to both forms of PTHrP and to PTH itself. As is the case with PTH, N-terminal fragments of PTHrP promote renal 1α-hydroxylation of vitamin D in vitro and in vivo (58,68). In contrast to the case in primary hyperparathyroidism, clinical observations indicate that low levels of 1,25-$(OH)_2$D are present in most patients with HHM (4), although this is not true in all cases (69). The reasons for this discrepancy remain unclear. It is possible that other factors released by tumors causing hypercalcemia may modify the capacity of the amino-terminal portion of PTHrP to stimulate the 1α-hydroxylase enzyme (70). Alternatively, the suppression of 1α-hydroxylase may be mediated by another region of the PTHrP molecule. It is noteworthy that tumors that cause the syndrome of oncogenic osteomalacia also contain PTH-like activity (71). Since patients with oncogenic osteomalacia show reduced renal absorptive capacity for phosphate, increased cAMP excretion, and markedly reduced serum 1,25-$(OH)_2$D levels, there is a possibility that these tumors secrete a similar PTH-like factor that in-

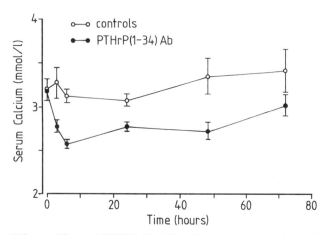

FIG. 2. Effect of PTHrP-(1–34) antiserum or normal rabbit serum (control) on serum calcium in an athymic mouse model of tumor-induced hypercalcemia due to a human squamous cell cancer.

hibits 1,25-$(OH)_2D$ production and phosphate reabsorption without stimulating bone resorption and hypercalcemia.

There is little doubt that PTHrP is the major, if not the sole, mediator of hypercalcemia in patients with the HHM syndrome. It is still possible that, in some cases, other bone resorbing factors contribute to the development of hypercalcemia on a humoral basis. A number of tumor-derived factors have been identified to be potent resorbers of bone: interleukin-1 (IL1), $TNF\alpha$ and -β, and transforming growth factor-α. PTHrP and IL1 can synergistically stimulate bone resorption in vitro and increase the serum calcium concentration in mice in vivo. (72). Production of IL1 has been identified in clonal cell lines established from squamous cell cancers associated with hypercalcemia and leukocytosis (73–75). The significance of these factors and their possible interplay with PTHrP should become clear as our knowledge of the role of cytokines in bone metabolism increases. This area is covered more completely in the chapter by Black and Mundy.

ROLE OF PARATHYROID HORMONE-RELATED PROTEIN (PTHrP) IN THE HYPERCALCEMIA OF CANCER

Further confirmation of the etiologic link between elevated levels of PTHrP and hypercalcemia associated with malignancy has been achieved by measurement of circulating levels by radioimmunoassay. Assays for PTHrP have provided further insight into the prevalence of PTHrP as a cause of hypercalcemia of cancer and have the potential to become diagnostically useful.

Despite their 60% homology over the first 13 amino acids, PTH and PTHrP are immunologically distinct. When the immunogenicities of the PTHrP and of human PTH-(1–34) sequences are predicted based on the assumptions of Welling et al. (76), the difference between the two is noted, particularly in the area of the greatest sequence homology. The first ten amino acids of PTH are poorly antigenic, in contrast to the N-terminal sequence of PTHrP, which is highly antigenic. From the earliest antisera raised against short amino-terminal sequences of PTHrP (52), it was clear that many antisera against PTHrP did not cross react with PTH. Subsequent experience confirmed this, and selection of antisera can provide reagents that do not cross react with PTH even at high concentrations (64).

The first radioimmunoassays (RIA) for PTHrP used antisera directed against the amino-terminal portion of the molecule. Several assays have been established that detect circulating levels of PTHrP with detection limits varying from 0.1 to 20 pmol/L. Radioimmunoassays and immunoradiometric assays have documented circulating levels of PTHrP in variable percentages of subjects with malignancy-associated hypercalcemia. A study using an affinity extraction RIA with an antiserum directed against PTHrP-(1–34) reported levels above the quoted normal range of up to 2.5 pM in 55% of patients with unselected cancer-associated hypercalcemia and in 85% of patients with solid tumors without bone metastases. This study also reported plasma levels of PTHrP in 32% of normal subjects (77). A direct RIA (78) using PTHrP-(1–34) as standard with a detection limit of 0.1 ng/ml (20 pM) reported plasma levels up to 0.7 ng/ml (145 pM) in patients with malignancy and hypercalcemia, which is much higher than in any other RIA. Detection of PTHrP was also found in 5% of normal subjects and also in a significant number of patients with primary and secondary hyperparathyroidism. A two-site immunoradiometric assay for the 1–74 region of PTHrP (IRMA) with a detection limit of 1 pM reported low but detectable levels in 46% of normal subjects (normal range up to 5.1 pM) and elevated levels (above the upper limit of the quoted normal range) in 83% of patients classified as having HHM (79). Ratcliffe et al. (80) found elevated levels in 85% of unselected patients with hypercalcemia of malignancy using a two-site immunoradiometric assay for PTHrP-(1–86) with a detection limit of 0.2 pmol/L. Even with a very low detection limit, no circulating levels were detected in normal subjects or in patients with primary hyperparathyroidism with this assay. Similar results were reported by Pandian et al. (81) using a modified IRMA for PTHrP-(1–74) with antisera developed by Burtis et al. (79) that gave a substantial improvement in sensitivity to 0.1 pmol/L. Interestingly, this IRMA also did not measure PTHrP levels >1.5 pmol/L in normal subjects.

Although some assays report higher levels of PTHrP in normal subjects (78,82), the lack of knowledge of the circulating forms of PTHrP and the lack of an appropriate technique to correct for nonspecific protein effects on antibody binding to antigen make interpretation of these data difficult. Unlike the availability of serum or plasma from patients with hypoparathyroidism for use in PTH assays, there is no serum or plasma known not to contain PTHrP to correct for nonspecific protein effects on antigen–antibody binding in PTHrP assays. Results so far suggest that PTHrP circulates at extremely low levels in healthy subjects, if at all, and may be only rarely detected by N-terminal radioimmunoassays.

The possibility that PTHrP circulates and contributes to hypercalcemia in primary hyperparathyroidism is raised by the demonstration of PTHrP mRNA in parathyroid adenomas (83) and the demonstration of PTHrP by immunohistochemistry and Western blotting in parathyroid adenomas (84) and also in hyperplastic parathyroid tissue associated with chronic renal failure (84). However, circulating levels of PTHrP generally are not elevated in primary hyperparathyroidism. Only in the study of Henderson et al. (78) were elevated levels of PTHrP reported, in four of 20 patients with primary hyperparathyroidism. These results were not validated by immunoaffinity extraction, so it remains unclear whether this discrepancy can be explained by a different antibody detecting a circulating fragment or whether it is due to a nonspecific serum protein effect rather than specifically to PTHrP. Using a two-site IRMA against PTHrP-(1–74), Burtis et al. (79) measured PTHrP in blood samples from draining neck veins obtained during parathyroid surgery in two patients. No gradient between neck veins and peripheral levels was seen. In any event, it is clear that circulating levels of PTHrP in cancer-associated hypercalcemia are very much higher than those in hyperparathyroidism.

Applying strict validation procedures to samples giving results near the assay detection limit (2 pM), we have detected circulating PTHrP levels in 100% of patients with hypercalcemia associated with malignancy without bone metastases and in only one of 38 normal subjects by RIA using an antiserum against PTHrP-(1–40) (85) (Fig. 3). We have analyzed hypercalcemic patients with solid tumors other than of breast in two groups, according to presence or absence of bone metastases, as demonstrated by isotope scanning. Breast cancer patients with hypercalcemia were analyzed separately. In patients with hypercalcemia associated with solid tumors, and with no evidence of bone metastases, PTHrP was always detected in plasma (Fig.

3). PTHrP levels above those of normal subjects were also found in 75% of patients with hypercalcemia and metastatic malignancy to bone, from primary sources other than breast (Fig. 3). This latter group included several patients in whom the mechanism of hypercalcemia was likely to be humoral. Consistent with this is the finding that, in the metastatic group, all squamous cell cancer patients had elevated PTHrP levels, as did one patient with a pancreatic neuroendocrine tumor.

As has been indicated in clinical studies (4,9), the presence or absence of bone metastases, a feature that was used to distinguish between humoral and osteolytic mechanisms of hypercalcemia, can no longer be used to define the syndrome of HHM. A humoral mechanism for the hypercalcemia may still exist with metastatic bone disease. Of particular interest is the finding of elevated plasma levels of PTHrP in patients with hypercalcemia associated with breast cancer and bone metastases (78,85,86) (Fig. 3). Although nephrogenous cAMP was not assayed in these patients, the hypercalcemia in this situation has not generally been considered to have a humoral basis (8). It would be of value to reconsider ideas of the mechanisms of hypercalcemia in breast cancer. In four studies (87–90), patients with hypercalcemia of breast cancer have been identified who show biochemical features of HHM. Parathyroid hormone-related protein has been purified from a breast cancer (53), and we have found evidence by immunohistology and in situ hybridization for the presence of PTHrP in 60% of cases from an unselected

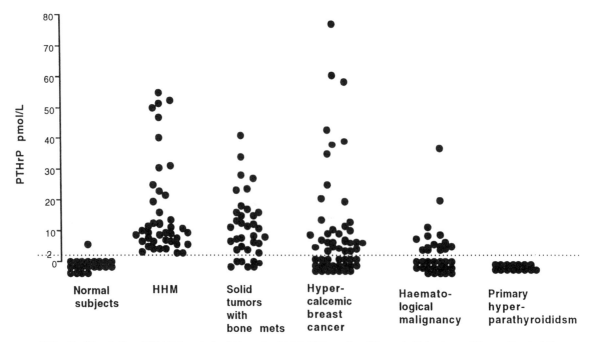

FIG. 3. Circulating PTHrP levels by N-terminal RIA (85) under different clinical conditions. *Dotted line* indicates assay detection limit.

series of breast cancers (91,92). We have also found an increased incidence of positive localization of PTHrP by immunohistochemistry in breast cancer bony metastases compared to other sites (6). All these observations focus on a possible role for PTHrP in malignant breast disease. One possibility of particular interest is that PTHrP production might contribute to the ability of breast cancers to erode bone and establish there as metastases.

In some normocalcemic patients with malignancy, levels close to the detection limit of this assay were found. We have shown by immunohistology that PTHrP was present in 100% of a series of squamous cell cancers of various origins (64). This suggests that further sensitivity is needed for PTHrP assays to be applied to the early identification of those patients with cancer, in whom circulating PTHrP levels are rising and who are therefore at risk for the development of hypercalcemia.

The development of RIAs that measure PTHrP in plasma has also resulted in the finding of elevated PTHrP levels in a proportion of patients with hematological malignancies and hypercalcemia (77–79). In our series of patients with hematological malignancies and hypercalcemia (Fig. 3), we found elevated PTHrP levels in cases of chronic myeloid leukemia, multiple myeloma, and B-cell non-Hodgkin's lymphoma. It is now well established that the retrovirus (HTLV-1) -associated adult T-cell leukemia/lymphoma often produces hypercalcemia associated with increased urinary excretion of cAMP, low-normal PTH levels, and reduced 1,25-$(OH)_2$D concentrations, as is the case in HHM associated with solid tumors. Parathyroid hormone-like biological activity is secreted by the neoplastic cells in vitro (93). Expression of PTHrP mRNA within HTLV-1-infected T cells in culture (94) has also been demonstrated, and immunohistochemical staining for PTHrP found in cells in lymph nodes involved with neoplastic tissue (95) in patients with HTLV-1-positive human adult T-cell leukemia/lymphoma. However, in cases of humoral hypercalcemia associated with both Hodgkin's and non-Hodgkin's lymphoma, elevated levels of 1,25-$(OH)_2$D and low levels of PTH in plasma have been consistently reported (18–24), as was discussed above. We have documented two cases of B-cell non-Hodgkin's lymphoma with hypercalcemia associated with elevated plasma levels of PTHrP as measured by N-terminal RIA (96). Plasma PTH and 1,25-$(OH)_2$D concentrations were suppressed below the normal range in these patients, as is the case in patients with solid tumors and HHM. Immunohistochemical staining demonstrated intracellular PTHrP in some of the neoplastic cells from a lymph node section in one of the cases. In another case of blastic transformation of chronic myeloid leukemia, elevated plasma levels of PTHrP were temporally related to the development of hypercalcemia, and a fall in PTHrP concentrations was associated with regression of disease following chemotherapy (97). These observations indicate that PTHrP-mediated humoral hypercalcemia occurs not only in association with solid tumors with or without skeletal secondaries but can also occur in association with hematological malignancies. In the latter, PTHrP-mediated hypercalcemia can extend not only to malignant processes involving the T-lymphocyte series but also to those involving the B-lymphocyte series and the myeloid series. It is possible that PTHrP has a role as local mediator of increased bone resorption in multiple myeloma and that it is at times produced in quantities sufficient to reach the circulation and produce an endocrine effect. Such a process could contribute to the osteoporosis in multiple myeloma as well as to the hypercalcemia.

The development of sensitive PTHrP assays has allowed a better understanding of its importance in hypercalcemia associated with different malignancies. Breast cancer is almost universally associated with bone metastases when hypercalcemia develops, and a high proportion of patients with hypercalcemia associated with this tumor have elevated PTHrP levels. Parathyroid hormone-related protein is produced by many tumor types, and a role in the development of bone metastases in breast cancer has been suggested (6). Other tumors not traditionally associated with humoral factor production, such as bowel cancer, can produce elevated PTHrP levels. Parathyroid hormone-related protein has a role in the pathogenesis of hypercalcemia in clear cell carcinoma of the ovary. All patients with hypercalcemia and squamous cell cancers have elevated levels of PTHrP regardless of whether bone metastases are present (85). Although less frequently than is the case for solid tumors, PTHrP also has a role in the hypercalcemia of hematological malignancy. It is now clear that the classification of hypercalcemia of malignancy in three syndrome classes no longer reflects distinct pathophysiological mechanisms.

In contrast to assays directed against the N-terminal portion of PTHrP, assays directed against the carboxy-terminal portion of the PTHrP molecule (79,98) show markedly elevated levels in patients with renal failure. This points out the similarity of PTHrP to native PTH with respect to metabolism of carboxy-terminal fragments that depend on renal mechanisms for their clearance. The accumulation of C-terminal fragments in renal failure suggests that PTHrP also originates in nonmalignant tissues. The source of PTHrP in the absence of malignancy remains unclear.

Specific and sensitive two-site, noncompetitive methods that measure intact PTH do not detect PTHrP (99–101). These assays have shown levels in tumor-induced hypercalcemia to be suppressed below the normal range in most patients, consistent with the inhibition of PTH secretion by hypercalcemia. Only three well-documented cases of true "ectopic" production of authentic PTH have been reported (102–104).

PLASMA CALCIUM LEVEL DOES NOT INFLUENCE TUMOR PRODUCTION OF PARATHYROID HORMONE-RELATED PROTEIN

The factors regulating the expression of the PTHrP gene are currently the subject of much interest. Consensus regulatory motifs for cAMP, 1,25-$(OH)_2$D, and glucocorticoids have been identified. Northern blot analysis of mRNA from control cells or from cells treated with 1,25-$(OH)_2$D or dexamethasone, or by transfection experiments using chimeric constructs, indicate that these agents decrease gene transcription (105,106). In contrast, agents that stimulate intracellular cAMP levels, such as calcitonin, increase mRNA levels for PTHrP (107) acting at the level of gene transcription. Both transforming growth factor-β (TGFβ) and estrogen have been shown to enhance PTHrP gene expression (108,109).

Ionized calcium in extracellular fluid is known to be the main physiologic regulator of PTH secretion (110,111). In addition to the rapid effects of ionized calcium on PTH secretion, hypercalcemia has been shown to reduce PTH mRNA levels, presumably reducing the long-term rate of hormone synthesis (112–114). Extracellular calcium concentrations have been varied over a wide range in animal studies (111) or using parathyroid cells in culture (115), demonstrating a sigmoidal relationship between PTH and calcium concentrations (see the chapter by Brown). This raises the question of whether ionized calcium concentrations regulate PTHrP production by tumors. The ability to measure PTHrP in plasma provided the opportunity to assess the response of tumor production of PTHrP to alterations in plasma calcium. The ability to measure intact PTH within and below a normal range also allowed us to study recovery of PTH secretion after prolonged suppression, such as has been done for recovery of endocrine function after suppression of hypothalamic–pituitary–adrenal and hypothalamic–pituitary–thyroid axis. The effect of lowering ionized calcium on circulating PTH and PTHrP was assessed in hypercalcemia of malignancy following treatment with the bisphosphonate pamidronate, in patients with PTHrP-mediated hypercalcemia (116). A rapid rise in PTH concentrations was seen in most patients after lowering ionized calcium (Fig. 4). In these patients with chronic hypercalcemia, PTH levels increased within 6 days, demonstrating a rapid recovery of parathyroid gland secretion of intact PTH, even following prolonged suppression. This is consistent with the observed rapid recovery of secretion of PTH following

surgical excision of a parathyroid adenoma (117). Posttreatment PTH levels rose above the upper limit of the normal range in some patients, even in the presence of normal ionized calcium concentrations. This is consistent with a rebound increase in PTH secretion in some patients. These findings may be explained by an increased responsiveness to a fall in calcium of parathyroid tissue that has been exposed to chronic hypercalcemia, with a shift in the "set point" (calcium concentration at which PTH secretion is half-maximal).

1,25-Dihydroxyvitamin D was not measured in this study, but 1,25-$(OH)_2$D levels have been found to be low in most cases of humoral hypercalcemia of malignancy (4). Since 1,25-$(OH)_2$D is known to inhibit transcription of the PTHrP gene (118), it is possible that the absence of inhibition in this group of patients may contribute to the rebound increase in PTH in response to lowering ionized calcium. This should be further examined by measuring 1,25-$(OH)_2$D levels before and after treatment with pamidronate. Alternatively, in the presence of continuing inhibition of bone resorption, higher circulating levels of PTH could be required for calcium homeostasis. In the clinical setting it is important to measure PTH levels in patients with hypercalcemia of malignancy prior to treatment with bisphosphonates, since the results after lowering plasma calcium could be misleading.

Parathyroid hormone-related protein concentrations and urinary cAMP excretion did not change significantly after lowering of plasma calcium (Figure 4). This is consistent with no response in tumor secretion of PTHrP to changes in ionized calcium, within the range of concentrations in the patients studied. These findings suggest an overriding and persistent effect of high circulating levels of PTHrP on cAMP production in the renal tubule in these patients, not influenced by the rise in PTH levels with correction of hypercalcemia. An increase in PTHrP secretion has been reported in a PTHrP-secreting rat parathyroid cell line with fetal cell characteristics, in response to lowering calcium concentrations in culture medium (119). Such an increase would be consistent with current evidence for PTHrP as a fetal hormone of the parathyroid gland (120,121), active in regulation of fetal plasma calcium concentrations (122,123). It is possible that this regulatory effect is not present in PTHrP-secreting cancers or that it does not take place within the range of calcium concentrations found in tumor-induced hypercalcemia. Studies of regulation of PTHrP secretion in tumor cell lines will no doubt shed further light on the regulatory processes affecting PTHrP secretion by cancer cells. These findings are also consistent with an increased sensitivity of parathyroid tissue to changes in ionized calcium following prolonged exposure to hypercalcemia.

It is noteworthy that following treatment with pamidronate, a fall in plasma calcium was observed in all

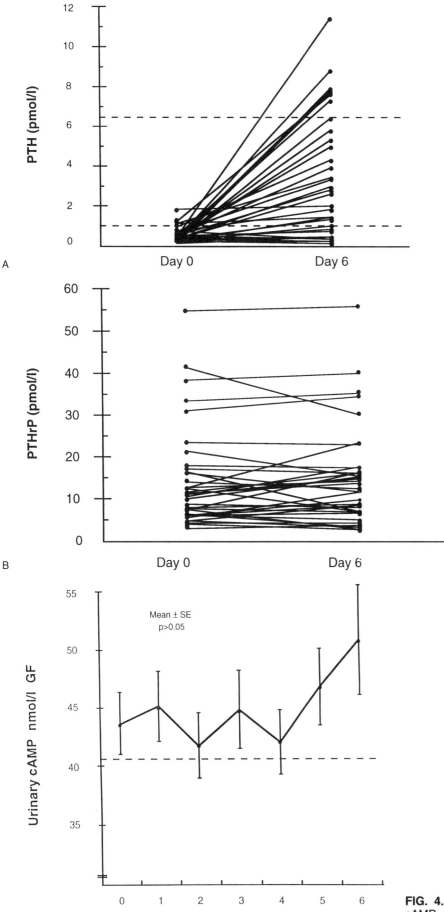

FIG. 4. PTH (**A**), PTHrP (**B**), and daily mean urinary cAMP excretion (**C**) following treatment with pamidronate. *Dashed lines* indicate normal range.

patients, but 40% remained hypercalcemic on the sixth day after treatment (116). The fall in ionized calcium indicates the importance of the contribution of increased bone resorption to the hypercalcemia that PTHrP mediates. The failure to correct ionized calcium in 40% of patients is likely to reflect the contribution of the humorally mediated renal tubular component of the hypercalcemia. This suggests that patients with tumors that produce high levels of PTHrP may respond less well to attempts to correct hypercalcemia with agents that block bone resorption, since the renal calcium conservation that PTHrP stimulates would remain unchanged following treatment with these agents. This was the subject of a further study (124).

PARATHYROID HORMONE-RELATED PROTEIN PREDICTS RESPONSE TO TREATMENT OF TUMOR-INDUCED HYPERCALCEMIA WITH BISPHOSPHONATES

Parathyroid hormone-related protein has potent effects on the renal tubule and on bone resorption. These actions are detected by a rise in the tubular calcium threshold and nephrogenous cAMP and a fall in the tubular phosphate threshold. Despite PTHrP having dual actions on bone and kidney, the agents available for treating hypercalcemia in cancer primarily reduce bone resorption. Pamidronate, a second-generation bisphosphonate, is a potent inhibitor of bone resorption, which has been used successfully in the treatment of hypercalcemia associated with cancer (125–127). Binding of pamidronate renders bone more resistant to osteoclastic resorption and also inhibits the recruitment and maturation of osteoclasts (128). However, pamidronate has no effect on the renal tubule. This agent is therefore effective against the bone-resorptive component of tumor-induced hypercalcemia, without any influence on the increased renal tubular calcium reabsorption that PTHrP produces. Calcitonin and perhaps mithramycin have a weak calciuric effect, but the main effect of these agents is also to inhibit bone resorption (129,130). A poor response to pamidronate occurs in cases of hypercalcemia of malignancy with evidence of renal tubular stimulation as indicated by a low tubular threshold for phosphate or a high threshold for calcium. (131). It is therefore not surprising that, in a study of patients with tumor-induced hypercalcemia, the PTHrP level was the best predictor of the calcemic response to pamidronate, with high levels correlating with poor response and vice versa (124) (Fig. 5). Other parameters that indirectly indicated the presence of a humoral factor also correlated with response. The presence of bone metastases on the other hand predicted a good response to treatment.

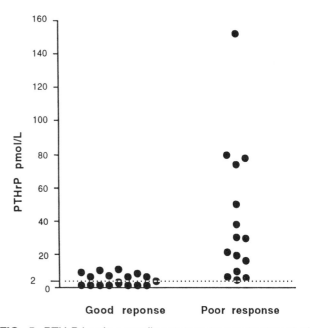

FIG. 5. PTHrP levels according to response to treatment of tumor-induced hypercalcemia with pamidronate. *Dotted line* indicates assay sensitivity.

Gurney et al. (124) established that plasma PTHrP levels predicted response to pamidronate in patients with solid tumors causing hypercalcemia. A clinical definition of response divided patients into good and poor response categories. Patients in whom the corrected calcium normalized and remained normal for >14 days were classified as good responders, while poor responders were those in whom the corrected calcium either failed to normalize or rose again within 14 days. Taking into account the length of response, rather than the acute fall in calcium level alone, may be a more clinically relevant definition of response and may give a better indication of the activity of antihypercalcemic agents. It is possible that high circulating PTHrP levels may have a more potent effect on bone resorption than locally released factors from skeletal deposits, explaining the poor response associated with high plasma levels of PTHrP. However, effective inhibition of bone resorption by pamidronate was demonstrated in patients who were poor responders, whereas complete correction of the tubular defect did not occur in these patients. This implies that the failure to inhibit the renal mechanism of hypercalcemia was the major cause of a poor response. A high PTHrP level was associated with a poor response (Fig. 5), which may relate to the failure to correct the renal component of hypercalcemia induced by this hormone.

Currently, the prediction of a poor response will not change clinical practice, because agents, other than loop diuretics, are not available that conveniently increase calcium excretion. The development of drugs that inhibit the tubular reabsorption of calcium (132), specific inhibitors of PTH or PTHrP action (133), antibodies to PTHrP (65), or inhibitors of PTHrP production may allow better control of hypercalcemia in these patients when used in combination with the available inhibitors of osteolysis. Although glucocorticoids are obvious candidates, of particular interest in this category may be the new analogs of vitamin D, which have low calcemic activity yet retain the property of inhibition of PTH gene expression. The first reported analog of this type was 22-oxa-1,25-$(OH)_2$D, or 22-oxacalcitriol (OCT) (134), which has been shown to inhibit expression of the PTH gene in vitro and in vivo (135) and is currently under investigation in the treatment of secondary hyperparathyroidism associated with chronic renal failure. Since 1,25-$(OH)_2$D is known to inhibit PTHrP gene expression (105), it is conceivable that 1,25-$(OH)_2$D analogs may have the same effect and hence offer a valuable option in addition to bisphosphonates in the treatment of PTHrP-mediated hypercalcemia.

PARATHYROID HORMONE-RELATED PROTEIN AS A CAUSE OF HYPERCALCEMIA IN NONMALIGNANT CONDITIONS

Parathyroid hormone-related protein-mediated hypercalcemia has also been described in a number of nonmalignant conditions. In patients with pheochromocytoma, hypercalcemia was reported in the absence of coexistent hyperparathyroidism (136), and pheochromocytomas have been shown to produce PTHrP (137). Hypercalcemia secondary to secretion of PTHrP from a pancreatic somatostatinoma has also been reported (138). Idiopathic infantile hypercalcemia (Williams' syndrome), an unusual syndrome consisting of multiple congenital defects including three major abnormalities—supravalvular aortic stenosis, "elfin-like" facies, and hypercalcemia during the first year of life (139,140)—may also be PTHrP mediated. Studies in affected children have demonstrated excessive circulating levels of 25-$(OH)_2$D after vitamin D administration (141), and elevated levels of 1,25-$(OH)_2$D have also been found in some children (142). However, no single, unifying hypothesis has yet emerged to explain these findings satisfactorily. Since large doses of vitamin D given to pregnant rabbits cause supravalvular aortic stenosis and dental abnormalities in the offspring, it seems that a disturbance of calcium homeostasis in utero is implicated in some way in this syndrome. In view of recent evidence for a role of PTHrP in fetal calcium metabolism (122,123), an investigation of the role for this hormone in Williams' syndrome seemed to be warranted. Elevated levels of PTHrP have been reported using a plasma extraction RIA in a small number of patients with this syndrome (143), suggesting that postnatal expression of PTHrP may play a significant role in the hypercalcemia of Williams' syndrome.

Hypercalcemia associated with benign breast hypertrophy and resolving following bilateral mastectomy has been documented (144,145), and PTHrP was demonstrated in breast tissue by immunohistochemistry in one of these cases (146). Readily assayable PTHrP levels were detected in plasma over a period of months in a pregnant patient with hypercalcemia, which continued during lactation (147). This provides an example of PTHrP released into the circulation by nonmalignant breast tissue, almost certainly producing a systemic effect.

PARATHYROID HORMONE-RELATED PROTEIN IN NORMAL PHYSIOLOGY

Parathyroid hormone-related protein has also been found to be expressed in placenta, in pregnant uterus, in the fetus at many locations, and in the lactating mammary gland. During pregnancy in mammals, large amounts of calcium are transferred across the placenta from the maternal to the fetal circulation to provide for the mineralization of the fetal skeleton (148). Evidence has been presented for a physiological role for PTHrP in regulating the transport of calcium from the maternal to the fetal circulation (122,123) and maintaining the fetus hypercalcemic with respect to the mother.

Immunohistochemical techniques and in situ hybridization have demonstrated PTHrP in placenta (Hayman et al., personal communication) (149), and PTHrP-like biological activity has been found in early placenta in sheep (122). Parathyroid hormone-related protein has also been localized by immunohistochemistry in a number of fetal tissues, including epithelia and parathyroid glands (121,150).

After birth, milk is the main source of calcium for the neonatal mammal. High concentrations of PTHrP are found in milk from a variety of mammalian species (151), and studies have also demonstrated PTHrP in the lactating mammary gland, where expression is induced by prolactin (152,153). During lactation, large amounts of calcium are transferred from the maternal circulation into milk (148). There is evidence that maternal bone loss occurs in lactation that is both PTH and vitamin D independent, suggesting the involvement of another, as yet unidentified, factor(s) in the altered calcium metabolism that accompanies lactation (154,155).

Parathyroid hormone-related protein is expressed in a variety of normal tissues in the adult, such as skin (156), central nervous system (157), pancreas (158), and uterus (159,160) (see also the chapter by Broadus and Stewart). Although the physiological role of PTHrP has yet to be defined, paracrine/autocrine roles in several locations seem likely. To date no evidence has been obtained for a classical endocrine role of PTHrP in the mammal (including man) after birth, except in cancer and perhaps in lactation.

To establish whether PTHrP reaches the maternal circulation when it is expressed in mammary tissue during lactation, in fetal tissues, or in the maternal reproductive tract during gestation, we have investigated circulating PTHrP levels in lactating women, in nonlactating controls, and also in pregnant women at all stages of gestation, using an RIA directed towards the N-terminal sequence of PTHrP (161). Circulating levels of PTHrP were detected in 63% of lactating mothers but in none of the nonlactating postpartum controls. The finding of readily measurable PTHrP concentrations in 12 of 19 lactating subjects suggests that PTHrP produced in the lactating breast can reach the circulation in quantities that could be sufficient to exert a conventional endocrine effect. The finding in this study of elevated levels of PTHrP in only a proportion of nursing mothers may be attributable to insufficient sensitivity of the RIA. In the adult, PTHrP is produced by the lactating mammary gland, and it has been shown in the rat that the induction of PTHrP mRNA in lactating tissue is due to increases in prolactin levels rather than to suckling per se (153). Maternal milk has also been shown to contain very high concentrations of PTHrP. We have found concentrations on the order of 20–200 nmol/liter in human milk (162). Since large amounts of maternal calcium must be available for delivery into milk during lactation, and this is associated with maternal bone loss and renal calcium conservation (154,155), PTHrP released by the lactating mammary gland could be the factor responsible for this endocrine effect. Some years ago, Brommage and DeLuca (154) suggested that the then uncharacterized "humoral hypercalcemia factor" might be the agent responsible for inducing bone mineral loss during lactation. Several observations support this hypothesis. In patients with hypoparathyroidism, requirements for calcium and vitamin D decline significantly during lactation (163,164). This observation could be explained by PTHrP reaching the maternal circulation and exerting endocrine effects. Suckling-associated increases in urinary phosphate and cAMP excretion have been reported in lactating rats (165), and a venous–arterial concentration gradient in plasma PTHrP was demonstrated across the mammary gland in the goat (166), supporting the notion that some of the PTHrP produced in mammary tissue is released systemically during suckling and produces an endocrine effect on the kidney. Using a plasma extraction assay, Khosla et al. (167) did not find levels of PTHrP above the normal range in subjects who were breast-feeding. This result may be explained by the different assay methodology used or alternatively by the fact that subjects in the latter study were only 2–3 days post partum.

The production of PTHrP by malignant breast tissue may be a reflection of the fact that the protein can be produced by the normal breast in lactation, just as its production by parathyroid adenomas may represent reexpression of its fetal origin. The finding of circulating levels of PTHrP during lactation is consistent with an endocrine role for this hormone in the physiology of lactation.

REFERENCES

1. Martin TJ, Atkins D. Biochemical regulators of bone resorption and their significance in cancer. *Essays Med Biochem* 1979;4:49–82.
2. Powell D, Singer FR, Murray TM, Minkin C, Potts JT. Nonparathyroid humoral hypercalemia in patients with neoplastic disease. *N Engl J Med* 1973;289:176–181.
3. Kukreja SC, Shermerdiak WP, Lad TE, Johnson PA. Elevated nephrogenous cyclic AMP with normal serum parathyroid hormone levels in patients with lung cancer. *J Clin Endocrinol Metab* 1980;51:167–169.
4. Stewart AF, Horst R, Deftos LJ, Cadman EC, Lang R, Broadus AE. Biochemical evaluation of patients with cancer-associated hypercalemia. Evidence for humoral and non-humoral groups. *N Engl J Med* 1980;303:1377–1383.
5. Rude RK, Sharp CF Jr, Fredericks RS, et al. Urinary and nephrogenous adenosine 3'5'-monophosphate in the hypercalemia of malignancy. *J Clin Endocrinol Metab* 1981;52:765–771.
6. Powell GJ, Southby J, Danks JA, et al. Localization of parathyroid hormone-related protein in breast cancer metastases: increased incidence in bone compared with other sites. *Cancer Res* 1991;51:3059–3061.
7. Legha SS, Powell K, Buzdar AU, Blumen-Schein GR. Tamoxifen-induced hypercalemia in breast cancer. *Cancer* 1981;47:2803–2806.
8. Mundy GR, Martin TJ. The hypercalemia of malignancy: pathogenesis and treatment. *Metabolism* 1982;31:1247–1277.
9. Ralston SH, Fogelman I, Gardiner MD, Boyle IT. Relative contribution of humoral and metastatic factors to the pathogenesis of hypercalemia in malignancy. *Br Med J* 1984;288:1405–1408.
10. Kubota K, Yanagisawa T, Kurabayashi H, et al. Hypercalemia associated with osteolytic lesions in the extramedullary blastic crisis of chronic myelogenous leukaemia: report of a case. *Blut* 1989;59:458–459.
11. Cohn SL, Morgan ER, Mallette LE. The spectrum of metabolic bone disease in lymphoblastic leukemia. *Cancer* 1987;59:346–350.
12. Kyle RA. Multiple myeloma: Review of 869 cases. *Mayo Clin Proc* 1975;50:29–40.
13. Mundy GR, Raisz LG, Cooper RA, Schechter GP, Salmon SE. Evidence for the secretion of an osteoclast stimulating factor in myeloma. *N Engl J Med* 1974;291:1041–1046.
14. Raisz LG, Luben RA, Mundy GR, Dietrich JW, Horton JE, Trummel CL. Effect of osteoclast activating factor from human leukocytes on bone metabolism. *J Clin Invest* 1975;56:408–413.
15. Garrett IR, Durie BGM, Nedwin GE, et al. Production of lymphotoxin, a bone-resorbing cytokine, by cultured human myeloma cells. *N Engl J Med* 1987;317:526–532.
16. Burt ME, Brennan MF. Incidence of hypercalemia and malignant neoplasm. *Arch Surg* 1980;115:704–707.
17. Canellos GP. Hypercalemia in malignant lymphoma and leukemia. *Ann NY Acad Sci* 1974;230:240–246.
18. Breslau NA, McGuire JL, Zerwekh JE, Frenkel EP, Pak CYC. Hypercalcaemia associated with increased serum calcitriol levels in three patients with lymphoma. *Ann Intern Med* 1984;100:1–7.
19. Rosenthal N, Insogna KL, Godsall JW, Smaldone L, Waldron JA, Stewart AF. Elevations in circulating 1,25-dihydroxyvitamin D in three patients with lymphoma-associated hypercalcaemia. *J Clin Endocrinol Metab* 1985;60:29–33.
20. Davies M, Hayes ME, Mawer EB, Lumb GA. Abnormal vi-

tamin D metabolism in Hodgkin's lymphoma. *Lancet* 1985;1:1186–1188.

21. Mudde AH, Van den Berg H, Boshuis PG, et al. Ectopic production of 1,25-dihydroxyvitamin D by B-cell lymphoma as a cause of hypercalcaemia. *Cancer* 1985;59:1543–1546.

22. Mercier RJ, Thompson JM, Herman GS, Messerschmidt GL. Recurrent hypercalcaemia and elevated 1,25-dihydroxyvitamin D levels in Hodgkin's disease. *Am J Med* 1988;84:165–168.

23. Jacobson JO, Bringhurst FR, Harris NL, Weitzman SA, Aisenberg AC. Humoral hypercalcemia in Hodgkin's disease. Clinical and laboratory evaluation. *Cancer* 1989;63:917–923.

24. Adams JS, Fernandez M, Gacad MA, et al. Vitamin D metabolite mediated hypercalcemia and hypercalcemia in patients with AIDS and non-AIDS associated lymphoma. *Blood* 1989;73:235–239.

25. Mason RS, Frankel T, Chan YL, Lissner D, Posen S. Vitamin D conversion by sarcoid lymph node homogenate. *Ann Intern Med* 1984;100:59–61.

26. Grossman B, Schechter GP, Horton JE, Pierce L, Jaffe E, Wahl L. Hypercalcaemia associated with T cell lymphoma-leukemia. *Am J Clin Pathol* 1981;75:149–155.

27. Kinoshita K, Kamihira S, Ikeda S, et al. Clinical, hematologic and pathologic features of leukemia T-cell lymphoma. *Cancer* 1982;50:1554–1562.

28. Bunn PA, Schechter GP, Jaffe E, et al. Clinical course of retrovirus associated adult T-cell lymphoma in the United States. *N Engl J Med* 1983;309:257–264.

29. Dodd RC, Winkler CF, Williams ME, et al. Calcitriol levels in hypercalcaemic patients with adult T-cell lymphoma. *Arch Intern Med* 1986;146:1971–1972.

30. Poiesz BJ, Ruscetti FW, Gazdar AF, Bunn PA, Minna JD, Gallo RC. Detection and isolation of type C retrovirus particles form fresh and cultured lymphocytes of a patient with cutaneous T-cell lymphoma. *Proc Natl Acad Sci USA* 1980;77:7415–7419.

31. Yoshida M, Miyoshi I, Hinuma Y. Isolation and characterisation of retrovirus from cell lines of human adult T-cell leukemia and its implication in the disease. *Proc Natl Acad Sci USA* 1982;79:2031–2035.

32. Clark JW, Gurgo C, Franchini G, et al. Molecular epidemiology of HTLVI-associated non-Hodgkin's lymphomas in Jamaica. *Cancer* 1988;61:1477–1482.

33. Fukumoto S, Matsumoto T, Ikeda K, et al. Clinical evaluation of calcium metabolism in Adult T-cell leukemia/lymphoma. *Arch Intern Med* 1988;148:921–925.

34. Zondek H, Petrow H, Siebert W. Die Bedeutung der Calcium-bestimmung im Blute fur die Diagnose der Nierreninsuffizientz. *Z Klin Med* 1923;99:129–132.

35. Case records of the Massachusetts General Hospital (Case 27401). *N Engl J Med* 1941;225:789–791.

36. Lafferty FW. Pseudohyperparathyroidism. *Medicine* 1966;45:247–260.

37. Berson AS, Yalow RS. Parathyroid hormone in plasma in adenomatous hyperparathyroidism, uremia and bronchogenic sarcoma. *Science* 1966;154:907–909.

38. Knill-Jones RP, Buckle RM, Parsons V, Caine RY, Williams R. Hypercalcaemia and increased parathyroid hormone activity in a primary hepatoma. Studies before and after hepatic transplantation. *N Engl J Med* 1970;282:704–708.

39. Greenberg PB, Martin TJ, Sutcliffe HS. Synthesis and release of parathyroid hormone by a renal carcinoma in cell culture. *Clin Sci* 1973;45:183–187.

40. Riggs BL, Arnaud CD, Reynolds JC, Smith LH. Immunological differentiation of primary hyperparathyroidism from hyperparathyroidism due to non-parathyroid cancer. *J Clin Invest* 1971;50:2079–2083.

41. Roof BS, Carpenter B, Fink DJ, Gordan GS. Some thoughts on the nature of ectopic parathyroid hormones. *Am J Med* 1971;50:686–691.

42. Benson RC, Riggs BL, Pickard BM, Arnaud CD. Immunoreactive forms of circulating parathyroid hormone in primary and ectopic hyperparathyroidism. *J Clin Invest* 1974;54:175–181.

43. Stewart AF, Insogna KL, Goltzman D, Broadus AE. Identification of adenylate-cyclase stimulating activity and cytochemical bioactivity in extracts of tumors from patients with humoral hypercalcemia of malignancy. *Proc Natl Acad Sci USA* 1983;80:1454–1458.

44. Nissenson RA, Strewler GJ, Williams RD, Leung SC. Activation of the PTH receptor adenylate cyclase complex by human renal carcinoma factor. *Cancer Res* 1985;45:5358–5368.

45. Goltzman D, Stewart AF, Broaus AE. Malignancy-associated hypercalcemia evaluation with a cytochemical bioassay for parathyroid hormone. *J Clin Endocrinol Metab* 1981;53:899–905.

46. Rodan SB, Insogna KL, Vignery AM-C, et al. Factors associated with humoral hypercalcemia of malignancy stimulate adenylate cyclase in osteoblastic cells. *J Clin Invest* 1983;72:1511–1515.

47. Simpson EL, Mundy GR, D'Souza SM, Ibbotson KJ, Bockman R, Jacobs JW. Absence of parathyroid hormone messenger RNA in non-parathyroid tumors associated with hypercalcemia. *N Engl J Med* 1983;309:325–330.

48. Strewler GJ, Williams RD, Nissenson RA. Human renal carcinoma cells produce hypercalcemia in the nude mouse and a novel protein recognized by parathyroid hormone receptors. *J Clin Invest* 1983;71:769–774.

49. Gkonos PJ, Hayes T, Burtis W, Jacoby R, McGuire J, Baron R, Stewart AF. Squamous carcinoma model of humoral hypercalcemia of malignancy. *Endocrinology* 1984;115:2384–2390.

50. Rosol TJ, Capen CC, Brooks CP. Bone and kidney adenylate cyclase-stimulating activity produced by a hypercalcemia canine adenocarcinoma line (CAC-8) maintained in nude mice. *Cancer Res* 1987;47:690–695.

51. Ikeda K, Matsumoto F, Fukumoto S, et al. A hypercalcemic nude rat model that completely mimics the human syndrome of humoral hypercalcemia of malignancy. *Calcif Tissue Int* 1988;43:97–102.

52. Moseley JM, Kubota M, Diefenbach-Jagger H, et al. Parathyroid hormone-related protein purified from a human lung cancer cell line. *Proc Natl Acad Sci USA* 1987;84:5048–5052.

53. Burtis WJ, Wu J, Bunch CM, et al. Identification of a novel 17,000-dalton parathyroid hormone-like adenylate cyclase-stimulating protein from a tumor associated with humoral hypercalcemia of malignancy. *J Biol Chem* 1987;262:7151–7156.

54. Suva LJ, Winslow GA, Wettenhall REH, et al. A parathyroid hormone-related protein implicated in malignant hypercalcemia: cloning and expression. *Science* 1987;237:893–896.

55. Mangin M, Webb AC, Dreyer BE, et al. Identification of a cDNA encoding a parathyroid hormone-like peptide from a human tumor associated with humoral hypercalcemia of malignancy. *Proc Natl Acad Sci USA* 1988;85:597–601.

56. Thiede MA, Strewler GA, Nissenson RA, Rosenblatt M, Rodan GA. Human renal carcinoma expresses two messages encoding a parathyroid hormone like peptide: evidence for the alternate splicing of a single copy gene. *Proc Natl Acad Sci USA* 1988;85:4605–4608.

57. Kemp BE, Moseley JM, Rodda CP, et al. Parathyroid hormone-related protein of malignancy: active synthetic fragments. *Science* 1987;238:1568–1570.

58. Horiuchi N, Caulfield MP, Fisher JE, et al. Similarity of synthetic peptide from human tumor to parathyroid hormone in vivo and in vitro. *Science* 1987;238:1566–1568.

59. Rodan SB, Noda M, Wesolowski G, Rosenblatt M, Rodan GA. Comparison of postreceptor effects of 1–34 human hypercalcemic factor and 1–34 human parathyroid hormone in rat osteosarcoma cells. *J Clin Invest* 1988;81:924–927.

60. Stewart AF, Mangin M, Wu T, et al. Synthetic human parathyroid hormone-like protein stimulates bone resorption and causes hypercalcemia in rats. *J Clin Invest* 1988;81:596–600.

61. Yates AJP, Gutierrez GE, Smoleus P, et al. Effects of a synthetic peptide of a parathyroid hormone-related protein on calcium homeostasis, renal tubular calcium reabsorption and bone metabolism in vivo and in vitro in rodents. *J Clin Invest* 1988;81:932–938.

62. Ebeling PR, Adam WR, Moseley JM, Martin TJ. Actions of parathyroid hormone-related protein on the isolated rat kidney. *J Endocrinol* 1988;12:45–52.

63. Zhou H, Leaver DD, Moseley JM, Kemp BE, Ebeling PR, Martin TJ. Actions of parathyroid hormone-related protein on the rat kidney in vivo. *J Endocrinol* 1989;122:227–235.

64. Danks JA, Ebeling PR, Hayman J, et al. Parathyroid hormone-related protein of cancer: immunohistochemical localization in cancers and in normal skin. *J Bone Mineral Res* 1989;4:273–278.

65. Kukreja SC, Schavin DH, Wimbuscus S, et al. Antibodies to parathyroid hormone-related protein lower serum calcium in athymic mouse models of malignancy associated hypercalcemia due to human tumors. *J Clin Invest* 1988;82:1798–1802.

66. Kukreja SC, Rosol TJ, Winbiscus SA, et al. Tumor resection and antibodies to parathyroid hormone-related protein cause similar changes on bone histomorphometry in hypercalcemia of cancer. *Endocrinology* 1990;127:305–310.

67. Ellis AG, Adam WR, Martin TJ. Comparison of the effects of parathyroid hormone (PTH) and recombinant PTH-related protein on bicarbonate excretion by the isolated perfused rat kidney. *J Endocrinol* 1990;126:403–408.

68. Fraher LJ, Hodsman AB, Jonas K, et al. A comparison of the in vivo bochemical responses to exogenous parathyroid hormone(1–34) [PTH-(1–34)] and PTH-related peptide-(1–34) in man. *J Clin Endocrinol Metab* 1992;75:417–423.

69. Yamamoto I, Kitamura N, Aoki J, Kawamura J, Dokoh S, Morita R, Torizuka K. Circulating 1,25-dihydroxyvitamin D concentrations in patients with renal cell carcinoma-associated hypercalcemia are rarely suppressed. *J Clin Endocrinol Metab* 1987;64:175–179.

70. Fukumoto S, Matsumoto T, Yamoto H, et al. Suppression of serum 1,25-dihydroxyvitamin D in humoral hypercalcemia of malignancy is caused by elaboration of a factor that inhibits renal 1,25-dihydroxyvitamin D_3 production. *Endocrinology* 1989;124:2057–2062.

71. Seshadri MS, Cornish CJ, Mason RS, Posen S. Parathyroid hormone-like activity in tumors from patients with oncogenic osteomalacia. *Clin Endocrinol* 1985;23:689–697.

72. Sato K, Fujii Y, Kasono K, et al. Parathyroid hormone-related protein and interleukin-I-alpha synergistically stimulate bone resorption in vitro and increase serum calcium concentration in mice in vivo. *Endocrinology* 1989;124:2172–2178.

73. Sato K, Fujii Y, Ono M, Nomura H, Shizume K. Production of interleukin 1-alpha like factor an colony-stimulating factor by a squamous cell carcinoma of the thyroid (T3M-5) derived from a patient with hypercalcemia and leukocytosis. *Cancer Res* 1987;47:6474–6480.

74. Sato K, Fujii Y, Kasono K, Tsishima T, Shizume K. Production of interleukin-1 alpha and parathyroid hormone-like factor by a squamous cell carcinoma of the esophagus (EC-GI) derived from a patient with hypercalcemia. *J Clin Endocrinol Metab* 1988;67:592–601.

75. Sato K, Fujii Y, Kakiuchi T, et al. Paraneoplastic syndrome of hypercalcemia and leukocytosis caused by squamous carcinoma cells (T3M-1) producing parathyroid hormone-related protein, interleukin 1 alpha, and granulocyte colony-stimulating factor. *Cancer Res* 1989;49:4740–4746.

76. Welling GW, Weijer WJ, van der Zee R, Welling-Wester S. Prediction of sequential antigenic regions in proteins. *FEBS Lett* 1985;188:215–218.

77. Budayr A, Nissenson RA, Klein RF, et al. Increased serum levels of a parathyroid hormone-like protein in malignancy-associated hypercalcemia. *Ann Intern Med* 1989;111:807–812.

78. Henderson JR, Shustik C, Kremer R, Rabbani SA, Hendy GN, Goltzman D. Circulating concentrations of Parathyroid hormone-like peptide in malignancy and hyperparathyroidism. *J Bone Mineral Res* 1990;5:105–113.

79. Burtis WJ, Brady TG, Orloff JJ, et al. Immunochemical characterization of circulating parathyroid hormone-related protein in patients with humoral hypercalcemia of cancer. *N Engl J Med* 1990;322:1106–1112.

80. Ratcliffe WA, Norbury S, Heath DA, Ratcliffe JG. Development and validation of an immunoradiometric assay of parathyrin-related protein in unextracted plasma. *Clin Chem* 1991;37:678–685.

81. Pandian MR, Morgan CH, Carlton E, Segre V. Modified immunoradiometric assay of parathyroid hormone-related protein: clinical application in the differential diagnosis of hypercalcemia. *Clin Chem* 1992;38:282–288.

82. Kao CK, Klee GG, Taylor RL, Heath H. Parathyroid hormone related peptide in plasma from patients with hypercalcemia and malignant lesions. *Mayo Clin Proc* 1990;65:1399–1406.

83. Ikeda K, Weir E, Mangin M, et al. Expression of messenger ribonucleic acids encoding a parathyroid hormone-like peptide in normal human and animal tissues with abnormal expression in human parathyroid adenomas. *Mol Endocrinol* 1988;2:1230–1235.

84. Danks JA, Ebeling PR, Hayman JA, et al. Immunohistochemical localization of parathyroid hormone-related protein in parathyroid adenoma and hyperplasia. *J Pathol* 1990;161:27–33.

85. Grill V, Ho P, Body JJ, et al. Parathyroid hormone-related protein: elevated levels both in humoral hypercalcemia of malignancy and in hypercalcemia complicating metastatic breast cancer. *J Clin Endocrinol Metab* 1991;73:1309–1315.

86. Bundred NJ, Ratcliffe WA, Walker RA, Coley S, Morrison JM, Ratcliffe JG. Parathyroid hormone related protein and hypercalcemia in breast cancer. *Br Med J* 1991;303:1506–1509.

87. Percival RC, Yates AJP, Gray RE, et al. Mechanisms of malignant hypercalcemia in carcinoma of the breast. *Br Med J* 1985;2:7766–7769.

88. Kimura S, Adchi I, Yamaguchi K, et al. Stimulation of calcium reabsorption observed in advanced breast cancer patients with hypercalcemia and multiple bone metastases. *Jpn J Cancer Res* 1985;76:308–314.

89. Isales C, Carangiu ML, Stewart AF. Hypercalcemia in breast cancer: reassessment of the mechanism. *Am J Med* 1987;82:1143–1147.

90. Gallacher SJ, Fraser WD, Patel U, et al. Breast cancer associated hypercalcemia: a reassessment of renal calcium and phosphate handling. *Ann Clin Biochem* 1990;27:551–556.

91. Southby J, Kissin MW, Danks JA, et al. Immunohistochemical localization of parathyroid hormone-related protein in human breast cancer. *Cancer Res* 1990;50:7710–7716.

92. Vargas SJ, Powell GJ, Gillespie MT, et al. Localization of parathyroid hormone-related protein mRNA expression in breast cancer and metastatic lesions by in situ hybridization. *J Bone Mineral Res* 1992;7:971–979.

93. Fukumoto S, Matsumoto T, Watanabe T, Takahashi H, Miyoshi I, Ogata E. Secretion of parathyroid hormone-like activity from human T-cell lymphotropic virus type I-infected lymphocytes. *Cancer Res* 1989;49:3849–3852.

94. Motokura T, Fukumoto S, Takahashi S, et al. Expression of parathyroid hormone-related protein in a human T cell lymphotrophic virus type 1-infected T cell line. *Biochem Biophys Res Commun* 1988;154:1182–1188.

95. Moseley JM, Danks JA, Grill V, Lister TA, Horton MA. Immunocytochemical demonstration of PTHrP protein in neoplastic tissue of HTLV-1 positive human adult T cell leukaemia/lymphoma: implications for the mechanism of hypercalcemia. *Br J Cancer* 1991;64:745–748.

96. Grill V, Seymour J, MacKenzie SL, Ho PMW, Martin TJ, Firkin F. Humoral hypercalcemia of malignancy mediated by parathyroid hormone-related protein in B-cell non Hodgkin's lymphoma. (Submitted for publication.)

97. Seymour J, Grill V, Lee N, Martin TJ, Firkin F. Humoral hypercalcemia of malignancy mediated by parathyroid hormone related protein in blastic crisis of chronic myeloid leukemia. Submitted for publication.

98. Kashara H, Tsuchiya M, Adachi R, Horikawa S, Tanaka S, Tachibana S. Development of a C-terminal region specific radioimmunoassay of parathyroid hormone-related protein. *Biomed Res* 1992;13:155–161.

99. Brown RC, Aston JP, Weekes I, Woodhead JS. Circulating

intact parathyroid measured by a two-site immunochemilu-minometric assay. *J Clin Endocrinol Metab* 1987;65:407–414.

100. Nussbaum SR, Zahradnik RJ, Lavigne JR, et al. Highly sensitive two-site immunoradiometric assay of parathyrin, and its clinical utility in evaluating patients with hypercalcemia. *Clin Chem* 1987;33:1364–1367.

101. Blind E, Schmidt-Gayk H, Scharla S, et al. Two-site assay of intact parathyroid in the investigation of primary hyperparathyroidism and other disorders of calcium metabolism compared with a mid-region assay. *J Clin Endocrinol Metab* 1988;67:353–360.

102. Schmelzer HJ, Hesch RD, Mayer H. Parathyroid hormone in a human small cell lung cancer. In: Haveman K, Sorensen G, Gropp C, eds. *Peptide hormones in lung cancer.* Berlin: Springer-Verlag, 1985;83–93.

103. Yoshimoto K, Yamasaki R, Sakai H, et al. Ectopic production of parathyroid hormone by small cell lung cancer in a patient with hypercalcemia. *J Clin Endocrinol Metab* 1989; 68:976–981.

104. Nussbaum SR, Gaz RD, Arnold A. Hypercalcemia and ectopic secretion of parathyroid hormone by an ovarian carcinoma with rearrangement of the gene for parathyroid hormone. *N Engl J Med* 1990;323:1324–1328.

105. Ikeda K, Lu C, Weir EC, Mangin M, Broadus AE. Transcriptional regulation of the parathyroid hormone-related protein gene by glucocorticoids and vitamin D in a human C-cell line. *J Biol Chem* 1989;264:15743–15746.

106. Lu C, Ikeda K, Deftos LJ, Gazdar AF, Mangin M, Broadus AE. Glucocorticoid regulation of parathyroid hormone-related protein gene transcription in a human neuroendocrine cell line. *Mol Endocrinol* 1989;3:2034–2039.

107. Rizzoli R, Sappino AP, Aubert ML, Bonjour JP. Effect of cAMP-stimulators on parathyroid hormone-related protein PTHrP release by a cultured lung squamous cell carcinoma. Abstracts of the Third International Workshop on Cells and Cytokines in Bone and Cartilage. *Calcif Tissue Int* 1990; 46(Suppl 2).

108. Kiriyama T, Gillespie MT, Glatz JA, Fukumoto S, Moseley JM, Martin TJ. TGFβ stimulation of parathyroid hormone-related protein: a paracrine regulator? *Mol Cell Endocrinol* 1993;92:55–62.

109. Thiede MA, Harm SC, Hasson DM, Gardner RM. In vivo regulation of parathyroid hormone-related peptide messenger ribonucleic acid in the rat uterus by 17β estradiol. *Endocrinology* 1991;28:2317–2323.

110. Sherwood LM, Potts JT Jr, Care AD, et al. Evaluation by radioimmunoassay of factors controlling the secretion of parathyroid hormone. Intravenous infusions of calcium and ethylenediamine tetraacetic acid in the cow and goat. *Nature* 1966;209:52–55.

111. Mayer GP, Hurst JG. Sigmoidal relationship between parathyroid hormone secretion rate and plasma concentrations in calves. *Endocrinology* 1978;102:1036–1042.

112. Russell J, Lettieri D, Sherwood LM. Direct regulation by calcium of cytoplasmic messenger ribonucleic acid coding for pre-proparathyroid hormone in isolated bovine parathyroid cells. *J Clin Invest* 1983;72:1851–1855.

113. Farrow SM, Karmali R, Gleed JH, Hendy GN, O'Riordan JLH. Regulation of pre prohormone messenger RNA and hormone synthesis in human parathyroid adenomata. *J Endocrinol* 1988;117:133–138.

114. Yamamoto M, Igarashi T, Murumatsu M, Fukagawa M, Motokura T, Ogata E. Hypocalcemia increases and hypercalcemia decreases the steady-state level of parathyroid hormone messenger RNA in the rat. *J Clin Invest* 1989;83:1053–1956.

115. Brown EM. Four-parameter model of the sigmoidal relationship between parathyroid hormone release and extracellular calcium concentration in normal and abnormal parathyroid tissue. *J Clin Endocrinol Metab* 1983;56:572–581.

116. Grill V, Murray RML, Ho PMW, et al. Circulating levels of PTH and PTHrP before and after treatment of tumor-induced hypercalcemia with pamidronate disodium. *J Clin Endocrinol Metab* 1992;76:1468–1470.

117. Brasier AR, Wang CA, Nussbaum SR. Recovery of parathyroid hormone secretion after parathyroid adenomectomy. *J Clin Endocrinol Metab* 1988;66:495–500.

118. Russell J, Lettieri D, Sherwood LM. Suppression by 1,25(OH)₂D₃ of transcription of the parathyroid hormone gene. *Endocrinology* 1986;119:2864–2866.

119. Zajac JD, Callaghan J, Eldridge C, et al. Production of parathyroid hormone-related protein by a rat parathyroid cell line. *J Mol Endocrinol Metab* 1989;67:107–112.

120. Abbas SK, Pickard DW, Illingworth D, et al. Measurement of parathyroid hormone-related protein in extracts of fetal parathyroid glands and placental membranes. *J Endocrinol* 1990;124:319–325.

121. McIsaac RJ, Caple IW, Danks JA, et al. Ontogeny of parathyroid hormone-related protein in the ovine parathyroid gland. *Endocrinology* 1991;129:757–764.

122. Rodda CP, Kubota M, Heath JA, et al. Evidence for a novel parathyroid hormone-related protein in fetal lamb parathyroid glands and sheep placenta: comparisons with a similar protein implicated in humoral hypercalcemia of malignancy. *J Endocrinol* 1988;117:261–271.

123. Abbas SK, Pickard DW, Rodda CP, et al. Stimulation of placental calcium transport by certain parathyroid hormone-related proteins. *Q J Exp Physiol* 1989;74:549–552.

124. Gurney H, Grill V, Martin TJ. Parathyroid hormone-related protein level predicts response to Pamidronate in the treatment of tumor-induced hypercalcemia. *Lancet* 1993;341:1611–1613.

125. Body JJ, Borkowski A, Cleeren A, Bijvoet OLM. Treatment of malignancy-associated hypercalcemia with intravenous aminohydroxypropylidenediphosphonate. *J Clin Oncol* 1986; 8:1177–1183.

126. Yates AJP, Murray RML, Jerums G, Martin TJ. A comparison of single and multiple intravenous infusions of APD in the treatment of hypercalcemia of malignancy. *Aust NZ J Med* 1987;17:387–391.

127. Thiebaud D, Jaeger B, Burckhard P. A single day treatment of tumor-induced hypercalcemia by intravenous APD. *J Bone Mineral Res* 1986;1:555–562.

128. Fleisch H. Diphosphonates: mechanisms of action and clinical applications. In Peck WA, ed. *Bone and mineral research.* Amsterdam: Exerpta Medica, 1983;319–329.

129. Ralston SH, Gardner MD, Dryburgh FJ, Jenkins AS, Cowan RA, Boyle IT. Comparison of aminohydroxypropylidene diphosphonate, mithramycin, and corticosteroids/calcitonin in treatment of cancer-associated hypercalcaemia. *Lancet* 1985; 2:907–910.

130. Bilezikian JP. Management of acute hypercalcemia. *N Engl J Med* 1992;326:1196–1203.

131. Gurney H, Kefford R, Stuart HR. Renal phosphate threshold and response to pamidronate in humoral hypercalcaemia of malignancy: see comments. *Lancet* 1989;2:241–244.

132. Hirschel SS, Caverzasio J, Bonjour JP. Inhibition of parathyroid hormone secretion and parathyroid hormone-independent diminution of tubular calcium reabsorption by WR-2721, a unique hypocalcemic agent. *J Clin Invest* 1985; 76:1851–1856.

133. Goldman ME, McKee RL, Caulfield MP, et al. A new highly potent parathyroid hormone antagonist: D-Trp12, Tyr34: bPTH-(7–34)NH2. *Endocrinology* 1988;123:2597–2599.

134. Murayama E, Miyamoto K, Kubodera N, Mori T, Matsunaga I. Synthetic studies of vitamin D3 analogues. VIII. Synthesis of 22-oxavitamin D3 analogues. *Chem Pharm Bull* 1986;34:4410–4413.

135. Brown AJ, Ritter CR, Finch JL, et al. The noncalcemic analogue of vitamin D, 22-oxacalcitriol, suppresses parathyroid hormone synthesis and secretion. *J Clin Invest* 1989; 84:728–732.

136. Stewart AF, Hoecker JL, Mallette LE, Segre GV, Amatruda T, Vignery A. Hypercalcemia in phaeochromocytoma. Evidence for a novel mechanism. *Ann Intern Med* 1985; 102:776–779.

137. Kimura S, Nishimura Y, Yamaguchi K, Nagasaki K, Shimada K, Uchida H. A case of pheochromocytoma producing parathyroid hormone-related protein and presenting

with hypercalcemia. *J Clin Endocrinol Metab* 1990;70: 1559–1563.

138. Williams EJ, Ratcliffe WA, Stavri G, Stamakis JD. Hypercalcemia secondary to secretion of parathyroid hormone related protein from a somatostatinoma of the pancreas. *Ann Clin Biochem* 1992;29:354–357.

139. Williams JCP, Barrat-Boyes BG, Lowe JB. Supravalvular aortic stenosis. *Circulation* 1961;24:1311–1318.

140. Black JA, Bonham Carter RE. Association between aortic stenosis and facies of severe infantile hypercalcaemia. *Lancet* 1963;2:745–748.

141. Taylor AB, Stern PH, Bell NH. Abnormal regulation of 25(OH)D in the Williams syndrome. *N Engl J Med* 1982; 306:972–975.

142. Garbedian M, Jacqz E, Guillozo H, et al. Elevated plasma 1,25-dihydroxyvitamin D concentrations in infants with hypercalcaemia and elfin faces. *N Engl J Med* 1985;312:948–952.

143. Langman CB, Budayr AA, Sailer DE, Strewler GJ. Nonmalignant expression of parathyroid hormone-related protein is responsible for idiopathic infantile hypercalcemia. *J Bone Mineral Res* 1992;7:S93.

144. Marx SJ, Zusman RM, Umiker WO. Benign breast dysplasia causing hypercalcemia. *J Clin Endocrinol Metab* 1977;45: 1049–1052.

145. Van Heerden JA, Gharib H, Jackson IT. Pseudohyperparathyroidism secondary to gigantic mammary hypertrophy. *Arch Surg* 1988;123:80–82.

146. Khosla S, van Heerden JA, Gharib IT, Danks JA, Hayman JA, Martin TJ. Parathyroid hormone-related protein and hypercalcemia secondary to massive mammary hyperplasia. *N Engl J Med* 1990;322:1157.

147. Lepre F, Grill V, Ho PMW, Martin TJ. Hypercalcemia in pregnancy and lactation due to parathyroid hormone-related protein. *N Engl J Med* 1993;328:666–667.

148. Garel JM. Hormonal control of calcium metabolism during the reproductive cycle in mammals. *Physiol Rev* 1987; 67:551–556.

149. Senior PV, Heath DA, Beck F. Expression of parathyroid hormone-related protein mRNA in the rat before birth: demonstration by hybridization histochemistry. *J Mol Endocrinol* 1991;6:281–290.

150. Moseley JM, Danks JA, Grill V, Southby J, Hayman JA, Horton MA. Immunohistochemical localization of parathyroid hormone-related protein in fetal tissues. *J Clin Endocrinol Metab* 1991;73:478–484.

151. Budayr AA, Halloran BP, King JC, Diepp D, Nissenson RA, Strewler GJ. High levels of a parathyroid hormone-like protein in milk. *Proc Natl Acad Sci USA* 1989;86:7183–7185.

152. Thiede MA, Rodan GA. Expression of a calcium-mobilizing parathyroid hormone-like peptide in lactating mammary tissue. *Science* 1988;242:278–280.

153. Thiede MA. The mRNA encoding a parathyroid hormone-like peptide is produced in mammary tissue in response to

elevations in serum prolactin. *Mol Endocrinol* 1989;3:1443–1447.

154. Brommage R, DeLuca HF. Regulation of bone mineral loss during lactation. *Am J Physiol* 1985;248:E182–E187.

155. Kent GN, Price RI, Gutteridge DH, et al. Human lactation: forearm trabecular bone loss, increased bone turnover, and renal conservation of calcium and inorganic phosphate with recovery of bone mass following weaning. *J Bone Mineral Res* 1990;55:361–369.

156. Hayman JA, Danks JA, Ebeling PR, Moseley JM, Kemp BE, Martin TJ. Expression of parathyroid hormone-related protein in normal skin and skin appendages. *J Pathol* 1989; 158:293–296.

157. Weir EC, Brines ML, Ikeda K, Burtis WJ, Broadus AE, Robbins RJ. Parathyroid hormone related peptide gene is expressed in the mammalian central nervous system. *Proc Natl Acad Sci USA* 1990;87:108–112.

158. Drucker DJ, Asa SL, Henderson J, Goltzman D. The parathyroid hormone-related peptide gene is expressed in the normal and neoplastic human endocrine pancreas. *Mol Endocrinol* 1990;3:1589–1595.

159. Thiede MA, Daifotis AG, Weir EC, et al. Intrauterine occupancy controls expression of the parathyroid hormone-related peptide gene in pre-term rat myometrium. *Proc Natl Acad Sci USA* 1990;87:6969–6973.

160. Paspaliaris V, Vargas SJ, Gillespie MT, et al. Oestrogen enhancement of the myometrial response to exogenous parathyroid hormone-related protein (PTHrP), and tissue localization of endogenous PTHrP and its mRNA in the virgin rat uterus. *J Endocrinol* 1992;134:415–425.

161. Grill V, Hillary T, Ho PMW, et al. Parathyroid hormone-related protein: a possible endocrine function in lactation. *Clin Endocrinol* 1992;37:405–410.

162. Law FMK, Moate PJ, Leaver DD, et al. Parathyroid hormone-related protein in milk and its correlation with bovine milk calcium. *J Endocrinol* 1991;128:21–26.

163. Rude RK, Haussler MR, Singer FR. Postpartum resolution of hypocalcemia in a lactating hypoparathyroid patient. *Endocrinol Jpn* 1984;31:227–233.

164. Caplan RH, Beguin EA. Hypercalcemia in a calcitriol-treated hypoparathyroid woman during lactation. *Obstet Gynecol* 1990;76:485–489.

165. Yamamoto M, Duong LT, Fisher JE, Thiede MA, Caulfield MP, Rosenblatt M. Suckling-associated increases in urinary phosphate and cAMP excretion in lactating rats may be a systemic effect of parathyroid hormone-related protein. *Endocrinology* 1992;129:2614–2622.

166. Ratcliffe WA, Thompson GE, Care AD, Peaker M. Production of parathyroid hormone-related protein by the mammary gland of the goat. *J Endocrinol* 1992;133:87–93.

167. Khosla S, Johansen K, Ory SJ, O'Brien PC, Kao PC. Parathyroid hormone-related peptide in lactation and in umbilical cord blood. *Mayo Clin Proc* 1990;65:1408–1414.

The Parathyroids, edited by J.P. Bilezikian,
M.A. Levine, and R. Marcus. Raven Press, Ltd.,
New York © 1994.

CHAPTER 19

Skeletal and Renal Actions of Parathyroid Hormone-Related Protein

Gordon J. Strewler and Robert A. Nissenson

At the time of its discovery, it was anticipated that parathyroid hormone-related protein (PTHrP) would mimic parathyroid hormone (PTH) in bone and kidney, because it was already clear that both peptides bound to and activated a common skeletal and renal receptor (1–3). Studies of the actions of PTHrP in the classic target tissues for PTH were immediately begun to determine whether PTHrP mimicked PTH as anticipated and to relate its actions to the pathogenesis of hypercalcemia in malignancy. These studies, some aspects of which are discussed in the previous chapter by Grill and Martin, have firmly established the paradigm that the acute skeletal and renal effects of PTHrP are similar to those of PTH itself.

However, the conclusion that PTH and PTHrP act alike raises the question of the physiological role of PTHrP in skeletal and renal systems. As discussed in previous chapters, PTHrP is thought in general to have predominately local rather than systemic actions in physiological circumstances. Since PTHrP is produced locally in skeletal tissues and in the kidney, it is a reasonable presumption that the hormone is physiologically active in these tissues. It may also be speculated that in kidney and bone the physiological effects of PTHrP are distinct, at least in part, from the effects of circulating PTH or infused peptides. As a peptide that acts via the PTH receptor, PTHrP would be redundant were it produced locally and without distinct tissue functions that cannot be fulfilled by its systemic

sister hormone, PTH. A new phase of the study of PTHrP in kidney and bone, the elucidation of its physiological roles in these tissues, is just underway. Already it is clear that PTHrP plays an essential role in the development of cartilage and bone and that PTH does not compensate for its absence.

This chapter first discusses the expression and developmental role of PTHrP in skeletal tissues and then summarizes the effects of PTHrP on bone remodelling, cellular aspects of PTHrP action in bone, and renal actions of PTHrP. The chapter concludes with a speculation regarding the physiological significance of PTH in kidney and bone and how its actions in these tissues are related to its actions in other systems.

DEVELOPMENTAL ROLE OF PARATHYROID HORMONE-RELATED PROTEIN IN CARTILAGE AND BONE

The strongest evidence for a developmental role of PTHrP in bone comes from recent work on the effects of targeted disruption of the *PTHrP* gene in the mouse. Karaplis and colleagues (3a) introduced a null mutation into the coding sequence of the *PTHrP* gene in mouse embryonic stem cells by the technique of homologous recombination and, by implanting blastocysts incorporating mutant cells, were able to breed mice that carried the *PTHrP* null mutation. Heterozygous null/+ mice appeared to be phenotypically normal, but null/null homozygotes (which did not express *PTHrP* from either allele) died in the peripartum period. Although the precise cause of death is not entirely clear, their only apparent abnormalities at day 18.5 (just prior to birth) were in the appendicular and axial skeleton. They had short limbs; heavily mineralized endochondral bones of the basilar skull with an abnormal

G. J. Strewler: Department of Medicine, University of California, San Francisco; and Endocrine Unit, Veterans Affairs Medical Center, San Francisco, California 94121.

R. A. Nissenson: Departments of Medicine and Physiology, University of California, San Francisco; and Endocrine Unit, Veterans Affairs Medical Center, San Francisco, California 94121.

domed contour of the vault (possibly resulting from upward pressure of the developing central nervous system in the face of premature mineralization of the skull base); and perichondrial ossification of the ribs, vertebrae, and other long bones. In the ribs the number of hypertrophic chondrocytes was increased compared to normal bones, and the outer cartilage layer was replaced by bone. This apparently represents an acceleration of the normal pattern of maturation and ossification. The organization of growth plates was also abnormal, with marked diminution of the zone of proliferation and disruption of its normal columnar architecture but a normal to abundant hypertrophic layer. Preliminary studies at earlier stages (days 14.5–15.5) indicate that the cartilaginous anlagen of the limb bones are already abnormally formed at a time before the growth plates have developed or mineralization has occurred.

In summary, the *PTHrP* null mutation appears to give rise to defects in chondrocyte function, a form of chondrodysplasia, with impaired endochondral bone formation; rhizomelic dwarfism; impaired chondrocyte proliferation in the growth plate; and premature ossification of the skull, vertebrae, and ribs. It is clear from these studies that PTHrP has an important developmental role in cartilage and bone. Presumably this role cannot be assumed by PTH.

Available knowledge regarding PTH and PTHrP in cartilage provides the backdrop for the PTHrP "gene knockout" experiment described above. During fetal life the *PTHrP* gene is expressed in immature cartilage and in zones of ossification. In the mouse, PTHrP mRNA is detected in perichondrium on day 16.5 by hybridization histochemistry, and expression of the gene drops as development proceeds (4). In the rat fetus, the PTHrP protein is detectable on day 13 by immunohistochemistry in condensing mesenchyme of the sclerotome and in immature cartilage of the early vertebral column, and the intensity of staining decreases with time until ossification, when chondrocytes and osteoblast-like cells become positive (5). In the limb bud the protein is present in condensing mesenchyme and immature cartilage (5), and PTHrP is also detectable by immunofluorescence in wing bud cartilage of the stage 27 chick embryo (S.A. Newman, G.J. Strewler, and R.A. Nissenson, unpublished data). The PTH/PTHrP receptor is also present in chick limb bud at this stage, and there is a marked cyclic adenosine monophosphate (cAMP) response to PTH (6). In micromass cultures of chick wing bud mesenchyme, exposure to chicken PTHrP-(1–34) accelerates differentiation to cartilage (S.A. Newman, G.J. Strewler, and R.A. Nissenson, unpublished data). This may be a cAMP-mediated effect, since cAMP analogs have long been known to accelerate chondrogenesis in this system (7). These fragmentary data suggest that a burst of endogenous PTHrP production may enhance

early stages of the formation of the cartilaginous anlage of endochondral bones.

At later stages PTHrP is present by immunohistochemistry in chondrocytes in zones of ossification in the rat and human fetus (5,8). In the chicken growth plate, PTHrP is identified immunohistochemically in the upper hypertrophic zone (K. Jensen, R. Rosier, R. Nissenson, G. Strewler, unpublished data). There is strong expression of the *PTHrP* gene in dental lamina of the teeth (4). No direct evidence is available that biologically active PTHrP is secreted from cells of early skeletal anlage, but bioactive PTHrP-like material is secreted from day 19 fetal rat limb bones and can be extracted from bone matrix (9,10). In addition, the PTH/PTHrP receptor is present in maturing chondrocytes of the growth plate by *in situ* hybridization (11) and in hypertrophic chondrocytes by receptor autoradiography (12).

There have been a number of studies of PTH action in cultured growth plate chondrocytes. These cells display a striking cAMP response to PTH, and PTH is a potent and effective mitogen, which also accelerates the incorporation of sulfate into proteoglycans (13,14). However, exposure to PTH decreases collagen synthesis and alkaline phosphatase activity. In addition, PTH can directly inhibit the mineralization of matrix by cultured rabbit growth plate chondrocytes, without affecting their proliferation (15). Interestingly, these effects of PTH are most prominant in embryonic growth plate chondrocytes and are absent in articular chondrocytes, which do not appear to express PTH-responsive adenylyl cyclase (14). It is conceivable that the effects of PTH observed in these cell culture systems reflect the physiological actions of PTHrP on the growth plate, since hypoparathyroidism is not associated with abnormalities of growth plate function, but knockout of the *PTHrP* gene is. Mesenchymal prechondrocytes, as do related developmental systems (e.g., myoblasts), tend to display an inverse relationship between proliferation and differentiation. One can speculate that null mutations of the *PTHrP* gene reduce the proliferative potential of the chondrocyte, giving rise to the decreased zone of proliferation. This could lead directly to the increase in hypertrophic chondrocytes and the premature mineralization that are observed in mice homozygous for the null mutation, or the presumed inhibition of mineralization by PTHrP could be independent of its effects on proliferation (15).

It is becoming clear that PTHrP is a key developmental regulator of skeletal tissues, one that acts at multiple points in the pathways of chondrogenesis and ossification. These are local effects for which circulating PTH apparently does not substitute. Some of the effects of PTHrP may occur in developmental periods before PTH secretion has matured. It is conceivable that parathyroid development is itself impaired in

PTHrP null/null homozygotes, although the glands are histologically normal. [PTHrP is expressed in the fetal parathyroid gland (4,8) but the functional significance of this is unknown.] It is also possible that certain cartilaginous sites of PTHrP action are not accessible to circulating PTH, but the receptor autoradiography studies of Barling and Bibby (12) suggest that the growth plate is readily accessible. Perhaps the effects of PTHrP on skeletal development require higher concentrations of hormone than are achieved in the circulation. Finally, it is possible that some of the skeletal actions of PTHrP involve a receptor distinct from the PTH/PTHrP receptor, which recognizes molecular determinants that are not shared by PTH. However, the effects of PTHrP and PTH described above were on chondrocytes obtained with cyclase-active amino-terminal peptide fragments of the hormones.

EFFECTS OF PARATHYROID HORMONE-RELATED PROTEIN ON BONE REMODELLING

Bone Resorption

During the purification of PTHrP, it was clear that bone resorbing activity copurified with adenylyl cyclase stimulating activity (16). When synthetic PTHrP became available, studies of its bone resorbing activity were immediately carried out to confirm that the peptides had the activity expected of them. The activity of synthetic hPTHrP-(1–34) (17–21), hPTHrP-(1–36) (22), hPTHrP-(1–40) (20), hPTHrP-(1–74) (23), and recombinant PTHrP-(1–141) (24) has been studied in bone explant systems. In fetal rat limb bone explants (17–20,22) and neonatal mouse calvaria (21), the potencies of PTHrP peptides and PTH-(1–34) are approximately equal. In these systems there is a tendency for shorter PTHrP peptides to be slightly less potent than longer ones and for bPTH-(1–34) to be more potent than hPTH-(1–34); in the extreme case, hPTHrP-(1–34) is reported to be ~5% as potent in the fetal rat limb bone assay as bPTH-(1–34) (20). However, in one study, recombinant hPTHrP-(1–141) was 100-fold less potent than bPTH-(1–34) in the fetal rat limb bone resorption assay (24).

In isolated rat osteoclasts, hPTHrP-(1–34), hPTHrP-(1–40), and hPTHrP-(1–84) are all about equipotent with PTH as inducers of bone resorption (25,26). Thus the bone resorbing activity of PTHrP resides in the adenylyl cyclase active domain in the 1–34 sequence and is presumably mediated by the classical PTH/PTHrP receptor. As is discussed elsewhere in this volume, PTH/PTHrP receptors have not been definitively demonstrated on osteoclasts, which are thought by many to utilize the osteoblast as an intermediary to respond to PTH peptides and other bone resorbing substances. In keeping with this view, neither amino-terminal nor full-length PTHrP peptides are active on isolated osteoclasts, except in the presence of osteoblasts, which possess the PTH/PTHrP receptor (25). PTHrP-(1–141) is reported to have biphasic effects on resorption in the presence of osteoblasts but to inhibit bone resorption in their absence, suggesting the existence of an inhibitory domain in the carboxyl-terminal region of PTHrP, as is discussed further below (27,28). In response to PTHrP-(1–74), SaOS-2 human osteosarcoma cells release an ~9 kDa peptide with bone resorbing activity, which is a candidate as the coupling factor between the osteoblast and the osteoclast (29).

When infused into rodents *in vivo*, PTHrP activates osteoclastic bone resorption (30–32) and produces hypercalcemia with approximately the same potency as PTH (17,18,30,32). In a recent study in normal humans the effects of a 12 hr infusion of hPTH-(1–34) at a dose of 8 pmol/kg · hr were compared to the effects of an equimolar or tenfold higher infusion of hPTHrP-(1–34) (33). The serum concentration of both peptides was measured during the infusions by radioimmunoassay. It was concluded that PTHrP-(1–34) has a shorter intravenous half-life in humans than PTH-(1–34) and is probably slightly less potent as a hypercalcemic factor (33). From the clinical perspective, however, it is clear that PTHrP fulfills the prediction that a potent hypercalcemic factor must circulate in patients with malignancy and hypercalcemia.

As is discussed in the chapter, "Parathyroid Hormone and Parathyroid Hormone-Related Protein as Polyhormones: Evolutionary Aspects and Neoclassical Actions, by Mallette, it has been suggested that PTHrP is a "polyhormone," which, like the ACTH/opiate precursor proopiomelanocortin, incorporates several different biological activities into different regions of the same protein. Fenton et al. (27,28) recently reported that the carboxyl-terminal domain of PTHrP contains a bone resorption-inhibitory activity. This activity was first detected in PTHrP-(107–139) (27) and subsequently was localized to a PTHrP-(107–111) peptide (28), which, unlike the remainder of the carboxyl terminus, is highly conserved among the human, rat, and chicken sequences. The 107–111 sequence lies directly carboxyl-terminal to a basic amino acid sequence that is a likely target for protease attack, and carboxyl-terminal fragments that are recognized by antibodies to PTHrP-(108–139) are detectable in the circulation. It is thus conceivable that fragments that circulate or that are produced locally contain the 107–111 sequence near their amino terminus. PTHrP-(107–139) inhibited bone resorption in isolated fetal rat limb explants and, like the physiological osteoclast inhibitor calcitonin, directly inhibited bone resorption by the isolated osteoclast. Thus PTHrP could be cleaved locally to release multiple active peptides. If this is confirmed in other laboratories, these observations raise the possibility that PTHrP has a complex, biphasic role in the regulation of bone remodelling. However, it has recently been reported that these peptides do not inhibit bone resorption in a different bone explant system (34), and more work will be required to elucidate the role of the carboxyl terminus.

Effects on Coupling of Bone Formation and Bone Resorption

It has been observed that patients with malignancies complicated by humoral hypercalcemia display markedly reduced bone formation in the presence of accelerated bone resorption (35). This contrasts to most other states of high bone resorption, including hyperparathyroidism, where coupled increases in bone formation lead to a high-turnover state. This finding raises the question of whether PTHrP might have a distinctive effect on bone remodelling, producing uncoupling of bone resorption and bone formation.

The effects of PTHrP on bone turnover have been investigated through subcutaneous infusion of PTHrP-(1–34) into parathyroidectomized rats (32) and infusion of PTHrP-(1–40) into nude mice (31). In both studies bone formation was increased, and the effects of PTHrP-(1–34) and hPTH-(1–34) were similar (32). When given to growing rats by daily subcutaneous injection, PTH-(1–34) increases bone formation and produces a net anabolic effect, with increased bone mass (36). In this model PTHrP-(1–34) is also anabolic but is less potent and less effective than hPTH-(1–34). However, given by daily subcutaneous injection, hPTHrP-(1–74) produced greater increases in femoral weight and calcium content in the rat than did bPTH-(1–34) (37). Thus PTHrP does not uncouple bone formation and resorption in rodent models, though its effects may differ subtly from those of PTH; the possibility that longer PTHrP peptides, which are probably similar to the principal circulating forms of PTHrP, are more anabolic than PTHrP-(1–34) has been suggested. However, it could be argued that the rodent is not the best model in which to investigate these issues, since human hypercalcemic tumors grown in the rodent induce marked increases in bone formation, in contrast to what has been reported in the human host (38).

Studies of PTHrP action on bone at the cellular level also have bearing on its effects on bone turnover. Like PTH itself, PTHrP inhibits the proliferation of rat osteosarcoma cells, an action that may be cAMP mediated (39,40). Given continuously, PTHrP-(1–34) and PTH-(1–34) both inhibit collagen synthesis in cultured fetal rat calvariae (41,42), but, given intermittently, PTHrP-(1–34) stimulates collagen synthesis in this system, as does PTH-(1–34) (41). The anabolic effect of

intermittent PTHrP administration may involve IGF-1 as a mediator, since this effect is blocked by neutralizing antibodies to insulin-like growth factor type I (IGF-I) (41). Addition of PTHrP to cultured osteosarcoma cells increases the release of multiple IGF binding proteins, which are capable of modulating IGF-I action (43). In all respects, these cellular effects of PTHrP on proliferation of bone cells, collagen synthesis, and growth factor secretion are essentially identical to the effects of PTH itself.

Neither the whole-animal effects of infusing PTHrP nor the cellular effects of PTHrP on bone offer a satisfactory explanation for the low bone formation rates observed in patients with malignancy. The effect of cancer on bone formation has many possible explanations that do not directly involve PTHrP. Indeed, it is notable that depressed bone formation rates occur in hypercalcemic patients with multiple myeloma, a neoplasm in which PTHrP levels are rarely increased (44). The uncoupling phenomenon could be a nonspecific effect of inanition, could be related to the suppressed 1,25-dihydroxycholecalciferol levels typical of malignancy-associated hypercalcemia (45), or could result from the secretion of another cytokine. For example, interleukin-1, which is sometimes cosecreted with PTHrP (46), inhibits osteoblast function.

Physiological Role of Parathyroid Hormone-Related Protein in Bone Remodelling

Although it is an attractive notion that PTHrP might have effects on bone remodelling in parallel with its effects on endochondral bone formation, it is not clear whether PTHrP has local effects on the postnatal skeleton. Although bioactive PTHrP-like material is secreted from day 19 fetal rat limb bone explants obtained near the end of the fetal period (9,10), nothing is known of its patterns of expression in postnatal bone. The *PTHrP* gene is expressed in a model osteoblast cell, SaOS-2 human osteosarcoma (47), but not in most rodent osteosarcoma cell lines. What the local effects of PTHrP might be is not readily predictable from available data and will not be easily determined, although localization of *PTHrP* gene expression and protein in postnatal bone would be a useful beginning.

RENAL ACTIONS OF PARATHYROID HORMONE-RELATED PROTEIN

Urinary Cyclic Adenosine Monophosphate Excretion

A portion of the cAMP that appears in the urine arises in renal tubular cells. In normal individuals, this "nephrogenous" cAMP is largely attributable to PTH receptor-mediated stimulation of renal tubular cAMP production in response to circulating PTH (48). The observation that NcAMP excretion is increased in a large proportion of patients with malignancy-associated hypercalcemia (MAH) despite normal or suppressed circulating levels of PTH suggested the presence of a humoral PTH-like factor capable of increasing renal tubular cAMP levels (45,49,50). Indeed, activation of adenylyl cyclase in renal plasma membranes was one of the bioassay systems in which PTH-like bioactivity was shown to be elaborated by human tumors (51,52). In a group of 28 patients with humorally based MAH, a significant correlation between circulating iPTHrP-(1–74) levels and urinary cAMP excretion was seen, suggesting a causal relationship (53). Urinary cAMP excretion was subsequently shown to be elevated in certain rodent models of MAH as well (54–57). Passive immunization with neutralizing PTHrP antibodies lowered urinary cAMP excretion in hypercalcemic rats bearing Rice-500 Leydig cell tumors (58) and in hypercalcemic nude mice bearing human squamous carcinomas (59).

The ability of exogenous PTHrP to alter urinary cAMP excretion in rats has been evaluated in several studies. PTHrP-(1–34) promotes enhanced cAMP excretion both in intact animals and in the isolated perfused kidney (18,19,60–63). In most studies, PTHrP-(1–34) displayed a potency similar to that of PTH-(1–34), although minor differences have been noted (see, e.g., 64). Recombinant PTHrP-(1–141) is also active and is equipotent with PTHrP-(1–34) (64). Studies in humans indicate that exogenous PTHrP-(1–34) increases urinary cAMP excretion and is equipotent with hPTH-(1–34) (33).

Renal Phosphate Handling

Serum phosphate levels are frequently reduced in patients with MAH, and thus the direct osteolytic activity of bone metastases cannot fully account for abnormalities in mineral ion homeostasis. This observation was one of the earliest indications that tumor cells might elaborate a humoral factor with PTH-like biological effects. Renal tubular reabsorption of phosphate is reduced in patients with humorally based MAH, and this reduction is comparable to that seen in patients with primary hyperparathyroidism (45). Hypercalcemic rats bearing the transplantable Leydig cell tumor excrete excess phosphate and are hypophosphatemic. Apical membranes from the proximal renal tubule of such animals display reduced sodium-dependent phosphate transport (65). The abnormalities in renal phosphate handling are ameliorated by passive immunization with neutralizing PTHrP antibodies (58).

Direct effects of exogenous PTHrP on renal phosphate handling have been examined both in vivo and in the opossum kidney (OK) cell model of the proximal nephron. Infusion of amino-terminal fragments of PTHrP into rats (17,19,62), lambs (66), or humans (33) produces phosphaturia and hypophosphatemia. In rat kidney, PTHrP-(1–74) and PTHrP-(1–141) inhibit phosphate reabsorption with a potency similar to that of PTHrP-(1–36) (63,64). The potencies of PTHrP peptides in these in vivo models do not differ markedly from those of bovine or human PTH-(1–34), although quantitative differences have been noted. Coadministration of the PTH receptor antagonist PTH-(7–34) blocks the phosphaturic effect of PTHrP-(1–34) in vivo (66,67). Analogous results have been obtained in studies of PTHrP inhibition of sodium-dependent phosphate uptake by OK cells in vitro (68–70).

Renal Calcium Handling

Stewart et al. (45) found that patients with MAH exhibited increased calcium excretion compared with patients with primary hyperparathyroidism and equivalent hypercalcemia. These findings led to the proposal that the putative tumor-derived "PTH-like" hypercalcemic factor might lack the anticalciuric action of PTH. However, subsequent studies have indicated that patients with MAH display renal calcium hyper-reabsorption, although perhaps to a lesser extent than in primary hyperparathyroidism. In the steady state, hypercalcemia in patients with MAH is maintained by excessive bone resorption, but it has been suggested that increased renal calcium reabsorption plays a significant role in maintaining hypercalcemia during the early phases of the MAH syndrome (71).

In thyroparathyroidectomized rats and in the isolated perfused rat kidney, amino-terminal fragments of PTHrP have been reported to be either equipotent to (18,72) or slightly more potent than (63,64) PTH-(1–34) in reducing urinary calcium excretion. Recombinant PTHrP-(1–141) and synthetic PTHrP-(1–74) elicit hypocalciuric actions similar to those of PTHrP-(1–34) (63,64). Evidence suggests that the calcium-sparing action of PTHrP may contribute significantly to hypercalcemia in rodent models of MAH, since hypercalcemia in rats bearing the Walker 256 carcinosarcoma and in rats chronically infused with PTHrP-(1–34) could not be normalized with antiresorptive bisphosphonates without the concomitant administration of drugs that inhibit renal calcium reabsorption (73).

Regulation of 25(OH)D-1-Hydroxylase

An interesting and puzzling aspect of mineral homeostasis in patients with MAH is the tendency for them to display low normal to frankly low levels of circulating 1,25-dihydroxyvitamin D_3 [$1,25(OH)_2D_3$], whereas patients with primary hyperparathyroidism and comparable hypercalcemia have generally elevated levels of $1,25(OH)_2D_3$ (45). Nonmutually exclusive explanations for low levels of $1,25(OH)_2D_3$ in MAH include the following: (a) PTHrP might differ from PTH in its ability to maintain 1-hydroxylase activity; (b) other tumor products might act as inhibitors of the 1-hydroxylase [or might increase the metabolic clearance of $1,25(OH)_2D_3$]; or (c) sequellae of malignant disease not present in patients with primary hyperparathyroidism (e.g., cachexia, immobilization) could influence vitamin D metabolism in patients with MAH.

Pertinent to the first possibility is the finding that administration of amino-terminal fragments of PTHrP in vivo increased in serum levels of $1,25(OH)_2D_3$ in rodents (31,74,75) and in humans (33). These increments did not differ from those produced by administration PTH-(1–34). Unfortunately, the effects of full-length PTHrP on serum levels of $1,25(OH)_2D_3$ were not evaluated. PTHrP-(1–34) injected subcutaneously elicited a potent stimulatory effect on 1-hydroxylase activity, as assessed in mouse renal tubules in vitro (76). Curiously, coadministration of maximally effective doses of PTH and PTHrP produced additive stimulation of the 1-hydroxylase. Thus PTHrP-(1–34) is clearly capable of reproducing the effects of PTH on the renal 1-hydroxylase, but it is possible that the two agents do not act by identical mechanisms.

A potentially important difference between MAH and primary hyperparathyroidism is that in the latter PTH is secreted in a pulsatile fashion, whereas in MAH PTHrP is presumably secreted continuously. The consequence of this difference for the responsivity of the 1-hydroxylase in renal target cells is unclear, but it is possible that continuous stimulation produces desensitization to PTHrP. If so, desensitization is response selective; the phosphaturic and hypocalciuric responses to PTHrP appear to be intact. It is of interest that chronic infusion of PTH into dogs and humans is reported to produce hypercalcemia, hypophosphatemia, and a *decrease* in plasma levels of $1,25(OH)_2D_3$; in dogs, EDTA administration normalizedserum calcium and raised $1,25(OH)_2D_3$ levels to the high-normal range (77). These findings are consistent with the possibility that continuous high-level stimulation of the PTH/PTHrP receptor, perhaps in concert with hypercalcemia, results in desensitization of the 1-hydroxylase response to PTHrP in MAH. Interestingly, rodents display increased $1,25(OH)_2D_3$ levels in response to continuous administration of PTH and in response to the development or implantation of tumors that elaborate PTHrP and elicit other features of the MAH syndrome (38).

A limited amount of data supports the presence of tumor-derived inhibitors of 1-hydroxylase activity in MAH. Ikeda et al. (78) reported that nude rats implanted with uterine cancer from a patient with MAH displayed biochemical features of the human syndrome, including suppressed plasma levels of $1,25(OH)_2D_3$. Fractionation of extracts of this tumor by reverse-phase high-performance liquid chromatography (HPLC) yielded two peaks of PTH-like bioactivity (adenylyl cyclase activation in osteosarcoma cells); one of these contained a factor capable of preventing PTH stimulation of $1,25(OH)_2D_3$ production by rat kidney cells in vitro (79). Fukumoto et al. (79) demonstrated that a second human tumor (squamous oral cavity cancer) implanted into nude rats produced increased levels of $1,25(OH)_2D_3$, and tumor extracts did not produce demonstrable inhibition of $1,25(OH)_2D_3$ production in vitro. These results are consistent with the possibility that a tumor-derived, circulating inhibitor of the renal 1-hydroxylase may contribute to suppression of $1,25(OH)_2D_3$ levels in a subset of patients with MAH. However, the identity and prevalence of this factor must be determined before its significance can be properly assessed.

Unlike patients with primary hyperparathyroidism, MAH patients frequently are bedridden and cachectic. There are no controlled studies that bear on the influence of factors such as nutritional status or immobilization on $1,25(OH)_2D_3$ levels in patients with MAH. Since these factors can influence vitamin D metabolism in other settings, they may be important determinants of $1,25(OH)_2D_3$ levels in some patients with MAH.

Other Renal Actions of Parathyroid Hormone-Related Protein

Acid–base balance frequently differs in patients with primary hyperparathyroidism vs. MAH. The former typically display mild hyperchloremic acidosis, whereas the latter often have mild hypokalemic alkalosis. PTH is well known to inhibit renal bicarbonate reabsorption, and this is probably the major factor contributing to acidosis. In the isolated perfused rat kidney, amino-terminal fragments of PTHrP mimic this effect of PTH, but PTHrP-(1–141) and PTHrP-(1–108) are reported to act somewhat differently. These peptides produced an initial inhibition of bicarbonate reabsorption, followed by a later decrease in bicarbonate excretion, and it is suggested that this later action of PTHrP may be responsible for alkalosis in MAH (80). This interesting idea awaits evaluation in human studies.

Several other known effects of PTH on the kidney are essentially reproduced by PTHrP. These include increases in renal glucose-6-phosphate dehydrogenase activity (81,82) and enhanced sodium excretion (63). PTH and PTHrP stimulate adenylyl cyclase and induce relaxation of renal vascular smooth muscle in vitro, and these actions are blocked by PTH receptor antagonists (83–85). Although relatively high concentrations of PTH and PTHrP are required to produce vascular effects, the PTHrP gene is expressed in vascular smooth muscle, and thus PTHrP may serve as a local modulator of renal vascular tone.

SIGNALLING BY PARATHYROID HORMONE-RELATED PROTEIN IN BONE AND KIDNEY

Early studies indicated that PTHrP-(1–34) binds the same receptor as PTH-(1–34) in cultured osteoblast-like osteosarcoma cells (86–89) and in renal plasma membranes (87,90). Each can displace the other in competitive binding experiments, and cross-linking studies in canine renal plasma membrane demonstrate that each labels a predominant 85 kDa receptor moiety (87). The two peptides display essentially identical potencies for activation of adenylyl cyclase in bone cells (21,86–89,91) and in opossum kidney cells (68). The details of signalling by the osteoblast PTHrP receptor have subsequently been studied in more detail. Besides their adenylyl cyclase response, osteosarcoma cells and opossum kidney cells exposed to PTHrP-(1–34) also respond with a calcium transient indistinguishable from that produced by PTH (92,93), despite early data to the contrary (94). It is now clear that the same PTH/PTHrP receptor can signal via both adenylyl cyclase and changes in intracellular calcium, in that both responses to PTHrP are conferred upon cells in which the recombinant receptor is expressed (95). This receptor does not appear to recognize peptide regions beyond the amino-terminal 1–34 domain; the effects of longer PTHrP peptides, up to PTHrP-(1–141), on the production of cAMP and of calcium transients are indistinguishable from those of PTHrP-(1–34) (92,93). However, the production of prostaglandin E_2 by SaOS-2 human osteosarcoma cells is stimulated considerably more by PTHrP-(1–141) than by PTHrP-(1–34) (96). This observation is consistent with subtle differences in recognition of different PTHrP peptides by a common receptor or with the possibility that a novel PTHrP receptor that binds determinants outside the 1–34 domain is coupled to phospholipase A_2 in osteosarcoma cells.

PERSPECTIVES

The actions of PTHrP in bone and kidney closely resemble the actions of PTH itself, largely accounting for the clinical syndrome produced by inappropriate humoral secretion of PTHrP from malignant neoplasms. In addition, there is preliminary evidence of activities residing in the mid- and carboxyl-terminal regions of PTHrP that are dissimilar to the actions of PTH. Much work will be required to confirm these results. Nonetheless, interest in this possibility is heightened by the recent finding of distinct intracellular pools of amino-terminal and midregion PTHrP peptides (97), which raises the possibility that region-specific peptides derived from PTHrP can be secreted independently.

The emerging developmental role of PTHrP in bone will undoubtedly be elaborated upon further in the next few years. The recent advent of reagents to measure PTHrP itself as well as its receptor and the recent availability of an experimental animal model with a null mutation in the *PTHrP* gene represent extremely valuable tools for this purpose. PTHrP is also present immunohistochemically in the developing urinary system. The mesonephros and subsequently the collecting tubule are stained; there is disagreement regarding whether the glomerulus and convoluted tubules are also positive (5,8,98). It seems possible that the expression of PTHrP in fetal kidney indicates a developmental role in the urogenital tract as well as in bone, even though gross urogenital anomalies were not noted in the PTHrP-less mouse. It is conceivable that subtle anomalies of renal development will be detected in further studies of these animals. It is also possible that the phenotype does not include obvious renal anomalies, because another factor, perhaps PTH itself, can compensate for the absence of PTHrP.

In contrast to its emerging developmental role, PTHrP's possible physiological role in postnatal bone remodelling or in the regulation of renal function remains to be clarified. This will undoubtedly be the subject of further investigation.

ACKNOWLEDGMENTS

The authors thank Henry Kronenberg and Gino V. Segre for providing data prior to publication.

REFERENCES

1. Strewler GJ, Nissenson RA. Peptide mediators of hypercalcemia in malignancy. *Annu Rev Med* 1990;41:35–44.
2. Broadus AE, Mangin M, Ikeda K, et al. Humoral hypercalcemia of cancer: identification of a novel parathyroid hormone-like. *N Engl J Med* 1988;319:556–563.
3. Martin TJ, Moseley JM, Gillespie MT. Parathyroid hormone-related protein: biochemistry and molecular biology. *Crit Rev Biochem Mol Biol* 1991;26:377–395.
3a. Karaplis AC, Tybulewicz V, Mulligan RC et al. Disruption of parathyroid hormone-related peptide gene leads to a multitude of skeletal abnormalities and perinatal mortality. *J Bone Mineral Res* 1992;7(Suppl 1):S93.

4. Senior PV, Heath DA, Beck F. Expression of parathyroid hormone-related protein mRNA in the rat before birth: demonstration by hybridization histochemistry. *J Mol Endocrinol* 1991;6:281–290.

5. Burton PB, Moniz C, Quirke P, et al. Parathyroid hormone-related peptide: expression in fetal and neonatal development. *J Pathol* 1992;167:291–296.

6. Parker CL, Biddulph DM, Ballard TA. Development of the cyclic AMP response to parathyroid hormone and prostaglandin E₂ in the embryonic chick limb. *Calcif Tissue Int* 1981; 33:641–648.

7. Solursh M, Reiter RS, Ahrens PB, Vertel BM. Stage- and position-related changes in chondrogenic response of chick embryonic wing mesenchyme to treatment with dibutyryl cyclic AMP. *Dev Biol* 1981;83:9–19.

8. Moseley JM, Hayman JA, Danks JA, et al. Immunohistochemical detection of parathyroid hormone-related protein in human fetal epithelia. *J Clin Endocrinol Metab* 1991.

9. Nijs-de Wolf N, Pepersack T, Corvilain J, Karmali R, Bergmann P. Adenylate cyclase stimulating activity immunologically similar to parathyroid hormone-related peptide can be extracted from fetal rat long bones. *J Bone Mineral Res* 1991;6:921–927.

10. Bergmann P, Nijs-de Wolf N, Pepersack T, Corvilain J. Release of parathyroid hormonelike peptides by fetal rat long bones in culture. *J Bone Mineral Res* 1990;5:741–753.

11. Lee K, Deeds JD, Bond AT, Jüppner H, Auou-Samra A-B, Segre GV. *In situ* localization of PTH/PTHrP receptor mRNA in the bone of fetal and young rats. *Bone* (in press).

12. Barling PM, Bibby NJ. Study of the localization of [³H]bovine parathyroid hormone in bone by light. *Calcif Tissue Int* 1985;37:441–446.

13. Koite T, Iwamoto M, Shimazu A, Nakashima K, Suzzuki F, Kato Y. Potent mitogenic effects of parathyroid hormone (PTH) on embryonic chick and rabbit chondrocytes. *J Clin Invest* 1990;85:629–631.

14. Crabb ID, O'keefe RJ, Puzas JE, Rosier RN. Differential effects of parathyroid hormone on chick growth plate and articular chondrocytes. *Calcif Tissue Int* 1992;50:61–66.

15. Kato Y, Shimazu A, Nakashima K, Susuki F, Kikko A, Iwamoto M. Effects of parathyroid hormone and calcitonin on alkaline phosphatase activity and matrix calcification in rabbit growth-plate chondrocyte cultures. *Endocrinology* 1990; 127:114–118.

16. Strewler GJ, Stern PH, Jacobs JW, et al. Parathyroid hormonelike protein from human renal carcinoma cells: structural and functional homology with parathyroid hormone. *J Clin Invest* 1987;80:1803–1807.

17. Horiuchi N, Caulfield MP, Fisher JE, et al. Similarity of synthetic peptide from human tumor to parathyroid hormone in vivo and in vitro. *Science* 1987;238:1566–1568.

18. Yates AJ, Gutierrez GE, Smolens P, et al. Effects of a synthetic peptide of a parathyroid hormone-related protein on calcium homeostasis, renal tubular calcium reabsorption, and bone metabolism in vivo and in vitro in rodents. *J Clin Invest* 1988;81:932–938.

19. Kemp BE, Moseley JM, Rodda CP, et al. Parathyroid hormone-related protein of malignancy: active synthetic fragments. *Science* 1987;238:1568–1570.

20. Raisz LG, Simmons HA, Vargas SJ, Kemp BE, Martin TJ. Comparison of the effects of amino-terminal synthetic parathyroid hormone-related peptide (PTHrP) of malignancy and parathyroid hormone on resorption of cultured fetal rat long bones. *Calcif Tissue Int* 1990;46:233–238.

21. Fukayama S, Bosma TJ, Goad DL, Voelkel EF, Tashjian AH Jr. Human parathyroid hormone (PTH)-related protein and human PTH: comparative biological activities on human bone cells and bone resorption. *Endocrinology* 1988;123:2841–2848.

22. Stewart AF, Mangin M, Wu T, et al. Synthetic human parathyroid hormone-like protein stimulates bone resorption and causes hypercalcemia in rats. *J Clin Invest* 1988;81:596–600.

23. Stewart AF, Elliot J, Burtis WJ, Wu T, Insogna KL. Synthetic parathyroid hormone-like protein-(1–74): biochemical and physiological characterization. *Endocrinology* 1989;124:642–648.

24. Thorikay M, Kramer S, Reynolds FH, et al. Synthesis of a gene encoding parathyroid hormone-like protein-(1–141): purification and biological characterization of the expressed protein. *Endocrinology* 1989;124:111–118.

25. Evely RS, Bonomo A, Schneider HG, Moseley JM, Gallagher J, Martin TJ. Structural requirements for the action of parathyroid hormone-related protein (PTHrP) on bone resorption by isolated osteoclasts. *J Bone Mineral Res* 1991;6:85–93.

26. Murrills RJ, Stein LS, Fey CP, Dempster DW. The effects of parathyroid hormone (PTH) and PTH-related peptide on osteoclast resorption of bone slices in vitro: an analysis of pit size and the resorption focus. *Endocrinology* 1990;127:2648–2653.

27. Fenton AJ, Kemp BE, Kent GN, et al. A carboxyl-terminal peptide from the parathyroid hormone-related protein inhibits bone resorption by osteoclasts. *Endocrinology* 1991;129:1762–1768.

28. Fenton AJ, Kemp BE, Hammonds RG Jr, et al. A potent inhibitor of osteoclastic bone resorption within a highly conserved pentapeptide region of parathyroid hormone-related protein; PTHrP[107–111]. *Endocrinology* 1991;129:3424–3426.

29. Morris CA, Mitnick ME, Weir EC, Horowitz M, Kreider BL, Insogna KL. The parathyroid hormone-related protein stimulates human osteoblast-like cells to secrete a 9,000 dalton bone-resorbing protein. *Endocrinology* 1990;126:1783–1785.

30. Thompson DD, Seedor JG, Fisher JE, Rosenblatt M, Rodan GA. Direct action of the parathyroid hormone-like human hypercalcemic factor on bone. *Proc Natl Acad Sci USA* 1988; 85:5673–5677.

31. Rosol TJ, Capen CC, Horst RL. Effects of infusion of human parathyroid hormone-related protein-(1–40) in nude mice: histomorphometric and biochemical investigations. *J Bone Mineral Res* 1988;3:699–706.

32. Kitazawa R, Imai Y, Fukase M, Fujita T. Effects of continuous infusion of parathyroid hormone and parathyroid hormone-related peptide on rat bone in vivo: comparative study by histomorphometry. *Bone Mineral* 1991;12:157–166.

33. Fraher LJ, Hodsman AB, Jonas K, et al. A comparison of the in vivo biochemical responses to exogenous parathyroid hormone-(1–34) [PTH-(1–34)] and PTH-related peptide-(1–34) in man. *J Clin Endocrinol Metab* 1992;75:417–423.

34. Sone T, Kohno H, Kikuchi H, et al. Human parathyroid hormone-related peptide-(107–111) does not inhibit bone resorption in neonatal mouse calvariae. *Endocrinology* 1992;131:2742–2746.

35. Stewart AF, Vignery A, Silverglate A, et al. Quantitative bone histomorphometry in humoral hypercalcemia of malignancy. *J Clin Endocrinol Metab* 1982;55:219–227.

36. Hock JM, Fonseca J, Gunness-Hey M, Kemp BE, Martin TJ. Comparison of the anabolic effects of synthetic parathyroid hormone-related protein (PTHrP) 1–34 and PTH 1–34 on bone in rats. *Endocrinology* 1989;125:2022–2027.

37. Weir EC, Terwilliger G, Sartori L, Insogna KL. Synthetic parathyroid hormone-like protein (1–74) is anabolic for bone in vivo. *Calcif Tissue Int* 1992;51:30–34.

38. Strewler GJ, Wronski TJ, Halloran BP, et al. Pathogenesis of hypercalcemia in nude mice bearing a human renal carcinoma. *Endocrinology* 1986;119:303–310.

39. Kano J, Sugimoto T, Fukase M, Fujita T. The activation of cAMP-dependent protein kinase is directly linked to the inhibition of osteoblast proliferation (UMR-106) by parathyroid hormone-related protein. *Biochem Biophys Res Commun* 1991.

40. Sugimoto T, Kano J, Fukase M, Fujita T. Second messenger signaling in the regulation of cytosolic pH and DNA synthesis by parathyroid hormone (PTH) and PTH-related peptide in osteoblastic osteosarcoma cells: role of Na+/H+ exchange. *J Cell Physiol* 1992;152:28–34.

41. Canalis E, McCarthy TL, Centrella M. Differential effects of continuous and transient treatment with parathyroid hormone related peptide (PTHrp) on bone collagen synthesis. *Endocrinology* 1990;126:1806–1812.

42. Klein-Nulend J, Fall PM, Raisz LG. Comparison of the effects of synthetic human parathyroid hormone (PTH)-(1–34)-related peptide of malignancy and bovine PTH-(1–34) on bone formation and resorption in organ culture. *Endocrinology* 1990;126:223–227.

43. Torring O, Firek AF, Heath H 3d, Conover CA. Parathyroid hormone and parathyroid hormone-related peptide stimulate insulin-like growth factor-binding protein secretion by rat osteoblast-like cells through an adenosine 3',5'-monophosphate-dependent mechanism. *Endocrinology* 1991;128:1006–1014.

44. Delmas PD, Demiaux B, Malaval L, Chapuy MC, Edouard C, Meunier PJ. Serum bone gamma carboxyglutamic acid-containing protein in primary hyperparathyroidism and in malignant hypercalcemia. *J Clin Invest* 1986;77:985–991.

45. Stewart AF, Horst R, Deftos LJ, Cadman EC, Lang R, Broadus AE. Biochemical evaluation of patients with cancer-associated hypercalcemia. *N Engl J Med* 1980;303:1377–1383.

46. Nowak RA, Morrison NE, Goad DL, Gaffney EV, Tashjian AH Jr. Squamous cell carcinomas often produce more than a single bone resorption-stimulating factor: role of interleukin-1 alpha. *Endocrinology* 1990;127:3061–3069.

47. Rodan SB, Wesolowski G, Ianacone J, Thiede MA, Rodan GA. Production of parathyroid hormone-like peptide in a human osteosarcoma cell line: stimulation by phorbol esters and epidermal growth factor. *J Endocrinol* 1989;122:219–227.

48. Broadus AE, Mahaffey JE, Bartter FC, Neer RM. Nephrogenous cyclic adenosine monophosphate as a parathyroid function test. *J Clin Invest* 1977;60:771–783.

49. Kukreja SC, Shemerdiak WP, Lad TE, Johnson PA. Elevated nephrogenous cyclic AMP with normal serum parathyroid hormone levels in patients with lung cancer. *J Clin Endocrinol Metab* 1980;51:167–169.

50. Rude RK, Sharp CF Jr, Fredericks RS, et al. Urinary and nephrogenous adenosine 3',5'-monophosphate in the hypercalcemia of malignancy. *J Clin Endocrinol Metab* 1981;52:765–771.

51. Strewler GJ, Williams RD, Nissenson RA. Human renal carcinoma cells produce hypercalcemia in the nude mouse and a novel protein recognized by parathyroid hormone receptors. *J Clin Invest* 1983;71:769–774.

52. Stewart AF, Insogna KL, Goltzman D, Broadus AE. Identification of adenylate cyclase-stimulating activity and cytochemical glucose-6-phosphate dehydrogenase-stimulating activity in extracts of tumors from patients with humoral hypercalcemia of malignancy. *Proc Natl Acad Sci USA* 1983;80:1454–1458.

53. Burtis WJ, Brady TG, Orloff JJ, et al. Immunochemical characterization of circulating parathyroid hormone-related protein in patients with humoral hypercalcemia of cancer. *N Engl J Med* 1990;322:1106–1112.

54. Sica DA, Martodam RR, Aronow J, Mundy GR. The hypercalcemic rat leydig cell tumor—a model of the humoral hypercalcemia of malignancy. *Calcif Tissue Int* 1983;35:287–293.

55. Spiegel AM, Saxe AW, Deftos LJ, Brennan MF. Humoral hypercalcemia caused by a rat leydig-cell tumor is associated with suppressed parathyroid hormone secretion and increased urinary cAMP excretion. *Hormone Metab Res* 1983;15:299–304.

56. Gkonos PJ, Hayes T, Burtis W, et al. Squamous carcinoma model of humoral hypercalcemia of malignancy. *Endocrinology* 1984;115:2384–2390.

57. Insogna KL, Stewart AF, Vignery MC, et al. Biochemical and histomorphometric characterization of a rat model for humoral hypercalcemia of malignancy. *Endocrinology* 1984;114:888–896.

58. Henderson J, Bernier S, D'Amour P, Goltzman D. Effects of passive immunization against parathyroid hormone (PTH)-like peptide and PTH in hypercalcemic tumor-bearing rats and normocalcemic controls. *Endocrinology* 1990;127:1310–1318.

59. Kukreja SC, Shevrin DH, Wimbiscus SA, et al. Antibodies to parathyroid hormone-related protein lower serum calcium in athymic mouse models. *J Clin Invest* 1988;82:1798–1802.

60. Rabbani SA, Mitchell J, Roy DR, Hendy GN, Goltzman D. Influence of the amino-terminus on in vitro and in vivo biological activity of synthetic parathyroid hormone-like peptides of malignancy. *Endocrinology* 1988;123:2709–2716.

61. Rizzoli R, Caverzasio J, Chapuy MC, Martin TJ, Bonjour JP. Role of bone and kidney in parathyroid hormone-related peptide-induced hypercalcemia in rats. *J Bone Mineral Res* 1989;4:759–765.

62. Ebeling PR, Adam WR, Moseley JM, Martin TJ. Actions of synthetic parathyroid hormone-related protein(1–34) on the isolated rat kidney. *J Endocrinol* 1989;120:45–50.

63. Scheinman SJ, Mitnick ME, Stewart AF. Quantitative evaluation of anticalciuretic effects of synthetic parathyroid hormonelike peptides. *J Bone Mineral Res* 1990;5:653–658.

64. Zhou H, Leaver DD, Moseley JM, Kemp B, Ebeling PR, Martin TJ. Actions of parathyroid hormone-related protein on the rat kidney in vivo. *J Endocrinol* 1989;122:229–235.

65. Sartori L, Insogna KL, Barrett PQ. Renal phosphate transport in humoral hypercalcemia of malignancy. *Am J Physiol* 1988;255:F1078–F1084.

66. Davicco MJ, Coxam V, Lefaivre J, Barlet JP. Parathyroid hormone-related peptide increases urinary phosphate excretion in fetal lambs. *Exp Physiol* 1992;77:377–383.

67. Horiuchi N, Hongo T, Clemens TL. The synthetic human tumor hypercalcemia factor is inhibited by a parathyroid hormone antagonist in rats in vivo. *J Bone Mineral Res* 1990;5:541–545.

68. Pizurki L, Rizzoli R, Moseley J, Martin TJ, Caverzasio J, Bonjour JP. Effect of synthetic tumoral PTH-related peptide on cAMP production and Na-dependent Pi transport. *Am J Physiol* 1988;255:F957–F961.

69. Muff R, Caulfield MP, Fischer JA. Dissociation of cAMP accumulation and phosphate uptake in opossum kidney (OK) cells with parathyroid hormone (PTH) and parathyroid hormone related protein (PTHrP). *Peptides* 1990;11:945–949.

70. Pizurki L, Rizzoli R, Bonjour JP. Inhibition by (D-Trp12, Tyr34)bPTH(7–34)amide of PTH and PTHrP effects on Pi transport in renal cells. *Am J Physiol* 1990;259:F389–F392.

71. Ralston SH, Boyce BF, Cowan RA, Gardner MD, Fraser WD, Boyle IT. Contrasting mechanisms of hypercalcemia in patients with early and advanced humoral hypercalcemia of malignancy. *J Bone Mineral Res* 1989;4:103–111.

72. Carney SL, Ray C, Ebeling PR, Martin TJ, Gillies AH. Synthetic human parathyroid hormone-related protein and rat renal electrolyte transport. *Mineral Electrolyte Metab* 1991;17:41–45.

73. Hurtado J, Esbrit P, Rapado A. Relative role of bone and kidney in the hypercalcemia associated with the rat Walker carcinosarcoma 256. *Eur J Cancer* 1991;27:76–79.

74. Walker AT, Stewart AF, Korn EA, Shiratori T, Mitnick MA, Carpenter TO. Effect of a parathyroid hormone-like peptides on 25-hydroxyvitamin D-1α-hydroxylase activity in rodents. *Am J Physiol* 1990;258:E297–E303.

75. Horiuchi N, Hongo T, Clemens TL. A 7–34 analog of the parathyroid hormone-related protein has potent antagonist and partial agonist activity in vivo. *Bone Mineral* 1991;12:181–188.

76. Nesbitt T, Drezner MK. Abnormal parathyroid hormone-related peptide stimulation of renal 25-hydroxyvitamin D-1-hydroxylase in Hyp mice: evidence for a generalized defect of enzyme activity in the proximal convoluted tubule. *Endocrinology* 1990;127:843–848.

77. Hulter HN, Halloran BP, Toto RD, Peterson JC. Long-term control of plasma calcitriol concentrations in dogs and humans. *J Clin Invest* 1985;76:695–702.

78. Ikeda K, Matsumoto T, Fukumoto S, et al. A hypercalcemic nude rat model that completely mimics human syndrome of humoral hypercalcemia of malignancy. *Calcif Tissue Int* 1988;43:97–102.

79. Fukumoto S, Matsumoto T, Yamoto H, et al. Suppression of serum 1,25-dihydroxyvitamin D in humoral hypercalcemia of malignancy is caused by elaboration of a factor that inhibits renal 1,25-dihydroxyvitamin D3 production. *Endocrinology* 1989;124:2057–2062.

80. Ellis AG, Adam WR, Martin TJ. Comparison of the effects of parathyroid hormone (PTH) and recombinant PTH-related protein on bicarbonate excretion by the isolated perfused rat kidney. *J Endocrinol* 1990;126:403–408.

81. Nakai M, Fukase M, Sakaguchi K, Noda T, Fujii N, Fujita T. Human parathyroid hormone related protein fragment-(1–34) had glucose-6-phosphate dehydrogenase activity on distal convoluted tubules in cytochemical bioassay. *Biochem Biophys Res Commun* 1988.

82. Loveridge N, Dean V, Goltzman D, Hendy GN. Bioactivity of parathyroid hormone and parathyroid hormone- like peptide: agonist and antagonist activities of amino-terminal fragments as assessed by the cytochemical bioassay and in situ biochemistry. *Endocrinology* 1991;128:1938–1946.

83. Winquist RJ, Baskin EP, Vlasuk GP. Synthetic tumor-derived human hypercalcemic factor exhibits parathyroid hormone-like vasorelaxation in renal arteries. *Biochem Biophys Res Commun* 1987;149:227–232.

84. Musso MJ, Plante M, Judes C, Barthelmebs M, Helwig JJ. Renal vasodilatation and microvessel adenylate cyclase stimulation by synthetic parathyroid hormone-like protein fragments. *Eur J Pharmacol* 1989;174:139–151.

85. Trizna W, Edwards RM. Relaxation of renal arterioles by parathyroid hormone and parathyroid hormone-related protein. *Pharmacology* 1991;42:91–96.

86. Jüppner H, Abou-Samra AB, Uneno S, Gu WX, Potts JT Jr, Segre GV. The parathyroid hormone-like peptide associated with humoral hypercalcemia of malignancy and parathyroid hormone bind to the same receptor on the plasma membrane of ROS 17/2.8 cells. *J Biol Chem* 1988;263:8557–8560.

87. Nissenson RA, Diep D, Strewler GJ. Synthetic peptides comprising the amino-terminal sequence of a parathyroid hormone-like protein from human malignancies. Binding to parathyroid hormone receptors and activation of adenylate cyclase in bone cells and kidney. *J Biol Chem* 1988;263:12866–12871.

88. Shigeno C, Yamamoto I, Kitamura N, et al. Interaction of human parathyroid hormone-related peptide with parathyroid hormone receptors in clonal rat osteosarcoma cells. *J Biol Chem* 1988;263:18369–18377.

89. Orloff JJ, Wu TL, Stewart AF. Parathyroid hormone-like proteins: biochemical responses and receptor interactions. *Endocr Rev* 1989;10:476–495.

90. Orloff JJ, Wu TL, Heath HW, Brady TG, Brines ML, Stewart AF. Characterization of canine renal receptors for the parathyroid hormone-like protein associated with humoral hypercalcemia of malignancy. *J Biol Chem* 1989;264:6097–6103.

91. Rodan SB, Noda M, Wesolowski G, Rosenblatt M, Rodan GA. Comparison of postreceptor effects of 1–34 human hypercalcemia factor and 1–34 human parathyroid hormone in rat osteosarcoma cells. *J Clin Invest* 1988;81:924–927.

92. Civitelli R, Martin TJ, Fausto A, Gunsten SL, Hruska KA, Avioli LV. Parathyroid hormone-related peptide transiently increases cytosolic calcium in osteoblast-like cells: comparison with parathyroid hormone. *Endocrinology* 1989;125:1204–1210.

93. Donahue HJ, Fryer MJ, Heath H 3d. Structure-function relationships for full-length recombinant parathyroid hormone-related peptide and its amino-terminal fragments: effects on cytosolic calcium ion mobilization and adenylate cyclase activation in rat osteoblast-like cells. *Endocrinology* 1990;126:1471–1477.

94. Yamada H, Tsutsumi M, Fukase M, Fujimori A, Yamamoto Y, Miyauchi A, Fujii Y, Noda T, Fujii N, Fujita T. Effects of human PTH-related peptide and human PTH on cyclic AMP production and cytosolic free calcium in an osteoblastic cell clone. *Bone Mineral* 1989;6:45–54.

95. Abou-Samra AB, Jüppner H, Force T, et al. Expression cloning of a common receptor for parathyroid hormone and parathyroid hormone-related peptide from rat osteoblast-like cells: a single receptor stimulates intracellular accumulation of both cAMP and inositol triphosphates and increases intracellular free calcium. *Proc Natl Acad Sci USA* 1992;890:2732–2736.

96. Mitnick M, Isales C, Paliwal I, Insogna K. Parathyroid hormone-related protein stimulates prostaglandin E_2 release from human osteoblast-like cells: modulating effect of peptide length. *J Bone Mineral Res* 1992;7:887–896.

97. Soifer NE, Dee KE, Insogna KL, et al. Parathyroid hormone-related protein. Evidence for secretion of a novel mid-region fragment by three different cell types. *J Biol Chem* 1992;267:18236–18243.

98. Burton PB, Moniz C, Quirke P, et al. Parathyroid hormone-related peptide in the human fetal uro-genital tract. *Mol Cell Endocrinol* 1990;69:R13–R17.

The Parathyroids, edited by J.P. Bilezikian, M.A. Levine, and R. Marcus. Raven Press, Ltd., New York © 1994.

CHAPTER 20

Assays for Parathyroid Hormone-Related Protein

Richard Kremer and David Goltzman

INTRODUCTION

In this chapter, which reviews assays for parathyroid hormone-related protein (PTHrP), we begin by discussing the role of bioassays in the discovery of PTHrP. In view of the importance of understanding the nature of the circulating forms of PTHrP in developing and applying assays in a rational manner, we next examine available information on the metabolism of PTHrP. We then describe the characteristics of "one-site" radioimmunoassays and two-site immunoradiometric assays reported in the literature. Examples of the utility of these assays in learning about aspects of the biology of PTHrP in studies in vitro are then reviewed. We next summarize available data concerning the application of these immunoassays to the study of human disorders, emphasizing malignancy, but also referring to other clinical conditions that have been investigated. Finally, we briefly discuss the applicability in animals in vivo of the immunoassays and of antisera developed for the assays in generating useful pathophysiological and pharmacologic information, which should be of relevance for understanding the role of PTHrP in humans.

R. Kremer: Department of Medicine, McGill University, and Royal Victoria Hospital, Montreal, Quebec, Canada H3A 1A1.

D. Goltzman: Departments of Medicine and Physiology, McGill University, and Calcium Research Laboratory, Royal Victoria Hospital, Montreal, Quebec, Canada H3A 1A1.

BIOASSAYS AND THEIR ROLE IN THE CHEMICAL IDENTIFICATION OF PARATHYROID HORMONE-RELATED PROTEIN

Identification of the hypercalcemic factor PTHrP, or parathyroid hormone (PTH)-like peptide (PLP), was achieved by careful observation and interpretation of in vivo and in vitro biological data accumulated over several decades (1–3). The search for a pathogenetic agent in malignancy-associated hypercalcemia was accompanied by recognition that other biochemical abnormalities, besides hypercalcemia, frequently occurred in these patients. These other features included hypophosphatemia, increased renal phosphate clearance, decreased fractional calcium excretion, and increased nephrogenous cyclic adenosine monophosphate (NcAMP) excretion. Overall, this constellation of biochemical alterations mimicked that seen in primary hyperparathyroidism. Despite the presence of these in vivo biological indices of increased PTH-like activity, a reduction in circulating concentrations of immunoreactive PTH was a consistent finding.

An in vitro cytochemical bioassay, initially developed for identification of PTH, was successful at measuring what we now know to be PTHrP in the plasma of patients with malignancy-associated hypercalcemia (4). This assay, based on stimulation of glucose 6-phosphate dehydrogenase activity (G6PD) in renal distal tubule cells, is exquisitely sensitive. Not only did it permit the initial measurement of PTHrP in human plasma but it also facilitated the demonstration that the PTH-like bioactivity detected in the plasma of hypercalcemic cancer patients was chromatographically and immunologically distinct from PTH (Fig. 1). This bioassay was later used to identify and to character-

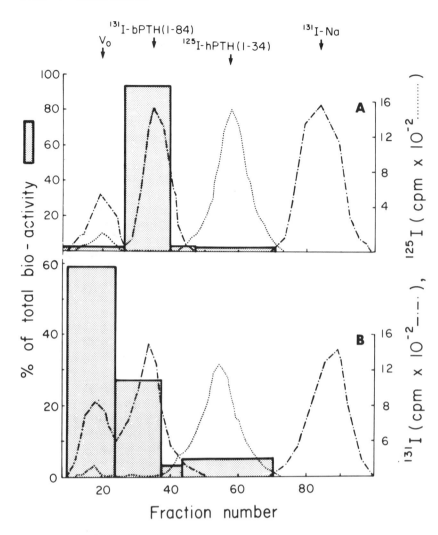

FIG. 1. Gel filtration analysis of cytochemical bioactivity in plasma from a patient with primary hyperparathyroidism (**A**) and from a patient with malignancy-associated hypercalcemia (MAH) (**B**). Vertical arrows from left to right denote, respectively, the elution position of the void volume (Vo), labeled intact PTH-(1–84), labeled active PTH-(1–34), and salt. Note that, in contrast to primary hyperparathyroidism, in MAH heterogeneous bioactive forms were observed. (Reprinted from ref. 42 with permission.)

ize PTHrP in extracts of tumors associated with hypercalcemia in vivo (5). In subsequent studies, both renal (6,7) and skeletal (8) in vitro adenylyl cyclase bioassays were shown to detect PTH-like bioactivity in extracts of tumors associated with this disorder and also in the conditioned medium of tumors grown in tissue culture. The activity in these in vitro assays could be inhibited by the synthetic PTH antagonist [Nle^{8,18},Tyr^{34}] bPTH-(3–34) NH$_2$, suggesting that the tumor-derived material was acting via PTH receptors despite the fact that it was not PTH.

In vivo PTH-like bioactivity of partially purified material extracted from human and rodent tumors, or from conditioned medium of rodent tumors, was then demonstrated (9). These extracts, when infused into parathyroidectomized rats, induced phosphaturia and increased urinary cAMP excretion and prevented the fall in serum calcium that occurred after parathyroidectomy. These in vivo bioassays therefore confirmed the PTH-like nature of the material identified by in vitro assays.

It was then possible, using the cytochemical bioassay, to identify PTH-like bioactivity in the conditioned medium of cultured *Xenopus* oocytes that had been microinjected with polyadenylated messenger RNA isolated from several different human and rodent tumors. This observation demonstrated that the bioactive material was indeed a secreted peptide (10). Ultimately, in vitro adenylyl cyclase bioassays were successfully employed to monitor the biochemical purification of tumor-derived material, and a short NH$_2$-terminal fragment of PTHrP was isolated and sequenced (6,11,12). The sequence was then employed, using molecular biological techniques, to clone cDNAs encoding PTHrP (13,14).

The deduced amino acid sequence of the initial PTHrP that was cloned from PTHrP cDNAs included a leader sequence, a "pro" sequence of ~36 amino acids, and a mature peptide of 141 residues. A high degree of homology with PTH was observed within the first 13 NH$_2$-terminal amino acids. This homology appeared to account for the PTH-like bioactivity of

PTHrP, resulting in the PTH-like biochemical abnormalities of malignancy-associated hypercalcemia. Further evidence to account for the similar bioactivities of these peptides was provided by the cloning of a common PTH/PTHrP receptor with which both ligands interact (15).

Nevertheless, differences between the manifestations of primary hyperparathyroidism and of malignancy-associated hypercalcemia are apparent. Osteoclastic bone resorption is enhanced in both disorders, but diminished bone formation, resulting in "uncoupling" of resorption and formation, is seen in malignancy-associated hypercalcemia (16–18). Additionally, in human subjects with malignancy-associated hypercalcemia plasma $1,25(OH)_2D_3$ concentrations are often decreased (3), whereas in primary hyperparathyroidism $1,25(OH)_2D_3$ concentrations are in the upper range of normal or actually elevated (19). The NH_2-terminal bioactive region of PTHrP can, however, increase 1α-hydroxylase activity when infused into human subjects (20). To account for these observations, it was recently suggested that other regions of the PTHrP molecule may modify the capacity of the NH_2-terminal region to increase 1α-hydroxylase activity and that other factors released by the tumor may inhibit 1α-hydroxylase activity (21). Finally, the severe hypercalcemia associated with the malignancy itself may inhibit 1α-hydroxylase activity.

Cloning of cDNAs encoding rat PTHrP, and subsequently other species of PTHrP, disclosed strong amino acid sequence homology with the human form of PTHrP up to approximately residue 110 (22–24). The highly conserved sequence between residues 13 and 110 may therefore be of functional importance, although the precise biological role or roles of this region is at present uncertain. A small carboxyl-terminal pentapeptide of PTHrP, PTHrP-(107–111), also called *osteostatin,* has been reported to act as a potent inhibitor of osteoclastic bone resorption in vitro (25). Whether such a small peptide acts as a systemic factor or is produced and/or metabolized locally by bone cells from a larger precursor is unknown.

In subsequent work, the gene structure of PTHrP in several species was elucidated (26–29) and revealed several important features. The gene was found to be a complex transcriptional unit spanning over 15 kilobases of DNA. The PTHrP and PTH genes share a common exonic organization, with separate axons encoding corresponding functional domains such as the leader and pro sequences. Together with other observations, this organizational format provided evidence that the PTHrP and PTH genes probably arose from a common ancestral gene. The human PTHrP gene consists of at least seven exons and is driven by several promoter sequences at the 5' end. At the 3' end, alter-

native splicing may occur resulting in three potential peptide isoforms of 139, 141, and 173 amino acids, each with a different COOH-terminal sequence. Consequently, peptide heterogeneity and messenger RNA transcript heterogeneity may result from both alternative splicing and alternative promoter utilization.

These studies therefore defined the precise chemical features of PTHrP, an essential step in the development of immunological methods of measurement. They proceeded from careful analysis of the biological issues related to malignancy-associated hypercalcemia, through the development of bioassays for in vivo and in vitro measurement of the pathogenetic entity, to the application of biochemical and molecular biological techniques for final identification of the novel mediator.

METABOLISM OF PARATHYROID HORMONE-RELATED PROTEIN

Knowledge of the precise nature of the circulating molecular forms of PTHrP is essential to the development and application of sensitive and specific radioimmunoassays. Considerable effort is therefore ongoing to define the molecular forms of PTHrP that may be produced, secreted, and metabolized.

In Vitro Studies: Parathyroid Hormone-Related Protein Synthesis Processing and Secretion

In addition to alternative splicing, which may lead to the production of three isoforms of human PTHrP, there is evidence to suggest that heterogeneous forms of PTHrP may also arise from posttranslational processing. Extracts of tumors have shown the presence of multiple PTHrP molecules of different sizes (30,31). Parathyroid tissue appears to produce a single immunoreactive PTHrP species which migrates with PTHrP 1–84 (32). The lactating mammary gland also produces PTHrP, which, (33) although not generally detected in the plasma of nursing mothers (34,35), is secreted at high levels into milk (34) from which it has subsequently been purified. NH_2-terminal forms of PTHrP in milk have been found to have molecular weights ranging from 9 to 21 kDa (36,37), which may represent different species ranging from the full-length molecule to smaller fragments.

A detailed analysis of the predicted amino acid sequences of the three major PTHrP isoforms reveals multiple potential sites of proteolysis. There are also two potential amidation consensus sites (38) as well as regions rich in serine and threonine residues, which are potential sites for o-glycosylation as has been reported in human keratinocytes (39). Recently Soifer et al. (40) studied the posttranslational processing of PTHrP in human renal carcinoma and rat insulinoma cells that were stably transfected with a human PTHrP cDNA encoding amino acids 1–141. Both cell lines produced at least three immunoreactive PTHrP species containing (1–36), (37–74), and (1–74) epitopes plus a novel midregion fragment starting at amino acid 38 with an approximate molecular weight of 7 kDa and distal cleavage sites at approximately amino acids 96–98 and 102–106. This midregion fragment was also shown to be secreted by normal human keratinocytes. The region between amino acids 38 and 106 is highly conserved among species. Over 80% of the secreted material described by Soifer et al. (40) was composed of the NH_2-terminal and mid-region fragment whereas only a small fraction contained (1–74) immunoreactivity. These results are in good agreement with experiments examining the processing of endogenous, internally labeled PTHrP in rat Leydig tumor cells in culture (41). The latter studies demonstrated the presence of three molecular forms of PTHrP comigrating with PTHrP-(1–36), PTHrP-(1–86), and PTHrP-(1–141) on high-pressure liquid chromatography (HPLC), and accounting for ~63%, ~30%, and ~7% of newly synthesized PTHrP, respectively. These studies demonstrated that the half-life of intact PTHrP-(1–141) is extremely short and suggest the presence of multiple secretory forms ranging from short NH_2-terminal fragments to the intact molecule. Whether the multiple forms described are generated in a tissue-specific fashion is not yet known. However, this extraordinarily intricate processing leading potentially to many different forms of PTHrP may confound substantially the development and interpretation of specific immunoassays. To add to this complexity, it is also likely that peripheral metabolism of PTHrP occurs, giving rise to additional forms. The issue of metabolic clearance has not yet been studied; this may also be a highly variable function of these different forms of PTHrP.

In Vivo Studies: Circulating Forms of Parathyroid Hormone-Related Protein

Initial in vivo studies in cancer patients used the cytochemical bioassay to demonstrate elevated plasma levels of PTH-like bioactivity in the absence of detectable immunoreactive PTH (4). Gel filtration analysis of bioactivity revealed a heterogenous profile, suggesting the presence of multiple bioactive fragments (42) (Fig. 1). More recently, immunoassays specific for selected epitopes of the molecule confirmed this apparent heterogeneity. Burtis et al. (43), using region-specific immunoassays, identified both NH_2- and COOH-terminal moieties in the circulation of cancer patients. Using a two-site immunoradiometric assay (IRMA),

an entity that concomitantly reacts with both PTHrP-(1–36) and PTHrP-(37–74) epitopes was detected together, along with a COOH-terminal-(109–138) fragment, which was present in equimolar concentrations. The full-length material, PTHrP-(1–141), appeared to be absent. Henderson et al. (44) reported the presence of PTHrP entities of ~6–7 kDa with a radioimmunoassay based on an NH_2-terminal antibody raised against PTHrP-(1–34). In addition, this study (44) and that of Burtis et al. (43) found species larger than the predicted full-length protein, suggesting that fragments or the intact form may aggregate in complexes with each other or with other proteins in the circulation, resulting in species of abnormally high molecular weight. Studies of gel filtration patterns of circulating PTHrP under denaturing conditions may help to resolve this issue. Finally, HPLC analysis of urine concentrates demonstrated the presence of 2–6 kDa immunoreactive PTHrP fragments using an antibody directed towards amino acids 126–144, suggesting that COOH-terminal fragments of PTHrP may be metabolized by the kidney (45).

These preliminary assessments point to the presence of heterogeneous forms of PTHrP in extracellular fluids. They will no doubt be refined as increased knowledge of the chemical nature of these forms becomes available, leading to the development of more sensitive and specific immunoassays.

PARATHYROID HORMONE-RELATED PROTEIN IMMUNOASSAYS

Radioimmunoassays

There appear to be major differences in the circulating forms of PTH and PTHrP. Considerably more is known about the secretion and metabolism of the PTH molecule, which is uniquely produced by parathyroid glands. The major glandular form is a single intact molecule, PTH-(1–84), which is also believed to be the only bioactive form in the circulation. Consequently, for PTH, efforts have centered on the development of specific immunoassays that recognize the intact molecule. Such efforts have been aided greatly by the development of two site IRMAs using two different antibodies, one of which recognizes an NH_2-terminal epitope and the other a COOH-terminal epitope. The two-site assay helps to ensure absolute specificity for the intact molecule. However, in contrast to PTH, secretion and metabolism of PTHrP are much less well understood and potentially far more complicated. First, in contrast to the human PTH gene, which encodes a single mature peptide, the human PTHrP gene has the potential to express three different isoforms. As was indicated above, each of these isoforms in turn has the potential to undergo complicated posttranslational processing and subsequently may be subject to further breakdown and metabolic clearance in sites outside the cell of synthesis. Additionally, in contrast to PTH, which is synthesized exclusively in parathyroid cells, PTHrP is produced by a wide variety of normal and malignant cells, each of which may exhibit tissue-specific expression and unique posttranslational processing. To add to this inordinately complex scheme, it is not known to what degree tumors of the same cell type express and process similar molecular forms. With these considerations in mind, and since the precise chemical natures of the heterogeneous forms of PTHrP are largely unknown, development of PTHrP immunoassays has been for the most part empirical to date. Nevertheless, since malignancy-associated hypercalcemia is characterized by the presence in the circulation of bioactive forms of PTHrP, and in view of the fact that structure–function studies of synthetic fragments indicated that such material must contain the amino-terminal region of the molecule, it seemed logical to focus initial efforts on the development of specific NH$_2$-terminal assays.

However, it must be remembered that other regions of the molecule may exhibit yet to be defined biological actions, which could contribute to the biochemical manifestations of malignancy-associated hypercalcemia or which could carry out noncalcemic-related changes and would therefore be of interest to measure. Furthermore, an unidentified subset of tumors may secrete inactive forms of the peptide, since histologically identical tumors may or may not be associated with hypercalcemia. Production of other non-NH$_2$-terminal molecular forms of PTHrP may also in theory provide useful information concerning the origin of a particular cancer or for monitoring response to treatment, i.e., as a tumor marker. Indeed, RIAs measuring midregion and inert COOH-terminal fragments of PTH have provided useful information in the past regarding the overall secretory activity of the parathyroid gland as well as the status of renal clearance mechanisms for PTH.

NH$_2$-Terminal Assays

The first NH$_2$-terminal RIA for PTHrP was that reported by Budayr et al. (46), employing a rabbit antiserum directed against PTHrP-(1–34) amide, which also served as a radioligand (Table 1). The tracer was labeled with chloramine T and purified with C$_{18}$ (octadecylsilyl silica; ODS) Sep-pak cartridges followed by reversed-phase HPLC. To eliminate nonspecific binding, this assay required large amounts of serum for extraction on an affinity column prior to measurement. Serum samples were stored at $-80°C$ until assay. The normal range was 1.4 ± 0.13 pmol/L with 68% of normal subjects having undetectable levels (<1.7 pmol/L). To define a normal range, large amounts of serum (30 ml) were immunoextracted and provided a mean level of 0.86 ± 0.17 pmol/L. More than one-half of the hypercalcemic cancer population studied by these investigators exhibited values above normal, with a mean of 6.2 pmol/L (range 2–49 pmol/L), whereas only ~10% of normocalcemic cancer patients demonstrated elevated values.

TABLE 1. *Assay characteristics and concentrations of PTHrP in normal subjects and cancer patients*

Type of assay	Sensitivity (pmol/L)	Antibody specificity	PTHrP concentrations (pmol/L)			Technical features
			Controls	↑ Ca^{++a}	→Ca^{++a}	
N-terminal RIA						
Budayr et al. (46)	1.7	PTHrP-(1–34)	0–2.5	2–49	0–7.5	Serum purified on an affinity column
Henderson et al. (44)	15	PTHrP-(1–34)	<15	15–245	15–105	Plasma directly assayed
Kao et al. (47)	2	PTHrP-(1–34)	2–5	2–85	2–3.7	Plasma purified on C$_2$ silica cartridges
Grill et al. (48)	2	PTHrP-(1–40)	<2	2.8–51.2	<2	Plasma directly assayed
Ratcliffe et al. (49)	1.5	PTHrP-(1–34)	0.35–5.7	2.7–41.3	N/A^b	Plasma purified on an affinity column
C-terminal RIA						
Burtis et al. (43)	2	PTHrP-(109–138)	<2	2.1–74	2–20	Plasma directly assayed
Midregion RIA						
Ratcliffe et al. (50)	57	PTHrP-(37–67)	270–680	150–1,570	N/A^b	Plasma directly assayed
IRMA						
Burtis et al. (43)	1	PTHrP-(1–74)	1–5.1	1.7–103	<5.1	Plasma directly assayed
Ratcliffe et al. (49)	0.23	PTHrP-(1–86)	<0.23	0.46–26.5	N/A^b	Plasma directly assayed

^{a}Cancer patients with hypercalcemia (↑ Ca^{++}) and normocalcemia (→Ca^{++}).
^{b}N/A, information not available.

Henderson et al. (44) (Fig. 2) described another NH₂-terminal RIA using a rabbit antiserum directed against human PTHrP-(1–34). [Tyr⁰] PTHrP-(1–34) was labeled by the lactoperoxidase method and employed as a tracer; PTHrP-(1–34) was used as a standard (Table 1). Plasma was collected in heparinized tubes, separated within 2 hr, and stored at $-20°C$. The sensitivity of this assay did not permit definition of the normal range, since ~95% of normal controls (37 of 39) had undetectable values. Consequently, most normal plasmas were assigned an arbitrary value based on the 95% confidence limit of <15 pmol/L (60 pg/ml). With this NH₂-terminal assay, ~40–50% of hypercalcemic cancer patients had elevated PTHrP values (ranging from 15 to 245 pmol/L), whereas only 10–30% of normocalcemic cancer patients had elevated PTHrP levels (ranging from 15 to 105 pmol/L). The levels reported with this assay were generally higher than those found by other groups and may reflect the specific moieties recognized by the different antisera.

Kao et al. (47) developed yet another NH₂-terminal RIA using a rabbit antiserum directed against human PTHrP-(1–34) amide, a [Tyr⁰]PTHrP-(1–34) tracer purified by reversed-phase HPLC, and PTHrP-(1–34) as standard (Table 1). This assay used EDTA plasma and required an extraction step with C_2 (silica) cartridges. No specific handling precautions were reported. Assay sensitivity was ~2 pmol/L, and PTHrP was measurable in 90% of normal subjects, with a mean of 3.1 $\pm$ 1 pmol/L (range 2–5 pmol/L). Again, ~50% of pa-

tients with cancer-associated hypercalcemia had elevated values with a range of 2–85 pmol/L.

An NH₂-terminal RIA developed by Grill et al. (48) used a goat antiserum against synthetic PTHrP-(1–40) and [Tyr⁰]PTHrP-(1–34) labeled with chloramine T and purified by reversed-phase HPLC as a tracer (Table 1). Recombinant PTHrP-(1–84) was employed as a standard in this assay, as opposed to PTHrP-(1–34), which was employed as a standard in the other three RIAs. Plasma was collected in chilled EDTA tubes containing protease inhibitors, separated within 60 min, and stored at $-20°C$ until assay. As in the RIA of Henderson et al. (44), no extraction step was used and >95% of normal control plasma (37/38) were undetectable (<2 pmol/L). All hypercalcemic cancer patients without bone metastases displayed elevated values (range 2.8–51.2 pmol/L), whereas none of the normocalcemic patients with squamous cell cancers had elevated PTHrP values.

Finally, an NH₂-terminal RIA developed by Ratcliffe et al. (49) employed a rabbit antiserum directed against PTHrP-(1–34) and [Tyr⁰]PTHrP-(1–34) as a tracer (Table 1). This was labeled with chloramine T and purified with C_{18} Sep-pak cartridges. Plasma was assayed either directly or after extraction with an affinity column containing monoclonal antibodies specific for amino acids 17–27 of PTHrP. Normal control values ranged from 13 to 760 pmol/L (mean 140 pmol/L) before extraction and only 0.35–5.7 pmol/L (mean 2.9 pmol/L) after extraction, suggesting the

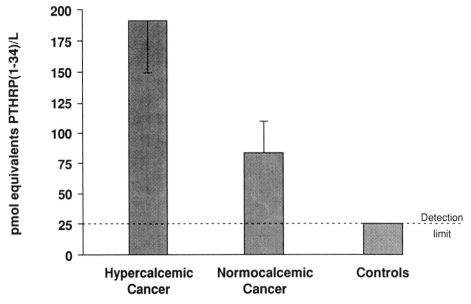

FIG. 2. Concentrations of immunoreactive PTHrP in cancer patients as determined by an NH₂-terminal (PTHrP 1–34) RIA. The dashed line represents the detection limit of the assay. Note that controls are reading below the detection limit and assigned an arbitrary value of <25 pmol/L. Approximately 60% of patients with cancer and hypercalcemia and 25% of patients with cancer and normocalcemia had values above 25 pmol/L. (Redrawn from ref. 44 with permission.)

presence of large amounts of cross-reacting material before plasma extraction. In nonextracted plasma, no significant differences in PTHrP values between control and hypercalcemic cancer patients were observed, but the latter group had clearly elevated concentrations after plasma extraction (mean 10.7 pmol/L, range 2.7–41.3 pmol/L). Nevertheless, the crossover between the two groups was inordinately high (~50%), suggesting that the specificity of the antibody was less than optimal.

All NH$_2$-terminal RIAs reported to date, therefore, measured elevated circulating PTHrP concentrations in a sizeable proportion of patients with cancer and hypercalcemia. Several studies have also reported elevated NH$_2$-terminal PTHrP concentrations in some normocalcemic cancer patients. However, the frequency of detection of PTHrP in normal individuals varied from assay to assay. NH$_2$-terminal bioactive forms of PTHrP therefore do indeed circulate in malignancy-associated hypercalcemia as was predicted by the earlier bioassays. Discrepancies among RIAs in the detection of NH$_2$-terminal PTHrP moieties in normocalcemic subjects may reflect differences in antibody sensitivity and/or epitope specificity. Whether these antibodies recognize only bioactive or also inert NH$_2$-terminal forms of PTHrP remains to be determined. Until the specific circulating entities with which the various antisera react are precisely identified, and until the standards used in the different RIAs correspond to the specific entities that are detected, it may be more accurate to refer to concentrations measured in terms of pM-equivalents/liter rather than in pmol/L.

COOH-Terminal Assays

Burtis et al. (43) reported a COOH-terminal RIA for PTHrP using a rabbit antiserum raised against [Tyr^{109}]PTHrP-(109–138), which was also used as a radioligand after labeling with the "Enzymobead" method (Table 1). Normal human plasma with no detectable PTHrP was supplemented with PTHrP 109–138 and used as a standard. Plasma was collected in heparinized tubes containing protease inhibitors and was stored at −70°C. Over 95% of normal controls (58/59) were undetectable in this assay (< 2p pmol/L), and all patients (30/30) with "classical" humoral hypercalcemia of malignancy (HHM) had detectable levels ranging from 2.1 to 74 pmol/L, with a mean value 23.9 ± 16.0 pmol/L. In addition, six of 23 normocalcemic cancer patients displayed increased concentrations of PTHrP. Patients with primary hyperparathyroidism did not differ significantly from controls, but patients with chronic renal failure and secondary hyperparathyroidism displayed markedly elevated concentrations in the range of those detected in hypercalcemic cancer patients (mean 79.6 ± 14.1 pmol/L).

To determine whether immunoreactivity was a function of "intact" circulating PTHrP or reflected the presence of COOH-terminal fragments, plasma from a number of hypercalcemic cancer patients was extracted using an anti-PTHrP-(1–36) affinity column. PTHrP 109–138 levels were virtually identical in the original plasma and in the column flow through, suggesting that COOH-terminal forms of PTHrP circulate in malignancy-associated hypercalcemia. Whether this material is produced in the parathyroid gland or at other sites in chronic renal failure will require further study.

Midregion Assay

Ratcliffe et al. (49) have developed an RIA using a rabbit antiserum directed against PTHrP-(37–67) (Table 1). This RIA had a detection limit of 57 pmol/L and gave detectable values for all control subjects, with a mean of 370 pmol/L. Patients with malignancy-associated hypercalcemia had significantly higher mean values (440 pmol/L), but there was a strong overlap between controls and hypercalcemic cancer patients, with only 30% of the latter showing concentrations above normal.

The capacity of these RIAs to detect NH$_2$-terminal, midregion, and COOH-terminal fragments of PTHrP in plasma therefore appears to confirm the presence of heterogeneous circulating PTHrP forms. Whether new generations of such assays will be useful for diagnosing malignancy-associated hypercalcemia or have a distinct role in identifying bioinert forms of PTHrP as tumor markers remains to be determined.

Immunoradiometric Assays

Two-site, noncompetitive IRMAs or "sandwich" immunoassays have also been developed for PTHrP. This method is based on the use of two antibodies recognizing different epitopes of the antigen (Fig. 3). The "capture" antibody, usually linked to a solid-phase matrix, is first allowed to react with the antigen. Addition of the second or "signal" antibody, which is radiolabeled, produces a "sandwich" complex. Both capture and signal antibodies must be present in excess concentration to ensure complete extraction of the antigen. In theory this technique allows specific assay of a particular molecular form of an analyte, since recognition of two specific sites is a prerequisite to measurement. Another practical advantage of IRMA methodology is improved sensitivity. Such assays have been developed to measure intact PTH-(1–84), providing great improvement in the specificity and

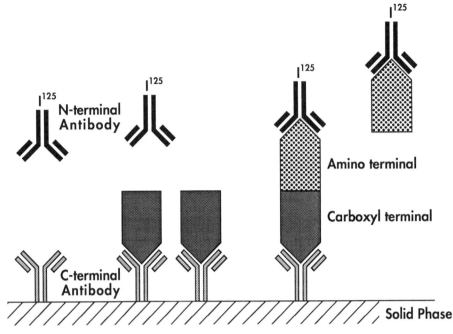

FIG. 3. Principle of the two-site immunoradiometric assay. The antigen reacts with a C-terminal antibody immobilized on a solid phase (capture antibody). Subsequently, an antibody labeled with ^{125}I and directed against the NH$_2$-terminal region of the peptide (signal antibody) is added and produces a "sandwich" complex. Both capture and signal antibodies are added in excess to ensure complete extraction of the antigen. Note that only circulating peptides reacting with both NH$_2$- and COOH-terminal antibodies can be measured. Excess labeled antibody, which is free or complexed to the NH$_2$-terminal fragments of the peptide, is removed during the washing procedure. In contrast to traditional RIAs, there is a direct linear relationship between the amount of antigen and the radioactive signal. Note that the capture and signal antibodies could be either COOH or NH$_2$ terminal.

clinical utility of PTH measurements. By eliminating the so-called serum blank effect, PTH IRMAs are exquisitely sensitive in differentiating normal from subnormal and elevated PTH concentrations. They are also clinically useful in malignancy-associated hypercalcemia inasmuch as they demonstrate suppressed intact PTH concentrations in this condition, a feature clearly important in the differential diagnosis of primary hyperparathyroidism and the hypercalcemia of cancer. Because very little is known about the metabolic fate of PTHrP, the development of specific IRMAs for that peptide can be based only on empirical assumptions.

Burtis et al. (43) developed an IRMA using PTHrP-(1–74) as an immunogen in rabbits to produce a polyclonal antiserum, which was then purified on affinity columns to enrich for antibodies recognizing either PTHrP-(1–74) or PTHrP-(1–36) (Table 1). The latter was radiolabeled and used as a signal antibody, whereas the former was used as a capture antibody. Improvement in assay sensitivity was moderate, but significant, compared to several previously described NH$_2$-terminal assays (detection limit ~1 pmol/L). Plasma was collected and stored as described for the COOH-terminal assay these investigators developed.

With this assay, ~50% of normal subjects had undetectable concentrations (<1 pmol/L). The normal range was 1.9 ± 1.6 pmol/L (range 1–5.1 pmol/L). Patients classified as having the "classical" syndrome of HHM, using the criterion of elevated nephrogenous cyclic AMP, had values ranging from 1.7 to 103 pmol/L, with a mean of 20.9 ± 21.8 pmol/L. However, a relatively large crossover existed between this group and the control group. Moreover, in contrast to results from several studies using NH$_2$-terminal assays, normocalcemic cancer patients did not differ significantly from normal controls.

More recently, Ratcliffe et al. (49,50) described an IRMA using a monoclonal capture antibody raised against PTHrP-(1–34) and a polyclonal rabbit antiserum raised against PTHrP-(37–67) as the signal "antibody" (Table 1). This assay is more sensitive than any of the previously described assays (detection limit 0.23 pmol/L). All control subjects were undetectable, indicating that circulating concentrations of the molecular species measured were much lower than the species measured with any previously reported immunoassay. Patients with malignancy-associated hypercalcemia, with or without bone metastases, all had detectable values, with a mean of 6.1 pmol/L (range

0.46–26.5 pmol/L). Immunoradiometric assays therefore have the potential of enhancing the specificity and sensitivity of PTHrP measurements and may be applied with greater success once the precise chemical natures of circulating PTHrP forms are elucidated.

APPLICATIONS OF THE PARATHYROID HORMONE-RELATED PROTEIN RADIOIMMUNOASSAY TO STUDIES IN VITRO

In contrast to PTH, PTHrP is expressed in a wide variety of normal and tumorous tissues. Using Northern blot hybridization and in situ hybridization techniques, mRNA encoding PTHrP has been identified in normal human keratinocytes (51–53), normal islet cells (54), lactating mammary glands (33,55), rat (56) and human (57) mammary epithelial cells, brain, fetal liver (51), fetal parathyroid (58), aortic smooth muscle (59), uterine smooth muscle (60), and normal human amnion (61). PTHrP is also expressed in a wide variety of tumor tissues (32,51,62,63) and in epithelial tumor cell lines (64), including squamous cell cancers, renal carcinoma (58,65), skin cancers (66), breast cancers (67), and parathyroid adenomas (63) as well as in human T-cell lymphotropic virus type 1 (HTLV1)-transformed lymphocytes (68), human osteosarcoma cells (69), and neuroendocrine tumor cells (see the chapter by Broadus and Stewart) (30). This wide tissue distribution is compatible with an autocrine/paracrine role for the peptide, a function likely to predominate over its endocrine role in normal tissues. Such a role has been suggested by recent experiments in human keratinocytes in which PTHrP acted as a potent antiproliferative (70,71) and prodifferentiating (72) factor. In normal postnatal animals, it appears to play no role as an endocrine factor in mediating calcium homeostasis (73), although it may subserve such a function during fetal life. In adults it appears that only during an extraordinary situation, such as cancer development and progression, does PTHrP play an endocrine role leading to hypercalcemia.

The development of RIAs for PTHrP greatly facilitated the study of its regulation in both normal and cancer cells in culture. The control of PTHrP released into conditioned medium by normal and neoplastic cell lines was initially monitored using bioassays. More recently, RIAs have been used in conjunction with the traditional bioassay systems to monitor the PTHrP response to various stimuli (52,53,56,57,74,75). Positive regulation of PTHrP expression and secretion by mitogenic stimuli such as epidermal growth factor (EGF) and fetal bovine serum (FBS) (52,53), along with inhibition by $1,25(OH)_2D_3$, has been demonstrated in normal human keratinocytes using these methods (Fig. 4). Furthermore, as opposed to the inhibitory in-

fluence of calcium on PTH secretion by parathyroid glands, PTHrP secretion by keratinocytes is enhanced by extracellular calcium. In contrast to the transcriptional effects of EGF and $1,25(OH)_2D_3$, no effects of calcium have been demonstrated at the level of PTHrP gene expression (53). Calcium also stimulates PTHrP production in transformed human keratinocytes (64), in rat Leydig tumor cells (76), and in a lung carcinoma cell line (77), but it inhibited PTHrP expression and secretion in a rat parathyroid cell line (78). With PTHrP RIAs, a variety of cell lines have been shown to increase PTHrP secretion in vitro in response to a number of factors, including phorbol esters (30,69), cAMP (79), calcitonin (80,81), the product of the Tax gene (82), and transforming growth factor-β (TGFβ) (83). In the same context, dexamethasone and testosterone (75) have been shown to reduce PTHrP secretion.

It should be emphasized that peptide growth factors are generally positive regulators of PTHrP production. This is exemplified in normal human keratinocytes, where EGF is essential for growth and is a potent positive stimulus for PTHrP production. In normal human mammary epithelial cells insulin-like growth factor-1 (IGF1), rather than EGF, is an absolute requirement for cell growth and is also more potent than EGF in stimulating PTHrP production (57).

The mechanism whereby PTHrP is produced in excess by tumor cells is not well understood at the present time but may be a function of abnormal gene regulation. This phenomenon has recently been studied in a model of tumor progression (64), in which PTHrP gene regulation and secretion were analyzed in the transition from the normal to the malignant phenotype. Normal human keratinocytes were established as a keratinocyte cell line following infection with human papilloma virus type 16 (HPK1A). This cell line was subsequently converted to the malignant phenotype (HPK1Aras) using an activated ras oncogene (84,85). In contrast to the established cells (HPK1A), which continued to produce PTHrP in a regulated manner, HPK1Aras cells expressed and secreted PTHrP in an autonomous fashion, i.e., in the absence of exogenous mitogenic factors such as EGF, and displayed resistance to the inhibitory effect of $1,25(OH)_2D_3$ (Fig. 4). Whether the unrestrained production of PTHrP demonstrated in vitro by cultured tumor cells is operative in vivo and results in the elevated circulating concentration noted in patients with squamous carcinoma remains to be elucidated.

The use of PTHrP RIAs for in vitro studies has therefore greatly facilitated examination of the regulation of PTHrP production by both normal and malignant cells in culture. Studies of this nature have the potential of disclosing potentially important control mechanisms in the regulation of PTHrP production in

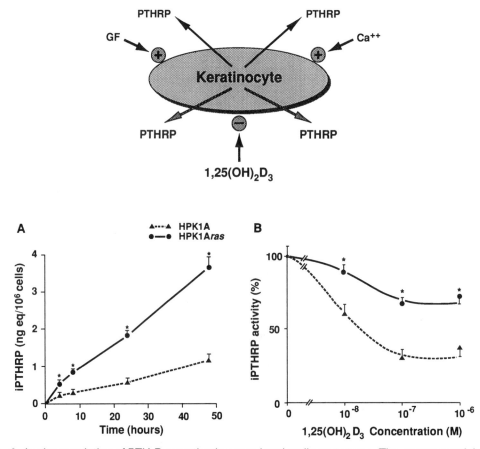

FIG. 4. *In vitro* regulation of PTHrP secretion in normal and malignant states. The *upper panel* depicts regulatory factors that operate in normal human keratinocytes. Growth factors (GF) and calcium (Ca^{++}) upregulate PTHrP secretion, whereas $1,25(OH)_2D_3$ inhibits this response. The *lower panels* compare the regulation of PTHrP in immortalized keratinocytes (HPKIA) vs. malignant keratinocytes (HPKIAras). **A:** Time course of PTHrP secretion in the absence of exogenous mitogenic growth factors, demonstrating that HPKIAras cells secrete far more PTHrP than HPKIA cells. **B:** Effects of $1,25(OH)_2D_3$ on EGF-stimulated PTHrP secretion in HPKIA and HPKIAras cells, showing that $1,25(OH)_2D_3$ is much more effective in inhibiting PTHrP secretion in HPKIA than in HPKIAras cultures. Significant difference from HPKIA (*$P < 0.01$). (Redrawn from ref. 64 with permission.)

vitro as well as critical mechanisms that might also operate in vivo.

APPLICATIONS OF THE PARATHYROID HORMONE-RELATED PROTEIN RADIOIMMUNOASSAY TO STUDIES IN VIVO

Human Studies

With the development of immunological techniques for measuring PTHrP, the possibility arose of applying those assays in vivo to obtain information regarding the biology of this peptide and its role in health and disease. In terms of the efficacy of available assays in diagnosing malignancy-associated hypercalcemia, initial reports suggested that NH_2-terminal RIAs lacked the sensitivity-required to measure low levels of PTHrP, and a large proportion of hypercalcemic cancer pa-

tients may have therefore escaped detection with such assays. Later studies using IRMAs demonstrated elevated levels of PTHrP in a far greater proportion of hypercalcemic cancer patients. Such improvement of diagnostic sensitivity (increased number of true positives) may reflect only arbitrary "cutoff" values imposed by the laboratory at the expense of a lower diagnostic specificity (increased number of false positives) as the value to discriminate between normal and abnormal results is reduced. On the other hand, a less sensitive assay (e.g., an NH_2-terminal RIA) has by necessity a higher "cutoff" value, which may translate into higher diagnostic specificity (less false positives) but potentially lower diagnostic sensitivity (a greater number of patients "escape" detection). This notion of trade off between diagnostic sensitivity and specificity has important implications for patient management. While the arbitrary cutoff, or upper limit of normal, may affect the number of patients correctly diagnosed, the issue becomes somewhat less critical if the same assay is used to monitor the effectiveness of therapeutic measures. In this case the patient may be used as his or her own control. Thus, in terms of the efficacy of available assays in monitoring malignancy-associated hypercalcemia, mounting evidence suggests that circulating concentrations do fall significantly after tumor ablation (surgical or chemical) (Fig. 5). Whether they are reduced into the "normal" range depends on the upper limit of normal assigned to the assay. It remains undetermined at present whether PTHrP is a good index of tumor recurrence, which would make it potentially useful as a tumor marker. This issue again rests with determination of the detection limit of the assay and the value ascribed to the upper limit of normal as well as with the assay specificity.

Circulating PTHrP Levels in Cancer Patients

Classification of Cancer Patients for Study

One criterion commonly used to define subgroups of patients with malignancy-associated hypercalcemia

has been the presence or absence of bone metastases (3). One group whose underlying mechanism was presumably local osteolytic hypercalcemia (LOH) comprised mainly patients harboring hematological malignancies or breast cancer. A second group, whose underlying mechanism of hypercalcemia was believed to be secretion by the tumor of a humoral factor with hypercalcemic activity (HHM), comprised mainly patients with epithelial and renal cancers (2,3,16,86–88). Although this distinction was initially useful in the conceptual approach, which ultimately resulted in the purification and identification of PTHrP, it is less useful in the pathogenetic and clinical senses. The occurrence of bone metastases (i.e., "LOH") does not exclude the presence of a systemic hypercalcemic factor, such as PTHrP, which may function locally. Furthermore, it seems likely that all malignancy-associated hypercalcemia, whether associated with a systematic circulating factor or not, is humoral in origin and could be called HHM. Additionally, several studies have reported a poor correlation between the presence or extent of bone metastases and the occurrence of hypercalcemia (89). The term LOH may also be inaccurate since it is uncertain whether hypercalcemia is ever due solely to osteolysis in the absence of altered renal

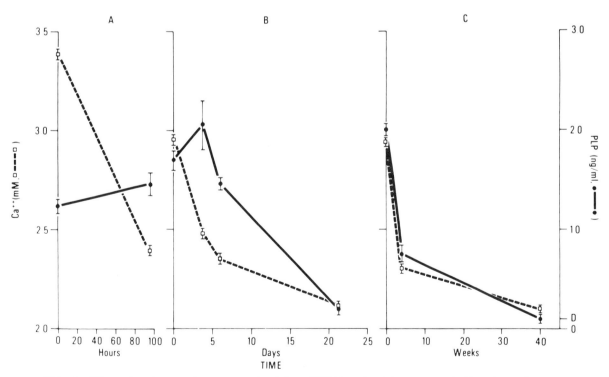

FIG. 5. Effect of antitumor therapy on circulating PTHrP and calcium concentrations in malignancy. **A:** Time course of PTHrP (PLP) and calcium concentrations after treatment of hypercalcemia in a patient with squamous carcinoma using saline, furosemide, and plicamycin (mithramycin). **B, C:** Time courses of PTHrP (PLP) and calcium concentrations in two hypercalcemic patients with breast cancer treated with chemotherapy which reduced tumor mass. All patients displayed a substantial lowering of serum calcium, but only the patients who sustained a reduction in tumor burden (**B, C**) had a concomitant decrease in plasma PTHrP. (Reprinted from ref. 74 with permission.)

handling of calcium. A more relevant pathogenetic consideration of malignancy-associated hypercalcemia, therefore, may be the presence or absence of elevated nephrogenous cAMP, as a reflection of the production and action of PTHrP by these tumors. In this respect it has been estimated that ~80% of unselected patients with malignancy-associated hypercalcemia (3) have such an abnormality.

The application of RIAs for PTHrP has resulted in the necessity to transfer breast cancer patients, whether or not they have skeletal metastases, out of the LOH classification. Indeed, the "humoral" nature of the hypercalcemia due to breast cancer had previously been predicted on the basis of studies of urinary phosphate and cAMP excretion (90,91). Additionally, hematological malignancies may not readily fall under an LOH classification. Thus certain types of lymphomas have been shown to produce both PTHrP (68) and $1,25(OH)_2D_3$ (19,92), adding to the complexity of potential underlying mechanisms of hypercalcemia in this condition. However, as the sensitivity and specificity of PTHrP immunoassays improve, it will be possible to classify malignancy-associated hypercalcemia patients more quickly and more accurately as PTHrP related or PTHrP unrelated, based on measurement of the causative agent per se. As improved methods of treating PTHrP overproduction are developed, such improved diagnostic accuracy should have therapeutic as well as pathogenetic importance.

Elevated PTHrP levels have been demonstrated in a number of normocalcemic cancer patients (44,46,47), an observation important from both a theoretical and a practical standpoint (Table 2). It is possible that, during the progression of malignancy, PTHrP secretion would increase to a point at which a critical threshold is attained, above which hypercalcemia ensues. A number of factors could underlie the progressive increased secretion, including an increase in cellular mass, an augmentation in locally produced growth factors that could stimulate PTHrP production, or deregulation of PTHrP gene expression. In theory, therefore, PTHrP might be secreted long before hypercalcemia occurs. Specific and sensitive PTHrP assays could then be used to detect the presence of tumors at an early stage and conceivably to predict those with the potential for developing hypercalcemic complications. Alternatively, the finding of elevated PTHrP concentrations in the absence of hypercalcemia might be due to the production of biologically inert fragments by tumors. Detection of such fragments might still be of clinical interest and utility, in that the fragments may serve as tumor markers to follow disease progression. It is also possible that other factors, in concert with PTHrP, are important in the overt expression of hypercalcemia in malignancy (see the chapter by Black and Mundy).

TABLE 2. *PTHrP levels in different histological types of malignancies*

| | Occurrence of elevated PTHrP in cancer patients (%) | | | |
| | Hypercalcemic subjects | | | Normocalcemic subjects |
Tumor type	BM (− & +)	BM (+)	BM (−)	
Solid tumors				
Mixed				
Budayr et al. (46)	51	N/A^c	85	10
Henderson et al. (44)	53	N/A	N/A	18
Kao et al. (47)	48	33	53	0
Grill et al. (48)	60	65^d	100	0
Burtis et al. (43)	85	0	N/A	9
Ratcliffe et al. (49)	100	N/A	N/A	N/A
Squamous cancers				
Budayr et al. (46)	85	N/A	N/A	N/A
Henderson et al. (44)	50	N/A	N/A	10
Kao et al. (47)	N/A^b	N/A	66	N/A
Grill et al. (48)	100	N/A	100	N/A
Renal cell cancer				
Budayr et al. (46)	60	N/A	N/A	N/A
Henderson et al. (44)	100	N/A	N/A	N/A
Kao et al. (47)	N/A^b	N/A	25	N/A
Breast cancer				
Budayr et al. (46)	50	N/A	N/A	N/A
Henderson et al. (44)	60	N/A	N/A	29
Kao et al. (47)	N/A^b	16	100	N/A
Hematological tumors				
Mixed				
Henderson et al. (44)	33	N/A^b	N/A^b	8
Lymphoma				
Budayr et al. (46)	0	N/A	N/A	N/A
Kao et al. (47)	80	N/A	N/A	N/A
Multiple myeloma				
Budayr et al. (46)	33	N/A	N/A	N/A
Kao et al. (47)	16	N/A	N/A	N/A

[a]Hypercalcemia of malignancy with ↑ NcAMP.
[b]Patients with (+) or without (−) bone metastases (BM).
[c]N/A, information not available.
[d]Solid tumors other than breast.

Relationship of Skeletal Metastases to Parathyroid Hormone-Related Protein Concentrations in Patients With Solid Tumors and Hypercalcemia

Employing NH_2-terminal RIAs, most assays of PTHrP in patients with malignancy-associated hypercalcemia revealed no more than a modest increase in the percentage of patients with elevated values when patients with bone metastases were excluded from the series studies (Table 2). Thus, in the study of Budayr et al. (46), 51% of patients with malignancy-associated hypercalcemia had elevated PTHrP values regardless of the presence of bone metastases. The number rose to ~85% when patients with bone metastases were excluded. In the study of Henderson et al. (44), 50% of unselected patients with malignancy-associated hypercalcemia, harboring a wide variety of histologic tumor types, had elevated PTHrP values. Grouping patients according to the presence or absence of bone metastases did not significantly alter those results. In the study of Kao *et al.* (47), ~48% of unselected patients with malignancy-associated hypercalcemia had elevated PTHrP values, a percentage that increased to ~53% when patients with bone metastases were excluded. Finally, in the study of Grill et al. (48), 100% of a group of patients with various solid tumors, excluding breast cancers, having no evidence of bone metastases, had elevated values of PTHrP (rangingfrom 2.8 to 51.2 pmol/L). In a second group, which included patients with solid tumors of the same type but having radiologic evidence of metastases, ~60% had elevated PTHrP levels, ranging from 4.9 to 47.5 pmol/L. In this study, all patients with squamous cancer, with or without bone metastases, had elevated PTHrP levels, whereas ~60% of hypercalcemic patients with breast cancer, almost all of whom had bone metastases (19/20), had elevated PTHrP values (ranging from 3.9 to 61.6 pmol/L).

Results are somewhat more conflicting when the two-site IRMA assays are considered. Burtis et al. (43), using a two-site assay specific for PTHrP-(1–74), found that 85% of 30 hypercalcemic cancer patients classified as HHM on the basis of elevated nephrogenous cyclic AMP had elevated PTHrP values (mean level 20.9 ± 21.8 pmol/L). In contrast, a group of patients, four with breast cancer, three with multiple myeloma, and one with undefined lung cancer, were classified as LOH on the basis of normal nephrogenous cAMP and extensive bone involvement and had normal PTHrP levels. On the other hand, Ratcliffe et al. (49), using a two-site assay specific for PTHrP-(1–86), found that, in an unselected group of patients with malignancy-associated hypercalcemia of various histological types and with advanced metastatic disease, all individuals had elevated PTHrP levels.

Consequently, it appears that many tumors produce PTHrP, which may contribute to hypercalcemia regardless of the presence or absence of skeletal metastases (Table 2). Whether different NH_2-terminal species of PTHrP are produced by tumors that differ histologically or in metastatic behavior is currently unknown.

Parathyroid Hormone-Related Protein Concentrations in Hematologic Malignancies Associated With Hypercalcemia

Hematological malignancies frequently associated with hypercalcemia include lymphoma, chronic myeloid and lymphoblastic leukemias, multiple myeloma, and adult T-cell leukemia. In multiple myeloma, a disorder characterized by extensive bone destruction, >30% of patients develop hypercalcemia (93). The mechanism postulated to explain the hypercalcemia associated with this disorder is production by the plasma cells of a group of cytokines collectively termed *osteoclast-activating factor* (OAF). These include interleukin-1 (IL1) and tumor necrosis factors-α and -β (TNFα and TNFβ), which are potent stimulators of osteoclastic bone resorption (see the chapter by Black and Mundy). Hypercalcemia is less common in lymphomas (both Hodgkin's and non-Hodgkin's). Circulating $1,25(OH)_2D_3$ is elevated in a number of lymphoma patients who are hypercalcemic without skeletal metastases and may play a pathogenetic role (19,94). In contrast, patients with adult T-cell leukemia/lymphoma show a high incidence of hypercalcemia. This disorder is caused by infection of T cells with human T cell lymphotropic virus type I (HTLV1). In addition to hypercalcemia, other associated biochemical abnormalities strongly indicate the presence of a circulating factor with PTH-like bioactivity (95). The demonstration of elevated PTHrP expression by T lymphocytes in culture after infection with HTLV1 supports this hypothesis (68).

Although no systematic evaluations of hematologic malignancies have been reported to date, patients with such disorders have been included in several studies (Table 2). Henderson et al. (44) reported that 33% of patients with hematological malignances had elevated PTHrP values, whereas Kao et al. (47) found four of five patients with lymphoma and one of six patients with multiple myeloma to have increased PTHrP concentrations. Burtis et al. (43) showed that two patients with lymphomas and elevated nephrogenous cAMP had increased PTHrP levels, while one patient with multiple myeloma and normal nephrogenous cAMP had a normal PTHrP value. The prevalence of elevated PTHrP levels in patients with unselected hematologic malignancies was not reported in that study. Finally, using a midregion assay recognizing PTHrP 50–69, another group has reported elevated concentrations of PTHrP in two patients with hypercalcemia and non-Hodgkin's lymphoma without bone metastases (96). It appears, therefore, that, despite frequent and extensive osseous metastases, many hematologic malignancies are associated with overproduction of PTHrP, suggesting a multifactorial basis for the hypercalcemia associated with these diseases.

Response to Treatment in Hypercalcemic Cancer Patients With Elevated Parathyroid Hormone-Related Protein Concentrations

Henderson et al. (44) reported that a reduction in the serum calcium concentration in a patient with malignancy-associated hypercalcemia did not significantly affect plasma immunoreactive PTHrP concentrations. However, reduction of tumor mass by chemotherapy in two other patients with malignancy-associated hypercalcemia did decrease circulating PTHrP levels (Fig. 5). Two recent studies examined the effect of the bisphosphonate pamidronate (Aredia), an inhibitor of bone resorption, in the treatment of cancer patients with hypercalcemia. The first study (96) demonstrated a significant decrease in PTHrP concentrations and hypercalcemia following treatment with pamidronate. Patients with hypercalcemia in the absence of bone metastases generally had higher initial concentrations of PTHrP and were relatively more resistant to pamidronate therapy. In a subsequent study by Grill et al. (97), 20 patients with solid tumors, hypercalcemia, and elevated PTHrP concentrations were examined. All patients treated with pamidronate responded with a decrease in ionized calcium. However, only 60% of those patients achieved normocalcemia, and no mention is made of whether the patients who did not achieve normocalcemia had higher initial PTHrP levels. This latter study, in contrast to the former report, demonstrated that PTHrP levels did not change significantly after treatment with pamidronate, despite a reduction in plasma calcium levels, suggesting that PTHrP production by tumors is not regulated by calcium in vivo.

Parathyroid Hormone-Related Protein During Pregnancy and Lactation

PTHrP has been detected in human placental tissue (33) and rat trophoblastic cells (98), raising the possibility that PTHrP plays a physiological role during pregnancy. It has been suggested that PTHrP may promote maternal calcium transfer across the placenta to maintain in the developing embryo hypercalcemia relative to the mother. Allgrove et al. (99) had previously demonstrated PTH-like bioactivity without PTH immunoreactivity in human umbilical cord blood, and it was subsequently shown that immunoassayable PTHrP is increased in cord blood (100). These findings may explain the apparent absence of skeletal defects in Di George syndrome, a disorder characterized by congenital absence of parathyroid glands. It is plausible that production of PTHrP by the placenta helps to maintain fetal calcium homeostasis in this disorder.

Expression of PTHrP mRNA has also been demonstrated in lactating mammary tissue (33), and PTH mRNA levels increase in response to suckling and to infusion of prolactin in nonlactating breast tissue (101). PTHrP was subsequently found to be extremely abundant in breast milk (34,36,37,55,102,103), where biochemical characterization revealed heterogeneity (36,37). It has been suggested, therefore, that PTHrP may play a role in the maturation of the newborn (or infant) digestive tract. However, no direct evidence in support of this thesis has yet been provided. The observation that PTHrP levels in bovine milk correlate with milk calcium concentration also suggests a local role for PTHrP in the transport of calcium across mammary epithelia (102). Increased circulating PTHrP concentrations have been documented in a lactating woman with massive breast hypertrophy and hypercalcemia, with normalization of the biochemical abnormalities following mastectomy (104). However, in general, circulating PTHrP concentrations in lactating women are essentially within the normal range (34,35), suggesting that PTHrP is not released into the maternal circulation under ordinary circumstances and therefore plays no endocrine role in maintaining normal blood calcium concentrations during lactation.

Parathyroid Hormone-Related Protein and Hyperparathyroidism

Parathyroid hormone-related peptide mRNA is easily detectable in parathyroid tissue of patients with primary adenomas or with hyperplasia secondary to renal failure (63,66). Immunohistochemical localization of PTHrP in human fetal parathyroids has also been demonstrated (105). Although several attempts have been made to measure PTHrP in the circulation of patients with primary hyperparathyroidism, only one report to date has revealed elevated PTHrP concentrations in a small number of these patients (44). On the other hand, two reports have demonstrated elevated levels of PTHrP in hyperparathyroidism secondary to chronic renal failure (43,44).

Idiopathic Infantile Hypercalcemia

Elevation of PTHrP in children with idiopathic infantile hypercalcemia (IHH) has been reported recently (106) from results of an NH₂-terminal RIA. However, William's syndrome which is phenotypically similar to IHH except for the presence of heart abnormalities was not characterized by elevated PTHrP levels.

Animal Studies

Several animal models of malignancy-associated hypercalcemia have been developed over the years in an effort to define the pathogenesis of the human syndrome. These models include both spontaneous and induced tumors in rodents and dogs as well as human tumors transplanted into athymic mice. Perhaps the most widely used, and therefore best defined, model is the Fischer rat bearing the Rice H500 Leydig cell tumor. This tumor, from which the rat PTHrP cDNA was cloned (23), occurs spontaneously in aged Fischer rats but can be successfully passaged by subcutaneous transplantation in younger animals. The nonmetastatic tumor grows rapidly in association with hypercalcemia, hypophosphatemia, increased urinary cAMP, renal phosphate wasting, and suppressed immunoreactive PTH (107–110). This constellation of biochemical abnormalities therefore closely mimics the syndrome of human malignancy-associated hypercalcemia. The Walker 256 carcinosarcoma, originating from a rat mammary gland, although less well characterized, has been shown to secrete PTH-like bioactivity, in the absence of PTH immunoreactivity, into conditioned medium when maintained in culture (111–113). Cutaneous squamous cell carcinoma induced by dimethylbenzanthracene treatment and adenocarcinoma of the anal sac in dogs (114,115) are also associated with hypercalcemia in vivo and appear to produce a factor with PTH-like bioactivity in vitro. Tumors of human and animal origin that have been transplanted into athymic mice include two human squamous carcinomas (116), a number of human renal carcinomas (117,118), and a canine adenocarcinoma (111). Although all these models demonstrated to some degree the biochemical abnormalities associated with malignancy-associated hypercalcemia, direct measurement of circulating PTHrP has been accomplished only in the Leydig cell tumor model (53,119).

Once antisera directed against the human (h)PTHrP molecule had been developed for use in PTHrP RIAs, they were also applied to passive immunization studies in rodents. Using athymic mice bearing human squamous carcinomas, Krukeja et al. (116) infused an antiserum directed against NH₂-terminal hPTHrP, which quickly reversed the hypercalcemia and the elevation of nephrogenous cAMP. Similar results were obtained by Henderson et al. (73) using the rat Leydig cell model, strongly implicating PTHrP as the humoral fac-

tor responsible for hypercalcemia in these models and providing evidence for a pathogenetic role for PTHrP in the syndrome of hypercalcemia associated with malignancy (Fig. 6).

Animal models have also been useful for examining the therapeutic efficacy of various agents in malignancy-associated hypercalcemia. In our laboratory we have recently taken advantage of our previous in vitro studies demonstrating the inhibitory effect of 1,25(OH)₂D₃ and vitamin D analogs on PTHrP gene expression and secretion (120,121) to study their potential usefulness in reducing serum calcium levels in vivo. A 1,25(OH)₂D₃ analog was found to have very low calcemic potency relative to 1,25(OH)₂D₃ when infused into control rats (53,122). In addition, when analyzed in vitro, this analog was ten to 100 times more potent than 1,25(OH)₂D₃ in inhibiting PTHrP produc-

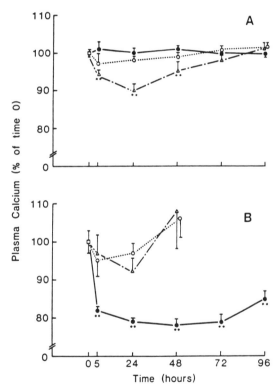

FIG. 6. Effect of passive immunization with PTHrP and PTH antisera on plasma calcium of normal rats and rats with hypercalcemia of malignancy. In normal rats (**A**) a moderate and transient decrease in plasma calcium was observed after injection of PTH antiserum (△) but not after injection of PTHrP antiserum (●) or normal preimmune rabbit serum (NRS) (○). In contrast, hypercalcemic rats implanted with the Leydig cell tumor H-500 (**B**) sustained a prolonged reduction in plasma calcium after injection of PTHrP antiserum (●) but not of PTH antiserum (△) or NRS (○). Consequently, PTH but not PTHrP appears to be the major modulator of plasma calcium homeostasis in the normal animals, whereas PTHrP is the major pathogenetic mediator in the hypercalcemia of malignancy. (Reprinted from ref. 73 with permission.)

tion in cancer cells (120) and was therefore chosen as a candidate for in vivo studies with hypercalcemic, tumor-bearing rats. After continuous infusion into Fischer rats bearing the Leydig cell tumor H500, a significant reduction in circulating PTHrP concentrations was demonstrated using an NH_2-terminal PTHrP RIA, with a concomitant reduction in plasma calcium levels (Fig. 7). These studies therefore indicate that the development of accurate methods for the measurement of PTHrP in humans can also be applied to animal studies, particularly of mammals, most likely because of the strong interspecies conservation of amino acid sequence within the NH_2-terminal two-thirds of PTHrP. Such assays appear to be useful both in defining the pathogenetic mechanisms underlying malignancy-as-sociated hypercalcemia and in assessing the therapeutic modalities to be used in its treatment.

SUMMARY

Rapid progress has been made in the development and application of immunologic methods of measurement of PTHrP since the elucidation of its primary structure. These developments have resulted in significant advances in our knowledge of the regulation of gene expression and metabolism of this hypercalcemic factor as well as of its central pathogenetic role in malignancy-associated hypercalcemia. Significant progress has yet to be made, however, in defining the exact nature of circulating molecular forms of PTHrP. Such progress should greatly facilitate the rational development of newer assays with even greater sensitivity and specificity and should markedly extend the clinical applicability of these assays to human disease.

ACKNOWLEDGMENTS

The authors thank Shafaat Rabbani and Geoffrey Hendy for important collaboration with parts of this work and Michael Sebag and Janet Henderson for essential contributions. They also extend their appreciation to Diane Allen, Gladys Chan, Judith Marshall, and Karuna Patel for excellent secretarial assistance. The research described in this chapter was funded by grants MT-10839 (R.K.) and MT-5775 (D.G.) from the Medical Research Council of Canada (MRC) and by the National Cancer Institute of Canada and the U.S. National Institutes of Health.

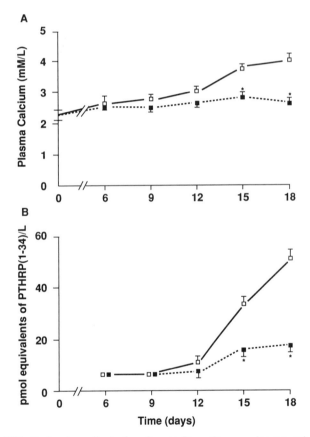

FIG. 7. In vivo effect of a vitamin D analog on plasma calcium and on PTHrP secretion in the rat Leydig cell tumor model. Tumor-bearing male Fischer rats were infused with a vitamin D analog (■) or vehicle (□) alone using Alzet osmotic minipumps implanted intraperitoneally. Blood was collected at timed intervals for PTHrP measurement using an NH_2-terminal RIA and for plasma calcium measurement. Control, vehicle-treated, tumor-bearing animals showed a progressive increase in both their plasma calcium (**A**) and immunoreactive PTHrP (**B**). In contrast, tumor-bearing animals infused with the vitamin D analog maintained near-normal plasma calcium (**A**) and PTHrP levels (**B**). Significant differences from control tumor bearing animals at each time point are represented by an asterisk ($P < 0.05$).

REFERENCES

1. Albright F. Case records of the Massachusetts General Hospital (case 27461). N Engl J Med 1941;225:789–791.
2. Lafferty FW. Pseudohyperparathyroidism. Medicine 1966; 45:247–260.
3. Stewart AF, Horst R, Deftos LJ, Cadman EC, Lang R, Broadus AE. Biochemical evaluation of patients with cancer-associated hypercalcemia. Evidence for humoral and non-humoral groups. N Engl J Med 1980;303:1377–1383.
4. Goltzman D, Stewart AE, Broadus AE. Malignancy-associated hypercalcemia: evaluation with a cytochemical bioassay for parathyroid hormone. J Clin Endocrinol Metab 1981;53:899–904.
5. Stewart AF, Insogna KL, Goltzman D, Broadus AE. Identification of adenylate cyclase-stimulating activity and cytochemical bioactivity in extracts of tumors from patients with humoral hypercalcemia of malignancy. Proc Natl Acad Sci USA 1983;90:1454–1458.
6. Stewart AF, Wu TL, Goumas D, Burtis WJ, Broadus AE. N-terminal amino acid sequence of two novel tumor-derived adenylate cyclase-stimulating proteins: identification of parathyroid hormone-like and parathyroid hormone-unlike domains. Biochem Biophys Res Commun 1987;146:672–678.
7. Strewler GJ, Williams RD, Nissenson RA. Human renal carcinoma cells produce hypercalcemic in the nude mouse and

a novel protein recognized by parathyroid hormone receptors. *J Clin Invest* 1983;71:769–774.

8. Rodan J, Insogna KL, Vignery AM, et al. Factors associated with humoral hypercalcemia of malignancy stimulate adenylate cyclase in osteoblastic cells. *J Clin Invest* 1983; 72:1511–1515.

9. Rabbani SA, Mitchell J, Roy DR, Kremer R, Bennett HPJ, Goltzman D. Purification of peptides with parathyroid hormone-like bioactivity from human and rat malignancies associated with hypercalcemia. *Endocrinology* 1986;118:1200–1210.

10. Broadus AE, Goltzman D, Webb AC, Kronenberg HM. Messenger RNA from tumors associated with humoral hypercalcemia of malignancy directs the synthesis of a secretory parathyroid hormone-like peptide. *Endocrinology* 1985;117:1661–1666.

11. Moseley JM, Kubota M, Diefenbach-Jagger H, et al. Parathyroid hormone-related protein purified from a human lung cancer cell line. *Proc Natl Acad Sci USA* 1987;84:5048–5052.

12. Strewler GJ, Stern PH, Jacobs JW, et al. Parathyroid hormone-like protein from human renal carcinoma cells. *J Clin Invest* 1987;80:1803–1807.

13. Suva LJ, Winslow GA, Wettenhall EH, et al. A parathyroid hormone-related protein implicated in malignant hypercalcemia: cloning and expression. *Science* 1987;237:893–896.

14. Mangin M, Webb AC, Dreyer BE, et al. Identification of a cDNA encoding a parathyroid hormone-like peptide from a human tumor associated with humoral hypercalcemia of malignancy. *Proc Natl Acad Sci USA* 1988;85:597–601.

15. Jüppner H, Abou-Samra A, Freeman M, et al. A G protein linked receptor for parathyroid hormone and parathyroid hormone-related peptide. *Science* 1991;254:1024–1026.

16. Stewart AF, Vignery A, Silvergate A, et al. Quantitative bone histomorphometry in humoral hypercalcemia of malignancy: uncoupling of bone cell activity. *J Clin Endocrinol Metab* 1982;55:219–227.

17. Insogna KL, Stewart AF, Vignery AM-C, et al. Biochemical and histomorphometric characterization of a rat model for humoral hypercalcemia of malignancy. *Endocrinology* 1984; 114:888–896.

18. Krukeja SC, Rosol RJ, Wimbiscus SA, et al. Tumor resection and antibodies to parathyroid hormone-related protein cause similar changes in bone histomorphometry in hypercalcemia of cancer. *Endocrinology* 1980;127:305–310.

19. Breslau NA, McGuire JL, Zerwekh JE, Frenkel EP, Pak CYC. Hypercalcemia associated with increased serum calcitriol levels in three patients with lymphoma. *Ann Intern Med* 1984;100:1–7.

20. Fraher LJ, Hodsman AB, Jonas K, et al. A comparison of the in vivo biochemical responses to exogenous parathyroid hormone-(1–34) [PTH-(1–34)] and PTH-related peptide-(1–34) in man. *J Clin Endo Metab* 1992;75:417–423.

21. Fukumoto S, Matsumoto T, Yamoto H, Kawashima Y, Tamaoki N, Ogata E. Suppression of serum 1,25(OH)$_2$D in humoral hypercalcemia of malignancy is caused by elaboration of a factor that inhibits renal 1,25 dihydroxyvitamin D production. *Endocrinology* 1989;124:2057–2062.

22. Yasuda T, Banville D, Rabbani SA, Hendy GN, Goltzman D. Rat parathyroid hormone-like peptide: comparison with the human homologue and expression in malignant and normal tissue. *Mol Endocrinol* 1989;3:518–525.

23. Mangin M, Ikeda K, Broadus AE. Structure of the mouse gene encoding the parathyroid hormone-related peptide. *Gene* 1990;95:195–202.

24. Schermer PT, Chan SDH, Bruce R, Nissenson RA, Wood WI, Strewler GJ. Chicken parathyroid hormone-related protein and its expression during embryologic development. *J Bone Mineral Res* 1991;6:149–155.

25. Fenton AJ, Kemp BE, Hammonds RG Jr, et al. A potent inhibitor of osteoclastic bone resorption within a highly conserved pentapeptide region of parathyroid hormone-related protein; PTHrP [107–111]. *Endocrinology* 1991;129:3424–3436.

26. Mangin M, Ikeda K, Dreyer BE, Broadus AE. Isolation and

27. Yasuda T, Banville D, Hendy GN, Goltzman D. Characterization of the human parathyroid hormone-like peptide gene. *Proc Natl Acad Sci USA* 1989;86:2408–2412.

28. Suva LJ, Mather KA, Gillespie MT, et al. Structure of the 5' flanking region of the gene encoding human parathyroid hormone-related protein (PTHrP). *Gene* 1989;77:95–105.

29. Karaplis AC, Yasuda T, Hendy GN, Goltzman D, Banville D. Gene-encoding parathyroid hormone-like peptide: nucleotide sequences of the rat gene and comparison with the human. *Mol Endocrinol* 1990;4:441–446.

30. Deftos LJ, Gazdar AF, Ikeda K, Broadus AE. The parathyroid hormone-related protein associated with malignancy is secreted by neuroendocrine tumors. *Mol Endocrinol* 1989; 3:503–508.

31. Brandt DW, Deftos LJ. All major lung cancer cell types produce parathyroid hormone-like peptide: heterogeneity assessed by HPLC. *J Bone Mineral Res* 1990;5(Suppl 2):S256.

32. Danks JA, Ebeling PR, Hayman JA, et al. Immunohistochemical localization of PTHRP in parathyroid adenoma and hyperplasia. *J Pathol* 1990;161:27–33.

33. Thiede M, Rodan GA. Expression of a calcium-mobilizing parathyroid hormone-like peptide in lactating mammary tissue. *Science* 1988;242:278–280.

34. Budayr AA, Halloran BP, King JC, Diep D, Nissenson RA, Strewler GJ. High levels of parathyroid hormone-like protein in milk. *Proc Natl Acad Sci USA* 1989;86:7183–7185.

35. Khosla S, Johansen KL, Ory SJ, O'Brien PC, Kao PC. Parathyroid hormone-related peptide in lactation and in umbilical cord blood. *Mayo Clin Proc* 1990;65:1408–1414.

36. Thurston AW, Cole JA, Hillman LS, et al. Purification and properties of parathyroid hormone-related peptide isolated from milk. *Endocrinology* 1990;126:1183–1190.

37. Stewart AF, Wu TL, Insogna KL, Milstone LM, Burtis WJ. Immunoaffinity purification of parathyroid hormone-related protein from bovine milk and human keratinocyte conditioned medium. *J Bone Mineral Res* 1991;6:305–311.

38. Orloff JJ, Wu TL, Stewart AF. PTH-like proteins, biochemical response receptor interactions. *Endocrine Rev* 1989;10: 476–495.

39. Wu TL, Soifer NE, Burtis WJ, Milstone LM, Stewart AF. Glycosylation of parathyroid hormone-related peptide secreted by human epidermal keratinocytes. *J Clin Endocrinol Metab* 1991;73:1002–1007.

40. Soifer NE, Dee KE, Insogna KL, et al. Parathyroid hormone related protein: evidence for secretion of a mid region fragment by three different cell types. *J Biol Chem* 1992; 267:18236–18243.

41. Haq M, Goltzman D, Rabbani SA. Biosynthesis and processing of endogenous parathyroid hormone related peptide (PTHRP) by the rat Leydig cell tumor H-500. *Biochemistry* 1993;32:4931–4937.

42. Goltzman D, Bennett HPJ, Koutsilieris M, Mitchell J, Rabbani SA, Rouleau MF. Studies on the multiple molecular forms of bioactive parathyroid hormone and parathyroid hormone-like substances. *Rec Progr Horm Res* 1986;42:665–703.

43. Burtis WJ, Brady TG, Orloff JJ, et al. Immunochemical characterization of circulating parathyroid hormone-related protein in patients with humoral hypercalcemia of cancer. *N Engl J Med* 1990;322:1106–1112.

44. Henderson JE, Shustik C, Kremer R, Rabbani SA, Hendy GN, Goltzman D. Circulating concentrations of parathyroid hormone-like peptide in malignancy and in hyperparathyroidism. *J Bone Mineral Res* 1990;5:105–113.

45. Imamura H, Sato K, Shizame K, et al. Urinary excretion of PTHRP fragments in patients with humoral hypercalcemia of malignancy and hypercalcemic tumor-bearing nude mice. *J Bone Mineral Res* 1991;6:77–84.

46. Budayr AA, Nissenson RA, Klein RF, et al. Increased serum levels of a parathyroid hormone-like protein in malignancy-associated hypercalcemia. *Ann Intern Med* 1989;111:807–812.

47. Kao PC, Klee GG, Taylor RL, Heath H III. Parathyroid hor-

mone-related peptide in plasma of patients with hypercalcemia and malignant lesions. *Mayo Clin Proc* 1990;65:1399–1407.

48. Grill V, Ho P, Body JJ, et al. Parathyroid hormone-related protein: Elevated levels both in humoral hypercalcemia of malignancy and in hypercalcemia complicating metastatic breast cancer. *J Clin Endocrinol Metab* 1991;73:1309–1315.

49. Ratcliffe WA, Norbury C, Stott RA, Heath DA, Ratcliffe JG. Immunoreactivity of plasma parathyrin-related peptide: three region specific radioimmunoassays and a two-site immunoradiometric assay compared. *Clin Chem* 1991;37:1781–1787.

50. Ratcliffe WA, Bowden SJ, Emly J, Hughes S, Ratcliffe JG. Production and characterization of monoclonal antibodies to the mid-region 37–67 sequence of parathyroid hormone-related protein. *J Immunol Methods* 1992;146:33–42.

51. Ikeda K, Weir EC, Mangin M, et al. Expression of messenger ribonucleic acids encoding a parathyroid hormone-like peptide in normal human and animal tissues with abnormal expression in human parathyroid adenomas. *Mol Endocrinol* 1988;2:1230–1236.

52. Kremer R, Henderson J, Gulliver W, Hendy GN, Goltzman D. EGF and 1,25 dihydroxycholecalciferol regulate PLP secretion in normal human keratinocytes. *J Bone Mineral Res* 1989;6(Suppl 1A):S195.

53. Haq M, Kremer R, Goltzman D, Rabbani RA. A vitamin D analogue (EB1089) inhibits parathyroid hormone related peptide production and prevents the development of malignancy-associated hypercalcemia in vivo. *J Clin Invest* 1993;91:2416–2422.

54. Drucker DJ, Asa SL, Henderson J, Goltzman D. The parathyroid hormone-like peptide gene is expressed in the normal and neoplastic human endocrine pancreas. *Mol Endocrinol* 1989;3:1589–1595.

55. Ratcliffe WA, Thompson GE, Care AD, Peaker M. Production of PTH-related protein (PTHrP) by the mammary gland of the goat. *J Endocrinol* 1991;129(Suppl):134.

56. Ferrari SL, Rizzoli R, Bonjour JP. Antagonistic effects of EGF and TGFβ on parathyroid hormone related protein (PTHRP) production by mammary epithelial cells. *J Bone Mineral Res* 1991;6(Suppl 1):S228.

57. Sebag M, Henderson J, Papavasiliou V, Goltzman D, Kremer R. Regulation of parathyroid hormone-related peptide expression (PTHRP) in normal human mammary epithelial cells. *J Bone Mineral Res* 1992;7(Suppl 1):S244.

58. Danks JA, Ebeling PR, Hayman J, et al. Parathyroid hormone-related protein: immunohistochemical localization in cancers and in normal skin. *J Bone Mineral Res* 1989;4:273–278.

59. Hongo TJ, Kupfer J, Enomoto H, et al. Abundant expression of parathyroid hormone related protein in primary rat arctic smooth muscle cells accompanies serum induced proliferation. *J Clin Invest* 1991;88:1841–1847.

60. Thiede MA, Daifotis AG, Weir EC, et al. Intrauterine occupancy controls expression of the parathyroid hormone-related peptide gene in preterm rat myometrium. *Proc Natl Acad Sci USA* 1990;87:6969–6973.

61. Brandt DW, Bruns ME, Bruns DW, Ferguson JE, Burton DW, Deftos LJ. Parathyroid hormone like protein (PLP) production in normal human amnion characterization of mRNA and protein species. *J Bone Mineral Res* 1992;7(Suppl 1):S236.

62. Martin TJ, Allan EH, Caple IW, et al. Parathyroid hormone-related protein: isolation, molecular cloning and mechanism of action. *Rec Progr Horm Res* 1989;45:467–506.

63. Danks JA, Ebeling PR, Hayman JA, et al. Immunohistochemical localization of parathyroid hormone-related protein in parathyroid adenoma and hyperplasia. *J Pathol* 1990;16:27–33.

64. Henderson J, Goltzman D, Sebag M, Rhim J, Kremer R. Dysregulation of parathyroid hormone-like peptide expression in a keratinocyte model of tumor cell progression. *Cancer Res* 1991;51:6521–6528.

65. Ikeda K, Mangin M, Dreyer BE, et al. Identification of transcripts encoding a parathyroid hormone-like peptide in mes-

66. Hayman JA, Danks JA, Ebeling PR, Moseley JM, Kemp BE, Martin TJ. Expression of parathyroid hormone-related protein in normal skin and in tumor of skin and skin appendages. *J Pathol* 1989;158:293–296.

67. Southby J, Kissin MW, Danks JA, et al. Immunohistochemical localization of parathyroid hormone-related protein in human breast cancer. *Cancer Res* 1990;50:7710–7716.

68. Motokura T, Fukumoto S, Takahashi S. Expression of PTH-rP in a human T-cell lymphotrophic virus type 1-infected T-cell line. *Biochem Biophys Res Commun* 1988;154:1182–1188.

69. Rodan SB, Wesolowdki G, Ianacone J, Thiede MA, Rodan GA. Production of parathyroid hormone-like peptide in a human osteosarcoma cell line: stimulation by phorbol esters and epidermal growth factor. *J Endocrinol* 1989;122:219–227.

70. Kaiser SM, Laneuville P, Rhim J, Kremer R, Goltzman D. Expression of antisense RNA for parathyroid hormone-like peptide enhances growth of human keratinocytes in culture. *J Bone Mineral Res* 1991;6(Suppl 1):S195.

71. Kaiser SM, Laneuville P, Rhim J, Kremer R, Goltzman D. Enhanced growth of a human keratinocyte cell line induced by anti-sense RNA for parathyroid hormone related peptide. *J Biol Chem* 1992;261:13623–13628.

72. Kaiser SM, Kremer R, Laneuville P, Rhim JS, Goltzman D. Inhibition of parathyroid hormone-related peptide expression by antisense RNA impedes differentiation of a human keratinocyte cell line. Paper presented at the *IX*th *International Congress of Endocrinology*, 1992.

73. Henderson J, Bernier S, D'Amour P, Goltzman D. Effects of passive immunization against parathyroid hormone (PTH)-like peptide on PTH in hypercalcemic tumor bearing rats and normocalcemic controls. *Endocrinology* 1990;127:1310–1318.

74. Henderson J, Shustik C, Kremer R, Rabbani S, Hendy GN, Goltzman D. Circulating concentrations of parathyroid hormone-like peptide in malignancy and in hyperparathyroidism. *J Bone Mineral Res* 1990;5:105–113.

75. Liu B, Goltzman D, Rabbani SA. Regulation of parathyroid hormone related peptide production in vitro by the rat hypercalcemic Leydig cell tumor H-500. *Endocrinology* 1993;132:1658–1664.

76. Rizzoli R, Bonjour JP. High extracellular calcium increases the production of a parathyroid hormone-activity by cultured Leydig tumor cells associated with humoral hypercalcemia. *J Bone Mineral Res* 1989;6:839–844.

77. Brandt DW, Pandol SJ, Deftos LJ. Calcium stimulates parathyroid hormone-like protein secretion: potentiation through a protein kinase c pathway. *J Bone Mineral Res* 1991;5(Suppl 2):A730.

78. Ikeda K, Weir EC, Sakaguchi K, et al. Clonal rat parathyroid cell line expresses parathyroid hormone-related peptide but not parathyroid hormone itself. *Biochem Biophys Res Commun* 1989;162:108–115.

79. Chan SDH, Strewler GJ, King KL, Nissenson RA. Expression of a parathyroid hormone-like protein and its receptor during differentiation of embryonal carcinoma cells. *Mol Endocrinol* 1990;4:638–646.

80. Deftos LJ, Hogue-Angeletti R, Chalberg C, Tu S. PTHrP secretion is stimulated by CT and inhibited by CgA peptides. *Endocrinology* 1989;125:563–565.

81. Rizzoli R, Sappino AP, Aubert ML, Bonjour JP. Effect of cyclic AMP-stimulators on parathyroid hormone-related protein (PTHRP) release by a cultured lungs cell carcinoma (BEN cells). *Calcif Tissue Int* 1990;46(Suppl 2):A58.

82. Watanabe T, Yamaguchi K, Takatsuki K, Osame M, Yoshida M. Constitutive expression of parathyroid hormone-related protein gene in human T cell leukemic virus type I (HTLVI) carriers and adult T cell leukemic patients that can be transactivated by HTLV-1 tax gene. *J Exp Med* 1990;172:759.

83. Kiriyama T, Gillensie MT, Glatz, et al. Regulation of parathyroid hormone-related protein (PTHRP) gene expression

senger RNAs from a variety of human and animal tumors associated with humoral hypercalcemia of malignancy. *J Clin Invest* 1988;81:2010–2014.

by transforming growth factor β-1. *J Bone Mineral Res* 1991;6(Suppl 1):S227.

84. Rhim JS, Jay G, Arnstein P, Price FM, Sanford KK, Aaronson SA. Neoplastic transformation of human epidermal keratinocytes by AD12-SV40 and kirsten sarcoma viruses. *Science* 1985;227:1250–1252.

85. Rhim JS, Park JB, Jay G. Neoplastic transformations of human keratinocytes by polybrene-induced DNA-mediated transfer of an activated oncogene. *Oncogene* 1989;4:1403–1409.

86. Godsall JW, Burtis WJ, Insogna KL, Broadus AE, Stewart AF. Nephrogenous cyclic AMP, adenylate cyclase-stimulating activity and the humoral hypercalcemia of malignancy. *Rec Progr Horm Res* 1986;42:705–750.

87. Powell D, Singer FR, Murray TM, Minkin C, Potts JT. Non parathyroid humoral hypercalcemia in patients with neoplastic diseases. *N Engl J Med* 1973;289:176–181.

88. Skrabanek P, McPartlin J, Powell D. Tumor hypercalcemia and ectopic hyperparathyroidism. *Medicine* 1980;58:262–265.

89. Ralston S, Fogelman I, Gardner MD, Boyle IT. Hypercalcemia and metastatic bone disease: is there a causal link? *Lancet* 1982;2:903–905.

90. Percival RC, Yates AJP, Grey RES, et al. Mechanism of malignant hypercalcemia in carcinoma of the breast. *Br Med J* 1985;291:776–779.

91. Ralston SH, Fogelman I, Gardiner MD, Boyle IT. Relative contribution of humoral and metastatic factors to the pathogenesis of hypercalcemia in malignancy. *Br Med J* 1984;288:1405–1408.

92. Rosenthal NR, Insogna KL, Godsall JW, Smaldone L, Waldron J, Stewart AF. Elevations in circulating 1,25 dihydroxyvitamin D in three patients with lymphoma associated hypercalcemia. *J Clin Endocrinol Metab* 1985;60:29–33.

93. Mundy GR, Martin TJ. The hypercalcemia of malignancy: pathogenesis and management. *Metabolism* 1982;31:1247–1277.

94. Adams JS, Fernandez M, Gacad MA, et al. Vitamin D metabolite-mediated hypercalcemia and hypercalciuria in patients with AIDS. *Blood* 1989;73:235–239.

95. Fukumoto S, Matsumoto T, Ikeda K, et al. Clinical evaluation of calcium metabolism in adult T-cell leukemia/lymphoma. *Arch Intern Med* 1988;148:921–925.

96. Dodwell DT, Abbas SK, Morton AR, Howell A. Parathyroid hormone-related protein and response to pamidronate therapy for tumor induced hypercalcemia. *Eur J Cancer* 1991;77:1629–1633.

97. Grill V, Murray RML, Ho PWM, et al. Circulating PTH and PTHRP levels before and after treatment of tumor induced hypercalcemia with pamidronate disodium (APD). *J Clin Endocrinol Metab* 1992;74:1468–1470.

98. Senior PV, Heath DA, Beck F. Expression of parathyroid hormone-related protein mRNA in the rat before birth: demonstration by hybridization histochemistry. *J Mol Endocrinol* 1991;6:281–290.

99. Allgrove J, Adami S, Manning RM, O'Riordan JLH. Cytochemical bioassay of parathyroid hormone in maternal and cord blood. *Arch Dis Child* 1985;60:110.

100. Hillman LS, Forte LR, Thorne PK, Johnson LS, Allen SH. Elevated PTH-related peptide in cord blood of term and premature neonates. *J Bone Mineral Res* 1990;5(Suppl):469.

101. Thiede MA. The mRNA encoding a parathyroid hormone-like peptide is produced in mammary tissue in response to elevations in serum prolactin. *Mol Endocrinol* 1989;3:1443–1447.

102. Law FMK, Moate PJ, Leaver DD, et al. Parathyroid hormone-related protein in milk and its correlation with bovine milk calcium. *J Endocrinol* 1991;128:21–27.

103. Ratcliffe WA, Green E, Emly J, et al. Identification and partial characterization of parathyroid hormone-related protein in human and bovine milk. *J Endocrinol* 1990;127:167–176.

104. Lepre F, Grill V, Danks JA, et al. Hypercalcemia in pregnancy and lactation due to parathyroid hormone-related protein production. *Bone Mineral* 1990;10:S317.

105. Loveridge N, Caple IW, Rodda C, Martin TJ, Care AD. Further evidence for a parathyroid hormone-related protein in fetal parathyroid glands of the sheep. *Q J Exp Physiol* 1988;73:781–784.

106. Langman CB, Budayr AA, Sailer DE, Strewler GJ. Non malignant expression of PTHRP is responsible for idiopathic infantile hypercalcemia. *J Bone Mineral Res* 1992;7(Suppl 1):S93.

107. Jacobs BB, Huseby RA. Neoplasms occuring in aged Fischer rats with special reference to testicular, uterine and thyroid tumors. *J Natl Cancer Inst* 1967;39:303–309.

108. Rice BF, Roth LM, Cole FE, et al. Hypercalcemia and neoplasia: biologic, biochemical, and ultrastructural studies of a hypercalcemia producing Leydig cell tumor of the rat. *Lab Invest* 1975;33:428–439.

109. Sica DA, Martodam RR, Aronow J, Mundy GR. The hypercalcemia rat leydig cell tumor. *Calcif Tissue Int* 1983;35:287–293.

110. Spiegel AM, Saxe AW, Deftos LJ, Brennan MF. Humoral hypercalcemia caused by a rat Leydig-cell tumor is associated with suppressed parathyroid hormone secretion and increased urinary cAMP excretion. *Horm Metab Res* 1983;15:299–304.

111. Scharla SH, Minne HW, Oswalk L, Lempert UG, Schmidt-Gayk H, Ziegler R. The hypercalcemia walker carcinosarcoma 256 of the rat causes an increase in serum 1,25 dihydroxyvitamin D₃. *Bone Mineral* 1989;6:155–164.

112. Minne HF, Rane S, Besswinkel S, Zieger R. The hypercalcemic syndrome in rats bearing the walker carcinoma 256. *Acta Endocrinol* 1975;78:613–624.

113. Scharla SH, Minne HW, Lempert UG, et al. Osteolytic activity of walker carcinoma 256 is due to parathyroid hormone-related protein (PTHRP). *Horm Metab Res* 1991;23:66–69.

114. Meuten DJ, Cooper BJ, Capen CC, Chew DJ, Dociba GJ. Hypercalcemia associated with an adenocarcinoma derived from the apocrine glands of the anal sac. *Vet Pathol* 1981;18:454–471.

115. Rosol TJ, Chew DJ, Lapen CC, Sherding RG. Acute hypocalcemia associated with infarction of parathyroid gland adenomas in two dogs. *J Am Vet Med Assoc* 1988;192:212–214.

116. Krukeja SC, Shevrin DH, Wimbiscus SA, et al. Antibodies to parathyroid hormone-related protein lower serum calcium in athymlic mouse models of malignancy-associated hypercalcemia due to human tumors. *J Clin Invest* 1988;82:1798–1802.

117. Strewler GJ, Wronski TJ, Halloran BP, et al. Pathogenesis of hypercalcemia in nude mice bearing a human renal carcinoma. *Endocrinology* 1986;119:303–310.

118. Weir EC, Insogna KL, Brownstein DG, Bander NH, Broadus AE. In vitro adenylate cyclase stimulating activity predicts the occurrence of humoral hypercalcemia of malignancy in nude mice. *J Clin Invest* 1988;81:818–821.

119. Gaich G, Burtis WJ. Measurement of circulating parathyroid hormone-related protein in rats with humoral hypercalcemia of malignancy using a two-site immunoradiometric assay. *Endocrinology* 1990;127:1444–1449.

120. Yu J, Rhim K, Goltzman D, Rabbani S, Kremer R. Vitamin D analogs as potential agents for the treatment of cancer associated hypercalcemia. Paper presented at the *84th Annual Meeting of the American Association for Cancer Research*, 1993;34:256.

121. Kremer R, Papavasiliou V, Henderson J, Rhim J, Goltzman D. Calcipotriol (MC903) is a potent inhibitor of parathyroid hormone-like peptide (PLP) expression in human keratinocytes. *J Bone Mineral Res* 1991;6(Suppl):S291.

122. Binderup L, Latini S, Kissmeyer A. New vitamin D₃ analogues with potent effects on cell growth regulation and immune responses: structure–activity studies. In: Norman AW, et al., eds. *Vitamin D: gene regulation, structure function analysis and clinical application* (Proceedings of the 8th workshop on vitamin D). Berlin: Walter De Gruyter, 1991;478–485.

The Parathyroids, edited by J.P. Bilezikian, M.A. Levine, and R. Marcus. Raven Press, Ltd., New York © 1994.

CHAPTER 21

Other Causes of Hypercalcemia

Local and Ectopic Secretion Syndromes

Karen Shipp Black and Gregory R. Mundy

The identification of a novel parathyroid hormone (PTH)-like factor produced by tumor cells that has amino acid homology to PTH and binds to the PTH receptor has naturally led to great interest in the potential role of this peptide in the causation of hypercalcemia of malignancy. Since the recombinant molecule appears to mimic the effects of PTH on calcium and bone metabolism in general, this has further stimulated interest in this factor as a mediator of humoral hypercalcemia. The biological effects it shares with PTH include the stimulation of both bone resorption and bone formation, increases of cyclic adenosine monophosphate (cAMP) production in renal tubular cells, enhanced renal tubular reabsorption of calcium, decreased renal tubular reabsorption of phosphate, and stimulation of the conversion of 25-dihydroxyvitamin D_3 [$25(OH)_2D_3$] to 1,25-dihydroxyvitamin D_3 [$1,25(OH)_2D_3$] (1–3). Recent studies indicate that this peptide, called parathyroid hormone-related protein (PTHrP) is present in increased amounts in the circulation of 70–80% of patients with humoral hypercalcemia of malignancy using currently available assays (5,6). If these assays accurately reflect the proportion of malignancy-associated hypercalcemia due to PTHrP, there may be as many as 20–30% of patients in whom PTHrP cannot account for the hypercalcemia. Moreover, since the same assays indicate that PTHrP is moderately elevated in 10–15% of cancer patients

without hypercalcemia, a small or moderate increase in PTHrP alone may be insufficient to cause hypercalcemia. In addition, the humoral hypercalcemic syndrome seen in many patients with malignancy cannot be ascribed solely to PTHrP excess. In many of these patients, circulating concentrations of $1,25(OH)_2D_3$ are reduced, bone formation is suppressed, and the patients develop a mild metabolic alkalosis, three observations diametrically opposite to what is seen in the syndrome PTHrP is thought to mimic, namely, primary hyperparathyroidism (7). For these reasons, the syndrome of hypercalcemia of malignancy is not a direct reflection of that expected from PTH or PTHrP excess (Table 1). In addition, recent studies using Chinese hamster ovarian cells transfected with human PTH or PTHrP indicate that the syndrome of PTHrP excess produced in this model in nude mice mimics exactly that caused by PTH excess, resembling the syndrome of primary hyperparathyroidism rather than the humoral hypercalcemia of malignancy (8,9).

For all these reasons, we believe that other tumor factors produced in excess in the humoral hypercalcemia of malignancy syndrome may in some patients be responsible for the hypercalcemia and in others may be responsible for modifying the biological effects of PTHrP on calcium and bone (Table 2). These factors include transforming growth factor-α, interleukin-1α and β, tumor necrosis factor and lymphotoxin, 1,25-dihydroxyvitamin D_3, interleukin-6, and prostaglandins of the F series. There may be additional factors that have not yet been identified. These factors may influence PTHrP to modify its effects on such target organs as bone and kidney. In the case of bone, these factors may enhance the effects of PTHrP to stimulate

K. S. Black and G. R. Mundy: Department of Medicine, Division of Endocrinology, University of Texas Health Science Center, San Antonio, Texas 78284.

TABLE 1. *Similarities and differences between humoral hypercalcemia of malignancy (HHM) and primary hyperparathyroidism (HPT)*

	HHM	HPT
Serum calcium	Increased	Increased
Serum phosphorus	Decreased	Decreased
Nephrogenous cAMP	Increased	Increased
$1,25-(OH)_2D_3$	Decreased	Increased
Bone resorption	Increased	Increased
Bone formation	Decreased	Increased
Acid/base	Met. alk.	Met. acid.

osteoclastic bone resorption but oppose the effects of PTHrP on osteoblasts. Similarly, they may oppose the effects of PTHrP on renal tubular cells to promote conversion of $25(OH)_2D_3$ to $1,25(OH)_2D_3$ and to promote bicarbonate excretion. Because these other factors are frequently produced together with PTHrP, and a considerable body of evidence is now accumulating to indicate that they may interact with PTHrP both in in vitro studies as well as in vivo, these factors, their effects on bone metabolism, and their potential role in hypercalcemia of malignancy are reviewed in this chapter. A complete discussion of PTHrP in the syndrome of hypercalcemia of malignancy is found in preceding chapters.

TRANSFORMING GROWTH FACTOR-α

Transforming growth factor-α (TGFα) is a 5 kD polypeptide that is homologous to epidermal growth factor (EGF) both by amino acid sequence and by conformation. It has 40% homology at the amino acid level with EGF and has a similar conformation (10,11). TGFα is encoded by a much larger precursor, which is about thirty times the size of the major secreted molecule (12,13), similar to the relationship between EGF and its much larger precursor. Release of TGFα from the cell may depend on a specific and novel protease (14). Larger forms of TGFα are present in the culture media of cells expressing TGFα. Pro-TGFα is glycosylated heterogeneously, which may account for the differing capacities of some cell types to secrete biologically active TGFα. Its normal tissue source remains unknown, but expression of TGFα has been detected in the bone marrow of 10-day-old rodent embryos (15).

TGFα binds to the EGF receptor and exerts biological effects through this receptor. It can exert its biological effects in soluble or membrane-bound form but obviously must be released first in soluble form to function in an endocrine manner. The release of pro-TGFα from the cell membrane via proteolysis is usually inefficient, and this may be an important site of regulation of its activity. Membrane-anchored pro-TGFα may be responsible for the interaction between cells expressing TGFα with other contiguous cells that possess EGF receptors. This may be a mechanism for activation of the target cell through cell–cell contact, a mechanism recently termed *juxtacrine stimulation* (16).

Effects of TGFα on Bone

TGFα causes increased osteoclast formation, bone resorption, and hypercalcemia. The effects of TGFα on osteoclasts have been demonstrated both in vivo and in vitro (17). It stimulates proliferation of osteoclast progenitors in human marrow cultures, increases osteoclast formation (18), and stimulates bone resorption in several different bone organ culture systems (19–22). The increased numbers of osteoclasts observed in mice bearing Chinese hamster ovarian (CHO) tumors secreting TGFα are small, and the nuclei are relatively few in number, (17), consistent with the major effect of this factor on osteoclast progenitors. TGFα is expressed in large amounts during embryonic development at a time when the bone marrow cavity is forming, suggesting that it might be important in the osteoclastic bone resorption necessary for the formation of the normal marrow cavity (23). TGFα also stimulates proliferation of cells with the osteoblast phenotype but inhibits their expression of differentiation markers (20).

TGFα may modulate the actions of other osteotropic factors on target cells. It impairs the effects of PTH and PTHrP to increase cAMP in bone cells and in renal cells (24–26). In contrast, it has synergistic effects with PTHrP to stimulate bone resorption in vitro and to cause hypercalcemia (27).

Evidence for a Role for Transforming Growth Factor-α in Hypercalcemia of Malignancy

Since TGFα is a tumor-derived growth regulatory factor that causes increased osteoclast formation, bone resorption, and hypercalcemia, it is likely to be an important mediator of bone destruction associated with solid tumors. The most convincing evidence that

TABLE 2. *Tumor-associated factors causing hypercalcemia*

PTHrP	TGF-α
IL-1α, IL-1β	PTH
IL-6	$1,25-(OH)_2 D_3$
TNF	Prostaglandins

tumor-derived TGFα may cause increased bone resorption and hypercalcemia in vivo comes from experiments in which CHO cells were transfected with the human TGFα gene and the tumor cells inoculated into nude mice, thus causing the formation of solid tumors which stably express TGFα (17). After four weeks, these mice became hypercalcemic, whereas mice bearing control tumors not producing TGFα remained normocalcemic. The control tumors were composed of CHO cells that had been transfected with the empty vector. The tumor-bearing mice also showed evidence of increased osteoclastic bone resorption as assessed by quantitative bone histomorphometry. To examine interactions between PTHrP and TGFα, mice bearing CHO tumors secreting TGFα were injected with PTHrP when they were still mildly hypercalcemic. These mice developed severe hypercalcemia, presumably a result of synergistic interactions between TGFα and PTHrP (27). Because these factors are often cosecreted by the same tumors, the interactions shown experimentally may be very important in the pathophysiology of the hypercalcemia of malignancy. These synergistic interactions between TGFα and PTHrP may occur because, in addition to its effects on bone resorption, PTHrP enhances renal tubular calcium reabsorption (28). Moreover, PTHrP and TGFα probably act at different sites in the osteoclast lineage (18). It is possible that TGFα enhances osteoclast precursor proliferation and that PTHrP simulates differentiation of committed progenitors. Since tumors often secrete other cytokines in addition to TGFα, TGFα may also have synergistic effects with these cytokines to cause hypercalcemia. It is not known whether TGFα activity alone is responsible for the hypercalcemia associated with many tumors, or if it acts to cause hypercalcemia only in conjunction with other factors or cytokines. In those tumors that secrete TGFα in sufficient quantities, it could conceivably be the sole etiologic agent. The bone-resorbing activity produced by some animal tumors associated with hypercalcemia can be blocked by antibodies to the EGF receptor (29,30), even in those tumors that also produce PTHrP. Since PTHrP and TGFα are often cosecreted by the same tumor (31,32), hypercalcemia in these cases could occur due to the combined effects under circumstances in which either one alone may not be sufficient.

TGFα is produced by many tumors, including squamous cell carcinomas of the lung, head, and neck, kidney, and breast cancers (33–37). Since each of these tumors is often associated with hypercalcemia, TGFα is likely playing a significant role in the pathophysiology of the hypercalcemia occurring with these tumors (21,38). TGFα production by breast cancer cells may be enhanced by treatment with estrogens (39,40), as can hypercalcemia (41).

INTERLEUKIN-1

Interleukin-1 is the most powerful peptide bone-resorbing factor known. Since it has been shown to be expressed by a number of different types of malignant cells, it is not surprising that it has been linked to the hypercalcemia of malignancy. There are two interleukin-1 molecules, interleukin-1α and interleukin-1β. Both are 17 kD peptides which share the same receptors and have apparently identical effects on bone cells and calcium metabolism both in vitro and in vivo (42). Both interleukin-1α and interleukin-1β are encoded by separate single copy genes in man (43–45). Interleukin-1β was first purified from active monocytes and was identified by its capacity to cause thymocyte proliferation. Stimulated human monocytes release interleukin-1β as the predominant form after cleavage by plasmin from the cell membrane (47). There are precursor forms of interleukin-1 that are membrane bound, including species of molecular weight 31 kD and 22 kD (46,47). The membrane-bound forms of interleukin-1 have been shown to be biologically active. This also suggests a role for interleukin-1 in biological effects mediated by cell–cell contact, such as those described above for TGFα. The membrane-bound form of interleukin-1 is predominantly interleukin-1α, in contrast to the circulating form in man, which is predominantly interleukin-1β (45).

Effects of Interleukin-1 on Bone

Interleukin-1 has been known to be a potent bone-resorbing factor in organ cultures for about 10 years. Gowen et al. (48) showed that partially purified interleukin-1 of human origin stimulated bone resorption in organ cultures of neonatal mouse calvariae. Heath et al. (49) found that purified porcine interleukin-1 resorbed bone in organ cultures of murine calvaria; Gowen and Mundy (50) found that recombinant human interleukin-1α and -β each had equivalent, powerful effects on bone resorption in similar organ culture systems. Dewhirst et al. (51) purified bone-resorbing activity from activated leukocyte culture supernatants and found by amino acid sequence that the purified factor was interleukin-1β. Although they concluded that interleukin-1 was solely responsible for bone resorption in activated leukocyte cultures, other bone-resorbing factors were not excluded.

These in vitro studies, supporting a role for interleukin-1 in bone resorption, were followed by studies in vivo. Interleukin-1 was administered to normal, intact mice by continuous infusion subcutaneously for 3 days via Alzet osmotic minipumps (42). A marked increase in systemic osteoclastic bone resorption was accompanied by hypercalcemia. Both interleukin-1α and interleukin-1β produced identical effects. In this model, interleukin-1 was more potent than PTH or tumor necrosis factor (TNF). Interleukin-1 was then examined in detail for its effects on bone as assessed by quantitative histomorphometry and on blood ionized calcium in normal mice following repeat subcutaneous injections (52,53). Immediately following injection of interleukin-1, a transient and modest decline in blood ionized calcium is seen. The transient reduction in blood ionized calcium is due to prostaglandin, since it can be ablated by treatment of the mice with doses of indomethacin that prevent prostaglandin synthesis. Following the transient decline in blood ionized calcium, the blood ionized calcium then steadily rises into the severe hypercalcemic range (53). Each time interleukin-1 was administered in bolus form, there was a transient decrease in blood ionized calcium before blood ionized calcium inevitably rose again. Because interleukin-1 may be produced and released in bolus form in patients with overwhelming infections, it is tempting to implicate a role for interleukin-1 in the hypocalcemia that is sometimes observed in patients with sepsis.

When interleukin-1 is continuously infused or given by repeated injection, profound hypercalcemia occurs. This is associated with a generalized increase in osteoclastic bone resorption. If interleukin-1 is administered subcutaneously, directly adjacent to bone, a marked inflammatory response is incited and is associated with bone resorption at the local bone site (52). The inflammatory response and local bone resorption can be prevented by treatment with inhibitors of prostaglandin synthesis such as indomethacin. However, the distant or systemic effects of interleukin-1 are not affected by indomethacin, and indomethacin has no effect on the level of blood ionized calcium (52,53). These data indicate that local effects of interleukin-1 on bone are, in part, mediated by prostaglandin but that the systemic effects are independent of prostaglandins.

The effects of interleukin-1 on cells in the osteoclast lineage have been studied in some detail. Interleukin-1 is a growth-regulatory factor for osteoclasts and acts at multiple steps (Fig. 1) (54). Its major effect may be to stimulate proliferation of osteoclast progenitors and to induce differentiation of committed progenitors to form multinucleated cells (55). In vitro, interleukin-1 has been shown to have an additional effect on activation of mature multinucleated cells to form resorption lacunae (56). These latter effects on osteoclasts are probably indirect and mediated through intermediate cells in the osteoblast lineage or through bone-lining cells (56). The molecular mechanisms responsible for these events remain unknown. Interleukin-1 resorbs bone in concentrations as low as 10^{-12} M alone and can stimulate bone resorption at even lower concentrations when it is administered in the presence of other cytokines (57).

There are several likely sources of interleukin-1 in both normal and pathological bone. In addition to tumor cells (58,59), interleukin-1 may be produced by immune cells in the bone cell microenvironment and also by bone cells with the osteoblast phenotype. The production of interleukin-1 by bone cells is not modulated by PTH but may be modulated by lipopolysaccharide (48). It is possible that other cytokines, estrogen, or various pathologic agents could also modulate the local production of interleukin-1 in bone.

There are two receptors for interleukin-1, an 80 kD receptor, which is present in athymic fibroblasts and

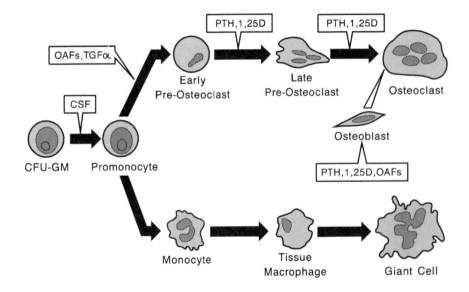

FIG. 1. Hypothetical model for osteoclast formation. Factors such as transforming growth factor-α, the colony-stimulating factors, and the osteoclast-activating factors, or OAFs (immune cell products such as interleukin-1 and tumor necrosis factor), act as regulatory growth factors on these mononuclear osteoclast precursors. Systemic hormones such as parathyroid hormone (PTH) and 1,25-dihydroxyvitamin D (1,25D) stimulate the differentiation process. The OAFs and the systemic hormones such as PTH and 1,25D can also work on the mature osteoclast (probably indirectly via other cells) to stimulate resorption. (Reprinted from ref. 54 with permission.)

T-lymphocytes, and a 60 kD receptor, which is present in cells of the monocyte–macrophage lineage. The availability of antibodies and antagonists to the interleukin-1 80 kD receptor has allowed clarification of the receptor mechanisms required for interleukin-1 to stimulate bone resorption (60,61). The interleukin-1 receptor antagonist is a naturally occurring endogenous peptide in the interleukin-1 family, which competes with interleukin-1 for binding to the 80 kD receptor (62–64). It also competes for some effects that are mediated through the 60 kD receptor. Neutralizing antibodies to the interleukin-1 80 kD receptor have also been developed. The receptor antagonist could be shown to inhibit hypercalcemia and bone resorption stimulated by interleukin-1 (9,65). When neutralizing antibodies to the 80 kD receptor were incubated with interleukin-1 in an organ culture assay, bone resorption was inhibited (60). These data suggest that a major receptor mechanism involved in the effects of interleukin-1 on bone is the 80 kD receptor.

It is possible that some of the effects of interleukin-1α and interleukin-β on bone are mediated by local generation of other cytokines. For example, interleukin-1 mediates its effects on bone resorption, in part, through local generation of prostaglandins of the E series (see above). Interleukin-1 is also a known inducer of interleukin-2, interferons-γ and -β, TNF, and interleukin-6 (66–68). In particular, the effects of TNF and IL-6 may be important for some of the effects of interleukin-1 on bone resorption. Interleukin-1 may work on bone directly, but generation of TNF and IL-6 may cause additional or even synergistic effects over and above those caused by interleukin-1. In fact, many of the actions of interleukin-1 on bone are similar to those of TNF (see above under Tumor Necrosis Factor-α).

Evidence for a Role for Interleukin-1 in Hypercalcemia of Malignancy

Interleukin-1 is produced by many tumors that are associated with bone destruction and hypercalcemia. The tumors are frequently associated with the production of PTHrP and TGFα. (58,59) Fried et al. (58) demonstrated that conditioned media harvested from two squamous cell carcinoma cell lines stimulated bone resorption in neonatal mouse calvarial organ cultures. Interleukin-1 was measured by its capacity to enhance thymocyte proliferation and induce prostaglandin synthesis. Fried et al. demonstrated that the bone-resorbing factor in the tumor cell conditioned media was interleukin-1α by using specific interleukin-1 enzyme-linked immunosorbent assays (ELISAs) and by showing that neutralizing antibodies to interleukin-

1α completely inhibited the bone-resorbing activity in the conditioned media. Sato et al. (59) found that a human esophageal carcinoma cell line (EC-GI) constitutively produced both interleukin-1α and PTHrP. They used interleukin-1α and PTHrP alone and together in vitro and noted dose-dependent effects on bone resorption. When interleukin-1 and PTHrP were administered alone or together in vivo, the combination caused hypercalcemia at doses that suggested synergistic effects (59).

Interleukin-1β has also been implicated in the hypercalcemia and bone destruction associated with myeloma. Cozzolino et al. (69) studied bone marrow aspirates from 12 patients with myeloma and found high concentrations of interleukin-1β in their culture supernatants but not in those of controls. These marrow cell supernatants also released a bone-resorbing factor that was similar in nature to the bone-resorbing activity released by activated peripheral blood leukocyte cultures. Cozzolino et al. showed that neutralizing antibodies to interleukin-1β blocked the bone-resorbing activity present in the marrow cell culture supernatants. Since the majority of the cells present in these marrow cell cultures were myeloma cells, the authors postulated that the mechanism by which myeloma stimulated bone resorption was through interleukin-1. Similar results with freshly isolated marrow cells derived from patients with myeloma were shown by Kawano et al. (70).

In spite of these data suggesting a role for interleukin-1β in myeloma, there is also evidence for other cytokines mediating bone destruction in this disease. Both lymphotoxin and interleukin-6 have been implicated (see below).

Evidence for a Role for Interleukin-1 in Disease States Other Than Hypercalcemia of Malignancy

Interleukin-1 is also likely involved in other pathological situations. In addition to a potential role as an important mediator of localized bone loss in chronic inflammatory diseases such as rheumatoid arthritis and periodontal disease, it has been suggested that interleukin-1 may play a pathogenetic role in some patients with osteoporosis. Pacifici et al. (71,72) have shown that unseparated peripheral blood mononuclear cells in patients with osteoporosis produce interleukin-1β in large amounts constitutively when examined in vitro. These investigators also found that patients treated with estrogen had a significant reduction in interleukin-1 production by the isolated peripheral blood monocytes. This work is controversial, however, because not all investigators have been able to reproduce the findings (73).

INTERLEUKIN-6

The cytokine interleukin-6 (IL-6) is a 26 kD polypeptide with pleotropic biological activities, some of which include the regulation of hematopoiesis and the host response to infection, inflammation, and malignancy (74). Interleukin-6 is produced by a variety of cells including T cells, monocytes, fibroblasts, and osteoblasts. Secretion of IL-6 by osteoblasts is induced by interleukin-1, PTH, TNF, and other osteotropic factors (75,76).

Effects of Interleukin-6 on Bone

Recent evidence suggests a role for IL-6 in the formation of osteoclasts (77–79). IL-6 acts on osteoclast progenitors to stimulate proliferation and formation of osteoclasts as well as on mature cells to stimulate osteoclastic bone resorption (55,80). Chinese hamster ovarian cells transfected with IL-6 cause hypercalcemia and increased bone loss when inoculated into nude mice (81).

IL-6 is produced by cells in the microenvironment of bone. For example, although resting osteoblasts produce little or no IL-6, IL-6 production is increased in a dose-dependent fashion in cultures treated with PTH (10^{-10}–10^{-7} M) (75). Production of IL-6 by cells of the osteoblast lineage can be enhanced by osteotropic factors such as interleukin-1, TNF, $1,25(OH)_2D_3$, and PTH (75). IL-6 is also produced by organ cultures of bone that have been stimulated with these bone-resorbing factors (75,76).

Stimulation of bone resorption by IL-6 in organ culture, either alone (77,79,82) or in concert with other cytokines (57,79), has been reported by some investigators but not by others (76). The discrepancies in these results may be due to differences in assay techniques or in concentrations of factors studied in the assays. For example, Lowik et al. (77) and Ishimi et al. (79) used bone cultures from embryonic rodents at relatively early stages in gestation. These organ cultures may have contained relatively more precursors in the osteoclast lineage than are present in the more widely used neonatal murine calvarial or fetal rat long bone assays. IL-6 may stimulate bone resorption by stimulating osteoclastogenesis (77,79), at least in part by increasing osteoclast number. Kurihara et al. (78) have shown that IL-6 stimulates the formation of multinucleated cells expressing the osteoclast phenotype in long-term human marrow cultures. These results are consistent with the hypothesis that IL-6 affects predominantly cells early in the osteoclast lineage. To determine interactions between IL-6 and other cytokines, IL-6 and interleukin-1 were studied together in

organ cultures. Concentrations of IL-6 that had no effect alone enhanced the bone-resorbing effects of interleukin-1 and TNF by two orders of magnitude (83). Neutralizing antibodies to IL-6 blocked the bone-resorbing effects of interleukin-1 and TNF in bone organ cultures. These data indicate that the effects of interleukin-1 and TNF on bone are dependent, at least in part, on the production of IL-6. Thus IL-6 appears to have two effects on bone resorption: low doses stimulate the growth and differentiation of osteoclast precursors, while high doses stimulate mature osteoclasts to resorb bone.

IL-6 may mediate some of its effects through the induction of other cytokines. It has been shown to enhance the effects of cytokines such as interleukin-3 and colony-stimulating factors (CSF) on the proliferation of multipotent hematopoietic progenitors (84). It may be significant that IL-6 shares some sequence homology (26%) with granulocyte-CSF (G-CSF).

Interleukin-6 in Hypercalcemia of Malignancy

IL-6 may play an important role in the pathophysiology of a number of paraneoplastic syndromes associated with solid tumors and with myeloma, including hypercalcemia. IL-6 has been demonstrated in most human tumors (85). Elevated IL-6 levels have been associated particularly with myeloma (86), in which it is likely to serve as a paracrine growth factor (86,87). Bataille et al. (86) have found that circulating concentrations of IL-6 are increased in patients with myeloma and particularly in those with very markedly increased tumor cell burdens, such as those occurring in plasma cell leukemia. In one patient, hypercalcemia was temporarily reversed by passive inoculation with IL-6 neutralizing antibodies (88). It is not clear whether the major effect in this study was on the tumor cells or on calcium metabolism, but these provocative results are of great interest. Recently, Yoneda et al. (89) have shown that neutralizing antibodies to IL-6 can lower serum calcium in hypercalcemic nude mice bearing a human squamous cell carcinoma expressing IL-6.

To determine if tumor-derived IL-6 can cause hypercalcemia, we have used CHO cells that were transfected with the cDNA for murine IL-6 (CHO/IL-6) and stably express this cytokine (81). We injected nude mice with these tumors and injected other nude mice to serve as controls with CHO cells that had not been transfected with IL-6 (CHO/−). The mice carrying tumors bearing CHO cells expressing IL-6 developed hypercalcemia in proportion to their circulating IL-6 levels and showed evidence of trabecular bone loss. Additionally, the CHO-IL-6 mice developed cachexia, thrombocytosis, and leukocytosis (Fig. 2), which were

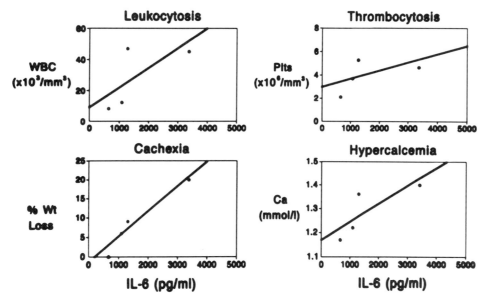

FIG. 2. Relationship between concentrations of IL-6 in serum of mice bearing CHO tumors expressing IL-6 and leukocytosis, cachexia, thrombocytosis, and hypercalcemia.

associated with rising IL-6 levels (81). These features associated with IL-6 could be abrogated by injections of IL-6 antibodies. The data indicate that tumor production of IL-6 may cause hypercalcemia, increased bone resorption, and other paraneoplastic syndromes. However, they do not identify whether the mechanism of action of IL-6 is direct or indirect. CHO tumor cells themselves do not produce interleukin-1 or TNF. To determine if there are important interactions between IL-6 and other cytokines, we inoculated mice bearing small CHO/IL-6 tumors with small amounts of interleukin-1. The mice bearing these tumors exhibited a marked increase in blood ionized calcium. Similar amounts of interleukin-1 had no effect of mice carrying CHO tumors not transfected with IL-6 (81). The data suggest synergistic effects between IL-6 and interleukin-1 causing hypercalcemia.

Interleukin-6 in Bone Disorders Other Than Hypercalcemia of Malignancy

Interleukin-6 may be an important mediator of bone resorption in other disease states, such as rheumatoid arthritis and periodontal disease, where bone resorption is associated with accumulations of chronic inflammatory cells (90). IL-6 has been found in the synovial fluid of patients with rheumatoid arthritis and other inflammatory arthritides (91). Recent evidence suggests that IL-6 may be involved in bone loss associated with estrogen deficiency. Girasole et al. (92) suggested that IL-6 production by bone cells may be

inhibited by estrogens. Later, this group showed that the bone loss in rodents associated with oophorectomy could be abrogated both by estrogen treatment and by neutralizing antibodies to IL-6 (93).

Goldring and coworkers (94) have reported that stromal cell elements from giant cell tumors of bone produce IL-6 and that interleukin-1 enhances production of IL-6 by these cells. Ohsaki et al. (95) used giant cells from giant cell tumors as a model to examine the role that IL-6 may play in osteoclastic bone resorption. They found that conditioned media from cultures of highly purified giant cells contained large amounts of IL-6. The giant cells expressed IL-6 mRNA and IL-6 receptors. In addition, the tumor stromal cells expressed IL-6 mRNA and very high amounts of IL-6. The formation of resorption lacunae on sperm whale dentine was blocked with neutralizing antibodies to IL-6. These data suggest an autocrine/paracrine role for IL-6 in the enhanced bone resorption induced by giant cell tumors of bone.

Roodman et al. (96) have shown also that IL-6 may play an important role in Paget's disease of bone. They showed that conditioned media from long-term bone marrow cultures obtained from patients with Paget's disease stimulated osteoclast-like multinucleated cell formation in normal marrow cultures and that at least part of this activity could be due to IL-6. Additionally, they showed that seven of eight bone marrow plasma samples taken from involved bones and 18 of 27 peripheral blood serum samples from Paget's disease patients had high levels of IL-6. Normal marrow plasma and peripheral blood serum had very low or absent levels of IL-6. The authors suggested that IL-6 produced by marrow and/or bone cells in patients with Paget's disease may be an autocrine/paracrine factor for pagetic osteoclasts and may in part be responsible for the increased osteoclast formation characteristically seen in the disease.

Recently, Strassmann et al. (97) found evidence for the involvement of IL-6 in the cachexia of cancer. They used C-26.IVX, a cell line derived from murine colon-26 adenocarcinoma. This cell line creates tumors that are readily transplantable and induce true cachexia in syngeneic hosts. The development or cachexia correlated with increasing IL-6 levels in the tumor-bearing mice, similar to our reported findings (81). Resection of the tumor by inoculation with monoclonal antibodies to murine IL-6 halted or prevented the development of cachexia. No TNF was detected in the tumors, and antimurine TNF antibodies were not able to decrease the cachexia significantly. Thus the evidence is strong that IL-6 mediates cancer cachexia in this model.

There is increasing evidence of an important role for IL-6 in many examples of pathologic bone resorption, and the elucidation of its role within the complex microenvironment of bone cells may provide information essential to our understanding of bone remodeling. The observation that IL-6 production by bone cells and by bone cultures may be regulated by osteotropic hormones also suggests that IL-6 could play an important physiological role in bone cell metabolism.

TUMOR NECROSIS FACTOR-α AND LYMPHOTOXIN

Tumor necrosis factor-α and lymphotoxin (TNFβ) are two closely related cytokines, which have equivalent effects on bone. They are both 18 kD peptides with considerable amino acid sequence homology. Both have been purified, cloned, and expressed in *Escherichia coli* (98,99). Both factors are multifunctional cytokines which are produced by activated monocytes or macrophages or by activated lymphocytes and lymphoid cell lines, respectively. Although they have separate single copy genes, they share the same receptor mechanism. Both molecules have identical overlapping biological effects, particularly on tumor cells, where they may either enhance or inhibit cell proliferation.

Effects of Tumor Necrosis Factor on Bone

Tumor necrosis factor has powerful effects on calcium metabolism and bone cell function. It increases the proliferation of osteoclast progenitors, stimulates differentiation of committed progenitors to form mature osteoclasts (55), and indirectly activates mature osteoclasts to form resorption lacunae (80). This effect was first shown in fetal rat long bones (100) and was later confirmed in neonatal mouse calvariae (101). The effects of TNF and TNFβ on bone organ cultures appear to be mediated through prostaglandins, since they can be blocked by inhibitors of prostaglandin synthesis (101).

Tumor Necrosis Factor in Hypercalcemia of Malignancy

Several lines of evidence indicate that TNF causes hypercalcemia in vivo (101,102). This has been demonstrated by repeated injections of TNF into normal mice (101) and by expression of TNF in CHO cells that have been transfected with the human TNF gene and inoculated into nude mice (102). Histology of bones from mice bearing CHO cells transfected with the TNF gene revealed a marked increase in osteoclastic bone resorption. These mice also became extremely cachectic. TNF inhibits lipoprotein lipase in vitro and has been linked to the cachexia associated with malignancy and chronic infections (103). TNF also appears to be a mediator of endotoxic shock (104).

Unlike TGFα, interleukin-1α, or IL-6, TNF is not commonly produced by solid tumors. However, it still may play an important role in the pathophysiology of some paraneoplastic syndromes, such as hypercalcemia and cachexia, because it is produced in excessive amounts by normal host cells. An important role for TNF production by host cells in the hypercalcemia associated with a human tumor has been clearly shown in the MH-85 squamous cell carcinoma of the maxilla (105,106). Tissue from this tumor, which was associated with hypercalcemia, leukocytosis, and cachexia in the patient, was explanted and inoculated into nude mice. Nude mice developed a transplantable tumor of the human cells associated with the same paraneoplastic features as those seen in the patient, namely, hypercalcemia, leukocytosis, and cachexia. When the tumor cells were established in continuous cell culture, they were also able to produce similar tumors in nude mice, with hypercalcemia, leukocytosis, and cachexia. We found that tumor-bearing nude mice had a fourfold increase in circulating concentrations of TNF but that the tumor cells themselves did not produce TNF. Working with the hypothesis that TNF was produced by host cells stimulated by the presence of the tumor, and that these host cells most likely were immune cells, Yoneda et al. (105) demonstrated that monocytes, macrophages, spleen cells, and cultured U937 human monocytic cells produced TNF following incubation with supernatant media harvested from the MH-85 tumor cell cultures. This supernatant media was partially purified, and the TNF-inducing factor was found to be a peptide factor that could not be ascribed to either granulocyte macrophage-CSF (GM-CSF) or IL-6. Furthermore, Yoneda et al. (106) found that removal of the spleen (a major source of immune cells in the nude mouse) from tumor-bearing nude mice led to a reduction in cachexia, leukocytosis, and, most significantly, hypercalcemia. Inoculation of hypercalcemic tumor-bearing mice with neutralizing antibodies to TNF also decreased blood ionized calcium (Fig. 3). These results show that, in this model of the hypercalcemia of malignancy caused by a human tumor, tumor cells stimulate normal host cells to produce TNF and that TNF is in turn responsible for some of the paraneoplastic syndromes associated with the tumor, including hypercalcemia.

The paraneoplastic syndromes of cachexia and hypercalcemia have also been demonstrated in other hypercalcemic tumor models, the rat Leydig tumor, and the A375 human melanoma (108,109). In these models, TNF is not produced by tumor cells, but rather tumor cells producing systemic mediators stimulate host immune cells to produce TNF. In nude mice bearing

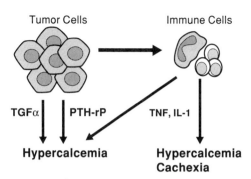

FIG. 4. Hypothesis for production of bone resorbing cytokines by normal immune cells in hypercalcemia of malignancy. (Reprinted from ref. 23 with permission.)

these tumors, TNF is increased at least four-fold in the circulation. In the A375 tumor, TNF production is induced by tumor cell production of CSF for the granulocyte-macrophage series (CSF-GM) (109). In the MH-85 tumor, CSF-GM and an apparently novel factor, TNF-inducing factor, are responsible for TNF production (107). It appears unlikely that TNF production by the tumor cells themselves is a cause of hypercalcemia of malignancy. Figure 4 shows a model for cytokine production by host cells contributing to hypercalcemia in conjunction with factors such as PTHrP and TGFα produced directly by tumor cells.

TNFβ (lymphotoxin) may play an important pathophysiological role in multiple myeloma. Using several myeloma cell lines derived from the myeloma cells of a patient who had osteolytic bone lesions and hypercalcemia, Garrett et al. (110) found that most of the bone-resorbing activity present in the culture media from this cell line could be inhibited by neutralizing antibodies to the cytokine lymphotoxin. They could not detect interleukin-1 in the cell culture media and concluded that the major bone-resorbing activity produced by human myeloma cell lines in established culture was lymphotoxin rather than interleukin-1β. Production of other cytokines such as interleukin-1 and IL-6 by other cells (such as marrow cells) may also be important in the osteoclastic bone resorption of myeloma. TNF, like interleukin-1 and IL-6, is probably involved in chronic inflammatory diseases, such as rheumatoid arthritis and periodontal disease, where it accumulates in the inflammatory fluids.

PROSTAGLANDINS AND OTHER ARACHIDONIC ACID METABOLITES

The prostaglandins are 20-carbon unsaturated fatty acids possessing a cyclopentane ring structure. They are one of a group of biologically active arachidonic acid metabolites, some of which have been implicated

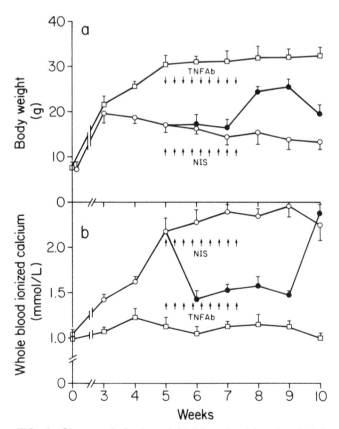

FIG. 3. Changes in body weight (**a**) and calcium levels (**b**) before and after injection of TNF Ab into MH-85-bearing (TNF-secreting) nude mice. □, Nontumor-bearing animals; ○, MH-85 tumor-bearing mice treated with nonimmune serum (NIS); ●, MH-85 tumor-bearing nude mice treated with TNF Ab. (Reprinted from ref. 107 with permission.)

as modulators of bone cell function. Arachidonic acid metabolites are produced by immune cells, by marrow cells, and by bone cells in the bone microenvironment. As is noted below, they are often produced locally in bone after treatment with peptide cytokines and growth factors.

Effects of Prostaglandins on Bone

Prostaglandins of the E series have long been implicated as bone-resorbing factors in many chronic inflammatory conditions, such as rheumatoid arthritis and periodontal disease. They are increased in the inflammatory fluids in patients with these conditions, and patients often obtain symptomatic relief by using prostaglandin inhibitors.

Klein and Raisz (111) first identified prostaglandins of the E series as stimulators of osteoclastic bone resorption. They tested their effects in fetal rat long bone organ cultures and demonstrated that prostaglandins were slow-acting but potent mediators of osteoclastic bone resorption in this organ culture system. Prostaglandins produced similar effects in neonatal calvarial cultures (112). They also enhance multinucleated cell formation in murine marrow cultures (113). However, the studies of Chenu et al. (114) revealed that prostaglandins of the E series are inhibitors of multinucleated cell formation in human marrow cultures. Roodman et al. (115) also did not show any stimulatory effects of prostaglandins of the E series on multinucleated cell formation in a baboon marrow culture system. Chenu et al. (114) postulated that the differences between the effects of prostaglandins of the E series in rodent and primate systems may be due to differences in the cellular composition of the marrow cultures. Prostaglandins mediate local effects on bone resorption but are probably not major mediators of systemic effects. Large systemic infusions of prostaglandins of the E series have caused mild elevations in the serum calcium, but only when enormous doses have been administered, which appear incompatible with either physiological or pathological situations (116).

Although prostaglandins of the E series stimulate bone resorption in organ culture systems, they cause transient contraction of osteoclast cell membranes, a phenomenon that has been associated with inhibition of bone resorption (117). However, this effect is transient, and the overall effect of prostaglandins on bone resorption is stimulatory. Prostaglandins of the E series have been shown to have both inhibitory and stimulatory effects on bone-forming cells in vitro (118). However, local administration is associated with a net increase in periosteal bone formation (119,120).

The effects of growth factors causing generation of prostaglandins depend on the bone organ culture system employed. Prostaglandin generation is more common in neonatal mouse calvariae than in fetal rat long bones. Growth factors such as the transforming growth factors stimulate bone resorption in fetal rat long bones by a nonprostaglandin-mediated mechanism but stimulate bone resorption in the neonatal mouse calvarial system via a prostaglandin-mediated mechanism (19,20,121,122).

Prostaglandins in Hypercalcemia of Malignancy

Tashjian et al. (112,123) provided evidence that prostaglandins may be important in the hypercalcemia associated with two animal models of the hypercalcemia of malignancy, the HSDM-1 mouse fibrosarcoma and the VX-2 rabbit carcinosarcoma. In both models, prostaglandins of the E series and hypercalcemia were produced by cultured tumor cells and inhibited by treatment of the animals with indomethacin. Some human tumors (e.g., breast cancer) are known to produce large amounts of prostaglandins in vitro. Prostaglandins were thus implicated as agents responsible for human hypercalcemia of malignancy. Several case reports of the successful use of indomethacin in the hypercalcemia of malignancy supported this notion (124). Seyberth et al. (125) reported successful treatment with indomethacin of patients with humoral hypercalcemia of malignancy who had increased urinary excretion of a metabolite of prostaglandins of the E series prior to treatment. However, the fall in serum calcium in these patients was unimpressive and difficult to distinguish from the effects that could be anticipated from volume expansion alone. Powles et al. (126) and Bennett et al. (127) showed that freshly isolated breast cancer cells contained large amounts of prostaglandins of the E series, which caused bone resorption when cocultured with organ cultures of neonatal mouse calvariae. However, in a follow-up study, Powles et al. (128) found that indomethacin had little effect on osteolytic bone destruction in the treatment of patients with metastatic breast cancer. Valentin et al. (129) found that both estrogens and antiestrogens markedly enhanced prostaglandin production and increased the bone-resorbing activity of cultured human breast cancer cells. Thus, prostaglandin production by these compounds may account for the induction or worsening of hypercalcemia in breast cancer patients treated with estrogens or antiestrogens. However, Eilon and Mundy (130) have found that established human breast cancer lines in culture do not release significant amounts of prostaglandins constitutively or cause bone resorption in a similar bioassay. The significance of prostaglandin secretion by breast cancer and the tumor cells in vitro remains uncertain. One problem in interpreting the data is that most cells may be stimulated to release prostaglandins by gentle manipulation such as detachment from tissue culture flasks or dispersal in cell cultures (131).

Mundy et al. (132) reported that treatment of humoral hypercalcemia of malignancy with indomethacin is usually ineffective. Since indomethacin profoundly inhibits prostaglandin synthesis in vivo, it is unlikely that prostaglandins are commonly involved in humoral hypercalcemia of malignancy as a major circulating factor. Even when involved, their role may be secondary to that of the primary agents responsible for osteoclastic activation.

It has been recognized for many years that some peptide factors, such as interleukin-1, TNF, EGF, and TGFα, stimulate bone resorption in organ cultures by generating synthesis of prostaglandins in the microenvironment of bone-resorbing cells. Endogenous prostaglandin production has been shown to mediate the bone-resorptive response to a number of different stimuli. Prostaglandins are probably produced in bone by normal cells in response to systemic factors. Serum complement increases prostaglandin E production and resorption in fetal rat long bones (133). Bacterial collagenases, phorbol esters, epidermal, fibroblast, and platelet-derived growth factors have all been found to stimulate bone resorption in mouse calvariae by a prostaglandin-mediated mechanism (134). However, only with interleukin-1 has it been shown that this may be an important phenomenon in vivo (52).

Evidence for Effects of Other Arachidonic Acid Metabolites on Bone

Bone resorption can also be stimulated by less stable precursors of prostaglandins of the E series, including endoperoxides (134,135). Arachidonic acid can also be metabolized by an alternative enzyme system, the lipoxygenase pathway, to produce leukotriene compounds. Some investigators (136,137) have reported bone resorption by leukotrienes in neonatal mouse calvariae, while others have not (138). Meghji et al. (136) reported that leukotrienes stimulate bone resorption at picomolar concentrations compared to prostaglandins, which produce resorption at nanomolar levels. Parker (139) showed that growth factors such as interleukin-1 and interleukin-2 induce production and secretion of leukotrienes. Gallwitz et al. (140) used C433 (stromal) cells derived from a giant cell tumor of bone to study the molecular mechanisms by which osteoclasts are induced to resorb bone. When C433 cells were stimulated with 1,25(OH)$_2$D$_3$ or PMA, they produced eicosanoids whose production was completely inhibited by specific inhibitors of the 5-lipoxygenase pathway. 5-Hydroxyeicosanoid production was confirmed by a number of parameters including gas chromatography/mass spectrometry and radioimmunoassay. Gallwitz et al. concluded that

products of the 5-lipoxygenase pathway produced by stromal cells derived from giant cell tumors of bone had the capacity to activate osteoclast-like cells in giant cell tumors of bone and normal osteoclasts by production of leukotrienes. They postulated that 5-lipoxygenase metabolites may represent a mechanism by which mononuclear stromal cells in human giant cell tumors communicate with giant cells and a possible means by which accessory cells and osteoclasts involved in normal bone resorption communicate. Gallwitz and his associates have also noted the unstable nature of the leukotrienes and have found that special precautions are necessary to maintain biological activity. The unstable nature of leukotrienes may explain why some investigators have not shown leukotriene-induced bone resorption. Recently, Bonewald et al. (141) showed that leukotrienes increased the number of resorption pits by rat osteoclasts on sperm whale dentine as well as bone resorption in organ cultures of neonatal mouse calvariae but not in fetal rat long bones. The bone-resorbing activity released by 1,25(OH)$_2$D$_3$-treated osteoblast-like cells was blocked by an inhibitor of 5-lipoxygenase. This suggests that osteoblastic cells may stimulate osteoclasts in part via production of 5-lipoxygenase metabolites. Mohammed et al. (142) found significant inhibition of tooth movement using the leukotriene inhibitor AA 861, although enhanced levels of prostaglandins remained. They postulated that inhibition of leukotriene synthesis may influence tooth movement and that prostaglandins and leukotrienes may mediate different steps in a series of events that initiates bone remodeling.

Involvement of lipoxygenase metabolites in localized bone destruction associated with inflamed and malignant tissues has been suggested by many investigators. These tissues include rheumatoid synovial tissue (143), inflamed gingival tissue (137), periodontal tissue (144), dental cysts (145), human oral cancers (146), and human bone marrow cells (147) as well as and in chronic myelocytic leukemia (147). It is likely that leukotrienes act as local rather than humoral mediators of bone resorption due to their instability and lack of storage forms in the tissues. Because these compounds are present in the inflammatory fluids of some diseases, they may have an ancillary role in the stimulation of bone resorption in diseases which cause accumulation of chronic inflammatory cells (137,144,148).

VITAMIN D METABOLITES

Although hypercalcemia of malignancy has many similarities to primary hyperparathyroidism, one of the most important differences is in the circulating levels of 1,25(OH)$_2$D. Most patients with hypercalcemia of malignancy have low serum 1,25(OH)₂D levels. In a series of 133 patients with hypercalcemia of malignancy, the mean circulating level of 1,25(OH)₂D was 22.5 pg/ml (normal 20–60 pg/ml) (149). Most of these patients have increased serum PTHrP. In contrast, the mean value in 50 patients with primary hyperparathyroidism was 72 pg/ml. The reason for this is unclear, given the similarities between PTH and PTHrP effects on the skeleton and the kidney.

Strewler et al. (150) have shown that rodent models of humoral hypercalcemia of malignancy (HHM) have increased 1,25(OH)₂D, and human HHM-associated tumors in nude mice also show increased 1,25(OH)₂D, in contrast to what the same tumors do in patients. Strewler et al. have postulated that these differences may reflect differences in receptor subtypes for PTH and PTHrP, tumor-derived inhibitors of renal 1α-hydroxylase, or effects of tumor-caused hypercalcemia on 1α-hydroxylase, the enzyme responsible for production of 1,25(OH)₂D. We believe another possible explanation is that the effects of PTHrP on target organs are modulated by other factors, such as interleukin-1, TGFα, and TNF, which are also produced by the tumors (27). Fukumoto et al. (151) hypothesized that low 1,25(OH)₂D levels may be due to a factor distinct from PTHrP. They purified extracts from tumors in athymic nude rats bearing human uterine cervical cancers and demonstrated two separate fractions, one of which contained parathyroid hormone-like biologic activity and one that suppressed 1α-hydroxylase activity in vitro. The factor that suppressed 1α-hydroxylase activity stimulated cAMP generation in renal tubular cells in vitro.

Increased serum 1,25(OH)₂D₃ levels are associated with the hypercalcemia seen in a few patients with some lymphomas, and in these cases PTH is not increased, and phosphate is not reduced (152–154). This finding contrasts with the vast majority of cases of hypercalcemia of malignancy, which are associated with suppressed 1,25(OH)₂D₃ levels and decreased gastrointestinal calcium absorption. The lymphoid malignancies associated with increased 1,25(OH)₂D₃ concentrations include adult T-cell lymphomas and Hodgkin's disease. Some of the cases of adult T-cell lymphoma have been associated with the human T-cell leukemia virus-1 (HTLV-1) type C retrovirus infections. Lymphoid cells infected with this virus can convert labeled 25-dihydroxyvitamin D to 1,25(OH)₂D in vitro (155). Hypercalcemia is relatively more common in lymphoproliferative disease than it is in patients with solid tumors, although there is some controversy over the relative frequency (156). Hypercalcemia is extremely common in patients with adult T-cell leukemia, developing in 50–100% of patients during the course of their disease (156). In a study involving 4,000 patients at the National Institutes of Health, 10.4% of patients with

lymphoproliferative disease had a plasma calcium > 11 mg/dl (2.75 mmol/liter), whereas in patients with solid tumors the frequency of hypercalcemia was 5.6% (157). Adams et al. (158) studied 16 patients with hypercalcemia and lymphoproliferative disorders prospectively. Eight of these patients (five with HTLV-1) had increased plasma 1,25(OH)₂D₃. In contrast, Motokura et al. (159) studied a large group of patients in Japan with HTLV-1-associated lymphoma and hypercalcemia and found evidence of elevated serum PTHrP (159) but no cases with increased 1,25(OH)₂D.

It is likely that lymphokines are also produced in malignant lymphoma associated with hypercalcemia. T-cell lymphomas produce a wide range of cytokines, and some studies indicate bone resorption by these tumor cells, which may be related to cytokine production (160).

Vitamin D metabolites are rarely if ever important in the pathophysiology of hypercalcemia associated with solid tumors. Although it was once suggested that breast cancer extracts may contain vitamin D-like sterols, this was later refuted (161,162). There is, however, one curious case report of a small cell lung cancer that was shown to produce 1,25(R)-dihydroxyvitamin D (41). This has not been described in any other patients.

PARATHYROID HORMONE

PTH is rarely increased and in fact almost always is suppressed in patients with hypercalcemia of malignancy. If PTH is increased, the patient usually has concomitant primary hyperparathyroidism (164). Tumors associated with hypercalcemia rarely express PTH mRNA (165), and there should be no cross reactivity between PTH and PTHrP in current radioimmunoassays. However, there have been several reported cases of nonparathyroid tumors producing PTH. Documented cases in which PTH is expressed in a nonparathyroid tumor include a small cell lung cancer (166), a primitive neuroectodermal tumor (167), and an ovarian carcinoma (168) (Table 3). Yoshimoto et al. (165) described severe hypercalcemia in a 70-year-old man who had a small cell carcinoma of the

TABLE 3. *Ectopic parathyroid hormone production by tumors*

1. Small cell lung cancer
   (Yoshimoto et al., 1989)
2. Primitive neuroectodermal tumor
   (Strewler et al., 1990)
3. Ovarian cancer
   (Nussbaum et al., 1990)

lung with multiple metastases. Elevated PTH levels were confirmed by three different PTH assays. There were substantial amounts of PTH in a liver metastasis, and PTH mRNA was expressed in the tumor. No PTHrP was detected in the blood or tumor. The parathyroid glands were histologically normal. No amplification of the PTH gene was detected in the tumor, suggesting that the ectopic transcription of PTH by the tumor cells may have resulted from loss or disruption of normal regulatory elements for the PTH gene or that an unknown factor(s) coded by a gene other than the PTH gene activated the transcription of the PTH gene. Strewler et al. (166) documented a case of ectopic PTH production associated with severe hypercalcemia in a malignant small cell tumor of primitive neuroectodermal origin in a 60-year-old man who presented in coma and had lytic lesions of the scapula and pelvis. Intact PTH levels were markedly elevated by a specific immunoradiometric assay (IRMA), and four normal parathyroid glands were identified. Northern analysis revealed strong expression of the hPTH gene and weak expression of the hPTHrP gene in the tumor. There was no evidence of a major clonal rearrangement of the hPTH gene. Serum levels of PTHrP were judged sufficient to cause hypercalcemia, but the authors believed that it was likely that secretion of PTH also played a role in the causation of the hypercalcemia. Nussbaum et al. (167) described the ectopic production of PTH associated with profound hypercalcemia in a woman with ovarian carcinoma. The presence of elevated PTH was confirmed by IRMA, a much higher serum PTH level in the tumor's venous effluent than in peripheral blood, an immediate decline in the serum PTH level and reversal of hypercalcemia after tumor resection, production of PTH by the cancer cells in culture, and elevated PTH mRNA in the tumor. Unlike the case in the patients previously described, a DNA rearrangement in the region of the promoter of the ectopically expressed PTH gene was present. In addition, the rearranged region was amplified, and this presumably led to overexpression of PTH by the tumor. Precisely how PTH overexpression occurred, whether by removal of negative regulatory elements or through the presence of positive regulatory elements in strategic positions, is unclear.

CONCLUSIONS

Many different tumor-derived and host-derived factors other than PTHrP, can cause hypercalcemia. These factors are likely to be important not only in those tumors in which PTHrP is not produced but also in these tumors in which PTHrP is produced. In addition to their potential even in causing or in fostering the development of hypercalcemia in malignancy, these factors may also be important particularly in local bone destruction associated with solid tumors and in other pathologic circumstances, such as chronic inflammatory diseases, Paget's disease, and osteoporosis. Insights into mechanisms by which these bone-active factors regulate osteoclast activity in abnormal circumstances should enhance our understanding of mechanisms of normal bone remodeling.

ACKNOWLEDGMENTS

The authors are grateful to Thelma Barrios for her excellent secretarial help. Work described in this review was supported in part by grants CA-40035, RR-013646, AR-07465, AR-39529, DE-08569, DK-45229, AR-28149 from the NIH and a Veterans Administration Merit Award. K.S.B. is a Research Associate of the Veterans Administration Hospital.

REFERENCES

1. Yates AJP, Gutierrez GE, Smolens P, et al. Effects of synthetic peptide of a parathyroid hormone-related protein on calcium homeostasis, renal tubular calcium reabsorption and bone metabolism in vivo and in vitro in rodents. *J Clin Invest* 1988;81:932–938.
2. Horiuchi N, Caulfield JP, Fisher JE, et al. Similarity of synthetic peptide from human tumor to parathyroid hormone in vivo and in vitro. *Science* 1987;238:1566–1568.
3. Kemp BE, Moseley JM, Rodda CP, et al. Parathyroid hormone-related protein of malignancy: active synthetic fragments. *Science* 1987;238:1568–1570.
4. Burtis WJ, Brady TG, Orloff J, et al. Immunochemical characterization of circulating parathyroid hormone-related protein in patients with humoral hypercalcemia of cancer. *N Engl J Med* 1990;322:1106–1112.
5. Henderson JE, Shustic C, Kremer R, Rabbani S, Hendy G, Goltzman D. Circulating concentrations of parathyroid hormone-like peptide in malignancy and in hyperparathyroidism. *J Bone Mineral Res* 1990;5:105–113.
6. Budayr AA, Nissenson RA, Klein RF, et al. Increased serum levels of a parathyroid hormone-like protein in malignancy-associated hypercalcemia. *Ann Intern Med* 1989;111:807–812.
7. Wills MR, McGowan GK. Plasma chloride levels in hyperparathyroidism and other hypercalcemic states. *Br Med J* 1964;1:1153–1156.
8. Guise TA, Chirgwin JM, Favarato G, Boyce BF, Mundy GR. Chinese hamster ovarian cells transfected with human parathyroid hormone-related protein cDNA cause hypercalcemia in nude mice. *Lab Invest* 1992;67:477–485.
9. Guise TA, Garrett IR, Bonewald LF, Mundy GR. The interleukin-1 receptor antagonist inhibits hypercalcemia mediated by interleukin-1. *J Bone Mineral Res* 1993;8:583–588.
10. Marquardt H, Todaro GJ. Human transforming growth factor: production by a melanoma cell line, purification, and initial characterization. *J Biol Chem* 1982;257:5220–5225.
11. Marquardt H, Hunkapiller MW, Hood LE, Todaro GJ. Rat transforming growth factor type I: Structure and relation to epidermal growth factor. *Science* 1984;223:1079–1082.

12. Lee DC, Rose TM, Webb NR, Todaro GJ. Cloning and sequence analysis of a cDNA for rat transforming growth factor α. *Nature* 1985;313:489–491.

13. Derynck R, Roberts AB, Winkler ME, Chen EY, Goeddel D. Human transforming growth factor α: Precursor structure and expression in E. coli. *Cell* 1984;38:287–297.

14. Bringman TS, Lindquist PB, Derynck R. Different transforming growth factor-alpha species are derived from a glycosylated and palmitoylated transmembrane precursor. *Cell* 1987;48:429–440.

15. Twardzik DR, Ranchalis JE, Todaro GJ. Mouse embryonic transforming growth factors related to those isolated from tumor cells. *Cancer Res* 1982;42:590–593.

16. Massague J. Transforming growth factor alpha. A model for membrane-anchored growth factors. *J Biol Chem* 1990; 265:21393–21396.

17. Yates AJ, Favarato G, Aufdemorte TB, et al. Expression of human transforming growth factor α by Chinese hamster ovarian tumors in nude mice causes hypercalcemia and increased osteoclastic bone resorption. *J Bone Mineral Res* 1992;7:847–853.

18. Takahashi N, MacDonald BR, Hon J, Mundy GR, Roodman GD. Recombinant human transforming growth factor alpha stimulates the formation of osteoclast-like cells in long-term human marrow cultures. *J Clin Invest* 1986;78:894–898.

19. Ibbotson KJ, Twardzik DR, D'Souza SM, Hargreaves WR, Todaro GJ, Mundy GR. Stimulation of bone resorption in vitro by synthetic transforming growth factor-alpha. *Science* 1985;228:1007–1009.

20. Ibbotson KJ, Harrod J, Gowen M, D'Souza SM, Smith DD, Mundy GR. Human recombinant transforming growth factor alpha stimulates bone resorption and inhibits formation in vitro. *Proc Natl Acad Sci USA* 1986;83:2228–2232.

21. Tashjian AH, Voelkel EF, Loyd W, Derynck R, Winkler M, Levine L. Actions of growth factors on plasma calcium. *J Clin Invest* 1986;78:1405–1409.

22. Stern PH, Krieger NS, Nissenson RA, et al. Human transforming growth factor alpha stimulates bone resorption in vitro. *J Clin Invest* 1985;76:2016–2020.

23. Mundy GR. Malignancy and hypercalcemia—humoral hypercalcemia of malignancy, hypercalcemia associated with osteolytic metastases. In: Dunitz, M, ed. *Calcium homeostasis: hypercalcemia and hypocalcemia,* London: Martin Dunitz, 1990;69–99.

24. Gutierrez GE, Mundy GR, Derynck R, Hewlett E, Katz MS. Inhibition of parathyroid hormone-responsive adenylate cyclase in clonal osteoblast-like cells by transforming growth factor α and epidermal growth factor. *J Biol Chem* 1987; 262:15845–15850.

25. Pizurki L, Rizzoli R, Caverzasio J, Bonjour J. Stimulation by parathyroid hormone-related protein and transforming growth factor α of phosphate transport in osteoblast-like cells. *J Bone Mineral Res* 1991;6:1235–1241.

26. Pizurki L, Rizzoli R, Caverzasio J, Bonjour J. Effect of transforming growth factor α and parathyroid hormone-related protein on phosphate transport in renal cells. *Am J Physiol* 1990;259:F929–F935.

27. Guise TA, Yoneda T, Yates AJ, Mundy GR. The combined effect of tumor-produced parathyroid hormone-related protein and transforming growth factor α enhance hypercalcemia in vivo and bone resorption in vitro. *J Clin Endocrinol Metab* (in press).

28. Yates AJP, Gutierrez GE, Smolens P, et al. Effects of a synthetic peptide of a parathyroid hormone-related protein on calcium homeostasis, renal tubular calcium reabsorption and bone metabolism. *J Clin Invest* 1988;81:932–938.

29. Ibbotson KJ, D'Souza SM, Smith DD, Carpenter G, Mundy GR. EGF receptor antiserum inhibits bone resorbing activity produced by a rat Leydig cell tumor associated with the humoral hypercalcemia of malignancy. *Endocrinology* 1985; 116:469–471.

30. Gutierrez GE, Mundy GR, Derynck R, Hewlett KL, Katz MS: Inhibition of parathyroid hormone-responsive adenylate cyclase in clonal osteoblast-like cells by transforming growth factor alpha and epidermal growth factor. *J Biol Chem* 1987;262:15845–15850.

31. Merryman JI, Rosol TJ, Brooks CL, Capen CC. Separation of parathyroid hormone-like activity from transforming growth factor-α and -β in the canine adenocarcinoma (CAC-8) model of humoral hypercalcemia of malignancy. *Endocrinology* 1989;124:2456–2463.

32. Insogna KL, Stewart AF, Morris CA, Hough L, Milstone L, Centrella M: Native and a synthetic analogue of the malignancy-associated parathyroid hormone-like protein have in vitro transforming growth factor-like properties. *J Clin Invest* 1989;83:1057–1060.

33. Gomella LG, Sargent ER, Wace TP, Anglarc P, Linehan WM, Kasio A. Expression of transforming growth factor alpha in normal human adult kidney and enhanced expression of transforming growth factors alpha and beta 1 in renal cell carcinoma. *Cancer Res* 1989;49:6972–6975.

34. Derynck R, Goeddel DV, Ullrich A, et al. Synthesis of messenger RNAs for transforming growth factors alpha and beta and the epidermal growth factor receptor by human tumors. *Cancer Res* 1987;47:707–712.

35. Smith JJ, Derynck R, Korc M. Production of transforming growth factor alpha in human pancreatic cancer cells: evidence for a superagonist autocrine cycle. *Proc Natl Acad Sci USA* 1987;84:7567–7570.

36. Arteaga CL, Hanauske AR, Clark GM, et al. Immunoreactive alpha transforming growth factor activity in effusions from cancer patients as a marker of tumor burden and patient prognosis. *Cancer Res* 1988;48:5023–5028.

37. Hanauske AR, Arteaga CL, Clark GM, et al. Determination of transforming growth factor activity in effusions from cancer patients. *Cancer* 1988;61:1832–1837.

38. Mundy GR, Ibbotson KJ, D'Souza SM: Tumor products and the hypercalcemia of malignancy. *J Clin Invest* 1985;76:391–395.

39. Lippman ME, Dickson RB, Bates S, et al. Autocrine and paracrine growth regulation of human breast cancer. *Breast Cancer Res Treat* 1986;7:59–70.

40. Salomon DS, Kidwell WR, Liu S. Presence of alpha TGF mRNA in human breast cancer cell lines and in human breast carcinomas. *Breast Cancer Res Treat* 1986;8:106A.

41. Galasko CSB, Burn JI. Hypercalcemia in patients with advanced mammary cancer. *Br Med J* 1971;3:573–577.

42. Sabatini M, Boyce B, Aufdemorte T, Bonewald L, Mundy GR. Infusions of recombinant human interleukins 1α and 1β cause hypercalcemia in normal mice. *Proc Natl Acad Sci USA* 1988;85:5235–5239.

43. Eastgate JA, Simons JA, Wood NC, Grinlenton TM, DiGiovine FS, Duff GW. Correlation of plasma interleukin-1 levels with disease activity in rheumatoid arthritis. *Lancet* 1988;2:706–709.

44. Elias JA, Chien P, Gustilo KM, Schreiber AD. Differential interleukin-1 elaboration by density-defined human monocyte subpopulations. *Blood* 1985;66:298–301.

45. Dinarello CA. Biology of interleukin-1. *FASEB J* 1988;2:108–115.

46. Lepe-Zuniga B, Gerg I. Production of intracellular and extracellular interleukin-1 by human monocytes. *Clin Immunol Immunopathol* 1984;31:222–230.

47. Watsuskina K, Tagusk M, Kovacs EV, Young HA, Oppenheim JJ. Intracellular localization of human monocyte-associated interleukin-1 activity and release of biologically active IL-1 from monocytes by trypsin and plasmin. *J Immunol* 1987;136:2883–2891.

48. Gowen M, Wood DD, Ihrie EJ, McGurie MK, Russell RG. An interleukin-1-like factor stimulates bone resorption in vitro. *Nature* 1983;306:378–381.

49. Heath JK, Saklatvala J, Meikle MC, Atkinson SJ, Reynolds JJ. Pig interleukin-1 (catabolin) is a potent stimulator of bone resorption in vitro. *Calcif Tissue Int* 1985;37:95–97.

50. Gowen M, Mundy GR. Actions of recombinant interleukin-1, interleukin-2 and interferon gamma on bone resorption in vivo. *J Immunol* 1986;136:2478–2482.

51. Dewhirst FE, Stashenko PP, Mole JE, Tsurumachi T. Puri-

fication and partial sequence of human osteoclast-activating factor: identity with interleukin-1 beta. *J Immunol* 1985; 135:2562–2568.

52. Boyce BR, Aufdemorte TB, Garrett IR, Yates AJP, Mundy GR. Effects of interleukin-1 on bone turnover in normal mice. *Endocrinology* 1989;125:1142–1150.

53. Boyce BR, Yates AJP, Mundy GR. Bolus injections of recombinant human interleukin-1 cause transient hypocalcemia in normal mice. *Endocrinology* 1989;125:2780–2783.

54. Mundy GR. Bone resorbing cells. In: Favus MJ, ed. *Primer on the metabolic bone disease and disorders of mineral metabolism,* 2nd Ed. New York: Raven Press; 1993:25–32.

55. Pfeilshifter J, Chenu C, Bird A, Mundy GR, Roodman GD. Interleukin-1 and tumor necrosis factor stimulate the formation of human osteoclast-like cells in vitro. *J Bone Mineral Res* 1989;4:113–118.

56. Thomson BM, Laklatvala J, Chambers T. Osteoblasts mediate interleukin-1 stimulation of bone resorption by rat osteoclasts. *J Exp Med* 1986;164:104–112.

57. Garrett IR, Black KS, Mundy GR. Interactions between interleukin-6 and interleukin-1 in osteoclastic bone resorption in neonatal mouse calvariae. *Calcif Tissue Int* 1990;46(Suppl 1):140A.

58. Fried RM, Voelkel EF, Rice RH, Levine L, Gaffney EV, Tashjian AH Jr. Two squamous cell carcinomas not associated with humoral hypercalcemia produce a potent bone resorption-stimulating factor which is interleukin-1α. *Endocrinology* 1989;125:742–751.

59. Sato K, Fujii Y, Kasono K, et al. Parathyroid hormone-related protein and interleukin-1α synergistically stimulate bone resorption in vitro and increase the serum calcium concentration in mice in vivo. *Endocrinology* 1989;124:2172–2178.

60. Garrett IR, Guise TA, Bonewald LF, Chizzonite R, Mundy GR. Evidence that interleukin-1 mediates its effects on bone resorption via the 80 kilodalton interleukin-1 receptor. *Calcif Tissue Int* 1993;52:438–444.

61. Arend WP, Joslin GF, Thompson RC, Hannum CH. An IL-1 inhibitor from human monocytes. Production and characterization of biologic preperties. *J Immunol* 1989;15:1851–1858.

62. Carter DB, Deibel MR, Dunn CJ, et al. Purification, cloning expression and biological characterization of an IL-1 receptor antagonist protein. *Nature* 1990;344:633–638.

63. Hannum CH, Wilcox CJ, Arend WP, et al. Purification, sequencing, and characterization of a human monocyte-derived interleukin-1 receptor antagonist (IL-1Ra). In: Oppenheim JJ, Powanda MC, Kluger MJ, Dinarello CA, eds. *Molecular and cellular biology of cytokines.* New York: Wiley-Liss, 1990;10A:287–292.

64. Eisenberg SP, Evans RJ, Brewer MT, et al. Sequencing, and expression of the cDNA for the human interleukin-1 receptor antagonist, IL-1Ra: Primary structure and functional expression from complementary DNA of a human interleukin-1 receptor antagonist. In: Oppenheim JJ, Powanda MC, Kluger MJ, Dinarello CA, eds. *Molecular and cellular biology of cytokines.* New York: Wiley-Liss, 1990;10A:293–298.

65. Seckinger P, Kaufmann MT, Dayer JM. An interleukin-1 inhibitor affects both cell-associated interleukin-1-induced T-cell proliferation and PGE$_2$ collagenase production by human dermal fibroblasts and synovial cells. *Immunobiology* 1990;180:316–327.

66. Billiau A, Van Dann J, Opdenakker G, Fibbe WE, Falkenburg JHF, Content J. IL-1 as a cytokine inducer. *Immunobiol* 1986;172:323–335.

67. Endres S, Van Der Meer JWM, Dinarello CA. IL-1 in the pathogenesis of fever. Editorial. *Eur J Clin Invest* 1987; 17:469–474.

68. Van Damme J, Cayphas S, Opdenakker G, Billiau A, Van Snick J. IL-1 and poly(rI)·poly(rC) induce production of a hybridoma growth factor by human fibroblasts. *Eur J Immunol* 1987;17:1–7.

69. Cozzolino F, Torcia M, Aldinucci D, et al. Production of in-

terleukin-1 by bone marrow myeloma cells. *Blood* 1989; 75:387–390.

70. Kawano M, Tanaka H, Ishikawa H, et al. Interleukin-1 accelerates autocrine growth of myeloma cells through interleukin-6 in human myeloma. *Blood* 1989;73:2145–2148.

71. Pacifici R, Rifas L, Teitelbaum S, et al. Spontaneous release of interleukin-1 from human blood monocytes reflects bone formation in idiopathic osteoporosis. *Proc Natl Acad Sci USA* 1987;84:4616–4620.

72. Pacifici R, Rifas L, McCracken R, et al. Ovarian steroid treatment blocks a postmenopausal increase in blood monocyte interleukin-1 release. *Proc Natl Acad Sci USA* 1989; 86:2398–2402.

73. Zarrabeitia MT, Riancho JA, Amado JA, Napal J, Gonzalez-macias J. Cytokine production by peripheral blood cells in postmenopausal osteoporosis. *Bone Mineral* 1991;14:161–167.

74. Kishimoto T. The biology of interleukin-6. *Blood* 1989;74:1–10.

75. Feyen JHM, Elford P, Di Padova FE, Trechsel U. Interleukin-6 is produced by bone and modulated by parathyroid hormone. *J Bone Mineral Res* 1989;4:633–638.

76. Al-Humidan A, Ralston S, Hughes D, et al. Interleukin-6 does not stimulate bone resorption in neonatal mouse calvariae. *J Bone Mineral Res* 1991;6:3–8.

77. Lowik C, Van der Pluijm G, Hoekman K, Aarden L, Bijvoet O, Papapoulos S. Parathyroid hormone and PTH-like protein stimulate interleukin-6 production by osteogenic cells: a possible role of interleukin-6 in osteoclastogenesis. *Biochem Biophys Res Commun* 1989;162:1546–1552.

78. Kurihara N, Bertolini D, Suda T, Akiyama Y, Roodman D. IL-6 stimulates osteoclast-like multinucleated cell formation in long term human marrow cultures by inducing IL-1 release. *J Immunol* 1990;144:4226–4230.

79. Ishimi Y, Miyaura C, Kin He C, et al. IL-6 is produced by osteoblasts and induces bone resorption. *J Immunol* 1990;145:3297–3303.

80. Thomson BM, Mundy GR, Chambers TJ. Tumor necrosis factors alpha and beta induce osteoblastic cells to stimulate osteoclastic bone resorption. *J Immunol* 1987;138:775–779.

81. Black K, Garrett IR, Mundy GR. Chinese hamster ovarian cells transfected with the murine interleukin-6 gene cause hypercalcemia as well as cachexia, leukocytosis and thrombocytosis in tumor-bearing nude mice. *Endocrinology* 1991; 128:2657–2659.

82. Linkhart TA, Linkhart SE, Strong D, Baylink DJ. Stimulation of IL-6 by normal human osteoblasts by IL-1 but not by PTH. *Endocrine Soc Abstracts* 1990;184:637A.

83. Black K, Mundy GR, Garrett IR. Tumors producing excessive interleukin-6 cause hypercalcemia in vivo, and interleukin-6 enhances the bone resorbing potency of interleukin-1 and tumor necrosis factor by two orders of magnitude in vitro. *J Bone Mineral Res* 1991;6(Suppl 1):813A.

84. Wong GC, Clark SC. Multiple actions of interleukin-6 within a cytokine network. *Immunol Today* 1988;9:137–139.

85. Tabibzadeh S, Poubouridis D, May L, Sehgal P. IL-6 immunoreactivity in human tumors. *Am J Pathol* 1989; 135:427–433.

86. Bataille R, Jourdan M, Zhang X, Klein B. Serum levels of IL-6, a potential myeloma cell growth factor, as reflection of disease severity in plasma cell dyscrasias. *J Clin Invest* 1989;84:2008–2011.

87. Klein B, Zhang ZG, Jourdan M, Bataille R. Cytokines involved in human multiple myeloma. *Monoclonal Gammapathies II* 1989;12:55–59.

88. Klein B, Wijdenes J, Jourdan M, Boiron J, Sang J, Bataille R. Monoclonal anti-IL-6 antibodies block myeloma cell proliferation in vivo. *Blood* 1991;78(Suppl 1):508A.

89. Yoneda T, Nakai M, Moriyama K, et al. Neutralizing antibodies to human interleukin-6 reverse hypercalcemia associated with a human squamous carcinoma. *Cancer Res* 1993;53:737–740.

90. Mundy GR. Immune system and bone remodeling. *Trends Endocrinol Metab* 1990;1:307–311.

91. Houssiau FA, Devogalaer JP, van Damme J, Nagant de Deuxchiasnes C, Van Snick J. Interleukin-6 in synovial fluid and serum of patients with rheumatoid arthritis and other inflammatory arthritides. *Arthritis Rheum* 1988;31:784–788.

92. Girasole G, Jilka R, Pusseri G, et al. 17β-estradial inhibits interleukin-6 production by bone marrow-derived stromal cells and osteoblasts in vitro: a potential mechanism for the antiosteoporotic effect of estrogens. *J Clin Invest* 1992; 89:883–891.

93. Jilka RL, Hangoc G, Girasole G, et al. Increased osteoclast development after estrogen loss: Mediation by interleukin-6. *Science* 1992;257:88–91.

94. Goldring SR, Kroop SF, Gorn AH, et al. Stromal cells from human giant cell tumors of bone: production of factors involved in recruitment and differentiation of osteoclasts. *J Bone Mineral Res* 1990;5(Suppl 2):79A.

95. Ohsaki Y, Takahashi S, Scarcez T, et al. Evidence for an autocrine/paracrine role for IL-6 in bone resorption by giant cells from giant cell tumors of bone. *Endocrinology* (in press).

96. Roodman GD, Kurihara N, Ohsaki Y, et al. Interleukin 6: a potential autocrine/paracrine factor in Paget's disease of bone. *J Clin Invest* 1992;89:46–52.

97. Strassmann G, Fong M, Kenney JS, Jacob CO. Evidence for the involvement of interleukin 6 in experimental cancer cachexia. *J Clin Invest* 1992;89:1681–1684.

98. Pennica D, Nedwin GE, Hayflick JS, et al. Human tumour necrosis factor: precursor structure expression, and homology to lymphotoxin. *Nature* 1984;312:724–729.

99. Gray PW, Aggarwal BB, Benton CV. Cloning and expression of cDNA for human lymphotoxin or lymphokine with tumor necrosis activity. *Nature* 1984;312:721–724.

100. Bertolini DR, Nedwin GE, Bringman TS, Mundy GR. Stimulation of bone resorption and inhibition of bone formation in vitro by human tumour necrosis factors. *Nature* 1986; 319:516–518.

101. Tashjian AH, Voelkel EF, Lazzaro M, Goad D, Bosma T, Levine L. Tumor necrosis factor α (cachectin) stimulates bone resorption in mouse calvaria via a prostaglandin-mediated mechanism. *Endocrinology* 1987;120:2029–2036.

102. Johnson RA, Boyce BF, Mundy GR, Roodman GD. Tumors producing human TNF induce hypercalcemia and osteoclastic bone resorption in nude mice. *Endocrinology* 1989; 124:1424–1427.

103. Torti FM, Dieckmann B, Beutler B, et al. A macrophage factor inhibits adipocyte gene expression: an in vitro model of cachexia. *Science* 1985;229:867–869.

104. Beutler BA, Milsark IW, Cerami A. Cachectin tumor necrosis factor: production, distribution and metabolic fate in vivo. *J Immunol* 1985;135:3972–3977.

105. Yoneda Y, Aufdemorte TB, Nishimura R, et al. Occurrence of hypercalcemia and leukocytosis with cachexia in a human squamous cell carcinoma of the maxilla in athymic nude mice. A novel experimental model of three concomitant paraneoplastic syndromes. *J Clin Oncol* 1991;9:468–477.

106. Yoneda T, Alsina MM, Chavez JB, Bonewald L, Nishimura R, Mundy GR. Evidence that tumor necrosis factor plays a pathogenetic role in the paraneoplastic syndromes of cachexia, hypercalcemia, and leukocytosis in a human tumor in nude mice. *J Clin Invest* 1991;87:977–985.

107. Yoneda T, Alsina M, Chavez J, Bonewald L, Nishimura R, Mundy G. Evidence that tumor necrosis factor plays a pathogenetic role in the paraneoplastic syndrome of cachexia, hypercalcemia and leukocytosis in a human tumor in nude mice. *J Clin Invest* 1991;87:977–985.

108. Sabatini M, Yates AJ, Garrett R, et al. Increased production of tumor necrosis factor by normal immune cells in a model of the humoral hypercalcemia of malignancy. *Lab Invest* 1990;63:676–681.

109. Sabatini M, Chaves J, Mundy GR, Bonewald LF. Stimulation of tumor necrosis factor release from monocytic cells by the A375 human melanoma via granulocyte-macrophage colony stimulating factor. *Cancer Res* 1990;50:2673–2678.

110. Garrett IR, Durie BGM, Nedwin GE, et al. Production of the bone resorbing cytokine lymphotoxin by cultured human myeloma cells. *N Engl J Med* 1987;317:526–532.

111. Klein DC, Raisz LG. Prostaglandins: stimulation of bone resorption in tissue culture. *Endocrinology* 1970;86:1436–1440.

112. Tashjian AH, Voelkel EF, Levine L, Goldhaber P. Evidence that the bone resorption-stimulating factor produced by mouse fibrosarcoma cells is prostaglandin E2: a new model for hypercalcemia of cancer. *J Exp Med* 1972;136:1329–1343.

113. Akatsu T, Takahashi N, Debari K, et al. Prostaglandins promote osteoclast-like cell formation by a mechanism involving cyclic adenosine 3′,5′-monophosphate in mouse bone marrow cell cultures. *J Bone Mineral Res* 1989;4:29–35.

114. Chenu C, Kukita T, Mundy GR, Roodman GD. Prostaglandin E2 inhibits formation of osteoclast-like cells in long-term human marrow cultures but is not a mediator of the inhibitory effects of transforming growth factor β. *J Bone Mineral Res* 1990;5:677–681.

115. Roodman GD, Ibbotson KJ, MacDonald BR, Kuehl TJ, Mundy GR. 1,25(OH)₂ vitamin D₃ causes formation of multinucleated cells with osteoclast characteristics in cultures of primate marrow. *Proc Natl Acad Sci USA* 1985;82:8213–8217.

116. Franklin RB, Tashjian AH. Intravenous infusion of prostaglandin E₂ raises plasma calcium concentration in the rat. *Endocrinology* 1975;97:240–243.

117. Chambers TJ, Ali NN. Inhibition of osteoclastic motility by prostaglandins I₂, E₁, E₂, and 6-oxo-E₁. *J Pathol* 1983; 139:383–397.

118. Chyun YS, Raisz LG. Stimulation of bone formation by prostaglandin E₂. *Prostaglandins* 1984;27:97–103.

119. Jee WS, Ueno K, Deng YP, Woodbury DM. The effects of prostaglandin E₂ in growing rats: increased metaphyseal hard tissue and cortico-endosteal bone formation. *Calcif Tissue Int* 185;37:148–157.

120. Jee WS, Ueno K, Kimmel DB, Woodbury DM, Price P, Woodbury LA. The role of bone cells in increasing metaphyseal hard tissue in rapidly growing rats treated with prostaglandin E₂. *Bone* 1987;8:171–178.

121. Raisz LG, Simmons HA, Sandberg AL, Canalasis E. Direct stimulation of bone resorption by epidermal growth factor. *Endocrinology* 1980;107:270–273.

122. Tashijian AH, Voelkel EF, Lazzaro M, et al. Alpha and beta transforming growth factors stimulate prostaglandin production and bone resorption in cultured mouse calvaria. *Proc Natl Acad Sci USA* 1985;82:4535–4538.

123. Tashjian AJ Jr. Prostaglandins, hypercalcemia and cancer. *N Engl J Med* 1975;293:1317–1318.

124. Ito H, Sanada T, Katamaya T, Shimazaki J. Letter: Indomethacin-responsive hypercalcemia. *N Engl J Med* 1975; 293:558–559.

125. Seyberth HW, Segre GV, Morgan JL, Sweetman BJ, Potts JT, Oates JA. Prostaglandins as mediators of hypercalcemia associated with certain types of cancer. *N Engl J Med* 1975;293:1278–1283.

126. Powles TJ, Dowsett M, Easty BN, Neville AM. Breast cancer osteolysis, bone metastases, and anti-osteolytic effect of aspirin. *Lancet* 1976;608–610.

127. Bennett A, McDonald AM, Simpson JS, Stamford IF. Breast cancer, prostaglandins, and bone metastases. *Lancet* 1975; 1:1218–1220.

128. Powles TJ, Muindi J, Coombes RC. Mechanisms for development of bone metastases and effects of anti-inflammatory drugs. In: Powles TJ, Bockman RS, Honn KV, Ramwell P, eds. *Prostaglandins and related lipids.* New York: Alan R. Liss, 1982;541–553.

129. Valentin A, Eilon G, Saez S, Mundy GR. Estrogens and antiestrogens stimulate release of bone resorbing activity by cultured human breast cancer cells. *J Clin Invest* 1985:75:726–731.

130. Eilon G, Mundy GR. Direct resorption of bone by human breast cancer cells in vitro. *Nature* 1978;276:726–728.

131. Hong SL, Polsky-Cynkin R, Levine L. Stimulation of prostaglandin biosynthesis by vasoactive substances in methyl-

cholanthrene-transformed mouse BALB-3T3. *J Biol Chem* 1976;251:776–780.

132. Mundy GR, Wilkinson R, Heath DA. Comparative study of available medical therapy for hypercalcemia of malignancy. *Am J Med* 1983;74:421–432.

133. Raisz LG, Sandberg AL, Goodson JW, Simmons HA, Mergenhagen SE. Complement-dependent stimulation of PG synthesis and bone resorption. *Science* 1974;185:789.

134. Tashjian AH, Rice JE, Sides K. Biological activities of prostaglandin analogues and metabolites on bone in organ culture. *Nature* 1977;266:645–647.

135. Raisz LG, Dietrich JW, Simmons HA, Seyberth HW, Hubbard WN, Oates JA. Effects of prostaglandin endoperoxides and metabolites and bone resorption in vitro. *Nature* 1977;267:532–535.

136. Meghji S, Sandy J, Scutt AM, Harvey W, Harris M. Stimulation of bone resorption by lipoxygenase metabolites of arachidonic acid. *Prostaglandins* 1988;36:139–149.

137. El Attar TMA, Lin HS. Relative conversion of arachidonic acid through lipoxygenase and cyclo-oxygenase pathways by homogenates of diseased periodontal tissues. *J Oral Pathol* 1983;12:7–10.

138. Belicl OM, Singer FR, Coburn JW. Prostaglandins: effect on plasma calcium concentration. *Prostaglandins* 1973;3:237–241.

139. Parker CW. Lipid mediators produced through the lipoxygenase pathway. *Annu Rev Immunol* 1987;5:65–84.

140. Gallwitz WE, Mundy GR, Oreffo ROC, Gaskell SJ, Bonewald LF. Purification of osteoclastotropic factors produced by stromal cells: identification of 5-lipoxygenase metabolites. *J Bone Mineral Res* 1991;61:457A.

141. Bonewald L, Garcia C, Gallwitz W, Qiao M, Arnett T, Mundy GR. Osteoclast stimulating activity produced by osteoblast-like cells is inhibited by a 5-lipoxygenase inhibitor. *J Bone Mineral Res* 1992;7(Suppl 1):882A.

142. Mohammed AH, Tatakis DN, Dziak R. Leukotrienes in orthodontic tooth movement. *Am J Orthol Dentofacal Orthop* 1989;95:231–237.

143. Dayer JM, Robinson DR, Krane SM. Prostaglandin production by rheumatoid synovial cells: Stimulation by a factor from human mononuclear cells. *J Exp Med* 1977;145:1399–1404.

144. El Attar TMA, Lin HS, Killoy WJ, Vanderhoek JY, Goodson JM. Hydroxy fatty acids and prostaglandin formation in diseased human periodontal pocket tissue. *J Period Res* 1986;21:169–176.

145. Harris M, Jenkins MV, Bennett A, Wills MR. Prostaglandin production and bone resorption by dental cysts. *Nature* 1973;245:213–215.

146. Porteder H, Matejka M, Ulrich W, Sinzinger D. The cyclooxygenase and lipoxygenase pathway in human oral cancer tissue. *J Max Facial Surg* 1984;12:145–147.

147. Stenke L, Lauren L, Reizenstein P, Lindren JA. Leukotriene production by fresh human bone marrow cells: evidence of altered lipoxygenase activity in chronic myelocytic leukaemia. *Exp Haematol* 1987;15:203–207.

148. Davidson EM, Rae SA, Smith MJ. Leukotriene B₄, a mediator of inflammation present in synovial fluid in rheumatoid arthritis. *Ann Rheum Dis* 1983;42:677–679.

149. Nussbaum S, Zahradrik R, La Vigne J, et al. Highly sensitive 2-site immunoradiometric assay of PTH and its clinical utility in evaluating patients with hypercalcemia. *Clin Chem* 1987;33:1364.

150. Strewler GJ, Wronski TJ, Halloran BP, et al. Pathogenesis of hypercalcemia in nude mice bearing a human renal carcinoma. *Endocrinology* 1986;119:303–310.

151. Fukumoto S, Matsumoto T, Yamoto H, et al. Suppression of serum 1,25-dihydroxyvitamin D in humoral hypercalcemia of malignancy is caused by elaboration of a factor that inhibits renal 1,25-dihydroxyvitamin D₃ production. *Endocrinology* 1989;124:2057–2062.

152. Breslau NA, McGuire JL, Zerwekh JC, Trenkel EP, Pak CYC. Hypercalcemia associated with increased serum calcitriol levels in three patients with lymphoma. *Ann Intern Med* 1984;100:1–7.

153. Rosenthal N, Insogna KL, Godsael JW, Smoldone L, Waldron JA, Stewart AL. Elevations in circulating 1,25 dihydroxyvitamin D in three patients with lymphoma-associated hypercalcemia. *J Clin Endocrinol Metab* 1985;60:29–33.

154. Davies M, Hages ME, Mawer EB, Lumb GA. Abnormal vitamin D metabolism in Hodgkin's lymphoma. *Lancet* 1985;1:1186–1188.

155. Fetchick DA, Bertolini DR, Sarin P, Weintraub ST, Mundy GR, Dunn JD. Production of 1,25-dihydroxyvitamin D by human T cell lymphotrophic virus-I transformed lymphocytes. *J Clin Invest* 1986;78:592–596.

156. Mundy GR. Hypercalcemia associated with hematologic malignancies. In: Dunitz, M, ed. *Calcium homeostasis: hypercalcemia and hypocalcemia.* London: Martin Dunitz, 1990; 100–115.

157. Burt ME, Brennan MF. Incidence of hypercalcemia in malignant neoplasms. *Arch Surg* 1980;115:704–707.

158. Adams JS, Fernandez M, Gacad MA, et al. Vitamin D metabolite-mediated hypercalcemia and hypercalciuria patients with AIDS- and non-AIDS-associated lymphoma. *Blood* 1989;73:235–239.

159. Motokura T, Fukumoto S, Matsumoto T, et al. Parathyroid hormone-related protein in adult T-cell leukemia-lymphoma. *Ann Intern Med* 1989;111:484–488.

160. Bertolini DR, Sarin P, Mundy GR. Production of macromolecular bone resorbing activity by human T cell leukemia virus (HTLV) transformed cell lines. *Calcif Tissue Int* 1984;36:284A.

161. Gordon GS, Cantino TJ, Erhardt L, et al. Osteolytic steroids in human breast cancer. *Science* 1966;151:1226–1228.

162. Haddad JG, Cowranz SJ, Avioli LV. Circulating phytosterols in normal females, lactating mothers, and breast cancer patients. *J Clin Endocrinol Metab* 1970;30:174–180.

163. Mundy GR. Hypercalcemia of malignancy. *Kidney Int* 1987; 31:142–155.

164. Simpson EL, Mundy GR, D'Souza SM, Ibbotson KJ, Bockman R, Jacobs JW. Absence of parathyroid hormone messenger RNA in non-parathyroid tumors associated with hypercalcemia. *N Engl J Med* 1983;309:325–330.

165. Yoshimoto K, Yamasaki R, Sakai H, et al. Ectopic production of parathyroid hormone by small cell lung cancer in a patient with hypercalcemia. *J Clin Endocrinol Metab* 1989; 68:976–981.

166. Strewler GJ, Budayr AA, Bruce RJ, Clark OH, Nissenson RA. Secretion of authentic parathyroid hormone by a malignant tumor. *Clin Res* 1990;38:462A.

167. Nussbaum SR, Gaz RD, Arnold A. Hypercalcemia and ectopic secretion of parathyroid hormone by an ovarian carcinoma with rearrangement of the gene for parathyroid hormone. *N Engl J Med* 1990;323:1324–1328.

The Parathyroids, edited by J.P. Bilezikian,
M.A. Levine, and R. Marcus. Raven Press, Ltd.,
New York © 1994.

CHAPTER 22

Acute Management of Hypercalcemia due to Parathyroid Hormone and Parathyroid Hormone-Related Protein

John P. Bilezikian and Frederick R. Singer

Hypercalcemia is a nearly universal manifestation in patients with primary hyperparathyroidism and is a common event in the later stages of some cancers. The clinical spectrum ranges from a few patients with symptomatic and perhaps life-threatening hypercalcemia that requires immediate treatment to a larger number of patients whose hypercalcemia is more mild and frequently asymptomatic. Widespread use of the multichannel screening test now accounts for the observation that a large percentage of hypercalcemic patients present without symptoms of this metabolic abnormality. The approach to the management of the hypercalcemic patient requires full knowledge of the principles of calcium homeostasis, a topic covered in the chapter by Brown. The approach to the patient also requires knowledge of the differential diagnosis of hypercalcemia and associated pathophysiologies and the clinical judgment to know when and how to administer appropriate therapy.

This chapter deals with the management of hypercalcemic patients who require immediate attention in the hospital. It focuses upon the management of acute hypercalcemia due to excess production of parathyroid hormone (PTH) or parathyroid hormone-related protein (PTHrP). Since acute hypercalcemia requiring urgent therapy is now uncommonly due to primary hyperparathyroidism (see chapter by Fitzpatrick), this discussion is most applicable to cancer-associated hy-

percalcemia due to PTHrP or other factors. However, the approach to any severely hypercalcemic individual, independent of etiology, is similar. Outpatient treatment of mild hypercalcemia due to asymptomatic primary hyperparathyroidism is considered in the chapter by Stock and Marcus.

DIFFERENTIAL DIAGNOSIS OF HYPERCALCEMIA

A classification of the differential diagnosis of hypercalcemia is provided in Table 1. The overwhelming majority (>90%) of hypercalcemic patients will be shown to have either primary hyperparathyroidism or a malignancy. Hypercalcemia requiring urgent therapy is caused most often by cancer, but severe primary hyperparathyroidism (acute parathyroid crisis) and the other etiologies noted in Table 1 require consideration at times. Thus the most simple and direct differential diagnosis of hypercalcemia is a distinction between these two most common causes. It is important not to assume that severe hypercalcemia is due to cancer, because when acute primary hyperparathyroidism is the cause it can be a clinical "lookalike."

The distinction between cancer-related hypercalcemia and primary hyperparathyroidism is usually not difficult and is readily confirmed by measurements of serum parathyroid hormone. Most patients with primary hyperparathyroidism have elevated concentrations of PTH and those with acute hyperparathyroid crisis have remarkably elevated levels of PTH (see the chapter by Fitzpatrick).

J.P. Bilezikian: Departments of Medicine and Pharmacology, College of Physicians and Surgeons, Columbia University, New York, New York 10032.

F.R. Singer: Osteoporosis and Metabolic Bone Diseases Program, St. John's Hospital and Health Center, Santa Monica, California 90404.

TABLE 1. *Differential diagnosis of hypercalcemia*

Primary hyperparathyroidism
    Sporadic (adenoma, hyperplasia, or carcinoma)
    Familial
        Isolated
        Cystic
        Multiple endocrine neoplasia type I or II
Malignancy
    Parathyroid hormone-related protein
    Excess production of 1,25(OH)₂D
    Other factors (cytokines, growth factors)
Nonparathyroid endocrine disorders
    Thyrotoxicosis
    Pheochromocytoma
    Acute adrenal insufficiency
    Vasointestinal polypeptide hormone-producing tumor
        (VIPoma)
Granulomatous diseases (1,25(OH)₂D excess)
    Sarcoidosis
    Tuberculosis
    Histoplasmosis
    Coccidiomycosis
    Leprosy
Medications
    Thiazide diuretics
    Lithium
    Estrogens/antiestrogens, testosterone in breast cancer
    Milk-alkali syndrome
    Vitamin A or D toxicity
Familial hypocalciuric hypercalcemia
Immobilization
Parenteral nutrition
Aluminum excess
Acute and chronic renal disease

In hypercalcemia of malignancy due to PTHrP and other nonparathyroid causes of hypercalcemia, the inhibition of parathyroid glandular activity is a normal physiologic response of parathyroid tissue. Virtually all patients with cancer-associated hypercalcemia have low or suppressed levels of intact PTH (1,2). Thus a good assay for parathyroid hormone will measure low or undetectable PTH in the circulation in patients with malignancy unless the patient has both cancer and primary hyperparathyroidism. If the PTH level is suppressed when hypercalcemia is present, the diagnosis of primary hyperparathyroidism becomes extremely unlikely. Practically, it is excluded. However, although suppressed PTH levels in hypercalcemia rules out primary hyperparathyroidism, they do not rule in malignancy, because a great many other causes of hypercalcemia are associated with suppression of parathyroid gland activity. Having ruled out primary hyperparathyroidism, one focuses more intently on malignancy in view of the fact that it is by far the most common cause of PTH independent hypercalcemia. The many other potential causes of hypercalcemia are considered only after malignancy has been ruled out or unless the history or physical examination suggests

that another explanation for the hypercalcemia is likely. In general, other endocrine disorders associated with hypercalcemia exhibit classical findings of the endocrine disorder.

The structure of PTHrP, which has limited chemical similarity to that of PTH, probably explains why the available radioimmunoassays for PTH do not detect it in the circulation. The only area of homology between PTHrP and PTH is the first 13 amino acids, where great homology exists. Thereafter, PTHrP diverges extensively from PTH (see the chapter by Chorev and Rosenblatt). The rest of the polypeptides of PTH and PTHrP are completely divergent from each other. The available radioimmunoassays for PTH, even those with amino-terminal specificity, recognize epitopes of the PTH molecule that are carboxy-terminal to the first 13 amino acids. Thus they do not detect PTHrP in the circulation but register the normal suppression of native PTH. Assays for PTHrP are now available with which the presence of this cause of cancer-related hypercalcemia can be confirmed sometimes by elevated levels in the circulation (3–7) (see the chapter by Kremer and Goltzman). Levels of PTHrP are not elevated in primary hyperparathyroidism but, with some assays, elevation of this protein may be found if renal failure is present (5).

The remaining cases of hypercalcemia, constituting only 10% of the total cases, are distributed among a great variety of other potential etiologies (Table 1). This is not just an academic discussion; in the occasional patient, one must search diligently among these many other possible etiologies. It is important to bear in mind these other disorders, especially in the patient who becomes a diagnostic problem.

An important clinical observation, which is quite useful in the differential diagnosis of symptomatic hypercalcemia, is the rapidity with which hypercalcemic symptoms and/or hypercalcemia develop. A normocalcemic state documented several weeks previously points to malignancy as a likely presenting cause of hypercalcemia. Review of prior calcium determinations in patients with primary hyperparathyroidism often reveals subtle hypercalcemia even over a period of years.

PATHOPHYSIOLOGY OF ACUTE HYPERCALCEMIA

The dominant process leading to severe hypercalcemia is the acceleration of calcium mobilization from bone due to activation of the osteoclast, a multinucleated, calcium-resorbing bone cell (8). The osteoclast can be activated by both local and/or systemic effects of various substances such as PTHrP. Osteoclast activation is a seminal pathophysiological feature of virtually all cases of marked hypercalcemia. Excessive absorption of calcium from the gastrointestinal tract is usually not a major factor, although it can contribute to hypercalcemia caused by exogenous or endogenous vitamin D excess. Hypercalcemia is manifested when calcium resorbed from bone into the extracellular space exceeds the homeostatic mechanisms that maintain normocalcemia. One of these, the suppression of PTH secretion by calcium, is obviously negated when the cause of increased bone resorption is PTH. In PTHrP-associated hypercalcemia, PTH secretion is suppressed, but PTHrP acts similarly to accelerate osteoclast-mediated bone resorption. When bone resorption is accelerated, the kidney becomes the major defense against hypercalcemia (9–11). When renal mechanisms are operating normally, the tendency for the serum calcium to rise is attenuated by greater urinary calcium excretion.

Severe hypercalcemia can be defined as a marked elevation in the serum calcium concentration (i.e., >14 mg/dl), which is usually associated with clinical features of hypercalcemia (see below). It is a manifestation of a series of pathophysiological events. Initially, factors that induce osteoclast-mediated bone resorption, such as PTH and PTHrP, also stimulate renal tubular reabsorption of calcium (12). Enhanced conservation of calcium impairs the efficiency of the kidneys to excrete the increased filtered load of calcium that is simultaneously released from bone. Second, hypercalcemia per se interferes with the renal mechanisms for reabsorption of sodium and water, leading to polyuria. The ensuing polyuria may not be matched by commensurate oral fluid intake because of anorexia and nausea, frequent symptoms of hypercalcemia. The result is extracellular volume depletion and a reduction in the glomerular filtration rate, which further increases the serum calcium concentration by increasing renal tubular calcium reabsorption. Hypercalcemia may also be exacerbated by immobilization of the severely ill patient, superimposing another stimulus for bone-related calcium loss. To a greater or lesser extent, these pathophysiological mechanisms are operative in virtually all patients who require hospitalization for hypercalcemia.

CLINICAL FEATURES OF HYPERCALCEMIA

An appreciation of the clinical features of hypercalcemia apart from its etiology is important, since this helps to determine decisions regarding instituting therapy for the hypercalcemia per se as well as possibly directing therapeutic approaches to the underlying problem. The signs and symptoms of hypercalcemia are listed in Table 2 and should not be confused with

TABLE 2. *Signs and symptoms of hypercalcemia*

General	Renal system
Weakness	Polyuria
Dehydration	Low urinary specific
Corneal and other ectopic	gravity
calcification	Reduced glomerular
Central nervous system	filtration rate
Impaired concentration	Flank pain
Depression	(nephrolithiasis)
Psychosis	Nephrocalcinosis
Altered consciousness	Cardiovascular system
(confusion, lethargy,	Hypertension
stupor, coma)	Shortened QT interval
Gastrointestinal tract	Digitalis sensitivity
Polydipsia	
Anorexia	
Nausea	
Vomiting	
Abdominal pain (pancreatitis,	
peptic ulcer)	
Constipation	

those of the underlying disorder. In the absence of clearcut features of hypercalcemia, measures to reduce the serum calcium may not be indicated, and therapy of hypercalcemia may distract the clinician from the underlying disorder. It is true that hypercalcemia is not always associated with a typical set of signs and symptoms that dictate whether the patient would improve with treatment. Quite commonly, various nonspecific complaints such as weakness and lethargy challenge our ability to define the specific cause of the symptomatology. Despite this, an attempt should be made to conclude whether the signs and symptoms of hypercalcemia are present in a given patient. If it is not possible to be certain, empiric but judicious therapy for the hypercalcemia is appropriate.

The clinical manifestations of hypercalcemia reflect disturbances in central nervous system, gastrointestinal, renal, and cardiovascular function (Table 2). Central nervous system dysfunction is most threatening to survival and ranges from mild impairment of cognitive function to coma. Gastrointestinal symptoms include anorexia, nausea and vomiting, constipation, and, rarely, abdominal pain due to pancreatitis. The symptoms of renal dysfunction are polyuria and polydipsia; patients who develop kidney stones may experience acute flank pain. The cardiovascular manifestations include hypertension, if intravascular volume is maintained, a shortened QTT interval on the electrocardiogram and greater sensitivity to digitalis. Not all patients have all of these symptoms. A number of factors account for the great clinical variability of hypercalcemic patients. These include the age of the patient, the presence of other medical problems, the duration of the hypercalcemia, and the rate of rise and the absolute level of the serum calcium. Therefore, in patients with moderate hypercalcemia, therapy should be based not only on the serum calcium concentration but also on the extent of symptomatology.

A particularly difficult situation is presented by the patient in whom hypercalcemia is not in the range that one would ordinarily treat aggressively (<12 mg/dl) but who exhibits central nervous system features that may be associated with hypercalcemia such as apathy, drowsiness, obtundation, or even coma. It is not possible to be certain that these changes in the sensorium are due to hypercalcemia, particularly in older patients with moderate hypercalcemia. This may be even more vexing in the younger patient who, in general, is more likely to tolerate the hypercalcemia. In this situation, it is important to seek other factors contributing to the symptomatology before attributing altered central nervous system function to hypercalcemia itself. On the other hand, it is entirely appropriate to suspect, when the serum calcium is in the moderately elevated range, 12–14 mg/dl, that altered central nervous system function is due to hypercalcemia. This is especially relevant in the individual who may also have other reasons for altered mental status. Correction of the hypercalcemia should improve central nervous system function if hypercalcemia is responsible for the symptomatology.

PRINCIPLES OF THERAPY FOR HYPERCALCEMIA

Hypercalcemia is a treatable metabolic abnormality, which need not always be directly treated. It often precedes the diagnosis of an underlying disorder that should be given more initial attention than the hypercalcemia. At the other end of the spectrum, hypercalcemia may present as a life-threatening disorder that demands vigorous therapy independent even of knowledge of the cause of the underlying disorder. Thus principles of therapy relate importantly to two elements: the underlying etiology and the severity of the hypercalcemia. When hypercalcemia is asymptomatic, attention should be directed to defining the etiology. In most patients, this would lead to a diagnosis of primary hyperparathyroidism. On the other hand, severe hypercalcemia associated with central nervous system symptoms demands that the hypercalcemia be treated first. An exception to this rule may be the patient with an incurable, disseminated malignancy in whom prolongation of life may be unkind.

THERAPY OF ACUTE HYPERCALCEMIA

The magnitude of the hypercalcemia is a key consideration when the decision to treat is imminent. If the serum total calcium concentration is >14 mg/dl (the upper limit of normal varies among laboratories but is generally ~10.2 mg/dl), a therapeutic plan to reduce the serum calcium is indicated, regardless of the presence of symptoms. The value of 14 mg/dl is based on the assumption that the serum albumin concentration is normal, but in hypercalcemic patients the serum albumin concentration may be increased because of dehydration or reduced because of chronic illness. A convenient rule of thumb is to adjust the serum total calcium concentration by 0.8 mg/dl for each 1 g/dl by which the serum albumin is increased or decreased (13). If the serum albumin concentration is increased, the serum total calcium concentration is adjusted downward; if the serum albumin concentration is reduced, the serum total calcium concentration is adjusted upward. When the serum calcium concentration is only moderately increased to 12–14 mg/dl, the clinical manifestations of hypercalcemia should dictate the type of therapy necessary and the dispatch with which it should be administered.

There are four basic goals in the therapy of hypercalcemia: to correct dehydration, to enhance renal excretion of calcium, to inhibit accelerated bone resorption, and to treat the underlying disorder. A summary of recommended approaches is provided in Table 3.

General Measures

Hydration

Administration of isotonic saline intravenously is the first step in the acute management of hypercalcemia. This can be done safely in the great majority of patients, since congestive heart failure is rare in this clinical setting. When the depleted intravascular volume is restored to normal, the serum calcium concentration will decline at least by the degree to which the

TABLE 3. *Management of hypercalcemia*

Repletion of extracellular fluid volume
  Saline infusion
Induction of facilitated calciuresis
  Saline infusion with furosemide (modest doses)
Inhibition of bone resorption
  Bisphosphonates
  Calcitonin
  Plicamycin
  Gallium nitrate
  Glucocorticoids
Miscellaneous
  Intravenous phosphate (not recommended)
  Dialysis
  Mobilization

calcium concentration was raised by the dehydration. The decrease in serum calcium usually amounts to 1.6–2.4 mg/dl, a substantial amount, but rarely does hydration alone lead to normalization of marked hypercalcemia (14). Expansion of intravascular volume is also helpful in that it begins to increase renal calcium clearance. First, the improved glomerular filtration rate leads to greater filtration of calcium. Second, increased proximal tubular sodium and calcium reabsorption, which has been mediated, in part, by the reduction in gromerular filtration rate (GFR), is returned towards normal. Third, as more sodium and water are presented to distal renal tubular sites, an obligatory calciuresis ensues. The rate of saline administration should be based on the severity of the hypercalcemia, on the extent of dehydration, and on judgment of the cardiovascular tolerance to volume loading. A widely used plan of action is to administer 2.5–4 liters isotonic saline daily, recognizing the need to adjust the rate of administration or to use judicious therapy with loop diuretics if symptoms and signs of fluid overload appear. The observation of an increasing urinary output during the initial hours of fluid repletion is an important guide to the adequacy of the fluid load and the ability of the patient to handle it.

Loop Diuretics (Furosemide)

In addition to hydration with saline, adjunctive diuretic therapy with furosemide has been effectively used in patients. There were two reasons to consider the use of a loop diuretic in the management of hypercalcemia before safe and effective agents were available to control bone resorption. The first was to facilitate further urinary calcium excretion. Loop diuretics, such as furosemide and ethacrynic acid, increase the calciuric effects of volume expansion by inhibiting calcium reabsorption in the thick ascending limb of the loop of Henle. Thiazide diuretics are contraindicated in this situation because they increase distal tubular reabsorption of calcium and may even exacerbate hypercalcemia. Volume repletion must precede use of furosemide because the drug's effect is dependent on delivery of calcium to the ascending limb. It is a key principle of diuretic therapy for hypercalcemia that normal hydration must first be established. It was reported in 1970 by Suki et al. (15) that intensive administration of furosemide, 80–100 mg every 1–2 hr, with fluid (10 liters or more in 24 hr) and electrolyte replacement based on urinary losses are an effective regimen for the acute treatment of hypercalcemia (15). Such an aggressive approach will lead to marked hypercalciuria, but it requires frequent measurement of water and electrolyte excretion. An already marginally

compensated patient can be destabilized further if losses of fluid and electrolytes, except for calcium, are not matched by adequate replacement therapy. Such intensive therapy with furosemide is not necessary in most patients. The second reason for considering therapy with a loop diuretic is to guard against the volume overload that may accompany saline administration. Concerns about volume overload are particularly relevant in older patients in whom cardiovascular function may be marginal. Under these circumstances, it is reasonable to administer modest doses of furosemide, for example, 10–20 mg intravenously every 6–12 hr, depending on the patient's capacity to handle the volume load. If fluid tolerance is not a major concern, furosemide should not be used but rather held in reserve should signs of fluid overload become apparent. In the patient with a history of cardiac disease, it is probably best not to exceed 2–3 liters of intravenous saline in a 24 hr period.

Inhibition of Bone Resorption

In most patients with a serum calcium concentration >12 mg/dl, saline infusion will produce a modest reduction but not normalization of hypercalcemia. Saline does not affect the major pathophysiological feature of hypercalcemia, which is excessive calcium mobilization from bone. Thus, it is usually necessary to use specific therapy to inhibit osteoclast-mediated bone resorption if the patient has severe symptoms of hypercalcemia or even if the serum calcium concentration remains moderately elevated after volume expansion. Such specific therapy is particularly indicated in a symptomatic patient whose initial serum calcium concentration is ≥14 mg/dl.

Well-controlled studies of the treatment of severe hypercalcemia are difficult, so some studies of osteoclast inhibitors are difficult to interpret because the extent of preceding saline and diuretic therapy was not always stated. The specific regimens found in the literature have been developed mainly in patients with hypercalcemia of cancer and acute primary hyperparathyroidism, disorders of greatest concern in this chapter. It is likely that other etiologies of hypercalcemia would be associated with similar responses to these agents. It is obvious, but should be remembered, that the specific means of inhibiting osteoclast-mediated bone resorption are not directed towards treating the underlying cause of the hypercalcemia. Management of hypercalcemia, thus, should not interdict the use of therapy for the cause of the hypercalcemia per se. It is also important to consider use of the least toxic agents to control bone resorption in patients who may also receive cytotoxic cancer therapies.

Bisphosphonates

The bisphosphonates are a family of compounds structurally related to a normal product of metabolism, pyrophosphate. Unlike the P-O-P bond in pyrophosphate, the bisphosphonates are characterized by a P-C-P backbone that renders them resistant to phosphatases. They bind to hydroxyapatite in bone and inhibit crystal dissolution (16,17). Their great affinity for bone surfaces and resistance to metabolic degradation produce an extremely long half-life in bone. They are excreted unchanged by the kidney. The major property shared by all bisphosphonates that has made them valuable agents for hypercalcemia is their inhibitory effect on osteoclasts. The mechanisms by which bisphosphonates impair osteoclast function are still not clarified but may involve inhibition of osteoclast differentiation as well as inhibition of cell function (18–22). Each bisphosphonate appears to have a somewhat different mechanism of osteoclast inhibition. The absorption of these compounds from the gastrointestinal tract is generally poor, averaging <5%. The main side effects of oral formulations are gastrointestinal. Intravenous administration of bisphosphonates is much more effective for acute hypercalcemia.

Three bisphosphonates are generally available: 1-hydroxyethylidene-1, 1-bisphosphonate (EHDP; etidronate); 3-amino-1, hydroxypropylidene-1, 1-bisphosphonate (APD; pamidronate); and dichloromethylene-bisphosphonate (Cl$_2$MBP; clodronate). Etidronate and pamidronate are approved for use in malignant hypercalcemia at this time in the United States. In addition to these three compounds, a new generation of more potent bisphosphonates is currently under investigation.

Etidronate is approved for administration in a daily dose of 7.5 mg/kg intravenously over 4 hr for 3 days. The drug is much more effective if given for up to 7 days. The serum calcium concentration begins to fall within 2 days after the first dose and reaches its nadir within 7 days (Fig. 1). The nadir is within the normal range in 33–80% of patients (23–29). Patients who are well hydrated before etidronate and who continue to receive intravenous fluids respond better (24,27). Whether etidronate should be given for a full 7 days depends on the level of the hypercalcemia after hydration and the response of the patient to the drug. Cessation of therapy is reasonable after 3 days if the patient shows a decline in serum calcium concentration after the first two or three doses by >2–3 mg/dl or if

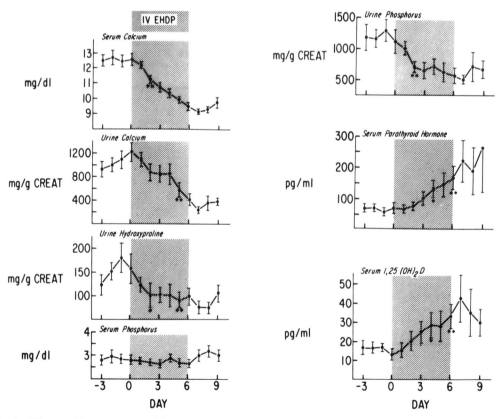

FIG. 1. Effects of intravenous etidronate (EHDP) therapy in hypercalcemia of malignancy. Mean responses ± SEM are shown for serum calcium and phosphorus concentration and urinary calcium and hydroxyproline excretion in 12 patients. (Adapted from ref. 27 with permission.)

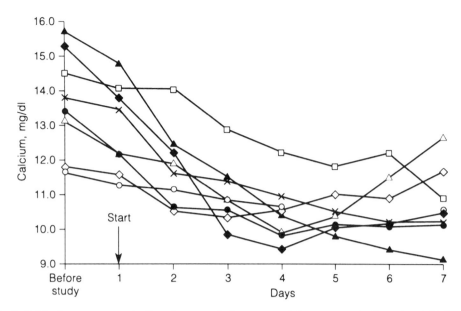

FIG. 2. Individual responses of albumin-corrected serum calcium concentrations in eight hypercalcemia cancer patients treated wtih a single 24 hr infusion of etidronate disodium. The patients were hydrated with intravenous saline for 48 hr prior to etidronate. (Reprinted from ref. 30 with permission.)

the serum calcium is close to the normal range. Persistent daily administration of etidronate until the serum calcium concentration has normalized theoretically could lead to a period of unwanted hypocalcemia. In a preliminary study, a single 24 hr infusion of 25 mg/kg etidronate proved to be highly effective and safe (30) (Fig. 2).

Biochemical evidence of the inhibition of bone resorption by etidronate (and other bisphosphonates) is provided by the decreases in urinary calcium and hydroxyproline excretion that accompany the reduction in serum calcium (Fig. 1). The duration of action of etidronate varies from days to several weeks, depending on the rate of underlying bone resorption and renal tubular reabsorption of calcium. In patients in whom parenteral administration of etidronate lowered the serum calcium concentration, oral administration given subsequently has not been nearly as effective as the intravenous therapy (24,27,29,31,32).

Etidronate treatment of hypercalcemia is safe, the only reported adverse effects being transient increases in serum creatinine and phosphate concentrations. While chronic administration of high doses of etidronate can impair bone formation and cause osteomalacia (33), short-term use apparently does not. This potential adverse effect of etidronate is not known to be shared by any other bisphosphonates currently in use or under investigation at dosages employed clinically.

Pamidronate is a much more potent bisphosphonate than etidronate, but it has more side effects. A variety of regimens have been utilized: slow, intravenous infusion of 15–45 mg daily for up to 10 days; single 2–24 hr intravenous infusion of doses of 30–90 mg (Fig. 3);

or oral administration 300 mg daily for months to 1,200 mg daily for up to 5 days. The recommended approach is 30–90 mg intravenously over 24 hr. The time course of the fall in serum calcium is similar to that in patients treated with etidronate. It is difficult to evaluate studies that have attempted comparisons between pamidronate and etidronate or among the several regimens of pamidronate (9,34–37), since dose-response curves were not established. The single dose regimen has been reported to lead to normalization of the serum calcium concentration in 70–100% of patients (38,39). The intravenous route is certainly preferred in view of the limited gastrointestinal tolerance of many patients with hypercalcemia and the gastrointestinal side effects that may be associated with oral administration of the drug (40). Oral pamidronate has also been used to attempt to prevent hypercalcemia in patients with cancer and bone metastases in whom hypercalcemia has not yet occurred (41). The adverse effects of parenteral pamidronate are limited to a mild, transient temperature elevation (<2°C), transient leukopenia, a small reduction in serum phosphate, and myalgias. These side effects occur in ~33% of patients.

Clodronate was one of the first bisphosphonates used to treat patients with malignant hypercalcemia (42–45). It can be administered intravenously in a dose of 4–6 mg/kg in 2–5 hr daily over 3–5 days or as a single infusion for 2–9 hr (46,47). Daily infusion may be associated with more prolonged normocalcemia. Oral clodronate is also quite effective and has few side effects, but the intravenous route is preferred in the setting of acute hypercalcemia. After intravenous administration, the serum calcium concentration declines at

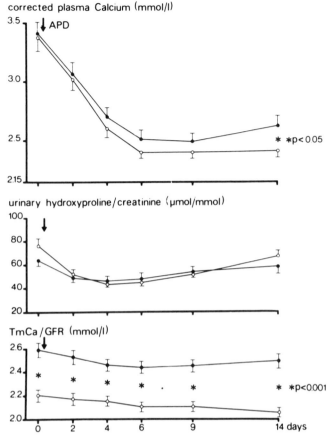

corrected plasma Calcium (mmol/l)

urinary hydroxyproline/creatinine (μmol/mmol)

TmCa/GFR (mmol/l)

FIG. 3. Comparison of plasma calcium, urinary hydroxyproline excretion, and TmCa/GFR (mean ± SEM) between 23 breast carcinoma patients (○) and 20 squamous cell carcinoma patients (●) treated with a single 24-hour infusion of pamidronate after rehydration with intravenous saline. The dose of pamidronate ranged from 30 to 90 mg (mean 56 and 57 mg, respectively). The increased renal tubular reabsorption of calcium in the squamous cell carcinoma patients may account for their higher plasma calcium at 14 days. (Reproduced from ref. 39, with permission.)

a rate typical for the bisphosphonates, with the initial substantial change occurring after 2 days and normocalcemia frequently occurring by 7 days. Similarly to pamidronate, clodronate has been reported to have the potential to reduce progression of skeletal metastases and to prevent the onset of hypercalcemia in patients with cancer who are at risk (48–51). Potential nephrotoxicity is avoided by slow infusion over a period of at least 2 hours. Concerns that the drug might be associated with leukemia led to suspension of clinical trials in the United States, but continuing use in other countries over the past 12 years has not substantiated this possibility (45).

Calcitonin

Calcitonin, the naturally occurring peptide hormone, should be the ideal therapy for hypercalcemia,

because it inhibits bone resorption and acutely increases renal calcium excretion. The drug is usually administered subcutaneously or intramuscularly in a dosage of 4 MRC units/kg every 12 hr. Doses as high as 8 MRC units/kg every 6 hr have been used. Among the major hypocalcemic agents available, calcitonin has the most rapid onset of action. The serum calcium concentration usually begins to decline within a few hours after therapy is initiated (52). This early effect may be related to its hypercalciuric action (53), although bone resorption is also rapidly inhibited. The nadir of the serum calcium concentration is reached within 12–24 hr but is often followed by a return towards initial hypercalcemic levels within 24–72 hr despite continued administration (54,55). Unlike the bisphosphonates and plicamycin, calcitonin is not a potent agent. The average maximal reductions in serum calcium seldom exceed 2 mg/dl. Thus, except in patients with mild hypercalcemia or in unusually responsive patients, the serum calcium is unlikely to become normal with calcitonin therapy alone (54–56).

Early studies of combination therapy with calcitonin and a glucocorticoid suggested that this was an effective regimen (54). However, subsequent studies failed to demonstrate that the combination of these agents was very effective, and at present it is not widely used (55–58). More impressive results have been reported when calcitonin is used in combination with a bisphosphonate. The simultaneous administration of calcitonin and pamidronate has been reported to cause a more rapid fall in serum calcium concentration than therapy with pamidronate alone, most likely due to calcitonin (59,60). Similar results were obtained with calcitonin and etidronate (61). The latter study utilized salmon calcitonin subcutaneously every 12 hr and produced normocalcemia in seven of nine patients, a result much superior to that with etidronate alone (Fig. 4).

Calcitonin is the safest antihypercalcemic agent. Side effects include mild, transient nausea; abdominal cramps; and flushing. True allergic reactions to salmon calcitonin, the preparation that has been used most widely, are quite rare. Human calcitonin, which is less potent than salmon calcitonin, has seldom been studied in the management of hypercalcemia.

Short-term use of calcitonin should be considered in the cancer patient with severe hypercalcemia because of its rapid onset of action and its safety profile. Simultaneous administration of a bisphosphonate would make likely more prolonged control of the hypercalcemic state. Another feature of calcitonin that should be borne in mind is the suggestion that it has potent analgesic properties (62). It has been reported to provide impressive relief in some patients with painful skeletal metastases.

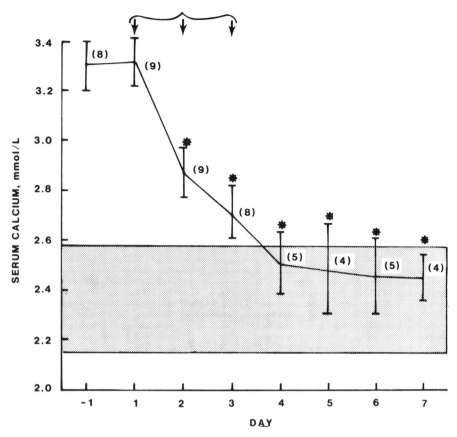

FIG. 4. Fall in the albumin-corrected serum calcium concentration during combined salmon calcitonin and etidronate therapy of nine patients with cancer. Each patient was hydrated with intravenous saline for at least 48 hr before treatment. Each received 7.5 mg/kg etidronate intravenously daily and 100 IU salmon calcitonin subcutaneously every 12 hr for 3 days. There was a significant fall in the serum calcium within 24 hr ($P < 0.001$). The *shaded area* is the normal range for serum calcium concentration. (Reprinted from ref. 61 with permission.)

Plicamycin (Mithramycin)

Plicamycin, an inhibitor of osteoclast RNA synthesis, is a potent therapy for hypercalcemia, which has been in clinical use for more than 20 years (63–66). It is given intravenously in a dose of 25 μg/kg over 4–6 hr. The dose can be repeated several times, although a single dose may normalize the serum calcium concentration. The serum calcium concentration begins to fall as early as 6 hr after administration of the drug. The maximal reduction occurs in 48–72 hr (Fig. 5). The duration of normocalcemia after a single dose of plicamycin is usually a few days and depends on the rate of ongoing bone resorption. Recurrent hypercalcemia can be retreated with plicamycin, but this should be done only in patients who are resistant to other therapies.

Plicamycin has disturbing side effects. Nausea is common and can be minimized by slow intravenous infusion. Care should be taken to avoid local extrava-sation of the drug, because irritation and cellulitis can result. Hepatic toxicity, manifested most often as transiently elevated serum aminotransferase concentrations, occurs in ~20% of patients (67). Nephrotoxicity (increased blood urea concentration, creatinine, and proteinuria) and thrombocytopenia can also occur (68), the latter especially in patients who have received previous chemotherapy or radiotherapy. These adverse effects are relatively unusual when plicamycin is given in the usual dosage for several courses but can occur after a single dose. With higher doses and repeated administration, these adverse effects become more likely. Concern for side effects has resulted in decreased use of plicamycin as other agents that are as effective but do not have the same potential for adverse consequences have become available. Contraindications to the use of plicamycin are overt hepatic or renal dysfunction, thrombocytopenia, or any coagulopathy.

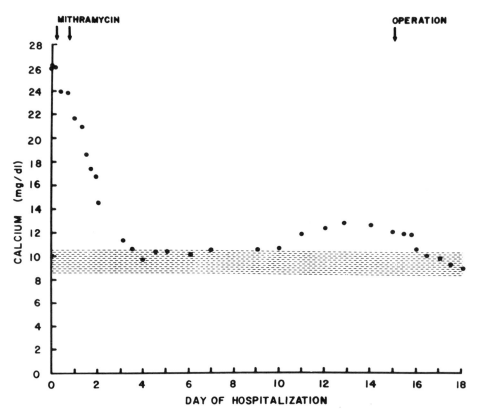

FIG. 5. Therapy of life-threatening hypercalcemia with mithramycin. The patient received two doses of mithramycin (25 μg/kg) 12 hr apart on the first day of admission. The calcium decreased into the normal range and did not return to life-threatening levels until the patient underwent successful parathyroidectomy.

Gallium Nitrate

Gallium nitrate is the agent most recently approved by the U.S. Food and Drug Administration for the parenteral therapy of hypercalcemia. It may inhibit bone resorption, in part, by reducing the solubility of hydroxyapatite cystals to which it adsorbs (69–71). In addition, a direct inhibitory action of gallium on osteoclasts has been observed (72). After gallium nitrate administration, reductions in urinary calcium and hydroxyproline excretion are found, confirming its action as an inhibitor of bone resorption (73). Gallium nitrate is approved for administration as a continuous intravenous infusion, 200 mg/m² in 1 liter of fluid daily for 5 days. The results of a controlled, double-blind study comparing maximum dose calcitonin with gallium nitrate showed normalization of the serum calcium concentration more frequently with gallium nitrate (75% vs. 31%) and for longer duration (6 days vs. 1 day). As in the case of bisphosphonates, the serum calcium concentration fell gradually and normocalcemia with gallium nitrate was not achieved until the 5 day infusion was completed (55). The nadir occurred

3 days later. In another study, it was found that gallium nitrate was more effective than etidronate given for 5 days (82% vs. 43% response rate) (74). However, in this report, the response rate to 5 days of therapy with etidronate was somewhat low in comparison to that in most other published reports. A potential toxicity of gallium nitrate is impaired renal function, manifested by an increase in serum creatinine. Other potential nephrotoxic agents such as aminoglycosides should be avoided at or around the time of gallium use. The patient's state of hydration should be well maintained and the drug should not be given to patients with renal insufficiency. Other reported side effects are hypophosphatemia and a small reduction inhemoglobin concentration (71,75). Although gallium nitrate appears to be an effective agent for the control of hypercalcemia, clinical experience with this drug is still quite limited. As greater experience is gained, it should become possible to evaluate this agent more completely in relation to other available therapeutic agents. In particular, it would be helpful to determine if shorter courses of therapy are also effective.

Glucocorticoids

Glucocorticoids can be effective calcium-lowering agents in limited groups of patients. For this purpose, 200–300 mg hydrocortisone, or its equivalent, is given intravenously daily for 3–5 days. In cancer patients, glucocorticoids are useful primarily in patients with hematological malignancies. They may act to inhibit the growth of neoplastic lymphoid tissue (76). In patients with lymphomas associated with increased 1,25(OH)$_2$D, glucocorticoids reverse hypercalcemia by lowering the level of the vitamin D metabolite (77). The same is true in sarcoidosis (78). In vitamin D intoxication, they may act on the target organ. In general, patients with nonhematological cancers do not respond to glucocorticoids (79). Primary hyperparathyroidism also is classically unresponsive to glucocorticoid administration (80).

Miscellaneous Therapy

Phosphate

Intravenous administration of sodium or potassium phosphate can produce a profound and rapid reduction in serum calcium concentrations. This treatment, however, is potentially very dangerous because of the possibility of deposition of calcium-phosphate complexes in blood vessels, lungs, and kidneys. Precipitation of these complexes has produced severe organ damage and even fatal hypotension in patients rapidly infused with high doses (81–83). The use of intravenous phosphate should be restricted, therefore, to patients with extreme, life-threatening hypercalcemia who are hypophosphatemic and in whom all other measures have failed. Oral phosphate is of little value in the emergency therapy of hypercalcemia, because its calcium-lowering activity is modest, and amounts >2 g daily are often associated with diarrhea. Oral phosphate should be reserved for settings of mild to moderate hypercalcemia associated with levels of serum phosphate that are frankly low or in the lower range of normal. The best rationale for its oral use is in patients with mild hypercalcemia due to primary hyperparathyroidism or in special circumstances surrounding the management of the secondary hyperparathyroidism of renal insufficiency (see the chapters by Stock and Marcus and by Coburn and Salusky).

Dialysis

In patients with significant renal failure, dialysis may be very effective in lowering the serum calcium concentration (84,85). Utilizing a low-calcium dialysate, either peritoneal dialysis or hemodialysis may be performed successfully.

Mobilization

Bed rest is associated with a significant increase in the rate of bone resorption as well as reduced bone formation. Therefore, patients should be encouraged to ambulate as soon as possible so that this contribution to the hypercalcemic state can be prevented.

Other Therapies

Prostaglandin synthetase inhibitors showed early promise in the control of malignant hypercalcemia in patients thought to have a prostaglandin-dependent mechanism of bone resorption (86,87). However, subsequent experience has not confirmed the value of this therapy, and these agents are now seldom used (88,89).

Amifostine, or *WR-2721*, is a chemoprotective agent that appeared to offer promise as an agent for control of hypercalcemia in primary hyperparathyroidism, particularly in patients with parathyroid carcinoma (90,91). The drug was shown to inhibit PTH secretion, to inhibit bone resorption, and to facilitate urinary calcium excretion (92–95). However, it became apparent that the potency was limited and that the effects were transient. Also, nausea, vomiting, somnolence, and hypotension were disturbing side effects (92,96,97).

Choice of Agent

The wide clinical spectrum of acute hypercalcemia prevents the use of a single therapeutic regimen for all hypercalcemic patients. It is necessary to tailor the therapy based on a consideration of the cause of the hypercalcemia, the clinical symptomatology of the patient, and the mode of action and potential side effects of the various agents. With mild hypercalcemia (serum calcium concentration <12 mg/dl), hydration with intravenous saline may be adequate therapy. Even in the presence of severe hypercalcemia, hydration with saline is the first step in management. If hypercalcemia is potentially life-threatening (>16 mg/dl) and is associated with clear symptomatology, more vigorous therapy is required along with saline. In this situation, the most rapidly acting osteoclast inhibitor, calcitonin, becomes a valuable drug. Because calcitonin alone seldom fully reverses hypercalcemia, immediate concurrent therapy should be considered. Based on safety profiles and efficacy, one of the bisphosphonates would be a good choice. Plicamycin should be considered in more difficult management situations. If the hypercalcemic state is likely to be sensitive to steroids, the concurrent administration of glucocorticoids is worthy of consideration. There are times when, despite the presence of marked hypercalcemia, the clinical appraisal does not lead to the same urgency to treat as in other situations. For example, in a patient whose serum calcium is high, >14 mg/dl, but who has only modest signs or symptoms of hypercalcemia and is otherwise stable, one might use a bisphosphonate, along with modest saline administration. The indications for the use of gallium nitrate are not yet clear; clinical experience with this drug is still quite limited. Side effects of gallium nitrate preclude its use when renal function is an issue or when potentially nephrotoxic antibiotics are being used. Finally, there is the rare patient in whom the serum calcium concentration is >20 mg/dl. Such a patient requires the most aggressive approach, with high rates of saline infusion, a bisphosphonate, calcitonin, and perhaps hydrocortisone as well if the patient has a hematologic malignancy.

THERAPY OF THE UNDERLYING DISORDER

In most hypercalcemic patients, successful management of acute hypercalcemia is followed by reappearance of hypercalcemia if definitive therapy of the underlying disorder is not possible. The availability of potent bisphosphonates now allows more long-term control of hypercalcemia even if definitive treatment fails. This is of considerable importance in that the patient whose serum calcium is now normal is still very much subject to the same pathophysiological mechanisms that originally produced the hypercalcemia. In patients with primary hyperparathyroidism, parathyroidectomy is nearly always successful in preventing recurrent hypercalcemia. Since most hypercalcemic cancer patients have advanced disease, a successful outcome for cancer therapy is much less likely. Nevertheless, satisfactory management of acute hypercalcemia allows time to plan a more definitive approach to the underlying disease.

ACKNOWLEDGMENTS

Some of the information presented in this chapter was obtained with partial support from NIH grant DK32333.

REFERENCES

1. Nussbaum SR, Zahradnik RJ, Lavigne JR, et al. Highly sensitive two-site immunoradiometric assay of parathyrin and its clinical utility in evaluating patients with hypercalcemia. *Clin Chem* 1987;33:1364–1367.

2. Broadus AE, Mangin M, Ikeda K, et al. Humoral hypercalcemia of cancer: identification of a novel parathyroid hormone-like peptide. *N Engl J Med* 1988;319:556–563.

3. Burtis WJ, Brady TG, Orloff JJ, et al. Immunochemical characterization of circulating parathyroid hormone-related protein in patients with humoral hypercalcemia of cancer. *N Engl J Med* 1990;322:1106–1112.

4. Budayr AA, Nissenson RA, Klein RF, et al. Increased serum levels of a parathyroid hormone-like protein in malignancy-associated hypercalcemia. *Ann Intern Med* 1989;111:807–812.

5. Henderson JE, Shustik C, Kremer R, Rabbani SA, Hendy GN, Goltzman D. Circulating concentrations of parathyroid hormone-like peptide in malignancy and in hyperparathyroidism. *J Bone Mineral Res* 1990;5:105–113.

6. Kao PC, Klee GG, Taylor RL, Heath H III. Parathyroid hormone-related peptide in plasma of patients with hypercalcemia and malignant lesions. *Mayo Clin Proc* 1990;65:1399–1407.

7. Bilezikian JP. Parathyroid hormone-related peptide in sickness and in health. *N Engl J Med* 1990;322:1151–1153.

8. Attie MF. Treatment of hypercalcemia. *Endocrinol Metab Clin North Am* 1989;18:807–828.

9. Harinck HIJ, Bijvoet OLM, Plantingh AST, et al. Role of bone and kidney in tumor-induced hypercalcemia and its treatment with bisphosphonate and sodium chloride. *Am J Med* 1987;82:1133–1142.

10. Nordin BEC. Plasma calcium and magnesium homeostasis. In: Nordin REC, ed: *Calcium, phosphate, and magnesium metabolism*. London: Churchill Livingstone, 1976;186–216.

11. Sleeboom HP, Bijvoet OL. Hypercalcaemia due to malignancy. Role of the kidney and treatment. *Contrib Nephrol* 1982;33:178–196.

12. Mundy GR. Hypercalcemia of malignancy revisited. *J Clin Invest* 1988;82:1–6.

13. Bilezikian JP. Management of acute hypercalcemia. *N Engl J Med* 1992;326:1196–1203.

14. Hosking DJ, Cowley A, Bucknall CA. Rehydration in the treatment of severe hypercalcemia. *Q J Med* 1981;200:473–481.

15. Suki WN, Yium JJ, Minden MV, et al. Acute treatment of hypercalcemia with furosemide. *N Engl J Med* 1970;283:836.

16. Fleisch H. Bisphosphonates: history and experimental basis. *Bone* 1987;8:S23–S28.

17. Fleisch H, Russell RGG, Bisaz S, et al. Diphosphonates inhibit hydroxyapatite dissolution in vitro and bone resorption in tissue culture. *Science* 1969;165:1262–1264.

18. Fast DK, Felix R, Dowse C, et al. The effects of diphosphonates on the growth and glycolysis of connective-tissue cells in culture. *Biochem J* 1978;172:97–107.

19. Felix R, Bettes J, Fleisch H. Effect of diphosphonates on the synthesis of prostaglandins in cultured calvaria cells. *Calcif Tissue Int* 1981;33:549–552.

20. Fleisch H. Bisphosphonates: a new class of drug in diseases of bone and calcium metabolism. In: Brunner KW, Fleisch H, Senn HJ, eds: *Recent results in cancer research, vol 116*, Berlin: Springer-Verlag, 1989;1–28.

21. Sato M, Grasser W. Effects of bisphosphonates on isolated rat osteoclasts as examined by reflected light microscopy. *J Bone Mineral Res* 1990;5:31–40.

22. Carrano A, Teitelbaum SL, Konsek JD, et al. Bisphosphonates directly inhibit the bone resorption activity of isolated avian osteoclasts in vitro. *J Clin Invest* 1990;85:456–461.

23. Ryzen E, Martodam RR, Troxell M, et al. Intravenous etidronate in the management of malignant hypercalcemia. *Arch Intern Med* 1985;145:449–452.

24. Hasling C, Charles P, Mosekilde L. Etidronate disodium in the management of malignancy-related hypercalcemia. *Am J Med* 1987;82(Suppl 2A):51–54.

25. Kanis JA, Urwin GH, Gray RES, et al. Effects of intravenous etidronate disodium on skeletal and calcium metabolism. *Am J Med* 1987;82(Suppl 2A):55–70.

26. Meunier PJ, Chapuy M-C, Delmas P, et al. Intravenous disodium etidronate therapy in Paget's disease of bone and hyper-

calcemia of malignancy: effects on biochemical parameters and bone histomorphometry. *Am J Med* 1987;82(Suppl 2A): 71–78.

27. Jacobs TP, Gordon AC, Silverberg SJ, et al. Neoplastic hypercalcemia: physiologic response to intravenous etidronate disodium. *Am J Med* 1987;82(Suppl 2A):42–50.

28. Singer FR. Role of the bisphosphonate etidronate in the therapy of cancer-related hypercalcemia. *Semin Oncol* 1990;2 (Suppl 5):34–39.

29. Singer FR, Ritch PS, Lad TE, et al. Treatment of hypercalcemia of malignancy with intravenous etidronate. *Arch Intern Med* 1991;151:471–476.

30. Flores JF, Singer FR, Rude RK. Effectiveness of a 24 hour infusion of etidronate disodium in the treatment of hypercalcemia of malignant disease. *Mineral Electrolyte Metab* 1991; 17:390–395.

31. Ringenberg QS, Ritch PS. Efficacy of oral administration of etidronate disodium in maintaining normal serum calcium levels in previously hypercalcemic cancer patients. *Clin Ther* 1987;9:1–8.

32. Schiller JH, Rasmussen P, Benson AB, et al. Maintenance etidronate in the prevention of malignancy-associated hypercalcemia. *Arch Intern Med* 1987;147:963–966.

33. Mautalen C, Gonzalez D, Blumenfeld EL, et al. Spontaneous fractures of uninvolved bones in patients with Paget's disease during unduly prolonged treatment with disodium etidronate. *Clin Orthop* 1986;207:150–155.

34. Thiebaud D, Portmann L, Jaeger P, et al. Oral versus intravenous AHP,BP(APD) in the treatment of hypercalcemia of malignancy. *Bone* 1986;7:247–253.

35. Cantwell BMJ, Harris A. Effect of single high dose infusions of aminohydroxypropylidine disphosphonate on hypercalcaemia caused by cancer. *Br Med J* 1987;294:467–469.

36. Ralston SH, Alzaid AA, Gallacher SJ, et al. Clinical experience with aminohydroxypropylidine bisphosphonate (APD) in the management of cancer-associated hypercalcaemia. *Q J Med* 1988;69:825–834.

37. Ritch PS. Treatment of cancer-related hypercalcemia. *Semin Oncol* 1990;2(Suppl 5):26–33.

38. Gucalp R, Ritch P, Wiernik PH, et al. Comparative study of pamidronate disodium and etidronate disodium in the treatment of cancer-related hypercalcemia. *J Clin Oncol* 1992; 10:134–142.

39. Thiebaud D, Jaeger P, Burckhardt P. Response to retreatment of malignant hypercalcemia with the bisphosphonate AHPrBP (APD): respective role of kidney and bone. *J Bone Mineral Res* 1990;5:221–226.

40. Fitton A, McTavish D. Pamidronate. A review of its pharmacological properties and therapeutic efficacy in resorptive bone disease. *Drugs* 1991;41:289–318.

41. van Holten-Verzantvoort AT, Bijvoet OLM, Hermans J, et al. Reduced morbidity from skeletal metastases in breast cancer patients during long-term bisphosphonates (APD) treatment. *Lancet* 1987;2:983–985.

42. Cohen AI, Koeller J, Davis TE, Citrin DL. IV dichloromethylene diphosphonate in cancer-associated hypercalcemia: a phase I–II evaluation. *Cancer Treat Rep* 1981;65:651–653.

43. Jacobs TP, Siris ES, Bilezikian JP, et al. Hypercalcemia of malignancy: treatment with intravenous dichloromethylene diphosphonate. *Ann Intern Med* 1981;94:312–316.

44. Shane E, Jacobs TP, Siris ES, et al. Therapy of hypercalcemia due to parathyroid carcinoma with intravenous dichloromethylene diphosphonate. *Am J Med* 1982;72:939–944.

45. Bonjour J, Rizzoli R. Clodronate in hypercalcemia of malignancy. *Calcif Tissue Int* 1990;46(Suppl):520–525.

46. Chapuy MC, Meunier PJ, Alexandre CM, Vignon EP. Effects of disodium dichloromethylene diphosphonate on hypercalcemia produced by bone metastases. *J Clin Invest* 1980; 65:1243–1247.

47. Douglas DL, Russell RGG, Preston CJ, et al. Effect of dichloromethylene diphosphonate in Paget's disease of bone and in hypercalcaemia due to primary hyperparathyroidism or malignant disease. *Lancet* 1980;1043–1047.

48. Siris ES, Sherman WH, Baquiran DC, et al. Effect of di-

chloromethylene diphosphonate on skeletal mobilization of calcium in multiple myeloma. *N Engl J Med* 1980;302:310–315.

49. Delmas PD, Charhon S, Chapuy MC, et al. Long-term effects of dichloromethylene diphosphonate (Cl₂MDP) on skeletal lesions in multiple myeloma. *Metab Bone Dis Rel Res* 1982; 4:163–168.

50. Jung A, Chantraine A, Donath A, et al. Use of dichloromethylene diphosphonate in metastatic bone disease. *N Engl J Med* 1983;308:1499–1501.

51. Elomaa I, Blomqvist C, Porkka L, et al. Diphosphonates for osteolytic metastases. *Lancet* 1985;1:1155–1156.

52. Silva O, Becker KL. Salmon calcitonin in the treatment of hypercalcemia. *Arch Intern Med* 1973;132:337–339.

53. Hosking DJ, Gilson D. Comparison of the renal and skeletal actions of calcitonin in the treatment of severe hypercalcaemia of malignancy. *Q J Med* 1984;53:359–368.

54. Binstock ML, Mundy GR. Effect of calcitonin and glucocorticoids in combination on the hypercalcemia of malignancy. *Ann Intern Med* 1980;93:269.

55. Warrell RP, Israel R, Frisone M, et al. Gallium nitrate for acute treatment of cancer-related hypercalcemia: a randomized, double-blind comparison to calcitonin. *Ann Intern Med* 1988;108:669–674.

56. Ralston SH, Gardner MD, Dryburgh FJ. Comparison of aminohydroxypropylidine diphosphonate, mithramycin, and corticosteroids/calcitonin in treatment of cancer-associated hypercalcemia. *Lancet* 1985;2:207–210.

57. Thiebaud D, Burckhardt P, Jaeger PH, et al. Effectiveness of salmon calcitonin administered as suppositories in tumor-induced hypercalcemia. *Am J Med* 1987;82:745–750.

58. Ralston SH, Gardner MD, Dryburgh FJ, et al. Comparison of aminohydroxypropylidene diphosphonate, mithramycin, and corticosteroids/calcitonin in treatment of cancer-associated hypercalcemia. *Lancet* 1985;2:907–909.

59. Thiebaud D, Jacquet F, Burckhardt P. Fast and effective treatment of malignant hypercalcemia. *Arch Intern Med* 1990;150:2125–2128.

60. Ralston SH, Alzaid AA, Gardner MD, Boyle IT. Treatment of cancer associated hypercalcemia with combined aminohydroxypropylidene diphosphonate and calcitonin. *Br Med J* 1986;292:1549–1550.

61. Fatemi S, Singer FR, Rude RK. Effect of salmon calcitonin and etidronate on hypercalcemia of malignancy. *Calcif Tissue Int* 1992;50:107–109.

62. Wisnecki LA. Salmon calcitonin in the acute management of hypercalcemia. *Calcif Tissue Int* 1990;46(Suppl):526–530.

63. Stewart AF. Therapy of malignancy-associated hypercalcemia. *Am J Med* 1983;74:475.

64. Perlia CP, Gubisch NJ, Cootter J, Edelberg D, Dederick MM, Taylor SG. Mithramycin treatment of hypercalcemia. *Cancer* 1970;25:389.

65. Minkin C. Inhibition of parathyroid hormone stimulated bone resorption in vitro by the antibiotic mithramycin. *Calcif Tissue Res* 1973;13:249–257.

66. Kiang DT, Loken MK, Kennedy BJ. Mechanism of the hypocalcemic effect of mithramycin. *J Clin Endocrinol Metab* 1979;48:341.

67. Green L, Donehower RC. Hepatic toxicity of low doses of mithramycin in hypercalcemia. *Cancer Treat Rep* 1984;68: 1379–1381.

68. Slavik M, Carter SK. Chromomycin A₂, mithramycin and olivomycin: antitumor antibiotics of related structure. 1975;12: 1–15.

69. Warrell RP Jr, Bockman RS, Coonley CJ, et al. Gallium nitrate inhibits calcium resorption from bone and is effective treatment for cancer-related hypercalcemia. *J Clin Invest* 1984;73:1487–1490.

70. Bockman RS, Boskey AL, Alcock N, et al. Gallium nitrate increases bone calcium and crystallite perfection of hydroxyapatite. *Calcif Tissue Int* 1986;39:376–381.

71. Warrell RP, Bockman RS. Gallium in the treatment of hypercalcemia and bone metastases. In: *Important advances in oncology*. Philadelphia: J.B. Lippincott, 1989;205–220.

72. Hall TJ, Chambers TJ. Gallium inhibits bone resorption by a direct action on osteoclasts. *Bone Mineral* 1990;8:211–216.
73. Warrell RP, Alcock NW, Bockman RS. Gallium nitrate inhibits accelerated bone turnover in patients with bone metastases. *J Clin Oncol* 1987;5:292–298.
74. Warrell RP, Murphy WK, Schulman P, O'Dwyer PJ, Heller G. A randomized double-blind study of gallium nitrate compared with etidronate for acute control of cancer-related hypercalcemia. *J Clin Oncol* 1991;9:1467–1475.
75. Warrell RP, Bosco B, Weinerman S, et al. Gallium nitrate for advanced Paget disease of bone: effectiveness and dose-response analysis. *Ann Intern Med* 1990;113:847–851.
76. Goodwin JS, Atluru D, Sierakowski S, et al. Mechanism of action of glucocorticosteroids: Inhibition of T cell proliferation and interleukin 2 production by hydrocortisone is reversed by leukotriene B4. *J Clin Invest* 1986;77:1244.
77. Breslau NA, McGuire JL, Zerwekh JE, et al. Hypercalcemia associated with increased serum calcitriol levels in three patients with lymphoma. *Ann Intern Med* 1984;100:1–7.
78. Sandler LM, Winearls CG, Fraher LJ, et al. Studies of the hypercalcemia of sarcoidosis: effect of steroids and exogenous vitamin D$_3$ on the circulating concentrations of 1,25-dihydroxyvitamin D$_3$. *Q J Med* 1984;53:165–180.
79. Percival RC, Yates AJP, Gray RES, et al. The role of glucocorticoids in the management of malignant hypercalcemia. *Br Med J* 1984;289:287.
80. Bilezikian JP. Hypercalcemic states. In: Coe FL, Favus MJ, eds. *Disorders of bone and mineral metabolism.* New York: Raven Press, 1992;493–522.
81. Shackney S, Hasson J. Precipitous fall in serum calcium, hypotension and acute renal failure after intravenous phosphate therapy for hypercalcemia. *Ann Intern Med* 1967;66:906–916.
82. Vernava AM, O'Neal LW, Palermo V: Lethal hyperparathyroid crisis: hazards of phosphate administration. *Surgery* 1987;102:942–948.
83. Carey RW, Schmitt GW, Kopald HH. Massive extraskeletal calcification during phosphate treatment of hypercalcemia. *Arch Intern Med* 1968;122:150–155.
84. Cardella CJ, Birkin BL, Rapoport A. Role of dialysis in the treatment of severe hypercalcemia: report of two cases successfully treated with hemodialysis and review of the literature. *Clin Nephrol* 1979;12:285–290.
85. Heyburn PJ, Selby PL, Peacock M, et al. Peritoneal dialysis in the management of severe hypercalcaemia. *Br Med J* 1980;280:525–526.
86. Brereton HD, Halushka PV, Alexander RW, et al. Indomethacin-responsive hypercalcemia in a patient with renal-cell adenocarcinoma. *N Engl J Med* 1974;291:83–85.
87. Seyberth HW, Segre GV, Morgan JL, et al. Prostaglandins as mediators of hypercalcemia associated with certain types of cancer. *N Engl J Med* 1975;293:1278–1283.
88. Brenner DE, Harvey HA, Lipton A. A study of prostaglandin E$_2$, parathormone and response to indomethacin in patients with hypercalcemia of malignancy. *Cancer* 1982;49:556–561.
89. Coombes RC, Neville AM, Bondy PK, et al. Failure of indomethacin to reduce hydroxyproline excretion or hypercalcemia in patients with breast cancer. *Prostaglandins* 1976;12:1027–1035.
90. Glover D, Riley L, Carmichael K, et al. Hypocalemia and inhibition of parathyroid hormone secretion after administration of WR-2721 (a radioprotective and chemoprotective agent). *N Engl J Med* 1983;309:1137–1141.
91. Glover DJ, Shaw L, Glick JH, et al. Treatment of hypercalcemia in parathyroid cancer with WR-2721, S-2-(3-aminopropylamino)ethyl-phosphorothioic acid. *Ann Intern Med* 1985;103:55–57.
92. Attie MF, Fallon MD, Spar B, et al. Bone and parathyroid inhibitory effects of S-2(3-aminopropylamino)ethylphosphorothioic acid. Studies in experimental animals and cultured bone cells. *J Clin Invest* 1985;75:1191–1197.
93. Fallon MD. Direct inhibition of osteoclast bone resorbing activity by WR-2721, a new hypocalcemic agent. *Calcif Tissue Int* 1984;36:481.
94. Hirschel-Scholz S, Caverzasio J, Bonjour JP. Inhibition of parathyroid hormone secretion and parathyroid hormone-independent diminution of tubular calcium reabsorption by WR-2721, a unique hypocalcemic agent. *J Clin Invest* 1985;76:1851–1856.
95. Hirschel-Scholz S, Caverzasio J, Rizzoli R, et al. Normalization of hypercalcemia associated with a decrease in renal calcium reabsorption in Leydig cell tumor-bearing rats treated with WR-2721. *J Clin Invest* 1986;78:319–322.
96. Hirschel-Scholz S, Jung A, Fischer JA, et al. Suppression of parathyroid secretion after administration of WR-2721 in a patient with parathyroid carcinoma. *Clin Endocrinol* 1985;23:313–318.
97. Glover D, Glick JH, Weiler C, et al. Phase I/II trials of WR-2721 and cisplatinum. *Int J Radiat Oncol Biol Phys* 1986;12:1509–1512.

The Parathyroids, edited by J.P. Bilezikian,
M.A. Levine, and R. Marcus. Raven Press, Ltd.,
New York © 1994.

CHAPTER 23

Parathyroid Growth

Normal and Abnormal

A. Michael Parfitt

INTRODUCTION AND BACKGROUND

Why Study Parathyroid Growth?

The functional performance of every endocrine gland requires delivery of the right number of hormone molecules into the circulation during each successive interval of the appropriate time scale. Total hormone secretion comprises the aggregate contribution of each cell and so depends not only on the average secretion per cell but also on the number of contributing cells. The regulation of cell number it seems should receive as much attention as the regulation of individual cell behavior, but in practice it is almost entirely ignored. For example, in a 2,700 page textbook of endocrinology (1), less than 1% of the material is concerned with the attainment and maintenance of gland size. Whether there are one hundred or one billion cells in a gland appears not to matter, and cell number is never considered explicitly in the description of feedback relationships. There are several reasons for this neglect. The rules of development normally ensure that each organ grows to the right size (2), so that adult cell number varies only over a three- to fourfold range. By contrast, hormone secretion by many endocrine glands can vary acutely over as much as a 100-fold range, which must reflect changes in the performance of individual cells. Another reason is that the endocrine glands are among the smallest of organs. Only the thyroid and the gonads can be palpated; the other glands

are inaccessible clinically, and estimation of their size by noninvasive methods is of varying precision, which is least for the parathyroid gland. Yet another reason is that people are attracted to endocrinology by their fascination with the hormones themselves and their mechanisms of secretion and action, rather than with the morphology of their glands of origin.

A neglect of gland size may be justified pragmatically if one's aim is restricted to understanding normal physiology but it involves neglect also of several interesting scientific questions. Why does the parathyroid gland need to be so much smaller than the other endocrine glands? Why is total parathyroid weight a much larger fraction of body weight in the chick (~10 mg/kg) (3) than in the rat (~1 mg/kg) (4)? Such questions lie within the realm of evolutionary biology, but their answers might well provide information relevant to medical science. At a more practical level, short-term changes in hormone secretion are of lesser magnitude than those in other glands and are not sustainable indefinitely; long-term changes, whether they are expressions of adaptation or of disease, invariably require changes in cell number as well as in individual cell function. Every parathyroid disorder considered in this book is a reflection of, or at least is associated with, characteristic changes in the number of functioning parathyroid cells. Understanding the mechanisms whereby parathyroid cells are able to change their number is essential to a full understanding of pathogenesis and is also relevant to both medical and surgical treatment. However, before these clinically important issues are approached, it is necessary to review concepts of normal organ and tissue growth, the regulation of cell number as the balance between cell proliferation and cell death, and the normal

A. M. Parfitt: Bone and Mineral Research Laboratory, Henry Ford Hospital, Detroit, Michigan 48202; and Department of Medicine, University of Michigan, Ann Arbor, Michigan 48109.

growth and turnover of parathyroid tissue. A central theme will be the close interrelationship between the regulation of hormone secretion and the regulation of cell number in the parathyroid glands.

Concepts of Growth

There is more to biological growth than increase in size; growth has been described as ". . . the study of change in an organism not yet mature" (5), which includes the processes of development and the determination of form, both external and internal. Relative growth is most rapid in utero, although for some tissues and organs absolute growth is more rapid after birth. It is useful to extend the scope of growth to cover also maintenance by turnover, repair, and regeneration (6). Growth can be studied at different levels of organization, both functional and structural. A functional unit, the smallest structure that can carry out a specific function by itself, may correspond to any structural level: whole organisms, organ, tissue, cell, or subcellular entity. In the endocrine system, functional units may be either multicellular, such as thyroid and ovarian follicles, or unicellular, as in the anterior pituitary and the testis. All functional units can increase or decrease in size—hyper- or hypotrophy, but only some can increase or decrease in number—hyper- or hypoplasia (7,8). During early development, hyperplasia, whether of individual cells or of functional units, precedes hypertrophy (2,9). After birth there is overlap between these different modes of growth, although in most organs significant hypertrophy is absent after the first 2 weeks, and at all ages hyperplasia is the main determinant of increase in size (10,11).

The basic instrument of growth is the cyclical process of cell replication and division. Despite spectacular advances in the understanding of this process (12), along with understanding of its stimulation by an ever larger number of growth factors (13), knowledge concerning growth regulation at higher levels of organization remains incomplete. In species of finite life span and determinate size, a growth target for the whole body and for each organ has to be specified very early in development (2,6), and approach toward the target has to be monitored and controlled in accordance with a characteristic growth curve. Precisely how such a "sizostat" (14) could function remains a mystery, but its rules of operation must be encoded somewhere in the genome. Many general theories of growth have been proposed, but none has become established. Almost 200 years ago, John Hunter concluded that growth was regulated by functional demand (15). This remains a sound principle of physiologic adaptation in mature organisms but cannot be the main explanation for developmental growth. During functional adaptation, hypertrophy is the initial response and may re-

main the only response if the work of the cell is mainly physical or if the functional unit is multicellular and of sufficient complexity that new ones cannot develop after birth, as for nephrons or lung alveoli (6,7). However, if the work of the cell is mainly biochemical, as in the endocrine glands, eventually hyperplasia will also develop.

It has several times been proposed that each organ or tissue secretes, in proportion to its size, an inhibitor of its own growth, now usually referred to as its *chalone* (15,16). Much evidence for the existence of chalones has been assembled (17), including feedback regulation of intestinal crypt cell proliferation in a manner consistent with the chalone concept (18), but no chalone has been fully characterized (16). A currently more popular theme is external control by means of tissue-specific stimulators, but most of these remain unidentified, and most known growth factors are ubiquitous in their distribution and sites of action (13). In some organs the same growth factors may be involved in developmental growth, regeneration after injury, and functional adaptation (19,20). In the pituitary and probably also in the glands under its control, the same hormones stimulate growth as well as hormone secretion (21), but at the appointed time growth stops, yet hormone secretion continues. There is evidence for central regulation of targeted whole body growth by a non growth hormone-dependent mechanism in the brain (14,22), but individual organs are more likely to be controlled locally by some widely distributed system, such as cells derived from the neural crest, lymphoid tissue (23), or vascular endothelium (24). The same growth factor could be used by different tissues, target specificity depending on autocrine or paracrine mechanisms (13), or on the constraints of the local microcirculation, but this would not explain how a predetermined size was chosen and reached. The possible role of parathyroid endothelium is mentioned below and is described in more detail in the chapters by Sakaguchi, Metz et al., and Friedman et al.

Patterns of Cell Renewal

All cells can be classified, on the basis of their current relationship to the cell cycle (Fig. 1), as cycling or non-cycling. Cycling cells are in one of the four stages of the cycle: G1, S, G2, or M. Noncycling cells may be in a resting state (G0) between one cycle and the next or no longer dividing because of terminal differentiation (16,25). From the standpoint of cell kinetics, all adult tissues are usually classified into one of three major types (16,25). Tissues such as nerve and cardiac muscle are nonreplicators, all cells having lost the capacity for division, perhaps as a consequence of the intracellular location of their end products (7). Tissues with a high rate of cell turnover (continuous replica-

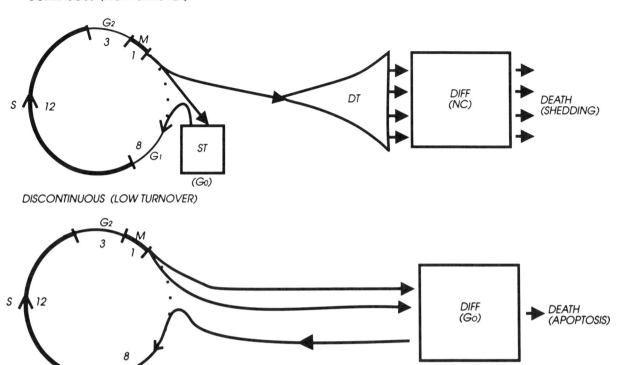

FIG. 1. Cell cycle in two types of tissue with respect to replication. The cell cycle comprises two periods of execution—DNA synthesis (S) and mitosis (M)—interrupted by two periods of preparation—gaps (G) 1 and 2. Durations (in hours) are chosen partly for convenience of illustration but are broadly representative of human nonneoplastic tissue (16). As well as duplication of the nucleus, the cycle involves duplication of all other constituents of the cell. The interrupted line between M and early G_1 is traversed only by continuously cycling cells. Other cells enter a quiescent state with respect to proliferation (G_0), the duration of which varies from days to decades in different tissues. Tissues in which replication is continuous (**top**) have high turnover, and a separate population of stem cells (St). Periodically, a stem cell switches from G_0 to G_1, and on average the mitosis leads to one new stem cell and one cell committed to differentiate. The commitment step is amplified by continuous cycling in a dividing transit (DT) compartment for a variable number of generations (two in this case). The differentiated cells (Diff) are noncycling (NC) and are eventually lost by shedding, or by sequestration, as in bone. Tissues in which replication is discontinuous (**bottom**) have low turnover and no stem cell or dividing transit compartments. Periodically, a differentiated cell switches from G_0 to G_1, and the result of the mitosis is two new differentiated cells. The addition of each new cell is balanced by loss of one old cell by apoptosis. It is this type of replication that occurs in the parathyroid gland.

tors) have a high rate of mitosis, which occurs initially in a functionally (and often anatomically) separate population of stem cells (Table 1). These cells, usually in G0, repeatedly but infrequently traverse the cell cycle, each complete cycle on the average producing one new cell committed to differentiate in a particular direction and one new stem cell. Renewal of stem cells probably depends on a stochastic balance between two types of symmetric cell division rather than on each stem cell division being asymmetric (26). The committed daughter cells undergo clonal expansion in a transit compartment for a variable number of generations (25,26). The number of terminally differentiated, nondividing but functionally active cells is maintained approximately constant by continuous shedding, either from the body (as in the skin or the intestinal mucosa) or into the circulation (as in the bone marrow).

By contrast, tissues with low cell turnover (discontinuous replicators or conditional renewal tissues) have a low rate of mitosis and no separate stem cell population (16,25) (Table 1). All cells of the tissue spend most of their time in G0 carrying out its normal function, but all have the potential for undergoing cell division. Periodically, a functioning cell enters the cell cycle ($G_0 \rightarrow G_1$), and the result of the mitosis is two new functioning cells. Cell balance is maintained by a few cells losing the capacity for division, eventually dying and being removed in some way. Mitosis can be stimulated by the need to regenerate (as in the liver) or by increased functional demand (as in endocrine glands) and occurs at random throughout the tissue. This concept has recently been challenged (27). Many organs traditionally classified as discontinuous replicators and lacking stem cells, including the liver (28),

TABLE 1. *Contrasting characteristics of two mechanisms for maintenance of adult tissue mass*

	Type of replication	
	Continuous	Discontinuous
Cell function	Poststem cells only	All cells
Cell life span	Short	Long
Mitosis		
Potential	Stem cells and transit cells only	All cells
Location	Often segregated	Scattered
Rate	High	Low[a]
Cell loss		
Mechanism	External[b] shedding	Internal[b] deletion
Rate	High	Low

[a]Can increase sharply in response to various stimuli.
[b]With respect to the tissue.

the submandibular gland, and the adrenal gland, may have to be reclassified as continuous replicators, with an anatomically discrete stem cell population. In each organ, after pulse administration of tritiated thymidine, serial examination for the appropriate frequency and duration has suggested that new cells originate in one region and are slowly displaced along a predictable trajectory. It is proposed that, in the liver, cell streaming occurs from the portal tract toward the hepatic vein; in the submandibular gland, from the intercalated toward the granular duct; and, in the adrenal gland, from the subcapsular region of the zona glomerulosa toward the zona reticularis (27). If the cell streaming concept is correct, the manner of cell renewal is the same in all tissues, and the categories in Table 1 differ in degree rather than in kind.

What is the mechanism of cell loss in tissues with a low rate of turnover and no obvious means of shedding cells? Except in pathologic situations in which the blood supply is jeopardized, it does not occur by necrosis. In recent years a nonnecrotic mechanism of cell deletion has been identified, referred to as *apoptosis* (29). This process normally affects scattered single cells and has characteristic histologic and ultrastructural features, beginning with condensation and disintegration of the nucleus, followed by breaking up of the whole cell into membrane-bound fragments of varying size, which are rapidly subjected to phagocytosis by adjacent cells. The remaining cells simply close ranks so that no gap is left by the deleted cell. The distinction between necrosis and apoptosis may be likened to the distinction between murder and suicide. Apoptosis is an active process dependent on altered gene expression, of which the molecular mechanisms are under intense investigation (30). Particularly relevant to the present discussion is that, whenever tissue that is hyperplastic as the result of endocrine stimulation undergoes involution, the process of cell loss occurs by apoptosis. This has been shown for the hyperplastic adrenal gland after with-

drawal of adrenocorticotropin (ACTH) (31), in the endometrium after withdrawal of estradiol in the normal menstrual cycle (32), in the breast after withdrawal of prolactin (33), and in the prostate after withdrawal of testosterone (34). Apoptosis is probably as important as mitosis in regulating the number of functioning cells in tissues and organs with normally low turnover (29,30,35).

NORMAL PARATHYROID GROWTH AND TURNOVER

Methods of Study

The most straightforward method of studying growth is to express some index of size, either weight or volume, as a function of age. Weight is preferred in that it is easier to measure accurately and is in general use in anatomy and pathology. Because of variation in tissue density, weight is a more accurate index of cell number than volume (= weight/density). A commonly used approximation is that 1 g tissue contains 2^{30} (= $1.094 \cdot 10^9$) cells (36). This disregards variation in cell size but in the parathyroid gland gives results very similar to total DNA content (37). Parathyroid tissue contains fat cells and a vascular connective tissue stroma as well as the parenchyma consisting of chief cells and their derivatives (see the chapter by LiVolsi). Parenchymal volume as a fraction of total volume can be measured by point counting on histologic sections (38), and parenchymal weight as a fraction of total weight can be derived from measurement of whole gland density, assuming a constant value for fat cell density (39). Estimated parenchymal weight provides a more accurate value for parenchymal cell number than total weight. Regrettably, even though "the best histological criterion (of diagnosis) is the weight of the gland" (40), weighing of parathyroid glands is frequently omitted, and only linear dimensions are recorded. The product of three dimensions (rectangular volume; RV) is significantly correlated with weight ($r = 0.81$) and can be used to estimate weight from the regression Wt (g) = 0.585 RV (cm^3) + 0.134 (41). The product of only two dimensions, measured in a representative section, also correlates quite well ($r = 0.76$) with weight (42).

If the parathyroid glands are very small, as in the rat, measurement of weight is less accurate because complete removal of extraneous tissue is more difficult, and measurement of volume is a good alternative. This can be obtained by means of the Cavalieri principle from serial sections that cover the entire length of the embedded gland. Volume can be calculated from the number of sections, the average distance between the sections, and the average cross-sectional area in the sections (38). For an unbiased estimate, it is necessary that the location of the first section with respect to the pole of the gland is selected randomly, but this precaution has usually been omitted. In the past, section area was measured by various planimetric and projection methods, but today point counting with systematic random sampling and an unbiased counting frame (38), digitization, or automated image analysis (43) would be used. The estimation of gland volume in this manner is essential for the most accurate distinction between hyperplasia (increase in cell number) and hypertrophy (increase in cell size). Average cell profile area can be measured in sections and average cell volume calculated on the basis of reasonable assumptions (44). More accurately, the number of cells or cell nuclei per unit volume of tissue can be obtained through the disector method (44). The distinction can also be approached biochemically, using total DNA as an index of cell number and total protein as an index of total cell mass; the protein/DNA ratio remains unchanged in hyperplasia but increases in hypertrophy (11,16).

Cell number, cell size, and tissue mass represent the "bottom line" of growth but give no information concerning mechanisms. For a complete description of cell cycle kinetics, the proportion of cycling cells (or growth fraction) and the durations of each phase of the cell cycle must be determined (16,25). Together these give the birth rate of new cells, from which can be calculated the rate of increase in tissue volume, usually expressed as potential doubling time (36). Comparison of this with the actual rate of tissue growth provides an indirect estimate of the rate of cell loss (25,29,36). The necessary methods are complex, are most appropriate for rapidly growing tissues, and have never been applied to the parathyroid gland. More generally useful is determination of the proportion of cells in one or more stages of the cell cycle (Table 2). The durations of S, G2, and M phases (Fig. 1) vary between fairly narrow limits among different tissues (16,25), and, if a representative value is assumed, the birth rate of new cells can be estimated, provided the rate of proliferation is stable and growth is slow (37,41). The first cell cycle marker to be used was the change in nuclear

morphology during mitosis (45). Prompt fixation for an adequate duration in fluid of the right pH is needed (46), and positive cells are much less frequent than with other cell cycle markers because the duration of mitosis is much shorter (Fig. 1). If mitosis is arrested, mitotic figures will be more frequent, but cell birth rate can no longer be estimated. There are currently more data on the prevalence of mitosis than of any other cell cycle phase in the parathyroid glands.

The most well established of such methods is identification of S-phase cells by radioautography after administration of tritiated thymidine (16,25,36). Much less satisfactory is measurement of thymidine incorporation into acid-insoluble macromolecules, the results of which are influenced not only by the rate of DNA synthesis but also by thymidine pool size, activity of thymidine kinase, utilization of the salvage pathway for pyrimidine biosynthesis, and diffusion of thymidine into dead or dying cells (19,47–49). These pitfalls are much more serious with acute in vitro experiments than with steady state in vivo measurements, and in parathyroid adenomas there is a good correlation between thymidine incorporation and the proportion of S-phase cells (37,50). S-phase cells can also be labeled by bromodeoxyuridine, a nonradioactive analog of thymidine that can be detected by immunostaining (51). Results can be obtained more quickly, but the method is less useful for following the migration of labeled cells or the recognition of subsequent division by the dilution of label intensity. More widely applicable are methods for the immunologic identification of other cell cycle markers (45), such as Ki67 or proliferating cell nuclear antigen (PCNA/cyclin). Not to be confused with the various cyclins identified as cell cycle regulators (52), PCNA/cyclin is an accessory factor for DNA polymerase δ and is expressed only in cycling cells, with greatest intensity during S phase (53). Since the information is already present in the nucleus, nothing has to be administered, and the method can be applied to paraffin-embedded sections and so to archival material.

Cells can be sorted according to their stage in the cycle by flow cytometry based on their content of DNA, which doubles between G0/G1 and G2/M phases and is intermediate in S phase (54). Despite the very large number of cells that can be counted, it is impossible to get accurate results when cell turnover is low and the growth fraction very small, because of cellular debris and other artefacts (55). In this circumstance, changes in DNA content are much more likely to reflect changes in ploidy than changes related to the cell cycle. Cells with a normal number of chromosomes are referred to as *diploid* or *euploid*. Cells with a diploid number increased exactly by a power of 2 are polyploid, most commonly tetraploid, and occasionally octaploid or of higher ploidy. Polyploidy is a normal occurrence in the liver and the heart. The mech-

TABLE 2. *Cell cycle markers*[a]

	Marker	Feature
Need either administration *in vivo* or cell survival *ex vivo* or *in vitro*	a. ³H-thymidine b. BrDU	Accepted standard Nonradioactive
Information already in nucleus	a. Mitosis b. Ki67 c. Cyclin/ PCNA	First to be used Fresh frozen tissue Archival tissue

[a]Except for mitosis, these markers mainly label S phase, but Ki67 and cyclin/PCNA may label a greater fraction of the cycle.

anism is unknown but presumably involves normal duplication of each chromosome, with failure of mitosis and cytokinesis. Such cells are, in effect, arrested in G2, a condition that may also represent a response to a growth stimulus that shares features of both hyperplasia and hypertrophy (16). Cells with an abnormal chromosome number that does not differ exactly by a power of 2 from the diploid number are aneuploid, either hypo- or hyperdiploid. This is the result of loss or duplication of individual chromosomes, a cytogenetic abnormality that is not related to normal cell replication (56).

Cell Number, Proliferation, and Loss as Functions of Age

The parathyroid glands appear abruptly during the fifth week of gestation (57). Based on the very small amount of fat present during growth (58) and a mean parenchymal cell density of 1.065 (39), the glands grow to a total parenchymal weight of ~3 μg at a crown–rump length of ~30 mm (57), corresponding to a gestational age of ~8 weeks (59). Weight increases quite slowly from 3 μg to 6 μg between 8 and 12 weeks, but then increases much more rapidly, growing to ~300 μg

(0.3 mg) between 12 and 18 weeks (57,60), and ~4 mg, corresponding to ~4.3 · 10⁶ cells, at birth (60,61). Based on interpolation and smoothing of quite sparse data (57,58,60,61), parathyroid growth appears to follow a sigmoid curve through the end of the first year of life, or up to 92 weeks of conceptional age (Fig. 2). The conversion of weight to cell number is only approximate, because in the rat parathyroid cell volume increases ~50% in the first 10 weeks of life (62). Similar sigmoid growth curves have been found for the adrenal, thyroid, and pituitary glands (63) but with the inflections occurring before rather than after birth. If the interpretation given in Fig. 2 is correct, absolute weight gain is most rapid at ~20 weeks after birth, although relative weight gain is most rapid at ~16 weeks of gestational age.

Parathyroid growth continues at the rate, established toward the end of the first year, of ~2.5–3.0 mg/year. The data are too few to demonstrate a second parathyroid growth spurt during adolescence, but in that such a spurt has been found in every organ and tissue for which sufficient data are available (64), it seems reasonable to assume that such a spurt would also occur in the parathyroid gland (Fig. 3). Growth then occurs progressively more slowly until the mature parenchymal weight is reached at age ~30 years (61,65). Total mature weight in white subjects has var-

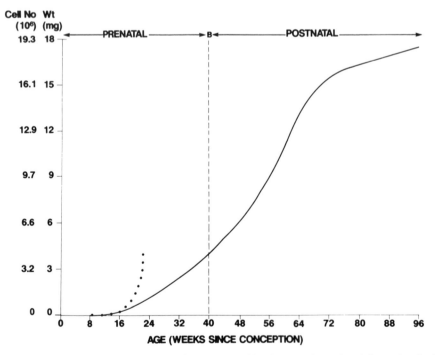

FIG. 2. Parathyroid growth curve during the first 2 years. Total parenchymal weight and calculated cell number are plotted as a function of age (in weeks) since conception. The cell number scale assumes that 1 mg tissue contains 1.074 · 10⁶ cells (36) and disregards modest changes in parathyroid cell volume during growth (61). A continuous curve was constructed based on data in references 57, 58, 60, and 61. *Dashed line* denotes time of birth (B); *dotted line* indicates predicted outcome of continued exponential growth at the peak rate found at 16 weeks.

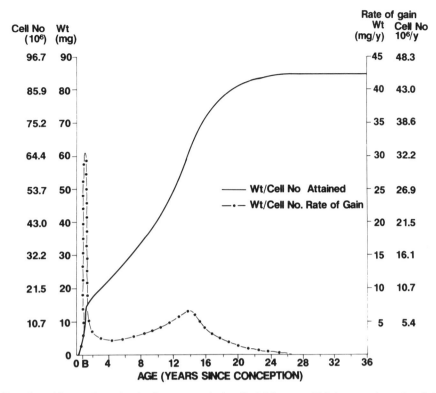

FIG. 3. Parathyroid growth and velocity curves during first 36 years. Total parenchymal weight and cell number, calculated as for Fig. 2, plotted as a function of age (in years) since conception (scales on the left). A continuous curve was constructed from data in references 57, 58, 60, and 65, assuming that there is an adolescent spurt centered at conceptional age 14 years. The *dotted line* is the first derivative of the growth curve and shows rate of absolute gain, or velocity, as a function of conceptional age (scales on the right). Note that the lifetime parathyroid growth curve consists of two successive sigmoid curves, the second one magnified on both axes. B, birth.

ied from ~85 mg (61,65,66) to ~95 mg (67,68), corresponding to a total cell number of 90–100 · 10⁶, with a coefficient of variation (CV; = SD/mean · 100) of ~30% (65), but there is no significant further change with increasing age (61,65,66). In different series, parathyroid weight in men has been less than (61), the same as (65), or more than (66,68) that in women. In three series (66,68,69), parathyroid weight has been significantly greater in black than in white subjects of both sexes, to a greater extent that could be accounted for by differences in body weight. Also in blacks, unlike the case in whites, there appear to be significant changes in parathyroid weight after attainment of maturity, with peak values in both sexes between the ages of 41 and 60 years (68).

During embryonic development, in organs and tissues that change in location or shape, as well as in size, or in which provisional structures must be replaced, growth is partly offset by apoptotic deletion of unwanted cells (29,30), but there is neither evidence nor apparent need for this process in the developing parathyroid gland. Assuming the absence of apoptosis, the first derivative of the growth curve, or growth ve-

locity, provides an estimate of the absolute frequency of mitoses associated with growth, which is about five times higher during the first year of life than at any other time (Fig. 3), presumably with a second, much smaller peak during the adolescent growth spurt. The absolute frequency of cell division depends on the number of cells present at a particular time and on the relative rate of cell division, or specific cell birth rate; the latter rate determines how frequently successive divisions occur in the same cell line. Disregarding turnover and considering only growth, this rate is most rapid during the second trimester of embryonic development, which is the only time of life when the interval between successive divisions is <1 month. The peak rate (3400%/year) occurs at ~16 weeks, when each cell is dividing about once every 10 days and the population doubling time is just over 1 week (Fig. 4). The specific birth rate then falls rapidly by more than tenfold to ~300%/year at birth, with a doubling time of ~3 months, continuing to fall to ~8%/year at age 9 years, with a doubling time of about 8 years. There is a modest increase in specific birth rate and a decrease in doubling time during the adolescent growth spurt,

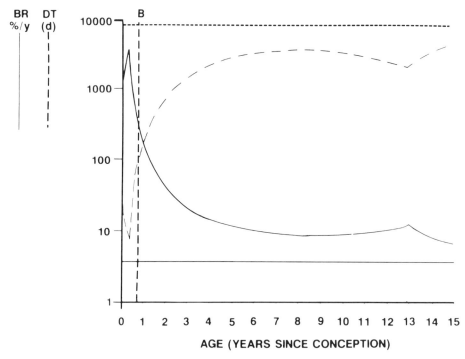

FIG. 4. Parathyroid relative growth and inferred doubling time during first 15 years. Cell birth rate (BR; %/year) and doubling time (DT, days) plotted on a logarithmic scale as functions of age (in years since conception), derived from the continuous curves illustrated in Figs. 2 and 3. The values are based only on growth and take no account of turnover. The relationship between the two variables is DT(day) = $\log_e 2/BR(\%/year) \cdot 100 \cdot 365$. The relationship is hyperbolic on a linear scale, but the curves are mirror images on a logarithmic scale. The *solid straight line* indicates the normal turnover rate in the adult gland, and the *dashed straight line* indicates the corresponding doubling time. B, birth.

after which the birth rate falls and the doubling time rises progressively toward the adult values, which are based solely on turnover, growth having ceased.

From the standpoint of cell turnover, the parathyroid glands are the least extensively studied tissue in the body; they are not mentioned in an otherwise comprehensive text (25). The rapid growth rate inferred from serial weights during embryonic development is supported by measurements of mitotic prevalence in 35–50 day guinea pig embryos (70). Assuming a duration of mitosis of 45 min (16), the mean value of 22.2/ 10^4 cells corresponds to a population doubling time of ~10 days, very similar to the inferred value of 7 days in the human. The prevalence of mitosis falls steadily after birth, although in the mouse a brief burst of mitosis occurs ~3 weeks after birth (71). Data on adult parathyroid glands are sparse, but it seems clear that they fall into the third category of discontinuous replicators (Table 1). The rate of mitosis is so low that no pathologist has had sufficient patience to count the prevalence of mitotic figures in normal human parathyroid tissue, and, in stimulated tissue, thymidine-labeled cells appear to be randomly dispersed (72), as would be expected in a tissue lacking a separate stem cell population. The prevalence of mitoses was 0.88/ 10^4 cells in the adult guinea pig, with a tendency to fall

with age (70), and 0.54/10^4 cells in the adult rat (73). Assuming the same duration of mitosis, these values correspond to average rates of cell turnover of 103%/ year and 63%/year and average cell life spans of 12 and 19 months, respectively. In humans, the reduction in parenchymal cell mass in the nonadenomatous glands of patients with primary hyperparathyroidism (74) and the proportion of labeled cells in such glands (50) suggest a normal rate of cell turnover of 2.8%/year and a cell life span of ~36 years (8). In all three species, the average cell life span is about one-half the usual life expectancy, so that, after cessation of growth, few parathyroid cells divide more than twice, and many do not divide at all, a characteristic feature of discontinuous replicators (75).

Even though cell turnover is very low, it contributes substantially to the total lifetime number of parathyroid mitoses (Fig. 5). Assuming that turnover-related mitoses occur at the same fractional rate throughout life, their rate of accumulation will increase with increasing size, reaching a maximum slope when adult size is attained at age 30 years. Growth-related mitoses follow the growth curve exactly and obviously predominate in early life, but they no longer occur when growth stops so that turnover-related mitoses predominate after age ~45 years and become a progressively

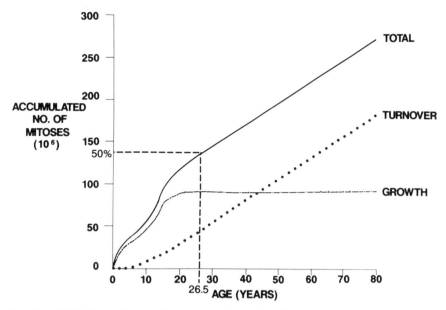

FIG. 5. Parathyroid lifetime mitoses. Accumulated number of mitoses as a function of age, growth-related (*dashed line*), turnover-related (*dotted line*), and total (*solid line*). Note that growth-related mitoses predominate during the first 20 years but that turnover-related mitoses predominate after about age 45 years. The *dashed right-angle lines* indicate that, for a life span of 80 years, the median parathyroid mitosis occurs at age 26.5 years; the median growth-related mitosis occurs at age 9.5 years, and the median turnover related mitosis at age 44 years.

larger fraction of the total with advancing age. In a life span of 80 years, the median growth-related mitosis occurs at age 9.5 years, the median turnover-related mitosis at age 44 years, and the median parathyroid mitosis of any kind at age 26.5 years (Fig. 5). Since adult parathyroid cell number does not change, the very slow rate of cell gain must be balanced by a correspondingly slow rate of cell loss. Although there is no direct evidence for the occurrence of apoptosis in the parathyroid glands, the very brief duration of this process makes it as difficult to find as mitosis (29), and the evidence presented earlier indicates that apoptosis is the likely mode of cell death in all endocrine glands. By analogy with many other tissues and organs (6,16,25,29), cell loss is presumably the primary event, and parathyroid cells somehow are occasionally triggered from G0 to G1 (Fig. 1) in order to maintain a stable cell number. Such a compensatory response occurs in all endocrine glands under the control of the hypothalamus or the pituitary (1), but its occurrence in a gland that has no known trophic hormone is more difficult to understand.

Physiological Influences on Parathyroid Growth

For the thyroid, adrenal, and reproductive glands, an important component of growth control resides in the pituitary (1); the relevant hormones are not only tropic but also trophic, and the same applies to the hy-pothalamic control of the pituitary (21). The parathyroid and pancreatic islets both lack a trophic hormone, and the variable they control (calcium and glucose, respectively) affects growth as well as hormone secretion. It is more difficult to establish the absence than the presence of something, but hypophysectomy has no effect on parathyroid size (76,77), any effects of growth hormone administration are mediated indirectly by increasing plasma phosphate (77), and the functions of individual pituitary cells are known in sufficient detail to leave no room for an undiscovered parathyrotrophic hormone (78). The association between pituitary and parathyroid disease in the multiple endocrine neoplasia type I (MEN-I) syndrome may reflect a pituitary origin for a novel parathyroid growth factor (see chapters by Metz et al. and Friedman et al.), but this is not a trophic hormone in the ordinary sense, and there is no evidence that it plays any role in normal physiology. The difference between the presence and the absence of a trophic hormone is illustrated by the responses to hemiresection. In the thyroid, compensatory hyperplasia is initiated promptly and briskly, with a 15-fold increase in mitotic prevalence within 2 days (79). In the parathyroid, however, the mitotic response is slow and of much smaller magnitude, with no more than a twofold increase (79,80), and may require simultaneous dietary calcium restriction for its unequivocal demonstration (79).

A hyperplastic response to a trophic stimulus is usually preceded by hypertrophy and by the ultrastructural appearances of increased secretory activity (81). The sequence of increased parathyroid hormone (PTH) secretion, cell hypertrophy, increased DNA synthesis, and increased mitosis has been demonstrated most convincingly within the first 48 hr after total nephrectomy (73,82,83) but is probably the characteristic mode of parathyroid growth response. The number of cells that contribute to total hormone secretion can also be increased by changing the relative durations of secretory activity and quiescence (84). The concept of a parathyroid secretory cycle, originally based on the ultrastructural distinction between dark and light chief cells (85), was challenged a few years ago as an artefact of the preparative method (86) but has recently been confirmed by the study of separated cells using the reverse hemolytic plaque method (87) and by the restriction of PTH mRNA expression to chief cells with large vesicular nuclei (88). This concept has several implications for the study of parathyroid growth. The response to an increased demand for PTH consists of a hierarchy of mechanisms that occur on successively longer time scales (84): release of stored hormone, decreased intracellular degradation of hormone, increased hormone biosynthesis, and decreased duration of secretory quiescence. Only if these mechanisms collectively are unable to meet the demand does hyperplasia become necessary. The first three of these mechanisms are ways of increasing hormone secretion by each contributing cell, but the last two are ways of increasing the number of contributing cells and represent the means whereby the parathyroid gland adds integral control to the proportional and derivative controls that suffice to meet most short-term needs (89).

Alternation of cells between secretory activity and quiescence also provides an explanation for a central paradox of parathyroid growth regulation. With few exceptions, a cell either executes its differentiated function or divides but does not do both at the same time (12,16). Consequently, when the stimulus to PTH secretion is most intense, some cells would have to disregard the stimulus, stop making PTH and, instead, get ready to divide. However, if secretion is cyclical, there will always be some cells able to respond to a proliferative stimulus without interrupting secretion. At the end of each quiescent period, the cell has the option of resuming secretion or entering the cell cycle (Fig. 6). Alternatively, if the cell streaming concept is correct, normal cell turnover is driven by cell production rather than by cell loss, the cells having a determinate life span. In response to increased functional demand, the stem cells would divide more frequently, but the differentiated cells would not be interrupted in their function. A structural basis for cell streaming is less evident in the parathyroid than in any of the other organs mentioned (27), but the three-dimensional ar-

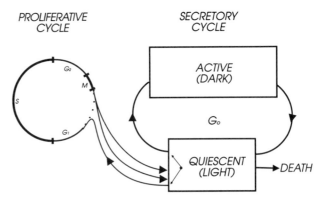

FIG. 6. Integration of proliferative cycle and secretory cycle in parathyroid cells. The chief cell alternates between periods of secretory activity and secretory quiescence with characteristic ultrastructural appearances (85); there are other stages in the secretory cycle that are omitted for simplicity of illustration. At the end of the period of secretory quiescence, the cell has the option of resuming secretion or switching from G_0 to G_1 to enter the proliferative cycle. The latter option is very rarely exercised in normal circumstances but is available if there is a need for more cells to contribute to hormone secretion, which cannot be met by a further increase in the duration of secretory activity relative to quiescence.

rangement of chief cells in relation to the capillaries and the stroma (88) should be reexamined from this standpoint, and the occurrence or not of streaming should be determined directly.

The notion that hypocalcemia stimulates parathyroid growth has a long history and is deeply embedded in current concepts regarding pathophysiology, but the occurrence of hyperplasia as well as hypertrophy has recently been challenged (91,92). Most of the earlier papers reported only gland volume (93), wet weight (94), or dry weight (95). An increase in organ size out of proportion to the degree of hypertrophy has often been claimed (96–98) but inadequately documented. In the most histologically complete study, the increase in parathyroid volume in response to dietary calcium restriction in young rats was due mainly to hypertrophy rather than to hyperplasia (92). Interpretation of such experiments is complicated by the ability of the rat to adapt to a low calcium intake with a large increase in calcitriol production by a PTH-independent mechanism (99,100). As is also discussed in the chapter by Sakaguchi, calcitriol has an effect, independent of calcium, of inhibiting parathyroid cell proliferation (91,101,102). It is unclear whether this effect is physiologically specific to the parathyroid gland or is simply part of a generalized antiproliferative action of calcitriol (103), but in either case it could mask the proliferative response to hypocalcemia (100). Only in one in vivo study has parathyroid hyperplasia, inferred from increased weight and unchanged protein/DNA ratio, developed concurrently with an increased serum calcitriol level (101). Another problem is that when, as has often been the case, deficiency of vitamin D as well as calcium has been induced (104), it may be impossible to determine the relative contributions of hypocalcemia and calcitriol deficiency to parathyroid hyperplasia.

The confounding effect of altered calcitriol biosynthesis in vivo can be circumvented by in vitro studies, but a major problem with cultured cells is their rapidity of growth, much faster even than the peak embryonic rate in vivo, with a doubling time of only 1–2 days (105). Consequently, the inability of calcium to inhibit serum-stimulated growth of cultured parathyroid cells (92) is unlikely to be of physiologic relevance. The most convincing results have been obtained with organ culture, in which lower ambient calcium concentrations have been accompanied by increased prevalence of both mitosis (106) and of S-phase cells labeled with tritiated thymidine (72). The failure to find this response consistently in vivo may reflect more than the suppressive effect of increased calcitriol levels. Why does parathyroid hyperplasia fail to occur (92), or to progress further (101), in hypocalcemic animals that are in serious need of more PTH? One possibility is that severe hypocalcemia has a generalized inhibitory effect on growth that includes the parathyroid gland, so that parathyroid cell number, although unchanged, may be increased in relation to body weight (92). Another possibility is that with severe hypocalcemia the duration of secretory quiescence is too short to permit the G0 → G1 switch to occur. In several in vitro studies, the effect of calcium has been biphasic, mild hypocalcemia stimulating and severe hypocalcemia inhibiting DNA synthesis (72,107,108), with a peak response occurring at ∼0.5 mmol/liter. Perhaps hyperplasia has evolved as a defense against hypocalcemia that is mild and chronic, rather than severe and acute, and so is more easily demonstrated in older animals that are growing more slowly.

Biological plausibility and the weight of experimental evidence both support the traditional view that hypocalcemia stimulates cell division as well as cell growth in the parathyroid gland. The greater effectiveness of this mechanism in countering mild, rather than severe, hypocalcemia is exemplified by the responses to hemiparathyroidectomy (79,80) and to pregnancy (4) and by the inverse correlation between plasma calcium and parathyroid weight in normal subjects (66,68). The mechanism of the proliferative effect of hypocalcemia is becoming clearer (see the chapter by Sakaguchi). There is evidence for an autocrine mechanism, whereby hypocalcemia increases both the production of acidic fibroblast growth factor (FGF) by parenchymal cells and the number of its surface receptors in the same cells (109). Less clear is a possible

paracrine mechanism. Parathyroid capillary endothelial cells release a factor that stimulates thymidine incorporation in parenchymal cells (110), but the endothelial cells do not respond to hypocalcemia (Brandi, personal communication). The link between hormone secretion and proliferation may be different in each endocrine gland or may reflect separate responses to the same intracellular signalling mechanism (107,111), but it remains an attractive concept that entry into the cell cycle is triggered by a fall in intracellular hormone concentration below a critical level when biosynthesis fails to keep pace with release (50). Such a relationship, for which there is evidence in the prolactin-secreting cells in the pituitary (112), could provide a common adaptive mechanism that was available to all endocrine cells.

ABNORMAL PARATHYROID GROWTH

Relationship Between Cell Number, Hormone Secretion, and Plasma Calcium

Unlike the pituitary and thyroid glands, in which abnormal growth can lead to space-occupying and pressure effects as well as hormonal effects, abnormal growth in the parathyroid gland is important only in that it contributes to abnormalities of hormone secretion. Implicit in the concept that parathyroid hyperplasia is the eventual long-term response to a sustained need for more PTH is the existence of an empirical, not just a formal, relationship between cell number and total hormone secretion. Indeed, as this author stated nearly 25 years ago, "if the secretory behavior of each individual cell in relation to its chemical environment is unaffected by the total number of cells . . ." then PTH secretion must be proportional to the number of contributing cells (113). Although an individual cell could communicate with adjacent cells by means of the mechanisms described in the chapter by Sakaguchi, the only way it could be influenced by the total number of cells is by the resultant changes in the composition of the blood, so that the proposition stated above still appears to be logically unassailable. However, in normal subjects, parathyroid parenchymal cell number has a CV of 30%, whereas plasma free calcium and, by inference, the average secretory set-point of parathyroid cells has a CV of <3% (89) (see the chapter by Brown).

Three main factors will obscure the relationship between total cell number and plasma free calcium within a population, based on the reciprocal functions that underlie the regulation of calcium homeostasis (114). The first factor concerns the control of PTH secretion as a dependent variable by calcium. PTH secretion by the same total number of cells will differ between subjects because of variations in set point (89) (see the chapter by Brown), maximum PTH secretion per cell or secretory capacity (115), and proportion of cells contributing to secretion (88). The response to calcium will also be modified by several other factors of lesser importance (89) (see chapter by Brown). The second factor is the clearance of secreted intact PTH. The plasma concentration of PTH produced by the same secretion rate will differ between subjects because of variations in the metabolic clearance rate (MCR) and volume of distribution (V_{dist}) (1). The third factor concerns the control of calcium as dependent variable by PTH. The plasma free calcium produced by the same circulating level of PTH will differ between subjects because of variation in the responses of target cells in bone and kidney to PTH (89) (see the chapter by Brown). Variation from all these sources is greater in patients with parathyroid disease than in normal subjects. However, in an individual, secretory set point and PTH secretory capacity are likely to remain reasonably stable, so that a change in active parathyroid cell number can be assumed, at least as a first approximation, to lead to a proportional change in hormone secretion, in response to the same values for plasma free calcium and for all other relevant variables. Likewise, if PTH MCR and V_{dist}, and target cell responses to PTH remain stable, the effect of a change in hormone secretion on plasma calcium will be predictable.

In all forms of hyperparathyroidism, three major mechanisms contribute in varying degrees to PTH hypersecretion. First, the secretory set point is increased (89) (see the chapter by Brown). Second, the proportion of active cells, reflecting the relative duration of secretory activity, is increased (88). Finally, the total number of parenchymal cells is increased. Together these latter two changes will increase the number of cells that contribute to hormone secretion at any time and so increase the aggregate PTH secretion by all glands proportionately at every level of plasma calcium. In terms of the sigmoid logistic model relating steady-state PTH secretion to steady-state plasma free calcium concentration (116) (Fig. 7), this will increase maximum total secretion, provided that individual values for this parameter are included, rather than setting maximum secretion to 100%, as is often done for ease of comparison between studies (116). Any combination of changes in these two fundamental quantities can be symbolized in the same two-dimensional diagram, a change in set point by a linear displacement along the abscissa, and a change in maximum total secretion, representing the number of secretory cells, by a proportional change along the ordinate (Fig. 7). To apply this model, it will initially be assumed that PTH MCR and V_{dist} are constant, so that there is a linear

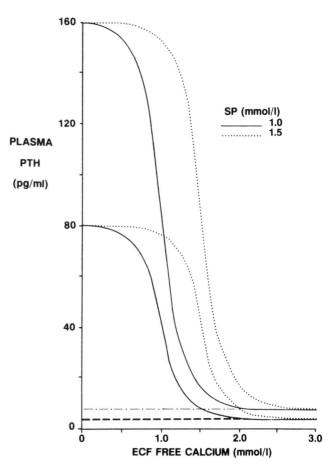

FIG. 7. Sigmoid relationship between PTH secretion (as reflected by plasma concentration) and ECF free calcium. The component not suppressible by calcium is assumed to be 5% of maximum secretion, indicated by the *dashed lines*. Four curves are shown, representing normal set point and normal number of secreting cells (*lower solid line*), increased set point and normal number of cells (*lower dotted line*), normal setpoint and increased number of cells (*upper solid line*), and increased setpoint and increased number of cells (*upper dotted line*). For clarity of depiction, the increase in set point (50%) is greater and the increase in number of cells (100%) is smaller than those usually found.

proportional relationship between PTH secretion and the circulating level of intact PTH.

The relative importance of increased set point and increased number of contributing cells can be estimated in terms of the reciprocal causality previously mentioned (114). The effect of calcium on PTH has already been examined. To this must now be added the effect of PTH on calcium (89). Based on mean values for plasma albumin-adjusted calcium and intact PTH at various levels of parathyroid function, the relationship is curvilinear such that the same successive increment in PTH produces successively smaller increments in calcium (81,89,114), and is modeled in Fig. 8 by an exponential approach to an asymptotic value. For clarity, the large between-person variances have

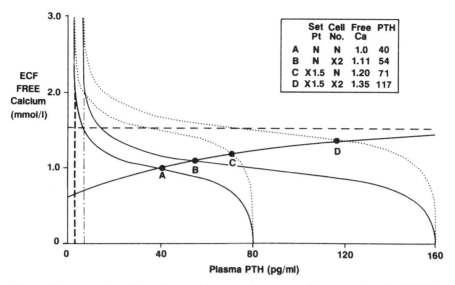

	Set Pt	Cell No.	Free Ca	PTH
A	N	N	1.0	40
B	N	X2	1.11	54
C	X1.5	N	1.20	71
D	X1.5	X2	1.35	117

FIG. 8. Effect of increases in cell number and/or set point on steady-state values for ECF free calcium and plasma PTH. Calcium (dependent variable) as a function of PTH (independent variable) is depicted by the *solid curved monotonic line,* based on published or personal values for adjusted total plasma calcium and intact PTH at various levels of parathyroid function (89). The *dashed line* represents the asymptotic value, estimated from the highest stable value for adjusted total plasma calcium found in patients with normal renal function of ∼ 3.5 mmol/liter. The four *solid circles* represent the intersection of this curve with the four versions of the sigmoid curve depicting plasma PTH (dependent variable) as a function of ECF free calcium (independent variable), taken from Fig. 7. The values for both variables corresponding to the points of intersection are given in the *inset.* For further details, see text.

been omitted; each relationship should be represented by a band rather than by a single line. System equilibrium is defined by the intersection of these two functional relationships in which dependent and independent variables are interchanged (114). Four versions of the sigmoid relationship between PTH and calcium are shown, taken from Fig. 7. They correspond to normal values for both set point and maximum secretion, increased set point with normal maximum secretion, increased maximum secretion with normal set point, and increased values for both determinants. The mean steady-state values for both variables corresponding to the four points of intersection are shown in the inset in Fig. 8, but the regions of intersection should be represented by areas rather than by points.

The superimposition of the curves confirms the conclusion drawn from earlier, less rigorous models (8,113), and what has long been inferred from both clinical and experimental (117) observations, that a relatively large increase in number of secretory cells has a lesser effect on PTH and calcium than a relatively smaller increase in set point (8). Several points require emphasis. First, because the proportion of active cells, as well as the number of cells, is increased, the increase in maximum secretion will be more than the increase in parathyroid size. Second, as cell number increases without an increase in set point, each cell operates ever more closely to its minimum capacity and is less able to defend against a rise in plasma cal-

cium (89). Third, a nonsuppressible component of PTH secretion (89,116) (see the chapter by Brown) is not a prerequisite for an effect of increasing cell number but increases the slope of that effect (8). Fourth, although an increase in set point alone will increase both plasma calcium and PTH levels, as set point increases without an increase in cell number, each cell will operate ever more closely to its maximum capacity and will be less able to defend against a fall in plasma calcium (89). With either abnormality alone, the biological advantage of operating on the central steep portion of the curve relating PTH secretion to calcium is blunted. This biologic advantage is partly restored when an increase in set point is combined with an increase in the number of secreting cells, as is found in most patients with primary hyperparathyroidism.

With this theoretical background in mind, the empirical relationships between cell number, hormone secretion, and plasma calcium can be examined. In all studies that included an adequate number of patients and covered a wide range of tumor size, there has been a highly significant correlation between tumor weight or volume and plasma calcium, with an average r value of about 0.6, ranging from 0.4 to 0.8 (118–124). The intervening correlations between weight (or volume) and plasma PTH level and between plasma PTH level and plasma calcium are equally or even more significant, although they are determined less frequently

(120,122,125–128). The most impressive correlation ($r = 0.98$) was found between the acute increase in plasma PTH in response to a standard hypocalcemic challenge and parathyroid volume (129). In other studies, the scatter about the regression line has invariably been wide, with about two-thirds of the variance in the level of plasma calcium unexplained by the regression on parathyroid weight or volume. Consequently, although the relationship is of biological and pathophysiological importance, it has been of little practical value to surgeons attempting to predict the characteristics of the tumor from preoperative measurements (124,126).

There are several reasons for the wide scatter. The slope relating plasma calcium to cell number is quite shallow (8), and all the relationships in the model have wide confidence intervals. Many of the numerous factors that disturb the relationship between cell number and plasma calcium have already been described, but two additional mechanisms, altered maximum secretory capacity and altered suppressibility, were not included in the model in order to maintain a manageable degree of complexity. Maximum secretory capacity varies much more between subjects in patients with parathyroid adenomas than in normals, with almost a tenfold range between the lowest and the highest values. Combining weight with various ultrastructural indices of hormone secretion significantly improved the correlation with PTH (125). In some patients, the slope relating PTH secretion to calcium is shallow and suppressibility is markedly impaired, such that the conventionally defined set point cannot be determined unless the ambient calcium concentration is raised to a much higher level than is usual (130). These abnormalities contribute to hypercalcemia in only a small proportion of patients (115) but contribute substantially to the variability between patients. Nevertheless, the empirical observations in patients with primary hyperparathyroidism support the conclusion from the theoretical analysis that, other things being equal, the more parathyroid cells, the greater the rate of hormone secretion and the higher the level of plasma calcium.

Primary Hyperparathyroidism: Disease Course as an Expression of Rate and Extent of Growth

Hypersecretion of PTH is usually classified as secondary or primary. Not all definitions of these qualifying terms are equally clear; for the purposes of this chapter, the former is a response to a sustained increase in demand for PTH that is extrinsic to the glands, whereas the latter is the expression of an intrinsic abnormality (131). In secondary hyperparathyroidism, plasma calcium is usually low or normal, and

parathyroid histology shows hyperplasia, whereas in primary hyperparathyroidism plasma calcium is usually high, and parathyroid histology usually shows adenoma (see the chapter by LiVolsi). However, classification according to the origin of the hyperparathyroid state makes more physiologic sense than classification according to the level of plasma calcium or the structure of the glands at the time when the condition is recognized (131,132). The designation of hyperparathyroidism as "primary" is otherwise not restrictive with respect to etiology; some cases of "primary" hyperparathyroidism are "secondary" to some etiologic agent, whether genetic (see the chapters by Arnold, Metz et al., and Friedman et al.) or environmental (41) (see the chapter by Mallette), which is not directly related to the demand for hormone secretion, and the proportion of such cases is likely to increase as further knowledge is gained.

Primary hyperparathyroidism has an extraordinarily wide range of clinical manifestations, encompassing severe, life-threatening hypercalcemia; moderate symptomatic hypercalcemia with osteitis fibrosa; mild hypercalcemia with nephrolithiasis; and even milder hypercalcemia in patients discovered fortuitously, many of whom are ostensibly asymptomatic and free of any obvious harmful consequences (see the chapters by Bilezikian and Silverberg and by Kleerekoper). Over the past 70 years, there has been a progressive increase in the apparent prevalence of the disease, accompanied by a progressive change in the relative frequency of these different syndromes. Prior to about 1935, almost all patients, whether the diagnosis was made at autopsy or during life, had osteitis fibrosa (133), the specific bone disease of primary hyperparathyroidism (134). The subsequent changes occurred in two stages. First, following the work of Albright et al. (135), more cases were found among patients with nephrolithiasis; the magnitude of increase is uncertain, but was probably more than tenfold (136,137). Second, following the widespread adoption of routine multichannel biochemical screening, more cases were found among patients who lacked any of the traditional indications for plasma calcium measurement. The magnitude of increase, after eliminating the backlog of undiagnosed patients, was about fourfold (138). At both stages, the increases were sustained and were accompanied by a rise rather than a fall in age at diagnosis (143) (Table 3). Consequently, only a small part of the 4-fold increase in apparent prevalence was due to interception of the same type of patient at an earlier age, and most of the increase was due to the discovery of cases that previously were never diagnosed, except very rarely by accident (140–143).

During the same period when the disease appeared to become both more prevalent and less severe, profound changes occurred in the characteristics of the

TABLE 3. *Primary hyperparathyroidism: mean age at diagnosis*

Authors	Reference	Year	Clue	Age (years)
Norris	133	1947	Osteitis fibrosa	43
Hellstrom and Ivemark	139	1962	Stones	49
Lloyd	119	1968	Stones	48
Mallette et al.	122	1974	Mixed	53
Mundy et al.	140	1980	Accidental	70

tumors, particularly in their size (Table 4). There was more than a tenfold decrease in geometric mean weight, and almost a 50-fold decrease in the weight of the largest tumor (119,126,133). This change provides a good explanation for the decline in disease severity, but, since the age at diagnosis was rising at the same time as tumor size was falling, there must also have been a large reduction in the average rate of growth. Initially, only the most rapidly growing and consequently largest tumors were diagnosed, and, at each stage of increased case finding, the disease population was expanded by the addition of patients whose tumors were growing more slowly, and so were smaller, despite their longer course. The relationship between tumor weight and disease course was first examined in detail by Lloyd (119). He began by dividing the patients into those with osteitis fibrosa (type 1), those with nephrolithiasis (type 2), and those with neither of these disease manifestations (type 3). This classification corresponded to the three stages in the history of the disease defined by the two mechanisms of increased case finding described earlier. The classification was not logically exhaustive, since a patient could have had both osteitis fibrosa and nephrolithiasis. Such patients have become progressively less common, and there were none in the particular series that was being studied.

The use of osteitis fibrosa as a criterion of classification has frequently been criticized on the grounds that osseous effects of excess PTH can be found in almost all patients if sought with the right methods (134,144). However, increased bone turnover and in-creased rate of loss of cortical bone are nonspecific, whereas osteitis fibrosa is a qualitatively different bone disorder that is specific to excess PTH secretion (134), and its presence is both a logical and an unambiguous index of a particular degree of disease severity that has existed for several years. Regrettably, many observers have failed to appreciate this crucial distinction and have reported the presence or absence of "bone disease" without qualification. The major characteristics of types 1 and 2 are compared in Table 5. As would be expected from the preceding discussion, and as previously observed many times (118,120, 122,123,145), every disease manifestation was more severe in type 1, with the exception of hypophosphatemia, which was masked by greater impairment of renal function. However, it was noted for the first time that the duration of symptoms was significantly shorter in type 1, indicating that it was not simply a more advanced form of type 2. The inverse relationship between weight of tumor and length of disease history, together with the substantial difference in tumor weights, immediately suggested that the fundamental difference between the two types was in the rate of tumor growth (119), an inference entirely consistent with the historical changes in the expression of the disease described earlier.

The notion that tumor growth rate is a major determinant of disease course and manner of presentation, although a commonplace of oncology, has been slow to find general acceptance among endocrinologists, despite numerous examples in other endocrine tumors. In hyperparathyroidism, tumors growing more

TABLE 4. *Historical changes in parathyroid adenoma weight*

	Norris (133)	Lloyd (119)	Rutledge et al. (126)
Period	1931–1945	1950–1965	1974–1984
Number	69[a]	98	68
Mean age (years)	43	48	56
Geometric mean wt (g)	6.44	1.26	0.58
Logarithmic SD[b]	3.2	3.4	2.2
Range (calculated)[c]	0.61–68	0.11–14.6	0.12–2.9
Range (observed)	0.40–120	0.15–26	0.10–2.6

[a]Excluding cases diagnosed at autopsy.
[b]Multiplier corresponding to SD on a linear scale.
[c]Geometric mean $\times / \div$ (logarithmic SD)^2.

TABLE 5. *Two types of primary hyperparathyroidism*[a]

	Type 1[b]	Type 2[c]
Number of cases	44	88
Tumor weight (geometric mean)	3.74 (2.69)[d]	0.65 (2.64)[d]
Range (observed)	0.7–26.0	0.15–3.5
Range (predicted)[e]	0.5–27.1	0.10–4.5
Length of history (years)	3.6 (4.8)	6.7 (7.2)
Plasma Ca (mmol/liter)	3.34 (0.60)	2.91 (0.20)

[a]Data from reference 119 and personal communication from the author.
[b]Presentation with osteitis fibrosa.
[c]Presentation with nephrolithiasis.
[d]Multiplier corresponding to SD on a linear scale.
[e]Geometric mean $\times/\div$ (logarithmic SD)^2.

rapidly lead to greater hormone hypersecretion, more severe hypercalcemia, and osteitis fibrosa, and tumors growing more slowly lead to less severe hypercalcemia, hormone secretion rarely attaining the level needed to produce osteitis fibrosa. The idea can be further developed in several directions. Some patients present with severe, life-threatening hypercalcemia of recent onset, so-called acute hyperparathyroidism or parathyroid crisis (146) (see the chapter by Fitzpatrick). Many such patients have had prior long-standing hyperparathyroidism of varying severity, often with osteitis fibrosa (acute superimposed upon chronic), but in others the crisis is the first manifestation of the disease, with a course too short for osteitis fibrosa to have developed (acute de novo). In either case, the hypercalcemia is of the progressive disequilibrium variety (147), often precipitated by intercurrent illness or surgery; the consequent immobilization and sodium depletion initiate several vicious circles that, uninterrupted, will lead to death. Extreme PTH hypersecretion is characteristic (146).

The pathogenesis is complex (146–150), but, since the tumors are generally large (151,152), and the duration of symptoms can be measured in weeks or months rather than in years, parathyroid growth is likely to have been unusually rapid, either abruptly accelerated (acute on chronic) or rapid from the outset (acute de novo). The importance of rapid growth is strengthened by the close resemblance between acute hyperparathyroidism and parathyroid carcinoma with respect to disease course, frequent presence of both osteitis fibrosa and nephrolithiasis (otherwise an unusual combination), manner of presentation, and severity of hypercalcemia (146,153) (see the chapter by Shane). Yet another resemblance is that the frequency

of both disorders has remained fairly stable, uninfluenced by the factors that have increased the frequency of diagnosis of hyperparathyroidism in general (146,154). In both conditions, geometric mean tumor weights are in the range of 4–10 g in representative series (151,152,155,156). The term atypical adenoma has been coined for tumors that resemble carcinomas, not only in clinical expression, but in histologic appearance (157), and in rapidity of regrowth following incomplete excision (154).

At the opposite end of the scale, in most patients in whom mild hypercalcemia is discovered fortuitously, indices of hormone hypersecretion and disease severity commonly remain stable for many years (158) (see the chapter by Kleerekoper), as would be expected if such patients were rarely diagnosed before the introduction of multichannel biochemical screening (143). Type 3 disease, as originally defined by Lloyd (119), thus includes patients at both ends of the growth scale, and, if the term is to be retained as a useful reminder of the historical evolution of the disease, it must be restricted to refer to patients who lack any of its traditional manifestations (see the chapter by Kleerekoper). Serial measurement of tumor size by noninvasive methods is obviously difficult and has never been accomplished in patients with primary hyperparathyroidism in whom surgical treatment has been withheld for any reason. Nevertheless, it is highly unlikely that the various determinants of hormone secretion would change proportionately in opposite directions, and the most reasonable explanation for long-term stability of hormone secretion is long-term stability of all its determinants, including cell number. Thus lack of disease progression implies that tumor growth has markedly slowed down or has even ceased altogether. The infrequency with which patients are intercepted during the transitional period when PTH and/or plasma calcium levels are increasing (158,159) implies that the duration of this period must, in most cases, be quite short (143).

An important question is whether it is only our perception of the disease that has changed, for the reasons given earlier, or whether the disease itself has changed. Most observers have taken the former view (142,160); after all, recognizing that there is more to an iceberg than its tip does not change the iceberg. Prior to the introduction of multichannel screening, nephrolithiasis was found in 80% of a large representative series (137); a fourfold increase in the apparent prevalence of primary hyperparathyroidism should have reduced the proportion of patients with nephrolithiasis to 20%. The proportions of 18% and 22% found in two recent series (160,161) suggest that the absolute incidence of nephrolithiasis due to hyperparathyroidism has not changed. Applying similar calculations to osteitis fibrosa is more problematic. If the absolute incidence of this remains unchanged, and the frequency of diagnosis has increased 4-fold from the time when osteitis fibrosa was present in almost all patients, it should occur in at least 2% of patients seen in current practice. Experience at Henry Ford Hospital suggests that the current prevalence is <1%; it was ~1% (1/97) and 1.7% (2/118) in two other recent series (160,161). These numbers are consistent with a modest reduction in the absolute frequency of osteitis fibrosa but are much too small for us to draw this conclusion with confidence. It has been suggested that osteitis fibrosa is less common than in the past, not just relatively but absolutely, as a result of improvement in vitamin D nutrition (162), an issue considered in more detail below in the discussion of the pathogenesis of different growth patterns.

Primary Hyperparathyroidism: Patterns of Growth and Implications for Pathogenesis

In his seminal paper, Lloyd (119) made three separate proposals. The first two, that there are large differences in growth rate between patients and that these differences contribute substantially to differences in clinical expression, are supported by all the available data and are consistent with accepted principles of clinical oncology (163,164). The third proposal, that the growth rates are bimodally distributed as a reflection of a basic difference in etiology, was more novel, has been more difficult to establish, and has largely been forgotten (or ignored) by contemporary students of the disease. The discovery that, in most patients with the mildest disease, tumor growth has probably ceased altogether suggests a more fundamental difference, not just in the rate but in the pattern of growth, because of a difference in the type of mutation (Fig. 9). The clinical course in these patients implies that growth is initially rapid but slows down progressively with time as an asymptotic value for tumor size is approached (37). This pattern of growth is often referred to as *gompertzian,* since the sigmoid curve can be described by the Gompertz function (165), but is referred to herein as *asymptotic growth,* the value of the asymptote differing between subjects.

Asymptotic growth is a feature of many tumors (36,163–167) but is usually the result of mechanisms that only rarely apply to the parathyroids. In rapidly growing malignant tumors, neoangiogenesis may occur too slowly to maintain adequate perfusion, leading to nutritional deprivation, hypoxia, and sometimes necrosis (166). Parathyroid tumors very occasionally undergo infarction by a similar mechanism, leading to temporary biochemical remission (168), but this is clearly not the explanation for growth retardation in patients with mild disease. In many tumors, benign as well as malignant, retardation and even cessation

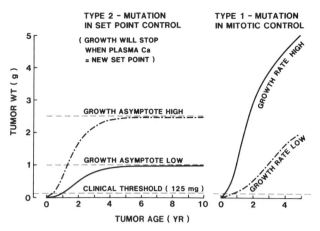

FIG. 9. Hypothetical growth curves of parathyroid adenomas corresponding to two types of mutation. In each case, a *solid line* depicts the more typical behavior and an *interrupted line* depicts the less typical behavior. For convenience of representation, the likely total duration of growth has been compressed. The clinical threshold is the weight of tumor below which detection is unlikely; the value chosen is close to the normal mean total weight and corresponds to ~27 doublings of a single cell (36). Type 2 tumors will grow exponentially until the clinical threshold is reached, after which growth will be progressively retarded as the asymptotic value corresponding to the new secretory set point is approached; the level of the growth asymptote will depend on the degree of increase in set point. Type 1 tumors will grow exponentially at a rate depending on the extent of progression along the neoplastic pathway. Eventually growth will be slowed by the same kinds of factors as in other neoplasms (163–167) but will rarely cease altogether.

of growth are the result of increased cell loss (36,165, 167), inferred because the observed doubling time is much longer than the potential doubling time deduced from cell kinetic studies (163,164). Most cell loss in tumors is due to apoptosis (167), but there is no evidence that this process is increased in parathyroid tumors (8), so retardation of their growth most likely is due to reduction in cell birth rate. In a minority of patients with parathyroid adenomas, growth becomes slower than it was at first but is sustained, so that, in the absence of treatment, the disease progresses in severity as the *extent* of growth increases in accordance with the *rate* of growth (Fig. 9). The classification based on this concept (Table 6) appears to be better able than the less complex previous scheme (119,131) to accommodate the variation in clinical and pathologic expression of primary hyperparathyroidism and to provide a framework for attempting to understand its molecular basis.

According to the current paradigm for neoplasia, most tumors originate from a single cell that has acquired a competitive growth advantage as the result of a somatic mutation and gives rise to a clone of cells, which at first are genetically and phenotypically iden-

TABLE 6. *Modified classification of clonal parathyroid tumors*

	Type (119)	
	1	2 and 3
Nature of mutation	Mitotic control	Set-point control
Manner of growth	Continuous	Asymptotic
Expression of variability[a]	Rate of growth	Plasma calcium
Clinical presentation[b]	Osteitis fibrosa	Nephrolithiasis (type 2)
	(Other factors)	(Other factors)
	Hypercalcemia	Fortuitous (type 3)

[a]Characteristic in which tumors of similar type may differ, depending on how large is the effect of the mutation.

[b]May be modified by environmental and life-style factors as well as by characteristics of the tumor.

TABLE 7. *Age at onset and age of adenoma in hyperparathyroidism*

	Etiology	
	Radiation (41)	Unknown (37)
No. of cases	56	63
Age at onset (years)	16.2[a] (9.3)	17.6[b] (3.8)
Age at operation (years)	55.7 (9.5)	55.0 (15.1)
Age of tumor (years)	39.5 (10.6)	37.4 (11.6)

[a]Age at exposure to external radiation. Data are mean (SD).

[b]Assuming that mutations have the same age distribution as mitoses (Fig. 5), so that age at median mitosis is the best estimate of age at mutation.

tical (12,169,170). The concept of clonality is not quite so straightforward as is often assumed. The definition of the founding cell of a clone may be ambiguous (169), monophenotypia does not necessarily imply monoclonality (171), and the founding cell of the population that has survived the process of clonal evolution (172) is not necessarily identical with the founding cell (or cells) from which the tumor originated (173). Despite these complexities, the concept of clonality has provided a useful starting point for the understanding of abnormal parathyroid growth. As with other benign endocrine tumors (174–176), parathyroid adenomas are usually monophenotypic, probably as the result of growth from a single mutant cell (177,178) (see the chapter by Arnold). The mutation may be the expression of one of several types of genetic abnormality (179) (see the chapters by Arnold, Metz et al., and Friedman et al.) or a consequence of exposure to external mutagens, such as therapeutic (41,180) or military (181,182) irradiation, but in most cases no such factor can be found. The mutation is generally assumed to initiate some form of neoplastic transformation, and mutations with such potential have been found in ~25% of cases (see the chapter by Arnold). Before considering an alternative possibility for the majority of cases in which such a mutation has not been found, some broader implications of clonality are examined here in relation to normal parathyroid growth.

DNA undergoes continuous damage and repair throughout life (12), but the perpetuation of a genetic or chromosomal abnormality as a mutation usually occurs only during mitosis (183,184). Consequently, the frequency of any mutation is the product of the probability of its occurrence at each mitosis (the mutagenic risk) and the frequency of mitosis (183–187). If mutagenic risk remains constant, and is the same for growth-related and turnover-related mitoses, then the

age distribution of the occurrence of any mutation should be the same as the age distribution of mitoses. Consequently, the best estimate of the age at which a mutation occurred is the age at the median parathyroid mitosis, counting only those that occurred early enough for a clinically detectable adenoma to have developed. Based on the maximum rate of parathyroid growth in utero, this would include any mitosis that occurred >1 year prior to diagnosis. By using the data in Fig. 5 in this manner, it is possible to estimate for a group of patients the mean age at the time of mutation and the mean age of the adenoma at the time of excision. Some results of such calculations are given in Table 7. Despite the numerous underlying assumptions, the mean values for both ages are very similar in patients with sporadic parathyroid adenomas (37) and in patients with radiation-associated hyperparathyroidism (41), in whom the age at exposure defines the earliest age at which the mutation could have occurred.

Assuming an origin from a single mutant cell, it is possible to estimate the number of doublings needed to produce a tumor of given weight (37), a useful first approach to studying the kinetics of growth even when doubling time is not constant. Dividing the required number of doublings into the estimated age of the tumor gives an upper limit to the doubling time, from which can be calculated the minimum cell birth rate needed to produce the tumor. This value will have little meaning in an individual case, but the mean value in groups of cases (Table 8) is four to eight times greater than the current cell birth rate at the time of tumor excision, both in sporadic (37) and in radiation-associated adenomas (41). The conclusion that cell birth rate must have slowed substantially supports the conclusion previously drawn from the usual course of the disease in current practice (Fig. 9). The cell birth rate is ten to 20 times lower than in other benign tumors, such as meningiomas (41); this appears to be a distinctive characteristic of parathyroid adenomas, not shared by any other tumor for which adequate data are

TABLE 8. Minimum cell birth rate in parathyroid adenomas

	Etiology[a]	
	Radiation	Unknown
Tumor weight (mg)	819[b] (2.63)[c]	827[b] (2.85)[c]
Number of doublings (N)[d]	29.7 (1.40)	29.7 (1.51)
Longest doubling time (years)[e]	1.33 (0.36)	1.27 (0.40)
Minimum birth rate (%/year)[f]	54.4[b] (1.37)[c]	58.7[b] (1.57)[c]

[a]As in Table 7.
[b]Geometric mean.
[c]Multiplier corresponding to SD on a linear scale.
[d]$\log_e$ Wt (g)/$\log_e$ 2 + 30.
[e]Age of tumor (from Table 7)/N.
[f]$\log_e 2/DT_{max} \cdot 100$.

available. Such extremely low rates of cell division, the prolonged duration of latency (Table 7), the virtual cessation of growth inferred from clinical studies (143), and the rarity of malignant transformation together suggest that many cases arise by a nonneoplastic mechanism (37,41).

Lloyd (119) suggested that type 1 tumors were true neoplasms but that type 2 tumors arose from hyperplastic foci of cells that were unusually responsive to the calcium demands of pregnancy and lactation, elaborating on a suggestion made earlier by Albright and Reifenstein (188). This concept was supported by evidence for polyphenotypia in parathyroid adenomas (174), but that evidence is open to an alternative interpretation and does not necessarily indicate polyclonality (189). The concept of focal hyperplasia can be reconciled with a monoclonal origin by means of the set point hypothesis, which proposes that the mutation involves one of the many proteins concerned in the recognition or transmembrane transport of calcium by the parathyroid cell (89) (see chapter by Brown), such that the mutant cell has an increase in secretory set point (37,41). Such a cell would respond to a normal extracellular free (ECF) calcium concentration in the same way as a normal cell responds to a low concentration (89) (see chapter by Mallette). It will maximize its rates of PTH biosynthesis and secretion, but to no avail. Sooner or later the mutant cell will divide, and the new clone of cells will grow exponentially until it is large enough to begin increasing the rate of hormone secretion by the whole gland. As the patient's ECF calcium rises, the rate of growth will slow down, and, when the value corresponding to the new set point is attained, there will be no stimulus to further growth (89). The rate of cell division in the mutant cells, rapid initially and slowing down with time, recapitulates on a longer time scale the changes that occur during normal development (Figs. 2–4).

The preceding discussion implies that a parathyroid cell can acquire a growth advantage in two different ways, a mutation in secretory set point control leading to asymptotic growth or a mutation in cell-cycle control leading to continuous growth (Table 6, Fig. 9). A parathyroid adenoma resulting from a set point mutation, although descriptively a tumor, would not be a neoplasm but a uniglandular focus of hyperplasia. This concept is supported by all the data reviewed but lacks direct confirmation. There are many potential candidates for a mutant protein that would increase the secretory set point by increasing the concentration difference for calcium across the parathyroid cell membrane (see the chapters by Brown and by Mallette), but none has been identified. Many characteristics of parathyroid adenomas that are consistent with, but do not establish, a dual etiology have already been mentioned, and there are several more. Histologic features of neoplasia, such as greater variability in size and shape of cells and nuclei and the presence of giant, multiple, and hyperchromatic nuclei, were commonly observed when only more severe disease was recognized (123,190) but are now only occasional findings (see chapter by LiVolsi). Histochemical or flow cytometric evidence of polyploidy and/or aneuploidy is found in a minority of patients but not in the majority (191–194) (see chapter by Mallette); differences in nuclear diameter greater than can be accounted for by proliferation or by ploidy (Table 9), suggest that type 1 tumors are more neoplastic than type 2 tumors (155,195). Hormone secretion is relatively autonomous in a small number of patients, both in vitro and in vivo, but is normally suppressible in most (115,196). In one large series, plasma calcium values were bimodally distributed, a majority of cases with a modal value of 3.6 mmol/liter and a minority with a modal value of 2.8 mmol/liter (197). However, whether it is the same patients who are atypical for all these different characteristics is not known.

TABLE 9. Parathyroid nuclear diameter

		Diameter (μm) (SD)
Normal	Diploid[a]	5.00 (3.30)
	Tetraploid[b]	6.3
	Octaploid[b]	7.9
Adenoma	Type II (n = 45)	5.64[c]
	Type I (n = 10)	6.68[d]
Carcinoma	(n = 18)	8.11[e] (1.39)

[a]Measured in 39 subjects (195).
[b]Calculated.
[c]Significantly different from normal diploid (P<0.01).
[d]Significantly different from type 2 (P<0.001).
[e]Significantly different from type 1 (P<0.001) (156). The increase in adenomas is much too great to be accounted for either by polyploidy or by the proportion of cycling cells.

The idea that there are two types of parathyroid tumor, hyperplastic and neoplastic, makes more sense from the available data than the current dogma that all parathyroid tumors are neoplasms, but three major questions remain to be answered. First, if a significant minority of cases do not have a secretory set point mutation, why is the set point increased in almost all cases? The usual answer is that rapid cell proliferation leads in some way to an altered secretory response to calcium (198), but the most rapid rate of cell division that has been measured at the time of tumor excision [44%/year (37)] is at least 300 times lower than the rate observed in cultured parathyroid cells (108). Consequently, rapid proliferation might lead to an increase in set point during the early phase of clonal expansion but is not a plausible explanation for a sustained increase in set point; an alternative is needed. Second, could differences in tumor growth rates and clinical expression depend not on differences in etiology but on differences in vitamin D nutrition? Both in France (199) and in India (Rao, personal communication), patients with primary hyperparathyroidism are more likely to have osteitis fibrosa if their serum levels of calcidiol and calcitriol are low. The most likely explanation is that calcitriol deficiency directly increases PTH secretion independent of any other factors (200), but, since calcitriol also has an antiproliferative effect on parathyroid cells (91,101,102), tumor growth rates could be enhanced by calcitriol deficiency. However, in England, the serum calcitriol level was positively correlated with immunoreactive PTH and was normal or increased in each of 11 patients with osteitis fibrosa, in whom the mean value tended to be higher than in patients with nephrolithiasis (201). Discussion of this issue will be resumed later.

The third, more fundamental, question is how can neoplastic transformation, a process widely believed to be restricted to the stem cells of tissues with rapid turnover, and their immediate progeny (12,16,25,163, 169,187), occur in a tissue with low turnover in which, unless the cell streaming concept is correct, there are no stem cells as ordinarily defined? Stem cells are susceptible to neoplastic transformation because of three characteristics: they retain indefinitely the ability to divide, they are capable of self-renewal, and their progeny rapidly proliferate, so that successive divisions occur at relatively short intervals (16,25,187). Parathyroid cells possess the first two of these characteristics, so that in this limited sense they are all stem cells. What is missing is the rapid proliferation, a deficit magnified by the small size of the glands. Traditional theories of carcinogenesis (187) were based on two sequential processes—initiation (by somatic mutation) and promotion (by stimulation of cell proliferation). This simple concept could apply to the colonic mucosa, in which cell turnover is at least 10^3 times higher than in the parathyroid glands (thymidine labeling index >5% (202) v <0.005% (37)). But in organs with low turnover, such as the liver, it has become evident that initiation must be preceded by an increase in cell proliferation, due either to an external mitogen or to the replacement of injured cells (183,184,186). The same need for amplification of the mutagenic risk by increased proliferation is evident in many other circumstances of tumorigenesis, both experimental (186,187) and clinical (185,202). The parathyroid glands have even lower turnover than the liver, and are even more in need of increased cell proliferation prior to neoplastic transformation.

In the normal parathyroid, the relative rate of cell division approaches that found in the dividing transit population of tissues, with rapid turnover for only a brief period around 16 weeks of conceptional age (Fig. 4), during which there probably occur the mutations that lead to the rare parathyroid tumor that presents in childhood (204). At other times the necessary population of rapidly dividing cells could be created by a nonneoplastic set point mutation. If a single cell grew exponentially to a 62.5 mg nodule (26 doublings) in 1 year, the necessary doubling time would be 2 weeks, the cell birth rate in the new clone of cells would be ~1,800%/year, and the total frequency of mitosis during that year would be increased 25-fold, with a corresponding increase in the risk of a subsequent mutation. In most cases, no further mutation would occur, growth would be asymptotic, and the asymptote would depend on the magnitude of the increase in set point. In a minority of cases, however, a neoplastic-type mutation would occur, leading to continuous growth, in some cases compounded by one or more further mutations leading to parathyroid carcinoma.

According to this concept, a mutation in set point control and a mutation in cell cycle control are not alternative but successive events, the former being a necessary preliminary to the latter, except when cell division is stimulated by some other means (Fig. 10), such as a germinal mutation (179), or by the initiation of secondary hyperparathyroidism; the latter sequence is referred to as *tertiary hyperparathyroidism,* a condition to be discussed in the next section. Polyclonal hyperplasia would also be the initial response to the putative MEN growth factor (110), the later occurrence of a mutation accounting for asymmetry of glandular enlargement (204), and for monoclonality of the largest glands. A novel feature of the set point hypothesis is that, in every other tissue in the body, a mutation that tended to decrease the intracellular calcium concentration would inhibit rather than stimulate growth (205) and would likely lead to malfunction and possibly death of the cell. Such mutations could be very common, but only in the parathyroid cell would they have a clinically detectable consequence. The new concept not only accounts for all the data suggesting nonneoplastic etiology but also answers each

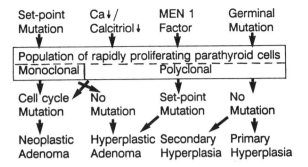

FIG. 10. Unified model of abnormal parathyroid growth. For reasons explained in the text, the first step is always the establishment of a population of rapidly proliferating cells, either monoclonal as the result of a set point mutation, or polyclonal as the result of stimulation by the circumstances leading to secondary hyperparathyroidism, or by the MEN-I growth factor, or as a consequence of one of the several genetic defects that can lead to primary hyperplasia. The rapidly proliferating cells are at increased risk of mutation. A set point mutation leading to monoclonal proliferation, followed by a cell cycle mutation, leads to a neoplastic adenoma causing type 1 primary hyperparathyroidism, and occasionally parathyroid carcinoma. A set point mutation, followed by no further mutation, leads to a hyperplastic adenoma causing type 2 primary hyperparathyroidism. Polyclonal proliferation as the expression of secondary hyperparathyroidism with no mutation leads to secondary hyperplasia, either diffuse or nodular; hypercalcemia may develop because of an acquired increase in secretory set point. Diffuse or nodular hyperplasia, followed by a mutation of either kind, leads to tertiary hyperparathyroidism.

of the three questions previously posed. It explains why an increase in secretory set point is found in almost all cases, provides a means whereby vitamin D deficiency may contribute to pathogenesis, and most importantly reconciles the occurrence of mutations in cell cycle control of the kind that can lead to neoplasia with the extremely low rate of cell division in the normal parathyroid gland.

Parathyroid Growth in Secondary and Tertiary Hyperparathyroidism

Secondary hyperparathyroidism, as defined in the previous section, can occur in a wide variety of circumstances, usually identified on the basis of physiologic reasoning and a sustained increase in blood levels of PTH, sometimes supported by histomorphometric, radiographic, and densitometric evidence of the skeletal effects of PTH excess. The circumstances are numerous (131) and include normal aging (206), dietary deficiency or malabsorption of calcium, renal wasting of calcium, pregnancy and lactation, Paget's disease (see the chapter by Siris and Canfield), pseudohypoparathyroidism (see the chapter by Levine et al.), vitamin D depletion both extrinsic and intrinsic (207), and impaired vitamin D metabolism at multiple levels. In

normal aging the pathogenesis of secondary hyperparathyroidism is multifactorial, and there is no evidence for a progressive age-related increase in parathyroid cell number (65). Presumably, the modest increase in PTH secretion (40% between ages 20 and 90 years) can be accommodated by the earlier members of the hierarchy described above (see under Physiological Influences on Parathyroid Growth). An alternative explanation is that values above the wide normal range in younger subjects, found in a small number of elderly persons (206), are the result of parathyroid microadenomas or hyperplastic nodules that occasionally occur in the absence of hypercalcemia (208). Qualitative evidence for parathyroid enlargement due to hyperplasia has been found in a few cases of rickets and osteomalacia at autopsy (209,210) and in a few cases of pseudohypoparathyroidism at diagnostic surgical exploration (211), but detailed information on abnormal parathyroid growth is available only for chronic renal failure (212) (see chapter by Martin and Slatopolsky). In this condition, PTH hypersecretion and parathyroid hyperplasia are initiated by hypocalcemia, and the stimulation is later augmented by calcitriol deficiency (200), but other factors contribute to the maintenance and progression of the growth disorder.

In unselected autopsy series of patients with renal failure published between 1926 and 1960 (212–215), before the wide availability of therapeutic regimens capable of substantially prolonging life, the degree of parathyroid enlargement was quite modest but was greater in patients dying from renal failure due to chronic glomerulonephritis than in those with less severe forms of renal disease (214) (Table 10). Individual values for combined parathyroid weight were log-normally distributed, and the geometric mean value was increased by ~65%; only ~40% of the values were >2 SD above the normal mean, whether arithmetic or geometric, although the highest values were far outside the normal range. Replacement of fat is an early stage of hyperplasia (214), but, even taking this into account, mean parenchymal weight could not have been increased by more than two- to threefold. In a more recent series, total parathyroid parenchymal weight was positively correlated with serum creatinine and was inversely correlated with renal weight, but hyperplasia could be detected histologically in patients without clinically manifested renal dysfunction (216).

In patients with rickets or osteomalacia as the main skeletal abnormality, the geometric mean parathyroid weight was similar to, and individual values were in the same range as, that in the unselected cases (215). However, in patients with osteitis fibrosa, there was very little overlap with the unselected cases; the geometric mean weight was increased >30-fold, and both the mean and range were much the same as for single adenomas causing osteitis fibrosa in primary hyperparathyroidism (Table 5). In recent years, parathyroid

TABLE 10. *Parathyroid weights in chronic renal failure*

Authors	Reference (year)	Feature	n	Geometric mean (SD)	Range (g)	Relative increase[a]
Pappenheimer and Wilens	213 (1935)	Unselected	27	0.148 (1.45)	0.067–0.433	1.36
Castleman and Mallory	214 (1937)	CGN[b]	12	0.301[c] (2.21)	0.12–0.863	2.74
Stanbury and Lumb	215[d] (1966)	Unselected	119	0.184 (2.23)	0.045–0.891[e]	1.67
		Rickets/OM[f]	10	0.158 (1.53)	0.071–0.281[e]	1.44
		Osteitis fibrosa[f]	26	3.517 (2.35)	0.78–12.0	31.9
Sivula et al.	217 (1979)	PTX	34	0.915 (3.88)	0.071–19.7	8.3
De Francisco et al.	219 (1985)	PTX				
		Diffuse	17	0.824 (1.86)	0.280–2.56	7.5
		Nodular	44	2.014 (2.16)	0.126–9.32	18.3
		Total	61	1.570 (2.30)	0.126–9.32	14.3
Krause and Hedinger	220 (1985)	PTX				
		Diffuse	17	1.509 (2.28)	0.2–7.5	13.7
		Nodular	22	3.523 (1.93)	0.8–10.1	32.0
		Total	39	2.434 (2.32)	0.2–10.1	22.1
Lloyd et al.	221 (1989)	PTX	16	3.920 (1.96)	0.91–17.2	35.6

[a]Assuming normal geometric mean (212) or median (65) of 0.110 g for all glands combined.
[b]Chronic glomerulonephritis, blood nonprotein nitrogen 105–300 mg/dl (normal 20–40).
[c]Some values estimated from rectangular volume.
[d]Including all cases previously published.
[e]Estimated from histograms.
[f]Based on skeletal histology at autopsy; OM, osteomalacia; PTX, parathyroidectomy, either total or subtotal.

weights have been published mainly for patients who were selected for surgical treatment, usually because of osteitis fibrosa or hypercalcemia or both (217–221) (Table 10). The values for total excised weight obviously reflect both historical changes and local variation in surgical policy but are in general quite similar to the total weights previously found at autopsy in patients with osteitis fibrosa. Although precise figures are not available, it seems reasonably certain that severe hyperparathyroidism remains much more frequent than in the prehemodialysis era, mainly because longer survival provides more time for the necessary parathyroid growth to occur.

In patients with hyperparathyroidism that was of severity sufficient to merit either individual publication of autopsy findings or selection for surgical treatment, the increase in parathyroid weight was so much greater than in unselected patients with chronic renal failure or in those with defective bone mineralization alone (Table 10) that the difference is likely to be qualitative as well as quantitative. The occurrence of hypercalcemia is often attributed to autonomy of hormone secretion, but the magnitude of the increase in parathyroid weight and its frequent correlation with both plasma calcium and PTH levels (218,221,222) indicate that it is not secretion but growth that is autonomous. In surgically resected parathyroid tissue, the rate of DNA synthesis is positively rather than negatively correlated with the level of plasma calcium (221) and so is behaving as the independent, rather than as the dependent, variable (114). Furthermore, the birth rate of new cells is higher than in primary parathyroid adenomas and is not significantly different from the min-

imum necessary birth rate, based on the weight of tissue removed and the estimated duration of renal failure (221). Evidently, cell proliferation had not slowed as in primary hyperparathyroidism but was still as rapid as when the glands first began to enlarge, soon after the onset of renal failure (216).

The secretory set point is usually increased in cells harvested from patients with secondary renal hyperplasia (223,224), so the abnormal growth could be driven by the same mechanism as in primary parathyroid adenomas with a set point mutation, with the difference that the majority of cells would be affected from the outset, not just a single cell. However, because of the many factors involved in chronic renal failure that impair the effectiveness of PTH in raising plasma calcium (see the chapter by Martin and Slatopolsky), the increase in total hormone secretion necessary to attain the new set point can be achieved only with an enormous increase in the number of secretory cells. Consequently, the asymptotic value for total gland size is much more difficult to reach than in primary hyperparathyroidism, accounting for the difference in growth behavior between the two disorders (221). In early renal failure, serum calcitriol levels are normal or only slightly reduced (224,225), so that hypocalcemia is the main stimulus to parathyroid cell proliferation, but, in advanced chronic renal failure, calcitriol levels are usually very low. The administration of calcitriol to such patients not only reduces PTH biosynthesis but also decreases the parathyroid secretory set point, so deficiency of calcitriol is a likely explanation for the increase in set point (200,224), and for the consequent acceleration of parathyroid growth that leads to osteitis fibrosa (221). This effect is probably augmented by the lower levels of calcitriol receptors in parathyroid cells from uremic patients (224,225).

Further insight into the mechanism of the growth disorder is provided by the histologic distinction between diffuse and nodular hyperplasia (see the chapter by LiVolsi). The nodules consist of cells that are more closely packed together, with larger nuclei and a greater prevalence of mitosis (219), more cycling cells by flow cytometry and greater depletion of calcitriol receptors (226). These characteristics account for the significantly greater increase in total parathyroid weight (Table 10) and for the continued growth, often rapid, of many parathyroid autografts (227). Detailed histochemical and immunocytochemical studies indicate similarity in gene expression between the cells in each nodule but differences between nodules (228). Each nodule could have arisen from a different single cell or, more likely, from a group of adjacent cells that themselves were the clonal descendants of a founding cell present during embryonic development. In this sense, nodular hyperplasia is multiclonal, in contrast to the polyclonality of diffuse hyperplasia and the monoclonality of adenomas. There can be as many as 100 nodules in four enlarged glands, so the likelihood that each nodule arose from a separate mutation is infinitesimally small. However, the secretory set point is higher in cells from the nodules than in cells from internodular tissue (229), so the growth advantage of the nodules could have the same explanation as for the clone of cells initiated by a set point mutation. Differences in set point between regions of the same gland could reflect intrinsic differences in responsiveness to calcitriol or differences in the extent of calcitriol receptor depletion.

The parathyroid growth response to chronic renal failure progresses through several stages. Diffuse secondary hyperplasia (polyclonal) is initiated by hypocalcemia, becomes more severe as the result of calcitriol deficiency, and leads eventually to osteitis fibrosa in many patients (215). Because of the additional effect of calcitriol deficiency to increase the parathyroid secretory set point, continued growth can lead to hypercalcemia (221); the hyperplasia becomes nodular (multiclonal) and the glandular enlargement asymmetric (230). The next stage is the emergence of an adenoma in one, or occasionally more than one, of the nodules, as the expression of a mutation in one of the cells undergoing the most rapid proliferation; the accumulation of 1.0 g of additional parathyroid tissue in five years requires a 100-fold increase in the frequency of mitosis. This sequence is referred to as *tertiary hyperparathyroidism* (231–236), a term often misapplied to patients with hypercalcemic secondary hyperparathyroidism but more accurately reserved for the disorder that combines in its etiology the hyperplasia of sec-

ondary hyperparathyroidism with the monoclonality of primary hyperparathyroidism (207,237). In addition to the usual histologic features of adenoma, nuclear diameter is increased to the same extent as in primary hyperparathyroidism (238). Furthermore, in two cases among six examined, there was loss of a tumor suppressor gene on chromosome 11 (239,240), a molecular defect with the potential for disrupting cell cycle control and found also in some primary parathyroid adenomas (see the chapter by Arnold). In other cases the mutation could lead to a further increase in secretory set point. The final and least common stage is malignant transformation leading to parathyroid carcinoma, an event reported in five patients on long-term hemodialysis (241–244), one of whom had previously undergone irradiation of the neck for laryngeal carcinoma (242).

Since long-term continued stimulation of parathyroid growth by chronic renal failure can culminate in neoplasia, either benign or malignant, the same would be expected in other circumstances, but the evidence is much less clear. Hypercalcemic hyperparathyroidism developed in some vitamin D-deficient migrants from India to England (245), but its anatomic basis remains unclear. A parathyroid adenoma was found in two such patients (246), but whether the incidence is increased in this population has not been established. In India, where vitamin D deficiency is common, parathyroid adenomas are rare and usually present with osteitis fibrosa (247), but in such patients the distinction between primary and tertiary hyperparathyroidism is difficult (248,249). Nevertheless, vitamin D deficiency increased the yield of radiation-induced parathyroid adenomas in rats (250), most likely by enhancing parathyroid cell proliferation. In intestinal malabsorption, secondary hyperparathyroidism has been demonstrated biochemically (207), but the histologic data are fragmentary (251). The apparent association between intestinal malabsorption and parathyroid adenomas has been described as tertiary hyperparathyroidism (232), but there was no evidence for hyperplasia of the other glands (252), as is found invariably in tertiary hyperparathyroidism due to renal failure. In the early stages of calcium malabsorption, serum calcitriol levels tend to be increased rather than decreased (253). This would delay the rise in secretory set point, which is probably necessary for the emergence of multiple foci of rapidly proliferating cells and increased mutagenic risk. Consequently, as has been suggested (252), growth would be stimulated only in the most responsive cells.

There is better evidence for tertiary hyperparathyroidism in patients with hypophosphatemic osteomalacia given long-term treatment with supplemental phosphate, which induces intermittent slight falls in plasma calcium and stimulation of PTH secretion (254). Hypercalcemic hyperparathyroidism has developed in 19 such patients (255–258), in whom parathyroid pathology encompassed the same spectrum of diffuse hyperplasia, nodular hyperplasia, and adenoma as in patients with chronic renal failure. Another similarity is that, in the three most recent cases, the secretory set point was increased (258); unlike the case in renal failure, the serum calcitriol levels were normal, but they tend to be low in the disease and to be affected little by treatment with calciferol (207,254). One of the three cases was treated only with calcitriol, but this compound seems to be more effective than calciferol in preventing the progression of parathyroid growth (254). Another therapeutic regimen causing short-term stimulation of PTH secretion is sodium fluoride administration (259). The author has observed the development of hypercalcemic hyperparathyroidism during prolonged treatment with sodium fluoride and its cure by removal of a parathyroid adenoma, but whether this was more than a coincidence is not clear. In summary, tertiary hyperparathyroidism definitely occurs in chronic renal failure and probably occurs in phosphate-treated osteomalacia. Its development in chronic vitamin D deficiency is plausible, but the evidence is suggestive rather than conclusive.

Therapeutic Implications of Parathyroid Growth

In primary hyperparathyroidism, a sustained fall in PTH secretion can at present be achieved only by ablation of surplus parathyroid tissue, usually by surgical resection (see the chapter by Norton et al.). There is currently no parathyroid counterpart to bromocriptine, which can produce shrinkage as well as reduced hormone secretion in many pituitary tumors (260). The rate of growth influences the timing of surgery, which is urgently needed in acute primary hyperparathyroidism; is mandatory but not immediately required in many patients with progressive disease; and can be delayed, sometimes indefinitely, in mild nonprogressive disease (143). Regarding secondary hyperparathyroidism, however, there is a long-standing and pervasive assumption that, if the initial stimulus to cell proliferation could be removed, the parathyroid glands would eventually return to their previous size. There are several bases for this assumption. First, a noninvasive reduction in size has for many years been easy to observe in the thyroid gland (1). Second, classical nutritional experiments that demonstrated cross-sectional differences in parathyroid growth (93) have often been misquoted as evidence for parathyroid involution. Third, the ultrastructural changes that accompany suppression of hormone synthesis and release by hypercalcemia (261) have been misinterpreted as evidence for suppression of growth. Nevertheless, it is far from certain that a nondestructive increase in cell loss is possible in human parathyroid glands. The

absence of a parathyrotrophic hormone appears to limit the capacity for involution as well as for growth.

The first indication that hyperplastic parathyroid glands regressed very slowly, if at all, came from the frequent persistence of PTH hypersecretion after renal transplantation (8). There are several causes for hypercalcemia in this situation, but in current practice the most common is hyperparathyroidism. Although sometimes this is described as tertiary hyperparathyroidism, in most patients only hyperplasia is found. Mild hypercalcemia can persist unchanged, with no tendency to resolve; if parathyroid involution is occurring in such patients, it is at a rate too low to be reflected by detectable changes in plasma calcium for up to 10 years (8). In primary hyperparathyroidism, the nonadenomatous parathyroid glands may show ultrastructural evidence of functional suppression (261), but the reduction in parenchymal cell mass is only ~10% (74), from which has been estimated a normal turnover rate of ~3%/year (8). In patients with nonparathyroid hypercalcemia, the parathyroid glands at autopsy are indistinguishable from normal glands in histologic appearance, in relative proportions of fat and parenchyma, and in size (42). Parathyroid cell number presumably reflects the balance between mitosis and apoptosis (8,35). Mitosis is stimulated by hypocalcemia and by calcitriol deficiency, and it would be a pleasing symmetry if apoptosis was stimulated by hypercalcemia and by calcitriol excess. The evidence reviewed above fails to support such an effect for hypercalcemia, but the status of calcitriol in this respect is less clear.

In chronic renal failure, calcitriol effectively suppresses PTH secretion and improves osteitis fibrosa, at least in the short term (see the chapter by Coburn and Salusky), but the long-term results are likely to depend on control of gland size rather than on control of hormone secretion. In patients on long-term hemodialysis, oral calcitriol pulse therapy induced a 40% reduction in parathyroid volume (measured by ultrasound) after 12 weeks (262), with most of the decrease occurring in the first 4 weeks; similar results have been reported independently (263). The shrinkage was much too rapid to be accounted for by even complete suppression of cell proliferation. The ultrasound method was reproducible, but its absolute accuracy is unknown, and the change could reflect reductions in vascularity and in cell size rather than in cell number. Nevertheless, the latter interpretation is supported by experiments in 3-month-old vitamin D-deficient chicks that received vitamin D replacement. There was good evidence for a reduction in parathyroid cell number, based on similar reductions in weight, protein, and DNA content (264); the change was detectable within 4 days and could have resulted only from apoptosis. In the clinical experiment, the large abrupt increase in serum calcitriol concentration produced by pulse therapy was likely crucial to the success of the regimen (265), since an abrupt decline in the level of the relevant trophic factor is necessary to induce apoptosis in tissues that are hyperplastic as a result of endocrine stimulation (29). If induction of apoptosis by calcitriol can be confirmed, a bromocriptine for the parathyroid glands may be at hand.

Parathyroid Growth in Hypoparathyroidsm

The parathyroid glands are difficult to find at autopsy even when they are normal in size, and there is only fragmentary information about their pathology when they are small. The available data in the various forms of idiopathic hypoparathyroidism are described in the chapters by LiVolsi, Sherwood and Santora, and Whyte. In surgical hypoparathyroidism, there has been almost no histologic examination, but an interesting paradox can be formulated on the basis of the course of parathyroid function in the absence of treatment. In many patients, the level of plasma calcium is higher than expected for the complete absence of PTH (265), there is a low but detectable level of intact PTH (266), and some recovery from EDTA-induced hypocalcemia is possible (267). Evidently some cells capable of secreting PTH remain, but depressed function persists. According to the model depicted in Figs. 7 and 8, because the relationship between cell number and plasma calcium is curvilinear, the fall in plasma calcium is proportionally less than the fall in cell number. Hormone secretion per cell is increased, and as cell number declines, each cell operates ever more closely to its upper limit with respect to hormone secretion. In these circumstances, why do not the remaining cells proliferate until normal function is restored? As mentioned earlier the effect of calcium on parathyroid cell proliferation is biphasic, and severe hypocalcemia is less effective than mild hypocalcemia. But this cannot be the whole explanation for the paradox, since even mild hypoparathyroidism can remain unchanged in severity for many years (265).

Except when all four glands are removed, which almost never happens with neck surgery for nonmalignant disease, there is no relationship between the development of hypocalcemia and the amount of parathyroid tissue in the surgical specimen (268). Rather than simple removal of some parathyroid tissue, there is interference with the blood supply of all four glands as the result of the surgical dissection and hemostasis (269). This occurs only in a small minority of patients, presumably because of individual differences in the precise location of the parathyroid glands and in the detailed anatomy of their blood supply. The progression of fibrosis is a likely explanation for the late occurrence of surgical hypoparathyroidism after a period of apparent recovery with normocalcemia (270), and

the parathyroid ischemia is a likely explanation for the development of apparently idiopathic hypoparathyroidism late in life (271). The susceptibility of parathyroid tissue to ischemia is indicated by uncertain survival after transplantation (227), and by spontaneous infarction in rapidly growing tumors (168). A subnormal degree of parathyroid function can be maintained by small islands of cells, but if separated by bands of fibrous tissue their viability will be precarious. Regeneration depends on neoangiogenesis as well as on chief cell proliferation (110), and both processes would be compromised by vascular injury, impaired circulation, and persistent fibrosis.

INTEGRATION OF PARATHYROID GROWTH AND HORMONE SECRETION

Increases in Set-Point and in Cell Proliferation— Further Examples

Both in primary and in hypercalcemic secondary hyperparathyroidism, cell proliferation is driven in large part by an increase in secretory set-point, the result either of a somatic mutation or of calcitriol deficiency. Three additional examples of this relationship merit brief discussion—normal embryonic development (272), familial hypocalciuric hypercalcemia (FHH) (see the chapter by Heath), and lithium-induced hypercalcemia (see the chapter by Mallette). The fetal parathyroid gland secretes PTH-related peptide (PTHrP) rather than PTH, but its secretory activity is regulated by calcium in the same manner as the adult parathyroid gland, except that the secretory set-point is higher than in the adult (272). The rapidity of embryonic parathyroid growth is consonant with a need to prevent fetal hypocalcemia (57) by supplying PTHrP to maintain normal placental calcium transport (273). This is probably an evolutionary rather than an individual functional adaptation, but proliferation could be driven in part by the increase in set-point.

In FHH, hypercalcemia is mild and nonprogressive. Urinary calcium excretion is normal, but is low relative to the plasma calcium, and tubular reabsorption of calcium is increased. Serum PTH levels are usually normal in childhood but increase slowly with time and are often above normal after age 30 (274). The secretory set-point determined in vivo by EDTA and calcium infusions is increased (196,275). The geometric mean for parathyroid parenchymal area in histologic sections was increased approximately three-fold, compared to a five-fold increase in other forms of primary hyperplasia, whether familial or sporadic (276). Parathyroid weights have been reported only in a few patients; the mean was increased about two-fold, but few individual glands weighed more than 75 mg (277). The mild hyperplasia represents the polyclonal (or multiclonal) expression of a germinal mutation (278). The data are consistent with a primary defect in membrane calcium transport affecting cells in the parathyroid gland, renal tubule, and possibly bone (89). In terms of the set-point hypothesis, a lesser degree of parathyroid enlargement is needed to satisfy the increased secretory set-point because the raised renal tubular set-point does not depend on increased PTH secretion (89).

Administration of lithium salts, usually for bipolar affective disorder, is in most patients followed within a few weeks by modest increases in plasma PTH and calcium levels, occasionally of sufficient magnitude to constitute hypercalcemia (279,280). Even a single dose of lithium carbonate increases the intact PTH level after two hours, with no change in ionized calcium (281). The early changes are reversible, but mild persistent hypercalcemia is found in about 15% of patients given prolonged treatment (279,280). The features of lithium-induced hypercalcemia are similar to those of FHH (280,282). Serum PTH levels are nonsuppressed or moderately raised, and tubular reabsorption of calcium is increased. Both short-term and long-term clinical studies indicate that lithium administration increases the PTH secretory set-point (282,283), a conclusion supported by the *in vitro* effects of lithium on cultured parathyroid cells, both bovine and human (279,280). As predicted by the set-point hypothesis, lithium administration stimulates parathyroid growth. Exposure to lithium increases tritiated thymidine uptake by cells cultured from parathyroid adenomas (284), and there is a significant increase in parathyroid volume measured by ultrasound in patients on long-term treatment (285). In lithium-induced hypercalcemia of sufficient severity to need surgical treatment, both hyperplasia and adenoma have been found (279,280,286). Adenoma tends to occur earlier in the course of lithium treatment than hyperplasia (287), suggesting that lithium promotes hyperplasia of normal parathyroid tissue and stimulates the growth of small adenomas already present (284).

A New Concept of Calcium Homeostasis

The consistency of the association between increased secretory set-point and increased cell proliferation suggests a new way of looking at plasma calcium homeostasis. According to this view, the controlled variable is not the plasma calcium itself, but rather the difference between the parathyroid secretory set-point (using the physiologic definition given earlier) and the prevailing plasma calcium level, with the target value for this variable being zero (Figure 11). If plasma calcium is below the set-point, the well-known short-term feedback loop is initiated; based on the hierarchy of mechanisms described earlier (see

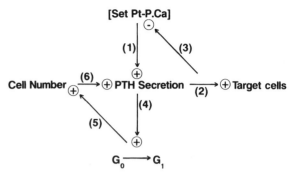

FIG. 11. Short-term and long-term loops in calcium homeostasis. The controlled variable is the difference between the parathyroid secretory set-point and the current level of plasma calcium, with a target value of zero. The signs indicate, for each step, the directional effect on the dependent variable of an increase in the independent variable. Steps 1, 2, and 3 constitute the short-term loop, and steps 4, 5, and 6 the long-term loop. Step 4 is initiated when PTH hypersecretion by individual cells is prolonged because a positive value of the controlled variable persists, but the mechanism is unknown. (For further details see text.)

the section on physiological influences on parathyroid growth and ref. 84), total hormone secretion by all glands is increased. Depending on the response of target cells in bone and in the renal tubule to higher PTH levels (89), plasma calcium rises, and the deviation from the set-point is eliminated. If this process is incompletely effective, there will be a sustained increase in demand for PTH, bringing into play a long-term feedback loop, whereby some parathyroid cells are triggered from the quiescent G0 state into the G1 stage of the cell cycle. The initiating signal may be a fall in PTH concentration in some critical intracellular compartment, augmented by the autocrine mechanism described earlier (see the section on physiological influences on parathyroid growth and ref. 109). The result will be an increase in the number of parathyroid cells, a consequent increase in total hormone secretion in response to the same stimulus, and a rise in plasma calcium toward the set-point. The cycle will be repeated until cell number has increased sufficiently to reduce the disturbing signal to trivial magnitude.

As mentioned earlier, the long-term loop adds integral control to the proportional and derivative controls that suffice for the short-term loop (89). This ensures that stimulated parathyroid cells need not long sustain maximum rates of hormone synthesis and secretion, in which state they cannot respond to an additional demand, but are returned to the steep central portion of the sigmoid curve where they can respond with greatest efficiency in either direction (89). The sustained increase in the controlled variable needed to initiate the long-term feedback loop can arise either because the plasma calcium is reduced or because the set-point is increased. Chronic hypocalcemia (if not due to hypo-

TABLE 11. *Comparison of different mechanisms of increase in set-point*

Disorder	Primary Adenoma	Secondary Hyperplasia	FHH[a]	Lithium Therapy
Set-point	↑	↑	↑	↑
Mechanism	Somatic Mutation	Calcitriol Deficiency	Germinal Mutation	Direct effect on cells
Affected cells	One clone	Nodules	All	All
PTH efficacy[b]	Normal	Reduced[c]	Increased[d]	Increased[d]
Cell increase	Moderate	Severe	Mild	Mild

[a]Familial hypocalciuric hypercalcemia; the situation in other forms of genetic primary hyperplasia is less clear
[b]in raising plasma calcium
[c]because of calcitriol deficiency and other effects of renal failure
[d]because of increase in tubular reabsorption of calcium.

parathyroidism) is the result of decreased efficacy of PTH in maintaining normocalcemia, for one of the reasons previously given (see the section on parathyroid growth in secondary and tertiary hyperparathyroidism), leading to diffuse secondary parathyroid hyperplasia. Depending on its cause, an increase in secretory set-point will affect a different population of cells and have different morphologic consequences (Table 11). If due to a somatic mutation, then only a single clone of cells will be affected, leading to primary or tertiary hyperparathyroidism (Figure 10). If due to calcitriol deficiency, some groups of cells may be affected more than others, leading to nodular secondary hyperplasia. If due to a germinal mutation or to an external agent such as lithium, all cells will be affected equally, leading to primary hyperplasia (Table 11).

There are significant differences between individuals in mean plasma calcium level, presumably reflecting small individual differences in parathyroid secretory set-point (89). There are also significant differences between families, implying that differences in set-point are genetically determined (89). According to the set-point hypothesis, there should be corresponding differences in cell number, and parathyroid weight should be positively correlated with plasma calcium level. But, in fact, the correlation is not positive but negative (66,68)! The patients available for sampling at autopsy probably encompassed a wide range of calcium and vitamin D nutrition, so that in this multiethnic population the variation in target cell responsiveness to PTH was large enough to dominate the reciprocal feedback relationship, allowing the observations to be reconciled with the set-point hypothesis. Whatever the molecular basis of the link between cell proliferation and hormone secretion in the parathyroid gland turns out to be, the set-point hypothesis, in conjunction with variation in the efficacy of PTH in raising plasma calcium (Table 11), accounts for the slowing down of growth in parathyroid adenomas, the persistence of rapid growth in secondary hyperplasia

with hypercalcemia, and the small extent of growth in FHH. Integration of the short-term loop governing hormone secretion and the long-term loop governing proliferation ensures that both in health and in disease, the parathyroid glands will attain the size needed to accomplish their biological purpose.

REFERENCES

1. DeGroot L, ed. *Endocrinology, 2nd ed.* Philadelphia: W.B. Saunders, 1989.
2. Wolpert L. *The triumph of the embryo.* Oxford: Oxford University Press, 1991.
3. Bloom W, Nalbandov AV, Bloom MA. Parathyroid enlargement in laying hens on a calcium-deficient diet. *Clin Orthop* 1960;17:206–209.
4. Sinclair JG. Size of the parathyroid glands of albino rats as affected by pregnancy and controlled diets. *Anat Rec* 1941; 80:479–496.
5. Falkner F, Tanner JM, eds. *Human growth. A comprehensive treatise, 2nd ed.* New York: Plenum Press, 1986.
6. Goss RJ. Modes of growth and regeneration. Mechanisms, regulation, distribution. In: Falkner F, Tanner JM, eds. *Human growth. A comprehensive treatise, 2nd ed.* New York: Plenum Press, 1986;3–26.
7. Goss RJ. The strategy of growth. In: Teir H, Rytömaa T, eds. *Control of cellular growth in adult organisms.* New York: Academic Press, 1967;3–27.
8. Parfitt AM. Hypercalcemic hyperparathyroidism following renal transplantation: differential diagnosis, management, and implications for cell population control in the parathyroid gland. *Mineral Electrolyte Metab* 1982;8:92–119.
9. Brasel JA, Gruen RK. Cellular growth. Brain, heart, lung, liver, and skeletal muscle. In: Falkner F, Tanner JM, eds. *Human growth. A comprehensive treatise, 2nd ed.* New York: Plenum Press, 1986;53–65.
10. Sands J, Dobbing J, Gratrix CA. Cell number and cell size: organ growth and development and the control of catch-up growth in rats. *Lancet* 1979;1:503–505.
11. Enesco M, Leblond CP. Increase in cell number as a factor in the growth of the organs and tissues of the young male rat. *J Embryol Exp Morphol* 1962;10:530–562.
12. Alberts B, Bray D, Lewis J, Raff M, Roberts K, Watson JD. *Molecular biology of the cell, 2nd ed.* New York: Garland Publishing, 1989.
13. Sporn MB, Roberts AB. *Peptide growth factors and their receptors I and II.* New York: Springer-Verlag, 1991.
14. Tanner JM. Catch-up and catch-down growth: a review. *Growth Genet Horm* 1987;3:8–11.

15. Goss RJ. Theories of growth regulation. In: Goss RJ, ed. *Regulation of organ and tissue growth.* New York: Academic Press, 1972;1–11.
16. Baserga R, ed. *The biology of cell reproduction.* Cambridge MA: Harvard University Press, 1985.
17. Bullough WS. *The dynamic body tissues.* New York: Scientific and Academic Editions, 1983.
18. Britton NF, Wright NA, Murray JD. A mathematical model for cell population kinetics in the intestine. *J Theor Biol* 1982;98:531–541.
19. Goodlad RA, Wright NA. Growth control factors in the gastrointestinal tract. *Bailliere's Clin Gastroenterol* 1990;4:97–118.
20. Fausto N, Mead JE. Biology of disease. Regulation of liver growth: protooncogenes and transforming growth factors. In: Rubin E, Damjanov I, eds. *Pathology reviews.* Clifton, NJ, Humana Press, 1990;3–12.
21. Ruvkun G. A molecular growth industry. *Nature* 1992; 360:711–712.
22. Mosier HD Jr, Jansons RA, Swingle KF, Dearden LC. Dissociation of catch-up growth control and neural control of growth hormone secretion in the stunted head-irradiated rat. *Pediatr Res* 1986;20:261–264.
23. Burch PRJ. Pathology, inference, and carcinogenesis. In: *Pathology annual, part 2, vol 15.* New York: Appleton-Century-Crofts, 1980;21–44.
24. Snow MHL. Control of embryonic growth rate and fetal size in mammals. In: Falkner F, Tanner JM, eds. *Human growth. A comprehensive treatise, 2nd ed.* New York: Plenum Press, 1986;67–82.
25. Wright N, Alison M, eds. *The biology of epithelial cell populations.* Oxford: Clarendon Press, 1984.
26. Lajtha LG. Stem cell concepts. In: Potten CS, ed. *Stem cells—their identification and characterisation.* New York: Churchill Livingstone, 1983;1–11.
27. Zajicek G. The time dimension in histology. *Methods Inform Med* 1987;26:1–2.
28. Zajicek G, Ariel I, Arber N. The streaming liver III. Littoral cells accompany the streaming hepatocyte. *Liver* 1988;8: 213–218.
29. Kerr JFR, Searle J, Harmon BV, Bishop CJ. Apoptosis. In: Potten CS, ed. *Perspectives on mammalian cell death.* Oxford: Oxford University Press, 1987;93–128.
30. Schwartzman RA, Cidlowski JA. Apoptosis: the biochemistry and molecular biology of programmed cell death. *Endocr Rev* 1993;14:133–151.
31. Wyllie AH, Kerr JFR, Macaskill AM, Currie AR. Adrenocortical cell deletion: the role of ACTH. *J Pathol* 1973; 111:85–94.
32. Hopwood D, Levison DA. Atrophy and apoptosis in the cyclical human endometrium. *J Pathol* 1976;119:159–166.
33. Ferguson DJP, Anderson DA. Morphological evaluation of cell turnover in relation to the menstrual cycle in the "resting" human breast. *Br J Cancer* 1981;44:177–181.
34. Kerr JFR, Searle J. Deletion of cells by apoptosis during castration-induced involution of the rat prostate. *Virchows Arch Abt B Zellpathol* 1973;13:87–102.
35. Kerr JFR, Wyllie AH, Currie AR. Apoptosis: a basic biological phenomenon with wide-ranging implications in tissue kinetics. *Br J Cancer* 1972;26:239–257.
36. Tannock IF. Principles of cell proliferation: Cell kinetics. In: DeVita VT, Hellman S, Rosenberg SA, eds. *Cancer. Principles and practice of oncology. vol 1, 3rd ed.* Philadelphia: J.B. Lippincott, 1989;3–13.
37. Parfitt AM, Willgoss D, Jacobi J, Lloyd HM. Cell kinetics in parathyroid adenomas: evidence for decline in rates of cell birth and tumour growth, assuming clonal origin. *Clin Endocrinol* 1991;35:151–157.
38. Gundersen HJG, Bendtsen TF, Korbo L, Marcussen N, Moller A, Nielsen K, Nyengaard JR, Pakkenberg B, Sorensen FB, Vesterby A, West MJ. Some new, simple and efficient stereological methods and their use in pathological research and diagnosis. *APMIS* 1988;96:379–394.
39. Åkerström G, Grimelius L, Johansson H, Pertoft H, Lundqvist H. Estimation of the parathyroid parenchymal

40. Bruining HA. *Surgical treatment of hyperparathyroidism.* Springfield, IL: Charles C. Thomas, 1971.
41. Parfitt AM, Braunstein GD, Katz A. Radiation-associated hyperparathyroidism: comparison of adenoma growth rates, inferred from weight and duration of latency, with prevalence of mitosis. *J Clin Endocrinol Metab* (in press).
42. Dufour DR, Marx SJ, Spiegel AM. Parathyroid gland morphology in nonparathyroid hormone-mediated hypercalcemia. *Am J Surg Pathol* 1985;9:43–51.
43. Grimelius L, Åkerström G, Johansson H, Lundqvist H. Estimation of parenchymal cell content of human parathyroid glands using the image analysing computer technique. *Am J Pathol* 1978;93:793–800.
44. Gundersen HJG, Bagger P, Bendtsen TF, et al. The new stereological tools: disector, fractionator, nucleator and point sampled intercepts and their use in pathological research and diagnosis. *APMIS* 1988;96:857–881.
45. Quinn CM, Wright NA. The clinical assessment of proliferation and growth in human tumours: evaluation of methods and applications as prognostic variables. *J Pathol* 1990;160: 93–102.
46. Baak JPA. Mitosis counting in tumors. *Hum Pathol* 1990; 21:683–685.
47. Cleaver JE. *Thymidine metabolism and cell kinetics.* Amsterdam: North Holland Publishing Co., 1967.
48. Maurer HR. Potential pitfalls of [³H]thymidine techniques to measure cell proliferation. *Cell Tissue Kinet* 1981;14:111–120.
49. Dickson RB, Aitken S, Lippman ME. Assay of mitogen-induced effects on cellular incorporation of precursors for scavenger, de Novo, and net DNA synthesis. *Methods Enzymol* 1987;146:329–340.
50. Lloyd HM, Jacobi JM, Willgoss D, Kearney J, Ward P. DNA synthesis and secretory activity in parathyroid adenomas. *Acta Endocrinol* 1981;96:70–74.
51. Hoshino T, Nagashima T, Murovic JA, Wilson CB, Davis RL. Proliferative potential of human meningiomas of the brain. A cell kinetics study with bromodeoxyuridine. *Cancer* 1986;58:1466–1472.
52. Murray AW, Kirschner MW. What controls the cell cycle. *Sci Am* 1991;3:56–63.
53. Galand P, Degraef C. Cyclin/PCNA immunostaining as an alternative to tritiated thymidine pulse labelling for marking S phase cells in paraffin sections from animal and human tissues. *Cell Tissue Kinet* 1989;22:383–392.
54. Raber MN, Barlogie B. DNA flow cytometry of human solid tumors. In: Melamed MR, Lindmo T, Mendelsohn ML, eds. *Flow cytometry and sorting, 2nd ed.* New York: Wiley-Liss, 1990;745–754.
55. Meyer JS, Coplin MD. Thymidine labeling index, flow cytometric S-phase measurement, and DNA index in human tumors. *Am J Clin Pathol* 1988;89:586–595.
56. Friedlander ML, Hedley DW, Taylor IW. Clinical and biological significance of aneuploidy in human tumours. *J Clin Pathol* 1984;37:961–974.
57. Norris EH. Anatomical evidence of prenatal function of the human parathyroid glands. *Anat Rec* 1946;96:129–141.
58. Roth SI. Anatomy of the parathyroid glands. In: DeGroot LJ, Cahill GF Jr, Martini L, et al. eds. *Endocrinology, vol 2, 1st ed.* New York: Grune & Stratton, 1979;587–592.
59. Corliss CE. *Patten's human embryology—elements of clinical development.* New York: McGraw-Hill, 1976.
60. Gilmour JR. The embryology of the parathyroid glands, the thymus and certain associated rudiments. *J Pathol Bacteriol* 1937;45:507–522.
61. Gilmour JR, Martin WJ. The weight of the parathyroid glands. *J Pathol Bacteriol* 1937;44:431–468.
62. Wild P, Manser EM. Ultrastructural morphometry of parathyroid cells in rats of different ages. *Cell Tissue Res* 1985;240:585–591.
63. Cheek DB. *Fetal and postnatal cellular growth—hormones and nutrition.* New York: John Wiley & Sons, 1975.
64. Cheek DB. *Human growth: body composition, cell growth,*

cell mass by density gradients. *Am J Pathol* 1980;99:155–164.

energy and intelligence. Philadelphia: Lea and Febiger, 1968.

65. Åkerström G, Grimelius L, Johansson H, Lundqvist H, Pertoft H, Bergstrom R. The parenchymal cell mass in normal human parathyroid glands. *Acta Pathol Microbiol Scand Section A* 1981;89:367–375.

66. Dufour DR, Wilkerson SY. Factors related to parathyroid weight in normal persons. *Arch Pathol Lab Med* 1983; 107:167–172.

67. Dekker A, Dunsford HA, Geyer SJ. The normal parathyroid gland at autopsy: the significance of stromal fat in adult patients. *J Pathol* 1979;128:127–132.

68. Ghandur-Mnaymneh L, Cassady J, Hajianpour MA, Paz J, Reiss E. The parathyroid gland in health and disease. *Am J Pathol* 1986;125:292–299.

69. Freeman W. The weight of the endocrine glands—biometrical studies in psychiatry. *Hum Biol* 1934;6:489–523.

70. Blumenthal HT. Aging processes in the endocrine glands of the guinea pig. *Arch Pathol* 1945;40:264–269.

71. Foster CL. Studies on the parathyroid of the mouse. 2. Some observations upon the postnatal cytological development of the normal gland, with particular reference to its mitotic activity and Golgi elements. *J Anat* 1946;80:171–178.

72. Lee MJ, Roth SI. Effect of calcium and magnesium on deoxyribonucleic acid synthesis in rat parathyroid glands in vitro. *Lab Invest* 1975;1:72–79.

73. Platt H. Mitotic activity in the parathyroid glands of the rat following bilateral nephrectomy. *J Pathol Bacteriol* 1950; 62:383–387.

74. Ejerblad S, Grimelius L, Johansson H, Werner I. Studies on the non-adenomatous glands in patients with a solitary parathyroid adenoma. *Uppsala J Med Sci* 1976;81:31–36.

75. Cameron IL. Cell renewal in the organs and tissues of the nongrowing adult mouse. *Texas Rep Biol Med* 1970;28:203–248.

76. Weymouth RJ. The cytology of the parathyroid glands of the rat after bilateral nephrectomy, administration of parathyroid hormone and hypophysectomy. *Anat Rec* 1957;127:509–526.

77. Engfeldt B. Studies on parathyroidal function in relation to hormonal influences and dietetic conditions. *Acta Endocrinol* 1950(Suppl 6):5:53–118.

78. Horvath E, Kovacs K. The adenohypophysis. In: Kovacs K, Asa SL, eds. *Functional endocrine pathology, vol 1*. Oxford: Blackwell Scientific Publications, 1991.

79. Ladizesky M, Diaz MC, Zeni S, Romeo HE, Cardinali DP, Mautalen CA. Compensatory parathyroid hypertrophy after hemiparathyroidectomy in rats feeding a low calcium diet. *Calcif Tissue Int* 1991;48:63–67.

80. Pavlov AV. Compensatory hypertrophy of the rat parathyroid glands. *Arch Anat Cytol Embryol* 1983;85:75–81.

81. Capen CC, Roth SI. Ultrastructural and functional relationships of normal and pathologic parathyroid cells. In: Ioachim HL, ed. *Pathobiology annual*. New York: Appleton-Century-Crofts, 1973;129–175.

82. Talmage RV, Toft RJ, Davis R. Parathyroid activity in nephrectomized rats. *Texas Rep Biol Med* 1960;18:298–308.

83. Hansson CG, Mathewson S, Norrby K. Parathyroid cell growth and proliferation in nephrectomised rats. *Pathol Eur* 1971;6:313–321.

84. Parfitt AM, Kleerekoper M. The divalent ion homeostatic system: physiology and metabolism of calcium, phosphorus, magnesium and bone. In: Maxwell M, Kleeman CR, eds. *Clinical disorders of fluid and electrolyte metabolism, 3rd ed*. New York: McGraw Hill, 1980;269–398.

85. Shannon WA Jr, Roth SI. An ultrastructural study of acid phosphatase activity in normal, adenomatous and hyperplastic (chief cell type) human parathyroid glands. *Am J Pathol* 1974;77:493–501.

86. Marti R, Wild P, Schraner EM, Mueller M, Moor H. Parathyroid ultrastructure after aldehyde fixation, high-pressure freezing, or microwave irradiation. *J Histochem Cytochem* 1987;35:1415–1424.

87. Fitzpatrick LA, Leong DA. Individual parathyroid cells are more sensitive to calcium than a parathyroid cell population. *Endocrinology* 1990;126:1720–1727.

88. Kendall CH, Roberts PA, Pringle JH, Lauder I. The expression of parathyroid hormone messenger RNA in normal and abnormal parathyroid tissue. *J Pathol* 1991;165:111–118.

89. Parfitt AM. Calcium homeostasis. In: Mundy GR, Martin TJ, eds. *Physiology and pharmacology of bone*. Heidelberg: Springer-Verlag, 1993;1–65.

90. Krstič R. Three-dimensional organization of the rat parathyroid glands. *Z Mikrosk Anat Forsch* 1980;94:445–450.

91. Kremer R, Bolivar I, Goltzman D, Hendy GN. Influence of calcium and 1,25-dihydroxycholecalciferol on proliferation and proto-oncogene expression in primary cultures of bovine parathyroid cells. *Endocrinology* 1989;125:935–941.

92. Wernerson A, Widholm SM, Svensson O, Reinholt FP. Parathyroid cell number and size in hypocalcemic young rats. *APMIS* 1991;99:1096–1102.

93. Stoerk HC, Carnes WH. The relation of the dietary Ca:P ratio to serum Ca and to parathyroid volume. *J Nutr* 1945;29:43–50.

94. Hurwitz S, Griminger P. The response of plasma alkaline phosphatase, parathyroids and blood and bone minerals to calcium intake in the fowl. *J Nutr* 1961;73:177–184.

95. Mueller GL, Anast CS, Breitenbach RP. Dietary calcium and ultimobranchial body and parathyroid gland in the chicken. *Am J Physiol* 1970;218:1718–1722.

96. Luce EM. The size of the parathyroids of rats, and the effect of a diet deficiency of calcium. *J Pathol* 1923;26:200–208.

97. Drake TG, Albright F, Castleman B. Parathyroid hyperplasia in rabbits produced by parenteral phosphate administration. *J Clin Invest* 1936;16:203–206.

98. Harrison M, Fraser R. The parathyroid glands and calcium deficiency in the rat. *J Endocrinol* 1960;21:207–211.

99. Trechsel U, Eisman JA, Fischer JA, Bonjour J-P, Fleisch H. Calcium-dependent, parathyroid hormone-independent regulation of 1,25-dihydroxyvitamin D. *Endocrinol Metab* 1980;2:E119–E124.

100. Parfitt AM, Willgoss D, Parikh N, Wilson P, Lloyd HM. Long term response of rats to dietary calcium restriction: Evidence for calcium dependent, parathyroid hormone independent, modulation of vitamin D metabolism. *J Bone Mineral Res* 4(Suppl 1):S252.

101. Szabo A, Merke J, Beier E, Mall G, Ritz E. 1,25(OH)$_2$ vitamin D$_3$ inhibits parathyroid cell proliferation in experimental uremia. *Kidney Int* 1989;35:1049–1056.

102. Ishimi Y, Russell J, Sherwood LM. Regulation by calcium and 1,25-(OH)$_2$D$_3$ of cell proliferation and function of bovine parathyroid cells in culture. *J Bone Mineral Res* 1990;5:755–760.

103. Holick MF, Adams JS. Vitamin D metabolism and biological function. In: Avioli LV, Krane SM, eds. *Metabolic bone disease and clinically related disorders, 2nd ed*. Philadelphia: W.B. Saunders, 1990;155–195.

104. Naveh-Many T, Silver J. Regulation of parathyroid hormone gene expression by hypocalcemia, hypercalcemia, and vitamin D in the rat. *J Clin Invest* 1990;86:1313–1319.

105. Brandi ML, Fitzpatrick LA, Coon HG, Aurbach GD. Bone parathyroid cells: cultures maintained for more than 140 population doublings. *Proc Natl Acad Sci USA* 1986;83: 1709–1713.

106. Raisz LG. Regulation by calcium of parathyroid growth and secretion in vitro. *Nature* 1963;197:1115–1117.

107. Willgoss D. *The role of cyclic nucleotides in parathyroid tissue*. MSc Thesis, University of Queensland, 1982.

108. Sakaguchi K, Santora A, Zimering M, Curcio F, Aurbach GD, Brandi ML. Functional epithelial cell line cloned from rat parathyroid glands. *Proc Natl Acad Sci USA* 1987; 84:3269–3273.

109. Sakaguchi K. Acidic fibroblast growth factor autocrine system as a mediator of calcium-regulated parathyroid cell growth. *J Biol Chem* 1992;34:24554–24562.

110. Brandi ML. Cellular models for the analysis of paracrine communications in parathyroid tissue. *J Endocrinol Invest* (in press).

111. Pawlikowski M. The link between secretion and mitosis in the endocrine glands. *Life Sci* 1982;30:315–320.

112. Jacobi JM, Lloyd HM. Modulation by dopamine antagonists

of DNA synthesis in the pituitary gland of the male rat. *Neuroendocrinology* 1981;33:97–100.

113. Parfitt AM. A theoretical model of the relationship between parathyroid cell mass and plasma calcium concentration in normal and uremic subjects: an analysis of the concept of autonomy and speculations on the mechanism of parathyroid hyperplasia. *Arch Intern Med* 1969;124:269–273.

114. Parfitt AM. Bone and plasma calcium homeostasis. *Bone* 1987;8:51–58.

115. Brown EM, Gardner DG, Brennan MF, et al. Calcium-regulated parathyroid hormone release in primary hyperparathyroidism: studies in vitro with dispersed parathyroid cells. *Am J Med* 1979;66:923–931.

116. Brown EM. Four-parameter model of the sigmoidal relationship between parathyroid hormone release and extracellular calcium concentration in normal and abnormal parathyroid tissue. *J Clin Endocrinol Metab* 1983;56:572–581.

117. Gittes RF, Radde IC. Experimental hyperparathyroidism from multiple isologous parathyroid transplants: homeostatic effect of simultaneous thyroid transplants. *Endocrinology* 1966;78:1015–1022.

118. Hodgkinson A. Biochemical aspects of primary hyperparathyroidism: an analysis of 50 cases. *Clin Sci* 1963;25:231–242.

119. Lloyd HM. Primary hyperparathyroidism: An analysis of the role of the parathyroid tumor. *Medicine* 1968;47:53–71.

120. Purnell DC, Smith LH, Scholz DA, Elveback LR, Arnaud CD. Primary hyperparathyroidism: a prospective clinical study. *Am J Med* 1971;50:670–678.

121. Wells SA Jr, Ketcham AS, Marx SJ, et al. Preoperative localization of hyperfunctioning parathyroid tissue: radioimmunoassay of parathyroid hormone in plasma from selectively catheterized thyroid veins. *Ann Surg* 1973;177:93–98.

122. Mallette LE, Bilezikian JP, Heath DA, Aurbach GD. Primary hyperparathyroidism: clinical and biochemical features. *Medicine* 1974;53:127–146.

123. Castleman B, Roth SI. Tumors of the parathyroid glands. Fascicle 14. In: Hartmann WH, Cowan WR, eds. *Atlas of tumor pathology, second series.* Bethesda, MD: AFIP 1978.

124. Saxe AW, Lincenberg S, Hamburger SW. Can the volume of abnormal parathyroid tissue be predicted by preoperative biochemical measurement? *Surgery* 1987;102:840–845.

125. Altenähr E, Arps H, Montz R, Dorn G. Quantitative ultrastructural and radioimmunologic assessment of parathyroid gland activity in primary hyperparathyroidism. *Lab Invest* 1979;31:303–312.

126. Rutledge R, Stiegel M, Thomas CG Jr, Wild RE. The relation of serum calcium and immunoparathormone levels to parathyroid size and weight in primary hyperparathyroidism. *Surgery* 1985;98:1107–1112.

127. Saadeh G, Licata A, Esselstyn C, Gupta M. Relationship of parathyroid adenoma volume and biochemical function. *Horm Res* 1989;32:142–144.

128. Ljunghall S, Hellman P, Rastad J, Åkerström G. Primary hyperparathyroidism: epidemiology, diagnosis and clinical picture. *World J Surg* 1991;15:681–687.

129. McCarron DA, Muther RS, Lenfesty B, Bennett WM. Parathyroid function in persistent hyperparathyroidism: relationship to gland size. *Kidney Int* 1982;22:662–670.

130. Marx SJ, Lasker RD, Brown EM, et al. Secretory dysfunction in parathyroid cells from a neonate with severe primary hyperparathyroidism. *J Clin Endocrinol Metab* 1986;62:445–449.

131. Parfitt AM, Kleerekoper M. Clinical disorders of calcium, phosphorus and magnesium metabolism. In: Maxwell M, Kleeman CR, eds. *Clinical disorders of fluid and electrolyte metabolism, 3rd. ed.* New York: McGraw-Hill, 1980;947–1152.

132. Reiss E, Canterbury JM. Spectrum of hyperparathyroidism. *Am J Med* 1974;56:794–799.

133. Norris EH. The parathyroid adenoma: A study of 322 cases. *Surg Gynecol Obstet* 1947;84:1–41.

134. Parfitt AM. The actions of parathyroid hormone on bone.

Relation to bone remodelling and turnover, calcium homeostasis and metabolic bone disease. III. PTH and osteoblasts, the relationship between bone turnover and bone loss, and the state of the bones in primary hyperparathyroidism. *Metabolism* 1976;25:1033–1069.

135. Albright F, Aub JC, Bauer W. Hyperparathyroidism: a common and polymorphic condition as illustrated by seventeen proved cases from one clinic. *J Am Med Assoc* 1934;102:1276–1287.

136. Goldman L, Gordan GS, Chambers EL Jr. Changing diagnostic criteria for hyperparathyroidism. *Ann Surg* 1957;146:407–416.

137. Keating FR Jr. Diagnosis of primary hyperparathyroidism. *J Am Med Assoc* 1961;178:547–555.

138. Heath H III, Hodgson SF, Kennedy M. Primary hyperparathyroidism: incidence, morbidity and potential economic impact in a community. *N Engl J Med* 1980;302:189–193.

139. Hellstrom J, Ivemark BI. Primary hyperparathyroidism, clinical and structural findings in 138 cases. *Acta Chir Scand* 1962;294(Suppl):1–113.

140. Mundy GR, Cove DH, Fisken R. Primary hyperparathyroidism: Changes in the pattern of clinical presentation. *Lancet* 1980;7:1317–1320.

141. Palmer M, Ljunghall S, Åkerström G, et al. Patients with primary hyperparathyroidism operated on over a 24-year period: temporal trends of clinical and laboratory findings. *J Chron Dis* 1987;40:121–130.

142. Heath H III. Clinical spectrum of primary hyperparathyroidism: evolution with changes in medical practice and technology. *J Bone Mineral Res* 1991;6:S63–S70.

143. Parfitt AM, Rao DS, Kleerekoper M. Asymptomatic primary hyperparathyroidism discovered by multi-channel biochemical screening. Clinical course and considerations bearing on the need for surgical intervention. *J Bone Mineral Res* 1991;6:S97–S101.

144. Parisien M, Silverberg SJ, Shane E, Dempster DW, Bilezikian JP. Bone disease in primary hyperparathyroidism. *Endocrinol Metab North Am Clin* 1990;19:19–34.

145. O'Riordan JLH, Adami S. Pathophysiology of hyperparathyroidism. *Horm Res* 1984;20:38–43.

146. Fitzpatrick LA, Bilezikian JP. Acute primary hyperparathyroidism. *Am J Med* 1987;82:275–282.

147. Parfitt AM. Equilibrium and disequilibrium hypercalcemia: new light on an old concept. *Metab Bone Dis Rel Res* 1979;1:279–293.

148. Thomas WC Jr, Wiswell JG, Connor TB, Howard JE. Hypercalcemic crisis due to hyperparathyroidism. *Am J Med* 1958;24:229–239.

149. Hehrmann R, Thiele J, Tidow G, Hesch R-D. Acute hyperparathyroidism. Clinical, laboratory and ultrastructural findings in a variant of primary hyperparathyroidism. *Klin Wochenschr* 1980;58:501–510.

150. Cundy T, Darby AJ, Berry HE, Parsons V. Bone metabolism in acute parathyroid crisis. *Clin Endocrinol* 1985;22:787–793.

151. Wang C-A, Guyton SW. Hyperparathyroid crisis. Clinical and pathologic studies of 14 patients. *Ann Surg* 1979;190:782–790.

152. Kelly TR, Zarconi J. Primary hyperparathyroidism: hyperparathyroid crisis. *Am J Surg* 1981;142:539–542.

153. Shane E, Bilezikian JP. Parathyroid carcinoma: a review of 62 patients. *Endocr Rev* 1982;3:218–226.

154. Fraker DL, Travis WD, Merendino JJ Jr, et al. Locally recurrent parathyroid neoplasms as a cause for recurrent and persistent primary hyperparathyroidism. *Ann Surg* 1991;213:58–65.

155. Jarman WT, Myers RT, Marshall RB. Carcinoma of the parathyroid. *Arch Surg* 1978;113:123–125.

156. Jacobi JM, Lloyd HM, Smith JF. Nuclear diameter in parathyroid carcinomas. *J Clin Pathol* 1986;39:1353–1354.

157. Levin KE, Galante M, Clark OH. Parathyroid carcinoma versus parathyroid adenoma in patients with profound hypercalcemia. *Surgery* 1987;101:649.

158. Rao DS, Wilson RJ, Kleerekoper M, Parfitt AM. Lack of biochemical progression or continuation of accelerated bone

loss in mild asymptomatic primary hyperparathyroidism: evidence for biphasic disease course. *J Clin Endocrinol* 1988;109:959–962.

159. Rudnicki M, Transbol I. Increasing parathyroid hormone concentrations in untreated primary hyperparathyroidism. *J Intern Med* 1992;232:421–425.

160. Bilezikian JP, Silverberg SJ, Shane E, Parisien M, Dempster DW. Characterization and evaluation of asymptomatic primary hyperparathyroidism. *J Bone Mineral Res* 1991;6:S85–S89.

161. Mitlak BH, Daly M, Potts JT Jr, Schoenfeld D, Neer RM. Asymptomatic primary hyperparathyroidism. *J Bone Mineral Res* 1991;6:S103–S110.

162. Kleeman CR, Norris K, Coburn JW. Is the clinical expression of primary hyperparathyroidism a function of the long-term vitamin D status of the patient? *Mineral Electrolyte Metab* 1987;13:305–310.

163. Steel GG. *Growth kinetics of tumors. Cell population kinetics in relation to the growth and treatment of cancers.* Oxford: Clarendon Press, 1977.

164. Shackney SE. Cell kinetics and cancer chemotherapy. In: Calabresi P, Schein PS, Rosenberg, eds. *Medical oncology: basic principles and clinical management of cancer.* New York: Macmillan, 1985; 41–60.

165. Laird AK. Dynamics of growth in tumors and in normal organisms. In: Perry S, ed. *Human tumor cell kinetics* (National Cancer Institute Monograph 30). Bethesda, MD: National Cancer Institute, 1969;15–29.

166. Sutherland RM. Importance of critical metabolites and cellular interactions in the biology of microregions of tumors. *Cancer* 1986;58:1668–1680.

167. Walker NI, Harmon BV, Gobe GC, Kerr JFR. Patterns of cell death. *Methods Achievements Exp Pathol* 1988;13:18–54.

168. Klimiuk PS, Mainwaring AR. Spontaneous biochemical remission in parathyroid carcinoma. *Br Med J* 1980;281:1394–1395.

169. Woodruff MFA. Tumor clonality and its biological significance. In: Klein G, Weinhouse S, eds. *Advances in cancer research, vol 50.* New York: Academic Press, 1988;197–229.

170. Fearon ER, Vogelstein B. A genetic model for colorectal tumorigenesis. *Cell* 1990;61:759–767.

171. Thomas GA, Williams D, Williams ED. The clonal origin of thyroid nodules and adenomas. *Am J Pathol* 1989;134:141–147.

172. Nowell PC. The clonal evolution of tumor cell populations. *Science* 1976;194:23–28.

173. Moore GW, Berman JJ. Cell growth simulations predicting polyclonal origins for "monoclonal" tumors. *Cancer Lett* 1991;60:113–119.

174. Jackson CE, Cerny JC, Block MA, Fialkow PJ. Probable clonal origin of aldosteronomas versus multicellular origin of parathyroid "adenomas." *Surgery* 1982;92:875–879.

175. Namba H, Matsuo K, Fagin JA. Clonal composition of benign and malignant human thyroid tumors. *J Clin Invest* 1990;86:120–125.

176. Klibanski A. Editorial: further evidence for a somatic mutation theory in the pathogenesis of human pituitary tumors. *J Clin Endocrinol Metab* 1990;71:1415A–1415C.

177. Arnold A, Staunton CE, Kim HG, Gaz RD, Kronenberg HM. Monoclonality and abnormal parathyroid hormone genes in parathyroid adenomas. *N Engl J Med* 1988;318:658–662.

178. Rosenberg CL, Kim HG, Shows TB, Kronenberg HM, Arnold A. Rearrangement and overexpression of D11S287E, a candidate oncogene on chromosome 11q13 in benign parathyroid tumors. *Oncogene* 1991;6;3:449–453.

179. Marx SJ. Etiologies of parathyroid gland dysfunction in primary hyperparathyroidism. *J Bone Mineral Res* 1991;6:S19–S24.

180. Katz A, Braunstein GD. Clinical, biochemical, and pathologic features of radiation-associated hyperparathyroidism. *Arch Intern Med* 1983;143:79–82.

181. Tsunoda T, Mochinaga N, Eto T, Maeda H. Hyperparathyroidism following the atomic bombing in Nagasaki. *Jpn J Surg* 1991;21:508–511.

182. Takeichi N, Dohi K, Ito H, et al. Parathyroid tumors in atomic bomb survivors in Hiroshima: a review. *J Radiat Res* 1991;82(Suppl):189–192.

183. Ames BN, Gold LS. Too many rodent carcinogens: Mitogenesis increases mutagenesis. *Science* 1990;249:970–971.

184. Cohen SM, Ellwein LB. Cell proliferation in carcinogenesis. *Science* 1990;249:1007–1011.

185. Albanes D, Winick M. Are cell number and cell proliferation risk factors for cancer? *JNCI* 1988;80:772–775.

186. Butterworth BE, Goldsworthy TL. The role of cell proliferation in multistage carcinogenesis. *Proc Soc Exp Biol Med* 1991;198:683–687.

187. Cohen SM, Ellwein LB. Genetic errors, cell proliferation, and carcinogenesis. *Cancer Res* 1991;51:6493–6505.

188. Albright F, Reifenstein EC. *The parathyroid glands and metabolic bone disease.* The Baltimore: Williams & Wilkins, 1948.

189. Stamberg J, Hirschfield L. Mitotic recombination can explain the apparent polyclonal origin of some tumors. *Cancer Genetics Cytogenet* 1987;27:5–8.

190. Castleman B, Mallory TB. The pathology of the parathyroid gland in hyperparathyroidism: a study of 25 cases. *Am J Pathol* 1935;11:73–91.

191. Bengtsson A, Grimelius L, Johansson H, Ponten J. Nuclear DNA-content of parathyroid cells in adenomas, hyperplastic and normal glands. *APMIS* 1977;85:455–460.

192. Levin KE, Chew KL, Ljung B-M, Mayall BH, Siperstein AE, Clark OH. Deoxyribonucleic acid cytometry helps identify parathyroid carcinomas. *J Clin Endocrinol Metab* 1988;67:779–784.

193. Shenton BK, Ellis H, Johnston IDA, Farndon JR. DNA analysis and parathyroid pathology. *World J Surg* 1990;14:296–302.

194. Obara T, Fujimoto Y, Yanaji Y, et al. Flow cytometric DNA analysis of parathyroid tumors. Implication of aneuploidy for pathologic and biologic classification. *Cancer* 1990;66:1555–1562.

195. Lloyd HM, Jacobi JM, Cooke RA. Nuclear diameter in parathyroid adenomas. *J Clin Pathol* 1979;32:1278–1281.

196. Gardin JP, Patron P, Fouqueray B, Prigent A, Paillard M. Maximal PTH secretory rate and set point for calcium in normal subjects and patients with primary hyperparathyroidism. *Mineral Electrolyte Metab* 1988;14:221–228.

197. Transbøl I. Hypercalcaemia—endocrine and metabolic aspects. With special reference to diagnosis and differential diagnosis. Thesis, University of Copenhagen, 1978.

198. LeBoff MS, Rennke HG, Brown EM. Abnormal regulation of parathyroid cell secretion and proliferation in primary cultures of bovine parathyroid cells. *Endocrinology* 1983;113:277–284.

199. Patron P, Gardin J-P, Paillard M. Renal mass and reserve of vitamin D: determinants in primary hyperparathyroidism. *Kidney Int* 1987;31:1174–1180.

200. Lopez-Hilker S, Galceran T, Chan Y-L, Rapp N, Martin KJ, Slatopolsky E. Hypocalcemia may not be essential for the development of secondary hyperparathyroidism in chronic renal failure. *J Clin Invest* 1986;78:1097–1102.

201. Thakker RV, Fraher LJ, Adami S, Karmali R, O'Riordan JLH. Circulating concentrations of 1,25-dihydroxyvitamin D_3 in patients with primary hyperparathyroidism. *Bone Mineral* 1986;1:137–144.

202. Terpstra OT, vanBlankenstein M, Dees J, Eilers GAM. Abnormal pattern of cell proliferation in the entire colonic mucosa of patients with colon adenoma or cancer. *Gastroenterology* 1987;92:704–708.

203. Allo M, Thompson NW, Harness JK, Nishiyama RH. Primary hyperparathyroidism in children, adolescents, and young adults. *World J Surg* 1982;6:771–776.

204. Marx SJ, Menczel J, Campbell G, et al. Heterogeneous size of the parathyroid glands in familial multiple endocrine neoplasia type 1. *Clin Endocrinol* 1991;35:521–526.

205. Lu KP, Means AR. Regulation of the cell cycle by calcium and calmodulin. *Endocr Rev* 1993;14:40–58.

206. Eastell R, Yergey AL, Vieira NE, Cedel SL, Kumar R,

Riggs BL. Interrelationship among vitamin D metabolism, true calcium absorption, parathyroid function, and age in women: evidence of an age-related intestinal resistance to 1,25-dihydroxyvitamin D action. *J Bone Mineral Res* 1991; 6:125–132.

207. Parfitt AM. Osteomalacia and related disorders. In: Avioli LV, Krane SM, eds. *Metabolic bone disease and clinically related disorders, 2nd ed.* Philadelphia: W.B. Saunders, 1990;329–396.

208. Åkerström G, Rudberg C, Grimelius L, et al. Histologic parathyroid abnormalities in an autopsy series. *Hum Pathol* 1986;17:520–527.

209. Ham AW, Littner N, Drake TGH, Robertson EC, Tisdall FF. Physiological hypertrophy of the parathyroids, its cause and its relation to rickets. *Am J Pathol* 1939;16:277–286.

210. Fraser R, Nordin BEC. Hyperparathyroidism and steatorrhoea. *Br Med J* 1956;12:1363.

211. Cope O, Barnes BA, Castleman B, Mueller GCE, Roth SI. Vicissitudes of parathyroid surgery: trials of diagnosis and management in 51 patients with a variety of disorders. *Ann Surg* 1961;154:491–508.

212. Gilmour JR. *The parathyroid glands and skeleton in renal disease.* London: Oxford University Press, 1947.

213. Pappenheimer AM, Wilens SL. Enlargement of the parathyroid glands in renal disease. *Am J Pathol* 1935;11:73–91.

214. Castleman B, Mallory TB. Parathyroid hyperplasia in chronic renal insufficiency. *Am J Pathol* 1937;553–573.

215. Stanbury SW, Lumb GA. Parathyroid function in chronic renal failure. *Q J Med* 1966;35:1–23.

216. Åkerström G, Malmaeus J, Grimelius L, Ljunghall S, Bergstrom R. Histological changes in parathyroid glands in subclinical and clinical renal disease. An autopsy investigation. *Scand J Urol Nephrol* 1984;18:75–84.

217. Sivula A, Kuhlbäck B, Kock B, Kahri A, Wallenius M, Edgren J. Parathyroidectomy in chronic renal failure. *Acta Chir Scand* 1979;145:19–25.

218. Malmaeus J, Grimelius L, Johansson H, Åkerström G, Ljunghall S. Parathyroid pathology in hyperparathyroidism secondary to chronic renal failure. *Scand J Urol Nephrol* 1984;18:157–166.

219. De Francisco AM, Ellis HA, Owen JP, et al. Parathyroidectomy in chronic renal failure. *Q J Med* 1985;55:289–315.

220. Krause MW, Hedinger CE. Pathologic study of parathyroid glands in tertiary hyperparathyroidism. *Hum Pathol* 1985; 16:772–784.

221. Lloyd HM, Parfitt AM, Jacobi JM, et al. The parathyroid glands in chronic renal failure: a study of their growth and other properties, based on findings in hypercalcemia patients. *J Lab Clin Med* 1989;114:358–367.

222. Johnson WJ, McCarthy JT, van Heerden JA, Serioff S, Grant CS, Kao PC. Results of subtotal parathyroidectomy in hemodialysis patients. *Am J Med* 1988;84:23–32.

223. Brown EM, Wilkson RE, Eastman RC, Pallotta J, Marynick SP. Abnormal regulation of parathyroid hormone release by calcium in secondary hyperparathyroidism due to chronic renal failure. *J Clin Endocrinol Metab* 1982;54:172–179.

224. Slatopolsky E, Lopez-Hilker S, Delmez J, Dusso A, Brown A, Martin KJ. The parathyroid–calcitriol axis in health and chronic renal failure. *Kidney Int* 1990;38:S41–S47.

225. Portale AA, Morris RC Jr. Pathogenesis of secondary hyperparathyroidism in chronic renal insufficiency. *Mineral Electrolyte Metab* 1991;17:211–220.

226. Akizawa T, Fukagawa M, Koshikawa S, Kurokawa K. Recent progress in management of secondary hyperparathyroidism of chronic renal failure. *Cur Opin Nephrol Hypertension* (in press).

227. Ellis HA. Fate of long-term parathyroid autografts in patients with chronic renal failure treated by parathyroidectomy: a histopathological study of autografts, parathyroid glands and bone. *Histopathology* 1988;13:289–309.

228. Oka T, Yoshioka T, Shrestha GR, et al. Immunohistochemical study of nodular hyperplastic parathyroid glands in patients with secondary hyperparathyroidism. *Virchows Arch Pathol Anat A* 1988;413:53–60.

229. Wallfelt CH, Larsson R, Gylfe E, Ljunghall S, Rastad J, Åkerström G. Secretory disturbance in hyperplastic parathyroid nodules of uremic hyperparathyroidism: implication for parathyroid autotransplantation. *World J Surg* 1988;12: 431–438.

230. Anderson TJ, Boyle IT. Autonomous nodular hyperplasia of the parathyroid glands. *J Pathol* 1971;105:211–214.

231. Golden A, Canary JJ, Kerwin DM. Concurrence of hyperplasia and neoplasia of the parathyroid glands. *Am J Med* 1965;38:562–578.

232. Davies DR, Dent CE, Watson L. Tertiary hyperparathyroidism. *Br Med J* 1968;3:395–399.

233. Kramer WM. Association of parathyroid hyperplasia with neoplasia. *Am J Clin Pathol* 1970;53:275–283.

234. Dominguez JM, Mautalen CA, Rodo JE, Barcat JA, Molins ME. Tertiary hyperparathyroidism diagnosed after renal homotransplantation. *Am J Med* 1970;49:423–428.

235. Ahmed KY, Varghese Z, Lange MJ, Lawrence DAS, Moorhead JF. Tertiary hyperparathyroidism with adenoma formation after renal transplantation. *Br Med J* 1978;7:92–93.

236. Kikuoka H, Emoto M, Yoshida T, et al. Development of parathyroid adenoma in a case of chronic renal failure suggesting tertiary hyperparathyroidism. *Endocrinol Jpn* 1982; 29:293–298.

237. Williams ED. Pathology of the parathyroid glands. *Clin Endocrinol Metab* 1974;3:285–303.

238. Banerjee SS, Faragher B, Hasleton PS. Nuclear diameter in parathyroid disease. *J Clin Pathol* 1983;36:143–148.

239. Falchetti A, Bale AE, Eubanks JH, et al. Use of a highly polymorphic locus on human chromosome 11q13 discloses allelic loss in parathyroid tissue from uremic patients. In: Cohn DV, Gennari C, Tasjian AH Jr, eds. *Calcium regulating hormones and bone metabolism.* Amsterdam: Elsevier, 1992;36–40.

240. Falchetti A, Bale AE, Amorosi A, et al. Progression of uremic hyperparathyroidism involves allelic loss on chromosome 11. *J Clin Endocrinol Metab* 1993;76:139–144.

241. Berland Y, Olmer M, Lebreuil G, Grisoli J. Parathyroid carcinoma, adenoma and hyperplasia in a case of chronic renal insufficiency on dialysis. *Clin Nephrol* 1982;18:154–158.

242. Ireland JP, Fleming SJ, Levison DA, Cattell WR, Baker LRI. Parathyroid carcinoma associated with chronic renal failure and previous radiotherapy to the neck. *J Clin Pathol* 1985;38:1114–1118.

243. Krishna GG, Mendez M, Levy B, Ritchie W, Marks A, Narins RG. Parathyroid carcinoma in a chronic hemodialysis patient. *Nephron* 1989;52:194–195.

244. Iwamoto N, Yamazaki S, Fukuda T, et al. Two cases of parathyroid carcinoma in patients on long-term hemodialysis. *Nephron* 1990;55:429–431.

245. Lumb GA, Stanbury SW. Parathyroid function in human vitamin D deficiency and vitamin D deficiency in primary hyperparathyroidism. *Am J Med* 1974;56:833–839.

246. Sultan AH, Bruckner FE, Eastwood JB. Association between prolonged dietary vitamin D deficiency and autonomous hyperparathyroidism. *Br Med J* 1989;299:236–237.

247. Kapur MM, Agarwal MS, Gupta A, Misra MC, Ahuja MMS. Clinical and biochemical features of primary hyperparathyroidism. *Indian J Med Res* 1985;81:607–612.

248. Keynes WM, Caird FI. Hypocalcaemic primary hyperparathyroidism. *Br Med J* 1970;1:208–211.

249. Dent CE, Jones PE, Mullan DP. Masked primary (or tertiary) hyperparathyroidism. *Lancet* 1975;1:1161–1164.

250. Wynford-Thomas V, Wynford-Thomas D, Williams ED. Experimental induction of parathyroid adenomas in the rat. *JNCI* 1983;70:127–134.

251. Dent CE. Hyperparathyroidism and steatorrhoea. *Br Med J* 1956;12:1546–1547.

252. Smith JF. Parathyroid adenomas associated with the malabsorption syndrome and chronic renal disease. *J Clin Pathol* 1970;23:362–369.

253. Clements MR, Davies M, Hayes ME, et al. The role of 1,25-dihydroxyvitamin D in the mechanism of acquired vitamin D deficiency. *Clin Endocrinol* 1992;37:17–27.

254. Glorieux FH. Vitamin D resistant hypophosphatemic rickets (VDRR): pathogenesis and medical treatment. In: Kleere-

koper M, Krane SM, eds. *Clinical disorders of bone and mineral metabolism.* New York: Mary Ann Liebert, Inc., 1989;425–432.

255. Kleerekoper M, Coffey R, Greco T, et al. Hypercalcemic hyperparathyroidism in hypophosphatemic rickets. *J Clin Endocrinol Metab* 1977;45:86–94.

256. Firth RG, Grant CS, Riggs BL. Development of hypercalcemic hyperparathyroidism after long-term phosphate supplementation in hypophosphatemic osteomalacia. Report of two cases. *Am J Med* 1985;78:669–673.

257. Reid IR, Teitelbaum SL, Dusso A, Whyte MP. Hypercalcemic hyperparathyroidism complicating oncogenic osteomalacia. Effect of successful tumor resection on mineral homeostasis. *Am J Med* 1987;83:350–354.

258. Rivkees SA, El-Hajj-Fuleihan G, Brown EM, Crawford JD. Tertiary hyperparathyroidism during high phosphate therapy of familial hypophosphatemic rickets. *J Clin Endocrinol Metab* 1992;75:1514–1518.

259. Larsen MJ, Melsen F, Mosekilde L, Christensen MS. Effects of a single dose of fluoride on calcium metabolism. *Calcif Tissue Res* 1978;26:199–202.

260. Bevan JS, Webbster J, Burke CW, Scanlon MF. Dopamine agonists and pituitary tumor shrinkage. *Endocr Rev* 1992;13:220–240.

261. Roth SI. Recent advances in parathyroid gland pathology. *Am J Med* 1971;50:612–622.

262. Fukagawa M, Okazaki R, Takano K, et al. Regression of parathyroid hyperplasia by calcitriol-pulse therapy in patients on long-term dialysis. *N Engl J Med* 1990;323:421–422.

263. Hyodo T, Ono K, Koumi T, et al. Can oral 1,25(OH)$_2$D$_3$ pulse therapy reduce parathyroid hyperplasia? *Nephron* 1991;59:171–172.

264. Henry HL, Taylor AN, Norman AW. Response of chick parathyroid glands to the vitamin D metabolites, 1,25-dihydroxycholecalciferol and 24,25-dihydroxycholecalciferol. *J Nutr* 1977;107:1918–1926.

265. Parfitt AM. The spectrum of hypoparathyroidism. *J Clin Endocr* 1972;152–158.

266. Wilson P, Kleerekoper M, Lillich R, Parfitt AM. Immunoradiometric assay for intact parathyroid hormone in the diagnosis of hypoparathyroidism. *J Bone Min Res* 1988;3(Suppl 1):S131.

267. Parfitt AM. The study of parathyroid function in man by EDTA infusion. *J Clin Endocr* 1969;29:569–580.

268. Girling JA, Murley RS. Parathyroid insufficiency after thyroidectomy. *Br Med J* 1967;1:1323.

269. Wade JSH, Goodall P, Deane L, et al. The course of partial parathyroid insufficiency after thyroidectomy. *Br J Surg* 1965;52:493.

270. Parfitt AM. Delayed recognition of postoperative hypoparathyroidism. *Med J Aust* 1967;1:702–708.

271. Parfitt AM. Idiopathic, surgical and other varieties of parathyroid hormone deficient hypoparathyroidism. In: DeGroot L, ed. *Endocrinology, 2nd ed.* Philadelphia: W.B. Saunders 1989:1049–1064.

272. Mallette LE. The parathyroid polyhormones: new concepts in the spectrum of peptide hormone action. *Endocr Rev* 1991;12:110–117.

273. Rodda CP, Caple IW, Martin TJ. Role of PTHrP in fetal and neonatal physiology. In: Halloran BP, Nissenson RA (eds). *Parathyroid hormone-related protein: normal physiology and its role in cancer.* Boca Raton, FL: CRC Press, 1992; 169–196.

274. McMurtry CT, Schranck FW, Walkenhorst DA, et al. Significant developmental elevation in serum parathyroid hormone levels in a large kindred with familian benign (hypocalciuric) hypercalcemia. *Am J Med* 1992;93:247–258.

275. Auwerx J, Demeats M, Bouillon R. Altered parathyroid set point to calcium in familian hypocalciuric hypercalcemia. *Acta Endocrinol (Copenh)* 1984;106:215–218.

276. Thorgeirsson U, Costa J, Marx SJ. The parathyroid glands in familial hypocalciuric hypercalcemia. *Hum Pathol* 1981;12:229–237.

277. Law Jr WM, Carney JA, Heath III H. Parathyroid glands in familial benign hypercalcemia (familial hypocalciuric hypercalcemia). *Am J Med* 1984;76:1021–1026.

278. Marx SJ, Bale AE, Brandi ML, Spiegel AM, Friedman E. The parathyroids in primary hyperparathyroidism: molecular biology and genetics give insights into broad areas of cell biology and endocrine pathophysiology. *Program and Abstracts:* Seventy-fifth Annual Meeting, Endocrine Society 1993(abstract):4.

279. Mallette LE, Eichhorn E. Effects of lithium carbonate on human calcium metabolism. *Arch Intern Med* 1986;146:770–776.

280. Larkins RG. Lithium and hypercalcaemia. *Aust NZ J Med* 1991;21:675–677.

281. Seely EW, Moore TJ, LeBoff MS, Brown EM. A single dose of lithium carbonate acutely elevates intact parathyroid hormone levels in humans. *Acta Endocrinol (Copenh)* 1989;121:174–176.

282. Christiansen C, Baastrup PC, Transbol I. Development of "primary" hyperparathyroidism during lithium therapy: longitudinal study. *Neuropsychobiol* 1980;6:280–283.

283. Shen F, Sherrard DJ. Lithium-induced hyperparathyroidism: an alteration of the "Set-Point." *Ann Int Med* 1982;96:63–65.

284. Saxe AW, Gibson G. Lithium increases tritiated thymidine uptake by abnormal human parathyroid tissue. *Surg* 1991;110:1067–1077.

285. Mallette LE, Khouri K, Zengotita H, Hollis BW, Malini S. Lithium treatment increases intact and mid region parathyroid hormone and parathyroid volume. *J Clin Endocrinol Metab* 1989;68:654–660.

286. McHenry CR, Rosen IB, Rotstein LE, Forbath N, Walfish PG. Lithiumogenic disorders of the thyroid and parathyroid glands as surgical disease. *Surg* 1990;108:1001–1015.

287. Nordenstrom J, Strigard K, Perbeck L, et al. Hyperparathyroidism associated with treatment of manic-depressive disorders by lithium. *Eur J Surg* 1992;158:207–211.

The Parathyroids, edited by J.P. Bilezikian, M.A. Levine, and R. Marcus. Raven Press, Ltd., New York © 1994.

CHAPTER 24

Molecular Basis of Primary Hyperparathyroidism

Andrew Arnold

GENERAL PRINCIPLES IN MOLECULAR ONCOLOGY

In recent years we have witnessed an explosion in our knowledge of the molecular basis of neoplasia. This revolution was spearheaded by work on various hematopoietic tumors, but major insights into solid tumor pathogenesis have become commonplace as well. However, knowledge of the molecular mechanisms underlying endocrine tumors in general and parathyroid tumors in particular is relatively undeveloped in comparison to that for lymphomas, leukemias, and colon and breast cancers. Existing information does suggest that many of the well-established general themes in tumor biology are quite applicable to parathyroid tumorigenesis, in spite of the generally nonmalignant status of these tumors. In addition, one molecular insight into parathyroid tumor development has had unexpectedly broad implications regarding nonparathyroid tumors and basic cell cycle biology.

It is now solidly established that cancer cells contain genetic damage that is central to the abnormal neoplastic phenotypes they characteristically exhibit. In addition to this damage to the actual base sequence in the DNA, certain "epigenetic" factors may also be important; these could include aberrant patterns of DNA methylation, hormonal influences on gene expression, or immune system stimulation. A critical feature of cancers is their clonal (monoclonal) nature; in other words, cancers arise from a single precursor cell, whose progeny of essentially identical daughter cells have a selective growth advantage and ultimately make up the clinically apparent tumor. An identical detailed pattern of DNA damage to key growth-regulating genes is typically seen in every cell of such a tumor, often identifying this clone uniquely and implying that many of the important underlying genetic events occurred early, before major proliferation (clonal expansion). The clonality of tumors also indicates that the summation/accumulation of factors needed to transform (or confer the malignant phenotype upon) a cell occurs only rarely in a large population of cells in a tissue. Within such a population of cells, the rare emergence of a transformed clone is consistent with the rare occurrence of certain key rate-limiting mutations and/or a requirement for the accumulation within one cell of multiple different damaging DNA alterations. The clonality of tumors does not, however, exclude an important role for field effects or generalized proliferative stimuli directed at the particular tissue as one of several factors contributing to tumorigenesis.

The molecular genetic heterogeneity underlying neoplasia should be emphasized. While certain tumor types might exist in which damage to only one gene is necessary and/or sufficient for transformation, the general rule appears to be that accumulating damage to multiple distinct genes, all within the same cell, is required for the ultimate expression of the neoplastic phenotype (1). Even after a clonal tumor is clearly established, increased genetic instability (a recognized property of many malignancies) still can alter other genes; subclones bearing these DNA derangements will emerge in this process of "clonal evolution" or tumor progression when they confer a more aggressive

A. Arnold: Endocrine Unit, Laboratory of Endocrine Oncology, Harvard Medical School; and Massachusetts General Hospital, Boston, Massachusetts 02114.

phenotype upon the cell or offer another selective advantage. Certain genes may be implicated in tumors of only one or a few cell types, while others may be involved in many different types of tumors (eg. p53). For most tumor types, however, it appears that no single gene will be both a necessary and a sufficient causative agent. More likely, disruption of certain biochemical pathways may be important unifying themes for the emergence of particular tumors, and different combinations of mutated genes may result in similar cellular and clinical consequences. Studies of oncogene additivity or cooperativity, and other functional studies, will help to shed light on these issues.

There are two broad categories of normal cellular genes in which clonal DNA damage contributes to neoplasia; these are protooncogenes and tumor-suppressor genes. Protooncogenes often have roles in the normal physiologic control of cellular growth, proliferation, or differentiation and may function by regulating protein phosphorylation, signal transduction, or gene transcription, for example. Damage to a protooncogene, converting or activating it to an "oncogene," usually causes a deregulation of expression of its normal protein product or the formation of an intrinsically abnormal product. Tumor-suppressor genes normally function to restrain cell proliferation and contribute to neoplasia through their functional inactivation. The types of somatic DNA derangements that can activate protooncogenes include chromosome translocations or inversions, point mutations, proviral insertions, and gene amplification. Inactivation of tumor-suppressor genes is typically accomplished by point mutation or deletion and may be inherited or incurred somatically. The causes of these types of oncogenic "hits" are not well understood. Environmental carcinogens such as ionizing irradiation or chemicals play a direct role in some instances, and errors in normal chromosomal recombinatory mechanisms also appear to occur, perhaps randomly. Many such changes tend to occur preferentially in mitotically active cells, and carcinogens may act either by direct mutagenizing of DNA or through augmentation of the mitotic rate, which secondarily increases the likelihood of an oncogenic chromosome aberrancy. Many excellent reviews are available to the reader interested in exploring these principles further (2–9).

Special Issues in Parathyroid Neoplasia

While the general principles described above are expected to hold true for the specific example of parathyroid neoplasia, a full molecular description of parathyroid tumorigenesis will ultimately have to explain a number of special features unique to the parathyroid model. Among these mysteries are the increased incidence of parathyroid tumors after exposure to neck irradiation, the heightened frequency with which hyperparathyroidism is found in postmenopausal women, the rarity of parathyroid cancer compared with the commonplace development of benign parathyroid tumors, and the relationship between excess cellular proliferation and the misadjusted set point linking ambient calcium level with parathyroid hormone (PTH) secretion in the tumor cells. Information relevant to these and other special issues is only beginning to be generated, but the continued application of modern methods certainly promises eventually to yield the required molecular/pathophysiologic synthesis.

CLONALITY OF PARATHYROID TUMORS

Much controversy and uncertainty has existed regarding the pathological etiologies and clinicopathologic categorization of hyperparathyroidism. Traditional distinctions between parathyroid adenoma and hyperplasia have been made on the basis of the number of abnormal, hypercellular parathyroid glands found in the patient, with single gland disease being defined as "adenoma." It can, however, occasionally be difficult to distinguish histologically a normal from a mildly hypercellular gland, and histological examination of a particular hypercellular gland offers no features clearly predictive of whether it is a solitary tumor or one of several in the patient (10,11). Multigland enlargement can nonuniformly affect an individual's parathyroid glands ("asymmetric hyperplasia"), even to the point of causing confusion between hyperplasia and adenoma. Whether "multiple adenomas" exist (i.e., together with at least one truly normal parathyroid gland in the patient) is therefore controversial (12–14).

Early studies of the clonal status of parathyroid tumors were designed to address some of these uncertainties. Assessment of X-chromosome inactivation patterns using the glucose-6-phosphate dehydrogenase (G6PD) protein polymorphism had indicated that parathyroid adenomas (single gland disease) were polyclonal as opposed to monoclonal growths (15,16). These data suggested that a parathyroid "adenoma" was really a highly asymmetric form fruste of multigland hyperplasia and were taken to support the surgical practice of routine bilateral neck exploration and/or subtotal parathyroidectomy for hyperparathyroidism. This hypothesis of the origins of parathyroid tumors did not encourage a search for the types of DNA damage (discussed above) characteristic of monoclonal tumors.

The clonal status of parathyroid adenomas was reevaluated several years later, again by X-chromosome inactivation analysis but using a DNA polymorphism-based method that avoids many of the pitfalls of the protein polymorphism method. It was determined that most and perhaps all parathyroid adenomas were in fact monoclonal tumors, i.e., that these glands were true neoplastic outgrowths of a single abnormal cell (17). Subsequent studies have resoundingly confirmed the monoclonality of parathyroid adenomas (18–21). This finding has been taken to support the surgical practice of resecting only the clearly enlarged, and therefore abnormal, gland when other glands are thought to be normal. As is covered in the chapter by Norton et al., a full bilateral exploration is still generally recommended because of the difficulties in distinguishing adenomatous from asymmetric hyperplastic disease at the time of parathyroid surgery. Also, even in the setting of a documented adenoma, the contralateral side could conceivably harbor another independent clonal adenoma, although such double adenomas are quite unusual (12,13,22). Parathyroid carcinomas, not surprisingly, are also monoclonal (23).

Even if one ignores the possible existence of multiple adenomas arising de novo, a finding of monoclonality in an enlarged parathyroid gland clearly cannot be viewed *in isolation* as diagnostic for single gland disease. It has now been established that, in most forms of parathyroid hyperplasia, which presumably begin with a stimulus for generalized (polyclonal) parathyroid cell proliferation affecting all the glands, monoclonal tumors can evolve in at least some of these glands. Monoclonal parathyroid tumors have been seen in familial multiple endocrine neoplasia type I (MEN-I) (19,20,24), in nonfamilial (sporadic) primary parathyroid hyperplasia (25), and in the secondary (or "tertiary") parathyroid hyperplasia of uremia (25,26). The clinical or pathophysiological significance of monoclonality in these settings remains to be determined. It is conceivable, for example, that such tumors may exhibit more pathological autonomy in PTH dysregulation as well as higher growth rates than do any truly hyperplastic (polyclonal) neighboring glands in the same patient.

SPECIFIC GENETIC ABNORMALITIES IN BENIGN PARATHYROID TUMORS

The determination that parathyroid adenomas are monoclonal neoplasms led to the expectation that these tumors, although benign, result from some of the same types of genetic damage that characterize clonal malignancies (17). This expectation is now shared for a subset of tumors, also found to be monoclonal, in patients with various forms of multigland "hyperplasia," discussed above. Identification of the particular genes whose tumor-specific activation or inactivation results in these clonal expansions is critical, since

building a detailed understanding of the molecular defects that underlie parathyroid neoplasia may ultimately lead to successes in diagnosis, pathologic classification, prevention, and/or treatment. Identifying these genes may also point to particular biochemical pathways of importance in regulating parathyroid cell proliferation, thus facilitating discovery of other genes of similar importance. So far, only one specific gene (*PRAD1*) has been convincingly incriminated in benign parathyroid tumorigenesis. Even this initial molecular insight, however, has been shown to have unexpectedly broad implications regarding basic cell cycle biology and human cancer, which speaks well for parathyroid tumors as potentially generalizable models of benign or well differentiated neoplasia. The principle of molecular heterogeneity predicts that still other parathyroid tumor genes exist, and there is strong evidence for at least one parathyroid tumor suppressor gene, which may soon be identified. These target areas for critical DNA damage, which confer a selective growth advantage upon the parathyroid cell in which they develop (i.e., the clonal precursor cell), are discussed in this section.

Activation of the *PRAD1* Oncogene

Initial cloning of PRAD1

DNA rearrangements, in the form of translocations and related chromosomal events, are among the best characterized types of clonal oncogenic genetic abnormalities (2). Very frequently, these rearrangements involve the tumor-specific juxtaposition of cellular protooncogenes with DNA sequences designed to regulate other genes; this may result in the overexpression or deregulated expression of the protooncogene, converting it to an oncogene. In fact, the cloning of DNA immediately adjacent to clonal chromosome breakpoints is an effective method for identification of new oncogenes. One example was the discovery of the *bcl-2* oncogene in follicular lymphomas with the t(14;18) chromosome translocation; *bcl-2* (on chromosome 18) is "activated" and overexpressed as a consequence of its relocation into the part of the immunoglobulin heavy chain gene, on chromosome 14, that contains sequences responsible for immunoglobulin's strong transcriptional activity in B-lymphoid cells (27). It is interesting to note that most oncogenes found to be activated in human cancer have been detected in hematopoietic tumors. While it is possible that chromosomal translocations occur more commonly in these tumors, the situation may also reflect technical advantages in performing cytogenetic analysis on hematopoietic compared with solid tumors. Improved cytogenetic methods should permit detection of more chromosome translocations in solid tumors, including parathyroid tumors, and thus provide searchlights for the identification of additional oncogenes.

The key initial observation in the identification of *PRAD1* was a band of abnormal size on a Southern blot of DNA from a single parathyroid adenoma, probed with a PTH genomic DNA fragment (17,28). This band was not present in the same patient's normal leukocyte control DNA and was thus tumor-specific and clonal. Relative intensities of this band compared with the remaining normal-size band suggested that the underlying DNA alteration affected one of the tumor's two PTH alleles and that the abnormality was present in every cell in the tumor. It had, therefore, presumably occurred in the original clonal progenitor cell of the tumor, likely conferring a selective growth advantage, and hence appeared worthy of additional investigation for its possible pathogenetic importance.

Southern analysis of this original adenoma revealed that the clonal alteration responsible for the observed abnormal band was a tumor-specific DNA rearrangement (28). The rearrangement separated the 5' regulatory region and noncoding exon I of the PTH gene from its coding exons. Different, non-PTH DNA was found to be placed adjacent to each PTH section (Fig. 1). In addition, the tumor possessed one intact PTH gene per cell, which appeared to be the source of PTH production by the adenoma. While a DNA rearrangement with this structure could have been tumorigenic in a few possible ways, it was hypothesized that, in analogous fashion to the immunoglobulin/ *bcl-2* model, the PTH gene regulatory region, which strongly drives tissue-specific gene expression in the parathyroid cell, could be activating the expression of a protooncogene brought under its influence by the rearrangement.

The DNA sequences of interest, lying adjacent to the PTH breakpoint, were then cloned from a genomic DNA library from this adenoma. From the PTH gene-positive bacteriophage inserts, subclones were made that contained only the breakpoint-adjacent non-PTH DNA. This "anonymous" single-copy DNA was mapped using somatic cell genetics and in situ hybridization, and was found to be normally located on chromosome 11 band q13. It was initially called *D11S287* (28). Because the normal chromosomal location of the PTH gene is also on chromosome 11, at 11p15, the simplest cytogenetic explanation for the observed tumor-specific DNA rearrangement was a pericentromeric inversion of chromosome 11 (Fig. 1). Although there were several oncogenes that had previously been mapped to 11q13, namely, *int-2, hst-1,* and *sea* as well as the *bcl-1* lymphoma translocation breakpoint, the newly cloned D11S287 region did not appear to be identical to any of these, as evidenced by restriction map comparisons and by direct clone to clone hybridization analysis. D11S287 subclones were then surveyed in attempts to detect an expressed gene or transcription unit in the region. One such probe, located ~1 kb from the breakpoint, detected a distinct 4.5 kb mRNA species on Northern blots (29). This mRNA was present in RNA from normal human parathyroid tissue, parathyroid adenomas without PTH/*D11S287* rearrangement, normal thyroid, and normal placenta. Thus, the transcript's presence was not highly cell type specific. Moreover, the same human D11S287 probe hybridized to mRNA of the same approximate size, withstanding stringent washing, on RNA blots from other species and tissues, including bovine lymph node, muscle, thyroid, and parathyroid and also mouse heart and liver (30). Most importantly, this sequence proved to be dramatically (15-fold) overexpressed in the original parathyroid adenoma from which the rearrangement had been cloned (29).

Additional independent parathyroid adenomas containing similar PTH rearrangement breakpoints were then detected; they also had D11S287 region breakpoints (29,31), which were seen to vary by as much as

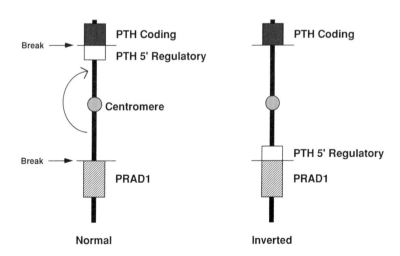

FIG. 1. Schematic diagram illustrating the DNA rearrangement involving the *PTH* gene and the *PRAD1* gene in a subset of parathyroid adenomas. Chromosomal inversion event deduced as the simplest cytogenetic mechanism consistent with the molecular details of this DNA rearrangement. (Reprinted from ref. 83 with permission.)

15 kb (29), and no other expressed genes were detectable in this 15 kb region. These additional cases also exhibited dramatic overexpression of the D11S287 transcription unit (29). Because of D11S287's involvement in clonal DNA rearrangements associated with gross abnormalities in its transcription, analogous to those in lymphoid neoplasia, this highly conserved sequence was considered further as a putative oncogene and was subsequently called *PRAD1*, for parathyroid adenomatosis 1.

Further Analysis of the Structure of PTH PRAD1 Rearrangements

After the cloning and analysis of the full-length complementary DNA (cDNA) representing *PRAD1* mRNA (discussed below), it was possible to define the complete intron/exon organization of the normal chromosomal *PRAD1* gene (32). The gene is oriented on 11q13 such that it is transcribed in a centromeric to telomeric direction, and contains five exons and four introns spanning ~15 kb. In the few parathyroid adenomas with well-characterized PTH/*PRAD1* rearrangements, the 11q13 breakpoints have occurred from 1 to 15 kb upstream of *PRAD1* exon I, leaving its exon-containing region and immediate promoter intact (Figure 2). Attached in these rearrangements to the *PRAD1* structural gene is the 5′ regulatory region, including noncoding exon I, of the PTH gene (Fig. 2). The remarkable up-regulation of *PRAD1* expression in these parathyroid tumors therefore appears to be driven by DNA sequences normally found in this upstream PTH gene vicinity. In fact, these rearrangements currently provide the strongest evidence for localizing the still-undefined tissue-specific enhancer of the PTH gene to its 5′ regulatory region, a common but by no means universal site for such sequences.

The presence of noncoding exon I of the PTH gene in the DNA rearranged upstream of *PRAD1* raised the possibility that a PTH exon I/*PRAD1* fusion mRNA might ensue and be transcribed from the PTH gene's own promoter. However, this does not appear to be the case. Analysis of the overexpressed *PRAD1* transcript (cDNA) from one such parathyroid tumor revealed normal *PRAD1* sequence at its 5′ end, with no contribution by the PTH gene (33). The rearranged *PRAD1*'s use of its own promoter could also predict that its overexpression might be insulated from signals such as 1,25-dihydroxyvitamin D [1,25-$(OH)_2$D] or hypercalcemia, which are inhibitory for PTH gene transcription. In addition, it appears that point mutations in *PRAD1* are not necessary for tumorigenesis, since the amino acid coding sequence of this overexpressed *PRAD1* cDNA was entirely normal (33).

Frequency of PRAD1 Involvement in Parathyroid Neoplasia

A still uncertain fraction of parathyroid adenomas (at least 5%) contain an activated form of the *PRAD1* oncogene. As was noted above, these adenomas bear tumor-specific DNA rearrangements that juxtapose the regulatory region of the PTH gene with the coding region of *PRAD1* (Fig. 1), resulting in dramatic overexpression/deregulation of *PRAD1* in the tumor cell (28,29,33). It is important to note that all the cases of

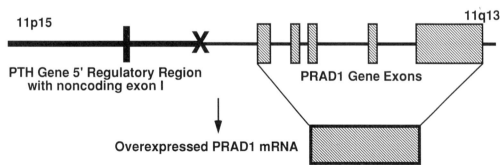

Overexpressed PRAD1 mRNA

Transcription starts with PRAD1's first exon, using its own promoter; coding sequence is normal. Active PRAD1 transcription is driven by tissue-specific enhancer(s) from the 5' PTH gene region.

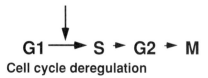

Cell cycle deregulation

FIG. 2. Directly observed molecular structure of the *PTH/PRAD1* DNA rearrangement and its functional consequences. (Reprinted from ref. 83 with permission.)

PTH/*PRAD1* rearrangement were identified by screening adenoma DNA with probes of PTH or *PRAD1* in the vicinity of their coding regions and with the use of a limited number of restriction endonucleases (17,28,29,31). However, the rearrangement breakpoints on 11q13 associated with overexpression of *PRAD1* in other tumors (discussed later below) are capable of occurring up to 120 kb upstream of the *PRAD1* gene (34), well out of the range of detection by Southern blotting. It is quite conceivable that PTH gene breakpoints could also vary considerably and have been missed by the previous approach; indeed, *PRAD1* expression could be deregulated in some parathyroid tumors by rearrangement with actively transcribed genes *other* than the PTH gene. For all these reasons, previous studies may not have given a full sense of the frequency with which *PRAD1* deregulation occurs in parathyroid neoplasia. Because overexpression of *PRAD1* may be a pathogenetic common denominator in tumors with widely varying DNA breakpoints, studies of *PRAD1 expression* in a large series of parathyroid tumors should help to resolve this issue. It should also be noted that neither DNA structure nor expression of *PRAD1* has been evaluated yet in the various forms of multiglandular disease, in which some enlarged glands are monoclonal.

The patients with parathyroid adenomas that have been clearly documented to have PTH/*PRAD1* rearrangement and *PRAD1* overexpression have exhibited typical clinical features of symptomatic hyperparathyroidism in comparison to the more common presentation of primary hyperparathyroidism today, which is asymptomatic. Patients with PTH/*PRAD1* rearrangement, however, have had unusually large adenomas (6–8 g), without any histologic features suggestive of malignancy (17,28,29,31). It remains to be seen whether this will prove to be a consistent feature of *PRAD1*-driven parathyroid disease.

PRAD1 *Gene Product as a Novel Cyclin*

The normal cDNA for *PRAD1* was cloned from a human placental cDNA library (30), screened with the original breakpoint-adjacent genomic fragment from 11q13 that had hybridized to a distinct transcript. Sequence of the cDNA revealed one long open reading frame, encoding a 295-amino-acid protein, and was also notable for a long 3'-untranslated region. The derived amino acid sequence was compared with all others in the computerized database, and no identities or strong homologies were present, indicating that the *PRAD1* protein was not closely related to any known protein or family. However, a weaker but consistent homology between *PRAD1* protein and the various

members of the cyclin classes of proteins, which have important roles in regulation of the cell cycle, was observed (Fig. 3) (30). In particular, a section of the *PRAD1* protein was 25% identical and 50% similar (conservative substitutions) to the best fitting part of human cyclin A, allowing for five gaps (30). The corresponding values for its comparison with human cyclin B were 24% and 47%. Cyclins A and B are more closely related to each other, with 42% identity. The *PRAD1* protein's best fitting region was an ~100-amino-acid stretch (amino acids 55–160), which matched within the so-called cyclin box, a 100–150-amino-acid domain of greatest conservation between all the known cyclins (Fig. 3). These other cyclins included A and B forms from yeast, clam, starfish, sea urchin, and *Drosophila; PRAD1* had similar homology to their cyclin box regions, e.g., 28% identity with *Drosophila* cyclin A and 31% identity with clam cyclin A. For comparison, human vs. clam cyclins A are 71% identical in their cyclin boxes (and, as is typical, quite dissimilar throughout their other regions). These sequence comparisons suggested that *PRAD1* was a novel cyclin, representing its own family distinct from the other families of cyclins (30). The recognition that *PRAD1* encoded a novel cyclin-type protein raised fascinating possibilities for its role in tumorigenesis, based on the role of cyclins in regulating progression through the cell division cycle (30,35).

The cell cycle comprises stages G1, S (DNA synthesis), G2, and M (mitosis). Progression through the cell cycle is regulated at two critical checkpoints, the G2–M border and a point in G1 (called START in *Saccharomyces* and the "restriction point" in mammalian cells) that enables the G1–S transition to proceed (36–38). Control of the G2–M transition is attained through a universal mechanism common to all eukaryotic cells. The key feature of M phase is the activation of a serine/threonine protein kinase, designated cdc2, p34^{cdc2}, p34, M-phase kinase, and others names, depending on the system of original study. Activation of cdc2 kinase induces mitosis through a process of phosphorylation of key proteins, which then lead to such events as chromosome condensation, cytoskeletal reorganization, nuclear envelope breakdown, and cell shape changes. The mitotic cyclins are another universal component of this system. First identified in dividing eggs of marine invertebrates, they are characterized by their accumulation throughout interphase until the G2–M transition and then their rapid destruction during mitosis. Mitotic cyclins are regulatory proteins, which must complex with cdc2 kinase to permit its activation and whose disappearance in M phase is necessary for kinase inactivation and exit from mitosis. Cyclins A and B each complex with cdc2, but the timing of their accumulation and destruction differ some-

```
human cyclin A:   MRAILVDWLVEVGEEYKLQNETLHLAVNYIDRFLSSMSVLRGKLQLVGTAAMLLASKFEEIYPPEVAEFVYITDDTYTK 288
                  || |*   |**|| || | **|   ||*||*|||||  *| ***|||*|** | *||| | |        ||**
pradl:            MRKIVATWMLEVCEEQKCEEEVFPLAMNYLDRFLSLEPVKKSRLQLLGATCMFVASKMKETIPLTAEKLCIYTDNSIRP 134
                  || |*  |**|| ||*|   |  |**|*|||||  *| ***|||*||* ||*|*|  | |        ||**  *
clam cyclin A:    MRCILVDWLVEVSEEDKLHRETLFLGVNYIDRFLSKISVLRGKLQLVGAASMFLAAKYEEIYPPDVKEFAYITDDTYTS 273

human cyclin A:   KQVLRMEHLVLKVLTFDLAAPTVNQFLTQYFLHQQPANCKVESL...AMFLGELSLIDADPYLKYLPSVIAGAA 359
                  **| || |** | **||| | *|* *  * |* * *   |    |    || ** ||**|***
pradl:            EELLQMELLLVNKLKWNLAAMTPHDFIEHFLSKMPEAEENKQIIRKHAQTFVALCATDVK.FISNPPSMVAAGS 207
                  ***| || |** | ***| |* | ||| |  *|** ** *  |  |* **  ||* ||**
clam cyclin A:    QQVLRMEHLILKVLTFDVAVPTTNWFCEDFL.KSCDADDK...LKSLTMFLTELTLIDMDAYLKYLPSITAAAA 343
```

```
human cyclin B:   MRAILIDWLVQVQMKFRLLQETMYMTVSIIDRFMQNNCVPKKMLQLVGVTAMFIASKYEEMYPPEIGDFAFVTDNTYTK 279
                  || |*  |***|   *  *| ***  *||*  * | | |||*| | ||*||| | |        |||*
pradl:            MRKIVATWMLEVCEEQKCEEEVFPLAMNYLDRFLSLEPVKKSRLQLLGATCMFVASKMKETIPLTAEKLCIYTDNSIRP 134
                  || |** |**|| *   |   ||*| *|||||| *|||*| * *|*||| | * * *     *| *
cdc13:            MRGILTDWLIEVHSRFRLLPETLFLAVNIIDRFLSLRVCSLNKLQLVGIAAALFIASKYEEVMCPSVQNFVYMADGGYDE 313

human cyclin B:   HQIRQMEMKILRALNFGLGRPLPLHFLRR.ASKIGEVDVEQHTL...AKYLMELTMLDYDMVHFPPSQIAAGA 348
                  ** |||* ** | * |*  | |*   ||* | * *  | * |   *   ||| *|||*
pradl:            EELLQMELLLVNKLKWNLAAMTPHDFIEHFLSKMPEAEENKQIIRKHAQTFVALCATDVKFISNPPSMVAAGS 207
                  ||*|| |  ** | *||| | *  || ***|*  | | |  |* | | ** ||| |**
cdc13:            EEILQAERYILRVLEFNLAYPNPMN....FLRRISKADFYDIQTRTVAKYLVEIGLLDHKLLPYPPSQQCAAA 382
```

```
pradl:            MRKIVATWMLEVCEEQKCEEEVFPLAMNYLDRFLSLEPVKKSRLQLLGATCMFVASKMKETIPLTA.....EKLCIYTD 129
                  || ** ***        |*  ||** |   *|   |||* | ****|| **    |    * ||  *
cln3:             MRFLIFDFIMYCHTRLNLSTSTLFLTFTILDKYSSRFIIKSYNYQLLSLTALWISSKFWDSKNRMATLKVLQNLC.CNQ 184

pradl:            NSIRPEELLQMELLLVNKLKWNLAAMTPHD.FIEHFLSKMPEAEENKQIIRKHAQTFVALCATDVKFISNPPSMVAAGS 207
                  ||* *   ||* *   | | *  ** | *|* ||   *  ** * |    * ||***      *
cln3:             YSIK..QFTTMEMHLFKSLDWSICQSATFDSYIDIFLFQSTSPLSPGVVL...SAPLEAFIQQKLALLNNAAGTAINKS 258
```

FIG. 3. Sequence homology in the "cyclin box" region between the predicted *PRAD1* protein and A-type cyclins (human and clam cyclin A, 32.2% and 33.6% identity, 56.6% and 59.2% similarity), B-type cyclins (human cyclin B and *Saccharomyces pombe cdc13*, 29.6% and 31.6% identity, 50.0% and 52.0 similarity) and one *S. cerevisiae* G1 cyclin (*cln3*, 19.1% identity, 44.1% similarity). Clam cyclin A and *S. pombe cdc13* homologies with *PRAD1* are representative of those found in their families; *cln3* is better aligned with *PRAD1* than is *cln1* or *cln2*. Identical amino acids, *vertical bars;* conservative substitutions, *asterisks.* Alignment was made with the assistance of the BESTFIT program, and conservative amino acids are grouped as follows: D,E,N,Q; H,K,R; A,G,P,S,T; I,L,M,V; F,W,Y. Amino acid numbers at right. (Reprinted from ref. 30 with permission.)

what. Cyclin B is unquestionably a mitotic cyclin, while the role of cyclin A in the cell cycle is less well established, probably functioning in S phase (39).

The G1–S transition is also a critical checkpoint, but has been less well characterized in higher eukaryotes than has mitotic control. The G1–S transition is also an attractive site for attack by an oncoprotein, since, once the cell enters S phase, it is committed to the rest of the cycle, culminating in mitosis. While cyclins are expected to participate in G1–S control, so-called GI cyclins, essential for this transition, have so far been clearly demonstrated only in yeast. These proteins, called *CLN1, CLN2,* and *CLN3 (DAF1),* have weak homology to the mitotic cyclins and associate with cdc2 kinase specifically at G1–S (40–43). The CLN1 and CLN2 peptides are virtually identical in their 100-amino-acid "cyclin box" domain (44), which is located more toward the N terminus than it is in mitotic cy-

clins. Comparing either CLN1 or CLN2 in this region with clam cyclin A showed 24% identity and less homology to cyclin B. Of interest, the *PRAD1* protein, like the CLN family but unlike cyclins A and B, has its cyclin box near its amino terminus. *PRAD1* is 19–20% identical and 24–25% similar to CLN1, CLN2, and CLN3; the homology extends beyond the cyclin box region.

The discovery of *PRAD1* thus raised the intriguing possibility that it might be a human G1 cyclin. Consistent with this possibility, *PRAD1* mRNA and protein levels begin to rise and also peak within G1, in 70N mammary epithelial cells (45) and fibroblasts (46) synchronized by serum starvation and subsequent addition of growth factors. The mouse homolog of *PRAD1* also appears to act in G1, and was in fact cloned as a macrophage cDNA specifically induced in G1 phase in response to colony-stimulating factor-1 (CSF-1) (47).

Perhaps the most convincing evidence that *PRAD1* is truly a functional cyclin was the demonstration that its cDNA could rescue mutant yeast deficient in G1 cyclins; introductions of *PRAD1* cDNA released these yeasts from cell cycle arrest in G1 (48,49) and was an alternative route to the cloning of *PRAD1*. However, because classical "mitotic cyclins" such as cyclin B can also rescue these G1 cyclin-deficient yeast, these data cannot be taken as proof that the *PRAD1* cyclin normally functions in G1 phase.

With the discovery of still other families of human cyclins, some of which are also candidate G1 cyclins, the picture has increased in complexity. *PRAD1*, now also known as *cyclin D1*, has been joined by other novel cyclins of the C and E families (49,50). In addition, two new cyclins quite closely related to *PRAD1*/cyclin D1 were isolated by low-stringency hybridization of the P cDNA; these members of the D-type cyclin family are known as *cyclin D2* and *cyclin D3* (45,51,52). Furthermore, multiple new cdc2-like kinases have been found, and it is not yet clear which of these cyclin-dependent kinases (cdk) are the physiologic partners for each novel cyclin. For example, the *PRAD1*/cyclin D1 protein has been found to be physically associated with cdk4 in a murine macrophage cell line (53) and with cdk2, cdk4, cdk5, PCNA, and an unknown 21 kD protein in a diploid fibroblast cell line (52). Similarly, the physiologic substrates for the presumed *PRAD1*/cyclin D1-activated kinase(s) have not yet been identified.

Another biochemical pathway in which *PRAD1*/cyclin D1 may participate involves the protein product of the retinoblastoma tumor suppressor gene *RB*. The RB protein appears to be an important regulator of the G1–S transition in the cell cycle and is phosphorylated in a cell cycle-dependent fashion (54). Early in G1, the hypophosphorylated form of pRB is thought to bind and sequester a variety of transcription factors such as E2F, which when released later in G1 (as pRB becomes highly phosphorylated) proceed to drive the cell into S phase. Thus active (hypophosphorylated) pRB has a growth-restraining effect, which can be seen by transfection of a plasmid expressing its cDNA into RB-negative, actively proliferating SAOS-2 cells, and results in a growth-arrested "flat cell" phenotype (55). Cotransfection of a *PRAD1*/cyclin D1-expressing plasmid along with RB partially reverses this flat cell phenotype (55). D-type cyclins have been shown to bind the RB protein in vitro and in cell lysates (53,56) and may be sequestered by pRB early in the cell cycle. This raises the interesting possibility that, in tumors, overexpression of *PRAD1*/cyclin D1 protein might act to titrate the available pRB binding sites, the functional equivalent of decreasing the amount of normal RB protein available for the sequestration of S phase-inducing transcription factors such as E2F during G1.

In spite of the emerging complexities involving cyclins, RB-related proteins, and cdk in cell cycle control, *PRAD1*/cyclin D1 stands out as the only cyclin strongly implicated as a human protooncogene (35,57). The sole additional description on a clonal cyclin gene abnormality in a human tumor has been an insertion of hepatitis B virus (HBV) DNA into the cyclin A gene in a single hepatoma (58,59). While its precise mechanisms of action remain to be worked out, overexpression or deregulated expression in the cell cycle of a candidate G1 cyclin such as *PRAD1* could quite conceivably accelerate the cell's progress through G1 into S phase, bypassing normal regulatory controls in committing it to divide, and also may be well tolerated by the cell during the remainder of the cycle. Such a mechanism would provide an appealing explanation for the benign nature of parathyroid adenomas, since it could yield excessive cellular proliferation without necessarily conferring the phenotypes of invasiveness or metastasis on the tumor cell.

Role of PRAD1 *in Other Human Tumors*

Interest in *PRAD1*s role with respect to oncogenesis has been intensified by its incrimination in other, non-parathyroid, human tumors (57). In a subset of B-cell lymphomas and leukemias, the upstream *PRAD1* gene region is rearranged with the immunoglobulin heavy-chain gene on chromosome 14. This t(11;14) translocation results in the marked overexpression of *PRAD1*, in a fashion analogous to the deregulated expression of oncogenes *c-myc* and *bcl-2* by their translocation into the immunoglobulin region in other types of B-cell lymphomas (60–62). Thus, *PRAD1* is overwhelmingly likely to be the so-called *bcl-1* oncogene, which had been presumed to exist but had eluded workers searching 11q13 in the vicinity of these translocation breakpoints for many years. The difficulty they had was due to the large distance, ~120 kb, between the original *bcl-1* translocation breakpoint and the first exon of *PRAD1*. It has recently been shown that centrocytic lymphomas, the B-cell tumor type that characteristically bears the t(11;14), may also have 11q13 breakpoints as close to *PRAD1* as they are in some parathyroid tumors, i.e., as near as 1 kb upstream (34). These data indicate that *PRAD1* expression can be modulated in tumors by the placement of a heterologous tissue-specific enhancer essentially anywhere within 120 kb 5' of the *PRAD1* gene.

In addition to being a B-cell lymphoma oncogene, *PRAD1* appears to be involved in human breast cancer and squamous cell cancer of the head, neck, and esophagus. In 15% of breast cancers and in up to 40% of the squamous cell tumors, a large stretch of DNA on 11q13 is amplified (present in extra copy number), but the particular gene whose amplification confers the selective growth advantage on the cell, i.e., the key oncogene in the region, has not been determined. *PRAD1* was shown to be consistently amplified in breast and squamous cell cancers, whenever any 11q13 amplification was present (63,64). Furthermore, *PRAD1* was abundantly expressed in these tumors, probably abnormally so; in contrast, the other genes that may be coamplified along with *PRAD1* typically exhibit poor expression (63). While there may be some complexities in the patterns of amplification in this region, perhaps signalling the existence of more than one relevant amplified oncogene (65,66), *PRAD1* is currently the best candidate for being a pathogenetically key breast and squamous cell cancer oncogene on 11q13.

Inactivation of a Putative Tumor Suppressor Gene on Chromosome 11

Considerable attention has been directed to the possibility that inactivation of a tumor suppressor gene on chromosome 11 plays a role in the pathogenesis of certain benign parathyroid tumors. The expected isolation of this gene (or genes) in the near future should yield valuable insights into the control of parathyroid cell proliferation.

Multiple Endocrine Neoplasia Type I

In 1988, the gene responsible for the MEN-I tumor predisposition syndrome was mapped by linkage analysis to the long arm of chromosome 11, in the general vicinity of the muscle phosphorylase *(PYGM)* gene (67). This finding initiated an extensive search of this region of 11q13, which is ongoing, for the specific "MEN-I gene" (see the chapters by Metz et al. and Friedman et al.). It should be noted that, while *PRAD1* also maps to 11q13, the tightest MEN-I-linked markers are located far upstream (centromeric) of *PRAD1*, probably several million base pairs away (60,63,68–72). The autosomal dominant inheritance pattern of MEN-I suggested the possibility that the MEN-I gene would prove to be a tumor suppressor gene, because of parallels with the paradigms of familial retinoblastoma and Li-Fraumeni syndromes, which involve inheritance of mutations in the *RB* and *p53* genes, respectively (54). Therefore, tumors from MEN-I patients were examined for evidence of somatic genetic events that could have inactivated one allele of a gene in this region and thereby unmask the inherited constitutional MEN-I mutation. In support of this hypothesis, "allelic loss" (or loss of heterozygosity) of polymorphic marker DNAs from chromosome 11 was initially found in two insulinomas from brothers with

MEN-I (67) and has been found in the majority of MEN-I-associated parathyroid tumors examined (19,20,24,73,74). The number of markers from different parts of chromosome 11 exhibiting allelic loss varied widely from tumor to tumor, but the region of overlap of these losses was consistent with the MEN-I region as determined by linkage analysis. Furthermore, when the parental origin of the tumor-specific, somatically lost allele could be determined, it derived from the clinically unaffected parent (20,24); this would be the expected pattern in the event that the retained chromosome contained an inherited mutant tumor suppressor gene (Fig. 4).

It is important to note that these tumor-specific allelic deletions from chromosome 11 are also markers of monoclonality, indicating that, despite the usual multigland involvement ("hyperplasia") found in MEN-I patients, their parathyroid tumors can be clonal. The inability to detect allelic loss of linked markers does not exclude the possibilities that both alleles of the true MEN-I gene have been clonally inactivated in a particular tumor or that critical clonal DNA damage exists at other genetic loci. Because available methods cannot prove that a parathyroid tumor is polyclonal, the frequency of monoclonality in hypercellular parathyroid glands in MEN-I remains uncertain and could be higher than the 58% figure recently reported in a large series (74). On the other hand, there has been no study in which all parathyroid glands removed from every patient have been systematically examined for allelic loss, and current information is biased toward examination of the larger gland(s) of individual patients. This selection bias could of course result in an overestimation of the true frequency of allelic loss in MEN-I-associated parathyroid tumors. Interestingly, the available data, generally derived from one or two resected glands per patient, do indicate that allelic loss on chromosome 11 is found more frequently in larger as contrasted with small tumors (74). This observation allows the speculation that monoclonal expansion of a parathyroid neoplasm, driven by loss of the remaining normal allele at the MEN-I locus, many follow an initial period of true polyclonal hyperplasia. It also remains unknown whether the presence of one mutant plus one normal copy of the "MEN-I gene" confers an abnormal proliferative phenotype on a parathyroid cell; such a situation could of course be the cause of a preliminary state of generalized true hyperplasia. Finally, it is worth noting that some, or even many, examples of familial primary hyperparathyroidism without other manifestations of MEN may well be variants of MEN-I. Cloning of the relevant tumor suppressor gene will permit more definitive tests of these hypotheses.

Brief mention should be made at this point of other inherited syndromes involving hyperparathyroidism.

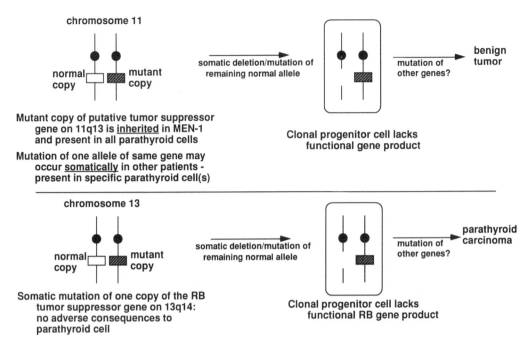

FIG. 4. Schematic diagram illustrating the hypothesized roles of inactivation of tumor suppressor genes as a contributory mechanism in parathyroid neoplasia. (Reprinted from ref. 83 with permission.)

Hyperparathyroidism is a component of MEN-IIa, although it is not as penetrant a feature in this syndrome as it is in MEN-I. The gene for which an inherited mutation predisposes to MEN-IIa has been mapped to chromosome 10, and it could function as a "classical" or variant parathyroid tumor suppressor gene. However, parathyroid and other MEN-IIa associated tumors have not been characterized by allelic losses of linked chromosome 10 markers (see the chapter by Gagel), so this issue remains in doubt pending the cloning of the responsible gene. Another syndrome, familial cystic parathyroid adenomatosis with ossifying fibromas of the jaw (see the chapter, "The Functional and Pathologic Spectrum of Parathyroid Abnormalities in Hyperparathyroidism," by Mallette), is clearly distinct genetically from either MEN syndrome (75,76). The primary responsible gene has not been isolated.

Sporadic Parathyroid Adenomas

The possibility that a chromosome 11-based tumor suppressor gene was involved in sporadic (nonfamilial) parathyroid adenomas was raised by two independent routes. In one, the cloning of parathyroid adenoma breakpoint-adjacent fragment D11S287 (eventually determined to be the location of *PRAD1*), described above, and its mapping to 11q13 initially led investigators to question whether D11S287 was part of a

known oncogene locus and thus to examine known 11q13 oncogenes for rearrangements in other parathyroid adenomas. One such locus tested was *INT-2,* the human homolog of a mouse mammary oncogene. Instead of finding an *int-2* rearrangement, however, investigators found tumor-specific allelic loss in one informative case (18). Subsequent study of polymorphic markers from all regions of chromosome 11 revealed that one allele of each was lost in this adenoma, indicating that an entire copy of the chromosome was somatically deleted from the tumor genome. Careful gene dosage analysis confirmed that this was a true deletion, unaccompanied by reduplication of the remaining chromosome, showing that monosomy 11 can be tolerated by a parathyroid cell and that only a single PTH gene copy per cell is sufficient to allow hyperparathyroid function by the adenoma (18). The observed allelic losses also confirmed the monoclonality of parathyroid adenomas and suggested that a tumor suppressor gene(s) important in the development of sporadic parathyroid neoplasia is located on chromosome 11 (18).

In the well-characterized *RB* tumor suppressor gene model, the sporadic (nonfamilial) counterpart of the familial retinoblastoma tumor results from the somatic inactivation/loss of both (initially normal) alleles of the *RB* gene in the clonal precursor cell. It therefore seemed reasonable to hypothesize that some sporadic parathyroid adenomas might evolve from a cell in which both copies of the putative MEN-I tumor suppressor gene became inactivated by somatic mechanisms (Fig. 4). Thus the mapping of the MEN-I gene to 11q13 (discussed above) was the other key result that focused attention on chromosome 11 as the possible site of a tumor suppressor gene for sporadic adenomas.

Study of considerable numbers of sporadic parathyroid adenomas has determined that allelic loss of chromosome 11 markers occurs in ~25% of the tumors (20,74). The true frequency of involvement of a chromosome 11 tumor suppressor gene could be even higher if some inactivating events/deletions are small. Unlike parathyroid tumors in MEN-I, sporadic adenomas with allelic losses of chromosome 11 do not tend to be larger than those without demonstrable allelic loss (74). Also in contrast to MEN-I-associated parathyroid tumors, the observed subchromosomal deletions in sporadic adenomas can occur in a complicated pattern and do not invariably encompass the mapped MEN-I gene region (74). Thus, while the still uncloned "MEN-I gene" is still the best candidate for also being the sporadic adenoma tumor suppressor gene expected on chromosome 11, the situation may be more complex, with inactivation of a different tumor suppressor gene(s) from this chromosome contributing to the proliferative phenotype in some cases.

Allelic losses of markers from chromosome 11 have also been demonstrated in two of 12 parathyroid glands removed from uremic patients (26). These data provided evidence that such tumors can be monoclonal and that inactivation of a chromosome 11 tumor suppressor gene(s) may contribute to the emergence of the clonal expansions on a background of true polyclonal hyperplasia. As was mentioned above, X-inactivation surveys of tumor clonality have indicated that a much higher proportion of hypercellular parathyroid glands from patients with uremic tertiary hyperparathyroidism as well as a minority of tumors from patients with nonfamilial primary multigland hyperplasia are monoclonal neoplasms (25, and unpublished data). Therefore, the chromosomal sites of most of the clonal oncogenic alterations in these tumors remain to be identified.

For sporadic parathyroid adenomas, the additional genes expected to participate in their development also remain unknown. Certain specific candidates such as *ras* (31), *p53* (23,77,78), and *RB* (23) do not appear to participate in any consistent fashion (or at all) in benign adenomas. Tumor cytogenetic analysis has not so far been very helpful in highlighting chromosomal target regions to be intensively searched for new parathyroid oncogenes or tumor suppressor genes. A cytogenetic translocation between chromosomes 1 and 5 has been reported in a single parathyroid adenoma (21), but it is unclear whether this was an isolated random occurrence or will be characteristic of a distinct subset of adenomas.

MOLECULAR PATHOGENESIS OF PARATHYROID CARCINOMA

The discovery that a cell cycle regulator, *PRAD1*, can be involved in parathyroid tumorigenesis has raised the possibility that still other genes with cell cyclase-regulatory functions also might contribute to parathyroid neoplasia. One example is *RB* (or *RB1*), the tumor suppressor gene implicated in retinoblastoma and certain other, often aggressive, human tumors (54). Current thoughts regarding *RB*'s participation in the cell cycle are discussed above in the section on *PRAD1*. Preliminary evidence suggests that complete inactivation of the *RB* tumor suppressor gene may be a key factor in the pathogenesis of most parathyroid carcinomas (23, also, Cryns and Arnold, unpublished), in contrast to benign adenomas and suggests that *RB* analysis should be evaluated as a possible diagnostic aid or prognostic indicator for parathyroid carcinoma. Other genes are also being assessed for their potential contributions to parathyroid carcinomatosis.

ECTOPIC SECRETION OF PARATHYROID HORMONE

Primary hyperparathyroidism is a biochemical diagnosis, and a rare cause of primary hyperparathyroidism is the ectopic secretion of PTH by nonparathyroid tumors. Older literature describing this as a common entity was confounded by nonspecificity in assays for PTH, and developing knowledge that led to the ultimate identification of PTHrP as the major cause of hypercalcemia of malignancy later placed the very existence of the true ectopic PTH syndrome in doubt. Recently, however, modern immunometric assays specific for PTH combined with molecular biological approaches have confirmed the occurrence of this syndrome, and the molecular basis for ectopic PTH production in one such case has been identified.

Because tumors may synthesize hormones without releasing them to cause an identifiable clinical syndrome, specific criteria have been recognized for documenting the diagnosis of a true ectopic hormone syndrome (79). These criteria have been solidly fulfilled for the diagnosis of one case of the ectopic PTH syndrome (80) and reasonable support for the diagnosis has been marshalled in two other reports (81,82). The latter two patients had metastatic small cell carcinomas, which synthesized PTH and PTH mRNA, in association with hypercalcemia, elevated serum PTH levels, and four grossly normal parathyroid glands. One of these tumors also produced PTHrP and was associated with elevated circulating levels of PTHrP (82). The former patient had elevated serum PTH (but not PTHrP) levels, four normal parathyroid glands, and an ovarian carcinoma whose PTH secretion was proven to be the cause of her hypercalcemia by a sevenfold increase in PTH concentration in the tumor's venous effluent, an immediate decline in serum PTH level as well as the development of hypocalcemia after tumor resection, the production of PTH by the ovarian carcinoma cells in culture, and the presence of PTH (but not PTHrP) mRNA in the tumor tissue (80). This ovarian cancer was the only nonparathyroid tumor responsible for hypercalcemia in >300 consecutive patients with a biochemical diagnosis of hyperparathyroidism (80).

Ectopic hormone production can be considered as an aberration in the tissue specificity of gene expression; it usually involves dysregulation of a normal hormone gene product. Tissue specificity of gene expression is controlled by DNA sequences called *enhancer*

and *silencer* elements, often located in the upstream regulatory region of a hormone gene, interacting with the particular mix of DNA binding proteins characteristic of that tissue type. Ectopic hormone production in a tumor could therefore result from an alteration in that tumor cell type's DNA binding protein environment (activating the intact enhancer of the hormone gene) or from a change in the enhancer/silencer region adjacent to the hormone structural gene (thereby conferring responsiveness to the DNA binding proteins typical of the tumor cell type).

In the ovarian carcinoma that ectopically produced PTH described above, a DNA rearrangement was present in the upstream regulatory region of the PTH gene (Fig. 5), replacing the gene's own control elements with DNA sequences that could interact with the ovarian cell's DNA binding proteins and thereby "inappropriately" activate PTH gene transcription (80). In ad-

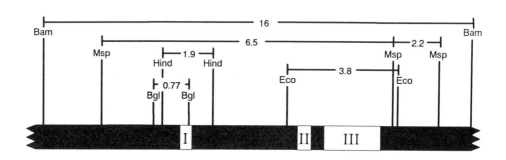

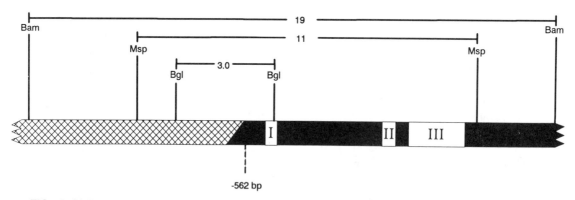

FIG. 5. Molecular pathology of the ectopic production of PTH by an ovarian cancer. Schematic diagram and restriction map of the rearranged and amplified *PTH* gene region (**bottom**) in the PTH-secreting ovarian tumor discussed in the text (80), compared with the normal *PTH* gene region (**top**). PTH exons I, II, and III are represented by *open bars,* normally present introns and flanking regions by *solid bars,* and the DNA placed upstream of PTH by the tumor-specific rearrangement by the *cross-hatched bar.* Restriction sites are labeled, and fragment sizes are shown in kilobases. For reasons of clarity and space, the map is not drawn to scale. The precise location of the breakpoint of the rearrangement was narrowed to a segment between the HindIII site at −562 bp (562 base pairs upstream of the start of exon I) and the normally present BglII site 150 bp further upstream (no longer present in the rearranged gene). Bam, Bam HI; Msp, Msp I; Hind, HindIII; Bgl, Bgl II; Eco, Eco RI. (Reprinted from ref. 80 with permission.)

dition, this PTH gene with its rearranged upstream regulatory region was amplified, i.e., was present at severalfold extra copy number, in the ovarian cancer cells, which almost certainly heightened the level of PTH production caused by the DNA rearrangement (80). The molecular mechanisms underlying other examples of the ectopic PTH syndrome remain to be elucidated.

SUMMARY

This is an exciting time for those interested in the molecular basis of the various forms of primary hyperparathyroidism. One oncogene involved in the development of parathyroid tumors, *PRAD1/cyclin D1*, has been discovered and is having a broad impact in oncology and cell cycle biology. An already recognized tumor suppressor gene, *RB*, has been linked to the pathogenesis of parathyroid carcinoma. Investigators are on the verge of isolating the MEN genes, which are sure to have important basic and clinical implications relevant to parathyroid and other endocrine diseases. Increasingly available are improved methods that will eventually permit the identification of still other parathyroid tumor-provoking genes that are certain to exist. Finally, there is reason to hope that the molecular basis of the relationship between abnormal parathyroid cell proliferation and abnormal hormonal regulatory function, plus other problems unique to parathyroid disease, will soon be elucidated.

REFERENCES

1. Fearon ER, Vogelstein B. A genetic model for colorectal tumorigenesis. *Cell* 1990;61:759–767.
2. Solomon E, Borrow J, Goddard AD. Chromosome aberrations and cancer. *Science* 1991;254:1153–1160.
3. Bishop JM. Molecular themes in oncogenesis. *Cell* 1991; 64:235–248.
4. Hunter T. Cooperation between oncogenes. *Cell* 1991;64:249–270.
5. Cross M, Dexter TM. Growth factors in development, transformation, and tumorigenesis. *Cell* 1991;64:271–280.
6. Cantley LC, Auger KR, Carpenter C, Duckworth B, Graziani A, Kapeller R, Soltoff S. Oncogenes and signal transduction. *Cell* 1991;64:281–302.
7. Lewin B. Oncogenic conversion by regulatory changes in transcription factors. *Cell* 1991;64:303–312.
8. Marshall CJ. Tumor suppressor genes. *Cell* 1991;64:313–326.
9. Liotta LA, Steeg PS, Stetler-Stevenson WG. Cancer metastasis and angiogenesis: an imbalance of positive and negative regulation. *Cell* 1991;64:327–336.
10. Black WC III, Utley JR. The differential diagnosis of parathyroid adenoma and chief cell hyperplasia. *Am J Clin Pathol* 1968;49:761–775.
11. Castleman B, Roth SI. Tumors of the parathyroid glands. In: Hartman WH, ed. *Atlas of tumor pathology.* Washington, DC: Armed Forces Institute of Pathology, 1978, Second series, fascicle 14.
12. Attie JN, Bock G, Auguste LJ. Multiple parathyroid adenomas: report of thirty-three cases. *Surgery* 1990;108:1014–1020.
13. Verdonk CA, Edis AJ. Parathyroid "double adenomas": fact or fiction? *Surgery* 1981;90:523–526.
14. Brothers TE, Thompson NW. Surgical treatment of primary hyperparathyroidism in early patients. *Acta Chir Scand* 1987; 153:175–178.
15. Fialkow PJ, Jackson CE, Block MA, Greenawald KA. Multicellular origin of parathyroid "adenomas." *N Engl J Med* 1977;297:696–698.
16. Jackson CE, Cerny JC, Block MA, Fialkow PJ. Probable clonal origin of aldosteronomas versus multicellular origins of parathyroid "adenomas." *Surgery* 1982;875:875–879.
17. Arnold A, Staunton CE, Kim HG, Gaz RD, Kronenberg HM. Monoclonality and abnormal parathyroid hormone genes in parathyroid adenomas. *N Engl J Med* 1988;318:658–662.
18. Arnold A, Kim HG. Clonal loss of one chromosome 11 in a parathyroid adenoma. *J Clin Endocrinol Metab* 1989;69:496–499.
19. Friedman E, Sakaguchi K, Bale AE, et al. Clonality of parathyroid tumors in familial multiple endocrine neoplasia type 1. *N Engl J Med* 1989;321:213–218.
20. Byström C, Larsson C, Blomberg C, et al. Localization of the MEN1 gene to a small region within chromosome 11q13 by deletion mapping in tumors. *Proc Natl Acad Sci USA* 1990; 87:1968–1972.
21. Örndal C, Johansson M, Heim S, et al. Parathyroid adenoma with t(1;5)(p22:q32) as the sole clonal chromosome abnormality. *Cancer Genet Cytogenet* 1990;48:225–228.
22. Salti GI, Fedorak I, Yashiro T, et al. Continuing evolution in the operative management of primary hyperparathyroidism. *Arch Surg* 1992;127:831–837.
23. Cryns VL, Arnold A. Retinoblastoma tumor suppressor gene deletions in human parathyroid neoplasia. *J Bone Mineral Res* 1992;7(Suppl 1):S101.
24. Thakker RV, Bouloux P, Wooding C, et al. Association of parathyroid tumors in multiple endocrine neoplasia type 1 with loss of alleles on chromosome 11. *N Engl J Med* 1989;321:218–224.
25. Arnold A, Brown M, Urena P, Gaz R, Drueke T, Sarfati E. X-inactivation analysis of clonality in primary and secondary parathyroid hyperplasia. *J Bone Mineral Res* 1992;7(Suppl 1):S153.
26. Falchetti A, Bale AE, Amorosi A, et al. Progression of uremic hyperparathyroidism involves allelic loss on chromosome 11. *J Clin Endocrinol Metab* 1993;76:139–144.
27. Korsmeyer SJ. Chromosomal translocations in lymphoid malignancies reveal novel protooncogenes. *Annu Rev Immunol* 1992;10:785–807.
28. Arnold A, Kim HG, Gaz RD, et al. Molecular cloning and chromosomal mapping of DNA rearranged with the parathyroid hormone gene in a parathyroid adenoma. *J Clin Invest* 1989;83:2034–2040.
29. Rosenberg CL, Kim HG, Shows TB, Kronenberg HM, Arnold A. Rearrangement and overexpression of D11S287E, a candidate oncogene on chromosome 11q13 in benign parathyroid tumors. *Oncogene* 1991;6:449–453.
30. Motokura T, Bloom T, Kim HG, et al. A novel cyclin encoded by a *bcl1*-linked candidate oncogene. *Nature* 1991;350:512–515.
31. Friedman E, Bale AE, Marx SJ, et al. Genetic abnormalities in sporadic parathyroid adenomas. *J Clin Endocrinol Metab* 1990;71:293–297.
32. Motokura T, Arnold A. The PRAD1/cyclin D1 proto-oncogene: genomic organization, 5' DNA sequence, and sequence of a tumor-specific rearrangement breakpoint. *Genes Chrom Cancer* (in press).
33. Rosenberg CL, Motokura T, Kronenberg HM, Arnold A. Coding sequence of the overexpressed transcript of the putative oncogene PRAD1/cyclin D1 in two primary human tumors. *Oncogene* 1993;8:519–521.
34. Williams ME, Swerdlow SH, Rosenberg CL, Arnold A. Chromosome 11 translocation breakpoints at the PRAD1 cyclin

gene locus in centrocytic lymphoma. *Leukemia* 1993;7:241–245.

35. Hunter T, Pines J. Cyclins and cancer. *Cell* 1991;66:1071–1074.

36. Nurse P. University control mechanism regulating onset of M-phase. *Nature* 1990;344:503–508.

37. Pardee AB. G_1 events and regulation of cell proliferation. *Science* 1989;246:603–608.

38. Reed SI. G1-specific cyclins: in search of an S-phase-promoting factor. *TIG* 1991;7:95–99.

39. Reed SI. The role of p34 kinases in the G1 to S-phase transition. *Annu Rev Cell Biol* 1992;8:529–561.

40. Lewin B. Driving the cell cycle: M phase kinase, its partners, and substrates. *Cell* 1990;61:743–752.

41. Cross FR. DAF1, a mutant gene affecting size control, pheromone arrest, and cell cycle kinetics of *Saccharomyces cerevisiae*. *Mol Cell Biol* 1988;8:4675–4684.

42. Reed SI, Wittenberg C. Mitotic role for the Cdc28 protein kinase of *Saccharomyces cerevisiae*. *Proc Natl Acad Sci USA* 1990;87:5697–5701.

43. Wittenberg C, Sugimoto K, Reed SI. G1-specific cylcins of S. cerevisiae: cell cycle periodicity, regulation by mating pheromone, and association with the $p34^{CDC28}$ protein kinase. *Cell* 1990;62:225–237.

44. Hadwiger JA, Wittenberg C, Rechardson HE, Lopes MDB, Reed SI. A family of cyclin homologs that control the G_1 phase in yeast. *Proc Natl Acad Sci USA* 1989;86:6255–6259.

45. Motokura T, Keyomarsi K, Kronenberg HM, Arnold A. Cloning and characterization of human cyclin D3, a cDNA closely related in sequence to the PRAD1/cyclin D1 proto-oncogene. *J Biol Chem* 1992;267:20412–20415.

46. Won KA, Xiong Y, Beach D, Gilman MZ. Growth-regulated expression of D-type cyclin genes in human diploid fibroblasts. *Proc Natl Acad Sci USA* 1991;89:9910–9914.

47. Matsushime H, Roussel MF, Ashmun RA, Sherr CJ. Colony-stimulating factor 1 regulates novel cyclins during the G1 phase of the cell cycle. *Cell* 1991;65:701–713.

48. Xiong Y, Connolly T, Futcher B, Beach D. Human D-type cyclin. *Cell* 1991;65:691–699.

49. Lew DJ, Dulic V, Reed SI. Isolation of three novel human cyclins by rescue of G1 cyclin (Cln) function in yeast. *Cell* 1991;66:1197–1206.

50. Koff A, Cross F, Fisher A, et al. Human cyclin E, a new cyclin that interacts with two members of the *CDC2* gene family. *Cell* 1991;66:1217–1228.

51. Inaba T, Matsushime H, Valentine M, Roussel MF, Sherr CJ, Look AT. Genomic organization, chromosomal localization, and independent expression of human cyclin D genes. *Genomics* 1992;13:565–574.

52. Xiong Y, Menninger J, Beach D, Ward DC. Molecular cloning and chromosomal mapping of *CCND* genes encoding human D-type cyclins. *Genomics* 1992;13:575–584.

53. Matsushime H, Ewen ME, Strom DK, Kato JY, Hanks SK, Roussel MF, Sherr CJ. Identification and properties of an atypical catalytic subunit ($p34^{PSK-J3}$/cdk4) for mammalian D type G1 cyclins. *Cell* 1992;71:323–334.

54. Weinberg RA. Tumor suppressor genes. *Science* 1991;254:1138–1146.

55. Hinds PW, Mittnacht S, Dulic V, Arnold A, Reed SI, Weinberg RA. Regulation of retinoblastoma protein functions by ectopic expression of human cyclins. *Cell* 1992;70:993–1006.

56. Dowdy SF, Hinds PW, Louie K, Reed SI, Arnold A, Weinberg RA. Physical interaction of the retinoblastoma protein with human D cyclins. *Cell* 1993;73:499–511.

57. Motokura T, Arnold A. Cyclin D and oncogenesis. *Curr Opinion Genet Dev* 1993;3:5–10.

58. Wang J, Chenivesse X, Henglein B, Bréchot C. Hepatitis B virus integration in a cyclin A gene in a hepatocellular carcinoma. *Nature* 1990;343:555–557.

59. Wang J, Zindy F, Chenivesse X, Lamas E, Henglein B, Bréchot C. Modification of cyclin A expression by hepatitis

60. Rosenberg CL, Wong E, Petty EM, et al. *PRAD1*, a candidate *BCL1* oncogene: mapping and expression in centrocytic lymphoma. *Proc Natl Acad Sci USA* 1991;88:9638–9642.

61. Withers DA, Harvey RC, Faust JB, Melnyk O, Carey K, Meeker TC. Characterization of a candidate *bcl-1* gene. *Mol Cel Biol* 1991;11:4846–4853.

62. Seto M, Yamamoto K, Iida S, et al. Gene rearrangement and overexpression of *PRAD1* in lymphoid malignancy with t(11;14)(q13;q32) translocation. *Oncogene* 1992;7:1401–1406.

63. Lammie GA, Fantl V, Smith R, et al. D11S287, a putative oncogene on chromosome 11q13, is amplified and expressed in squamous cell and mammary carcinomas and linked to BCL-1. *Oncogene* 1991;6:439–444.

64. Schuuring E, Verhoeven E, Mooi WJ, Michalides RJAM. Identification and cloning of two overexpressed genes. U21B31/*PRAD1* and *EMS1*, within the amplified chromosome 11q13 region in human carcinomas. *Oncogene* 1992;7:355–361.

65. Proctor AJ, Coombs LM, Carins JP, Knowles MA. Amplification at chromosome 11q13 in transitional cell tumours of the bladder. *Oncogene* 1991;6:789–795.

66. Szepetowski P, Courseaux A, Carle GF, Theillet C, Gaudray P. Amplification of 11q13 DNA sequences in human breast cancer: D11S97 identifies a region tightly linked to BCL1 which can be amplified separately. *Oncogene* 1992;7:751–755.

67. Larsson C, Skogseid B, Oberg K, Nakamura Y, Nordenskjold M. Multiple endocrine neoplasia type I gene maps to chromosome 11 and is lost in insulinoma. *Nature* 1988;332:85–87.

68. Petty EM, Arnold A, Marx SJ, Bale AE. A pulse-field gel electrophoresis (PFGE) map of twelve loci on chromosome 11q11–q13. *Genomics* 1993;15:423–425.

69. Janson M, Larsson C, Werelius B, et al. Detailed physical map of human chromosomal region 11q12–13 shows high meiotic recombination rate around the *MEN1* locus. *Proc Natl Acad Sci USA* 1991;88:10609–10613.

70. Larsson C, Weber G, Kvanta E, et al. Isolation and mapping of polymorphic cosmid clones used for sublocalization of the multiple endocrine neoplasia type 1 (MEN1) locus. *Hum Genet* 1992;89:187–193.

71. Nakamura Y, Larsson C, Julier C, et al. Localization of the genetic defect in multiple endocrine neoplasia type 1 within a small region of chromosome 11. *Am J Hum Genet* 1989;44:751–755.

72. Julier C, Nakamura Y, Lathrop M, et al. A detailed genetic map of the long arm of chromosome 11. *Genomics* 1990;7:335–345.

73. Radford DM, Ashley SW, Wells SA Jr, Gerhard DS. Loss of heterozygosity of markers on chromosome 11 in tumors from patients with multiple endocrine neoplasia syndrome type 1. *Cancer Res* 1990;50:6529–6533.

74. Friedman E, De Marco L, Gejman PV, et al. Allelic loss from chromosome 11 in parathyroid tumors. *Cancer Res* 1992;52:6804–6809.

75. Mallette LE, Malini S, Rappaport MP, Kirkland JL. Familial cystic parathyroid adenomatosis. *Ann Intern Med* 1987;107:54–60.

76. Jackson CE, Norum RA, Boyd SB, et al. Hereditary hyperparathyroidism and multiple ossifying jaw fibromas: a clinically and genetically distinct syndrome. *Surgery* 1990;108:1006–1013.

77. Cryns V, Thor A, Louis D, Benedict W, Arnold A. Tumor suppressor gene abnormalities in human parathyroid carcinoma. *J Bone Mineral Res* 1993;8:S148.

78. Yoshimoto K, Iwahana H, Fukuda A, Sano T, Saito S, Itakura M. Role of *p53* mutations in endocrine tumorigenesis: mutation detection by polymerase chain reaction-single strand conformation polymorphism. *Cancer Res* 1992;52:5061–5064.

79. Sherwood LM. Paraneoplastic endocrine disorders: ectopic hormone syndromes. In: DeGroot LJ, ed. *Endocrinology*, 2nd ed., vol 3. Philadelphia: W. B. Saunders, 1989;2550–2599.

80. Nussbaum SR, Gaz RD, Arnold A. Hypercalcemia and ectopic secretion of parathyroid hormone by an ovarian carcinoma with rearrangement of the gene for parathyroid hormone. *N Engl J Med* 1990;323:1324–1328.

81. Yoshimoto K, Yamasaki R, Sakai H, et al. Ectopic production of parathyroid hormone by small cell lung cancer in a patient with hypercalcemia. *J Clin Endocrinol Metab* 1989;68:976–981.

82. Strewler GJ, Budayr AA, Clark OH, Nissenson RA. Production of parathyroid hormone by a malignant nonparathyroid tumor in a hypercalcemic patient. *J Clin Endocrinol Metab* 1993;76:1373–1375.

83. Arnold A. Molecular genetics of parathyroid gland neoplasia. *J Clin Endocrinol Metab* (in press).

The Parathyroids, edited by J.P. Bilezikian, M. Levine, and R. Marcus. Raven Press, Ltd., New York © 1994.

CHAPTER 25

The Functional and Pathologic Spectrum of Parathyroid Abnormalities in Hyperparathyroidism

Lawrence E. Mallette

Primary enlargement and hyperfunction of one or more parathyroid glands produces the clinical syndrome of primary, or hypercalcemic, hyperparathyroidism. Secondary, or compensatory, hyperparathyroidism begins as a normal and appropriate response to hypocalcemia or decreased 1,25-dihydroxyvitamin D [$1,25(OH)_2D$] levels, but the excess of parathyroid hormone (PTH) may become so great that it produces its own set of complications. These are common clinical problems that may present in subtle or florid form. Parathyroid enlargement may also exist in the face of a normal serum calcium value, either in the form of a nonfunctional parathyroid neoplasm or with PTH excess when the hypercalcemia is prevented by a concomitant metabolic problem. This chapter reviews the pathophysiology of the syndromes in which parathyroid enlargement and hyperfunction occur, focusing on the variety of pathological changes that are observed in the parathyroid glands.

THE CLINICAL SYNDROME OF PRIMARY HYPERPARATHYROIDISM

Primary PTH excess may be produced by a parathyroid adenoma, parathyroid hyperplasia, or a parathyroid carcinoma. The ectopic production of authentic PTH by a nonparathyroid malignancy can mimic primary hyperparathyroidism but it is rare (1,2). The clinical manifestations of primary parathyroid hyper-

function are reviewed in the chapter, "Clinical Presentation of Primary Hyperparathyroidism," by Bilezikian et al. and elsewhere (3–6) but are summarized briefly here.

Biochemical Changes

The chief biochemical manifestation of primary PTH excess is hypercalcemia. The excess PTH acts on the renal tubule to produce a relative retention of calcium, an increase in urinary cyclic adenosine monophosphate (cAMP) excretion, a low or low-normal serum phosphate value, and a high or high-normal serum chloride value. As a result of the low serum phosphate and high PTH values, serum $1,25(OH)_2D$ values may be increased or inappropriately normal for the hypercalcemia. Maintenance or enhancement of both intestinal calcium absorption and bone resorption by the $1,25(OH)_2D$ contributes to the hypercalcemia. Markers of bone remodeling are often increased in concentration, including serum alkaline phosphatase and osteocalcin (markers of bone formation) and urinary hydroxyproline and collagen cross-link residues (markers of bone resorption). Many of these changes are non-specific, but measurement of serum PTH values serves as a convenient and more specific diagnostic tool (see the chapter by Nussbaum and Potts). Serum PTH values will be elevated in > 90% of patients with a parathyroid adenoma if measurement is made with an adequately sensitive midregion-specific radioimmunoassay (RIA) or immunoradiometric assay for intact PTH (7,8).

L. E. Mallette: Division of Endocrinology and Metabolism, Baylor College of Medicine, Houston, Texas 77030.

Symptoms and Signs

The clinical signs and symptoms of primary hyperparathyroidism are myriad. Skeletal involvement may be minimal or marked. Skeletal symptoms may range from vague diffuse bone pain or arthralgias to a severe deforming bone disease (osteitis fibrosa et cystica), seen only in the patients with the most severe excess of PTH. Nephrolithiasis occurs in ~15-20% of cases. Gastrointestinal complications of primary hyperparathyroidism include peptic ulcer disease, perhaps due in part to the calcium-mediated increase in serum gastrin values (9), and pancreatitis. Neurologic complications include neurogenic muscle atrophy with proximal muscle weakness (10), a decrease in mentation, and depression. The risks for gout and pseudogout are probably increased, and anemia may occur in severe cases (11).

A few unusual manifestations of parathyroid tumors have been reported, including polycythemia vera (12) or pancytosis (13) and intractable fever and intense headache (14). In each case, the parathyroid tumor appeared to be responsible, since the complication remitted after its resection.

Masked Primary Hyperparathyroidism

A rare presentation of parathyroid adenomas is the syndrome of masked primary hyperparathyroidism (15–18), in which the hypercalcemia is prevented (masked) by a concomitant metabolic problem such as malabsorption of vitamin D or hypothyroidism. One of my patients had primary hyperparathyroidism masked by simple vitamin D deficiency from habitual wearing of full body clothing, including a veil as fulfillment of religious requirements, and an unwillingness to take vitamin supplements. One study reported 17 patients in whom hypercalcemia developed while under treatment for hypothyroidism due to Hashimoto's thyroiditis, including four in whom it appeared as early as 2 months after starting treatment, suggesting that preexisting hyperparathyroidism had been masked by the hypothyroid state (19). Since hyperthyroidism can increase the severity of hypercalcemia in primary hyperparathyroidism (20), it is not surprising that hypothyroidism might lower serum calcium concentration.

Patients with masked hyperparathyroidism usually present with weakness, bone pain, a marked elevation of serum alkaline phosphatase, and severe hypophosphatemia, with normal or low serum ionized calcium concentration (15). The serum PTH value is markedly elevated. Muscle weakness is attributable to PTH excess, hypophosphatemia, or both. Bone histomorphometry reveals a mixture of hyperparathyroid bone disease and osteomalacia. Vitamin D or L-thyroxine replacement will unmask the hypercalcemia, confirming the diagnosis.

Theoretically, the hypercalcemia due to primary parathyroid hyperplasia might also become masked, but this situation would will be impossible to differentiate from longstanding secondary hyperparathyroidism with tertiary changes in the hyperplastic glands (see below). Thus, masked primary hyperparathyroidism can be diagnosed only when an adenoma is the cause of the hyperparathyroidism. In the management of these patients, it may then be difficult to decide how long to wait for the newly appearing hypercalcemia to resolve before exploring for a parathyroid adenoma, since tertiary hyperparathyroidism might slowly resolve. Parathyroid ultrasonography to differentiate between parathyroid hyperplasia and adenoma may help with this decision.

PARATHYROID ADENOMA

Definition

The parathyroid adenoma is a solitary benign parathyroid gland tumor. Most parathyroid adenomas are hyperfunctional, as manifested by an increased serum concentration of PTH and hypercalcemia. Histologic examination of a single enlarged parathyroid gland cannot distinguish unequivocally between an adenoma and a hyperplastic gland. The distinction can be made only when resection of a single enlarged gland permanently restores serum calcium and PTH values to normal.

Etiology

Known and Suspected Causes of the Parathyroid Adenoma

A few discrete causes of the parathyroid adenoma have been recognized, but the majority of parathyroid adenomas remain idiopathic. Aging increases the incidence of adenomas in man (21) and in rat (22), but what events might mediate this effect of aging is unknown. The pesticide Rotenone increased the incidence of parathyroid adenomas in male Fisher rats (22), but epidemiologic studies have not yet examined for a link between chemical toxins and adenomas in man.

Ionizing radiation increases the incidence of parathyroid adenomas. The lag phase for tumor induction, 30–40 years, is greater than for radiation-induced thyroid lesions (23–28). Adenomas will develop in between 4% and 11% of patients who receive head and neck irradiation. The risk seems to be minimal at an absorbed radiation dose <300 rads, but the incidence may approach 66% among those receiving >1,200 rads (24). The hypercalcemia seems to be mild in most patients with presumptive radiation-induced hyperparathyroidism, but many of these subjects were found by way of recall screening examinations while asymptomatic. Their biochemical changes are typical for primary hyperparathyroidism; the only apparently unique feature of radiation-associated adenomas is a more fibrotic histologic appearance (29). The ability of calcium to suppress PTH secretion (see below) has apparently not been studied in a group of radiation-associated parathyroid adenoma patients. The irradiated patient is of course more likely to manifest an associated skin, thyroid, and salivary gland malignancy (30).

At least 30 cases of primary hyperparathyroidism occurring during long-term lithium treatment have been reported, raising the suspicion that lithium might be able to induce parathyroid adenomas in certain susceptible individuals (31). Hypercalcemia was noted in most of these patients only after many months of lithium treatment. Some were asymptomatic, but others had experienced a worsening of psychiatric symptoms, representing an acquired refractoriness to lithium therapy. Parathyroidectomy allowed resumption of lithium therapy in 17 of the patients without a recurrence of hypercalcemia and often restored responsiveness of the psychiatric disorder to lithium. A generalized stimulus such as lithium should produce parathyroid hyperplasia, which was found in six recently reported cases, but adenomas were found in the remaining 11 surgery cases. We have shown that lithium in the usual doses does constitute a stimulus to parathyroid function and growth. Circulating intact and midregion PTH values and parathyroid volume estimated by ultrasonography were increased in a series of patients after an average of 8 years of lithium treatment (32). The increase in parathyroid size was not limited to a single gland but also was not uniform, representing an asymmetric form of hyperplasia. The parathyroid adenomas reported in some of the surgery patients might instead have represented the largest of four asymmetrically hyperplastic glands, but the possibility that some were true adenomas, either induced by lithium or occurring coincidentally with the usual cause, cannot be discounted.

Cellular Defect of the Parathyroid Adenoma: A Model for Adenoma Formation

The most common cellular defect identifiable in parathyroid adenomas is an increase in the calcium value needed to inhibit PTH secretion, i.e., a shift in the calcium inhibitory set point (33). From this obser-

vation one can construct a hypothetical model to explain the genesis of the parathyroid adenoma and its usual clinical course (34,35). By this clonal expansion model, the adenoma originates when a single parathyroid cell undergoes a change in its calcium inhibitory set point. The altered cell perceives itself to be in a hypocalcemic environment and begins to hypersecrete and divide. The progeny of this altered cell becomes the growing adenoma. After this clone expands sufficiently, the increased cell mass will be secreting enough PTH to increase serum calcium. The serum calcium value will rise slowly until it has reached the new set point of the abnormal clone. At this point the stimulus to cell proliferation has been removed, since the cells now perceive themselves to be in a normocalcemic environment, and the adenoma ceases to grow.

One of the attractions of this hypothesis is that it can explain the observed clinical course of the usual parathyroid adenoma, in which the calcium values rise over a period of a few weeks or months, but then remains relatively stable during years of follow-up. What objective findings support this clonal expansion model? There are two lines of evidence in addition to the shifted set point. First, parathyroid adenomas in many cases have been shown to be clonal in nature, either by studies of X-chromosome inactivation in tumors from women (36) or by study of restriction fragment length polymorphisms for chromosome 11 markers (36–38; see also the chapter by Arnold). Second, the rate of cell division in various tumors can be estimated by thymidine labeling in vitro. Cells from resected parathyroid adenomas show a very slow rate of cell division, far too slow for the tumor to have formed during the life of the patient unless cell division had been more rapid earlier in the evolution of the tumor (34,35). This implies that clonal expansion has slowed significantly by the time the adenoma is resected. The simplist explanation is that cell division slowed because serum calcium had reached the new set point. Alternately one would need to hypothesize that the increase in tumor bulk had somehow induced autocrine or paracrine factors that inhibited cell division. Cells prepared from the hyperplastic glands of renal failure patients show a faster rate of cell division, more in line with that of other neoplasms, suggesting that the stimulus for cell proliferation was still present at the time of resection.

How does the shift in sensitivity to extracellular calcium occur? One hypothesis draws upon observations from fetal metabolism. The mammalian fetus is "hypercalcemic" relative to the mother, with serum ionized calcium values that are 15–40% higher (39,40). Parathyroidectomy of the fetal lamb will abolish this gradient (40). The fetal parathyroid gland must therefore be driving the placental calcium pump. If fetal serum calcium concentrations are regulated through changes in fetal parathyroid function (a hypothesis not yet tested directly), the fetus's parathyroid set point for calcium would be higher than that of the adult's. One might then hypothesize that the shifted set point in the adenoma represents a reversion to the calcium sensing mechanism of the fetal parathyroid cell (41).

How might the calcium sensing mechanism be altered, either in the adenoma or in the fetal parathyroid gland or in both? The parathyroid cell probably senses the ambient calcium value by way of a "calcium receptor" on its cell surface (42). There are several lines of evidence for such a receptor. First, increasing the ambient calcium ion concentration depolarizes the parathyroid cell membrane far more than would be predicted simply from the change in electromotive force calculated from the altered ion concentrations. This observation can most easily be explained by postulating the presence of a cell surface divalent cation receptor capable of regulating membrane potential (43). Second, an acute increase in extracellular calcium will cause a "spike and plateau" pattern in the parathyroid cytosolic calcium value, probably resulting from mobilization of intracellular calcium stores and resembling that induced in other cell types by secretagogues known to interact with cell surface receptors (43–45). Third, several substances that bind to the parathyroid cell surface can alter cytosolic calcium values and/or PTH release. These include lectins (46), naturally occurring antibodies (47), and monoclonal antibodies (48,49). These factors may be interacting directly or indirectly with a cell membrane calcium receptor. Fourth, flow dialysis studies give evidence for stereospecific calcium binding sites on the parathyroid cell membrane with a K_d that is near the normal serum calcium value and one that is not found in other cell membranes (50) (see also the chapter by Brown).

These observations lead to the hypothesis that a change in calcium set point could arise from an alteration in the number or configuration of cell membrane calcium receptors or in the intracellular signaling resulting from receptor occupancy. Early evidence of altered cell surface properties in parathyroid adenomas was provided by Woltering and coworkers (51), who found that ~90% of adenomas had lost their cell surface ABO (H) markers. Recent studies have used monoclonal antibodies thought to be specific for the parathyroid calcium receptor. Normal parathyroid cells show intense and uniform immunofluorescent staining with these antibodies, but cells from parathyroid adenomas gave a reduced and heterogeneous staining (52). The mechanism by which the putative change in calcium receptor number or distribution occurs must now be ascertained, and it must be determined whether there is a similar alteration in the receptor in fetal parathyroid cells.

The clonal-expansion hypothesis based on a shift in calcium set point probably will not account for all parathyroid adenomas. Clinical evidence suggests that parathyroid adenomas represent a heterogeneous category. Not all parathyroid adenomas remain responsive to ambient calcium (33). Some adenomas seem to grow rapidly and continuously and produce steadily rising serum calcium and PTH values. These tumors may account for many cases of osteitis fibrosa et cystica. Thus, it is likely that other mechanisms of neoplasia are operative in ~10% of cases and await discovery.

Alterations in chromosomal structure or rearrangements of DNA that activate an oncogene or inactivate a tumor suppressor gene have been postulated as one such mechanism. Chromosomal abnormalities in adenomas have been suggested by studies of nuclear DNA content (reviewed below), which indicate that ~13% of adenomas are aneuploid, the remainder being diploid or diploid with a component of tetraploid cells. An unusual DNA rearrangement was characterized in detail in one parathyroid adenoma (53). This rearrangement separated the 5' flanking region of the PTH gene on chromosome 11 from its coding exons and placed the coding region near DNA that normally maps to 11q13, a marker for several nearby oncogenes and for the multiple endocrine neoplasia-I (MEN-I) gene locus, which may represent a tumor suppressor gene (see below). Deletion of one allele of the MEN-I locus on chromosome 11 can be detected in perhaps one-third of sporadic adenomas (38,54). Adenomas with allelic losses on chromosome 11 are larger than those without (1,105 mg vs. 356 mg) (38), but the mechanism by which this rearrangement contributes to tumorigenesis remains to be demonstrated. This point is covered in the chapter by Arnold in greater detail.

Treatment

The parathyroid adenoma can be cured only by removal or destruction, but medical measures may ameliorate some adverse metabolic effects.

Parathyroid Surgery

Parathyroid surgery is effective. Its success rate when performed by an experienced parathyroid surgeon approaches 98% (55,56) (see the chapter by Norton et al.). The incidence of recurrent hyperparathyroidism in the first 5–8 years after resection of a parathyroid adenoma is ~0.6%, or about 1 in 200, and probably less if familial cases are excluded (4). Parathyroid surgery is also safe, its risk being essentially that of a general anesthetic plus the rare occurrence of recurrent laryngeal nerve palsy or total hypoparathyroidism.

To determine that surgery has been curative, one must demonstrate normal or low serum calcium and PTH values a few weeks later. The persistence of increased PTH values has been reported in a fraction of adenoma patients who are normocalcemic after resection of the adenoma (57–59), but in my experience this reflects (a) secondary hyperparathyroidism related to a decrease in serum calcium within the normal range, (b) renal insufficiency, which causes retention of PTH fragments that react in the midregion and carboxyterminal PTH RIAs (8), or (c) a false-positive RIA result caused by interfering substances in the patient's serum (60).

Hungry Bone Syndrome

Early postoperative hypocalcemia is common. It may indicate hypoparathyroidism, either transient or permanent, signaled by high serum phosphate and low PTH values, or it may occur because of the "hungry bone syndrome," with an appropriate rise in PTH. The hungry bone syndrome occurs in patients in whom severe hyperparathyroidism has markedly accelerated skeletal remodeling. Removing the excess PTH rapidly lowers the resorptive activity, but bone formation continues for several weeks (the duration of an osteoblast lifespan) at each of the increased number of remodeling sites. Intense skeletal uptake of calcium occurs, producing hypocalcemia and a compensatory increase in PTH secretion by the remaining parathyroid glands. Serum phosphate concentration remains low, because of skeletal uptake of phosphate and phosphaturia induced by the PTH. Serum alkaline phosphatase activity may increase for a few days during this healing phase as a sign of increased osteoblast activity, and the patient may experience a transient increase in bone pain. The low serum phosphate and high PTH activate renal 1-α-hydroxylation of $25(OH)_2D$ (61), and the rise in serum $1,25(OH)_2D$ concentration enhances intestinal calcium absorption, so that oral calcium supplements are often useful in minimizing the hypocalcemia.

If renal insufficiency prevents the rise in $1,25(OH)_2D$ values, oral administration of calcitriol may be needed to help restore effective calcium absorption. Relative hypoparathyroidism or hypomagnesemia derived either from skeletal uptake of magnesium or from renal tubular damage by severe preoperative hypercalcemia (62) can also make oral correction of hypocalcemia difficult in this setting.

The hungry bones phenomenon may also occur in patients from whom not all the hyperfunctioning parathyroid tissue was resected, specifically those with a nonresected hyperplastic gland, a missed second parathyroid adenoma, or metastatic parathyroid carcinoma. In this case, the intense skeletal uptake of calcium may lower serum calcium values temporarily into the normal range or below, but PTH values will remain elevated even when calcium has normalized, and hypercalcemia will eventually recur.

The hungry bone syndrome persists for a variable time, and residual parathyroid tissue that may have become ischemic during the surgery may recover slowly. To accommodate this variability, the patient with an adenoma is declared cured only when normal serum calcium values are present after 6 months of postoperative follow-up (63).

Nonsurgical Ablation

Nonsurgical ablation of the parathyroid adenoma can be accomplished, but is reserved for cases when surgical intervention is not feasible or has failed. Currently available techniques include transarterial catheter ablation (see the chapter by Doppman).

Medical Measures

Medical treatment cannot yet ablate the adenoma or effectively inhibit its function. One hope for this would be to target the parathyroid cell membrane calcium receptor with a high-affinity agonist, either a long-lived antibody or stereospecific drug. Other cell types might also utilize this receptor; however, and the consequences of long-term interaction with it would have to be assessed. For example, the osteoclast is capable of sensing the ambient calcium level and may carry the calcium receptor (64). If the latter is true, a parallel inhibition of the osteoclast might ensue, and the long-term consequences of low bone remodeling would need careful assessment. Medical therapies for primary hyperparathyroidism, proposed for use when surgery is contraindicated, refused, or deemed unnecessary, represent attempts to reduce morbidity of the chronic biochemical abnormality, as discussed in the chapter by Stock and Marcus and elsewhere (4,6,65–68).

Histology

Common Findings

Many sources illustrate the usual histologic appearance of the parathyroid adenoma (69–71) (see the chapter by LiVolsi).

Histologic Variants of the Adenoma

Not all parathyroid adenomas are of the chief cell or mixed variety. Rare variants include the oxyphil adenoma, the cystic adenoma, and the lipoadenoma. To this author's knowledge, water-clear cell adenomas have not yet been reported.

Oxyphil parathyroid adenomas are usually nonfunctional. The oxyphilic staining characteristic results from the presence of a large number of mitochondria (70). Nonfunctional oxyphil adenomas stain positively for PTH by immunofluorescence (72) but do not secrete enough hormone to cause hypercalcemia, probably correlating with the fact that electron microscopy of normal oxyphil cells shows few secretory granules (70). With age, the normal human parathyroid gland develops clusters or nodules of oxyphil cells, which are nonfunctional and probably should not be classed as neoplasms (70). Exactly how large an oxyphilic nodule should be to receive the diagnosis of oxyphil adenoma, however, is not clear. When a nonfunctional oxyphil adenoma occurs within the thyroid, histologic differentiation from a thyroid Hürthle cell tumor can be difficult, but staining for PTH and thyroglobulin will be diagnostic (73).

The oxyphil adenoma may cause primary hyperparathyroidism, but only 23 functional oxyphil adenomas were reported to 1981 (73,74). The functional oxyphil adenoma differs in that it does contain secretory granules. There are no unique biochemical changes associated with the functional oxyphil adenoma, however, and it is usually diagnosed histologically after routine resection done to treat hyperparathyroidism.

Parathyroid adenomas occasionally show cystic changes, which are traditionally attributed to local infarcts (70). Small pseudofollicles are common in adenomas and should not be confused with cysts. The presence of one or two isolated cysts within an adenoma may be attributable to infarction, especially if hemosiderin laden macrophages are seen in and near the cyst. This tumor should be labeled a *parathyroid adenoma with cystic change*. A rare parathyroid adenoma will be riddled with multiple cysts of varying sizes, giving it a Swiss-cheese appearance, but without hemosiderin or other evidence of prior infarction. This is a true "cystic parathyroid adenoma." Cystic adenomas may be familial (see below) and are an indication for family screening.

Parathyroid adenomas usually contain little interspersed fat tissue, unlike the normal parathyroid gland, but some may contain a large amount of fat. One palpable but nonfunctional parathyroid adenoma was reported histologically to show a large amount of interspersed fat and was labeled a *parathyroid hamartoma* (75). Other parathyroid tumors with a similar histologic appearance, but functional, have since been described (76,77) and were variously termed *lipadenoma, lipoadenoma,* or *adenolipoma.* The genesis of the fatty tissue component is unknown. There are no recognized clinical findings that predict such a tumor preoperatively, but it seems likely that the appearance of such a tumor on sonography or magnetic resonance imaging (MRI) might be distinctive.

MULTIPLE PARATHYROID ADENOMAS

Definition

A second or rarely a third parathyroid adenoma can develop in the same patient, either at the same time (synchronously) or at different times (metachronously) (69,78–80). The diagnosis of synchronous double adenomas is made when two enlarged and at least two normal parathyroid glands are documented at the same operation. Proving that nonresected parathyroid glands are of normal size is difficult, however, so one must hold in reserve the possibility that asymmetric hyperplasia is at fault. A diagnosis of synchronous triple adenomas will always be suspect, since this anatomic finding would more likely represent hyperplasia. It would be impossible to prove that the single normal-sized gland was normal without resecting or extensively biopsying it, with the attendant risk of hypoparathyroidism. Triple parathyroid adenomas thus can be diagnosed with certainty only when the adenomas are metachronous.

For the diagnosis of metachronous adenomas, resection of the first adenoma should restore normocalcemia and normal PTH values for at least 6 months before the recurrence is detected. With strict criteria, the incidence of multiple adenomas was 1.7–1.9% (78,79). Attie et al. (80) observed that in seven published series multiple adenomas were said to account for 3.9% of 2,123 cases of primary hyperparathyroidism, probably reflecting use of less stringent criteria (80). The double adenomas were synchronous in 28 of 865 patients (3.2%) and metachronous in five of 865 (0.58%), and the delay before appearance of the second adenoma was 3–18 years (80). This incidence of metachronous second adenoma is the same as the rate of recurrence after surgical resection of a parathyroid adenoma that this author has estimated from the literature (0.6%) (4).

Etiology

Multiple parathyroid adenomas may be familial (see below), but no other specific cause has been reported. All patients with multiple adenomas should undergo thorough family screening. I have suggested the term *adenomatosis* be applied when a familial condition predisposes to metachronous double or triple adenomas (81). The cellular defects leading to the occurrence of sporadic or familial multiple parathyroid adenomas are unknown and will be difficult to establish in view of the rarity of this condition.

Treatment

The only cure for multiple parathyroid adenomas is surgical resection of each lesion. Each metachronous adenoma will require its own operation. Synchronous double adenomas need to be detected at first operation. This can usually be accomplished by routine bilateral neck exploration or by selective bilateral explorations in cases when preoperative ultrasonographic examination suggests bilateral disease (by surgeons who prefer the unilateral approach for the majority of cases). Parathyroid surgery is discussed extensively in the chapter by Norton et al. Long-term postoperative follow-up of patients with synchronous double adenomas is important, both to help establish the diagnosis (normal calcium homeostasis demonstrated at six months after surgery) and to detect a metachronous third adenoma at the earliest possible time.

Histology

The histologic appearance of each of the double parathyroid adenomas is not remarkable, except in families with cystic parathyroid adenomatosis (discussed below) (81).

PARATHYROID CARCINOMA

The clinical syndrome produced by the parathyroid carcinoma is discussed in the chapter by Shane. Parathyroid carcinoma is rare, accounting for <1% of all parathyroid neoplasms (82,83). Unlike most adenomas, it shows unrestrained growth, is often palpable, and usually presents with severe hypercalcemia. Additionally it tends to be locally invasive and often has the ability to metastasize. The tumor tends to recur months or years after its primary resection, either locally or with metastasis to bone, lung, liver, or adrenal. The major morbidity is usually from severe hyperparathyroidism rather than tumor mass, so that aggressive surgery to reduce the whole body tumor burden, even if not curative, may benefit the patient by controlling the hyperparathyroidism.

A few parathyroid carcinomas are classed as nonfunctional since they do not cause hypercalcemia (70,84). They present as a neck or mediastinal mass and can be identified postoperatively by their histologic appearance. Normal serum PTH values have

been reported in a few of these cases, but the origin of the tumor can usually be proved by immunostaining to show the presence of PTH and absence of thyroglobulin (84–87). Electron microscopy of these tumors would be of interest to seek evidence of abnormalities in the secretory apparatus. Measurement of serum PTH with assays of varying specificity might be used to test whether the tumor secretes fragments of PTH that lack calcemic activity. Assays for serum human chorionic gonadotropin (hCG) subunits, calcitonin, and other peptides should also be done in these cases, since the carcinoma might secrete these without PTH (see below). Measurement of these peptides or of inactive PTH fragments could then serve as a useful index of tumor bulk.

Etiology

The cellular abnormalities causing the unrestrained growth of the parathyroid carcinoma and its ability to metastasize will be difficult to determine because the lesion is rare. Study of the expression of various oncogenes is indicated. One parathyroid carcinoma was shown to express receptors for platelet-derived growth factor-β (88). Abnormal expression of such a receptor might convert a normal constituent of the milieu of the tumor into a continuous stimulus to growth. Unfortunately, no control parathyroid tissues were examined in this report.

The ability of melanomas, stomach and colon carcinomas, and other malignancies to invade capillary basement membranes and metastasize is determined in part by the ability to synthesize type IV collagenase (89–92) and is enhanced by decreased secretion of tissue inhibitors of this collagenase (93). Study of type IV collagenase and its inhibitors in a series of parathyroid carcinomas, adenomas, and hyperplastic glands would be of interest.

Possible etiologies of the parathyroid carcinoma include familial syndromes (reviewed below) and environmental insults. Exposure of animals to chemical carcinogens produced parathyroid hyperplasia (94), but no parathyroid carcinomas were reported. Radiation of experimental animals can produce parathyroid carcinomas, parathyroid adenomas, or hyperplasia (95–98). One report has suggested an increased incidence of parathyroid carcinoma in humans after irradiation. In a series of 1,550 consecutive parathyroid surgery patients, ten patients had a known history of head and neck irradiation, and three of the ten had a parathyroid carcinoma (99). At least three other cases of parathyroid carcinoma have been reported in radiation-exposed patients (29,100,101), but it cannot be concluded from these data alone that radiation is a definite risk factor.

Parathyroid tumors that seem to be locally invasive or show histologic changes suggestive of parathyroid carcinoma may develop in patients with chronic renal failure, but it is not clear that these are carcinomas (102). Metastasis was reported in only one case, and this patient had previously received neck irradiation (29).

Treatment

The only cure is surgical. Recognition of the carcinoma at the time of initial operation and its proper resection en bloc is the best hope for cure. These tumors tend to be hard and to be fibrosed to surrounding structures, sometimes the only clue that one is dealing with a carcinoma. Attempts to free up the tumor or a rupture of its capsule are sure to produce local recurrence.

Recurrences or metastases can be treated with aggressive debulking surgery. Antiresorptive agents (plicamycin, bisphosphonates, or calcitonin) can help control the hypercalcemia and minimize the impact on the skeleton, although they have little if any antitumor activity. Parathyroid carcinoma has been regarded as resistant to nonsurgical modalities. Radiation therapy has not been effective (83,103). Chemotherapy should be considered, however, for the patient whose surgical options have elapsed. Three different patients have now been reported to respond. One had a 5 month remission of pulmonary metastases and hypercalcemia after cyclophosphamide, fluorouracil, and dacarbazine (104). Two had partial remissions of nonfunctioning parathyroid carcinomas, one after cyclophosphamide, methotrexate, adriamycin, and lomustine (CCNU) (105) and the other after cyclophosphamide, methotrexate, mitoxandrone, and CCNU (85).

Histology

The histologic features thought to distinguish the parathyroid carcinoma from the adenoma were synthesized by Schantz and Castleman (106) and are reviewed in the chapters by LiVolsi and by Shane. These included a trabecular or palisading pattern in the arrangement of parenchymal cells, mitotic figures in parenchymal cells, thick fibrous bands coursing through the tumor, and invasion of the capsule or blood vessels by tumor cells. The likelihood of malignancy increases roughly in proportion to the number of these features present, but no one feature is diagnostic. The presence of cellular pleomorphism or nuclear atypia is not helpful in differentiating parathyroid adenoma from carcinoma, since adenomas often contain regions that show significant pleomorphism, atypical cells, or both (106),

and the cellular pattern is usually more uniform in carcinomas than in adenomas (70,82).

It is difficult or impossible to distinguish invasion of the capsule from simple entrapment of a nest of parathyroid cells within the capsule (107,108). Thus capsular invasion does not identify the tumor as a carcinoma unless it has progressed into the surrounding tissue. The presence of parenchymal cells within a vessel is no longer regarded as a valid criterion of endocrine malignancy, unless they are clearly located beyond the boundaries of the tumor (107,109). Van Heerden et al. (82) concluded that a trabecular arrangement of parathyroid cells is probably the least helpful criterion, whereas the most helpful may be a "fibrous, inflammatory-like reaction." Thick, fibrous trabeculae may be found in parathyroid adenomas, however, especially those developing after neck irradiation (29).

The presence of mitoses in a parathyroid tumor originally was considered almost diagnostic for carcinoma, since mitoses are rare in benign parathyroid glands (106). Mitoses can occur, however, in benign parathyroid lesions; Lawrence (71) found "very small numbers" of mitoses in 1 of 35 parathyroid adenomas and in three of 18 hyperplastic glands from renal failure patients. Quantification of the mitoses may be helpful diagnostically. In another series, two of 17 adenomas and two of ten hyperplastic glands contained more than one mitosis per ten high-power microscopic fields, but none showed more than four mitoses per ten high-power fields (110). Additional quantitative studies are needed, but for now the presence of mitoses probably should not be taken as evidence for parathyroid carcinoma unless there are more than four mitoses per ten high-power fields.

Several factors might influence the number of mitoses in the parathyroid glands. Mitoses should be more frequent if the gland is actively growing at the time it is resected. This might apply to the parathyroid glands of a renal failure patient or an adenoma that was resected during its period of active clonal expansion or after serum calcium has been lowered below the new set point by medical treatment. A study is needed to determine whether the number of observed mitoses does in fact correlate with the clinical stage of the adenoma (difficult to determine) or with preoperative treatment. In a prospective study, preoperative treatments could be assigned at random either to maintain or to lower serum calcium for a few days before surgery. The degree of tetraploidy of the tumor (see below) and its rate of tritiated thymidine incorporation (34) could also be monitored in this study. Until better diagnostic criteria are developed, long-term postsurgical follow-up for the rare patients with severe primary hyperparathyroidism or tumors with suspicious histology is mandatory so that any recurrence can be detected early.

PRIMARY PARATHYROID HYPERPLASIA

Definition and Clinical Features

Hypercalcemic hyperparathyroidism can be caused by an idiopathic generalized enlargement of the parathyroid glands, primary parathyroid hyperplasia. Water-clear cell hyperplasia was recognized first (111), and primary chief cell hyperplasia was described more than 20 years later (112). The clinical presentation of primary parathyroid hyperplasia is indistinguishable from that of the parathyroid adenoma.

Etiology

Hereditary syndromes, especially MEN-I, account for roughly one-half of the cases of primary parathyroid hyperplasia. The etiology of sporadic primary parathyroid hyperplasia is not known, but the stimulus must be a generalized one. In MEN-I a circulating mitogenic factor has been identified, but it seems unlikely that this factor accounts for any of the sporadic cases. The parathyroid cell's inhibitory set point for calcium is usually normal in sporadic parathyroid hyperplasia (33), although more studies are needed. Hyperplastic parathyroid glands, but not parathyroid adenomas, may have high-affinity binding sites for epidermal growth factor (113), but whether occupancy of these putative receptors will stimulate function or growth of the parathyroid cells has not been reported.

Might a circulating antibody stimulate generalized parathyroid growth? An antibody that inhibits PTH secretion has been identified in patients with waxing and waning hypoparathyroidism (47,114). By analogy to Graves' disease, an antibody directed toward a different part of the calcium receptor might be able to stimulate PTH secretion and cell division.

Treatment

The usual surgical approach to parathyroid hyperplasia has been a near total parathyroidectomy (see chapter by Norton et al.), the goal being to secure normal calcium homeostasis by leaving in situ an ~120 mg viable remnant of the most normal-appearing parathyroid gland. Transcervical thymectomy is an essential part of this surgery, to minimize the number of missed supernumerary glands (115,116). The incidence of hypoparathyroidism after this approach is ~10%, with a similar incidence of persistent or recurrent hyperparathyroidism (117). A recurrence necessitates a second operation through the scar tissue from the first, so the risk of injury to the recurrent laryngeal nerve is increased, as is the incidence of postoperative hypoparathyroidism, which may approach 25% (117).

A better method is total parathyroidectomy with transcervical thymectomy and grafting of autogenous parathyroid tissue to a muscle in the forearm (118–121). The autogenous graft comprises 10 to 20 fragments of tissue, approximately 1 × 2 mm each, prepared by carefully slicing the most normal appearing parathyroid gland, which has been chilled to increase its firmness to facilitate cutting. Ten individual pockets are prepared in the muscle, and each receives one or two parathyroid fragments, after which the muscle sheath is closed with a loop of nonresorbable suture to prevent extrusion and to mark the site. These grafts survive by diffusion of oxygen from the muscle capillary bed until they receive their own capillary ingrowth at ~10–20 days (119). During the period of temporary aparathyroidism, the patient must be managed closely to avoid tetany. Oral administration of calcitriol and calcium supplements is used for ~4–6 weeks to keep serum calcium values between 8.0 and 9.0 mg/dl. The incidence of permanent hypoparathyroidism after autogenous grafting is probably below 1% (118). Late graft failure has not yet been reported.

Serum PTH must be measured on the first or second day after surgery to prove that the parathyroidectomy was complete. A normal or elevated early postoperative PTH value shows that a missed parathyroid gland remains in situ in the neck or mediastinum, and this gland must be dealt with first in the event of recurrent hyperparathyroidism. If the postoperative PTH value was low as expected, recurrent hyperparathyroidism will direct attention to the graft, a portion of which can be resected with the patient under local anesthesia.

The recurrence rate is relatively low in sporadic cases of primary parathyroid hyperplasia, so that parathyroid autogenous grafting offers mainly the advantage of a lower incidence of hypoparathyroidism. In MEN-I, however, the recurrence rate is high (117,121), and autogenous grafting is the procedure of choice. Thus preoperative identification of MEN-I patients is important. Any patient found by preoperative ultrasonography to have parathyroid hyperplasia should undergo a full preoperative assessment (and detailed family screening) to rule out occult MEN-I.

Histology

Chief cell hyperplasia is the most common variety. Oxyphil cell hyperplasia has not been reported to my knowledge. Water-clear cell hyperplasia was reported in ~4% of cases of primary hyperparathyroidism in the early Massachusetts General Hospital series, but now appears to be rare (69,70). The reason for its virtual disappearance is unknown. These patients seemed prone to present with nephrolithiasis (70), but it is not known whether this is a feature peculiar to water-clear cell hyperplasia or whether the apparent association derived from the fact that these early series were compiled at a time when stone clinic populations were being screened for hypercalcemia soon after the discovery of stone disease as a complication of hyperparathyroidism.

Cystic parathyroid hyperplasia causing hypercalcemic hyperparathyroidism has been reported at least twice (122,123). One patient had four parathyroid cysts, two associated with hyperplastic nodules of parathyroid tissue. The other patient had four hyperplastic glands, two with multiple cystic spaces. In neither case was the family history reported, so one might wonder whether one or both of these patients had familial cystic parathyroid adenomatosis (see below). Fat tissue is usually missing from hyperplastic parathyroid glands, but lipohyperplasia, a form of parathyroid hyperplasia, in which each gland has a generous component of fat tissue, has been reported as a cause of hypercalcemic hyperparathyroidism in a few cases (77).

SECONDARY PARATHYROID HYPERPLASIA

Definition

Secondary hyperplasia of the parathyroid glands arises as a compensatory response to hypocalcemia or a deficiency of $1,25\text{-OH}_2\text{D}$ or its action. The associated clinical syndrome is termed *secondary hyperparathyroidism* or *compensatory hyperparathyroidism*.

Clinical Manifestations

Symptoms that may occur in patients with secondary hyperparathyroidism can be categorized as (a) those of the underlying disease; (b) those of hypocalcemia, including circumoral and acral paresthesias and carpopedal spasm; (c) neuromuscular symptoms, especially proximal muscular weakness (124); and (d) the pain of hyperparathyroid bone disease or the concomitant osteomalacia. Children also may manifest growth retardation and clinical rickets.

Hypocalcemia, hypophosphatemia, or both are present in secondary hyperparathyroidism of nonrenal origin, and serum alkaline phosphatase activity of bone origin is usually increased by the time the diagnosis is made. Hyperchloremic acidosis is almost always present, since the renal tubular maximum for bicarbonate reabsorption has been reduced by both the excess PTH and the hypocalcemia.

To seek the cause of hypocalcemia or hypophosphatemia, measurement of serum ionized calcium, 25-hydroxyvitamin D, $1,25(\text{OH})_2\text{D}$, and PTH are needed.

Almost by definition, hypocalcemia or low serum $1,25\text{-OH}_2\text{D}$ values or both should be present, since these are the factors to which the parathyroid gland responds. Serum PTH values will be increased if the PTH assay is sensitive enough at least to discriminate between normal and slightly elevated values.

Serum 25-hydroxyvitamin D concentrations correlate well with overall vitamin D nutrition. A more sensitive means to detect mild degrees of hypocalcemic hyperparathyroidism, however, is to measure serum ionized calcium and PTH values, which will often be abnormal before the 25-hydroxyvitamin D value reaches its lower normal limit. Ionized calcium measurement may demonstrate mild hypocalcemia when total serum calcium values are still normal.

Circulating $1,25(\text{OH})_2\text{D}$ is not always decreased in concentration in compensatory hyperparathyroidism. It may instead be increased if there is resistance to $1,25(\text{OH})_2\text{D}$ action (as with a defective vitamin D receptor) or after instituting treatment of vitamin D deficiency. As vitamin D deficiency develops, three factors drive renal $1\text{-}\alpha$-hydroxylation: the rise in PTH, the fall in serum phosphate, and possibly the fall in serum calcium. Thus, serum $1,25(\text{OH})_2\text{D}$ values are maintained until the vitamin deficiency is severe. With institution of treatment, a small increment in the serum 25-hydroxyvitamin D concentration will produce a great increase in $1,25(\text{OH})_2\text{D}$ synthesis (125). Serum values will increase above normal until the physiologic need for increased intestinal calcium absorption has resolved.

Etiology

Hypocalcemia has been regarded traditionally as the proximate cause of secondary parathyroid hyperplasia, but deficiency of $1,25(\text{OH})_2\text{D}$ also stimulates PTH secretion and proliferation of parathyroid cells and is an important factor in many types of secondary parathyroid hyperplasia. Low $1,25(\text{OH})_2\text{D}$ levels decrease the sensitivity of the parathyroid cell to calcium (126) and, as in hypocalcemia, will increase prepro-PTH mRNA levels (127–130). How these changes might be coupled to a proliferative response is not known.

Deficiency of $1,25(\text{OH})_2\text{D}$ action may occur because of deficiency or malabsorption of vitamin D itself, increased hepatic catabolism or enterohepatic losses of vitamin D and 25-hydroxyvitamin D, defects in the hepatic 25-hydroxylation of vitamin D, defects in the renal 1α-hydroxylation of 25-hydroxyvitamin D, or resistance to $1,25(\text{OH})_2\text{D}$ action.

The parathyroid glands in secondary hyperparathyroidism show generalized chief cell hyperplasia, but nodules eventually develop. This change may correlate with the development of a degree of secretory autonomy. An increase in the calcium inhibitory set point of glands with nodular hyperplasia that were removed from renal failure patients has been demonstrated (131,132). This functional autonomy may progress to the point of producing hypercalcemia, a situation that has been called *tertiary hyperparathyroidism.* Clinically it is hard to say exactly when the transition to tertiary hyperparathyroidism occurs or, in a given patient with hypercalcemia, to exclude all other factors that might contribute to hypercalcemia, such as a recent improvement in phosphate restriction or vitamin D status (133). For these reasons, Oliver Cope (134), who originated the term *tertiary hyperparathyroidism,* later suggested that it be abandoned in favor of a more precise description of the exact clinical situation.

Treatment

The most effective treatment of secondary hyperparathyroidism is to correct the predisposing condition, when possible. Adequate amounts of 1,25(OH)$_2$D, calcium, and phosphate should be provided to allow the skeleton to heal and the parathyroid hyperplasia to regress (treatment is discussed in detail in the chapter by Coburn and Salusky).

Histology

The histology of secondary hyperparathyroidism is that of generalized chief cell hyperplasia. For unclear reasons, the right side parathyroid glands tend to be slightly more enlarged than the left (135). Nodular changes occur later and become especially prominent in patients with autonomous or hypercalcemic ("tertiary") hyperparathyroidism (136).

UNUSUAL SECRETORY PRODUCTS OF PARATHYROID TUMORS

Secretory Products

The normal adult parathyroid gland secretes the products of at least two genes, the PTH and chromogranin A (CgA) genes. PTH is synthesized as a preprohormone and is released after cleavage of the "pro-" piece. The resulting main secretory product is a straight-chain 84-amino-acid peptide, intact PTH, or PTH (1–84). Fragments of the PTH molecule are also secreted, most of which are truncated at both ends in humans (137). The more biologically important of these truncations is probably the cleavage of at least 27 amino acids from the amino-terminal end, the region responsible for the calcemic action of the hormone.

Intact PTH is secreted as an inverse sigmoidal function of the ambient calcium concentration. Serum calcium concentration also governs the secreted ratio of intact PTH to PTH fragments (138,139). Hypocalcemia increases the percentage of intact hormone, while hypercalcemia decreases it. Teleologically, it is sensible to emphasize secretion of the calcium elevating hormonal species when hypocalcemia prevails, but the mechanisms by which this adjustment is accomplished are not understood. An important factor may be the dwell time of the secretory granule within the parathyroid cell before secretion, but alterations in proteolytic activity have not been excluded.

Deficiency of 1,25-OH$_2$D promotes PTH synthesis and secretion, at least in part by rendering the gland less sensitive to the extracellular ionized calcium concentration, and, as in hypocalcemia, will promote parathyroid cell division and the development of parathyroid hyperplasia. Other factors such as catecholamines can stimulate the acute release of PTH but do not seem to increase hormone synthesis or produce a sustained rise in secretion (140). These factors are not known to have any importance in the genesis or function of the parathyroid adenoma.

A second parathyroid secretory product was identified by chromatography of parathyroid culture media and initially termed *parathyroid secretory protein-I* (141,142). This same protein was independently found as a secretory product of other peptide-secreting tissues and the adrenal medulla and is now called *chromogranin A* (143,144). The parathyroid version of this glycoprotein differs from the chromogranin A of other tissues chiefly in the degree of tyrosine sulfation and carbohydrate composition. It is a large molecule of ≈ 450 amino acids and is costored and cosecreted with PTH (see the chapter by Cohn et al.).

The concentration of chromogranin A in serum is increased in many patients with tumors of chromaffin cell origin and is sometimes increased in parathyroid adenoma patients (144,145). The chomogranin A level in hyperparathyroid patients, however, may be of islet cell origin, since resection of the hyperfunctional parathyroid tissue decreases plasma chromogranin A values only in patients with the Zollinger-Ellison syndrome, in which a fall in serum calcium is known to reduce the pathological gastrin secretion (146).

The function of chromogranin A is not known. It contains the sequences for pancreastatin, β-granin, and chromostatin, and in different species contains eight to ten conserved pairs of basic amino acids, suggesting that it may serve as a hormone precursor. Pancreastatin can inhibit low-calcium-stimulated bovine or porcine PTH secretion, but bovine and porcine parathyroid cells do not secrete detectable amounts of pancreastatin (147,148). In bovine parathyroid cells, a conserved Lys-Arg site at residues 114–115 is used to generate a β-granin-like peptide that is secreted. This peptide also has the ability to inhibit low-calcium-stimulated PTH secretion and must be considered a potential autocrine regulator of parathyroid function (149). Peripheral measurements of β-granin immunoreactivity in hyperparathyroid patients have not to this author's knowledge been reported. The third biologically active peptide, chromostatin, will inhibit nicotine stimulated secretion of catecholamine by adrenal cells but does not affect PTH secretion (148).

A final class of proteins that can be secreted by normal parathyroid tissue is the plasminogen activators. Hyperplastic human parathyroid glands from renal insufficiency patients secrete tissue-type plasminogen activator (tPA), while normal bovine parathyroid cells secrete a similar enzyme, urokinase-type plasminogen activator (uPA) (150). Calcium regulates the secretion of tPA or uPA by these cells exactly in parallel with that of PTH. Other tissues are known to secrete tPA in one species and uPA in another species. These plasminogen activators are postulated to play a role as autocrine regulators of growth, matrix remodeling, or angiogenesis by interacting with factors present in the extracellular milieu, for example, by releasing or activating latent proteases or growth factors in the matrix. Activation of basic fibroblast growth factor might account for the angiogenesis that can be stimulated by parathyroid tissue (150,151). The potential secretion of tPA by human parathyroid adenomas and carcinomas will be a fertile field for investigation. Might the fibrotic reaction observed around the parathyroid carcinoma be caused by secretion of high levels of tPA?

Normal or abnormal parathyroid tissue may synthesize or secrete other peptides. Fetal parathyroid glands of some species are rich in PTHrP (152,153), but in situ hybridization studies failed to detect PTHrP mRNA in the fetal rat parathyroid (154). Nevertheless, rat parathyroid cell lines that secrete PTHrP instead of PTH have been established (155,156). The expression of PTHrP in normal parathyroid glands of human adults is suppressed, as judged either by immunochemical staining or assay of gland extracts. PTHrP messenger RNA (mRNA) may be overexpressed in parathyroid adenomas (157,158), and the peptide itself can often be identified in parathyroid adenomas by immunohistochemical staining for PTHrP-(1–34) and PTHrP-(50–69) though not for PTHrP-(106–141) (159). Parathyroid extracts, however, contain 100-fold less PTHrP than PTH immunoreactivity (158). The cells that stain for PTHrP in adenomas tend to be found in nodules or clusters, usually in areas that contain a high number of oxyphil cells (160). Immunohistochemical stains for PTHrP were negative in parathyroid glands from six patients with primary parathyroid hyperplasia (159), but the peptide could be detected in extracts by immunoassay, again in very low abundance relative to

PTH (158). PTHrP is probably rarely secreted by pathologic human parathyroid tissue in sufficient quantity to contribute to hypercalcemia, since serum PTHrP values are very rarely increased in patients with primary hyperparathyroidism (161–163). Study of the rare functional oxyphil adenoma for PTHrP secretion would be of interest.

Other peptides not normally associated with the parathyroid gland at any stage of development have been identified in parathyroid tumors. Parathyroid carcinomas may occasionally secrete calcitonin (164). Calcitonin gene-related peptide (CGRP) can be identified in parathyroid glands, but only in the capsule and in nerve fibers apposed directly to parathyroid parenchymal cells (165). It has been hypothesized that CGRP might be a mediator of neural influences of PTH secretion. Secretion of CGRP by a parathyroid parenchymal cell or by parathyroid tumors to this author's knowledge has not been reported.

Gastrin (both G-17 and G-34) has been found in parathyroid adenomas by RIA of tumor extracts or by immunohistochemistry. In one study gastrin was found histochemically in adenomas from four of 11 patients, located in cytoplasmic vesicles in scattered parathyroid cells (166), but it seems unlikely that gastrin is ever secreted by parathyroid tumors in sufficient quantities to have systemic effects.

Somatostatin was found in six of 21 parathyroid adenomas and in a parathyroid carcinoma (167). Again, it seems unlikely that somatostatin is ever secreted from parathyroid tumors in quantities large enough to act systemically, but somatostatin was reported to suppress PTH secretion in vivo and in vitro (168), suggesting a possible autocrine role for the peptide. Little further study of this question has been carried out, but octreotide treatment of a patient with parathyroid hyperplasia was recently reported to normalize serum calcium and to reduce serum PTH values markedly (68).

Parathyroid carcinomas may secrete both subunits of hCG (169,170). Six of eight patients with MEN-I and islet cell tumors had high serum α-subunit concentrations, with an additional increase in β-hCG in one case. In >50 patients with primary hyperparathyroidism caused by adenoma or hyperplasia, circulating hCG subunits were normal. Thus, the finding of an elevated α- or β-hCG level in a hypercalcemic patient would suggest either parathyroid carcinoma or MEN-I with an islet cell tumor. Whether sporadic islet cell tumors make hCG was not reported.

One parathyroid carcinoma secreting β-hCG was glucocorticoid responsive (170). The administration of prednisolone, 30 mg daily for 4 days, suppressed both serum PTH (to normal) and β-hCG (nearly to normal). Perhaps the genes for PTH and β-hCG had somehow come under the influence of an inhibitory glucocorticoid response element, a hypothesis that could be tested with modern techniques. It is not known whether glucocorticoid responsiveness will always correlate with β-hCG secretion, so suppression should probably be attempted in other cases of parathyroid carcinoma with or without β-hCG secretion. Control of hypercalcemia would be beneficial in the management of the patient, even if there were no tumoristic effect. This is one situation in which normalization of serum calcium by glucocorticoid would not rule out primary hyperparathyroidism.

Eleven of 28 patients with parathyroid adenomas were reported to have high serum pancreatic polypeptide values, which decreased to normal in ten of the patients after successful parathyroidectomy (171). Although nine of 19 human parathyroid culture media contained immunoreactive pancreatic polypeptide (172), the fact that there was a parallel fall in serum gastrin and pancreatic polypeptide after parathyroidectomy suggests a pancreatic rather than a parathyroid origin for the peptide in serum (171). Patients with MEN-I may show increased pancreatic polypeptide levels or increased pancreatic polypeptide release after a test meal, a change that may be the earliest biochemical manifestation of the trait, even before hypercalcemia appears (173). Basal pancreatic polypeptide values have little specificity or sensitivity, however, since levels were increased in 54% of MEN-I patients with islet cell tumors and in patients with hepatic metastases of sporadic islet cell tumors (174).

PARATHYROID CYSTS

Parathyroid tissue can give rise to a fluid-filled structure, the parathyroid cyst. The nature of the cyst can be identified by showing that its fluid contains a higher PTH concentration than a simultaneous serum sample or that the cyst wall contains islands of parathyroid parenchyma (175). The parathyroid cyst should be differentiated from a cystic parathyroid adenoma (an otherwise solid adenoma containing numerous small cystic areas), and from a parathyroid adenoma with cystic change (an adenoma in which one or two nodules have infarcted to form cystic areas) (69,70) (Table 1).

The parathyroid cyst may present as a mass, as a cause of hypercalcemic hyperparathyroidism, or as an incidental finding during neck surgery or an imaging procedure carried out for an unrelated indication. It may be mistaken for a thyroid nodule or other cervical mass or may appear on a chest radiograph as a mediastinal mass (176–178).

Unlike parathyroid adenomas, parathyroid cysts are more common in men, with a male to female ratio of ~1.6 (179). Overall they are rare, but their exact inci-

TABLE 1. *Tentative classification of parathyroid cysts*

Ontogenous parathyroid cyst	Contains clear colorless fluid; thin wall containing smooth muscle; wall sometimes contains elements of thymic or lymphoid tissue or small nests of parathyroid cells separate from the single layer of lining cells
Coalescence parathyroid cyst	Lining layer more than one cell thick; fluid serous or serosanguineous; if arising in an adenoma, may have own pseudocapsule, separate from capsule of adenoma
Parathyroid pseudocyst	Variant of the adenoma with cystic change; here a single infarcted area occupies most of the adenoma volume; fluid is brown; fluid and adjacent tissue usually contain hemosiderin-laden macrophages; wall is of fibrous tissue often admixed with nests of parathyroid cells
Differentiate from	
Parathyroid adenoma	One-half or more will harbor a few small pseudofollicles
Cystic parathyroid adenoma	Parechyma of adenoma studded with multiple small cysts
Adenoma with cystic change	Adenoma with one or more areas of prior infarction, each leaving a cyst filled with brown fluid

dence is debatable, varying from 0.08% to 3.4% in various series (Table 2).

Classification of Parathyroid Cysts

There is probably more than one type of parathyroid cyst. This author has proposed classifying them into three categories based on the presumptive mechanism of cyst formation (102) (Table 1). The mechanism of parathyroid cyst formation will require more study before final adoption of these categories.

Ontogenous Parathyroid Cysts

The ontogenous parathyroid cyst is one that develops from vestigial remnants of the third or fourth branchial clefts (175). It is an encapsulated, thin-walled cyst containing a clear, colorless ("water-clear") fluid and is lined with a single layer of cuboidal cells resting

TABLE 2. *Observed incidence of parathyroid cysts*

Authors (reference)	Type of observation	Incidence (%)
Welti (180)	12,000 thyroid operations	0.08
Randel et al. (181)	235 abnormal parathyroids seen by sonography	0.4
Gilmour (182)	428 autopsies for study of parathyroid anatomy	2.8
Calandra et al. (183)	325 patients undergoing parathyroid operations	3.4

on smooth muscle. The lining cells have the appearance of parathyroid parenchymal cells by light microscopy and presumably secrete PTH, which can be measured in the cyst fluid in moderately increased levels. The ontogenous cyst is thought to develop as an anomaly during embryological development. By electron microscopy, its lining cells resemble those cells that line the microscopic cysts (pseudofollicles or "acinal units") present in normal parathyroid glands and adenomas. Both cell types have few secretory organelles and show microvilli and terminal bars at the luminal surface (22,70,184), and both are thought to be derived from the lining cells of the canals of Kürsteiner, the embryonic ducts that connect the thymic and parathyroid primordia of branchial pouches 3 and 4 during development.

The wall of the ontogenous parathyroid cyst often contains separate islands of parathyroid tissue, another possible source for the PTH within the cyst, and may contain other elements derived from branchial pouches 3 or 4, specifically islands of thymic or lymphoid tissue. Ontogenous cysts may very rarely cause primary hyperparathyroidism, when an island of parathyroid cells in the cyst wall has undergone adenomatous change.

Coalescence Parathyroid Cysts

The coalescence parathyroid cyst has been assumed to form via the "coalescence of microcysts" within an otherwise normal parathyroid gland or an adenoma. It may be lined with cells similar to those lining the ontogenous cyst, but the lining layer will be several cells thick and should not rest on a layer of smooth muscle. This may be the type of cyst that contains clear yellow (serous) or serosanguineous fluid. A coalescence cyst arising in an adenoma will be associated with primary hyperparathyroidism and may have a fibrous pseudocapsule separate from the capsule of the adenoma (185). The coalescence cyst may enlarge considerably relative to the original parathyroid adenoma, which may be pushed aside and appear as a "remnant" of parathyroid tissue (though of increased total weight) in the cyst wall. If the cyst arises in a normal gland, there will be less associated parathyroid tissue, the

patient will be normocalcemic, and the pseudocapsule of the cyst and the capsule of the gland may be indistinguishable.

It is unclear how a group of microcysts might coalesce to form a large cyst. This author has proposed an alternate hypothesis in which this parathyroid cyst is indeed derived from a microcyst or acinal unit, but not by coalescence. It may form after one of the lining cells has undergone a functional or neoplastic transformation that causes it to secrete more "pseudofollicular" fluid than normal or to proliferate more rapidly. Either change would serve as the driving force to enlarge the cyst. If this neoplastic change happened also to increase the set point for inhibition by calcium, it might increase cell proliferation enough to cause an adenoma.

Parathyroid Pseudocysts

The third presumptive mechanism for parathyroid cyst formation is infarction within a parathyroid adenoma. If small infarctions have produced several cystic areas, the lesion should be labeled an adenoma with cystic change. A large infarction, however, might produce a single large cyst occupying most of the volume within the parathyroid capsule. This "parathyroid pseudocyst" will usually be associated with primary hyperparathyroidism, unless the infarction had obliterated essentially the entire adenoma (parathyroid apoplexy). Parathyroid pseudocysts will have a thick "wall" made up of the residual parathyroid tissue, often admixed with fibrous scar tissue (185). The cyst cavity may appear to have a fibrous lining, but this may be minimally or not at all organized and probably represents the remnant of fibrous trabeculae around the nodule that infarcted. The parathyroid pseudocyst should be filled with turbid, bloody, or brown fluid, and its fluid or wall should contain hemosiderin-laden macrophages from the previous infarction.

Parathyroid pseudocysts may grow quite large and become far larger than the adenoma from which they originated (177,178). The mechanism of this enlargement is unknown. Differentiation between pseudocysts and coalescence cysts of this size might be difficult.

Treatment

Parathyroid cysts discovered incidentally during surgery may be cured by resection. The parathyroid origin, in fact, may be discovered retrospectively from the histologic findings. Nonfunctional cysts may be discovered during fine needle aspiration (FNA) of a presumed thyroid nodule. Aspiration of clear colorless fluid is essentially diagnostic of a parathyroid cyst (186), since other cervical cysts essentially never contain clear and colorless fluid. Measurement of PTH and thyroxine or thyroglobulin in the water-clear fluid can confirm the diagnosis but may not be essential (186). If the fluid is serous, serosanguineous, or brown, the lesion may be of either thyroid or parathyroid origin, although thyroid cysts are far more common. The diagnosis must be made either by hormonal analysis or surgery.

What should be done when fluid is encountered during FNA of an apparent thyroid mass? First, aspirate all the cyst fluid to collapse the cyst completely and lessen the chances of fluid reaccumulating. Next, determine whether a palpable mass remains after cyst evacuation. If so, the mass must be subjected to FNA for cytology as with any other thyroid mass. If no residual mass is palpable, time will tell whether the patient is cured or the cyst will refill. A thyroid cyst that refills is more likely to harbor a thyroid carcinoma and should be resected after either the first or the second recurrence. In contrast, a nonfunctional parathyroid cyst may be treated by repeated aspirations (187). Thus further management of the recurrent cyst may depend on its tissue of origin. Hormone measurement on the cyst fluid may then be helpful in confirming the need for surgery.

This author uses the following cost-effective strategy. The initial fluid from any cervical cyst is centrifuged and the supernatant frozen for possible hormonal analysis later. The pellet may be sent for microscopic evaluation, which usually shows only macrophages but is occasionally of diagnostic use. Many thyroid cysts will never refill, so the aspiration is curative, and routine hormonal analysis would be an unnecessary expense. If the cyst does eventually refill, however, it is reaspirated, but the supernatant fraction of the original fluid is sent for measurement of thyroxine or thyroglobulin (and PTH if the fluid is colorless or if thyroglobulin is not elevated). Why use the first rather than second fluid? I have observed in several cases that the PTH or thyroxine concentration was much higher in the initial fluid, giving a clearer diagnosis.

Some palpable parathyroid cysts will be functional, i.e., will cause primary hyperparathyroidism. Cysts that cause hypercalcemia should probably be treated by surgical resection instead of aspiration. Our group did observe a decline in serum PTH values after each of several aspirations of a functional parathyroid cyst, but surgery was eventually required (178). An increase in severity of hypercalcemia after cyst aspiration was noted in another case (188). It is also of hypothetical concern that spillage of cells might occur from the cyst during aspiration. If the spilled cells had the adenoma phenotype, they might implant and cause a recurrence as parathyromatosis (see below). This author could find only one case of a parathyroid carcinoma reported in association with a parathyroid cyst, but this was probably a carcinoma with cystic change rather than a true parathyroid cyst (189). Nevertheless, verification of normocalcemia should probably precede FNA of any neck mass.

SUPERNUMERARY PARATHYROID GLANDS

The majority of humans have four parathyroid glands, one pair each from the third and fourth branchial pouches. During embryological development, one or more of the parathyroid glands may fragment, producing one or more supernumerary glands. Anatomical studies involving dissection to locate parathyroid glands suggest an incidence of supernumerary glands of 2.5–5% (190–192), including six or more glands in 1.2% of cases (192). Åkerström and colleagues distinguished the "proper" supernumerary gland, i.e., one located well away from the other glands (5%), from the rudimentary gland, a small gland ~5 mg in weight lying immediately, next to a larger one (2%); and from the split gland, two or more approximately equal-sized glands lying immediately next to each other (6%).

Studies using anatomic dissection may underestimate the true incidence of supernumerary glands, since parathyroid glands in an abnormal location or of smaller size will be more easily overlooked, and since efforts might slacken after the fourth gland is found. In a postmortem study, cervical vascular latex injections followed by block dissections showed five or more parathyroid glands in nine of 45 subjects (20%) (193). In five of the nine cases, the supernumerary gland was thought to be "accessory," leaving four cases of proper supernumerary glands, an incidence of 8.9%. Surgical series in patients with hyperplasia also suggest an incidence of supernumerary glands of >10%, the hyperplastic glands being easier to locate than normal-sized glands in anatomic studies (194).

The incidence of supernumerary parathyroid glands thus lies somewhere between 2.5% and 20% and certainly is high enough to influence surgical practice. Specifically, in cases of parathyroid hyperplasia, the surgeon must always seek supernumerary glands. In practical terms, this means that the dissection does not stop when the fourth parathyroid gland is found. A thorough dissection of the thyroid bed should be completed and a transcervical thymectomy performed as an integral part of the operation (115,116,192). Intrathyroidal or subcapsular parathyroid glands should also be sought (see below).

Some humans may have only three parathyroid glands, but the incidence of this finding is not over 3% (192). Many doubt that only three glands were present in these cases, since the combined parathyroid weight is lower in the subjects with only three glands (192). Probably the prosector in anatomic studies simply failed to locate the fourth gland or the blood supply of the fourth hyperplastic gland became disrupted during surgery. The ability of the surgeon to locate only three glands is not necessarily a bad prognostic sign, however, assuming that a thorough exploration has been performed. We reported two subjects with MEN-I who were cured of hyperparathyroidism after resection of only three hyperplastic parathyroid glands (119).

PARATHYROMATOSIS

A parathyroid gland may also disperse into multiple small nodules during embryological development (192,195), perhaps an exaggeration of the tendency to split to form supernumerary glands. In one reported case, there were 11 separate nodules of parathyroid tissue. If the subject with multiple nodules develops parathyroid hyperplasia, each nodule may enlarge and begin to contribute to the PTH excess. The occurrence of multiple hyperplastic parathyroid nodules has been termed *parathyromatosis* (196). Originally, two patients were reported, including one with no prior neck surgery, who must be presumed to have had an exaggerated embryological fragmentation of one parathyroid gland. Resection of multiple parathyroid nodules failed to restore normocalcemia in either case, but three similar patients in a later report were cured of hypercalcemia by resection of a wide area of adipose tissue bearing hyperplastic parathyroid nodules (195). This phenomenon may actually have been described earlier and interpreted to represent a low-grade parathyroid carcinoma (197). Cure of these three patients, together with the anatomical observations of Åkerström, help to refute this supposition.

A different mechanism may produce a similar anatomic situation. Rupture of the capsule of a parathyroid adenoma in the operative field may be followed by regrowth of multiple nodules of adenomatous parathyroid tissue months or years later, with a recurrence of hyperparathyroidism (198,199). Rupture of a functional parathyroid cyst can produce the same compli-

cation (200), as can rupture of a parathyroid carcinoma (198). This phenomenon reflects the ability of parathyroid tissue in small fragments to survive by diffusion of nutrients and later to induce capillary ingrowth, the same ability that allows an autogenous parathyroid graft to survive. Thus it is mandatory that meticulous care be taken during surgical manipulation of any parathyroid tumor to avoid rupture of its capsule. Since it may be impossible to know histologically whether the original tumor was a parathyroid carcinoma, the discovery of numerous small parathyroid nodules during cervical reexploration will mandate a wide resection to maximize the chance of complete cure. For clarity, the development of multiple parathyroid nodules after parathyroidectomy might be termed *postsurgical parathyromatosis,* and the occurrence of hyperplasia in a congenitally disbursed or fragmented parathyroid gland might be called *ontogenous parathyromatosis.*

ECTOPIC PARATHYROID GLANDS

Location of Ectopic Parathyroid Glands as Determined by Parathyroid Embryology

Parathyroid glands are frequently found in an ectopic location. In two reported series, abnormal parathyroid glands were found in other than the expected locations in 242 of 1216 consecutive parathyroid operations (20%) (201,202). Locating an abnormal ectopic parathyroid gland for resection can be difficult for the surgeon.

The ectopic locations of parathyroid glands can usually be explained by considering the pathways of parathyroid gland migration during embryonic development (203). The inferior parathyroid gland (parathyroid III) develops from the third branchial pouch in conjunction with the thymus and migrates toward the thorax with the thymus. At a variable point along the way, parathyroid III separates from the thymus and ceases migration. This usually places it in the adult just at, below, or posterior to the inferior thyroid pole (61%). Approximately 17% will lie on the anterior surface of the thyroid lobe, closely attached to the thyroid capsule (192).

If separation of parathyroid III from the thymus is delayed, it may descend into the thorax with the thymus. Anatomic studies suggested an incidence of intrathymic parathyroid glands of ~2%, but the true incidence is probably higher, based on the fraction of adenomas found there. The source of the intrathymic blood supply may depend on the level at which the descending parathyroid III finds itself when angiogenesis begins. The arterial blood supply of an intrathymic adenoma often arises from the inferior thyroid artery and occasionally arises from the internal mammary artery or rarely another mediastinal vessel.

In contrast, separation of parathyroid III may occur early, leaving it near the origin of the third pharyngeal pouch, high in the neck, often in association with a remnant of thymus (204). This "undescended parathymus" occurs <1% of the time (3/312 inferior parathyroid glands in one study) (191). These high cervical glands may (a) be displaced laterally and present as a palpable mass, (b) associate with the carotid sheath, or (c) migrate posteriorly to present as a lateral pharyngeal mass (205).

The superior parathyroid gland (parathyroid IV) develops from the dorsal portion of the fourth pharyngeal pouch, and the lateral thyroid anlage develops from its ventral portion. Since the lateral thyroid anlaga merge with the midline thyroid anlage, rather than descending, parathyroid IV usually remains nearby, coming to lie in the adult ~1 cm cranial to the crossing of the inferior thyroid artery and recurrent laryngeal nerve (80%) (192). Parathyroid IV will be located above the superior thyroid pole only 0.8% of the time. Probably because it begins as a more dorsal structure, abnormal migration of the parathyroid gland IV may place it in the retroesophageal or retropharyngeal position (1%) (192) or in the posterior superior mediastinum.

Intrathyroidal Parathyroid Adenomas or Hyperplasia

A strict definition of the intrathyroidal parathyroid gland is that it is situated totally within the thyroid, surrounded on all sides by thyroid parenchyma (191, 206,207). Some mammals routinely have parathyroid glands in an intrathyroidal location, but this location is rare in man.

There is disagreement about which parathyroid glands are more likely to be found within the thyroid. Wang (206) reported that four of four intrathyroidal parathyroids were of superior origin, and thought that this was expected, since they arose in proximity to the lateral thyroid anlage. Åkerström et al. (192) also found no inferior parathyroid glands in a true intrathyroidal position, while 0.2% of superior parathyroid glands were intrathyroidal (192). Several inferior glands located anteriorly were hidden deep in a groove of a nodular thyroid gland, but were considered to lie within the thyroid capsule and not in a true intrathyroidal location. Other observers have thought that intrathyroidal parathyroid adenomas are usually of inferior origin. Seven of eight intrathyroidal glands were of inferior origin in the Wheeler et al. (207) series, and Esselstyn (208) reported that, among 1,200 cases of hyperparathyroidism, all the intrathyroidal parathy-

roid glands were of inferior origin. The question remains open.

Mediastinal Parathyroid Tumors

Approximately 5% of parathyroid adenomas are found in the mediastinum. Approximately 95% of these are associated with the thymus and take their blood supply from the inferior thyroid artery. Intrathymic parathyroid glands usually can be resected safely by a transcervical thymectomy (through the collar incision used for the neck exploration). A few mediastinal parathyroid adenomas, either in the thymus or below, derive their blood supply from an internal mammary artery or elsewhere (209) and often must be resected by thoracotomy, which has traditionally employed sternotomy. When an adenoma lies anteriorly, however, it can be resected by a parasternal approach involving resection of a rib segment without a sternal incision (210). Mediastinal parathyroid glands outside the thymus represent ~0.2% of all parathyroid glands and are usually located in midmediastinum, away from the body of the thymus and often near the great vessels. Several groups have reviewed their experience with intrathoracic parathyroid tumors (211–215) and report their experience with various surgical approaches and preoperative localization techniques. Sternotomy was required in 1.3% in one series of 522 cases (213).

Other Locations

Parathyroid adenomas may be located in the alimentary submucosa, of the esophagus (216), the hypopharynx (217), or the pharynx (218). In one case a pharyngeal parathyroid adenoma was shown to be connected to the mucosa by a small duct (persistent ductus pharyngobrachialis) (218). Parathyroid glands may also become trapped within the vagus or phrenic nerve (218). A rare parathyroid may migrate laterally, into the lateral triangle of the neck. Such lateral parathyroids are usually supernumerary and may be formed when the carotid artery splits a superior parathyroid anlage that has taken a more lateral course of descent (219).

Parathyroid glands are generally found above the level of the hyoid bone or below the diaphragm only in association with a teratoma. A parathyroid gland was found in an epignathus on the posteriolateral wall of the nasopharynx (220). A parathyroid gland of normal size (2 mm diameter) was found within thyroid tissue in a vaginal wall teratoma and identified by its histologic appearance (221). This author is not aware of any other examples of parathyroid glands below the diaphragm.

Treatment: Selective Use of Localization Procedures

The experienced parathyroid surgeon can find most displaced parathyroid tumors at the first operation without specific preoperative localizing information. This task is facilitated by a systematic search and a working knowledge of frequent "hiding places" and how to approach them surgically (see chapter by Norton et al.). When surgery has failed to locate the ectopic parathyroid gland, localization procedures can be employed (see chapter by Doppman).

DOMINANT FAMILIAL ENDOCRINOPATHIES WITH PRIMARY PARATHYROID HYPERFUNCTION

Several hereditary syndromes that include primary hyperparathyroidism have been identified (Table 3), and at least three have been shown to be genetically distinct (MEN-I, MEN-II, and cystic parathyroid adenomatosis). Other hereditary endocrine syndromes and variants involve the parathyroid gland only sporadically (Table 4) (102).

Multiple Endocrine Neoplasia

Multiple endocrine neoplasia-I and -II are discussed at length in the chapters by Metz et al., Friedman et al., and Gagel.

Cystic Parathyroid Adenomatosis With Fibroosseous Jaw Tumors

In 1987 we described a father and three sons who at early ages developed severe hypercalcemia (total se-rum calcium values ranged as high as 14.7 mg/dl) due to a single parathyroid adenoma (225). Three members of this family developed recurrent hypercalcemia from a second parathyroid adenoma 6–10 years later, while the fourth had become hypoparathyroid after his first operation. Review of the pathological specimens showed that each parathyroid tumor was a cystic adenoma. Cysts were also present in these subjects' resected normal parathyroid glands, an unusual finding in those under age 35 years (70). The inheritance suggested but did not prove an autosomal dominant trait. We termed this syndrome *cystic parathyroid adenomatosis,* using the term *adenomatosis* to indicate the tendency to develop multiple adenomas, usually metachronously.

Urinary calcium was elevated in the four subjects, and one originally presented with nephrolithiasis. Three other first-degree relatives of affected subjects were hypercalcemic. They were not available for detailed study, but two proved to be hypocalciuric. The third refused urine collection but had a normal serum PTH value. These observations suggested a possible relationship of this syndrome to benign familial (hypocalciuric) hypercalcemia.

Three of the four adenoma patients also had undergone resection of ossifying fibromas of the mandible or maxilla. These jaw tumors were not the brown tumors of severe hyperparathyroidism, since they contained no osteoclasts even though they were resected while severe hyperparathyroidism was present. We suggested that the jaw tumors might be an integral part of the syndrome, but that data from other families with cystic adenomas were needed before the fibromas could be definitively included.

Several years earlier, a syndrome of familial parathyroid adenomas with fibroosseous jaw tumors had been described (226,227). At this author's suggestion, the parathyroid histology of this family was reexamined and showed that their adenomas were in fact cystic (228). Thus the two presumably unrelated families

TABLE 3. *Familial endocrinopathies that include primary hyperparathyroidism*

Dominant traits	Syndromes of recessive or uncertain inheritance
Multiple endocrine neoplasia I	Recessive familial parathyroid adenomas
Multiple endocrine neoplasia IIa	Familial parathyroid hyperplasia with nephropathy and neuropathy
Familial cystic parathyroid adenomatosis with fibroosseous jaw tumors	Familial parathyroid hyperplasia with intrathyroidal parathyroid glands
Dominant isolated familial parathyroid adenomas	Familial parathyroid hyperplasia with colon polyps or carcinoma
Dominant isolated familial parathyroid hyperplasia	Familial parathyroid hyperplasia with parathyroid carcinoma
Dominant parathyroid carcinomas (with atypical adenomas)	
Benign familial (hypocalciuric) hypercalcemia with hyperparathyroidism	

TABLE 4. *Hereditary multiple endocrine neoplasia syndromes with minimal or uncertain parathyroid involvement*

Syndromes of dominant inheritance	Syndromes of recessive or uncertain inheritance
Variants of multiple endocrine neoplasia-II (map to chromosome 10)	Myxomas, spotty pigmentation and nodular adrenal, testicular, or pituitary tumors (222)
Multiple endocrine neoplasia-IIa with lichen amyloidosis (282)	Gastric leiomyosarcoma, extraadrenal paraganglioma, pulmonary chondroma (223)
Familial medullary carcinoma (no pheochromocytoma or hyperparathyroidism)	Extraadrenal parangangliomas and pituitary adenoma (may include primary parathyroid hyperplasia and may have dominant inheritance with partial penetrance) (224)
Multiple endocrine neoplasia-IIb (mucosal neuromas)	
Von Hipple-Lindau's disease (CNS and retinal angiomas, renal cell carcinoma, pheochromocytoma, visceral cysts, and islet cell tumors)	
Familial pheochromocytoma (no thyroid, CNS, or retinal lesions)	
Familial papillary thyroid carcinoma	
Familial arrhenoblastoma and thyroid adenoma	

probably have the same syndrome, of which the fibroosseous jaw tumors can be regarded as an integral part. Our group is evaluating the genetics of this syndrome and so far have evidence that it is not carried near the respective loci for MEN-II or MEN-I on chromosome 10 or 11 (228).

The literature revealed five other families who may have the same trait, although the parathyroid histology was not described fully enough to determine whether the adenomas were cystic (229–332). Three of these five families included at least one patient with a parathyroid carcinoma, suggesting that this syndrome might require consideration as a potential cause of parathyroid carcinoma. The cellular basis for the development of these adenomas, for their cystic nature, and for their possible occasional malignant transformation must be established.

Until further evidence is available, the parathyroid adenomas in this syndrome should be regarded surgically as premalignant, so care must be taken to resect them intact and to avoid using them for grafts when possible. The proper surgical management of this syndrome is still evolving, but a few tentative principles can be listed. At least in our family, the parathyroid adenomas seemed more often to involve inferior parathyroid glands (81). Furthermore, parathyroid carcinomas (at least sporadic ones) seem to occur almost exclusively in the inferior parathyroid glands (233,234). Thus, this author recommends bilateral inferior parathyroidectomy (and transcervical thymectomy) at the first operation. Total parathyroidectomy with autogenous grafting of one or both superior parathyroid glands might also be considered.

Dominant Isolated Familial Parathyroid Adenomas

Parathyroid adenomas with apparently dominant transmission but without accompanying jaw tumors or other endocrinopathy have been reported in a few families, although usually only in two consecutive generations. In at least two such families, the parathyroid adenomas were cystic (235,236), suggesting a variant of the familial cystic parathyroid adenomatosis syndrome with low penetrance of the jaw fibroma component. This hypothesis may become testable when the genetic locus of the cystic adenoma–jaw fibroma syndrome has been found. In at least one family, the adenomas were not cystic (237), so a separate syndrome may exist.

Dominant Isolated Familial Parathyroid Hyperplasia

Several families have been described who seemed to show only primary parathyroid hyperplasia. Unless the family is large, it is difficult to exclude the presence of MEN-I, and at least three of these families have later been found to have MEN-I (238,239).

Dominant Isolated Familial Parathyroid Carcinoma

Primary hyperparathyroidism occurred in three siblings and their uncle (240). Their mother had died at age 31 years with features suggesting severe hyperparathyroidism. There was no evidence for parathyroid hyperplasia, hypercalcemia being relieved by resection of parathyroid carcinomas in two patients and an atypical adenoma in two. No other endocrine tumors and no evidence of parathyroid hyperplasia was found. Chromosomal abnormalities were identified in one of the carcinomas (reciprocal translocation between chromosomes 3 and 4, trisomy 7, and a pericentric inversion in chromosome 9). Tumor DNA from one carcinoma and one adenoma showed no loss of heterozygosity of chromosome 11, no evidence of *ras* gene mutations, and no PTH gene rearrangements.

Benign Familial (Hypocalciuric) Hypercalcemia With Hyperparathyroidism

Benign familial (hypocalciuric) hypercalcemia (FHH) is an autosomal dominant syndrome marked by the lifelong elevation of free and total serum calcium values and relative hypocalciuria (241,242). This syndrome is discussed in detail in the chapter by Heath.

Most patients with FHH have normal serum PTH values (242,243) and parathyroid size as estimated by ultrasonography is normal (244). In some FHH families, however, elevated serum PTH concentrations occur in a high percentage of affected members, the incidence rising with age (245,246). To explain this variant, one might hypothesize that the increased renal retention of calcium has not raised serum calcium quite enough to overcome the decreased parathyroid sensitivity to calcium, so that generalized parathyroid hyperplasia occurs. These patients may develop a hypophosphatemic osteomalacia, that can serve as an indication for parathyroid surgery (246).

Neonatal Severe Primary Hyperparathyroidism

Infants may be born with severe hypercalcemic hyperparathyroidism, with both life-threatening hypercalcemia and severe bone disease. The syndrome of neonatal severe primary hyperparathyroidism is different from the neonatal hyperparathyroidism that is seen in infants born to hypocalcemic mothers, where the hyperparathyroidism develops in utero as a secondary response to hypocalcemia and is manifested postnatally as transient mild or moderate hypercalcemia that resolves spontaneously as the parathyroid hyperplasia involutes.

Clinical Manifestations

Serum calcium values in severe neonatal primary hyperparathyroidism have ranged from ~13 mg/dl to >20 mg/dl. Serum PTH values were measured in several cases and found to be high, although not always as elevated as might be expected. Many patients have also shown slightly elevated or high-normal serum magnesium levels and low urinary calcium values. Clinical signs include lethargy, muscular hypotonia, and severe skeletal deformities, including a narrow thorax, sometimes with spontaneous rib fractures, bowed long bones, craniotabes, and radiographic osteopenia. As often occurs when hyperparathyroidism develops while the epiphyses are open, the changes of rickets are seen on radiographs. There is also radiographically evident subperiosteal resorption of bone, and histologic examination of bone may show typical osteitis fibrosa et cystica (247). As with rickets, morbidity often derives from respiratory complications of the thoracic deformity. The syndrome is often fatal, especially if parathyroid surgery is delayed in the face of severe muscular weakness or increasing serum calcium values.

Etiology

The earliest reports found that the syndrome was associated with parathyroid hyperplasia but not adenoma (248). Marx and coworkers (247) recognized that many of these patients were members of families affected with FHH. In one of their cases, both parents were affected members of separate FHH kindreds, suggesting that homozygosity for FHH could be a cause of the syndrome (247). Cooper and colleagues (249) reported another patient who was apparently homozygous for FHH because of parental consanguinity. They demonstrated that the infant's parathyroid glands in vitro showed poor suppresibility by calcium (249).

In other cases, however, only one parent has had FHH, suggesting that another genetic (presumably recessive) or environmental factor must be acting synergistically with the FHH trait to generate the severe degree of hyperparathyroidism. This factor remains unidentified but must be operative in only a small percentage of FHH births.

In some reported cases, including three of the four patients Marx et al. (247) reported, the father was the affected parent, the mother being normocalcemic. Here the usual activity of the placental calcium pump would place the fetal serum calcium value below the presumably higher fetal parathyroid set point and produce parathyroid hyperplasia. In this model, however, the hyperplasia and the bone disease that had developed in utero should resolve gradually after birth, leaving the infant with only the usual features of FHH. This situation is analogous to the hyperparathyroidism that develops in the normal fetus of a hypocalcemic mother. Marx et al. (247) found no evidence of excess fetal wastage in FHH pregnancies of normocalcemic mothers, suggesting that this mechanism alone is not the cause of the severe neonatal hyperparathyroid syndrome.

How then would one explain the occasional case of severe neonatal hyperparathyroidism in this situation? One might postulate that another factor prevented the placental calcium pump from increasing the calcium gradient sufficiently. Studies of placental weight and histology would be of interest but may not be technically feasible, since the syndrome may be recognized hours to days after birth. Another hypothesis would be that some other factor, such as a subclinical form of FHH in the mother, had shifted the fetal parathyroid set point even further from normal. Detailed study of the calcium inhibitory set point of parathyroid glands from severely affected, but apparently heterozygous, neonates and dynamic in vitro studies of maternal parathyroid function would be of great interest.

There are probably other causes of severe neonatal hyperparathyroidism, unrelated to FHH. Several reported cases seemed to show recessive transmission or represented the sporadic occurrence of a similar neonatal syndrome (247).

Treatment

In neonates with severe hypercalcemia and marked skeletal deformities, aggressive respiratory support and treatment can be lifesaving, since the skeletal deformity may eventually resolve. Parathyroidectomy can be lifesaving in the most severe cases and should not be delayed (250). Since repeated parathyroid operations have sometimes been required because of early return of severe hypercalcemia after subtotal parathyroidectomy, some authors have advocated deliberate total parathyroidectomy (247,249), with the understanding that lifelong treatment of hypoparathyroidism will then be needed. A possible alternative approach would be total parathyroidectomy with parathyroid autogenous grafting. This seemed satisfactory in one case, but only 6 weeks of postoperative follow-up was available, and later graft-dependent recurrence was a concern (249).

The presence of skeletal hyperparathyroid changes in FHH offspring is itself not an indication for parathyroid exploration, unless accompanied by severe hypercalcemia. At least two patients with FHH-associated neonatal hyperparathyroidism with significant skeletal changes but mild hypercalcemia (11.2 and 11.4 mg/dl) have been reported to survive and their skeletal deformities to heal without parathyroid surgery (251,252). These patients, however, clearly did not have the full syndrome of severe neonatal primary hyperparathyroidism.

Histology

Histologic examination of the parathyroid glands in severe neonatal hyperparathyroidism usually shows chief cell hyperplasia (247), but one patient had water-clear cell hyperplasia of four glands (253).

PRIMARY HYPERPARATHYROIDISM IN FAMILIAL SYNDROMES OF RECESSIVE OR UNCERTAIN INHERITANCE

Recessive Isolated Familial Parathyroid Adenomas

Apparently recessive familial parathyroid adenomas were reported in each of three offspring of a nonconsanguineous marriage. There was no other evidence of endocrine tumors and no hypercalcemia or hyperpara-

thyroidism in other members of a large extended family (254).

Recessive Isolated Familial Parathyroid Hyperplasia

Several reports have described recessive syndromes of isolated primary parathyroid hyperplasia with other associations not including endocrine tumors.

Familial Parathyroid Hyperplasia With Nephropathy and Neuropathy

A familial syndrome of primary parathyroid hyperplasia with nephropathy and neural deafness was reported in five of six children born to a marriage between first cousins (255). Three of the five had primary parathyroid hyperplasia, three had renal failure, and all five had sensorineural deafness. Female patients were equally as severely affected as males, and the absence of hematuria distinguished the syndrome from Alport's syndrome, which is usually an X-linked illness. The hyperparathyroidism was of early onset, being diagnosed at ages 9, 18, and 22 years.

Familial Parathyroid Hyperplasia With Intrathyroidal Parathyroid Locations

A familial syndrome of primary parathyroid hyperplasia with a tendency for intrathyroidal location of one or more parathyroid glands has been reported (256). A mother and two of her six children were affected. The age of onset was early in the two sons, at ~22 years of age, and was uncertain in the mother, who presented with staghorn calculi at age 49 years. In two of the three affected subjects, one of the hyperplastic parathyroid glands was located within the substance of the thyroid. A review of large series of hyperparathyroidism in the literature in which location of the abnormal gland(s) was specified suggested that an intrathyroidal location was more common in familial cases (10.4%) than in sporadic ones (4.2%). The family was not large enough to allow the mode of inheritance to be determined or to exclude the possibility of an associated endocrinopathy.

Familial Parathyroid Hyperplasia With Colon Polyps or Carcinoma

Primary parathyroid hyperplasia was associated with polyps and carcinoma of the colon in two brothers (257). The colon malignancy appeared 12 and 36 years before the hypercalcemia. A sister also had undergone resection of a colon carcinoma but refused calcium measurement. Both parents had expired of a malignancy (lung or breast) in the fifth or sixth decade. This association was probably more than a chance occurrence. Data from three large series found that 7% of 244 patients with primary hyperparathyroidism also had a history of colon cancer, while matched controls had a 5% incidence of colon cancer, not a significant difference (257). Colonic polyposis is also associated with familial papillary thyroid cancer (258–260), but these families have not been found to have a high incidence of parathyroid hyperplasia.

Familial Parathyroid Hyperplasia With Parathyroid Carcinoma

Our group described a family among whom parathyroid hyperplasia occurred in three siblings, without evidence of other endocrine tumors, with one of the siblings also having a parathyroid carcinoma (261). A pancreatic carcinoma, visualized in the mother at laparotomy but not biopsied, had followed a rapid clinical course, making it unlikely to have been of islet cell origin. The parathyroid carcinoma presented as a hard nodule fixed to the thyroid, with severe hypercalcemia (14.7 mg/dl). In addition to thyroid invasion, it showed fibrosis, a trabecular growth pattern, and venous invasion. Persistent hypercalcemia which progressively worsened led to three further operations, at which, respectively, were resected (a) a hyperplastic right inferior parathyroid gland, (b) a hyperplastic right superior parathyroid gland displaced to the posterior superior mediastinum, and (c) a large mass of nodules adherent to the trachea at the site of the initial thyroid resection plus multiple nodules studded along the entire left paratracheal area from upper thyroid cornu to upper thymic pole. These nodules microscopically contained numerous mitoses but more importantly had invaded muscle, confirming that this was a local recurrence of a carcinoma rather than parathyromatosis, as was proposed in a later review (233).

A similar syndrome of parathyroid hyperplasia and carcinoma has been reported in at least two other families, each with two affected siblings (262,263). The parathyroid carcinoma did not metastasize in any of the five patients, the diagnosis of carcinoma being based on local recurrence of tumor or histologic findings or both. Only one of the five parathyroid carcinoma patients in these three families died during the reported follow-up period (122). He succumbed to severe hypercalcemia hyperparathyroidism, the cause of which was presumed to be further recurrence of carcinoma, but neither left-side parathyroid gland was ever identified.

The inheritance of this syndrome is uncertain. Two families could not be screened adequately, but in one family both parents and two other siblings were normocalcemic (262). Thus a dominant trait has not been

excluded. The syndrome is rare enough that it may take many years to track down its genetic basis.

It is possible that one or more of these families had a variant of the cystic parathyroid adenomatosis–fibroosseous jaw tumor syndrome, which may also be associated with parathyroid carcinoma (see above). Two of the four patients examined via mandibular radiographs had mandibular tumors (261,262), although biopsy of one lesion showed increased osteoclastic activity that excluded an ossifying fibroma (262). There was at least one recurrence of hypercalcemia in each patient at a time that would have been compatible either with appearance of a metachronous adenoma or progression of hyperplasia in a previously minimally affected gland. The published histologic studies of the carcinomas showed mild cystic changes in only one of the five cases (261), but the cysts in the original adenoma might have been lost after a carcinoma developing in situ had spread throughout the gland. We should examine all parathyroid tissue in future cases in such families carefully for cystic change.

Once such a family has been identified, the surgical treatment of this syndrome should probably employ the same approach used for the cystic adenomatosis–jaw tumor syndrome. Since any enlarged parathyroid gland might represent or harbor a carcinoma, biopsy of enlarged parathyroids should be avoided and enlarged parathyroid glands handled with extreme caution. Bilateral inferior parathyroidectomy should probably be routine. Autogenous parathyroid grafting of the most normal-appearing superior parathyroid gland might be considered in preference to subtotal parathyroidectomy, even with the increased chance of later malignant change. It is not clear whether metastasis would be more likely to occur from a gland fragment left at the original site in the neck or from a transplant in the forearm, but the forearm site would be more accessible should the parathyroid remnant develop aggressive behavior.

NEWER METHODS FOR EXAMINATION OF PARATHYROID LESIONS

Fine Needle Aspiration

The emergence of the technique of FNA for cytological evaluation of thyroid nodules has ensured that interest would also arise in the cytopathology of parathyroid lesions. When FNA of a thyroid lesion happens to sample a parathyroid lesion, knowledge of parathyroid cytopathology would be helpful. Image-guided FNA has also been tested as a tool for the preoperative confirmation of the location of parathyroid lesions. This section discusses the technical aspects of parathyroid FNA, summarizes the expected cytopathologic findings, and addresses the indications and precautions for parathyroid FNA.

Sampling Technique

Almost all enlarged parathyroid glands causing hyperparathyroidism are small relative to the thyroid. Most are deeply placed, and few are palpable. Blind attempts at parathyroid FNA will thus have a low yield. With the use of imaging techniques such as ultrasonography or computed tomograph (CT) scans to guide needle placement, it is possible to obtain transcutaneous aspirates from enlarged parathyroid glands (264,265). The small amount of fluid taken into the needle by capillary action or aspiration may be examined cytologically or by RIA.

Cytopathologic Examination of Cervical Aspirate

Slides may be prepared from guided parathyroid aspirations for cytopathologic examination by the same method as for thyroid FNA cytology (266). It may be difficult cytologically to differentiate clusters of parathyroid cells from thyroid cell clumps (267,268), sometimes leading to an erroneous diagnosis of thyroid neoplasm (268). Based on a series of 21 parathyroid aspirates, Davey and colleagues (266) reported that the parathyroid aspirate could best be recognized by examining the cell grouping and the characteristics of the nuclei. Fragments from thyroid colloid nodules or thyroid adenomas are usually monolayered with uniformly spaced cells. The form typical of a parathyroid cell group is a "thick, often branching, fragment with frayed edges," with irregularly spaced cells, requiring multiple planes of focus. This typical irregular grouping was seen in 18 of the 21 parathyroid aspirates, but not in two atypical adenomas or in one case of parathyroid hyperplasia. Microfollicular cell clusters, typical of cellular thyroid adenomas, were seen only in rare parathyroid aspirates.

The parathyroid cell nucleus is round, with smooth borders and regular, coarse granular chromatin, a bit like that of mature lymphocytes and unlike the fine chromatin pattern of benign thyroid nuclei; nucleoli are rare (266). The average nuclear diameter ranges from 6 to 7 μm in most parathyroid samples, smaller than for most thyroid adenomas or carcinomas. These nuclear criteria were not met in all parathyroid specimens, however. One hyperplastic parathyroid and the two atypical parathyroid adenomas had greater nuclei diameters, 7.4, 7.4, and 10 μm, and the two atypical adenomas showed frequent nucleoli. Thus atypical parathyroid lesions may be difficult to differentiate from thyroid lesions cytologically.

Differentiation of parathyroid oxyphil cells from thyroid Hürthle cells is also important. Both show abundant, granular cytoplasm, but the oxyphil cell nuclei will have the same coarse chromatin pattern as the parathyroid chief cells and will lack the nucleoli expected in the Hürthle cell (266). Unfortunately, nuclei of parathyroid carcinomas may contain prominent nucleoli (269).

Parathyroid specimens often [seven of ten times (266)] contain fragments of dense hyaline material, resembling the colloid that is usually taken as a sign of thyroid origin of an aspirate. The parathyroid colloid-like material, however, stains blue-green with Papanicolaou stain, with only the center of larger fragments being eosinophilic as is thyroid colloid. The nuclear chromatin pattern is a more reliable sign than the colloid staining pattern, however. Fibrillary or laminar structures staining with Congo red and thus resembling amyloid are sometimes found in parathyroid aspirates (266). The nature of this material is not known, but amyloid material can sometimes be seen in histologic sections of parathyroid lesions (70).

Immunochemical staining of the cytologic specimen for PTH and thyroglobulin is probably the most definitive means of differentiating thyroid from parathyroid lesions (72,270).

Radioimmunoassay of Cervical Aspirate

For PTH RIA, the contents of the sampling needle may be washed into a known volume of sterile water, usually 1.0 ml (264,265). A known volume of acetic acid solution may be added (usually 100 μl of 1 M acetic acid) to minimize adsorption and degradation of intact PTH. Some investigators have sonicated the solution briefly to disrupt cells, but this is probably not necessary. The solution is mixed well and stored frozen until analysis via a standard PTH RIA (264,271). A blank sample of water-acetic acid (without tissue aspirate) should be included in the assay run to verify the zero reference binding value. Even the small volume of aspirate from a parathyroid gland often has such a high PTH concentration that the dilution in water–acetic acid may be insufficient to bring the binding value onto the RIA standard curve, and further dilution may be required. Thyroid or muscle aspirates contain no significant PTH immunoreactivity (264). Thus, a lesion visualized on ultrasonography or CT scan can be identified by RIA as of parathyroid origin, but data are too few to estimate sensitivity and specificity.

Rarely, a parathyroid cyst may be aspirated during FNA (178,272). This aspirate may be of sufficient volume to be stored safely without dilution. Successful assay may require a manyfold dilution, however, since parathyroid cyst fluid often contains very high PTH concentrations.

Indications for Parathyroid Fine Needle Aspiration

Parathyroid gland verification by FNA is not indicated as a routine preoperative procedure, in view of the high success rate of initial operations by experienced parathyroid surgeons. FNA is contraindicated in a patient with presumptive primary hyperparathyroidism when the nodule in the thyroid bed is palpably firm or hard or when the serum calcium value is above ~13 mg/dl, since these signs increase the chance of parathyroid carcinoma or atypical adenoma. The nodule will have to be resected en bloc regardless of the results of FNA, and one should take no chance of implanting one of these lesions to produce postsurgical parathyromatosis. FNA of thyroid carcinoma clearly does not lead to local spread or implantation, but no such data are available for the parathyroid carcinoma, which is less amenable to nonsurgical modalities than thyroid carcinoma. One patient has been reported to experience a local recurrence of parathyroid carcinoma after FNA but had undergone a core biopsy at the same time (273).

The need for sure preoperative knowledge of the location of the adenoma is the indication for parathyroid FNA. This will usually be for a patient with a strong need for surgery because of severe hyperparathyroidism but who has a high anesthetic risk or who has undergone previous unsuccessful parathyroid surgery (264). Here FNA can substitute for the more laborious and higher risk procedures of arteriography and selective venous sampling for PTH RIA. Since only a few patients meet these criteria, most centers will gain little experience with the FNA technique, and it would be wise for most patients in need of FNA to be referred to a specialized center with experience in the technique.

Aspiration Biopsy of Osseous Lesions

Patients with severe hyperparathyroidism may present with lytic bone lesions. When these occur in a patient with a palpable neck mass, with severe hyper-calcemia, or with recurrent primary hyperparathyroidism, one concern is that the lytic lesions might represent a metastasis of parathyroid carcinoma. It may be possible to identify parathyroid carcinoma in a lytic bone lesion by aspiration biopsy (269). The cell types that would normally be expected from aspiration of a brown tumor of osteitis fibrosa et cystica would include "multinucleated osteoclast-type giant cells" and "spindly or fibrillary cells with single, ovoid nuclei, probably of stromal origin" (274). Aspiration of a metastasis instead will show cells that resemble those aspirated from the primary parathyroid lesion. Actually, any parathyroid cells recovered from bone would by definition be carcinoma. Surgical attack on an osseous metastasis would probably be indicated to help reduce the body's tumor burden, especially since the number of osseous metastases may be low and the tumor usually is only slowly progressive.

Analysis of Nuclear DNA Content

Profiling of nuclear DNA content has been used to study parathyroid lesions. It might be hoped that information about DNA content might be useful for four purposes (Table 5): (a) In a patient with one definitely enlarged and one borderline large parathyroid gland, it would be useful to determine (perhaps with a biopsy) whether a questionably enlarged parathyroid gland represents a small second adenoma. (b) When only two parathyroid glands are enlarged, there is a need to differentiate between asymmetric parathyroid hyperplasia and double parathyroid adenomas. (c) When the serum calcium is very high or the tumor shows atypical or suspicious histologic features, a definitive diagnosis by DNA profiling would be useful. (d) When the histology strongly suggests parathyroid carcinoma, it might be useful to predict the likelihood of local recurrence or metastatic behavior of the neoplasm.

A profile of the number of nuclei with various quantities of DNA can be constructed after measuring the intensity of the signal for each of several hundred stained nuclei. The first study of parathyroid nuclear

TABLE 5. *Possible uses for DNA profiling of parathyroid tumors*

Potential differentiations	Discrimination
Normal gland vs. small second adenoma (one gland large, second gland borderline large)	Probably not possible (normal sized glands proliferative in adenoma patient)
Hyperplasia vs. double adenomas (two enlarged and two normal sized glands)	Not yet possible (disagreement on fraction of hyperplastic glands proliferative)
Carcinoma vs. adenoma (very high calcium and suspicious tumor)	Some value (aneuploidy favors carcinoma, but apparent adenomas may be aneuploid)
Aggressive vs. indolent carcinoma (histologic diagnosis of carcinoma)	Good discrimination (aneuploid tumors more likely to recur or metastasize)

DNA content used cell imprints of parathyroid glands ("touch preps") stained for DNA and studied by microscopic fluorimetry (275). Subsequent studies have used flow cytometry, since the automated technique allows quantitation of thousands rather than a few hundred nuclei and since specimens from previous cases can be studied after special processing of the paraffin-embedded tissue. The results published to date do not agree on every point (Table 6), possibly because different techniques and criteria have been applied and the exact source of the glands has not always been specified. Nevertheless, interesting findings have emerged.

The first study defined a diploid tissue as one in which at least 98% of the nuclei have a diploid DNA content, with the remaining nuclei (<2%) showing a tetraploid DNA content (presumably undergoing replication but having not yet divided). In this study all normal parathyroid glands (n = 19) and all parathyroid glands with chief cell hyperplasia (12 primary and 12 secondary) were diploid. In contrast all parathyroid adenomas (n = 24) showed an increased frequency of tetraploid nuclei, ranging from 2% to 50%. An increase in tetraploidy was termed a *proliferative change* (Table 6), since it might be expected in a tissue with an increased rate of cell division. A few nuclei of ploidy higher than four were found in several adenomas but never in normal or hyperplastic glands. Since very few nuclei were aneuploid (showing an uneven multiple of the diploid DNA value), the authors surmised that the nuclear atypia often seen in adenomas was usually a manifestation of hyperdiploidy. They concluded that nuclear DNA content could differentiate the adenoma from normal or hyperplastic parathyroid glands, with ≥ 2% hyperdiploidy signifying an adenoma.

Later studies, although using varying criteria for tetraploidy and aneuploidy, have confirmed that many adenomas show a large tetraploid component (Table 6). None of these studies, however, found 100% of the adenomas with increased tetraploidy, the values instead ranging from a high of 80% to 20%. Only three of the studies found that parathyroid adenomas (one-sixth to one-eighth of the time) had a significant percentage of aneuploid nuclei (Table 6). The lack of agreement among studies raises questions about the true incidence of tetraploidy and aneuploidy and about the reasons for the discrepancies. The explanation may well be technical, based on difference in tissue

TABLE 6. *Nuclear DNA histograms of normal and abnormal parathyroid glands*[a]

Authors (Reference)	Normal parathyroid glands			Parathyroid adenomas			Hyperplastic parathyroids			Parathyroid carcinomas			Percentage tetraploidy used for cutoff to define "proliferative"
	Diploid	Proliferative	Aneuploid	Diploid	Proliferative	Aneuploid	Diploid	Proliferative	Aneuploid	Diploid	Proliferative	Aneuploid	
Bengtsson et al. (275)[b]	19	0	0	0	24	0	24	0	0	0	0	0	2% of nuclei tetraploid
Irvin and Bagwell (58)	17	0	0	10	38	1	0	0	0	0	0	0	3% of nuclei tetraploid
	34[c]	14[c]	0[c]										
	1[d]	7[d]	0[d]										
Bowlby et al. (276)	9	0	0	41	12	3	25	2[f]	0	0	1	1	15% of nuclei tetraploid
Irvin et al. (59)	12[e]	17[e]	1[e]	1	30	6	0	10	1	0	0	0	6% of nuclei tetraploid
Levin and Klemi (277)	6	0	0	9	22	1	0	0	0	0	3	6	Not quantitative; "proliferative shoulder" on DNA histogram
Joensuu et al. (278)	0	0	0	27	13	14	0	0	0	0	0	0	11% of nuclei tetraploid
Obara et al. (279)	0	0	0	(28)[g]	?	1	(15)[g]	?	0	(11)[g]	?	5	Distinction not made
Shenton et al. (280)	21	0	0	14	20	5[h]	20	0	3[h]	0	1	3	25% of nuclei tetraploid

[a]Diploid, DNA histogram shows a minimal component of hyperploidy; proliferative, DNA histogram shows a "proliferative shoulder" or a significant component of tetraploidy (percentage used for cutoff differs; see last column); aneuploid, DNA histogram shows a significant peak with an uneven ploidy number.
[b]DNA content by microscope fluorimetry. All later studies used flow cytometry.
[c]Normal sized glands from adenoma patients; normal histologic appearance.
[d]Normal sized glands from adenoma patients; hyperplastic histologic appearance.
[e]Normal sized glands from adenoma patients; histologic appearance not specified.
[f]Two of ten parathyroid glands with primary hyperplasia showed increased tetraploidy.
[g]The 28, 15, and 11 glands were non-aneuploid (diploid or proliferative), but the division was not given.
[h]Aneuploid component stated to be hypodiploid.

preparation methods and completeness of disaggregation, but geographic differences in the type of patients under study cannot be ruled out.

Later studies have confirmed that normal parathyroid glands are diploid (Table 6). Irvin and Bagwell (58) observed in two studies, however, that normal-sized parathyroid glands from adenoma patients often showed increased tetraploidy. In one study increased tetraploidy was seen in seven of eight parathyroid glands that were histologically hypercellular and 14 of 48 glands that were histologically normal (58). This observation to this author's knowledge was the first evidence for a more widespread parathyroid abnormality in patients with parathyroid adenomas. At least one other group has since confirmed that normal-sized glands from adenoma patients cannot be distinguished from hyperplastic or adenomatous parathyroid glands by DNA flow cytometry (281) (data not in form suitable for summary in Table 6). If confirmed, this observation would have implications about the etiology of the parathyroid adenoma. Possibly the studies that found only diploid normal glands examined mainly normal glands from thyroid surgery cases (the number of thyroid cases vs. parathyroid cases with normal glands often was not given).

More study is needed, however, Irvin et al. (59) reported that many hyperplastic glands, like adenomas, also show a high percentage of tetraploid nuclei and occasionally even a significant aneuploid component, an observation at odds with observations of three other groups (275,276,280). Unfortunately these studies often give no information about the current intensity of calcitriol treatment in renal cases; radiation history; concomitant drugs such as lithium; or whether the patients had sporadic primary hyperplasia or familial hyperplasia, MEN, or uremia as the underlying cause. Until the disagreement about tetraploidy in normal and hyperplastic parathyroid glands is resolved, we cannot use DNA quantification to help differentiate normal glands from small adenomas or hyperplastic glands (Table 5).

The three studies that found increased aneuploidy in one-fourth to one-sixth of parathyroid adenomas (Table 6) would suggest that DNA measurements might not be useful for detecting the parathyroid carcinoma. Four other studies, however, found that aneuploidy was largely restricted to the parathyroid carcinoma (Table 6), and two of these studies suggested that aneuploidy in the parathyroid carcinoma is a sign of poor prognosis.

Bowlby et al. (276) first reported aneuploidy in a parathyroid carcinoma (one of two cases studied). Levin et al. (277) found that four of nine carcinomas were aneuploid, including two that had been diagnosed histologically as atypical adenomas but later proved to have metastasized. Shenton et al. (280) found four of four parathyroid carcinomas to be aneuploid, with ploidy indices of 1.2, 2.9, 3.0, and 3.2 (normal 0.85–1.1). Obara et al. (279) found that five of 16 parathyroid carcinomas were aneuploid. In these four studies combined, only ten of 155 adenomas were aneuploid, including five adenomas in the Shenton et al. study that showed aneuploidy of the hypodiploid variety (ploidy indices in the 0.80–0.89 range). These studies suggest that DNA profiles may be able to predict malignancy of parathyroid lesions, but the reasons why the three other studies found a high frequency of aneuploid adenomas must be explained and the hypodiploidy of some adenomas confirmed. Technical problems may have produced false-positive aneuploidy results in some studies, or potentially malignant tumors with aneuploidy may have been classified as adenomas, or the biology of the adenoma might truly be different in the various locales.

Flow cytometry by itself clearly will not be the gold standard for diagnosis of parathyroid malignancy, since not all carcinomas are aneuploid and since not all aneuploid tumors will recur, but cytometry might at least supplement the histologic findings. Cytometry may also provide an index of aggressiveness of the carcinoma. Levin et al. (277) found that three of four aneuploid parathyroid carcinomas recurred vs. only one of five that were not aneuploid. Obara et al. (279) reported that four of five aneuploid carcinomas had recurred or metastasized, whereas only four of 11 diploid carcinomas had shown a local recurrence (no metastases), with two of those four patients apparently cured by a second local operation (3–6 years of follow-up).

Would the routine determination of ploidy values for parathyroid tumors alter clinical practice? The primary surgical management of the tumor would not be altered, for two reasons. First, it is probable that normal and abnormal glands cannot be differentiated in the patient with a parathyroid adenoma. Second, intraoperative biopsy of an obviously enlarged parathyroid gland for flow cytometry is not advisable, because biopsy might increase the chance of local recurrence of a low-grade malignancy or atypical adenoma.

Cytometry might be helpful in a patient with hyperplasia for whom autogenous grafting is planned, to help identify the most normal gland for implantation, but no data are yet available to show that visual inspection of the glands would not lead to the same choice. The duration of postoperative follow-up might be lengthened if cytometry suggested an aneuploid component in an apparent adenoma. Since metastatic or recurrent parathyroid carcinoma may not become evident for months or years, a patient with an aneuploid parathyroid tumor should probably be followed closely for years rather than for the usual 6–12 months.

ACKNOWLEDGMENTS

This study was supported by the Department of Veterans Affairs.

REFERENCES

1. Nussbaum SR, Gaz RD, Arnold A. Hypercalcemia and ectopic secretion of parathyroid hormone by an ovarian carcinoma with rearrangement of the gene for parathyroid hormone. *N Engl J Med* 1990;323:1324–1328.
2. Yoshimoto K, Yamasaki R, Sakai H, et al. Ectopic production of parathyroid hormone by a small cell lung cancer in a patient with hypercalcemia. *J Clin Endocrinol Metab* 1990; 68:976–983.
3. Mallette LE, Bilezikian JP, Heath DA, Aurbach GD. Primary hyperparathyroidism, clinical and biochemical features. *Medicine* 1974;53:127–146.
4. Mallette LE. Primary hyperparathyroidism: an update on incidence, etiology, diagnosis and treatment. *Am J Med Sci* 1987;293:239–249.
5. Heath DA. Primary hyperparathyroidism. Clinical presentation and factors influencing clinical management. *Endocrinol Metab Clin North Am* 1989;18:631–646.
6. Mallette LE. Is surgery necessary for the asymptomatic patient with primary hyperparathyroidism? Negative. In: Barnes HV, ed. (Gitnick G, series ed. vol 4.) *Debates in medicine*, Vol 4. St. Louis: Mosby-Year Book, 1991;126–141.
7. Endres DB, Villanueva R, Sharp CF Jr, Singer FR. Measurement of parathyroid hormone. *Endocrinol Metab Clin North Am* 1989;18:611–630.
8. Mallette LE, Gagel RF. Parathyroid hormone and calcitonin. In: Favus M, ed. *Primer on metabolic bone diseases and disorders of mineral metabolism*. Kelseyville, CA: American Society for Bone and Mineral Research, 1990;65–70.
9. Zaniewski M, Jordan PH Jr, Yip B, Thornby JI, Mallette LE. Serum gastrin level is increased by chronic hypercalcemia of parathyroid or nonparathyroid origin. *Arch Intern Med* 1986;146:478–482.
10. Patten BM, Bilezikian JP, Mallette LE, Prince A, Engel WK, Aurbach GD. Neuromuscular disease in primary hyperparathyroidism. *Ann Intern Med* 1974;80:182–193.
11. Mallette LE. Anemia in hypercalcemic hyperparathyroidism, renewed interest in an old observation. *Arch Intern Med* 1977;137:572–573.
12. Weinstein RS. Parathyroid carcinoma associated with polycythemia vera. *Bone* 1991;12:237–239.
13. Ziv Y, Rubin M, Lombrozo R, Rapoport D, Dintsman M. Primary hyperparathyroidism associated with pancytosis. *N Engl J Med* 1985;313:187.
14. Blair DC, Fekety FR. Primary hyperparathyroidism presenting as fever of unknown origin with unremitting headache. *Ann Intern Med* 1979;91:575–576.
15. Keynes WM. Hypocalcaemic primary hyperparathyroidism. *Br Med J* 1970;1:208–211.
16. Frame B, Foroozanfar F, Patton RB. Normocalcemic primary hyperparathyroidism with osteitis fibrosa. *Ann Intern Med* 1970;73:253–257.
17. Heath DA, Wills MR. Normocalcaemic primary hyperparathyroidism with osteitis fibrosa. *Postgrad Med J* 1971; 47:815–817.
18. Dent CE, Jones PE, Millam DP. Masked primary (or tertiary) hyperparathyroidism. *Lancet* 1975;1:1161–1164.
19. Calandra DB, Shah K, Lawrence AM, Paloyan E. Hyperparathyroidism unmasked by the treatment of hypothyroidism secondary to Hashimoto's thyroiditis. *Surgery* 1984; 96:1015–1018.
20. Arem R, Lim-Abrahan MA, Mallette LE. Concomitant Graves' disease and primary hyperparathyroidism. Influence of hyperthyroidism on serum calcium and parathyroid hormone. *Am J Med* 1986;80:693–698.
21. Heath H III, Hodgson SF, Kennedy MA. Primary hyperparathyroidism: incidence, morbidity, and potential impact in a community. *N Engl J Med* 1980;302:189–193.
22. Capen CC, Rosol TJ. Recent advances in the structure and function of the parathyroid gland in animals and the effects of xenobiotics. *Toxicol Pathol* 1989;17:333–345.
23. Tisell LE, Carlsson S, Lindberg S, Ragnhult I. Autonomous hyperparathyroidism: a possible late complication of neck radiotherapy. *Acta Chir Scand* 1976;142:367–373.
24. Tisell LE, Hansson G, Lindberg S, Ragnhult I. Hyperparathyroidism in persons treated with X-rays for tuberculous cervical adenitis. *Cancer* 1977;40:846–854.
25. Okerlund MD, Beckmann A, Galante M, Hunt T. Radiation-induced parathyroid tumors following head and neck radiation in childhood. *Clin Res* 1978;26:191A.
26. Takeichi N, Dohi K, Ito H, Hara H, Usui T, Yokoro K. Parathyroid tumors in atomic bomb survivors in Hiroshima: first report of surgical cases, 1956-1988. *Hiroshima J Med Sci* 1991;40:75–77.
27. Tsunoda T, Mochinaga N, Eto T, Maeda H. Hyperparathyroidism following the atomic bombing in Nagasaki. *Jpn J Surg* 1991;21:508–511.
28. Fujiwara S, Sposto R, Ezaki H, et al. Hyperparathyroidism among atomic bomb survivors in Hiroshima. *Radiat Res* 1992;130:372–378.
29. Ireland JP, Fleming SJ, Levison DA, Cattell WR, Baker LR. Parathyroid carcinoma associated with chronic renal failure and previous radiotherapy to the neck. *J Clin Pathol* 1985; 38:1114–1118.
30. Katz A, Braunstein GD. Clinical, biochemical, and pathologic features of radiation-associated hyperparathyroidism. *Arch Intern Med* 1983;143:79–82.
31. Mallette LE. Acute and chronic effects of lithium on human calcium metabolism. *Lithium* 1991;2:209–226.
32. Mallette LE, Khouri K, Zengotita H, Hollis BW, Malini S. Lithium treatment increases intact and midregion parathyroid hormone and parathyroid volume. *J Clin Endocrinol Metab* 1989;68:654–660.
33. Brown EM, Gardner DG, Brennan MF, et al. Calcium-regulated parathyroid hormone release in primary hyperparathyroidism. Studies in vitro with dispersed parathyroid cells. *Am J Med* 1979;66:923–931.
34. Lloyd HM, Parfitt AM, Jacobi JM, et al. The parathyroid glands in chronic renal failure: A study of their growth and other properties made on the basis of findings in patients with hypercalcemia. *J Lab Clin Med* 1989;114:358–367.
35. Parfitt AM, Willgoss D, Jacob J, Lloyd HM. Cell kinetics in parathyroid adenomas: evidence for decline in rates of cell birth and tumour growth, assuming clonal origin. *Clin Endocrinol* 1991;35:151–157.
36. Arnold A, Staunton CE, Kim HG, Gaz RD, Kronenberg HM. Monoclonality and abnormal parathyroid hormone genes in parathyroid adenomas. *N Engl J Med* 1988;318:658–662.
37. Friedman E, Sakaguchi K, Bale AE, et al. Clonality of parathyroid tumors in familial multiple endocrine neoplasia type 1 (published erratum: *N Engl J Med* 1989;321:1057). *N Engl J Med* 1989;321:213–218.
38. Sandelin K, Larsson C, Falkmer UG, Farnebo LO, Grimelius L, Nordenskjold M. Morphology, DNA ploidy and allele losses on chromosome 11 in sporadic hyperparathyroidism and that associated with multiple neoplasia, type 1. *Eur J Surg* 1992;158:199–206.
39. Pitkin RM. Calcium metabolism in pregnancy and the perinatal period: a review. *Am J Obstet Gynecol* 1985;151:99–109.
40. Care AD, Caple IW, Abbas SK, Pickard DW. The effect of fetal thyroparathyroidectomy on the transport of calcium across the ovine placenta of the fetus. *Placenta* 1986;7:417–424.
41. Mallette LE. The parathyroid polyhormones: New concepts

in the spectrum of peptide hormone action. *Endocr Rev* 1991;12:110–117.

42. Brown E, Enyedi P, LeBoff M, Rotberg J, Preston J, Chen C. High extracellular Ca^{2+} and Mg^{2+} stimulate accumulation of inositol phosphates in bovine parathyroid cells. *FEBS Lett* 1987;218:113–118.

43. Lopez-Barneo J, Armstrong CM. Depolarizing response of rat parathyroid cells to divalent cations. *J Gen Physiol* 1983;82:269–294.

44. Douglas WW. Stimulus-secretion coupling: variations on the theme of calcium-activated exocytosis involving cellular and extracellular sources of calcium. *Ciba Found Symp* 1978; 54:61–90.

45. Nemeth EF, Scarpa A. Intracellular Ca^{2+} and regulation of secretion in parathyroid cells. *FEBS Lett* 1986;203:15–19.

46. Ota K, Poras A, Sherwood LM. The effects of concanavalin A on parathyroid hormone (PTH) release and adenylate cyclase activity in isolated bovine parathyroid cells. Washington, DC: The Endocrine Society, Abstract No. 450, 1980; 187.

47. Posillico JT, Wortsman J, Srikanta S, Eisenbarth GS, Mallette LE, Brown EM. Parathyroid cell surface autoantibodies that inhibit parathyroid hormone secretion from dispersed human parathyroid cells. *J Bone Mineral Res* 1986; 1:475–483.

48. Posillico JT, Srikanta S, Eisenbarth GS, Quaranta V, Kajiji S, Brown EM. Binding of monoclonal antibody (4F2) to its cell surface antigen on dispersed adenomatous parathyroid cells raises cytosolic calcium and inhibits parathyroid hormone secretion. *J Clin Endocrinol Metab* 1987;64:43–50.

49. Nygren P, Gylfe E, Larsson R, et al. Modulation of the Ca^{2+}-sensing function of parathyroid cells in vitro and in hyperparathyroidism. *Biochim Biophys Acta* 1988;968:253–260.

50. Wolf F, Scarpa A. Calcium binding by parathyroid cell plasma membranes. *Cell Calcium* 1987;8:171–183.

51. Woltering E, Emmott R, Jabadpoor N, Marx S, Brennan M. ABO (H) cell surface antigens in parathyroid adenoma and hyperplasia. *Surgery* 1981;90:1–9.

52. Juhlin C, Rastad J, Klareskog L, Grimelius L, Åkerström G. Parathyroid histology and cytology with monoclonal antibodies recognizing a calcium sensor of parathyroid cells. *Am J Pathol* 1989;135:321–328.

53. Arnold A, Kim HG, Gaz RD, et al. Molecular cloning and chromosomal mapping of DNA rearranged with the parathyroid hormone gene in a parathyroid adenoma. *J Clin Invest* 1989;83:2034–2040.

54. Marx SJ. Etiologies of parathyroid gland dysfunction in primary hyperparathyroidism. *J Bone Mineral Res* 1991;2 (Suppl 2):S19–S24.

55. Brennan MF. Reoperation for suspected hyperparathyroidism. In: Kaplan EL, ed. *Surgery of the thyroid and parathyroid glands.* New York: Churchill Livingstone, 1983;168–176.

56. Farley DR, van Heerden JA, Grant CS. Are concomitant surgical procedures acceptable in patients undergoing cervical exploration for primary hyperparathyroidism? *Mayo Clin Proc* 1991;66:681–685.

57. Attie JN, Wise L, Mir R, Ackerman LV. The rationale against routine subtotal parathyroidectomy for primary hyperparathyroidism. *Am J Surg* 1978;136:437–445.

58. Irvin GL, Bagwell CB. Identification of histologically undetectable parathyroid hyperplasia by flow cytometry. *Am J Surg* 1979;138:567–571.

59. Irvin GL III, Taupier MA, Block NL, Reiss E. DNA patterns in parathyroid disease predict postoperative parathyroid hormone secretion. *Surgery* 1988;104:1115–1120.

60. Mallette LE, Nammour H. False elevation of the midregion PTH value. Inhibition of tracer binding by heterophilic antibody in patient serum (abstract). *J Bone Mineral Res* 1987;2(Suppl 1):102.

61. Gonzalez-Villapando C, Porath A, Berelowitz M, Marshall L, Favus MJ. Vitamin D metabolism during recovery from severe osteitis fibrosa cystica of primary hyperparathyroidism. *J Clin Endocrinol Metab* 1980;51:1180–1183.

62. Jones CTA, Sellwood RA, Evanson JM. Symptomatic hypomagnesaemia after parathyroidectomy. *Br Med J* 1973; 3:391–392.

63. Clark OH, Way LW, Hunt TK. Recurrent hyperparathyroidism. *Ann Surg* 1976;184:391–402.

64. Shankar VS, Bax CM, Alam AS, Bax BE, Huang CL, Zaidi M. The osteoclast Ca^{2+} receptor is highly sensitive to activation by transition metal cations. *Biochem Biophys Res Commun* 1992;187:913–918.

65. Bilezikian FP. The medical management of primary hyperparathyroidism. *Ann Intern Med* 1982;96:198–202.

66. Broadus AE, Magee JS, Mallette LE, et al. A detailed evaluation of oral phosphate therapy in selected patients with primary hyperparathyroidism. *J Clin Endocrinol Metab* 1983;56:953–961.

67. Marcus R. Estrogens and progestins in the management of primary hyperparathyroidism. *Endocrinol Metab Clin North Am* 1989;18:715–722.

68. Miller D, Edmonds MW. Hypercalcemia due to hyperparathyroidism treated with a somatostatin analogue. *Can Med Assoc J* 1991;145:227–228.

69. Kay S. The abnormal parathyroid. *Hum Pathol* 1976;7:127–138.

70. Castleman B, Roth SI. *Tumors of the parathyroid glands. Atlas of tumor pathology. second series, fascicle 14.* Washington, DC: Armed Forces Institute of Pathology, 1978:1–94.

71. Lawrence DAS. A histologic comparison of adenomatous and hyperplastic parathyroid glands. *J Clin Pathol* 1978; 31:626–632.

72. Civantos F. Parathyroid hormone. In: Nadji M, Morales AR, eds. *Immunoperoxidase techniques: a practical approach to tumor diagnosis.* Chicago: American Society of Clinical Pathologists Press, 1986;69–70.

73. Sandler R, Jourdain LM, Damjanov I. Functioning oxyphil parathyroid adenoma. *Ann Clin Lab Sci* 1981;2:180–183.

74. Arnold BM, Kovacs K, Horvath E, Murray TM, Higgins HP. Functioning oxyphil cell adenoma of the parathyroid gland: evidence for parathyroid secretory activity of oxyphil cells. *J Clin Endocrinol Metab* 1974;38:458–462.

75. Ober WH, Kaiser GH. Hamartoma of the parathyroid. *Cancer* 1958;11:601–606.

76. Abul-Haj SK, Conklin H, Hewitt WC. Functioning lipoadenoma of the parathyroid gland. *N Engl J Med* 1962;266:121–123.

77. Straus FH II, Kaplan EL, Nishiyama RH, Bigos ST. Five cases of parathyroid lipohyperplasia. *Surgery* 1983;94:901–905.

78. Verdonk CA, Edis AJ. Parathyroid "double adenomas": fact or fiction? *Surgery* 1981;90:523–526.

79. Harness JK, Ramsburg SR, Nishiyama RH, Thompson NW. Multiple adenomas of the parathyroids: do they exist? *Arch Surg* 1979;114:468–474.

80. Attie JN, Bock G, Auguste L. Multiple parathyroid adenomas: report of thirty-three cases. *Surgery* 1990;108:1014–1020.

81. Mallette LE, Malini S, Rappaport MP, Kirkland JL. Familial cystic parathyroid adenomatosis. *Ann Intern Med* 1987; 107:54–60.

82. van Heerden J, Weiland L, ReMine W, Walls J, Purnell D. Cancer of the parathyroid gland. *Arch Surg* 1979;114:475–480.

83. Shane E, Bilezikian J. Parathyroid carcinoma: A review of 62 patients. *Endocr Rev* 1982;3:216–226.

84. Anderson BJ, Samaan NA, Vassilopoulou-Sellin R, Ordonez NG, Hickey RC. Parathyroid carcinoma: features and difficulties in diagnosis and management. *Surgery* 1983;94:905–915.

85. Murphy MN, Glennon PG, Diocee MS, Wick MR, Cavers DJ. Nonsecretory parathyroid carcinoma of the mediastinum. Light microscopic, immunocytochemical, and ultrastructural features of a case, and review of the literature. *Cancer* 1986;58:2468–2476.

86. Baba H, Kishihara M, Tohmon M, et al. Identification of parathyroid hormone messenger ribonucleic acid in an ap-

parently nonfunctioning parathyroid carcinoma transformed from a parathyroid carcinoma with hyperparathyroidism. *J Clin Endocrinol Metab* 1986;62:247–252.

87. Yamashita H, Noguchi S, Murakami N, Toda M, Adachi M, Daa T. Immunohistological study of nonfunctional parathyroid carcinoma. Report of a case. *Acta Pathol Jpn* 1992; 42:279–285.

88. Funa K, Papanicolaou V, Juhlin C, et al. Expression of platelet-derived growth factor beta-receptors on stromal tissue cells in human carcinoid tumors. *Cancer Res* 1990;50:748–753.

89. Thompson EW, Reich R, Martin GR, Albini A. Factors regulating basement membrane invasion by tumor cells. *Cancer Treat Res* 1988;40:239–249.

90. Hoyhtya M, Hujanen E, Turpeenniemi-Hujanen T, Thorgeirsson U, Liotta LA, Tryggvason K. Modulation of type-IV collagenase activity and invasive behavior of metastatic human melanoma (A2058) cells in vitro by monoclonal antibodies to type-IV collagenase. *Int J Cancer* 1990;46:282–286.

91. Goldberg GI, Eisen AZ. Extracellular matrix metalloproteinases in tumor invasion and metastasis. *Cancer Treat Rep* 1991;53:421–440.

92. Levy AT, Cioce V, Sobel ME, et al. Increased expression of the Mr 72,000 type IV collagenase in human colonic adenocarcinoma. *Cancer Res* 1991;51:439–444.

93. Ponton A, Coulombe B, Skup D. Decreased expression of tissue inhibitor of metalloproteinases in metastatic tumor cells leading to increased levels of collagenase activity. *Cancer Res* 1991;51:2138–2143.

94. Verdeal K, Erturk E, Rose DP. Endometrial adenomatous hyperplasia and carcinoma and multiple endocrinopathies in rats exposed to N-nitrosomethylurea. *Anticancer Res* 1986; 6:5–10.

95. Potter GD, Lindsay S, Chaikoff IL. Induction of neoplasms in rat thyroid glands by low doses of radioiodine. *Arch Pathol* 1960;69:257–267.

96. Warren S, Chute RN. Radiation-induced osteogenic sarcoma in parabiont rats. *Lab Invest* 1963;12:1041–1045.

97. Berdjis CC. Parathyroid diseases and irradiation. *Strahlentherapie* 1972;143:48–62.

98. Makarewicz CR. Radiation and thyroid cancer. *JAMA* 1984; 251:1280.

99. Christmas TJ, Chapple CR, Noble JG, Milroy EJ, Cowie AG. Hyperparathyroidism after neck irradiation. *Br J Surg* 1988;75:873–874.

100. Smith JF, Coombs RRH. Histological diagnosis of carcinoma of the parathyroid gland. *J Clin Pathol* 1984;37:1370–1378.

101. Mashburn MA, Chonkich GD, Chase DR, Petti GHJ. Parathyroid carcinoma: two new cases—diagnosis, therapy, and treatment. *Laryngoscope* 1987;97:215–218.

102. Mallette LE. Hyperparathyroidism: The spectrum of parathyroid tumors in primary and secondary hyperparathyroidism. In: Mazzaferri EL, Samaan NA, eds. *Endocrine tumors.* Boston: Blackwell Scientific Publications, Inc. (in press).

103. Holmes EC, Morton DL, Ketcham AS. Parathyroid carcinoma: a collective review. *Ann Surg* 1969;169:631–640.

104. Bukowsky RM, Sheeler L, Cunningham J, Esselstyn C. Successful combination chemotherapy for metastatic parathyroid carcinoma. *Arch Intern Med* 1984;144:399–400.

105. Chahinian AP, Holland J, Nieburgs NE, Marinescu A, Geller SA, Kirschner PA. Metastatic nonfunctioning parathyroid carcinoma: ultrastructural evidence of secretory granules and response to chemotherapy. *Am J Med Sci* 1981;282:80–84.

106. Schantz A, Castleman B. Parathyroid carcinoma. A study of 70 cases. *Cancer* 1973;31:600–605.

107. Black BK, Ackerman LV. Tumors of the parathyroid: a review of twenty-three cases. *Cancer* 1950;3:415–444.

108. McKeown PP, McGarity WC, Sewell CW. Carcinoma of the parathyroid gland: is it overdiagnosed? *Am J Surg* 1984; 147:292–298.

109. Rosai J. Parathyroid glands. In: Rosai J, eds. *Ackerman's surgical pathology,* 7th ed. St. Louis: C.V. Mosby, 1989; 449–466.

110. Snover DC, Foucar K. Mitotic activity in benign parathyroid disease. *J Clin Pathol* 1981;75:345–347.

111. Albright F, Bloomberg E, Castleman B, Churchill ED. Hyperparathyroidism due to a diffuse hyperplasia of all parathyroid glands rather than to a parathyroid adenoma of one gland. Clinical studies on three such cases. *Arch Intern Med* 1934;54:315–329.

112. Cope O, Keynes WM, Roth SI, Castleman B. Primary chief-cell hyperplasia of the parathyroid glands: a new entity in the surgery of hyperparathyroidism. *Ann Surg* 1958;148: 375–387.

113. Duh QY, Gum ET, Sancho JJ, Levin KE, Raper SE, Clark OH. Epidermal growth factor receptors in parathyroid tumors. *J Surg Res* 1986;40:569–573.

114. Wortsman J, Posillico JT, Brown EM, Eisenbarth GS, Mallette LE. Case 34-1987: comments concerning a new syndrome of idiopathic hypoparathyroidism (letter). *N Engl J Med* 1988;318:857.

115. Freeman JB, Sherman BM, Mason EE. Transcervical thymectomy: an integral part of neck exploration for hyperparathyroidism. *Arch Surg* 1976;111:359–364.

116. Clark OH, Duh Q. Primary hyperparathyroidism. A surgical perspective. *Endocrinol Metab Clin North Am* 1989;18:701–714.

117. Rizzoli R, Green J III, Marx SJ. Primary hyperparathyroidism in familial multiple endocrine neoplasia type 1. Long-term follow-up of serum calcium levels after parathyroidectomy. *Am J Med* 1985;78:467–474.

118. Wells SA Jr, Farndon JR, Dale JK, Leight GS, Dilley WG. Long-term evaluation of patients with primary parathyroid hyperplasia managed by total parathyroidectomy and heterotopic autotransplantation. *Ann Surg* 1980;192:451–458.

119. Mallette LE, Eisenberg K, Wilson H, Noon G. Studies of the evolution of autogenous parathyroid graft function. *Surgery* 1983;93:254–259.

120. Malmaeus J, Benson L, Johansson H, et al. Parathyroid surgery in the multiple endocrine neoplasia type I syndrome: choice of surgical procedure. *World J Surg* 1986;10:668–672.

121. Mallette LE, Blevins T, Jordan PH, Noon GP. Autogenous parathyroid grafts for generalized primary parathyroid hyperplasia: contrasting outcome in sporadic hyperplasia versus multiple endocrine neoplasia type I. *Surgery* 1987; 101:738–745.

122. Clark OH. Hyperparathyroidism due to primary cystic parathyroid hyperplasia. *Arch Surg* 1978;113:748–750.

123. Fallon MD, Haines JW, Teitelbaum SL. Cystic parathyroid hyperplasia. *Am J Clin Pathol* 1982;77:104–107.

124. Mallette LE, Patten BM, Engel KA. Neuromuscular disease in secondary hyperparathyroidism. *Ann Intern Med* 1975; 82:474–482.

125. Adams JS, Clemens TL, Parrish JA, Holick MF. Vitamin-D synthesis and metabolism after ultraviolet irradiation of normal and vitamin-D-deficient subjects. *N Engl J Med* 1982; 306:722–725.

126. Delmes J, Tindira CA, Grooms P, Dusso A, Windus DW, Slatopolsky E. Parathyroid hormone suppression by intravenous 1,25-dihydroxyvitamin D: a role for increased sensitivity to calcium. *J Clin Invest* 1989;83:1349–1355.

127. Russell J, Lettieri D, Sherwood LM. Supression by 1,25(OH)₂D3 of transcription of the pre-proparathyroid hormone gene. *Endocrinology* 1986;119:2864–2866.

128. Russell J, Sherwood LM. The effects of 1,25-dihydroxyvitamin D, and high calcium on transcription of the pre-proparathyroid hormone gene are direct. *Trans Assoc Am Physicians* 1987;100:256–262.

129. Silver J, Naveh MT, Mayer H, Schmelzer HJ, Popovtzer MM. Regulation by vitamin D metabolites of parathyroid hormone gene transcription in vivo in the rat. *J Clin Invest* 1986;78:1296–1301.

130. Yamamoto M, Igarashi T, Muramatsu M, Fukagawa M, Motokura T, Ogata E. Hypocalcemia increases and hypercal-

cemia decreases the steady-state level of parathyroid hormone messenger RNA in the rat. *J Clin Invest* 1989;83:1053–1056.

131. Brown EM, Wilson RE, Eastman RC, Marynick SP. Abnormal regulation of PTH release by calcium in secondary hyperparathyroidism due to chronic renal failure. *J Clin Endocrinol Metab* 1982;54:172–179.

132. Rudberg C, Åkerström G, Ljunghall S, et al. Regulation of parathyroid hormone release in primary and secondary hyperparathyroidism—studies in vivo and in vitro. *Acta Endocrinol* 1982;101:408–413.

133. Somerville PJ, Tiller DJ, Evans RA. What is tertiary hyperparathyroidism? *Aust NZ J Med* 1975;5:551–556.

134. Case records of the Massachusetts General Hospital. *N Engl J Med* 1978;298:266–274.

135. McCarron DA, Lenfesty B, Narasimhan N, Barry JM, Vetto RM, Bennett WM. Anatomical heterogeneity of parathyroid glands in posttransplant hyperparathyroidism. *Am J Nephrol* 1988;8:388–391.

136. Krause MW, Hedinger CE. Pathologic study of parathyroid glands in tertiary hyperparathyroidism. *Hum Pathol* 1985;16:772–784.

137. Marx SJ, Sharp ME, Krudy A, Rosenblatt M, Mallette LE. Radioimmunoassay for the middle region of human parathyroid hormone: studies with a radioiodinated synthetic peptide. *J Clin Endocrinol Metab* 1981;53:76–84.

138. Hanley DA, Ayer LM. Calcium-dependent release of carboxyl-terminal fragments of parathyroid hormone by hyperplastic human parathyroid tissue in vitro. *J Clin Endocrinol Metab* 1986;63:1075–1079.

139. D'Amour P, Palardy J, Bahsali G, Mallette LE, DeLéan A, Lepage R. The modulation of circulating parathyroid hormone immunoheterogeneity in man by ionized calcium concentration. *J Clin Endocrinol Metab* 1992;74:525–532.

140. Heath H III. Biogenic amines and the secretion of parathyroid hormone and calcitonin. *Endocr Rev* 1980;1:319–338.

141. Kemper B, Habener JF, Rich A, Potts JT Jr. Parathyroid secretion: Discovery of a major calcium-dependent protein. *Science* 1974;184:167–169.

142. Cohn DV, Morrisey JJ, Hamilton JW, Shofstall RE, Smardo FL, Chu LLH. Isolation and partial characterization of secretory protein I from bovine parathyroid glands. *Biochemistry* 1981;20:4135–4140.

143. Ahn TG, Cohn DV, Gorr SU, Ornstein DL, Kashdan MA, Levine MA. Primary structure of bovine pituitary secretory protein I (chromogranin A) deduced from the cDNA sequence. *Proc Natl Acad Sci USA* 1987;84:5043–5047.

144. Levine MA, Dempsey MA, Helman LJ, Ahn TG. Expression of chromogranin-A messenger ribonucleic acid in parathyroid tissue from patients with primary hyperparathyroidism. *J Clin Endocrinol Metab* 1990;70:1668–1673.

145. O'Connor DT, Deftos LJ. Secretion of chromogranin A by peptide-producing endocrine neoplasms. *N Engl J Med* 1986;314:1145–1151.

146. Nanes MS, O'Connor DT, Marx SJ. Plasma chromogranin-A in primary hyperparathyroidism. *J Clin Endocrinol Metab* 1989;69:950–955.

147. Drees BM, Hamilton JW. Pancreastatin and bovine parathyroid cell secretion. *Bone Mineral* 1992;17:335–346.

148. Fasciotto BH, Gorr S, Cohn DV. Autocrine inhibition of parathyroid cell secretion requires proteolytic processing of chromogranin A. *Bone Mineral* 1992;17:323–333.

149. Drees BM, Rouse J, Johnson J, Hamilton JW. Bovine parathyroid glands secrete a 26-kDa N-terminal fragment of chromogranin-A which inhibits parathyroid cell secretion. *Endocrinology* 1991;129:3381–3387.

150. Bansal DD, MacGregor RR. Calcium-regulated secretion of tissue plasminogen activator and parathyroid hormone from human parathyroid cells. *J Clin Endocrinol Metab* 1992;74:266–271.

151. Saxe A. Angiogenesis of human parathyroid tissue. *Surgery* 1984;96:1138–1143.

152. Rodda DP, Kubota M, Heath JA, et al. Evidence for a novel parathyroid hormone-related protein in fetal lamb parathyroid glands and sheep placenta: comparisons with a similar protein implicated in humoral hypercalcaemia of malignancy. *J Endocrinol* 1988;117:261–271.

153. Loveridge N, Caple IW, Rodda C, Martin TJ, Care AD. Further evidence for a parathyroid hormone-related protein in fetal parathyroid glands of sheep. *Q J Exp Physiol* 1988;73:781–784.

154. Senior PV, Heath DA, Beck F. Expression of parathyroid hormone-related protein mRNA in the rat before birth: demonstration by hybridization histochemistry. *J Mol Endocrinol* 1991;6:281–290.

155. Ikeda K, Weir EC, Sakaguchi K, et al. Clonal rat parathyroid cell line expresses a parathyroid hormone-related peptide but not parathyroid hormone itself. *Biochem Biophys Res Commun* 1989;162:108–115.

156. Zajac JD, Callaghan J, Eldridge C, et al. Production of parathyroid hormone-related protein by a rat parathyroid cell line. *Mol Cell Endocrinol* 1989;67:107–112.

157. Ikeda K, Arnold A, Mangin M, et al. Expression of transcripts encoding a parathyroid hormone-related peptide in abnormal human parathyroid tissues. *J Clin Endocrinol Metab* 1989;69:1240–1248.

158. Docherty HM, Ratcliffe WA, Heath DA, Docherty K. Expression of parathyroid hormone-related protein in abnormal human parathyroids. *J Endocrinol* 1991;129:431–438.

159. Danks JA, Ebeling PR, Hayman JA, et al. Immunohistochemical localization of parathyroid hormone-related protein in parathyroid adenoma and hyperplasia. *J Pathol* 1990;161:27–33.

160. Matsushita H, Hara M, Nakazawa H, Shishiba Y, Matuhasi T. The presence of immunoreactive parathyroid hormone-related protein in parathyroid adenoma cells. *Acta Pathol Jpn* 1992;42:35–41.

161. Budayr AA, Nissenson RA, Klein RF, et al. Increased serum levels of a parathyroid hormone-like protein in malignancy-associated hypercalcemia. *Ann Intern Med* 1989;111:807–812.

162. Burtis WJ, Brady TG, Orloff JJ, et al. Immunochemical characterization of circulating parathyroid hormone-related protein in patients with humoral hypercalcemia of cancer. *N Engl J Med* 1990;322:1106–1112.

163. Henderson JE, Shustik C, Kremer R, Rabbani SA, Hendy GN, Goltzman D. Circulating concentrations of parathyroid hormone-like peptide in malignancy and in hyperparathyroidism. *J Bone Mineral Res* 1990;5:105–113.

164. Manente P, Cecchettin M, Infantolino D, Foscolo G, Conte N. Apparently nonfunctioning metastases of parathyroid carcinoma. *Tumori* 1987;73:191–193.

165. Zabel M, Biela-Jacek I, Surdyk J, Dietel M. Studies on localization of calcitonin gene-related peptide (CGRP) in the thyroid-parathyroid complex. *Virchows Arch Pathol Anat A* 1987;411:569–573.

166. Fabri PJ, Gower WRJ, Weber C, Tuttle S. Hyperparathyroid glands contain G-17 and G-34 gastrin. *J Surg Res* 1986;41:333–337.

167. Weber CJ, Marangos PJ, Richardson S, et al. Presence of neuron-specific enolase and somatostatin in human parathyroid tissues. *Surgery* 1985;98:1008–1012.

168. Hargis GK, Williams GA, Reynolds WA, et al. Effect of somatostatin on parathyroid hormone and calcitonin secretion. *Endocrinology* 1978;102:745–750.

169. Stock JL, Weintraub BD, Rosen SW, Aurbach GD, Spiegel AM, Marx SJ. Human chorionic gonadotrophin subunit measurement in primary hyperparathyroidism. *J Clin Endocrinol Metab* 1982;54:57–63.

170. Chng SL, Krishnan MM, Ramachandran, Chan CH, Zain Z. Parathyroid carcinoma with steroid-suppressible plasma immunoreactive parathyroid hormone and human chorionic gonadotrophin. *Singapore Med J* 1990;31:83–84.

171. Strodel WE, Vinik AI, Eckhauser FE, Thompson NW. Hyperparathyroidism and gastroenteropancreatic hormone levels. *Surgery* 1985;98:1101–1106.

172. Weber CJ, Modlin I, DiBella F, et al. Pancreatic polypeptide immunoreactivity in human parathyroid culture media. *J Surg Res* 1983;35:421–425.

173. Skogseid B, Eriksson B, Lundquist G, et al. Multiple endo-

crine neoplasia type 1: a 10-year prospective screening study in four kindreds. *J Clin Endocrinol Metab* 1991;73: 281–287.

174. Langstein HN, Norton JA, Chiang B, et al. The utility of circulating levels of human pancreatic polypeptide as a marker for islet cell tumors. *Surgery* 1990;108:1109–1116.

175. Turner A, Lampe HB, Cramer H. Parathyroid cysts. *J Otolaryngol* 1989;18:311–313.

176. Cruse CW, Daouk AA. Mediastinal parathyroid cysts: report of a case and review of the literature. *Am J Surg* 1978; 135:714–716.

177. Buchanan G, Gregory MM. Giant functioning cervicomediastinal parathyroid cyst. *Ann Otol* 1979;88:545–549.

178. Ramos-Gabatin A, Mallette LE, Bringhurst FR, Draper MW. Functional mediastinal parathyroid cyst. Dynamics of parathyroid hormone secretion during cyst aspirations and surgery. *Am J Med* 1985;79:633–639.

179. Clark OH. Parathyroid cysts. *Am J Surg* 1978;135:395–402.

180. Welti H. A propos des kystes parathyroidiens. *Mem Acad Chir* 1946;72:33–35.

181. Randel SB, Gooding GA, Clark OH, Stein RM, Winkler B. Parathyroid variants: US evaluation. *Radiology* 1987;165: 191–194.

182. Gilmour JR. The normal histology of the parathyroid glands. *J Pathol Bacteriol* 1939;48:187–222.

183. Calandra DB, Shah KH, Prinz RA, et al. Parathyroid cysts: a report of eleven cases including two associated with hyperparathyroid crisis. *Surgery* 1983;94:887–892.

184. Miyauchi A, Kakudo K, Fujimoto T, Onishi T, Takai S. Parathyroid cyst: analysis of the cyst fluid and ultrastructural observations. *Arch Pathol Lab Med* 1981;105:497–499.

185. Albertson DA, Marshall RB, Jarman WT. Hypercalcemic crises secondary to a functioning parathyroid cyst. *Am J Surg* 1981;141:175–177.

186. Oertel YC, Wargotz ES. Diagnosis of parathyroid cysts. *Am J Clin Pathol* 1987;88:252.

187. Clark OH, Okerlund MD, Cavalieri RR, Greenspan FS. Diagnosis and treatment of thyroid, parathyroid, and thyroglossal duct cysts. *J Clin Endocrinol Metab* 1979;48:983–988.

188. Kobayashi A, Kuma K, Matsuzuke F. Exacerbation of hypercalcemia after needle biopsy of a parathyroid cyst. *Ann Intern Med* 1989;110:326–327.

189. Wright JG, Brangle RW. Carcinoma in a parathyroid cyst. *Illinois Med J* 1985;168:98–100.

190. Gilmour JR. The gross anatomy of the parathyroid glands. *J Pathol Bacteriol* 1938;46:133–149.

191. Wang CA. The anatomic basis of parathyroid surgery. *Ann Surg* 1976;183:271–275.

192. Åkerström G, Malmaeus J, Bergström R. Surgical anatomy of human parathyroid glands. *Surgery* 1984;95:14–21.

193. Delattre J, Flament JB, Palot JP, Pluot M. Les variations des parathyroides. *J Chir* 1982;119:633–641.

194. Meakins JL, Milne CA, Hollomby DJ, Goltzman D. Total parathyroidectomy: parathyroid hormone levels and supernumerary glands in hemodialysis patients. *Clin Invest Med* 1984;7:21–25.

195. Reddick RL, Costa JC, Marx SJ. Parathyroid hyperplasia and parathyromatosis (letter). *Lancet* 1977;1:549.

196. Palmer JA, Brown WA, Kerr WH, Rosen IB, Watters NA. The surgical aspects of hyperparathyroidism. *Arch Surg* 1975;110:1004–1007.

197. Barnes BA, Cope O. Carcinoma of the parathyroid glands. *J Am Med Assoc* 1961;178:556–559.

198. Åkerström G, Rudberg C, Grimelius L, Rastad J. Recurrent hyperparathyroidism due to perioperative seeding of neoplastic or hyperplastic parathyroid tissue. *Acta Chir Scand* 1988;154:549–552.

199. Fitko R, Roth SI, Hines JR, Roxe DM, Cahill E. Parathyromatosis in hyperparathyroidism. *Hum Pathol* 1990;21: 234–237.

200. Rattner DW, Marrone GC, Kasdon E, Silen W. Recurrent hyperparathyroidism due to implantation of parathyroid tissue. *Am J Surg* 1985;149:745–748.

201. Sarfati E, De Ferron P, Gossot D, Assens P, Dubost C. Para-

202. Hooghe L, Kinnaert P, Van Geertruyden J. Surgical anatomy of hyperparathyroidism. *Acta Chir Belg* 1992;92:1–9.

203. Granberg P, Cedermark B, Farnebo L, Hamberger B, Werner S. Parathyroid tumors. *Curr Probl Cancer* 1985;9:1–52.

204. Edis AJ, Purnell DC, van Heerden JA. The undescended "parathymus." An occasional cause of failed neck exploration for hyperparathyroidism. *Ann Surg* 1979;190:64–68.

205. Deeb ZE, Trible WM, Page R, Fernandez MG. Parathyroid tumors as lateral pharyngeal masses: report of a case. *Ann Otol Rhinol Laryngol* 1976;85:86–89.

206. Wang C. Hyperfunctioning intrathyroid parathyroid gland: a potential cause of failure in parathyroid surgery. *J R Soc Med* 1981;74:49–52.

207. Wheeler MH, Williams ED, Wade JSH. The hyperfunctioning intrathyroidal parathyroid gland: a potential pitfall in parathyroid surgery. *World J Surg* 1987;11:110–114.

208. Esselstyn CB Jr. Invited commentary. *World J Surg* 1987; 11:114.

209. Geelhoed GW, Krudy AG, Doppman JL. Long-term followup of patients with hyperparathyroidism treated by transcatheter staining with contrast agent. *Surgery* 1983;94:849–862.

210. Schlinkert RT, Whitaker MD, Argueta R. Resection of select mediastinal parathyroid adenomas through an anterior mediastinotomy. *Mayo Clin Proc* 1991;66:1110–1113.

211. Nudelman IL, Deutsch AA, Reiss R. Primary hyperparathyroidism due to mediastinal parathyroid adenoma. *Int Surg* 1987;72:104–108.

212. Roblot P, Alcalay M, Azais O, Jardel P, Gouet, Bontoux D. Ectopic parathyroid adenoma vascularized by the internal mammary artery. *Am J Med* 1987;83:382–393.

213. McHenry C, Walsh M, Jarosz H, et al. Resection of parathyroid tumor in the aorticopulmonary window without prior neck exploration. *Surgery* 1988;104:1090–1094.

214. Dubost CI, Bouteloup PY. Mediastinal exploration by sternotomy in surgery of hyperparathyroidism. 36 cases. *J Chir* 1988;125:631–637.

215. Obara T, Fujimoto Y, Tanaka R, et al. Mid-mediastinal parathyroid lesions: preoperative localization and surgical approach in two cases. *Jpn J Surg* 1990;20:481–486.

216. Sloane JA. Parathyroid adenoma in submucosa of esophagus. *Arch Pathol Lab Med* 1978;102:242–243.

217. Joseph MP, Nadol JB, Pilch BZ, Goodman ML. Ectopic parathyroid tissue in the hypopharyngeal mucosa (pyriform sinus). *Head Neck Surg* 1982;5:70–74.

218. Gilmour JR. Some developmental abnormalities of the thymus and parathyroids. *J Pathol Bacteriol* 1941;52:213–218.

219. Udekwu AO, Kaplan EL, Wu T, Arganini M. Ectopic parathyroid adenoma of the lateral triangle of the neck: report of two cases. *Surgery* 1987;101:114–118.

220. Willis RA. Teratomas. In: *The pathology of the tumors of children.* (Cameron R, Wright GP, eds. Pathological monographs, vol 2.) Springfield, IL: Charles C. Thomas, 1962;76–92.

221. Kurman RJ, Prabha AC. Thyroid and parathyroid glands in the vaginal wall: report of a case. *Am J Clin Pathol* 1973;59:503–507.

222. Carney JA, Gordon H, Carpenter PC, Shenoy BV, Go VLW. The complex of myxomas, spotty pigmentation, and endocrine overactivity. *Medicine* 1985;64:270–283.

223. Carney JA. The triad of gastric epithelioid leiomyosarcoma, functioning extra adrenal paraganglioma and pulmonary chondroma. *Cancer* 1979;43:374–382.

224. Mallette LE. Dominant familial syndromes with endocrine hyperfunction—an additional syndrome? *Med Hypoth* 1992; 38:364–367.

225. Mallette LE, Malini S, Rappaport MP, Kirkland JL. Familial cystic parathyroid adenomatosis. *Ann Intern Med* 1987; 107:54–60.

226. Jackson CE. Hereditary hyperparathyroidism associated with recurrent pancreatitis. *Ann Intern Med* 1958;49:829–836.

227. Jackson CE, Boonstra CE. The relationship of hereditary

hyperparathyroidism to endocrine adenomatosis. *Am J Med* 1967;43:727–734.

228. Jackson CE, Norum RA, Boyd SB, et al. Hereditary hyperparathyroidism and multiple ossifying jaw fibromas: a clinically and genetically distinct syndrome. *Surgery* 1990;108: 1006–1013.

229. Kennett S, Pollick H. Jaw lesions in familial hyperparathyroidism. *Oral Surg* 1971;31:502–510.

230. Dinnen JS, Greenwood RH, Jones JH, Walker DA, Williams ED. Parathyroid carcinoma in familial hyperparathyroidism. *J Clin Pathol* 1977;30:966–975.

231. Rosen IB, Palmer JA. Fibroosseous tumors of the facial skeleton in association with primary hyperparathyroidism: an endocrine syndrome or coincidence? *Am J Surg* 1981; 142:494–498.

232. Warnakulasuriya S, Markwell BD, Williams DM. Familial hyperparathyroidism associated with cementifying fibromas of the jaws in two siblings. *Oral Surg* 1985;59:269–274.

233. Flye MW, Brennan MF. Surgical resection of metastatic parathyroid carcinoma. *Ann Surg* 1981;193:425–435.

234. Cohn K, Silverman M, Corrado J, Sedgewick C. Parathyroid carcinoma: the Lahey Clinic experience. *Surgery* 1985;98: 1095–1100.

235. Grevsten S, Grimelius L, Thorén L. Familial hyperparathyroidism. *Upsala J Med Sci* 1974;79:109–115.

236. Sandler LM, Moncrieff MW. Familial hyperparathyroidism. *Arch Dis Child* 1980;55:146–147.

237. Allo M, Thompson NW. Familial hyperparathyroidism caused by solitary adenomas. *Surgery* 1982;92:486–490.

238. Jung RT, Davie M, Grant AM, Jenkins D, Chalmers TM. Multiple endocrine adenomatosis (type I) and familial hyperparathyroidism. *Postgrad Med J* 1978;54:92–94.

239. Marx SJ, Attie MF, Levine MA, Spiegel AM, Downs RW, Lasker RD. The hypocalciuric or benign variant of familial hypercalcemia: clinical and biochemical features in fifteen kindreds. *Medicine* 1981;60:397–412.

240. Streeten EA, Weinstein LS, Norton JA, et al. Studies in a kindred with parathyroid carcinoma. *J Clin Endocrinol Metab* 1992;75:362–366.

241. Marx SJ. Familial hypocalciuric hypercalcemia. *N Engl J Med* 1980;303:810–811.

242. Heath H III. Familial benign (hypocalciuric) hypercalcemia. *Endocrinol Metab Clin North Am* 1989;18:723–740.

243. Marx SJ, Spiegel AM, Brown EM, et al. Circulating parathyroid hormone activity: familial hypocalciuric hypercalcemia versus typical primary hyperparathyroidism. *J Clin Endocrinol Metab* 1978;47:1190–1197.

244. Law WM Jr, James EM, Charboneau JW, Purnell DC, Heath H III. High-resolution parathyroid ultrasonography in familial benign hypercalcemia (familial hypocalciuric hypercalcemia). *Mayo Clin Proc* 1984;59:155–159.

245. Gilbert F, D'Amour P, Gascon-Barré M, et al. Familial hypocalciuric hypercalcemia: Description of a new kindred with emphasis on its difference from primary hyperparathyroidism. *Clin Invest Med* 1985;8:78–84.

246. McMurtry CT, Schranck FW, Walkenhorst DA, et al. Significant developmental elevation in serum parathyroid hormone levels in a large kindred with familial benign (hypocalciuric) hypercalcemia. *Am J Med* 1992;93:247–258.

247. Marx SJ, Attie MF, Spiegel AM, Levine MA, Lasker RD, Fox M. An association between neonatal severe primary hyperparathyroidism and familial hypocalciuric hypercalcemia in three kindreds. *N Engl J Med* 1982;306:257–264.

248. Mühlethaler JP, Schärer K, Antener I. Akuter hyperparathyreoidismus bei primärer nebenschilddrüsenhyperplasie. *Helv Pediatr Acta* 1967;22:529–557.

249. Cooper L, Wertheimer J, Levey R, et al. Severe primary hyperparathyroidism in a neonate with two hypercalcemic parents: Management with parathyroidectomy and heterotopic autotransplantation. *Pediatrics* 1986;78:263–268.

250. Marx SJ, Spiegel AM, Levine MA, et al. Familial hypocalciuric hypercalcemia: the relation to primary parathyroid hyperplasia. *N Engl J Med* 1982;307:416–426.

251. Eftekhari F, Yousefzadeh DK. Primary infantile hyperparathyroidism: clinical, laboratory, and radiographic features in 21 cases. *Skel Radiol* 1982;8:201–208.

252. Page LA, Haddow JE. Self-limited neonatal hyperparathyroidism in familial hypocalciuric hypercalcemia. *J Pediatr* 1987;111:261–264.

253. Steinmann B, Gnehm HE, Rao VH, Kind HP, Prader A. Neonatal severe primary hyperparathyroidism and alkaptonuria in a boy born to related parents with familial hypocalciuric hypercalcemia. *Helv Pediatr Acta* 1984;39:171–186.

254. Law WM Jr., Hodgson SF, Heath H III. Autosomal recessive inheritance of familial hyperparathyroidism. *N Engl J Med* 1983;309:650–652.

255. Edwards BD, Patton MA, Dilly SA, Eastwood JB. A new syndrome of autosomal recessive nephropathy, deafness, and hyperparathyroidism. *J Med Genet* 1989;26:289–293.

256. Colon-Zorba GE, Aguilo F Jr, Vazquez-Quintana E. A syndrome of familial intrathyroidal primary parathyroid hyperplasia: case reports and critical review of literature. *PR Health Sci J* 1986;5:55–63.

257. Feig DS, Gottesman IS. Familial hyperparathyroidism in association with colonic carcinoma. *Cancer* 1987;60:429–432.

258. Delamarre J, Capron JP, Armand A, Dupas JL, Deschepper B, Davion T. Thyroid carcinoma in two sisters with familial polyposis of the colon. Case reports and review of the literature. *J Clin Gastroenterol* 1988;10:659–662.

259. Herrera L, Carrel A, Rao U, Castillo N, Petrelli N. Familial adenomatous polyposis in association with thyroiditis. Report of two cases. *Dis Colon Rectum* 1989;32:893–896.

260. Reed MW, Harris SC, Quayle AR, Talbot CH. The association between thyroid neoplasia and intestinal polyps. *Ann R Coll Surg England* 1990;72:357–359.

261. Mallette LE, Bilezikian JP, Ketcham AS, Aurbach GD. Parathyroid carcinoma in familial hyperparathyroidism. *Am J Med* 1974;57:642–648.

262. Frayha RA, Nassar VH, Dagher F, Salti IS. Familial parathyroid carcinoma. *Leb Med J* 1972;25:299–309.

263. Leborgne J, Neel L, Buzelin F, Malvy P. Cancer familial des parathyroides. Intérêt de l'angiographie dans le diagnostic des récidives loco-régionales. Considérations á propos de deux cas. *J Chir* 1975;109:315–326.

264. Doppman JL, Krudy AG, Marx SJ, et al. Aspiration of enlarged parathyroid glands for parathyroid hormone assay. *Radiology* 1983;148:31–35.

265. Bergenfelz A, Forsberg L, Hederstrom E, Ahren B. Preoperative localization of enlarged parathyroid glands with ultrasonically guided fine needle aspiration for parathyroid hormone assay. *Acta Radiol* 1991;32:403–405.

266. Davey DD, Glant MD, Berger EK. Parathyroid cytopathology. *Diagn Cytopathol* 1986;2:76–80.

267. Löwhagen T, Sprenger E. Cytologic presentation of thyroid tumors in aspiration biopsy smear. A review of 60 cases. *Acta Cytol* 1974;18:192–197.

268. Friedman M, Shimaoka K, Lopez CA, Shedd DP. Parathyroid adenoma diagnosed as papillary carcinoma of thyroid on needle aspiration smears. *Acta Cytol* 1983;27:337–340.

269. Sulak LE, Brown RW, Butler DB. Parathyroid carcinoma with occult bone metastases diagnosed by fine needle aspiration cytology. *Acta Cytol* 1989;33:645–648.

270. Winkler B, Gooding GA, Montgomery CK, Clark OH, Arnaud C. Immunoperoxidase confirmation of parathyroid origin of ultrasound-guided fine needle aspirates of the parathyroid glands. *Acta Cytol* 1987;31:40–44.

271. Mallette LE, Tuma SN, Berger RE, Kirkland J. Radioimmunoassay for the middle region of human parathyroid hormone using an homologous antiserum with a carboxy-terminal fragment of bovine PTH as radioligand. *J Clin Endocrinol Metab* 1982;54:1017–1024.

272. Duber C, Hinkel E, Moll R, Rothmund M. Preoperative diagnosis of cystic parathyroid adenoma by ultrasonic-guided fine-needle puncture and parathormone determination. *Deutsch Med Wochenschr* 1986;111:943–945.

273. de la Garza S, Flores-de la Garza E, Hernandez-Batres F. Functional parathyroid carcinoma. Cytology, histology, and ultrastructure of a case. *Diagn Cytopathol* 1985;1:232–235.

274. Watson CW, Unger P, Kaneko M, Gabrilove JL. Fine needle aspiration of osteitis fibrosa cystica. *Diagn Cytopathol* 1985;1:157–160.

275. Bengtsson A, Grimelius L, Johanssen H, Pentén J. Nuclear DNA-content of parathyroid cells in adenomas, hyperplastic and normal glands. *Acta Pathol Microbiol Scand* (Sect A) 1977;85:455–460.

276. Bowlby LS, De Bault LE, Abraham SR. Flow cytometric DNA analysis of parathyroid glands. Relationship between nuclear DNA and pathologic classifications. *Am J Pathol* 1987;128:338–344.

277. Levin KE, Chew KL, Britt-Marie L, Mayall BH, Clark OH. Deoxyribonucleic acid cytometry helps identify parathyroid carcinomas. *J Clin Endocrinol Metab* 1988;67:779–784.

278. Joensuu H, Klemi P. DNA aneuploidy in adenomas of endocrine organs. *Am J Pathol* 1988;132:145–151.

279. Obara T, Fujimoto Y, Kanaji Y, et al. Flow cytometric DNA analysis of parathyroid tumors. Implication of aneuploidy for pathologic and biologic classification. *Cancer* 1990;66:1555–1562.

280. Shenton BK, Ellis H, Johnston ID, Farndon JR. DNA analysis and parathyroid pathology. *World J Surg* 1990;14:296–301.

281. Rosen IB, Musclow E. DNA histogram of parathyroid tissue in determining extent of parathyroidectomy. *Surgery* 1985;98:1024–1030.

282. Gagel RF, Levy ML, Donovan DT, Alford BR, Wheeler T, Tschen JA. Multiple endocrine neoplasia type 2a associated with cutaneous lichen amyloidosis. *Ann Intern Med* 1989;111:802–806.

The Parathyroids, edited by J.P. Bilezikian, M.A. Levine, and R. Marcus. Raven Press, Ltd., New York © 1994.

CHAPTER 26

Clinical Presentation of Primary Hyperparathyroidism

John P. Bilezikian, Shonni J. Silverberg, Flore Gartenberg, Tae-Sook Kim, Thomas P. Jacobs, Ethel S. Siris, and Elizabeth Shane

Primary hyperparathyroidism is a common endocrine disorder. It is characterized by the excessive and incompletely regulated secretion of parathyroid hormone (PTH) from one or more parathyroid glands. The major actions of PTH, to mobilize calcium from bone, to conserve calcium in the kidney, and indirectly to increase gastrointestinal calcium absorption, lead to one of the major biochemical hallmarks of the disease, hypercalcemia. Another major sign of the disorder is an elevated level of PTH, now readily detected by accurate assays for the hormone. Advances in evaluation of metabolic bone diseases by sensitive, newly available circulating and urinary markers of calcium metabolism have permitted a more detailed assessment of patients who do not appear to be suffering from overt clinical consequences of primary hyperparathyroidism. In addition, bone densitometry and analysis of bone by quantitative histomorphometry have provided direct insight into important current features of the disease. The result is a profile of primary hyperparathyroidism that not only is quite different from earlier historical descriptions but also requires consideration of a new set of issues insofar as the clinical management of the disease is concerned.

Because primary hyperparathyroidism is the major clinical disorder of the parathyroids, it is fitting that this disorder be the focus of an extensive discussion covering over 14 chapters in this volume that each deal with many important individual issues. This chapter

introduces many of these issues in describing major clinical features of primary hyperparathyroidism. The evolving clinical spectrum of primary hyperparathyroidism is considered also, with a retrospective view of what used to be more typical presentations of the disease. Frequent cross-references will facilitate easy access to other chapters for readers who may want to explore some of these points in greater depth.

PREVALENCE AND INCIDENCE

It is remarkable that within the lifetimes of many endocrinologists, most notably the senior ones, primary hyperparathyroidism has been transformed from an extremely rare endocrine disorder to one of the most common. In the 1930s and 1940s, primary hyperparathyroidism was appreciated virtually always in the context of a most unusual disorder with characteristic skeletal features known as osteitis fibrosa cystica. In fact, it was said in those days that "the x-ray findings proved to be so characteristic that chemical analysis was needed only for confirmation" (1). Other features of the historical summary of primary hyperparathyroidism by Oliver Cope in 1966 point out aptly how these patients invariably deteriorated with a particularly pernicious bone disease. Studies of the famous sea captain Charles Martell by Bauer and colleagues (2,3) and the work of the Viennese surgeon Mandl (4) gave great impetus to the correct idea that primary hyperparathyroidism is caused by abnormal function of parathyroid tissue and that removal of the offending adenoma leads to correction of the hypercalcemia. Despite the facts that the disorder used to be rare and that the first series of patients with primary hyperparathyroidism described in 1934 included only 17 patients (5), it was evident even in those days that the incidence of

J. P. Bilezikian: Departments of Medicine and Pharmacology, College of Physicians and Surgeons, Columbia University, New York, New York 10032.

S. J. Silverberg, F. Gartenberg, T. S. Kim, T. P. Jacobs, E. S. Siris, E. Shane: Department of Medicine, Division of Endocrinology, College of Physicians and Surgeons, Columbia University, New York, New York 10032.

the disease was, in part, a function of how high one's index of suspicion was for it. For example, Raymond Keating, whose work at the Mayo Clinic helped to establish modern concepts of the disease, was dispatched to the Massachusetts General Hospital in 1942 specifically to learn how the physicians there seemed to recognize patients fairly readily (Aub, Bauer, Albright, and Cope had seen 67 patients by this time), while the experience at the Mayo Clinic was much more limited. After this tutorial in Boston, Keating returned to the Mayo Clinic and, with a clear intention to uncover the disease, saw more patients with primary hyperparathyroidism in the next year than he had seen in the preceding 15 years (6). This early experience makes a point that has been relived in the modern era. In the absence of serendipity or incidental discovery, the disorder is not readily diagnosed without a high index of suspicion.

The dramatic change in the incidence of primary hyperparathyroidism occurred in the late 1960s and early 1970s, due primarily to the introduction of the multichannel autoanalyzer. Documentation of this change comes from the work of Heath and his colleagues as well as from other groups (7–11). Incidence figures among residents of Rochester, Minnesota, increased nearly fivefold in the first year after the multichannel screening profile became routinely available (1974–1975). Thereafter, allowing for the "catch-up" detection factor in that first year, the incidence figures continued to show an impressive fourfold increase in comparison to the premultichannel autoanalyzer era (12) (Table 1).

It is difficult to estimate true incidence figures for primary hyperparathyroidism (13), but the experience in Rochester, Minnesota, of 27.7 per 100,000 person-years is essentially identical to figures from Sweden (9) and from Birmingham, England (8). On the basis on these figures, an estimate of ~100,000 new cases of primary hyperparathyroidism per year in the United States is likely to be accurate.

The prevalence of primary hyperparathyroidism (the proportion of the population affected with the disease at a given point in time) is higher than earlier estimates of incidence (the number of *new* cases diagnosed over a specified period of time). Prevalence

estimates have been as high as 1 in 100 (14), but 1 per 1,000 would appear to be closer to the true prevalence rate (15).

Primary hyperparathyroidism occurs throughout life, but the incidence peaks in the middle years. Women predominate over men by a 2:1–3:1 margin. The disease is recognized most commonly in women who are in the first postmenopausal decade, between ages 50 and 60 years. It is perhaps because of the effects of estrogens to oppose some of the skeletal actions of PTH that the disease may surface clinically when estrogen levels fall. There do not appear to be any well-established predisposing factors for the development of primary hyperparathyroidism, but a history of irradiation to the neck and upper chest area in childhood is obtained in as many as 15–25% of patients with the disease (16,17). Rarely, primary hyperparathyroidism after ^{131}I therapy for thyroid disease has been reported (18). Exciting new insights into the molecular bases of some cases of primary hyperparathyroidism are covered in the chapter by Arnold (19). Newer concepts of parathyroid cell growth properties in primary hyperparathyroidism are presented in the chapter by Parfitt (20).

PATHOLOGY

Most patients with primary hyperparathyroidism (80–85%) harbor a single adenoma; the other three glands are normal. The adenoma is described histologically as a confluence of parathyroid cells that may be associated with a rim of normal tissue at the margins. The usual size of the adenoma is ~0.5–1.0 g, although abnormal glands distinctly smaller or larger are seen. Even the smaller adenomas, <0.5 g, are usually much larger than normal parathyroid glands, which are ~25–35 mg. Cystic elements in an adenomatous gland may call attention to a rare familial variant of primary hyperparathyroidism, cystic parathyroid adenomatosis (21). Details of the histopathology of primary hyperparathyroidism are covered in the chapter by LiVolsi and of unusual variants in the chapter, "The Functional and Pathologic Spectrum of Parathyroid Abnormalities in Hyperparathyroidism," by Mallette.

Approximately 15–20% of patients with primary hy-

TABLE 1. *Average annual incidence rates for primary hyperparathyroidism in Rochester, Minnesota, before addition of calcium measurement to serum chemistry panel (1/1/65–6/30/74) and afterward (7/1/74–12/31/76)[a]*

	Time interval	Years	No. cases	Average annual incidence [new diagnoses (mean ± SD) per 100,000 population per year]
Before	1/1/65–6/30/74	9.5	39	7.8 ± 1.2
After	7/1/74–6/30/75	1	28	51.1 ± 9.6
	7/1/75–12/31/76	1.5	23	27.7 ± 5.8

[a]Note that the latter period is divided to illustrate "catch-up" diagnosis. Reprinted from Heath (12) with permission of the publisher.

perparathyroidism have a pathologic process involving all four parathyroid glands. Four-gland hyperplasia may occur sporadically and is more likely to be seen in younger individuals. This pathology is also seen in conjunction with multiple endocrine neoplasia Types I or II (see chapters by Metz et al., Friedman et al., and by Gagel). The extent to which each parathyroid gland is involved may vary from a gland that is abnormal only by the most subtle histological clues (i.e., diminished fat content) to others that are so grossly enlarged that they look like adenomas. The correct distinction between hyperplastic and adenomatous disease is important because the surgical approach is defined, in part, by the pathology (see chapter by Norton et al.). As was noted in the chapters by LiVolsi and by Norton et al., the success of this distinction depends upon readily available, accurate histological appraisal at the time of parathyroid surgery. Other variants of these basic pathologic types of primary hyperparathyroidism are covered in the chapter, "The Functional and Pathologic Spectrum of Parathyroid Abnormalities in Hyperparathyroidism," by Mallette.

The rarest form of primary hyperparathyroidism is parathyroid carcinoma (22,23). In that primary hyperparathyroidism has changed in its clinical presentation from a disorder with invariable signs and symptoms to one of asymptomatic hypercalcemia, it is not surprising that the diagnosis of parathyroid carcinoma is made much less frequently relative to the hyperparathyroid population. Recent incidence figures place parathyroid carcinoma as a cause of primary hyperparathyroidism in well under 1% of all patients with primary hyperparathyroidism. For patients suspected of having parathyroid carcinoma from their rather distinctive clinical presentation (see chapter by Shane), the gross appearance and the pathology of the parathyroid tissue removed become key elements in the diagnosis.

CLASSICAL CLINICAL MANIFESTATIONS OF PRIMARY HYPERPARATHYROIDISM

Physical Findings

The most noteworthy aspect of the physical examination in primary hyperparathyroidism is that the examination is not noteworthy. There are usually no abnormal physical findings specifically related to the disease. Hypertension, which is frequently seen, has not been established to be related directly to primary hyperparathyroidism (see below). Calcium-phosphate deposition in the medial and lateral limbic margins of the cornea (band keratopathy) is seen now only rarely and virtually only by ophthalmologic slit-lamp examinations. Enlarged parathyroid tissue is usually palpable only when parathyroid carcinoma is present. The neurological examination, which used to be of interest

in the days when the neuromuscular manifestations of primary hyperparathyroidism were often seen (see below), is now invariably normal.

Symptoms and Signs

The symptoms and signs of primary hyperparathyroidism are, in part, related to those of hypercalcemia per se. The clinical features of hypercalcemia as well as its differential diagnosis are covered in the chapter by Bilezikian and Singer (24). In this regard, the extent to which patients may be symptomatic is related directly to whether the hypercalcemia is in the range usually associated with specific symptomatology. It should be recalled that the symptoms of hypercalcemia are a function of the rate of rise of the serum calcium as well as the actual level. In addition, symptoms of hypercalcemia vary from patient to patient. Most patients with mild primary hyperparathyroidism and calcium levels within 1 mg/dl of the upper limits of normal do not have features that can readily be attributed to the hypercalcemia per se.

Specific manifestations of primary hyperparathyroidism are those traditionally viewed as features of the disease itself. Along with the dramatic increase in the incidence of this disease, its clinical presentation has also undergone a major change. Nevertheless, primary hyperparathyroidism may still be associated with a number of different clinical presentations (Table 2) (25).

Classic Radiological Manifestations of Bone Disease Associated With Primary Hyperparathyroidism

The classic bone disease of primary hyperparathyroidism is osteitis fibrosa cystica (Fig. 1). When symptomatic, osteitis fibrosa cystica is experienced by patients as bone pain. Pathological fractures may occur. Overt bone resorption caused by excessive concentrations of PTH is associated with several typical radiological signs. Subperiosteal bone resorption of the distal phalanges is the most sensitive radiological sign of

TABLE 2. *Clinical presentations of primary hyperparathyroidism*

Asymptomatic hypercalcemia
Bone or stone disease
Other recognized complications (neuromuscular, gastrointestinal, articular, hematologic, central nervous system)
Acute primary hyperparathyroidism
Parathyroid carcinoma
Familial primary hyperparathyroidism
Familial cystic parathyroid adenomatosis
Neonatal hyperparathyroidism
Multiple endocrine neoplasia type I or II

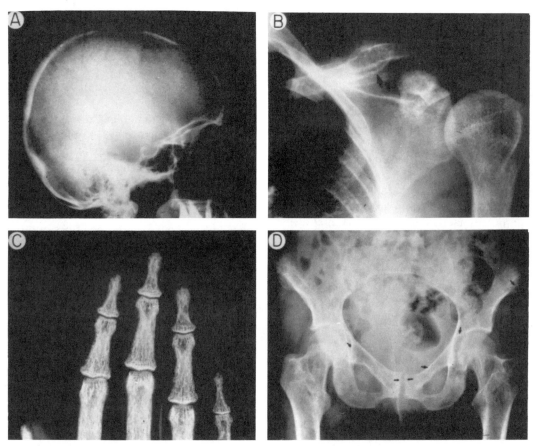

FIG. 1. Classical radiographic manifestations of primary hyperparathyroidism. The salt and pepper appearance of the skull (**A**), distal tapering of the clavicle (**B**), resorption of the distal phalanges (**C**), and cysts in the pelvis (**D**) are seen.

primary hyperparathyroidism. It is appreciated best on the radial side of the middle phalanges. Similar radiological changes may be present in the skull in the form of a motheaten or salt-and-pepper pattern. The distal one-third of the clavicles may appear to be tapered. Local destructive lesions, bone cysts, and "brown tumors" in the long bones and pelvis constitute other skeletal manifestations of the disease. Brown tumors are collections of osteoclasts intermixed with poorly mineralized woven bone. Nonspecific generalized skeletal demineralization is sometimes evident in the absence of these other features of hyperparathyroid bone disease. Both nonspecific demineralization and the specific radiological manifestations outlined above reflect the catabolic skeletal actions of PTH.

Stone Disease

Kidney stones constitute another classic manifestation of primary hyperparathyroidism. Although the incidence of nephrolithiasis in primary hyperparathyroidism has diminished along with the incidence of

bone disease, stones nevertheless are still seen. Most series now place the incidence of kidney stones at 15–20% of all patients with primary hyperparathyroidism (see the chapter by Klugman et al.) (25–27). Because nephrolithiasis is such an important complication of primary hyperparathyroidism and because primary hyperparathyroidism is such a common disorder, it is still advisable to investigate the possibility of primary hyperparathyroidism in any patient who develops a kidney stone. It is even worth screening the population of stone sufferers for this possibility despite the fact that only ~2–5% of stone formers will be shown to have primary hyperparathyroidism (28). Besides nephrolithiasis, the kidneys may be affected in other ways. Deposition of calcium-phosphate crystals throughout the renal parenchyma, a process known as *nephrocalcinosis*, may occur. Nephrocalcinosis may or may not be associated with frank stones and/or a reduction in creatinine clearance. Hypercalciuria defined as a total urinary calcium excretion of >250 mg (women) or >300 mg (men) occurs in up to 35–40% of patients with primary hyperparathyroidism (29). The hypercalciuria is caused by the greater load of filtered calcium, which exceeds the capacity of the kidney to reabsorb it despite the conserving actions of PTH on renal calcium handling. Whether hypercalciuria is related to or places patients at risk for stone disease is discussed in the chapter by Klugman et al. Some patients with primary hyperparathyroidism will show reduced creatinine clearance without stones, hypercalciuria, nephrocalcinosis, or other predisposing factors.

Involvement of Other Organs

Primary hyperparathyroidism has the potential to involve organ systems besides the skeleton and the kidneys. The common complaints of weakness and easy fatigueability used to be associated, in an earlier time, with a particular neuromuscular syndrome characterized histologically by atrophy of type II muscle fibers (30,31). Recent experience suggests that the weakness and easy fatigueability sometimes ascribed to the hyperparathyroid syndrome are no longer associated with overt neurological findings (32). However, in detailed electromyographical studies of muscles in primary hyperparathyroidism, abnormalities are still reported (33).

The gastrointestinal tract may also appear to be a target of the hyperparathyroid state. Historically, peptic ulcer disease was regarded as a frequent complication. It is now seen predominantly with the MEN-I Syndrome, in which primary hyperparathyroidism and peptic ulcer disease may coexist. Aside from this specific association, there is continuing debate over a pathophysiological link between these two relatively common disorders (34). Similarly, the association between primary hyperparathyroidism and acute pancreatitis, apart from that related to hypercalcemia per se, remains to be established (35).

Gout or pseudogout may affect the articular system of those with primary hyperparathyroidism. Older patients with asymptomatic chondrocalcinosis of the knees and bones of the wrist may be at risk for the development of pseudogout (36,37). The anemia of primary hyperparathyroidism, characterized by normocytic and normochromic indices (38), is an unusual finding, occurring only when other systemic manifestations of primary hyperparathyroidism are also present.

Hypertension has been thought for many years to be a complicating feature of primary hyperparathyroidism. The experience of Heath et al. (7), in which there seems to be a greater incidence of hypertension among those with primary hyperparathyroidism in comparison to a control population, is in agreement with the experience of others (39–42). However, most patients do not experience a significant reduction in the blood pressure after successful parathyroid surgery (43,44). The neuropsychiatric manifestations of primary hy-

perparathyroidism are the subject of great debate and much uncertainty. In part, this is because the symptomatology is exceedingly nonspecific. Affective disorders, anxiety, cognitive difficulties, and somatization exemplify the kinds of manifestations that have been ascribed to the hyperparathyroid syndrome. Certainly most clinicians who care for patients with primary hyperparathyroidism agree that such symptoms are sometimes elicited from or volunteered by their patients. Moreover, some reports are intriguing for an apparent reversal of these symptoms after successful parathyroid surgery. Ljunghall and his colleagues (45–48) have investigated this problem in a series of impressive studies attempting to quantify this symptom complex using psychopathological rating scales before and after surgery. Their work, which suggests an association, has not been generally appreciated by others (49,50). Also pertinent to this discussion are attempts to study the potential reversibility of these symptoms after successful parathyroid surgery, a subject mired in great uncertainty (see the chapter by Kleerekoper). It is unclear to what extent patients with primary hyperparathyroidism have manifestations that can be ascribed with certainty to a neuropsychiatric complex specifically due to primary hyperparathyroidism.

CLINICAL MANIFESTATIONS OF PRIMARY HYPERPARATHYROIDISM: THEN AND NOW

It is obvious that the clinical manifestations of primary hyperparathyroidism have changed dramatically over the past 40 years. A comparison of several series makes this point well. The series published by Cope (1), which is typical of the preautoanalyzer years, reviewed the experience of the first 343 cases at the Massachusetts General Hospital up to 1965. Heath and colleagues (7,12) and Mallette et al. (51) report an experience that straddles a 10 year period when the autoanalyzer became widely used. The experience of Silverberg and colleagues (26,27) exemplifies the more modern clinical presentation of primary hyperparathyroidism in the 1980s and 1990s. These comparisons are shown in Table 3. The frequency of specific radiological manifestations of primary hyperparathyroidism dropped from 23% in the Cope series to 10–14% in the Heath and Mallette series, to a remarkably low 2% in the Silverberg series. In fact, hyperparathyroid bone disease is now so rarely seen that most clinicians dispense with routine radiological assessment of primary hyperparathyroidism. Also noteworthy is the drop in the incidence of nephrolithiasis among these series. In the Cope series, stone disease was very common, occurring in 57% of all cases. In the Heath and Mallette series, the incidences of stone disease were 51% and

TABLE 3. *Changing profile of primary hyperparathyroidism*

	Cope (1) (1930–1965)	Heath et al. (7) (1965–1974)	Mallette et al. (51) (1965–1972)	Silverberg et al. (1986–1993)
Nephrolithiasis (%)	57	51	37	19.5
Skeletal disease (%)	23	10	14	2
Hypercalciuria (%)	NR[a]	36	40	39
Asymptomatic (%)	0.6	18	22	80

[a]Not reported.

37%, respectively. In the Silverberg series, the incidence dropped further to 19%, an incidence similar to the report of Nikkil et al. (52). Hypercalciuria was not noted in the Cope series, but it is interesting that the incidence of this feature of primary hyperparathyroidism did not change from an incidence of 36% reported by Heath and colleagues to ~40% reported by Mallette et al. to 39% reported by Silverberg et al. (29). Other possible manifestations of note such as pancreatitis and peptic ulcer disease are too infrequent in any of the series to make meaningful comparisons or to detect any trends.

It is thus clear that the profile of primary hyperparathyroidism, insofar as the well-established clinical manifestations of the disease are concerned, has changed dramatically. If potential manifestations of primary hyperparathyroidism (hypertension, neuropsychiatric abnormalities, etc.) are excluded from consideration, simply because we do not yet know whether they are specific for the hyperparathyroid process, one reaches the conclusion that the vast majority of patients seen with primary hyperparathyroidism today (~80%) are asymptomatic. The definition of asymptomatic primary hyperparathyroidism was stated best by Heath et al. (53): "well-documented primary hyperparathyroidism in which there are neither complications nor symptoms that are clearly and commonly attributable to either hypercalcemia or parathyroid hormone excess."

BIOCHEMICAL MANIFESTATIONS OF PRIMARY HYPERPARATHYROIDISM

The presence of hypercalcemia is an essential part of the biochemical definition of primary hyperparathyroidism. Most often, the serum calcium concentration is not >1 mg/dl above the upper limits of normal (Table 4). However, in marked contrast to the mild hypercalcemia characteristic of most patients with primary hyperparathyroidism, life-threatening hypercalcemia can still occur. This entity, which is known as *acute primary hyperparathyroidism* (also as *parathyroid poisoning* or *parathyroid crisis*) has a distinctive presen-

TABLE 4. *Baseline serum indices in 97 patients with primary hyperparathyroidism*

	All patients[a]	Normal range
Calcium (mg/dl)	11.1 ± 0.1	8.7–10.7
Phosphorus (mg/dl)	2.8 ± 0.1	2.5–4.5
Alk. phos. (IU/liter)	114 ± 5	<100
Magnesium (mg/dl)	2.0 ± 0.1	1.8–2.4
N-PTH (pg/ml)	30.0 ± 1.5	8–24
MM-PTH (pg/ml)	771 ± 64	50–330
IRMA-PTH (pg/ml)	119 ± 7	10–65
25-(OH)D (ng/ml)	19 ± 1	9–52
1,25-(OH)$_2$D (pg/ml)	54 ± 2	16–60

[a]Mean age 55 ± 1 years.

tation (54) (see the chapter by Fitzpatrick). On the extreme other hand, there are very rare patients with normal serum calcium values who have primary hyperparathyroidism. The designation *normocalcemic primary hyperparathyroidism* for these patients is probably not accurate, because hypercalcemia invariably surfaces in these patients over time or is seen intermittently. If both the total and ionized serum calcium concentrations are normal, it is exceedingly difficult to make the diagnosis of primary hyperparathyroidism.

Another important feature of the biochemical definition of primary hyperparathyroidism is elevated circulating levels of PTH. Improved assays to detect intact PTH in the circulation with immunoradiometric and immunochemiluminometric techniques have not only served to establish the diagnosis of primary hyperparathyroidism with greater certainty but have also served to exclude virtually all other causes of hypercalcemia. The assays in common use in the United States detect elevated levels of PTH in patients with primary hyperparathyroidism ~90% of the time. If multiple samples are obtained in patients who eventually are shown to have primary hyperparathyroidism, the incidence of elevated levels is even higher. This subject is covered in greater detail in the chapter by Nussbaum and Potts.

The serum phosphorus level is usually in the lower range of normal. It is frankly below normal, <2.5 mg/

dl, in only 25% of all patients. In the absence of significant renal insufficiency, it is distinctly unusual for the serum phosphorus to be >3.5 mg/dl in primary hyperparathyroidism. The serum chloride is usually >103 mEq/liter (55). Lafferty has used the serum chloride, calcium, and phosphorus as well as the hematocrit to derive a discriminant function to distinguish primary hyperparathyroidism from other causes of hypercalcemia. Similarly, Lind and Ljunghall (56) have employed the serum chloride, alkaline phosphatase, and albumin. Although this approach is undoubtedly valid, the improved diagnostic utility of currently available assays for PTH makes discriminant analysis useful only in those very unusual patients for whom the differential diagnosis of hypercalcemia is exceedingly difficult.

In our recent experience, the serum alkaline phosphatase activity was modestly but significantly elevated, 114 ± 5 IU/liter (normal <100). When correlated with more specific markers of bone formation, such as the osteocalcin level (see the chapter by Deftos), it is clear that the total alkaline phosphatase is a bone marker in primary hyperparathyroidism. The implications of this finding for the presence of bone involvement in asymptomatic primary hyperparathyroidism are described below. The 25-hydroxyvitamin D level tends to be in the lower range of normal, while the 1,25-dihydroxyvitamin D [1,25(OH)$_2$D] level tends to be in the upper range of normal (Table 4). In 30–35% of patients, the 1,25(OH)$_2$D level is frankly elevated (57), illustrating a physiological action of PTH to stimulate the production of 1,25(OH)$_2$D. When hyperparathyroidism is associated with marked hypercalcemia, the 1,25(OH)$_2$D level may be suppressed, mimicking the profile seen in hypercalcemia of malignancy. In this unusual situation, it would appear that the inhibitory effects of hypercalcemia on 1,25(OH)$_2$D production override the stimulatory effects of PTH (58).

Urinary indices in primary hyperparathyroidism are shown in Table 5. Total urinary calcium excretion in most patients with primary hyperparathyroidism is at the upper limits of the normal range, 248 mg total excretion, or 240 mg/g creatinine. Urinary calcium excretion is elevated in 39% of all patients. Excretion of urinary pyridinium cross-links of collagen is in the upper range of normal for pyridinoline and is frankly elevated for the collagen cross-link with more specificity for bone, deoxypyridinoline (Table 5) (59,60). Urinary collagen cross-link excretion reflects bone resorption (see the chapter by Deftos). Similar to use of the osteocalcin measurement, the use of a more specific marker of bone metabolism, such as urinary pyridinium crosslink excretion, has implications for detection of bone involvement in patients with asymptomatic primary hyperparathyroidism.

TABLE 5. *Baseline urinary indices in 97 patients with primary hyperparathyroidism*

Urine index	All patients[a]	Normal range
Calcium	248 ± 14	
Calcium/creat (mg/g)	240 ± 11	<250
Phosphorus (mg/dl)	753 ± 34	
Cyclic AMP (nmol/dl)	3.9 ± 0.2	3.9 ± 1.1
Hydroxyproline (mg/day)	39 ± 2	<40 mg/day
Pyridinoline (nmol/mmol creatinine)	46.8 ± 2.7	<51.8
Deoxypyridinoline (nmol/mmol creatinine)	17.6 ± 1.3	<14.6

ASSESSMENT OF PRIMARY HYPERPARATHYROIDISM WITH NEWER APPROACHES

The increased incidence of asymptomatic primary hyperparathyroidism presents a dilemma to the clinician. On the one hand, one could argue that this increased incidence merely reflects enhanced recognition of the disease because of the widespread availability of the multichannel screening test and that patients being identified now represent part of a cohort of patients who were present but unrecognized even in the days of Fuller Albright. The argument continues that these patients could just as well be returned to that unrecognized cohort, because it is only the unusual patient who surfaces with overt clinical complications of the disease. This approach suggests a rather benign natural history of primary hyperparathyroidism in most patients. On the other hand, we are faced with the knowledge of the potential destructiveness of hyperparathyroidism at its target organs. Recognition of the disease in milder form might be an opportunity to examine more carefully at the time of diagnosis questions such as whether the disease process has already affected the skeleton and whether it progresses over time. These as yet unanswered questions highlight the need to gain greater insight into the course of primary hyperparathyroidism, an area explored in the chapter by Kleerekoper. These issues also highlight the need to establish guidelines for parathyroid surgery based on knowledge more certain than is currently available. The availability of sensitive techniques to monitor the skeleton has given us an opportunity to address some of these issues in patients who have asymptomatic primary hyperparathyroidism.

Bone Densitometry in Primary Hyperparathyroidism

Bone density was measured at three sites to evaluate areas enriched in cortical bone (distal radius), cancellous bone (vertebral spine), and a mixture of both (the hip region) (26,27). At the distal radius, bone density was <80% of age- and sex-matched control values in 58% of our patients. The actual value at this site (0.54 ± 0.1 g/cm) was only 79% of the expected mean value. In contrast, at the lumbar spine, bone mineral density was relatively well preserved. Only 13% of patients had lumbar bone density <80% of age- and sex-matched control values. The actual value (1.07 ± 0.03 g/cm²) was within 5% of the expected mean. The values for the hip region were midway between data obtained for the spine and those for the distal radius (Fig. 2). Pfeilschifter et al. (61) recently confirmed these findings. Among 38 patients with primary hyperparathyroidism, bone mineral density was reduced much more markedly at the radius than at the lumbar spine. At the lumbar spine, bone mineral density was greater in those with only mildly elevated PTH levels. There was a strong association between total serum alkaline phosphatase and low bone mineral z scores (61). These results indicate that, in mild primary hyperparathyroidism, reductions in cortical bone density are seen regularly and that the cancellous bone is relatively well preserved. This is of particular importance for several reasons. First, it is consistent with the impression that PTH has effects to mobilize calcium from cortical sites before it impacts negatively on the cancellous skeleton. In patients with more marked elevations in PTH, reductions in bone density at cancellous sites would be expected to be seen. Second, significant reductions in cortical bone are detectable before any radiological manifestations are apparent. Third, the preservation of cancellous bone may be of particular importance in that primary hyperparathyroidism is a disease that disproportionately affects postmenopausal women. Women in their postmenopausal years are at risk for bone loss due to estrogen deficiency, which occurs

first in the cancellous bone of the spine. Thus the early effects of primary hyperparathyroidism on vertebral cancellous bone appear to be opposite to those of estrogen deficiency. Moreover, a characteristic pattern of bone densitometry in primary hyperparathyroidism is the opposite of the early changes seen in postmenopausal osteoporosis, namely, more significant loss at a cortical site, exemplified by the distal radius, than at a cancellous site, such as the spine. These observations have several important implications. They support data suggesting that the anabolic actions of PTH can be appreciated at the spine (62) and that, in some protocols, this anabolic effect occurs at the expense of a loss of cortical bone (63). They also have implications for the potential use of parathyroid hormone as a therapeutic agent for postmenopausal osteoporosis (see the chapter by Marcus). The observations also have bearing on the indications for parathyroid surgery in postmenopausal women with primary hyperparathyroidism (see the chapter by Bilezikian).

Bone Histomorphometry in Primary Hyperparathyroidism

The results obtained by bone densitometry have been supported by a direct analysis of the bone biopsy by quantitative histomorphometry (64–68). Bone biopsy results are consistent with a loss of cortical bone and preservation of cancellous bone. The measurements included both static and dynamic parameters of bone as well as a newer approach, strut analysis. The work of Parisien et al. has shown that static parameters of bone such as osteoid surface, osteoid volume, and eroded surface are all elevated in both men and women with primary hyperparathyroidism compared to normal values. Dynamic parameters of bone turnover (mineralizing surface and bone formation rate) are also elevated. Consistent with observations made via bone densitometry, indices that describe cancellous bone architecture are preserved in primary hyperparathyroidism. These parameters include cancellous bone volume, trabecular number, and trabecular separation. On the other hand, cortical thickness is significantly decreased in biopsies from patients with primary hyperparathyroidism. These data support the idea that patients with primary hyperparathyroidism have increased bone turnover, thinning of cortical bone, and increased cancellous bone volume. The striking maintainence of trabecular plates further supports the idea that the hyperparathyroid process protects cancellous bone. By strut analysis, this preservation appears to be based on an architectural maintenance of connectivity between and among trabecular plates (see the chapter by Parisien et al.)

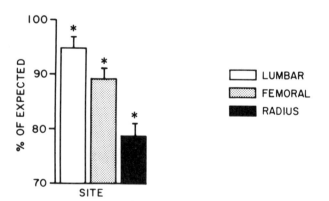

FIG. 2. Bone densitometry in primary hyperparathyroidism. Three different sites, radius, femoral neck, and lumbar spine, are shown in comparison to expected values for age-, sex-, and ethnicity-matched normal subjects. Divergence from expected values is different at each site ($P = 0.0001$). (Reprinted from ref. 26 with permission.)

Fracture Incidence in Primary Hyperparathyroidism

These observations might lead to certain predictions about fracture incidence in primary hyperparathyroidism. It is generally agreed that, as bone mass decreases, there is a rise in the incidence of fractures (69). Certainly in the form of primary hyperparathyroidism seen many years ago, generalized osteopenia and fractures were regularly appreciated (70). In the disease as it is seen today, however, the skeleton appears to be targeted selectively, with cortical sites being the focus of the catabolic actions of PTH, and cancellous sites being a focus of its anabolic actions. At this phase of the disease (if indeed, the disease has phases), one might expect that, in the primary hyperparathyroidism seen today, fracture incidence is not increased at the spine, whereas fracture of the distal radius or other cortical sites might depend, in part, on the degree to which there has been a reduction in bone mineral density at those site(s). Unfortunately, very little information is available. Wilson et al. (71) reported on 174 patients with primary hyperparathyroidism in whom there was no increased incidence of vertebral fractures. In contrast, Peacock and colleagues (72,73) have reported an increased incidence of both vertebral and cortical fractures in patients with primary hyperparathyroidism. In Peacock's series, however, both cortical and cancellous bone were reduced, suggesting that these patients may have had more bone involvement than the patients seen by Wilson et al. (71). Other studies have argued for (74,75) or against (76) an increase in fracture incidence in primary hyperparathyroidism. In a retrospective series, Melton et al. (77) recently reported the observation that fracture incidence was increased in patients *before* the diagnosis was made but that, afterwards, there was no difference in fracture incidence between hyperparathyroid subjects and a control group. One of the major areas in need of investigation is the matter of fracture incidence in primary hyperparathyroidism as well as information pertinent to changes in bone mineral density and fracture incidence following successful parathyroidectomy.

BONE AND STONE DISEASE IN PRIMARY HYPERPARATHYROIDISM

Older concepts of primary hyperparathyroidism included the teaching that concurrent bone and stone disease is rare (5,70,78,79). It was believed that patients who hyperabsorbed calcium from the gastrointestinal tract were predisposed to stones, whereas those who did not show gastrointestinal hyperabsorp-

tion of calcium were predisposed to bone disease. Recently, evidence for and against these older notions has been presented (78,79).

The hypothesis of two distinct pathophysiological groupings of patients with primary hyperparathyroidism is difficult to test now because overt, radiologically evident bone disease has become rare. Thus concomitant, overt skeletal disease and stone disease are seen usually only in the special situations of acute primary hyperparathyroidism and parathyroid cancer (see the chapters by Fitzpatrick and by Shane). However, since recent data indicate that hyperparathyroid bone involvement can be detected in a large number of patients with asymptomatic primary hyperparathyroidism when more sensitive methods (bone densitometry and quantitative bone histomorphometry) are employed, it is useful to reconsider this hypothesis.

In our experience, cortical demineralization occurs to the same extent and with the same frequency in patients with and without nephrolithiasis (29) (Fig. 3). Moreover, the pattern of skeletal demineralization of cortical sites was similar in stone formers and in the entire cohort of hyperparathyroid subjects. Bone densitometric analysis provided further evidence against a pathophysiological distinction between bone disease and stone disease in primary hyperparathyroidism. Urinary calcium excretion correlated negatively with forearm bone mineral density, suggesting that at least a component of urinary calcium excretion reflects events occurring in bone (Fig. 4). These detailed studies thus fail to confirm the classic teaching that bone disease and stone disease are mutually exclusive man-

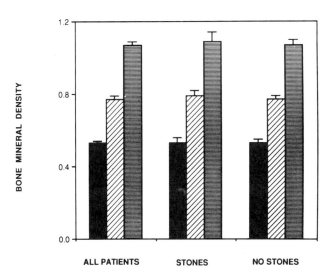

FIG. 3. Bone mineral density by at the forearm (*solid bars,* g/cm), femoral neck (*diagonally hatched bars,* g/cm²), and lumbar spine (*horizontally hatched bars,* g/cm²). Values are shown as mean ± SEM for the entire cohort and the subgroups with and without nephrolithiasis. (Reprinted from ref. 29 with permission.)

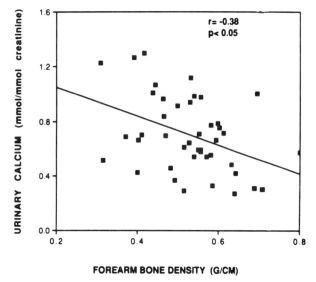

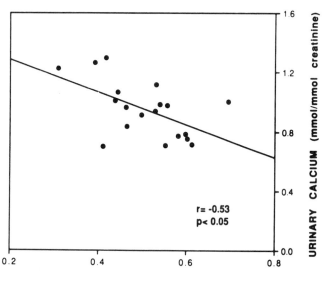

FIG. 4. Correlation of urinary calcium excretion per mmol creatinine with forearm bone mineral density in the entire cohort of hyperparathyroid subjects (*top*) and a subgroup with hypercalciuria (*bottom*). (Reprinted from ref. 29 with permission.)

ifestations of primary hyperparathyroidism. Another view of this issue is presented in the chapter by Parfitt.

WHAT HAS HAPPENED TO THE PRIMARY HYPERPARATHYROIDISM OF OLD? HOW CAN WE ACCOUNT FOR THE PRIMARY HYPERPARATHYROIDISM OF TODAY?

How can we account for the clear increase in the incidence of primary hyperparathyroidism and the concomitant reduction in the symptomatic presenta-

tion of this disease? In one view, this disorder is merely being detected earlier than it used to be. Thus, the old-fashioned presentation of primary hyperparathyroidism, accompanied by specific symptomatology, does not have a chance to develop, and asymptomatic primary hyperparathyroidism predominates among the many other potential presentations of the disease. There are several problems with accepting this idea completely. If primary hyperparathyroidism is simply being detected at an earlier stage, one might expect that the average age of the patient at diagnosis would be younger now than before. This is not clearly the case. However, the well-recognized trend towards an aging population may explain why this disease is discovered so frequently in older individuals and may confound the analysis of this point. Moreover, if the predominance of asymptomatic disease is due solely to earlier detection, one would predict that many of those asymptomatic patients who are followed conservatively without surgery would demonstrate progression to overt clinical disease. Unfortunately, a sufficient number of patients have not been followed for a sufficiently long period of time to test this point. With very incomplete longitudinal data in patients with asymptomatic primary hyperparathyroidism, it is not possible to predict whether and in what ways the disease will progress. Some information is available, however, to suggest that, over a limited period of time (within 5 years), progressive bone disease is uncommon (80). With respect to bone densitometry, it will require a longer period of observation to know whether there is any progression over time. Other, incomplete longitudinal data suggest that patients with primary hyperparathyroidism do not appear to show worsening hypercalcemia, increasing levels of PTH, or worsening circulating markers of bone formation and bone resorption (81) (see the chapter by Kleerekoper).

Another critical area in which more information is needed is a potential protective effect of the hyperparathyroid process on the cancellous skeleton. Data available from bone histomorphometry are based on cross-sectional results only. Serial bone biopsies in patients who do or do not undergo parathyroidectomy are critically needed to address the issues of progression of bone disease as well as its potential reversibility.

Finally, if the increased incidence of asymptomatic primary hyperparathyroidism is simply a matter of early detection, patients with "old-fashioned" primary hyperparathyroidism should still be seen with a certain, albeit reduced, incidence. This reasoning is based on the fact that the multichannel screening test is not available to everyone. There are many parts of the world where regular access to medical care is unavailable. In addition, not everyone who could gain access to such screening tests takes advantage of their availability. Among these populations, patients would be expected to surface only when symptoms develop. However, it appears that the "old-fashioned" presentations of primary hyperparathyroidism have become extremely unusual. It is not known whether this population still exists but is obscured by the many more patients with asymptomatic disease. However, this presentation appears to be uncommon in both tertiary referral centers and general care centers. Perhaps a more global epidemiological view is necessary, one that would analyze data from both medically underserved and more industrialized countries. While very little information is available on this point, it is curious that, in several reports from South America, the disease does seem to present more along classical lines (82). In Malaysia, an experience amounting only to 12 patients in 11 years showed patients presenting late with complications of bone and stone disease to be most common (83). A similar, "old-fashioned" presentation of primary hyperparathyroidism has been reported from the former West Germany (84).

Consideration of these questions about asymptomatic primary hyperparathyroidism raises another possibility, namely, that the disease itself has changed. Perhaps the predominance of asymptomatic disease in our population is a reflection of different etiologies or environmental or nutritional factors. One speculative example might suffice. Residents of many Western countries supplement the diet with vitamin D. Thus vitamin D stores are more likely to be replete now than in the past. It is conceivable that the high normal or frankly elevated levels of $1,25(OH)_2D$ routinely seen in primary hyperparathyroidism could serve to limit the extent to which PTH levels are elevated by virtue of the effect of $1,25(OH)_2D$ to control PTH gene transcription. Moreover, sufficient vitamin D might protect against some of the skeletal effects of vitamin D deficiency in conjunction with elevated levels of PTH. In France, primary hyperparathyroidism is more likely to present with *osteitis fibrosa cystica* if levels of vitamin D metabolites are low (85). This hypothesis thus suggests that the disease itself has changed along with development of a technology that has improved recognition. Whether we are in the midst of an evolving disease process in part responsible for the changing clinical profile of primary hyperparathyroidism or whether we are seeing merely a disorder that is showing its clinical features more accurately now than in the past are issues that await further study.

SUMMARY

Primary hyperparathyroidism, a common endocrine disorder, now presents most frequently as an asymp-

tomatic disease. This is a picture markedly different from earlier descriptions of the disease, from before the widespread use of the multichannel autoanalyzer, when symptoms and signs were the rule rather than the exception. The disease no longer appears to be one of "stones, bones, and groans." However, the evolving clinical profile of primary hyperparathyroidism leads to a number of key questions that cannot be answered by the older literature on this disease. Many of these questions can be addressed only by continued clinical studies into some of the issues raised in this chapter. To name but a few examples, we need more information about the natural history of the disease, the incidence of fracture, as well as the putative neuropsychiatric manifestations. Greater insight into the relationship between the hyperparathyroid process and postmenopausal bone loss, especially insofar as the cancellous spine is concerned, is essential. Moreover, information is needed on the course of patients who undergo parathyroid surgery as well as those who are followed conservatively. With additional studies, providing more information in these critical areas, we should be in a position to refine more clearly currently accepted guidelines for surgery versus medical management for primary hyperparathyroidism.

ACKNOWLEDGMENTS

Some of the information contained in this chapter was obtained with support from NIH grants DK 32333 and AR 39191.

REFERENCES

1. Cope O. The story of hyperparathyroidism at the Massachusetts General Hospital. *N Engl J Med* 1966;21:1174–1182.
2. Bauer W. Hyperparathyroidism: distinct disease entity. *J Bone Joint Surg* 1933;15:135–141.
3. Bauer W, Federman DD. Hyperparathyroidism epitimized: case of Captain Charles E. Martell. *Metabolism* 1962;11:21–22.
4. Mandl F. Therapeutiscle Versuch bei Ostitis fibrosa generalisata mittels Extirpation lines Epithelkoperchentumon. *Wien Klin Wochenschr* 1925;50:1343–1344.
5. Albright F, Aub JC, Bauer W. Hyperparathyroidism common and polymorphic condition as illustrated by seventeen proved cases from one clinic. *J Am Med Assoc* 1934;102:1276–1287.
6. Keating FR Jr, Cook EN. Recognition of primary hyperparathyroidism: analysis of 24 cases. *J Am Med Assoc* 1945;129:994–1002.
7. Heath H III, Hodgson SF, Kennedy M. Primary hyperparathyroidism: incidence, morbidity and potential economic impact in a community. *N Engl J Med* 1980;302:189–193.
8. Mundy GR, Cove DH, Fisken R. Primary hyperparathyroidism: changes in the pattern of clinical presentation. *Lancet* 1980;1:1317–1320.
9. Stenstrom G, Heedman P. Clinical findings in patients with hypercalcemia: a final investigation based on biochemical screening. *Acta Med Scand* 1974;195:473–477.

10. Aitken RE, Bartley PC, Bryant SJ, Lloyd HM. The effect of multiphasic biochemical screening on the diagnosis of primary hyperparathyroidism. *Aust NZ J Med* 1975;5:224–226.
11. Trigonis C, Hamberger B, Farnebo LO, Abarca J, Granberg PO. Primary hyperparathyroidism. Changing trends over fifty years. *Acta Chir Scand* 1983;149:675–679.
12. Heath H III. Clinical spectrum of primary hyperparathyroidism: evolution with changes in medical practice and technology. *J Bone Mineral Res* 1991;6(Suppl 2):S63–S70.
13. Melton LJ III. Epidemiology of primary hyperparathyroidism. *J Bone Mineral Res* 1991;6(Suppl 2):S25–S30.
14. Palmer M, Jakobsson S, Akerstrom G, Ljunghall S. Prevalence of hypercalcaemia in a health survey: a 14-year follow-up study of serum calcium values. *Eur J Clin Invest* 1988; 18:39–46.
15. Boonstra CE, Jackson CE. Serum calcium survey for hyperparathyroidism: results in 50,000 clinic patients. *Am J Clin Pathol* 1971;55:523–526.
16. Beard CM, Heath H III, O'Fallon WM, Anderson JA, Earle JD, Melton LJ III. Therapeutic radiation and hyperparathyroidism: a case-control study in Rochester, Minn. *Arch Intern Med* 1989;149:1887–1890.
17. Cohen J, Gierlowski TC, Schneider AB. A prospective study of hyperparathyroidism in individuals exposed to radiation in childhood. *JAMA* 1990;264:581–584.
18. Bondeson AG, Bondeson L, Thompson NW. Hyperparathyroidism after treatment with radioactive iodine: not only a coincidence? *Surgery* 1989;106:1025–1027.
19. Parfitt AM, Willgoss D, Jacobi J, Lloyd M. Cell kinetics in parathyroid adenomas: evidence for decline in rates of cell birth and tumor growth, assuming clonal origin. *Clin Endocrinol* 1991;35:151–157.
20. Arnold A, Staunton CE, Kim HG, Gaz RD, Kronenberg HM. Monoclonality and abnormal parathyroid hormone genes in parathyroid adenomas. *N Engl J Med* 1988;318:658–662.
21. Mallette LE, Malini S, Rappaport MP, Kirkland JL. Familial cystic parathyroid adenomatosis. *Ann Intern Med* 1987;107:54–60.
22. Shane E, Bilezikian JP. Parathyroid carcinoma In: Williams CJ, Krikorian JC, Green MR, Raghavan D, eds. *Textbook of uncommon cancer.* New York: Wiley, 1988;763–771.
23. Wynne AG, van Heerden J, Carney JA, Fitzpatrick LA. Parathyroid carcinoma: clinical and pathological features in 43 patients. *Medicine* 1992;71:197–205.
24. Bilezikian JP. Management of acute hypercalcemia. *N Engl J Med* 1992;326:1196–1203.
25. Fitzpatrick L, Bilezikian JP. Primary hyperparathyroidism. In: Becker KL, ed. *Principles and practice of endocrinology and metabolism.* Philadelphia: JB Lippincott, 1990;430–437.
26. Silverberg SJ, Shane E, DeLaCruz L, et al. Skeletal disease in primary hyperparathyroidism. *J Bone Mineral Res* 1989;4:283–291.
27. Bilezikian JP, Silverberg SJ, Shane E, Parisien M, Dempster DW. Characterization and evaluation of asymptomatic primary hyperparathyroidism. *J Bone Mineral Res* 1991;6(Suppl I) 585–589.
28. Fuss M, Pepersack T, Corvilain J, et al. Infrequency of primary hyperparathyroidism in renal stone formers. *Br J Urol* 1988;62:4–6.
29. Silverberg SJ, Shane E, Jacobs TP, et al. Nephrolithiasis and bone involvement in primary hyperparathyroidism. *Am J Med* 1990;89:327–334.
30. Aurbach GD, Mallette LE, Patten BM, Heath DA, Doppman JL, Bilezikian JP. Hyperparathyroidism: recent studies. *Ann Intern Med* 1973;79:566–581.
31. Patten BM, Bilezikian JP, Mallette LE, Prince A, Engel WK, Aurbach GD. The neuromuscular disease of hyperparathyroidism. *Ann Intern Med* 1974;80:182–194.
32. Turken SA, Cafferty M, Silverberg SJ, et al. Neuromuscular involvement in mild, asymptomatic primary hyperparathyroidism. *Am J Med* 1989;87:553–557.
33. Joborn C, Rastad J, Stalberg E, Akerstrom G, Ljunghall S. Muscle function in patients with primary hyperparathyroidism. *Muscle Nerve* 1989;12:87–94.
34. Linos DA, vanHeerdan JA, Abboud CF, Edis AJ. Primary

35. Bess MA, Edis AJ, vanHeerden JA. Hyperparathyroidism and pancreatitis. Chance or a causal association? *JAMA* 1980;243:246–247.
36. Bilezikian JP, Aurbach GD, Connor TB, et al. Pseudogout following parathyroidectomy. *Lancet* 1973;1:445–447.
37. Geelhoed GW, Kelly TR. Pseudogout as a clue and complication in primary hyperparathyroidism. *Surgery* 1989;106:1036–1041.
38. Mallette LE. Anemia in hypercalcemic hyperparathyroidism, renewed interest in an old observation. *Arch Intern Med* 1977;137:572–573.
39. Ringe JD. Reversible hypertension in primary hyperparathyroidism—pre- and postoperative blood pressure in 75 cases. *Klin Wochenschr* 1984;62:465–469.
40. Broulik PD, Horky K, Pacovsky V. Blood pressure in patients with primary hyperparathyroidism before and after parathyroidectomy. *Exp Clin Endocrinol* 1985;86:346–352.
41. Rapado A. Arterial hypertension and primary hyperparathyroidism. *Am J Nephrol* 1986;6(Suppl 1):49–50.
42. Diamond TW, Botha JR, Wing J, Meyers AM, Kalk WJ. Parathyroid hypertension. A reversible disorder. *Arch Intern Med* 1986;146:1709–1712.
43. Sancho JJ, Rouco J, Riera-Vidal R, Sitges-Serra A. Long-term effects of parathyroidectomy for primary hyperparathyroidism on arterial hypertension. *World J Surg* 1992;16:732–735.
44. Lind L, Jacobsson S, Palmer M, Lithell H, Wengle B, Ljunghall S. Cardiovascular risk factors in primary hyperparathyroidism: a 15-year follow-up of operated and unoperated cases. *J Intern Med* 1991;230:29–35.
45. Joborn C, Hetta J, Johansson H, et al. Psychiatric morbidity in primary hyperparathyroidism. *World J Surg* 1988;12:476–481.
46. Joborn C, Hetta J, Frisk P, Palmer M, Akerstrom G, Ljunghall S. Primary hyperparathyroidism in patients with organic brain syndrome. *Acta Med Scand* 1986;219:91–98.
47. Alarcon RD, Franceschini JA. Hyperparathyroidism and paranoid psychosis case report and review of the literature. *Br J Psychiatr* 1984;145:477–486.
48. Ljunghall S, Jakobsson S, Joborn C, Palmer M, Rastad J, Akerstrom G. Longitudinal studies of mild primary hyperparathyroidism. *J Bone Mineral Res* 1991;6(Suppl 2):S111–S116.
49. Brown GG, Preisman RC, Kleerekoper MD. Neurobehavioral symptoms in mild primary hyperparathyroidism: related to hypercalcemia but not improved by parathyroidectomy. *Henry Ford Med J* 1987;35:211–215.
50. Cogan MG, Covey CM, Arieff AI, Wisniewski A, Clark OH. Central nervous system manifestations of hyperparathyroidism. *Am J Med* 1978;65:963–970.
51. Mallette LE, Bilezikian JP, Heath DA, Aurbach GD. Hyperparathyroidism: a review of 52 cases. *Medicine* 1974;53:127–147.
52. Nikkil MT, Saaristo JJ, Koivula TA. Clinical and biochemical features in primary hyperparathyriodism. *Surgery* 1989;105:148–153.
53. Heath H III, Oh S, Peacock M. Clinical spectrum of primary hyperparathyroidism: discussion. *J Bone Mineral Res* 1991;6 (Suppl 2):583.
54. Fitzpatrick LA, Bilezikian JP. Acute primary hyperparathyroidism. *Am J Med* 1987;82:275–282.
55. Lafferty FW. Differential diagnosis of hypercalcemia. *J Bone Mineral Res* 1991;6(Suppl 2):S51–S59.
56. Lind L, Ljunghall S. Serum chloride in the differential diagnosis of hypercalcemia. *Exp Clin Endocrinol* 1991;98:179–184.
57. Vieth R, Bayley TA, Walfish PG, Rosen IB, Pollard A. Relevance of vitamin D metabolite concentrations in supporting the diagnosis of primary hyperparathyroidism. *Surgery* 1991;110:1043–1046.
58. Shakes JL, Krawczyk KW, Findling JW. Primary hyperparathyroidism and severe hypercalcemia with low circulating 1,25-dihydroxyvitamin D. *J Clin Endocrinol Metab* 1990;71:1305–1309.

59. Seibel MJ, Gartenberg F, Silverberg SJ, Ratcliffe A, Robins SP, Bilezikian JP. Urinary hydroxypyridinium crosslinks of collagen as markers of bone resorption in primary hyperparathyroidism. *J Clin Endocrinol Metab* 1992;74:481–486.
60. Seibel MJ, Robins SP, Bilezikian JP. Urinary pyridinium crosslinks of collagen: specific markers of bone resorption in metabolic bone disease. *Trends Endocrinol Metab* 1992;3: 263–270.
61. Pfeilschifter J, Siegrist E, Wuster C, Blind E, Ziegler R. Serum levels of intact parathyroid hormone and alkaline phosphates correlate with cortical and trabecular bone loss in primary hyperparathyroidism. *Acta Endocrinol* 1992;127: 319–323.
62. Slovik DM, Rosenthal DF, Doppert SH, et al. Restoration of spinal bone in osteoporotic men by treatment with human parathyroid hormone (1–34) and 1,25 dihydroxyvitamin D. *J Bone Mineral Res* 1986;1:377–381.
63. Slovik DM, Neer RM, Potts JT Jr. Short-term effects of synthetic human parathyroid hormone (1–34) administration on bone mineral metabolism in osteoporotic patients. *J Clin Invest* 1981;68:1261–1271.
64. Parisien MV, Silverberg SJ, Shane E, de la Cruz L, Lindsay R, Bilezikian JP, Dempster DW. The histomorphometry of bone in primary hyperparathyroidism: preservation of cancellous bone structure. *J Clin Endocrinol Metab* 1990;70:930–938.
65. Parisien M, Mellish RWE, Silverberg SJ, et al. Maintenance of cancellous bone connectivity in primary hyperparathyroidism: trabecular strut analysis. *J Bone Mineral Res* 1992;7: 913–920.
66. Parisien MV, Silverberg SJ, Shane E, Dempster DW, Bilezikian JP. Bone disease in primary hyperparathyroidism. *Endocrinol Metab Clin North Am* 1990;19:19–34.
67. Christiansen P, Steiniche T, Vesterby A, Mosekilde L, Hessov I, Melsen F. Primary hyperparathyroidism: iliac crest trabecular bone volume, structure, remodeling, and balance evaluated by histomorphometric methods. *Bone* 1992;13:41–49.
68. Delling G. Bone morphology in primary hyperparathyroidism. *Appl Pathol* 1987;5:147–159.
69. Newton-John HF, Morgan DB. The loss of bone with age, osteoporosis and fractures. *Clin Orthop* 1970;71:229–252.
70. Albright F, Reifenstein EC. *The parathyroid glands and metabolic bone disease*. Baltimore: Williams & Wilkins, 1948.
71. Wilson RJ, Rao DS, Ellis B, Kleerekoper M, Parfitt AM. Mild asymptomatic primary hyperparathyroidism is not a risk factor for vertebral fractures. *Ann Intern Med* 1988;109:959–962.
72. Peacock M, Horsman A, Aaron JE, Marshall DH, Selby PL, Simpson M. The role of parathyroid hormone in bone loss. In: Christiansen C, et al., eds. *Osteoporosis I*. Glostrup Hospital, Denmark: Department of Clinical Chemistry, 1984;463–467.
73. Peacock M. Interpretation of bone mass determinations as they relate to fracture: implications for asymptomatic primary hyperparathyroidism. *J Bone Mineral Res* 1991;6(Suppl 2):S77–S82.
74. Dauphine RT, Riggs BL, Scholz DA. Back pain and vertebral crush fractures: an unrecognized mode of presentation for primary hyperparathyroidism. *Ann Intern Med* 1975;83:365–367.
75. Larsson K, Lindh E, Lind L, Persson I, Ljunghall S. Increased fracture risk in hypercalcemia. Bone mineral content measured in hyperparathyroidism. *Acta Orthop Scand* 1989; 60:268–270.
76. Lafferty FW, Halsay CA. Primary hyperparathyroidism: a review of the long-term surgical and non-surgical morbidities as a basis for a rational approach to treatment. *Arch Intern Med* 1986;149:789–796.
77. Melton LJ 3d, Atkinson EJ, O'Fallon WM, Heath H 3d. Risk of age-related fractures in patients with primary hyperparathyroidism. *Arch Intern Med* 1992;152:2269–2273.
78. Broadus AE, Horst RL, Lang R, Littledike ET, Rasmussen H. The importance of circulating 1,25(OH)₂D in the pathogenesis of hypercalciuria and renal stone formation in primary hyperparathyroidism. *N Engl J Med* 1980;302:421–426.
79. Pak CYC, Nicar MJ, Peterson R, Zerwekh JE, Snyder W. Lack of unique pathophysiologic background for nephrolithiasis in primary hyperparathyroidism. *J Clin Endocrinol Metab* 1981;53:536–542.
80. Rao DS, Wilson RJ, Kleerekoper M, Parfitt AM. Lack of biochemical progression or continuation of accelerated bone loss in mild asymptomatic primary hyperparathyroidism: evidence for biphasic disease course. *J Clin Endocrinol Metab* 1988;67:1294–1298.
81. Silverberg SJ, Gartenberg F, Bilezikian JP. Primary hyperparathyroidism protects cancellous bone density in postmenopausal women. *J Bone Mineral Res* 1992;7(Suppl):813a.
82. Leite MOR, Correa PHS, Jorgetti V, Batalha JFR, Pereira RC, Mechica JB, Borelli A. Dynamic bone histomorphometry in hyperparathyroidism. *J Bone Min Res* 1990;5(Suppl 2) 664a.
83. Meah FA, Tan TT, Taha A, Khalid BA. Primary hyperparathyroidism—a surgical review of 12 cases. *Med J Malaya* 1991;46:144–149.
84. Dotzenrath C, Goretzki PE, Roher HD. West Germany: still an underdeveloped country in the diagnosis and early treatment of primary hyperparathyroidism? *World J Surg* 1990;14: 660–661.
85. Patron P, Gardin J-P, Paillard M. Renal mass and reserve of vitamin D. Determinants in primary hyperparathyroidism. *Kidney Int* 1987;31:1174–1180.

The Parathyroids, edited by J.P. Bilezikian,
M.A. Levine, and R. Marcus. Raven Press, Ltd.,
New York © 1994.

CHAPTER 27

Clinical Course of Primary Hyperparathyroidism

Michael Kleerekoper

The natural history of primary hyperparathyroidism (PHPT) as it used to be recognized is well documented in the early medical reports of this disease. Beginning with Mandl's Viennese tram conductor (1) and seaman Captain Charles Martel in Boston (2), the earliest patients came to medical attention invariably because of a severely progressive bone disease, osteitis fibrosa cystica. After the first 50 or so patients had undergone successful parathyroidectomy (PTX), Albright (3) observed that almost 80% of the patients also gave a history of recurrent nephrolithiasis. A diligent search in stone-forming patients uncovered many more patients with PHPT who had no clear-cut evidence of osteitis fibrosacystica or other metabolic bone disease. Serum calcium in these stone-forming patients tended to be lower than in patients with the bone disease, and they were less prone to the neurologic complications of severe hypercalcemia. These observations led Lloyd (4) eventually to classify PHPT into two distinct types; type I, with large glands associated with severe, symptomatic hypercalcemia, and bone disease; and type II, with smaller glands, less severe hypercalcemia, and stone disease (discussed in more detail in the chapter by Parfitt). Lloyd noted that, while many patients with type I disease gave a history of stones, there was apparently little overlap in the opposite direction. He postulated that the natural history of PHPT was related to the growth of the tumorous parathyroid tissue, that some tumors were destined from their origin to grow rapidly and to produce a more severe disturbance

of calcium homeostasis, while the rest were inherently less aggressive in their growth and clinical consequences. Patients with types I and II PHPT were easy to recognize at presentation and were routinely referred for PTX at that time. Thus the natural histories of these classical forms of the disease are well described historically. It is difficult to improve on those classical descriptions.

These observations predated the introduction of automated biochemistry in medical practice, which heralded a new era for PHPT (and many other disorders such as hyperuricemia and hypercholesterolemia), in which a biochemical diagnosis could be firmly established well in advance of any relevant clinical symptoms. It would appear from the author's personal experience and review of the literature that the classical bone disease of PHPT as described by Lloyd (type I) is now quite a rare medical condition. Many series also report a reduced prevalence of PHPT among kidney stone formers (5), suggesting that type II PHPT also has become less common. In the preceding chapter by Bilezikian et al., the modern clinical presentations of PHPT were described. The question addressed in this chapter is, what do we know about the natural history of PHPT as it presents today? Is today's predominant form of PHPT simply a benign variant of early presentations (types I or II), or does it represent a new entity, type III PHPT, as was postulated by Lloyd et al. (6), with its own natural history? One way to address this question is to relate the current observations to what is known about symptoms and signs, serum calcium, bone disease, and nephrolithiasis in the classic forms of the disease. Some material covered in the chapter by Bilezikian et al. is presented again here to provide the proper setting to this chapter, namely, the clinical course of PHPT.

M. Kleerekoper: Division of Endocrinology, Wayne State University School of Medicine, Detroit, Michigan 48201.

NONTRADITIONAL SYMPTOMS AND SIGNS

Primary hyperparathyroidism detected by chance as part of a routine biochemical screening program has been termed *asymptomatic PHPT*. For many subjects, this term could be quite inappropriate, because the medical visit that resulted in the biochemical screen was prompted by symptoms. These symptoms may not be completely unrelated to PHPT. Thus serendipitously found PHPT is more properly classified as two entities: (a) totally asymptomatic and (b) PHPT manifesting symptoms not traditionally linked either to PHPT or to hypercalcemia.

The true prevalence of totally asymptomatic PHPT can be determined only by measuring serum calcium and parathyroid hormone (PTH) in all members of a selected cohort and ascertaining the proportion of identified patients who are asymptomatic. With the changing delivery of health care, one can anticipate that more truly asymptomatic subjects will undergo a biochemical screen on an annual or biannual basis. There is no reason to suspect that this will alter the prevalence of serendipitously detected PHPT. It will, however, become important to monitor separately the natural history of the disease in this group from that in those in whom the biochemical screen was obtained on the basis of symptoms. At present there are no data to allow any comments on the possible differing natural histories of these two types of "asymptomatic" PHPT.

In those patients with PHPT in whom symptoms are present, it will not be possible to determine which symptoms resulted from PHPT until a randomized, controlled, clinical trial of PTX has been completed. We could then ascertain which of the symptoms were alleviated by successful PTX. One must be mindful, however, that symptoms not being alleviated by PTX does not mean that they are not the result of PHPT.

CLINICAL PRESENTATION AND COURSE OF NONSPECIFIC MANIFESTATIONS OF PRIMARY HYPERPARATHYROIDISM

Neuropsychiatric Manifestations

Pending the outcome of these ideal studies, for which there is great need, increasing anecdotal information indicates that many patients with serendipitously detected PHPT indeed have symptoms. These symptoms tend to be vague and nonspecific, but some authorities believe that they do result from PHPT and are apparently alleviated by PTX. These nonspecific symptoms can be classified under the general rubric of neuropsychiatric disorders: pain, weakness, lassitude, anxiety, depression, etc. (Fig. 1) (7). Unfortunately, this has been a particularly difficult area to study in a quantitative manner. As a result, the literature has not

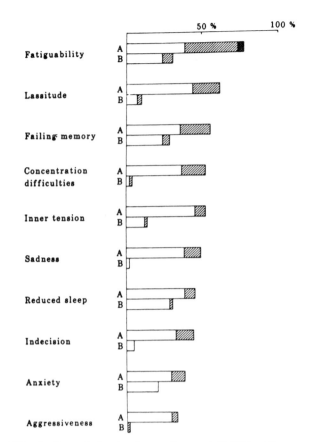

FIG. 1. Neurobehavioral symptoms of PHPT, while vague and nonspecific, are quite prevalent. In this series, there was substantial improvement following successful PTX, but, as is detailed in the text, this is not always the case. *Top panel* is before surgery, *bottom panel* post-PTX. *Unshaded bars* represent moderate or periodical symptoms, *shaded bars* represent more severe symptoms. (Reproduced from ref. 7 with permission.)

led to clear conclusions. In 1987, we reported our observations on 34 patients with PHPT referred from the author's metabolic bone disease clinic for formal psychiatric interview and neuropsychologic testing (8). While every patient with PHPT seen during a 30 month period was invited to participate in this study, several declined to do so, introducing a marked self-selection bias into the observations. Three patients had kidney stones, two had peptic ulcers, and the remainder had a variety of medical conditions not thought to be related to PHPT or were entirely "asymptomatic" (seven patients). The mean serum calcium in this group was 11.5 ± 1.0 mg/dl. There was excellent agreement (82%) between the psychiatric interview and the psychometric studies. Results of this study are summarized in Table 1. Follow-up observations were obtained in ten patients 6 months after successful PTX (serum calcium 11.7 ± 1.0 preoperatively, 9.2 ± 0.9 postoperatively) and after 6 months of conservative follow-up without surgery in nine patients (serum calcium 11.0 ± 1.0 and 10.7 ± 0.8 at baseline and follow-

TABLE 1. *Psychiatric and psychometric evaluation in 34 patients with PHPT[a]*

I. Psychiatric findings (%)	Serum calcium (mg/dl)	
No behavioral disorders (29)	10.9 ± 0.9	
Affective disorders (32)	11.3 ± 0.7	
Brain dysfunction (39)	12.2 ± 1.2	
II. Psychometric study	Correlation with serum calcium	P
Tapping score	-0.33	<0.05
Fluid intelligence	-0.45	<0.01
Short-term memory distractor	-0.36	<0.05
Trail making	0.39	<0.05

[a]Mean serum calcium was lower in those without neurobehavioral abnormalities than in those with subjective and objective findings of disease (I), and there was a significant relationship between individual components of the psychometric evaluation and the serum calcium (II). Only the depression scale of the MMPI did not correlate with the serum calcium. (Data from ref. 8.)

up, respectively). Despite the expected significant reduction in serum calcium following PTX, and improvement in some neurobehavioral abnormalities, we observed no improvement in functioning for those behavioral domains that were correlated with the serum calcium at the time of initial testing. Cogan et al. (9) made similar observations in seven subjects undergoing PTX for PHPT. Their subjects had abnormal encephalograms preoperatively, with significant improvement postoperatively. Most had abnormal psychologic tests preoperatively, with no improvement when retested an average of 3.6 months after surgery. Joborn and her colleagues (10) reported self-rated psychiatric symptoms in 30 patients with PHPT referred for surgery, 38 subjects detected in a health screening with 15 years of mild hypercalcemia and presumed PHPT, and 38 normocalcemic control subjects. Using the Hopkins Symptom Checklist (HSCL-56), the patients presenting for surgery had the highest mean score and the control subjects the lowest score (89.1 ± 20.1, 76.6 ± 17.0, 73.8 ± 16.0 for the three groups, respectively). One year postoperatively, the score had improved to 73.2 ± 13.7 ($P < 0.001$). In the nonoperated subjects and in the controls, 6 months of oral vitamin D (1 µg alphacalcidol daily) or placebo had no effect on the HSCL score, despite a 0.05 mmol/liter increase in serum calcium in the vitamin D-treated group (compared to placebo). McAllion and Paterson (11) reported on 15 patients undergoing a standardized psychiatric interview before and 3 months after PTX. Thirteen of the patients had less psychiatric morbidity postoperatively, with improvement most marked in symptoms of fatigue, depression, irritability, sleep disturbance, and lack of concentration. However, the levels of intellectual impairment and anxiety were unchanged by surgery. An additional 21 patients with PHPT of 2–7 years' duration, regarding whom an independent decision had been made to follow without surgery, underwent the same standardized psychiatric interview. The results were not different from the postoperative results in the treated group. In the entire

group of 37 unoperated patients with PHPT, there was no relationship between the psychiatric findings and either serum calcium or parathyroid hormone levels.

Overall, the prevalence of neuropsychiatric abnormalities in patients with PHPT appears to be greater than the prevalence of similar illnesses in outpatient medical settings (12), but the reported prevalence varies widely (Table 2). This is undoubtedly a function of the rigor with which such symptoms were sought in the various studies. Of particular importance to this discussion on the natural history of asymptomatic PHPT is the failure of PTX to correct these abnormalities. The reports of these neurobehavioral symptoms being "cured" by PTX have generally paid insufficient attention to the appropriate control group (7,25,26). The improvement we noted in our unoperated group, despite the stability of the hypercalcemia, suggests that there is a learning response for many of these psychometric tests and that improvement following surgery might simply be a repeat-testing phenomenon.

It is possible and, in fact, quite reasonable to assume that patients with vague, nonspecific symptoms would be more likely than truly asymptomatic subjects to present for a "routine" physical examination or biochemical profile. However, if so many studies with appropriate controls demonstrate an increased prevalence of psychiatric dysfunction, we can conclude that neurobehavioral symptoms are a common part of the symptom complex in otherwise asymptomatic PHPT and that there is a cause and effect relationship between the disease and the symptoms. If, as we demonstrated in our small study, there is a relationship between the severity of the hypercalcemia and the severity of psychometric abnormalities, one would expect that the symptoms would not be progressive if the severity of hypercalcemia is not progressive. However, there is no consensus about a relationship between neurobehavioral findings and serum calcium (26). Of particular concern is the failure of PTX to alter consistently the results of the psychometric studies. Against this background of very limited formal data,

TABLE 2. *Case series studies of psychiatric symptoms in hyperparathyroidism and other hypercalcemic disorders*[a]

Authors/reference	Year	No. of cases	Neuro-psychiatric symptoms n(%)	Types of symptoms
Ettinger (13)	1947	30	7 (14)	"Psychic changes"
St. Goar (14)	1957	45	3 (7)	"Pronounced emotional symptoms"
Cope (15)	1960	230	2 (1)	"Mental disturbance"
Hellstrom and Ivermark (16)	1962	138	11 (8)	Nervous disorders, depression
Karpati and Frame (17)	1964	33	14 (42)	Anxiety, tension, irritability, depression, confusional state
Henson (18)	1966	34	8 (24)	Depression, anxiety, loss of energy, paranoia
Watson (19)	1968	200	8 (4)	"Mental symptoms," "psychological disorders"
Salahudeen et al. (20)	1968	30	3 (10) 7 (23)	Depression, loss of energy, thought disorder, paranoia, disoriented
Petersen (21)	1968	54	36 (65)	Impairment of memory, neurasthenic personality changes, affective disturbance, acute organic psychosis with disorientation, delerium, confusion, paranoid ideas
Mallette et al. (22)	1974	57	19 (33)	Decreased memory for recent events, irritability, depression; one case psychotic, one case delerious
Palmer (23)	1983	110[b]	25 (23)	Poor memory, anxiety, depression, hysterical personality, organic brain syndrome
Joborn et al. (24)	1986	441	102 (23)	Depression, anxiety, psychosis, organic brain syndrome, minor cerebral impairment

[a]Reprinted from ref. 8 with permission.
[b]Regarding neuropsychiatric symptoms, the first entry is the number of patients who presented as psychotic, and the second entry is the number of patients who gave a history of depression and loss of energy.

we must consider the large volume of anecdotal data regarding the benefits of PTX in relieving these non-traditional symptoms. All of us caring for large numbers of patients with PHPT can recall many patients who underwent PTX for reasons other than control of symptoms and who claim to feel "much better" following the surgery. This statement is often made even by patients who claimed to be asymptomatic preoperatively. Thus, when PHPT is truly detected serendipitously in patients presenting for a health check-up as part of their ongoing routine, subtle neurobehavioral symptoms may well go unrecognized by both patient and physician.

For now, it would seem reasonable for physicians evaluating patients with PHPT to develop, with their colleagues in psychiatry, a brief list of questions that would allow one to determine quickly whether the patient has any of these neurobehavioral symptoms. If these are present, the patient should be alerted to the possibility that some of this symptomatology may improve following successful PTX. This should then enter into the physician–patient decision concerning the indications for PTX and should be evaluated without regard to more objective data concerning the need for surgery. If patients are to be followed conservatively, the responses to these questions should become part of the ongoing monitoring, with worsening of these symptoms being regarded as an indication of disease progression. It is clear that formal studies of these neurobehavioral aspects of PHPT must become an integral part of planned studies evaluating the natural history PHPT and the effect of PTX. However, formal psychiatric consultation of psychometeric testing for individual patients is not recommended outside the confines of such research studies.

Hypertension

When PHPT is complicated by renal impairment, or severe hypercalcemia, or is present as part of a multiple endocrine neoplasia (MEN) syndrome that includes either pheochromocytoma or hyperaldosteronism, hypertension is a common feature in the overall clinical picture. Hypertension is also reported to be more prevalent in mild, asymptomatic PHPT patients than in appropriately matched control groups (27–29). There are also reports of amelioration of hypertension following successful PTX (27,28,30), but this is not a universal observation (31–34). Nonetheless, it has been extremely difficult to show a cause and effect relationship between PHPT and hypertension. Several years ago, Brinton et al. (35) reported a small series of subjects with PHPT and hypertension with and without increased plasma renin activity (PRA). Amelioration of hypertension was observed only in that subset of patients with high renin hypertension preoperatively, although PTX corrected the hypercalcemia in all, and PTX restored the PRA to normal in those with an initially elevated level. Ganguly et al. (36) could not confirm any association between the renin–angiotensin–aldosterone system and hypertension in PHPT, but their study was also quite small. It is possible that there is a small subset of patients with PHPT in whom hypertension is an integral part of the disease process and in whom PTX may be curative of the hypertension. If they could be identified correctly at the time of diagnosis, then the hypertension could be categorized as part of the natural history of this form of PHPT.

Carbohydrate Intolerance

There have been attempts to link carbohydrate intolerance and frank diabetes mellitus to PHPT (37,38), but the association is very much more tenuous than the previous association between hypertension and PHPT (39). Until more prospective information is available, diabetes in a patient with PHPT should be treated independently of the parathyroid disease and vice versa. One should not consider the presence or absence of diabetes when making individual clinical decisions concerning the potential benefits of PTX, and one should be reluctant to attribute any post-PTX improvement in the control of the diabetes to the surgery.

Clinical Course and Presentations of Other Nontraditional Aspects of Primary Hyperparathyroidism

Peptic ulcer disease and pancreatitis do not appear to be part of the syndrome of mild PHPT, and there is even uncertainty about the validity of the association between these two clinical entities and types I and II

PHPT (40–46). The neuromuscular complications of types I and II PHPT are not seen in the mild form of the disease. In a detailed neurologic study of 42 patients with a mean serum calcium of 11.1 ± 0.1 mg/dl, Turken et al. (47) found no consistent pattern of abnormalities either on physical examination or on electromyography, and creatine phosphokinase levels were normal in all subjects. Joborn et al. (48) studied 18 randomly selected patients with PHPT and concluded that, as a group, the patients had slight but significant impairment of the muscle function, a finding that the authors speculated might be responsible for the "fatigue" that is apparently so prevalent in this disease.

Asymptomatic Primary Hyperparathyroidism and Cancer

There are several reports of an increased occurrence of nonparathyroid cancers in patients with PHPT (49,50). Whether there is a cause and effect relationship (i.e., are calcium and/or PTH potential mitogens in human subjects?) has not been established. In patients with hypercalcemia detected unexpectedly on a biochemical profile, the most important cause of the hypercalcemia to exclude is hypercalcemia associated with malignancy. It is uncommon for malignant disease patients to present with mild, unanticipated hypercalcemia, but, as with all things in medicine, the more diligently one searches for a particular disease, the more likely one is to find it. Thus the association between PHPT and cancer may simply reflect the more diligent search for cancer in patients with hypercalcemia. This chance association might also work in the other direction; i.e., patients with known malignancy who are found to be hypercalcemic are more likely to have a measurement of PTH to confirm that the hypercalcemia resulted from PHPT and was not related to the cancer. Another possible mechanism for a chance association between PHPT and cancer results from the frequency with which clinically silent thyroid malignancies are found during the neck exploration for PTX. Regarding 948 such operations performed during a 40 year period, Attie and Vardham (51) reported a 26% prevalence of associated thyroid lesions, with 31 of them being nonmedullary thyroid carcinomas. In our institution, we have evaluated the possible association between PHPT and cancer, and, among those patients in whom the malignancy did not predate the diagnosis of PHPT, thyroid malignancies were the most prevalent (52). Even though thyroid carcinoma detected at PTX may have occurred for reasons totally unrelated to PHPT, it would seem prudent for surgeons carefully to examine the exposed thyroid gland for possible malignancy whenever PTX is performed.

However, it may be premature to conclude that the increased frequency with which cancer is detected in patients with PHPT is simply a chance association. In Posen et al.'s (53) follow-up study of a large cohort of patients undergoing successful or unsuccessful PTX as well as patients followed without surgery, there was a lower incidence of malignancy among those in whom PTX was curative of the PHPT.

The potential importance of these observations cannot be overemphasized. If properly conducted surveillance programs do indicate a higher likelihood of cancer in patients with PHPT, then the current philosophy that there are patients with mild, asymptomatic PHPT who never need surgical cure of their disease will have to be reevaluated. As with most other aspects discussed in this chapter, this is an area where our knowledge base is quite deficient.

COURSE OF HYPERCALCEMIA AND OTHER SERUM CHEMISTRIES IN PRIMARY HYPERPARATHYROIDISM

Calcium Levels Without Surgery in Primary Hyperparathyroidism

Not surprisingly, the mean level of serum calcium in surgically confirmed cases of PHPT decreased in the first several years after the introduction of automated biochemical profiling (Table 3). Mitlak et al. (56) reported that, among 100 consecutive cases diagnosed between 1972 and 1983, 85% had a serum calcium <3.0 mmol/liter. Heath and Heath (57) reported a series of 113 patients undergoing PTX between 1980 and 1989 in whom mean serum calcium was 2.87 ± 0.43 mmol/liter. An additional 92 patients followed for >5 years without surgery had a mean serum calcium of 2.81 ± 0.17 mmol/liter at diagnosis and 2.73 ± 0.20 mmol/liter at latest follow-up. In our series of 174 patients initially diagnosed during the 10 year period 1976–1985, the mean serum calcium was 2.77 ± 0.09 mmol/liter

(58). Bilezikian et al. (59) reported an identical mean value in a group of 97 subjects recently recruited into a study on the natural history of mild PHPT.

As has been discussed in earlier chapters, PHPT appears to result from a resetting of the level at which the parathyroids respond to the serum calcium. Once this has developed, the control of serum calcium appears to be normal, with very minor fluctuations over many years of observation (Fig. 2) (60).

The serum calcium is so well regulated in PHPT that patients who develop a second illness that might independently be associated with hypercalcemia, e.g., thyrotoxicosis or granulomatous disease, do not appear to have aggravation of the hypercalcemia. This is illustrated in part by the patient whose data are presented in Figure 3. The constancy of the serum calcium, clearly independent of progression or regression of the skeletal metastases, is typical and diagnostic of PHPT, not hypercalcemia complicating her breast cancer. Similarly, there is no apparent adverse effect of dietary calcium on the serum calcium in PHPT, and oral calcium supplements do not result in accelerated hypercalcemia. Tohme et al. (61) did report, however, that the rise in serum calcium in response to a fixed oral calcium load (25 mg/kg) was slightly greater in PHPT compared to normal (0.34 ± 0.06 vs. 0.53 ± 0.10 mg/dl), and there was less suppression of circulating levels of amino-terminal PTH fragment. Nonetheless, it is probably unwise to restrict dietary calcium intake in patients with PHPT, in that this could result in a "secondary" hyperparathyroidism, with increased PTH synthesis and secretion (see the chapter by Stock and Marcus). While not aggravating the hy-

TABLE 3. *Serum calcium¹ (mmol/l)*

Period	Series Iᵃ (n)	Series IIᵇ (n)
1953–64	3.05 ± 0.45 (32)	2.90 ± 0.51 (75)
1965–70	2.87 ± 0.34 (83)	2.86 ± 0.33 (200)
1971–75	2.82 ± 0.27 (165)	2.83 ± 0.39 (276)
1976–82	2.88 ± 0.25 (161)	2.77 ± 0.25 (345)

The mean level of serum calcium in reported series of cases of PHPT has fallen progressively in the years following the introduction of automated biochemical profiling. This is particularly evident when the serum calcium has been corrected for protein binding.

¹adapted from references 54 and 55
ᵃcalcium not corrected for protein binding
ᵇcalcium corrected for protein binding

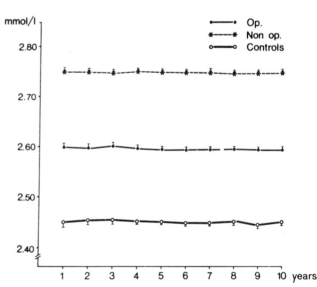

FIG. 2. Serum calcium in untreated, mild PHPT is stable over many years of observation. (Reprinted from ref. 60 with permission.)

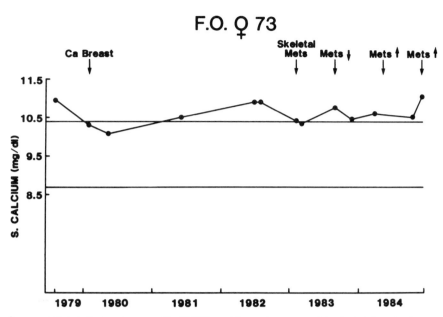

FIG. 3. Serum calcium in a woman with PHPT and breast cancer with skeletal metastases was relatively stable during many years of observation, despite periodic development and remission of the metastases. This is characteristic of the stable hypercalcemia of PHPT and strongly suggests that the skeletal metastases were not contributing to the hypercalcemia.

percalcemia, it would tend to exaggerate any adverse effect of the PTH on the skeleton, which, in the absence of adequate dietary calcium, becomes the major source of calcium in the circulation.

While intercurrent illness and dietary calcium intake have little effect on serum calcium in PHPT, except in those unusual circumstances discussed above, this is not the case for several therapeutic agents. The relationship of thiazide diuretics and lithium to the pathogenesis and/or detection of PHPT is well reported but poorly understood. Some studies have suggested that both these drugs cause the de novo development of PTH hypersecretion and PHPT. Others have suggested that patients receiving these drugs had very mild PHPT that was aggravated or "unmasked" by the therapy. Ideally, the diagnostic evaluation for possible PHPT should be deferred until the patient has not taken thiazides or lithium for 3 months. This is an arbitrary wash-out period and is often impractical, particularly for patients on lithium, for which there are fewer substitute medications. If it is not possible to find a temporary therapeutic substitute for thiazides or lithium, the diagnostic evaluation should proceed while therapy is continued. If the PTH is clearly elevated, this supports a diagnosis of PHPT. Similarly, suppressed PTH in the face of hypercalcemia is indicative of a nonparathyroid cause. The real diagnostic dilemma occurs for those patients on one of these medications, with mild hypercalcemia, in whom PTH is still within the normal range or very modestly elevated. Not surprisingly, this is often the clinical situation, and every effort should again be made to discontinue the medication temporarily.

Thiazides, apparently by inhibiting urine calcium excretion, result in a mild rise in the serum calcium, usually <0.05 mmol/liter, which may be sufficient in subjects with minimal disease biochemically to become overtly hypercalcemic for the first time. The counterargument has been raised that only patients with preexisting PHPT develop hypercalcemia while taking thiazide diuretics. There are few formal studies directly addressing the magnitude of the rise in serum calcium in patients with known PHPT. Farquhar et al. (62) studied 13 patients with known PHPT who were taking thiazides intermittently for periods of up to 18 months. During an average follow-up of 5.3 years, the authors could not detect any significant difference in either albumin-corrected or ionized calcium for periods in which patients were on or off thiazides. While this finding requires careful verification, it may be appropriate to withhold thiazides whenever possible in patients known to have PHPT. However, both the disease and the use of the drug are so common among the elderly that, if there was a marked and consistent effect on serum calcium, physicians would expect to encounter accelerated hypercalcemia far more frequently than is currently the case. It should be added parenthetically that thiazides may in fact be safer for a patient with PHPT than more potent loop diuretics, with their greater tendency towards dehydration and worsening hypercalcemia on that basis.

A cause and effect relationship between lithium

therapy for affective disorders and the development of hyperparathyroidism is more clearly established. Several series have shown that there is a duration-dependent tendency for lithium-treated patients to develop hypercalcemic hyperparathyroidism, with the usual history being one of therapy for 10 years or more (63,64). Additionally, there is an apparently greater likelihood of parathyroid hyperplasia or multiple adenoma being found at PTX in lithium-treated patients (63,65) than is seen in either sporadic PHPT or radiation-induced PHPT (66). Saxe and Gibson (67) demonstrated that lithium increases tritiated thymidine uptake in dispersed cells taken from patients with parathyroid adenoma (not treated with lithium prior to the diagnosis of PHPT). Other studies using dispersed bovine parathyroid cells have indicated that lithium results in a decrease in low calcium-stimulated PTH release but a potentiation of PTH release at physiologic concentrations of extracellular calcium (68). In a perfusion experiment using normal parathyroid tissue from patients undergoing thyroid surgery and hyperplastic parathyroid tissue removed from patients with renal osteodystrophy, Birnbaum et al. (69) demonstrated an increased release of intact PTH in normocalcemic conditions. This could not be demonstrated in human parathyroid tissue obtained from patients with single gland adenoma. Following a single oral dose of 600 mg lithium carbonate to nine normal subjects, Seely et al. (70) demonstrated a significant rise in serum levels of intact PTH but no significant change in the serum ionized calcium levels. Mallette et al. (71) demonstrated that, compared to normal subjects, patients with affective disorders treated with lithium for <6 months had a higher mean serum ionized calcium, but there were no differences in plasma intact or midregion PTH. In subjects treated with lithium for >3 years, plasma PTH and parathyroid gland volume were significantly higher than in controls. Thus chronic lithium therapy appears to stimulate parathyroid cell growth and PTH secretion, leading, after long-term therapy, to hypercalcemic parathyroid hyperplasia, i.e., PHPT. However, as is the case with thiazide therapy, there is no evidence that lithium therapy per se alters the natural history of the disease in patients with sporadic adenomatous PHPT.

Acute Hypercalcemic Crisis

There are reports of patients with longstanding, mild hypercalcemia developing acute hypercalcemic crises. In the author's experience, on those few occasions when this has occurred, it has always been in the setting of an elderly patient developing an acute, unrelated illness complicated by dehydration. Even in that setting, acute hypercalcemic crisis is uncommon.

Nonetheless, as Fitzpatrick and Bilezikian (73) pointed out in their recent review of parathyroid crises that 25% of patients with this acute form of the disease have a history of mild hypercalcemia, often of many years duration (see also chapter by Fitzpatrick). Corsello et al. (74) reported five cases treated over a 2 year period, including a 35-year-old man in whom PTX revealed a parathyroid carcinoma. Uncommon as this complication might be, some have pointed to this as a reason to recommend elective PTX at the time of diagnosis in otherwise healthy, particularly elderly, patients with serendipitously detected PHPT.

Course of Other Biochemical Markers in Primary Hyperparathyroidism

There is ample documentation that the other biochemical abnormalities so characteristic of PHPT are stable during long-term follow-up of mild, asymptomatic PHPT patients (72). Of particular importance is the lack of evidence that this type of PHPT is associated with progressive renal impairment, at least as measured by serum creatinine, blood urea nitrogen, or endogenous creatinine clearance. Serum alkaline phosphatase, both total and bone specific, is also stable during several years of follow-up, suggesting lack of progression of PTH-mediated bone disease, as is discussed in detail below. Serum inorganic phosphate and the tubular maximum reabsorption of phosphate (TmP) are also very stable, but this is quite characteristic of all forms of PHPT, independent of the clinical and biochemical severity of the disease. Data on long-term stability of PTH in this form of PHPT are quite limited and difficult to interpret because of frequent changes in the methods for measuring serum PTH over the past several years. When expressed in terms of a percentage of the upper limit of normal for a particular assay, the data suggest that there is not a progressive increase in serum PTH levels (72). This could be predicted from the observed set point change but the otherwise normal relationship between serum calcium and PTH synthesis and secretion and the long-term stability of serum calcium in this disease. As was discussed above, lithium-induced PHPT may be an exception to this general observation, along with those rare cases of acute hypercalcemic crises complicating seemingly mild, asymptomatic PHPT.

In this mild form of the disease, the parathyroid glands are generally too small to be routinely detected by the various imaging techniques (see the chapter by Doppman), so there are no reliable data on parathyroid gland growth. However, given the stability of all the other objective measurements of parathyroid hypersecretion, it could be legitimately concluded that progressive gland growth must be absent, or very slow in mild, asymptomatic PHPT (see the chapter by Parfitt).

Course of Biochemical Markers of Primary Hyperparathyroidism Following Successful Parathyroidectomy

The typical biochemical profile of primary hyperparathyroidism as it presents today is covered in the preceding chapter by Bilezikian et al. It is of interest that, despite the asymptomatic nature of the presentation vis-á-vis bone disease, the total alkaline phosphatase concentration is mildly elevated. In addition, more specific markers of bone formation (bone-specific alkaline phosphatase and osteocalcin) as well as markers of bone resorption (collagen crosslinks, pyridinoline, and deoxypyridinoline) are elevated. Postoperatively, these markers return to normal with a time course that reflects the rapid reduction in the rate of bone resorption and the more slowly normalizing preoperative accelerated rate of bone formation. This is discussed in more detail in the chapter by Deftos.

CLINICAL PRESENTATION AND COURSE OF CLASSIC MANIFESTATIONS OF PRIMARY HYPERPARATHYROIDISM

Parathyroid Bone Disease

Osteitis fibrosa cystica, the classic form of parathyroid bone disease, is rarely encountered in PHPT now, although it remains a clinical problem in the secondary hyperparathyroidism of patients with end-stage renal disease complicated by renal osteodystrophy. In contrast, many patients with asymptomatic PHPT do exhibit asymptomatic bone disease if this is sought diligently. A small proportion of patients, well under 10%, will have radiographic evidence of PTH excess on carefully obtained hand radiographs examined with a magnifying glass (75). A larger proportion of patients is likely to have histologic changes compatible with, but not necessarily diagnostic of, PTH excess on transiliac needle bone biopsy (76). Many more patients, possibly the majority, will have skeletal demineralization when investigated with the more sensitive noninvasive methods for measuring bone mass. Several studies have indicated, based on these bone densitometry studies and confirmed histologically, that there is preferential loss of cortical bone, with relative sparing of cancellous bone (77–79). Why this should be the case is unknown, but studies with synthetic PTH as a potential therapy for osteoporosis have demonstrated an increase in cancellous bone volume with-

out any significant changes in cortical bone volume or porosity (80–82). This osteotrophic action of PTH on cancellous bone in osteoporosis might explain the apparent preferential sparing of cancellous bone in PHPT, but it would not explain the preferential loss of cortical bone. Moreover, PTH therapy appears to be effective only when administered intermittently, with no appreciable effects observed with continuous infusions of PTH (83). In PHPT, hypersecretion of PTH appears to be continuous rather than intermittent. These paradoxical effects of PTH on the skeleton are among the more important questions for which answers are needed regarding both PHPT and osteoporosis.

Data from the author's unit indicates that most patients with mild, asymptomatic PHPT have documented bone loss at the time of diagnosis; that is, the mean bone mass is significantly lower than in appropriate controls (72). This bone loss does not appear to be progressive, at a rate faster than the bone loss associated with normal aging, if the disease is left untreated. Furthermore, there is little restoration of the cortical bone following successful PTX, with most of the gain evident within 6 months of surgery (84). On the other hand, more impressive changes are seen postoperatively in the bone mineral density in the lumbar spine. This is a curious observation in view of the fact that the lumbar region, enriched in cancellous bone, appears to be relatively well protected by PTH in PHPT. The higher turnover rate of cancellous bone and the filling in, postoperatively, of the expanded remodeling space at this region could account for these observations.

"Clinical consequences of bone loss in PHPT: fractures," an early paper by Dauphine et al. (85), reported an increased prevalence of vertebral fractures in patients with this mild form of PHPT, but several more recent studies have failed to confirm this observation (86,87). When vertebral fracture is the starting point for the studies, PHPT is a rare finding, although all authorities continue to recommend measurement of serum calcium as part of the routine screening for all newly diagnosed cases of osteoporosis. Our series of over 600 consecutive patients referred to our metabolic bone disease clinic for evaluation of bone loss with or without vertebral fracture (88) failed to uncover a single case of PHPT. Similarly, Johnson et al. (89) did not find a single case of PHPT in >300 consecutive cases of osteoporosis. It is reasonable to conclude that this form of PHPT does not predispose patients to spinal osteoporosis and may in fact offer some protection against it because of the sparing of cancellous bone. Interestingly, Melton et al. (90) recently reported that patients with PHPT had sustained more fractures prior to the diagnosis than did a control population, but during >1,000 person-years of follow-up, survival free of new fracture was the same in the two groups. This is in keeping with our observation that significant bone loss appears to have occurred at some time prior to the diagnosis of PHPT but that, once the diagnosis is established, accelerated bone loss is not seen. One explanation for this phenomenon is that the skeleton is the source of the extra calcium in the circulation as a new steady state is being established during the initial stages of PHPT but that, once established, the higher serum levels of calcium are maintained by mechanisms that do not involve the skeleton. This would be in keeping with the concept that the skeleton plays little role in the maintenance of serum calcium under normal physiologic conditions.

There are insufficient data to form any valid conclusions about a relationship between PTH-mediated cortical bone loss and an increased occurrence of long bone or proximal femur fractures. It would seem logical to anticipate this devastating consequence of progressive loss of cortical bone, but PHPT is not a dominant feature in any series of hip fracture patients, and hip fractures are not a dominant feature in any series of elderly patients with PHPT. This strongly suggests that, as is the case with PHPT and vertebral fractures, long bone and proximal femur fractures and not a feature of untreated PHPT. If this is substantiated by long-term prospective studies, it may provide important clues to the pathogenesis of osteoporotic hip fractures. One of the favored current hypotheses for this pathogenesis is that the aging kidney has impaired production of calcitriol and that the resultant compensatory increase in PTH secretion results in cortical bone loss and hip fractures. One important difference between this scenario and the situation in PHPT is the (often) increased production of calcitriol in PHPT. A recent study from France has suggested that only small doses of vitamin D (800 units/day) are sufficient to suppress PTH secretion and to decrease the likelihood of osteoporotic hip fracture (91). Thus high PTH with low calcitriol might predispose to hip fracture, while high PTH with normal or elevated calcitriol might be protective. Though still quite speculative, this hypothesis deserves evaluation. Regrettably it is unlikely to be studied extensively, since most centers caring for many patients with PHPT are so concerned (appropriately so) about the potential for continued cortical bone loss in untreated PHPT to result in hip fracture that they have adopted a policy of recommending PTX in all subjects with a measured low bone mass. Given the limited reversibility of PTH-mediated bone loss, one cannot really afford to reserve this recommendation for those in whom serial measurement of bone mass demonstrates progressive loss. In brief, bone loss is common in mild, asymptomatic PHPT, but progressive bone loss (greater than can be accounted for by age alone) is uncommon. The clinical significance of this bone loss is probably more theoretical than real, but it seems prudent to err on the side of conservatism.

Clinical Course of Stone Disease in Primary Hyperparathyroidism

Stone disease in PHPT is covered in the chapter by Klugman et al. Regarding those patients with stone disease, it would seem that the incidence is reduced following successful PTX. Certainly, urinary calcium excretion is reduced following surgery. Thus, despite uncertainty in attributing stone disease in patients with PHPT to the hyperparathyroid state per se (two common disorders are likely to occur with some regularity in the same patient), it appears reasonable to do so based on these data.

Long-Term Longitudinal Course of Primary Hyperparathyroidism

What is needed at this time is a long-term, prospective, multisite study of the course of PHPT. Such a study should take into account the key needs regarding this disease which have been covered above. The long-term incidence of fractures, potential progressive changes in bone mineral density, development of stone disease, and neuropsychiatric elements are all areas for which long-term data are lacking. In addition, a matched group of subjects who undergo parathyroid surgery is needed to determine to what extent these long-term manifestations, if any, are reversible.

SUMMARY AND CONCLUSIONS

The earliest clinical descriptions of PHPT point to an inexorably progressive, crippling, and sometimes fatal metabolic bone disease (type I PHPT). Later writings highlighted nephrolithiasis as a common feature of this disease, and it subsequently became apparent that more patients with PHPT in fact have stone disease without skeletal involvement (type II PHPT). Three decades ago, the introduction of automated, screening biochemical profiles that included serum calcium led to the serendipitous discovery of PHPT in large numbers of patients who had no clinical evidence of either metabolic bone or stone disease, so-called asymptomatic PHPT. This review has developed the hypothesis that this constitutes a distinct clinical entity, type III PHPT, with few clinical features in common with the other two types and little evidence of progression to either type I or type II except in rare cases. An unknown proportion of subjects is truly asymptomatic when the diagnosis is confirmed biochemically, and they appear to remain asymptomatic during many years of observation. In those patients with symptoms, the major clinical manifestation appears to be a constellation of vague and nonspecific neurobehavioral symptoms that were not traditionally thought to be related to PHPT. The prevalence of these symptoms is significantly greater than in control populations, strongly suggesting a cause and effect relationship to PHPT. However, most of them are not predictably improved by successful PTX, leaving this potential relationship to PHPT unresolved. Hypertension is more prevalent in type III PHPT than in the population at large, but this too is unpredictably ameliorated by PTX, and the mechanisms linking PHPT and hypertension are not clear. Diabetes mellitus, peptic ulcer disease, and pancreatitis, all traditionally linked to PHPT, probably are not more prevalent in this mild form of the disease than in the population at large. A link between PHPT and an increased likelihood of nonparathyroid malignancies has been suggested from several observational studies, but here too the link is tenuous. If such a link is established more fully in the less common type I and type II forms of PHPT, this would constitute a compelling reason for early diagnosis and cure of the type II disease. Finally, newer methods of measuring bone mass indicate that this disease is characterized by disproportionate loss of cortical bone, with preservation of cancellous bone. The clinical consequence of this is that patients with type III PHPT are, to some extent at least, protected from developing vertebral fractures. The fear, of course, is that these same patients are at increased risk for developing the more catastrophic hip fractures that are so prevalent in older women, the group with the highest prevalence of type III PHPT. However, there is as yet no documentation that this fear is justified.

Inexplicably, all these manifestations of type III PHPT appear to be present when the disease is first discovered in an individual patient but show little evidence of progression if the disease remains untreated. Similarly, the major biochemical abnormalities (hypercalcemia, hypophosphatemia, increased total and bone-specific alkaline phosphatase, increased PTH) are also present when the disease is first detected and in general show little progression with time. Thus the natural history of type III PHPT, once the diagnosis has been established, is one of a very mild clinical disease, with little objective or subjective evidence of progression if left untreated. An uncertain proportion of patients feel "better" after successful PTX (including many who claimed to be totally asymptomatic prior to surgery), yet it has been difficult to demonstrate that this is more than a "placebo" effect of surgery. Perhaps more importantly, when there is more subjective evidence of end-organ damage from mild PHPT, as is the case with the cortical bone loss, successful PTX has a very limited effect on reversing the bone loss. Clearly, much of the natural history of type III PHPT develops before the disease is serendipitously diagnosed. For now, any comments on this remain purely speculative.

REFERENCES

1. Mandl F. Therapeutiscle Versuch bei Ostitis fibrosa generalisata mittels Extirpation lines Epithelköperchentumon. *Wien Klin Wochenschr* 1925;50:1343–1344.
2. Cope O. The story of hyperparathyroidism at the Massachusetts General Hospital. *N Engl J Med* 1966;21:1174–1182.
3. Albright F. Page out of history of hyperparathyroidism. *J Clin Endocrinol Metab* 1948;8:637–657.
4. Lloyd HM. Primary hyperparathyroidism: an analysis of the role of the parathyroid tumor. *Medicine* 1968;47:53–71.
5. Fischer JA, Bronner F, Coburn J. Parathyroid hormone. In: Bronner, Coburn, eds. *Disorders of mineral metabolism,* Vol. II. New York: Academic Press, 1982;271–358.
6. Lloyd HM, Jacobi JM, Cooke RA. Nuclear diameter in parathyroid adenomas. *J Clin Pathol* 1979;32:1278–1281.
7. Joborn C, Hetta J, Johansson H, Rastad J, Agren H, Akerstrom G, Ljunghall S. Psychiatric morbidity in primary hyperparathyroidism. *World J Surg* 1988;12:476–481.
8. Brown GG, Preisman RC, Kleerekoper MD. Neurobehavioral symptoms in mild primary hyperparathyroidism: related to hypercalcemia but not improved by parathyroidectomy. *Henry Ford Med J* 1987;35:211–215.
9. Cogan MG, Covey CM, Arieff AI, Wisniewski A, Clark OH. Central nervous system manifestations of hyperparathyroidism. *Am J Med* 1978;65:963–970.
10. Joborn C, Hetta J, Lind L, Rastad J, Akerstrom G, Ljunghall S. Self-rated psychiatric symptoms in patients operated on because of primary hyperparathyroidism and in patients with long-standing mild hypercalcemia. *Surgery* 1989;105:72–78.
11. McAllion SJ, Paterson CR. Psychiatric morbidity in primary hyperparathyroidism. *Postgrad Med J* 1989;65:628–631.
12. Cavanaugh S, Wettstein RM. Prevalence of psychiatric morbidity in medical populations. In: Grinspoon L, ed. *Psychiatry update, the American Psychiatric Association annual review,* Vol. 3. Washington, DC: American Psychiatric Press 1984;187–215,279–281.
13. Ettinger L. Hyperparathyroidism and mental changes. *Nord Med* 1942;4:15(S1-5).
14. St. Goar WT. Gastrointestinal symptoms as a clue to the diagnosis of primary hyperparathyroidism: a review of 45 cases. *Ann Intern Med* 1957;46:102–118.
15. Cope O. Hyperparathyroidism: diagnosis and management. *Am J Surg* 1960;99:394–403.
16. Hellstrom J, Ivermark BI. Primary parathyroidism. *Acta Chir Scand* 1962;294(Suppl.):5–113.
17. Karpati G, Frame B. Neuropsychiatric disorders in primary hyperparathyroidism. *Arch Neurol* 1964;10:387–397.
18. Henson RA. The neurological aspects of hypercalcemia: with special reference to primary hyperparathyroidism. *J R Coll Phys London* 1966;1:41–50.
19. Watson L. Clinical aspects of hyperparathyroidism. *Proc R Soc Med* 1968;61:1123.
20. Salahudeen AK, Thomas TH, Sellars L, et al. Hypertension and renal dysfunction in primary hyperparathyroidism: effect of parathyroidectomy. *Clin Sci* 1989;76:289–296.
21. Peterson P. Psychiatric disorders in primary hyperparathyroidism. *J Clin Endocrinol Metab* 1968;28:1491–1495.
22. Mallette LE, Bilezikian JP, Heath DA, Aurbach GD. Primary hyperparathyroidism: Clinical and biochemical features. *Medicine* 1974;53:127–146.
23. Palmer FJ. The clinical manifestation of primary hyperparathyroidism. *Comp Ther* 1983;9:56–64.

24. Joborn C, Hetta J, Palmer M, Akerstrom G, Ljunghall S. Psychiatric symptomatology in patients with primary hyperparathyroidism. *Upsala J Med Sci* 1986;91:77–87.

25. Joborn C, Hetta J, Frisk P, Palmer M, Akerstrom G, Ljunghall S. Primary hyperparathyroidism in patients with organic brain syndrome. *Acta Med Scand* 1986;219:91–98.

26. Alarcon RD, Franceschini JA. Hyperparathyroidism and paranoid psychosis case report and review of the literature. *Br J Psychiatr* 1984;145:477–486.

27. Diamond TW, Botha JR, Wing J, Meyers AM, Kalk WJ. Parathyroid hypertension. A reversible disorder. *Arch Intern Med* 1986;146:1709–1712.

28. Broulik PD, Horky K, Pacovsky V. Blood pressure in patients with primary hyperparathyroidism before and after parathyroidectomy. *Exp Clin Endocrinol* 1985;86:346–352.

29. Nainby-Luxmoore JC, Langford HG, Nelson NC, Watson RL, Barnes TY. A case-comparison study of hypertension and hyperparathyroidism. *J Clin Endocrinol Metab* 1982;55:303–306.

30. Ringe JD. Reversible hypertension in primary hyperparathyroidism—pre- and postoperative blood pressure in 75 cases. *Klin Wochenschr* 1984;62:465–469.

31. Jones DB, Jones JH, Lloyd HJ, Lucas PA, Wilkins WE, Walker DA. Changes in blood pressure and renal function after parathyroidectomy in primary hyperparathyroidism. *Postgrad Med J* 1983;59:350–353.

32. Bradley EL III, Wells JO. Primary hyperparathyroidism and hypertension. *Am Surg* 1983;49:569–570.

33. Sancho JJ, Rouco J, Riera-Vida R, Sitges-Serra A. Long-term effects of parathyroidectomy for primary hyperparathyroidism on arterial hypertension. *World J Surg* 1992;16:732–736.

34. Dominiczak AF, Lyall F, Morton JJ, et al. Blood pressure, left ventricular mass and intracellular calcium in primary hyperparathyroidism. *Clin Sci* 1990;78:127–132.

35. Brinton GS, Jubiz W, Lagerquist LD. Hypertension in primary hyperparathyroidism: the role of renin-angiotensin system. *J Clin Endocrinol Metab* 1975;41:1025–1029.

36. Ganguly A, Weinberger MH, Passmore JM, et al. The renin-angiotensin-aldosterone system and hypertension in primary hyperparathyroidism. *Metabolism* 1982;31:595–600.

37. Taylor WH. The prevalence of diabetes mellitus in patients with primary hyperparathyroidism and among their relatives. *Diabet Med* 1991;8:683–687.

38. Ljunghall S, Palmer M, Akerstrom G, Wide L. Diabetes mellitus, glucose tolerance and insulin response to glucose in patients with primary hyperparathyroidism before and after parathyroidectomy. *Eur J Clin Invest* 1983;13:373–377.

39. Bannon MP, vanHeerden JA, Palumbo PJ, Ilstrup DM. The relationship between primary hyperparathyroidism and diabetes mellitus. *Ann Surg* 1988;207:430–433.

40. Linos DA, vanHeerden JA, Abboud CF, Edis AJ. Primary hyperparathyroidism and peptic ulcer disease. *Arch Surg* 1978;113:384–386.

41. Watson RG, vanHeerden JA, Grant CS, Klee GG. Postoperative hypermylasemia, pancreatitis, and primary hyperparathyroidism. *Surgery* 1984;96:1151–1157.

42. Sitges-Serra A, Alonso M, deLecea C, Gores PF, Sutherland DE. Pancreatitis and hyperparathyroidism. *Br J Surg* 1988;75:158–160.

43. Prinz RA, Aranha GV. The association of primary hyperparathyroidism and pancreatitis. *Am Surg* 1985;51:325–329.

44. vanLanschot JJ, Bruining HA. Primary hyperparathyroidism and pancreatitis. *Netherlands J Surg* 1984;36:38–41.

45. Paloyan D, Simonowitz D, Paloyan E, Snyder TJ. Pancreatitis associated with primary hyperparathyroidism. *Am Surg* 1982;48:366–368.

46. Bess MA, Edis AJ, van Heerden JA. Hyperparathyroidism and pancreatitis. Chance or a causal association? *JAMA* 1980;243:246–247.

47. Turken SA, Cafferty M, Silverberg SJ, et al. Neuromuscular involvement in mild, asymptomatic primary hyperparathyroidism. *Am J Med* 1989;87:553–557.

48. Joborn C, Rastad J, Stalberg E, Akerstrom G, Ljunghall S. Muscle function in patients with primary hyperparathyroidism. *Muscle Nerve* 1989;12:87–94.

49. Wajngot A, Werner S, Granberg PO, Lindvall N. Occurrence of pituitary adenomas and other neoplastic diseases in primary hyperparathyroidism. *Surg Gynecol Obstet* 1980;151:401–403.

50. Farr HW, Fahey TJ Jr, Nash AG, Farr CM. Primary hyperparathyroidism and cancer. *Am J Surg* 1973;126:539–543.

51. Attie JN, Vardhan R. Association of hyperparathyroidism with nonmedullary thyroid carcinoma: review of 31 cases. *Head Neck* 1993;15:20–23.

52. Kambouris AA, Ansari MR, Talpos GT. Primary hyperparathyroidism and associated neoplasms. *Henry Ford Med J* 1987;35:207–210.

53. Posen S, Clifton-Bligh P, Reeve TS, Wagstaffe C, Wilkinson M. Is parathyroidectomy of benefit in primary hyperparathyroidism? *Q J Med* 1985;54:241–251.

54. Palmer M, Ljunghall S, Akerstrom G, et al. Patients with primary hyperparathyroidism operated on over a 24-year period: temporal trends of clinical and laboratory findings. *J Chronic Dis* 1987;40(2)121–130.

55. Hedback G, Oden A, Tisell LE. The influence of surgery on the risk of death in patients with primary hyperparathyroidism. *World J Surg* 1991;15:399–407.

56. Mitlak BH, Daly M, Potts JT Jr, Schoenfeld D, Neer RM. Asymptomatic primary hyperparathyroidism. *J Bone Mineral Res* 1991;6(Suppl. 2):S103–S124.

57. Heath DA, Heath EM. Conservative management of primary hyperparathyroidism. *J Bone Mineral Res* 1991;6(Suppl. 2):S117–S124.

58. Parfitt AM, Rao DS, Kleerekoper M. Asymptomatic primary hyperparathyroidism discovered by multichannel biochemical screening: clinical course and considerations bearing on the need for surgical intervention. *J Bone Mineral Res* 1991;6(Suppl. 2):S97–S101.

59. Bilezikian JP, Silverberg SJ, Shane E, Parisien M, Dempster DW. Characterization and evaluation of asymptomatic primary hyperparathyroidism. *J Bone Mineral Res* 1991;6(Suppl. 2):S85–S89.

60. Christensson TAT. Primary hyperparathyroidism—pathogenesis, incidence and natural history. *Prog Surg* 1986;18:34–44.

61. Tohme JF, Bilezikian JP, Clemens TL, Silverberg SJ, Shane E, Lindsay R. Suppression of parathyroid hormone secretion with oral calcium in normal subjects and patients with primary hyperparathyroidism. *J Clin Endocrinol Metab* 1990;70:951–956.

62. Farquhar CW, Spathis GS, Barron JL, Levin GE. Failure of thiazide diuretics to increase plasma calcium in mild primary hyperparathyroidism. *Postgrad Med J* 1990;66:714–716.

63. Nordenstrom J, Strigard K, Perbeck L, Willems J, Bagedahl-Strindlund M, Linder J. Hyperparathyroidism associated with treatment of manic-depressive disorders by lithium. *Eur J Surg* 1992;158:207–211.

64. McHenry CR, Rosen IB, Rotstein LE, Forbath N, Walfish PG. Lithiumogenic disorders of the thyroid and parathyroid glands as surgical disease. *Surgery* 1990;108:1001–1005.

65. Krivitzky A, Bentata-Pessayre M, Sarfati E, Gardin JP, Callard P, Delzant G. Multiple hypersecreting lesions of the parathyroid glands during treatment with lithium. *Ann Med Intern* 1986;137:118–122.

66. Rao SD, Frame B, Miller MJ, Kleerekoper M, Block MA, Parfitt AM. Hyperparathyroidism following head and neck irradiation. *Arch Intern Med* 1980;140:205–207.

67. Saxe AW, Gibson G. Lithium increases tritiated thymidine uptake by abnormal human parathyroid tissue. *Surgery* 1991;110:1067–1077.

68. McHenry CR, Racke F, Meister M, et al. Lithium effects on dispersed bovine parathyroid cells grown in tissue culture. *Surgery* 1991;110:1061–1066.

69. Birnbaum J, Klandorf H, Giuliano A, VanHerle A. Lithium stimulates the release of human parathyroid hormone in vitro. *J Clin Endocrinol Metab* 1988;66:1187–1191.

70. Seely EW, Moore TJ, LeBoff MS, Brown EM. A single dose of lithium carbonate acutely elevates intact parathyroid hormone levels in humans. *Acta Endocrinol* 1989;121:174–176.

71. Mallette LE, Khouri K, Zengotita H, Hollis BW, Malini S. Lithium treatment increases intact and midregion parathyroid

hormone and parathyroid volume. *J Clin Endocrinol Metab* 1989;68:654–660.

72. Rao DS, Wilson RJ, Kleerekoper M, Parfitt AM. Lack of biochemical progression or continuation of accelerated bone loss in mild asymptomatic primary hyperparathyroidism: evidence for biphasic disease course. *J Clin Endocrinol Metab* 1988;67:1294–1298.

73. Fitzpatrick LA, Bilezikian JP. Acute primary hyperparathyroidism. *Am J Med* 1987;82:275–282.

74. Corsello SM, Folli G, Crucitti F, et al. Acute complications in the course of "mild" hyperparathyroidism. *J Endocrinol Invest* 1991;14:971–974.

75. Hayes CW, Conway WF. Hyperparathyroidism. *Radiol Clin North Am* 1991;29:85–96.

76. Parisien M, Silverberg SJ, Shane E, et al. The histomorphometry of bone in primary hyperparathyroidism: preservation of cancellous bone structure. *J Clin Endocrinol Metab* 1990; 70:930–938.

77. Kleerekoper M, Villanueva AR, Mathews CHE, Rao DS, Pumo B, Parfitt AM. PTH mediated bone loss in primary and secondary hyperparathyroidism. In: Frame B, Potts J Jr, eds. *Clinical disorders of bone and mineral metabolism.* Amsterdam: Excerpta Medica, 1983;200–203.

78. Silverberg SJ, Shane E, Jacobs TP, et al. Nephrolithiasis and bone involvement in primary hyperparathyroidism. *Am J Med* 1990;89:327–334.

79. Delmas PD, Meunier PJ, Faysse E, Saubier EC. Bone histomorphometry and serum bone gla-protein in the diagnosis of primary hyperparathyroidism. *World J Surg* 1986;10:572.

80. Slovik DM, Rosenthal DF, Doppert SH, et al. Restoration of spinal bone in osteoporotic men by treatment with human parathyroid hormone (1–34) and 1,25 dihydroxyvitamin D. *J Bone Mineral Res* 1986;1:377–381.

81. Hesch RD, Busch V, Rokop M, Delling G, Rittinghaus EF. Increase of vertebral density by combination therapy with pulsatile 1–38 HPTH and sequential addition of calcitonin nasal spray in osteoporotic subjects. *Calcif Tissue Int* 1987; 44:176–180.

82. Reeve J, Bradbeer JN, Arlot M, et al. LPTH 1–34 treatment of osteoporosis with added hormone replacement therapy: biochemical, kinetic, and histological responses. *Osteo Int* 1991;1:162–170.

83. Podbesek R, Edouard C, Meunier PJ, et al. Effects of two treatment regimes with synthetic human parathyroid hormone fragment on bone formation and the tissue balance of trabeculated bone in greyhounds. *Endocrinology* 1983;112:1000–1006.

84. Martin P, Bermann P, Sillet C. Partially reversible osteopenia after surgery for primary hyperparathyroidism. *Arch Intern Med* 1986;146:689–691.

85. Dauphine RT, Riggs BL, Scholz DA. Back pain and vertebral crush fractures: an unrecognized mode of presentation for primary hyperparathyroidism. *Ann Intern Med* 1975;83:365–367.

86. Wilson RJ, Rao DS, Ellis B, Kleerekoper M, Parfitt AM. Mild asymptomatic primary hyperparathyroidism is not a risk factor for vertebral fractures. *Ann Intern Med* 1988;109:959–962.

87. Lafferty FW, Halsay CA. Primary hyperparathyroidism: A review of the long-term surgical and non-surgical morbidities as a basis for a rational approach to treatment. *Arch Intern Med* 1986;149:789–796.

88. Kleerekoper M, Peterson E, Nelson D, et al. Identification of women at risk for developing postmenopausal osteoporosis with vertebral compression fractures: role of history and single photon absorptiometry. *Bone Mineral* 1989;7:171–186.

89. Johnson BE, Lucasey B, Robinson RG, Lukert BP. Contributing diagnoses in osteoporosis. *Arch Intern Med* 1989;149: 1069–1072.

90. Melton LJ III, Atkinson EJ, O'Fallon WM, Heath H III. Risk of age-related fractures in patients with primary hyperparathyroidism. *Arch Intern Med* 1992;152:2269–2273.

91. Chapuy MC, Arlot ME, DuBoeuf F, et al. Vitamin D and calcium to prevent hip fractures in elderly women. *N Engl J Med* 1992;327:1637–1642.

The Parathyroids, edited by J.P. Bilezikian, M.A. Levine, and R. Marcus. Raven Press, Ltd., New York © 1994.

CHAPTER 28

Markers of Bone Turnover in Primary Hyperparathyroidism

Leonard J. Deftos

Parathyroid hormone (PTH) increases bone resorption and bone formation, the latter by direct stimulation of osteoblasts and the former by the indirect stimulation of osteoclasts (1). The degree of involvement of the skeleton in primary hyperparathyroidism (PHPT) can, therefore, be assessed by the measurement in blood (serum or plasma) and urine of the products of skeletal metabolism that reflect osteoblast-mediated bone formation and osteoclast-mediated bone resorption (2). These products can come from bone cells and bone matrix. Bone matrix components reflect bone resorption. Osteoblast products reflect bone formation, and osteoclast products reflect bone resorption, as these two cell types mediate these two processes. The major osteoblast products that are clinically useful indices of bone formation are alkaline phosphatase (AP), type I procollagen, and bone gla (γ-carboxyglutamic acid) protein (BGP) (also known as osteocalcin; OC). The major osteoclast product that is useful for assessment of skeletal metabolism is tartrate-resistant acid phosphatase (TRAP). The major components of bone matrix that can be measured are type I procollagen, collagen cross-links, and hydroxyproline and hydroxylysine. These proteins and their derived peptides are the targets for biochemical and immunochemical assays that are currently used and are being developed further to detect and characterize skeletal involvement in PHPT and other metabolic bone diseases (Table 1).

Because highly sensitive immunoassays now facilitate the early diagnosis of mild PHPT, the presence of the parathyroid abnormality is often documented before there is clinically advanced involvement of the skeleton (3). Accordingly, early defects in skeletal me-

tabolism may produce only mild changes in these biochemical measurements. Thus sensitivity as well as specificity of biochemical indices for skeletal involvement in PHPT are usually intermediate between those that accompany the dramatic changes of Paget's disease and the more subtle abnormalities of osteoporosis.

Each biochemical test has its advantages and disadvantages (4–7). While specificity and sensitivity are both important characteristics for a marker of skeletal metabolism, sensitivity is especially important to identify early bone involvement in PHPT. Establishing the presence of bone involvement in PHPT has the important implications for therapy that are discussed in other chapters in this volume (Fig. 1).

ALKALINE PHOSPHATASE

The measurement of serum AP enzyme activity continues to be a useful biochemical test for skeletal assessment in PHPT (7). In most studies of patients with PHPT, AP correlates with the other direct and indirect biochemical indices of skeletal involvement (8–10). Thus AP is positively correlated with levels of serum PTH, calcium, BGP, and procollagen peptides and with levels of urinary hydroxyproline, hydroxylysine, and collagen-derived pyridinium cross-links. AP also correlates with histomorphometric and calcium kinetic studies of increased bone formation. Finally, AP shows an inverse correlation with densitometric assessment of bone mass in most studies of PHPT.

Despite these relationships, the clinical utility of AP measurements in the patient with PHPT is limited (8–10). The previously mentioned correlations with other indices of skeletal involvement are present but generally are too weak to be useful in an individual patient.

L. J. Deftos: Department of Medicine, University of California San Diego and; San Diego Veterans Affairs Medical Center, San Diego, California 92161.

TABLE 1. *Biochemical markers of bone formation and bone resorption*

Bone formation	Bone resorption
Bone alkaline phosphatase (BAP)	Bone acid phosphatase (TRAP)
Bone gla protein (Osteocalcin)	Free gla (gammacarboxyglutamic acid)
Collagen related products	Collagen related products
Procollagen I extension peptides	Amino acids
Amino-terminal (N)	Hydroxyproline glycoside
Carboxy-terminal (C)	Galactosyl hydroxylysine
	Cross-links
	Pyridinoline (pyr) [hydrolysylpyridinoline (hp)]; PYD
	Deoxypyridinoline (d-pyr) [lysylpyridinoline (lp)]; DPD

This is not surprising, in that the skeleton is only one of the tissues that contributes to total serum AP activity. Because total serum AP activity reflects AP synthesized from a variety of different tissues, AP measurement lacks specificity. The clinical impact of this lack of specificity is clearly evident in the patient with both skeletal and liver disease, in whom routine testing can not distinguish the source of the serum AP. Moreover, in patients with only modest biochemical abnormalities, any changes in AP from bone can be obscured by the small contribution bone makes to the circulating pool of the enzyme. In addition to being only weakly correlated with other measurements of disease activity, AP measurements in PHPT are commonly within the normal range (8–10). Thus the relationships that are found between AP and disease activity in group studies are often not useful in identifying skeletal involvement in the individual patient with PHPT.

In an attempt to improve the specificity and the sensitivity of serum AP assays, techniques have been developed to differentiate bone alkaline phosphatase from other isoenzymes, especially from liver (7). These isoenzymes differ only in their posttranslational modification, as they are all encoded by a single gene (11). Many biochemical procedures have been developed to identify the bone-specific form of AP (BAP) in serum. Although these procedures have improved the specificity of measurements for BAP, they remain technically difficult and have not had wide acceptance. These techniques rely on the use of differentially effective activators and inhibitors of AP enzymatic activity (heat, phenylalanine, and urea) and separation by electrophoresis (4–6). In general, the assays have slightly enhanced the specificity of this marker, but most of the assays remain relatively nonspecific for bone and are technically cumbersome.

Substantial improvement in measuring BAP could be obtained by using antibodies that recognize the bone but not the liver and kidney isoenzymes (12,13). Such approaches have recently become possible with the development of immunochemical assays for BAP (12–14). These assays rely upon the specificity of antibodies generated against unique epitopes of BAP. In one procedure, two separate radioimmunoassays (RIAs) are used to increase specificity for serum BAP (14). One of the RIAs utilizes an antibody that recognizes BAP and liver AP equally; the other RIA uses an antibody that has a fivefold greater affinity for BAP than for the liver isoenzyme. The serum concentration of BAP can be calculated from the results of the two RIAs. This method appears to give better clinical correlations between skeletal disease and AP measurement than does enzymatic measurement of AP in patients with PHPT (14).

A recently developed assay that uses two BAP-specific antibodies now provides a more direct and novel approach to the measurement of BAP (12,13). These two antibodies recognize distinct BAP epitopes and show minimal cross-reactivity for other types of alkaline phosphatase. These two antibodies are used in a two-site immunoradiometric "sandwich" assay

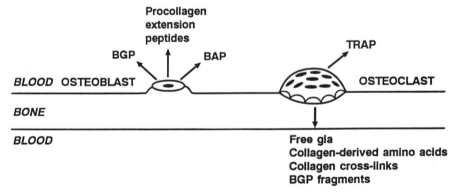

FIG. 1. Schematic representation of the cellular and skeletal sources of markers for bone formation and resorption.

(IRMA) that has specificity only for BAP. In the IRMA assay, a "capture antibody" is bound to a polystyrene bead, and the second antibody, the "detector," is radioactively labeled with ^{125}I. The antibody-coated bead is incubated with the serum sample and the other labelled antibody, and after a specified interval the complex is then washed. Levels of immunoactive BAP in the unknown sample are determined by comparison of the number of radioactive counts in the tube with a standard curve of BAP extracted from human osteoblast cells. This assay has <15% cross-reactivity with liver AP. In addition to this specificity, the two-site IRMA is rapid and convenient compared to standard RIA formats (13).

In preliminary studies, the IRMA procedure for BAP appears to be more clinically useful than other AP assays in patients with PHPT (15). BAP was elevated above normal in more patients with PHPT than was total serum AP activity and BAP correlated with other indices of skeletal activity, including bone mineral density of trabecular bone sites. Although total AP was somewhat elevated on average, BAP was more clearly above the upper limit of normal. As for total AP, serum levels of BGP and urinary hydroxyproline were only modestly elevated. BAP and total AP correlated with each other and with parathyroid hormone (PTH). BAP, but not total AP, correlated with 1,25-dihydroxyvitamin D [1,25(OH)$_2$D] and urinary collagen cross-links. Neither BAP nor total AP was correlated with serum calcium, BGP, or urinary hydroxyproline. In contrast to BAP, BGP did not correlate with any index of bone turnover. Unlike BAP, urinary hydroxyproline correlated with serum calcium. In addition, BAP correlated with bone mineral density of the lumbar spine and the femoral neck but not with that of the radius. None of the other indices of bone turnover (total AP, BGP, urinary hydroxyproline) correlated with any densitometric measurement. These data indicate that BAP is a more sensitive index of bone involvement in PHPT than either total AP, BGP, or urinary hydroxyproline. The correlation of BAP with densitometry at sites with significant trabecular composition suggests that BAP is a marker of increased trabecular bone formation. Further improvements in BAP assay procedures should enhance the clinical utility of this measurement in PHPT and other metabolic bone diseases.

BONE GLA PROTEIN

Measurement of bone gla protein (BGP) has become increasingly useful in studies of bone metabolism. BGP, also called *osteocalcin* (OC), is the major non-collagen protein of bone (4–6). BGP, so called because of the presence of glutamic acid residues that have been posttranslationally modified by addition of a γ-carboxyl group, has 49 amino acids and is produced exclusively by the osteoblast. The function of BGP is not known, although considerable effort has been directed toward investigating a role for BGP in bone formation and/or resorption. Nevertheless, the essentially exclusive production of BGP by the osteoblast makes the measurement of serum BGP valuable for assessing skeletal metabolism.

The rationale for the assay of serum BGP is that production of BGP provides an index of bone formation (4). As an osteoblast product, BGP represents the activity of the cell responsible for bone formation. Thus it is assumed that increased bone formation is associated with increased serum BGP concentrations. This hypothesis is generally supported by clinical studies of BGP. However, it is also possible that certain forms of BGP are indices of bone resorption. This possibility is based on the notion that BGP is incorporated into bone matrix and that, when the matrix is resorbed, BGP is released into serum (4,5). The forms of BGP entrapped in and then released from bone matrix are likely to be fragments of the molecule. Although most BGP measurements are believed to reflect bone formation, some data, discussed below, support the hypothesis that BGP can, under certain circumstances, be a marker of resorption.

Radioimmunoassays for BGP have proved to be clinically useful in the assessment and management of patients with PHPT (14,16–19). Serum BGP concentrations are typically elevated in such patients. In most of these patients, serum BGP measurements correlate with other indices of bone formation, such as serum total AP, bone histomorphometry, bone scans, calcium kinetic studies, and densitometric imaging procedures (14–19). Therefore, BGP provides useful biochemical information that can assist in the management of patients with PHPT; BGP is increased when bone formation is increased, and, unlike serum total AP activity, BGP is specific for bone (Table 2).

BGP seems to offer diagnostic advantages over total AP in the evaluation of patients with PHPT. BGP responds more rapidly than total AP to parathyroidectomy, changing within hours to reflect perturbations in skeletal homeostasis (9). In one study of PHPT, BGP measurements also seemed to provide a more sensitive index of altered bone metabolism than did AP measurements (17). Preparathyroidectomy BGP measurements were elevated significantly above normal for both men and women, whereas AP levels were abnormally elevated only in women. In these patients, BGP and AP were significantly greater in women than in men before as well as after treatment. Although postoperative levels of both BGP and AP declined postoperatively for men and women, the decrease in BGP levels was significant for BGP in women only. In an-

TABLE 2. *Plasma BGP and serum total alkaline phosphatase and calcium measurements in 11 men and 12 women with primary hyperparathyroidism before and after parathyroidectomy (PTX)[a]*

	Pre-PTX			Post-PTX		
	Ca (mg/dl)	BGP (ng/ml)	AP (IU/liter)	Ca (mg/dl)	BGP (ng/dl)	AP (IU/liter)
Men						
Mean	12.10[c]	16.5[c]	64	8.56[b]	14.3[c]	62
SE	0.36	1.7	6.8	0.27	1.9	8.2
Women						
Mean	11.90[c]	35[c,d]	98[c,d]	8.19[b]	26[b–d]	90[c,d]
SE	0.29	6.1	12	0.20	4.2	13

[a]Reprinted from ref. 17 with permission.
[b]Significantly ($P < 0.001$) lower than preoperative value.
[c]Significantly ($P < 0.05–0.001$) higher than normal.
[d]Significantly ($P < 0.05–0.005$) greater than male values.

other study of PHPT, serum levels of BGP were elevated in 55% of the patients, whereas the serum levels of total AP were increased in only 45% of the patients (19). In 25% of the patients, the serum levels of BGP, but not those of total AP, were increased; by contrast, in 15% of patients, the activity of total AP phosphatase was elevated, but the serum BGP levels were normal. In all patients with PHPT, a significant positive correlation could be found between the serum BGP levels and the levels of serum PTH and the serum creatinine levels. In contrast, no significant correlations could be established between the serum BGP levels and age, serum calcium, and serum phosphorus. In this study, in accordance with previous reports (14), positive correlations were found between the serum levels of BGP and total AP; nevertheless, 25% of the patients with PHPT had increased serum BGP levels but normal serum total AP levels. These data for PHPT indicate that in general BGP is a more sensitive parameter of bone formation than is total AP.

Although BGP seems to be a more sensitive and specific index of bone formation than the enzymatic measurement of total AP in PHPT, recent studies sustain certain controversies about the utility of BGP assays (20). These studies reveal further complexities in BGP production and metabolism. Whereas most laboratories report higher BGP concentrations in males than in females, only some laboratories have reported a circadian pattern for serum BGP (4–6, 21–23). Inconsistent results have been reported for BGP levels across the menopause, across the menstrual cycle, and during pregnancy (24–27). By contrast, significant increases in BGP have been reported during the gonadal changes of puberty (28). Although some of the published discrepancies regarding BGP levels may represent clinical or biological differences, others may represent technical differences in the RIAs (29). Newer assay formats may help to resolve some of these prob-

lems (29–31). These methods of measuring BGP include assays based on human BGP, enzyme-linked assays, and two-site assays.

Several laboratories have reported the detection of immunochemically heterogenous fragments of BGP in urine and in serum (32,33). However, these measurements have not been applied extensively to PHPT. Two-site BGP assays confirm the immunochemical heterogeneity of circulating BGP, and this heterogeneity is manifest even with immunoassays specific for the same region of the molecule (31). Such two-site assay procedures may be useful to distinguish native BGP from BGP fragments. The measurement of BGP propeptide could theoretically resolve yet another species of BGP. However, this BGP precursor has not been detected in sera of normal subjects or patients with PHPT (34).

COLLAGEN PRODUCTS

Bone Formation

Type I collagen is a major product of the osteoblast (2). Collagen is synthesized as a precursor molecule, procollagen, that contains both amino- and carboxy-terminal extensions (35–38). After the soluble high-molecular-weight precursor molecule procollagen is secreted from the cell, endoproteolytic cleavage removes extension peptides at both the amino and the carboxyl termini to form the mature insoluble collagen chain that is incorporated into bone matrix. Type I procollagen is cleaved first at the amino terminus and then at the carboxyl terminus (Fig. 2). The extension peptides, known as amino- and carboxyl-terminal procollagen propeptides, are produced in a stoichiometric ratio. They are released into the extracellular fluid; however, a portion of the amino-terminal propeptide is

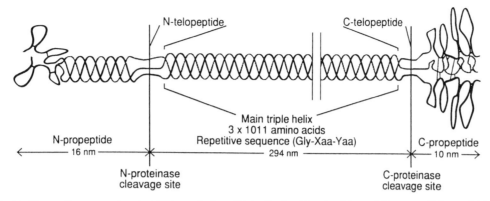

FIG. 2. The collagen molecule (294 nm in length) is flanked by the N- and C-propeptides, which are cleaved during the extracellular processing. The central main triple helix is made of 337 Gly-Xaa-Yaa repeats. The mature molecule conserves two short nontriple helical domains (N- and C-telopeptides), which contain cross-linking sites. (Reproduced from ref. 52 with permission.)

probably also incorporated into bone. The carboxyl-terminal propeptide of type I procollagen is a trimeric glycoprotein stabilized by interchain disulfide bonds and has a molecular mass of ~100 kilodaltons (kDa). The amino-terminal propeptide of type I procollagen is a smaller, globular protein with a molecular mass of ~64–70 kDa and may circulate as the full molecule or as fragments; it has no interchain disulfide bonds to stabilize its trimeric structure.

Because these procollagen extensions are cleaved before collagen becomes incorporated as a fibril into bone matrix, measurement of these peptides can theoretically serve as an index of osteoblast activity and bone formation. In fact, immunoassays based on antibodies for the terminal extension of type I procollagen can serve this purpose (35–38). Alternatively, the procollagen peptides could represent the resorptive cleavage and release from bone of the intact molecule. Acute studies of hormone-induced changes in procollagen peptides support the former hypothesis, that bone formation, and not bone resorption, determines circulating concentrations of the extension peptides (36). The measurement of procollagen extension peptides provides yet another serum marker for bone formation. Although these assays have clinical value, recent studies in PHPT patients have shown that both serum BGP and serum BAP are more sensitive than procollagen extension peptides for detection of abnormal bone metabolism in these patients (38).

Bone Resorption

Whereas the peptidic derivatives of procollagen reflect bone formation, the major amino acid components of collagen, hydroxyproline and hydroxylysine, are derived from the osteoclast-driven catabolism of collagen and, thus, reflect bone resorption (2). Specificity for resorption is due to the fact that free hydroxyproline released during degradation of collagen cannot be reutilized for collagen synthesis. The measurement of urinary, and in some cases serum, hydroxyproline has long been used to assess bone resorption (4–6). However, despite improved methodology, assays of collagen-derived hydroxyproline and hydroxylysine remain technically difficult procedures that are not suitable for routine clinical use. In addition, these measurements are not specific indices for bone but, rather, are influenced by collagen in the diet and by a variety of nonskeletal diseases that involve collagen. The fact that urinary hydroxyproline has rather low sensitivity and specificity for bone is also due in part to the fact that hydroxyproline is released when both newly synthesized and mature collagen are metabolized (2). In addition, hydroxyproline is derived from the total body collagen pool, including skin and noncollagen proteins. Finally, excreted hydroxyproline represents only a small fraction of collagen catabolism. Thus urinary hydroxyproline lacks both specificity and sensitivity as a marker of bone metabolism. As a consequence, urinary hydroxyproline excretion correlates poorly with bone resorption as assessed by calcium kinetics or bone histomorphometry. Like hydroxyproline, hydroxylysine that is released during bone resorption cannot be reutilized; it represents a posttranslational modification of lysine residues incorporated in collagen. There are some data suggesting that urinary hydroxylysine excretion is a more sensitive marker of bone resorption than urinary hydroxyproline. Nevertheless, the lack of sensitivity and specificity of both of these urinary collagen catabolites for bone diminishes their clinical value in the assessment of patients with PHPT as well as other skeletal diseases (2,4–6).

γ-Carboxyglutamic Acid

γ-Carboxyglutamic acid results from the vitamin K-dependent posttranslational modification of glutamic acid residues in at least two bone proteins, BGP and matrix gla protein (5,39). Because of this skeletal origin, the measurement in serum and urine of free gla has been proposed as an index of bone resorption. However, gla is not specific for bone but is also present in some coagulation factors and plasma proteins. Because of this mixed origin, serum or urine free gla is not sensitive enough to assess changes in bone resorption that accompany skeletal diseases, especially the subtle changes of PHPT.

CROSS-LINKS

Other markers for collagen turnover may be more promising for assessing bone resorption (40). Pyridinoline (PYD) and deoxypyridinoline (DPD), also called hydroxylysylpyridinoline (HP) and lysylpyridinoline (LP), respectively, are the two nonreducible pyridinium cross-links present in the mature form of collagen (2,40). This posttranslational covalent cross-linking step, based on the action of lysyl oxidase on lysine and hydroxylysine residues, is unique to collagen and elastin molecules. To establish more sensitive and specific indices for bone resorption, assays for the measurement of urinary PYD and DPD have been developed (41–45). The lysine cross-link DPD is found mainly in bone and dentin. Urinary DPD is thus considered to be derived almost exclusively from the skeleton, because turnover of dentin is negligible. In contrast, the hydroxylysine cross-link, PYD, also is a major cross-link in type II collagen of cartilage as well as type I bone collagen. Importantly, both of these pyridinium cross-links are completely absent from skin.

It has been shown in healthy individuals that urinary excretion of the two cross-links is in approximately the same ratio as that found in bone (40). These compounds are released only when mature collagen is degraded. This observation suggests that bone resorption accounts for the majority of both pyridinium cross-links in urine. In osteoporosis the concentrations of urinary PYD and DPD are highly correlated with bone resorption, and there is a significant correlation between urinary excretion of pyridinium cross-links and bone resorption as assessed by iliac crest biopsy (41–43).

Measurements of DPD and PYD have found recent application in studies of PHPT (45). Urinary concentrations of PYD and DPD were determined in a group of patients with untreated or surgically treated PHPT. Mean urinary excretions of PYD and DPD were significantly higher in patients with untreated PHPT than

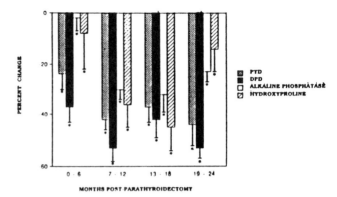

FIG. 3. Relative changes of urinary PYD, DPD, hydroxyproline (OPH), and serum alkaline phosphatase (AP) after successful parathyroidectomy. Values represent percent change as compared to the last preoperative measurement (baseline value). $P < 0.05$. Error bars denote SEM. (From ref. 45 with permission.)

in normal subjects. In patients undergoing successful parathyroidectomy, mean urinary concentrations of PYD and DPD became significantly lower than in the untreated patient population and were similar to those in normal controls (Fig. 3). The reduction, more pronounced for DPD than for PYD, was accompanied by significant changes in serum total alkaline phosphatase. Although mean levels of urinary hydroxyproline were lower in the treated than in the untreated group, this difference was not statistically significant. A subgroup of the patients with PHPT was followed longitudinally for up to 2 years after successful parathyroidectomy. Mean urinary concentrations of both cross-link compounds decreased significantly within 6 months in these patients and as early as 2 weeks after surgery in individual patients compared to presurgical baseline values. These changes preceded a reduction in serum alkaline phosphatase and urinary hydroxyproline by ~6 months. Thus the changes in PYD and DPD responded more rapidly to surgical treatment of PHPT than did the other biochemical measurements of skeletal metabolism. These promising observations will be confirmed and extended in additional studies of collagen cross-links in patients with PHPT as well as other skeletal diseases.

ACID PHOSPHATASE

Acid phosphatase has been proposed as a potential marker of bone resorption (2). This premise is based on the observation that, analogous to alkaline phosphatase and osteoblasts, osteoclasts contain a large amount of acid phosphatase activity and they secrete this enzyme when actively resorbing bone. Serum activity of bone acid phosphatase thus is thought to represent the activity of the cell responsible for bone resorption, the osteoclasts. In some studies, there appears to be a correlation between the rate of bone resorption and the serum acid phosphatase activity (46). However, both biochemical and cellular considerations complicate the enzymatic assay for acid phosphatase and the interpretation of its results. The serum acid phosphatase activity derived from osteoclasts must be distinguished from that derived from other tissue sources, notably prostate, pancreas, and blood cells (2). This is usually accomplished by analysis of the mobility of bone acid phosphatase on acrylamide gel and by the resistance of its activity to the inhibitor tartrate. Thus bone acid phosphatase is usually referred to as *tartrate-resistant acid phosphatase* (TRAP) (46). However, some question remains about the osteoclast specificity of TRAP. This form of the enzyme may also be present in the mononuclear precursors of osteoclasts, and a closely related acid phosphatase has been isolated from the uterus, from the spleen of patients with hairy cell leukemia, and from the liver in patients with Gaucher's disease (48–50). Furthermore, significant TRAP activity has recently been detected in the osteoblast and osteocyte (51).

There have been only limited studies of TRAP activity in patients with skeletal diseases (46–51). Elevated serum levels of this presumed osteoclast-specific marker have been demonstrated in patients with Paget's disease, skeletal metastases, and osteopetrosis as well as PHPT (46,51). These observations are consistent with the hypothesis that serum TRAP is a marker for osteoclastic bone resorption (2,51). Preliminary application of an enzyme-linked immunosorbent assay (ELISA) for TRAP to sera from patients with metabolic bone disease revealed that normal individuals had measurable amounts of the immunoreactive TRAP and that patients with PHPT had elevated levels of this immunoreactive material in their sera (51). Measurement of immunoreactive TRAP thus shows considerable promise as an index of osteoclast activity. Recent progress in understanding the molecular biology, biochemistry, and immunochemistry of TRAP should lead to the development of novel and clinically applicable procedures for assessing bone resorption by measurement of this osteoclast product in patients with PHPT and skeletal disease (48,50).

SUMMARY

Continued progress in basic and clinical studies of skeletal metabolism has elucidated the cellular and molecular mechanisms that regulate bone formation and bone resorption (Fig. 1). Understanding these mechanisms has also led to the development of clinically useful biochemical and immunochemical tests that can be used to distinguish between the contributions of formation and resorption in normal and abnormal skeletal metabolism. Application and refine-

ment of these tests will continue to assist in the diagnosis and management of patients with PHPT and other skeletal diseases.

ACKNOWLEDGMENTS

This work was supported by the National Institutes of Health, National Cancer Institute, and the RR&D Service of the Department of Veterans Affairs.

REFERENCES

1. Aurbach GD, Marx SJ, Spiegel AM. Parathyroid hormone calcitonin, and the calciferols. In: Wilson JD, Foster DW, eds. *Textbook of endocrinology, 8th Ed,* Vol 27. Philadelphia: W.B. Saunders, 1992;1397–1476.
2. Deftos LJ and Glowacki J. Mechanisms of bone metabolism. In: Kem DC, Frohlich E, eds. *Pathophysiology, 3rd Ed.* Philadelphia: J.B. Lippincott, 1984;445–468.
3. Deftos LJ, Parthemore JG, Stabile BE. Management of primary hyperparathyroidism. *Annu Rev* 1993;44:19–26.
4. Deftos LJ. Bone protein and peptide assays in the diagnosis and management of skeletal disease. *Clin Chem* 1991;37:1143–1148.
5. Delmas PD. Biochemical markers of bone turnover: methodology and clinical use in osteoporosis. *Am J Med* 1991;91:169–174.
6. Parfitt AM. Serum markers of bone formation in parenteral nutrition patients. *Calcif Tissue Int* 1991;49:143–145.
7. Moss DW. Perspectives in alkaline phosphatase research. *Clin Chem* 1992;38:2486–2492.
8. Pfeilschifter J, Siegrist E, Wüster C, Blind E, Ziegler R. Serum levels of intact parathyroid hormone and alkaline phosphatase correlate with cortical and trabecular bone loss in primary hyperparathyroidism. *Acta Endocrinol* 1992;127:319–323.
9. Minisola S, Scarnecchia L, Carnevale V, et al. Clinical value of the measurement of bone remodeling markers in primary hyperparathyroidism. *J Endocrinol Invest* 1989;12:537–543.
10. Torres R, De La Pirera C, Papado A. Osteocalcin and bone remodeling in Paget's disease of bone, primary hyperparathyroidism, hypercalcemia of malignancy and involutional osteoporosis. *Scand J Clin Invest* 1989;49:279–285.
11. Weiss MJ, Junal R, Henthorn PS, Kadesch T, Harris H. Structure of the human liver/bone/kidney alkaline phosphatase gene. *J Biol Chem* 1988;263:12002–12010.
12. Hill CS, Wolfert RL. The preparation of monoclonal antibodies which react preferentially with human bone alkaline phosphatase and not liver alkaline phosphatase. *Clin Chim Acta* 1989;186:315–320.
13. Deftos LJ, Wolfert RL, Hill CS. Bone alkaline phosphatase in Paget's disease. *Hormone Metab Res* 1991;23:515–561.
14. Duda RJ, O'Brien JF, Katzman JA, Peterson JM, Mann KG, Riggs BL. Concurrent assays of circulating bone Gla-protein and bone alkaline phosphatase: effects of sex, age, and metabolic bone disease. *J Clin Endocrinol Metab* 1988;5:1–7.
15. Silverberg SJ, LJ Deftos, Kim T, Hill CS. Bone alkaline phosphatase in primary hyperparathyroidism. *J Bone Mineral Res* 1991;6:A624.
16. Price PA, Parthemore JG, Deftos LJ. New biochemical marker for bone metabolism. Measurement by radioimmunoassay of bone gla protein in the plasma of normal subjects and patients with bone disease. *J Clin Invest* 1980;66:878–883.
17. Deftos LJ, Parthemore JG, Price PA. Changes in plasma bone Gla protein during treatment of bone disease. *Calcif Tissue Int* 1982;34:121–124.
18. Eastell R, Delmas PD, Hodgson S, Eriksen EF, Mann KM, Riggs BL. Bone formation rate in older normal women: con-

current assessment with bone histomorphometry, calcium kinetics, and biochemical markers. *J Clin Endocrinol Metab* 1988;67:741–748.

19. Pietschmann P, Niederle B, Anvari A, Woloszczuk W. Serum osteocalcin levels in primary hyperparathyroidism. *Klin Wochenschr* 1991;69:351–353.

20. Tracy RP, Andrianorivo A, Riggs BL, Mann KG. Comparison of monoclonal and polyclonal antibody-based immunoassays for osteocalcin: a study of sources of variation in assay results. *J Bone Mineral Res* 1990;5:451–461.

21. Markowitz ME, Dimarino-Nardi J, Gasparini F, Fishman K, Rosen JF, Seanger P. Effects of growth hormone therapy on circadian osteocalcin rhythms in idiopathic short stature. *J Clin Endocrinol Metab* 1989;69:420–425.

22. Pietschmann P, Resch H, Woloszczuk W, Willvonseder R. A circadian rhythm of serum osteocalcin levels in postmenopausal osteoporosis. *Eur J Clin Invest* 1990;20:310–312.

23. Nielsen HK, Brixen K, Mosekilde L. Diurnal rhythm in serum activity of wheatgerm lectin-precipitable alkaline phosphatase temporal relationships with the diurnal rhythm of serum osteocalcin. *Scand J Clin Lab Invest* 1990;50:851–856.

24. Rico H, Coastales C, Cabranes JA, Escudero M. Lower serum osteocalcin levels in pregnant drug users and their newborns at the time of delivery. *Obstet Gynecol* 1990;75:998–1000.

25. Rodin A, Duncan A, Quartero WP, et al. Serum concentrations of alkaline phosphatase isoenzymes and osteocalcin in normal pregnancy. *J Clin Endocrinol Metab* 1989;68:1123–1127.

26. Hill CS, Wolfert R. The preparation of monoclonal antibodies which react preferentially with human bone alkaline phosphatase. *Clin Chim Acta* 1989;186:315–320.

27. Nielsen HK, Brixen K, Bouillon R, Mosekilde L. Changes in biochemical markers of osteoblastic activity during the menstrual cycle. *J Clin Endocrinol Metab* 1990;70:1431–1437.

28. Riis BJ, Krabbe S, Christiansen C, Catherwood BD, Deftos LJ. Bone turnover in male puberty. A longitudinal study. *Calcif Tissue Int* 1985;37:213–217.

29. Delmas PD, Price PA, Mann KG. Validation of the bone Gla protein (osteocalcin) assay. *J Bone Mineral Res* 1990;5:3–4.

30. Garnero P, Grimaux M, Demiaux B, Preaudat C, Seguin P, Delmas PD. Measurement of serum osteocalcin with a human-specific two-site immunoradiometric assay. *J Bone Mineral Res* 1992;7:1389–1398.

31. Deftos LJ, Wolfert RL, Hill CS, Burton DW. Two-site assays for bone gla protein (BGP) demonstrate immunochemical heterogeneity for the intact molecule. *Clin Chem* 1992;38:2318–2321.

32. Gundberg CM, Weinstein RS. Multiple immunoreactive forms of osteocalcin in uremic serum. *J Clin Invest* 1986;77:1762–1767.

33. Taylor AK, Linkhart S, Mohan S, Christensen RA, Singer FR, Baylink DJ. Multiple osteocalcin fragments in human urine and serum as detected by a midmolecule osteocalcin radioimmunoassay. *J Clin Endocrinol Metab* 1990;70:467–472.

34. Gundberg CM, Clough ME. The osteocalcin propeptide is not secreted in vivo or in vitro. *J Bone Mineral Res* 1989;7:73–80.

35. Simon LS, Krane SM, Wortman PD, Drane IM, Kovitz KL. Serum levels of types I and III procollagen fragments in Paget's disease of bone. *J Clin Endocrinol Metab* 1984;58:110–115.

36. Simon LS, Slovik DM, Neer RM, Krane SM. Changes in serum levels of type I and III procollagen extension peptides during infusion of human parathyroid hormone fragment. *J Bone Mineral Res* 1988;3:241–246.

37. Parfitt AM, Simon LS, Villanueva AR, Krane SM. Procollagen type 1 carboxyterminal extension peptide in serum as a marker of collagen biosynthesis in bone. Correlation with iliac bone formation rates and comparison with total alkaline phosphatase. *J Bone Mineral Res* 1987;2:427–436.

38. Eberling PR, Peterson JM, Riggs BL. Utility of type I procollagen propeptide assays for assessing abnormalities in metabolic bone diseases. *J Bone Mineral Res* 1992;7:1243–1250.

39. Hale JE, Fraser JD, Price PA. Identification of matrix gla protein in cartilage. *J Biol Chem* 1988;253:5820–5824.

40. Eyre D. Editorial: new biomarkers of bone resorption. *J Clin Endocrinol Metab* 1992;74:470A–475A.

41. Hanson DA, Weis MAE, Bollen A-M, Maslan SL, Singer FR, Eyre DR. A specific immunoassay for monitoring human bone resorption: quantitation of type I collagen cross-linked n-telopeptides in urine. *J Bone Mineral Res* 1992;7:1251–1258.

42. Bettica P, Moro L, Robins SP, et al. Bone-resorption markers galactosyl hydroxylysine, pyridinium crosslinks, and hydroxyproline compared. *Clin Chem* 1992;38:2313–2318.

43. Seibel MJ, Robins SP, Bilezikian JP. Urinary pyridinium crosslinks of collagen: specific markers of bone resorption in metabolic bone disease. *TEM* 1992;3:263–267.

44. Beardsworth LJ, Eyre DR, Dickson IR. Changes with age in the urinary excretion of lysyl- and hydroxylysylpyridinoline, two new markers of bone collagen turnover. *J Bone Mineral Res* 1990;5:671–676.

45. Seibel MJ, Gartenberg F, Silverberg SJ, Ratcliffe A, Robins SP, Bilezikian JP. Urinary hydroxypyridinium cross-links of collagen in primary hyperparathyroidism. *J Clin Endocrinol Metab* 1992;74:481–486.

46. Lam KL, Dannaher C, Letchford S, Eastlund T. Tartrate-resistant acid phosphatase in serum of cancer patients. *Clin Chem* 1984;30:457.

47. Allen SH, Nuttleman PR, Ketcham CM, Roberts RM. Purification and characterization of human bone tartrate-resistant acid phosphatase. *J Bone Mineral Res* 1989;4:47–55.

48. Stephan JJ, Lau KHW, Mohan S, Singer FR, Baylink DJ. Purification and N-terminal amino acid sequence of the tartrate-resistant acid phosphatase form human osteoclastoma—evidence for a single structure. *Biochem Biophys Res Commun* 1990;168:792–800.

49. Lau KHW, Stephan JJ, Yoo A, Mohan S, Baylink DJ. Evidence that tartrate-resistant acid phosphatases from osteoclastomas and hairy cell leukemia spleen are members of a multigene family. *Int J Biochem* 1991;23:1237–1244.

50. Ek-Rylander B, Bill P, Norgard M, Nilsson S, Andersson A. Cloning, sequence, and development expression of a type 5, tartrate-resistant, acid phosphatase of rat bone. *J Biol Chem* 1991;266:24684–24689.

51. Kraenzlin ME, Lau KHW, Liang L, et al. Development of an immunoassay for human serum osteoclastic tartrate-resistant acid phosphatase. *J Clin Endocrinol Metab* 1990;71:442.

52. Van Der Rest M. Collagens of bone. In: Hall BK, ed. *Bone vol 3: bone matrix and bone specific products.* Boca Raton, FL: CRC Press, 1991;192.

The Parathyroids, edited by J.P. Bilezikian,
M.A. Levine, and R. Marcus. Raven Press, Ltd.,
New York © 1994.

CHAPTER **29**

Histomorphometric Analysis of Bone in Primary Hyperparathyroidism

May Parisien, David W. Dempster, *Elizabeth Shane, and John P. Bilezikian

Primary hyperparathyroidism is recognized now as a relatively common disorder that is often asymptomatic (1–6). Reports of the devastating effects of excess parathyroid hormone (PTH) secretion on the skeleton are considered to be part of the history of the disease (7–12). Severe bone involvement is now distinctly uncommon. However, in spite of this now well-established clinical trend, the question of bone involvement and fracture risk in modern primary hyperparathyroidism is still an important issue (13–18). The use of bone densitometry has helped to focus attention on the extent and sites of bone loss in mild, asymptomatic primary hyperparathyroidism, especially with regard to involvement of the two major skeletal compartments, cortical and cancellous bone (6,19–24). Application of the technique of bone histomorphometry has also provided new information on the effects of mild primary hyperparathyroidism on the skeleton. This chapter reviews the histomorphometric characteristics of bone involvement in primary hyperparathyroidism and considers them in light of current concepts of normal and abnormal bone remodeling.

BONE HISTOMORPHOMETRY: STATIC AND DYNAMIC INDICES

Microscopic examination of bone biopsied from the iliac crest after in vivo tetracycline labeling permits separate assessments of cortical and cancellous bone, a clear advantage over noninvasive methods of bone mass measurement, which can provide only indirect information in this regard. Bone histomorphometry allows accurate evaluation not only of bone mass and turnover but also of bone microarchitecture. Although primarily a research tool, this sensitive technique has clinical applications in selected disorders, such as primary hyperparathyroidism, where it allows the detection of abnormalities of bone turnover, even in asymptomatic subjects showing no radiologic evidence of bone disease (6). In spite of limitations inherent in the small size of the bone biopsy sample and regional variations between skeletal sites, the iliac crest site is generally considered to be representative of both the structure and the metabolic processes that affect the entire skeleton (25–27).

A number of indices are utilized in bone histomorphometry to measure bone mass, architecture, and turnover (Table 1). Cancellous bone volume measures the amount of trabecular bone relative to the total amount of tissue in the cancellous space (bone and bone marrow). Cortical width measures the thickness of the cortical envelope. Evaluation of bone turnover in the cancellous compartment relies on a number of other variables (Table 1): (a) osteoid surface is the fraction of trabecular surfaces covered by unmineralized bone matrix (osteoid); (b) osteoid volume is the proportion of cancellous bone represented by osteoid; (c) eroded surface is the fraction of trabecular surfaces showing signs of osteoclastic resorption. In addition, dynamic indices are obtained when tetracycline is administered to the patient in two time-spaced doses before the biopsy is obtained. Tetracycline is avidly taken up by bone and is deposited at sites of active bone formation, where it is readily visualized via fluorescence microscopy. Dynamic indices are as fol-

E. Shane and J. P. Bilezikian: Departments of Medicine and Pharmacology, *Division of Endocrinology, College of Physicians and Surgeons, Columbia University, New York, New York 10032.

M. Parisien, D. W. Dempster: Department of Pathology, College of Physicians and Surgeons, Columbia University, New York, New York 10032; and Regional Bone Center, Helen Hayes Hospital, West Haverstraw, New York 10993.

TABLE 1. *Histomorphometric indices of bone mass, architecture and turnover*

Cancellous bone volume	Cn BV/TV	%
Cortical width	Ct.Wi	um
Trabecular number	Tb.N	/mm
Trabecular thickness	Tb.Th	um
Trabecular separation	Tb.Sp	um
Marrow space star volume	V*m.space	mm3
Total strut length*	TSL	mm/mm2
Node number*	N.Nd	/mm2
Terminus number*	N.Tm	/mm2
Node to node strut*	Nd.Nd	mm/mm2
Node to terminus strut*	Nd.Tm	mm/mm2
Node to terminus ratio*	N.Nd/ N.Tm	
Terminus to terminus strut*	Tm.Tm	mm/mm2
Osteoid surface	OS/BS	%
Osteoid volume	OV/BV	%
Eroded surface	ES/BS	%
Mineralizing surface	MS/BS	%
Bone formation rate (tissue level)	BFR/BS	um3/um2/day
Mineral apposition rate	MAR	um/day
Adjusted apposition rate	Aj.AR	um3/um2/day

*See Figure 4.

lows: (a) mineralizing surface is the extent of tetracycline-labeled surface relative to the total trabecular surface; (b) bone formation rate (tissue-based) is the volume of mineralized bone formed per unit of bone surface per day; bone formation rate is derived from the measurement of the mineralizing surface and the calculation of the rate of mineral apposition; (c) adjusted apposition rate is the volume of mineralized bone formed per unit of osteoid-covered bone surface per day. Other variables of bone structure have been applied successfully to the study of cancellous bone architecture. These variables include trabecular number, trabecular thickness, trabecular separation, and more recently, marrow star volume (25,28–32). All these indices are obtained using manual stereological methods or computer-assisted or automated image-analysis technology. The values obtained are compared to those of age- and sex-matched controls from the relevant normal population.

BONE TURNOVER IN PRIMARY HYPERPARATHYROIDISM

An increase in the rate of bone turnover is the hallmark of skeletal involvement in primary hyperparathyroidism (33). Among histomorphometric studies performed over 20 years ago, the classic studies of Meunier, Melsen, Mosekilde, and colleagues have contributed importantly to our present understanding of bone turnover in this disease (34–38). More recent studies conducted over the past decade have con-

firmed the accelerated rate of bone remodeling in primary hyperparathyroidism (39–47). In a group of subjects with mild primary hyperparathyroidism, there was a two- to threefold increase in the values of static and dynamic turnover indices (Fig. 1). Moreover, osteoid surface, osteoid volume, mineralizing surface, and tissue-based bone formation rate correlated well with levels of PTH as determined by mid-molecule radioimmunoassay. Eroded surface and mineralizing surface correlated well with serum calcium and urinary adenosine monophosphate (AMP) levels, respectively (46). These correlations are highly reflective of the response of the skeleton to PTH, in spite of only minimal clinical manifestations and the complete absence of radiological signs of bone disease (6,46). Further quantitative evidence of PTH action on bone was provided by correlations between PTH or 1,25-dihydroxyvitamin D [1,25(OH)$_2$D] and static and dynamic indices of bone turnover (41,47,48).

BONE MASS IN PRIMARY HYPERPARATHYROIDISM

Cortical Bone

Recent studies employing densitometric techniques to measure bone mass have shown a decrease in bone density at the appendicular skeleton in primary hyperparathyroidism (6,20–23). A reduction at this site, which is made up primarily of cortical bone, is in keeping with physiological actions of PTH to set preferentially on cortical bone. Further documentation of cortical bone loss was obtained by analysis of biopsy specimens of iliac crest bone in which several studies, including our own, have shown that cortices are thinner (Fig. 2) (46,49,50) or excessively porous in primary hyperparathyroidism (48). A catabolic effect of excessive PTH secretion on cortical bone was also suggested in van Doorn et al.'s 1989 study (48) by the positive correlation between circulating levels of intact PTH and cortical porosity.

Cancellous Bone

In spite of a substantial increase in bone turnover, cancellous bone volume is maintained in primary hyperparathyroidism (23,38–42,44,46–48,50,51). Of great interest is the finding that cancellous bone volume is actually higher than normal in primary hyperparathyroidism (42,46,48,52). The mean volume of cancellous bone of subjects with primary hyperparathyroidism exceeded control values by more than 2 SD in 32% of the patients in Delling's (42) study and in 26% in our study (46) (Fig. 2). An increase in cancellous bone volume was reflected in greater compressive strength, tra-

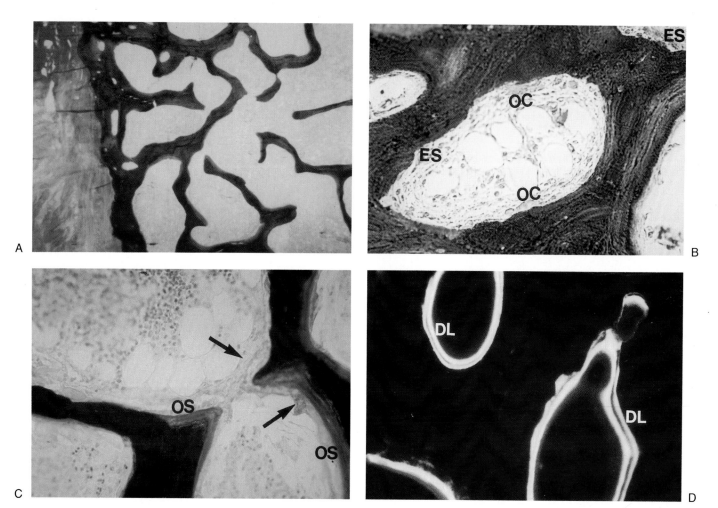

FIG. 1. Low-power photomicrograph illustrating the extended osteoid surface (stained red) on mineralized trabecular surfaces (stained green). **(A)** Original magnification ×6. Extended eroded surface (ES) appearing as irregular scalloped surface covered by osteoclasts (OC) **(B).** Original magnification ×25. Extended osteoid surface (OS) seen at higher magnification peritrabecular fibrosis (*arrows*) **(C).** Original magnification ×25. Goldner's trichrome. Extended double tetracycline labels (DL) seen by fluorescence microscopy covering trabecular surfaces **(D).** Unstained section. Original magnification ×25.

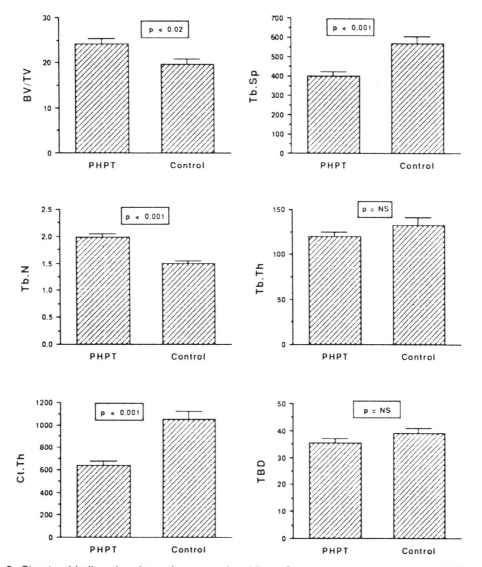

FIG. 2. Structural indices in primary hyperparathyroidism. Comparison between patients (PHPT) and controls. Values are expressed as mean ± SEM. (Reprinted from ref. 46 with permission.)

becular ash weight, and maximum stress in iliac biopsy cores of patients with primary hyperparathyroidism (53). These observations support the view that elevated levels of endogenous PTH, in modest amounts, as occurs in mild primary hyperparathyroidism, exert a dual action on bone, with a preferential loss of cortical bone and conservation of cancellous bone (46). Clinical data from our work reinforce this concept, as shown by the general maintenance of bone mineral density in the spine, which is well endowed with cancellous bone, as compared to a substantial decline of bone mineral density at the distal radius, a site rich in cortical bone (6) (see chapter by Bilezikian et al.). A critical clinical correlate of these observations relates to the incidence of fracture of cancellous bone in primary hyperparathyroidism. Unfortunately, this area lacks adequate data. The few published studies, how-

ever, show no increase in the rate of fracture after diagnosis and conservative treatment of primary hyperparathyroidism (16,17).

BONE STRUCTURE IN PRIMARY HYPERPARATHYROIDISM

Conventional Indices of Bone Structure

With the recognition that bone structure, in addition to bone mass, is an important determinant of bone strength, quantitative analysis of bone microarchitecture in the iliac biopsy specimen has begun to make significant contributions to our understanding of metabolic bone disease. Through primary measurements of cancellous bone area and bone perimeter, the major

TABLE 2. *Parameters characterizing the iliac trabecular bone structure in primary hyperparathyroidism compared with normal controls matched for age and sex.*

	PHP patients			Normal controls		
	All	Males	Females	All	Males	Females
Trabecular bone volume (BV/TV, %)	20.6 ± 7.1	21.3 ± 4.2 (20)	20.3 ± 8.0 (47)	21.5 ± 8.7	21.8 ± 7.2 (10)	21.3 ± 9.3 (20)
Trabecular thickness (T.Th, μm)*	124 ± 33	117 ± 21 (21)l	127 ± 48 (45)	139 ± 32[a]	135 ± 33 (10)	141 ± 32 (20)
Mean trabecular plate density (MTPD, μm⁻¹)*	1.33 ± 0.36	1.44 ± 0.29 (20)	1.28 ± 0.38 (44)	1.22 ± 0.42	1.26 ± 0.26 (10)	1.20 ± 0.49 (20)
Intertrabecular distance (IT.D, μm)*	648 ± 154	628 ± 140 (20)	659 ± 160 (40)	632 ± 156	650 ± 126 (10)	623 ± 172 (19)
Marrow space star volume (V*$_{m,space}$·mm³)*	14.4 ± 14.0	7.2 ± 5.0 (11)	17.6 ± 15.6 (24)	15.9 ± 14.5	13.8 ± 12.2 (8)	18.2 ± 17.5 (7)

MTPD equals the trabecular number and ITD equals the trabecular separation. Reprinted from ref. 47, with permission.

determinant of the increase in bone volume in our study of patients with primary hyperparathyroidism showed a greater number of trabeculae with a reciprocal decrease in trabecular separation. In addition, trabecular plates were somewhat thinner than in normal subjects (46,52) (Fig. 2). When these indices were evaluated as a function of age, distinctly different patterns between hyperparathyroid and control subjects were seen. Cancellous bone volume declined in both groups. However, trabecular number did not decline with age in hyperparathyroid subjects, in contrast to normal individuals. Moreover trabecular separation increased as a function of age in the normal subjects but not in the patients with primary hyperparathyroidism. Finally, trabecular thickness did not change in the control group but showed an age-related decline in the hyperparathyroid subjects. These observations clearly

suggest that modestly elevated levels of PTH can retard the normal processes of aging on the microarchitecture of bone.

The profile of structural changes that we observed with age in normal subjects conforms to that previously described by Wakamatsu and Sissons (28) and later by Parfitt et al. (29). This profile is the basis for the proposed mechanism of bone loss with aging in normal subjects, particularly in women. According to this mechanism, bone is lost by way of increased spacing between the trabeculae, without significant reduction in plate thickness (28). Parfitt et al. (29) later (1983) refined this concept and postulated that, with age, cancellous bone is lost by the removal of entire trabecular units through enhanced resorption, resulting in increased intertrabecular separation without significant reduction in plate thickness.

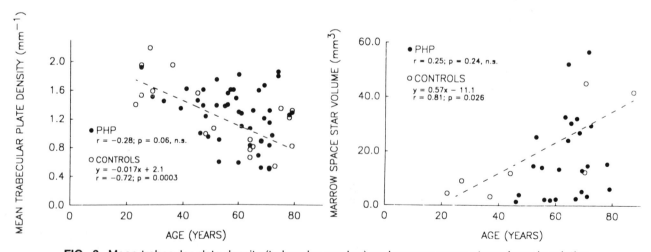

FIG. 3. Mean trabecular plate density (trabecular number) and marrow space star volume in relation to age in women with primary hyperparathyroidism and normal subjects. A decrease in trabecular number and increase in marrow space star volume with age are observed in the control groups (*dashed lines*) but not in the patients. (Modified from ref. 47 with permission.)

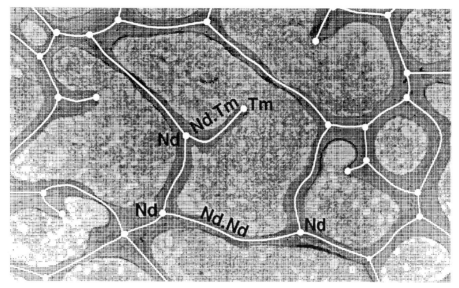

FIG. 4. Nodes, termini, and trabecular struts are superimposed on the photomicrograph of the iliac crest biopsy of a subject with primary hyperparathyroidism. Abbreviations: Nd, node; Tm, terminus; Nd.Nd, node to node strut; and Nd.Tm, node to terminus strut. (Reprinted from ref. 51 with permission.)

The age-related pattern of bone loss in hyperparathyroid subjects differs dramatically from that which occurs in normal subjects (30,46). In primary hyperparathyroidism, cancellous bone structure appears to be preserved through the maintenance of trabecular plates, which remain connected despite age-related thinning (46). This concept is supported by recent findings of Christiansen et al. (47). This pattern of bone loss is more consistent with the normal aging pattern observed in men as opposed to women (28,29,54–57). However, although two independent groups have now reported trabecular thinning in this disease, it should be noted that Delling (42) found that trabecular thickness was increased.

In the recent study of Christiansen et al. (47) involving 69 patients with primary hyperparathyroidism, normal cancellous bone volume was observed with no disturbance of the normal cancellous network. Normal bone structure was clearly maintained in spite of apparently more severe disease in this population, as judged by higher values of serum calcium and the greater percentage of complications than reported in other studies of mild primary hyperparathyroidism (16,46). Quantitative analysis of bone structure indicated normal trabecular microarchitecture, with no decrease in cancellous bone volume or trabecular number, as shown in Table 2. The only abnormality was the presence of significantly thinner plates than normal, with no change in intertrabecular separation (47). Furthermore, there was an age-related decline of can-

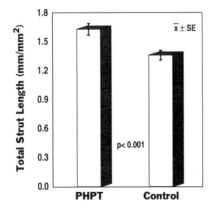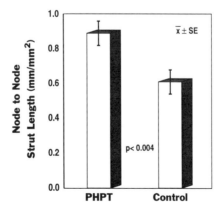

FIG. 5. Bar graphs representing the values of total strut length **(left),** an index of the amount of cancellous bone, and node to node strut length **(right),** an index of trabecular connectivity in patients with primary hyperparathyroidism and control subjects. (Reprinted from ref. 51 with permission.)

TABLE 3. *Correlations between age and variables expressing connectivity in PHPT and controls*[a]

Age	TSL (mm/mm²)	N.Nd (/mm²)	N.Tm (/mm²)	N.Nd/N.Tm	Nd.Nd (mm/mm²)	Nd.Tm (mm/mm²)	Tm.Tm (mm/mm²)
PHPT							
r	−0.38	−0.28	0.014	−0.08	−0.35	−0.0009	0.114
P	0.020	NS	NS	NS	0.032	NS	NS
Control							
r	−0.44	−0.42	0.117	−0.46	−0.43	−0.077	0.205
P	0.030	0.043	NS	0.033	0.033	NS	NS

[a] N.Nd, node number; N.Tm, terminus number; TSL, total strut length; N.Nd/N.Tm, node to terminus ratio; Nd.Nd, node to node strut length; Nd.Tm, node to terminus strut length; Tm.Tm, terminus to terminus strut length. Values are mean ± SD. (Reprinted from ref. 51 with permission.)

cellous bone volume in both patients and controls, with preservation of the normal architecture in hyperparathyroid subjects but a contrasting loss of structure with age in the controls (47) (Fig. 3), confirming previous findings (28–30,46).

Indices of Connectivity: Trabecular Strut Analysis

Examination of iliac crest bone biopsies from patients with primary hyperparathyroidism suggests that the plates are remarkably well connected. The technique of two-dimensional trabecular strut analysis has permitted quantitative assessment of this observation. Two-dimensional strut analysis permits quantification of the number of connecting points or nodes between trabecular segments, the free ends of unconnected trabeculae or termini, the relative lengths of trabecular struts showing various degrees of connectivity, and the total length of all the trabecular struts (58,59) (Fig. 4).

With this method it can be appreciated that indices of connectivity are greater in patients with primary hyperparathyroidism. Total strut length, node number, and node-to-node strut lengths are all greater in the hyperparathyroid subjects (Fig. 5). These findings are consistent with higher cancellous bone volume and greater degree of trabecular connectivity in primary hyperparathyroidism patients than in normal individuals. Moreover, total strut length, an index of the amount of cancellous bone, declined with age, confirming the age-related loss of cancellous bone volume in both hyperparathyroidism and control subjects. However, while a loss of trabecular connectivity was shown in the controls, no such decline was observed in the hyperparathyroid group (51) (Table 3).

MECHANISM OF MAINTENANCE OF BONE VOLUME AND STRUCTURE

It now seems well-established that in primary hyperparathyroidism, cancellous bone volume is normal or increased despite higher bone turnover. Mechanisms

for the maintenance of normal bone balance bone type are the subjects of speculation. Delling (42) has suggested that intact coupling between erosion and formation together with increases in the activity and life-span of osteoblasts maintain intact bone structure. Baron and Magee (43) suggest a coupled and balanced increase in bone turnover. Eriksen (45) proposes, through reconstruction of the remodeling sequence in primary hyperparathyroidism, that the activation frequency of remodeling cycles is increased with decreased final erosion depth and wall thickness of completed structural units, resulting in normal or increased bone balance. Formation period is not significantly different from normal. According to this model, a smaller amount of bone is exchanged during the remodeling sequence, which is compensated for at the tissue level by increased bone turnover (Fig. 6). The trend toward a reduction in cancellous bone volume (reversible bone loss) is attributed to the expansion of the remodeling space (45). This mechanism contrasts with that observed in hyperthyroidism, in which normal erosion depth and decreased estimated completed wall thickness result in a net negative balance between erosion and formation at each remodeling cycle. This process is compounded in hyperparathyroidism by the reduction in bone formation period and the increased activation frequency resulting in increased trabecular perforation and irreversible bone loss (44,45).

Christiansen et al.'s (47) recent study of primary hyperparathyroidism shows increased activation frequency with a corresponding decrease in the extent of the quiescent surface, which further documented expansion of the remodeling space. In this study, however, there was no difference in the final depth of erosion or in the final amount of bone deposited at the bone remodeling unit (wall thickness) between patients and controls and, hence, no change in bone balance or in cancellous bone volume (47). These observations support the concept of "reversible bone loss" in primary hyperparathyroidism. In a previous study, the increase in cancellous bone volume following successful parathyroidectomy in a small subset of patients

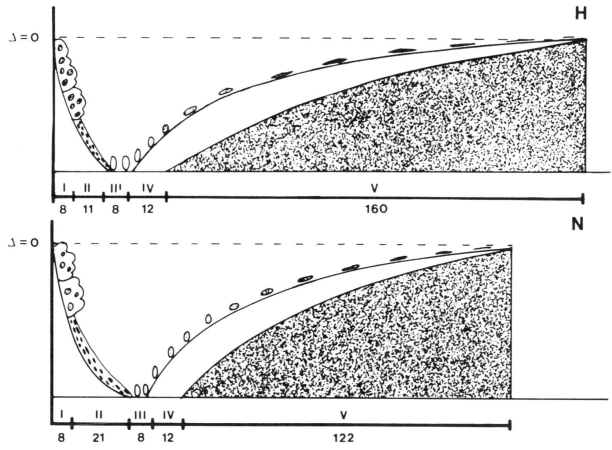

FIG. 6. Complete remodeling sequences in primary hyperparathyroidism (*H*) and age- and sex-matched normal controls (*N*). (From ref. 44 with permission.)

was attributed to normalization of bone turnover and consequent reduction of an expanded remodeling space (60). Similarly, in a recent study by Silverberg et al. (61), postmenopausal hyperparathroid women treated by parathyroidectomy and followed over a 3 year period showed an increase over baseline values in bone density at the spine and hip, an increase that could also be attributable to a postoperative decrease in the remodeling space.

What is the mechanism at the cellular level for maintenance of trabecular connectivity, and how does one reconcile the paradox that trabecular plates become thinner but remain connected with the increased turnover state of primary hyperparathyroidism? The plate thinning reported in the Christiansen et al. (47) study and the age-related attenuation of plates observed in our study (46) could well be consequences of a twofold increase in activation frequency with substantial enlargement of the remodeling space. If one considers the stochastic model of Reeve (62), the increase in birth rate of teams of osteoclasts would greatly increase the probability of erosion on opposite sides of a plate and hence of plate perforation (55,63). The likelihood of such perforation might be further increased

by the coincidental occurrence of deep erosion on thin plates (64). This might be expected from the known aggressive behavior of the osteoclast in the more severe form of primary hyperparathyroidism. However, a lesser degree of osteoclastic activity is suggested in the milder, more common form of the disease (44). Under these circumstances, the resulting reduction in the final depth of erosion might offer a mechanism whereby trabecular plates would be protected against perforation (63). This protective mechanism would be operative despite the predisposition to plate thinning caused by the greater activation frequency. A correlative mechanism of protection, inferred from the pattern of "tunneling resorption" of the more severe disease, would be that osteoclasts alter their behavior under the influence of excessive endogenous PTH secretion. They appear to change direction, eroding in a direction parallel to the long axis of the trabecular plate rather than to penetrate in perpendicular fashion across the full thickness of the plate. In doing so, the osteoclasts create long furrows in the interior of the trabecular plate (Fig. 7) (12,33,65,66). This mechanism is compatible with Eriksen's finding of decreased erosion depth (44,45). Under conditions of moderate PTH

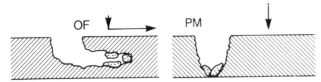

FIG. 7. Two morphologically different types of increased bone resorption in severe primary hyperparathyroidism (osteitis fibrosa; OF) and in the postmenopausal state (PM). In OF, the osteoclasts have eroded more deeply into the bone and then changed direction to undermine the surface by dissecting intratrabecular resorption. In PM, the osteoclasts have eroded a deeper than normal cavity on the way to complete perforation of the trabecular plate. The predominant direction of osteoclast movement is perpendicular to the surface. (Modified from ref. 66 with permission.)

excess, the change in osteoclast behavior would result in a more tangential pattern of "sweeping erosion," quantitatively translated by more shallow erosion lacunae, thereby allowing the plates to remain connected, though they are thinner than normal.

Paradoxically, under the influence of PTH, osteoclasts are thought to exhibit more aggressive behavior along the corticomedullary junction, where they appear to erode more deeply and extensively. This is the presumed mechanism underlying the thinning of cortices observed in primary hyperparathyroidism (46,50). These findings suggest that the effects of PTH on osteoclast recruitment and/or activity are different when cortical and cancellous envelopes are compared.

An anabolic action of PTH on bone is suggested by the histological evidence of increased bone forming surfaces and mineral apposition rate following intermittent administration of PTH to rats (67), an effect that is not altered by antiresorptive agents (68). Furthermore, while continuous exposure to PTH causes inhibition of collagen synthesis in cultured fetal rat calvariae (69,70), transient exposure to PTH stimulates collagen synthesis (71). This anabolic effect is presumably the basis for the increased bone density and calcium accretion observed after chronic administration of PTH to rats (72). In human subjects with primary hyperparathyroidism, the development of osteosclerosis in the axial skeleton and femora of adults (73–79) and in the long bone metaphyses of children (80–85) are further evidence of this anabolic response. An even more compelling argument is the greater bone density and increase in new bone accretion (by ^{47}Ca kinetic studies) as well as the histomorphometric evidence of increased cancellous bone volume following treatment of osteoporotic subjects with PTH-(1–34) (86–90) as discussed in the chapter by Marcus. More recently, convincing evidence of increased cancellous bone volume and trabecular connectivity was shown in a rat experimental model of osteoporosis after administration of PTH-(1–34) (91,92).

CLINICAL RELEVANCE OF HISTOMORPHOMETRIC FINDINGS IN PRIMARY HYPERPARATHYROIDISM

The relevance of the maintenance of cancellous bone mass as well as structural integrity in primary hyperparathyroidism with regard to sites of potential fracture deserves consideration. The suitability of the iliac crest as a representative site to study cancellous bone compared to more directly relevant sites such as the spine has been previously noted (25,31,59,93–96). The concordance between indices of bone mass and structure at these two sites in normal subjects (31,59), supported by the maintenance or even increase of trabecular connectivity (51) and greater compressive strength and ash weight at the iliac crest in primary hyperparathyroidism (53), suggests the strong possibility that cancellous architecture and strength are maintained at the spine as well. This maintenance is further supported by the positive correlations found in women with primary hyperparathyroidism between conventional indices of bone mass and structure and bone density measurements at the lumbar spine, a site of high cancellous bone composition, but not at the hip and forearm (97,98).

Postmenopausal Women With Primary Hyperparathyroidism

Data supporting the idea that cancellous bone is protected in primary hyperparathyroidism have particular relevance for postmenopausal women, who are at increased risk for cancellous bone loss due to estrogen deficiency. If mild primary hyperparathyroidism is a relative protector of the cancellous skeleton, will postmenopausal women with primary hyperparathyroidism show better indices of cancellous bone mass and architecture than normal postmenopausal women without primary hyperparathyroidism?

To study this issue, we have compared a group of postmenopausal women with primary hyperparathyroidism with a cohort of healthy postmenopausal women. When the two groups were matched by age and by number of years after the menopause, cancellous bone volume was greater in hyperparathyroid women than in women without primary hyperparathyroidism. Trabecular number did not show the age-related decline observed in the normal population (99). This finding is of great clinical significance, in that trabecular number has been found to be a better discriminator than cancellous bone volume when distinguishing between those subjects with vertebral fractures and normal subjects (54). These data are consistent with previous histomorphometric studies (100,101). In the study of Courpron et al. (100), cancellous bone volume, although slightly decreased in premenopausal women, remained normal in postmenopausal women and in men with primary hyperparathyroidism. In a corroborating study by Charhon et al. (101), wall thickness, the final amount of bone deposited at the unit of bone remodeling, was normal in postmenopausal women and in men but was slightly decreased in premenopausal women. Additional confirmation of these findings is provided by Christiansen et al.'s (47) study, in which cancellous bone volume, was slightly higher although not significantly different in women older than age 50 years are in their normal counterparts. Furthermore, wall thickness, while significantly decreased in women younger than age 50 years, remained normal in those older than age 50 years.

The demonstration of greater trabecular connectivity in a heterogeneous group of patients with primary hyperparathyroidism is strong evidence that cancellous integrity is maintained in primary hyperparathyroidism with the consequent likelihood that fracture risk is decreased (51). It would be more convincing to document these findings in a more homogeneous population of postmenopausal women with primary hyperparathyroidism. However, to this end, we have compared a subset of 16 postmenopausal women with hyperparathyroidism with osteoporotic and healthy postmenopausal women matched by the number of years since menopause. Cancellous bone volume and indices of connectivity were the lowest in the osteoporotic group and highest in the hyperparathyroid subjects. The converse was true for indices of disconnectivity. These findings indicate that in osteoporosis there is an irreversible loss of bone with deterioration of trabecular architecture due to loss of connectivity, whereas in primary hyperparathyroidism there is maintenance of the architectural integrity of cancellous bone, with normal or even greater plate connectivity (102).

If bone mass and structure are predictive of bone strength, the evidence available thus far clearly supports the concept that mild primary hyperparathyroidism exerts a protective effect on cancellous bone. Whether postmenopausal women with this disease are less susceptible to vertebral fracture and whether there is truth in the logical assumption of a greater risk of peripheral fractures await confirmation by long-term, randomized, controlled, clinical trials.

ACKNOWLEDGMENTS

Some of the work covered in this chapter was supported, in part, by NIH grants AR 41386, DK 32333, AR 39191, and RR 00645

REFERENCE

1. Heath H, Hodgson SF, Kennedy MA. Primary hyperparathyroidism incidence, morbidity, and potential economic impact in a community. *N Engl J Med* 1980;302:189–193.
2. Mundy GR, Cove DH, Fisken R. Primary hyperparathyroidism: changes in the pattern of clinical presentation. *Lancet* 1980;1:1318–1320.
3. Mallette LE, Bilezikian JP, Heath DA, Aurbach GD. Primary hyperparathyroidism: clinical and biochemical features. *Medicine* 1974;53:127–146.
4. Lafferty FW. Primary hyperparathyroidism: changing clinical spectrum, prevalence of hypertension, and discriminant analysis of laboratory tests. *Arch Intern Med* 1981;141:1761–1766.
5. Sudhaker RD. Primary hyperparathyroidism: changing patterns in presentation and treatment decisions in the eighties. *Henry Ford Hosp Med J* 1985;33:194–197.
6. Silverberg SJ, Shane E, De La Cruz L, et al. Skeletal disease in primary hyperparathyroidism. *J Bone Mineral Res* 1989; 4:283–291.
7. von Recklinghausen F. Die fibrose oder deformirende Ostitis, die Osteomalacie und die carcinose in gengensitigen. In: Beziehungen, ed. *Festschrift Rudolf Virchow*. Berlin: G. Reiner, 1891.
8. Mandl R. Therapeutisher verusch bei ostitis fibrosa generalizata mittels extirpation eines epithelkorperchen tumors. *Wien Klin Wochenschr* 1925;38:1383–1384.
9. Albright F, Aub JC, Bauer W. Hyperparathyroidism: a common and polymorphic condition as illustrated by seventeen proven cases from one clinic. *J Am Med Assoc* 1934; 102:1276–1287.
10. Albright F, Reifenstein EC. *The parathyroid glands and metabolic bone disease*. Baltimore: Williams and Wilkins, 1948.
11. Schajowicz F. *Tumors and tumor-like lesions of bones and joints*. Berlin: Springer Verlag, 1981.
12. Uehlinger E. Osteofibrosis deformans juvenilis. *Virchows Arch* 1940;306:255.
13. Dauphine RT, Riggs BL, Scholz DA. Back pain and vertebral crush fractures: an unemphasized mode of presentation for primary hyperparathyroidism. *Ann Intern Med* 1975;83: 365–367.
14. Kochersberger G, Buckley NJ, Leight GS. What is the clinical significance of bone loss in primary hyperparathyroidism? *Arch Intern Med* 1987;147:1951–1953.
15. Peacock M, Horsman A, Aaron JE, Marshall DH, Selby PL, Simpson M. The role of parathyroid hormone in bone loss. In: Christiansen C, Arnaud CD, Nordin BEC, Parfitt AM, Peck WA, Riggs BL, eds. *Osteoporosis* (Proceedings of the Copenhagen International Symposium on Osteoporosis, June 3–8, 1984). Copenhagen: Aalborg Stiftsbogtrykkeri, 1984;463–467.
16. Wilson RJ, Rao DS, Ellis B, Kleerekoper M, Parfitt AM. Mild asymptomatic primary hyperparathyroidism is not a risk factor for vertebral fractures. *Ann Intern Med* 1988; 109:959–962.
17. Melton LJ III, Atkinson EJ, O'Fallon WM, Heath H III. Risk of age-related fractures in patients with primary hyperparathyroidism. *Arch Intern Med* 1992;152:2269–2273.
18. NIH Consensus Development Conference Statement on Primary Hyperparathyroidism. *J Bone Mineral Res* 1991;6:s9–s13.
19. Seeman E, Wahner HW, Offord KP, Kumar R, Johnson WJ, Riggs BL. Differential effects of endocrine dysfunction on the axial and the appendicular skeleton. *J Clin Invest* 1982;69:1302–1309.
20. Richardson ML, Pozzi-Mucelli RS, Kanter AS, Kolb FO, Ettinger B, Genant HK. Bone mineral changes in primary hyperparathyroidism. *Skel Radiol* 1986;15:85–95.
21. Martin P, Bergmann P, Gillet C. Partially reversible osteopenia after surgery for primary hyperparathyroidism. *Arch Intern Med* 1986;146:689–691.
22. Rao DS, Wilson RJ, Kleerekoper M, Parfitt AM. Lack of biochemical progression or continuation of accelerated bone

loss in mild asymptomatic primary hyperparathyroidism: evidence for biphasic disease course. *J Clin Endocrinol Metab* 1988;67:1294–1298.

23. Kleerekoper M, Villaneuva AR, Mathews CHE, Rao DS, Pumo B, Parfitt AM. PTH mediated bone loss in primary and secondary hyperparathyroidism. In: Frame B, Potts JT, eds. *Clinical disorders of bone and mineral metabolism.* Amsterdam: Excerpta Medica, 1983;200–203.

24. Hesp R, Tellez M, Davidson L. Trabecular and cortical bone in the radii of women with parathyroid adenoma. *Bone Mineral* 1987;2:301–310.

25. Dempster DW. Relationship between the iliac crest bone biopsy and other skeletal sites. In: Kleerekoper M, Krane SM, eds. *Clinical disorders of bone and mineral metabolism.* New York: Mary Ann Liebert, 1989;247–252.

26. Parfitt AM. The physiologic and clinical significance of bone histomorphometric data. In: Recker RR, ed. *Bone histomorphometry: techniques and interpretation.* Boca Raton, FL: CRC Press, 1983;143–223.

27. Cosman F, Schnitzer MB, McCann PD, Parisien MV, Dempster DW, Lindsay R. Relationships between quantitative histologic measurements and noninvasive assessments of bone mass. *Bone* 1992;13:237–242.

28. Wakamatsu E, Sissons HA. The cancellous bone of the iliac crest. *Calcif Tissue Res* 1969;4:147–161.

29. Parfitt AM, Mathews HE, Villaneuva AR, Kleerekoper M, Frame B. Relationships between surface, volume, and thickness of iliac trabecular bone in aging and in osteoporosis. Implications for the microanatomic and cellular mechanisms of bone loss. *J Clin Invest* 1983;72:1396–1409.

30. Parisien MV, McMahon D, Pushparaj N, Dempster DW. Trabecular architecture in iliac crest bone biopsies: intra-individual variability in structural parameters and changes with age. *Bone* 1988;9:289–295.

31. Dempster DW, Ferguson-Pell M, Mellish RWE, et al. Relationship between bone structure in the iliac crest and bone structure and strength in the lumbar spine. *Osteoporosis Int* 1993;3:90–96.

32. Vesterby A. Star volume of marrow space and trabeculae in iliac crest. Sampling procedure and correlation to star volume of first lumbar vertebra. *Bone* 1991;12:33–38.

33. Parisien M, Silverberg SJ, Shane E, Dempster DW, Bilezikian JP. Bone disease in primary hyperparathyroidism. *Endocrinol Metab Clin* 1990;19:19–34.

34. Riggs BL, Kelly PJ, Jowsey J, Keating FR. Skeletal alterations in hyperparathyroidism: determination of bone formation, resorption and morphologic changes by microradiography. *J Clin Endocrinol Metab* 1965;25:777–783.

35. Byers PD, Smith R. Quantitative histology of bone in hyperparathyroidism: its relation to clinical features, x-ray, and biochemistry. *Q J Med* 1971;160:471–486.

36. Wilde CD, Jaworski ZF, Villaneuva AR, Frost HM. Quantitative histological measurements of bone turnover in primary hyperparathyroidism. *Calcium Tissue Res* 1973;12:137–142.

37. Meunier PJ, Vignon G, Bernard J. Clinical aspects of metabolic bone disease. In: Frame B, Parfitt AM, Duncan H, eds. *Quantitative bone histology as applied to the diagnosis of hyperparathyroid states.* Amsterdam: Excerpta Medica, 1973;215–221.

38. Mosekilde L, Melsen F. A tetracycline-based histomorphometric evaluation of bone resorption and bone turnover in hyperthyroidism and hyperparathyroidism. *Acta Med Scand* 1978;204:97–102.

39. Melsen F, Mosekilde L. The role of bone biopsy in the diagnosis of metabolic bone disease. *Orthop Clin North Am* 1981;12:571–601.

40. Delmas PD, Meunier PJ, Faysse E, Saubier EC. Bone histomorphometry and serum bone gla-protein in the diagnosis of primary hyperparathyroidism. *World J Surg* 1986;10:572–578.

41. de Vernejoul MC, Benamount MP, Cancela L. Hyperparathyroidie primitive vue en rhumatologie: Signes cliniques et relations entre les signes histologiques osseux et les parametres biologiques. *Rev Rhum* 1988;55:489–494.

42. Delling G. Bone morphology in primary hyperparathyroidism. A qualitative and quantitative study of 391 cases. *Appl Pathol* 1987;55:147–159.

43. Baron R, Magee SS. Estimation of trabecular bone resorption by histomorphometry: evidence for a prolonged reversal phase with normal resorption in post menopausal osteoporosis and coupled increased resorption in primary hyperparathyroidism. In: Frame B, Potts JT, eds. *Clinical disorders of bone and mineral metabolism.* Amsterdam: Excerpta Medica, 1983;191–195.

44. Eriksen EF, Mosekilde L, Melsen F. Trabecular bone remodeling and balance in primary hyperparathyroidism. *Bone* 1986;7:213–221.

45. Eriksen EF. Normal and pathological remodeling of human trabecular bone: Three dimensional reconstruction of the remodeling sequence in normals and in metabolic bone disease. *Endocrine Rev* 1986;7:379–408.

46. Parisien M, Silverberg SJ, Shane E, et al. The histomorphometry of bone in primary hyperparathyroidism: Preservation of cancellous bone structure. *J Clin Endocrinol Metab* 1990;70:930–938.

47. Christiansen P, Steiniche T, Vesterby A, Mosekilde L, Hessov I, Melsen F. Primary hyperparathyroidism: iliac crest trabecular bone volume, structure, remodeling, and balance evaluated by histomorphometric methods. *Bone* 1992;13:41–49.

48. van Doorn L, Lips P, Netelenbos JC, Hackengt WHL. Bone histomorphometry and serum intact PTH(1–84) in hyperparathyroid patients. *Calcif Tissue Int* 1989;44S:N36.

49. Parfitt AM. Accelerated cortical bone loss: primary and secondary hyperparathyroidism. In: Uhthoff H, Stahl E, eds. *Current concepts of bone fragility.* Berlin: Springer-Verlag, 1986;279–285.

50. Parfitt AM. Surface specific bone remodeling in health and disease. In: Kleerekoper M, ed. *Clinical disorders of bone and mineral metabolism.* New York: Mary Ann Liebert, 1989;7–14.

51. Parisien M, Mellish RWE, Silverberg SJ, et al. Maintenance of cancellous bone connectivity in primary hyperparathyroidism: trabecular strut analysis. *J Bone Mineral Res* 1992;7:913–919.

52. Parisien M, Dempster DW, Shane E, Silverberg S, Lindsay R, Bilezikian JP. Structural parameters of bone biopsies in primary hyperparathyroidism. In: Takahashi HE, ed. *Bone morphometry* (Proceedings of the Fifth International Congress on Bone Morphometry, Niigata, Japan). New York: Smith-Gordon, 1988;228–231.

53. Mosekilde Le, Mosekilde L. Iliac crest trabecular bone compressive strength and ash weight is increased in moderate primary hyperparathyroidism. In: Takahashi HE, ed. *Bone morphometry* (Proceedings of the Fifth International Congress on Bone Morphometry, Niigata, Japan). New York: Smith-Gordon, 1988;483.

54. Kleerekoper M, Villaneuva AR, Stanciu J, Rao DS, Parfitt AM. The role of three-dimensional trabecular microstructure in the pathogenesis of vertebral compression fractures. *Calcif Tissue Int* 1985;37:594–597.

55. Parfitt AM. Trabecular bone architecture in the pathogenesis and prevention of fracture. *Am J Med* 1987;82:68–72.

56. Aaron JE, Makins NB, Sagreiya K. The microanatomy of trabecular bone loss in normal aging men and women. *Clin Orthop Rel Res* 1987;215:260–267.

57. Mellish RWE, Garrahan NJ, Compston JE. Age-related changes in trabecular width and spacing in human iliac crest biopsies. *Bone Mineral* 1989;6:331–338.

58. Garrahan N, Mellish R, Compston J. A new method for the two-dimensional analysis of bone structure in human iliac crest biopsies. *J Microsc* 1986;142:341–349.

59. Mellish RWE, Ferguson-Pell MW, Cochran GVB, Lindsay R, Dempster DW. A new method for the two-dimensional analysis of bone structure in human iliac crest biopsies. *J Bone Mineral Res* 1991;6:689–696.

60. Christiansen R, Steiniche T, Mosekilde Le, Hessov I, Melsen F. Primary hyperparathyroidism: changes in trabecular bone remodeling following surgical treatment evaluated by histomorphometric methods. *Bone* 1990;11:75–79.

61. Silverberg SJ, Gartenberg F, Bilezikian JP. Primary hyper-

parathyroidism protects cancellous bone density in post-menopausal women. *J Bone Mineral Res* 1992;7(Suppl 1):s296 (Abstract 813).

62. Reeve J. A stochastic analysis of iliac trabecular bone dynamics. *Clin Orthop* 1986;213:264–278.

63. Parfitt AM. Implications of architecture for the pathogenesis and prevention of vertebral fracture. *Bone* 1992;13:S41–S47.

64. Compston JE, Mellish RWE, Croucher P, Newcombe R, Garrahan NJ. Structural mechanisms of trabecular bone loss in man. *Bone Mineral* 1989;6:339–350.

65. Parfitt AM. Oliver I, Villanueva ADR. Bone histology in metabolic bone disease. *Orthop Clin North Am* 1979;10:329–345.

66. Parfitt AM. Relationship to the amount and structure of bone, and the pathogenesis and prevention of fractures. In: Riggs BL, Melton LJ III, eds. *Osteoporosis, etiology, diagnosis, and management.* New York: Raven Press, 1988; 45–93.

67. Tam CS, Heersche JNM, Murray TM, Parsons JA. Parathyroid hormone stimulates the bone apposition rate independently of its resorptive action: differential effects of intermittent and continuous administration. *Endocrinology* 1982; 110:506.

68. Hock JM, Hummert JR, Boyce R, Fonseca J, Raisz LG. Resorption is not essential for the stimulation of bone growth by hPTH-(1–34) in rats in vivo. *J Bone Mineral Res* 1989;4:449.

69. Kream BE, Rowe RW, Gworek SC, Raisz LG. Parathyroid hormone alters collagen synthesis and procollagen mRNA levels in fetal rat calvariae. *Proc Natl Acad Sci USA* 1980;77:5654.

70. Vargas SJ, Raisz LG. Simultaneous assessment of bone resorption and formation in cultures of 22-day fetal rat parietal bones: Effects of parathyroid hormone and prostaglandin E2. *Bone* 1990;11:61.

71. Canalis E, Centrella M, Burch W, McCarthy TL. Insulin-like growth factor I mediates selective anabolic effects of parathyroid hormone in bone cultures. *J Clin Invest* 1989; 83:60.

72. Kalu DN, Pennock J, Doyle FH, Foster GV. Parathyroid hormone and experimental osteosclerosis. *Lancet* 1970;27: 1363.

73. Doyle FH. Some quantitative radiological observations in primary and secondary hyperparathyroidism. *Br J Radiol* 1966;39:161–167.

74. Ellis K, Hostim RJ. The skull in hyperparathyroid bone disease. *Am J Roentgenol* 1960;83:732.

75. Jaffe HL. Hyperparathyroidism (Recklinghausen's disease of bone). *Arch Pathol* 1933;16:63.

76. Aitken RE, Kerr JL, Lloyd HM. Primary hyperparathyroidism with osteosclerosis and calcification in articular cartilage. *Am J Med* 1964;37:813–820.

77. Eugenidis N, Olah AJ, Haas HG. Osteosclerosis in hyperparathyroidism. *Radiology* 1972;105:265.

78. Genant HK, Baron JM, Straus FH, Paloyan E, Jowsey J. Osteosclerosis in primary hyperparathyroidism. *Am J Med* 1975;59:104.

79. van Holsbeeck M, Roex L, Favril A, Burssens D, Baert AL. Osteosclerosis in primary hyperparathyroidism. *Fortschr Rontgenstr* 1987;147:690–691.

80. Dresser R. Osteitis fibrosa cystica associated with parathyroid over activity. *Am J Roentgenol Radium Ther Nucl Med* 1933;30:596.

81. Albright F, Baird PC, Cope D, Bloomberg E. Studies on the physiology of the parathyroid glands IV. Renal complication of hyperparathyroidism. *Am J Med Sci* 1934;187:49.

82. Aub JC. Lack of effect of parathyroid gland on growth of bone. Case presentation. In: *Association Proceedings 26th Annual Meeting Atlantic City June 8–9, 1942.* Endocrinology, 1942;(Suppl):1024.

83. Shallow TA, Fry KE. Parathyroid adenoma. Occurrence in father and daughter. *Surgery* 1948;24:1020–1025.

84. Adam A, Ritchie D. Hyperparathyroidism with increased bone density in the areas of growth. *J Bone Joint Surg* 1954;37B:257.

85. Lloyd HM, Aitken RE, Ferrier TM. Primary hyperparathyroidism resembling rickets of late onset. *Br Med J* 1965; 2:853.

86. Reeve J, Meunier PJ, Parsons JA, et al. Anabolic effect of human PTH on trabecular bone in involutional osteoporosis: a multicenter trial. *Br Med J* 1980;280:1340.

87. Reeve J, Arlot M, Bernat M, et al. Calcium-47 kinetic measurements of bone turnover compared to bone histomorphometry in osteoporosis: the influence of human parathyroid fragment (hPTH 1–34) therapy. *Metab Bone Dis Rel Res* 1981;3:23–30.

88. Reeve J, Arlot M, Bernat M, et al. Treatment of osteoporosis with human parathyroid hormone fragment 1–34: a positive final tissue balance in trabecular bone. *Metab Bone Dis Rel Res* 1980;(Suppl 2):355.

89. Slovik DM, Rosenthal DI, Doppelt SH, et al. Restoration of spinal bone in osteoporotic men by treatment with human parathyroid hormone (1–34) and 1,25-dihydroxyvitamin D. *J Bone Min Res* 1986;1:377.

90. Neer RM, Slovik D, Doppelt S, et al. The use of parathyroid hormone plus 1,25-dihydroxyvitamin D to increase trabecular bone in osteoporotic men and postmenopausal women. In: Christiansen C, Johansen JS, Riis BJ, eds. *Osteoporosis.* Copenhagen: Osteopress, 1987;829–835.

91. Shen V, Dempster DW, Mellish RWE, Birchman R, Horbert W, Lindsay R. Effects of combined and separate intermittent administration of low-dose human parathyroid hormone fragment (1–34) and 17B-estradiol on bone histomorphometry in ovariectomized rats with established osteopenia. *Calcif Tissue Int* 1992;50:214–220.

92. Shen V, Dempster DW, Birchman R, Xu R, Lindsay R. Loss of cancellous bone mass and connectivity in ovariectomized rats can be restored by combined treatment with parathyroid hormone and estradiol. *J Clin Invest* 1993;91:2479–2480.

93. Meunier PJ, Courpron P. Iliac trabecular bone volume in 236 controls: representativeness of iliac samples. In: Jaworski ZFG, ed. *Proceedings of the first workshop on bone morphometry.* Ottawa: University of Ottawa Press, 1976;100–105.

94. Podenphant J, Gotfredsen A, Nilas L, Norgaard H, Braendstrup O. Iliac crest biopsy: Representativity for the amount of mineralized bone. *Bone* 1986;7:427–430.

95. Mosekilde L, Viidik A, Mosekilde L. Correlation between the compressive strength of iliac and vertebral trabecular bone in normal individuals. *Bone* 1985;6:291–295.

96. Mosekilde L, Mosekilde L. Normal vertebral body size and compressive strength: Relations to age and to vertebral and iliac trabecular bone compressive strength. *Bone* 1986;7: 207–212.

97. Parisien M, Dempster DW, Silverberg SJ, et al. Relationship between bone mass as assessed by densitometry and by histomorphometry in primary hyperparathyroidism. *J Bone Mineral Res* 1990;5:137.

98. Parisien M, Cosman F, Silverberg SJ, et al. Relationship between bone mass by densitometry and by histomorphometry in primary hyperparathyroidism and in osteoporosis. *Bone Mineral* 1992;17(Suppl 1):214.

99. Parisien M, Recker R, Silverberg SJ, et al. Cancellous bone structure in postmenopausal women with primary hyperparathyroidism. In: Christiansen C, Overgaard K, eds. *Third International Symposium on Osteoporosis, October 14–20, 1990.* Copenhagen: Osteopress, 1990;1139–1140.

100. Courpron P, Meunier P, Bressot C, Giroux JM. Amount of bone in iliac crest biopsy: significance of the trabecular bone volume. Its values in normal and in pathological conditions. In: Meunier PJ, ed. *Proceedings.* Lyon: Second International Bone Histomorphometry Workshop, 1976;39–53.

101. Charhon SA, Edouard CM, Arlot ME, Meunier PJ. Effects of parathyroid hormone on remodeling of iliac trabecular bone packets in patients with primary hyperparathyroidism. *Clin Orthop Rel Res* 1982;162:255–263.

102. Parisien M, Mellish RW, Schnitzer M. Cancellous bone structure in postmenopausal women: comparison among osteoporosis of primary hyperparathyroidism and normals. *J Bone Mineral Res* 1992;7:S114.

The Parathyroids, edited by J.P. Bilezikian,
M. Levine, and R. Marcus. Raven Press, Ltd.,
New York © 1994.

CHAPTER 30

Nephrolithiasis in Primary Hyperparathyroidism

Vanessa A. Klugman, Murray J. Favus, and Charles Y. C. Pak

The initial patient with primary hyperparathyroidism who underwent successful parathyroidectomy by Mandl (1) may have had kidney stone as well as severe bone disease. While earlier patients were described who had bone disease and nephrocalcinosis (2), it was not until 1930 that Barr and Bugler (3) called attention to the association between renal calculus and primary hyperparathyroidism. Severe primary hyperparathyroidism without clinical or radiographic evidence of bone disease was first described in 1937 by Albright, Sulkowitch, and Bloomberg (4). The primary clinical manifestation of these patients was kidney stone, either with or without nephrocalcinosis. Although clinical experience is now dominated by a large subgroup of asymptomatic patients with mild disease, renal stone remains the single most common presenting manifestation in patients with symptomatic primary hyperparathyroidism.

CLINICAL PRESENTATION

Stone Disease

The clinical manifestations of stone formation and passage observed in patients with primary hyperparathyroidism are indistinguishable from those of other types of calcium nephrolithiasis. The initial phase of stone formation, the early growth of crystals on the surfaces of renal papillae or within the urinary collect-

ing system, is usually asymptomatic. Anchored stones may become manifest with gross or microscopic hematuria alone. However, those that pass into the renal pelvis and urinary tract may obstruct the flow of urine and cause severe acute renal colic.

The pain usually begins gradually in the flank or lower anterior abdomen and increases with time. As the stone moves, so does the location of the pain. Stones at the junction of the ureter and bladder cause dysuria and urinary frequency. Pain from stones located in the lower portion of the ureter can radiate to the ipsilateral testicle or vulva, mimicking genital disease. Stone passage, either spontaneous or by surgical removal, rapidly alleviates the pain.

Clinical Presentation of Primary Hyperparathyroidism

In the past, clinical descriptions of primary hyperparathyroidism have emphasized bone disease and nephrolithiasis as primary complications of the disease. Studies in the 1930s by Albright and colleagues (8) showed that bone and stone disease usually do not occur in the same patient. They proposed that differences in calcium intake might explain the two clinical presentations of the disorder. Furthermore, they suggested that bone disease might occur more commonly in patients with an inadequate calcium intake and predisposition to negative calcium balance, whereas stone disease might occur in patients with normal or excessive calcium intake and neutral or positive calcium balance.

Hodgkinson (7) confirmed Albright's finding that patients with primary hyperparathyroidism and stone disease maintain neutral external calcium balance.

V.A. Klugman, M.J. Favus: Department of Medicine, The University of Chicago, Chicago, Illinois 60637.

C.Y.C. Pak: Department of Internal Medicine, Division of Mineral Metabolism, University of Texas Southwestern Medical Center, Dallas, Texas 75235.

Conversely, Dent et al. (9) found no difference between the dietary calcium intake of patients presenting with bone disease and those with stone disease. Dent et al. proposed that the parathyroid glands might produce two hormones, one that causes hypercalcemia and another that affects bone and is nephrotoxic. Mallette et al. (6) found that patients with osteitis fibrosa had a brief period of symptoms before diagnosis, high serum calcium and immunoreactive parathyroid hormone (PTH) levels, and large tumors. In contrast, patients with nephrolithiasis tended to show moderate hypercalcemia, a longer duration of symptoms, and perhaps a more slowly growing tumor mass. Lloyd (5) also found that patients with clinically evident bone disease had higher serum calcium levels, lower urine calcium excretion, and a shorter duration of symptoms compared to those with kidney stones.

Peacock (10) found higher intestinal calcium absorption rates in patients with kidney stone than in those without stones, so it is possible that patients with stones were able to preserve bone mass through increased calcium absorption, while those without stones developed bone disease because of lower intestinal calcium absorption rates and increased bone resorption.

Patron et al. (11) found that, among 306 patients with documented primary hyperparathyroidism, those with overt bone disease had a mean serum PTH level four times greater than that in those who presented with kidney stones. Patients with bone disease also had lower circulating 1,25-dihydroxyvitamin D [1,25(OH)$_2$D] levels and diminished calciuric responses to a standard oral calcium load. These observations suggest that, in patients with bone disease, PTH hypersecretion might be due to lack of PTH suppression by the low to normal circulating 1,25-(OH)$_2$D levels. Relative vitamin D deficiency, also noted in patients with bone disease as indicated by low circulating 25-hydroxyvitamin D levels, could contribute to the low 1,25-(OH)$_2$D levels. In one patient with severe primary hyperparathyroidism, osteitis fibrosa, and normal serum 1,25-(OH)$_2$D level, increasing daily doses of intravenous 1,25-(OH)$_2$D (calcitriol) over several days doubled circulating 1,25-(OH)$_2$D and decreased PTH levels by 46% without changing the serum calcium concentration. Thus serum calcitriol levels in patients with bone disease may be insufficient to suppress PTH hypersecretion by individual cells independent of serum calcium.

Stone Types

Renal calculi in patients with primary hyperparathyroidism are similar in composition to calculi from non-hyperparathyroid patients. These calculi may contain pure calcium oxalate, mixed calcium phosphate and calcium oxalate, or pure calcium phosphate (brushite) (Table 1). Patients with primary hyperparathyroidism differ from those with idiopathic hypercalciuria by having a greater percent of calcium phosphate or brushite stones (12) (Fig. 1). Using chemical analysis of stones from 33 patients, Hellstrom and Ivemark (13) found that 15% contained only calcium oxalate, 48% were composed of a combination of calcium oxalate and calcium phosphate, and 36% were composed of pure calcium phosphate.

Lagergren and Ohrling (14) found a similar frequency of pure calcium phosphate stones and calcium phosphate with a small admixture of calcium oxalate. Ten patients had calcium oxalate stones, and two had ammonium magnesium phosphate stones. Thus two-thirds of their patients had calculi composed purely or predominantly of calcium phosphate.

Hodgkinson and Marshall (15) analyzed the composition of stones passed by 23 patients with primary hyperparathyroidism and found the portion of calcium phosphate to be considerably higher than in calcium containing stones from stone formers without hyperparathyroidism. The increased phosphate content was thought to be due to the renal effects of PTH to increase urine phosphate excretion and raise urine pH. Peacock et al. (16) also found that most hyperparathyroid stone formers produced stones composed mainly of calcium phosphate (20–80%), with calcium oxalate and magnesium ammonium phosphate making up the remainder.

However, in a recent series of patients with primary hyperparathyroidism and renal stones reported by Parks et al. (17), the majority of patients (20/31) formed calcium oxalate stones. For the others, two had pure calcium phosphate, two a mixture of calcium

TABLE 1. Composition of kidney stones in primary hyperparathyroidism[a]

Series	No.	CaOx	CaPO$_4$	CaOx/CaPO$_4$	MgNH$_4$PO$_4$	CaOx/U
Hellstrom (1950)	33	5 (15)	12 (36)	8 (48)	—	—
Lagergren (1959)	33	10 (30)	13 (40)	8 (24)	2 (6)	—
Coe (1980)	31	20 (64)	2 (6)	2 (6)	1 (3)	5 (16)

[a]No. is number of stone formers with hyperparathyroidism; values are number of each type of stone (percent of total).

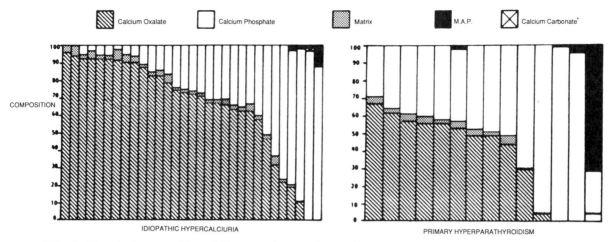

FIG. 1. Chemical composition of 30 stones from patients with idiopathic hypercalciuria and 14 stones from patients with primary hyperparathyroidism. All patients are males. M.A.P., magnesium ammonium phosphate. Note that no patient with primary hyperparathyroidism had a pure calcium oxalate stone. (Reprinted from ref. 12 with permission.)

phosphate and oxalate, five a mixture of calcium oxalate and uric acid, one calcium oxalate and cystine, and one a struvite (ammonium-magnesium phosphate) stone. Taken together, these series indicate that stones in patients with primary hyperparathyroidism vary from pure calcium phosphate to pure calcium oxalate or are a mixture of the two.

PREVALENCE OF STONES

Common Primary Hyperparathyroidism

The frequency of stone disease in primary hyperparathyroidism varies among series (Table 2). The incidence has been noted to decrease since the condition was first described because of the increasing numbers of asymptomatic patients discovered by routine biochemical screening. In 1937, Albright and Reifenstein (8) reported that 80% of their patients with primary hyperparathyroidism had renal calculi. A series of 171 patients with primary hyperparathyroidism evaluated at the Mayo Clinic (18) was composed of twice as many women as men. No clinical findings or biochemical tests distinguished those with stone disease from those without. Fifty-nine percent developed urologic complications, including nephrolithiasis in 46%, nephrocalcinosis in 5%, and impairment of renal function in 8%. Calcification of the papillary tips was not included in this evaluation, so the incidence of nephrocalcinosis may have been underestimated. Nephrolithiasis accompanied all cases of nephrocalcinosis. Active stone disease as documented by new stone passage, appearance on X-ray, or passage of gravel within a year prior to parathyroidectomy, was present in only 10.5% of patients. The prevalence of nephrolithiasis in

15 series of patients published since 1961 (Table 2) varied from 7 to 78%, with an average incidence of 41%. From these and other series, it appears that nephrolithiasis is currently the most frequent complication of primary hyperparathyroidism.

The incidence of primary hyperparathyroidism in patients presenting with nephrolithiasis has on the other hand remained quite stable. The occurrence of primary hyperparathyroidism among all stone formers in series published since 1960 ranges from 3% to 13%, with an average of ~7% (19). Thus, the frequency of

TABLE 2. *Prevalence of renal stones in patients with primary hyperparathyroidism*

Series	No. of patients	Percentage with stones[a]
Keating (1961)	380	64
Hodgkinson (1963)	50	68
Cope (1966)	343	57
Pyrah (1966)	68	40
Lloyd (1968)	138	59
Purnell (1971)	171	51
Pratley (1973)	60	78
Mallette (1974)	57	39
Broadus (1979)	50	42
Mundy (1980)	111	7
Siminovitch (1981)	448	41
Ranni-Sivula (1985)	289	11
Deaconson (1987)	258	28
Lafferty (1989)	100	18
Silverberg (1990)	62	18
Total	2,585	41

[a]The percentages may reflect a small contribution of patients with nephrocalcinosis but without nephrolithiasis, in that some series did not clearly distinguish those findings. (Adapted and reprinted from ref. 19 with permission.)

primary hyperparathyroidism as a cause of stone disease in patients presenting with nephrolithiasis is rather low.

Mild Primary Hyperparathyroidism

In recent years routine screening of serum calcium levels with automated biochemical techniques has led to the increased diagnosis of asymptomatic primary hyperparathyroidism. For middle-aged adults, the annual incidence is 100–200 cases per 100,000 population, which accounts for approximately 60,000 new cases diagnosed each year in the United States (20). Primary hyperparathyroidism is being recognized more frequently, and the clinical presentation is changing. At the Mayo Clinic, the frequency of stone disease in patients with primary hyperparathyroidism has decreased from 51% to 4% following the advent of routine measurement of serum calcium in the late 1960s (21).

Multiple Endocrine Neoplasia Type I

Multiple endocrine neoplasia type I (MEN-I) is an autosomal dominant disorder characterized by benign tumors of the parathyroid, pancreatic islet, and anterior pituitary cells. Of patients with this disorder, 95% present with hyperparathyroidism, and fewer than one-third have either gastrinoma or prolactinoma. The clinical manifestations of primary hyperparathyroidism in MEN-I are very similar to those in sporadic cases of primary hyperparathyroidism, with a few important exceptions. Patients with MEN-I tend to appear at a younger age (20–40 years), and the sex ratio does not favor females (22). In addition, parathyroid hyperfunction in MEN-I is generally multiglandular, with hyperplasia of all four glands. Series of patients with primary hyperparathyroidism reported from academic medical centers include ~50% with asymptomatic hypercalcemia, up to 50% with nephrolithiasis, and <10% with clinical bone disease.

Multiple Endocrine Neoplasia Type IIa

Multiple endocrine neoplasia type IIa (MEN-IIa) syndrome is characterized by medullary carcinoma of the thyroid, pheochromocytoma, and parathyroid hyperplasia. This disorder is also inherited as an autosomal dominant trait. In contrast to the frequent appearance of hyperparathyroidism in MEN-I, hypercalcemia occurs in only 10% of patients with MEN-IIa (23). Histologically proven parathyroid hyperplasia may be found in 40–50% of patients and remains clinically silent in most. Because of the mild nature of the primary hyperparathyroidism, patients with MEN-IIa can best be managed conservatively, in contrast to the surgical approach recommended for MEN-I.

Familial Hypocalciuric Hypercalcemia

Familial hypocalciuric hypercalcemia (FHH) is an autosomal dominant disorder characterized by hypercalcemia and relative hypocalciuria that begins in infancy or early childhood and follows a benign course (24). Patients with FHH are usually asymptomatic, lack typical manifestations of primary hyperparathyroidism, and maintain a stable hypercalcemia. The rate of nephrolithiasis in FHH is the same as in the general population.

Familial Hyperparathyroidism

The occurrence of two or more cases of isolated primary hyperparathyroidism in one kindred, while less common than the familial MEN syndromes, is referred to as *familial hyperparathyroidism*. In a study of 29 families with presumed familial hyperparathyroidism (25), 83 of the 261 members studied had surgically proven hyperparathyroidism, with multiglandular parathyroid enlargement demonstrated in 42. Fifty-seven percent (47/83) had either nephrocalcinosis or nephrolithiasis. Inheritance consistent with an autosomal dominant pattern was found in most families, although recently a family has been described with an autosomal recessive pattern of inheritance and multiple recurrent large adenomas.

DIAGNOSIS

Diagnosis of Primary Hyperparathyroidism

The approach to the diagnosis of primary hyperparathyroidism is discussed in the chapter, "Clinical Presentation of Primary Hyperparathyroidism," by Bilezikian et al.

Differential Diagnosis of Hypercalcemia and Nephrolithiasis

Primary hyperparathyroidism is the most common of the several diseases that may present with hypercalcemia and stone formation (Table 3). Other causes include vitamin D intoxication, sarcoidosis and other active granulomatous diseases, milk alkali syndrome, thyrotoxicosis, and immobilization. All can be distinguished from primary hyperparathyroidism by normal or suppressed serum PTH levels. All patients may have hypercalciuria unless renal failure supervenes.

TABLE 3. *Causes of hypercalcemia and nephrolithiasis*

Primary hyperparathyroidism
Thyrotoxicosis (spontaneous and iatrogenic)
Vitamin D intoxication
Milk alkali syndrome
Immobilization
Sarcoidosis

PATHOGENESIS OF ABNORMAL URINE CHEMISTRY

Parathyroid hormone excess may increase or decrease the urinary excretion of several ions and may alter the urinary formation product and activity product ratio, resulting in urine that favors crystallization of urinary calcium salts (Table 4).

Hypercalciuria

The pathogenetic risk factors responsible for stone formation in primary hyperparathyroidism remain unclear. Hypercalciuria (24 hr urine calcium excretion >250 mg for women and $\geq$ 300 mg for men) is frequently encountered in patients with hyperparathyroidism and has been implicated in the pathogenesis of renal stone formation (26). Excess calcium in the urine may come from increased intestinal absorption increased bone resorption, or from both. As a result, ultrafilterable calcium increases and may be sufficient to exceed distal tubular reabsorptive capacity. Increased intestinal calcium absorption has been documented in primary hyperparathyroidism using metabolic balance, double isotope of Ca, and fecal excretion of radiolabeled Ca (27) methodologies. 1,25-Dihydroxyvitamin D is the major stimulator of intestinal calcium absorption, and PTH stimulates its synthesis in the renal proximal tubule (28). In addition, low serum phosphate concentrations, caused by PTH inhibition of proximal tubular phosphate reabsorption, may also stimulate 1,25(OH)$_2$D synthesis (28). In support of a regulatory role of 1,25(OH)$_2$D in the increased intestinal calcium absorption, Kaplan et al. (27) found that

TABLE 4. *Metabolic causes of stone formation in primary hyperparathyroidism*

Hypercalciuria
Reduced urinary inhibitory activity
Increased urinary promoter activity
Reduced urinary pyrophosphate
Low urine citrate excretion
Reduced urinary magnesium
Hyperuricosuria
Mild renal tubular acidosis

the mean plasma concentration of 1,25(OH)$_2$D was greater in 18 patients with primary hyperparathyroidism than in normal subjects and was highly positively correlated with fractional calcium absorption.

Increased intestinal calcium absorption and elevated calcitriol levels were found in some but not all hyperparathyroid stone formers. In a study by Peacock (10), patients with primary hyperparathyroidism and stone disease uniformly displayed an increase in fractional intestinal calcium absorption. Broadus et al. (29) also attributed stone formation to increased intestinal calcium absorption and calcitriol excess. Among 50 unselected patients with primary hyperparathyroidism, 22 had a history of one or more kidney stones. An abnormal response to a calcium load test (>0.20 mg calcium per 100 ml glomerular filtration) was associated with a greater serum 1,25(OH)$_2$D level, a higher incidence of stones, and a higher 24 hr urinary calcium excretion compared to patients showing a normal response (<0.20 mg calcium per 100 ml glomerular filtration) to the calcium load test. Fasting urine calcium excretion was not different between the groups. Patients with greater calcium absorption and more marked hypercalciuria had greater parathyroid suppression as determined by suppression of nephrogenous cyclic adenosine monophosphate (cAMP). Broadus et al. concluded that patients with elevated serum 1,25(OH)$_2$D levels, increased intestinal absorption, and greater parathyroid suppression are predisposed to stone formation by their more marked hypercalciuria.

In contrast, Pak et al. (30) found no significant difference in 1,25(OH)$_2$D levels, intestinal calcium absorption, urinary calcium excretion, height of serum calcium and PTH concentrations, serum phosphate level, or bone density between stone forming and non-stone nonforming patients. Both groups had elevated fasting urinary calcium excretion and low bone mineral density. From these data, Pak et al. concluded that there was no unique pathophysiological background for nephrolithiasis in primary hyperparathyroidism.

The discrepancy between the studies of Pak et al. and Broadus et al. may have resulted in part from differences in patient classification. Broadus et al. initially separated patients with primary hyperparathyroidism on the basis of intestinal calcium absorption using the indirect method of incremental increase in urinary calcium after an oral calcium load. In contrast, Pak et al. compared data from stone formers with those from patients without stone disease.

Among 62 patients with primary hyperparathyroidism, 18% of whom were stone formers, Silverberg et al. (31) found a strong positive correlation between urinary calcium excretion and serum 1,25(OH)$_2$D levels. However, as in the study of Pak et al., stone formers and non-formers did not differ with respect to serum PTH, calcium, phosphorus, or $1,25(OH)_2D$ or in urinary calcium excretion.

Mild hypercalcemia may be associated with significant hypercalciuria and stone formation. Parks et al. (17) found that, in patients with surgically documented hyperparathyroidism, the serum calcium levels were between 10.2 and 10.8 mg/dl, just above the upper limit of normal of 10.1 mg/dl. However, urine calcium excretion exceeded normal in most patients and was markedly elevated in some patients in whom hypercalcemia was extremely mild. Thus one cannot assume that mild hypercalcemia is accompanied by only mild hypercalciuria.

Elevated serum $1,25(OH)_2D$ levels have been reported in some hyperparathyroid stone formers (11) but not in others (32). The latter study did not control calcium intake, while other studies that have reported serum $1,25(OH)_2D$ levels have used a restricted calcium intake. Serum $1,25(OH)_2D$ is sensitive to dietary calcium restriction in patients with primary hyperparathyroidism (33), and diet therefore could account for the elevated $1,25(OH)_2D$ levels in some series reported.

A second source of elevated urine calcium is bone resorption. PTH increases osteoclastic bone resorption, which results in the release of both mineral constituents and bone matrix protein degradation products. As a result, serum calcium and phosphate concentrations and urinary hydroxyproline excretion increase (34). In 26 patients, urinary calcium excretion exceeded net intestinal calcium absorption (35). In addition, fasting urinary calcium excretion is elevated in the majority of patients. Thus hypercalciuria is partly the result of an excessive skeletal mobilization of calcium.

Silverberg et al. (31) found elevated levels of urinary hydroxyproline and a negative correlation between urinary calcium excretion and forearm bone density in hyperparathyroid subjects with hypercalciuria, including stone formers (Fig. 2). Thus it appears that bone resorption contributes to the hypercalciuria observed in patients with hyperparathyroidism.

Inhibitors and Promoters

Reduced urinary inhibitory activity and/or increased promoter activity could contribute to the predilection for stone formation in primary hyperparathyroidism. Pak and Holt (36) found that the urine of patients with hyperparathyroidism was significantly more supersaturated with respect to calcium oxalate and brushite ($CaHPO_4 \cdot 2H_2O$) as expressed by the activity product ratio (APR) compared to normal subjects without stones. Urine APR was higher in patients with stones

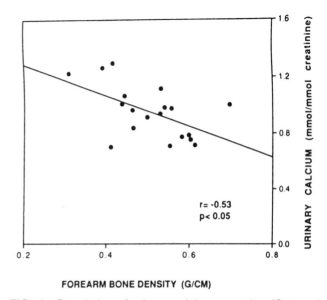

FIG. 2. Correlation of urinary calcium excretion (Ca/mmol creatinine) with forearm bone mineral density in a subgroup of hypercalciuric patients with hyperparathyroidism. (Reprinted from ref. 31 with permission.)

than in those without stones. The urinary formation product ratio (FPR), an inhibitor activity against spontaneous nucleation of brushite and calcium oxalate, was reduced in patients with primary hyperparathyroidism compared to values in normal subjects. Following parathyroidectomy, both urinary APR and FPR returned toward normal. These studies indicate that the urine of patients with primary hyperparathyroidism is supersaturated with respect to stone forming constituents and shows an increased propensity for crystallization of stone forming calcium salts. These findings are consistent with either excess urine promoters or reduced inhibitors leading to stone formation in primary hyperparathyroidism. However, physicochemical presentation in urine of stone forming patients with primary hyperparathyroidism has not been rigorously compared to that of non-formers. Moreover, promoter excess or inhibitor deficiency has not been documented by direct analysis. Thus the propensity to form stones cannot be understood on the basis of present knowledge of urinary inhibitors and promoters.

Pyrophosphate is a naturally occurring urinary inhibitor of the crystallization of calcium oxalate and calcium phosphate. Measurements of urinary excretion of pyrophosphate in patients with hyperparathyroidism have been reported to be either not different from normal (37) or increased (38). Studies have found no significant change in pyrophosphate excretion following surgical removal of the adenoma (39). The reasons for the difference between the findings in these studies remains obscure.

Citrate is a natural urinary inhibitor of crystallization of calcium salts through its formation of soluble calcium citrate complexes. Citrate is also a direct inhibitor of crystal growth of calcium phosphate and nucleation of calcium oxalate. Alvarez-Arroyo (40) and Smith et al. (41) reported that hyperparathyroid kidney stone formers showed lower urinary citrate excretion than did patients without stones, apparently due to increased tubular reabsorption of citrate.

Magnesium inhibits calcium oxalate crystallization by complexing oxalate. Low urinary magnesium in relation to calcium is a common finding in hyperparathyroid stone formers and may contribute to the development of calcium oxalate stones (42). Others have found low urinary Mg/Ca ratios in primary hyperparathyroidism, which appear to correct postoperatively to normal (43). However, normalization of the Mg/Ca ratio is a function of changes in urinary calcium excretion, since low urinary magnesium is uncommon in primary hyperparathyroidism.

"Consumption" of normal urine inhibitors may occur with hypercalciuria. Zerewekh et al. (44) found that hypercalciuria induced by calcium supplementation in stone formers decreased the urinary formation product ratio, probably by complexing of negatively charged urinary inhibitors by calcium. Other evidence suggesting an alteration in crystal growth inhibitors comes from observations that urine of hyperparathyroid stone formers contains crystals that are larger due to enhanced aggregation rather than crystal growth (45). Thus stone forming urine may contain promoters of crystal growth or substances that block the effects of crystal growth inhibitors found in normal urine.

Hyperuricosuria

Hyperuricosuria has been linked to calcium oxalate crystal formation through induction of epitaxial growth of calcium oxalate crystals by uric acid or Na urate or adsorption of naturally occurring inhibitors (46,47). There is, however, no convincing evidence that urinary uric acid excretion is elevated in patients with primary hyperparathyroidism. Broulek et al. (48) found that hyperparathyroid patients have lower urate clearance than controls. Ljunghall and Akerstrom (49) found a reduction in the clearance of urate and a rise in serum urate concentrations that normalized postoperatively. The fasting urine excretion of urate was slightly higher in stone formers preoperatively, whereas there were no significant differences for the 24 hr before or after surgery. Thus disturbances of urate metabolism are not likely to be important in the pathogenesis of renal stones in primary hyperparathyroidism.

Acidosis

Hereditary, type I distal renal tubular acidosis (RTA) typically presents with a nonanion gap hyperchloremic acidosis, medullary nephrocalcinosis, calcium phosphate nephrolithiasis, and osteopenia. Pure calcium phosphate stones develop in this environment as a consequence of the alkaline urine, decreased citrate excretion, and hypercalciuria secondary to enhanced bone resorption and impaired renal tubular reabsorption of calcium. Because patients with primary hyperparathyroidism have an increased incidence of calcium phosphate stones, acidification defects have been considered in the pathogenesis of stones in this disorder. Primary hyperparathyroidism may be associated with a proximal RTA, which, unlike the distal RTA, has not been associated with stone formation. It is clear that a mild hyperchloremic acidosis may occur in patients with hyperparathyroidism, but its frequency is debated. Muldowney et al. (50) described four patients with primary hyperparathyroidism who had hyperchloremic acidosis; however, all the patients had impaired renal function. Because hypercalcemic nephropathy itself can impair renal acidification, the cause of acidosis in these patients is unclear. Among 13 patients with primary hyperparathyroidism studied by Coe (51), only two had metabolic acidosis. Blood chloride and CO_2 concentrations rose after parathyroidectomy, and the serum PTH level was not significantly correlated with either. Thus, PTH is unlikely to be an important regulator of renal acid excretion. Whether metabolic acidosis occurs in primary hyperparathyroidism was challenged by Hulter and Peterson (52), who found a mild transient acidosis, which subsequently was replaced by a sustained mild alkalosis associated with increased urine proton excretion. In addition, PTH does not typically alter urinary pH (36). Therefore, there is little evidence to favor sustained acidosis as an important factor in the pathogenesis of nephrolithiasis in primary hyperparathyroidism.

TREATMENT

Surgical Treatment of Hyperparathyroidism

Stone Recurrence After Parathyroidectomy

For asymptomatic patients, the decision whether to treat hyperparathyroidism medically or surgically is controversial (see chapters by Bilezikian et al., "Clinical Presentation of Primary Hyperparathyroidism," Kleerekoper, and Bilezikian, "Guidelines for the Medical or Surgical Management of Primary Hyperparathyroidism"), but there is agreement about the value of surgery in patients who form stones. McGeown (53) followed 56 patients for 1–5 years following parathyroidectomy. Prior to parathyroidectomy, 99 stones were formed in 401 patient-years, whereas, in the post-parathyroidectomy period, only eight stones were formed in 158 patient-years. Deaconson et al (54) also observed a decline in the rate of new stone formation after surgical correction of primary hyperparathyroidism from 0.36 to 0.02 new stones formed per patient per year. Two of the four patients with recurrent stones had persistent hypercalcemia and evidence of persistent or recurrent hyperparathyroidism.

Parks et al. (17) described similar findings in 48 patients with primary hyperparathyroidism and renal stones. The only patient with stone recurrence post-operatively was the only one who remained hypercalciuric following parathyroidectomy. On the other hand, Posen et al. (55) observed a 50% recurrence rate of new stone formation or passage of an existing stone after surgery among 77 hyperparathyroid patients followed for 7–8 years. Patients with no previous history of renal calculi were unlikely to form stones postoperatively even if they remained hypercalcemic and hypercalciuric. Thus parathyroidectomy results in a virtual disappearance of first-onset stone formation.

Resolution of stone disease is less certain in patients with parathyroid hyperplasia than in those with adenomas. Siminovitch et al. (56) observed 448 patients who underwent surgery for presumed hyperparathyroidism. Of the 72 patients with active stone disease, 48 were found to have adenomas, 18 had hyperplasia, and six had normal glands. Patients with adenomas had no recurrent calculi, whereas 50% of those with normal glands and 45% of those with hyperplasia had recurrent stone formation. Similarly, Johannsen et al. (57) found that patients with adenomas had no recurrent calculi after parathyroidectomy, whereas recurrent calculi developed in 25% of the patients with parathyroid hyperplasia and in 48% of those with normal parathyroid glands.

Metabolic Changes After Surgery

Successful parathyroidectomy decreases serum calcium levels to normal, which, in the majority of patients, leads to resolution of hypercalciuria (58). It has been estimated that, of the 5–10% of patients who continue to form stones after surgery, 90% have some form of hypercalciuria (59). Occurrence of hypercalciuria after parathyroidectomy may be as high as 30% (60). Parks et al. (17) found that, in 66 patients with renal stones and primary hyperparathyroidism, urine calcium, urine oxalate, and urine calcium oxalate concentration product ratio (CPR) returned to normal after surgery in males. In contrast, in women, urine oxalate and the calcium oxalate CPR returned to normal, but the urine calcium levels did not. Hypercalciuria persisted in seven of 17 women even though the serum calcium level was normal.

The cause of this persistent hypercalciuria despite normocalcemia remains unknown, but it is probably multifactorial. Breslau et al. (61) have suggested coexistence of absorptive (idiopathic) hypercalciuria as the underlying etiology of the recurrent hypercalciuria observed in some patients after surgery. In five such patients, serum PTH and calcium levels returned to normal, but serum $1,25(OH)_2D$ remained elevated in four. Four of the patients had recurrent stones and persistent elevation in fractional intestinal ^{47}Ca absorption. Thus absorptive hypercalciuria and primary hyperparathyroidism may occur together, and absorptive hypercalciuria may persist after surgery. Absorptive hypercalciuria was also suggested in a patient with persistent hypercalciuria postparathyroidectomy, in whom hypercalciuria was abolished with dietary calcium restriction (62). This would not be expected to lower urine calcium excretion if it were the result of a renal calcium leak or secondary to bone resorption.

An alternative mechanism for persistent hypercalciuria after parathyroidectomy is so-called renal hypercalciuria. Bordier et al. (63) and Maschio et al. (64) described patients with apparent normocalcemic hyperparathyroidism, in whom persistent hypercalciuria after parathyroid surgery resulted from a primary renal calcium leak. This leak led initially to a state of secondary hyperparathyroidism and eventually to autonomous or tertiary hyperparathyroidism. It appears therefore that recurrent stones can occur despite cure of the clinical hyperparathyroidism. The etiology may be secondary to underlying absorptive or renal hypercalciuria. All patients should therefore have urinary calcium excretion evaluated after parathyroidectomy.

Although successful surgery for hyperparathyroidism corrects serum and urine calcium abnormalities, Pak (65) observed that urinary calcium decreased significantly after parathyroidectomy without significant changes in urinary phosphate, oxalate, magnesium, sodium, potassium, uric acid, or pH. The urinary activity product ratio (state of saturation) of brushite $(CaHPO_4 \cdot 2H_2O)$ and calcium oxalate decreased significantly due primarily to decreased urinary calcium. In addition, the urinary formation product ratio of calcium oxalate, the minimum supersaturation required for spontaneous nucleation, increased significantly after parathyroidectomy (Fig. 3). Therefore, surgery restores the normal urinary environment with

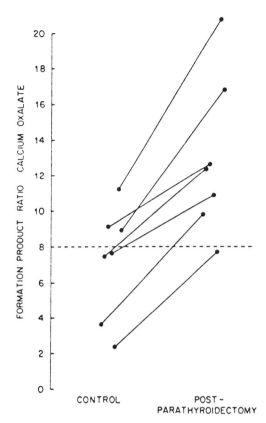

FIG. 3. Effect of parathyroidectomy on the urinary formation product ratio of calcium oxalate in seven patients with primary hyperparathyroidism. Each line represents measurements in an individual patient before (control) and after parathyroidectomy. *Dashed line* represents value in synthetic medium devoid of known inhibitors and promoters. (Reprinted from ref. 65 with permission.)

respect to saturation and inhibitor and/or promoter activity.

Medical Treatment of Hyperparathyroidism

Curative surgery is indicated for patients with primary hyperparathyroidism and renal stones. Medical treatment outcome is less certain and should be reserved for patients who refuse surgery, who are unable to withstand general anesthesia, or who require a temporizing measure prior to surgery. Several medical therapies have been assessed, with few shown to be of clear value in reducing serum or urine calcium and diminishing stone formation (Table 5).

Fluid Intake

Because low urine volume has been considered a risk factor in the development of renal stones (66), high fluid intake is recommended in patients with renal

TABLE 5. *Medical therapy of primary hyperparathyroidism and kidney stones*

High fluid intake
Dietary restriction
  Sodium
  Protein
  Calcium
Cellulose phosphate
Diuretics
Inhibitors of PTH secretion
  Propranolol
  Cimetidine
Antiresorptive agents
  Estrogen
  Bisphosphonates
  Phosphate

stones. Pak et al. (67) suggested that the high fluid intake may be effective through dilution of stone forming constituents as well as decreased urinary saturation of stone salts. Urinary dilution by high fluid intake assessed both in vitro and in vivo in stone formers and controls revealed that both forms of urinary dilution resulted in a significant reduction of urinary APR (state of saturation) of calcium phosphate, calcium oxalate, and monosodium urate. In addition, the formation product ratio (minimum supersaturation needed to elicit spontaneous nucleation) of calcium oxalate significantly increased. Thus the propensity for crystallization of calcium salts is decreased by dilution of the urine, resulting in a beneficial role of increased fluid intake in the management of nephrolithiasis.

Dietary Protein Restriction

High dietary protein intake, estimated by excretion of urinary urea nitrogen, and urinary calcium may be highly correlated in some patients with recurrent nephrolithiasis (68,69). Moreover, stone formers appeared to be more sensitive to the calciuric action of protein, and increments in dietary protein resulted in a greater increment in calciuria in patients with recurrent nephrolithiasis than in controls. Urinary oxalate and uric acid may increase along with calcium excretion following ingestion of a protein load (70), and the increases may persist for as long as the increased dietary protein is maintained. Protein may also increase calcium oxalate stone formation through changes in the excretion of various promoters and inhibitors. Wasserstein et al. (68) found that protein ingestion results in hypocitrituria in patients with recurrent stones, whereas protein restriction increases urinary citrate excretion. Thus the hypocitrituria often found in patients with recurrent nephrolithiasis may be the result of a high-protein diet.

Sodium Restriction

The renal tubular handling of calcium and sodium is closely related such that factors that promote natriuresis also increase urinary calcium excretion. A large epidemiologic study showed that urinary sodium excretion directly correlated with urinary calcium excretion (68). Dietary sodium intake may therefore be a risk factor for hypercalciuria and for calcium oxalate kidney stone formation. Moreover, patients with recurrent stones and hypercalciuria were more sensitive to the hypercalciuric action of dietary sodium. Muldowney et al. (71) suggested that dietary sodium restriction may have a role in the management of hypercalciuria in mild hyperparathyroid patients when parathyroidectomy is contraindicated. For example, moderate dietary sodium restriction decreases 24 hr urine calcium excretion in primary hyperparathyroidism patients.

Calcium Restriction

Calcium restriction has been used commonly in patients with primary hyperparathyroidism to control hypercalcemia and reduce hypercalcuria. While severe restriction of dietary calcium may reduce urine calcium excretion, it may also result in negative calcium balance (72) and hyperoxaluria by increasing intestinal oxalate absorption.

Cellulose Phosphate

This resin binds dietary calcium in the intestinal lumen and prevents absorption. Cellulose phosphate decreases urinary calcium excretion in patients with primary hyperparathyroidism and may thus be important in preventing stones (73). Urinary hydroxyproline levels, however, tend to increase, so bone resorption may be increased. Thus long-term use of cellulose phosphate is contraindicated.

Diuretic Therapy

Diuretics should be used with caution in patients with primary hyperparathyroidism. Because of the reversible loss of urine concentrating ability due to the hypercalciuria, excessive fluid loss or decreased fluid intake could result in dehydration and lead to a further increase in blood calcium level. Thiazide diuretics particularly should be avoided; they may increase hypercalcemia by increasing distal tubular calcium reabsorption (74). Thiazide-induced hypercalcemia tends to occur in patients with nonsuppressible parathyroid glands as in primary hyperparathyroidism.

Loop diuretics such as furosemide, with adequate sodium intake, may facilitate urinary calcium excretion and therefore may be a useful short-term measure in decreasing serum calcium until surgery is performed. However, furosemide should not be used over the long term; it increases urinary calcium excretion, may increase the risk of further stone formation, and may worsen negative calcium balance.

Inhibitors of Parathyroid Hormone Secretion

An agent that inhibits the secretion of parathyroid hormone would be extremely useful in primary hyperparathyroidism. β-Adrenergic catecholamines stimulate PTH secretion (75), and the beta blocker propranolol can block catecholamine-stimulated PTH secretion. Short-term in vivo studies in animals and humans have shown that β-receptor agonists stimulate PTH secretion and that this response can be eliminated by propranolol. Caro et al. (76) observed a variable decrease in serum PTH and calcium levels with propranolol in eight patients with primary hyperparathyroidism, with a marked response in two patients and marginal or no response in the remainder. Other reports have failed to demonstrate a decline in serum calcium during propranolol administration (75,77).

The stimulatory action of histamine to increase PTH secretion can be inhibited by the H_2 receptor antagonist cimetidine. Sherwood et al. (78) reported a significant decrease in serum PTH levels with cimetidine in 12 patients with primary hyperparathyroidism. However, subsequent studies have not confirmed these initial findings (79,80). Thus the therapeutic trials to date have failed to identify an inhibitor of PTH secretion that may be useful as medical therapy for primary hyperparathyroidism.

Antiresorptive Therapy

Inhibition of osteoclastic bone resorption is another medical strategy to control the hypercalcemia and hypercalciuria of primary hyperparathyroidism.

Estrogens

Estrogens are inhibitors of PTH-stimulated osteoclastic activity and can reduce bone resorption. Gallagher and Nordin (81) showed that estrogen administration successfully decreased serum calcium and urine calcium and hydroxyproline excretion in a group of women with primary hyperparathyroidism. They therefore attributed the effects of estrogen to the inhibition of PTH-induced bone resorption. Marcus et al. (82) observed a reduction in serum calcium and urinary calcium excretion for up to 2 years in ten patients treated with estrogen. Temporary interruption of therapy was associated with return of hypercalcemia to untreated levels within 2–3 days, but this resolved quickly with resumption of estrogen therapy. Urinary hydroxyproline and serum alkaline phosphatase decreased during estrogen therapy, suggesting a decrease in bone formation and resorption rates. Serum PTH and 1,25-$(OH)_2D$ levels and urine cAMP excretion did not change with treatment. These data indicate that estrogen inhibits the skeletal actions of PTH but does not secondarily stimulate parathyroid function and, therefore, does not alter the course of the disease. None of the previous studies has addressed the effect of estrogen therapy on stone formation in particular. Therefore, estrogen therapy may provide an alternative to surgical cure for postmenopausal females who are unwilling or unable to undergo parathyroidectomy (see the chapter by Stock and Marcus).

Bisphosphonate Therapy

Bisphosphonates are related synthetic analogs of endogenous pyrophosphate. They bind with high affinity to bone crystal hydroxyapatite and inhibit its dissolution and growth. Perhaps more importantly, bone resorption is inhibited by a direct action to suppress osteoclastic activity (83). Ethane hydroxy-1,1-diphosphonate (EHDP) was the first bisphosphonate to be investigated in primary hyperparathyroidism. Serum calcium was not reduced by EHDP therapy, although 5 weeks of EHDP decreased urine calcium and hydroxyproline (84). Urine calcium increased after 6 months of therapy, suggesting that the decrease in bone resorption may be transient.

Dichloromethylene diphosphonate (Cl_2 MDP, clodronate), which does not inhibit skeletal mineralization, decreased serum calcium and urinary calcium and hydroxyproline excretion in each of the 14 primary hyperparathyroidism patients treated (85).

3-Amino-1-hydroxypropylidine-1,1-diphosphonate (APD) is similar to clodronate in that it inhibits bone resorption at doses that do not alter mineralization. APD rapidly reduced serum calcium to normal in two patients with primary hyperparathyroidism (86). Clearly, more studies are needed before a role, if any, for APD or other newer bisphosphonates can be established in treatment of hyperparathyroid stone disease.

Phosphate Therapy

A decrease in urinary calcium following phosphate administration to hypercalciuric patients was first described by Albright et al. (87). Subsequently, Gold-smith and Ingbar (88) confirmed that phosphate reduces urine calcium excretion and also noted that administration of intravenous or oral phosphate reduced hypercalcemia in 20 patients with hypercalcemia of diverse etiology. A number of side effects including renal failure and dystrophic calcification have limited the use of this approach, however. Phosphate decreases serum calcium levels by shifting extracellular fluid calcium into bone and also by inhibiting PTH-mediated bone resorption and stimulating osteoblastic bone formation.

Purnell et al. (89) treated 14 patients with primary hyperparathyroidism who were surgical failures with moderate doses (1,000–2,500 mg) of elemental phosphorus daily. They concluded that patients with moderate disease (mean serum calcium 12.5 mg/dl), particularly those with prior renal impairment, were not good candidates for phosphate therapy and were at risk for worsening of renal function and/or rapid progression of hyperparathyroidism. However, patients with mild primary hyperparathyroidism (mean serum calcium 10.8 mg/dl) had no side effects of therapy, and the metabolic activity of renal stone complications appeared to be controlled.

Broadus et al. (90) found that 1 year of oral phosphate therapy in ten patients with primary hyperparathyroidism and elevated serum 1,25$(OH)_2D$ levels significantly decreased circulating 1,25$(OH)_2D$, calciuric response to an oral calcium tolerance test, and urine calcium excretion on an unrestricted calcium diet. Six of the ten patients had a history of renal stones, and none formed new renal stones during the course of the treatment. Although phosphate appears to reverse intestinal calcium hyperabsorption, serum PTH levels increase and may aggravate the state of bone resorption.

The indications for phosphate therapy remain uncertain. Even though urinary calcium excretion is reduced, the efficacy in reducing stone formation has not been determined. In addition, phosphate may accelerate renal impairment in patients with serum calcium levels >11.5 mg/dl and in those with established renal insufficiency.

REFERENCES

1. Mandl F. Therapeutischer versuch bei einem falle von ostitis fibrosa generalisata mittels extirpation eines epithelkorperchentumors. *Z Chir* 1926;53:260–264.
2. Davies-Colley N. Bones and kidneys from a case of osteomalacia in a girl aged 13. *Trans Pathol Soc London* 1884; 35:285–297.
3. Barr DP, Bulger HA. The clinical syndrome of hyperparathyroidism. *Am J Med Sci* 1930;179:471–473.
4. Albright F, Sulkowitch HW, Bloomberg E. Further experience in diagnosis of hyperparathyroidism, including discussion of cases with minimal degree of hyperparathyroidism. *Am J Med Sci* 1937;193:800–812.

5. Lloyd HM. Primary hyperparathyroidism: an analysis of the role of the parathyroid tumor. *Medicine* 1968;47:53–71.
6. Mallette LE, Bilezikian JP, Heath DA, et al. Primary hyperparathyroidism: clinical and biochemical features. *Medicine* 1974;53:127–146.
7. Hodgkinson A. Biochemical aspects of primary hyperparathyroidism: an analysis of 50 cases. *Clin Sci* 1963;25:231–236.
8. Albright F, Reifenstein EC. *The parathyroid glands and metabolic bone disease*. Baltimore: Williams and Wilkins, 1948:393.
9. Dent CE, Hartland BV, Hicks J, et al. Calcium intake in patients with primary hyperparathyroidism. *Lancet* 1961;2:330–338.
10. Peacock M. Renal stone disease and bone disease in primary hyperparathyroidism and their relationship to the action of parathyroid hormone on calcium regulation. In: *Calcium regulating hormones, proceedings of the fifth parathyroid conference*. Amsterdam: Excerpta Medica, 1975;78.
11. Patron P, Gardin JP, Poullard M. Renal mass and reserve of vitamin D: determinants in primary hyperparathyroidism. *Kidney Int* 1987;31:1176–1180.
12. Rose AG. Primary hyperparathyroidism. In: Wickham JEA, Buck AC, eds. *Renal tract stone: metabolic basis and clinical features*. London: Churchill Livingstone, 1990;401–413.
13. Hellstrom J, Ivemark BI. Primary hyperparathyroidism: clinical and structural findings in 138 cases. *Acta Chir Scand* 1962;294:Suppl. 1.
14. Lagergren C, Ohrling H. Urinary calculi composed of pure calcium phosphate. *Acta Chir Scand* 1959;117:335–341.
15. Hodgkinson A, Marshall RW. Changes in the composition of urinary tract stones. *Invest Urol* 1975;13:131–135.
16. Peacock M, Marshall RW, Roberston WG, et al. Renal stone formation in primary hyperparathyroidism and idiopathic stone disease; diagnosis, etiology and treatment. In: Finlayson B, Thomas WC, eds. *Colloquium on renal lithiasis*. University Press of Florida 1976;339–355.
17. Parks J, Coe F, Favus M. Hyperparathyroidism in nephrolithiasis. *Arch Intern Med* 1980;140:1479–1481.
18. Purnell DC, Smith LH, Scholz DA, et al. Primary hyperparathyroidism: a prospective clinical study. *Am J Med* 1971;50:670–678.
19. Broadus A. Nephrolithiasis in primary hyperparathyroidism. In: Coe F, Brenner B, Stein J, eds. *Nephrolithiasis*. New York: Churchill Livingstone, 1980.
20. Heath H III, Hodgson SF, Kennedy MA. PHPT: incidence, morbidity and potential economic impact in a community. *N Engl J Med* J 1980;302:189–193.
21. Hodgson SF, Heath H III. Asymptomatic primary hyperparathyroidism: treat or follow? *Mayo Clin Proc* 1981;56:521–523.
22. Marx SJ, Vinek AI, Sanken RJ, et al. Multiple endocrine neoplasia type I: assessment of laboratory tests to screen for the gene in a large kindred. *Medicine* 1986;65:226–261.
23. Scheinke RN. Genetic aspects of multiple endocrine neoplasia. *Annu Rev Med* 1986;35:25–31.
24. Marx SJ, Brandu ML. Familial primary hyperparathyroidism. In: Peck WA, ed. *Bone and mineral research*, Vol. 5. Amsterdam: Elsevier, 1987;375–407.
25. Goldsmith RE, Sizemore G, Falme E, et al. Familial hyperparathyroidism. *Ann Intern Med* 1976;84:36–43.
26. Coe FL, Parks JL, Asplin JR. The pathogenesis and treatment of kidney stones. *N Engl J Med* 1992;327:1141–1152.
27. Kaplan RA, Haussler MR, Deftos LJ, et al. The role of 1,25 dihydroxy vitamin D in the mediation of intestinal hyperabsorption of calcium in primary hyperparathyroidism and absorptive hypercalciuria. *J Clin Invest* 1977;59:756–760.
28. Henry HL, Norman AW. Metabolism of vitamin D. In: Coe FL, Favus MJ, eds. *Disorders of bone and mineral metabolism*. New York: Raven Press 1992;149–162.
29. Broadus AE, Horst RL, Lang R, et al. The importance of circulating 1,25 dihydroxy vitamin D in the pathogenesis of hypercalciuria and renal stone formation in primary hyperparathyroidism. *N Engl J Med* 1980;302:421–425.
30. Pak CY, Nicar MJ, Peterson R, et al. A lack of unique pathophysiologic background for nephrolithiasis of primary hyperparathyroidism. *J Clin Endocrinol Metab* 1981;53:536–542.
31. Silverberg SJ, Shane E, Jacobs TP, et al. Nephrolithiasis and bone involvement in primary hyperparathyroidism. *Am J Med* 1990;89:327–334.
32. Thakker RV, Fraher LJ, Adami S, et al. Circulating concentrations of 1,25 dihydroxy vitamin D in patients with primary hyperparathyroidism. *Bone Mineral* 1986;1:137.
33. Insogna KL, Mitnick ME, Stewart A, et al. Sensitivity of the parathyroid hormone 1,25 dihydroxy vitamin D axis to variations in calcium intake in patients with primary hyperparathyroidism. *N Engl J Med* 1985;313:1126–1130.
34. Fitzpatrick LA, Coleman DT, Bilezikian JP. The target tissue actions of parathyroid hormone. In: Coe FL, Favus MJ, eds. *Disorders of bone and mineral metabolism*, vol. 6. Raven Press, 1992;123–148.
35. Pak CY, Ohata M, Lawrence EC, et al. The hypercalciurias: causes, parathyroid functions, and diagnostic criteria. *J Clin Invest* 1976;54:387–400.
36. Pak CYC, Holt K. Nucleation and growth of brushite and calcium oxalate in urine of stone formers. *Metabolism* 1976; 25:665–673.
37. Russell RGG, Hodgkinson A. The urinary excretion of inorganic pyrophosphate in hyperparathyroidism, hyperthyroidism, Paget's disease and other disorders of bone metabolism. *Clin Sci* 1969;36:435–443.
38. Avioli LV, McDonald JE, Singer RA. Excretion of pyrophosphate in disorders of bone metabolism. *J Clin Endocrinol* 1965;25:912–915.
39. Lewis AM, Thomas WC, Tomita A. Pyrophosphate and the mineralizing potential of urine. *Clin Sci* 1966;30:389–397.
40. Alvarez-Arroyo MV, Traba ML, Rapado A, et al. Role of citric acid in primary hyperparathyroidism with renal lithiasis. *Urol Res* 1992;20:88–90.
41. Smith LH, Vandenberg CJ, Wilson DM, et al. Urolithiasis in primary hyperparathyroidism. *Abstracts of the American Society of Nephrology*. 1977;109A.
42. Sutton RAL, Watson L. Urinary excretion of calcium and magnesium in primary hyperparathyroidism. *Lancet* 1969: 1000–1003.
43. Johannson G, Danielson BG, Ljunghall S. Magnesium homeostasis in mild to moderate primary hyperparathyroidism. *Acta Chir Scand* 1980;146:85–91.
44. Zerewekh JE, Hwang TIS, Poindexter J, et al. Modulation by calcium of the inhibitor activity of naturally occurring urinary inhibitors. *Kidney Int* 1988;33:1005–1008.
45. Koide T, Yoshioka T, Oka T, et al. Promotive effect of urines from patients with primary hyperparathyroidism calcium oxalate crystal aggregate. In: Walker V, Sutton RAL, Cameron EC, Pak CYC, Robertson WA, eds. *Urolithiasis*. New York: Plenum Press, 1989;109–111.
46. Lonsdale K. Human stones. *Science* 1968;159:1199–1207.
47. Pak CYC, Holt K, Zerewekh JK. Attenuation by sodium urate of the inhibitory effect of glycosaminoglycans on calcium oxalate nucleation. *Invest Urol* 1979;17:138–141.
48. Broulek PD, Stepan JJ, Pacovsky V. Primary hyperparathyroidism and hyperuricemia are associated but not correlated with indicators of bone turnovers. *Clin Chim Acta* 1987; 170:195–200.
49. Ljunghall S, Akerstrom G. Urate metabolism in primary hyperparathyroidism. *Urol Int* 1982;37:73–78.
50. Muldowney JP, Carroll DV, Donohoe JF, et al. Correction of renal bicarbonate wastage by parathyroidectomy. *Q J Med* 1971;160:487–498.
51. Coe FL. Magnitude of metabolic acidosis in primary hyperparathyroidism. *Arch Intern Med* 1974;134:202–205.
52. Hulter HN, Peterson JC. Acid–base homeostasis during chronic PTH excess in humans. *Kidney Int* 1985;28:187–192.
53. McGeown MG. Effect of parathyroidectomy on the incidence of renal calculi. *Lancet* 1961;1:586–587.
54. Deaconson TF, Wilson SD, Lemann J. The effect of parathyroidectomy on the recurrence of nephrolithiasis. *Surgery* 1987;102:910–912.
55. Posen S, Clifton-Bligh P, Reeve TS, et al. Is parathyroidectomy of benefit in primary hyperparathyroidism? *Q J Med* 1985;215:241–251.
56. Siminovitch JMP, Caldwell BE, Straffen RA. Renal lithiasis

and hyperparathyroidism: diagnosis, management and prognosis. *J Urol* 1981;126:720–722.

57. Johannsen H, Thoren L, Werner I, et al. Normocalcemic hyperparathyroidism, kidney stones and idiopathic hypercalciuria. *Surgery* 1975;77:691–696.

58. Kaplan RA, Snyder WH, Stewart A, et al. Metabolic effects of parathyroidectomy in asymptomatic primary hyperparathyroidism. *J Clin Endocrinol Metab* 1976;42:415–426.

59. Siminovitch JMP, James RE, Esselsytne CBJ, et al. The effect of parathyroidectomy in patients with normocalcemic calcium stones. *J Urol* 1980;123:335–337.

60. Fabris A, Ortalda V, D'Angelo A, Giannin S, Maschio G. Biochemical and clinical studies after parathyroidectomy in primary hyperparathyroidism. In: Walker V, Sutton RAL, Cameron EC, Pak CYC, Robertson WG, eds. *Urolithiasis*. New York: Plenum Press, 1989;637–640.

61. Breslau NA, Pak CYC. Combined primary hyperparathyroidism and absorptive hypercalciuria: clinical implication. In: Walker V, Sutton Ral, Cameron EC, Pak CYC, Robertson WG, eds. *Urolithiasis*. New York: Plenum Press, 1989;627–630.

62. Muir JW, Baker LRI. Hypercalciuria and recurrent urinary stone formation despite successful surgery, for primary hyperparathyroidism. *Br Med J* 1978;738:1–3.

63. Bordier P, Ryckewort A, Gueris J. On the pathogenesis of so called idiopathic hypercalciuria. *Am J Med* 1977;63:398–408.

64. Maschio G, Vecchioni R, Tessitore N. Recurrence of autonomous hyperparathyroidism in calcium nephrolithiasis. *Am J Med* 1980;68:607–609.

65. Pak CYC. Effect of parathyroidectomy on crystallization of calcium salts in urine of patients with primary hyperparathyroidism. *Invest Urol* 1979;17:140–148.

66. Robertson WG. Risk factors in calcium stone disease. In: Brackis G, Finlayson B, eds. *International urinary stone conference*. Nettleton, MA: PSG Publishing Co., 1979;12.

67. Pak CYC, Sakhaee K, Crowther C, et al. Evidence justifying a high fluid intake in treatment of nephrolithiasis. *Ann Intern Med* 1980;93:36–39.

68. Wasserstein AG, Stolley PD, Soper KA, et al. Case–control study of risk factors for idiopathic calcium nephrolithiasis. *Mineral Electrolyte Metab* 1987;13:85–95.

69. Goldfarb S. Dietary factors in the pathogenesis and prophylaxis of calcium nephrolithiasis. *Kidney Int* 1988;34:544–555.

70. Robertson WG, Heyburn PJ, Peacock M. The effect of high animal protein intake on the risk of calcium stone-formation in the urinary tract. *Clin Sci* 1979;57:285–288.

71. Muldowney FP, Freaney R, Muldowney EP, et al. Hypercalciuria in parathyroid disorders: effect of dietary sodium control. *Am J Kidney Dis* 1991;17:323–329.

72. Coe FL, Favus MJ, Crocket T, et al. Effects of low calcium diet on urine calcium excretion, parathyroid function and serum 1,25(OH)$_2$D levels in patients with idiopathic hypercalciuria and in normal subjects. *Am J Med* 1982;72:25–32.

73. Pak CYC, Delea CS, Bartter FC. Successful treatment of recurrent nephrolithiasis with cellulose phosphate. *N Engl J Med* 1976;290:175–180.

74. Duarte CG, Winnaker JL, Becker KL, et al. Thiazide induced hypercalcemia. *N Engl J Med* 1971;15:828–830.

75. Kukreja SC, Johnson PA, Ayala G, et al. Role of calcium and beta-adrenergic system in control of parathyroid hormone secretion. *Proc Soc Exp Biol Med* 1976;151:320–328.

76. Caro JF, Castro JH, Glennon JA. Effect of long term propranolol administration on parathyroid hormone and calcium concentration in primary hyperparathyroidism. *Ann Intern Med* 1979;91:740–741.

77. Monson JP, Beer M, Boucher BJ, et al. Propranolol in primary hyperthyroidism. *Lancet* 1979;1:884.

78. Sherwood JK, Ackroyd FW, Garcia M. Effect of cimetidine on circulating parathyroid hormone in primary hyperparathyroidism. *Lancet* 1980;1:616–620.

79. Palmer FJ, Sawyers TM, Wierzbinski SJ. Cimetidine and hyperparathyroidism. *N Engl J Med* 1980;302:692.

80. Awoke S, Lawrence GD. Cimetidine and hyperparathyroidism. *Lancet* 1980;1:1134.

81. Gallagher JC, Nordin BEC. Treatment with estrogens of primary hyperparathyroidism in post-menopausal women. *Lancet* 1972;1:503–507.

82. Marcus R, Modvig P, Crim M, et al. Conjugated estrogens in the treatment of post menopausal women with hyperparathyroidism. *Ann Intern Med* 1984;100:633–640.

83. Fleisch H, Felix R. Diphosphonates. *Calcif Tissue Int* 1979;27:91–94.

84. Kaplan RA, Gero WB, Poindexter C. Metabolic effects of diphosphonate in primary hyperparathyroidism. *J Clin Pharmacol* 1977;17:410–419.

85. Shane E, Baquiran DC, Bilezikian JP. Effect of dichloromethylene diphosphonate on serum and urinary calcium in primary hyperparathyroidism. *Ann Intern Med* 1981;95:23–27.

86. Mundy GR, Wilkinson R, Heath DA. Comparative study of available medical therapy for hypercalcemia of malignancy. *Am J Med* 1983;74:421–432.

87. Albright F, Bauet W, Claflin D, et al. Studies in parathyroid physiology. *J Clin Invest* 1932;11:411–435.

88. Goldsmith RS, Ingbar SH. Inorganic phosphate treatment of hypercalcemia of diverse etiologies. *N Engl J Med* 1966;274:1.

89. Purnell DC, Scholz DA, Smith LH, et al. Treatment of primary hyperparathyroidism. *Am J Med* 1974;56:800–810.

90. Broadus AE, Magee JS, Mallette LE. A detailed evaluation of oral phosphate therapy in selected patients with primary hyperparathyroidism. *J Clin Endocrinol Metab* 1983;56:953–961.

The Parathyroids, edited by J.P. Bilezikian,
M.A. Levine, and R. Marcus. Raven Press, Ltd.,
New York © 1994.

CHAPTER 31

Medical Management of Primary Hyperparathyroidism

John L. Stock and Robert Marcus

Surgery is the treatment of choice for patients with symptomatic primary hyperparathyroidism (PHP) (1–3). Although the role of medical management for asymptomatic PHP is still controversial (3), there are subsets of symptomatic patients who clearly benefit from medical rather than surgical intervention. These include patients who refuse surgery, are too ill for surgery, have had unsuccessful previous neck explorations (4), or have inoperable parathyroid carcinoma (5,6). Occasionally, a trial of medical therapy to normalize the serum calcium concentration can assist the patient and physician in deciding whether symptoms are related to hypercalcemia (7). Patients may require stabilization of severe hypercalcemia prior to surgery (4). In its most extreme form, this has been called *parathyroid crisis* or *acute PHP* (see the chapter by Fitzpatrick) (8).

This chapter describes the nonsurgical modalities available for the treatment of PHP. After an introduction to the general principles of medical care for patients with PHP, specific agents that decrease parathyroid hormone (PTH) action and/or decrease PTH secretion are discussed.

GENERAL PRINCIPLES

The general principles of medical treatment of symptomatic hypercalcemia in PHP are the same as those for the treatment of symptomatic hypercalcemia

of any etiology (9,10). Patients with PHP may be volume depleted due to decreased oral intake and increased renal losses of free water. Immediate rehydration and treatment of nausea and vomiting followed by saline diuresis usually result in a prompt fall in the serum calcium concentration. The acute treatment of hospitalized patients with intravenous saline and furosemide has been well studied (9,11), but the value of salt and water loading and chronic oral furosemide in the outpatient setting is not well documented. Potential complications of this therapy include congestive heart failure if salt loading is too vigorous, prerenal azotemia with worsening of hypercalcemia if excessive diuretics are used, and other electrolyte abnormalities (see the chapter by Bilezikian and Singer) (12,13).

Thiazides and related diuretics, including metolazone and indapamide, actually decrease calcium excretion at distal tubular sites and should be discontinued in patients with PHP (12,13). Lithium carbonate may also decrease urinary calcium excretion (14), and direct effects of the drug on the parathyroid glands may contribute further to hypercalcemia. Short-term administration of lithium carbonate decreases the sensitivity of parathyroid cells to inhibition by calcium; chronic administration of this drug may predispose to development of parathyroid adenomas (14). At the least, lithium toxicity, if present, should be corrected in any patient with PHP, but the discontinuation of this psychotropic drug is often problematic and depends on the underlying psychiatric diagnosis and other available options for therapy.

Immobilization is known to result in hypercalciuria and hypercalcemia as a consequence of increased bone resorption and decreased bone formation (15), and patients with PHP should be instructed to avoid sustained bed rest and to increase their general levels of activity. Although the hypercalcemia of PHP is pre-

J. L. Stock: Endocrinology Division, The Medical Center of Central Massachusetts, Worcester, Massachusetts 01605.

R. Marcus: Department of Medicine, Stanford University School of Medicine, Stanford, California 94305; and Aging Study Unit, Veterans Affairs Medical Center, Palo Alto, California 94304.

dominantly related to increased bone resorption, a component of the hypercalcemia may be sensitive to diet. Some patients with PHP show hyperabsorption in a calcium tolerance test, hypercalciuria, and elevated 1,25-dihydroxyvitamin D_3 [1,25(OH)$_2$D$_3$] levels (16). However, in another study of 18 unselected patients with PHP, a high (1,000 mg)-calcium diet suppressed PTH and 1,25(OH)$_2$D$_3$ levels in some subjects (17). Thus the benefits of a low-calcium diet might include a lower urinary calcium excretion in certain patients, but should be balanced by a concern about bone loss. The benefit of a higher calcium diet might be to suppress parathyroid function and thus theoretically delay progression of disease in a subset of patients, but could be offset by an increase in urinary calcium excretion in some of these subjects. There are currently no long-term studies that allow one individually to tailor dietary recommendations, and we suggest a moderate intake of dietary calcium in most patients with PHP.

SPECIFIC PHARMACOLOGIC THERAPY

Phosphate

Albright et al. (18) described the use of oral phosphate for the treatment of PHP in 1932. In elegant metabolic studies of three patients, he attributed the fall in serum calcium levels and urinary calcium excretion with phosphate therapy to the rise in the Ca × P product in the serum. He also predicted the theoretical dangers of such therapy: "parathyroid poisoning," or the deposition of calcium deposits in the kidney and other organs with resultant uremia, as well as the risk of producing phosphate kidney stones. In 1966 Goldsmith and Ingbar (19) described the short-term use of oral phosphate in four patients with PHP, with a resultant decline in the serum calcium concentration in all and actual normalization of the serum calcium concentration in one subject. More recently, 14 subjects with persistent or recurrent PHP were given 1.0–2.5 g elemental phosphorus daily by mouth for up to 51 months (20). In seven patients with serum calcium levels >11.0 mg/dl, the serum calcium normalized in one, decreased in four, and was unchanged in two after 1 month of therapy. Although these effects were generally sustained with more long-term treatment, an increase in serum creatinine levels was noted in three patients. In those patients affected by nephrolithiasis, there appeared to be a palliative effect on the disease progression. In patients with milder disease and a serum calcium concentration <11.0 mg/dl, phosphate treatment had no effect on serum calcium or creatinine levels. The mechanisms of the effects of oral phosphate therapy were investigated in a series of ten patients with PHP and elevated serum levels of

1,25(OH)$_2$D$_3$ who received 1,500 mg elemental phosphorus daily for 1 year (21). Phosphate treatment led to a decrease in serum 1,25(OH)$_2$D$_3$ levels, the calciuric response to an oral calcium tolerance test, and urinary calcium excretion, suggesting a decrease in calcium hyperabsorption in these subjects (Fig. 1). No untoward clinical events were noted, but circulating immunoreactive PTH and nephrogenous cyclic adenosine monophosphate (cAMP) excretion increased. No definitive skeletal effects were documented other than a trend toward a reduction in bone turnover in

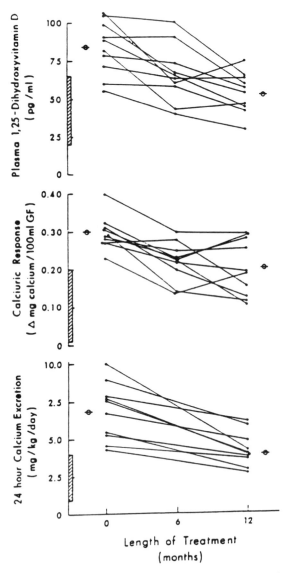

FIG. 1. Effect of oral phosphate (1,500 mg elemental phosphorus daily) on the plasma 1,25(OH)$_2$D$_3$ concentration, calciuric response to an oral calcium tolerance test, and 24 hr calcium excretion (mg per kg/day) in ten patients with PHP. (Subjects consumed a 1,000 mg calcium diet.) The *hatched bars* adjoining the ordinates represent normal ranges, and the *circles with slashes* are the mean values. (Reprinted from ref. 21 with permission.)

those patients with increased bone resorption before therapy. These results suggest that the effect of phosphate therapy to lower serum calcium is more complex than just a lowering of the Ca × P product and includes also a decrease in calcium absorption mediated by the fall in 1,25(OH)₂D₃ and probable complex effects on bone metabolism.

The conclusion from these studies is that oral phosphate therapy may have a role in the treatment of a few, select patients with PHP, but the long-term consequences on renal function and bone metabolism are still not well established. An additional concern is the possibility of ectopic calcification in other soft tissues such as lung, gastric mucosa, blood vessels, and myocardium (22).

Estrogens and Progestins

Other pharmacologic therapies that lower the serum and/or urinary calcium excretion in patients with PHP may be divided into two categories: those that act primarily by inhibiting the effects of parathyroid hormone on bone resorption or those that decrease parathyroid hormone secretion.

Drugs or hormones that inhibit the effects of PTH on bone resorption have been most effective in treating PHP. A salutary effect on calcium metabolism may be noted in postmenopausal women with PHP treated with estrogen-replacement therapy. In 1972 Gallagher and Nordin (23) gave ten such women ethinyl estradiol (50 μg/day, 3 weeks out of 4) for up to 1 year and noted gradual decreases in fasting plasma calcium concentration and in urinary calcium and hydroxyproline excretion, suggesting an inhibitory effect of estrogen on PTH-mediated bone resorption (Fig. 2). A follow-up study of eight women confirmed these findings and also documented an improved calcium balance and a decrease in bone mineralization and resorption rates in most subjects (24).

In 1984 Marcus et al. (25) treated 14 postmenopausal women with conjugated estrogen (0.625–2.5 mg/day) for up to 1 year. Four women also received cyclic medroxyprogesterone acetate. Ten subjects responded with a decrease in serum calcium levels. There were no changes noted in serum PTH or 1,25(OH)₂D₃ levels, or in urinary cAMP excretion. Decrements in the serum alkaline phosphatase activity and urinary hydroxyproline and calcium excretion suggested that estrogen inhibited the effects of PTH on bone turnover. Iliac crest bone biopsy specimens in subjects responding to estrogen showed maintenance of bone volume but no significant change in hyperosteoidosis after 1 year of therapy. A few subjects demonstrated typical minor side effects of estrogen, including breast tenderness, vaginal bleeding, and mild increases in blood pressure. Ten year follow-up data on these subjects was recently reported (26). Of the ten initial responders, seven continued to have normal serum calcium levels and urinary calcium excretion, although three of them elected to have parathyroidectomy because of their desire to stop regular surveillance. One subject stopped estrogen because of concerns about malignancy, and two were lost to follow-up.

Selby and Peacock (27) reported a series of 17 postmenopausal women with PHP treated with ethinyl estradiol (30 μg/day) for 3 weeks. Despite a decrease in serum calcium concentrations and in fasting urinary calcium and hydroxyproline excretion, there were no changes in serum levels of PTH, calcitonin, or calculated free 1,25(OH)₂D₃ or in urinary cAMP excretion. Except for a small increase in the calculated free 1,25(OH)₂D₃ concentration, these metabolic changes were maintained for a longer 3 month follow-up period. These results confirmed the efficacy of estrogen in the treatment of the biochemical abnormalities of

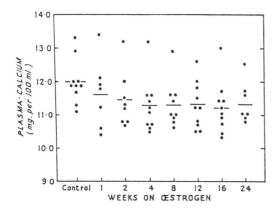
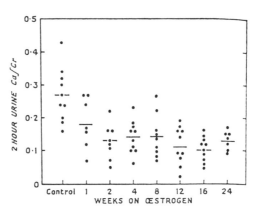

FIG. 2. Effects of ethinyl estradiol (50 μg/day, 3 weeks out of 4) on the plasma calcium concentration **(left)** and on the fasting urine calcium/creatinine ratio in ten postmenopausal women with PHP **(right)**. (Reprinted from ref. 23 with permission.)

PHP and suggested that their action was mediated by resetting the threshold for PTH secretion.

Transdermal estrogen appears to be effective in slowing bone loss in postmenopausal women with osteoporosis (28) but has not been studied in patients with PHP. Estrogen analogs with lower estrogenicity have been used to treat PHP. The synthetic stilbestrol derivative cyclofenil was given to six women and two men with PHP for 5–13 weeks, and reductions in serum calcium and urinary calcium and hydroxyproline were noted (29). Methallenestril was given to six postmenopausal women with PHP for 5–24 weeks with similar results (30). The antiestrogen tamoxifen was given to a postmenopausal patient with PHP and breast cancer, and a decrease in the activity of alkaline phosphatase and serum ionized calcium and an upward trend in PTH concentration were noted (31). Other studies in postmenopausal women have documented the agonistic effects of tamoxifen on bone (32) and lipids (33) and beneficial effects of tamoxifen on cardiovascular mortality (34). Further investigation of tamoxifen in the treatment of postmenopausal women with PHP who are not candidates for estrogen-replacement therapy is warranted.

Progestins may also have similar effects on bone and mineral metabolism in patients with PHP. Selby and Peacock (27) treated 11 postmenopausal women with the androgenic progestin norethindrone (5 mg/day) and found the same beneficial effects as noted above in their group treated with ethinyl estradiol. Horowitz et al. (35) treated 20 postmenopausal women with PHP with the same regimen of norethindrone for 3 months, with no apparent side effects and confirmed the decrease in serum calcium and urinary calcium excretion. There was no change in calcium absorption, and forearm mineral density increased. A 2 year follow-up was reported for 15 of these women. Fat-corrected forearm bone mineral content increased 1.9% per year, with most of the gain occurring in the first 6 months (Fig. 3) (36). This increase might simply represent a reduction in the remodeling space, in which case it would not be expected to continue. Longer term studies will be necessary to define fully these effects on bone mass.

The beneficial effects of progestins may be limited to those agents with androgenic properties. Marcus (26) reported that serum calcium and phosphorus concentrations, alkaline phosphatase activity, and urinary calcium and hydroxyproline excretion were unchanged in six women and two men treated with the nonandrogenic C-21 progestin medroxyprogesterone acetate (10 mg/day for 2 months followed by 20 mg/day for 2 months).

The risk-benefit equation for determining the use of hormonal replacement therapy is complex. Unopposed estrogen increases the risk of endometrial hy-

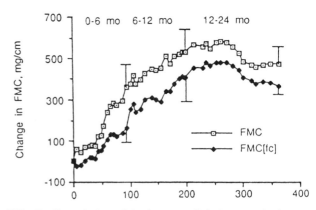

FIG. 3. Cumulative plot of sequential changes in forearm mineral content (FMC) and fat-corrected FMC (FMC[fc]) in 15 postmenopausal women with PHP treated with norethindrone (5 mg/day). Each line segment represents an individual case, in which change in FMC is plotted against duration of observation in months. Shown are standard errors for the cumulative sum rates of change between 0 and 6 months, 6 and 12 months, and 12 and 24 months. (Reprinted from ref. 36 with permission.)

perplasia and carcinoma. The effect of estrogen on the incidence of breast cancer is controversial (37). The reduction in serum phosphorus levels as a result of estrogen (or progestin) therapy raises the theoretical risk of osteomalacia (26).

The benefits of estrogen replacement therapy include reduction of symptoms of estrogen deficiency, such as hot flashes and vaginal atrophy; improvement in the lipid profile; and decreased risk of ischemic heart disease (38) as well as the lowering of serum calcium levels and urinary calcium excretion. Progestins may adversely affect the lipid profile and cardiovascular risk. As with estrogen, they may lower serum calcium levels and urinary calcium excretion, and already there are data showing their benefit in decreasing bone turnover. Given this complexity, the use of hormonal therapy should be individualized, based on an assessment and discussion with the patient of risk and benefit. Further prospective, controlled trials investigating the effects of estrogen, tamoxifen, and progestins on mineral metabolism, bone density and histomorphometry, cardiovascular morbidity, and risk of breast cancer are needed to resolve these issues.

Bisphosphonates

Bisphosphonates are pyrophosphate analogs that bind to hydroxyapatite and inhibit osteoclastic bone resorption. These drugs have been used for many years in the treatment of Paget's disease and more recently in the management of hypercalcemia of malignancy and osteoporosis (39). Chronic oral use of bisphosphonates in patients with PHP would theoretically be limited by their poor absorption and potential for causing osteomalacia (39). However, several new bisphosphonate analogs, which are more potent and cause fewer mineralization abnormalities, may become therapeutic options in the medical management of PHP.

Etidronate (EHDP), the first widely available bisphosphonate, was given to six patients with PHP by Kaplan et al. in 1977 (40). After 5 weeks of a relatively high oral dose (20 mg/kg/day), the serum calcium concentration decreased in only one subject, and this was not maintained after 6 months of treatment. The urinary calcium excretion decreased in three patients, and this was maintained in two of them after 6 months of treatment. There was a significant decrease in urinary hydroxyproline excretion in all subjects, which was more sustained at 6 months. There were no significant changes in serum PTH levels, urinary cAMP excretion, fractional calcium absorption, or bone density of the distal radius measured by single photon absorptiometry. Due to the inefficacy of EHDP in correcting hypercalcemia, there has been little further interest in its use in the management of PHP, other than a case report of a patient who responded to intermittent administration of a lower dose (5 mg/kg) (41).

Clodronate (Cl$_2$MDP), a more potent, second-generation bisphosphonate with little effect on bone mineralization, is currently available in Europe for the treatment of hypercalcemia. Shane et al. (42) treated 14 patients with PHP with Cl$_2$MDP by mouth (1.6 g/day) for 12 weeks in a double-blind, placebo-controlled, crossover design. The mean serum calcium concentration dropped significantly from 11.5 mg/dl to 10.8 mg/dl during treatment and remained below initial pretreatment levels 3 months after drug was discontinued (Fig. 4). There were also significant declines in urinary excretion of calcium and hydroxyproline, and no changes in serum PTH or urinary cAMP excretion were observed. Douglas et al. (43) treated nine patients with Cl$_2$MDP by mouth (1.0–3.2 g/day) for 2–32 weeks in an open study design. There were significant decreases in serum calcium levels to the upper normal range and in urinary calcium and hydroxyproline excretion into the normal range. The fall in serum calcium concentration was not sustained in three subjects who were followed for more than 19 weeks. Similar results were found by Hamdy et al. (44), who treated 20 PHP patients with Cl$_2$MDP (0.8–1.6 g/day by mouth) for 8 weeks. As in the previous study, the serum calcium levels tended to increase in the 12 patients who were treated with a more prolonged, 12 week course of therapy, despite a sustained fall in the parameters of bone resorption. Adami et al. (45) also noted a temporary and inconsistent effect of Cl$_2$MDP on serum calcium levels in 27 patients with PHP treated with Cl$_2$MDP by mouth or parenterally for up to 180 days. The drug appeared most effective in those subjects with marked bone resorption, and prolonged therapy was associated with a rise in serum PTH concentrations. These studies consistently suggest a partial short-term effect of Cl$_2$MDP on serum calcium levels related to an inhibition of bone resorption. The incompleteness of this effect most likely relates to the unopposed effect of PTH on renal tubular resorption of calcium. The consistent late rise in serum calcium concentrations may be due to a secondary decrease in bone formation, which has not been substantiated, as well as to a further increase in renal tubular calcium reabsorption due to the rise in circulating PTH (44,45). Thus, Cl$_2$MDP does not appear to be very useful in the long-term management of hypercalcemia of PHP, although its partial short-term effects on serum calcium

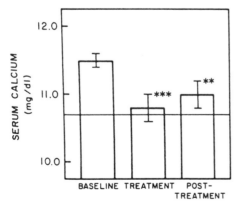 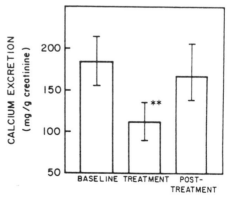

FIG. 4. Effects of Cl$_2$MDP (1.6 g/day by mouth) on the serum calcium concentration and urinary calcium excretion in 14 patients with PHP. The values shown represent the means (±SEM) for the entire group of patients. Mean treatment values for serum calcium ($P < 0.001$) and urinary calcium excretion ($P < 0.01$) and mean posttreatment serum calcium levels were significantly different from baseline. The *horizontal line* indicates the upper limits of normal for serum calcium concentration (10.7 mg/dl). (Reproduced from ref. 42 with permission.)

levels suggest a possible role for the intravenous use of this drug in the acute management of life-threatening hypercalcemia before surgery.

Similar transient effects of lowering the serum calcium in PHP have been noted with pamidronate (APD), another second-generation bisphosphonate. Schmidli et al. (7) treated ten patients with mild PHP with a single intravenous dose of APD (30 mg) in a randomized single-blind, placebo-controlled, crossover design. The serum calcium concentration decreased in nine of the ten subjects, and a decrease in urinary calcium excretion and an increase in circulating serum PTH were noted after 7 days. Although there were no changes in hypercalcemic symptoms, muscle strength, cognitive function, or blood pressure in these patients with mild PHP, this approach might be useful in surgical candidates for whom it is not clear whether their symptoms are related to the hypercalcemia. Jansson et al. (46) treated nine elderly PHP patients with a single intravenous infusion of APD (15–60 mg) (46). Six of the patients had severe hypercalcemia, and three were in hypercalcemic crisis, due in one instance to parathyroid carcinoma. After 1 week, seven patients were normocalcemic or mildly hypocalcemic and two patients had serum calcium levels at the upper limits of normal (Fig. 5). Monthly infusions in two patients for up to 9 months maintained serum calcium levels at the upper limit of normal. There have been other reports of the successful acute treatment of parathyroid crisis using intravenous infusion of APD (47). Although transient elevations in body temperature and decrease in lymphocyte counts are described after APD treatment of patients with hypercalcemia of malignancy, minimal side effects were noted in subjects with PHP. There are few studies investigating the chronic use of APD in PHP, although animal experiments suggest a protective effect on bone loss (48).

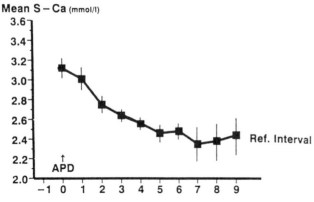

FIG. 5. Mean serum calcium concentration (± SEM) before and after a single intravenous infusion of APD (15–60 mg) in nine patients with PHP. (Reprinted from ref. 46 with permission.)

However, chronic use of APD will be limited because it is unlikely to become available as an oral agent.

Of the currently available bisphosphonates, APD appears to be the most effective in the acute management of the hypercalcemia associated with PHP. The long-term benefits of other second-generation bisphosphonates in the medical management of PHP are promising but not yet proven. A third generation of bisphosphonates, now entering clinical trials, may become useful in the treatment of PHP.

Calcitonin

The peptide hormone calcitonin inhibits osteoclastic bone resorption and increases renal calcium excretion. Human calcitonin and the more potent fish-derived calcitonins have been successfully used to treat hypercalcemia, particularly in patients with malignancy, taking advantage of their rapidity of action and good safety profile (9). However, their general use has been limited by low potency and short-lived effects. Torring et al. (49) treated 13 patients with histologically confirmed PHP with salmon calcitonin by either intranasal or intramuscular administration. Intramuscular calcitonin (100 IU) lowered the mean blood ionized calcium concentration for up to 12 hr, but three subjects did not respond. Intranasal administration of up to 400 IU calcitonin led to only minimal decreases in blood ionized calcium levels, with no overall effect after 24 hr on integrated blood calcium levels. Stone et al. (50) administered salmon calcitonin to 20 patients with biochemical evidence for PHP, either by a single intramuscular injection (100 IU) or by daily intravenous infusion over 5 days (100 IU/day). The serum calcium concentrations were slightly but significantly lower after 5 days in both groups. The response to the intravenous infusions was greater than that to the single intramuscular injection, possibly because of the enhanced renal effects of intravenous calcitonin. The expected attenuation of the hypocalcemic response with time was noted after only 2 days of infusions. These studies suggest that the chronic use of calcitonin for the treatment of PHP would be limited by its low potency, short-term efficacy, and inconvenient routes of administration.

Pharmacologic Agents That Decrease PTH Secretion

Pharmacologic agents that decrease PTH secretion should theoretically correct most of the manifestations of PHP. This approach is more disease-specific than the maneuvers described earlier, which deal primarily with the consequences of PTH action on bone and/or kidney. In reality, however, these agents have been less effective and more problematic than those that inhibit bone resorption and/or the renal reabsorption of calcium.

Based on animal models suggesting sympathetic nervous system control of PTH secretion, Kukreja et al. in 1975 (51) showed that injections of the β-adrenergic agonists isoproterenol and epinephrine in man increased and injections of the β-adrenergic antagonist propranolol decreased circulating PTH, although neither significantly affected serum calcium concentrations. Brown et al. (52), working in Dr. Aurbach's laboratory, demonstrated the presence of β-adrenergic receptors in parathyroid cells obtained from human parathyroid adenomas and hyperplastic glands. Most subsequent studies failed to show any consistent effects of propranolol on serum concentrations of PTH or calcium in patients with PHP (53–55) or in normal individuals (55). The lack of importance of the sympathetic nervous system in parathyroid regulation in vivo (55) or pathologic changes in PHP causing a loss of responsiveness to β-adrenergic agents (53) have been offered as explanations for these consistently negative results.

Documentation of functional H_2 receptors for histamine in pathologic parathyroid tissue (56) led to attempts to treat PHP with the H_2 receptor antagonist cimetidine. Although a preliminary study of 12 patients showed a normalization of the serum PTH and a variable decrease in the serum calcium concentration (57), subsequent efforts have shown consistently negative results (58–62). Similarly, although there is in vitro evidence for serotonergic modulation of parathyroid function, treatment of PHP with the serotonin antagonist cyproheptadine has not been successful (63).

More recently, the demonstration that $1,25(OH)_2D_3$ directly inhibits PTH gene transcription (64) led to a clinical trial of the analog 1α-hydroxyvitamin D_3 in 31 patients with mild PHP (65). Circulating levels of PTH were only transiently lowered when 1α-hydroxyvitamin D_3 was given in high doses and the serum calcium concentration increased. In a preliminary report, $1,25(OH)_2D_3$ (3–6 μg/week by intravenous injection for 8–10 weeks) was administered to nine postmenopausal women with PHP (66). The circulating serum PTH decreased in all patients and the serum calcium levels decreased by 20–22% in the six patients who responded. Decrements in fasting urinary calcium excretion and urinary deoxypyridinium cross-link excretion were also noted. These preliminary results suggest that parenterally administered $1,25(OH)_2D_3$ might be effective in decreasing parathyroid gland function and lowering the serum calcium levels in PHP. Analogs of $1,25(OH)_2D_3$, such as 22-oxacalcitriol, which suppress PTH secretion but do not have calcemic activity (67), offer another potential approach to the treatment of PHP.

In 1983 Glover et al. (68) demonstrated that the ra-

dioprotective organic thiophosphate agent WR-2721 inhibited PTH release from dispersed bovine parathyroid cells in vitro. This drug administered intravenously has been used successfully in the treatment of hypercalcemia of malignancy, including parathyroid carcinoma, where its use is accompanied by a decrease in PTH levels (68–70). In a preliminary report, seven patients with PHP received a single dose of WR-2721 (400 mg by intravenous injection), and the mean serum calcium concentration dropped significantly from 11.6 to 10.6 mg/dl after 24 hr, but in the absence of a significant change in circulating PTH (71). Thus, in addition to its possible effects on PTH secretion, WR-2721 may cause a PTH-independent inhibition of renal tubular calcium reabsorption (67). The late Dr. Maurice Attie, after training in Dr. Aurbach's laboratory, also demonstrated direct inhibitory effects of WR-2721 on bone resorption (72). The multiple sites of action of this drug may explain its increased efficacy compared with other agents, which only inhibit PTH secretion. However, it is unlikely that WR-2721 will ever become an attractive medical approach to PHP because of debilitating side effects, including nausea, vomiting, somnolence, and hypotension (68).

SPECIFIC SITUATIONS

Parathyroid Crisis

Although most patients with PHP have chronic mild hypercalcemia, concomitant dehydration, immobilization, other intercurrent illnesses, or drug therapy, occasionally lead to severe, potentially life-threatening hypercalcemia (8) (see the chapter by Fitzpatrick). The approach to lowering the serum calcium concentration in a patient with parathyroid crisis is similar to the approach to life-threatening hypercalcemia of any etiology (see the chapter by Bilezikian and Singer). In addition, parathyroid surgery should follow correction of the hypercalcemia as soon as the patient's condition permits.

Although the usual nonspecific measures of rehydration and diuresis are helpful and should be part of any initial therapeutic approach to severe hypercalcemia, specific pharmacologic agents are also beneficial in decreasing the effects of PTH on bone and/or kidney. Intravenous infusions of the bisphosphonate APD have been used successfully to lower the serum calcium in several patients with parathyroid crisis (46,47). As was previously discussed, parenteral administration of salmon calcitonin might safely achieve a rapid, albeit short-lived and incomplete, improvement of hypercalcemia (73). The intravenous administration of gallium nitrate inhibits PTH-mediated bone resorption. This drug has been used to treat severe hypercalcemia associated with parathyroid carcinoma (74). Experience with gallium nitrate, however, is limited. The potential for nephrotoxicity necessitates maintenance of hydration and avoidance of concomitant use of other nephrotoxic drugs (9). Plicamycin (mithramycin) administered intravenously also decreases PTH-mediated bone resorption by inhibiting osteoclast function. Plicamycin has been effective in the treatment of parathyroid crisis (75) and in the control of hypercalcemia associated with parathyroid carcinoma (76), but its prolonged use is limited by the potential for nephrotoxicity and thrombocytopenia (9). Phosphate administered intravenously has also been used to treat parathyroid crisis but is dangerous because of the risk of ectopic calcification in blood vessels, lungs, and kidney, which may lead to organ failure and fatal hypotension (9).

Pregnancy

Clinically apparent PHP is unusual during pregnancy, but it has been described in association with maternal pancreatitis and hypercalcemic crisis as well as with neonatal hypocalcemia and tetany (77,78). Parathyroidectomy during the second trimester has been suggested for women with progressive symptoms (77,79) and by others for all patients with PHP (80). Medical therapy has been proposed for patients with mild hypercalcemia, although the specific risks to the fetus of untreated mild maternal hypercalcemia have not been well documented. The use of oral phosphate has been described in several pregnant women who were not surgical candidates (81). In one case report, intravenous administration of magnesium to treat preeclampsia in a patient with PHP and acute pancreatitis also normalized the serum calcium concentration (78). Most of the usual pharmacologic agents used to treat hypercalcemia have not been studied during pregnancy. Anecdotal experience suggests that a nonsurgical, nonpharmacological approach to mild PHP in pregnancy is safe and well tolerated.

SUMMARY AND CONCLUSIONS

There is currently no ideal long-term medical management for PHP. The best studied treatment has been estrogen, which remains an excellent option for selected postmenopausal women. The potent orally administered second- and third-generation bisphosphonates appear to be promising. There are currently several potential options for short-term medical treatment of PHP in patients who need therapy before surgery, in parathyroid crisis, or with parathyroid carcinoma: a second-generation bisphosphonate, parenteral administration of calcitonin, or plicamycin.

Even if an effective long-term therapy is developed for PHP, issues of cost and compliance must be addressed given the relatively inexpensive and effective surgical treatment available. There have been no prospective randomized clinical trials assessing the clinical benefit, cost-benefit, or cost-effectiveness of any surgical or medical treatment for PHP (3,82). Most of the cost estimates of this disease have not included a specific cost for a potential pharmacologic therapy. The expense of follow-up testing, combined with drug treatment, would be interesting to compare to the expense of surgery (82,83). Such a cost-benefit analysis would also have to take into consideration the potential risks of surgery, the availability of expert parathyroid surgeons, and the prospects of unsuccessful parathyroid surgery in hospitals that are not fortunate enough to have those with requisite surgical expertise.

As a minimum, patients whose PHP would ordinarily lead to surgery but who do not undergo parathyroidectomy should be followed similarly to patients with mild, asymptomatic PHP (3). This would include semiannual follow-up until lack of disease progression has been established and then annual follow-up evaluations. Along with interval history and physical examination, serum calcium and creatinine levels, creatinine clearance, 24 hr urinary calcium excretion, and bone density determinations are recommended. More frequent monitoring for potential side effects is tailored to the individual and to the pharmacologic therapy, if any, being used.

Compliance with long-term medical follow-up is also an issue. No long-term prospective data have satisfactorily addressed this point, yet, in most reported series of patients with asymptomatic PHP, a small but significant percentage of subjects are lost to follow-up. Heath and Heath (84) found that 13 of 122 of their conservatively managed, mostly asymptomatic patients with PHP seen over a 10 year period in Birmingham, England, were lost to follow-up. Of 142 patients with mild, asymptomatic PHP in Rochester, Minnesota, who were followed prospectively for 10 years by Scholz and Purnell (85), ten refused follow-up evaluations and nine others could not be traced. Marcus reported that only four of the ten estrogen-responsive patients originally reported (25) were controlled on therapy 5 years later (26). Three well-controlled patients elected to undergo surgery because they wanted to stop regular surveillance, one subject discontinued estrogen because of concerns about malignancy, and two patients were lost to follow-up.

When data on compliance become available, it will be important to consider whether an expected "dropout" rate is acceptable and who exactly is "dropping out." If it is likely that asymptomatic patients who show no manifestations of disease except mildly abnormal biochemical indices are the ones most likely to be lost to follow-up, studies will be needed to ascertain whether this lack of compliance is detrimental. One could argue that this conservative, nonsurgical approach to patients with asymptomatic PHP can tolerate a certain dropout rate because, after all, before the multichannel analyzer, these patients were all unknown or undiscovered and were not followed. Presumably, the great majority of these patients who never came to medical attention never suffered adverse consequences of PHP.

Definitive recommendations for long-term medical management of PHP must await well-controlled, prospective studies of specific medical therapies compared to surgery. The clinical application of recently developed specific PTH antagonists (86) and vitamin D analogs (67), as well as the development of other more potent pharmacologic agents that block the action of PTH at multiple sites, hold the greatest promise for future approaches to PHP.

REFERENCES

1. Clark OH, Wilkes W, Siperstein AE, Duh Q-Y. Diagnoses and management of asymptomatic hyperparathyroidism: safety, efficacy, and deficiencies in our knowledge. *J Bone Mineral Res* 1991;6(Suppl 2):S135–S152.
2. Wells SA Jr. Surgical therapy of patients with primary hyperparathyroidism: long-term benefits. *J Bone Mineral Res* 1991;6(Suppl 2):S143–S149.
3. Consensus Development Conference Panel. Diagnosis and management of asymptomatic primary hyperparathyroidism: Consensus Development Conference Statement. *Ann Intern Med* 1991;114:593–597.
4. Editorial. Medical management of primary hyperparathyroidism. *Lancet* 1984;2:727–728.
5. McCance DR, Kenny BO, Sloan JM, Russell CFJ, Hadden DR. Parathyroid carcinoma: a review. *J R Soc Med* 1987; 80:505–509.
6. Shane E, Bilezikian JP. Parathyroid carcinoma: a review. *Endocr Rev* 1982;3:218–226.
7. Schmidli RS, Wilson I, Espiner EA, Richards AM, Donald RA. Aminopropylidine diphosphonate (APD) in mild primary hyperparathyroidism: effects on clinical status. *Clin Endocrinol* 1990;32:293–300.
8. Fitzpatrick LA, Bilezekian JP. Acute primary hyperparathyroidism. *Am J Med* 1987;82:275–282.
9. Bilezekian JP. Management of acute hypercalcemia. *N Engl J Med* 1992;326:1196–1203.
10. Shane E. Medical management of asymptomatic primary hyperparathyroidism. *J Bone Mineral Res* 1991;6(Suppl 2):S131–S134.
11. Suki WN, Yium JJ, von Minden M, Saller-Hebert C, Eknoyan G, Martinez-Maldonado M. Acute treatment of hypercalcemia with furosemide. *N Engl J Med* 1970;283:836–840.
12. Stier CT, Itskovitz HD. Renal calcium metabolism and diuretics. *Annu Rev Pharmacol Toxicol* 1986;26:101–116.
13. Sutton RAL. Diuretics and calcium metabolism. *Am J Kidney Dis* 1985;5:4–9.
14. Mallette LE, Eichhorn E. Effects of lithium carbonate on human calcium metabolism. *Arch Intern Med* 1986;146:770–776.
15. Stewart AF, Adler M, Byers CM, Segre GV, Broadus AE. Calcium homeostasis in immobilization: an example of resorptive hypercalciuria. *N Engl J Med* 1982;306:1136–1140.
16. Broadus AE, Horst RL, Lang R, Littledike E, Rasmussen H. The importance of circulating 1,25-dihydroxyvitamin D in the pathogenesis of hypercalciuria and renal stone formation in primary hyperparathyroidism. *N Engl J Med* 1980;302:421–426.
17. Insogna KL, Mitnick ME, Stewart AF, Burtis WJ, Mallette LE, Broadus AE. Sensitivity of the parathyroid hormone-1,25-dihydroxyvitamin D axis to variations in calcium-intake in patients with primary hyperparathyroidism. *N Engl J Med* 1985;313:1126–1130.
18. Albright F, Baver W, Claflin D, Cockrill JR. Studies in parathyroid physiology. III. The effect of phosphate ingestion in clinical hyperparathyroidism. *J Clin Invest* 1932;11:411–435.
19. Goldsmith RS, Ingbar SH. Inorganic phosphate treatment of hypercalcemia of diverse etiologies. *N Engl J Med* 1966; 274:1–7.
20. Purnell DC, Scholz DA, Smith LM, et al. Treatment of primary hyperparathyroidism. *Am J Med* 1974;56:800–809.
21. Broadus AE, Magee JS, Mallette LE, et al. A detailed evaluation of oral phosphate therapy in selected patients with primary hyperparathyroidism. *J Clin Endocrinol Metab* 1983; 56:953–961.
22. Vernava AM III, O'Neal LW, Palermo V. Lethal hyperparathyroid crisis: hazards of phosphate administration. *Surgery* 1987;102:941–948.
23. Gallagher JC, Nordin BEC. Treatment with oestrogens of primary hyperparathyroidism in post-menopausal women. *Lancet* 1972;1:503–507.
24. Gallagher JC, Wilkinson R. The effect of ethinyloestradiol on calcium and phosphorus metabolism of post-menopausal women with primary hyperparathyroidism. *Clin Sci Mol Med* 1973;45:785–802.
25. Marcus R, Madvig P, Crim M, Pont A, Kosek J. Conjugated estrogens in the treatment of postmenopausal women with hyperparathyroidism. *Ann Intern Med* 1984;100:633–640.
26. Marcus R. Estrogens and progestins in the management of primary hyperparathyroidism. *J Bone Mineral Res* 1991; 6(Suppl 1):S125–S129.
27. Selby PL, Peacock M. Ethinyl estradiol and norethinedrone in the treatment of primary hyperparathyroidism in postmenopausal women. *N Engl J Med* 1986;314:1481–1485.
28. Lufkin EG, Wahner HW, O'Fallon WM, et al. Treatment of postmenopausal osteoporosis with transdermal estrogen. *Ann Intern Med* 1992;117:1–9.
29. Herbai G, Ljunghall S. Treatment of primary hyperparathyroidism with cyclofenil—a synthetic stilbestrol derivative with minimal feminizing effects. *Horm Metabol Res* 1984; 16:374–376.
30. Herbai G, Ljunghall S. Normalization of hypercalcemia of primary hyperparathyroidism by treatment with methallenestril, a synthetic oestrogen with low oestrogenicity. *Urol Int* 1983;38:371–373.
31. Kristensen B, Mouridsen HT, Holmegaard SN, Transbol AI. Amelioration of postmenopausal primary hyperparathyroidism during adjuvant tamoxifen for breast cancer. *Cancer* 1989;64:1965–1967.
32. Love RR, Mazess RB, Barden HS, et al. Effects of tamoxifen on bone mineral density in postmenopausal women with breast cancer. *N Engl J Med* 1992;326:852–856.
33. Bagdade JD, Wolter J, Subbaiah PV, Ryan W. Effects of tamoxifen treatment on plasma lipids and lipoprotein lipid composition. *J Clin Endocrinol Metab* 1990;70:1132–1135.
34. McDonald CC, Stewart HJ. Fatal myocardial infarction in the Scottish adjuvant tamoxifen trial. *Br Med J* 1991;303:435–437.
35. Horowitz M, Wishart J, Need AG, Morris H, Philcox J, Nordin BEC. Treatment of postmenopausal hyperparathyroidism with norethindrone. Effects on biochemistry and forearm mineral density. *Arch Intern Med* 1987;147:681–685.
36. Wishart J, Horowitz M, Need A, Chatterton B, Nordin BEC. Treatment of postmenopausal hyperparathyroidism with norethindrone. Long-term effects on forearm mineral content. *Arch Intern Med* 1990;150:1951–1953.
37. Steinberg KK, Thacker SB, Smith J, et al. A meta-analysis of the effect of estrogen replacement therapy on the risk of breast cancer. *JAMA* 1991;265:1985–1990.
38. Stampfer MJ, Colditz GA, Willett WC, et al. Postmenopausal

estrogen therapy and cardiovascular disease. Ten year follow-up from the Nurses' Health Study. *N Engl J Med* 1991; 325:756–762.

39. Fleisch H. Bisphosphonates—history and experimental basis. *Bone* 1987;8(Suppl 1):S23–S28.

40. Kaplan RA, Geho WB, Poindexter C, Haussler M, Dietz GW, Pak CYC. Metabolic effects of diphosphonate in primary hyperparathyroidism. *J Clin Pharmacol* 1977;17:410–419.

41. Licata AA, O'Hanlon E. Treatment of hyperparathyroidism with etidronate disodium. *JAMA* 1983;249:2063–2064.

42. Shane E, Baquiran DC, Bilezikian JP. Effects of dichloromethylene diphosphonate on serum and urinary calcium in primary hyperparathyroidism. *Ann Intern Med* 1981;95:23–27.

43. Douglas DL, Kanis A, Paterson AD, et al. Drug treatment of primary hyperparathyroidism: use of clodronate disodium. *Br Med J* 1983;286:587–590.

44. Hamdy NAT, Graz RES, McCloskey E, et al. Clodronate in the medical management of hyperparathyroidism. *Bone* 1987; 8(Suppl 1):S69–S77.

45. Adami S, Mian M, Bertoldo F, et al. Regulation of calcium-parathyroid hormone feedback in primary hyperparathyroidism: effects of bisphosphonate treatment. *Clin Endocrinol* 1990;33:391–397.

46. Jansson S, Tisell L-E, Lindstedt G, Lundberg P-A. Disodium pamidronate in the preoperative treatment of hypercalcemia in patients with primary hyperparathyroidism. *Surgery* 1991; 110:480–486.

47. Evans RA. Aminohydroxypropylidene diphosphonate treatment of hypercalcemic crisis due to primary hyperparathyroidism. *Aust NZ J Med* 1987;17:58–59.

48. Mitlak BH, Rodda CP, von Deck MD, Dobrolet NC, Neer RM, Nussbaum SR. Pamidronate reduces PTH-mediated bone loss in a gene transfer model of hyperparathyroidism in rats. *J Bone Mineral Res* 1991;6:1317–1321.

49. Torring O, Bucht E, Sjostedt U, Sjoberg HE. Salmon calcitonin treatment by nasal spray in primary hyperparathyroidism. *Bone* 1991;12:311–316.

50. Stone MD, Marshall DH, Hosking DJ, Garcia-Himmelstine CG, White DA, Worth HG. Comparison of low dose intramuscular and intravenous salcatonin in the treatment of primary hyperparathyroidism. *Bone* 1992;13:265–271.

51. Kukreja SC, Hargis GK, Bowser EN, Henderson WJ, Fisherman EW, Williams GA. Role of adrenergic stimuli in parathyroid hormone secretion in man. *J Clin Endocrinol Metab* 1975;40:478–481.

52. Brown EM, Gardner DG, Windeck RA, Hurwitz S, Brennan MF, Aurbach GD. β-adrenergically stimulated adenosine 3′,5′-monophosphate accumulation in and parathyroid hormone release from dispersed human parathyroid cells. *J Clin Endocrinol Metab* 1979;48:618–626.

53. Caro JF, Castro JH, Glennon JA. Effect of long-term propranolol administration on parathyroid hormone and calcium concentration in primary hyperparathyroidism. *Ann Intern Med* 1979;91:740–741.

54. Kukreja SC, Williams GA, Vora NM, Hargis GK, Bowser EN, Henderson WJ. Parathyroid hormone secretion in primary hyperparathyroidism: retained control by calcium with impaired control by β-adrenergic system. *Mineral Electrolyte Metab* 1980;3:98–103.

55. Ljunghall S, Rudberg C, Akerstrom G, Wide L. Effects of beta-adrenergic blockade on serum parathyroid hormone in normal subjects and patients with primary hyperparathyroidism. *Acta Med Scand* 1982;211:27–30.

56. Brown EM. Histamine receptors on dispersed parathyroid cells from pathologic human parathyroid tissue. *J Clin Endocrinol Metab* 1980;51:1325–1329.

57. Sherwood JK, Ackroyd FW, Garcia M. Effect of cimetidine on circulating parathyroid hormone in primary hyperparathyroidism. *Lancet* 1980;1:616–619.

58. Williams GA, Longley RS, Bowser EN, et al. Parathyroid hormone secretion in normal man and in primary hyperparathyroidism: role of histamine H₂ receptors. *J Clin Endocrinol Metab* 1981;52:122–127.

59. Robinson MF, Hayles AB, Heath H III. Failure of cimetidine

to affect calcium homeostasis in familial primary hyperparathyroidism (multiple endocrine neoplasia type I). *J Clin Endocrinol Metab* 1980;51:912–914.

60. Fisken RA, Wilkinson R, Heath DA. The effects of cimetidine on serum calcium and parathyroid hormone levels in primary hyperparathyroidism. *Br J Clin Pharmacol* 1982;14:701–705.

61. Wiske PS, Epstein S, Norton JA Jr, Bell NH, Johnston CC Jr. The effects of intravenous and oral cimetidine in primary hyperparathyroidism. *Horm Metab Res* 1983;15:245–248.

62. Kristoffersson A, Dahlgren S, Jarhult J, Wahlby L. Cimetidine does not correct circulating calcium and parathyroid hormone in primary hyperparathyroidism. *J Endocrinol Invest* 1983;6:489–491.

63. Gedik O, Usman A, Telatar F, Adalar N, Koray Z. Failure of cyproheptadine to affect calcium homeostasis and PTH levels in primary hyperparathyroidism. *Horm Metab Res* 1983; 15:616–618.

64. Silver J, Naveh-Many T, Mayer H, Schmelzer HJ, Popovtzer MM. Regulation by vitamin D metabolites of parathyroid hormone gene transcription in vivo in the rat. *J Clin Invest* 1986;78:1296–1301.

65. Lind L, Wengle B, Sorensen OH, Wide L, Akerstrom G, Ljunghall S. Treatment with active vitamin D (alpha calcidol) in patients with mild primary hyperparathyroidism. *Acta Endocrinol* 1989;120:250–256.

66. Wassif W, Nyan O, Moniz C, Parsons V. Intravenous 1,25 dihydroxy-cholecalciferol reduces serum calcium in primary hyperparathyroidism. *J Bone Mineral Res* 1991;6(Suppl 1): S176 (abstract).

67. Brown AJ, Ritter CR, Finch JL, et al. The normocalcemic analogue of vitamin D, 22-oxacalcitriol suppresses parathyroid hormone synthesis and secretion. *J Clin Invest* 1989; 84:728–732.

68. Glover D, Riley L, Carmichael K, et al. Hypocalcemia and inhibition of parathyroid hormone secretion after administration of WR-2721 (a radioprotective and chemoprotective agent). *N Engl J Med* 1983;309:1137–1141.

69. Glover DJ, Shaw L, Glick JH, et al. Treatment of hypercalcemia or parathyroid cancer with WR-2721, S-2-(3-aminopropylamino) ethyl-phosphorothioic acid. *Ann Intern Med* 1985; 103:55–57.

70. Hirschel-Scholz S, Jung A, Fischer A, Trechsel U, Bonjour J-P. Suppression of parathyroid secretion after administration of WR-2721 in a patient with parathyroid carcinoma. *Clin Endocrinol* 1985;23:313–318.

71. Morita M, Higashi K, Tajiri J, Sato T. S-2-(3-aminopropylamino)ethylphosphorothioic acid (WR-2721) in primary hyperparathyroidism. *Ann Intern Med* 1985;103:961 (letter).

72. Attie MF, Fallon MD, Spar B, Wolf JS, Slatopolsky E, Goldfarb S. Bone and parathyroid inhibitory effects of S-2(3-aminopropylamino)ethylphosphorothioic acid. *J Clin Invest* 1985; 75:1191–1197.

73. Sjoberg HE, Hjern B. Acute treatment with calcitonin in primary hyperparathyroidism and severe hypercalcemia of other origin. *Acta Chir Scand* 1975;141:90–95.

74. Warrell RP Jr, Issacs M, Alcock NW, Bockman RS. Gallium nitrate for treatment of refractory hypercalcemia from parathyroid carcinoma. *Ann Intern Med* 1987;107:683–686.

75. Perlia CP, Gubisch NJ, Wolter J, Edelberg D, Dederick MM, Taylor SG III. Mithramycin treatment of hypercalcemia. *Cancer* 1970;25:389–394.

76. Trigonis C, Cedermark B, Willems J, Hamberger B, Granberg P-O. Parathyroid carcinoma—problems in diagnosis and treatment. *Clin Oncol* 1984;10:11–19.

77. Kelly TR. Primary hyperparathyroidism during pregnancy. *Surgery* 1991;110:1028–1034.

78. Rajala B, Abbasi RA, Hutchinson HT, Taylor T. Acute pancreatitis and primary hyperparathyroidism in pregnancy: treatment of hypercalcemia with magnesium sulfate. *Obstet Gynecol* 1987;70:460–462.

79. Croom RD III, Thomas CG Jr. Primary hyperparathyroidism during pregnancy. *Surgery* 1984;96:1109–1118.

80. Kristoffersson A, Dahlgren S, Lithner F, Jarhult J. Primary hyperparathyroidism in pregnancy. *Surgery* 1985;97:326–330.

81. Montoro MN, Collea JV, Mestman JH. Management of hyperparathyroidism in pregnancy with oral phosphate therapy. *Obstet Gynecol* 1980;55:431–434.
82. Melton LJ III. Epidemiology of primary hyperparathyroidism. *J Bone Mineral Res* 1991;6(Suppl 2):S25–S29.
83. Heath H III, Hodgson SF, Kennedy MA. Primary hyperparathyroidism: incidence, morbidity, and potential economic impact in a community. *N Engl J Med* 1980;302:189–193.
84. Heath DA, Heath EM. Conservative management of primary hyperparathyroidism. *J Bone Mineral Res* 1991;6(Suppl 2):S117–S120.
85. Scholz DA, Purnell DC. Asymptomatic primary hyperparathyroidism: 10-year prospective study. *Mayo Clin Proc* 1981;56:473–478.
86. Rosenblatt M. Peptide hormone antagonists that are effective in vivo: lessons from parathyroid hormone. *N Engl J Med* 1986;315:1004–1013.

The Parathyroids, edited by J.P. Bilezikian,
M.A. Levine, and R. Marcus. Raven Press, Ltd.,
New York © 1994.

CHAPTER 32

Surgical Management of Hyperparathyroidism

Jeffrey A. Norton, Murray F. Brennan, and Samuel A. Wells, Jr.

HISTORY OF PARATHYROID PHYSIOLOGY, DISEASE, AND SURGERY

In 1880 a Swedish student named Ivar Sandstrom first described the parathyroid glands in several animal species, including man (1). In 1891 Gley removed parathyroid glands from animals and noted that subsequently the animals developed tetany (2). In 1909 MacCallum and Voegtlin noted that tetany could be treated by an infusion of calcium salts (3).

In 1891 von Recklinghausen described a characteristic disease of bone that was later found to be caused by hyperparathyroidism (4). In 1904 Askanasy studied a woman with severe bone pain and spontaneous fractures who was noted to have osteitis fibrosa cystica and parathyroid neoplasia at autopsy. In 1907 Erdheim studied several patients who had died of severe bone disease and also had parathyroid hyperplasia. He concluded that the observed parathyroid hyperplasia was secondary to the bone disease (5). Thereafter, most views held that all parathyroid tumors, whether single or multiple, developed to compensate for osseous disease. This theory was not challenged until 1915, when Schlagenhaufer argued that it was unlikely that compensatory hypertrophy would occur in a single parathyroid gland. Therefore, he stated that some parathyroid tumors were primary and that the observed bony changes were secondary (6). Schlagenhaufer's theory was confirmed in 1925 by Mandl, who removed an en-

larged parathyroid gland from a Viennese streetcar conductor (7). The patient had hypercalcemia, hypercalciuria, and radiographic evidence of generalized osteitis fibrosa cystica as well as a broken leg. After surgery, all the signs and symptoms resolved, and the patient became pain free and ambulatory. However, 6 years later, he developed recurrent disease. The patient underwent a repeat surgical procedure, which was unsuccessful. His disease progressed, and he died 3 years later. Subsequent autopsy failed to demonstrate any additional abnormal parathyroid tissue.

The first operation for parathyroid disease in the United States was performed at the Massachusetts General Hospital in 1926. The patient was a merchant marine captain, Charles Martell, with severe bone disease. Unfortunately, the abnormal gland was in the chest and was not found until the seventh operation in 1932 (8). He subsequently died of tetany during a procedure to remove a kidney stone that was impacted in the ureter. The first successful operation for parathyroid disease was performed at Barnes Hospital in St. Louis in 1929. I. Y. Olch removed a parathyroid tumor and used the term *hyperparathyroidism* to describe the disease (9). In 1934 Albright and others noted an association of parathyroid bone disease with renal stones and then identified a group of patients who had hyperparathyroidism with renal disease (either calculi or nephrocalcinosis) but no evidence of bone disease (10).

In 1925 Collip first prepared biologically active parathyroid extracts (11). In 1959 Gerald Aurbach used phenol extraction to isolate and purify parathyroid hormone (PTH) (12). In 1963, Berson, Yalow, Aurbach, and Potts developed a radioimmunoassay for PTH (13).

J. A. Norton, S. A. Wells: Department of Surgery, Washington University School of Medicine, St. Louis, Missouri 63110.

M. F. Brennan: Department of Surgery, Memorial Sloan Kettering Cancer Center, New York, New York 10025.

CLINICAL FEATURES AND INDICATIONS FOR SURGERY

The clinical and laboratory features of primary hyperparathyroidism are reviewed in detail in other chapters of this volume, as are diagnostic features and special laboratory tests. This chapter focuses on the features particularly important in planning for parathyroid surgery.

Indications for Surgery

Patients with primary hyperparathyroidism tend to have one of three forms of presentation: (a) asymptomatic hypercalcemia, (b) renal disease with nephrolithiasis or nephrocalcinosis, and/or (c) bone disease. Patients with bone disease from primary hyperparathyroidism generally have more severe hypercalcemia, fatigue, debility, bone pain, weight loss, and rarely pathological fracture and may have acute hyperparathyroidism with distinct hyperparathyroid crisis. Surgical intervention is clearly indicated for distinct, significant symptoms or signs of the disease (14,15) (Table 1). Hyperparathyroid-induced bone disease, evident as bone cysts, brown tumors, or subperiosteal resorption on X-ray, clearly warrants neck exploration and parathyroidectomy. Documented demineralization of the spine, determined by bone densitometry, warrants correction of the disease, as do documented renal forms of the disease, including nephrolithiasis, nephrocalcinosis, and impaired renal function with marked calciuria. Gastrointestinal manifestations of primary hyperparathyroidism including pancreatitis and peptic ulcer disease are also considered to be indications for surgery. Other indications for surgery include distinct neuromuscular or musculoskeletal symptoms such as proximal muscle weakness and chondrocalcinosis with pseudogout. Moderate to severe hypercalcemia (serum calcium level >12 mg/dl) is another indication for surgery, because these individuals may be at risk for hyperparathyroid crisis.

The best treatment for totally asymptomatic patients is still a subject of controversy (14). There is certainly no urgent need for surgery in this group. Regular follow-up of individuals managed medically is necessary to guard against progression of hyperparathyroidism. Studies indicate that some proportion of patients with apparently asymptomatic primary hyperparathyroidism will develop signs and symptoms with long-term follow-up (see the chapter by Kleerekoper) (16). Furthermore, an unknown proportion of asymptomatic patients may have or will develop more subtle symptoms of primary hyperparathyroidism such as memory loss, personality change, inability to concentrate, exercise fatigue, back pain, and other symptoms that are difficult to document but may totally disappear following successful surgery (15). Studies demonstrate that vague neuromuscular symptoms such as weakness are prevalent (20–60%) in patients with primary hyperparathyroidism and that successful surgery improves these symptoms in most patients (17).

In general, neck exploration is indicated for all patients with biochemical evidence of primary hyper-

TABLE 1. *Signs or symptoms of primary hyperparathyroidism that may warrant surgery*

Organ system	Sign or symptom	
	Indicated	? Indicated[a]
Skeletal	Decreased bone density Pain Pathological fracture Bone cysts Brown tumors Osteitis fibrosa cystica	Gout and pseudogout Nonspecific arthralgias
Renal	Renal colic Nephrolithiasis Nephrocalcinosis	Decreased creatinine clearance
Gastrointestinal	Peptic ulcer disease Pancreatitis	
Neurological		Emotional lability Slow mentation Poor memory Depression Easy fatigability
Neuromuscular	Proximal muscle weakness Muscle atrophy	
Other		Ectopic calcification Anemia

[a]Sign or symptom is controversial. Some may not consider it a true indication for surgery.

parathyroidism (elevated serum level of calcium and PTH) and documented signs or symptoms of the disease (Fig. 1). In young asymptomatic patients with primary hyperparathyroidism, surgery is recommended, since there is a low operative risk, and, with a long temporal exposure to primary hyperparathyroidism, these patients may be at greater risk for developing significant symptoms. In apparently asymptomatic older individuals with primary hyperparathyroidism, careful observation and follow-up are recommended, with surgery reserved for patients who develop signs and symptoms. Progression may be documented by reduced bone mineral density on serial studies, rising serum calcium level >12 mg/dl, or rising levels of bone-specific alkaline phosphatase (Fig. 1).

Clues to Pathology

Certain signs or symptoms may be helpful in predicting specific types of parathyroid pathology. Parathyroid adenoma is essentially never palpable, but parathyroid carcinoma is palpable in ~50% of patients

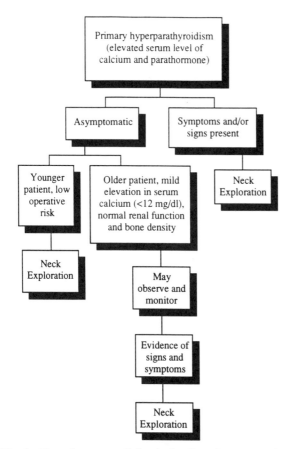

FIG. 1. Flow diagram outlining indications for surgery in patients with clear biochemical evidence of primary hyperparathyroidism.

(18,19). Markedly elevated serum levels of PTH and calcium may also suggest parathyroid carcinoma (18,19). The knowledge that an individual patient is a member of a kindred with multiple endocrine neoplasia type I or type 2a (MEN-1 or MEN-2a) indicates that the individual has parathyroid hyperplasia as a cause of hyperparathyroidism (20,21). Furthermore, there may be a wide variance in the size of the abnormal parathyroid glands in patients with HPT and MEN-I such that knowledge that an individual patient has the syndrome will aid in performance of the appropriate operation (22). Multiple lipomas are sometimes seen in patients with MEN-1, although lipomas are common and are not specific for MEN-1. There are no physical signs characteristic of MEN-2a. Recent studies have characterized the hereditary genetic defect in patients with MEN-1 and MEN-2a (see the chapters by Metz et al., Friedman et al., and Gagel). Genetic linkage studies have mapped the locus for MEN-2a to the pericentromeric region of chromosome 10 (23,24) and for MEN-1 to the long arm of chromosome 11 (25). When the precise gene locus for each of these syndromes is isolated, it will be possible to determine whether an individual patient has MEN. Currently, the disease gene has not been cloned.

Familial hypocalciuric hypercalcemia (FHH) is inherited as an autosomal dominant trait. Patients with FHH usually have asymptomatic hypercalcemia and hypocalciuria (see chapter by Heath) (26–29). The hypocalciuria differentiates it from hyperparathyroidism because patients with hyperparathyroidism are more likely to have hypercalciuria. In patients with FHH, surgery is rarely successful in correcting hypercalcemia and is contraindicated. Without 24 hr urinary calcium laboratory analyses, the only useful clue to this diagnosis is a family history of unsuccessful parathyroidectomy and/or the occurrence of hypercalcemia recognized prior to age 10 years (26–28). In such cases, measurement of urinary calcium excretion and detection of relative hypocalciuria should lead to postponing surgery and testing for mild hypercalcemia in close relatives.

Hyperparathyroid Crisis

Hyperparathyroid crisis is an unusual state of accelerated hyperparathyroidism producing anorexia, fatigue, polyuria, polydipsia, muscle weakness, vomiting, dehydration, decrease in renal function, severe hypercalcemia, altered mental status, confusion, coma, and if untreated death (see chapter by Fitzpatrick) (30,31). Hypercalcemia may have been noted in the past but not treated. Usually there is no apparent cause for acute hyperparathyroidism. However, crisis may be precipitated by bacterial or viral infection, trauma, or recent surgery. It is almost always attributable to adenoma, but parathyroid carcinoma can also cause it (19).

Acute parathyroid crisis affects males as often as females. It is usually associated with a markedly elevated plasma PTH level and significant bone disease as indicated by elevated serum levels of alkaline phosphatase. These patients also experience significant hypocalcemia postoperatively, and this is called the *hungry bone syndrome* (32).

Parathyroid crisis is a clinical emergency that requires vigorous medical management in preparation for surgery. The major defect is dehydration, and rapid hydration with intravenous normal saline usually reduces the hypercalcemia. Once fluid has been administered and adequate hydration has been accomplished, intravenous furosemide will further reduce the hypercalcemia. Furosemide should not be used until the patient is well hydrated. In patients with low serum concentration of phosphate, normal renal function, and moderate hypercalcemia, oral phosphate may also be effective. While attention and efforts are directed at lowering hypercalcemia, the diagnosis of hyperparathyroidism is established by measuring plasma levels of PTH. If hydration and treatment with furosemide are ineffective at reducing serum levels of calcium to <12 mg/dl, treatment with bisphosphonates, plicamycin, calcitonin, or gallium nitrate may be used (see the chapter, "Acute Management of Hypercalcemia due to Parathyroid Hormone- and Parathyroid Hormone-Related Protein," by Bilezikian) (31). In most cases, once the clinical condition has been stabilized with rehydration, one can complete the preoperative evaluation, confirm the diagnosis, and proceed with surgery.

PREOPERATIVE LOCALIZATION OF PARATHYROID GLANDS

Parathyroid Localization Before Initial Surgery

Ultrasound (US), computed tomography (CT), magnetic resonance imaging (MRI), and technetium/thallium scanning (thall/tech) have each been advocated by some for localization of parathyroid adenomas (see chapter by Doppman) (Table 2). Some recommend the use of noninvasive imaging studies to guide exploration in patients undergoing initial surgery. However, most experienced parathyroid surgeons attempt to identify all four parathyroid glands at the initial operation and can reliably do so with minimal morbidity (33–37). If the surgeon chooses to find and/or biopsy each parathyroid gland, preoperative localization studies do not have a significant impact on the conduct of the initial operation (38,39). Prospective studies (38,39) have evaluated this question, and each of the studies found preoperative localization to be of minor significance. Serpell et al. (40) demonstrated that correct preoperative radiographic localization of parathyroid adenoma did not even decrease the length of time of the operation.

Because these studies are expensive and are not as effective as having an experienced parathyroid surgeon (86–100%) (Table 3) in detecting abnormal parathyroid glands, imaging studies are not recommended in patients undergoing initial explorations. Localizing studies should be reserved for cases in which reoperation is necessary. Reoperations for primary hyperparathyroidism are technically more difficult, may seek a gland that is located ectopically, and are associated with more potential complications such that

TABLE 2. *Noninvasive radiographic studies for parathyroid glands[a]*

Method	Sensitivity (%)		Advantages	Disadvantages
	Initial	Reoperation		
Ultrasound	72 (57–100)[b]	46 (25–63)	Images glands adjacent or within thyroid	Observer dependent, misses mediastinal and posterior glands
Tech/Thall scintigraphy	47 (38–56)	58 (50–68)	Computer based	Misses glands removed from thyroid
Computed tomography	79 (56–89)	60 (50–77)	Observer independent anterior and posterior mediastinum	Cost
Magnetic resonance	69 (60–78)	69 (65–75)	No radiation, similar to CT, abnormal glands appear bright on T_2	Cost, images less distinct

[a]Data are from references 39,41,76,77,127–149.
[b]Number is mean; range is in parenthesis.

TABLE 3. *Results and complications of initial exploration and reoperation for primary hyperparathyroidism*

	n	Success (%)	Long-term hypoparathyroidism (%)	Vocal cord paralysis (%)	Mortality
Initial operation for adenoma					
Patow et al. (43)	77	—	—	1.3	—
Piemonte et al. (59)	71	94	2.8	0	0
Tibblin et al. (65)	102	100	2	0	0
Russel et al. (34)	90	95	—	—	—
McGarity et al. (151)	193	93	0	0	0
Russell and Edis (33)	500	92	2	<1	<1
Rudberg et al. (60)	441	84	3.4	—	1.8
Bruining (152)	562	96	—	—	—
Initial operation for hyperplasia					
Edis et al. (50)	55	87	5.4	—	—
Block et al. (51)	44	86	—	—	—
Reoperation					
Brennan and Norton (64)	106	96	—	<1	1.9
Patow et al. (43)	163	—	—	4.9	—
Edis et al. (153)	51	84	30	1.9	0
Cheung et al. (154)	83	85	9.6	1.2	1.2
Granberg et al. (155)	53	83	13	3.7	0
Bruining et al. (152)	562	96	1.2	—	—
Grant et al. (63)	157	88	14	3.8	0

correct preoperative identification of the abnormal tissue greatly improves the chances for a successful outcome. Pending the development of improved noninvasive imaging studies with fewer false-negative results that could be more widely applicable, localization studies should be reserved for patients undergoing repeat neck exploration.

Parathyroid Gland Localization Before Repeat Surgery

In patients with persistent or recurrent hyperparathyroidism, the chance of successful repeat surgery is reduced (29,41,42), and the incidence of complications is greater (43) (Table 3). Therefore, a maximum effort at precise preoperative parathyroid gland localization is necessary, commencing with noninvasive studies including a battery of studies (US, CT, MRI, technetium/thallium parathyroid scan) and proceeding, if noninvasive imaging is equivocal, to invasive studies. Some rely on the technetium/thallium scan and proceed to reoperation if that study is positive. Currently, the combination of the four noninvasive techniques, plus aspiration by direct-needle puncture for PTH assay in equivocal cases (44,45), will localize an abnormal gland in approximately three-fourths of patients requiring repeat surgery (46). The invasive procedures can be saved for the remainder of patients, and these studies usually provide some useful information (47). In centers where experienced invasive imaging is not available, the decision to proceed to a repeat operation rather than to referral should be based on the experience of the surgeon performing the initial operation and the operative findings at that initial operation. For example, the need for accurate localization following an initial operation in which four normal glands were identified by an experienced surgeon is greater than the need following brief exploration by an inexperienced surgeon in which no glands were identified.

One important consideration in the interpretation of any radiographic localization technique is that identification of a single abnormal parathyroid gland does not exclude the existence of one or more additional abnormal parathyroid glands in other locations. In fact, imaging studies seldom, if ever, localize multiple abnormal parathyroid glands. This should be remembered in interpretation of radiographic imaging results because approximately 30 percent of patients undergoing reoperations will have hyperplasia with multiple abnormal glands (42,48). This high incidence of hyperplasia must be considered by both the surgeon and the radiologist when interpreting the results of parathyroid localization studies.

Strategy of Radiographic Localization

Preoperative localization studies add expense, do not shorten operative time, and are not as sensitive as an experienced surgeon (see chapter by Doppman). The results of reoperations, following either unsuccessful initial operations or the development of recurrent hyperparathyroidism, are less satisfactory. In these patients, preoperative radiologic localization

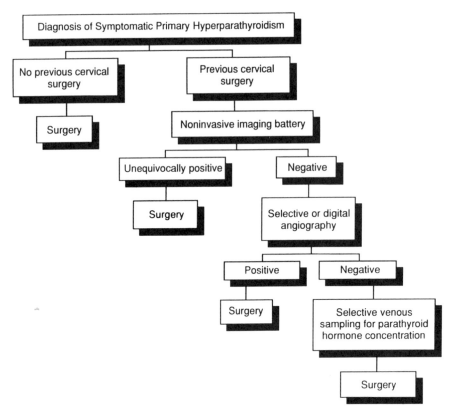

FIG. 2. Flow diagram outlining a suggested radiological localization strategy for patients with primary hyperparathyroidism undergoing reoperations. Noninvasive imaging battery includes ultrasound, CT, MR, and technetium/thallium scintigraphy.

studies are necessary and helpful (Fig. 2). We recommend the use of each of the four noninvasive imaging studies as an initial imaging cluster. If two studies appear independently to identify the same site harboring the presumed abnormal parathyroid gland, we proceed to repeat exploration based on the results of these studies. If the noninvasive studies are equivocal, we perform digital subtraction or standard arteriography. Because angiography has few false-positive results, if it is positive, we perform surgery. If the angiography is negative, we recommend selective venous sampling of the neck and mediastinal veins for localization by high levels of PTH. Selective venous samplings provides regional localization in most patients, with few false-positive results.

There are two basic points to bear in mind when radiologic imaging studies are used in patients with primary hyperparathyroidism. First, these imaging studies do not identify normal parathyroid glands. The precise identification of normal glands is required for the unequivocal diagnosis of the abnormal gland. Second, imaging studies seldom identify multiple abnormal parathyroid glands and these are limited when the primary hyperparathyroidism is caused by hyperplasia of multiple abnormal glands.

SURGICAL MANAGEMENT OF PRIMARY HYPERPARATHYROIDISM

Surgery is the mainstay of treatment for patients with primary hyperparathyroidism. Operations for primary hyperparathyroidism are called *neck explorations* because the surgeon has two missions. First, the surgeon must identify and determine the cause of primary hyperparathyroidism. This intraoperative determination may be difficult in that there are usually four parathyroid glands and three or four possible etiologies of primary hyperparathyroidism, and the pathologist may not be able to distinguish normal from abnormal glands or the type of abnormal gland. Second, dependent on intraoperative assessment of the etiology, the surgeon must execute the appropriate operation. The operation should ensure the highest probability of establishing a normal serum level of calcium, minimize the likelihood of eventual development of recurrent disease, and avoid complications. This section attempts to discipher the complexities of parathyroid surgery.

The possible etiologies of primary hyperparathyroidism are adenoma (83%), hyperplasia (15%), double adenoma (1 to 2%), and carcinoma (<1%) (49–54).

Whether "double adenomas" represent true double adenomas or hyperplasia is not clear. To simplify the possible diagnoses, we prefer to classify double adenoma and hyperplasia as multiple gland disease. Double adenoma as an etiology of primary hyperparathyroidism probably does occur; some patients have maintained long-term normal serum levels of calcium following complete resection of two abnormal glands (55,56). In any case, patients with double adenoma are rare. A family history of parathyroid disease, hypercalcemia, or associated endocrinopathies is important to identify by careful questioning, because, if the history is positive, the etiology of primary hyperparathyroidism is more likely to be hyperplasia. A history of neck irradiation should be sought and may also be pertinent. If the history is positive, the diagnosis is more likely to be an adenoma.

Before performing a neck exploration, the surgeon must be certain of the diagnosis of primary hyperparathyroidism and have the necessary skill to identify normal and abnormal parathyroid glands. As was discussed above for initial operations, localization procedures are unnecessary and even potentially hazardous (57), because the abnormal gland or glands can be correctly identified at the initial exploration without preoperative localization in ~85–95% of patients (33,58,58–61) (Table 3). Patients must be aware of complications related to parathyroid surgery. Recurrent laryngeal nerve injury and resultant vocal cord paresis or paralysis occurs in <1% of initial operations but in >5 percent of repeat operations for primary hyperparathyroidism (35,43). Fortunately, voice impairment associated with recurrent laryngeal nerve injuries is usually temporary, and full recovery may be seen at 3–6 months of follow-up. Hypoparathyroidism is a complication that seldom occurs following initial procedures (35) but does occur in 3–16% of individuals following reoperations (43,48,62–64). A final undesired result is unsuccessful surgery, which is defined as persistently elevated serum levels of calcium postoperatively. Initial explorations are unsuccessful in between 5% and 15% of cases (33,58–61,65) and in repeat procedures between 10% and 28% of cases (43,48, 62–64) (Table 3). The success rate of parathyroid surgery is closely related to the skill of the parathyroid surgeon.

Anatomy

The ability to identify and to distinguish normal and abnormal parathyroid glands at surgery is essential. Parathyroid glands can vary in color from a pale yellow to a golden or reddish-brown (66). Normal glands are very thin, and the consistency is soft and pliable (66). Yellowish-white color is commonly associated with normal glands that have a high fat content (66). Reddish-brown color and dense consistency (they sink in saline solution) reflect a high parenchymal nonfat cell content in the abnormal gland.

The typical parathyroid gland is oval or bean-shaped; however, normal and abnormal parathyroid glands can vary in size and shape. Eighty-three percent are bean-shaped; 11% are more elongated, like a cigar; 5% are bilobated, like a horseshoe; and 1% are multilobated, like a fern (66). This understanding of potential differences in shape is critical to the surgeon, who must meticulously dissect and remove the entire abnormal gland. If the gland is fractured during the operation, parathyroid cells would be left behind, leading to "seeding" and recurrent hypercalcemia. Normal glands tend to be flat and ovoid. With enlargement, they become globular. Measurements of a normal gland range from 5 to 7 mm × 3 to 4 mm × 0.5 to 2 mm. The typical normal gland that is trimmed of fat weighs 30–50 mg. The combined weight of all four parathyroid glands is 90–130 mg. The superior glands are usually smaller than the inferior glands (36). Most parathyroid glands are supplied by a solitary artery and vein and are suspended by a small vascular pedicle enclosed in an envelope of fatty tissue (67).

Typically, there are four parathyroid glands. Autopsy series demonstrate that four glands are found in 90% of subjects, five glands in 4%, and three glands in 5% (68). It may be that the identification of only three glands in these studies indicated a failure to identify correctly a fourth gland. In studies done by serial sectioning of embryos, at least four parathyroid glands were found in every specimen (50,68). Approximately 5% of humans have more than four glands (69). Supernumerary glands and fragments of glands are generally distributed within the thymus. The working hypothesis is that all individuals have four parathyroid glands.

Although the distribution of parathyroid glands may deviate extensively, the location of glands can be determined from knowledge of embryology (67). Originating from the fourth pharyngeal pouch (70), the superior parathyroid glands are commonly located along the posterior surface of the upper two-thirds of the thyroid gland (92%) (49,66) (Fig. 3A). Frequently, superior parathyroid adenomas will migrate posteriorly, underneath the inferior thyroid artery, to a position beside the esophagus (49). Ligation of the superior thyroid artery and complete mobilization of the superior thyroid pole are not necessary to expose the superior parathyroid glands, but the investing fascia connecting the lateral portion of the thyroid lobe to the carotid sheath must be incised. The location of the superior glands is relatively constant, and these glands can usually be identified more rapidly than the inferior glands. The superior parathyroid glands are symmetrically located in 80% of individuals such that identification of

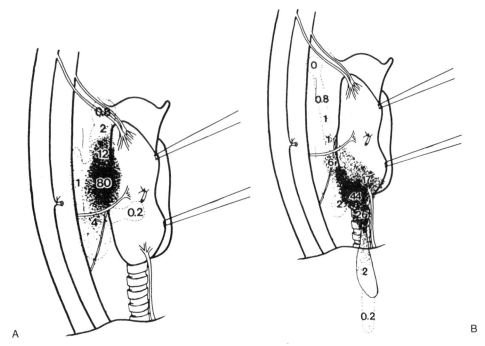

FIG. 3. Locations of the superior (**A**) and inferior (**B**) parathyroid glands. The more common locations are indicated by the darker shading. (Reprinted from ref. 66 with permission.)

one gland is a clue to the location of the other gland on the other side of the neck. Superior parathyroid adenomas may have a unique relationship to the recurrent laryngeal nerve, such that the nerve is embedded in the anteromedial capsule of the adenoma (71), or the gland can be rounded and tucked into the tight space where the recurrent laryngeal nerve enters the larynx. Superior parathyroid adenomas are generally posterolateral to the recurrent laryngeal nerve and superior to the inferior thyroid artery.

The inferior parathyroid glands have a more variable distribution than the superior (Fig. 3B). With the thymus, they originate from the third pharyngeal pouch (70). As the thymus migrates caudally, the lower glands migrate with it until they reach the lower pole of the thyroid gland. Seventeen percent of inferior parathyroid glands are directly contiguous with the inferior border of the thyroid; 44% are within 1 cm of the inferior border of the thyroid; 26% are within the superior horn of the thymus; and 2% are in the mediastinal thymus (66,67). The remainder either are within the thyroid or an undescended parathyroid gland in the upper neck near the carotid bifurcation (72). This variable anatomical distribution makes the inferior glands more difficult to locate than the superior parathyroid glands. An inferior parathyroid adenoma is generally bordered posteriorly and laterally by the recurrent laryngeal nerve (71) and is inferior to the inferior thyroid artery.

General Technique of Exploration

The goal of surgery is to identify each parathyroid gland and to remove any abnormal gland(s). We recommend either biopsy of each gland to prove that what has been identified is indeed parathyroid tissue or biopsy of any gland that is in doubt. In patients with a single enlarged gland and three identified normal glands, biopsy of all normal glands may not be mandatory and may increase the risk of temporary hypocalcemia. The manner of parathyroid biopsy is very important. Parathyroid glands may be encircled in a complete envelope of fat (halo sign) (37). The single small artery and vein form a long discrete vascular pedicle. It is mandatory to dissect gently the whitish-yellow fat away from the more brown parathyroid gland and to biopsy the side opposite to the blood supply. Parathyroid glands should be handled with fine forceps, since they are fragile, and the blood supply may be disrupted (36).

General endotracheal anesthesia is usually used, although regional anesthesia may be used effectively (73,74). The patient is positioned with the neck extended to expose maximally the cervical structures (Fig. 4A). A transverse cervical incision is made 2 cm superior to the sternal notch (Fig. 4B). The platysma is also incised (Fig. 5A), and subplatysmal flaps are raised cephalad to the thyroid notch (Fig. 5B) and caudad to the sternal notch. The Mahorner retractor fa-

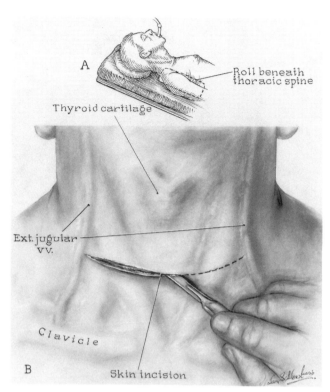

FIG. 4. A: Diagram to demonstrate proper positioning of a patient undergoing parathyroid surgery. **B:** Skin incision of a patient undergoing an initial operation for primary hyperparathyroidism. The cervical incision is made two centimeters above the sternal notch. (Reprinted from ref. 36 with permission.)

cilitates exposure. The fascia between the strap muscles is opened in the midline with electrocautery (Fig. 6).

After the strap muscles are separated from the thyroid gland and the thyroid is exposed, the exposed lobe is elevated and rotated medially to visualize the critical area posterior to the thyroid. The recurrent laryngeal nerve and inferior thyroid artery must be carefully exposed (Figs. 7, 8). The inferior thyroid artery generally courses superficial to the recurrent laryngeal nerve (65%), but the relationships can vary considerably, and the exact opposite may be true. The recurrent laryngeal nerve lies in the tracheoesophageal groove. On the right side it travels at a more oblique angle slightly lateral to the trachea, where it is more susceptible to injury (75). Furthermore, rarely, it is direct rather than recurrent on the right side (36). A recommended method to identify the location of each recurrent laryngeal nerve is to remember its relationship to the inferior cornu of the thyroid cartilage (75). One centimeter anteriomedial to the inferior cornu will mark the point where the recurrent laryngeal nerve enters the larynx.

Exploration of the neck for parathyroid glands requires meticulous hemostatic technique. Bleeding al-

ters the color of surrounding tissues and makes identification of normal or abnormal parathyroid glands more difficult. As was mentioned above, parathyroid glands may be correctly identified by their relationship to the recurrent laryngeal nerve and the inferior thyroid artery. The upper glands are usually posterior and lateral to the recurrent laryngeal nerve and superior to the inferior thyroid artery (Fig. 7), while the lower glands are usually anteromedial to the nerve and inferior to the artery (Fig. 8). Since the upper glands are most constant in location, they are identified first. If the upper glands are biopsied and found to be normal but the lower glands cannot be located, then both superior horns of the thymus in the lower neck should be dissected and removed. Seventeen percent of inferior glands will be found within the cervical horn of the thymus. If the inferior gland is still not found, then the thyroid lobe on the side of the missing gland may be removed. Thyroid lobectomy should be considered only after three normal parathyroid glands have been identified by biopsy, the superior horn of the thymus has been removed, a usual location inferior to the thyroid along the trachea has been dissected, and a search has been conducted high along the carotid sheath for a parathymic parathyroid (72). Three percent of the inferior parathyroid glands will be found either within the thyroid lobe or underneath a cleft in its surface (49). Ultrasound may be used during the operation before thyroid lobectomy to determine whether a suspicious sonolucent mass lesion (parathyroid adenoma) is present within the thyroid (76,77). A recent report suggests that it is possible to remove mediastinal parathyroid adenomas that are within the thymus from the neck using a special retractor (78). The exact role of this maneuver during initial operations has not been defined, but it enables the surgeon to resect the most common site for "ectopic" inferior parathyroid glands without resorting to open median sternotomy. This new maneuver should be considered when inferior parathyroid adenomas have not been identified and superior glands have been found to be normal by biopsy.

Failure of the initial exploration, even with diligent search of the areas noted above, calls for terminating the procedure. Reevaluation of the patient and localization procedures should then be performed before the second operation (Fig. 2). Reoperations for primary hyperparathyroidism usually focus on the neck, but in some patients median sternotomy may be necessary (79). In one series of 33 patients who underwent median sternotomy as part of reoperation for primary hyperparathyroidism, as many as 30% did not have abnormal parathyroid tissue located in the mediastinum (80). Of the abnormal mediastinal glands found, most were discovered in the thymus (64%), indicating the importance of total thymectomy whenever the mediastinum is explored for primary hyperparathyroidism

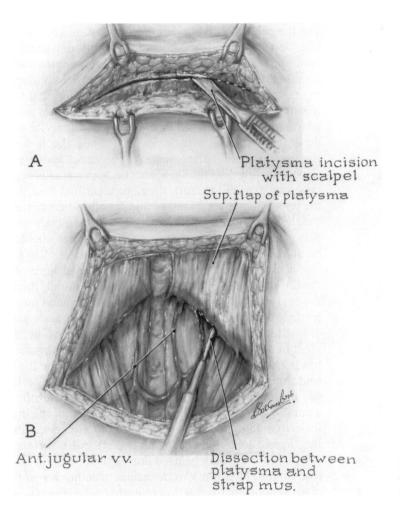

A

Platysma incision
with scalpel
Sup. flap of platysma

B

Ant. jugular v.v.

Dissection between
platysma and
strap mus.

FIG. 5. After incision of the platysma (**A**), superior and inferior flaps are developed with the cautery (**B**). (Reprinted from ref. 36 with permission.)

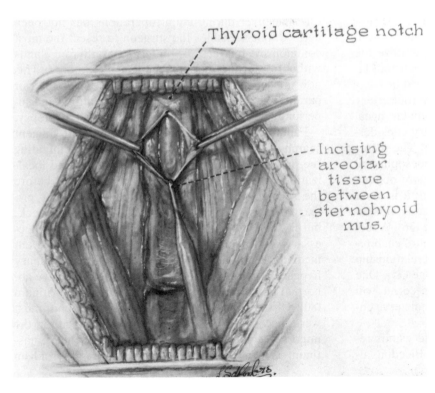

Thyroid cartilage notch

Incising
areolar
tissue
between
sternohyoid
mus.

FIG. 6. Separation of the pretracheal fascia and strap muscles in the midline. (Reprinted from ref. 36 with permission.)

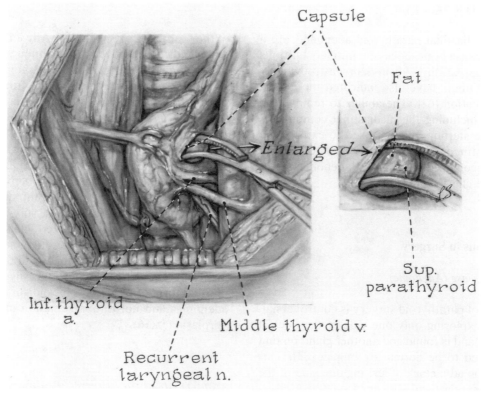

FIG. 7. Identification of a left superior parathyroid adenoma. The thyroid gland is elevated with a bab-cock clamp. The investing thyroid fascia is opened posterior to the upper pole of the left lobe. A left upper parathyroid adenoma is identified superior to the inferior thyroid artery and posterolateral to the recurrent laryngeal nerve. The left recurrent laryngeal nerve is shown in its usual location within the tracheoesophageal groove and posterior to the inferior thyroid artery. (Reprinted from ref. 36 with permission.)

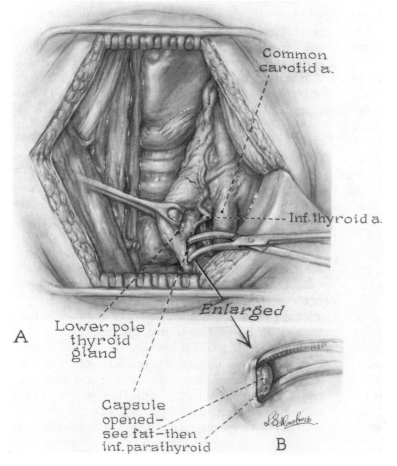

FIG. 8. Identification of a left inferior parathyroid adenoma. The thyroid gland is elevated with a bab-cock clamp. A left lower parathyroid adenoma is identified inferior to the inferior thyroid artery and anteromedial to the recurrent laryngeal nerve. Al-though the inferior parathyroid gland can be located in other positions (see Fig. 3), this is the most common position for a left inferior parathyroid adenoma. (Reprinted from ref. 36 with permission.)

(80). Missed mediastinal parathyroid adenomas are a more common cause of unsuccessful initial operations for primary hyperparathyroidism than was previously expected (81). Others have also indicated the importance of this location (62). The ability to remove the entire thymus (including the mediastinal component) by elevating the sternum may be used to explore the anterior mediastinum less invasively and to remove heretofore unrecognized parathyroid adenomas without entering the chest (82).

Specific Situations in Surgery

Single Gland Disease (Adenoma)

The strategy of parathyroid surgery is controversial. Some suggest exploring only one side of the neck if one abnormal gland is found and another gland on that side is confirmed to be normal by biopsy (83). This approach has the advantage of leaving one side of the neck free from surgery and thus untraumatized. However, this strategy may lead to occasional failure in patients with unrecognized multiple-gland disease. Furthermore, how does the surgeon choose which side of the neck to explore? If the side without the adenoma is selected, the opposite side will have to be explored.

In contrast to this very selective strategy, a much more aggressive strategy is advocated by Paloyan, who recommends three and one-half gland parathyroidectomy in all patients with primary hyperparathyroidism (84,85). This approach is based on the notion that multiglandular disease is much more common than is generally recognized. Such a view is certainly a minority one. Long-term follow-up of patients treated with this more radical approach is comparable to that in other series, but a higher (3%) incidence of permanent hypoparathyroidism is reported (85). This approach cannot be recommended because the majority of patients who have a single adenoma as a cause of hyperparathyroidism will be subject to resection of most of their normal parathyroid tissue and a high incidence of hypoparathyroidism.

The most common strategy of parathyroid surgery is to identify visually all four parathyroid glands and to ascertain by biopsy that one gland is normal while the single abnormal gland is removed (37,86,87). This approach holds for the initial operation. In the case of repeat parathyroid surgery, visualization of apparently normal parathyroid tissue is more routinely followed by biopsy (42,48,64,88,89). Even an experienced parathyroid surgeon has to recognize that identification of a normal parathyroid gland by inspection alone is inconclusive. We, thus, recommend bilateral neck exploration with visual identification *and* biopsy of each

of the four parathyroid glands. Any enlarged or abnormal glands are removed (36). Although the usefulness of the biopsy is emphasized, pathologists may find it difficult to differentiate normal from hypercellular parathyroid tissue (36) or hyperplasia from adenoma. Certainly most pathologists can reliably determine whether biopsied tissue is parathyroid or not. It is just as important for an experienced parathyroid pathologist to be part of the operative team as it is for an experienced parathyroid surgeon to be performing parathyroid surgery. In the rare event that two of four glands are enlarged (52), most surgeons will resect both, leaving the normal-sized glands undisturbed except for biopsy. This operative management has proven to be very satisfactory, without the development of recurrent hypercalcemia, suggesting that this unusual form of hyperparathyroidism is due to double adenomas and not a representation of four-gland hyperplasia (55,56).

Multiple-Gland Disease (Hyperplasia)

In typical multiple gland disease, generalized four-gland enlargement or hyperplasia, surgical management is more demanding, and the results are less satisfactory. The two recommended surgical procedures for multiple-gland disease are either subtotal (three and one-half gland) parathyroidectomy or four-gland parathyroidectomy with immediate autograft. The results of subtotal three and one-half gland parathyroidectomy have been variable. There is a 13% incidence of persistent hypercalcemia (50), an 11–16% incidence of recurrent hypercalcemia (60,86,87), and a 5–15% incidence of permanent hypocalcemia or hypoparathyroidism (50,85,87,90,91). Moreover, in patients with multiple endocrine neoplasia type I, subtotal parathyroidectomy led to a recurrence rate of 50% by 12 years after surgery (20,92). These data led Wells et al. (93) to suggest total parathyroidectomy with autotransplantation rather than subtotal parathyroidectomy for patients with hyperplasia. Results for 21 patients with parathyroid hyperplasia have been reported (94,95). Twenty patients (95%) developed hypocalcemia immediately postoperatively and required vitamin D and calcium replacement. One patient had persistent disease secondary to a fifth hyperplastic gland (5%). Within 2 months postoperatively, 20 of 20 grafted patients with postoperative hypocalcemia developed a detectable PTH gradient between the grafted and the nongrafted arms, indicating normal autograft function, and each was then able to discontinue oral vitamin D and calcium replacement therapy. However, two of ten patients with nonfamilial hyperplasia and seven of 11 with familial hyperplasia developed evidence of recurrent hypercalcemia with long-term follow-up. Four patients with recurrent hypercalcemia underwent subtotal graft resection under local anesthesia, and each was again rendered normocalcemic. The advantage of the autograft is well illustrated in that recurrent hypercalcemia due to a hyperfunctioning tissue at the graft site can be managed readily by reducing the amount of graft tissue via a local procedure.

The recommended approach to nonfamilial parathyroid hyperplasia is subtotal (three and one-half gland) parathyroidectomy, leaving ~30–50 mg of the most normal-appearing parathyroid gland in the neck. The tissue left in the neck is marked with a surgical clip. The incidence of persistent hypercalcemia or hypocalcemia will be low, but the incidence of recurrent hypercalcemia will be between 10% and 20% with long-term follow-up (60). For familial parathyroid hyperplasia, especially that occurring in MEN-I, total four-gland parathyroidectomy, including removal of as much thymic tissue as possible, and immediate parathyroid autograft to the nondominant forearm, if four glands are pathologically proven to be removed, is an acceptable procedure in experienced hands. Since the incidence of recurrent hypercalcemia is high (38–64%) (38,96–98), a portion of the transplanted tissue is easily removed under local anesthesia. When patients develop recurrent hypercalcemia following three and one-half gland subtotal parathyroidectomy, resection of the remaining abnormal gland and cryopreservation of removed parathyroid tissue are required (89). It is important to delay reimplantation of hyperplastic, cryopreserved tissue until it is certain that all parathyroid tissue has been removed (95). Unfortunately, function of grafted, cryopreserved parathyroid tissue appears to be less successful than freshly transplanted tissue. Only 50–70% of human cryopreserved autografts function normally, in contrast to fresh grafts, which function normally virtually always (99,100).

Secondary and Tertiary Hyperparathyroidism

Nearly every patient with advanced renal disease maintained on chronic dialysis has evidence of parathyroid-induced bone disease, with elevated serum levels of PTH. The progression of secondary hyperparathyroidism in these individuals should be minimized by using a dialysate calcium concentration of 3.5 mEq/liter, oral calcium supplementation, dietary restriction of phosphorus (<600 mg/day), phosphate binding antacids, and vitamin D analogues to promote intestinal absorption of calcium and to control PTH production (101). These measures can control second-

ary hyperparathyroidism in most individuals. Parathyroidectomy is used for the remaining small number of patients in whom secondary hyperparathyroidism is far advanced and for whom the time required to achieve metabolic control will lead to unacceptable, further worsening of the bone disease. *Tertiary hyperparathyroidism* refers to an advanced stage of secondary hyperparathyroidism in which the parathyroid tissue has become autonomous.

Potential indications for parathyroidectomy in patients with chronic renal failure and autonomous hyperplastic parathyroid glands (tertiary hyperparathyroidism) include (a) hypercalcemia in prospective renal transplant patients; (b) pathological features secondary to renal osteodystrophy; (c) symptoms secondary to hyperparathyroidism, including pruritus, bone pain, and extensive soft-tissue calcification, and calciphylaxis; (d) hypercalcemia in patients with well-functioning renal transplants; and (e) calcium × phosphate product >70 (102,103). Improvements in medical management as listed above and covered further in the chapter by Coburn have reduced these complications in many patients so that surgery is needed less often.

Because patients with secondary hyperparathyroidism always have hyperplasia, there is controversy regarding whether to perform a subtotal parathyroidectomy (101) or a total parathyroidectomy with immediate autograft (94,104). Johnson et al. (101) recommend subtotal (three and one-half gland) parathyroidectomy and report that this procedure affords complete relief of the hyperparathyroidism and its symptoms in patients who were unresponsive to medical therapy. Others recommend total (four-gland) parathyroidectomy, with immediate parathyroid autograft (94). In one study of 30 patients, 80% showed symptomatic relief. Although most patients developed immediate postoperative hypoparathyroidism, the autograft functioned in 87% of patients at 20 months of follow-up, and these patients could be withdrawn from supplemental calcium or vitamin D.

It is particularly important to avoid permanent hypoparathyroidism in these patients, in that this may increase the likelihood of aluminum-related bone disease (102). Although many surgeons recommend subtotal parathyroidectomy for secondary hyperparathyroidism, we perform total parathyroidectomy with immediate autograft. In our experience, repeat neck explorations in these patients with recurrent secondary hyperparathyroidism have been extremely difficult. The difficulty and complexity of further neck surgery in this group and the well-documented excellent results with total parathyroidectomy and autotransplant (94,104) make it the procedure of choice for these patients. Immediate autograft of a small amount (20 fragments, 50 mg total weight) of the resected tissue is placed in the nondominant forearm.

Reoperations for Primary Hyperparathyroidism

The complexity of repeat neck surgery for primary hyperparathyroidism makes it imperative to reconfirm the original diagnosis, to reconfirm the indication for surgery, and to attempt precise preoperative localization (Fig. 2) (42,48). The prior operative record and pathology reports should be carefully reviewed. The surgeon who performed the initial operation should be questioned to obtain as much technical information as possible. An operative record that notes that a normal gland was identified, but not biopsied, is of little value, because lymph nodes or fatty tissue can often be mistaken for parathyroid glands. Differentiation between upper and lower glands can also be unclear unless four structures are identified in the context of the surgery: the superior parathyroid glands, the inferior parathyroid glands (each biopsied), the recurrent laryngeal nerve, and the inferior thyroid artery.

The results of the initial operation and the data from the localization procedures should be used to plan the reexploration. For example, if two abnormal parathyroid glands have been removed and there is a family history of hypercalcemia, then hyperplasia is likely, and the goal of the reoperation is to remove the two remaining abnormal glands. A biopsy-proven normal gland found at the time of initial surgery and radiologic localization studies suggesting a mediastinal adenoma would prompt a direct approach to the identified abnormal parathyroid gland either by a transcervical approach (78) or by median sternotomy (80,81). Designing the operation, right-side, left-side, or median sternotomy, all or any, can be done only when all the information is assembled and evaluated. For repeat neck surgery, we use an alternative approach in the neck, along the medial border of the sternocleidomastoid muscle instead of between the strap muscles (42,48,89). This requires a separate approach on each side of the neck. Intraoperative ultrasound (IOUS) using an 10-MHz transducer may be performed after the right or left side of the neck is exposed. In our experience, IOUS can image most abnormal glands during reoperations (76,77). It is especially helpful for intrathyroidal, intrathymic, and paraesophageal parathyroid adenomas (77).

Intraoperative determination of urinary cyclic adenosine 3',5'-monophosphate (UcAMP) levels allows rapid monitoring of parathyroid status during parathyroid surgery (105,106). Excretion of UcAMP is a rapidly changing index of parathyroid function and represents the direct influence of circulating biologically active PTH on the renal tubule (107–109). With a usually constant clearance of creatinine during surgery, the availability of a rapid radioimmunoassay for cAMP (within 6 min) can be used to determine intraoperative PTH secretion. A rapid reduction in UcAMP in association with removal of parathyroid tissue ensures that the tissue removed was responsible for the hyperparathyroidism.

Generally, after successful removal of a single parathyroid adenoma or adequate resection of multiple hyperplastic glands, cAMP excretion begins to fall immediately and reaches the normal range within 0.5 to 1.5 hr after removal of all abnormal tissue (105). Recent studies have demonstrated similar results by measuring intraoperative levels of intact PTH during parathyroid operations (see the chapter by Nussbaum and Potts) (106,110). These studies demonstrate that measurement of intact PTH may be preferable to measurement of cAMP because plasma PTH levels decline more rapidly, only 15 min following resection of a parathyroid adenoma (106,110). Furthermore, the rate of decline is less in patients with hyperplasia, and this may prove to be useful as an additional intraoperative means of diagnosing hyperplasia (110). These intraoperative maneuvers are limited to the centers that have access to such rapid measurements of UcAMP and PTH.

Intraoperative functional studies of PTH and UcAMP concentration only complement surgical skill and histopathologic information. They have the potential for providing additional guidance regarding the extent and degree of neck exploration necessary for a successful outcome. However, in our careful prospective analysis of UcAMP determinations (111), false-negative results (three of 25 patients) or technical difficulties may be encountered. This information thus should serve only as an adjunct to standard judgement. Furthermore, for the patient to benefit maximally from this intraoperative high technology, the surgeon and associates should use this methodology on every case instead of intermittently on more difficult cases. Currently, these determinations are not a standard of care and should be viewed only as experimental adjuncts to surgery. Determination of their exact role, if any, and ultimate usefulness awaits prospective studies.

Finally, it should be remembered that, at reoperations for primary hyperparathyroidism, the majority of abnormal glands can be removed through a cervical incision (62,82) (Fig. 9). Abnormal parathyroid glands may be located in the retroesophageal area or posteriorly along the tracheoesophageal groove, the most common position for elusive glands (42,48,49,62). They may also be intrathyroidal (77,112), or they may be in an undescended parathymic remnant high in the carotid sheath (72,113). If these abnormal glands are not in the neck, they may be in the thymus or behind the aortic arch (67,80). Slow, meticulous exploration in a bloodless field is generally necessary to find these "ectopic" glands (Fig. 9).

Cryopreservation of removed parathyroid tissue during reoperations is indicated. One cannot predict

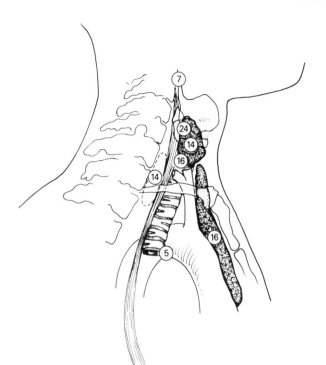

FIG. 9. Location of abnormal parathyroid glands found during reoperations for primary hyperparathyroidism. Number refers to the percentage of glands found at each location. (Reprinted from ref. 48 with permission.)

from prior records for any patient whether any normal parathyroid tissue remains in the neck. In our experience with reoperations on 175 patients, 35% left the hospital taking vitamin D medication and 43% taking supplemental calcium. Twenty-two patients (12%) ultimately were found to be permanently hypoparathyroid and required cryopreserved autologus parathyroid grafts (64). This agrees with other published reports suggesting that the rate of hypoparathyroidism following reoperative parathyroid surgery is between 2.7% and 16% (48). Cryopreservation and delayed autografting are a standard approach, although the overall success rate with delayed cryopreserved grafts is only 50–60% (99).

Repeat parathyroid surgery remains a major challenge. It is clear that the operative risk increases with each reexploration. However, with careful attention to confirmation of diagnosis and to prior operative records, with judicious use of preoperative localization techniques, and with postoperative autografting, a successful outcome may be achieved in ~90% of patients (48,64) (Table 3).

Parathyroid Carcinoma

Parathyroid carcinoma should be included in the differential diagnosis of patients with primary hyperparathyroidism when the patient has a very high serum

level of calcium (>14 mg/dl); evidence of recurrent tumor at the same site where an abnormal gland was previously removed (19,114); a fixed, hard, palpable neck mass (19,115), or hoarseness of voice (see chapter by Shane). It is difficult to assess accurately the spectrum of clinical presentation, degree of malignancy, and prognosis of parathyroid carcinoma. The incidence is rare, and patients appear to be diagnosed at an earlier stage as a result of earlier detection of hypercalcemia. A major problem in these patients is failure to identify properly the correct pathological diagnosis during the operation and, therefore, failure to perform adequate resection of the carcinomatous parathyroid tissue along with the ipsilateral lobe of the thyroid (116). Unequivocal pathological features of parathyroid carcinoma include the identification of mitoses in several high-power microscopic fields; fibrous bands or desmoplasia; and evidence of distant metastases or direct local invasion of the capsule, adjacent structures, and blood vessels (115) (see chapters by LiVolsi and Shane). However, not all patients with parathyroid carcinoma will have all these features, so the diagnosis must be ascertained from clinical as well as pathological evidence (19). Furthermore, there appears to be variability in the natural history of patients with parathyroid cancer. Some show dissemination rapidly and have a poor prognosis (117,118), while others tend to show only local recurrence and experience long disease-free intervals with a reasonable long-term prognosis (19,115).

Reports in the literature of single cases tend to emphasize more serious tumors, either more intrinsically malignant or of longer standing, with clear evidence of extraglandular spread at initial operation. The cancer usually invades along the tracheoesophageal groove, and the patient, thus, may present with hoarseness secondary to a recurrent laryngeal nerve injury. At neck exploration, the carcinomatous tissue appears gray, with a thick, hard capsule. Based on suspicion of parathyroid cancer (mass, local recurrence, high serum level of calcium), we recommend wide excision including thyroid lobectomy in continuity with the tumor (119). If the surgeon has a reason to doubt the diagnosis, incisional biopsy of tumor extrinsic from the main tumor mass, either within lymph nodes or invading local strap muscle, will provide clear evidence of cancer. Recurrent laryngeal nerve injury, either from the tumor itself or from the surgeon attempting to resect the tumor mass completely with the ipsilateral thyroid lobe, is probable and occurs in 75% of patients (19). Locally recurrent benign parathyroid adenomas may occur and be confused with parathyroid carcinomas. Recurrent adenomas generally present with a longer disease-free interval, a lower serum level of calcium, and a history of either incomplete resection or "spillage" of benign cells at the time of initial surgery (19). Nevertheless, both locally recurrent parathyroid adenoma and cancer appear to respond favorably to aggressive local resection, and most patients can be rendered either hypo- or normocalcemic for a reasonable period of time (19,120). Once disease has spread to distant sites, surgery plays a less prominent role in treatment. However, resection of pulmonary metastases has been attempted (118), but with minimal long-term gain. In patients with distant metastases, chemotherapy has been utilized, with minimal benefit (117). Therapy for these patients has been directed primarily at controlling the severe hypercalcemia (31).

Parathyroid Transplantation

Possible clinical indications for autotransplantation at the time of surgery for primary hyperparathyroidism or delayed transplantation with cryopreserved tissue for either primary or secondary parathyroid hyperplasia or reexploration for persistent or recurrent hyperparathyroidism have all been reviewed (99,100,121). The function of parathyroid autografts immediately transplanted is nearly 100% (99,121). The function of delayed cryopreserved autografts varies from 50% (99) to 80% (42,95,100). Immediate autografts of either adenoma (122) or hyperplastic glands (95) may lead to recurrent hypercalcemia and may require partial reexcision. Cryopreserved abnormal

parathyroid tissue has not appeared to result in recurrent disease but has a higher likelihood of inadequate function (100,123). In vitro studies demonstrating reasonable function of cryopreserved parathyroid tissue do not appear to correlate with outcome of human grafts.

The procedure for parathyroid transplantation and cryopreservation is as follows. Maintain the tissue on the operating table, chilled, in sterile saline. Slice the tissue into slivers 1 × 1 × 3 mm in size (Fig. 10). For immediate autografting, 20 pieces are implanted into the brachioradialis muscle of the forearm (Fig. 11). Care is taken not to induce bleeding, and each implantation site is closed with fine silk suture. Should graft-dependent hyperparathyroidism subsequently develop, a portion of the total graft site in the brachioradialis muscle can be removed under local anesthesia. For cryopreservation, the parathyroid slivers are put into 3 ml glass vials, ten pieces each, with 1.5 ml of solution containing 10% dimethylsulfoxide (DMSO), 10% autologous serum, and 80% tissue culture media. The vials are immediately placed in an automated freezing chamber and programmed to freeze 1°C per minute to −80°C. The vials are then stored in a liquid nitrogen freezer. For transplantation, the slivers are rapidly thawed in a 37°C water bath until crystals are visible; then, tissue is washed three times in tissue culture media to remove DMSO, and the parathyroid fragments are brought immediately on ice to the operating room and autografted into the brachioradialis muscle as described above (Fig. 11).

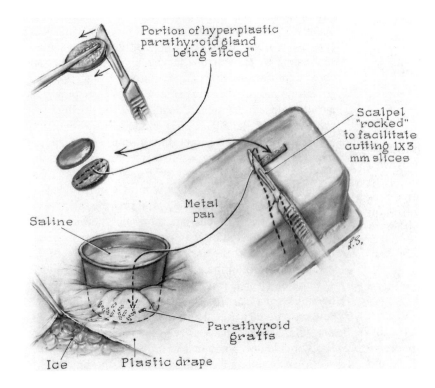

FIG. 10. Operative method of cryopreservation and transplantation of abnormal hyperplastic parathyroid tissue. Abnormal gland is sliced into small fragments (1 × 2 mm) and kept in iced saline. (Reprinted from ref. 36 with permission.)

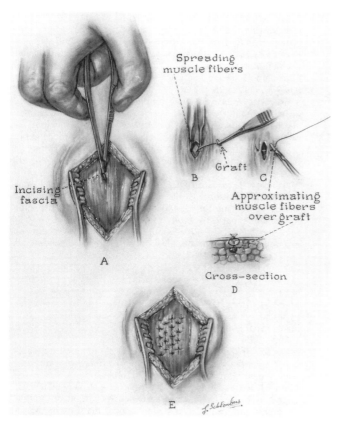

FIG. 11. Twenty fragments are grafted into small pockets in the nondominant brachioradialis muscle of the forearm. Each graft is marked with a suture to facilitate future identification of grafted site. (Reprinted from ref. 36 with permission.)

POSTOPERATIVE MANAGEMENT

Successful parathyroidectomy leads to dramatic changes in calcium metabolism. Levels of serum calcium usually reach a nadir on the second or third postoperative day, but may take even longer to fall in patients with renal disease. Most patients who have undergone successful surgery for primary hyperparathyroidism will have some (albeit mild) symptoms of hypocalcemia and may develop a positive Chovstek's sign. Routine postoperative measurements of serum calcium will track the calcium concentration. The need for calcium is guided primarily by the serum level of calcium, which should be maintained >8 mg/dl. Initially, dietary calcium is utilized to maintain serum levels of calcium. However, dietary calcium, primarily from milk products, is sometimes problematical because of lactose intolerance in some adults and the large phosphate load that may result in hyperphosphatemia. Alternatively, elemental calcium may be given in oral doses of 1–2 g/day. Most patients show a temporary hypocalcemia that rather quickly is restored as the normal parathyroid glands, left behind, begin to function. Too aggressive supplemental calcium in the early post-operative phase may delay restoration of normal parathyroid function, which depends upon the response to mild hypocalcemia.

If symptoms of hypocalcemia are severe and the patient appears to be on the verge of tetany (this occurs most frequently in patients with "hungry bone syndrome"), the clinician may need to treat with intravenous calcium. The distinction between transient hypoparathyroidism and the hungry bone syndrome is made clinically, the latter usually associated with more severe and more prolonged hypocalcemia. In addition, the hungry bone syndrome, which is characterized by rapid deposition of calcium into bone, will be associated with detectable PTH levels, whereas the transient hypoparathyroidism is associated with reduced levels of PTH (see the chaper by Nussbaum and Potts). These symptoms can usually be corrected rapidly with the infusion of 2 mg/kg of elemental calcium over 15 min. Symptoms will return unless a more prolonged infusion is used. Approximately 15 mg/kg of elemental calcium is then infused over 24 hr with one-half of the total amount administered in the initial 6 hr. Serum levels of calcium should be monitored during the infusion, and infusion rates and amounts can be adjusted accordingly. Only ~13% of patients will have major symptoms of hypoparathyroidism following surgery. These patients appear to be ones who are older; have higher preoperative serum levels of calcium, PTH, alkaline phosphatase and urea nitrogen; and have large adenomas removed at surgery (32). Underlying hyperparathyroid bone disease is usually present. These patients are typically the ones who require intravenous calcium. Most patients do not need this type of calcium replacement, because primary hyperparathyroidism only rarely presents in this way now.

When hypocalcemia persists, despite maximal oral replacement of calcium, vitamin D may be necessary (124). We use 1,25-dihydroxyvitamin D_3 [$1,25(OH)_2D_3$] (calcitriol), which is the major biologically active metabolite of vitamin D_3. This drug is recommended because it acts rapidly and has a short half life. The usual initial dose of calcitriol in this setting is 1 μg/day given in divided dosage. The dose can be increased to 2 μg/day or decreased to 0.5 μg/day depending on the response in serum levels of calcium and phosphorus. In general, the lowest possible dose that produces normal serum levels should be utilized. Serum levels of calcium should be monitored weekly following discharge to adjust oral calcium and calcitriol doses further.

Some patients with severe forms of primary hyperparathyroidism, including altered renal function and bone resorption, may demonstrate worsening kidney function in the postoperative period (125). The exact etiology is not known. However, the complication appears temporarily, and kidney function reverses within several days. Specific joint complaints may also occur in a small proportion of patients following successful parathyroidectomy. Pseudogout develops in ~5% of individuals, and examination of joint fluid demonstrates calcium phosphate crystals (126). These patients usually respond to a short course of indomethacin. Bone remineralization following parathyroid surgery may cause a significant reduction in serum levels of magnesium. Hypomagnesemia may contribute to the development of tetany in patients following parathyroidectomy. It inhibits secretion of PTH by the remaining parathyroid glands and exacerbates symptoms of hypocalcemia. Patients with serum magnesium levels <2.0 mg/dl should be treated with magnesium. The usual dosage of magnesium is ~50 mM/day in divided doses.

REFERENCES

1. Sandstrom I. On a new gland in man and several mammals (gladulae parathyroideae). *Upsala Lak Foren Forh* 1879; 15:441.
2. Gley E. Sur es fonctions du corps thyroide. *CR Soc Biol* 1891;43:841.
3. MacCallum WB, Voegtlin C. On the relation of tetany to the parathyroid glands and to calcium metabolism. *J Exp Med* 1909;11:118.
4. von Recklinghausen FD. Die Fibrose oder deformierte ostitis, die osteomalacie und die Osteoplastische carcinose in ihren gegenseitigen Beziehungen. *Festschr Rud Virchos* 1891;1:89.
5. Erdheim J. Uber epithelkorperchenbefunde bei osteomalacie. *SB Akad Wiss Math Naturw Cl* 1907;116:311.
6. Schlagenhaufer F. Zwei falleron parathyroidratumoren. *Wien Klin Wochenschr* 1915;28:1362.
7. Mandl F. Therapeutischer Versuch bei einem Falle von Ostitis fibrosa generalisata mittels exstirpation eines epithelk orperchen Tumors. *Zentrabl Chir* 1926;5:260.
8. Richardson EP, Aub JC, Bauer W. Parathyroidectomy is oseomalacia. *Ann Surg* 1929;90:730.
9. Barr DP, Bulger MA. The clinical syndrome of hyperparathyroidism. *Ann J Med Sci* 1930;179:449.
10. Albright F, Baird PC, Cope O, Bloomberg E. Studies in the physiology of the parathyroid glands: Renal complications of hyperparathyroidism. *Am J Med Sci* 1934;197:49.
11. Collip JB. The extraction of a parathyroid hormone that will prevent or control parathyroid tetany and which regulates the level of blood calcium. *J Biol Chem* 1928;63:293.
12. Aurbach GD. Isolation of parathyroid hormone after extraction with phenol. *J Biol Chem* 1959;234:3179.
13. Berson SA, Yalow RS, Aurbach GD, Potts JT. Immunoassay of bovine and human parathyroid hormone. *Proc Natl Acad Sci USA* 1963;49:613.
14. Potts JT Jr, Ackerman IP, Barker CF, et al. Diagnosis and management of asymptomatic primary hyperparathyroidism: consensus development conference statement. *Ann Intern Med* 1991;114:593.
15. Norton JA. Controversies and advances in primary hyperparathyroidism. *Ann Surg* 1992;215:297.
16. Scholz DA, Purnell DC. Asymptomatic primary hyperparathyroidism: 10 year prospective study. *Mayo Clin Proc* 1981;56:473.
17. Delbridge LW, Marshman D, Reeve TS, Crummer P, Posen S. Neuromuscular symptoms in elderly patients with hyperparathyroidism: improvement with parathyroid surgery. *Med J Aust* 1988;149:74.
18. Shane E, Bilezikian JP. Parathyroid carcinoma: a review of 62 patients. *Endocr Rev* 1982;3:218.
19. Fraker DL, Travis WD, Merendino JJJ, et al. Locally recurrent parathyroid neoplasms as a cause for recurrent and persistent primary hyperparathyroidism. *Ann Surg* 1991;213:58.
20. Rizzoli R, Green J III, Marx SJ. Primary hyperparathyroidism in familial multiple endocrine neoplasia type I: long-term follow-up of serum calcium levels after parathyroidectomy. *Am J Med* 1985;78:467.
21. Keiser HR, Beaven MA, Doppman J, et al. Sipple's syndrome: Medullary thyroid carcinoma, pheochromocytoma and parathyroid disease. *Ann Intern Med* 1973;78:561.
22. Marx SJ, Menczel J, Campbell G, Aurbach GD, Spiegel AM, Norton JA. Heterogeneous size of the parathyroid glands in familial multiple endocrine neoplasia type 1. *Clin Endocrinol* 1991;35:521.
23. Matthew CGP, Easton DF, Nakamura Y, Ponder BAJ, and MEN2a International Collaborative Group. Presymptomatic screening for multiple endocrine neoplasia type 2A with linked DNA markers. *Lancet* 1991;337:7.
24. Simpson NE, Kidd KK, Goodfellow PJ, et al. Assignment of multiple endocrine neoplasia type 2A to chromosome 10 by linkage. *Nature* 1987;328:528.
25. Larsson C, Skogseid B, Öberg K, Nakamura Y, Nordenskôld M. Multiple endocrine neoplasia type 1 gene maps to chromosome 11 and is lost in insulinoma. *Nature* 1988;332:85.
26. Marx SJ, Stock JL, Attie MF, et al. Familial hypocalciuric hypercalcemia: recognition among patients referred after unsuccessful parathyroid exploration. *Ann Intern Med* 1980;92:351.
27. Marx SJ, Speigel AM, Levine MA, et al. Familial hypocalciuric hypercalcemia: The relation to primary parathyroid hyperplasia. *N Engl J Med* 1982;307:416.
28. Marx SJ, Attie MF, Levine MA, Spiegel AM, Downs RW Jr, Lasker RD. The hypocalciuric or benign variant of familial hypercalcemia: clinical and biochemical features in fifteen kindreds. *Medicine* 1981;60:397.
29. Levin KE, Clark OH. The reasons for failure in parathyroid operations. *Arch Surg* 1989;124:911.
30. Fitzpatrick LA, Bilezikian JP. Acute primary hyperparathyroidism: A review of 48 patients. *Am J Med* 1987;82:272.
31. Bilezikian JP. Management of acute hypercalcemia. *N Engl J Med* 1992;326:1196.
32. Brasier AR, Nussbaum SR. Hungry bone syndrome: Clinical and biochemical predictors of its occurrence after parathyroid surgery. *Am J Med* 1988;84:654.
33. Russell CF, Edis AJ. Surgery for primary hyperparathyroidism: experience with 500 consecutive cases and evaluation of the role of surgery in the asymptomatic patient. *Br J Surg* 1982;69:244.
34. Russell CFJ, Laird JD, Ferguson WR. Scan-directed unilateral cervical exploration for parathyroid adenoma: A legitimate approach? *World J Surg* 1990;14:406.
35. Cowie AGA. Morbidity in adult parathyroid surgery. *JR Soc Med* 1982;75:942.
36. Wells SA, Leight GF, Ross A. Primary hyperparathyroidism. *Curr Probl Surg* 1980;17:398.
37. Thompson NW, Vinik AI. The technique of initial parathyroid exploration and reoperative parathyroidectomy. In: Thompson NW, Vinik AI, eds. *Endocrine surgery update.* New York: Grune and Stratton, 1983;368.
38. van Heerden JA, James EM, Caselle PR, et al. Small part ultrasonography in primary hyperparathyroidism. *Ann Surg* 1982;195:774.
39. Brewer WH, Walsh JW, Newsome HH Jr. Impact of sonography on surgery for primary hyperparathyroidism. *Am J Surg* 1983;145:270.
40. Serpell JW, Campbell PR, Young AE. Preoperative localization of parathyroid tumours does not reduce operating time. *Br J Surg* 1991;78:589.
41. Levin KE, Gooding GAW, Okerlund M, et al. Localizing studies in patients with persistent or recurrent hyperparathyroidism. *Surgery* 1987;102:917.
42. Carty SE, Norton JA. Management of patients with persistent or recurrent primary hyperparathyroidism. *World J Surg* 1991;15:716.

43. Patow CA, Norton JA, Brennan MF. Vocal cord paralysis and reoperative parathyroidectomy. *Ann Surg* 1986;203:282.

44. Doppman JL, Krudy AG, Marx SJ, et al. Aspiration of enlarged parathyroid glands for parathyroid hormone assay. *Radiology* 1983;148:31.

45. Bergenfelz A, Forsberg L, Hederström E, Ahrén B. Preoperative localization of enlarged parathyroid glands with ultrasonically guided fine needle aspiration for parathyroid hormone assay. *Acta Radiol* 1991;32:403.

46. Miller DL, Doppman JL, Shawker TH, et al. Localization of parathyroid adenomas in patients who have undergone surgery. Part I. Noninvasive imaging methods. *Radiology* 1987;162:133.

47. Miller DL, Doppman JL, Krudy AG, et al. Localization of parathyroid adenomas in patients who have undergone surgery. Part II. Invasive procedures. *Radiology* 1987;162:138.

48. Lange JR, Norton JA. Surgery for persistent or recurrent primary hyperparathyroidism. *Curr Pract Surg* 1992;4:56.

49. Thompson NW, Eckhauser F, Harness J. Anatomy of primary hyperparathyroidism. *Surgery* 1982;92:814.

50. Edis AJ, van Heerden JA, Scholz DA. Results of subtotal parathyroidectomy for primary chief cell hyperplasia. *Surgery* 1979;86:462.

51. Block MA, Frame B, Keerekoper M, et al. Surgical management of persistence or recurrence after subtotal parathyroidectomy for primary hyperparathyroidism. *Am J Surg* 1979; 138:561.

52. Harness JK, Ramsburg SR, Nishiyama RH, et al. Multiple adenomas of the parathyroids, do they exist? *Arch Surg* 1979;114:468.

53. Wang CA. Hyperparathyroidism due to primary hyperplasia. *Ann Surg* 1982;195:384.

54. Verdonk CA, Edis AJ. Parathyroid double adenomas, fact or fiction? *Surgery* 1981;90:523.

55. Attie JN, Bock G, Auguste L-J. Multiple parathyroid adenomas: report of thirty-three cases. *Surgery* 1990;108:1014.

56. Roses DF, Karp NS, Sudarsky LA, Valensi QJ, Rosen RJ, Blum M. Primary hyperparathyroidism associated with two enlarged parathyroid glands. *Arch Surg* 1989;124:1261.

57. Brennan MF, Doppman JL, Krudy AG, et al. Assessment of the techniques for preoperative gland localization in patients undergoing reoperations for hyperparathyroidism. *Surgery* 1982;91:6.

58. Poole GV Jr, Albertson DA, Myers RT. Causes of the failed cervical exploration for primary hyperparathyroidism. *Am Surg* 1988;54:553.

59. Piemonte M, Miani P, Bacchi G. Parathyroid surgery in primary hyperparathyroidism: an update. *Arch Otorhinolaryngol* 1989;246:324.

60. Rudberg C, Akerström G, Palmer M, et al. Late results of operation for primary hyperparathyroidism in 441 patients. *Surgery* 1986;99:643.

61. Lavelle MA. Parathyroid adenoma stained with methylene blue. *J R Soc Med* 1980;73:462.

62. Wang C. Parathyroid re-exploration. A clinical and pathological study of 112 cases. *Ann Surg* 1977;186:140.

63. Grant CS, van Heerden JA, Charboneau JW, James EM, Reading CC. Clinical management of persistent and/or recurrent primary hyperparathyroidism. *World J Surg* 1986; 10:555.

64. Brennan MF, Norton JA. Reoperation for persistent and recurrent hyperparathyroidism. *Ann Surg* 1985;201:40.

65. Tibblin S, Bondeson A-G, Bondeson L, Ljungberg O. Surgical strategy in hyperparathyroidism due to solitary adenoma. *Ann Surg* 1984;200:776.

66. Akerstrom G, Malmaeus J, Bergstrom R. Surgical anatomy of human parathyroid glands. *Surgery* 1984;95:14.

67. Wang CA. The anatomic basis of parathyroid surgery. *Ann Surg* 1975;183:271.

68. Alveryd A. Parathyroid glands in thyroid surgery. *Acta Chir Scand* 1968;389:1.

69. Wang CA, Mahaffey JE, Axelrod L, et al. Hyperfunctioning supernumary parathyroid glands. *Surg Gynecol Obset* 1979; 148:711.

70. Gilmour JR. The embryology of the parathyroid glands, the thymus and certain associated rudiments. *J Pathol* 1937; 45:507.

71. Pyrtek LJ, Painter RL. An anatomic study of the relationship of the parathyroid glands to the recurrent laryngeal nerve. *Surg Gynecol Obstet* 1964;119:509.

72. Edis AJ, Purnell DC, van Heerden JA. The undescended parathymus: An occasional cause of failed neck exploration of hyperparathyroidism. *Ann Surg* 1979;190:64.

73. Saxe A, Brown E, Hamburger SW. Thyroid and parathyroid surgery performed with patient under regional anesthesia. *Surgery* 1988;103:415.

74. Crile G Jr. Letter to the editor. *Surgery* 1989;105:455.

75. Wang CA. The use of the interior cornu of the thyroid cartilage in identifying the recurrent laryngeal nerve. *Surg Gynecol Obstet* 1975;140:91.

76. Norton JA, Shawker TH, Jones BL, et al. Intraoperative ultrasound and reoperative parathyroid surgery: An initial evaluation. *World J Surg* 1986;10:631.

77. Kern KA, Shawker TH, Doppman JL, et al. The use of high-resolution ultrasound to locate parathyroid tumors during reoperations for primary hyperparathyroidism. *World J Surg* 1987;11:579.

78. Wells SA, Cooper JD. Closed mediastinal exploration in patients with persistent hyperparathyroidism. *Ann Surg* 1991; 214:555.

79. Nathanials EK, Nathaniels AM, Wang C. Mediastinal parathyroid tumors. A clinical and pathological study of 84 cases. *Ann Surg* 1970;171:165.

80. Norton JA, Schneider PD, Brennan MF. Median sternotomy in reoperations for primary hyperparathyroidism. *World J Surg* 1985;9:807.

81. Doherty GM, Doppman JL, Miller DL, et al. Results of a multidisciplinary strategy for management of mediastinal parathyroid adenoma as a cause of persistent primary hyperparathyroidism. *Ann Surg* 1992;215:101.

82. Wells SA Jr, Copper JD. Closed mediastinal exploration in patients with persistent hyperparathyroidism. *Ann Surg* 1991;214:555.

83. Ribblin SA, Bondeson A, Ljungberg O. Unilateral parathyroidectomy due to single adenoma. *Ann Surg* 1982;195:245.

84. Paloyan E, Lawrence AM, Baker WH, Strauss FH. Near-total parathyroidectomy. *Surg Clin North Am* 1969;49:43.

85. Paloyan E, Lawrence AM, Oslapas R. Subtotal parathyroidectomy for primary hyperparathyroidism: Long-term results in 292 patients. *Arch Surg* 1983;118:425.

86. Satava RMJ, Beahrs OH, Scholz DA. Success rate of cervical exploration for hyperparathyroidism. *Arch Surg* 1975; 110:625.

87. McGarity WC, Bostwick J. Technique for parathyroidectomy. *Ann Surg* 1976;42:657.

88. Brennan MF, Marx SJ, Doppman J, et al. Results of reoperation for persistent and recurrent hyperparathyroidism. *Ann Surg* 1981;194:671.

89. Saxe AW, Brennan MF. Strategy and technique of reoperative parathyroid surgery. *Surgery* 1981;89:417.

90. Castleman B, Cope O. Primary parathyroid hyperplasia. *Bull Hosp Joint Dis* 1951;12:368.

91. Castleman B, Schantz A, Roth S II. Parathyroid hyperplasia in primary hyperparathyroidism. *Cancer* 1976;38:1668.

92. Lamers CBHW, Froeling PGAM. Clinical significance of hyperparathyroidism in familial multiple endocrine adneomatosis type I (MEA I). *Am J Med* 1979;66:422.

93. Wells SA, Ellis GJ, Gunnells JC, et al. Parathyroid autotransplantation in primary parathyroid hyperplasi. *N Engl J Med* 1976;295:57.

94. Romanus ME, Farndon R, Wells SA Jr. Transplantation of the parathyroid glands. In: Johnston IDA, Thompson NW, eds. *Endocrine surgery.* Stoneham, MA: Butterworth Publishers, 1983;25–40.

95. Wells SA Jr, Farndon JR, Dale JK, et al. Long-term evaluation of patients with primary parathyroid hyperplasia managed by total parathyroidectomy and heterotopic autotransplantation. *Ann Surg* 1980;192:451.

96. Fisher MR, Higgins CB, Andereck W. MR imaging of an intrapericardial pheochromocytoma. *J Comput Assist Tomogr* 1985;9:1103.
97. Scheible W, Deutsch AL, Leopold GR. Parathyroid adenoma: accuracy of preoperative localization by high resolution real time sonography. *J Clin Ultrasound* 1981;9:325.
98. Chaudhuri TK, Shirazi SS, Condon RE. Radioisotope scan—a possible aid in differentiating retained gastric antrum from Zollinger-Ellison syndrome in patients with recurrent peptic ulcer. *Gastroenterology* 1973;65:697.
99. Senapati A, Young AE. Parathyroid autotransplantation. *Br J Surg* 1990;77:1171.
100. Brunt LM, Sicard GA. Current status of parathyroid autotransplantation. *Semin Surg Oncol* 1990;6:115.
101. Johnson WJ, McCarthy JT, van Heerden JA, Sterioff S, Grant CS, Kao PC. Results of subtotal parathyroidectomy in hemodialysis patients. *Am J Med* 1985;84:23.
102. Andress DL, Ott SM, Maloney NA, Sherrard DJ. Effect of parathyroidectomy on bone aluminum accumulation in chronic renal failure. *N Engl J Med* 1985;312:468.
103. Clark OH. Secondary hyperparathyroidism. In: Clark OH, ed. *Endocrine surgery of the thyroid and parathyroid glands*. St. Louis: CV Mosby, 1985;241.
104. Kaye M, D'Amour P, Henderson J. Elective total parathyroidectomy without autotransplant in end-stage renal disease. *Kidney Int* 1989;35:1390.
105. Norton JA, Brennan MF, Saxe AW, et al. Intraoperative urinary cyclic adenosine monophosphate as a guide to successful reoperative parathyroidectomy. *Ann Surg* 1984;200:389.
106. Nussbaum SR, Thompson AR, Hutcheson BA, Gaz RD, Wang C. Intraoperative measurement of parathyroid hormone in the surgical management of hyperparathyroidism. *Surg* 1988;104:1121.
107. Broadus AE. Nephrogenous cyclic AMP. *Rec Progr Horm Res* 1981;36:667.
108. Broadus AE, Mahaffey JE, Barter FC, Neer RM. Nephrogenous cyclic adenosine monophosphate as a parathyroid function test. *J Clin Invest* 1977;60:667.
109. Spiegel AM, Marx SJ, Brennan MF, et al. Parathyroid function after parathyroidectomy: Evaluation by measurement of urinary cyclic AMP. *Clin Endocrinol* 1981;15:65.
110. Bergenfelz A, Nordén NE, Ahrén B. Intraoperative fall in plasma levels of intact parathyroid hormone after removal of one enlarged parathyroid gland in hyperparathyroid patients. *Eur J Surg* 1991;157:109.
111. Darling GE, Marx SJ, Spiegel AM, Aurbach GD, Norton JA. Prospective analysis of intraoperative and postoperative urinary cyclic adenosine 3′,5′-monophosphate levels to predict outcome of patients undergoing reoperations for primary hyperparathyroidism. *Surg* 1988;104:1128.
112. Wang CA. Hyperfunctioning intrathyroid glands: a potential cause of failure in parathyroid surgery. *J R Soc Med* 1981;74:49.
113. Fraker DL, Doppman JL, Shawker TH, Marx SJ, Spiegel AM, Norton JA. Undescended parathyroid adenoma: an important etiology for failed operations for primary hyperparathyroidism. *World J Surg* 1990;14:342.
114. Wang C, Gaz RD. Natural history of parathyroid carcinoma. Diagnosis, treatment, and results. *Am J Surg* 1985;149:522.
115. Schantz A, Castleman B. Parathyroid carcinoma: a study of 70 cases. *Cancer* 1973;31:600.
116. Cohn K, Silverman M, Corrado J, Sedgewick C. Parathyroid carcinoma: the Lahey Clinic experience. *Surgery* 1985;98:1095.
117. Calandra DB, Chejfec G, Foy BK, et al. Parathyroid carcinoma: biochemical and pathologic response to DTIC. *Surgery* 1984;96:1132.
118. Flye MW, Brennan MF. Surgical resection of metastatic parathyroid carcinoma. *Ann Surg* 1981;193:425.
119. van Heerden JA, Weiland LH, Re Mine WH, et al. Cancer of the parathyroid glands. *Arch Surg* 1979;114:475.
120. Haff RC, Ballinger WF. Causes of recurrent hypercalcemia after parathyroidectomy for primary hyperparathyroidism. *Ann Surg* 1971;173:884.
121. Edis AJ, Linos DA, Kao PC. Parathyroid autotransplantation at the time of reoperation for persistent hyperparathyroidism. *Surgery* 1980;88:588.
122. Brennan MF, Brown EM, Marx SJ, et al. Recurrent hyperparathyroidism from an autotransplanted parathyroid adenoma. *N Engl J Med* 1978;299:1057.
123. Niederle B, Roka R, Brennan MF. The transplantation of parathyroid tissue in man: Development, indications, techniques, and results. *Endocr Rev* 1982;3:345.
124. Reichel H, Koeffler HP, Norman AW. The role of the vitamin D endocrine system in health and disease. *N Engl J Med* 1989;320:980.
125. Mallette LE, Bilezikian JP, Heath DA, Aurbach GD. Primary hyperparathyroidism: Clinical and biochemical features. *Medicine* 1974;53:127.
126. Bilezikian JP, Aurbach GD, Connor TB, et al. Pseudogout after parathyroidectomy. *Lancet* 1973;1:445.
127. Muhr C, Ljunghall S, Akerstrom G, et al. Screening for multiple endocrine neoplasia syndrome (type I) in patients with primary hyperparathyroidism. *Clin Endocrinol* 1984;20:153.
128. Krudy AG, Shawker TH, Doppman JL, et al. Ultrasonic parathyroid localization in previously operated patients. *Clin Radiol* 1984;35:113.
129. Reading CC, Charboneau JW, James EM, et al. Postoperative parathyroid high-frequency sonography: Evaluation of persistent or recurrent hyperparathyroidism. *AJR* 1985;144:399.
130. Simeone JF, Mueller PR, Feriucci JT, et al. High resolution real time sonography with a parathyroid. *Radiology* 1981;141:745.
131. Reading CC, Charboneau JW, James EM, et al. High resolution parathyroid sonography. *AJR* 1982;139:539.
132. Stein BL, Wexler MJ. Preoperative parathyroid localization: a prospective evaluation of ultrasonography and thallium-technetium scintigraphy in hyperparathyroidism. *Can J Surg* 1990;33:175.
133. Okerlund MD, Sheldon K, Corpuz S, et al. A new method with high sensitivity and specificity for localization of abnormal parathyroid glands. *Ann Surg* 1984;200:381.
134. Sandrock D, Merino MJ, Norton JA, Neumann RD. Parathyroid imaging by Tc/Tl scintigraphy. *Eur J Nucl Med* 1990;16:607.
135. Skibber JM, Reynolds JC, Spiegel AM, et al. Computerized technetium/thallium scan and parathyroid reoperation. *Surgery* 1985;98:1077.
136. Doppman JL, Brennan MF, Kohler JO, et al. CT scanning for parathyroid localization. *J Comput Assist Tomogr* 1977;1:30.
137. Doppman JL, Krudy AG, Brennan MF, et al. CT appearance of enlarged parathyroid glands in the posterior-superior mediastinum. *J Comput Assist Tomogr* 1982;6:1099.
138. Sommer B, Welter HF, Spelsberg F, et al. Computed tomography for localizing enlarged parathyroid glands in primary hyperparathyroidism. *J Comput Assist Tomogr* 1982;6:521.
139. Stark DD, Gooding JW, Moss AA, et al. Parathyroid scanning by computer tomography. *Radiology* 1983;148:297.
140. Stark DD, Gooding JW, Moss AA, et al. Parathyroid imaging: Comparison of high resolution CT and high resolution sonography. *AJR* 1983;141:633.
141. Auffermann W, Guis M, Tavares NJ, Clark OH, Higgins CB. MR signal intensity of parathyroid adenomas: Correlation with histopathology. *AJR* 1989;153:873.
142. Jenkins BJ, Newell MS, Goode AW, Boucher BJ, Monson JP, Brown CL. Impact of conventional and three-dimensional thallium-technetium scans on surgery for primary hyperparathyroidism. *J R Soc Med* 1990;83:427.
143. Spritzer CE, Gefter WB, Hamilton R, Greenberg BM, Axel L, Kressel HY. Abnormal parathyroid glands: high-resolution MR imaging. *Radiology* 1987;162:487.
144. Peck WW, Higgins CB, Fisher MR, Ling M, Okerlund MD, Clark OH. Hyperparathyroidism: comparison of MR imaging with radionuclide scanning. *Radiology* 1987;163:415.
145. Winzelberg GG, Hydovitz JD, O'Hara KR, et al. Parathyroid adenomas evaluated by Tl-201/Tc-99m pertechnetate

subtraction scintigraphy and high-resolution ultrasonography. *Radiology* 1985;155:231.

146. Ferlin G, Camerani M, Conte N, et al. New perspectives in localizing enlarged parathyroids by technetium/thallium subtraction scan. *J Nucl Med* 1983;24:438.

147. Young AE, Gaunt JI, Croft DN, et al. Location of parathyroid adenoma by thallium 201 and technetium-99m subtraction scanning. *Br Med J* 1983;286:1384.

148. Carmalt HL, Gillett DJ, Chu J, Evans RA, Kos S. Prospective comparison of radionuclide, ultrasound, and computed tomography in the preoperative localization of parathyroid glands. *World J Surg* 1988;12:830.

149. Krubsack AJ, Wilson SD, Lawson TL, Collier BD, Hellman RS, Isitman AT. Prospective comparison of radionuclide, computed tomographic, and sonographic localization of parathyroid tumors. *World J Surg* 1986;10:579.

150. Grunberger G, Weiner JL, Silverman R, Taylor S, Gorden P. Factitious hypoglycemia due to surreptitious administration of insulin: Diagnosis, treatment and long-term follow-up. *Ann Intern Med* 1988;108:252.

151. McGarity WC, Mathews WH, Fulenwider JR, Isaacs JW, Miller DA. The surgical management of primary hyperparathyroidism. *Ann Surg* 1981;193:794.

152. Bruining HA, van Houten H, Jettmann JR, Lamberts SWJ, Birkenhager JC. Results of operative treatment of 615 patients with primary hyperparathyroidism. *World J Surg* 1981;5:85.

153. Edis AJ, Sheedy PF II, Beahrs OH, van Heerden JA. Results of reoperation for hyperparathyroidism, with evaluation of preoperative localization studies. *Surgery* 1978; 84:384.

154. Cheung PSY, Borgstrom A, Thompson NW. Strategy in reoperative surgery for hyperparathyroidism. *Arch Surg* 1989; 124:676.

155. Granberg P-O, Johansson G, Lindvall N, et al. Reoperation for primary hyperparathyroidism. *Am J Surg* 1982;143:296.

The Parathyroids, edited by J.P. Bilezikian,
M.A. Levine, and R. Marcus. Raven Press, Ltd.,
New York © 1994.

CHAPTER 33

Preoperative Localization of Parathyroid Tissue in Primary Hyperparathyroidism

John L. Doppman

In patients with primary hyperparathyroidism and unsuccessful initial surgery, localization studies have made a significant contribution to the success of subsequent operations. In a review of a large series of patients from the Mayo Clinic reported prior to the use of preoperative localization studies (1975) (1), the success of reoperative surgery was only 62% compared to a 95% success rate in patients undergoing their initial operation. Relying heavily on localization studies, the success rate in 107 consecutive patients at the NIH undergoing reoperative surgery was 97%, comparable to the results in patients undergoing initial surgery (2). There is unanimous agreement concerning the need for preoperative localization in patients undergoing reoperation for primary hyperparathyroidism. The first section of this chapter describes a strategy for localization studies in such patients and the results to be expected. Controversy exists concerning the need to perform preoperative localization studies in patients undergoing their initial operation for primary hyperparathyroidism. In the second section of this chapter, the advantages and disadvantages of preoperative localization in the context of initial surgery will be considered.

LOCALIZATION STUDIES IN PATIENTS UNDERGOING REOPERATIVE SURGERY FOR PRIMARY HYPERPARATHYROIDISM

The need for localization studies in patients undergoing reoperative parathyroid surgery is undisputed. The noninvasive studies—ultrasound, thallium/tech-

netium subtraction scintigraphy, computed tomography (CT), and magnetic resonance imaging (MRI)—are performed first. Table 1 summarizes the strengths and weaknesses of each procedure. Ultrasound and thallium/technetium scanning are best for eutopic lesions in and about the thyroid gland, whereas CT and MRI are more effective in detecting ectopic glands in the anterior mediastinum and tracheoesophageal groove.

With all four noninvasive techniques, there is a significant number of false-positive studies ranging from 15% to 18%. We require two positive noninvasive studies at the same site for definitive localization. In an earlier report of our experience in 1987, 70% of patients had one positive study, but only 30% of patients had two such positive studies (3). In our more recent experience, ~60% of patients have two positive noninvasive studies, the improvement being due to the contribution of MRI in confirming ectopic locations detected by CT scanning. The sequence of performing the noninvasive studies is not critical. Because ultrasound and thallium/technetium scanning are least invasive and least expensive, we perform them first. None of the noninvasive studies will establish the diagnosis of hyperplasia with any reliability, each generally visualizing only the dominant hyperplastic gland. Thallium/technetium scanning, CT, and MRI rarely visualize adenomas smaller than 1 cm.

Features of Noninvasive Localization Tests

Thallium/Technetium Imaging

The principle of thallium/technetium scanning is based on the subtraction of the technetium image, which identifies only the thyroid gland, from the thal-

J. L. Doppman: Department of Radiology, National Institutes of Health, Bethesda, Maryland 20892.

TABLE 1. *Characteristics of noninvasive parathyroid imaging modalities[a]*

Characteristic	US Ultrasound	Th/Tc Thallium/Technetium	CT	MRI
Sensitivity to lesion size	+	+ + +	+ + +	+ + +
Areas best visualized	Juxtathyroid Intrathyroid Undescended	Juxtathyroid	Mediastinum TE[b] groove	Mediastinum TE groove
Areas poorly visualized	Mediastinum TE[b] groove	Mediastinum TE groove	Juxtathyroid	Juxtathyroid
Other		Poor resolution Radiation to thyroid	Requires IV contrast Radiation to thyroid	
Availability	+ + +[c]	+ + +	+ + +	+ +
Operator dependency	+ + +	+	+	+
Risk	0	0	Low[d]	0
Cost	+	+	+ +	+ + +

[a]Modified from ref. 22 with permission.
[b]Tracheosophageal.
[c]A 10 MHz small parts tranducer is required for optimum results.
[d]Iodinated intravenous contrast material essential.

lium image, which labels both thyroid and parathyroid glands. Figure 1 demonstrates a typical positive scan for an adenoma adjacent to the lower pole of the right thyroid lobe. Thallium/technetium scanning is most effective for cervical adenomas adjacent to the thyroid gland. Mediastinal glands can be imaged by this technique but they must be distinguished from activity in the cardiac blood pool. A new agent for imaging the parathyroid glands, technetium-99m-Sestamibi has recently been introduced. Developed as a myocardial imaging agent, this compound is taken up by the parathyroids as well as thyroid tissue but persists for a longer duration in the parathyroid glands. It has been used by O'Doherty et al. (4) in combination with 99-Tc-pertechnetate imaging as a substitute for thallous chloride, with an improved sensitivity and ability to demonstrate multiple hyperplastic glands. Taillifer et al. (5) have recently introduced a double-phase study using technetium-99m-Sestamibi alone, with the 2–3 hr delayed scan demonstrating parathyroid tissue only. If these preliminary findings are confirmed in larger series, technetium-99m-Sestamibi may become the agent of choice for imaging parathyroid tumors.

Ultrasound

Ultrasound is particularly sensitive to the presence of intrathyroidal parathyroid glands, a diagnosis difficult to confirm with the other noninvasive approaches. When an intrathyroidal parathyroid gland is suspected, aspiration for parathyroid hormone (PTH) lev-

els under ultrasound control (6) is recommended to avoid arteriography and venous sampling.

Computed Tomography

Computed tomography should always be performed during a dynamic injection (1–2 cc/sec) of iodinated contrast material. Nonionic contrast material should be used because it is less likely to cause patient motion due to burning or nausea and vomiting. Modern scanners generally allow one to scan from above the angle of the mandible to the level of the carina during maximal contrast enhancement. Although this is rare, parathyroid glands can lie in the aortopulmonary window (Fig. 2), and scanning should be extended to this level in problem cases. Parathyroid venous sampling will often give a clue to the location of an adenoma in the aortopulmonary window, a site that is not excluded by a previous sternotomy and thymectomy. Glands in the aortopulmonary window are generally best approached by a left thoracotomy, especially if the patient has previously undergone an exploration of the anterior mediastinum through a standard sternotomy incision.

Magnetic Resonance Imaging

Magnetic resonance imaging is the latest of the noninvasive imaging modalities. Parathyroid adenomas have intermediate signal intensity similar to muscle on

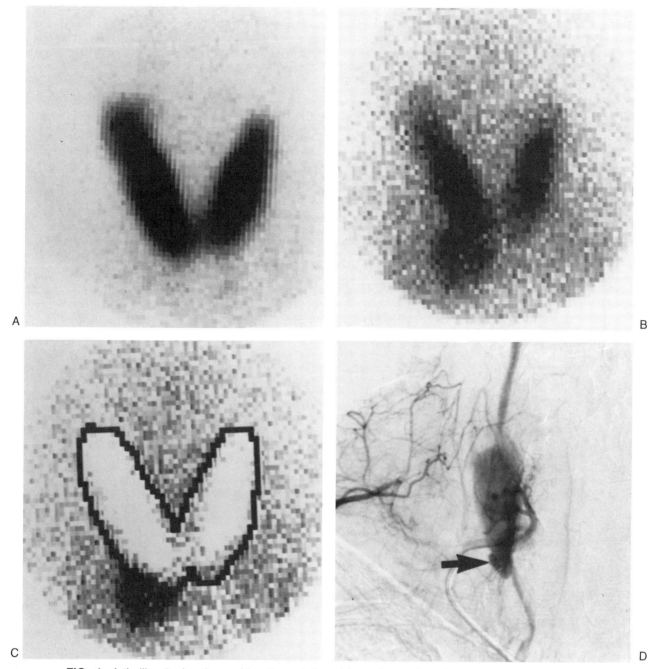

FIG. 1. A thallium/technetium subtraction scintigraphic study consists of a technetium scan labeling thyroid (**A**), a thallium scan labeling thyroid and parathyroid (**B**), and the subtracted image identifying a right inferior parathyroid adenoma (**C**). The arteriogram shows good correlation of adenoma (*arrow* in **D**) with scintigraphic studies.

T1-weighted images and are bright on T2-weighted and short time-of-inversion recovery (STIR) sequences (7–9). Although parathyroid adenomas are enhanced following gadopentate dimeglumine (10) (Magnavist; Berlex, Wayne, NJ), use of this expensive paramagnetic contrast material is generally not necessary when fat-suppressed pulse sequences are available. T2 images are helpful for glands in the juxtathyroid location, but, in the anterior mediastinum, bright adenomas disappear into the bright signal of the surrounding fat and thymic tissue. In our experience, STIR or other fat-suppressed sequences have been particularly helpful in detecting parathyroid adenomas in ectopic locations. Presaturation pulses can be used to eliminate the bright flow-related artifacts in the arterial and venous system.

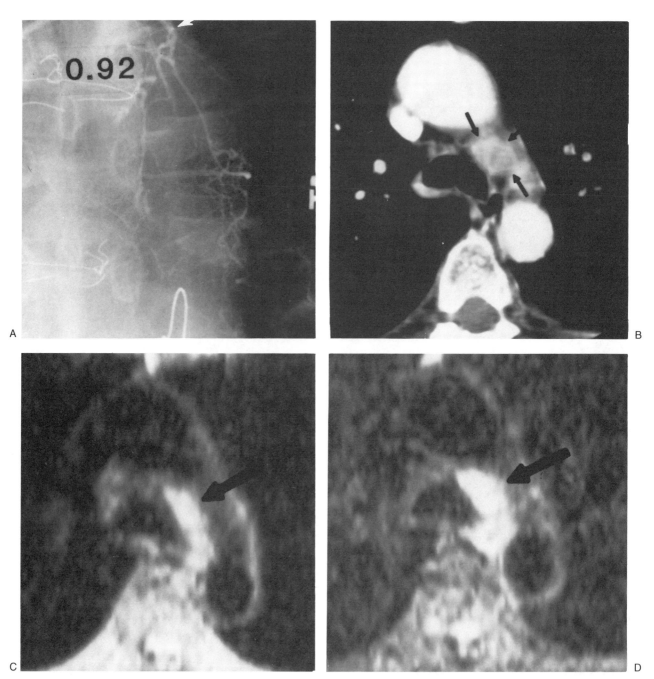

FIG. 2. This 58-year old woman underwent multiple cervical as well as a mediastinal explorations with thymic resection, but continued to be hypercalcemic with disabling nephrolithiasis. Initially all noninvasive studies as well as parathyroid arteriography were interpreted as normal. Venous sampling demonstrated a small but significant (fourfold) step-up in a left thymic vein (*arrow* in **A**), indicating a mediastinal location (peripheral 0.21 PTH pg/ml). Computed tomography was considered suspicious for a mass in the aortopulmonary window (*arrows* in **B**), but it could not be separated from the top of the pulmonary artery. However, MRI with T2-weighted (*arrow* in **C**) and especially with fat-suppressed STIR (*arrow* in **D**) sequences demonstrated a mass of increased signal intensity in the aortopulmonary window. A 2.5 cm adenoma was removed by a left thoracotomy (surgical follow-up courtesy of Dr. Samuel Wells, Washington University, St. Louis, MO).

Aspiration of Parathyroid Tissue Suspected From One Noninvasive Technique

When ultrasound or CT shows a suspicious lesion not confirmed by a second noninvasive technique, direct aspiration of the lesion to measure PTH levels will often eliminate the necessity of proceeding to invasive procedures such as arteriography and venous sampling (6). One passes the 23 gauge needle under ultrasound or CT control back and forth through the suspicious mass, applying gentle suction to the attached syringe. Upon withdrawing the needle, one aspirates 1 ml of albumin through the needle into the syringe and measures the concentration of PTH in the specimen (Fig. 3).

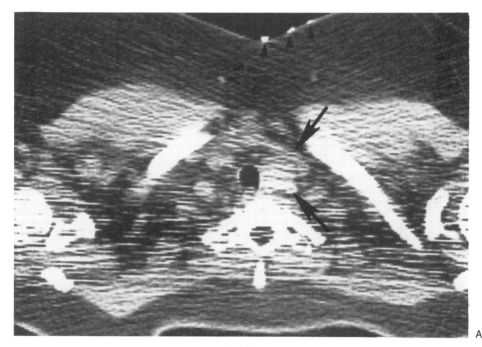

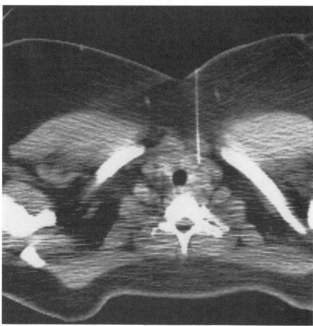

FIG. 3. There is a suspicious mass just to the left of the trachea below the left thyroid lobe (*arrows* in **A**) in a very obese patient with previous unsuccessful surgery. Neither ultrasound nor thallium/technetium scanning identified the mass, probably because of the marked obesity. Note the barium markers (*arrowheads* in **A**) on the anterior neck that assist in directing the needle. Needle aspiration (**B**) was performed for PTH level. Measurement revealed very high levels of PTH in the aspirate, and a left peritracheal adenoma was subsequently removed.

PTH levels are usually astronomically high, and the diagnosis is thus very specific. When successful this is more direct and less expensive than cytological examination of the aspirate. Although an experienced cytologist can distinguish thyroid from parathyroid tissue easily, the distinction between thyroid and parathyroid adenomas cannot always be made cytologically. In a review of our last 40 aspirations, the sensitivity was 75%, with no false positives. A negative aspiration has no meaning, in that 25% of surgically proven parathyroid adenomas had a negative aspiration. We have aspirated lesions in the tracheoesophageal groove and the anterior mediastinum under CT control with no morbidity. In a single instance, a postaspiration intraadenomal hemorrhage led to remission of the primary hyperparathyroidism (Fig. 4). However, the deliberate attempt to ablate parathyroid tissue by direct injection of ethanol into the adenoma (11,12) is not recommended. It is difficult to control reflux of alcohol into surrounding tissues, which contain the recurrent laryngeal nerve and other vital structures. The direct percutaneous injection of ethanol into cervical adenomas has been associated with an unacceptable frequency of transient and permanent recurrent nerve injuries and in my opinion is never justified in patients with well localized adenomas and no previous surgery. Under special circumstances, injection of ethanol into intrathyroidal parathyroid adenomas can be safely performed because of the protective effect of surrounding thyroid tissue (13). Direct ethanol injection may be an acceptable technique to palliate secondary hyperparathyroidism in severely ill patients with chronic renal failure (14), but as a primary treatment for cervical adenomas its effectiveness and safety have not been demonstrated.

Invasive Localization Tests: Arteriography and Selective Venous Sampling

Parathyroid arteriography and selective venous sampling are the ultimate invasive studies for parathyroid localization in patients who have had previous surgery (15). In our experience, ~35–40% of patients will require arteriography, and ~20% will require venous sampling (an unequivocally positive parathyroid arteriogram in a patient with known adenoma does not require venous sampling). Parathyroid arteriography requires selective injection of the internal mammary arteries, the thyrocervical trunks, and the common carotid arteries. The internal mammary arteries and thyrocervical trunks are injected first, because there is a slight but definite risk when performing common carotid artery injections in this middle-aged population. When the thyrocervical and internal mammary arteriograms do not reveal the adenoma, common carotid injections are performed to exclude an undescended parathyroid gland. Digital subtraction angiography is

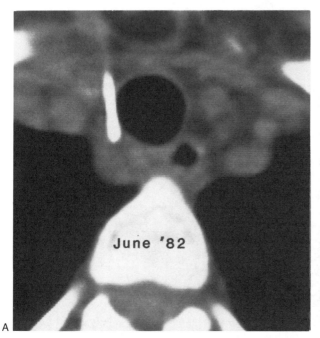 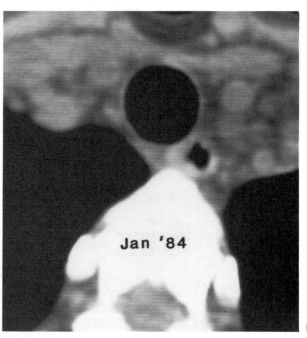

FIG. 4. Computed tomography demonstrates needle aspiration of a typical ectopic superior adenoma in the right tracheoesophageal groove (**A**). The patient developed discomfort in the neck and hypocalcemia following the positive aspiration, probably due to hemorrhage within the adenoma. Two years later the adenoma has disappeared and the patient remains normocalcemic (**B**).

used with dilute contrast agent to lessen neurotoxicity. Contrary to a widely held opinion, there is no risk to the cervical spinal cord when injecting the thyrocervical, trunk. Blood supply to the cervical spinal cord arises from the costocervical, not from the thyrocervical, trunk, and the two should not be confused by an experienced angiographer. In over 1,000 selective injections of the thyrocervical trunk, I have visualized only a single instance of blood supply to the cervical spinal cord.

At arteriography, parathyroid glands appear as homogeneous dense areas of enhancement (Fig. 5). Large, nonhomogeneous staining areas and a compatible clinical history (severe hypercalcemia, rapidly progressive course) may suggest the diagnosis of parathyroid carcinoma, but localization is generally not a problem in that carcinomas tend to recur at the site of the initially resected tumor. Adenomas in the anterior mediastinum may have a descending blood supply from the thyrocervical trunk or may be fed by the thymic branch of the internal mammary artery. Glands with a blood supply from the internal mammary artery may be more difficult to extract by cervical thymectomy but are particularly well suited for transcatheter ablation (16,17). If the catheter can be wedged into the artery feeding the adenoma, a prolonged injection of contrast results in dense staining of the gland. We use ionic contrast material and repeat the procedure three or four times until a long-lasting dense opacification is achieved (Fig. 6). Persistence of the stain on a CT examination 24 hr later has in our experience invariably been associated with cure of hyperparathyroidism.

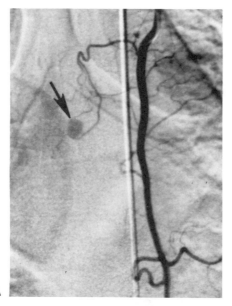

A

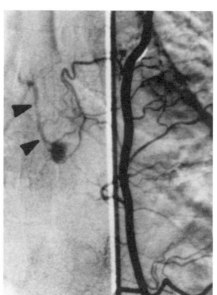

B

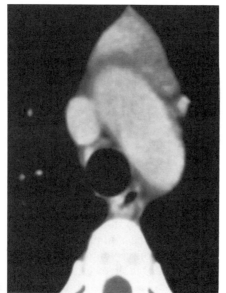

C

FIG. 5. This 19-year-old woman underwent unsuccessful neck exploration for hypercalcemia. Selective left internal mammary arteriogram demonstrates a densely enhancing parathyroid adenoma in the anterior mediastinum (*arrow* in **A**) supplied by the thymic branch. Delayed films identified venous drainage (*arrowheads* in **B**) into the left thymic vein, but venous sampling would not be necessary with such a pathognomonic arteriogram. Note that this gland is not visible by CT (nor by any noninvasive localizing study) because it is contained within a water density thymic gland. The adenoma was successfully treated by staining (see text) (**C**).

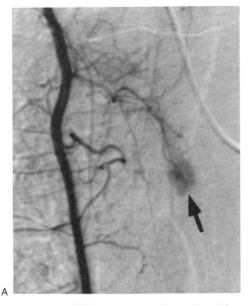

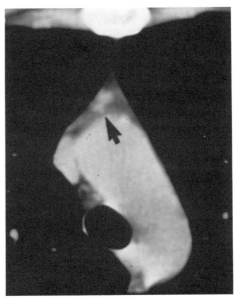

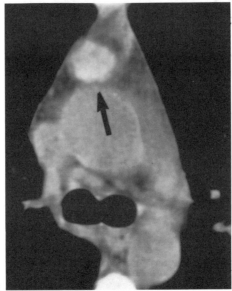

FIG. 6. Right internal mammary arteriogram demonstrates a parathyroid adenoma in the anterior mediastinum (*arrow* in **A**). CT was positive (*arrow* in **B**), but the patient elected to undergo staining rather than sternotomy. Note the persistent staining and swelling of the adenoma at 24 hr (*arrow* in **C**). Such findings at 24 hr are almost always associated with permanent ablation, as in this patient (follow-up 6 years).

Only minimal discomfort is associated with staining, and this technique obviates the need for a sternotomy. We have stained over 30 glands, with only a single significant morbidity, a severe vasovagal reaction. Unsuccessful staining does not compromise subsequent surgery (18), unlike direct alcohol injection, which tends to fix glands to surrounding critical structures in the neck and renders subsequent surgical excision more difficult.

Venous sampling for elevated levels of PTH remains the final and often the only positive study in patients with multiple, competently performed previous operations. Positive venous sampling often leads to detection of an adenoma on reviewing the noninvasive studies (Fig. 7). Venous sampling does not demonstrate the adenoma but directs the surgeon to the area (right

neck, left neck, mediastinum) in which the adenoma lies. Successful venous sampling is compromised by the previous performance of a thyroidectomy, because access to parathyroid venous drainage is dependent on the larger thyroid veins. Unilateral thyroidectomy is frequently performed at the initial exploration when no adenoma is found and a gland is missing on one side. The incidence of intrathyroidal parathyroid adenomas is <5% in our experience, and they can be excluded with 100% accuracy with the use of intraoperative ultrasound (19). There is little reason, therefore, for performing a hemithyroidectomy at the time of an unsuccessful parathyroid exploration. Following thyroidectomy, venous drainage of cervical parathyroid glands is diverted into the vertebral vein, which should always be sampled in difficult cases. Para-

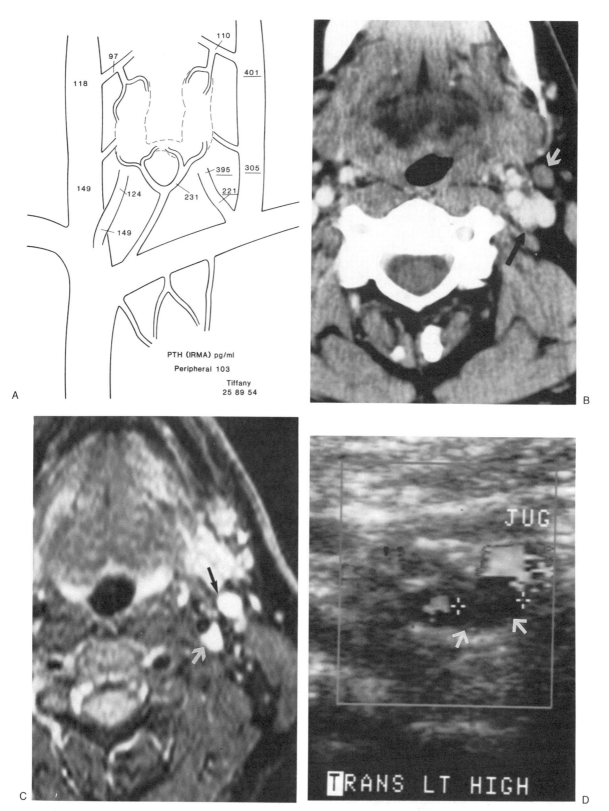

FIG. 7. This 35-year-old man had undergone three previous neck operations and one mediastinal exploration without correcting his hypercalcemia. On ultrasound, CT, and MRI, no lesion was seen, although multiple anterior cervical "lymph nodes" were noted bilaterally. Parathyroid venous sampling showed increasing levels (underscored) of PTH as one ascended the left internal jugular and left vertebral veins, indicating a left-sided undescended parathyroid gland (**A**). Review of the CT scan revealed an enhancing mass between the left internal carotid artery and the left jugular vein (*black arrow* in **B**). Note that this lesion enhances as compared to the lymph node anterior to the left internal jugular vein (*white arrow* in **B**). On MRI, both the parathyroid adenoma (*white arrow* in **C**) and the lymph node lateral to the internal jugular vein (*black arrow* in **C**) appear bright and cannot be distinguished, but the results of parathyroid venous sampling assured us the lesion was high in the left neck. A repeat ultrasound examination demonstrated a hypoechoic mass within the carotid sheath between the carotid artery and jugular vein. (*white arrows* in **D**). The patient was cured by a simple vertical incision just anterior to the left midsternocleidomastoid muscle, avoiding the heavily scarred original operative site.

thyroid venous sampling requires experience; such problem cases should be referred to institutions performing this study. We obtain venous gradients such as those shown in Fig. 7 in >90% of patients sampled.

In our experience, undescended parathyroid glands constitute ~10% of all reoperative cases but are particularly common among referrals from experienced parathyroid surgeons (20,21). The undescended or parathymic parathyroid gland lies adjacent to the carotid bifurcation and is readily visualized by ultrasound, CT, and MRI, provided that these studies are performed high enough in the neck. These glands classically lie immediately in front of the carotid bifurcation (Fig. 8) but may occur within the carotid sheath posterior to the jugular vein (Fig. 7). Embryologically, these glands remain at the level of the branchial cleft from which they originate and are difficult to reach from a classical transverse cervical incision. Noninvasive studies routinely must be carried above the angle of the mandible to visualize these glands. Distinguishing them from lymph nodes is particularly difficult. Both undescended parathyroid glands and cervical lymph nodes appear bright on T2-weighted and STIR sequences and are usually indistinguishable by ultrasound. Doppler color flow imaging shows evidence of blood flow in adenomas but not in lymph nodes. The presence of multiple masses favors a diagnosis of lymph nodes, but direct aspiration for PTH levels or venous sampling can confirm the diagnosis of an undescended parathyroid gland. Once established, a small incision anterior to the midportion of the sternocleidomastoid muscle permits removal of the gland without going through the original transverse cervical incision.

In summary, the noninvasive techniques—ultrasound, thallium/technetium subtraction scintigraphy, CT, and MRI—should be performed initially for parathyroid localization in patients who have undergone previous neck surgery. For definitive localization, two positive studies at the same site are required because of the high incidence (15–18%) of false-positive studies. If only a single noninvasive study is positive, the diagnosis can often be confirmed by direct aspiration of the suspicious nodule under control of the appropriate imaging modality. When noninvasive studies are negative (40% of all reoperative cases), parathyroid arteriography and venous sampling should be performed. Using this algorithm, we have achieved a 97% success rate in a series of 107 consecutive reoperative cases (2). Blind thyroidectomies and sternotomies following a negative cervical exploration are no longer justified with the current sophisticated localization techniques. A close collaboration between endocrinologist, radiologist, and surgeon is essential to ensure a successful outcome.

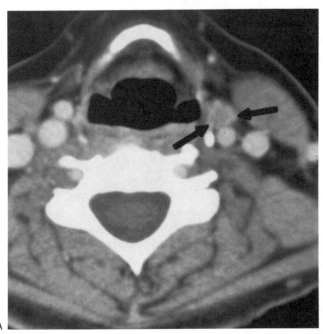 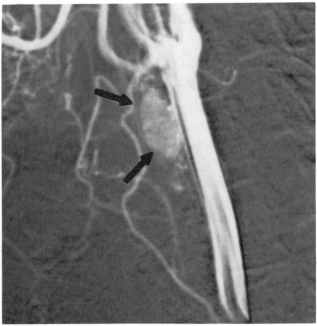

A

B

FIG. 8. Note the undescended adenoma (*arrows* in **A**) immediately anterior to the carotid artery at the level of the lateral pharyngeal pouch, from which parathyroid glands arise. Lateral left carotid arteriography demonstrates the "undescended" position of the adenoma (*arrows* in **B**).

LOCALIZATION STUDIES IN PATIENTS UNDERGOING INITIAL SURGERY FOR PRIMARY HYPERPARATHYROIDISM

There is a growing tendency for physicians to recommend one or several noninvasive localizing studies prior to initial surgery in patients with primary hyperparathyroidism. A review of 15 recent studies reported in the literature revealed eight recommending localization procedures and seven seeing no need for preoperative localization (22). Ultrasound and thallium/technetium scanning, because of their noninvasiveness and low cost, are generally the initial procedures of choice, but both CT and even MRI are sometimes performed when the ultrasound and thallium/technetium examinations are negative. The arguments used to support these studies are that preoperative localization 1) shortens operating time and 2) prevents failed operations. Although most surgeons, when armed with a positive preoperative ultrasound study, explore the positive side first, few perform a unilateral exploration at the time of the initial surgery for fear of overlooking four-gland hyperplasia or double adenomas. Thus limiting surgery to one side of the neck is not an argument supporting preoperative localization.

At the recent NIH Consensus Conference dealing with asymptomatic hyperparathyroidism, I reviewed the results from several large (>25 patients) series of patients undergoing noninvasive localizing studies (ultrasound, thallium/technetium scanning, CT, and MRI) prior to successful surgery (22–28). Only series published after 1985 were included, because the state of the art for ultrasound, thallium/technetium scanning, and CT has remained relatively stable during this period. Interestingly, the initial descriptions for each imaging modality were often unduly optimistic. Edis and Evans (29) reported 100% sensitivity (ten of ten successfully localized adenomas) in the first study using high-resolution ultrasound and predicted that advances in ultrasonic instrumentation would soon enable us to image normal glands. Similarly, the first description (30,31) of thallium/technetium subtraction scintigraphy stated a sensitivity of 95% (20 of 21 successfully localized tumors). These initial optimistic results have not been sustained in larger series. Table 2 summarizes the true-positive and false-positive rates of ultrasound, thallium/technetium scanning, CT, and MRI as reported in several large series of surgically proven cases. Sensitivity varied between 60% and 70%, with a false-positive rate for all studies of ~15%. Although some investigators report a higher sensitivity with a specific modality, it often occurred at the expense of an increased false-positive rate. Workers from a few institutions reported superior sensitivities using a modality with which they had extensive experience, but the purpose of the study was to evaluate the results that could be expected in institutions with broad experience with parathyroid localization but without dedication to a single modality. The NIH experience is not included, because very few patients are seen at the NIH before their initial surgery.

The sensitivity of 60–70% with a false-positive rate of 15% must be contrasted with widely reported surgical success rates of 90–95% in patients undergoing initial operations (1,32). In addition, studies that have monitored operating times or surgical success rates have not been able to establish a significant difference between patients without and with preoperative localization. Serpell et al. (28) evaluated 50 patients with thallium/technetium scanning. Although the sensitivity of the scintigraphy study in their hands was outstanding (68%), operating times were the same in patients with successful (90 min) and failed (80 min) preoperative localization. Wilson et al. (26) compared their surgical results in 100 patients undergoing all four localizing studies (ultrasound, thallium/technetium, CT, and MRI) with 100 patients in whom no localization studies were performed. Operating times were similar in both groups (107 vs. 104 min) and the success rates were indistinguishable (97% vs. 96%). There has never been a well-controlled study showing a decrease in operating time or improvement in surgical success attributable to preoperative localization in patients undergoing initial surgery.

Is there any evidence that preoperative localization prevents those 5–8% unsuccessful initial operations? Several reviews have addressed the causes of failed initial surgery (33,34). The most common cause is the failure of the surgeon to recognize hyperplasia. However, all noninvasive localizing studies perform poorly in distinguishing hyperplasia from adenoma, usually disclosing only the largest of the hyperplastic glands. The second most common cause for failed initial surgery was glands in ectopic locations, particularly in the tracheoesophageal groove and anterior mediastinum. Such glands are usually demonstrated by CT and MRI, but ultrasound and thallium/technetium scanning, the two most commonly recommended noninvasive screening studies, perform poorly in these

TABLE 2. *Sensitivity and false-positive rate of noninvasive localizing studies[a]*

	Sensitivity (%)	False-positive rate (%)
Ultrasound	65	12.5
Thallium/Tc scintigraphy	55	13.5
CT	63	—
MRI	74	18

[a]Modified from ref. 22 with permission.

areas. Bruining et al. (33) list inexperience of the surgeon as a cause for a significant number of failed initial operations. The confidence of the clinician engendered by a positive preoperative localization study may encourage referral to a less experienced surgeon, but 15% of patients with positive noninvasive localization will have unanticipated hyperplasia requiring resection of 3.5 glands, and at least 15% will have false-positive results unless two studies are positive at the same site. Therefore, 30% of anticipated "simple adenomectomies" will be complex, requiring an experienced parathyroid surgeon.

Clinicians sometimes express the fear that failure to conduct localizing studies prior to initial surgery exposes them to medicolegal liability in the 5–10% of patients with failed initial operations. It is difficult to justify performing unindicated localization in 90% of patients when there is strong evidence that preoperative localization does not prevent surgical failures. The current emphasis on cost containment should lead to standards for the diagnostic workup of primary hyperparathyroidism, based on the scientific evidence, not only excluding the necessity of but refusing to compensate for such studies. The only localization study needed by a patient undergoing initial parathyroid surgery is to locate an experienced parathyroid surgeon.

REFERENCES

1. Savata RM Jr, Beahrs OH, Scholz DA. Success rate of cervical exploration for hyperparathyroidism. *Arch Surg* 1975;110:625–628.
2. Carty SE, Norton J. Management of patients with persistent or recurrent primary hyperparathyroidism. *World J Surg* 1991;15:716–723.
3. Miller DL, Doppman JL, Krudy AG, et al. Localization of parathyroid adenomas in patients who have undergone surgery. Part I. Non-invasive imaging methods. *Radiology* 1987;162:133–137.
4. O'Doherty MJ, Kettle AG, Wells P, Collins EC, Coakley AJ. Parathyroid imaging with Technetium-99m-Sestamibi: preoperative localization and tissue uptake studies. *J Nucl Med* 1992;33:313–318.
5. Taillifer R, Boucher Y, Potvin C, Lambert R. Detection and localization of parathyroid adenomas in patients with hyperparathyroidism using a single radionuclide imaging procedure with technetium-99m-Sestamibi (double phase study). *J Nucl Med* 1992;33:1801–1807.
6. Doppman JL, Shawker TH, Krudy AG, et al. Aspiration of enlarged parathyroid glands for parathyroid hormone assay. *Radiology* 1983;148:31–35.
7. Peck WW, Higgins CB, Fisher MR, et al. Hyperparathyroidism: comparison of MR imaging with radionuclide scanning. *Radiology* 1987;163:415–420.
8. Kneeland JB, Krubsack AJ, Lawson TL, et al. Enlarged parathyroid glands: high resolution local coil MR imaging. *Radiology* 1987;162:143–146.
9. Auffermann W, Gooding GAW, Okerlund MD, et al. Diagnosis of recurrent hyperparathyroidism: comparison with MR imaging with other imaging techniques. *Am J Roentgenol* 1988;150:1027–1033.
10. Seelos KC, DeMarco R, Clark OH, et al. Persistent and recurrent hyperparathyroidism: assessment with gadopentate dimeglumine-enhanced MR imaging. *Radiology* 1990;177:373.
11. Karstrup S, Transbol I, Holm HH, Glenthoj A, Hegedus L. Ultrasound-guided chemical parathyroidectomy in patients with primary hyperparathyroidism: a prospective study. *Br Radiol* 1989;62:1037–1042.
12. Karstrup S, Holm HH, Granthoj A, et al. Non-surgical treatment of primary hyperparathyroidism with sonographically guided percutaneous injection of ethanol: results in a selected series of patients. *Am J Roentgenol* 1990;154:1087–1090.
13. Charboneau JW, Hay ID, van Heerden JA. Persistent primary hyperparathyroidism: successful ultrasound-guided percutaneous ethanol ablation of an occult adenoma. *Mayo Clin Proc* 1988;63:913–917.
14. Solbiati L, Giangrande AL, DePra L, et al. Percutaneous ethanol injection of parathyroid tumors under US guidance: treatment for secondary hyperparathyroidism. *Radiology* 1985;155:607–610.
15. Miller DL, Doppman JL, Krudy AG, et al. Localization of parathyroid adenomas in patients who have undergone surgery. Part II. Invasive procedures. *Radiology* 1987;162:138–141.
16. Doppman JL. The treatment of hyperparathyroidism by transcatheter techniques. *Cardiovasc Intervent Radiol* 1980;3:268–281.
17. Miller DL, Doppman JL, Chang R, et al. Angiographic ablation of parathyroid adenomas: lessons from a 10-year experience. *Radiology* 1987;165:601–607.
18. Doherty GM, Doppman JL, Miller DL, et al. Results of the multidisciplinary strategy in managing mediastinum parathyroid adenoma as the cause of persistent primary hyperparathyroidism. *Ann Surg* 1992;215:101–106.
19. Kern KA, Shawker TH, Doppman JL, et al. The use of high-resolution ultrasound to locate parathyroid tumors during reoperations for primary hyperparathyroidism. *World J Surg* 1987;11:579–585.
20. Doppman JL, Shawker TH, Krudy AG, et al. Parathymic parathyroid, CT, US, and angiographic findings. *Radiology* 1985;157:419–423.
21. Fraker DL, Doppman JL, Shawker TH, Marx SJ, Spiegel AM, Norton JA. Undescended parathyroid adenoma: an important etiology for failed operations for primary hyperparathyroidism. *World J Surg* 1990;14:342–348.
22. Doppman JL, Miller DL. Localization of parathyroid tumors in patients with asymptomatic hyperparathyroidism and no previous surgery. *J Bone Mineral Res* 1991;6:S153–S158.
23. Krubsack AJ, Wilson SD, Lawson TL, et al. Prospective comparison of radionuclide, computed tomographic, sonographic and magnetic resonance localization of parathyroid tumors. *Surgery* 1989;106:639–646.
24. Roses DF, Sudarsky LA, Sanger J, Raghavendra BN, Reede DL, Blum M. The use of preoperative localization of adenomas of the parathyroid glands by thallium/technetium subtraction scintigraphy, high-resolution ultrasonography and computed tomography. *Surg Gynecol Obstet* 1989;168:99–105.
25. Uden P, Aspelin P, Berglun J, et al. Preoperative localization and unilateral parathyroid surgery. *Acta Chir Scand* 1990;156:29–35.
26. Wilson SD, Hoffmann RG, Cerletty JM, et al. Parathyroidectomy for primary hyperparathyroidism: the influence of preoperative localizing studies on cure rate and operating time. Paper presented at the 1991 Annual Meeting Society for Endocrine Surgeons, San Jose, California, March, 1991.
27. Carlson GL, Farndon JR, Clayton B, Rose PG. Thallium isotope scintigraphy and ultrasonography: comparative studies of localization techniques in primary hyperparathyroidism. *Br J Surg* 1990;77:327–329.
28. Serpel JW, Campbell PR, Young AE. Preoperative localization of parathyroid tumors does not reduce operating time. *Br J Surg* 1991;78:589–590.
29. Edis AJ, Evans PC Jr. High resolution real time ultrasonog-

raphy and preoperative localization of parathyroid tumors. *N Engl J Med* 1979;301:532–534.
30. Ferlin G, Borsato N, Perelli R. Technetium/thallium subtraction scan. A new method in preoperative localization of parathyroid enlargement. *Eur J Nucl Med* 1981;6A:12.
31. Ferlin G, Borsato, Camerani M. New perspectives in localizing enlarged parathyroid glands by technetium/thallium subtraction scan. *J Nucl Med* 1983;24:438–441.
32. Thompson N. Localization studies of patients with primary hyperparathyroidism. *Br Med J* 1988;75:97–98.
33. Bruining HA, Birkenhager JC, Ong GL, Lamberts SWJ. Causes of failure in operations for hyperparathyroidism. *Surgery* 1987;101:562–565.
34. Levin KE, Clark OH. The reasons for failure in parathyroid operations. *Arch Surg* 1989;124:911–915.
35. Young AE, Gaunt JI, Croft DN, et al. Location of parathyroid adenoma by thallium 201 and technetium 99M subtractions scanning. *Br Med J* 1983;286:1384–1386 [adenoma was localized in 20 of 21 cases].

The Parathyroids, edited by J.P. Bilezikian, M.A. Levine, and R. Marcus. Raven Press, Ltd., New York © 1994.

CHAPTER 34

Guidelines for the Medical or Surgical Management of Primary Hyperparathyroidism

To Operate or Not to Operate

John P. Bilezikian

In the preautoanalyzer era, when primary hyperparathyroidism was appreciated virtually exclusively in the context of symptomatic disease, surgery was always indicated. Removal of the offending adenoma or hyperplastic tissue invariably led to correction of the hypercalcemia and normalization of the parathyroid hormone (PTH) level. Surgery is still the only definitive therapy for primary hyperparathyroidism. In the hands of a surgeon with expertise and interest in parathyroidectomy, cure is achieved >90% of the time (1). If there are no contraindications, surgery for primary hyperparathyroidism in any of its modern presentations is always a reasonable course of action. However, the most common presentation of primary hyperparathyroidism now is an asymptomatic one, in which patients have neither signs nor symptoms that can be clearly attributed to the disease (2). The serendipitous discovery of asymptomatic primary hyperparathyroidism in many patients has raised important questions about the advisability of surgery in all patients. If the natural history of the disease were known with regard to who is likely to develop complications and who is likely to remain asymptomatic, one could be more secure in making decisions about surgery. No surgery using general anesthesia can be undertaken lightly. Of greater concern is the fact that not all surgeons who operate on patients with primary hyperparathyroidism enjoy the high operative success rates of those who are experts in the operation. Finally, there can be complications of surgery per se (see the chapter by Norton et al.). A general rule is that surgery of any kind is performed only when indicated, but, regarding patients with primary hyperparathyroidism, for whom is surgery indicated?

Simply stated, the dilemma is who among the large number of patients seen with primary hyperparathyroidism should be advised to undergo parathyroid ectomy and who can be safely advised to be monitored without surgery? Uncertainty about the management of primary hyperparathyroidism as it presents today led to an important Consensus Development Conference on the Diagnosis and Management of Asymptomatic Primary Hyperparathyroidism, which was held at the National Institutes of Health, October 29–31, 1990. The proceedings of this conference were published in the *Journal of Bone and Mineral Research* (3) and in summary form elsewhere (4,5). Based on our current knowledge, guidelines were recommended for surgical or medical management of primary hyperparathyroidism. This chapter summarizes the views expressed at that conference as well as other pertinent issues related to this topic.

It should be emphasized that this is an uncertain area; our knowledge of the course of primary hyperparathyroidism as it is seen today is incomplete. The guidelines are based on our current knowledge and are likely to be modified as additional information relevant to this area becomes available.

J. P. Bilezikian: Departments of Medicine and Pharmacology, College of Physicians and Surgeons, Columbia University, New York, New York 10032.

WHO SHOULD BE REFERRED FOR SURGERY?

It is clear that patients who have symptoms directly attributable to primary hyperparathyroidism are candidates for surgery. It is important to recognize that some patients with asymptomatic primary hyperparathyroidism may also meet guidelines for surgery. In fact, a significant number of patients with asymptomatic primary hyperparathyroidism will meet one or more currently accepted surgical guidelines. Thus, in our experience, whereas only ~20% of patients with primary hyperparathyroidism are symptomatic, and therefore are surgical candidates, an additional 30–40% of asymptomatic patients also meet guidelines for surgery. Overall, about one-half of all patients will meet criteria for surgery (Fig. 1). Guidelines for surgery are summarized in Table 1.

Definite Indications for Surgery

1. *Serum calcium >1 mg/dl above the upper limits of normal.* No great insight has led to this rather arbitrary designation of a calcium level above which most clinicians would be more comfortable recommending surgery. However, it is in the range of mild hypercalcemia, within 1 mg/dl of the upper limits of normal, that most patients are asymptomatic both of the hyperparathyroidism and of the hypercalcemia. As the serum calcium rises above this concentration, symptoms of hypercalcemia per se and of primary hyperparathyroidism become more likely. Among laboratories in the United States, the upper limit of normal ranges between 10.2 and 10.7 mg/dl. Depending on the laboratory, therefore, levels of serum calcium exceeding 11.2 (if the upper of limit of normal is 10.2) or 11.7 (if the upper limit of normal is 10.7) would be sufficient to recommend for surgery. Certainly, anyone with a serum calcium consistently >12.0 mg/dl would meet this guideline.

2. *Hypercalciuria.* The 24 hr urinary collection for calcium excretion should be obtained on a diet that is not >1 g calcium and is not supplemented with calcium. The Consensus Development Conference suggested a value of 400 mg for total urinary calcium excretion as unequivocally qualifying as hypercalciuria. However, many definitions of hypercalciuria would place the upper limit at 250 mg total excretion for women and 300 mg total excretion for men. As has been noted in the chapter by Klugman et al. and in other studies (6), there is no clear relationship between primary hyperparathyroidism and hypercalciuria insofar as nephrolithiasis is concerned. Nevertheless, it may be more likely for a patient with hypercalciuria to be predisposed towards kidney stones, nephrocalcinosis, or reduced renal function. Thus patients with primary hyperparathyroidism and hypercalciuria are candidates for parathyroid surgery.

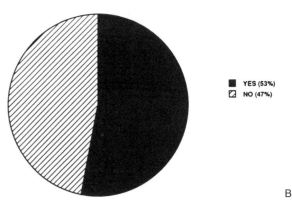

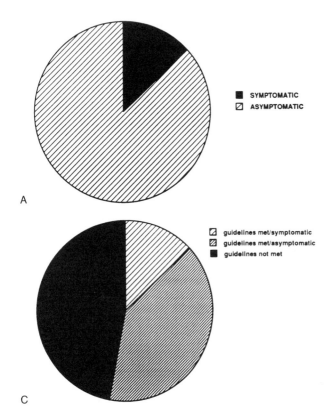

FIG. 1. Distribution of patients with primary hyperparathyroidism. **A:** Prevalence of symptoms in 100 patients with primary hyperparathyroidism (PHPT). The graph indicates that the majority of patients today have asymptomatic primary hyperparathyroidism (see text for definition). **B:** Even though the majority of patients are asymptomatic, approximately one-half of the patient population meet one or more guidelines for surgery (see Table 1). **C:** Among the group of patients who meet one or more guidelines for surgery, the majority are asymptomatic.

TABLE 1. *Guidelines for surgery in primary hyperparathyroidism*

Definite	Relative
Serum calcium >1 mg/dl above the upper limits of normal	Classic neuromuscular or neuropsychiatric manifestations
Hypercalciuria	Peptic ulcer disease or pancreatitis
Nephrolithiasis or nephrocalcinosis	Hypertension
Reduced creatinine clearance (in absence of other cause)	Age <50 years
Specific radiographic manifestations of primary hyperparathyroidism (osteitis fibrosa cystica)	
Substantial reduction in bone mineral density	
Episode of acute primary hyperparathyroidism	

3. *Nephrolithiasis or nephrocalcinosis.* A well-documented history of a kidney stone is a rather straightforward indication for surgery. One could argue, of course, that nephrolithiasis need not be pathophysiologically related to primary hyperparathyroidism. Indeed, in some cases, one may be dealing with the coincidental occurrence of two common disorders. Moreover, about 7% of the stone-forming population will be shown to have primary hyperparathyroidism (7-8). Nevertheless, the association of primary hyperparathyroidism and stone disease is so well established that it would seem reasonable to consider a stone in any patient with primary hyperparathyroidism to be an indication for surgery. Similarly, the process of calcium deposition in the parenchyma of the kidney, nephrocalcinosis, is an indication for surgery. Nephrocalcinosis cannot be excluded without abdominal radiography or ultrasound examination of the abdomen.

4. *Reduced creatinine clearance in the absence of any other cause.* If the creatinine clearance is reduced by >30% from age- and sex-adjusted norms, without any other apparent cause, most clinicians would follow through with a recommendation for surgery. It is true, however, that renal function, as reflected in the creatinine clearance, generally does not improve after successful surgery (9). Nevertheless, without any other explanation, one is justifiably concerned that renal function could deteriorate further without successful parathyroid surgery.

5. *Overt bone disease.* In those few individuals who have radiologically evident parathyroid bone disease, surgery should be performed. This presentation accounts for fewer than 5% of patients with the disease.

6. *Reduced bone mineral density.* The preferential loss of cortical bone in primary hyperparathyroidism has been reviewed (see the chapters by Bilezikian,

"Clinical Presentation of Primary Hyperparathyroidism," and Parisien et al.). If bone mineral density of the distal radius, a site enriched in cortical bone, is reduced 2 SD below age- and sex-matched control values (z score < -2), most experts would agree that surgery is strongly indicated. The subject of changes at cancellous sites is more complicated and is discussed in a separate section (see below).

7. *An episode of acute primary hyperparathyroidism.* Approximately 25% of patients who develop acute primary hyperparathyroidism have a history of mild hypercalcemia (see the chapter by Fitzpatrick) (10). For this group as well as the vast majority of patients with acute primary hyperparathyroidism whose disease is first manifested by this dramatic presentation, surgery is clearly indicated.

Possible Other Indications for Surgery

1. *Classic neuromuscular or neuropsychiatric manifestations.* The neuromuscular manifestations of primary hyperparathyroidism are now seen only in more advanced cases (11). On the other hand, neuropsychiatric manifestations continue to be a subject of great concern (12–15). Although nonspecific, these manifestations may occasionally be so compelling that it is hard not to conclude that the patient is symptomatic (for discussion, see the chapters by Bilezikian et al., "Clinical Presentation of Primary Hyperparathyroidism," and by Kleerekoper). This is an area in which quantitative data are still inconclusive.

2. *Gastrointestinal manifestations: peptic ulcer disease and pancreatitis.* Although the association between primary hyperparathyroidism and peptic ulcer disease is not well established except in the setting of multiple endocrine neoplasia type I, it is reasonable to be concerned about a pathophysiological relationship (16). The association may be merely coincidental, or it may be based on the effects of calcium on gastric acid production or other mechanism. The presence of peptic ulcer disease should be regarded as a relative indication for surgery. Similarly, the association between primary hyperparathyroidism and pancreatitis, which is well established in situations in which the serum calcium is markedly elevated, might conceivably play a role even when the serum calcium is only modestly elevated (17). In the absence of other clear predisposing factors, hyperparathyroid patients with acute pancreatitis should be seriously considered for surgery.

3. *Hypertension.* Here, again, the presence of hypertension is not clearly a specific manifestation of the hyperparathyroid process. However, studies reviewed earlier suggest that there may be a greater incidence of hypertension among patients with primary hyperparathyroidism compared to control populations (18–22). Even if hypertension is regarded to be a feature of pri-

mary hyperparathyroidism, the hypertension does not usually remit after successful surgery (23,24). Whether the hypertension is easier to treat after normocalcemia has been achieved is unclear.

4. *Age over 50 years.* Patients who are under 50 years old at the time of diagnosis are generally recommended for parathyroidectomy even if they have no other indications for surgery. The reason for this recommendation is that younger patients are more likely eventually to experience a complication of primary hyperparathyroidism. There are, however, no data to support this view at the present time.

Other Considerations Affecting Surgery for Primary Hyperparathyroidism

There are patients who do not meet any of the criteria described above but who nevertheless do not want to live with their disease. If, after being completely informed, these patients prefer to undergo parathyroid surgery, and no contraindications exist, it is hard to argue against this choice. On the other hand, there are patients who meet one or more guidelines for surgery who, either because of extenuating medical circumstance or for strong personal reasons, do not undergo parathyroid surgery. These final points illustrate the importance of close physician–patient interaction at this point of decision making.

CHOICE OF SURGEON

The topic of surgery is covered completely in the chapter by Norton et al. The only point to restate here is that, when the decision is made in favor of parathyroid surgery, it is important to refer the patient to a surgeon whose mastery of this potentially difficult operation is unquestioned. Major medical centers tend to have one or two surgeons who regularly perform parathyroidectomy and have become familiar with the nuances of the operation. Expert parathyroid surgeons, in fact, are so successful that they locate abnormal parathyroid tissue with only rare failures and certainly more commonly than any preoperative localization tests that are currently available (see the chapters by Norton et al. and by Doppman).

WHO CAN BE FOLLOWED SAFELY WITHOUT SURGERY?

It is the consensus of most experts that there are patients for whom a nonsurgical approach to primary hyperparathyroidism can be taken without undue risk. Characteristics of this group are listed in Table 2. The serum calcium concentration is not >1 mg/dl above the upper limits of normal. Urinary calcium excretion

TABLE 2. *Asymptomatic primary hyperparathyroidism in which surgery is not clearly the treatment of choice*

Serum calcium within 1 mg/dl of the upper limits of normal
Normal urinary calcium excretion
No nephrolithiasis and no nephrocalcinosis
No substantial reduction in bone mineral density
No other clearly attributable symptoms or signs
Age >50 years

is normal. These patients are without any other renal manifestations of primary hyperparathyroidism, have bone mineral densities that are within normal limits, and feel well. Many of them do not complain of fatigue, nor do they have a sense that they are "slowing down," features that may suggest that the nonspecific features of primary hyperparathyroidism are present. They have no history of peptic ulcer disease or pancreatitis. These patients are followed regularly as described below.

Primary Hyperparathyroidism in Postmenopausal Women

This group of patients deserves special consideration because of the potential combined effects of estrogen deficiency and PTH excess on the skeleton. At first glance, one would be tempted to recommend surgery for all postmenopausal women with primary hyperparathyroidism because PTH excess and estrogen deficiency can each be responsible for bone loss. With the two together, bone loss could be even worse. However, our observations (25–27) and those of others (28,29) have shown clearly that, in primary hyperparathyroidism, the cancellous bone at risk in the face of estrogen deficiency is not generally reduced. The typical pattern of bone mineral density is relative preservation of bone mass at a site of cancellous bone, the lumbar spine (see the chapters by Bilezikian, "Clinical Presentation of Primary Hyperparathyroidism," and Parisien et al.). One could argue that, in some postmenopausal women with primary hyperparathyroidism, cancellous bone is protected by PTH from the adverse effects of estrogen deficiency. This idea is supported by the effects of PTH to increase cancellous bone density in postmenopausal women without primary hyperparathyroidism (30,31). Thus, in postmenopausal women with primary hyperparathyroidism who have normal lumbar bone mineral density, a nonsurgical approach may be particularly attractive. Opting against surgery for these patients would be reasonable if cortical bone is not significantly reduced and no other surgical guidelines are met.

A more complicated issue arises in postmenopausal women whose lumbar spine density is below normal.

If the reduction is associated with concomitant, and usually more substantial, reductions at the distal radius, it is possible that this presentation represents a more advanced stage of primary hyperparathyroidism. Alternatively, reduced lumbar spine bone mineral density could reflect the effects of estrogen deficiency (cancellous bone loss) along with the adverse effects of PTH (cortical bone loss). In this case, the hyperparathyroid process is not sufficiently effective to counteract the deleterious effect of estrogen deficiency on cancellous bone. In a given individual who shows reductions at both sites, it is difficult to distinguish between these two possibilities without obtaining a bone biopsy. Histomorphometric analysis of the bone biopsy specimen can be very helpful here in that it can distinguish readily between the effects of PTH and those of estrogen deficiency on cancellous bone.

Another presentation of postmenopausal women with primary hyperparathyroidism that deserves special consideration is the unusual combination of normal cortical bone with reduced cancellous bone. The likelihood in this case is that the effect of estrogen deficiency has predominated at cancellous sites and that the hyperparathyroid state has not successfully counteracted the adverse effects of estrogen deficiency. This situation would reflect someone who has sustained postmenopausal bone loss and then has developed early primary hyperparathyroidism. One would expect to find very little evidence for hyperparathyroidism if a bone biopsy were to be obtained and analyzed in this situation.

When bone mineral density of the lumbar spine is reduced in postmenopausal women, with or without a concomitant reduction in cortical bone, a strong argument could be made for parathyroid surgery. Parathyroid hormone is unlikely to be showing protective effects on the cancellous spine in these patients. Reversal of the hyperparathyroidism might well be associated with early gains in bone mineral density of the cancellous skeleton (32). Moreover, one might expect that therapeutic regimens to address non-PTH-related postmenopausal bone loss might be more effective after successful parathyroidectomy.

This discussion assumes that bone mineral density at both the lumbar spine and the distal radius is measured. Although the distal radius is the most sensitive site to monitor in primary hyperparathyroidism (because it comprises primarily cortical bone), the proper approach to the postmenopausal woman with primary hyperparathyroidism depends also on knowing the state of the cancellous skeleton. Thus bone mineral density measurements at both the distal radius and the lumbar spine are to be recommended strongly, at least during the initial evaluation of the postmenopausal woman with primary hyperparathyroidism. For completeness, bone mineral density of the hip region is also of interest. The hip region is an area of more

mixed composition, comprising both cancellous and cortical elements compared to the radius or lumbar spine, which are enriched in either cortical or cancellous bone, respectively. Thus, for the purpose of this discussion, knowledge of bone mineral density at hip sites is not a key to deciding on who is a candidate for surgery. On the other hand, there is great interest in the hip region as a site of potential fracture. Without this information, the picture is less complete than it would otherwise be. We have all seen patients in whom, for inexplicable reasons, the spine and forearm bone mineral density are normal but that in the hip region it is significantly reduced. These patients are probably surgery candidates.

HOW SHOULD PATIENTS BE FOLLOWED IF THEY ARE NOT TO UNDERGO PARATHYROID SURGERY?

It is assumed that all patients who are not to undergo surgery for primary hyperparathyroidism can be, and will be, followed adequately. This is a very important point because of our incomplete knowledge about the natural history of primary hyperparathyroidism. Table 3 summarizes recommendations for monitoring patients who do not undergo parathyroid surgery.

Patients should be seen every 6 months for routine testing of the serum calcium concentration. Use of a multichannel analyzer for this purpose provides the serum inorganic phosphorus concentration and the alkaline phosphatase activity as well. It is not necessary to repeat measurements of PTH. Yearly monitoring of bone density is recommended. The technique of dual-energy X-ray absorptiometry, which is now in widespread use, includes use of software to measure both cortical (distal radius) and cancellous bone (lumbar spine). These machines are now sufficiently precise to permit significant changes to be observed from year to year. One could argue that the distal radius is the most important site to monitor, since any change due to primary hyperparathyroidism is likely to be seen there first. With the exception of postmenopausal women, single site monitoring of the distal radius is reasonable. However, for postmenopausal women with primary hyperparathyroidism, the author recommends yearly monitoring at both the distal radius and the lumbar spine.

TABLE 3. *Management of primary hyperparathyroidism during surveillance*

Serum calcium measurement every 6 months
Urinary calcium determination yearly
Creatinine clearance measurement yearly
Bone mineral density determination yearly

The Consensus Development Conference recommended that monitoring of bone mineral density at the distal radius could be discontinued once it was ascertained that there was no significant change occurring (3). Observations of Rao et al. (33) suggest that patients may not show any significant change in bone mineral density over 4 years of monitoring. However, changes are likely to be small, if any, over time, and it is recommended that monitoring be continued for at least 4 years before concluding that bone mass is not changing.

Yearly measurements of urinary calcium excretion and creatinine clearance are also recommended as part of the monitoring process. Whether attention should be paid to the possibility of nephrocalcinosis or silent nephrolithiasis by obtaining periodic abdominal radiography and/or ultrasound measurements is debatable. The Consensus Development Conference recommended abdominal radiographs to detect occult stones and nephrocalcinosis.

The challenge of following patients with asymptomatic primary hyperparathyroidism should not be underemphasized. Patients should be fully informed that we do not know the natural history of this disease, in a given patient, and that it is vital that the patient be monitored as indicated above. Many studies have amply demonstrated how difficult it is to follow patients successfully over the years. Some have even advocated that surgery be a more serious consideration for patients who wish not or refuse to be followed.

MANAGEMENT OF PRIMARY HYPERPARATHYROIDISM DURING SURVEILLANCE

General guidelines to the medical management of primary hyperparathyroidism are covered completely in the chapter by Stock and Marcus and elsewhere (34,35). Principles of medical management include maintenance of adequate hydration at all times, ambulation (avoidance of immobilization), and a diet that is neither restricted nor excessive in calcium. The choice of a diuretic agent, if necessary for another medical condition, is a particular concern. Certainly, thiazide diuretics should be avoided because of their effects of raising the serum calcium. However, loop diuretics such as furosemide are also problematic because of their tendency to cause dehydration. All patients should be properly educated about the signs and symptoms of hypercalcemia. Should any features of hypercalcemia develop, immediate medical attention should be sought. Other pertinent topics in this section, such as the use of estrogens in postmenopausal women with primary hyperparathyroidism, oral phosphate, and newer bisphosphonates are covered in the chapter by Stock and Marcus.

WHEN DOES A PATIENT WHO IS FOLLOWED FOR ASYMPTOMATIC PRIMARY HYPERPARATHYROIDISM BECOME A SURGICAL CANDIDATE?

The rationale for monitoring a patient with primary hyperparathyroidism who does not meet surgical guidelines is that we do not know whether the disease is progressive and, if it is, who might begin to show objective adverse consequences of the disease. Thus patients who are followed conservatively could become surgical candidates over time. The indications for changing to a recommendation for surgery are summarized in Table 4. Certainly the development of hypercalcemia >1 mg/dl above the upper limits of normal and the development of hypercalciuria are two reasons for proceeding with surgery. If the patient were to sustain an episode of acute primary hyperparathyroidism, surgery would be definitely recommended. In addition, if the kidneys are affected by a kidney stone, nephrocalcinosis, or a worsening creatinine clearance, in the absence of any other cause, surgery is clearly indicated. If there is a significant decline in bone mass at the distal radius, one would favor intervention. Changes in bone mass at the lumbar spine require considerations discussed above for postmenopausal women with primary hyperparathyroidism. The development of significant and classical neuromuscular manifestations of primary hyperparathyroidism constitutes another change in status that would favor a recommendation of surgery. If some of the nonspecific neuropsychiatric features associated with primary hyperparathyroidism become manifest and compelling, one might well justify surgery. This is sometimes a difficult decision to make in a patient who otherwise is completely asymptomatic. On the other hand, there is substantial anecdotal and other published information (13) that certainly suggests that, in some patients, marked improvement in some of these neuropsychiatric manifestations occurs after successful parathyroid surgery.

Finally, there are patients who themselves decide that they would prefer not to be followed and/or simply would like to proceed with surgery. Respecting this desire, and fully aware that we are dealing with a dis-

TABLE 4. *Development of surgical indications in asymptomatic patients who are being followed medically*

Hypercalcemia consistently >1 mg/dl above the upper limits of normal
Hypercalciuria or worsening renal function
Nephrolithiasis or nephrocalcinosis
Significant decline in bone mass
An episode of acute primary hyperparathyroidism
Classic neuromuscular features
Compelling nonspecific symptomatology (neuropsychiatric manifestations)

order whose biochemical manifestations should be completely curable by successful surgery, the physician may well go along with this change in approach.

SUMMARY

Until we know more about the natural history of primary hyperparathyroidism and gain more insight into those patients who are destined to develop complications of the disease, we are left with a set of guidelines to help us decide what is the wisest decision for our patients. It seems at this time that there are patients with mild disease who are asymptomatic and do not meet any surgical guidelines. These patients constitute ~50% of all patients with primary hyperparathyroidism. It seems reasonable to forego surgery in these patients, recognizing that, without definitive cure by parathyroidectomy, these patients must be monitored regularly.

When more certain information is available about the natural history of primary hyperparathyroidism as it presents today, we will be better positioned to develop more definitive guidelines. Until that time, however, the suggestions given in this chapter are agreed to by most experts in the field as useful in dealing with a disease that continues to present challenges in management and therapy.

ACKNOWLEDGMENTS

Some of the information contained in this chapter was obtained with support by NIH grants DK 32333 and AR 39191.

REFERENCES

1. Wells SA Jr. Surgical therapy of patients with primary hyperparathyroidism: long term benefits. *J Bone Mineral Res* 1987;6(Suppl 2):S143–S149.
2. Bilezikian JP, Silverberg SJ, Shane E, Parisien M, Dempster DW. Characterization and evaluation of asymptomatic primary hyperparathyroidism. *J Bone Mineral Res* 1991;6(Suppl 2):585–589.
3. Potts JT Jr, Fradkin JE, Aurbach JD, Bilezikian JP, Raisz LG. Proceedings of the NIH Consensus Development Conference on diagnosis and management of asymptomatic primary hyperparathyroidism. *J Bone Mineral Res* 1991;6(Suppl 2):S1–S165.
4. Consensus Development Conference Panel. Diagnosis and management of asymptomatic primary hyperparathyroidism: Consensus Development Conference Statement. *Ann Intern Med* 1991;114:593–597.
5. Potts JT Jr. Management of asymptomatic hyperparathyroidism. A report on the NIH Consensus Development Conference. *Trends Endocrinol Metab* 1992;3:376–379.
6. Silverberg SJ, Shane E, Jacobs TP, et al. Nephrolithiasis and bone involvement in primary hyperparathyroidism. *Am J Med* 1990;89:327–334.
7. Fuss M, Pepersack T, Corvilain J, et al. Infrequency of primary hyperparathyroidism in renal stone formers. *Br J Urol* 1988;62:4–6.
8. Broadus A. Nephrolithiasis in primary hyperparathyroidism. In: Coe F, Brenner B, Stein J, eds. *Nephrolithiasis*. New York: Churchill Livingstone, 1980.
9. Silverberg SJ, Shane E, DeLaCruz L, et al. Skeletal disease in primary hyperparathyroidism. *J Bone Mineral Res* 1989; 4:283–291.
10. Fitzpatrick LA, Bilezikian JP. Acute primary hyperparathyroidism. *Am J Med* 1987;82:275–282.
11. Turken SA, Cafferty M, Silverberg SJ, et al. Neuromuscular involvement in mild, asymptomatic primary hyperparathyroidism. *Am J Med* 1989;87:553–557.
12. Joborn C, Hetta J, Johansson H, Rastad J, Agren H, Akerstrom G, Ljunghall S. Psychiatric morbidity in primary hyperparathyroidism. *World J Surg* 1988;12:476–481.
13. Ljunghall S, Jakobsson S, Joborn C, Palmer M, Rastad J, Akerstrom G. Longitudinal studies of mild primary hyperparathyroidism. *J Bone Mineral Res* 1991;6(Suppl 2):S111–S116).
14. Brown GG, Preisman RC, Kleerekoper MD. Neurobehavioral symptoms in mild primary hyperparathyroidism: related to hypercalcemia but not improved by parathyroidectomy. *Henry Ford Hosp Med J* 1987;35:211–215.
15. Cogan MG, Convey CM, Arieff AI, Wisniewski A, Clark OH. Central nervous system manifestations of hyperparathyroidism. *Am J Med* 1978;65:963–970.
16. Linos DA, vanHeerdan JA, Abboud CF, Edis AJ. Primary hyperparathyroidism and peptic ulcer disease. *Arch Surg* 1978;113:384–386.
17. Bess MA, Edis AJ, vanHeerdan JA. Hyperparathyroidism and pancreatitis. Chance or a causal association? *JAMA* 1980;243:246–247.
18. Bauer W, Federman DD. Hyperparathyroidism epitimized: case of Captain Charles E. Martell. *Metabolism* 1962;11:21–22.
19. Ringe JD. Reversible hypertension in primary hyperparathyroidism—pre- and postoperative blood pressure in 75 cases. *Klin Wochenschr* 1984;62:465–469.
20. Broulik PD, Horky K, Pacovsky V. Blood pressure in patients with primary hyperparathyroidism before and after parathyroidectomy. *Exp Clin Endocrinol* 1985;86:346–352.
21. Rapado A. Arterial hypertension and primary hyperparathyroidism. *Am J Nephrol* 1986;6(Suppl 1):49–50.
22. Diamond TW, Botha JR, Wing J, Meyers AM, Kalk WJ. Parathyroid hypertension. A reversible disorder. *Arch Intern Med* 1986;146:1709–1712.
23. Sancho JJ, Rouco J, Riera-Vidal R, Sitges-Serra A. Long-term effects of parathyroidectomy for primary hyperparathyroidism on arterial hypertension. *World J Surg* 1992;16:732–735.
24. Lind L, Jacobsson S, Palmer M, Lithell H, Wengle B, Ljunghall S. Cardiovascular risk factors in primary hyperparathyroidism: a 15-year follow-up of operated and unoperated cases. *J Intern Med* 1991;230:29–35.
25. Parisien MV, Silverberg SJ, Shane E, et al. The histomorphometry of bone in primary hyperparathyroidism: preservation of cancellous bone structure. *J Clin Endocrinol Metab* 1990;70:930–938.
26. Parisien M, Mellish RWE, Silverberg SJ, et al. Maintenance of cancellous bone connectivity in primary hyperparathyroidism: trabecular strut analysis. *J Bone Mineral Res* 1992;7:913–920.
27. Parisien MV, Silverberg SJ, Shane E, Dempster DW, Bilezikian JP. Bone disease in primary hyperparathyroidism. *Endocrinol Metab Clin North Am* 1990;19:19–34.
28. Delling G. Bone morphology in primary hyperparathyroidism. *Appl Pathol* 1987;5:147–159.
29. Christiansen P, Steiniche T, Vesterby A, Mosekilde L, Hessov I, Melsen F. Primary hyperparathyroidism: iliac crest trabecular bone volume, structure, remodeling, and balance evaluated by histomorphometric methods. *Bone* 1992;13:41–49.
30. Slovik DM, Neer RM, Potts JT Jr. Short-term effects of synthetic human parathyroid hormone (1–34) administration on bone mineral metabolism in osteoporotic patients. *J Clin Invest* 1981;68:1261–1271.
31. Slovik DM, Rosenthal DF, Doppert SH, et al. Restoration of

spinal bone in osteoporotic men by treatment with human parathyroid hormone (1–34) and 1,25-dihydroxyvitamin D. *J Bone Mineral Res* 1986;1:377–381.

32. Silverberg SJ, Gartenberg F, Bilezikian JP. Primary hyperparathyroidism protects cancellous bone density in postmenopausal women. *J Bone Mineral Res* 1992;7(Suppl): 813a.

33. Rao DS, Wilson RJ, Kleerekoper M, Parfitt AM. Lack of biochemical progression or continuation of accelerated bone loss in mild asymptomatic primary hyperparathyroidism: evidence for biphasic disease course. *J Clin Endocrinol Metab* 1988;67:1294–1298.

34. Shane E. Medical management of asymptomatic primary hyperparathyroidism. *J Bone Mineral Res* 1991;6(Suppl 2): S131–S134.

35. Marcus R. Estrogens and progestins in the management of primary hyperparathyroidism. *J Bone Mineral Res* 1991;6 (Suppl 2):S125–S130.

The Parathyroids, edited by J.P. Bilezikian,
M.A. Levine, and R. Marcus. Raven Press, Ltd.,
New York © 1994.

CHAPTER 35

Parathyroid Carcinoma

Elizabeth Shane

Parathyroid carcinoma is an uncommon cause of parathyroid hormone-dependent hypercalcemia, with ~290 cases reported in the English-language literature between 1930 and 1992. In most series, this entity accounts for <1% of patients with primary hyperparathyroidism (1–8). The collective published experience with this rare neoplasm has provided a distinctive clinical profile that differs in a number of respects from that of benign primary hyperparathyroidism (4,6). The distinguishing features of parathyroid carcinoma assume even greater prominence when viewed within the current context of primary hyperparathyroidism as it commonly presents today (9–13). In this chapter, the clinical features, natural history and prognosis of parathyroid cancer are reviewed. Surgical approaches to parathyroid cancer are outlined as well as medical therapies of the hypercalcemia that accompanies recurrent or metastatic disease. Since the ultimate prognosis depends to a major extent on successful resection of the tumor at the time of the initial operation, major emphasis is placed upon those features of parathyroid carcinoma that help to differentiate it from primary hyperparathyroidism due to benign adenomatous or hyperplastic disease.

ETIOLOGY AND PATHOGENESIS

The etiology of parathyroid cancer is unknown. No clear pattern of predisposing factors has emerged in the cases described thus far. Although there have been a number of reports of carcinoma occurring within an adenoma or a hyperplastic parathyroid gland (14–21), Shantz and Castleman (2), in an extensive review of 70 cases, found no evidence for malignant transformation of previously pathologic tissue. Parathyroid carcinoma

has also been described in several patients with end-stage renal disease; all demonstrated hyperplasia of other parathyroid glands (14,22–27), and one had a history of prior neck irradiation (23). Carcinoma has been reported in association with familial hyperparathyroidism (28–32). In one such case, chromosomal abnormalities commonly observed in other solid tumors were identified (32). The disease may be somewhat more common in Japan than in Western countries; in one series, parathyroid carcinoma was found in 5% of patients with primary hyperparathyroidism (33).

CLINICAL FEATURES

The clinical features of parathyroid carcinoma (1–8) are due primarily to the effects of excessive secretion of parathyroid hormone (PTH) by the functioning tumor rather than to infiltration of vital organs by tumor mass. Thus signs and symptoms of hypercalcemia often dominate the clinical picture, with contributions from typical hyperparathyroid bone disease and features of renal involvement, such as nephrolithiasis or nephrocalcinosis. The challenge to the clinician rests in differentiating between hyperparathyroidism due to parathyroid carcinoma and that due to its much more common benign counterpart. It is of great importance that parathyroid carcinoma be considered in the differential diagnosis of PTH-dependent hypercalcemia, since the morbidity and mortality associated with this diagnosis are substantial, and optimal outcomes are associated with complete resection of the tumor at the time of the initial operation (1–8,34). Too often the diagnosis of parathyroid carcinoma is made in retrospect, when hypercalcemia recurs due to local spread of tumor or distant metastases.

There are several features of patients with primary hyperparathyroidism that when present, should suggest a malignant rather than a benign etiology. There is no association of gender with parathyroid carci-

E. Shane: Department of Medicine, Division of Endocrinology, College of Physicians and Surgeons, Columbia University, New York, New York 10032.

noma. The ratio of affected women to men is 1:1 in most series compared to primary hyperparathyroidism, for which there is a marked female predominance (3–4:1). Most authors have noted the average age of the patient with parathyroid carcinoma to be in the fifth decade (1,3,6), ~10 years younger than typical patients with primary hyperparathyroidism, who most often present in their fifties or sixties (9,10,13). In contrast, a recent review of the Mayo Clinic experience indicated that the average age of their patients was somewhat greater [54 years (8)]. Thus considerations of gender and age are of little help in evaluating the individual patient.

Since the advent of the multichannel autoanalyzer, the clinical profile of primary hyperparathyroidism, due to benign adenomatous or hyperplastic disease, has changed. Today, primary hyperparathyroidism usually presents with mild hypercalcemia (within 1 mg/dl above the upper limit of normal) that frequently is asymptomatic and often is discovered during a routine evaluation or during the investigation of an unrelated complaint (see the chapter, "Clinical Presentation of Primary Hyperparathyroidism," by Bilezikian et al.) (9,10,13). In contrast, the serum calcium level of most patients with parathyroid carcinoma is much higher, generally >14 mg/dl or 3–4 mg/dl above the upper limit of normal (1–8). Moreover, this more marked elevation is almost invariably associated with the typical signs and symptoms of hypercalcemia. The most frequent complaints are fatigue, weakness, weight loss, anorexia, nausea, vomiting, polyuria, and polydipsia. Other common presenting symptoms, characteristic of a severely hyperparathyroid state, include bone pain, fractures, and renal colic. When reported, PTH levels have ranged from three to ten times above the upper limit of normal for the assay employed. Extremely high levels of PTH are unusual in primary hyperparathyroidism, in which circulating concentrations are commonly less than twice normal. Alkaline phosphatase activity is also higher in patients with parathyroid carcinoma than in those with primary hyperparathyroidism, in which levels are generally in the vicinity of the upper limit of the normal range (12). Patients with parathyroid carcinoma may have elevated levels of α and β subunits of human chorionic gonadotropin, whereas patients with primary hyperparathyroidism do not (35).

A palpable neck mass has been reported in from 30% to 76% of patients with parathyroid carcinoma. This important clinical finding constitutes another striking difference between benign and malignant parathyroid disease, since a palpable neck mass is distinctly unusual in primary hyperparathyroidism (34). In addition, recurrent laryngeal nerve palsy in a patient with primary hyperparathyroidism who has not had previous neck surgery is also very suggestive of parathyroid cancer.

The classical targets of PTH, kidney and skeleton, are affected with greater frequency and severity in parathyroid carcinoma (1–8) than is commonly observed in the modern presentation of benign primary hyperparathyroidism. Most recent series of primary hyperparathyroidism report the prevalence of renal involvement, including nephrolithiasis, nephrocalcinosis, and impaired glomerular filtration, to be <20% (9,12). In contrast, renal colic is a frequent presenting complaint in patients with parathyroid carcinoma. The prevalence of nephrolithiasis was 56% and the prevalence of renal insufficiency was 84% in one recent series (8). These figures are somewhat higher than in previous reports, in which the prevalence of renal involvement generally has ranged from 32% to 60%. Bone pain and pathologic fractures are also common features of parathyroid cancer. Overt radiologic signs of hyperparathyroid skeletal disease, such as osteitis fibrosa cystica, subperiosteal bone resorption, "salt and pepper" skull, and absent lamina dura, as well as less specific signs, such as diffuse spinal osteopenia, are commonly seen in parathyroid carcinoma (44–91%). In contrast, patients with benign primary hyperparathyroidism rarely have skeletal complaints, and specific radiologic signs are found in <5% of patients (9,10,12). It is also important to note the high incidence of concomitant bone and stone disease that occurs in parathyroid cancer, whereas simultaneous renal and overt skeletal involvement are distinctly unusual in primary hyperparathyroidism. In addition to the kidneys and the skeleton, other systems are frequently affected. Recurrent severe pancreatitis, peptic ulcer disease, and anemia occur with greater frequency in patients with malignant disease than in those with benign primary hyperparathyroidism.

Parathyroid carcinoma shares many clinical features with acute primary hyperparathyroidism (parathyroid crisis; see the chapter, "Acute Primary Hyperparathyroidism," by Fitzpatrick). In view of the marked elevations of serum calcium and PTH that are common in patients with parathyroid crisis, the diagnosis of parathyroid cancer should be considered. While the distinction between these two entities is not possible preoperatively, it is important to bear the diagnosis in mind, because the surgical approaches differ.

A summary of features that might lead one to suspect parathyroid cancer in a patient with hypercalcemia and elevated PTH level is given in Table 1. It should be noted, however, that some patients with benign primary hyperparathyroidism present with more severe disease than is commonly seen today. In such patients, the distinction between benign and malignant disease may be even more difficult to make on clinical grounds, in that profound hypercalcemia, renal disease, and osteitis fibrosa or diffuse osteoporosis may occur, and concomitant kidney and bone disease may even be present (34). However, it is preferable to have

TABLE 1. *Parathyroid carcinoma and benign primary hyperparathyroidism: typical features*

	Parathyroid carcinoma	Primary hyperpara-thyroidism
Female:male ratio	1:1	3.5:1
Average age (years)	48	55
Asymptomatic (%)	<5	>80
Serum calcium (mg/dl)	>14	Within 1 mg/dl of the upper limit of normal
Parathyroid hormone	Markedly elevated	Mildly elevated
Palpable neck mass	Common	Rare
Renal involvement[a] (%)[a]	32–60	4–18
Skeletal involvement[b] (%)[b]	34–91	<5
Concomitant renal and skeletal involvement	Common	Rare

[a]Includes nephrolithiasis, nephrocalcinosis, and impaired renal function in the absence of any other etiology.

[b]Includes osteitis fibrosa, subperiosteal resorption, "salt and pepper" skull, and diffuse osteopenia on plain radiographs.

a high index of suspicion for parathyroid carcinoma when these features are present than to miss the opportunity for surgical cure by failing to consider it in the differential diagnosis.

PATHOLOGY

Several operative findings have been described that, when present, help to distinguish benign parathyroid adenomas from parathyroid carcinoma. The typical parathyroid adenoma is usually of soft consistency, round or oval in shape, and of a reddish-brown color. In contrast, parathyroid carcinoma is frequently described as a lobulated, firm to stony-hard mass. In ~50% of cases, it is surrounded by a dense, fibrous, greyish-white capsule, which adheres tenaciously to adjacent tissues and makes the tumor difficult to separate from contiguous structures. If there is gross infiltration of adjacent thyroid, nerve, muscle, or esophagus or obvious cervical node metastases, the diagnosis of carcinoma is not difficult. However, any one or all of these operative findings may be absent, and the examination of frozen sections is of little value in distinguishing benign from malignant disease.

As is the case with many endocrine neoplasms, the histopathologic distinction between benign and malig-

nant parathyroid tumors is difficult. In 1973 Schantz and Castleman (2), based on an analysis of 70 cases of parathyroid carcinoma, established a set of criteria for the pathologic diagnosis of this malignancy. These histologic features are (a) uniform sheets of (usually chief) cells arranged in a lobular pattern, separated by dense fibrous trabeculae; (b) capsular or vascular invasion; and (c) mitotic figures within tumor parenchymal cells, which must be distinguished from endothelial cell mitoses. Unfortunately, none of these features is pathognomonic of parathyroid carcinoma. Several features—namely, dense fibrous trabeculae, trabecular growth pattern, mitoses, and capsular invasion—have been found in parathyroid adenomas (34). Capsular and vascular invasion appears to correlate best with subsequent tumor recurrence (see the chapter by LiVolsi) (34).

Several other histologic techniques have been investigated to improve further the accuracy of diagnosing parathyroid carcinoma. Electron microscopy of parathyroid cancer tissue reveals nuclear and mitochondrial alterations and evidence of increased secretory activity but does not appear to be of value in distinguishing benign from malignant tumors (36–39). Nuclear diameter appears to be greater in parathyroid carcinomas than in adenomas (2,40,41), but this index is not very useful in individual cases. Measurement of nuclear DNA content by flow cytometry may be of some value both in establishing the diagnosis of parathyroid carcinoma and in predicting the invasive potential of the tumor. Mean nuclear DNA content is greater and an aneuploid DNA pattern is more common in parathyroid carcinoma than in adenomas; when present, aneuploidy appears to be associated with a poorer prognosis (42,43).

NATURAL HISTORY

Parathyroid carcinoma is an indolent, albeit tenacious, tumor with rather low malignant potential. It tends to recur locally at the operative site and to spread to contiguous structures in the neck. Metastases occur late in the course of the disease and spread via both lymphatic and hematogenous routes. Cervical nodes (30%) and lung (40%) are involved most commonly, followed by liver (10%). Occasional involvement of bone, pleura, pericardium, and pancreas has been reported.

MANAGEMENT

Surgery

The single most effective therapy for parathyroid carcinoma is complete resection of the primary lesion at the time of the initial operation, when extensive local invasion and distant metastases are less likely (34). For this reason both preoperative suspicion and intraoperative recognition are of paramount importance. Patients whose clinical presentation is suggestive of parathyroid carcinoma warrant thorough exploration of all four parathyroid glands, since parathyroid carcinoma has been reported to coexist with benign adenomas or hyperplasia (14–21,34,43). When the gross pathologic findings suggest malignancy, the following steps should be taken: en bloc removal of the lesion together with the ipsilateral thyroid lobe and isthmus; skeletonization of the trachea; and removal of any contiguous tissues to which the tumor adheres. Great care must be exercised to avoid rupture of the capsule of the gland, which increases the likelihood of local seeding of the tumor. If the recurrent laryngeal nerve is involved with tumor, it must be resected. Tracheoesophageal, paratracheal, and upper mediastinal lymph nodes should be excised, but an extensive lateral neck dissection is indicated only when there is spread to the anterior cervical nodes.

The situation becomes more complex when the diagnosis is made in the early postoperative period on the basis of pathology. This is particularly so in view of the controversy that exists regarding the histopathologic diagnosis of parathyroid carcinoma. If the gross characteristics of the lesion were typical of a parathyroid cancer, and if the subsequent pathology appears to be aggressive, with extensive vascular or capsular invasion, or if the patient remains hypercalcemic, reexploration of the neck is indicated. The structures adjacent to the tumor site should be resected in the manner described above. If none of these features is present, but the diagnosis is made on the basis of the microscopic characteristics, immediate reoperation may not be necessary, since a simple complete resection of the tumor is often curative. Such a patient must be observed carefully with frequent measurements of PTH and serum calcium levels.

The postoperative management of a patient with parathyroid cancer must include careful attention to the serum calcium level. As calcium and phosphorus are deposited into the skeleton, symptomatic hypocalcemia ("hungry bone syndrome") may ensue and should be regarded as a sign that the surgery has been successful. The hypocalcemia may be severe and protracted, requiring large doses of intravenous calcium. Sufficient supplemental calcium and calcitriol should be prescribed to maintain the serum calcium at the low end of the normal range. As the bones heal and the remaining parathyroid glands recover, the requirement for calcium will decrease, permitting gradual reduction of the doses of calcium and calcitriol. After this point, serum calcium and PTH levels should be monitored every 3 months.

The management of recurrent or metastatic parathyroid carcinoma reflects the rather indolent biology of this cancer and, in contrast to management of many other tumors, is primarily surgical. Since even very small tumor deposits may produce sufficient PTH to cause severe hypercalcemia, significant palliation may result from resection of lesions in the neck, lymph nodes, lungs, or liver. Many situations have been described in which resection of such lesions has resulted in periods of normocalcemia that range from months to years. Even if surgery is only palliative, amelioration of the hypercalcemia may result making its control more amenable to medical therapies.

In patients with recurrent hypercalcemia, localization studies should be performed prior to reoperation. Careful palpation of the neck should be performed, since recurrence occurs earliest and most often at the original site, and such tumors are frequently palpable. The initial procedure should be ultrasonography of the neck with a 10 MHz real-time small-parts scanner, since this detects small tumors in the neck, particularly when adjacent to or within the thyroid gland (34). Thallium 201-technetium 99m scanning is useful in locating tumors in the neck and upper mediastinum. Thallium 201 is also helpful for situations in which the thyroid has been partially or completely resected or when pulmonary metastases are suspected. Computerized tomography (CT) and magnetic resonance imaging (MRI) are useful adjuncts to ultrasonography in evaluation of the neck and are superior for detection of distant metastases in the chest or abdomen. If noninvasive testing does not yield results, arteriography or selective venous catheterization may be useful. Recurrent carcinoma in the neck should be treated with wide excision of the involved area, including the regional lymph nodes and other involved structures. Accessible distant metastases should also be resected when possible.

Radiation Therapy

Parathyroid carcinoma is not a radiosensitive tumor. In the occasional situation, radiation to the neck after surgery for recurrence may be helpful in preventing tumor regrowth (34), and recently an apparent cure (10 years) of locally invasive parathyroid carcinoma with radiation therapy was reported (8). However, the use of radiation therapy to control tumor growth and to decrease hormone production has been ineffective in the majority of cases in which it has been attempted (2,4).

Chemotherapy

Because of the rarity of parathyroid carcinoma, few investigators have sufficient numbers of patients to permit large-scale clinical research trials. Thus complete investigations of the utility of a given therapy do not exist, and experience is usually limited to scattered case reports. It is with these unavoidable limitations in mind that the following comments should be interpreted.

Attempts to control tumor burden with chemotherapy have been disappointing. Several regimens (nitrogen mustard; vincristine, cyclophosphamide, and actinomycin D; Adriamycin, cyclophosphamide and 5-fluorouracil; and Adriamycin alone) have been ineffective (44–46). Two patients have been treated with synthetic estrogens with some success (47,48). A single patient with pulmonary metastases responded to treatment with dacarbazine, 5-fluorouracil, and cyclophosphamide with a decrease in PTH and normalization of serum calcium for 13 months (49). Another patient responded to dacarbazine alone with a brief but significant decline in her serum calcium level (50). An 18 month remission, with regression of a mediastinal mass and pleural effusion, was induced in a patient with a nonfunctioning parathyroid carcinoma by a regimen consisting of methotrexate, doxorubicin, cyclophosphamide, and lomustine (51). Such approaches warrant further investigation.

Management of Hypercalcemia

When parathyroid carcinoma has become widely disseminated and surgical resection is no longer effective, the prognosis is poor. However, even at this juncture, relatively prolonged survival (5 years) is possible. The therapeutic goal at this point is to control the hypercalcemia, which, because of the extremely elevated PTH levels and the intensity of the associated bone resorption, may be a difficult and frustrating task (52).

The acute hypercalcemia of parathyroid carcinoma is treated in the same way as hypercalcemia due to any other cause (see the chapter by Bilezikian and Singer) (53,54). Management includes infusion of saline to restore fluid volume and to enhance urinary calcium excretion and loop diuretics to increase calciuresis further. Such measures rarely suffice, however, and addition of agents that interfere with osteoclast-mediated bone resorption is always necessary.

Calcitonin both inhibits osteoclast-mediated bone resorption and increases urinary calcium excretion. However, it lowers serum calcium transiently, if at all, in most patients with parathyroid carcinoma (3,49,55–58). It has been effective in a single patient when used in doses of 200–600 MRC units per day in combination with glucocorticoids (300 mg hydrocortisone) (59) and in occasional patients when used alone (60).

Plicamycin (mithramycin) is a specific inhibitor of bone resorption and lowers serum calcium levels in parathyroid carcinoma (61). It is administered intravenously at a dose of 25 μg/kg over 4–8 hr, which may be repeated at daily intervals for up to 7 days until the serum calcium falls to the acceptable range (52–54). Unfortunately, complete normalization of the serum calcium is often not achieved, and the effectiveness of the drug not only is transient but diminishes with repeated courses. Conversely, the toxic effects of plicamycin on the liver, kidneys, and bone marrow increase with the number of exposures. Although it has been effective and without significant side effects in a single patient when used in smaller doses (12.5 μ/kg), in general plicamycin therapy should be reserved for therapy of life-threatening hypercalcemia while surgically accessible metastases are sought or for those patients whose hypercalcemia can be controlled in no other way.

The bisphosphonates are another group of drugs that inhibit osteoclast-mediated bone resorption. Several of these drugs have shown some promise in the therapy of parathyroid carcinoma. Clodronate (Cl_2MDP) lowers serum calcium in patients with parathyroid carcinoma when administered intravenously (56,62,63). It is widely available in Europe and the United Kingdom, but it is not available in the United States. Etidronate has also been shown to lower serum calcium transiently in parathyroid cancer patients (64). It is administered intravenously over a 2 hr period at a dose of 7.5 mg/kg and may be repeated daily or until the serum calcium falls to normal for a maximum of 7 days. Although the drug is available in an oral form, it is not effective in patients with parathyroid carcinoma, and even the intravenous preparation may not normalize the serum calcium. Another more potent bisphosphonate, pamidronate, is now widely available for intravenous use. When infused for periods ranging from 2 to 24 hr and in doses ranging from 45 to 90 mg/day, pamidronate has been at least transiently effective in lowering serum calcium levels in several patients with parathyroid cancer (65–67). New and more potent bisphosphonates are being investigated actively in the United States and soon may become available for the treatment of hypercalcemia of malignancy, including that due to parathyroid cancer.

Gallium nitrate is another anticalcemic drug that appears to inhibit bone resorption by preventing dissolution of hydroxyapatite crystals (68). Gallium nitrate lowered serum calcium in two patients with parathyroid carcinoma (68). It is administered as a continuous 24 hr infusion at a dose of 200 mg/m²/day for up to 5 days. Significant toxicities include elevation of the serum creatinine potentiated by volume depletion and the concomitant use of potentially nephrotoxic drugs. It is not clear whether gallium nitrate is going to prove useful in the management of chronic hypercalcemia due to parathyroid cancer.

Oral phosphate in doses up to 2 g/day may decrease serum calcium by 1–2 mg/dl. Its effect is rather modest, so it is generally not used in parathyroid carcinoma.

WR-2721 [5-,2-,(3-aminorpropyl)amino] ethylphosphorothoric acid is a hypocalcemic agent that acts by inhibiting PTH secretion and bone resorption. It has been shown to lower PTH levels and serum calcium levels in parathyroid carcinoma (69,70). Severe toxicities limit its use (see the chapter by Stock and Marcus).

PROGNOSIS

The prognosis of parathyroid carcinoma is quite variable. No one characteristic correlates predictably with outcome. Early recognition and complete resection at the time of the initial surgery carry the best prognosis. The average time between surgery and the first recurrence is ~3 years, although intervals of up to 20 years have been reported. Once the tumor has recurred, complete cure is unlikely, although prolonged survival is still common under these circumstances with palliative surgery. Five year survival rates vary from 40% to 69%.

REFERENCES

1. Holmes EC, Morton DL, Ketcham AS. Parathyroid carcinoma: a collective review. *Ann Surg* 1969;169:631–640.
2. Schantz A, Castleman B. Parathyroid carcinoma: a study of 70 cases. *Cancer* 1973;31:600–605.
3. Shane E, Bilezikian JP. Parathyroid carcinoma: A review of 62 patients. *Endocr Rev* 1982;3:218–226.
4. Cohn K, Silverman M, Corrado J, Sedgewick C. Parathyroid carcinoma: The Lahey Clinic experience. *Surgery* 1985; 98:1095–1110.
5. Wang C, Gaz R. Natural history of parathyroid carcinoma: Diagnosis, treatment, and results. *Am J Surg* 1985;149:522–527.
6. Shane E, Bilezikian JP. Parathyroid carcinoma. In: Williams CJ, Krikorian JC, Green MR, Raghaven D, eds. *Textbook of uncommon cancer*. New York: John Wiley and Sons, 1987; 763–771.
7. Obara T, Fujimoto Y. Diagnosis and treatment of patients with parathyroid carcinoma: an update and review. *World J Surg* 1991;15:738–744.
8. Wynne AG, Van Heerden J, Carney JA, Fitzpatrick LA. Parathyroid carcinoma: clinical and pathological features in 43 patients. *Medicine* 1992;71:197–205.
9. Heath H III, Hodgson SF, Kennedy MA. Primary hyperparathyroidism: incidence, morbidity, and potential economic impact in a community. *N Engl J Med* 1980;302:189–193.
10. Silverberg SJ, Shane E, de la Cruz L, et al. Skeletal disease in primary hyperparathyroidism. *J Bone Mineral Res* 1989; 4:283–291.
11. Parisien M, Silverberg SJ, Shane E, Bilezikian JP. Bone disease in primary hyperparathyroidism. *Endocrinol Metab Clin North Am* 1990;19:19–34.
12. Silverberg SJ, Shane E, Jacobs TP, et al. Nephrolithiasis and bone involvement in primary hyperparathyroidism. *Am J Med* 1990;89:327–334.
13. Bilezikian JP, Silverberg SJ, Shane E. Primary hyperparathy-roidism in the 1980s. In: Kleerekoper M, Krane S, eds. *Clinical disorders of bone and mineral metabolism*. New York: Mary Anne Liebert, 1989;359–365.
14. Berland Y, Olmer M, Lebreuil G, Grisoli J. Parathyroid carcinoma, adenoma and hyperplasia in a case of chronic renal insufficiency on dialysis. *Clin Nephrol* 1982;18:154–158.
15. Haghighi P, Astarita RW, Wepsic T, Wolf PL. Concurrent primary parathyroid hyperplasia and parathyroid carcinoma. *Arch Pathol Lab Med* 1983;107:349–350.
16. Desch CE, Arsensis G, May AG, Amatruda JM. Parathyroid hyperplasia and carcinoma within one gland. *Am J Med* 1984;77:131–134.
17. Kramer WH. Association of parathyroid hyperplasia with neoplasia. *Am J Clin Pathol* 1970;53:275–283.
18. Murayama T, Kawabe K, Tagami M. A case of parathyroid carcinoma concurred with hyperplasia: an electron microscopic study. *J Urol* 1977;118:126–127.
19. Guazzi A, Gabrielli M, Guadagni G. Cytologic features of a functioning parathyroid carcinoma: a case report. *Acta Cytol* 1982;26:709–713.
20. Parham GP, Orr JW. Hyperparathyroidism secondary to parathyroid carcinoma in pregnancy: a case report. *J Reprod Med* 1987;32:123–125.
21. Aldinger KA, Hickey RC, Ibanez ML, et al. Parathyroid carcinoma: a clinical study of seven cases of functioning and two cases of nonfunctioning parathyroid cancer. *Cancer* 1982; 49:388–397.
22. Sherlock DJ, Newman J, Holl-Allen RTJ. Parathyroid carcinoma presenting as tertiary hyperparathyroidism. *Postgrad Med J* 1985;61:243–244.
23. Ireland JP, Fleming SJ, Levison DA, Cattell WR, Baker LRI. Parathyroid carcinoma associated with chronic renal failure and previous radiotherapy to the neck. *J Clin Pathol* 1985; 38:1114–1118.
24. Kodama M, Ikegami M, Imanishi M, et al. Parathyroid carcinoma in a case of chronic renal failure on dialysis. *Urol Int* 1989;44:110–112.
25. Iwamoto N, Yamazaki S, Fukuda T, et al. Two cases of parathyroid carcinoma in patients on long-term hemodialysis. *Nephron* 1990;55:429–431.
26. Greenberg A, Piraino BM, Brun FJ. Hypercalcemia in patients with advanced chronic renal failure not yet requiring dialysis. *Am J Nephrol* 1989;9:205–210.
27. Krishna GG, Mendez M, Levy B, Ritchie W, Marks A, Narins RG. Parathyroid carcinoma in a chronic hemodialysis patient. *Nephron* 1989;52:194–195.
28. Frayha RA, Nassar VH, Dagher F, Salti IS. Familiar parathyroid carcinoma. *Leban Med J* 1972;25:299–309.
29. Dinnen JS, Greenwood RH, Jone JH, Walker DA, Williams ED. Parathyroid carcinoma in familial hyperparathyroidism. *J Clin Pathol* 1977;30:966–975.
30. Mallette LE, Bilezikian JP, Ketcham AS, Aurbach GD. Parathyroid carcinoma in familial hyperparathyroidism. *Am J Med* 1974;57:642–648.
31. Leborgne J, LeNeel JC, Brizelin F, Malvy P. Cancer familiar des parathyroids. *J Chir* 1975;109:315–326.
32. Streeten EA, Weinstein LS, Norton JA, et al. Studies in a kindred with parathyroid carcinoma. *J Clin Endocrinol Metab* 1992;75:362–366.
33. Fujimoto Y, Obara T, Ito Y, Kanazawa K, Aiyoshi Y, Nobori M. Surgical treatment of ten cases of parathyroid carcinoma: importance of an initial en bloc tumor resection. *World J Surg* 1984;8:392–400.
34. Levin KE, Galante M, Clark OH. Parathyroid carcinoma versus parathyroid adenoma in patients with profound hypercalcemia. *Surgery* 1987;101:647–660.
35. Stock JL, Wientraub BD, Rosen SW, Aurbach GD, Spiegel AM, Marx SJ. Human chorionic gonadotropin subunit measurement in primary hyperparathyroidism. *J Clin Endocrinol Metab* 1982;54:57–63.
36. Holck S, Pedersen NT. Carcinoma of the parathyroid gland. A light and electron microscopic study. *Acta Pathol Microbiol Scand* 1981;89:297–302.
37. de la Garza S, de la Garza EF, Batres FH. Functional para-

thyroid carcinoma: Cytology, histology and ultrastructure of a case. *Diagn Cytopathol* 1985;1:232.

38. Smith JF, Coombs RRH. Histological diagnosis of carcinoma of the parathyroid gland. *J Clin Pathol* 1984;37:1370–1378.

39. Obara T, Fujimoto Y, Yamaguchi K, et al. Parathyroid carcinoma of the oxyphil cell type. A report of two cases, light and electron microscopic study. *Cancer* 1985;55:1482–1489.

40. Jacobi JM, Lloyd HM, Smith JF. Nuclear diameter in parathyroid carcinomas. *J Clin Pathol* 1986;39:1353–1354.

41. Lloyd HM, Jacobi JM, Cooke RA. Nuclear diameter in parathyroid adenomas. *J Clin Pathol* 1979;32:1278–1281.

42. Levin KE, Chew KL, Ljung BM, Mayall BH, Siperstein AE, Clark OH. Deoxyribonucleic acid flow cytometry helps identify parathyroid carcinomas. *J Clin Endocrinol Metab* 1988;67:779–784.

43. Obara T, Fujimoto Y, Hirayama A, et al. Flow cytometric DNA analysis of parathyroid tumors with special reference to its diagnostic and prognostic value in parathyroid carcinoma. *Cancer* 1990;65:1789–1793.

44. Golden A, Canary JJ, Kerwin DM. Concurrence of hyperplasia and neoplasia of the parathyroid gland. *Am J Med* 1965;38:562–578.

45. Anderson BJ, Samaan NA, Vassilopoulou-Sellin R, Ordonez NG, Hickey RC. Parathyroid carcinoma: features and difficulties in diagnosis and management. *Surgery* 1983;94:906–915.

46. Grammes CF, Eyerly RC. Hyperparathyroidism and parathyroid carcinoma. *South Med J* 1980;73:814–816.

47. Sigurdsson G, Woodhouse NJY, Taylor S, Joplin GF. Stilboestrol diphosphate in hypercalcemia due to parathyroid carcinoma. *Br Med J* 1973;1:27–28.

48. Goepfert H, Smart CR, Rochlin DB. Metastatic parathyroid carcinoma and hormonal chemotherapy: case report and response to Hexestrol. *Ann Surg* 1966;164:917–918.

49. Bukowski RM, Sheeler L, Cunningham J, Esselstyn C. Successful combination chemotherapy for metastatic parathyroid carcinoma. *Arch Intern Med* 1984;144:399–400.

50. Calandra DB, Chejfec G, Foy BK, Lawrence AM, Paloyan E. Parathyroid carcinoma: biochemical and pathologic response to DTIC. *Surgery* 1984;96:1132–1137.

51. Chahinian AP, Holland JF, Nieburgs HE, Marinescu A, Geller Sa, Kirschner PA. Metastatic nonfunctioning parathyroid carcinoma: ultrastructural evidence of secretory granules and response to chemotherapy. *Am J Med Sci* 1981;282:80–84.

52. Shane E. Parathyroid carcinoma. In: Bardin CW, ed. *Current therapy in endocrinology and metabolism*. St. Louis: Mosby-Yearbook, (in press).

53. Bilezikian JP. Management of acute hypercalcemia. *N Engl J Med* 1992;326:1196–1203.

54. Shane E. Hypercalcemia. In: *ASBMR primer on metabolic bone disease,* 2nd ed. New York: Raven Press 1993;153–155.

55. Dubost C, Jehanno C, Lavergne A, Charpentier YL. Successful resection of intrathoracic metastases from two patients with parathyroid carcinoma. *World J Surg* 1984;8:547–551.

56. Jungst D. Disodium clodronate effective in management of severe hypercalcemia caused by parathyroid carcinoma. *Lancet* 1984;1:1043.

57. Lake MS, Kahn SE, Favus MJ, Bermes EW. Case report: clinical pathological correlations in a case of primary parathyroid carcinoma. *Ann Clin Lab Sci* 1984;14:458–463.

58. Trigonis C, Cedermark B, Willems J, Hamberger B, Granberg PO. Parathyroid carcinoma—problems in diagnosis and treatment. *Clin Oncol* 1984;10:11–19.

59. Au WYW. Calcitonin treatment of hypercalcemia due to parathyroid carcinoma: synergistic effect of prednisone on long-term treatment of hypercalcemia. *Arch Intern Med* 1975;135:1594–1597.

60. Edelson GW, Kleerekoper M, Talpos GB, Zarbo R, Saeed-Uz-Zafar M. Mucin-producing parathyroid carcinoma. *Bone* 1992;13:7–10.

61. Singer FR, Neer RM, Murray TM, Keutmann HT, Deftos LJ, Potts JT Jr. Mithramycin treatment of intractable hypercalcemia due to parathyroid carcinoma. *N Engl J Med* 1970;283:634–636.

62. Jacobs TP, Siris ES, Bilezikian JP, Baquiran DC, Shane E, Canfield RE. Hypercalcemia of malignancy: treatment with intravenous dichloromethylene diphosphonate. *Ann Intern Med* 1981;94:312–316.

63. Shane E, Jacobs TP, Siris ES, et al. Therapy of hypercalcemia due to parathyroid carcinoma with intravenous dichloromethylene diphosphonate. *Am J Med* 1982;72:939–944.

64. Jacobs TP, Gordon AC, Gundberg CM, et al. Neoplastic hypercalcemia: physiologic response to intravenous etidronate. *Am J Med* 1987;82:42–52.

65. Mann K. Oral bisphosphonate therapy in metastatic parathyroid carcinoma. *Lancet* 1985;1:101–102.

66. Sandelin K, Thompson NW, Bondeson L. Metastatic parathyroid carcinoma: Dilemmas in management. *Surgery* 1992;110:978–988.

67. Weinstein RS. Parathyroid carcinoma associated with polycythemia vera. *Bone* 1991;12:237–239.

68. Warrell RP, Isaacs M, Alcock NW, Bockman RS. Gallium nitrate for treatment of refractory hypercalcemia from parathyroid carcinoma. *Ann Intern Med* 1987;197:683–686.

69. Hirschel-Scholtz S, Jung A, Fischer JA, Trechsel U, Bonjour JP. Suppression of parathyroid secretion after administration of WR-2721 in a patient wtih parathyroid carcinoma. *Clin Endocrinol* 1985;23:313–318.

70. Glover DJ, Shaw L, Glick JH, et al. Treatment of hypercalcemia in parathyroid cancer with WR-2721, S-2-(3-aminopropylamino) ethyl-phosphorothioic acid. *Ant Int Med* 1985;103:55–57.

The Parathyroids, edited by J.P. Bilezikian, M.A. Levine, and R. Marcus. Raven Press, Ltd., New York © 1994.

CHAPTER 36

Acute Primary Hyperparathyroidism

Lorraine A. Fitzpatrick

Prior to the development of multichannel autoanalyzers, primary hyperparathyroidism (HPT) was an infrequent diagnosis and was often associated with clear manifestations of end-organ disease (1,2). Older clinical descriptions of primary HPT were associated with symptoms related to the effects of parathyroid hormone (PTH) on kidney and bone. Acute, severe hypercalcemia (parathyroid poisoning, parathyroid intoxication, or parathyroid crises) was described as a possible complication of primary HPT. Although acute primary HPT appears to be seen in a smaller percentage of patients with primary HPT, this is due most likely to the tremendous increase in the number of patients who present with asymptomatic HPT. With increasing frequency, primary HPT presents as asymptomatic hypercalcemia; however, severe, life-threatening, symptomatic hypercalcemia is still sometimes described (3). Acute primary hyperparathyroidism is associated with high rates of morbidity and mortality.

A recent review of 48 cases of acute primary HPT emphasized the life-threatening nature of the hypercalcemia (3). Invariably, marked signs and symptoms were present. Some of the highest serum calcium levels reported in the literature have been attributed to acute primary HPT. Although primary HPT is rare, the number of cases in the medical literature and the curable nature of the disorder suggest that this disease must be considered in the differential diagnosis of hypercalcemia.

RISK OF DEVELOPING ACUTE PRIMARY HYPERPARATHYROIDISM

The incidence of acute primary HPT is difficult to assess. At Loyola Medical Center, ten patients from among 325 consecutive cases of surgically proven primary hyperparathyroidism developed acute primary hyperparathyroidism. Nine of these patients had a single adenoma (4). Among 90 cases of primary hyperparathyroidism treated surgically between 1975 and 1985 in Athens, Greece, one case of hyperparathyroid crisis was identified (5).

The risk of development of hypercalcemic crisis in patients with untreated primary hyperparathyroidism is low. Only one patient among a group of 47 patients followed over a 5-year interval developed acute primary HPT (6). In a prospective series of patients at the Mayo Clinic followed for 10 years, only one of 142 patients, or 0.7%, developed acute primary HPT (7). Neither series identified a specific parameter to predict accurately the likelihood of progression to severe hypercalcemia.

DEMOGRAPHICS

In one series, the age at the time of clinical presentation of acute primary HPT was the same or slightly lower than the average age of patients with primary HPT (Table 1) (3,8,9). This is in contrast to expected findings; patients who are elderly and immobile and with a higher likelihood of compromised renal function might be expected to be at increased risk for the development of acute primary HPT. Ages ranged from 27 to 82 years, and distribution by decade was fairly constant. No correlation was noted between serum calcium concentrations and age ($r = 0.11$; $P > 0.05$). The ratio of affected women to men (1.1:1.0) was similar to the distribution in parathyroid carcinoma (Table 2) (10–12) but markedly different from the gender ratio in recent series of primary HPT (8,9).

LABORATORY EVALUATION

In one series, serum calcium levels were as high as 26.3 mg/dl, with an average level of 17.5 mg/dl (3). In

---

L. A. Fitzpatrick: Department of Medicine, Mayo Clinic and Mayo Foundation, Rochester, Minnesota 55905.

TABLE 1. *Acute primary hyperparathyroidism vs. routine primary hyperparathyroidism*

	Acute	Routine	
	(Fitzpatrick and Bilezikian)	Heath et al.	Silverberg et al.[a]
Period of review	1974–1981	1974–1976	Longitudinal ongoing study
Number of cases	48	51	97
Female/male ratio	1.1:1.0	3.6:1	3.2:1
Average age (years)	55	62	55
Serum calcium (mg/dl)	17.5	10.8	11.1
Renal involvement (%)	69	4	18
Skeletal involvement (%)	53	20	1–2
Asymptomatic (%)	0	51	—

[a]Includes patients with bone mineral density <80% of normal.

another series, the serum calcium concentrations ranged from 15.0 to 17.6 mg/dl (4). Serum calcium levels were indistinguishable from levels noted in patients with parathyroid carcinoma (Table 2) (3,10–12). Serum phosphate levels were in the low-normal range, and severe hypophosphatemia was not common (3).

Of particular note were the strikingly elevated levels of PTH, averaging 20 times normal levels. Extremely high levels of PTH in association with marked hypercalcemia are strongly suggestive of acute primary HPT (3) or parathyroid carcinoma (10). Hypercalcemia associated with nonparathyroid malignancy or of other etiologies is notable for suppressed levels of PTH (13). In asymptomatic primary HPT, a two- to threefold elevation of serum PTH is present (14), and, in parathyroid carcinoma, PTH levels at presentation are markedly elevated (ten times the upper limit of normal) (10). Thus PTH levels are useful in distinguishing malignancy-associated or asymptomatic primary HPT from acute primary HPT, but these markedly elevated levels of PTH do not rule out the possibility of parathyroid carcinoma. The distinction between acute HPT due to a benign adenoma and parathyroid carcinoma is important in that a surgical approach to the patient de-

pends on the nature of the lesion. A history of mild hypercalcemia within 10 years in up to 25% of patients presenting with acute primary HPT has been noted (2). This history is extremely useful in the differential diagnosis of the disorder. Intervening illness, perhaps with associated bed rest, may catalyze increased mobilization of calcium from bone and play a role in the development of the acute parathyroid crisis: Eleven patients had undergone surgery; two had viral illnesses; two had pneumonia; and one each had diabetic ketoacidosis, trauma, and urinary tract infection (2). A recently reported case was thought to be precipitated by herpes zoster infection (15), and, in another report, a 50-year-old woman developed acute hypercalcemia due to HPT after head and intraabdominal trauma (16).

TARGET ORGAN MANIFESTATIONS

Most subjects with acute primary HPT have some manifestation of renal involvement. Among 29 patients for whom clinical documentation was adequate, 20 (69%) had nephrolithiasis or nephrocalcinosis (3).

TABLE 2. *Acute primary hyperparathyroidism vs. parathyroid carcinoma*

	Acute primary hyperparathyroidism	Parathyroid carcinoma		
	(Fitzpatrick and Bilezikian)	Shane et al.	Wang	Wynne et al.
Period of review	1974–1984	1968–1981	1948–1983	1920–1990
Number of cases	48	62	28	43
Female/male ratio	1.1:1.0	1.2:1.0	1:1	1:1
Average age (years)	55	48	45	54
Serum calcium (mg/dl)	17.5	15.5	13.7	14.6
Renal involvement (%)	69	60	64	56
Skeletal involvement (%)	53	55	46	91
Asymptomatic (%)	0	2	4	7

Radiologic criteria of primary HPT included subperiosteal resorption of the distal phalanges, overt osteitis fibrosa cystica, "salt and pepper" skull, or diffuse activity on bone scan. Nineteen of 36 patients (53%) had documented skeletal disease (3). The percentage of patients with skeletal involvement is markedly increased compared to current estimates of overt skeletal manifestations in primary HPT (1–2%) (9). In association with the skeletal findings, alkaline phosphatase concentration averaged twice the upper limit of normal in patients with acute primary HPT. This is unusual for the typical patient with HPT, in whom the average serum alkaline phosphatase is only minimally elevated. A high frequency (50%) of both renal and skeletal involvement was observed in ten of 20 patients for whom sufficient information was available (3). The presentation of concurrent renal and overt skeletal disease is unusual in patients with HPT.

The death of a patient with acute primary HPT has revealed further information regarding the calcium dynamics of the disorder (17). Based on the urinary calcium excretion, the amount of calcium loss from bone during the period of acute parathyroid crisis was estimated to be ~2 g/day. Histologic appearance of bone was remarkable for the low level of bone formation despite a massive increase in osteoclastic activity. Trabecular osteoid surface was at the lower limit of normal, and osteoid consisted of only one lamella. No active osteoblasts were noted, and no woven bone was visible. Trabecular bone volume was slightly reduced. In this patient, immunoreactive PTH was extremely elevated, as was serum calcium at 5.1 mmol/liter. The histologic appearance of bone in this patient suggested marked activation of basic multicellular units of bone. Subperiosteal erosions of the phalanges and clavicles were absent in this patient, although the length of time necessary for these characteristic radiographic signs of hyperparathyroid bone disease to develop is unknown. The authors emphasize that there was no compensatory increase in bone formation and suggest that there was marked dissociation between bone resorption and bone formation in this patient (17). This pathological appearance distinguishes the bone histology from the patient with acute HPT (if this patient is representative) from the bone histology in routine primary HPT patients. In primary HPT, bone formation and bone resorption are increased (see chapter by Parisien et al.). One might speculate that the inhibition of bone formation in acute HPT may contribute to the marked hypercalcemia.

OUTCOME

Among a series of patients studied between 1960 and 1986, there were no preoperative deaths, a gratifying result of medical management including rapid rehydra-tion and correction of electrolyte disorders (18). Three perioperative deaths (6%) among 48 cases (2) is a great improvement from the 59% mortality observed prior to 1970. This decrease in mortality may be due to earlier recognition, refined preoperative medical management, and improved surgical techniques. Recently, a nonoperative approach to ablate a parathyroid adenoma in a patient with acute HPT has been described. A single parathyroid adenoma was treated by direct instillation of 96% ethanol under ultrasonic guidance. Recurrence of the hypercalcemia required repeat injections 1 year later (19). Further studies will be necessary to assess the feasibility and safety of this technique.

PATHOLOGY

Review of the pathology of tissue obtained from patients with acute HPT revealed parathyroid adenomas exclusively, except in one patient who appeared to have multiple gland involvement (3). Among another series of 57 patients with serum calcium > 13.0 mg/dl, 28% had multiglandular involvement (20). At Loyola Medical Center, one in ten patients with acute primary HPT had multiglandular involvement at surgery (4). Although cysts are not commonly noted on pathologic examination of the parathyroid glands (see chapter by LiVolsi), two cases of parathyroid cysts were noted in patients with acute primary HPT (21). In an additional report, Albertson and coworkers (22) described hypercalcemic crisis due to the presence of a large functioning parathyroid cyst.

Ultrastructural analyses of parathyroid glands associated with acute HPT revealed unique features in comparison to atrophic contralateral glands. The cell nucleus is enlarged, with increased numbers of pores and abundant rough endoplasmic reticulum. Conspicuous interdigitations of the plasma membrane, increased number of mitochondria, and extensive Golgi apparatus are also present. These features are consistent with the markedly increased function of the parathyroid cell associated with acute HPT (23).

PATHOPHYSIOLOGY

This unusual presentation of parathyroid disease is marked by extreme hypercalcemia and associated target tissue manifestation. The mechanism(s) by which a seemingly "ordinary" case of primary hyperparathyroidism develops into a life-threatening medical emergency remains unknown. However, several pathophysiologic factors may be suspected from the various case studies.

One hallmark of parathyroid crisis is the extraordinary elevations of PTH. Levels 20 times normal values have been described (3) and are much greater than the 1.5–2.0-fold elevation of PTH measured in patients with primary hyperparathyroidism. Although one might predict that renal impairment may contribute to the increased circulating levels of PTH, the N-terminal fragment may be as elevated as the C-terminal, renal-cleared fragment (3). These high levels of PTH suggest that there is a marked increase in the secretion of PTH from the abnormal parathyroid gland. The pathology of the parathyroid gland itself reflects this increased secretory rate (23). With rare exceptions, the single adenoma found at surgery has not been compromised by infarction or rupture leading to massive release of PTH into the systemic circulation.

The physiological effects of excessive PTH production are manifested on target organs. Reported urinary calcium concentrations are extremely elevated. In bone, massive osteoclast activity reflects the rapid bone resorption and extreme hypercalcemia noted in acute primary hyperparathyroidism. In one case study that evaluated the histological appearance of bone (7), the lack of formation suggests that bone resorption and formation are dissociated.

A history of mild hypercalcemia was present in 25% of patients in one series (3). An additional common denominator to many cases is an intervening illness, which may precipitate the disorder. One could hypothesize that bed rest associated with an acute illness may catalyze increased mobilization of calcium from bone. Such an illness may also be associated with mild dehydration, and the volume contraction that occurs could compromise renal function. These features, however, do not in completely account for the marked elevation in PTH levels.

ACUTE PARATHYROID CRISIS IN PREGNANCY

Management of maternal hyperparathyroidism during pregnancy is usually based on the patient's symptoms, severity of the disease, and gestational age of the fetus (see the chapter by Marcus and Stock). A few cases of acute parathyroid crisis have been described during pregnancy (24–26). Although most patients underwent surgical removal of a parathyroid adenoma, acute primary HPT has been described in which medical management resulted in a favorable outcome (25).

In an unusual case, a 34-year-old female developed acute primary hyperparathyroidism several days postpartum. She was admitted to the hospital at 39 weeks of gestation due to polyhydramnios, and she spontaneously delivered a healthy 3070 mg infant at 40 weeks gestation. Postpartum, she developed progressive weakness and nausea. On the third postpartum day, serum calcium was >20 mg/dl, phosphate was 1.9 mg/dl. Further evaluation revealed subperiosteal resorption on hand radiographs and a "pepper pot" appearance and resorption around the teeth on skull X-rays. Her condition deteriorated rapidly, and she was treated medically with intravenous fluids, hydrocortisone, and phosphates. Hemodialysis was performed on day 5, and respiratory failure was managed with intermittent positive pressure ventilation. Neck exploration revealed a 3 g parathyroid tumor in the left pole of the thyroid gland, and laparotomy was performed due to gross distension of the abdomen. Acute pancreatitis was treated with drainage. On the following day, shock intervened, and resuscitation was unsuccessful. On pathological examination, two normal parathyroid glands were identified. Metastatic calcification was noted in kidney tubules, myocardium, pulmonary vessel walls, and bronchial walls.

A serum sample obtained at 16 weeks of gestation was retrieved, and the patient was found to have had an elevated serum calcium (11.6 mg/dl). The authors suggest that the increased need of the fetus for calcium and physiological hypoalbuminemia may have protected the patient in the peripartum period. In an animal model, advanced pregnancy has provided protection against administration of PTH in toxic doses; this protection did not extend to the postpartum period (27). A similar situation may have occurred in this unfortunate woman with acceleration of calcium mobilization and increased serum concentration of calcium in the postpartum period.

OTHER ASSOCIATIONS WITH ACUTE PRIMARY HYPERPARATHYROIDISM

An extraordinarily rare combination of endocrine emergencies, acute primary HPT and thyrotoxicosis, has been described in one patient (28). Asymptomatic hyperparathyroidism in a patient with thyrotoxicosis is a relatively uncommon condition; other authors have described an incidental occult parathyroid adenoma in a patient with a preexisting thyroid disorder (29,30). This 32-year-old female was diagnosed with Graves' disease and treated with radioactive iodine. After 3 months, she was admitted to a psychiatric hospital with the diagnosis of depression. Her medical evaluation revealed emesis, constipation, perioral and digital numbness, and serum calcium 14 mg/dl. On transfer to a medical facility, serum calcium rose to 15 mg/dl, and diffuse demineralization was noted on hand radiographs. Serum calcium remained markedly elevated in spite of treatment with intravenous fluids (400 ml/hr), prednisolone (30 mg bid), and phosphorus (750 mg tid). For her thyroid disorder (T_4 = 19.1 µg/dl; T_3 = 361 ng/dl), the patient was treated with propranolol, saturated solution of potassium iodide and propylthiouraul. On hospital day 11, she underwent neck exploration and a $2 \times 2 \times 3$ cm right upper parathyroid adenoma weighing 6 g was removed, and a bilateral subtotal thyroidectomy was performed. Postoperatively, the patient required intravenous calcium gluconate; her serum calcium reached a nadir of 4.6 mg/dl. The authors emphasize the need to render the patient euthyroid prior to surgical treatment of hyperparathyroidism.

ANIMAL MODELS OF ACUTE PRIMARY HYPERPARATHYROIDISM

In 1926, the administration of large amounts of parathyroid extract to dogs produced anuria, renal failure, and death. Calcium deposits were present in soft tissues throughout the animal (31). These experiments, which provided insight into the pathophysiology of primary hyperparathyroidism, were extended by Hulter and colleagues (32). These investigators proposed that chronic alterations in plasma calcium concentrations would alter the response of plasma calcitriol concentrations to PTH. Intact dogs underwent continuous intravenous PTH infusion for 12 days, with sustained hypercalcemia and hypophosphatemia. Plasma calcitriol concentrations decreased significantly.

Recently, Wilson and colleagues (33) developed an in vivo model of hyperparathyroidism. A cDNA encoding human prepro-PTH was cloned into a replication-defective retroviral vector. The retrovirus containing the PTH gene was then transfected into a retroviral packaging cell line. Harvested virus was used to infect RAT-1 fibroblasts. The RAT-1 fibroblasts were injected into the peritoneal cavity of syngeneic Fisher rats. A severe and progressive rise in human PTH levels and a rise in serum calcium occurred in these animals. This model allowed histological evaluation of bone and kidney in severe hyperparathyroidism. Marked osteoclastic bone resorption and extensive osteitis fibrosa cystica were observed. Nephrocalcinosis was present on histologic examination of the kidneys (33). This model mimics acute primary hyperparathyroidism in the rapidity of the development of hypercalcemia and may help to provide further insight into the pathogenesis of acute parathyroid disease.

TREATMENT

Definitive treatment of acute HPT is surgical extirpation of the abnormal parathyroid gland or glands (Figs. 1,2). However, treatment of severe, life-threatening hypercalcemia must be instituted and is similar to therapy of acute hypercalcemia of other causes (34) (see chapter by Bilezikian and Singer). In two recently reported cases, acute hypercalcemia occurring several

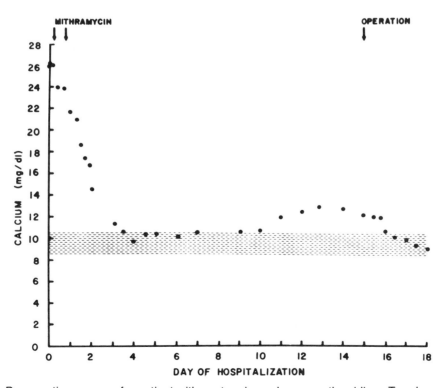

FIG. 1. Preoperative course of a patient with acute primary hyperparathyroidism. Two doses of mithramycin (25 μg/kg) 12 hr apart were administered for life-threatening hypercalcemia. The serum calcium levels remained stable until the diagnosis of primary hyperparathyroidism was confirmed and the patient underwent successful parathyroidectomy. The *shaded area* represents the normal range of the serum calcium concentration.

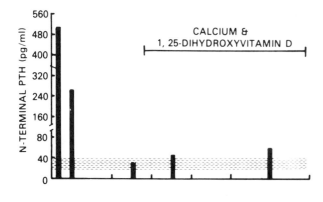

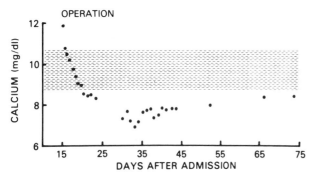

FIG. 2. Postoperative course of the same patient following successful parathyroidectomy. The decline in N-terminal PTH (**top**) levels was monitored in sequence with the postoperative decline in serum calcium levels (**bottom**). Calcium (1 g daily) and 1,25(OH)$_2$D (0.25 μg three times daily) were administered over the times indicated. *Shaded areas* in both panels indicate the normal range of the N-terminal PTH and calcium concentration respectively.

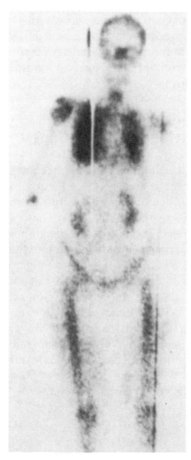

FIG. 3. Pulmonary calcinosis in a patient with acute primary hyperparathyroidism. Hypercalcemic crisis occurred due to a large mediastinal parathyroid adenoma. (Reprinted from ref. 36 with permission.)

days after cholecystectomy (35) or splenectomy (16) was successfully temporized with the administration of intravenous pamidronate [(3-amino-1-hydroxypropylidene)-1-1-bisphosphonic acid (APD)] prior to surgical removal of the parathyroid adenoma.

The use of intravenous phosphates in acute HPT is contraindicated. Extensive systemic calcinosis precipitated by phosphates can occur pre- or postoperatively (36,37) (see Fig. 3). Intravascular precipitation of calcium-phosphate salts may cause pulmonary insufficiency, vascular calcification, hypotension, and death.

SUMMARY

Acute primary hyperparathyroidism is a reversible, curable, and life-threatening disorder. Although the pathophysiology is not well understood, several factors are common to many reported cases. Age and gender are not risk factors. An antecedent history of primary hyperparathyroidism has been confirmed in several cases (3,26), although the risk of development of acute toxicity among the asymptomatic hyperparathyroid population is low (6,7). An incapacitating ill-

ness, perhaps associated with bed rest, is frequently associated with acute primary HPT. The immobilization that occurs during intercurrent illness may foster mobilization of calcium from bone, aggravating the hypercalcemic state. Remarkable elevations of PTH suggest that the hallmark of the disorder is uncontrolled PTH secretion. PTH levels are elevated to a much greater extent than can be accounted for by impairment of kidney function alone.

Recognition of acute HPT, rapid diagnosis, aggressive medical management, and successful surgery can result in a favorable outcome. The fact that the diagnosis can be readily distinguished from other causes of hypercalcemia and the fact that the disorder is curable mean that this disorder must be considered in any patient with life-threatening hypercalcemia.

ACKNOWLEDGMENTS

The author thanks Dr. Bart Clarke for his helpful review of the manuscript and Ms. Jennifer Hultgren for her excellent secretarial assistance.

REFERENCES

1. Fitzpatrick LA. Is surgery necessary for the asymptomatic patient with primary hyperparathyroidism? In: Gitnick F, Barnes HV, Duffy TP, Lewis RP, Winterbauer RH, eds. *Debates in medicine, 4th ed.* Chicago: Mosby-Year Book, 1991;114–157.
2. Fitzpatrick LA, Bilezikian JP. Primary hyperparathyroidism. In: Becker KL, ed. *Principles and practice of endocrinology and metabolism.* Philadelphia: J.B. Lippincott, 1990;430–437.
3. Fitzpatrick LA, Bilezikian JP. Acute primary hyperparathyroidism. *Am J Med* 1987;82:275–282.
4. Maselly MJ, Lawrence AM, Brooks M, et al. Hyperparathyroid crisis. Successful treatment of ten comatose patients. *Surgery* 1981;90:741–760.
5. Nudelman IL, Deutsch AA, Reiss R. Primary hyperparathyroidism due to mediastinal parathyroid adenoma. *Int Surg* 1987;72:104–108.
6. Corlew DS, Bryda SL, Bradley EL, DiGirolamo M. Observations on the course of untreated primary hyperparathyroidism. *Surgery* 1985;98:1064–1071.
7. Scholz DA, Purnell DC. Asymptomatic primary hyperparathyroidism: 10-year prospective study. *Mayo Clin Proc* 1981;56:473–478.
8. Heath H, Hodgson SF, Kennedy MA. Primary hyperparathyroidism: incidence, morbidity, and potential economic impact in a community. *N Engl J Med* 1980;4:189–193.
9. Bilezikian JP, Silverberg SJ, Shane E, Parisien M, Dempster D. Characterization and evaluation of asymptomatic primary hyperparathyroidism. *J Bone Mineral Res* 1991;6(Suppl 2):S85–S90.
10. Wynne AG, van Heerden J, Carney JA, Fitzpatrick LA. Parathyroid carcinoma: clinical and pathologic features in 43 patients. *Medicine* 1992;71:197–205.
11. Shane E, Bilezikian JP. Parathyroid carcinoma: a review of 62 patients. *Endocr Rev* 1982;3:218–226.
12. Wang C, Gaz RD. Natural history of parathyroid carcinoma: diagnosis, treatment and results. *Am J Surg* 1979;149:522–527.
13. Martin TJ, Grill V. Hypercalcemia in cancer. *J Steroid Biochem Mol Biol* 1992;43:123–129.
14. Kao PC, Jiang N, Klee G, Purnell DC. Development and validation of a new radioimmunoassay for parathyrin (PTH). *Clin Chem* 1982;28:69–74.
15. Phillips P. Letter to the editor: herpes zoster-induced acute hyperparathyroid crisis. *Clin Infect Dis* 1992;14:1270–1271.
16. Canivet JL, Damas P, Lamy M. Posttraumatic parathyroid crisis and severe hypercalcemia treated with intravenous bisphosphonate (APD). Case report. *Acta Anaesthesiol* 1990;41:47–50.
17. Wang CA, Gaz RD. Bone metabolism in acute parathyroid crisis. *Clin Endocrinol* 1985;22:787–793.
18. Sarfati E, Desported L, Gossot D, Dubost C. Acute primary hyperparathyroidism: experience of 59 cases. *Br J Surg* 1989;76:979–981.
19. Karstrup S, Lohela P, Apaja-Sarkkinen M, Borgmastars H, Holopeinen O. Non-operative inactivation of a parathyroid tumour in a patient with hypercalcaemic crisis. *Acta Med Scand* 1988;224:187–188.
20. Bizard JP, Quiévreux, Carnaille B, Proye C. Formes toxiques de l'hyperparathyroïdie primaire (57 observations) Réappréciation de leur définition et de leur substratum anatomopathologique. *Lyon Chir* 1992;88:117–122.
21. Calandra DB, Shah KH, Prinz RA, et al. Parathyroid cysts: a report of eleven cases including two associated with hyperparathyroid crisis. *Surgery* 1983;94:887–892.
22. Albertson DA, Marshall RB, Jarman WT. Hypercalcemic crisis secondary to a functioning parathyroid cyst. *Am J Surg* 1981;141:175–177.
23. Thiele J. The human parathyroid chief cell—a model for polypeptide hormone producing endocrine unit as revealed by various functional and pathological conditions. A thin section and freeze-fracture study. *J Submicrosc Cytol* 1986;18:205–220.
24. Clark D, Seeds JW, Cefalo RC. Spontaneous cervical hematoma: a rare manifestation of parathyroid adenoma. *Surgery* 1981;89:697–700.
25. Thomason JL, Sampson MB, Farb HF, Spellacy WN. Pregnancy complicated by concurrent primary hyperparathyroidism and pancreatitis. *Obstet Gynecol* 1981;57:34S–36S.
26. Matthias GSM, Helliwell TR, Williams A. Postpartum hyperparathyroid crisis. Case report. *Br J Obstet Gynaecol* 1987;94:807–810.
27. Lehr D, Krukowski M. Prevention of myocardial necrosis by advanced pregnancy. *J Am Med Assoc* 1961;1781:823–826.
28. Piccione W, Selenkow HA, Cady B. Management problems in coexisting parathyroid crisis and florid thyrotoxicosis. *Surgery* 1984;96:1009–1014.
29. Attie JN, Estrin J, Khafif RA, Dweck F. Parathyroid adenomas discovered incidentally during explorations of the thyroid. *Am J Surg* 1967;114:538–542.
30. Frame B, Durham RH. Simultaneous hyperthyroidism and hyperparathyroidism. *Am J Med* 1959;27:824–828.
31. Albright F, Reifenstein EC. *The parathyroid glands and metabolic bone disease.* Baltimore: Williams & Wilkins, 1948.
32. Hulter HN, Halloran BP, Toto RD, Peterson JC. Long-term control of plasma calcitriol concentration in dogs and humans. Dominant role of plasma calcium concentration in experimental hyperparathyroidism. *J Clin Invest* 1985;76:695–702.
33. Wilson JM, Grossman M, Thompson AR, et al. Somatic gene-transfer in the development of an animal-model for primary hyperparathyroidism. *Endocrinology* 1992;130:2947–2954.
34. Bilezikian JP. Management of acute hypercalcemia. *N Engl J Med* 1992;326:1196–1203.
35. Evans RA. Aminohydroxypropylidene diphosphonate treatment of hypercalcemic crisis due to primary hyperparathyroidism. *Aust NZ J Med* 1987;17:58–59.
36. Khafif RA, Delima C, Silverberg A, Frankel R, Groopman J. Acute hyperparathyroidism with systemic calcinosis. Report of a case. *Arch Intern Med* 1989;149:681–684.
37. Vernava AM, O'Neal LW, Palermo V. Lethal hyperparathyroid crisis: hazards of phosphate administration. *Surgery* 1987;102:941–948.

The Parathyroids, edited by J.P. Bilezikian, M.A. Levine, and R. Marcus. Raven Press, Ltd., New York © 1994.

CHAPTER 37

Multiple Endocrine Neoplasia Type I

Clinical Features and Management

David C. Metz, Robert T. Jensen, Allen E. Bale, Monica C. Skarulis, Richard C. Eastman, Lynette Nieman, Jeffrey A. Norton, Eitan Friedman, Catharina Larsson, Andrea Amorosi, Maria-Luisa Brandi, and Stephen J. Marx

DEFINITIONS

Multiple endocrine neoplasia syndrome is a term that encompasses several "syndromes" with little or no etiologic relation to each other. This term literally includes all cases with neoplasia in more than one endocrine gland. For example, it includes cases with sporadic tumor in two endocrine organs (such as a thyroid adenoma and an adrenocortical adenoma). Even

D. C. Metz: Department of Medicine, Division of Gastroenterology, Hospital of the University of Pennsylvania, University of Pennsylvania, Philadelphia, Pennsylvania 19104.

R. T. Jensen: Digestive Diseases Branch, National Institute of Diabetes, Digestive, and Kidney Diseases, National Institutes of Health, Bethesda, Maryland 20892.

A. E. Bale: Department of Genetics, Yale University School of Medicine, New Haven, Connecticut 06510.

M. C. Skarulis: Division of Intramural Research, National Institute of Diabetes, Digestive, and Kidney Diseases, National Institutes of Health, Bethesda, Maryland 20892.

R. C. Eastman: Diabetes Branch, National Institute of Diabetes, Digestive, and Kidney Diseases, National Institutes of Health, Bethesda, Maryland 20892.

L. Nieman: Developmental Endocrinology Branch, National Institute of Child Health and Human Development, National Institutes of Health, Bethesda, Maryland 20892.

E. Friedman, C. Larsson: Department of Clinical Genetics, Karolinska Hospital, S-10401, Stockholm, Sweden.

M. Brandi, A. Amorosi: Endocrine Section, Department of Clinical Physiopathology, University of Florence Medical School, 50139 Florence, Italy.

J. A. Norton: Department of Surgery, Washington University School of Medicine, St. Louis, Missouri 63110.

S. J. Marx: Genetics and Endocrinology Section, National Institute of Diabetes, Digestive, and Kidney Diseases, National Institutes of Health, Bethesda, Maryland 20892.

a case with a sporadic tumor, secreting a growth factor [such as adrenocorticotropic hormone (ACTH)] that caused secondary "tumor" in another endocrine gland (in this case, the adrenal cortex), would be included.

The terms *multiple endocrine neoplasia types I, II, and III* have a narrower scope. Multiple endocrine neoplasia type I (MEN-I) is a syndrome that can be expressed as tumors of the parathyroid, pancreatic islets, anterior pituitary, and certain other tissues. It is often hereditary; most or all familial cases and most sporadic cases are believed to be caused by mutation in one gene, the *men1* gene. Some sporadic cases will undoubtedly prove to have other causes. Earlier terms for MEN-I have included multiple endocrine adenoma, multiple endocrine adenomatosis, multiple endocrine adenopathy, pluriglandular syndrome, and Wermer's syndrome (1).

Multiple endocrine neoplasia type II (MEN-II) differs from MEN-I. It is caused by mutation in the *men2* gene and is expressed as neoplasms of the calcitonin-secreting (or parafollicular) cells in the thyroid (C cells), the adrenal medulla, and the parathyroid glands (2). It can be subdivided as MEN-IIa and MEN-IIb, or these subgroups can be termed *MEN-II* and *MEN-III*, respectively; the second term of either pair is a syndrome of marfanoid body habitus with combinations of neoplasms of C cells, adrenal medulla, and peripheral nerves (the latter causing characteristic mucosal neuromas). Primary hyperparathyroidism is rarely, if ever, a feature of MEN-IIb/MEN-III. MEN-I may have a pathophysiology unrelated to MEN-II; while MEN-I is caused by loss of function at the *men 1* locus, MEN-II results from a gain of function (activation) of the *men 2* (*ret* oncogene) gene on chromosome 10 (4).

HISTORY

Erdheim (5) is generally credited with the first description of MEN-I. He described in 1903 the autopsy of a patient with acromegaly, eosinophilic adenoma of the pituitary, and four enlarged parathyroid glands. Cushing and Davidoff in 1927 (6) and Lloyd in 1929 (7) reported the autopsy of a patient with tumors of the three principal MEN-I components, parathyroid, pancreas, and pituitary. In 1939 Rossier and Dressler (8) first reported these features in a kindred. They reported sisters with kidney stones; one had Cushing's syndrome, the other hypoglycemic attacks and parathyroid adenomas. The first substantive review of MEN-I was published by Underdahl et al. in 1953 (9). They reviewed six published cases and added eight additional cases. Though familial occurrence was under consideration in several of these cases, it was not recognized as an integral feature of the disease. In 1953 and 1954 Moldower and colleagues (10,11) reported MEN-I in a kindred. Also in 1954, Wermer (12) reported a kindred with features of MEN-I in five members. He suggested that the trait was caused by an autosomal dominant gene with high penetrance; MEN-I is sometimes referred to as *Wermer's syndrome*. Though severe ulcer diathesis was accepted as a feature in several of these early reports, the central features of sporadic gastrinoma were only delineated between 1955 and 1961 (13–15). Prolactinoma was accepted as a feature of MEN-I shortly after proof of the existence of prolactin in humans in 1971 (16,17).

Advances in knowledge about the expression of MEN-I between 1960 and 1980 largely paralleled the development of radioimmunoassays (RIAs) for the various peptides that circulate at high levels in MEN-I [i.e., parathyroid hormone (PTH), gastrin, insulin, prolactin, etc. (16,18,19)]. Historical advances in management of MEN-I are too extensive to recount, since they span so many topics in endocrine therapeutics. Some of the important milestones include the development of parathyroidectomy for primary hyperparathyroidism around 1925 (20), total gastrectomy for gastrinoma around 1961 (13), H_2 histamine receptor antagonists as effective pharmacotherapy for Zollinger-Ellison syndrome in 1977, improved microsurgery for pituitary tumor, and ergot agonists as effective pharmacotherapy for prolactinoma in 1982 (21). The number of reports and reviews of MEN-I (1,22–24) seems disproportionate to its rather low incidence. Interest in MEN-I has been consistently high because MEN-I spans multiple divisions of endocrinology and because studies of MEN-I might provide insight into the etiology of more common cases of sporadic hyperfunction in any single endocrine tissue.

In 1988, Larsson et al. (3) used genetic linkage analysis to establish the chromosomal region carrying the *men1* gene; they showed simultaneously that a tumor in MEN-I probably develops by inactivation of the normal copy of the *men1* gene in one or more tumor precursor cells. This study initiated a new phase in MEN-I research, deriving insights from sophisticated molecular biologic and genetic methods.

CLINICAL AND PATHOLOGICAL EXPRESSION OF MULTIPLE ENDOCRINE NEOPLASIA TYPE I

Clinical Features

Parathyroids: Primary Hyperparathyroidism in Multiple Endocrine Neoplasia Type I

Primary Hyperparathyroidism as the Most Common Endocrinopathy in Multiple Endocrine Neoplasia Type I

Primary hyperparathyroidism is the most common expression of *men1* (Table 1) (25–29). However, the reported rates for disease in other target tissues have varied widely in review articles. The prevalence rate for any feature of MEN-I is closely tied to the biases in patient selection and to the methods used to test patients for that feature (Table 1).

An autopsy-based evaluation concluded that, in every adult, MEN-I is expressed as macro- and microscopic tumors simultaneously in all three target organs, the parathyroids, pancreas, and anterior pituitary (25). This conclusion, however, must be tempered by the biases inherent in that review. This was an analysis of 32 autopsy reports in the medical literature from 1953 to 1978. Many of those autopsy reports were published because of the very unusual discovery of multiple endocrine tumors in several organs.

Ballard et al. (26) in 1964 published a detailed review of MEN-I, recognizing most of its important features. They reported pancreatic islet tumor in 81% and pituitary tumor in 65% of cases. These very high prevalences reflect their biased case-accrual method. Ballard et al. reviewed findings in one large kindred plus published reports of kindreds or interesting cases. Since this was prior to the era of radioimmunoassay development and widespread use of accurate serum calcium measurements, cases were recognized and, in particular, reported only if they had rather severe clinical endocrinopathies. More importantly, isolated case reports had been published principally to show striking involvement of several endocrine glands.

More recent reviews based on subjects with any clinically recognizable endocrinopathy in large MEN-I kindreds have continued to find a very high prevalence of hyperparathyroidism (in 87–97% of cases expressing any feature of MEN-I), with lower hyper-

TABLE 1. *The expressions of MEN-I depend on the methods to derive indices of disease expression and on the biases in patient selection*

| | Portion of affected cases with hyperfunction in a tissue | | |
Reference	Parathyroid (%)	GI-endocrine axis (%)	Anterior pituitary (%)
Majewski and Wilson (25)[a]	100	100	100
Ballard et al. (26)[b]	87	81	65
Marx et al. (27)[c]	97	32	16
Vasen et al. (28)[d]	87	64	27
Skogseid et al. (29)[e]	90	75	19

[a]Review of 32 autopsies published with detailed description between 1953 and 1978. All subjects were older than age 24 years.

[b]Detailed biochemical testing in some members of one large kindred (14 well-studied affected members) and 74 single case reports or well-studied members of small kindreds from the literature up to 1964 (i.e., mainly prior to development of radioimmunoassays).

[c]Tabulation of 198 affected members in 21 large kindreds from literature up to 1982.

[d]Fifty-two affected members in 11 families seen between 1974 and 1989 at two hospitals in The Netherlands. Patients received standard endocrine testing and were not tested in a systematic serial manner.

[e]Thirty-two affected members in four kindreds seen between 1981 and 1991 at one hospital in Sweden. All patients received extensive testing that included challenge tests, imaging tests, and serial testing.

function rates in other target organs—pancreatic islet hyperfunction in 32–75% and anterior pituitary hyperfunction or neoplasm in 16–40% (27–30) (Table 1).

DNA testing (genetic linkage analysis) can now identify *menI* gene carriers with a high degree of reliability in some kindreds (see below). Thus silent carriers are now identifiable. The true rates for age-dependent target tissue expression should soon be established.

Clinical Features of Primary Hyperparathyroidism in Multiple Endocrine Neoplasia Type I

The clinical features of primary hyperparathyroidism in MEN-I reproduce most of the features of sporadic primary hyperparathyroidism (30–34). These include a prolonged early stage of asymptomatic hypercalcemia, generally low morbidity, slow if any progression of symptoms and signs, and high likelihood of amelioration through parathyroidectomy by an experienced surgeon. An impression that a disproportionally high incidence of urolithiasis is characteristic of MEN-I has not been confirmed in one detailed analysis (31).

As with sporadic adenoma, MEN-I occasionally presents as a clinically severe form with hypercalcemic crisis, osteitis fibrosa cystica, or acute pancreatitis (24). Parathyroid cancer has been described in one case of MEN-I (35).

Some features of primary hyperparathyroidism differ in cases of MEN-I vs. sporadic parathyroid adenoma (Table 2). These features are emphasized herein.

Onset Age. There have been reports of primary hyperparathyroidism at ages of 4, 8, and 12 years, in MEN-I (29,32). Betts et al. (32) reported hypercalcemia between ages 8 and 11 years in six members of an MEN-I family. The prevalence of primary hyperparathyroidism increases with age, approaching 100% after age 50 years in MEN-I (36). Clinically important primary hyperparathyroidism is extremely rare in those under age 15 years in MEN-I. One study with serial testing found a mean age for onset of primary hyperparathyroidism at 18 years (in seven cases of MEN-I converting from normocalcemic to hypercalcemic during serial screening) (29). Too few subjects reported in the literature developed a first onset of hypercalcemia during prospective screening to establish the average onset age for expression of primary hyperparathyroidism in MEN-I.

The average age for onset of hypercalcemia seems to be ~25 years (36). This is far younger than that for sporadic parathyroid adenoma (37) and is in good accord with the "two-hit" mechanism for neoplasia. Knudson (38) developed the "two-hit" concept to explain epidemiological features in hereditary vs. sporadic tumor caused by mutations in one gene, for example, retinoblastoma. Somatic mutation must inactivate both normal copies ("two hits") of a growth suppresser-type gene to allow a clone precursor cell to develop into a tumor. For the hereditary variant, one copy of this gene is already inactivated in every cell by transmission in the germline; thus only the second copy of the gene must become inactivated ("one hit") in one cell to allow it to grow into a clonal tumor. Sporadic tumor, requiring two stochastic hits in a tumor clone precursor cell, will develop later than hereditary tumor, requiring only one hit.

TABLE 2. *Distinguishing features in three categories of primary hyperparathyroidism*

Feature	Sporadic adenoma	Multiple endocrine neoplasia type I	Familial hypocalciuric hypercalcemia (FHH)
Transmission	Sporadic	Autos. dom.	Autos. dom.[c]
Hypercalcemia onset age (year)	50–60	25	0 (at birth)
Sex ratio (F:M)	3:1	1:1	1:1
Calcium in urine	High	High	Normal to low
Magnesium in serum	Low to normal	Low to normal	Normal to high
Parathyroid hormone in serum	High	High	Normal (high in 10–15%)
Endocrine tumors outside of the parathyroids	No	Often	No
Adverse interaction with gastrinoma	No	Yes	No
Parathyroid glands pathology	Adenoma, single	Adenoma, multiple	Hyperplasia, mild
Surgical result[a]			
Immediate cure (%)	95	92	2
Persistence (%)	5	8	98
Hypopara (%)[b]	2	5	2
Late recur (%)	2	50 +	NA[c]

[a]Neonatal severe primary hyperparathyroidism can result from a double dose of *fhh* alleles; thus this rare trait can be considered as autosomal recessive. In other cases, neonates with severe primary hyperparathyroidism have only one parent known to carry an *fhh* allele, and the pathophysiology of the severe trait is not fully understood (27).

[b]The estimated surgical results are for a center using appropriate preoperative evaluation of the patient and of the family and having an experienced parathyroid surgeon. In this table, hypoparathyroidism is treated as a "cure," though it is clearly less desirable than euparathyroidism. Note also that hypoparathyroidism in sporadic adenoma or MEN-I can sometimes be reversed with a cryopreserved autograft of pathologic parathyroid tissue.

[c]NA, not applicable, since virtually no operations lead to transient normocalcemia in FHH.

Female:Male Gender Ratio. Unlike sporadic parathyroid adenoma, with a 3:1 female-to-male gender ratio (37), primary hyperparathyroidism in MEN-I has a similar prevalence in females and males.

Interaction With Zollinger-Ellison Syndrome. Primary hyperparathyroidism exacerbates the expression of Zollinger-Ellison syndrome (see below). Cure of primary hyperparathyroidism in MEN-I can decrease the dosage requirement for antisecretory drugs and can occasionally cause remission of all biochemical features of Zollinger-Ellison syndrome. However, because of excellent gastric acid control by antisecretory medications, concomitant Zollinger-Ellison syndrome is rarely a sufficient indication for parathyroidectomy in MEN-I.

Appearance of the Parathyroid Glands. The most common finding in sporadic primary hyperparathyroidism is a single adenoma. Though there is controversy about the possibility of microscopic abnormality in the remaining glands (39,40), this is unimportant in the current context. Multiple parathyroid glands are enlarged in association with primary hyperparathyroid in MEN-I, and the enlargement is usually quite asymmetric (41,42) (Fig 1); commonly one or two glands are normal or minimally enlarged. Very rarely, three glands are normal-sized in a patient with primary hyperparathyroidism and MEN-I (41,42).

Outcomes of Parathyroid Surgery. The outcomes of parathyroidectomy differ between MEN-I-associated and sporadic primary hyperparathyroidism (31,42–46). First, because more than one parathyroid gland is generally overactive in the primary hyperparathyroidism of MEN-I, there is an increased prevalence of persistent postoperative hyperparathyroidism. Hyperparathyroidism persists after surgery in 40–60% of MEN-I cases operated on by inexperienced parathyroid surgeons (43) and in 0–25% operated on by experienced surgeons (42,43,46). A postoperative persistence rate of 0% was found in several small series (42,43); all surgeons may experience occasional failures with current methods. Second, because of the need for more extensive parathyroid resection and concomitantly a wider exploration, the prevalence of postoperative hypoparathyroidism is also increased, being 0–30% (42,44,46). Third, the incidence of postoperative recurrent primary hyperparathyroidism is strikingly high in MEN-I. While postoperative recurrence is very rare (~3%) in sporadic primary hyperparathyroidism (47), it increases with time after apparently successful parathyroidectomy, reaching 50% within 12 years in MEN-I (Fig. 2) (43). Rarely, an MEN-I patient has had prolonged postoperative hypoparathyroidism (partial hypoparathyroidism), subsequently has become euparathyroid, and later has developed recurrent primary

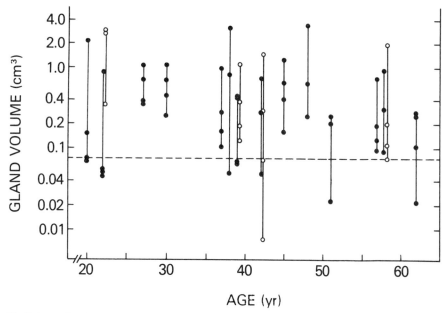

FIG. 1. Multiple endocrine neoplasia type I cases show heterogeneous enlargement of the parathyroid glands at initial parathyroid exploration. Data are from initial operation at the NIH for 18 patients with primary hyperparathyroidism and familial MEN-I. The volumes of all four parathyroid glands within an operation are connected by a vertical line. The *dashed line* shows the upper limit of normal gland volume (0.075 cm³, equivalent to 75 mg mass) (41).

hyperparathyroidism (46) (S.J.M. and J.N., unpublished observations). True recurrent primary hyperparathyroidism has a far lower incidence in sporadic primary parathyroid "hyperplasia" than in MEN-I (48). The high recurrence rate after "successful" parathyroidectomy in MEN-I in contrast to the stability of established primary hyperparathyroidism in MEN-I indicates that the iatrogenic hypo- or normocalcemia may promote the emergence of a new parathyroid tumor in MEN-I. These considerations justify approaches to parathyroid surgery that are specific for MEN-I (see below) (Fig. 2).

Gastrointestinal Manifestations of Multiple Endocrine Neoplasia Type I

In comparison to sporadic endocrine tumors of the upper gastrointestinal tract, tumors in patients with MEN-I develop at a younger age, are almost always multiple, and may arise in the setting of other endocrinopathies (24,49,50). It is generally believed that >95% of MEN-I patients who develop enteropancreatic neuroendocrine tumors will already have developed hyperparathyroidism by the time they present with their gastrointestinal tumor (24,49). Classically, hyperparathyroidism manifests in the third decade of life, whereas enteropancreatic tumors develop later and become clinically apparent in the fourth or fifth decades (49,50). However, recent evidence suggests that Zollinger-Ellison syndrome may in fact be the first

clinical manifestation of MEN-I in a small proportion of patients (51).

Unless the tumors are nonfunctional, the clinical presentation of enteropancreatic neuroendocrine tumors in patients with MEN-I is almost always due to excessive hormone release by the tumor (49,52,53). Therefore, in contrast to nonfunctional tumors, many

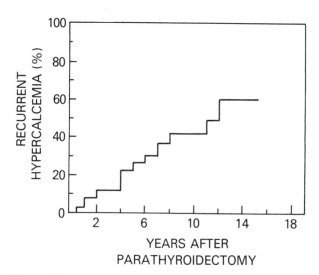

FIG. 2. The fraction of patients with recurrent primary hyperparathyroidism increases with time after parathyroidectomy. Data are from a retrospective series of 41 MEN-I patients who had undergone "successful" subtotal parathyroidectomy at many hospitals (243).

functional tumors tend to present earlier, when they are small (52,53). It is not uncommon for certain functional tumors (especially gastrinomas and insulinomas) to present when they are so small that they cannot be detected by routine abdominal imaging modalities (24,49,54). Under these circumstances, the only indication of a gastrointestinal neuroendocrine tumor is the endocrine syndrome itself. Symptoms or signs of local enlargement or infiltration (back pain, jaundice, abdominal mass, left-side portal hypertension) or metastatic diseases (cachexia, hepatomegaly) may rarely occur at presentation (49,52,53,55).

With regard to the various types of enteropancreatic neuroendocrine tumors in MEN-I, gastrinomas (see next section) are the most common functional endocrine tumors, occurring in up to 54% of all patients with MEN-I (Table 3) (24,49,52,53). Insulinomas (see below) are the next most common, occurring in up to 21% of patients with MEN-I (24,49). Glucagonomas (~3%), VIP-omas (~1%), GRF-omas (no estimates available), and somatostatinomas (no estimates available) have also been well described in patients with MEN-I (see below) (24,49). Conversely, MEN-I occurs in ~20% of patients with the Zollinger-Ellison syndrome, in 4% of patients with insulinomas, and in 33% of patients with GRF-omas (24,49,52,53,56,57). However, nonfunctional neuroendocrine tumors (approximately three-fourths of which are PP-omas; see below) are probably the most common enteropancreatic neuroendocrine tumors in MEN-I (24,49,50,53,57,58). Precise data on their prevalence are not available, since MEN-I patients without functional endocrine syndromes are generally not subjected to routine surgery (53,57,58). Furthermore, patients with MEN-I appear to be predisposed to the development of various other enteropancreatic neuroendocrine tumors, including gastric ECL-omas (see below), which may have an association with Zollinger-Ellison-induced hypergastrinemia (59,60) as well as other varieties of neuroendocrine carcinoid tumors (see below) (24). At least 5% and up to 13% of patients with Zollinger-Ellison syndrome and MEN-I have gastric ECL-omas, some of which are invasive (59–61).

It is important to note that patients with MEN-I may

TABLE 3. *Enteropancreatic neuroendocrine tumors in multiple endocrine neoplasia type I*

Tumor	Syndrome	% with MEN-I	% of MEN-I	Signs/symptoms	Location	Hormone
Gastrinoma	Zollinger-Ellison syndrome	20	50	Abdominal pain, diarrhea, reflux symptoms	Duodenum > 80%?	Gastrin
Insulinoma	Insulinoma	4	21	Hypoglycemia	Pancreas >97%	Insulin
Glucagonoma	Glucagonoma	Rare	3	Rash, anemia, diabetes/glucose intolerance, weight loss, thromboembloic disease	Pancreas	Glucagon
VIP-oma	Verner-Morrison, pancreatic cholera, WDHA	rare	1	Severe watery diarrhea, hypokalemia	Pancreas 90% Other 10%	Vasoactive intestinal peptide
GRF-oma	GRFoma	33	Unknown	Acromegaly	Pancreas	Growth hormone-releasing factor
Somatostatinoma	Somatostatinoma	Unknown	Unknown	Diabetes mellitus, cholelithiasis, diarrhea, steatorrhea	Pancreas 56%, duodenum or jejunum 44%	Somatostatin
PP-oma	PPoma	Unknown	60–100	No proven endocrine symptoms, weight loss, abdominal mass, hepatomegaly	Pancreas	Pancreatic polypeptide released but no symptoms are due to PP hypersecretion
Nonfunctional	Nonfunctional pancreatic endocrine tumor	Unknown	Unknown	Same as PP-oma	Pancreas	None secreted but various peptides synthesized
Gastric ECL-oma	Gastric carcinoid tumor	90–100	5–10	None	Stomach, duodenum	None
Carcinoid tumor	Carcinoid	See text	See text	Flushing, palpitations, wheezing, diarrhea, cramping	See text	Serotonin (5-HT), histamine, prostaglandins, tachykinins, kinins

manifest more than one different enteropancreatic malignancy at the same time and may even manifest multihormonal endocrine syndromes due either to the production of more than one hormone by a single tumor or, more commonly, to the presence of more than one variety of functional primary tumor (24,49). Furthermore, a patient may develop one clinical neuroendocrine tumor syndrome at one point in time and then develop another syndrome later (24,49). Finally, it must also be stressed that it is essential for the clinician to establish whether an enteropancreatic neuroendocrine tumor is occurring sporadically or whether it is occurring in association with MEN-I syndrome, because the management of patients with neuroendocrine tumors in the setting of MEN-I differs significantly from that of patients with sporadic disease (24,49,52,53,62).

Zollinger-Ellison Syndrome and Gastrinoma in Patients with Multiple Endocrine Neoplasia Type I

Gastrinomas are gastrin-secreting tumors that generally originate in the pancreas or proximal duodenum (59,62,63). Although gastrin also exerts effects on other tissues, all the usual initial manifestations of the Zollinger-Ellison syndrome can be explained on the basis of gastrin's ability to stimulate gastric acid secretion and induce gastric parietal cell hypertrophy (64,65). When initially described (14), the diagnostic triad included (a) a non-β islet cell tumor of the pancreas; (b) gastric acid hypersecretion; and (c) severe, often fatal peptic ulcer disease. With an increasing awareness of the disease in recent years, fulminant and complicated peptic ulcer disease is seen less commonly, and associated effects of gastric acid hypersecretion (gastroesophageal reflux disease, diarrhea, etc.) are more readily recognized (52,53).

In patients with both the sporadic and MEN-I-associated forms of Zollinger-Ellison syndrome, the vast majority of all gastrinomas (>85%) occur in the region of the duodenum or head of the pancreas in an area described as the "gastrinoma triangle" (66,67). This area is defined by the junction of the cystic and common bile ducts superiorly, the junction of the second and third portions of the duodenum inferiorly, and the junction of the neck and body of the pancreas medially (67). In patients with MEN-I and Zollinger-Ellison syndrome, gastrinomas, like insulinomas and other enteropancreatic neuroendocrine tumors, were initially thought to occur primarily in the pancreas (24,49). However, recent evidence suggests that MEN-I-associated gastrinomas may occur almost exclusively in the duodenum (49,52,53,64,68). This is in contrast to the more common sporadic gastrinomas, which are believed to occur in the pancreas in 40–80% of cases (52,59,66,67,69). Moreover, most cases of MEN-I-as-

sociated gastrinoma are believed to occur in the setting of multiple, microscopic submucosal lesions (62), whereas sporadic gastrinomas are generally believed to be solitary. It has been proposed by some (52,59,70) but not others (52,59,71,72) that MEN-I-associated gastrinomas are less likely to be malignant than those that occur sporadically. This conclusion has been questioned because patients with MEN-I and Zollinger-Ellison syndrome present at an earlier age than their sporadic counterparts (49,52,53,71,73). As more is being learned about MEN-I syndrome in general and as the overall management of these patients improves, it is becoming clearer that patients with MEN-I and Zollinger-Ellison syndrome do develop gastrinomas that metastasize to the liver (52,59,73) and that metastatic disease occurs commonly enough that it effects overall management of these patients.

Gastrinomas generally present during adulthood and most cases are diagnosed after 40 years of age (49,52,59). It is generally believed that MEN-I-associated Zollinger-Ellison syndrome presents at an earlier age than sporadic Zollinger-Ellison syndrome and that >95% of the patients with MEN-I-associated disease will already have evidence of hyperparathyroidism at the time of their initial presentation with Zollinger-Ellison syndrome (24,49,53,71,73). However, recent studies have suggested that Zollinger-Ellison syndrome can either present concomitantly with or even precede the hyperparathyroidism in patients with MEN-I-associated disease (51). In one recent study of 28 patients with Zollinger-Ellison syndrome and MEN-I (51), 30% of patients were initially thought to have the sporadic form of Zollinger-Ellison syndrome. The mean time to the subsequent diagnosis of MEN-I was >5 years (51). These patients were ultimately diagnosed accurately after repeated evaluation for hyperparathyroidism (51). Zollinger-Ellison syndrome has been described in early childhood (74), but pediatric cases almost invariably have the sporadic form of the disease.

The autonomous release of gastrin, the resultant increase in the number of parietal cells, and the gastric acid hypersecretion secondary to hyperstimulation of parietal cells are responsible for the principal symptoms of the gastrinoma syndrome. In various large series, the mean time to diagnosis after the development of initial symptoms is 6.4 years (52,53,75). The major clinical manifestations of Zollinger-Ellison syndrome at presentation are listed in Table 4 (52,59). In early studies, 18% of patients presented with severe complications of acid peptic disease, such as perforation or gastrointestinal bleeding (52,53,76,77). Today, these presentations are less common, but they still occur. In a recent large series of gastrinoma patients, 7% of cases presented with perforation (77).

Abdominal pain, indistinguishable from that occurring with idiopathic acid peptic disease (75), is the ma-

TABLE 4. *Clinical features of Zollinger-Ellison syndrome*[a]

Sign/symptom	Frequency (%)
Abdominal pain	24–93
Dysphagia/pyrosis	31–61
Pain and diarrhea	30–55
Diarrhea only	7–35
Ulcer complications (bleeding/perforation)	17–18
Gastric rugal hypertrophy	Unknown

[a]Data from references 52, 53, 59, 76–79.

jor presenting symptom in the vast majority of patients (52,53,75). In contrast to earlier studies (52,59,76,78), in more recent studies (52,59,79), symptoms of gastroesophageal reflux (e.g., heartburn, dysphagia, pyrosis) are seen in up to two-thirds of Zollinger-Ellison syndrome patients. However, gastroesophageal reflux disease is also not a distinguishing feature (52,59,79). Diarrhea, which can either occur alone (in up to 35% of patients) or together with abdominal pain (in up to 55% of patients), can be a feature that distinguishes Zollinger-Ellison syndrome from idiopathic acid peptic disease (52,59,75,76). Seven percent to 35% of patients with Zollinger-Ellison syndrome have diarrhea as the only presenting symptom (52,53). It is unclear why some patients do not manifest abdominal pain or gastroesophageal reflux disease despite a very high acid output. The diarrhea is due to (a) excessive secretion of fluid into the bowel lumen, which overwhelms the absorptive capacity; (b) inactivation of pancreatic digestive enzymes and precipitation of bile acids by the acidic pH within the duodenal lumen; and (c) mucosal ulceration and inflammation caused by unbuffered gastric acid reaching the proximal small bowel (52,53,73,80,81). Direct, gastrin-induced fluid secretion by the small bowel mucosa, once thought to be a causative factor in the generation of diarrhea in these patients (82), has now been disproved, because the diarrhea disappears once gastric acid hypersecretion has been controlled either surgically or with antisecretory medications despite continued high serum gastrin levels (52,53). Because the diarrhea in Zollinger-Elli-

son syndrome is secretory in nature, it will not respond to fasting. However, a response to nasogastric suction does occur and is pathognomonic of the disease (52,53).

It has been claimed previously that, in comparison to idiopathic acid-peptic disease, peptic ulcers in the Zollinger-Ellison syndrome are often multiple, are located further along the small bowel, and are more likely to be complicated by hemorrhage or perforation at presentation (52,53,75,76). Although some patients do present with atypical ulcer disease, in most patients with Zollinger-Ellison syndrome, including those with MEN-I-associated disease, acid peptic disease is indistinguishable from idiopathic acid peptic disease (52,53).

Occasionally patients with Zollinger-Ellison syndrome come to the attention of the physician when an upper gastrointestinal barium study (usually performed in the workup for abdominal pain) demonstrates gastric rugal hypertrophy (52,53,83). While this finding is suggestive of the disease (especially if it occurs in the setting of documented peptic ulceration or gastric acid hypersecretion), there are many other causes of hypertrophic folds (e.g., Menetrier's disease, gastric carcinoma, or lymphoma) that make it a nonspecific finding.

Diagnosis and Differential Diagnosis. Patients with MEN-I or a family history suggestive of MEN-I should be screened for Zollinger-Ellison syndrome with at least one fasting serum gastrin determination during a period when they are known to be producing gastric acid if they develop either clinical or laboratory features suggestive of the disease (Table 5). However, screening should be limited to patients with suggestive clinical or laboratory features because, among *men1* gene carriers, Zollinger-Ellison syndrome has a penetrance of only 30–50% by age 50 years (24,49,52,53). Suggestive clinical features include the development of signs or symptoms of persistent gastric acid hypersecretion such as heartburn, pyrosis, peptic ulceration, persistent abdominal pain, or diarrhea (Table 5). In addition, Zollinger-Ellison syndrome should also be considered in MEN-I patients who develop clinical fea-

TABLE 5. *Features that suggest the development of the Zollinger-Ellison syndrome in a patient with multiple endocrine neoplasia type I*

Clinical signs/symptoms	Laboratory features
Due to gastric acid hypersecretion 　gastroesophageal reflux (heartburn, pyrosis) 　peptic ulcer or persistent abdominal pain 　persistent diarrhea Complications of gastric acid hypersecretion 　iron deficiency anemia or upper gastrointestinal bleeding 　perforation, penetration or bleeding from a peptic ulcer 　peptic esophageal stricture formation	Peptic ulcer on endoscopy or X-ray Gastric rugal hypertrophy on endoscopy or X-ray Elevated fasting serum gastrin level Hepatomegaly or multiple hepatic masses on imaging studies Abdominal mass on imaging studies

tures suggestive of complications from long-standing gastric acid hypersecretion such as iron deficiency anemia, upper gastrointestinal bleeding, perforation or penetration of existing peptic ulcers, and peptic esophageal stricture formation (Table 5). Finally, because gastrinomas are the most common functional enteropancreatic neuroendocrine tumors in patients with MEN-I (24,49,52,53) and because metastatic disease is now being recognized more commonly in patients with MEN-I and Zollinger-Ellison syndrome (52,59,73), the development of an enlarged liver on physical examination should raise the possibility of the development of Zollinger-Ellison syndrome in this group of patients as well (Table 5). With regard to laboratory features that suggest the development of Zollinger-Ellison syndrome in patients with MEN-I, endoscopic or X-ray documentation of a peptic ulcer or hypertrophic gastric folds requires that Zollinger-Ellison syndrome be sought carefully (Table 5). Similarly, documentation of an elevated fasting serum gastrin level in a known MEN-I patient who is producing gastric acid requires that Zollinger-Ellison syndrome be considered (Table 5). Finally, documentation of diffuse hepatomegaly or multiple hepatic masses or an abdominal mass on abdominal imaging studies (Table 5) requires that Zollinger-Ellison syndrome be considered, because gastrinomas are the most common functional neuroendocrine tumors that occur in MEN-I patients (24,49, 52,53) and metastatic gastrinomas do occur in these patients (52,59,73). A number of studies have been proposed to be useful in establishing the diagnosis of Zollinger-Ellison syndrome, once the disease is clinically suspected, including measurement of basal (BAO) and maximal (MAO) acid output, fasting serum gastrin determinations, and various gastrin provocative tests (52,53).

Acid output measurements. The BAO in normal individuals is <10 mEq/hr for males and <5.6 mEq/hr for females (84). The generally used acid secretory criterion for Zollinger-Ellison syndrome is a BAO (in the absence of previous gastric acid-reducing surgery) of 15 mEq/hr (for both genders) (52,53). This criterion will identify from 66% to 99% of all patients with Zollinger-Ellison syndrome and will exclude 90% of patients with idiopathic ulcer disease (52,53). However, the utility of acid output measurements alone for the diagnosis of Zollinger-Ellison syndrome in the setting of MEN-I is limited. The extent of gastric acid hypersecretion in patients with MEN-I and Zollinger-Ellison syndrome may vary with the degree of hypercalcemia due to the presence of associated hyperparathyroidism (85). After surgical correction of hypercalcemia and hyperparathyroidism, BAO may even return to the normal range, despite the continued presence of Zollinger-Ellison syndrome (Fig. 3). Furthermore, gastric acid output can also be elevated in

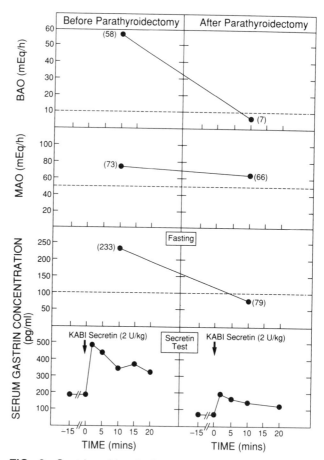

FIG. 3. Gastric acid output measurements, fasting serum gastrin levels, and secretin test results in an MEN-I patient with hyperparathyroidsm and Zollinger-Ellison syndrome before and after parathyroidectomy. Basal acid output (BAO), maximal acid output (MAO), fasting serum gastrin level (FSG), and secretin provocative testing results are illustrated in order from top downwards. The *dashed lines* represent the upper limits of normal for the BAO, MAO, and FSG levels. The *left panels* illustrate results obtained before parathyroidectomy and the *right panels* illustrate results obtained after parathyroidectomy. In this example, successful parathyroidectomy with correction of hypercalcemia resulted in normalization of the BAO, FSG, and secretin provocative testing results.

another hypersecretory state, which is much more common than Zollinger-Ellison syndrome, idiopathic hypersecretion (86). Idiopathic hypersecretion, a condition in which serum gastrin is not elevated, is so much more common than Zollinger-Ellison syndrome (it occurs in up to 25% of all patients with peptic ulcer disease) that measurement of BAO alone will never permit the definitive diagnosis of Zollinger-Ellison syndrome to be made even in the absence of MEN-I or hyperparathyroidism (52,53). Consequently, a BAO above 15 mEq/hr alone only suggests the possibility of Zollinger-Ellison syndrome and should prompt the physician to perform additional diagnostic tests. The criterion generally used to define basal gastric acid hypersecretion in patients who have previously undergone acid-reducing surgery is 5 mEq/hr (52,53,87).

The MAO, measured after the subcutaneous administration of pentagastrin (6 μg/kg), has been shown to correlate closely with the parietal cell mass (52,53,64). In patients with Zollinger-Ellison syndrome, the MAO is also high and is a reflection of the parietal cell hypertrophy resulting from chronic hypergastrinemia (52,53,64). However, there is such a large variation in MAO that it cannot be used as a reliable secretory criterion with which to define Zollinger-Ellison syndrome (52,53,73,80). A BAO/MAO ratio above 0.6 is also said to be indicative of Zollinger-Ellison syndrome, but measurements of the BAO/MAO ratio add little more to the diagnosis of Zollinger-Ellison syndrome than the measurement of BAO alone (52,53,73,80). Unfortunately, gastric analysis is not routinely available in most laboratories at present. In general, a fasting gastric juice pH value above 3.0 in a patient who is not taking any antisecretory medications rules out the Zollinger-Ellison syndrome (52,53,88). A gastric juice pH below 3.0 does not establish the diagnosis, and formal gastric analysis or provocative testing (see below) is therefore required. The recent widespread use of the H^+,K^+-ATPase inhibitor omeprazole makes the interpretation of gastric acid output measurements more difficult. This potent antisecretory agent has a prolonged duration of action, so patients should be withdrawn from therapy for at least 1 week (probably even 2 weeks) to be certain that a significant residual inhibitory effect is not still present when gastric acid output measurements are made (89).

Fasting serum gastrin measurements. As was mentioned above, the diagnosis of Zollinger-Ellison syndrome cannot rest solely on gastric acid output measurements. The diagnosis depends on proving autonomous gastrin secretion by the tumor that does not respond to normal physiologic control mechanisms (i.e., hypergastrinemia in the presence of increased gastric acid production) (52,53). With only rare exceptions (<1%) (83), gastrinoma patients have elevated fasting serum gastrin measurements at the time of initial presentation (88). However, at least two determinations should be made on different days and then averaged because the serum gastrin levels can fluctuate.

The presence of gastric acid hypersecretion in association with fasting hypergastrinemia is highly suggestive of Zollinger-Ellison syndrome (52,53). With one exception (see below), if the fasting serum gastrin level is >1,000 pg/ml and the patient is producing any gastric acid (in this case a gastric juice pH value of <3.0 will suffice), the diagnosis of Zollinger-Ellison syndrome is ensured and no further testing is required (52,53,80,88). Approximately one-third of patients will be diagnosed this way (52,53). The remaining two-thirds of patients who have hypergastrinemia from 100 to 1,000 pg/ml will require provocative testing to rule out the other causes of hypergastrinemia that can mimic Zollinger-Ellison syndrome (52,53).

All the causes of hypergastrinemia (Table 6) should be considered in the differential diagnosis of Zollinger-Ellison syndrome. The causes of hypergastrinemia can be divided into those that are physiological and secondary to hypo- or achlorhydria and those that are inappropriate and associated with gastric acid hypersecretion. Achlorhydria rules out the diagnosis of Zollinger-Ellison syndrome unless the patient is taking large doses of histamine H_2-receptor antagonists or an H^+,K^+-ATPase inhibitor (52,53). Because the use of antisecretory agents has increased so dramatically in recent years, drug-induced achlorhydria is probably the most common cause of hypergastrinemia at present (Table 6). Moreover, it must be stressed that drug-induced physiologic hypergastrinemia and gastrinoma-induced inappropriate hypergastrinemia can coexist in the same patient (89). Therefore, to diagnose the Zollinger-Ellison syndrome accurately, fasting serum gastrin determinations should be made at a time when the patient is known to be producing gastric acid (i.e., in the absence of large doses of antisecretory agents). Although hypergastrinemia commonly occurs in chronic renal failure (Table 6), acid secretion is usually depressed, and a BAO of >15 mEq/hr is highly unlikely (52,53). Unless the patient has an acid output >15 mEq/hr with hypergastrinemia and a positive secretin stimulation test, the working diagnosis should be chronic renal failure without Zollinger-Ellison syndrome (52,53); localization studies involving contrast agents should be deferred, since they may precipitate total renal shutdown from contrast dye. Other important causes of physiological hypergastrinemia (Table 6)

TABLE 6. *Causes of fasting hypergastrinemia*

Achlorhydria/hypochlorhydria	Inappropriate (with gastric acid production)
Medications (histamine H_2-receptor antagonists, omeprazole)	Retained gastric antrum syndrome
Chronic renal failure	Small bowel resection
Atrophic gastritis (including pernicious anemia)	Chronic gastric outlet obstruction
Postvagotomy/gastric resection	Antral G-cell hyperplasia or hyperfunction
	Zollinger-Ellison syndrome

(52,53,59,75–78) include hypo/achlorhydria secondary to atrophic gastritis with or without pernicious anemia and vagotomy- or gastrectomy-induced hypergastrinemia (Table 6).

There are a number of causes of inappropriate hypergastrinemia in addition to the Zollinger-Ellison syndrome (Table 6). The retained gastric antrum syndrome in which, after a Billroth II gastrectomy, some antral tissue is retained in the afferent loop and excluded from the flow of gastric acid is the only condition in which hypergastrinemia in the presence of gastric acid production can be associated with fasting serum gastrin levels >1,000 pg/ml (52,53). This rare condition can be diagnosed by performing a ^{99m}Tc-pertechnetate scan, which localizes to gastric tissue, and Zollinger-Ellison syndrome can be ruled out by a negative secretin stimulation test (52,53). Patients with massive small bowel resection can usually be excluded by history if this diagnosis is considered. Classically the period of hypergastrinemia and gastric acid hypersecretion in these patients is short (52,53). Chronic gastric outlet obstruction should respond to prolonged nasogastric suction and antral decompression so that in these cases the hypergastrinemia and gastric acid hypersecretion should also be reversible (52,53). If the hypergastrinemia and gastric acid hypersecretion fail to respond to prolonged nasogastric suction, the patient may have Zollinger-Ellison syndrome with the outlet obstruction secondary to deforming ulcer disease (52,53). In these cases the secretin stimulation test is likely to be positive. As is alluded to below, antral G-cell hyperplasia/hyperfunction is believed by some (92,93) but not others (52,53,90) to mimic the Zollinger-Ellison syndrome closely. It must also be stressed that hyperparathyroidism with Zollinger-Ellison syndrome in the setting of MEN-I has been shown to be associated with an elevated fasting serum gastrin, which may subsequently resolve after parathyroidectomy (Fig. 3) (85).

Provocative testing. The provocative tests that have been proposed in the diagnosis of Zollinger-Ellison syndrome include the secretin stimulation test, the calcium infusion test, and the standard meal test (52,53,90,93). The most useful provocative test is the *secretin stimulation test,* in which 2 U/kg Kabi secretin is injected i.v. and the gastrin response is measured 2, 5, 10, 15, and 20 min after having obtained two basal values beforehand (52,53,94). A positive test is accompanied by an increase in the serum gastrin concentration of >200 pg/ml and is seen in 87% of Zollinger-Ellison syndrome patients (52,53,94). Using Kabi secretin, the only cause of a false-positive test is achlorhydria, which is readily excluded by measuring the gastric juice pH (94). The extent of hypercalcemia due to MEN-I-associated hyperparathyroidism in patients with Zollinger-Ellison syndrome may influence

the result of the secretin stimulation test. In one study (85), the secretin test became normal in 20% of patients with MEN-I, hyperparathyroidism, and Zollinger-Ellison syndrome after successful parathyroidectomy (Fig. 3).

The *calcium infusion test* involves the continuous infusion of calcium gluconate [54 mg/kg/hr 10% calcium gluconate (5 mg Ca^{2+}/kg/hr) for 3 hr], with serial measurements of serum calcium (to document an effect) and serum gastrin (to measure the response) at 120, 150, and 180 min after having obtained two baseline measurements beforehand (52,53,94). A positive test is defined as an increase in the serum gastrin concentration of >395 pg/ml and is seen in 56% of Zollinger-Ellison syndrome patients (52,53,94). An increase in the serum gastrin concentration of <395 pg/ml can only be considered negative for gastrinoma if the serum calcium increased by more than 0.75 mM (1.5 mEq/liter) (94). Contraindications to the calcium infusion test include hypercalcemia prior to the start of the test as well as a history of cardiac arrhythmias (52,53,94). For this reason, the calcium infusion test is not commonly employed in patients with MEN-I, since they commonly have hyperparathyroidism and hypercalcemia as well. Use of the calcium infusion test for diagnostic purposes should be limited to patients strongly suspected of having a gastrinoma who already have had a negative secretin stimulation test because the calcium infusion test is both cumbersome to perform and more likely to be associated with significant side effects than the secretin stimulation test (52,53). However, the calcium infusion test will be positive in one-third of cases with primarily sporadic disease who have a negative secretin stimulation test, leaving only 9% of gastrinoma patients who have both a negative secretin stimulation test and calcium infusion test (52,53). The percentage of patients with Zollinger-Ellison syndrome and MEN-I with a negative secretin test who would have a positive calcium infusion test after successful parathyroidectomy is unknown.

Antral G-cell hyperplasia or hyperfunction should be considered in those patients with mild hypergastrinemia and hyperchlorhydria but with negative secretin and calcium provocative tests. The importance of G-cell hyperplasia/hyperfunction lies in its potential ability to mimic Zollinger-Ellison syndrome (52,53, 90). Certain authorities have suggested that antral G-cell hyperplasia/hyperfunction may occur more frequently in patients with MEN-I (92,93). However, this association has been strongly questioned recently (90). Furthermore, there currently is controversy regarding the very existence of this entity (52,53). If antral G-cell hyperplasia/hyperfunction is suspected, it is suggested that a *standard meal test* be done. The standard meal test involves measuring the gastrin response 30, 60, and 90 min after the ingestion of a standardized meal containing 30 g protein, 20 g fat, and 25 g carbohydrate, having obtained two basal gastrin values immediately beforehand (93). A positive test, thought to exclude Zollinger-Ellison syndrome, is defined as an increase in the serum gastrin concentration >100% (52,53,90). Unfortunately the meal test is positive in up to 30% of patients with Zollinger-Ellison syndrome, so that a positive meal test in a patient with negative secretin and calcium infusion tests is not helpful in distinguishing Zollinger-Ellison syndrome from antral G-cell hyperplasia/hyperfunction in either the presence or the absence of MEN-I syndrome (52,53,90). Any MEN-I patient with documented gastric acid hypersecretion and hypergastrinemia but with negative secretin and calcium infusion tests should still be considered as having Zollinger-Ellison syndrome even if the standard meal test is positive. Some groups have reported that antral G-cell quantitation following endoscopic biopsy permits the identification of antral G-cell hyperplasia (95). However, experience with this technique is limited in Zollinger-Ellison syndrome and in other conditions that may mimic antral G-cell hyperplasia clinically.

Insulinoma

Diagnosis. Insulinomas with symptomatic hypoglycemia are found in from 10% (96) to 26% (97) of patients with MEN-I but are infrequently the presenting manifestation of the syndrome (98) (Tables 1, 3). Of all patients presenting with insulinoma, fewer than 10% have MEN-I (99,100); however, >60% of hypoglycemic patients with multiple-cell adenomas have MEN-I (99). Patients typically present with fasting hypoglycemia. The median age of onset of insulinoma in MEN-I is the third decade, in contrast to fifth decade in sporadic cases (101). The male to female sex ratio is 1:1 in both sporadic and MEN-I-associated insulinoma.

In sharp contrast to sporadic insulinoma, ~80% of cases of MEN-I insulinoma are associated with multifocal islet disease (1,99,101). A spectrum of primary pancreatic pathology has been described in MEN-I, including multiple adenomas, adenoma with microadenomatosis, adenoma with β-cell hyperplasia, nesidioblastosis (islet cells arising from exocrine ducts), and multicentric β-cell carcinoma (57,102). Most studies suggest that insulin-induced hypoglycemia in MEN-I patients is due to discreet, albeit multiple, adenomas as opposed to diffuse microscopic pancreatic lesions (57). Tumors tend to be small, 0.2–4 cm (103–105), with 90% being 2 cm (106) and numerous (mean 7.4) (104); they frequently escape detection by conventional radiographic procedures. The tumors tend to be

evenly distributed throughout the pancreas, although some series have reported a greater frequency in the head of the pancreas (105). The high surgical cure rate for insulinoma in MEN-I may be an indicator that only one adenoma is sustaining the high blood insulin levels.

Immunohistochemistry of resected adenomas reveals a spectrum of antibody staining (57). In addition to insulin, tumors frequently stain positive for pancreatic polypeptide, glucagon, serotonin, somatostatin, and vasoactive intestinal peptide. Of all islet cell tumors resected from MEN-I patients, regardless of the clinical syndrome, insulin immunostaining is positive in 66–70% (57,107). Immunohistochemistry shows hormone storage but does not establish that an adenoma is causing high blood levels of a peptide hormone.

Patients frequently present with symptoms of neuroglycopenia, often demonstrating deterioration in school performance and precipitation of symptoms after participating in sports (104). Once hypoglycemia is suspected, fasting hypoglycemia should be rigorously documented, and then other etiologies of hypoglycemia should be excluded. These include hypoglycemia due to prescribed medications; prescription or pharmacy error; surreptitious use of insulin, sulfonylureas, or other hypoglycemic agents; severe liver dysfunction; renal failure; severe wasting; primary and secondary adrenal insufficiency; and in children growth hormone deficiency. Supervised fasting is the best test for establishing fasting hypoglycemia. The fast should be continued until the time of symptomatic hypoglycemia (plasma glucose <40 mg/dl). Most patients with symptomatic insulinoma develop hypoglycemia after 48 hr of fasting; the test should be extended to 72 hr if symptomatic hypoglycemia does not occur. Glucose, insulin, C peptide, and proinsulin fraction or concentration should be obtained specifically at the time of hypoglycemia (108). In addition, it is prudent to measure antiinsulin antibodies in all patients and antiinsulin receptor antibodies in selected patients. The single most valuable diagnostic finding is an insulin concentration above 6 μU/ml at the time of hypoglycemia. This establishes (in the absence of antiinsulin antibodies) that hypoglycemia is insulin mediated, but it is also seen in patients using insulin or sulfonylureas surreptitiously and in patients with antiinsulin receptor antibody-mediated hypoglycemia.

Measurement of C-peptide concentration at the time of hypoglycemia is helpful in evaluating the etiology of insulin-mediated hypoglycemia. C-peptide is suppressed (<1.2 ng/ml) in patients using insulin surreptitiously, and is usually elevated in insulinoma and in patients ingesting sulfonylureas. Surreptitious use of insulin or sulfonylurea should be excluded in all patients with hypoglycemia and ruled out prior to invasive studies. Caution is required in interpreting positive sulfonylurea assays performed by high-performance liquid chromatography (HPLC), since false-positive elevations have been observed. Confirmation by gas chromatography–mass spectroscopy is available for first-generation sulfonylureas through some laboratories, but not for second-generation agents.

Measurement of the proinsulin fraction is often helpful in diagnosis. In normal individuals, ~20% of the immunoreactive insulin is proinsulin-like (109). A proinsulin fraction of >30% has been noted in 80–90% of insulinomas (106,110,111) and if found is presumptive evidence of insulinoma. Radioimmunoassays (RIAs) specific for proinsulin (112) have simplified the measurement of this fraction and may replace the more tedious gel filtration column method. Caution should be used in interpreting negative results, since the new RIAs have not yet been validated for this application.

Various approaches have been used to avoid supervised fasting and to simplify the diagnosis of insulinoma. These include measurement of the ratio of immunoreactive insulin to plasma glucose when plasma glucose is <60 mg/dl and various dynamic tests of insulin secretion. Unfortunately, insulin/glucose ratios are frequently nondiagnostic in patients with proven insulinoma and should not be relied upon. Dynamic tests of insulin secretion with tolbutamide, glucagon, C-peptide suppression by insulin infusion, or calcium stimulation have also been employed and are often diagnostic, but these tests too are often normal in patients with proven insulinoma.

Once the diagnosis of insulinoma is confirmed, in MEN-I, preparation must be made for surgical approach by preoperative tumor localization. Since there are no large published series on localization of insulinoma in MEN-I, the approach must be guided partly by the experience in sporadic insulinomas (Table 7) (113). Conventional radiographic techniques such as computer-assisted tomography, ultrasound, and selective pancreatic angiography tend to underestimate the number of lesions in the MEN-I patient's pancreas and have significant false-negative and false-positive rates

(114). Magnetic resonance imaging has not added significantly to the preoperative evaluation. Preoperative localization of insulinoma is much more important in MEN-I than in sporadic cases because of the likelihood of encountering several associated islet tumors that are not oversecreting insulin. Percutaneous transhepatic sampling of the pancreatic venous drainage with measurement of insulin is powerful in determining the regions of functioning β-cell tumors, thus guiding the extent and region of surgical intervention; this may be the single best preoperative study (115). Newer methods such as selective arterial injection of calcium with hepatic venous sampling and endoscopic ultrasound are presently being evaluated (113). Preoperative studies and palpation at the time of surgical exploration are complimented by the use of intraoperative ultrasound, which enables the surgeon to visualize nonpalpable tumors, particularly in the head of the pancreas, as well as to determine the relation of adenomas to critical structures such as the pancreatic duct, influencing the surgical approach to these tumors (116,117). This procedure is the most useful test for finding sporadic insulinoma, but has not been fully validated in MEN-I, where a high "false-positive" rate (from adenomas not causing hyperinsulinemia) should be expected.

Miscellaneous Other Enteropancreatic–Neuro-Endocrine Tumors in Patients with Multiple Endocrine Neoplasia Type I

Glucagonoma. Glucagonomas are glucagon-secreting tumors that originate in the pancreas (91,118–120). The glucagonoma syndrome is the autonomous secretion of glucagon resulting in a specific dermatitis, weight loss, glucose intolerance, and anemia (118–120) (Table 8). Wilkinson (121) first described the rash as migratory necrolytic erythema in 1973, and Mallinson et al. (122) are credited with specifically establishing the association of the rash with a glucagon-secreting tumor of the pancreas in 1974.

TABLE 7. *Radiographic localization of sporadic insulinoma[a]*

Radiographic study	Percentage of successfully localized insulinomas	
	NIH experience (%)	Range in literature (%)
Ultrasound	26	0–62
CT	17	11–73
MRI	25	0–25
Angiography	35	41–67
Transhepatic portal venous sampling	77	64–100
Intraoperative ultrasound	92	75–100

Data from reference 110.

TABLE 8. *Clinical features of the glucagonoma syndrome*[a]

Sign/symptom	Frequency (%)
Migratory necrolytic erythema	64–90
Glucose intolerance or diabetes mellitus	83–90
Weight loss	56–96
Hypoaminoacidemia	26–90
Anemia	44–85
Thromboembolism	12–35
Psychiatric disturbance	Uncommon
Diarrhea	15
Abdominal pain	12

[a]Data from references 118–121, 123, 124, 131.

Glucagonomas occur in ~3% of all MEN-I syndrome patients (24,49). However, glucagonoma patients only rarely have MEN-I (Table 3) (24,49). Glucagonomas generally present in middle age or later (119,120). The glucagonoma syndrome has not been described in children or adolescents, and only 16% of cases occur before the age of 40 years (119,120). Almost all glucagonomas originate in the pancreas, characteristically in the body and tail (119,120). They are usually large at presentation (118,123) (average size is 5–10 cm, but a glucagonoma of 35 cm has been documented), and multiple tumors are unusual (up to 12% in one series of "sporadic" cases) (120,124). Malignancy is common, with 50–80% of cases having evidence of metastatic spread at presentation (119,120).

Glucagon is a 29-amino-acid peptide, which acts primarily to antagonize the effects of insulin, the release of which it also stimulates (125,126). Its primary action is catabolic in that it acts to increase blood glucose levels by stimulating glycogenolysis and gluconeogenesis (123,126). The latter effect results in a decrease of serum amino acids (123,126,127). As well as causing lipolysis directly, glucagon also antagonizes lipolysis indirectly because it stimulates insulin release (125). The net effect is to supply substrate for gluconeogenesis, but ketonemia is rare (126). In addition, glucagon inhibits gastric and pancreatic secretion and inhibits gastrointestinal motility (125). The symptoms of the glucagonoma syndrome are due to the known actions of glucagon. The clinical presentation does not appear to be different in the setting of MEN-I or sporadic disease.

Migratory necrolytic erythema is the most specific symptom, but it is not seen in all cases (119,120,123). It may precede the ultimate diagnosis by as much as 18 years (mean delay of ~7 years), because it tends to come and go and because it may be misdiagnosed as a wide range of other dermatological conditions (120,124). The rash [seen in 64–90% of cases (119,120)] has a predilection for areas of friction, including intertrigenous zones, the extremities, perineum, buttocks, or face. It initially appears as erythematous areas, which later become raised with central blister formation. The blisters rupture, crust, and finally heal with hyperpigmentation in 1–3 weeks (120,125). The skin biopsy characteristically shows superficial spongiosis and necrosis with deeper blister formation. Mononuclear inflammatory cell infiltration and fusiform keratinocytes with pyknotic nuclei are commonly seen. These changes are best seen on biopsy of early skin lesions (121,122). Whether hyperglucagonemia per se is responsible for the rash is unclear (123). Similar lesions following prolonged exogenous glucagon administration have been observed in some patients (128) but not in others (123). The hypoaminoacidemia characteristic of the glucagonoma syndrome, as well as zinc deficiency, has been implicated, since correction of the hypoaminoacidemia (123,129) and treatment with zinc (123) have been shown to be associated with healing of the rash without affecting serum glucagon concentrations (123). Associated integumentary abnormalities include alopecia, nail dystrophy, and angular stomatitis (119,120).

Hyperglycemia occurs commonly (up to 90% of cases), but not universally, in patients with the glucagonoma syndrome (Table 8) (119,120,123,124,130). On average, the onset of diabetes mellitus precedes the diagnosis of the glucagonoma syndrome by 5 years (120). This is of importance in patients with MEN-I because Cushing's syndrome (see below) is a far more common cause of hyperglycemia in this population than is glucagonoma. Patients with documented glucagonomas who do not develop glucose intolerance are probably protected by an effective insulin response to glucagon-induced catabolism (120,124). Weight loss, which can be severe (up to 30 kg), is a common feature (56–96% of patients). The weight loss does not correlate with tumor size (123,124,126,127) and is reversible by exogenous somatostatin analog (131,132), suggesting that it is due to the catabolic effects of glucagon itself. Hypoaminoacidemia, seen in 26–90% of patients (124,128), is probably due to a direct hormone effect, since administration of exogenous glucagon decreases plasma amino acid concentrations (127,137), whereas glucagon deficiency (following total pancreatectomy or secondary to exogenous somatostatin) increases plasma amino acid concentrations (131,138). Plasma concentrations of amino acids are frequently <25% of normal (122,124,137). Other less common features of the glucagonoma syndrome include a normochromic, normocytic anemia in up to 85% of cases (120,123), thromboembolic phenomena in up to 35% (119,120), neuropsychiatric disturbances (119,120,122), diarrhea (120), and nonspecific abdominal pain (120).

Diagnosis and differential diagnosis. Since most patients present with the skin rash, glucagonoma is often suspected from this typical feature (119,120). However, as was mentioned above, the skin rash is often misdiagnosed (127). More importantly, the typical glucagonoma rash also occurs in other hyperglucagonemic conditions, such as cirrhosis (123). Occasionally, the syndrome is considered when a patient presents with a large abdominal mass associated with diabetes mellitus and weight loss (119,120). Demonstration of an elevated plasma glucagon level is highly suggestive of the diagnosis, but a level >1,000 pg/ml (normal <150 pg/ml) is required (120) for firm diagnosis. In practice, this is rarely a problem, because a diagnostic-range plasma glucagon level occurs in 70–90% of cases (120,124). Provocative testing (e.g., with glucose) does not provide reliable information and should therefore not be attempted even in patients with moderately elevated glucagon levels <1,000 pg/ml (118). Other conditions that can cause a moderate increase in plasma glucagon levels [although not >500 pg/ml (120,123)] include chronic renal insufficiency, hepatic insufficiency, prolonged fasting, diabetic ketoacidosis, acute pancreatitis, acromegaly, septicemia, severe burns, exercise, and familial hyperglucagonemia (119,123,135,136). Familial hyperglucagonemia is an asymptomatic condition associated with an increased percentage of high-molecular-weight glucagon in the plasma (136). These conditions can usually be excluded on clinical grounds.

VIP-oma. VIP-omas are VIP-secreting tumors that, in adults, usually originate in the pancreas (141,142). The VIP-oma syndrome occurs as a result of high blood VIP levels, which cause severe watery diarrhea, hypokalemia, and hypochlorhydria (Table 9) (130,139–142).

Most VIP-omas occur sporadically, and only ~1% of all VIP-omas occur in patients with MEN-I (Table 3) (24,49,142). In adults, >80% of VIP-omas occur in the pancreas (137,138). VIP-omas occasionally originate in intestinal carcinoids or pheochromocytomas (143). Only ~5% of adult VIP-omas originate in a ganglioneuroma or ganglioneuroblastoma (138). However, when children present with the VIP-oma syndrome, it is almost always due to an extrapancreatic ganglioneuroma or ganglioneuroblastoma (138). VIP-omas are almost always solitary (98%) (137,138) and are usually

large (>3 cm) (137,138). Three-fourths occur in the pancreatic tail (137,138). More than 60% are malignant, and 37–68% of patients have metastases at the time of presentation or surgical intervention (137,138). VIP-omas in adults generally present in the fourth or fifth decade of life (138,140). In children, the mean age is from 2 to 4 years, with all cases occurring before age 10 years (138,140).

Vasoactive intestinal peptide is a 28-amino-acid peptide that interacts with high-affinity receptors on small intestinal mucosal cells as well as on cells of a number of other tissues (144). Activation of VIP receptors leads to an increase in cellular adenylyl cyclase and cAMP (144). In intestinal cells, net fluid and electrolyte secretion is the end result (144). In addition, VIP also increases gluconeogenesis. Another peptide, originally isolated from porcine intestine, which also stimulates intestinal secretion, is peptide histidine isoleucine (PHI) (145). The human equivalent of PHI is peptide histidine methionine (PHM), a 27-amino-acid peptide (144), which shares a common precursor peptide with VIP, prepro-VIP/PHM-27, and recent studies show that both peptides are cosecreted by VIP-oma cells (144). PHM-like immunoreactivity has been found in 92% of VIP-omas (145), and PHM has been implicated as contributing to the diarrhea in some VIP-oma patients (144,147). However, PHM is 32 times less potent than VIP, and in recent studies VIP levels were elevated in all cases of VIP-oma (147). It is now generally accepted that the VIP-oma syndrome occurs as a result of unregulated VIP secretion, because the actions of VIP can account for most of the clinical manifestations of the syndrome (144), because VIP levels are elevated in virtually all cases of the VIP-oma syndrome (144), and because continuous infusion of VIP to reach plasma VIP levels typical of the VIP-oma syndrome produces watery diarrhea in normal individuals within 7 hr (141). VIP-omas in the setting of MEN-I have been well described (24,114,142). The clinical presentation does not appear to be different from that occurring in the setting of sporadic disease.

The major manifestation is profound watery diarrhea (seen in 100% of cases), leading to hypokalemia and dehydration (Table 9) (130,138,148,149). Despite the severity of the symptomatology, delays of up to 4 years prior to diagnosis have been described (130,138). The syndrome is also called the *Verner-Morrison syndrome* after those who originally described the disease (130), as well as the *WDHA syndrome*, which stands for watery diarrhea, hypokalemia, and achlorhydria (130,150). Although the term *pancreatic cholera* aptly describes the symptoms as well as the cellular mechanism of the diarrhea (cAMP mediated) (139), it is an inaccurate term, since, as was mentioned above, not all VIP-omas occur in the pancreas (138). The stool has the appearance of weak tea (139). Stool output

TABLE 9. *Clinical features of the VIP-oma syndrome*[a]

Sign/symptom	Frequency (%)
Secretory diarrhea	100
Hypokalemia	90–100
Dehydration	100
Hypochlorhydria	70–76
Hyperglycemia	18–50
Hypercalcemia	25–50
Flushing	20
Dilated, atonic gallbladder	Unknown

[a]Data from references 138, 140–142, 150, 151.

does not decrease with fasting, and, classically, there is no osmolar gap (151). Early in the syndrome, the diarrhea can be mild and intermittent (138,143,150). However, with time, it becomes constant and profound (>1 liter/day and up to 8 liters/day), leading to hypokalemia, dehydration, shock, and renal failure (137,138,148,151). It has been proposed that a stool volume of <700 ml/day is insufficiently severe for the diagnosis of VIP-oma syndrome (142,152). Associated symptoms include flushing episodes in 20% of patients (Table 9); electrolyte abnormalities; dehydration, which may cause a multitude of nonspecific symptoms, such as lethargy, nausea, vomiting, muscle weakness, and cramping; and others (138,150). Hypokalemia (Table 9) (130,138–140) occurs in virtually all patients on presentation and is a reflection of the severity of the diarrhea (138,150). Stool potassium losses can exceed 300 mEq/liter (154). Hypochlorhydria rather than true achlorhydria (since most patients respond to pentagastrin or histamine stimulation) occurs in three-fourths of patients (Table 9) (130,138,149). The hypochlorhydria is most likely due to a direct inhibitory action of VIP on gastric acid secretion (138,144,150,155). Hypercalcemia is seen in up to 50% of cases and may possibly be a result of an endocrine product of the tumor itself. Of course in MEN-I it can reflect associated hyperparathyroidism (24,49,138). Glucose intolerance and hyperglycemia are also commonly seen (Table 9) (138,149).

Diagnosis and differential diagnosis. The diagnosis of VIP-oma is established by the presence of a high-volume, secretory diarrhea in the presence of a pancreatic endocrine tumor, ideally with documentation of elevated serum concentration of VIP (normal <170 pg/ml) (130,138,140,148,151). However, for a definitive diagnosis, all three criteria must be met (138, 148,151). The volume of the diarrhea is always >700 ml/day and is >3 liters/day in >80% of patients (138,148,151). There is seldom controversy in the case of a patient with a proven pancreatic tumor. In a recent study of 29 patients with VIP-oma, the mean serum VIP level was 956 pg/ml (range 225–1850 pg/ml) (140).

There are no reliable provocative tests for the diagnosis of the VIP-oma syndrome, so that in the occasional patient, with only mildly elevated VIP levels, it may not be possible to make a definitive diagnosis. However, in two recent large series (138,140), there was no overlap in VIP levels between normal individuals and patients with VIP-oma, suggesting that even mildly elevated levels of VIP should be considered significant. Vasoactive intestinal peptide levels can fluctuate and should thus be measured during periods when the patient is having diarrhea (140,148).

The differential diagnosis of the VIP-oma syndrome includes all causes of secretory diarrhea (151,156). However, because of the severity of the diarrhea, the major considerations include the pseudo-VIP-oma syndrome, chronic laxative abuse, and the Zollinger-Ellison syndrome (49,148,151,157). The pseudo-VIP-oma syndrome consists of high-volume, secretory diarrhea, but without an elevated VIP level, and can mimic the VIP-oma syndrome closely. In Zollinger-Ellison syndrome, the serum gastrin level is elevated and the diarrhea responds to nasogastric suction and control of gastric acid hypersecretion with antisecretory medications (52,59,73). Recent studies have demonstrated that laxative abuse as the cause of a high-volume, secretory diarrhea can be reliably excluded by measuring serum VIP levels (138,148,150).

GRF-omas. GRF-oma is an endocrine tumor that secretes growth hormone-releasing factor (GRF) (158, 159). The GRF-oma syndrome is a result of high blood GRF levels, which cause acromegaly (158,159).

GRF-oma is a rare tumor; however, when present, it commonly occurs in association with the MEN-I syndrome (~30%) (56,160,161) (Table 3). Most GRF-omas occur in the lung (53%) (56). The remaining tumors occur in the pancreas (30%) or small intestine (10%) (56). Pancreatic GRF-omas are usually found in the pancreatic tail (56). Patients with GRF-omas are younger than patients with other pancreatic endocrine tumors (mean age 38 years) (56). GRF-omas are often multiple (30%), large (<6 cm), and metastatic (<30%) at the time of presentation (56,162). However, there

TABLE 10. *Clinical features of the somatostatinoma syndrome*[a]

Sign/symptom	Pancreatic tumors (%)	Intestinal tumors (%)	Range for all tumors (%)
Diabetes mellitus	95	21	55–63
Gallbladder disease	94	43	65–70
Diarrhea	97	36	35–68
Steatorrhea	83	12	35–52
Hypochlorhydria	86	17	33–70
Weight loss	90	44	19–75

[a]Data from references 158, 159, 174, 175.

does not appear to be a relationship between tumor size and the presence or absence of metastatic disease (56). Approximately 65% of GRF-omas are associated with a tumor causing another hormonal syndrome (56,163). Most commonly the primary syndrome is Zollinger-Ellison syndrome (40%) (56,163). In addition, Cushing's syndrome occurs in ~40% of patients with GRF-omas (56,163).

Growth hormone-releasing factor is a 44-amino-acid peptide with structural similarity to VIP (158). It is a potent stimulant of growth hormone release (158). Excessive production of GRF by the tumor results in somatotroph hyperplasia and continued release of growth hormone by the pituitary gland (164). The end result of excessive growth hormone release is acromegaly (164).

Classically, in both the general population as well as in the MEN-I population, acromegaly results from a growth hormone-producing pituitary tumor (see below) (56,164,165). The features of acromegaly in GRF-oma are indistinguishable from those that occur with classical acromegaly (56,165). In cases of pancreatic GRF-omas, there is commonly a long delay (mean 5.3 years) following the diagnosis of acromegaly before the pancreatic cause is recognized (56). In addition, patients with pancreatic GRF-omas can present with features of other associated endocrine syndromes or with features of local tumor enlargement (see below under nonfunctional tumors) (56).

Diagnosis and differential diagnosis. GRF-oma should be suspected in any patient with a known pancreatic endocrine tumor who develops features suggestive of acromegaly. GRF-oma should be considered especially in patients with Zollinger-Ellison syndrome, ACTH-producing pancreatic endocrine tumor, or MEN-I syndrome because of its known associations with these syndromes (56,163). However, it must be stressed that GRF-oma is a rare cause of acromegaly (<2% of cases) (165). The diagnosis is confirmed by demonstrating an elevated plasma level of GRF (162,166,167). In classical acromegaly, GRF levels are not elevated >191 pg/ml (164). Consequently, it has been suggested that a plasma GRF level of >300 pg/ml is highly suggestive of a GRF-oma (56,162). Plasma growth hormone and insulin-like growth factor type I (IGF-I) levels are elevated in both classical acromegaly and GRF-omas and are therefore not useful in distinguishing one from the other (164). Similarly, provocative tests for growth hormone release, which are routinely used in the diagnosis of acromegaly, are also not useful in distinguishing between classical acromegaly and GRF-oma (164,165). These tests are useful in confirming the presence of acromegaly regardless of its cause.

Somatostatinoma. Somatostatinoma is a somatostatin-secreting tumor that occurs in the pancreas or proximal small bowel (152,153). On the basis of the known physiological effects and the earlier documentation of two endocrine tumors (positive for somatostatin histochemically) found incidentally during elective cholecystectomy in 1977, a proposed somatostatinoma syndrome was described in 1979 (168,169).

Approximately one-half of cases of somatostatinoma are associated with other endocrinopathies, including MEN-I, as well as MEN-II (152). However, the percentage of MEN-I patients who develop somatostatinoma is unknown. Somatostatinoma usually occurs in a middle-aged individual (mean age at presentation 51–53 years) (152,153). From 56% to 75% of somatostatinomas occur in the pancreas (168,169), and most of these occur in the pancreatic head (66–77%) (152,153). The location of extrapancreatic somatostatinomas appears to follow the distribution of the somatostatin-producing D cells of the upper gastrointestinal tract such that they occur primarily in the proximal duodenum (43%) or ampulla of Vater (48%), although, to date, no hypersecreting gastric somatostatinoma has yet been described (152). Somatostatinoma has also been found in the cystic duct (5%) and jejunum (5%) (152). Most somatostatinomas are solitary (90%) (153). At the time of presentation, most somatostatinomas are large [average size in one series 4.9 cm (153)], and metastases to lymph nodes or the liver are frequently found (>80%) (152,153). Somatostatinoma commonly occurs as a secondary hormonal syndrome. In one series 20% of patients had concomitant insulinoma (153).

Somatostatin is a naturally occurring tetradecapeptide (14 amino acids) with multiple inhibitory effects on the gastrointestinal tract (170). It also occurs in a larger, 28-amino-acid form (170). Native somatostatin is known to (a) inhibit the release of numerous gastrointestinal hormones, (b) decrease both basal and stimulated gastric acid secretion, (c) decrease gallbladder contractility and bile flow, (d) decrease pancreatic enzyme and fluid secretion, and (e) decrease absorption of lipid, D-xylose, vitamin B_{12}, and folate (170). Somatostatin has a mixed action on intestinal motility (170). All these factors contribute to the various clinical aspects of the somatostatinoma syndrome.

The features of the somatostatinoma syndrome given in early reports included mild diabetes mellitus, gallbladder disease, weight loss, and anemia (168,169), but, later, diarrhea, steatorrhea, and hypochlorhydria were added (Table 10). It must be stressed that the symptom complex attributable to the somatostatinoma syndrome is both mild and nonspecific in most patients (153). In addition, the clinical effects of the syndrome appear to be more common in pancreatic than in duodenal somatostatinoma (Table 10) (152). Diabetes mellitus (seen in ~60% of cases) is most likely due to the inhibition of pancreatic insulin release (152,153) and may also reflect replacement of normal pancreatic tissue in some cases (153). The diabetes is mild, and ketosis, although it has been described, is unusual (152,153). Since native somatostatin inhibits gallbladder contraction (170), it has been proposed that the cholelithiasis seen in ~65% of patients with pancreatic or duodenal somatostatinoma is a result of prolonged biliary stasis (152,153). The diarrhea (up to ten stools/day) and steatorrhea (up to 76 g/day) of the somatostatinoma syndrome are probably multifactorial in cause (153). Diarrhea and steatorrhea are each seen in >35% of cases and in turn contribute to the weight loss occurring in up to 75% of somatostatinoma patients (153). Hypochlorhydria is seen in up to 70% of cases (153).

Diagnosis and differential diagnosis. In most cases, somatostatinoma has been discovered by intraabdominal imaging in the workup for abdominal pain, bleeding, or diarrhea or at the time of exploratory laparotomy performed for cholecystectomy (152,153). The diagnosis of somatostatinoma is then made after documentation of an elevated somatostatin-like immunoreactivity in plasma and/or an increased number of D cells by immunohistochemical stains of tumor tissue (153). Because of the nonspecific, often mild symptoms preceding the diagnosis, somatostatinoma is commonly large and/or metastatic when initially diagnosed (152,153). In the future, the diagnosis of somatostatinoma at an earlier stage of the disease, prior to the development of a large tumor and/or metastatic disease, will require an awareness of the various components of the clinical syndrome, routine availability of a reliable plasma somatostatin assay, and a reliable provocative test (153,171,172). Presently, plasma somatostatin assays are complicated and are not routinely available, and no reliable provocative test has yet been developed (171). Elevated plasma somatostatin levels have also been described in a variety of other apudomas, including medullary thyroid carcinoma, small cell cancer of the lung, pheochromocytoma, and paraglanglioneuromas (153).

PP-omas and Nonfunctional Pancreatic Endocrine Tumors. PP-oma is a pancreatic polypeptide (PP)-secreting tumor that usually originates in the pancreas (103,173–176). Despite the fact that PP-omas secrete excessive amounts of PP, they are not associated with any recognizable endocrine syndrome (i.e., they are clinically silent with regard to hormonal effects) (152,174). Nonfunctional endocrine tumors of the pancreas are also not associated with any recognizable endocrine syndrome (49,103,152,174). With both these pancreatic endocrine tumor types, symptoms are due entirely to the presence of the tumor itself (49). Following the discovery of PP and the development of reliable serum PP assays, it is now believed that as many as 70–80% of all apparently nonfunctional pancreatic islet tumors are actually PP-omas (152).

PP-omas and nonfunctional tumors are probably the most common neuroendocrine tumors that occur in patients with MEN-I syndrome (Table 3) (24,49,175). However, because these tumors do not cause any hormonal symptoms and because these patients do not routinely undergo exploratory surgery, their true incidence in this population is unknown (24,49). With sporadic disease, multiple tumors are rare. Therefore, if more than one clinically silent endocrine tumor of the pancreas is found, MEN-I should be strongly considered (57,58). PP-omas and nonfunctional endocrine tumors of the pancreas are more commonly found in the pancreatic head (>70%) and are usually large at the time of presentation (72% >5 cm) (91,103). Malignancy is common, occurring in 64–92% of cases (91,103,104). Up to 75% of clinically silent endocrine tumors of the pancreas are PP-omas in that they produce elevated serum PP levels (174). Early studies (57,58,91) suggested that serum PP levels correlated with the presence of MEN-I syndrome in patients with pancreatic endocrine tumors (see below), although this association has now been largely refuted (393).

PP-omas and nonfunctional neuroendocrine tumors cannot be differentiated from functional neuroendocrine tumors on histological, electron microscopic, or immunohistochemical grounds (152,174,176). In addition, the pathological distinction between PP-omas and nonfunctional tumors (i.e., elevated serum levels of PP) has not been found to be of any clinical significance (163).

It is unclear why PP-omas are not associated with symptoms due to the elevated levels of plasma PP, since, in animal studies, PP has numerous effects, including inhibition of pancreatic exocrine secretion, relaxation of gallbladder smooth muscle, inhibition of stimulated gastric acid secretion, stimulation of small bowel fluid and electrolyte secretion, and prokinetic effects on gastrointestinal motility (177,178). Some authors have proposed a PP-oma syndrome based on the known physiological effects of PP, since clinical symptoms attributable to the known actions of PP have been observed in a small number of patients with PP-omas (177,178). However, in numerous other studies, no correlation was observed between the expected effects in patients with elevated PP levels and the absence of these effects in patients without elevated PP levels (103,176,393).

PP-omas and nonfunctional neuroendocrine tumors generally present after 40 years of age, although cases have been described in patients as young as age 20 years (103,152,173). The major presenting symptoms are abdominal pain (in 36% of cases) and jaundice (in 28%) (173). Other less common presentations include gastrointestinal bleeding from isolated gastric varices

(55,173). In 16% of cases, nonfunctional tumors are discovered incidentally during abdominal surgery for unrelated illness (173).

Diagnosis and differential diagnosis. In patients with sporadic disease, PP-omas and nonfunctional neuroendocrine tumors must be distinguished from the far more common adenocarcinoma of the pancreas, which has a significantly worse prognosis (152). In MEN-I, PP-omas and nonfunctional endocrine tumors of the pancreas are relatively more common. Plasma PP levels, when elevated, may be helpful in making this distinction (152). In a study of 53 cases of pancreatic adenocarcinoma, not one case was associated with an elevated plasma PP level (152). However, the absence of an elevated plasma PP level does not rule out the possibility of a nonfunctional pancreatic endocrine tumor (103,152,173), and elevated PP levels also occur in a number of other situations such as old age, various inflammatory conditions, bowel resection, alcohol abuse, chronic renal failure, and diabetes, so an elevated PP level does not establish that a pancreatic endocrine tumor is the source (152,179,181, 182). An atropine suppression test was developed to address this problem (180,183,184). This test involves the intramuscular administration of 1 mg atropine followed by measurement of the plasma PP response (183,184). Autonomous PP release (i.e., PP-oma) is characterized by a failure to suppress PP levels following atropine administration, whereas PP elevations from other causes are characterized by a suppression of PP levels to at least 50% of baseline (184). The utility of the atropine suppression test has yet to be definitely established.

Miscellaneous Gastrointestinal Tumor Syndromes. Cushing's syndrome occurs commonly in patients with MEN-I. In one series (185), it occurred in 20% of patients with Zollinger-Ellison syndrome and MEN-I, and in all cases it was due to an ACTH-producing tumor of the pituitary gland (see below). In this situation the disease is usually mild (70,185,186). Alternatively, Cushing's syndrome can also result from ectopic ACTH production by foregut carcinoid tumors (see above). Furthermore, severe Cushing's syndrome resulting from ectopic ACTH production by widely metastatic pancreatic endocrine tumors has also been described (180,185,187). Although this has been best described in the setting of long-standing sporadic Zollinger-Ellison syndrome (185), it appears to be rare in patients with Zollinger-Ellison syndrome and MEN-I, except perhaps in association with GRF-omas, where it occurs in ~40% of cases (56,163). Isolated Cushing's syndrome from a pancreatic endocrine tumor without any other clinically apparent hormonal syndrome is extremely rare (186).

Paraneoplastic hypercalcemia due to release of both an immunoreactive PTH or PTH-like substance as well as other unidentified nonimmunoreactive hypercalcemic substances has been documented in late-stage endocrine tumors of the pancreas with liver metastases (188,189). A neurotensin-producing tumor has been described, and a neurotensinoma syndrome presenting with diarrhea, hypokalemia, weight loss, diabetes, cyanosis, hypotension, and flushing has been proposed, although most authorities believe that this is not a distinct syndrome (49,152,180,190,191). No association of these latter two syndromes with MEN-I is known.

Carcinoid Tumors of Bronchi and Thymus

Carcinoid tumors may be classified as derived from embryonic foregut, midgut, or hindgut tissue (192). The foregut tumors occur in the bronchi, thymus, stomach, pancreas, and duodenum.

The anatomic distribution of carcinoid tumors in MEN-I differs from that in sporadic carcinoid tumors. In a review of 2,837 cases of sporadic carcinoids, Godwin (193) noted a 12% incidence of bronchial carcinoid and a <5% incidence of other foregut tumors, while ~55% were hindgut tumors. By contrast, a 69% incidence of foregut tumors was noted in association with MEN-I carcinoid tumors (194). Thus foregut tumors, normally representing a small percentage of overall carcinoid tumors, are an increased fraction of carcinoid tumors in MEN-I.

Foregut carcinoid tumors occur with low or high penetrance in MEN-I kindreds. In one family, three of five affected individuals had bronchial carcinoid tumors (195). Carcinoid tumors have not been a feature in most MEN-I kindreds, however, being present in only ~7% of MEN-I patients. This percentage may reflect the lack of specific screening for this manifestation. Most bronchial carcinoid tumors were identified on necropsy or after evaluation of an asymptomatic mass on X-ray. An abnormal chest X-ray, back pain, chest pain, or dyspnea prompted evaluations leading to the diagnosis of thymic carcinoid tumors. A few thymic carcinoid tumors have been resected during mediastinal exploration for ectopic parathyroid tissue or during routine transcervical thymectomy incidental to parathyroidectomy.

In contrast to midgut carcinoid tumors, which are associated with the carcinoid syndrome, foregut carcinoid tumors produce this syndrome less commonly. However, an atypical carcinoid tumor syndrome, characterized by severe facial flush, lacrimation, headache, and bronchoconstriction, may occur. The biologic cause of these signs is unknown. The foregut carcinoid tumors do not, in general, secrete serotonin (5-hydroxytryptamine, 5-HT). They may secrete histamine and 5-hydroxytryptophan (5-HTP), which is metabolized to 5-hdyroxyindoleacetic acide (5-HIAA) and can be measured in the urine.

Bronchial and thymic carcinoid tumors may elaborate neuroendocrine peptides other than serotonin, including ACTH (196,197) GHRH (198), calcitonin, bombesin, neurotensin, somatostatin, gastrin-releasing peptide, and gastrin (195). Clinical syndromes of GHRH and ACTH excess have been only rarely reported in MEN-I but are part of the differential diagnosis in an MEN-I patient with Cushing's syndrome or acromegaly (199). Sporadic bronchial carcinoid tumors have been designated as typical or atypical based on morphologic features. Typical carcinoid tumors are benign and express serotonin and α-human chorionic gonadotropin (hCG) less frequently than do atypical carcinoid tumors, which tend to be malignant (200). Despite the fact that this histochemical evaluation may predict the prognosis of these tumors, it has been performed very rarely with intrathoracic carcinoid tumors in MEN-I patients.

Foregut carcinoid tumors in MEN-I differ from sporadic carcinoid tumors in anatomic distribution. In one large review, 40% were bronchial, 35% were thymic, 20% were duodenal, and 5% were gastric, with most of the latter being ECL-omas (194). This compares with a 75% rate of bronchial carcinoid tumors and <2% of thymic carcinoid tumors among sporadic cases (193).

In contrast to the even sex distribution of sporadic bronchial carcinoid tumors (201), 79% of bronchial carcinoid tumors associated with MEN-I occur in women, and the age at diagnosis is lower (42 vs. 52 years). The rate of malignancy (26%) (194) is similar to that of sporadic cases (22%) (202).

Men represent ~90% of sporadic thymic carcinoid tumor cases, with a mean age of diagnosis of ~40 years (203,204). Similar gender (91% men) and age (37 years) associations are found in MEN-I thymic carcinoid tumors (194,205). Mediastinal carcinoid tumors

have a high propensity for malignancy (~90%) in MEN-I and are more aggressive than bronchial carcinoid tumors when malignant.

Carcinoid Tumors of the Gastrointestinal Tract

Carcinoid tumors are relatively benign-appearing tumors of neuroendocrine origin that originate in the gastrointestinal tract, lung, or gonads. They are structurally indistinguishable from other enteropancreatic neuroendocrine tumors, with the result that the term *carcinoid tumor* is often used loosely to describe all tumors of neuroendocrine origin whether they give rise to the carcinoid tumor syndrome or not (49,59). The carcinoid tumor syndrome occurs as a result of unregulated secretion of a variety of vasoactive amines by certain carcinoid tumors, but not all carcinoid tumors produce functionally active amines (49, 206,207).

Carcinoid tumors account for 1.5% of all gastrointestinal tract tumors (206,207), and the carcinoid tumor syndrome is the most common functional enteropancreatic neuroendocrine tumor syndrome in the general population (49,53,59). More than 90% of all sporadic carcinoid tumors occur in the gastrointestinal tract. The most common sites of origin are the mid- and hindgut, which together account for >80% of all carcinoid tumors (49,206,207).

The specific site of origin for a particular carcinoid tumor is important because the natural history and likelihood of functionality differ from site to site (Table 11) (24,49,60,206,207). Carcinoids of the appendix account for 30–40% of those in the general population but are unusual in MEN-I syndrome (24,208). They are generally asymptomatic, only rarely give rise to the carcinoid tumor syndrome, and only rarely metastasize (49,206,207). These tumors are often discovered only following routine appendectomy for what appears

TABLE 11. *Characteristics of gastrointestinal carcinoid tumors dependent on site of origin*[a]

Characteristic	Site of origin		
	Foregut	Midgut	Hindgut
Frequency in general population	4	75	19
Frequency in MEN-I	Common	Intermediate	Rare
Carcinoid syndrome	Variable	Common	Rare (if metastatic)
Metastatic disease	Rare	Rare (appendix) Common (ileum)	Rare (rectal) Common (colon)
Serotonin (5-HT) production	Variable	Yes	No
Urinary 5-HIAA	Variable	Yes	No
5-HTP production	Yes	Variable	No
Histamine production	Yes	No	No

[a]Abbreviations: 5-HT, 5-hydroxytryptamine; 5-HIAA, 5-hydroxyindoleacetic acid; 5-HTP, 5-hydroxytryptophan. Data from references 49, 59, 206–209.

to be an uncomplicated attack of appendicitis (49,209). The small intestine is the second most common site for carcinoid tumors in the general population (49). Carcinoid tumors at this site have been described in patients with MEN-I (24,208). These tumors generally occur in the terminal ileum, are often aggressive, and commonly metastasize to the liver, where they cause the carcinoid tumor syndrome (see below) in 10–40% of cases (49,206,207). The presence of metastatic disease has been shown to correlate closely with the size of the primary tumor (49,209). Rectal and other hindgut carcinoid tumors constitute <25% of all carcinoid tumors in the general population, and no specific relationship between hindgut carcinoid tumors and MEN-I syndrome has yet been described. Only very rarely are hindgut carcinoid tumors associated with the carcinoid tumor syndrome, since they generally do not produce significant amounts of functionally active vasoactive substances (49,206,207). Rectal carcinoid tumors metastasize only occasionally, whereas cecal and left and right colonic carcinoid tumors are characteristically more aggressive (49,206,207).

The Carcinoid Tumor Syndrome. Carcinoid tumors secrete a variety of vasoactive amines as well as a number of peptide hormones, depending on their site and precise cell of origin (49,206,207). The term *carcinoid tumor syndrome* is generally used to refer to the constellation of signs and symptoms believed to result from the action of a variety of vasoactive amines (49,206,207). This syndrome is characterized by episodes of flushing, diarrhea, abdominal cramping, wheezing, dyspnea, and palpitations (49,207). The carcinoid tumor syndrome generally occurs with functional mid- and hindgut carcinoid tumors only after the development of liver metastases, whereas it can occur with bronchial carcinoid tumors without the presence of liver metastases (49,206,207). This difference may occur because, in the case of mid- and hindgut carcinoids, tumor products are secreted into the portal venous system and are metabolized by the liver before they reach the general circulation (49,206).

Episodic flushing is the hallmark of the carcinoid tumor syndrome although flushing may be absent in up to one-third of cases (206,207). It is important to note that the typical pattern of flushing differs according to the site of the primary tumor (49). This difference may be due to the different hormonal products that are produced by tumors at different sites (49,206,207). The typical flush is erythematous and involves the head, neck, and upper chest. Bronchial carcinoid tumors are characteristically associated with more prolonged and severe flushing episodes than are described with mid- and hindgut carcinoid tumors, and they are also more commonly associated with lacrimation, periorbital edema, and salivation (206,207). The flush associated with functional gastric carcinoid tumors is character-

istically bright red and patchy, with sharply delineated serpentine borders that coalesce as the flush spreads (49,206,207). Palpitations and tremulousness commonly accompany the onset of flushing episodes. The carcinoid tumor syndrome is characteristically not associated with hypertension, and a decrease in blood pressure is typically described (206,207). Gastrointestinal and pulmonary manifestations commonly accompany the flushing episode (49,206,207). In addition, pellagra-like skin lesions, telangiectasias of the face and neck, and left- or right-sided cardiac murmurs (depending on the site of amine origin) are characteristic in patients with long-standing disease (49,206,207). The attacks are due to the release of a variety of vasomotor substances by the tumor, including 5-HT, which is the major substance responsible for the carcinoid tumor syndrome (49,206,207). Other vasoactive tumor products include 5-hydroxytryptophan (5-HTP), histamine, catecholamines, kinins, tachykinins, and prostaglandins (Table 11) (49,206,207).

Diagnosis and differential diagnosis. The carcinoid tumor syndrome is best diagnosed by documenting increased 24 hr urinary excretion of the various carcinoid tumor products or their metabolites (49,206, 207). 5-Hydroxyindoleacetic acid (5-HIAA) is the major urinary metabolite of 5-HT (49,206,207). Increased excretion of 5-HIAA (>10 mg/24 hr) is the biochemical hallmark of the carcinoid tumor syndrome in the vast majority of cases, although occasionally (especially with certain foregut tumors), the tumor lacks the necessary enzymes to convert 5-HTP to 5-HT, with the result that 5-HIAA is not produced (Table 11) (49,206,207). Urinary 5-HIAA levels >10 mg/24 hr have been described with certain 5-HT-containing foods (e.g., walnuts, pineapple, bananas), with drugs that increase 5-HT levels (e.g., phenothiazines), and rarely with other gastrointestinal conditions such as malabsorption secondary to sprue or intestinal obstruction (49,206,207). Other causes of flushing that should be considered in the differential diagnosis of the carcinoid tumor syndrome include systemic mastocytosis, the menopausal syndrome, and medullary carcinoma of the thyroid (49,206,207). Urinary 5-HIAA levels would not be expected to be elevated in these conditions.

Gastric ECL-omas in Patients With Multiple Endocrine Neoplasia Type I

The human gastric oxyntic mucosa is populated by six different endocrine cell types (60,212). Histamine-secreting enterochromaffin-like cells (ECL cells) make up 30–50% of this cell population, whereas the remaining cell types include the enterochromaffin (EC), D, P, K_1, and X cells (60,212). Gastric oxyntic endocrine cells give rise to two types of gastric carcinoid tumors (60). Non-ECL-cell carcinoids (see above) are generally sporadic lesions, have no specific association with either hypergastrinemia or MEN-I syndrome, and are not discussed further here. ECL-cell carcinoid tumors (ECL-omas) are gastric endocrine carcinoid tumors that arise from ECL cells and are associated with hypergastrinemia and the MEN-I syndrome (60,83).

In recent years, there has been significant interest regarding the association between hypergastrinemia and ECL-omas (60,61). It is now generally believed that prolonged hypergastrinemia causes chronic ECL-cell stimulation, leading to progressive ECL hyperplasia and ultimately ECL-omas (60,61,212). In animal studies, ECL-cell hyperplasia is proportional to the degree of hypergastrinemia induced by a variety of methods including gastric fundectomy, exogenous gastrin infusion, or drug-induced achlorhydria (53,59,61). Progression from diffuse ECL-cell hyperplasia through linear and micronodular hyperplasia to carcinoid tumors has been observed by several investigators (60,61), and a hyperplasia–neoplasia sequence similar to the adenoma–carcinoma sequence that has been described for carcinoid of the colon has been postulated (210).

ECL-cell hyperplasia and carcinoid tumors of the stomach have been reported to occur in human hypergastrinemic conditions such as pernicious anemia or Zollinger-Ellison syndrome (60,61). As many as 5% of patients with pernicious anemia develop gastric carcinoid tumors (60,61,210,211). However, not all hypergastrinemic states are associated with ECL-omas. ECL-omas are particularly common in patients with Zollinger-Ellison syndrome associated with MEN-I syndrome but occur only rarely in patients with sporadic Zollinger-Ellison syndrome (59–61). In one study, 16 Zollinger-Ellison syndrome patients with gastric carcinoid tumors were identified (61). Sufficient information was available to determine the MEN-I status in 15 of these patients, and 14 of them also had MEN-I syndrome (59–61). One study suggested that ~5% of all patients with MEN-I and Zollinger-Ellison syndrome develop gastric carcinoids (63), although other studies have suggested a prevalence as high as 13% (212). In contrast, gastric carcinoid tumors occur in 0.6% of patients with sporadic Zollinger-Ellison syndrome (59,61). Because the sporadic form of Zollinger-Ellison syndrome occurs four times more commonly than the inherited form of the disease, these data suggest that gastric ECL-omas are at least 100 times more common in patients with the hereditary form of Zollinger-Ellison syndrome than in patients with the sporadic form of the disease. It is unknown at present whether ECL-omas also occur in patients with MEN-I who do not have Zollinger-Elli-

son syndrome and who are not hypergastrinemic. It has been postulated that a circulating factor other than gastrin, such as the factor that can stimulate parathyroid growth in patients with MEN-I (213), may be responsible or coresponsible with gastrin for producing ECL-omas in these patients (214).

There is no hormonal syndrome that has been associated with ECL-omas, and the true natural history of gastric ECL-omas in patients with MEN-I is unknown for a number of reasons. First, long-term survival has only recently improved in these patients. Previously, the long-term prognosis was poor, with many patients dying of various complications of MEN-I syndrome, and follow-up was relatively short (24,49). Second, many patients with Zollinger-Ellison syndrome and MEN-I previously underwent total gastrectomy for control of gastric acid hypersecretion because, until recently, effective medical therapy was unavailable (52,53). Third, the association of MEN-I with gastric ECL-omas has only recently been described, and only a relatively small number of cases have been systematically evaluated (60,61). Therefore, only limited long-term data from a relatively small number of patients are available. Numerous investigators have demonstrated that gastric carcinoid tumors commonly invade the muscularis mucosa (60,215), but whether these tumors metastasize and, if so, the exact percentage that do so and the resultant overall prognosis are not yet known.

Diagnosis and Differential Diagnosis. Because they are generally asymptomatic, gastric ECL-omas are usually discovered during endoscopic examination for another indication (e.g., follow-up of Zollinger-Ellison syndrome). Figure 4 (top) illustrates the stomach of a typical MEN-I patient with Zollinger-Ellison syndrome and gastric ECL-omas. These submucosal lesions are indistinguishable from other mucosal or submucosal gastric lesions endoscopically. The definitive diagnosis of gastric ECL-omas requires histological examination, including immunohistochemical stains, to confirm the neuroendocrine origin of the constituent cells (215). This may be difficult to achieve because of the submucosal location of the tumors. A recent study demonstrated the utility of fine-needle aspiration cytology in identifying submucosal gastroduodenal lesions of neuroendocrine origin in patients with Zollinger-Ellison syndrome (Fig. 4, middle and bottom) (216). ECL cells can be distinguished histologically from non-ECL oxyntic endocrine cells using the Sevier-Munger technique, which selectively identifies the argyrophylic ECL cells (60,215). This distinction may be of extreme importance, since it appears that ECL-cell carcinoid tumors are significantly less aggressive than non-ECL-cell sporadic carcinoid tumors despite the fact that the latter tumors are known to invade the muscular layer of the stomach (60).

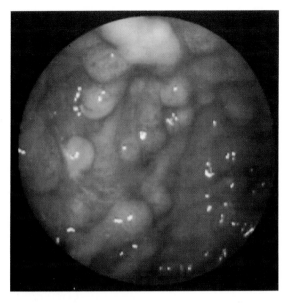

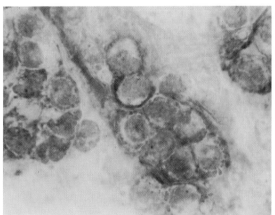

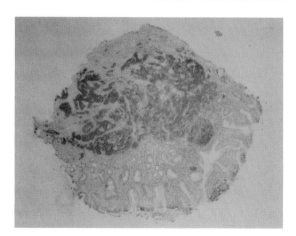

FIG. 4. Gastric ECL-omas in a patient with MEN-I and hypergastrinemia from the Zollinger-Ellison syndrome. The *top panel* is an endoscopic photograph of the gastric corpus showing multiple submucosal nodules, which were shown to be ECL-omas histologically. The *middle panel* illustrates the immunohistochemical stain for chromogranin-A (magnification ×1,000) of cells obtained by fine-needle aspiration of one of the nodules in the top panel. In this example, the chromogranin-A stain is positive in the cytoplasm (brown color), confirming a neuroendocrine origin of cells in the fine-needle aspirate. The *bottom panel* illustrates the immunohistochemical stain for chromogranin (magnification ×32) of one of the nodules in the top panel, which was removed by snare polypectomy. In this example, the chromogranin-A stain is positive (brown color), confirming a neuroendocrine origin for the nodule.

Expressions of "Tumor Markers" in Multiple Endocrine Neoplasia Type I

Neuroendocrine tumor cells contain various chromogranins, neuron specific enolase, synaptophysin, and specific hormonal products, including various peptides and amines. These substances can be targeted histochemically using specific antibodies to these substances, and, in recent years, immunohistochemical staining techniques utilizing these antibodies have been developed (91,176,217,218). In addition, these substances can also be detected in the serum using radioimmunoassay techniques (218,219).

The *chromogranin* family of proteins, chromogranins A, B, and C, are acidic and soluble proteins that are costored with peptides and amines in the granules of endocrine cells (218,220). They make up 87% of the total soluble protein of chrommaffin granules (221). Elevated serum levels of chromogranin A have been documented in patients with enteropancreatic neuroendocrine tumors (218,221). Despite utility for confirming an endocrine origin for a specific tumor, serum chromogranin levels are not helpful in determining whether a particular tumor is malignant or not, nor in distinguishing between MEN-I-associated vs. sporadic endocrine tumor.

Elevated levels of serum hCG or either of its subunits, α-hCG or β-hCG, have been proposed to correlate with malignancy in patients with enteropancreatic neuroendocrine tumors (219,222). However, because of conflicting results from another series (223), the utility of hCG-subunit measurements as an indicator of malignancy in patients with endocrine tumors of the pancreas remains to be definitively established. In addition, there is no evidence to date suggesting that hCG levels can distinguish between MEN-I-associated and sporadic tumor.

Specific hormonal products (e.g., pancreatic polypeptide, gastrin, glucagon, VIP) are essential in the diagnosis of endocrine tumor syndromes in that, by definition, the diagnosis depends (among other criteria) on elevated serum levels of the hormone that causes the syndrome. It has also been proposed that elevated plasma levels of PP are more likely to be associated with MEN-I tumors, suggesting that PP levels can be used to differentiate between MEN-I-associated and sporadic disease (57,58,91). However, recent studies have suggested that this is not true; high PP levels have been shown to occur with similar frequency in patients with MEN-I-associated or sporadic neuroendocrine tumor (393). In addition to the native hormone, various precursors, such as progastrin and proinsulin, as well as peptide fragments, such as NH_2- and COOH-terminal gastrin fragments, have been detected in the plasma of patients with enteropancreatic neuroendocrine tumors (59,224,225). Although it has been proposed that prohormone-to-hormone ratios or peptide fragment analysis may provide information regarding the malignancy or growth potential of certain pancreatic endocrine tumors such as insulinoma or gastrinoma (224,226,227), at present it is unclear whether analyses of this type will provide clinically useful information for most peptide-secreting tumors (49,59).

Anterior Pituitary Tumors

Knowledge of the true incidence of pituitary tumors in MEN-I syndrome is limited by the rarity of the condition and the paucity of studies using state-of-the-art radiographic techniques and radioimmunoassays for pituitary products to screen kindreds. Keeping these caveats in mind, the incidence of pituitary tumor varies from 0 to 100% in affected members of well-documented kindreds (228,229), suggesting marked differences in the phenotypic expression of the syndrome; 106 of 303 patients from MEN-I kindreds reported since 1967 had pituitary tumors (195,228–232) (see also Table 1). This 35% incidence contrasts with the 74% incidence of pituitary involvement reported by Ballard in 1964 (26). However, the latter figure was based primarily on necropsy material and on case reports. The pituitary abnormality may be the first manifestation of MEN-I, and for this reason screening with prolactin levels has been recommended (233,234).

While the sex distribution of MEN-I patients is divided evenly between males and females, the percentage of women with pituitary abnormalities in MEN-I is approximately double that in men. This may be accounted for by the common occurrence of prolactinoma, whose clinical symptoms may be more easily recognized in women. The successful detection of four prolactinomas in men (but not women) using screening serum prolactin measurements supports this speculation (228). The age at the time of diagnosis of pituitary tumors reported in kindreds ranged from 17 (235) to 65 (228) years, with a mean of ~40 years (228,236,237). The age range reported in sporadic patients with pituitary tumors is similar, 13–75 years (238).

Do MEN-I tumors differ from sporadic pituitary tumors? Table 12 summarizes data on (a) the prevalence of tumor type in unselected patients at the Mayo Clinic (238), (b) 106 patients with pituitary tumor from MEN-I kindreds and sporadic cases with additional pancreatic or parathyroid involvement, and (c) 40 patients with MEN-I syndrome found in a retrospective unselected review of 1,500 pituitary adenomas surgically resected at the Mayo Clinic (238). The latter study represents the only large-scale evaluation of immunohistochemical reactivities in these patients. In contrast to the data from the kindreds, the sex distribution was even in this group (18:22, males:females).

TABLE 12. *Hormonal production by pituitary adenomas with and without multiple endocrine neoplasia type I syndrome treated surgically at the Mayo Clinic (238) and by pituitary adenomas in 106 multiple endocrine neoplasia type I patients*

	MEN-I/Mayo No (%)	MEN-I literature[a] No (%)	Without MEN-I/ Mayo (%)
Prolactin	16 (41)	81 (76)	30
GH	4 (12)	8 (8)	10
Gh-PRL	6 (15)	3 (3)	5
Plurihormonal	9 (22)	—	10
ACTH			11
Active	2 (5)	4 (4)	
Silent	1 (2)	1 (1)	
Hyperplasia	1 (2)	1 (1)	n/a
LH/FSH	0	1 (1)	7–15
TSH	0	1 (1)[b]	1
Null cell/nonsecreting	3 (7)	7 (6)	20
Other	0		0–6

[a]Data from references 195, 230–232, 235, 239–248.
[b]Biochemical and clinical features were compatible with TSH-secreting tumor; immunohistochemistry revealed GH and PRL as well as TSH (248).

As compared to the Mayo Clinic experience with sporadic pituitary tumors (Table 12), the overall distribution of tumor types is altered in MEN-I; there are fewer gonadotropin and null-cell tumors, and more plurihormonal and prolactin-producing tumors. About one-third of the Mayo Clinic MEN-I patients had clinical features of acromegaly, and 41% had prolactinomas, compared to 11% and 76% incidences of these conditions respectively, in the MEN-I literature review group. Immunohistochemical data suggest that the incidence of plurihormonal tumors is greater in patients with MEN-I, and it is possible that some of the tumor classified in other studies as secreting solely prolactin in fact represent plurihormonal tumors. Although the overall incidence of surgically resected macroadenomas was not different from that in the general population (238), data are not available to evaluate whether the incidence of unresected macroadenomas is increased in MEN-I. Earlier reports of an increased rate of macroadenomas may represent an ascertainment bias. Multicentric tumors occur, possibly at increased number (229,249).

The clinical presentation of pituitary tumors does not differ from the presentation in patients without MEN-I. Symptoms of mass effect, usually headache, visual field loss, and hypopituitarism, and/or symptoms and signs of excessive hormone production call attention to a pituitary abnormality. Galactorrhea, amenorrhea, and/or infertility are common presentations in women with prolactinoma. MEN-I patients with prolactinoma may have primary amenorrhea or secondary amenorrhea before the age of 20 years (237). In men, hypogonadism and mass effect may be the only signs of prolactinoma. The biochemical diagnosis is made in the usual fashion: prolactin levels >300 ng/ml indicate prolactinoma, while elevated values of 40–60 ng/ml may indicate compression of the stalk or prolactinoma. Intermediate values may be seen in either condition, depending on the assay used.

The protean manifestations of sporadic Cushing's syndrome are unchanged in the setting of MEN-I. The diagnosis is established by demonstration of increased glucocorticoid levels or diminished response to glucocorticoid feedback as evidenced by increased urine cortisol excretion or inability to suppress cortisol <5μg/dl at 8:00 AM after administration of 1 mg dexamethasone 9 hr earlier. The differential diagnosis is essentially unchanged. Pituitary-dependent ACTH excess due to an ACTH-secreting adenoma or corticotrope hyperplasia has been described (Table 12). Ectopic ACTH secretion from a bronchial carcinoid tumor has been reported (199). Cushing's syndrome resulting from primary neoplasm of the adrenal gland has also been reported in a few patients (250). The differential diagnosis begins with measurement of plasma ACTH. Values <10 pg/ml identify ACTH-independent Cushing's syndrome, and localization of the adrenal disease may then be accomplished with CT scan (251,252). If more than one nodule is seen, iodocholesterol scanning should be performed to identify functioning masses. Forms of Cushing's syndrome that are ACTH dependent, either corticotropinoma or ectopic ACTH secretion, can be differentiated by their peripheral (253) or petrosal venous (254) responses to corticotropin-releasing hormone (CRH) or by dexamethasone stimulation (255).

Luteinizing hormone (LH) and follicle-stimulating hormone (FSH) showed a paradoxical increase after thyrotropin-releasing hormone (TRH) administration in the sole MEN-I patient with gonadotropin and α subunit-secreting tumor, as has been described in other such patients without MEN-I (256,257). The patient with the thyroid-stimulating hormone (TSH)-secreting tumor demonstrated an increased α subunit-to-TSH molar ratio, and no TSH response after TRH administration, both diagnostic of this type of tumor (248).

What is the appropriate evaluation for pituitary tumors in patients with MEN-I? A careful history, with attention to reproductive function (menstrual dates, galactorrhea, fertility in women, and potency and libido in men), weight gain, headaches, or change in hand size may suggest an expanding mass, prolactinoma, Cushing's syndrome, or acromegaly. Physical examination should evaluate the visual fields and check for signs of hormonal excess. There is no clear consensus on whether all patients should undergo pituitary imaging in the absence of suggestive clinical signs. Biochemical screening, especially for prolactin, may be more cost effective but will not detect all tumors. It is reasonable to investigate members of an MEN-I kindred more closely when any member has pituitary involvement, since some kindreds have particularly high penetrance for pituitary tumor.

If a pituitary tumor is discovered, three considerations guide the therapeutic approach. First, is the tumor a macroadenoma? If so, is there evidence for mass effects, such as visual field defects or local invasion of the cavernous sinus? Second, is there clinical evidence of hormonal hypersecretion? Third, is there evidence for hypopituitarism?

To answer these questions, a number of baseline tests should be performed, including high-quality imaging of the sella, preferably using magnetic resonance imaging and gadolinium contrast, to delineate the size and possibly the invasiveness of the tumor. Patients with suprasellar extension should undergo formal testing of the visual fields. If not previously obtained, basal plasma GH and prolactin and urine free cortisol may demonstrate hormone excess. Patients without clinical evidence of hormonal hypersecretion may be screened for gonadotropin-secreting tumor with basal and TRH-stimulated LH, LH-β LH-α, and FSH. Baseline thyroid function tests (free T4 and TSH) will identify patients with central hypothyroidism (low free T4) and the rare patient with TSH-secreting tumors (elevated free T4 and normal TSH). A plasma cortisol value >18 μg/dl obtained 30–60 min after cortrosyn injection (250 μg, i.v.) excludes adrenal insufficiency.

Tumors Outside the Parathyroid, Gastrointestinal-Endocrine, and Anterior Pituitary Tissues

Primary Thyroid Neoplasms

Ballard (26) described thyroid adenoma as an occasional feature of MEN-I, and there have been periodic reports of this association but no careful analysis to establish that this is anything but a chance association. Allelic loss from chromosome 11 (which carries the *men1* gene and several other tumor suppressor genes) was common in sporadic follicular tumors of the thyroid but not in sporadic papillary thyroid tumor (258), suggesting that follicular thyroid neoplasms might also be expressed as a specific component of MEN-I.

Primary Adrenocortical Neoplasms

Syndromes of primary oversecretion of adrenal steroid hormones have been a rather uncommon association in MEN-I. Several cases have shown hypercortisolism or hyperaldosteronism (259). When there is glucocorticoid excess in MEN-I, it usually results from pituitary oversecretion of ACTH (260). Often adrenal enlargement is biochemically silent in MEN-I (261). Adrenocortical cancer has been reported once (262), and we have encountered two more cases (S.J.M. and J.N., unpublished observations).

Lipoma

Lipoma has a widely recognized association with MEN-I, having been reported in ~20% of cases (27). The lipomas in MEN-I may occur anywhere; they are often multiple, and they may be small or large and cosmetically disturbing. When removed, they typically do not recur. Large visceral lipomas are occasionally noted incidental to abdominal imaging or at laparotomy.

Other Neoplasms

The incidence rates of other tumors in MEN-I are not known. A tabulation of associated tumors in 200 case reports did not reveal other neoplasms with unusually high incidence (24).

Intrafamilial Homogeneity or Heterogeneity in Expressions of Multiple Endocrine Neoplasia Type I

Isolated Primary Hyperparathyroidism

Several kindreds reported initially as isolated familial primary hyperparathyroidism were shown to have MEN-I on further follow-up (27). However, in two extremely large kindreds, there have been no (263) or very few (27,264) disorders outside the parathyroid. In one, the "isolated hyperparathyroidism" showed genetic linkage to 11q13, the locus of the *men1* gene (263). There are also several other forms of familial primary hyperparathyroidism not caused by the *men1* gene (see below).

Variable Aggressiveness of Gastrinoma

The typical MEN-I kindred has a high penetrance of primary hyperparathyroidism and a somewhat lower and later penetrance of Zollinger-Ellison syndrome. Gastrinoma may be particularly aggressive or particularly mild (29) in some kindreds, or even in some branches of extended kindreds. Such claims have been anecdotal, but the possibility of unusual interactions of the *men1* gene with other genes or with environmental factors requires careful evaluation.

Prolactinoma Variant

Several large kindreds have shown features quite different from those of typical MEN-I. Hershon et al. (265) reported a large kindred with a very high penetrance of prolactinoma but no case of gastrinoma. There is a cluster of several similar kindreds in Canada (266,267). In the latter cluster, there was also an unusually high expression of carcinoid tumor. We reported absence of gastrinoma in a large MEN-I kindred (268); prolactinoma was later diagnosed in many members (S.J.M., unpublished observations). Genetic linkage analysis has established that the MEN-I trait is linked to 11q13 in the largest of these three "prolactinoma variant" kindreds or clusters (274). Further testing established that gastrinoma did occur in this MEN-I variant kindred, albeit with a low prevalence (8%) (269).

Insulinoma Variant

Other MEN-I kindreds seem to have a disproportionate expression of insulinoma, with little if any gastrinoma (27). Skogseid et al. (29) have shown linkage of this trait to 11q13 in one such kindred; this kindred had a pronounced excess of tumors oversecreting insulin and proinsulin, and the GI-endocrine neoplasms showed a high propensity to metastasize.

TREATMENT AND RESPONSES TO TREATMENT

Treatment of Parathyroid Tumors

Intervention vs. Nonintervention

The proper treatment for primary hyperparathyroidism is controversial (270). Symptomatic disease usually justifies surgical treatment (271). However, different groups take divergent approaches to cases with asymptomatic primary hyperparathyroidism. Since primary hyperparathyroidism is more difficult to manage surgically in MEN-I than in sporadic cases, most centers apply more restrictive criteria to undertake surgery in MEN-I than in sporadic cases.

Medical Supervision: Nonintervention

In theory, the primary hyperparathyroidism in MEN-I could be more aggressive than in sporadic cases; it begins earlier, and new tumor clones may continue to form. For this reason there is a need to compare the prognosis of untreated primary hyperparathyroidism in MEN-I and in sporadic cases. Without this information, the current guidelines for treatment of hyperparathyroidism are similar in sporadic and MEN-I-associated cases. Many patients with asymptomatic primary hyperparathyroidism are candidates for supervision without any treatment; this is appropriate in a higher proportion of MEN-I cases.

Patients with MEN-I require periodic follow-up for the pleiomorphic features of their disorder. Thus concomitant monitoring of the hyperparathyroidism is convenient. We (S.J.M., unpublished observations) have followed one MEN-I patient for >20 years without progression of asymptomatic primary hyperparathyroidism.

Pharmacotherapy

As new pharmacologic options are explored, for example, potent bisphosphonates, noncalcemic analogs of vitamin D (272), and selective calcium channel blockers (277), these might become suitable for application to the mild hyperparathyroidism that is common in MEN-I.

Factors Influencing the Decision for Parathyroidectomy

The decision about parathyroidectomy in MEN-I must take into account the following considerations. (a) Severe symptoms or signs of primary hyperparathyroidism always warrant parathyroidectomy unless there are clear contraindications. (b) Most cases of primary hyperparathyroidism in MEN-I can be diagnosed at an early and asymptomatic stage. Parathyroid surgery is more difficult at this stage because the glands, being only modestly enlarged, are harder to find. (c) Parathyroid surgery is more difficult for MEN-I than for sporadic disease. There may be four and rarely even five or six parathyroid tumors. If the diagnosis is not recognized or if the surgeon is not experienced, the operation might be concluded too early. The multiplicity of parathyroid tumors increases the likelihood that at least one tumor will be abnormally located in any patient with MEN-I. (d) Amelioration of primary hyperparathyroidism might slow the progression of some or even all MEN-I-associated endocrinopathies (274). This is highly speculative, and it is probably incorrect with regard to residual parathyroid tissue. Successful treatment of hyperparathyroidism in MEN-I decreases the previously elevated serum levels of gastrin (275) and of chromogranin A (280). It has been suggested that the decrease in circulating chromogranin A reflects decreased secretory activity of enterochromaffin-like cells of the stomach (277). In many endocrine tissues, measures that decrease secretion rate also decrease growth rate. There are currently no data, such as serial indices of tumor mass, indicating that parathyroidectomy slows tumor development or progression in any of the tissues affected by MEN-I.

Special Approaches That May Be Beneficial at Initial Parathyroid Surgery in Multiple Endocrine Neoplasia Type I

There are many special considerations that can help optimize surgical approaches to hyperparathyroidism in MEN-I (271).

Experienced Surgeon. Two of the most critical factors for successful surgery are recognition preoperatively that the patient has MEN-I and involvement of an experienced parathyroid surgeon.

No need for noninvasive preoperative gland imaging. We cannot overemphasize the importance of having an experienced surgeon. Noninvasive preoperative gland imaging has not been shown to lead to shorter operative times or to higher success rates at initial parathyroid surgery in MEN-I.

Extensive Initial Exploration. The surgeon should try to identify all four parathyroid glands with biopsy confirmation. The strongest determinant of surgical success has been biopsy confirmation of identification of four glands (43,279). The parathyroid glands are more difficult to identify at subsequent operations, and reoperations carry extra morbidity because of additional difficulty in identifying critical structures (mainly the recurrent laryngeal nerves) that may be imbedded in scar.

Resection of All but 50 mg of the Most Normal-appearing Parathyroid Tissue. There are several approaches to a successful subtotal parathyroidectomy in MEN-I. Some surgeons prefer not to remove normal-appearing parathyroid glands and to minimize the amount of trauma caused by a biopsy (281). Most prefer to remove three and one-half glands, leaving 50 mg of the most normal-appearing tissue. The remaining tissue can be left attached to its natural pedicle or it can be autografted to another site (see below).

Transcervical Thymectomy. Transcervical thymectomy should be attempted at initial parathyroid exploration in all patients with MEN-I and no prior neck operation. The thymus may contain one or more parathyroid glands, parathyroid nests, MEN-I-associated anterior mediastinal carcinoid tumor, or the precursor cells for such a tumor (279).

Intraoperative Ultrasound. If four parathyroid glands are not identified, intraoperative ultrasound may aid in locating a remaining tumor. Intraoperative ultrasound is particularly valuable to detect parathyroid tumor within the thyroid gland (282).

Parathyroid Autograft with Fresh Tissue. Wells et al. (283) showed that total parathyroidectomy with fresh autograft could treat so-called primary parathyroid hyperplasia (see the chapter by Norton et al.). The goal is to resect all abnormal and normal parathyroid glands. Approximately 50 mg of the most normal-appearing parathyroid tissue is then minced into 2 × 1 × 1 mm segments and autografted into 20–25 pockets in the brachioradialis muscle of the nondominant arm. Each pocket is closed with a nonresorbable suture. Seven of 23 MEN-I patients (32%) remained hypoparathyroid after receiving a fresh autograft for MEN-I (284). Parathyroid autografts for MEN-I in other series have encountered lower rates of postoperative hyperparathyroidism. Successful total parathyroidectomy, even with a fresh autograft, is manifested by a period of hypoparathyroidism for 3–6 weeks after surgery. If this does not occur, then the patient has residual parathyroid tissue in the neck or chest. We recommend maintaining the serum calcium at the lower limit of normal with calcium and a rapidly acting vitamin D analog during this 1–2 month period of autograft "maturation." There is no evidence that iatrogenic hypocalcemia increases the graft success rate. Total parathyroidectomy with autograft has the benefit of removing all parathyroid tissue from the neck (it is hoped) so that, if a late recurrence develops, the overactive tissue will be readily accessible in the graft bed. Considering the high recurrence rate after subtotal parathyroidectomy in MEN-I, a similarly high recurrence rate should be anticipated after treatment with an autograft. In one series, graft-dependent recurrence was found in four of six cases with MEN-I but in none of nine cases with sporadic hyperplasia (285). In another series of 23 MEN-I patients with average postoperative follow-up of 6 years, five developed recurrent hyperparathyroidism (279). From analysis of PTH step-ups in the graft effluents, the authors speculated that recurrent hyperparathyroidism arose principally from residual parathyroid tissue in the neck or chest.

Cryopreservation of Parathyroid Tissue. Parathyroid tissue can be cryopreserved with relatively simple procedures. The tissue can then be stored indefinitely. It can be used as an autograft if the patient becomes hypoparathyroid, whether or not this outcome had been intended (see below for deliberate total parathyroidectomy at initial operation in MEN-I). The frozen tissue could also be used if the patient becomes hypoparathyroid many years later after a repeat parathyroidectomy. These cryopreservation methods have not yet reached their theoretical potential of 100% viable tissue. In our experience (J.N. and S.J.M.), parathyroid cryopreservation has led to a successful autograft in only ~65% of patients.

Parathyroid Autograft With Cryopreserved Tissue. The general principles are similar to those with fresh autografts. The graft procedure is postponed for 3–6 months to confirm that the patient shows "total" hypoparathyroidism. If not, no autograft is placed. Late recurrent primary hyperparathyroidism after cryopreserved grafts seems to be very rare in MEN-I (J.N. and S.J.M., unpublished observations). This may reflect damage to the cryopreserved tissue or a lower mass of functioning parathyroid tissue than after a standard subtotal parathyroidectomy.

Parathyroid Reoperation

The most common reason for persistent hyperparathyroidism in MEN-I is failure to identify and remove (subtotally) four parathyroid glands during initial surgery (43). Less frequently, persistent hyperparathyroidism reflects one or more tumors in unusual locations. True recurrent primary hyperparathyroidism usually is attributable to a tumor that grows from a "normal" gland or from a gland remnant; remnants, to the extent the original gland was pathologic, should have a higher propensity to induce recurrence.

The principles in management of parathyroid reoperation are generally the same whether or not the patient has MEN-I (271,286) (however, see below for intraoperative PTH assay, a method that is particularly valuable in MEN-I). Some of the more critical issues are summarized briefly here.

Efforts should be made to review surgery notes, histologic slides, and pathology reports from previous parathyroid operations. Even with these measures, it is always difficult to predict how many parathyroid tumors will be encountered.

We recommend preoperative parathyroid gland imaging for all patients with MEN-I who need parathyroid reoperation (287–289). However, in a previously operated patient with MEN-I, it is rarely possible to image more than one enlarged gland preoperatively (S.J.M. and J.N., unpublished observations).

A careful operative plan should be based on the extent of prior surgery and interpretation of the preoperative tumor localization studies. If a tumor mass is identified high in the neck or low in the chest, an in-

cision is directed at that area. If a tumor is tentatively localized to the neck or if no tumor is localized, a full repeat neck operation may be planned with the possibility to do a sternotomy if a parathyroid tumor is not found in the neck.

At present the best way to diagnose inadequate resection of parathyroid tumor or tumors intraoperatively is through intraoperative PTH immunoassay with ultrashort turnaround time (15 min) (see the chapter by Nussbaum and Potts; 290). This is particularly valuable during parathyroid reoperations in MEN-I, wherein there is otherwise uncertainty about how many parathyroid tumors must be removed. Similar turnaround time and results have also been possible for the RIA of urinary cAMP intraoperatively (291). The intact PTH assay can be easier to interpret in that it can have a much wider dynamic range than assay of urinary cAMP. This highly specialized capability is currently under evaluation in a few centers but is too demanding for use at initial operation in MEN-I.

Enteropancreatic Neuroendocrine Tumors, Including Gastrointestinal Carcinoid Tumors and Gastric ECL-omas

Both the endocrine syndrome as well as the tumor itself must be addressed in order to manage MEN-I patients with enteropancreatic neuroendocrine tumors appropriately. If present, the endocrine syndrome must be addressed first because it often causes severe, life-threatening disease (292–296). With control of the endocrine syndrome, attention must be given to the tumor itself, since many of these tumors are malignant, and in recent years tumor growth has become an important determinant of long-term survival in many patients (292,297–298).

Management of the Endocrine Syndrome in Patients with Multiple Endocrine Neoplasia Type I

Management of the endocrine syndrome is not required for ECL-omas, PP-omas, and nonfunctional enteropancreatic neuroendocrine tumors (including nonfunctional mid- and hindgut carcinoid tumors), because they are not associated with an endocrine syndrome *per se*. However, as was mentioned above, the presence of an endocrine syndrome with other enteropancreatic neuroendocrine tumors can cause life-threatening disturbances of normal physiology, so that specific management of the endocrine syndrome is required. This is especially true for gastrinoma, insulinoma (see below), glucagonoma and VIP-oma (292–296). In these situations, therapy is aimed at controlling the tumor activity or the specific end-organ responses in each syndrome (292,297,298), and the specific treatments for each syndrome differ.

Medical Management

Control of gastric acid hypersecretion in Zollinger-Ellison syndrome. Gastric acid hypersecretion can be effectively controlled in virtually all patients with Zollinger-Ellison syndrome using histamine H_2-receptor antagonists (provided that sufficient medication is prescribed) or H^+,K^+-ATPase inhibitors (297–300). At present, the major role for H_2-receptor antagonists in Zollinger-Ellison syndrome is as intravenous agents (see below) (299,300).

H^+,K^+-ATPase inhibitors, such as lansoprazole or omeprazole, which inhibit the final common step in acid formation by the gastric parietal cell, have recently become available in the United States (297, 298,300,302). These drugs have been shown to be effective in all gastrinoma patients, including those with gastrinoma complicated by severe gastroesophageal reflux disease or previous partial gastrectomy (300–302). Moreover, unlike the case with histamine H_2-receptor antagonists, H^+,K^+-ATPase inhibitors have also been shown to be effective in all MEN-I patients with Zollinger-Ellison syndrome regardless of whether they also have hyperparathyroidism (300–302). H^+,K^+-ATPase inhibitors are now the oral antisecretory agents of choice in patients with Zollinger-Ellison syndrome because of their high potency, long duration of action, lack of significant long-term side effects, and ease of administration (300–302). We currently recommend starting with 60 mg omeprazole twice daily in MEN-I patients who have Zollinger-Ellison syndrome (twice the usual starting dose for sporadic gastrinoma patients). The reason for starting with a higher dose in MEN-I patients is that they commonly have hyperparathyroidism-induced hypercalcemia in association with the Zollinger-Ellison syndrome. The hypercalcemia itself contributes to gastric acid output and also renders the patient less sensitive to antisecretory therapy (303,304). The improved sensitivity to oral antisecretory therapy following successful parathyroidectomy is illustrated in Fig. 5. In the example shown, 150 mg oral ranitidine was much more effective in reducing acid secretion for up to 8 hr after administration following normalization of serum calcium. Once instituted, the dose of antisecretory therapy should be titrated with gastric acid output for effective control of gastric acid hypersecretion (300–302), because the presence or absence of symptoms of gastric acid hypersecretion is not useful as a guide to assess whether acid output is effectively controlled (300,305). Previous studies have shown that acid output should be maintained <10 mEq/hr in the last 1 hr before the next dose of medication (<5 mEq/hr in pa-

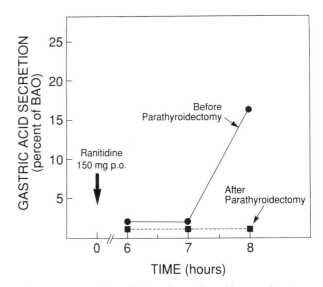

FIG. 5. Improved sensitivity of gastric acid secretion to antisecretory therapy following successful parathyroidectomy in a patient with MEN-I and Zollinger-Ellison syndrome. Gastric acid secretion is expressed as the percentage of the basal acid output (BAO) as determined pre- and postoperatively. In this example, following 150 mg oral ranitidine, both the degree of inhibition of acid secretion and the duration of the inhibition of acid secretion improved postoperatively.

tients with previous partial gastrectomy or severe gastroesophageal reflux disease) (300,301). In our experience, acid output can be controlled in all MEN-I patients with Zollinger-Ellison syndrome with twice daily oral omeprazole (300–302).

For reasons that are not yet clear, the efficacy of omeprazole improves over the first few days of administration (300–302). It has recently been shown that, once acid output has been controlled in patients with gastrinoma, the long-term maintenance dose can be reduced significantly in most patients without compromising acid output control, provided that acid output is monitored closely during dose reduction attempts (306). However, the same study (306) also showed that MEN-I patients with Zollinger-Ellison syndrome are less likely to tolerate dose reduction than patients with sporadic disease. The need for rapidly controlling acid output in the initial stages of illness precludes starting omeprazole at a reduced dose (306). We currently recommend that patients with MEN-I and Zollinger-Ellison syndrome be started on 60 mg of omeprazole twice daily and then, once acid output is effectively controlled, the dose can be titrated downwards using endoscopy and acid output measurements as guides (306).

The major reasons for attempting to reduce the long-term maintenance dose of omeprazole are expense and to limit the potential risks of a superimposed, secondary, physiological hypergastrinemia as a result of drug-induced achlorhydria (297,298,300–302,307). Long-term administration of high doses of omeprazole and other potent antisecretory agents to rats resulted in the development of gastric ECL-omas, some of which were invasive (295,307). Most authorities believe that this is due to achlorhydria-induced hypergastrinemia, which results in stimulation of ECL cells and culminates in ECL-oma development (295,307). This association is also discussed above in the section on gastric ECL-omas in patients with MEN-I. There has been concern that increased ECL-oma formation could occur with long-term use of omeprazole in gastrinoma patients (300–302). However, Zollinger-Ellison syndrome patients treated with omeprazole for up to 4 years have not been shown to have a higher incidence of ECL-omas compared with those who have not been treated with omeprazole (308). A recent analysis (301) showed that ECL-omas are almost always seen in patients with MEN-I-associated disease and not in patients with sporadic gastrinoma, so the presence of MEN-I syndrome, rather than the specific antisecretory therapy utilized, appears to be the important predisposing factor in ECL-oma development (297,298,301,308).

Intravenous antisecretory therapy should be utilized when patients are unable to take food or medication by mouth. In addition to the routine indications for i.v. therapy that occur in the general population, MEN-I patients also require i.v. antisecretory therapy during surgery for other possible indications, including parathyroid, pituitary, enteropancreatic, or adrenal resections. Intravenous omeprazole is extremely effective (309), but it is not yet available in the United States. Therefore, in perioperative patients or in patients who cannot take oral medications for any other reason, intravenous histamine H_2-receptor antagonists should be used (309,310). Doses for both intravenous and oral histamine H_2-receptor antagonists must also be titrated to acid output to ensure adequate control (299,300,310). If they are used in equipotent doses, there are no significant differences in efficacy or safety between the three histamine H_2-receptor antagonists available in the United States, although gynecomastia is a concern in male patients who receive cimetidine chronically (299,300). It is preferable to administer intravenous histamine H_2-receptor antagonist therapy by continuous intravenous infusion rather than by intermittent bolus dose administration (299,300,310). For ranitidine, we currently recommend starting with an i.v. bolus injection of 100–150 mg followed immediately by a continuous intravenous ranitidine infusion (300,310). If the effective oral ranitidine dose for the specific patient is known, the infusion rate should be started at 100% of the daily oral dose, since this rate will be effective in 95% of patients, thereby limiting the need for subsequent titrations to maintain efficacy (300,310). If the effective oral ranitidine dose is not known, the infusion rate should be started at 1 mg/kg/hr. The infusion rate should then be titrated upwards in 0.5 mg/kg/hr increments, with repeated acid output measurements every 4 hr to verify the effect, until effective control of acid output has been achieved (300,310). A ranitidine infusion rate of 1.5 and 2.5 mg/kg/hr effectively controls acid output in 84% and 100% of patients, respectively (310). Once the patient has resumed eating, oral therapy can be reinstituted at the previously effective dose, provided it is overlapped briefly with the intravenous infusion. The same general recommendations pertain for cimetidine, although three to four times higher doses are required because cimetidine is three to four times less potent than ranitidine (310). The long-acting somatostatin analog octreotide (see below) is also extremely effective in the control of gastric acid hypersecretion, although its use is limited for this application by the need for subcutaneous injections two or even three times daily and by associated effects such as cramping, steatorrhea, or gallstone formation (297,298,300).

Control of the carcinoid tumor syndrome. Until recently a variety of different medications (e.g., 5-HT antagonists, such as methysergide maleate, cyproheptadine, or ketanserin; combinations of histamine H_1- and H_2-receptor antagonists; corticosteroids; prochlorperazine; phenoxybenzamine; methyldopa; and cholestyramine), alone or in combination, have been used for the management of the various components of the carcinoid tumor syndrome (292,311,312). Responses, to varying degrees, have been described with all these agents, although the long-acting somatostatin analog octreotide (see below) is now considered to be the drug of choice because of its improved efficacy over alternative therapies (292,313,314). Interferon-α has also been reported to be effective in reducing symptoms as well as 24 hr urinary 5-HIAA levels in a significant number of patients with the carcinoid tumor syndrome (292,315). Supportive measures include the provision of a nutritious diet containing nicotinamide supplementation but excluding serotonin-containing foods that may precipitate episodes of flushing and diarrhea (292). High fluid intake to ensure adequate hydration has also been recommended, and symptomatic measures to control cardiac or respiratory disease are often required (292).

Control of the glucagonoma syndrome. Migratory necrolytic erythema in patients with glucagonoma may respond to normalization of amino acid levels, oral zinc therapy, and even glucose or normal saline infusions (316,317). Currently, octreotide is the drug of choice (see below). In addition, glucagonoma patients are generally poor operative risks because of their poor nutritional status resulting from the catabolic effects of glucagon combined with glucose intolerance (318,319). If surgery is contemplated, blood transfusions, total parenteral nutrition, and control of hyperglycemia have all been recommended for the preoperative period (296,317).

Control of the high-output diarrhea in the VIP-oma syndrome. The primary initial concern in the management of VIP-oma patients is to replace volume losses and to correct acid–base and electrolyte abnormalities (154,295,320–324). Fluid requirements as high as 5 liters/day and potassium requirements as high as 350 mEq/day are not unusual (154,320–322). A common cause of death is renal failure (321–323), and congestive heart failure, related to uncorrected hypokalemia, has also been described. Until recently a variety of different medications that either reduce renal wasting of fluid and electrolytes or inhibit intestinal secretion (e.g., high-dose steroids, clonidine, angiotensin II, norepinephrine, indomethacin, lithium carbonate, phenothiazines, propranolol, metoclopramide, and loperamide) were used for the medical management of the diarrhea (146,295,320,322,324–326). Responses, to varying degrees, have been described with all these agents, although specific information is lacking, since all reported series have been small. The long-acting somatostatin analog octreotide (see below) is now considered to be the drug of choice because of its improved efficacy over alternative therapies (313,314).

Control of the somatostatinoma syndrome. The somatostatinoma syndrome differs from other pancreatic endocrine tumors in that the agent most commonly employed for medical management of these tumors (octreotide, see below) is a somatostatin receptor agonist and therefore cannot be used for control of somatostatinoma. Consequently, medical therapy of the somatostatinoma syndrome is limited to symptomatic management of the diabetes (either oral agents or low-dose insulin) and nutritional deficiencies (total parenteral nutrition) (327,328).

Medical Management with Octreotide. Somatostatin has a number of potentially beneficial effects in the management of most pancreatic endocrine tumor syndromes. Somatostatin inhibits the release of many hormones from endocrine cells, including pancreatic islet cells, and in addition has specific end-organ inhibitory effects on gastric acid secretion, pancreatic exocrine secretion, intestinal absorption, and gastrointestinal motility (329–332). Administration of native somatostatin by continuous infusion to a number of patients with functional endocrine tumors of the pancreas demonstrated symptomatic improvement in patients with insulinoma, gastrinoma, glucagonoma, and VIP-oma (322,331–334). However, because of its extremely short half-life, somatostatin has limited therapeutic efficacy (313,334,335).

Recently, a long-acting synthetic octapeptide analog of somatostatin, octreotide acetate (Sandostatin), has been developed (313,335). In addition to having a du-

ration of action that is 33 times longer than that of native somatostatin, octreotide is also extremely potent. For example, in the rat, octreotide is 70-fold more potent in inhibiting growth hormone release, threefold more potent in inhibiting insulin release, 23-fold more potent in inhibiting glucose release, and 80-fold more potent in inhibiting acid secretion than native somatostatin (313,334–335). Because of its longer duration of action ($t_{1/2}$ 100 min), octreotide can be given by intermittent subcutaneous injection two or three times daily (313,335). Octreotide is usually started at a dose of 50–150 μg two or three times daily, and the dose can be increased up to 450 μg three times per day (313,335).

In *gastrinoma*, octreotide effectively inhibits gastric acid output in most patients by a direct effect on parietal cells as well as by inhibiting gastrin production by the tumor (297,298,313). One of the potential benefits of octreotide in patients with gastrinoma is decreased serum gastrin level, limiting the potential long-term side effects of chronic hypergastrinemia (i.e., the potential for ECL-cell hyperplasia and gastric carcinoid tumor formation) (297,298,300,313). However, because the incidence of gastric carcinoids appears to be low and because extremely effective oral gastric acid antisecretory agents are readily available, the use of long-term octreotide for this application is limited by the need for repeated subcutaneous injections and by the potential side effects of long-term therapy (e.g., gallstones and steatorrhea) (297,298,300,313). Short-term use in *insulinoma* (see section below) has demonstrated an improvement in symptoms in at least 50% of patients, with a reduction in plasma insulin levels occurring in 65% (313). Octreotide has been shown to be extremely effective in controlling *carcinoid* tumor syndrome symptoms (335–337). Flushing improved in 85% of cases (disappearing completely in 50%), and diarrhea improved in 75% of cases (disappearing completely in 25%) (335–337). In addition, 24 hr urinary 5-HIAA levels were reduced by >50% in 68% of cases and were normalized in 5% (335–337). Octreotide decreases plasma glucagon levels in 80–90% of patients with *glucagonoma* and normalizes plasma glucagon levels in 10–20% (313,314). The rash improves in 90% of patients and disappears completely in 30% (313,314). The weight loss and diarrhea seen in the glucagonoma syndrome also improved in most patients (313,314). Plasma VIP levels and symptoms improve dramatically in most patients with *VIP-oma* (>75%) within 24 hr of commencing therapy (313,314,335). In one study, the diarrhea was totally abolished by octreotide in 65% of patients (313). In another study, only 10% of patients had a complete response, but the diarrhea decreased in 90% of patients and the response was maintained for at least 6 months (314). However, there have been reports of patients becoming refractory to increasing doses of octreotide. These patients may respond to combined therapy with octreotide and glucocorticoids (295,313,337). In patients with *GRF-omas,* octreotide has been useful in controlling the symptoms of growth hormone excess as well as in reducing the levels of circulating growth hormone and IGF-I for up to 4 months; therefore, it is the drug of choice for the management of the endocrine syndrome in these patients (292,313,338–340). Octreotide either significantly suppresses or normalizes growth hormone and IGF-I levels in almost all cases of GRF-oma, and in some cases reduction in the size of the pituitary gland has been documented as well (292,313,338,340,341). It appears that the major site of action of octreotide in patients with acromegaly due to GRF-omas is the pituitary gland and not the pancreatic endocrine tumor itself (338). Some (338,339), but not others (313), have reported that octreotide is useful in the management of *ectopic ACTH production* by pancreatic endocrine tumor. Octreotide may also be beneficial in controlling nonspecific symptoms of fatigue and abdominal pain, as was demonstrated in four patients with nonfunctional endocrine tumors of the pancreas (313). However, its routine use in patients with *PP-oma* or *nonfunctional endocrine tumor* of the pancreas as well as for gastric and duodenal carcinoid tumors is not recommended. Similarly, as was mentioned above, the use of octreotide in patients with *somatostatinoma* is not recommended. Octreotide has been given to one somatostinoma patient (313). The serum somatostatin level was unaltered following two 200 μg doses, but the postprandial increase in somatostatin concentration was abolished (313).

Side effects of octreotide are generally not severe enough to warrant discontinuation of therapy. Most patients experience pain at the injection site and occasionally postprandial hyperglycemia is noted (313,314). Steatorrhea, a common finding, is usually not limiting at lower doses but may become a problem with high doses (313,335). Gallbladder dysfunction especially with gallstone formation is a potential concern (313,335). There is only a limited experience with long-term therapy using octreotide for enteropancreatic neuroendocrine tumors. Since gallstones develop slowly, it is unclear at present whether this potential side effect is likely to cause significant morbidity. In addition, tachyphylaxis may also become a problem in patients who receive prolonged octreotide therapy. Some patients appear to develop increasing dose requirements with time (313,344). However, the ideal method for establishing dose requirements has not yet been ascertained, and, until this has been formalized, it will not be possible to assess the true potential for tachyphylaxis. At present the dose is increased progressively until a clinical response is obtained and then is increased again if break-

through occurs (313). Preliminary reports suggest that octreotide may inhibit directly the growth of a small percentage of tumors (292,345). The potential antitumor effect of octreotide is below in the section on management of the tumor.

Surgical Management of the Endocrine Syndrome. The role of surgery in the management of the entero-pancreatic neuroendocrine syndrome in patients with MEN-I is limited by the availability in recent years of safe and effective pharmacological agents (300,301, 313,334,345) as well as by the low likelihood of surgical cure of the endocrine syndrome in these patients. Surgical extirpation of the tumor itself is discussed in the next section, although it must be recognized that removal of the source of the excessive hormone production, if successful, would in theory be the ideal approach for management of the endocrine syndrome. In practice, however, surgical removal of the primary tumor to cure the endocrine syndrome is frequently not feasible in patients with MEN-I either because liver metastases already are present (especially with regard to the carcinoid tumor syndrome, glucagonoma, and VIP-oma) or because there are multiple primary tumors (especially with gastrinoma) at the time of initial presentation with the hormonal syndrome (292,346, 347). An exception to this rule of thumb in patients with MEN-I is the insulinoma syndrome, in which primary removal is indicated because the tumor is solitary and benign in >85% of cases (see below).

In patients with MEN-I and Zollinger-Ellison syndrome, the endocrine syndrome can be addressed surgically by targeting the gastrin end-organ, namely, the stomach. However, because of the availability of safe and effective medical agents and because of the morbidity associated with the surgical procedures required, surgery is limited for this application as well. Total gastrectomy, once the mainstay of therapy in these patients, is now indicated only in the rare situation in which a patient is unable or is unwilling to take medications (300). The role of parietal cell vagotomy (PCV) is controversial (297,298,300). Although PCV reduces the subsequent dose requirements for adequate control of acid output, it will not entirely prevent the subsequent need for any medical therapy in all patients. The potency of omeprazole and the recognition that it can be used in lower doses argue against the routine use of PCV in patients with Zollinger-Ellison syndrome and MEN-I (297,298).

In contrast to the role for abdominal surgery, a possible role for the control of gastric acid hypersecretion exists for parathyroidectomy in MEN-I patients with hyperparathyroidism and Zollinger-Ellison syndrome (299). Prior to the availability of omeprazole, gastric acid hypersecretion itself was an indication for parathyroidectomy in patients with MEN-I (297,298,300, 303), because successful parathyroidectomy increased the sensitivity to therapy with histamine H_2-receptor antagonists (Fig. 5) (303,304). Hyperparathyroid-induced hypercalcemia is no longer an absolute indication for parathyroidectomy in this setting, since omeprazole permits effective control of gastric acid output even in the presence of hypercalcemia (303,304). We currently recommended that all patients with MEN-I, hyperparathyroidism, and Zollinger-Ellison syndrome be considered for parathyroidectomy, since correction of the hypercalcemia will ameliorate the manifestations of the Zollinger-Ellison syndrome in most cases (297,298,303) and may even result in apparent disappearance of the Zollinger-Ellison syndrome completely (Fig. 3). It must also be stressed that patients with MEN-I who have undergone effective surgery for hyperparathyroidism are still at risk for recurrent parathyroid disease (292,297,298,346). For this reason, MEN-I patients with Zollinger-Ellison syndrome and previously treated hyperparathyroidism should continue with effective, potent antisecretory therapy (i.e., omeprazole) long term and should be screened regularly via serum calcium levels so that recurrent hypercalcemia can be recognized rapidly prior to the development of uncontrolled gastric acid hypersecretion.

Management of the Tumor

The natural history of metastatic insulinoma, VIP-oma, glucagonoma, somatostatinoma, and GRF-oma in both sporadic and MEN-I-associated disease is not clear; until recently, no effective medical therapy was available for the hormone excess state, and patients frequently succumbed to complications arising from the hormonal excess per se (292,297,298,346). Now that effective therapy (octreotide, etc.) for the hormone excess is available, it is likely that an increasingly important determinant of long-term survival in these patients will be the malignant potential of the tumor itself (292,297,298,346). This has been convincingly shown with gastrinomas, for which effective antihormonal therapy has been available for >20 years (297,298). Fifty to seventy percent of deaths in patients with metastatic gastrinoma are due to tumor progression (292,345,348,349). In various studies on unoperated gastrinoma, the overall 5 year survival with metastatic disease ranges from 20% to 75% (20–30% at 10 years) (292,297,298,350). Furthermore, a number of studies (292,297,298,350) have shown that long-term survival is related to extent of disease. In one recent study of 92 patients with sporadic gastrinoma (351), patients in whom no tumor was found at exploratory laparotomy had a 5 year survival approaching 100%, whereas those with liver metastases had a 5 year survival of ~20% (351). Recent evidence suggests that these facts apply both to the sporadic as well as to

MEN-I-associated disease. In contrast to some studies (292,297,298,352,353) suggesting that islet cell tumors in the setting of MEN-I were less likely to metastasize to the liver, a number of other studies (346,354–356) have suggested that this is not true and that death from metastatic disease is a real consideration in both MEN-I-associated and sporadic cases. These data can probably be extrapolated to other noninsulinoma enteropancreatic neuroendocrine tumors, including glucagonoma, VIP-oma, somatostatinoma, GRF-oma, and midgut carcinoid tumors as well, because the percentage of patients with malignant disease is similar to that found in gastrinoma (292,297,298,346). Therefore, if the tumor is likely to be fully resectable, this should be attempted early since, except for insulinoma (see below), these tumors have a high likelihood of being malignant (60–90%), and, if they are treated early, there should be a better chance of curing the disease.

However, there are a number of reasons not to operate on patients with enteropancreatic neuroendocrine tumors, especially those with MEN-I. It is inadvisable to operate on a patient whose endocrine syndrome is well controlled by medical therapy and who is unlikely to outlive the tumor due to age or concomitant medical illness. In addition, patients with widely metastatic disease are generally unlikely to benefit from surgery (292,297,298,346). For this reason, it is essential to exclude liver metastases in any patient in whom surgery is being contemplated. Furthermore, whereas localized insulinoma and VIP-oma are potentially curable in the patient with or without MEN-I, at present, gastrinomas (the most common functional pancreatic endocrine tumor in patients with MEN-I) are not easily cured surgically (297,298, 347,357,358). Although controversy regarding the correct approach to patients with gastrinomas in the setting of MEN-I exists, many authorities believe that these patients should not have surgery because the likelihood of cure is extremely low (297,298,347, 357,358). This issue is discussed in more detail below. Finally, so little is known about the natural history of gastric ECL-omas, which are commonly seen in MEN-I-associated disease, that there is no evidence available yet to justify a surgical approach in these cases. Many of these tumors are known to be at least locally invasive; however, whether these tumors actually represent a significant mortality or morbidity risk remains to be established.

Determining the Extent of Enteropancreatic Neuroendocrine Disease. The major goals for determining the extent of disease are to localize the enteropancreatic neuroendocrine tumor and to identify patients with widespread metastases who are unlikely to benefit from attempts at surgical resection (292,297,298, 327). Enteropancreatic neuroendocrine tumors spread first to local and regional lymph nodes and from there generally to the liver (292,297,298). Bone metastases generally occur late in the course of disease, and distant metastases to the lungs, brain, or other sites are extremely rare (292,297,298). Therefore, the primary concern in determining the extent of disease is to establish whether liver metastases have developed. The most valuable imaging modalities for this purpose are MRI and the selective abdominal arteriogram (with or without provocation) (292,297,298,256), and no patient should be taken to surgery without having first undergone both of these studies or their equivalent. In addition, because both MRI and selective abdominal arteriography occasionally miss liver metastases (359,360), bone scanning should be performed if both studies are negative. If all three of these modalities suggest the presence of localized and resectable disease, other localizing modalities (see below) should be utilized to aid the surgeon in locating primary tumors, which are often small and difficult to find at operation and which, especially in the case of MEN-I-associated disease, may even be multiple (292,297,298,361). Most surgical series of pancreatic endocrine tumors include a significant percentage of patients in whom no tumor is found at surgery (292,297,348,351,362,363). However, with recent improvements in tumor localization techniques, the percentage of patients in whom no tumor is found can be expected to decline. Patients with liver metastases should undergo surgical resection only under special circumstances, which are discussed below in the section on the management of patients with metastatic disease. A brief discussion of the utility of the various available imaging modalities follows.

Traditional radiological procedures (ultrasound, CT, MRI, and bone scan) that are useful for tumors in general are also the primary initial localization methods employed for enteropancreatic neuroendocrine tumors (292,297,298). The "gold standard" is angiography, and selective angiography provides the most complete information (292,297,298).

Ultrasonography is useful as an initial test (364,365). There is no radiation risk, and it localizes from 10% to 20% of primary tumors and documents from 14% to 20% of liver metastases in the case of insulinoma and gastrinoma (365,366). Occasionally, ultrasound detects extrapancreatic gastrinomas that are not seen using other modalities (365). There have not been any detailed studies on the utility of ultrasound in other endocrine tumor types. Computed tomography scanning is the initial imaging modality of choice, because it can identify pancreatic lesions that are poorly visualized by ultrasound (because of intervening bowel gas) and MRI (because of motion artifacts arising from the aorta) (297,298,359). Computed tomography scanning localizes 20–40% of primary pancreatic insulinomas and gastrinomas and from 35–74% of liver metastases from insulinoma or gastrinomas (297,298,359). The localization rate of MRI for primary endocrine tumors

of the pancreas is similar to that of ultrasound or CT scanning (297,298,367,368). However, its major contribution in the workup for enteropancreatic neuroendocrine tumors is to document liver metastases (297,298,367,368). A recent study (368) found that the sensitivity of MRI, in comparison to other noninvasive imaging modalities, for diagnosing liver metastases was higher (e.g., 83% for gastrinomas), but the specificity was slightly lower (e.g., 88% for gastrinomas), because MRI was unable to distinguish between hypervascular endocrine tumor metastases and liver hemangiomata. As was mentioned above, bone metastases occur late in the course of disease in patients with metastatic enteropancreatic neuroendocrine tumors (369). Invariably, liver metastases are already present (292,297,298,369). However, bone scanning is useful in certain circumstances such as in determining whether attempted resection of isolated liver metastases is likely to be successful or whether an attempt at regional intrahepatic therapy should be considered in patients with widely metastatic liver disease who have not responded to peripheral chemotherapy. Angiography is useful for localizing both primary tumors as well as liver metastases and is essential in all patients prior to surgery to prevent unnecessary operations in patients who may have unresectable disease not identified by other imaging modalities (292,297, 298,360,370–372). Selective abdominal angiography localizes from 50% to 90% of primary insulinomas and from 33% to 86% of primary gastrinomas (292,297, 298,360,371,372). The difference in localization rates for primary insulinomas and gastrinomas is most likely a reflection of their different anatomical locations; angiography is likely to be more useful for pancreatic primary tumors than for extrapancreatic primary tumors. Angiography will detect up to 86% of all enteropancreatic neuroendocrine tumors that have metastasized to the liver (292,297,298,360,371,372), and in one study a combination of CT scanning plus selective angiography detected 98% of all hepatic metastases (360). Recently, selective angiography has been combined with provocative hormonal testing (see below).

The major limiting factor in the ability of traditional imaging modalities to localize endocrine tumors is tumor size (359,360). For example, using any of the standard imaging modalities (ultrasound, CT scanning, selective angiography, or MRI) <10% of tumors smaller than 1 cm, 30–40% of tumors 1–3 cm, and 70–80% of tumors larger than 3 cm were detected (292,297, 298,359,360). Furthermore, traditional imaging modalities are also of limited use in MEN-I patients because they fail to provide functional localization. For example, MEN-I patients with Zollinger-Ellison syndrome are now known generally to have multiple microscopic duodenal primary gastrinomas (292,297,298,357,373). Not only are these lesions commonly not visualized using traditional imaging modalities (297,298), but it is also likely that traditional imaging modalities may localize a second enteropancreatic neuroendocrine tumor type (e.g., a pancreatic PP-oma), which, despite being readily imaged, is not responsible for the hormonal syndrome being evaluated (292,297,298,361). Angiographically directed hormone sampling techniques and radiolabeled hormone scans have recently been developed to permit functional localization of enteropancreatic neuroendocrine tumors (374–376). Moreover, angiographically directed hormone sampling techniques, such as portal venous sampling for hormonal gradients or stimulation with various provocative agents during angiography followed by hormonal sampling, are not limited by tumor size and may therefore improve the ability to localize tumors preoperatively. Intraoperative localizing techniques (e.g., hand-held ultrasound probes or intraoperative endoscopy with transillumination) are also useful in the localization of small endocrine tumors not visualized preoperatively (377,378).

By detecting a gradient at a specific location along the portal vein or one of its tributaries, portal venous sampling (PVS) for gastrin localizes 73% of gastrinomas (379). However, because of their typical distribution within the upper GI tract, gastrinomas invariably localize to the duodenum/pancreatic head region (364,381), limiting the utility of the test for precise localization. Despite this limitation, functional localization is important in Zollinger-Ellison syndrome patients with MEN-I who are being considered for surgery in that it confirms the presence of one or more functional gastrinomas as opposed to another functional or nonfunctional tumor type in the region of interest. Because insulinomas are more variably distributed in the pancreas, PVS for insulin to localize insulinomas may be of more use for precise functional localization (see below). The utility of PVS for localization of other enteropancreatic neuroendocrine tumors both in MEN-I and in sporadic disease has not been determined.

Angiography with selective intraarterial secretion injection and gastrin determination in hepatic venous samples permits selective provocation for gastrinoma localization in tandem with standard angiography (382,383). The technique requires the additional placement of hepatic venous catheters for gastrin sampling in response to the arterial secretin stimulation (383). Preliminary data suggest that this technique is as good as PVS for localizing primary gastrinomas (384). One potential benefit of this technique over PVS is the ability to identify the presence of liver metastases by documenting a gastrin response to secretin administration directly into the hepatic artery. A similar provocative test using calcium to stimulate insulin release from insulinoma has also been developed (see below) (385).

A type of radionuclide scanning utilizes the fact that neuroendocrine cells commonly have somatostatin receptors (374). In one study of 15 pancreatic endocrine tumors, all 15 contained somatostatin receptors (386). Pancreatic endocrine tumors can be localized by injecting radiolabeled octreotide and then performing standard nuclear imaging (375). The utility of this technique remains to be defined.

Intraoperative ultrasound (IOUS) using a hand-held transducer to examine the pancreas and other potential sites for enteropancreatic neuroendocrine tumors has been shown to be very useful in the detection of these tumors (377); IOUS localizes 90% of all insulinomas and 83% of all gastrinomas (377). This modality is not able to detect gastrinomas as well as it is able to detect insulinomas, because it is less sensitive for extrapancreatic as compared to intrapancreatic lesions. The combination of PVS and intraoperative ultrasound will allow pancreatic primary tumors to be found at operation in virtually 100% of patients even if preoperative imaging studies are negative (377). Recently, intraoperative endoscopic ultrasound (as well as endoscopic transillumination) of the duodenum has been used to localize tumors in a small number of patients (378,382). The utility of this instrument in the detection of duodenal wall endocrine tumors remains to be assessed.

Management of Nonmetastatic Disease. As was mentioned above, all MEN-I patients with potentially resectable functional enteropancreatic neuroendocrine tumors should probably be considered for curative surgery. This is particularly true for insulinoma (see below), carcinoid tumor, glucagonoma, and VIP-oma, all of which are likely to derive benefit both with regard to the tumor itself and with regard to the tumor syndrome should surgery be successful. The approach to MEN-I patients with Zollinger-Ellison syndrome is less well defined because of the multiplicity of duodenal primary tumors (373) and because of the uncertainties regarding the prospects of long-term cure as a result of surgical intervention (292,297,357,387). The controversy regarding how best to approach MEN-I patients with apparently localized Zollinger-Ellison syndrome ranges from the opinions of certain authorities (388,389), who believe that all patients should undergo surgery, to the opinions of others (381), who believe that none should undergo surgery. Still others (292,297,390) believe that certain subgroups of patients (those patients believed to be more at risk over the long term) should undergo surgery because of recent evidence suggesting that Zollinger-Ellison syndrome in the setting of MEN-I is not a more benign disease than that occurring in the sporadic setting, as was previously thought.

In contrast to earlier studies (292,297,361,391) suggesting that gastrinomas in the setting of MEN-I could occur in both the pancreas and the duodenum, a recent study (373) provided strong evidence that virtually all gastrinomas in the setting of MEN-I occur in the duodenum. Therefore, it is possible that surgical cure of the Zollinger-Ellison syndrome in patients with MEN-I could be achieved by performing a pancreaticoduodenectomy (a Whipple's procedure) on all MEN-I patients with localized disease, as has been suggested by at least one authority (388). However, it is unknown at present whether such extensive surgery is actually more likely to achieve cure than simple tumor enucleation, which is the standard current approach (293,297,348,351,364). The increased morbidity and mortality associated with a pancreaticoduodenectomy instead of a less aggressive enucleation procedure would be justified only if the chances of long-term cure were significantly higher with the more aggressive surgical approach, and this too is unknown at present. With regard to the possibility of performing less aggressive surgery in all patients with MEN-I and Zollinger-Ellison syndrome, one proponent of this approach (389) has documented normal postoperative fasting serum gastrin levels in ten of 11 patients who came to surgery (91%). However, only three of 11 patients (27%) had negative secretin stimulation tests postoperatively, so it is not clear whether simple enucleation of all neuroendocrine tumor tissue found at surgery will cure the vast majority of MEN-I patients with Zollinger-Ellison syndrome (292,297,298,347). Finding a tumor does not mean that it is functional, nor that it is the only functional gastrinoma present (388). It is unknown whether partial tumor resection (i.e., unsuccessful simple enucleation) will limit the likelihood of a patient later developing metastatic disease.

The major argument against a standardized nonoperative approach toward patients with MEN-I and localized Zollinger-Ellison syndrome is that this approach does nothing to prevent the later development of metastatic disease, which can ultimately lead to death at an early age from tumor growth. Recent studies have shown that tumor growth in MEN-I patients with gastrinoma does occur, and that death from metastatic disease is a real possibility (293,297,358).

Serum PP level has been suggested as a predictor of the presence of a resectable tumor (390). However, a recent study showed no correlation between serum PP levels and the presence or absence of a tumor at surgery (393). These data suggest that PP levels are not useful in predicting which MEN-I patients with Zollinger-Ellison syndrome are likely to benefit from surgery. Others have suggested that PVS be used to identify patients likely to benefit from surgery (389). However, PVS cannot distinguish between lesions located in the pancreatic head or the proximal duodenal submucosa, nor can it distinguish between primary tumors and regional lymph node metastases, and it is also unable to provide information on the number of functional lesions that exist in a particular patient (372,379). Moreover, a subgroup of patients with

MEN-I and Zollinger-Ellison syndrome were subjected to surgery based on the results of PVS, and none of those patients was cured. Finally, it has also been suggested that patients with imagable tumors who have a strong family history of aggressive disease be considered for surgical resection.

Data from carcinoid tumors (292,336) suggest that the likelihood of developing liver metastases is associated with the size of the primary lesion. Furthermore, aggressive surgery in patients with large pancreatic masses may have a beneficial effect on overall survival (396). For these reasons, we currently operate only on MEN-I patients with Zollinger-Ellison syndrome who also have a large pancreatic mass (>3 cm) regardless of whether the mass itself is believed to be the functional tumor or not. With this approach in a recent study (396), 50% of the patients who underwent surgery had invasive or metastatic disease, suggesting an association between tumor size and metastases for pancreatic neuroendocrine tumors. However, it has not been established whether this approach will increase life expectancy.

In contrast to the surgical approach recommended for the tumors mentioned above, a "wait and see" approach is currently advised for ECL-omas, since surgery (partial or total gastric resection) is likely to be associated with significant morbidity. Information is insufficient at present to justify surgery; the natural history of ECL-omas is unknown. Despite the fact that larger lesions are easily removed endoscopically (292), the multiplicity of these lesions in many patients with MEN-I (Fig. 5) makes this approach impractical.

Because of the uncertainties associated with abdominal surgery in MEN-I patients with enteropancreatic neuroendocrine tumors, we currently believe that abdominal surgery should be performed only on these patients within the setting of a clinical trial and only by surgeons who are experienced in dealing with MEN-I. Prior to surgery, all patients should receive pneumococcal vaccine in anticipation of a possible splenectomy, which is sometimes necessary during distal pancreatic resections (292,297,298,351). In patients with gastrinomas or somatostatinoma, a bowel preparation preoperatively is also required in anticipation of a possible duodenotomy (292,297,298,351). It is essential that the surgery be done by a surgeon who is experienced in operating on patients with endocrine tumors of the pancreas (292,297,298,351). As was described above, intraoperative ultrasound and transillumination of the duodenum are extremely helpful to the experienced surgeon in locating pancreatic and duodenal tumors, respectively. Intraoperative ultrasound may also permit the identification of malignant infiltration thereby permitting the appropriate resection to be done (370,377).

At exploration, the liver should be carefully examined for metastatic disease (292,297,298,351). The entire abdomen, especially the pancreas, proximal small intestine, common bile duct region, peripancreatic tissues, and retroperitoneum, must be carefully explored for evidence of the tumor (301,351). This approach requires an extended Kocher maneuver (301). Even if a tumor is found, the entire abdomen still must be examined, because there may be more than one tumor causing the disease, and there may be other tumors (especially if the patient is likely to have MEN-I) (292,297,298,353,361,394). Isolated small insulinomas (see below) should be enucleated, since they are rarely malignant. Isolated noninsulinoma tumors in the pancreatic body or tail should be removed en bloc by distal pancreatectomy, since they are often malignant (292,297,298,351). Noninsulinoma lesions of the pancreatic head require careful enucleation only, since a more aggressive resection (e.g., a Whipple's procedure) has not been shown to provide an increased benefit that outweighs the increased risk of morbidity associated with more aggressive surgery (292,297,298, 351). If an isolated, resectable liver metastasis is found at surgery, it should be removed. In the event that no tumor is found, blind resection of the pancreas is not recommended, and total pancreatectomy is contraindicated (351). Because of the distribution of pancreatic endocrine tumors within the pancreas itself and because, in some syndromes, enteropancreatic neuroendocrine tumors are commonly extrapancreatic in location, wide resections may not cure the disease and may leave the patient with additional morbidity from pancreatic insufficiency.

As methods for tumor localization improve, and as surgeons develop more experience with the methods to find and safely remove enteropancreatic neuroendocrine tumors, results of surgery can be expected to improve. In a recent study of 73 patients with sporadic gastrinoma 58% of patients were free of disease immediately postoperatively, and 30% remained disease-free at 5 years (351). However, using the surgical approach described above, no patients with MEN-I-associated gastrinoma have been cured (347). There have been reports of both long-term surgical cure and subsequent relapses in patients with glucagonomas (318,319). However, it is difficult to assess the percentage of patients whose tumors can be resected likely to be cured surgically, because, in the available studies, most glucagonomas were already metastatic at the time of surgery (296,316,319,395). Information is limited regarding surgical cure rates of the remaining enteropancreatic neuroendocrine tumors. It is likely that cure rates for the other tumors will be similar to those for sporadic gastrinomas, because their malignancy rates and likelihood of multiplicity are similar.

Management of Metastatic Disease. Patients with widely metastatic disease will require life-long medical management of the endocrine syndrome (omeprazole in the case of gastrinoma, octreotide for the other tumors), since surgery will not cure the endocrine syndrome (292,297,298,301). The role of debulking operations in an attempt to limit both the hormonal drive of the endocrine syndrome as well as the rate at which metastatic disease progresses is controversial (292, 297,298,393). In general, patients with widely metastatic disease should not be subjected to surgery, since the overall prognosis (5 year survival as low as 20% for gastrinomas) does not warrant it. Although most authorities agree that treatment directed against metastatic disease is indicated, controversy exists about when to start therapy and about which modalities to use (292,297,298). The reasons for a lack of consensus are that these tumors are often slow-growing, that patients often feel well once the hormonal excess is controlled, and that the available treatment strategies are toxic and are not uniformly effective (292,297, 298). All patients should have a confirmed tissue diagnosis before any of the potentially toxic therapeutic modalities discussed below is introduced.

Chemotherapy. Various chemotherapy regimens have been used in the treatment of metastatic enteropancreatic neuroendocrine tumors (292,297,298). Most studies have considered all pancreatic neuroendocrine tumors as a group or included them in series with metastatic carcinoid tumors, so that it is difficult to determine whether the response rates differ among neuroendocrine tumor types (292,297,298). Some results suggest that not all enteropancreatic neuroendocrine tumors respond equally to chemotherapy (292). For example, the response rate of gastrinomas to streptozotocin is low (5–40%) (396,397,400), whereas the response rate of VIP-omas to streptozotocin was reported to be as high as 90% in one study (400). Dacarbazine (DTIC) appears to be especially effective for glucagonomas (336) but ineffective in other metastatic pancreatic endocrine syndromes (358). The reason for these differences is unclear, because these tumors are all histologically similar, and there is no relationship between the endocrine syndrome and the immunohistochemistry of tissue specimens (297,298,394, 398). It is also unclear at present whether chemotherapy response rates differ in patients with or without MEN-I.

Streptozotocin appears to be the best single agent in the treatment of metastatic enteropancreatic neuroendocrine tumors, with objective remissions in 41–60% of cases (292,399,400). Streptozotocin plus 5-fluorouracil and/or doxorubicin has been reported to cause objective responses in 5–80% of patients, with a mean response rate of 40% (292,315,336,399,401). The combination of streptozotocin plus 5-fluorouracil has been more effective than streptozotocin alone (63% vs. 36%). Therefore, this regimen, with or without doxorubicin, is the current therapy of choice for metastatic enteropancreatic neuroendocrine tumors (402). In one study (402), streptozotocin and 5-fluorouracil caused a complete response in 33% of patients. However, a more recent study (401) demonstrated that combination therapy with streptozotocin and doxorubicin was more effective than that with streptozotocin and 5-fluorouracil. Streptozotocin causes significant side effects (403). Nausea and vomiting are extremely common (397), but with the recent availability of the 5-HT$_3$ inhibitor ondansetron, this is no longer a major problem. Renal toxicity occurs in 20–40% of patients, and severe, usually reversible, renal insufficiency can occur (399,404). All patients should be carefully monitored by 24 hr urine measurements for protein and creatinine clearance before each cycle of therapy. As with most chemotherapy, doses may need to be modified to prevent bone marrow depression (404). Patients who are receiving doxorubicin should have a baseline cardiac ejection fraction measurement and should be monitored for the development of cardiotoxicity, although this is unusual with the doses used. Alopecia is common when doxorubicin is used.

Because of the toxicity and generally poor response rates to chemotherapy, some investigators believe that routine chemotherapy should not be given unless the patient is symptomatic from metastatic disease and has clear evidence of tumor progression on imaging studies (292,297,298). Other agents have recently been investigated in an attempt to develop better therapeutic approaches to these tumors.

Interferon. The use of human leukocyte interferon (3–6 million units daily) was assessed in 22 patients with various pancreatic endocrine tumors, many of whom had already failed chemotherapy (405). The overall response rate (decrease of >50% in tumor size or hormone level) was 77%, and VIP-oma patients appeared to respond best (405). A decrease in tumor size was noted in 27% of patients (all of whom had already failed chemotherapy) (405). In a recent study of 12 patients with metastatic gastrinoma, interferon-α (5 million units daily) was found to carry only a marginal benefit (403). In this study (403); tumor size remained stable in about one-third of patients for up to 21 months of treatment. The interferon was well tolerated by most patients (403). To date, there has been only one study examining the use of combination chemotherapy plus interferon in patients with metastatic pancreatic endocrine tumors (406). In this study, a partial response to doxorubicin plus interferon was reported in only three of 16 patients (406). However, there is precedent for a synergistic antitumor effect of interferon and chemotherapeutic agents in the treatment of other gastrointestinal tumors (407,408). In particular, combination interferon and 5-fluorouracil has been more effective than either agent alone in the treatment of metastatic colorectal cancer (407). Although the overall toxicity is unlikely to be significantly higher than with each regimen alone, the potential for synergistic bone marrow depression will have to be carefully assessed. In addition, combination interferon plus 5-fluorouracil has resulted in severe diarrhea, dehydration, sepsis, and death in and least two patients with colorectal cancer (408). This may have been a result of using doses of 5-fluorouracil much higher than those likely to be used for pancreatic endocrine tumor therapy, although this issue will require further study before it can be established whether the potential benefits of combination interferon plus chemotherapy outweighs the potential risks.

Octreotide. Octreotide may be useful in controlling tumor growth in some patients with metastatic endocrine tumors of the pancreas (292,313,344). A number of animal studies have demonstrated that somatostatin analog can inhibit the growth of various tumors (409,410). Preliminary results in humans with carcinoid and other endocrine tumors suggest an overall response rate (decrease in tumor size) of <20% (292,313). However, this poor response may be a dose-dependent phenomenon, and the dose required to inhibit tumor growth consistently (if in fact this is possible) may be much higher than the dose required for hormonal control. This issue requires further study.

Regional therapies. Hepatic artery embolization or ligation has been used effectively in many patients with enteropancreatic neuroendocrine tumors, including carcinoid tumors that have metastasized to the liver (292,336,411,412). Reports of symptomatic improvement range from 14% in one study (411) to as high as 80–90% in others (336,412–413). Intrahepatic artery streptozotocin has also been shown to be effective in isolated patients with large tumor loads in the liver causing symptoms (336,414). In some cases, interferon has been utilized in addition to regional therapy modalities (336). Combination hepatic artery embolization plus postocclusion chemotherapy has been reported to cause a complete symptomatic response in 64% of patients and may be more beneficial than either regional treatment modality alone (336,412). It must be recognized that these highly invasive approaches are only palliative and that side effects may be severe (411,412). Because these tumors grow slowly, regional palliation may provide significant long-lasting symptom relief in carefully selected patients (411). Regional therapy should be considered in patients with uncontrolled hormonal syndromes who are no longer responsive to other treatment modalities. By the time patients are being considered for regional hepatic therapies, bone metastases (369) may be present, so regional therapy may be of limited value in controlling metastatic spread. However, hepatic artery embolization with or without interferon or chemotherapy may be very helpful in decreasing plasma hormone levels, making control of symptoms easier in patients with severe symptoms of hormonal excess no longer responsive to octreotide.

Debulking surgery. As was mentioned above, the role of debulking surgery (i.e., surgical removal of all resectable tumor) in the control of metastatic disease is controversial (292,297,298,393). Proponents of debulking maintain that removal of tumor tissue decreases the hormone levels in patients with endocrine tumors of the pancreas, making it easier to control the hormonal syndrome medically, and also decrease the rate at which metastatic disease progresses (316, 327,362,393,415,418). Debulking surgery has been recommended in patients with VIP-omas (327), glucagonomas (316,362), somatostatinomas (417), and intestinal carcinoid tumors (336); it may lead to a marked improvement in symptoms. Recently, the successful resection of all metastatic gastrinoma has been reported in three of 20 patients with extensive disease, two of whom subsequently appeared to be cured (396). However, it remains to be proved whether the potential long-term benefit of such therapy outweighs the risks, especially in patients whose endocrine syndrome is easily controlled with medical therapy. It is possible that patients with widely metastatic disease and severe endocrine symptoms who have not responded to chemotherapy and octreotide (i.e., those who have exhausted all the available therapeutic modalities) may benefit from debulking surgery. Debulking surgery should be considered in patients with uncontrolled hormonal syndromes that are no longer responsive to other treatment modalities.

Insulinoma Treatment

The multiplicity of islet cell tumors and the inherent abnormalities of the pancreatic islet in MEN-I (419) underly the controversy regarding the surgical approach to these patients. All agree that surgical treatment is the most effective therapy available. The goals of surgical management of insulinoma are alleviation of potentially life-threatening hypoglycemic events and preservation of pancreatic endocrine and exocrine function. Many investigators regard subtotal pancreatectomy (85%) and enucleation of any other detectable lesions in the pancreatic head as the appropriate surgical approach in both adults and children (420). Some advocate removal of as much of the pancreas as possible to avoid future tumors from developing, although the prevention of such metachronous pancreatic syndromes is purely speculative. Recurrence of

hypoglycemia after initial operative therapy may be as high as 42% (420), indicating that the initial surgery is often inadequate. In our experience recurrence has been far lower.

Pharmacotherapy of insulinoma is limited but should be tried in all patients prior to surgery to establish a possible therapeutic option. Patients with life-threatening hypoglycemia who do not respond to preoperative trial of medical therapy are candidates for more extensive surgery, particularly if no lesions are identified at surgery, while more limited surgery is an option if hypoglycemia can be treated medically. The mainstay of medical therapy is diazoxide (421). Diazoxide decreases insulin concentrations as well as decreases glucose utilization rates as demonstrated by euglycemic clamp technique, suggesting that it may decrease peripheral tissue sensitivity to insulin (274).

Several studies have demonstrated variable degrees of success with somatotostatin analogs in the treatment of benign and malignant insulinoma (422,423). Despite suppression of insulin levels, episodes of clinically significant hypoglycemia may continue due to concomitant suppression of counterregulatory hormones (424). There are a few uncontrolled reports in the literature describing successful alleviation of hypoglycemia with diphenylhydantoin (425,426), calcium channel blockers (43,280,426), and beta blockers (427) in small numbers of patients with insulinoma. These therapies, in concert with frequent small feedings are unsatisfactory in most patients and can be associated with significant side effects, the most serious of which is hypoglycemia that can result in permanent neurological damage.

Treatment of Bronchial and Thymic Carcinoid Tumors

Surgery remains the mainstay of treatment of bronchial and thymic carcinoid tumors. Although conservative surgery for bronchial carcinoid tumor was associated with excellent survival, regardless of lymph node involvement (428), others have shown that node involvement predicts a poorer long-term survival. Likewise, because of the malignant nature of thymic carcinoid tumors, resection with careful nodal dissection is recommended. While mediastinal radiation is not universally advocated for lymph node involvement, possibly because of the relatively indolent nature of these tumors, some centers employ it routinely (429).

While streptozotocin and interferon-α have been used as chemotherapy for malignant foregut carcinoid tumors, each has been of limited utility in decreasing tumor growth or symptoms in this setting. Similarly, histamine antagonists and somatostatin analogs may reduce serotonin production and may decrease flushing, if present, but have limited ability to reduce tumor mass (400).

Pituitary Tumor Treatment

The treatment of pituitary tumors in MEN-I does not differ from the treatment of sporadic pituitary tumors; treatment includes surgical and X-ray extirpation and medications. Generic considerations pertinent to transsphenoidal surgery and radiation therapy and the relative utility of these approaches in each tumor type are discussed in this section.

Transsphenoidal resection of a pituitary tumor is advisable for treatment of mass effects on the optic system, to remove or to debulk aggressive tumors (usually in conjunction with radiation therapy), or as definitive treatment of hormonal excess. The goal of surgery is to remove the adenoma selectively and to preserve as much normal pituitary tissue as possible. The mortality of transsphenoidal surgery should be 1% or less (431). Perioperative diabetes insipidus, cerebrospinal fluid leak, and/or meningitis are uncommon (<10%). Permanent complications include diabetes insipidus, injury to the carotid arteries, nasal injury, optic nerve damage, injury to nerves of the cavernous sinus (causing ptosis or diplopia), and partial or complete hypopituitarism. These occur in <5% of patients after initial resection of a microadenoma, but are more common after resection of larger tumors or larger amounts of normal pituitary tissue (or stalk), or after repeat surgery (432,433).

Radiation therapy is, in general, a palliative measure to prevent further tumor growth; tumoral hormone secretion may decrease also. Conventional radiation therapy, delivered at a total dose of 4,500 cGY (rad) in 25 fractional doses over 35 days using a three-field technique, avoids the complications of optic neuritis and cortical necrosis associated with larger total and fractional doses (434). Temporal hair loss at the time of therapy, and hypopituitarism, which may develop many years later, are the main side effects. TSH deficiency is seen in 10–20% and gonadotropin deficiency in 33–50% of patients evaluated 6–15 years after treatment with 4,500 cGY for Cushing's disease or acromegaly (435,436).

Radiosurgery of the pituitary gland using heavy charged particles has been available at a few centers since the 1950s. The limited reports, using three or four fractionated doses (60–150 Gy) over 5 days and a stereotactic system for dose localization within 0.3 mm, indicate response rates for Cushing's syndrome and acromegaly similar to those after conventional radiation therapy (437–439). Side effects include visual field defects and transient partial third nerve palsies (<10%) and endocrine deficiency (~30%).

What is the approach to specific tumor types? Controversy exists regarding the optimal therapy for the patient who does not have a hormone excess syndrome, visual system abnormalities, or evidence of an invasive tumor. We adopt a "watch and wait" approach that requires education of the patient regarding the signs of pituitary apoplexy; meticulous interval evaluation (initially every 6 months) of tumor size, visual integrity, and hormone deficiency; and prompt intervention if deterioration is noted. This strategy presumes that the morbidity and mortality of surgical and radiation therapies outweigh the risk of progression, and that follow-up can be diligent and reasonable in expense to the patient. As the natural history of these tumors in a given patient is difficult to predict, early ("prophylactic") intervention is an alternative choice.

Tumors without a clinical syndrome of hormone excess (gonadotropin-secreting, null-cell, or silent types) can require intervention because of tumor growth. Medical therapy with bromocriptine at high doses (20 mg/day) occasionally reduces tumor size in nonfunctioning tumors (440). Surgical and/or radiation therapy is used for invasive tumors. Prompt surgical decompression may reverse new visual field loss.

The treatment choices for prolactinoma differ depending on the tumor size and patient gender. Untreated, sporadic microadenomas either progress, regress, or remain stable, each outcome occurring in about one-third of patients (441). Thus, surgery is not required to prevent predictable tumor growth; moreover, recurrence is common after surgical resection. For these reasons, and given the excellent response to dopamine agonists, surgery is rarely the treatment of choice for a small prolactinoma. Restoration of gonadal function is important to prevent loss of bone mass (442) and to allow fertility. However, observation alone may be chosen if a women has withdrawal bleeding after progesterone, the bone density is normal, and fertility is not desired. Such patients require interval evaluation to assess tumor size, bone density, and clinical symptoms; similarly, periodic follow-up and testosterone administration (100 mg i.m. every 2 weeks) may be sufficient for the man with a microadenoma. Medical therapy is the treatment of choice for women desiring fertility and for those at risk for bone demineralization (especially with coexisting hyperparathyroidism). Dopamine agonists, bromocriptine or pergolide, normalize prolactin levels in this setting in nearly all patients, providing return of menses and fertility (443). Compliance problems associated with the usual effective three times daily doses of bromocriptine (2.5 mg tid) are not encountered with pergolide, taken once daily (25–75 μg). Side effects of these compounds include nausea, and postural hypotension, which may be reduced by taking them with food or before bed, and by gradual increase in the dose.

The natural history of larger prolactinomas is less well documented, but it is unlikely that a significant proportion regress spontaneously. While the treatment options include periodic follow-up as detailed above, many of these tumors present with symptoms referable to size or growth so that intervention is often required. Medical treatment may reduce both tumor size and prolactin secretion, if the dose of bromocriptine can be increased to 30 mg/day; side effects limit this approach, however (444). Long-acting injectible preparations of bromocriptine, while currently investigational, work as well or better with only transient side effects after each injection (445). Surgical intervention is an alternative in this setting, but normalization of prolactin is uncommon, and recurrence occurs in up to 90% of patients (446–448). In general, prolactin values normalize in a minority of patients after radiation therapy alone, and the full effects of radiotherapy may take years to appear. Combination strategies of bromocriptine, surgery, and/or radiation therapy that overcome the deficiencies of each approach when used alone are employed for patients with more aggressive tumors.

Surgical resection of GH-secreting tumors normalizes GH levels (by the criterion of <5 ng/ml) in only one-half of patients (449–451). A successful outcome is associated with microadenomas and basal GH levels <40 ng/ml, both of which are uncommon in acromegaly. Radiation therapy alone slowly reduces GH values to <5 ng/ml in 69% of patients by 10 years (436), which compares favorably with surgical outcome at 10 years. Although surgery produces a quicker decline in GH values, radiation therapy avoids surgical morbidity. Bromocriptine therapy improves clinical symptoms in ~70% of patients but normalizes GH values in far fewer (452) and has relatively little effect on tumor size (453). Therefore, the agent is not indicated as primary treatment but may be useful as adjunctive therapy after radiation or with octreotide. Octreotide, a long-acting somatostatin analog, suppresses GH secretion in most patients with pituitary-dependent acromegaly at s.c. doses of 100 μg every 8 hr. However, some patients require much larger doses (6 mg/day s.c., or continuous i.v. infusion), and some do not respond at all (454). The agent reduces tumor size in some patients (455), an effect that may be useful in preoperative preparation (456). In that GH secretion resumes on discontinuation of medical therapy, one attractive strategy is to administer octreotide after radiation therapy until the full effects of radiation are achieved. Impaired glucose tolerance and gallstone formation are side effects of long-term administration.

Transsphenoidal resection is the preferred treatment of corticotropinomas with minimal suprasellar extension (457). The initial cure rate in this setting is as high as 89% in the hands of an experienced neurosurgeon but is lower in less experienced hands, with a second operation, or when removal of a macroadenoma or invasive tumor is attempted (431,456,458). Radiation therapy and adrenolytic agents are equally acceptable alternative approaches in the latter situations.

Although radiation therapy alone induces remission in only a minority of adults with sporadic Cushing's syndrome (459), it is effective in up to 80% of children treated before reaching the age of 18 years (460). The response of adults is improved to between 53% and 69% by the adjuvant use of metyrapone, aminoglutethimide, ketoconazole, or mitotane (435,461,462). The doses and side effects of these agents have been reviewed elsewhere (463). Medical therapy is initiated with radiation therapy and is increased as needed to normalize cortisol values; subsequent monitoring is necessary to reduce and possibly discontinue the medication. Because corticotrope tumors increase ACTH production to overcome cortisol blockade, medical therapy alone is rarely effective in Cushing's disease. If the patient has failed transsphenoidal surgery, bilateral adrenalectomy, preferably via two flank incisions, provides rapid resolution of hypercortisolism (464). Adjunctive prophylactic radiation to the sella to prevent Nelson syndrome, while controversial, is commonly used (465).

Surgical resection and radiotherapy cured the TSH-secreting adenoma reported in a single patient with MEN-I (466). When the tumor is aggressive, octreotide may control further growth and hormone production in a sporadic TSH-secreting tumor.

Other Tumors

The incidence of "other tumors" in patients with MEN-I is similar to that in the control population except for the following diagnoses: lipoma, thyroid adenoma, and adrenal cortical adenoma. Lipomas should be excised for cosmetic reasons or for symptoms related to a fatty mass. Thyroid nodules should be evaluated by aspiration cytology (467), and a thyroid lobectomy should be performed if the aspiration is suspicious for or diagnostic of cancer (468). In our experience, thyroid nodules in MEN-I are usually benign and are not usually treated. Adrenal cortical lesions should be evaluated just as any "incidentaloma" (469). If the tumor appears to be benign and nonfunctional, no treatment is necessary. If the patient has symptoms or signs of hormonal excess related to it, adrenalectomy may be necessary. Cancer of the adrenal can occur in these patients, but it is rare and requires adrenalectomy. The classic "other tumors" associated with MEN-I, thyroid adenoma, adrenal cortical adenoma, and lipoma, usually do not require surgical therapy. However, the presence of mass symptoms, evidence of excessive hormonal production, or presence of cancer are indications for surgery. Careful surveillance is necessary in the management of these tumors.

General Principles for Follow-Up of *men1* Gene Carriers

Men1 gene carriers can be ascertained through either of two mechanisms. First, they can be ascertained because they express diagnostic clinical features of MEN-I. Second they can be ascertained by genetic linkage analysis, if the kindred is suitable (see below). A third method, direct DNA testing for mutations of the *men1* gene, will probably become the ascertainment method of choice within ~5 years, following cloning of the *men1* gene.

The physician and patient must address three broad and interacting issues in follow-up of MEN-I. These are treatment of established disease expressions, monitoring for progression of disease, and counseling of the patient and family. We cover counseling separately (see below).

Treatment of Established Expressions of Multiple Endocrine Neoplasia Type I

We have described above the clinical features and management strategy for the organ disturbances in MEN-I. The overriding principle in treatment is that each established expression must be handled as a distinct disorder in its own right. There is only one important known interaction between two MEN-I-related disease expressions, the exacerbation of Zollinger-Ellison syndrome by primary hyperparathyroidism.

Monitoring for Increased Aggressiveness of an Established Expression of Multiple Endocrine Neoplasia Type I

As with treatment of any individual expression of MEN-I (see above), monitoring of an untreated or partially treated expression must follow the general principles developed for each disorder. Expense and local availability of tests may require modifications of the plan.

Untreated hyperparathyroidism justifies monitoring parathyroid indices annually (serum calcium, creatinine, alkaline phosphatase, and PTH), urine calcium and urinalysis annually, and bone mass less frequently.

Zollinger-Ellison syndrome justifies acid testing to verify the correctness of antisecretory dosage at least once annually. The patient needs a dose of antisecretory drug to keep acid output <10 mEq/liter

before the next dose (<5 mEq/liter if the patient has had prior acid reduction surgery). Endoscopy should be done if acid control has not been satisfactory as judged from acid testing, suspicion of poor compliance, or gastrointestinal symptoms. Future developments may lead to recommendations about periodic efforts to localize and remove an offending tumor (see above). At present we do not recommend this in Zollinger-Ellison syndrome with MEN-I.

Prolactinoma warrants monitoring serum prolactin annually. For microprolactinoma, pituitary imaging should follow the same guidelines as in MEN-I patients without prolactinoma. For macroprolactinoma, pituitary imaging and visual field testing should be done annually.

The less common expressions of MEN-I can be followed-up in manners analogous to these more common expressions.

Monitoring for New Expressions or for True Recurrence of "Cured" Expressions

Because of the pleiomorphic and stochiastic expressions of MEN-I, comprehensive monitoring for new expressions would be prohibitively expensive and possibly too invasive (470–472). Some patients can receive quite extensive monitoring in the context of a national registry or a research protocol, and this should be accepted if it seems in the patient's interest.

We provide general guidelines below for gene carriers not expressing the endocrinopathy in question, but these must be interpreted in the context of locally available methods and their accompanying expense. Sometimes symptoms (such as those of Zollinger-Ellison syndrome) will present before an increase of the trophic hormone has been detected.

Parathyroids: If the patient is not hypoparathyroid, serum calcium (preferably ionized calcium) should be measured about once per year. Serum intact PTH should be measured every 5 years. Approximately equal numbers of patients will show borderline elevation of only one of the two (PTH or calcium). Since this is a mild and early expression not requiring intervention, little is gained from the added expense of monitoring PTH as often as calcium. Parathyroid gland imaging should not be used for diagnosis of primary hyperthyroidism in any cases.

Pituitary: Prolactin should be measured about every 3 years. Pituitary imaging should be done initially and then every 10 years, preferably via MRI. Other pituitary axes (ACTH/cortisol, GH/IGF-I) need not be measured unless symptoms or signs suggest their overfunction.

GI–endocrine axis: The intensity and methods for monitoring the GI–endocrine axis in MEN-I are currently controversial and potentially expensive. In general, yearly measurement of fasting gastrin is sufficient. High gastrin values should lead to confirmation and then evaluation of acid status and perhaps a secretin challenge test (see above). Pancreatic polypeptide measurement at baseline and after challenges is under investigation, but this cannot currently be recommended outside a research protocol. We do not recommend routine testing with other peptides (chromogranin A, human glycoprotein α subunit, insulin/proinsulin). Periodic imaging of the abdomen should be done only if the medical and surgical team is prepared to treat abnormal findings in asymptomatic cases. This can be accomplished most cost effectively via CT.

APPLICATION OF GENETIC LINKAGE TO DIAGNOSIS

DNA analysis is used in prenatal diagnosis, carrier detection, and presymptomatic diagnosis for a variety of hereditary disorders (473). The main application of DNA-based methods in MEN-I has been in presymptomatic diagnosis. Because of the age-dependent penetrance, most individuals carrying the gene do not develop clinical manifestations until at least the third decade. Biochemical screening at 5 year intervals after age 15 years is recommended for all family members at risk, because effective therapy is available for most manifestations of the disease, and early detection may reduce morbidity (472). DNA-based methods can distinguish, among MEN-I families, individuals who carry the gene from those who are not gene carriers and need not undergo routine biochemical screening. Presymptomatic diagnosis may also benefit at-risk individuals who wish to know whether they carry the gene before planning a family. Many of those who are in the child-bearing years have not yet reached the age at which symptoms appear, and DNA studies can identify those who are gene carriers.

The same methods that are used for presymptomatic diagnosis can also be applied to prenatal diagnosis. However, termination of pregnancy is rarely considered because of MEN-I. In general, prenatal diagnosis is applied to disorders in which affected individuals are likely to die in the neonatal period or are severely disabled from birth or early childhood and have a limited life expectancy. Prenatal diagnosis may also be considered in some adult-onset disorders that have a particularly severe and disabling course (e.g., Huntington's disease). For most patients with MEN-I, the onset is in the middle years, and the physical burden of the disease may be quite minor. On the other hand, individuals in whom disabling medical symptoms began in the second or third decade of life or who have had a rela-

tive with a particularly severe course might be more apt to consider termination of pregnancy. Unless there is good evidence that the disorder in a particular family is consistently more or less severe than average, individuals should be counseled on the average burden of the disease to obtain a more balanced view. For those who choose to proceed with prenatal diagnosis, fetal cells can be obtained through either amniocentesis, in which a sample of amniotic fluid is removed transabdominally at 16–17 weeks of gestation, or chorionic villus sampling, in which a placental biopsy is obtained either transcervically at 9–12 weeks of gestation or transabdominally at a slightly later gestational age. Amniocentesis gives a diagnosis at a later stage because the procedure itself is done later in pregnancy and because the few cells obtained are usually cultured for 2 weeks before sufficient DNA can be extracted for diagnostic studies. The tissue obtained from chorionic villus sampling can be used directly for diagnosis without culturing so that a diagnosis is obtained much earlier. Chorionic villus sampling carries a higher risk of miscarriage than amniocentesis (1/100 vs. 1/200) and may also be associated with an increased risk of birth defects. In the future, it may be possible to sort fetal cells for testing from a sample of maternal blood.

For an increasing number of hereditary disorders, isolation of the disease gene has set the stage for accurate mutation-specific diagnosis (474); i.e., analysis of the DNA allows for detection of the exact alteration that causes the disease. An example is sickle cell disease, in which the same single base change is always responsible for the disease, and the mutation is easily detected due to its alteration of the recognition site for a restriction endonuclease (475). Because the gene for *men1* has not yet been identified, mutation-specific diagnosis remains a prospect for the future. Even with identification of the gene, mutation-specific diagnosis may remain problematic because nearly every kindred may have a unique mutation; and many of the mutations may be single base changes. Finding a unique point mutation can be very time consuming, and distinguishing a missense mutation from a normal variant can be particularly difficult.

Genetic linkage can be used as an indirect method of diagnosis when a disease gene has not yet been isolated or the disease-causing mutation cannot be identified (473). This method exploits the tendency for genes that lie close together on a chromosome (linked genes) to cosegregate in families. Normal human cells contain two copies of each chromosome (except X and Y). In the gonads, however, cells undergo "meiotic" division to generate gametes with only one copy of each chromosome. For any pair of genes that lie on different chromosomes, meiosis results in random distribution in the resulting gametes, leading to independent segregation in offspring. Genes that are close together on the same chromosome tend to remain "linked" during gametogenesis, so traits related to these genes cosegregate in families. If a gene having several possible forms (such as the ABO gene, with the three possible alleles, A, B, or O) is known to lie close to a disease gene, then the disease can be tracked through a family by its cosegregation with one of the alleles of the linked polymorphism (Fig. 6).

Genetic recombination affects the accuracy of linkage-based diagnosis. Genes that lie on the same chromosome but are separated by more than ~100,000 base pairs undergo a measurable amount of recombination during meiosis, allowing them to separate from one another (Fig. 7) (476). The rate of recombination between two genes is roughly proportional to the physical distance between them. On average, 1% recombination corresponds to a distance of 1 million base pairs, but the relationship between recombination and physical distance becomes nonlinear with loci that are separated by more than a few million base pairs, because double recombination becomes a factor (476). Mathematical formulae to compensate for double recombination convert percentage recombination to "centiMorgans" (cM), which correlate more closely with actual physical distance. Even with this correction, map distances determined by linkage do not correspond exactly to physical distance, because some regions of the genome undergo more recombination per unit length than others. In fact there appears to be excess recombination between polymorphisms in the *men1* region (477). In predictive testing, the accuracy of the diagnosis decreases as the rate of recombination between the disease gene and linked polymorphism increases. Estimates of the recombination rate are derived from research studies of affected families. Because of limitations in the amount of data and the complexity of human pedigree structure, statistical analysis is critical in distinguishing true linkage from

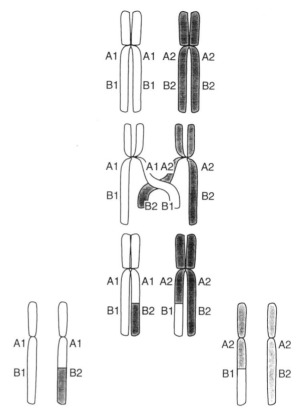

FIG. 7. Crossing-over during meiosis. Meiosis is the process through which gametes are formed by two sequential cell divisions. Prior to the first meiotic division, DNA synthesis has been completed so that each chromosome consists of two identical sister chromatids. A single cross-over event between homologous chromosomes during the first meiotic division is shown. The second meiotic division results in the formation of four different types of gametes. Two of the resulting gametes (the solid white and the solid gray) are nonrecombinant; e.g., they have the same alleles that were present on one of the original chromosomes. The other two gametes are recombinants; e.g., they contain parts of both original chromosomes and therefore have new combinations of alleles (A1 with B2 and A2 with B1).

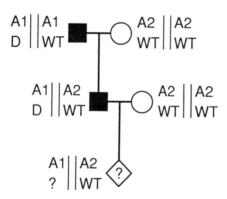

FIG. 6. Cosegregation of a disease gene, D, with the A1 allele of a linked RFLP. The child in question would be expected to have the disease because he inherited the A1 allele from his affected parent.

cosegregation attributable to random chance. Results of linkage analysis are reported as a maximum LOD score, often abbreviated "z," and a corresponding "θ," indicating the best estimate of recombination rate between the genes being tested (476). A LOD score ≥3 indicates that there is significant evidence for linkage, and higher LOD scores correspond to more precise estimates of recombination. In a clinical laboratory setting in which linkage is being applied to presymptomatic testing, the recombination estimates should be derived from a large series of observations, preferably observations from more than one laboratory. Using linkage analysis the gene for MEN-I was shown to map near the polymorphic marker *pygm*, which is located near the centromere of chromosome 11q (43). This chromosomal location was confirmed by several groups, and additional linked markers have been identified (479–481). Several polymorphisms show little or no recombination with the *men1* gene, with supporting LOD scores on the order of 10. Based on the resulting genetic map, predictions can be made about the affection status of young, at-risk individuals (478). Linkage-based diagnosis can be applied only to families. In contrast to mutation-specific diagnosis, with which DNA from any single individual can be tested, linkage requires samples from several family members. In MEN-I, at least two affected individuals in addition to those seeking presymptomatic diagnosis must be typed for a linked polymorphic marker to determine which allele is cosegregating with the disease. Typically the affected and the unaffected parents of the individuals undergoing presymptomatic diagnosis plus one other affected family member are typed for linked polymorphic markers. The allelic contribution of the unaffected parent is "subtracted" from the genotype of the offspring, and the remaining allele is the affected parent's contribution. The disease-associated marker is the one shared by the two affected family members (Fig. 8). Linkage cannot be used for diagnosis of the offspring of sporadic cases of MEN-I because there is no way to determine which is the disease-associated allele.

The affected parent must be informative (heterozygous) for a linked polymorphism to determine whether he transmitted the disease-associated allele or the allele corresponding to the normal gene. Variable number of tandem repeats (VNTR) polymorphisms are useful in this regard because they have many alleles, and nearly every one is heterozygous. At least three such polymorphisms, *pygm*, D11S97, and D11S427, are closely linked to *men1*. Generally, several poly-

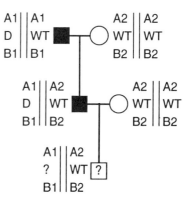

FIG. 9. Multipoint linkage analysis in DNA-based diagnosis. Polymorphic loci A and B flank the disease gene, D. Although neither A nor B is closely linked to D, when A1 and B1 are transmitted from an affected parent to a child, it is very likely that the disease gene will also be transmitted. Simultaneous recombination between A1 and D and B1 and D would be required for the wild-type (WT) gene to be transmitted on a chromosome bearing A1 and B1.

morphisms are typed to provide an accurate diagnosis. In those cases in which a marker showing <1% recombination with the disease gene is informative, diagnosis based on this marker alone may be adequate. More accurate diagnosis can be obtained using a group of linked markers ("multipoint analysis"). Knowledge of the location of a disease gene within a group of polymorphisms allows for the use of flanking markers in diagnosis. If a carrier parent transmits the disease-associated alleles from polymorphisms on both sides of the disease gene, then the probability that the disease gene has been transmitted is very high (Fig. 9). Under these circumstances, closely linked polymorphisms and precise estimates of recombination rates are less important than in the case when diagnosis is based on a single polymorphism. With the large number of highly polymorphic markers on proximal chromosome 11q, nearly every member of an MEN-I family can be diagnosed with a high degree of accuracy.

GENETIC COUNSELING

Most of the manifestations of MEN-I are related to the endocrine system, and the long-term medical management of this disease usually falls to generalists or endocrinologists. However, genetic consultation is indicated for the purpose of explaining the inheritance pattern of the disease to affected individuals and their relatives and discussing the consequences for future generations. In addition, clinical geneticists and genetic counselors may be more familiar than other medical practitioners with DNA-based diagnostic testing and the reproductive issues arising from its availability. A patient-oriented booklet for counseling members of MEN-I families is available from the NIH. Because

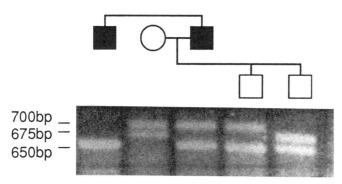

FIG. 8. Polymerase chain reaction analysis of DNA for presymptomatic diagnosis of MEN-I based on close linkage to *pygm*. Members of an MEN-I kindred were typed for a *pygm* short tandem repeat polymorphism. The carrier father shares a 650 bp allele with his affected brother, indicating that the disease is cosegregating with this allele in the kindred. Both children have a 650 bp allele that must have come from their father. Their mother transmitted a 700 bp to the first child and a 675 bp allele to the second child. Both are at high risk of developing clinical manifestations of MEN-I.

multiple endocrine neoplasia type I is an autosomal dominant disorder, an individual who is affected has a 50% chance of passing the disease on to his or her offspring. There is an equal chance that a child will not inherit the abnormal gene, and both the child and his children should be free of the disorder. Because the *men1* gene is not on the X or Y chromosome, the transmission of the disease is not influenced by gender. Multiple endocrine neoplasia type I is typical of dominant disorders in that it shows some variability in clinical manifestations, with different individuals having somewhat different endocrinologic features. Although the onset of symptoms may not occur until late in life, most gene carriers do eventually develop the medical problems related to the disease ("age-dependent penetrance"). As a result, the trait is usually transmitted through a kindred from parent to child, with no skipped generation. Family members who have been carefully evaluated and do not show any clinical signs by the fifth or sixth decade of life are probably free of disease and would not be expected to transmit the trait to their children. Occasionally autosomal dominant disorders arise as a result of a new mutation; i.e., a genetically normal parent may transmit a mutated, defective gene to his or her offspring. The frequency of such sporadic cases in late-onset diseases is very low, and cases that appear to be sporadic more likely represent nonpaternity or failure to identify the disease in mildly affected relatives. In this regard an important part of genetic counseling is obtaining medical records on a patient's parents and other family members to help distinguish whether they are affected with the disease. For a truly sporadic case, the risk to each offspring is still near 50%, but the risk that other family members will bear children with MEN-I is negligible.

REFERENCES

1. Lips CJM, Vasen HFA, Lamers CBHW. Multiple endocrine neoplasia syndromes. *CRC Crit Rev Oncol Hematol* 1984;2:117–184.
2. Gagel RF. Multiple endocrine neoplasia type II. This volume.
3. Larsson C, Skogseid B, Öberg K, Nakamura Y, Nordenskjöld M. Multiple endocrine neoplasia type 1 gene maps to chromosome 11 and is lost in insulinoma. *Nature* 1988;332:85–88.
4. Mulligan LM, Kwok JB, Healey CS, et al. Germ-line mutations of the RET protooncogene in multiple endocrine neoplasia type 2A. *Nature* 1993;363:458–460.
5. Erdheim J. Zur normalen und pathologischen histologie der glandula thyroidea, parathyroidea, und hypophysis. *Beitr Z Pathol Anat* 1903;33:158–236.
6. Cushing H, Davidoff LM. In: *The pathologic findings in four autopsied cases of acromegaly. With a discussion of their significance. Monograph 22.* New York: The Rockefeller Institute for Medical Research, 1927.
7. Lloyd PC. A case of hypophyseal tumor with associated tumor like enlargement of the parathyroids and islands of Langerhans. *Bull Johns Hopkins Hosp* 1929;45:1.
8. Rossier PH, Dressler M. Familiare erkankung inner-skretorischer drusen kombiniert mit ulcuskrankheit. *Schweiz Med Wochenschr* 1939;20:95.
9. Underdahl LO, Woolner LB, Black BM. Multiple endocrine adenomas: report of eight cases in which the parathyroids, pituitary and pancreatic islets were involved. *J Clin Endocrinol* 1953;13:20.
10. Moldawer MP. Case records of the Massachusetts General Hospital, case 39501. *N Engl J Med* 1953;249:990.
11. Moldawer MP, Nardi GL, Raker JW. Concomitance of multiple adenomas of the parathyroids and pancreatic islet cells with tumor of the pituitary; a syndrome with familial incidence. *Am J Med Sci* 1954;228:190.
12. Wermer P. Genetic aspects of adenomatosis of endocrine glands. *Am J Med* 1954;16:363.
13. Schmid JR, Labhart A, Rossier PH. Relationship of multiple endocrine adenomas to the syndrome of ulcerogenic islet cell adenomas (Zollinger-Ellison). Occurrence of both syndromes in one family. *Am J Med* 1961;31:343.
14. Zollinger RM, Ellison EH. Primary peptic ulceration of the jejunum associated with islet cell tumors of the pancreas. *Ann Surg* 1955;142:702–723.
15. Gregory RH, Tracy HJ, French JM, Sircus W. Extraction of a gastrin-like substance from a pancreatic tumor in a case of Zollinger-Ellison syndrome. *Lancet* 1960;1:1040.
16. Malarkey WB. Prolactin and the diagnosis of pituitary tumors. *Annu Rev Med* 1979;30:249–258.
17. Lewis UJ, Singh RNP, Seavey BK. Human prolactin: isolation and some properties. *Biochem Biophys Res Commun* 1971;44:1169–1176.
18. Yalow RS. Radioimmunoassay: a probe for the fine structure of biologic systems. *Science* 1978;200:1236–1245.
19. Nussbaum SR, Potts JT Jr. Immunoassays for parathyroid hormone 1–84 in the diagnosis of hyperparathyroidism. *J Bone Mineral Res* 1991;6(Suppl. 2):S43–S50.
20. Albright F, Ellsworth R. *Uncharted seas.* Portland, ME: Kalmia Press, 1990.
21. Bevan JS, Webster J, Burke W, Scanlon MF. Dopamine agonists and pituitary tumor shrinkage. *Endocrine Rev* 1992;13:220–240.
22. Brandi ML, Marx SJ, Aubarch GD, Fitzpatrick LA. Familial multiple endocrine neoplasia type I: a new look at pathophysiology. *Endocrine Rev* 1987;8:391–405.
23. DeLellis RA, Ayal Y, Tischler A, Lee A, Wolfe HJ. Multiple endocrine neoplasia (MEN) syndromes: cellular origins and interrelationships. *Int Rev Exp Pathol* 1986;28:164–198.
24. Eberle F, Grün R. Multiple endocrine neoplasia, type I (MEN I). In: *Advances in internal medicine and pediatrics.* Frick P, Harnack G-A, Kochsiek K, Martini GA, Prader A, eds. New York: Springer-Verlag, 1981;77–149.
25. Majewski JT, Wilson SD. The MEA-I syndrome: an all or none phenomenon? *Surgery* 1979;86:475–484.
26. Ballard HS, Frame B, Hartsock RJ. Familial multiple endocrine adenoma-peptic ulcer complex. *Am J Med* 1964;43:481–516.
27. Marx SJ, Spiegel AM, Levine MA, et al. Familial hypocalciuric hypercalcemia: the relation to primary parathyroid hyperplasia. *N Engl J Med* 1982;307:416–426.
28. Vasen HFA, Lamers CBHW, Lips CJM. Screening for multiple endocrine neoplasia syndrome type I. *Arch Intern Med* 1989;149:2717–2722.
29. Skogseid B, Eriksson B, Lundqvist G, et al. Multiple endocrine neoplasia type 1: a 10-year prospective screening study in four kindreds. *J Clin Endocrinol Metab* 1991;73:281–287.
30. Samaan NA, Ouais S, Ordonez N, Choksi UA, Sellin RV, Hickey RC. Multiple endocrine syndrome type 1. *Cancer* 1989;64:741–752.
31. Lamers C, Froeling PGAM. Clinical significance of hyperparathyroidism in familial multiple endocrine adenomatosis type I (MEA I). *Am J Med* 1979;66:422–424.
32. Betts JB, O'Malley BP, Rosenthal FD. Hyperparathyroidism: a prerequisite for Zollinger-Ellison syndrome in multiple endocrine adenomatosis type 1—report of a further family and a review of the literature. *Q J Med* 1980;73:69–76.

33. Bilezikian JP, Silverberg SJ, Shane E. Clinical presentation of primary hyperparathyroidism. This volume.

34. Kleerekoper M. Clinical course of primary hyperparathyroidism. This volume.

35. Shepherd JJ. Latent familial multiple endocrine neoplasia in Tasmania. *Med J Aust* 1985;142:395–397.

36. Marx SJ, Vinik AI, Santen RJ, Floyd JC Jr, Mills JL, Green J. Multiple endocrine neoplasia type I: assessment of laboratory tests to screen for the gene in a large kindred. *Medicine* 1986;65:226–241.

37. Heath H III, Hodgson S, Kennedy MA. Primary hyperparathyroidism: incidence, morbidity, and potential economic impact in a community. *N Engl J Med* 1980;302:189–225.

38. Knudson AG. Mutation and cancer: statistical study of retinoblastoma. *Proc Natl Acad Sci USA* 1971;68:820–823.

39. Black WC III, Utley JR. The differential diagnosis of parathyroid adenoma and chief cell hyperplasia. *Am J Clin Pathol* 1968;49:761–775.

40. Ghandur-Mnaymneh L, Kimura N. A histopathologic definition with a study of 172 cases of primary hyperparathyroidism. *Am J Pathol* 1984;115:70–83.

41. Marx SJ, Menczel J, Campbell G, Aurbach GD, Spiegel AM, Norton JA. Heterogeneous size of the parathyroid glands in familial multiple endocrine neoplasia type I. *Clin Endocrinol* 1991;35:521–526.

42. Hellman P, Skogseid B, Juhlin C, Akerstrom G, Rastad J. Findings and long-term result of parathyroid surgery in multiple endocrine neoplasia type I. *World J Surg* 1992;16:718–723.

43. Rizzoli R, Green J III, Marx SJ. Primary hyperparathyroidism in familial multiple endocrine neoplasia type I. *Am J Med* 1985;78:468–473.

44. van Heerden JA, Kent RB III, Sizemore GW, Grant CS, ReMine WH. Primary hyperparathyroidism in patients with multiple endocrine neoplasia syndromes. *Arch Surg* 1983;118:533–535.

45. Malmaeus J, Benson L, Johansson H, et al. Parathyroid surgery in the multiple endocrine neoplasia type I syndrome: choice of surgical procedure. *World J Surg* 1986;10:668–672.

46. Prinz RA, Gamvros OI, Sellu D, Lynn JA. Subtotal parathyroidectomy for primary chief cell hyperplasia of the multiple endocrine neoplasia type I syndrome. *Ann Surg* 1981;193:26–29.

47. Rudberg C, Akerstrom G, Palmer M, et al. Late results of operation for primary hyperparathyroidism in 441 patients. *Surgery* 1986;99:643–651.

48. Mallette LE, Blevins T, Jordan PH, Noon GP. Autogenous parathyroid grafts for generalized primary parathyroid hyperplasia versus multiple endocrine neoplasia type I. *Surgery* 1987;101:738–744.

49. Norton JA, Levin B, Jensen RT: Principles and practice of oncology. In: *Cancer*, 4th ed. DeVita VT, Hellman S, Rosenberg SA, eds. Philadelphia: JB Lippincott, 1993; 1335–1435.

50. Bone HG. Diagnosis of the multiglandular endocrine neoplasias. *Clin Chem* 1990;36:711–718.

51. Benya RV, Metz DC, Fishbeyn VA, Strader DB, Orbuch M, Jensen RT. Gastrinoma can be the initial presentation for patients with multiple endocrine neoplasia type 1 (MEN-1). *Gastroenterology* 1993;104:A42.

52. Jensen RT, Gardner JD. Gastrinoma. In: *The Pancreas: Biology, Pathobiology, and Diseases*, 2nd ed. Go VLW, Gardner JD., DiMagno EP, et al., eds. New York: Raven Press, 1993.

53. Metz DC, Jensen RT: Endocrine tumors of the pancreas. In: *Bockus gastroenterology*. Haubrich WB, Berk F, Schaffner JE, eds. Philadelphia: WB Saunders, 1993.

54. Galiber HK, Reading CC, Charboneau JW. Localization of pancreatic insulinoma: comparison of pre- and intraoperative US with CT and angiography. *Radiology* 1988;166:405–410.

55. Metz DC, Benjamin SB. Islet cell carcinoma of the pancreas presenting as bleeding from isolated gastric varices. *Dig Dis Sci* 1991;36:241–244.

56. Sano T, Asa SL, Kovacs K. Growth hormone releasing factor-producing tumors: clinical, biochemical and morphological manifestations. *Endocrine Rev* 1988;9:357–373.

57. Thompson NW, Lloyd RU, Nishiyama RN. MEN-1 pancreas: a histological and immunohistochemical study. *World J Surg* 1984;8:561–568.

58. Kloppel G, Sillemar S, Stamm B, Hacki WH, Heitz PN. Pancreatic lesions and hormonal profile in pancreatic tumors in multiple endocrine neoplasia type I. *Cancer* 1986;57: 1824–1831.

59. Jensen RT, Gardner JD. Zollinger-Ellison syndrome: clinical presentation, pathology, diagnosis and treatment. In: *Peptic ulcer and other acid-related diseases*. Dannenberg A, Zakim D, eds. New York: Academic Research Association, 1991; 117–211.

60. Maton PN, Dayal Y. Clinical implication of hypergastrinemia. In: *Peptic ulcer and other acid-related diseases*. Dannenberg A, Zakim D, eds. New York: Academic Research Association, 1991;213–246.

61. Frucht H, Maton PN, Jensen RT. Use of omeprazole in patients with Zollinger-Ellison syndrome. *Dig Dis Sci* 1991; 36:394–404.

62. Pipeleers-Marichial M, Somers G, Willems G. Gastrinomas in the duodenum of patients with multiple endocrine neoplasia type 1 and the Zollinger-Ellison syndrome. *N Engl J Med* 1990;322:723–727.

63. Norton JA, Doppman JL, Jensen RT. Curative resection in Zollinger-Ellison syndrome: results of a 10 year prospective study. *Ann Surg* 1992;215:8–18.

64. Neuburger P, Lewin M, Bonfils S. Parietal and chief cell population in four cases of the Zollinger-Ellison syndrome. *Gastroenterology* 1972;63:937–942.

65. Kaye M, Thodes J, Beck P. Gastric secretion in duodenal ulcer with particular reference to the diagnosis of Zollinger-Ellison syndrome. *Gastroenterology* 1970;58:476–481.

66. Norton JA, Doppman JL, Collen MJ. Prospective study of gastrinoma localization and resection in patients with Zollinger-Ellison syndrome. *Ann Surg* 1986;204:468–479.

67. Stabile BE, Morrow DJ, Passaro E Jr. The gastrinoma triangle: operative implications. *Am J Surg* 1984;147:25–32.

68. Norton JA, Jensen RT. Unresolved issues in the management of patients with Zollinger-Ellison syndrome. *World J Surg* 1991;15:151–159.

69. Zollinger RM, Ellison EH, Fabri PJ, Johnson J, Sparks J, Carey LC. Primary peptic ulceration of the jejunum associated with islet cell tumors: twenty-five year appraisal. *Ann Surg* 1980;192:422–430.

70. Oberg K, Skogseid B, Eriksson B. Multiple endocrine neoplasia type 1. *Acta Oncol* 1989;28:383–387.

71. Zollinger RM. Gastrinoma factors influencing prognosis. *Surgery* 1985;97:49–54.

72. Podevin P, Ruszniewski P, Mignon M. Management of multiple endocrine neoplasia type 1 (MEN 1) in Zollinger-Ellison syndrome. *Gastroenterology* 1990;98:A230.

73. Jensen RT, Gardner JD, Raufman J-P. Zollinger-Ellison syndrome: current concepts and management. *Ann Intern Med* 1983;98:59–75.

74. Wilson SD. The role of surgery in children with Zollinger-Ellison syndrome. *Surgery* 1982;92:682–692.

75. Stage JG, Stadil R. The clinical diagnosis of the Zollinger-Ellison syndrome. *Scand J Gastroenterol* 1971;14(Suppl. 53):79–91.

76. Bonfils S, Landor JH, Mignon M. Results of surgical management in 92 consecutive patients with Zollinger-Ellison syndrome. *Ann Surg* 1981;194:692–697.

77. Waxman I, Gardner JD, Jensen RT, Maton PN. Peptic ulcer perforation as the presentation of Zollinger-Ellison syndrome. *Dig Dis Sci* 1991;36:19–24.

78. Ellison EH, Wilson SD. The Zollinger-Ellison syndrome reappraisal and evaluation of 260 registered cases. *Ann Surg* 1964;160:512–530.

79. Miller LS, Vinayek R, Frucht H, Gardner JD, Jensen RT, Maton PN. Reflux esophagitis in patients with Zollinger-Ellison syndrome. *Gastroenterology* 1990;98:341–346.

80. Isenberg JI, Walsh JH, Grossman MI. Zollinger-Ellison syndrome. *Gastroenterology* 1973;65:140–165.

81. Shimoda SS, Saunders DR. Rubin C. The Zollinger-Ellison syndrome with steatorrhea: mechanisms of fat and vitamin B 12 malabsorption. *Gastroenterology* 1968;55:705–715.
82. Moshal MG, Broitman SA, Zamcheck N. Gastrin and absorption: a review. *Am J Clin Nutr* 1970;23:336–342.
83. Yonda RJ, Ostroff JW, Ashbaugh CD, Guis MS, Goldberg HI. Zollinger-Ellison syndrome with a normal screening gastrin level. *Dig Dis Sci* 1989;34:1929–1932.
84. Feldman M: Gastric secretion. In: *Gastrointestinal disease.* Sleisenger MH, Fordtran JS, eds. Philadelphia: WB Saunders, 1983;541–548.
85. Norton JA, Cornelius MJ, Doppman JL. Effect of parathyroidectomy in patients with hyperparathyroidism and multiple endocrine neoplasia type I. *Surgery* 1987;102:958–966.
86. Collen MJ, Sheridan MJ. Definition for idiopathic gastric acid hypersecretion. *Dig Dis Sci* 1991;36:1371–1376.
87. Maton PN, Frucht H, Vinayek R, Wank SA, Gardner JD, Jensen RT. Medical management of patients with Zollinger-Ellison syndrome who have had previous gastric surgery: a prospective study. *Gastroenterology* 1988;94:294–299.
88. Wolfe MM, Jensen RT. Zollinger-Ellison syndrome. *N Engl J Med* 1987;317:1200–1209.
89. Metz DC, Pisegna JR, Fishbeyn VA, Benya RV, Jensen RT. Current maintenance doses of omprazde in Zollinger-Ellison syndrome are too high. *Gastroenterology* 1992;103:1498–1508.
90. Frucht H, Howard JM, Stark HA. Prospective study of meal provocative gastrin testing in patients with Zollinger-Ellison syndrome. *Am J Med* 1989;87:528–536.
91. Kloppel G, Heitz PU. Pancreatic endocrine tumors. *Pathol Res Pract* 1988;183:155–175.
92. Ganguli PC, Polak JM, Pearse AGE, Elder JB, Hegarty M. Antral-gastrin-cell hyperplasia in peptic-ulcer disease. *Lancet* 1974:1288–1289.
93. Taylor IL, Calam J, Rotter JI. Family studies of hypergastrinemic hyperpepsinogenemic I duodenal ulcer. *Ann Intern Med* 1981;95:421–425.
94. Frucht H, Howard JM, Slaff JE. Secretin and calcium provocative tests in patients with Zollinger-Ellison syndrome: a prospective study. *Ann Intern Med* 1989;111:713–722.
95. Lewin KJ, Yana K, Ulrich I, Elashoff JD, Walsh JH. Primary gastrin-cell hyperplasia. *Am J Surg Pathol* 1984;8:821–832.
96. Galbut DL, Markowitz AM. Insulinoma: diagnosis, surgical management and long term follow-up. Review of 41 cases. *Am J Surg* 1980;139:682–690.
97. Croisier JC, Azerad E, Lubetzki J. L'adenomatse polyendocrinienne. A propos d'une observation peronelle et revenue de la litterature. *Semin Hop Paris* 1971;47:494–525.
98. Jadoul M, Koppeschaar HPF, Bax MA, et al. Insulinomas in MEN-1 patients: Early detection and treatment of insulinomas in patients with the multiple endocrine neoplasia syndrome type-1. *Netherlands J Med* 1990;37:95–102.
99. Service FJ, Nelson RL. Insulinoma. *Compr Ther* 1980;6:70–74.
100. Stefanini P, Carboni M, Patrassi N. Surgical treatment and prognosis of insulinoma. *Clin Gastroenterol* 1974;3:697–709.
101. Service FJ, McMahon MM, O'Brien PC, Ballard DJ. Functioning insulinoma—Incidence, recurrence, and long term survival of patients: a 60 year study. *Mayo Clin Proc* 1991;66:711–719.
102. Harrison TS, Fajans SS, Floyd JC, et al. Prevalence of diffuse pancreatic beta islet cell disease with hyperinsulinism: Problems in recognition and management. *World J Surg* 1984;8:583–589.
103. Eckhauser FE, Cheung PS, Vinik A, Strodel WE, Lloyd R, Thompson NW. Nonfunctioning malignant neuroendocrine tumors of the pancreas. *Surgery* 1986;100:978–988.
104. Rasbach DA, van Heerden JA, Telander RL, Grant CS, Carney A. Surgical management of hyperinsulinism in the multiple endocrine neoplasia type I syndrome. *Arch Surg* 1985;123:584–589.
105. Pasieka JL, McLoed MK, Thompson NW, Burney RE. Surgical approach to insulinomas. Assessing the need for preoperative localization. *Arch Surg* 1992;127:442–447.

106. van Heerden JA, Edis AJ, Service FJ. Surgical aspects of insulinomas. *Ann Surg* 1992;189:677–682.
107. Samaan NA, Quais S, Ordonez NG, Chosksi UA, Sellin RV, Hickey RC. Multiple endocrine syndrome type 1. Clinical, laboratory findings and management in five families. *Cancer* 1989;64:741–752.
108. Eastman RC, Kahn CR. Hypoglycemia. In: *Diagnostic endocrinology.* Moore WT, Eastman RC, eds. Toronto: BC Decker, 1990;183–199.
109. Gorden P, Roth J, Freychet P, Kahn R. The circulating proinsulin-like components. *Diabetes* 1972;21:673–677.
110. Doherty GM, Doppman JL, Shawker TH, et al. Results of a prospective strategy to diagnose, localize and resect insulinomas. *Surgery* 1991;110:989–997.
111. Gutman RA, Lazarus NR, Penhos JC, Fahans S, Recant LR. Circulating pro-insulin material in patients with functioning insulinomas. *N Engl J Med* 1971;284:1003–1008.
112. Cohen RM, Givens BD, Licinio J, et al. Proinsulin radioimmunoassays in the evaluation of insulinomas and familial hyperproinsulinemia. *Metabolism* 1986;35:1137–1146.
113. Doppman JL, Miller DL, Chang R, Shawker TH, Gorden P, Norton JA. Insulinomas: localization with selective intraarterial injection of calcium. *Radiology* 1991;178:237–241.
114. Sheppard BC, Norton JA, Doppman JL, Maton PN, Gardner JD, Jensen RT. Management of islet cells tumors in patients with multiple endocrine neoplasia: A prospective study. *Surgery* 1989;106:1108–1117.
115. Vinik A, Delbridge L, Moattari AR, Cho K, Thompson NW. Transhepatic portal vein catheterization for localization of insulinomas: a ten year experience. *Surgery* 1991;109:1–11.
116. Grant CS, van Heerden JA, Charboneau JW, James EM, Reading CC. Insulinoma: the value of intraoperative ultrasonography. *Arch Surg* 1988;123:843–848.
117. Norton JA, Cromack DT, Shawker TH, et al. Intraoperative ultrasonographic localization of islet cell tumors. A prospective comparison to palpation. *Ann Surg* 1988;207:160–168.
118. Boden G. Glucagonomas and insulinomas. *Gastroenterol Clin North Am* 1989;18:831–845.
119. Leichter SB. Clinical and metabolic aspects of glucagonoma. *Medicine* 1980;59:100–113.
120. Guillausseau PJ, Guillausseau C, Villet R. Les glucagonomas. Aspect Clinques, biologiques, Anatomo-pathologiques et therapeutiques (Revue general de 130 cas). *Gastroenterol Clin Biol* 1982;6:1029–1041.
121. Wilkinson DS. Necrolytic migratory erythema with carcinoma of the pancreas. *Trans St. John's Hosp Dermatol Soc* 1973;59:244.
122. Mallison CN, Bloom SR, Warin AP. A glucagonoma syndrome. *Lancet* 1974;2:1–5.
123. Holst JJ. Hormone producing tumors of the gastrointestinal tract. In: *Glucagon-producing tumors.* Cohen S, Soloway RD, eds. New York: Churchill Livingstone, 1985;57–84.
124. Stacpoole PW. The glucagonoma syndrome: clinical features, diagnosis and treatment. *Endocrine Rev* 1981;2:347–361.
125. Bataille D. The gastrointestinal system. In: *Handbook of physiology. Section 6.* Makhlouf GM, ed. Bethesda, MD: American Physiological Society, 1989;455–474.
126. Boden G, Wilson RM, Owen OE. Effects of chronic glucagon excess on hepatic metabolism. *Diabetes* 1978;27:643–648.
127. Holst JJ, Helland S, Ingemansson S. Functional studies in patients with glucagonoma syndrome. *Diabetologia* 1979;17:151–156.
128. Barber SG, Hamer JD. Skin rash in patients receiving glucagon. *Lancet* 1976;2:1138.
129. Norton JA, Kahn CR, Schiebinger R. Amino acid deficiency and the skin rash associated with glucagonoma syndrome. *Ann Intern Med* 1979;91:213–215.
130. Verner JV, Morrison AB. Endocrine pancreatic islet disease with diarrhea: report of a case due to diffuse hyperplasia of non beta islet tissue with a review of 54 additional cases. *Arch Intern Med* 1974;133:492–500.
131. Maton PN, Gardner JD, Jensen RT. Use of long-acting somatostatin analogue SMS 201-995 in patients with pancreatic islet cell tumors. *Dig Dis Sci* 1989;34:28S–37S.

132. Dunne MJ, Fletcher R, Hofker PH, Shui J. Somatostatin and gastroenteropancreatic endocrine-tumors: therapeutic characteristics. In: *Somatostatin in the treatment of GEP endocrine tumors.* O'Dorisio TM, ed. Berlin: Springer-Verlag, 1987;93–113.

133. Boden G, Rezvani I, Owen OE. Effects of glucagon on plasma amino acids. *J Clin Invest* 1984;73:785–793.

134. Boden G, Master RW, Rezvani I. Glucagon deficiency and hyperaminoacidemia after total pancreatectomy. *J Clin Invest* 1980;65:706–716.

135. McGavran MH, Unger RH, Recant L. A glucagon-secreting alpha-cell carcinoma of the pancreas. *N Engl J Med* 1966; 274:1408–1413.

136. Palmer JP, Werner PL, Benson JW. Dominant inheritance of large molecular weight immunoreactive glucagon. *J Clin Invest* 1978;61:763–769.

137. Welbourn RB, Wood SM, Polak JM, Bloom SR. Pancreatic endocrine tumors. In: *Gut hormones.* Bloom SR, Polak JM, eds. New York: Churchill Livingstone, 1981;547–554.

138. Long RG, Bryant MG, Mitchell SJ, Adrian TE, Polak JM, Bloom SR. Clinicopathological study of pancreatic and ganglioneuroblastoma tumors secreting vasoactive intestinal polypeptide (Vipomas). *Br Med J* 1981;282:1767–1771.

139. Matsumoto KK, Peter JB, Schultze RG. Water diarrhea and hypokalemia associated with pancreatic islet cell adenoma. *Gastroenterology* 1966;50:231–242.

140. Mekhjian H, O'Dorisio TM. VIPoma syndrome. *Semin Oncol* 1987;14:282–291.

141. Kane MG, O'Dorisio TM, Krejs GJ. Production of secretory diarrhea by intravenous infusion of vasoactive intestinal peptide. *N Engl J Med* 1983;309:1482–1485.

142. Namihara Y, Achord JL, Subramony C. Multiple endocrine neoplasia, type 1, with pancreatic cholera. *Am J Gastroenterol* 1987;82:794–797.

143. Capella C, Polak JM, Butta R. Morphologic patterns and diagnostic criteria of VIP-producing endocrine tumors. A histologic, histochemical, ultrastructural and biochemical study of 32 cases. *Cancer* 1983;52:1860–1874.

144. Laburthe M, Amiranoff B. Peptide receptors in intestinal epithelium. In: *The gastrointestinal system, section 6: handbook of physiology.* Makhlouf GM, ed. Bethesda, MD: American Physiological Society, 1989;215–243.

145. Bloom SR, Christofides ND, Yiangan T. Peptide histidine isoleucine (PHI) and Verner-Morrison syndrome. *Gut* 1983; 4:473.

146. Yamashiro Y, Yamamoto K, Sato M. Loperamide therapy in a child with VIPoma-associated diarrhea. *Lancet* 1982;1: 1413.

147. Krejs GJ. Comparison of the effect of VIP and PHI on water and ion movement in the canine jejunum in vivo. *Gastroenterol Clin Biol* 1984;8:868.

148. Krejs GJ. VIPoma syndrome. *Am J Med* 1987;82(Suppl. 5B):37–48.

149. Bloom SR, Long RG, Bryant MG. Clinical, biochemical and pathological studies on 62 VIPomas. *Gastroenterology* 1980; 78:1143.

150. O'Dorisio TM, Mekhjian H, Gaginella TS. Medical therapy of VIPomas. *Endocrinol Metab Clin North Am* 1989;18:545–556.

151. Krejs GJ, Walsh JH, Morawski BA. Intractable diarrhea: intestinal perfusion studies and plasma VIP concentrations in patients with pancreatic Pomas cholera syndrome and surreptitious ingestion of laxatives and diuretics. *Am J Dig Dis* 1977;22:280–292.

152. Vinik AI, Strodel WE, Eckhauser FE, Moattari AR, Lloyd R. Somatostatinomas, pomas and neurotensinomas. *Semin Oncol* 1987;14:263–281.

153. Boden G, Shimoyama R. Hormone-producing tumors of the gastrointestinal tract. In: *Somatostatinoma.* Cohen S, Soloway RD, eds. New York: Churchill Livingstone, 1985;85–100.

154. Maton PN, O'Dorisio TM, Howe B. Effect of the long-acting somatostatin analogue (SMS 201–995) in a patient with pancreatic cholera. *N Engl J Med* 1985;312:17–21.

155. Holm-Bentzen M, Schulta A, Fahrenkrug J. Effect of VIP

156. on gastric acid secretion in man. *Hepatogastroenterology* 1980;27(Suppl.):126–134.

156. Krejs GJ, Fordtran JS. *Diarrhea in gastrointestinal diseases.* Philadelphia: WB Saunders, 1983.

157. Morris AI, Turnberg LA: Surreptitious laxative abuse. *Gastroenterology* 1979;77:780–786.

158. Rivier J, Spress J, Thorner M, Vale W. Characterization of a growth-hormone releasing factor from a human pancreatic islet cell tumor. *Nature* 1982;300:276–278.

159. Thorner M, Perryman RI, Cronin MJ. Somatotroph hyperplasia. *J Clin Invest* 1982;70:965–975.

160. Asa SL, Singer W, Kovacs K. Pancreatic endocrine tumor producing growth hormone-releasing hormone associated with multiple endocrine neoplasia type 1 syndrome. *Acta Endocrinol* 1987;115:331–337.

161. Barkan AL, Shenker Y, Grekin RJ. Acromegaly from ectopic GHRH secretion by malignant carcinoid tumor: successful treatment with long-acting somatostatin analogue. SMS. *Cancer* 1986;61:221–226.

162. Sano T, Yamasaki R, Saito H. Growth hormone-releasing hormone (GHRH) secreting pancreatic tumor in a patient with multiple endocrine neoplasia type 1. *Am J Surg Pathol* 1987;11:810–819.

163. Donow C, Pipeleers-Marichial M, Stamm B, Heitz PU. Pathologie des insulinoms und gastrinoms. Lokalisation, gruke, mulizentrizitat, Association mit der Multiplenendokrinen Neiplasie type 1 und malignitat. *Deutsch Med Wochenschr* 1990;115:1386–1391.

164. Barkan AL. Acromegaly: diagnosis and therapy. *Endocrinol Metab Clin North Am* 1989;18:277–310.

165. Thorner M, Frohman LA, Leong DA. Extrahypothalamic GRF secretion is a rare cause of acromegaly. Plasma GRF in 177 acromegalic patients. *J Clin Endocrinol Metab* 1984; 59:846–849.

166. Price DE, Absolom SR, Davidson K, Bolia A, Bell PRF, Howlett TA. A case of multiple endocrine neoplasia: hyperparathyroidism, insulinoma, GRF-oma, hypercalcitonemia and intractable peptic ulceration. *Clin Endocrinol* 1992;37: 187–188.

167. Dayal Y, Lin HD, Tallberg K, Reichlin BAS, DeLellis RA, Wolfe JH. Immunocytochemical demonstration of growth hormone-releasing factor in gastrointestinal and pancreatic endocrine tumors. *Am J Clin Pathol* 1986;85:13–23.

168. Larsson LI, Hirsch MA, Holst JJ. Pancreatic somatostatinoma clinical features and physiologic implications. *Lancet* 1977;1:666–668.

169. Ganda OP, Weir GC, Soeldner JS. Somatostatinoma: a somatostatin-containing tumor of the endocrine pancreas. *N Engl J Med* 1977;296:963–967.

170. Yamada T, Chiha T. The gastrointestinal system. In: Makhlouf GM, ed. *Somatostatin, section 6: handbook of physiology.* Bethesda, MD: American Physiological Society, 1979; 431–453.

171. Pipeleers D, Couturier E, Gepts W. Five cases of somatostatinoma: clinical heterogeneity and diagnostic usefulness of basal and tolbutamide-induced hypersomatostatinemia. *J Clin Endocrinol Metab* 1983;56:1236–1242.

172. Krejs GJ, Orci L, Conlon M. Somatostatinoma syndrome (biochemical, morphological, and clinical features). *N Engl J Med* 1979;301:285–292.

173. Kent RB, van Heerden JA, Weiland LH. Nonfunctioning islet cell tumors. *Ann Surg* 1981;193:185–190.

174. O'Dorisio TM, Vinik AI. Pancreatic polypeptide and mixed peptide-producing tumors of the gastrointestinal tract. In: *Contemporary issues in gastroenterology.* Cohen S, Soloway RD, eds. Edinburgh: Churchill Livingstone, 1984;117–128.

175. Takahashi H, Nakano K, Adachi Y. Multiple nonfunctional pancreatic islet cell tumor in multiple endocrine neoplasia type 1; a case report. *Acta Pathol Jpn* 1988;38:667–682.

176. Heitz PU, Kasper M, Polak JM, Kloppel G. Pancreatic endocrine tumors: immunocytochemical analysis of 125 tumors. *Hum Pathol* 1982;13:163–271.

177. Walsh JH. Physiology of the gastrointestinal tract. In: *Gastrointestinal hormones.* Johnson LR, ed. New York: Raven Press, 1987;181–254.

178. Taylor IL. Pancreatic polypeptide family: pancreatic polypeptide, neuropeptide Y, and peptide YY. In: *Gastrointestinal system, section 6: handbook of physiology*. Makhlouf GM, ed. Bethesda, MD: American Physiological Society, 1989;475–543.

179. Hayes MMM. Report of a pancreatic polypeptide producing islet-cell tumor of the pancreas causing the watery diarrhea, hypokalemia, achlorhydria syndrome in a 55-year-old Zimbabwean African male. *Central African J Med* 1980;26:195–197.

180. Vinik AI, Moattari AR. Treatment of endocrine tumors. *Endocrinol Metab Clin North Am* 1989;18:483–518.

181. Berger D, Crowther FC, Floyd JC, Pek C, Fajans SS. Effect of age on fasting plasma levels of pancreatic hormones in men. *J Clin Endocrinol Metab* 1978;47:1183–1189.

182. Lamers CBHW, Diemel LM, van Leer E, Van Leusen R, Peetoom JJ. Mechanism of elevated serum pancreatic polypeptide in chronic renal failure. *J Clin Endocrinol Metab* 1982;55:922–926.

183. Schwartz T. Atropine suppression test for pancreatic polypeptide. *Lancet* 1978;2:43–44.

184. Adrian TE, Uttenthal LO, Williams SJ, Bloom SR. Secretion of pancreatic polypeptide in patients with pancreatic endocrine tumors. *N Engl J Med* 1986;315:287–291.

185. Maton PN, Gardner JD, Jensen RT. Cushing's syndrome in patients with Zollinger-Ellison syndrome. *N Engl J Med* 1986;315:1–5.

186. Clark ES, Carney JA. Pancreatic islet cell tumor associated with Cushing's syndrome. *Am J Surg Pathol* 1984;8:917–924.

187. Eriksson B, Oberg K, Skogseid B. Neuroendocrine pancreatic endocrine tumors. *Acta Oncol* 1989;28:373–377.

188. Cryer PE, Hill GJ. Pancreatic islet cell carcinoma with hypercalcemia and hypergastrinemia. *Cancer* 1976;3876:2217–2221.

189. Bresler L, Boissel P, Conroy T, Grosdidier J. Pancreatic islet cell carcinoma with hypercalcemia: complete remission 5 years after surgical excision and chemotherapy. *Am J Gastroenterol* 1991;86:635–638.

190. Feurle GE, Helmstaedter V, Tischbirek K. A multihormonal tumor of the pancreas producing neurotensin. *Dig Dis Sci* 1981;26:1125–1133.

191. Gutniak M, Rosenqvist U, Grimelius L. Report on a patient with watery diarrhea syndrome caused by a pancreatic tumour containing neurotensin, encephalin and calcitonin. *Acta Med Scand* 1980;208:95–100.

192. Williams ED. The classification of carcinoid tumors. *Lancet* 1963;1:238–239.

193. Godwin JD II. Carcinoid tumors: an analysis of 2837 cases. *Cancer* 1975;36:560–569.

194. Duh Q-Y. Carcinoids associated with multiple endocrine neoplasia syndromes. *Am J Surg* 1987;154:142–148.

195. Farhangi M, Taylor J, Havey A, O'Dorisio TM. Neuroendocrine (carcinoid) tumor of the lung and type I multiple endocrine neoplasia. *South Med J* 1987;80:1459–1462.

196. Pass HI, Doppman JL, Nieman L. Management of the ectopic ACTH syndrome due to thoracic carcinoids. *Ann Thorac Surg* 1990;50:52–57.

197. Doppman JL, Pass HI, Nieman LK. Detection of ACTH-producing bronchial carcinoid tumors: MR imaging vs CT. *AJR* 1991;156:39–43.

198. Glikson M, Gil-Ad I, Calun E, Dresner R. Acromegaly due to ectopic growth hormone-releasing hormone secretion by a bronchial carcinoid tumour. Dynamic hormonal responses to various stimuli. *Acta Endocrinol* 1991;125:366–371.

199. Amano S, Hazama F, Haebara H. Ectopic ACTH-MSH producing carcinoid tumor with multiple endocrine hyperplasia in a child. *Acta Pathol Jpn* 1978;28:721–730.

200. Bonato M, Cerati M, Pagani A, Papotti M. Differential diagnostic patterns of lung neuroendocrine tumours. A clinico-pathological and immunohistochemical study of 122 cases. *Virchows Arch A Pathol Anat Histopathol* 1992;420:201–211.

201. Pal V, Frigyes K, Attila C. Surgical treatment of bronchial carcinoid tumours. Radical surgery prognosis. *Int J Surg* 1991;76:98–100.

202. Harpole DHJ, Feldman JM, Buchanan S, Young WG, Wolfe WG. Bronchial carcinoid tumors: a retrospective analysis of 126 patients. *Ann Thorac Surg* 1992;54:50–55.

203. Salyer WR, Salyer DC, Eggleston JC. Carcinoid tumors of the thymus. *Cancer* 1976;37:958–973.

204. Wick MR, Scott RE, Li C-Y, Carney JA. Carcinoid tumor of the thymus. A clinicopathologic report of seven cases with a review of the literature. *Mayo Clin Proc* 1980;55:246–254.

205. Zeiger MA, Swartz SE, MacGillivray DC, Linnoila I, Shakir M. Thymic carcinoid in association with MEN syndromes. *Am J Surg* 1992;58:430–434.

206. Thompson GB, van Heerden JA, Martin JK, Scutt AJ, Ilstrup DM, Carney JA. Carcinoma of the gastrointestinal tract: presentation, management and prognosis. *Surgery* 1985;98:1054–1062.

207. Godwin JD. Carcinoid tumors. An analysis of 2837 cases. *Cancer* 1975;36:560–569.

208. Croisier J-C, Azerad E, Lubetski J. L'adenomatose polyendocrinienne (syndrome de Wermer). Revue de la litterature. *Semin Hop Paris* 1971;47:494–519.

209. Moertel CG. An odyssey in the land of small tumors. *J Clin Oncol* 1987;5:1503–1522.

210. Lehtola J, Karttunen T, Krekala I. Gastric carcinoids with minimal or no macroscopic lesion in patients with pernicious anemia. *Hepatogastroenterology* 1985;32:72–76.

211. Stockbrugger RW, Menon CG, Bielby JOW. Gastroscopic screening in 80 patients with pernicious anemia. *Gut* 1983;24:1141–1147.

212. Jensen RT. Gastrinoma as a model for prolonged hypergastrinemia in man. In: *Gastrin*. Walsh JH, ed. New York: Raven Press, 1993.

213. Brandi ML, Aurbach GD, Fitzpatrick LA, et al. Parathyroid mitogenic activity in plasma from patients with familial multiple endocrine neoplasia type 1. *N Engl J Med* 1986;314:1287–1293.

214. Maton PN, Lack EE, Collen MJ. The effect of Zollinger-Ellison syndrome and omperazole therapy on gastric endocrine cells. *Gastroenterology* 1990;99:943–950.

215. Solcia E, Bordi C, Creutzfeldt W. Histopathological classification of nonantral gastric endocrine growths in man. *Digestion* 1988;41:185–200.

216. Benya RV, Metz DC, Hijazi YM, Fishbeyn VA, Pisegna JR, Jensen RT. Fine needle aspiration cytology for the evaluation of submucosal nodules in patients with zollinger-ellison syndrome. *Am J Gastroenterol* 1993;88:258–265.

217. Wilander E. Diagnostic pathology of gastrointestinal and pancreatic neuroendocrine tumors. *Acta Oncol* 1989;28:363–369.

218. Eriksson B, Arnberg H, Oberg K. A polyclonal antiserum against chromogranin A and B—a new sensitive marker for neuroendocrine tumors. *Acta Oncol* 1990;122:145–155.

219. Eriksson B, Oberg K. Peptide hormones as tumor markers in neuroendocrine gastrointestinal tumors. *Acta Oncol* 1991; 30:477–484.

220. Vyberg M, Horn T, Francis D, Askaa J. Immunocytochemical identification of neuron-specific enolase, synaptophysin, chromogranin and endocrine granule constituent in neuroendocrine tumors. *Acta Histochem* 1990;38:S179–S181.

221. Eriksson B, Arnberg H, Oberg K. Chromogranins—new sensitive markers for neuroendocrine tumors. *Acta Oncol* 1989;28:325–329.

222. Kahn CR, Rosen SW, Weintraub BD, Fajans SS, Gorden P. Ectopic production of chorionic gonadotropin and its subunits by islet cell tumors. *N Engl J Med* 1977;297:565–569.

223. Bardram L, Agner T, Hagen C. Levels of alpha subunits of gonadotropin can be increased in Zollinger-Ellison syndrome, both in patients with malignant tumors and apparently benign disease. *Acta Endocrinol* 1988;118:135–141.

224. Comi R, Gorden P. The exocrine pancreas: biology, pathobiology and disease. In: *Insulinoma*. Go VLW, ed. New York: Raven Press, 1986;745–761.

225. Creutzfeldt W, Arnold R, Creutzfeldt C, Deuticke U, Frerichs H, Track NS. Biochemical and morphological investigations of 30 human insulinomas. *Diabetologia* 1973;9:217–231.

226. Johnson J, Fabri PJ, Lott JA. Serum gastrins in Zollinger-

Ellison syndrome: identification of localized disease. *Clin Chem* 1980;26:867–870.

227. Kothary PC, Fabri PJ, Gower W, O'Dorisio TM, Ellis J, Vinik A. Evaluation of NH₂-terminus gastrins in gastrinoma syndrome. *J Endocrinol Metab* 1986;62:970–974.

228. Vasen HF, Lamers CB, Lips CJ. Screening for the multiple endocrine neoplasia syndrome type I. A study of 11 kindreds in The Netherlands. *Ann Intern Med* 1989;149:2717–2722.

229. Hershon KS, Kelly WA, Shaw CM, Schwartz R, Bierman EL. Prolactinomas as part of the multiple endocrine neoplastic syndrome type 1. *Am J Med* 1983;74:713–720.

230. Manes JL, Taylor HB. Thymic carcinoid in familial multiple endocrine adenomatosis. *Arch Pathol* 1973;95:252–255.

231. Carlson HE, Levine GA, Goldberg NJ, Hershman JM. Hyperprolactinemia in multiple endocrine adenomatosis, type 1. *Arch Intern Med* 1978;138:1807–1808.

232. Marx SJ, Spiegel AM, Brown EM, Aurbach GD. Family studies in patients with primary parathyroid hyperplasia. *Am J Med* 1977;62:698–706.

233. Vandeweghe M, Braxel K, Schutyser J, Vermeulen A. A case of multiple endocrine adenomatosis with primary amenorrhoea. *Postgrad Med J* 1978;54:618–622.

234. Davies M, Klimiuk PS, Adams PH, Lumb GA, Large DM, Anderson DC: Familial hypocalciuric hypercalcaemia and acute pancreatitis. *Br Med J* 1981;282:1023–1025.

235. Samaan NA, Ouais S, Ordonez NG, Choksi UA, Sillin RV, Hickey RC. Multiple endocrine syndrome type I. Clinical, laboratory findings, and management in five families. *Cancer* 1989;64:741–752.

236. Skogseid B, Eriksson B, Lundqvist G. Multiple endocrine neoplasia type 1: a 10-year prospective screening study in four kindreds. *J Clin Endocrinol Metab* 1991;73:281–287.

237. Oberg K, Skogseid B, Eriksson B. Multiple endocrine neoplasia type 1 (MEN-1). *Acta Oncol* 1989;28:383–387.

238. Scheithauer BW, Laws J, Kovacs K, Horvath E, Randall RV, Carney JA. Pituitary adenomas of the multiple endocrine neoplasia type I syndrome. *Semin Diagn Pathol* 1987;4:205–211.

239. Vasen HF, Lamers CB, Lips CJ. Screening for the multiple endocrine neoplasia syndrome type I. A study of 11 kindreds in the Netherlands. *Arch Int Med* 1989;149:2717–2722.

240. Bear JC, Briones UR, Fahey JF, Farid NR. Variant multiple endocrine neoplasia I (MEN I Burin): further studies and non-linkage to HLA. *Hum Hered* 1985;35:15–20.

241. Bahn RS, Scheithauer BW, Van HJ, Laws EJ, Horvath E, Gharib H. Nonidentical expressions of multiple endocrine neoplasia, type I, in identical twins. *Mayo Clin Proc* 1986; 61:689–696.

242. Snyder NI, Scurry MT, Deiss WP. Five families with multiple endocrine adenomatosis. *Ann Intern Med* 1972;76:53–58.

243. Craven DE, Goodman D, Carter JH. Familial multiple endocrine adenomatosis. Multiple endocrine neoplasia, type I. *Arch Intern Med* 1972;129:567–569.

244. Johnson GJ, Summerskill WHJ, Anderson VE, Keating FJ. Clinical and genetic investigation of a large kindred with multiple endocrine adenomatosis. *N Engl J Med* 1967;277: 1379–1385.

245. Farnid NR, Buehler S, Russell NA, Maroun FB, Allerdice P, Smyth HS. Prolactinomas in familial multiple endocrine neoplasia syndrome type I. Relationship to HLA and carcinoid tumors. *Am J Med* 1980;69:874–880.

246. Prosser PR, Karam JH, Townsend JJ, Forsham PH. Prolactin-secreting pituitary adenomas in multiple endocrine adenomatosis, type I. *Ann Intern Med* 1979;91,1:41–44.

247. Scheithauer BW, Laws ER Jr, Kovacs K, Horvath E, Randall RV, Carney JA. Pituitary adenomas of the multiple endocrine neoplasia type I syndrome. *Semin Diagn Pathol* 1987;4:205–211.

248. Wynne AG, Gharib H, Scheithauer BW, Davis DH, Freeman SL, Horvath E. Hyperthyroidism due to inappropriate secretion of thyrotropin in 10 patients. *Am J Med* 1992;92:15–24.

249. Banik S, Hasleton PS, Lyon RL. An unusual variant of multiple endocrine neoplasia syndrome: a case report. *Histopathology* 1984;8:135–144.

250. Sawano S, Shishiba Y, Shimizu T. Hyperparathyroidism associated with Cushing's syndrome due to an adrenal cortical adenoma. *Endocrinol Jpn* 1990;37:255–260.

251. Fig LM, Gross MD, Shapiro B. Adrenal localization in the adrenocorticotropic hormone-independent Cushing syndrome. *Ann Intern Med* 1988;109:547–553.

252. Perry RR, Nieman LK, Cutler GJ. Primary adrenal causes of Cushing's syndrome. Diagnosis and surgical management. *Ann Surg* 1989;210:59–68.

253. Nieman LK, Chrousos GP, Oldfield EH, Avgerinos PC, Cutler GBJ, Loriaux DL. The ovine corticotropin-releasing hormone stimulation test and the dexamethasone suppression test in the differential diagnosis of Cushing's syndrome. *Ann Intern Med* 1986;105:862–867.

254. Oldfield EH, Doppman JL, Nieman LK. Petrosal sinus sampling with and without corticotropin-releasing hormone for the differential diagnosis of Cushing's syndrome. *N Engl J Med* 1991;325:897–905.

255. Flack MR, Oldfield EH, Cutler GBJ. Urine free cortisol in the high-dose dexamethasone suppression test for the differential diagnosis of the Cushing syndrome. *Ann Intern Med* 1992;116:211–217.

256. Daniels M, Newland P, Dewar JH, White MC, Taylor PK. Gonadotrophin secretion in vitro by cells of a pituitary tumor from a patient with multiple endocrine neoplasia type I. *Clin Endocrinol* 1992;36:475–480.

257. Snyder NI, Scurry MT, Deiss WP Jr. Five families with multiple endocrine adenomatosis. *Ann Intern Med* 1972;76:53–58.

258. Matsuo K, Tang SH, Fagin JA. Allelotype of human thyroid tumors: loss of chromosome 11q13 sequences in follicular neoplasms. *Mol Endocrinol* 1991;5:1873–1879.

259. Skogseid B, Larsson C, Lindgren P-G, et al. Clinical and genetic features of adrenocortical lesions in multiple endocrine neoplasia type 1. *J Clin Endocrinol Metab* 1992;75:76–81.

260. Maton PN, Gardner JD, Jensen RT. Cushing's syndrome in patients with the Zollinger-Ellison syndrome. *N Engl J Med* 1986;315:1–5.

261. Skogseid B, Larsson C, Lindgran PG, et al. Clinical and genetic features of adrenocortical lesions in multiple endocrine neoplasia type I. *J Clin Endocrinol Metab* 1992;75:76–81.

262. Houdelette P, Chagnon A, Dumotier J, Marthan E. Corticosurrenalome malin dans le cadre d'un syndrome de Wermer. *J Chir* 1989;126:385–387.

263. Kassem M, Xu C, Brask S, Eriksen EF, Mosekilde L, Kruse T. Familial isolated primary hyperparathyroidism. *J Bone Mineral Res* 1992;7(Suppl. 1):s249.

264. Goldsmith RE, Sizemore GW, Chen I, Zalme E, Altemeier WA. Familial hyperparathyroidism description of a large kindred with physiologic observations and a review of the literature. *Ann Intern Med* 1976;842:36–43.

265. Hershon KS, Kelly WA, Shaw CM, Schwartz R, Bierman EL. Prolactinomas as part of the multiple endocrine neoplastic syndrome type 1. *Am J Med* 1983;74:713–720.

266. Farid NR, Buehler S, Russell NA, Maroun FB, Allerdice P, Smith HS. Prolactinomas in familial multiple endocrine neoplasia syndrome type I. *Am J Med* 1980;69:874–880.

267. Bear JC, Urbina RB, Fahey JF, Farid NR. Variant multiple endocrine neoplasia I (MEN I-Burin): further studies and non-linkage to HLA-1. *Hum Hered* 1985;35:15–20.

268. Marx SJ, Powell D, Shimkin P, et al. Familial hyperparathyroidism: mild hypercalemia in at least nine members of a kindred. *Ann Intern Med* 1973;78:371–377.

269. Green J, Farid N. Natural history and management of a prolactinoma variant of multiple endocrine neoplasia type 1. *Program & Abstracts of the 72nd Annual Meeting of the Endocrine Society,* 1990 (Abstract).

270. Potts JT Jr, ed. Proceedings of the NIH consensus development conference on diagnosis and management of asymptomatic primary hyperparathyroidism. *J Bone Mineral Res* 1991;6(Suppl 2).

271. Norton JA, Brennan MF, Wells SA. Surgical management of primary hyperparathyroidism. This volume.

272. Bikle DD. Clinical counterpoint: vitamin D: new actions, new analogs, new therapeutic potential. *Endocrin Rev* 1992;13:765–783.

273. Fox J, Hadfield S, Petty BA, Nemeth EF. A first generation calcimimetic compound (NPS R-568) that acts on the parathyroid cell calcium receptor: a novel therapeutic approach for hyperparathyroidsim. *J Bone Min Res* 1993;8(Suppl 1): s181.

274. Eberle F, Grün R. Multiple endocrine neoplasia, type I (MEN I). In: *Advances in internal medicine and pediatrics*. Frick P, Harnack G-A, Kochsiek K, Martini GA, Prader A, eds. New York: Springer-Verlag, 1981;77–149.

275. Norton JA, Cornelius MJ, Doppman JL, Maton PN, Gardner JD, Jensen RT. Effect of parathyroidectomy in patients with hyperparathyroidism, Zollinger-Ellison syndrome, and multiple endocrine neoplasia type I: a prospective study. *Surgery* 1987;102:958–966.

276. Nanes MS, O'Connor DT, Marx SJ. Plasma chromogranin-A in primary hyperparathyroidism. *J Clin Endocrinol Metab* 1989;69:950–955.

277. Stabile BE, Howard TJ, Passaro E Jr., O'Connor DT. Source of plasma chromogranin A elevation in gastrinoma patients. *Arch Surg* 1990;125:451–453.

278. Rizzoli RE, Murray TM, Marx SJ, Aurbach GD. Binding of radioiodinated bovine parathyroid hormone-(1–84) to canine renal cortical membranes. *Endocrinology* 1983;112:1303–1312.

279. Malmaeus J, Benson L, Johansson H, et al. Parathyroid surgery in the multiple endocrine neoplasia type I syndrome: choice of surgical procedure. *World J Surg* 1986;10:668–672.

280. Prinz RA, Gamvros OI, Sellu D, Lynn JA. Subtotal parathyroidectomy for primary chief cell hyperplasia of the multiple endocrine neuroendoplasia type I syndrome. *Ann Surg* 1981;193:26–29.

281. Kaplan EL, Bartlett S, Sugimoto J, Fredland A. Relation of postoperative hypocalcemia to operative techniques: deleterious effect of excessive use of parathyroid biopsy. *Surgery* 1982;92:827–834.

282. Norton JA, Shawker TH, Jones BL, et al. Intraoperative ultrasound and reoperative parathyroid surgery: an initial evaluation. *World J Surg* 1986;10:631–639.

283. Wells SA Jr, Farndon JR, Dale JK, Leight GS, Dilley WG. Long-term evaluation of patients with primary parathyroid hyperplasia managed by total parathyroidectomy and heterotopic autotransplantation. *Ann Surg* 1980;192:451–457.

284. Hellman P, Skogseid B, Juhlin C, Akerstrom G, Rastad J. Findings and long-term result of parathyroid surgery in multiple endocrine neoplasia type 1. *World J Surg* 1992;16:718–723.

285. Mallette LE, Blevins T, Jordan PH, Noon GP. Autogenous parathyroid grafts for generalized primary parathyroid hyperplasia versus multiple endocrine neoplasia type I. *Surgery* 1987;101:783–744.

286. Norton J, Aurbach GD, Marx SJ, Doppman JL. Surgical management of hyperparathyroidism. In: *Endocrinology*. DeGroot LJ, ed. Philadelphia: WB Saunders, 1989;1013–1031.

287. Miller DL, Doppman JL, Krudy AG, et al. Localization of parathyroid adenomas in patients who have undergone surgery. Part II. Invasive procedures. *Radiology* 1987;162:138–141.

288. Miller DL, Doppman JL, Shawker TH, et al. Localization of parathyroid adenomas in patients who have undergone surgery. Part I. Noninvasive imaging methods. *Radiology* 1987;162:133–137.

289. Doppman J. Preoperative localization of parathyroid tissue in primary hyperparathyroidism. This volume.

290. Nussbaum SR, Potts JT Jr. Immunoassays for parathyroid hormone 1–84 in the diagnosis of hyperparathyroidism. *J Bone Mineral Res* 1991;6(Suppl. 2):S43–S50.

291. Norton JA, Brennan MF, Saxe AW, et al. Intraoperative urinary cyclic adenosine monophosphate as a guide to successful reoperative parathyroidectomy. *Ann Surg* 1984;200:389–395.

292. Norton JA, Levin B, Jensen RT. Principles and practice of oncology. In: *Cancer*. DeVita VT, Hellman S, Rosenberg SA, eds. Philadelphia: JB Lippincott, 1993.

293. Jensen RT, Gardner JD. Zollinger-Ellison syndrome: clinical presentation, pathology, diagnosis and treatment. In: *Peptic ulcer and other acid-related diseases*. Dannenberg A, Zakim D, eds. New York: Academic Research Association, 1991: 117–211.

294. Waxman I, Gardner JD, Jensen RT, Maton PN. Peptic ulcer perforation as the presentation of zollinger-ellison syndrome. *Dig Dis Sci* 1991;36:19–24.

295. O'Dorisio TM, Mekhjian H, Gaginella TS. Medical therapy of VIPomas. *Endocrinol Metab Clin North Am* 1989;18:545–556.

296. Vinik AI, Moattari AR. Treatment of endocrine tumors. *Endocrinol Metab Clin North Am* 1989;18:483–518.

297. Jensen RT, Gardner JD. Gastrinoma. In: *The exocrine pancreas*. Go VLW, Brooks FP, DiMagno EP, eds. New York: Raven Press, 1993.

298. Metz DC, Jensen RT. Endocrine tumors of the pancreas. In: *Bockus gastroenterology*. Haubrich WB, Berk F, Schaffner JE, eds. Philadelphia: WB Saunders, 1993.

299. Howard JM, Chremos AN, Collen MJ. Famotidine, a new potent long acting histamine H2-receptor antagonist: comparison with cimetidine and ranitidine in the treatment of Zollinger-Ellison syndrome. *Gastroenterology* 1985;88:1026–1033.

300. Metz DC, Pisegna JR, Fishbeyn VA, Benya RV, Jensen RT. Control of gastric acid hypersecretion in the management of patients with Zollinger-Ellison syndrome. *World J Surg* (in press).

301. Frucht H, Maton PN, Jensen RT. Use of omeprazole in patients with Zollinger-Ellison syndrome. *Dig Dis Sci* 1991; 36:394–404.

302. Maton PN, Vinayek R, Frucht H. Long term efficacy and safety of omeprazole in patients with Zollinger-Ellison syndrome: a prospective study. *Gastroenterology* 1989;97:827–836.

303. Norton JA, Cornelius MJ, Doppman JL. Effect of parathyroidectomy in patients with hyperparathyroidism and multiple endocrine neoplasia type I. *Surgery* 1987;102:958–966.

304. McCarthy DM, Peikin SR, Lopatin RN. Hyperparathyroidism: a reversible cause of cimetidine-resistant gastric hypersecretion. *Br Med J* 1979;1:765–766.

305. Raufman J-P, Collins SM, Pandol S. Reliability of symptoms in assessing control of gastric acid secretion in patients with Zollinger-Ellison syndrome. *Gastroenterology* 1983;84:108–113.

306. Metz DC, Pisegna JR, Fishbeyn VA, Benya RV, Jensen RT. Current maintenance doses of omeprazole in Zollinger-Ellison syndrome are too high. *Gastroenterology* 1992;103:1498–1508.

307. Maton PN, Dayal Y. Clinical implication of hypergastrinemia. In: *Peptic ulcer and other acid-related diseases*. Dannenberg A, Zakim D, eds. New York: Academic Research Association, 1991;213–246.

308. Maton PN, Lack EE, Collen MJ. The effect of Zollinger-Ellison syndrome and omeprazole therapy on gastric endocrine cells. *Gastroenterology* 1990;99:943–950.

309. Vinayek R, Frucht H, London JF. Intravenous omeprazole in patients with Zollinger-Ellison syndrome undergoing surgery. *Gastroenterology* 1990;99:10–16.

310. Metz DC, Jensen RT. Zollinger-Ellison syndrome. In: *Consultations in gastroenterology*. Snape WJ, eds. Philadelphia: WB Saunders, 1993.

311. Thompson GB, van Heerden JA, Martin JK, Scutt AJ, Ilstrup DM, Carney JA. Carcinoma of the gastrointestinal tract: presentation, management and prognosis. *Surgery* 1985;98:1054–1062.

312. Godwin JD. Carcinoid tumors. An analysis of 2837 cases. *Cancer* 1975;36:560–569.

313. Maton PN, Gardner JD, Jensen RT. Use of long-acting somatostatin analogue SMS 201-995 in patients with pancreatic islet cell tumors. *Dig Dis Sci* 1989;34:28S–37S.

314. Dunne MJ, Fletcher R, Hofker PH, Shui J. Somatostatin and gastroenteropancreatic endocrine-tumors: therapeutic characteristics. In: *Somatostatin in the treatment of GEP endocrine tumors*. O'Dorisio TM, ed. Berlin: Springer-Verlag, 1987;93–113.

315. Oberg K, Eriksson B. Medical treatment of neuroendocrine gut and pancreatic tumors. *Acta Oncol* 1989;28:425–431.
316. Holst JJ. Hormone producing tumors of the gastrointestinal tract. In: *Glucagon-producing tumors.* Cohen S, Soloway RD, eds. New York: Churchill Livingstone, 1985; 57–84.
317. Norton JA, Kahn CR, Schiebinger R. Amino acid deficiency and the skin rash associated with glucagonoma syndrome. *Ann Intern Med* 1979;91:213–215.
318. Leichter SB. Clinical and metabolic aspects of glucagonoma. *Medicine* 1980;59:100–113.
319. Guillausseau PJ, Guillausseau C, Villet R. Les glucagonomas. Aspect cliniques, biologiques, anatomo-pathologiques et therapeutiques (Revue general de 130 cas). *Gastroenterol Clin Biol* 1982;6:1029–1041.
320. Welbourn RB, Wood SM, Polak JM, Bloom SR. Pancreatic endocrine tumors. In: *Gut hormones.* Bloom SR, Polak JM, eds. New York: Churchill Livingstone, 1981;547–554.
321. Verner JV, Morrison AB. Endocrine pancreatic ilset disease with diarrhea: report of a case due to diffuse hyperplasia of non beta islet tissue with a review of 54 additional cases. *Arch Intern Med* 1974;133:492–500.
322. Mekhjian H, O'Dorisio TM. VIPoma syndrome. *Semin Oncol* 1987;14:282–291.
323. Verner JV, Morrison AB. Islet cell tumor and a syndrome of refractory watery diarrhea and hypokalemia. *Am J Med* 1958;25:374–380.
324. Long RG, Bryant MG, Mitchell SJ, Adrian TE, Polak JM, Bloom SR. Clinicopathological study of pancreatic and ganglioneuroblastoma tumors secreting vasoactive intestinal polypeptide (Vipomas). *Br Med J* 1981;282:1767–1771.
325. Charney AN, Donowitz M. Prevention and reversal of cholera enterotoxin-induced intestinal secretion by methyl prednisolone induction of Na$^+$-K$^+$-ATPase. *J Clin Invest* 1976; 57:1590–1599.
326. Rao MB, O'Dorisio TM, George JM. Angiotensin II and norepinephrine antagonize the effect of vasoactive intestinal peptide on rat ileum and colon. *Peptides* 1984;5:291–294.
327. Vinik AI, Strodel WE, Eckhauser FE, Moattari AR, Lloyd R. Somatostatinomas, VIPomas and neurotensinomas. *Semin Oncol* 1987;14:263–281.
328. Boden G, Shimoyama R. Hormone-producing tumors of the gastrointestinal tract. In: *Somatostatinoma.* Cohen S, Soloway RD, eds. New York: Churchill Livingstone, 1985;85–100.
329. Yamada T, Chiha T. The gastrointestinal system. In: *Somatostatin, section 6: handbook of physiology.* Makhlouf GM, ed. Bethesda, MD: American Physiological Society, 1979; 431–453.
330. Walsh JH. Physiology of the gastrointestinal tract. In: *Gastrointestinal hormones.* Johnson LR, ed. New York: Raven Press, 1987;181–254.
331. Adrian TE, Barnes AJ, Long RG. The effect of somatostatin analogs on secretion of growth, pancreatic and gastrointestinal hormones in man. *J Clin Endocrinol Metab* 1981; 53:675–681.
332. Konturek SJ, Kewcien N, Obtuowicz W. Effects of somatostatin-14 and somatostatin-28 on plasma hormonal and gastric secretory response to cephalic and gastrointestinal stimulation. *Scand J Gastroenterol* 1985;20:31–38.
333. Vyberg M, Horn T, Francis D, Askaa J. Immunocytochemical identification of neuron-specific enolase, synaptophysin, chromogranin and endocrine granule constituent in neuroendocrine tumors. *Acta Histochem* 1990;38:S179–S181.
334. Pless J, Bauer W, Briner U. Chemistry and pharmacology of SMS 201-995, a long-acting octapeptide analogue of somatostatin. *Scand J Gastroenterol* 1974;21(Suppl. 119):54–64.
335. Kvols LK, Buck M, Moertel CG. Treatment of metastatic islet cell carcinoma with a somatostatin analogue (SMS 201-995). *Ann Intern Med* 1987;107:162–168.
336. Moertel CG. An odyssey in the land of small tumors. *J Clin Oncol* 1987;5:1503–1522.
337. Kvols LK, O'Connell MJ, Schutt AJ, Rubin AJ, Hahn RG. Treatment of the malignant carcinoid syndrome: evaluation

338. Price DE, Absolom SR, Davidson K, Bolia A, Bell PRF, Howlett TA. A case of multiple endocrine neoplasia: hyperparathyroidism, insulinoma, GRF-oma, hypercalcitonemia and intractable peptic ulceration. *Clin Endocrinol* 1992;37: 187–188.
339. Benya RV, Metz DC, Fishbeyn VA, Strader DB, Orbuch M, Jensen RT. Gastrinoma can be the initial presentation for patients with multiple endocrine neoplasia type 1 (MEN-1). *Gastroenterology* (in press).
340. Melmed S, Ziel FH, Braustein GD. Medical management of acromegaly due to ectopic production of GHRH by carcinoid tumor. *J Clin Endocrinol Metab* 1988;67:395–399.
341. Thorner M, Frohman LA, Leong DA. Extrahypothalamic GRF secretion is a rare cause of acromegaly. Plasma GRF in 177 acromegalic patients. *J Clin Endocrinol Metab* 1984; 59:846–849.
342. Lamberts SWJ, Tilanus HW, Klooswijk AIJ, Bruining HA, Van der Lely AJ, de Jong FH. Successful treatment with SMS 201-995 of Cushing's syndrome caused by ectopic adrenocorticotropin secretion from a metastatic gastrin-secreting pancreatic islet cell carcinoma. *J Clin Endocrinol Metab* 1988;67:1080–1085.
343. Ruszniewski P, Giarard F, Benamouzing R, Mignon M, Bonfils S. Long-acting somatostatin treatment of paraneoplastic Cushing's syndrome in a case of Zollinger-Ellison syndrome. *Gut* 1988;29:838–842.
344. Koelz A, Kraenzlin M, Gyr K. Escape of the response to a long-acting somatostatin analogue (SMS 201-995) in patients with VIPoma. *Gastroenterology* 1987;92:527–531.
345. Maton PN. Octreotide acetate and islet cell tumors. *Gastroenterol Clin North Am* 1989;18:897–922.
346. Bone HG. Diagnosis of the multiglandular endocrine neoplasias. *Clin Chem* 1990;36:711–718.
347. Sheppard BC, Norton JA, Doppman JL, Maton PN, Gardner JD, Jensen RT. Management of islet cells tumors in patients with multiple endocrine neoplasia: a prospective study. *Surgery* 1989;106:1108–1117.
348. Bonfils S, Landor JH, Mignon M. Results of surgical management in 92 consecutive patients with Zollinger-Ellison syndrome. *Ann Surg* 1981;194:692–697.
349. Fox PS, Hofmann JW, Wilson SD, DeCosse JJ. Surgical management of the Zollinger-Ellison syndrome. *Surg Clin North Am* 1974;54:395–407.
350. Malagelada JR, Edis AJ, Adson MA. Medical and surgical options in the management of patients with gastrinoma. *Gastroenterology* 1983;84:1524–1532.
351. Norton JA, Doppman JL, Jensen RT. Curative resection in Zollinger-Ellison syndrome: results of a 10 year prospective study. *Ann Surg* 1992;215:8–18.
352. Wermer P. Endocrine adenomatosis: peptic ulcer in a large kindred. *Am J Med* 1963;35:205–221.
353. Oberg K, Skogseid B, Eriksson B. Multiple endocrine neoplasia type 1. *Acta Oncol* 1989;28:383–387.
354. Zollinger RM. Gastrinoma factors influencing prognosis. *Surgery* 1985;97:49–54.
355. Podevin P, Ruszniewski P, Mignon M. Management of multiple endocrine neoplasia type 1 (MEN 1) in Zollinger-Ellison syndrome. *Gastroenterology* 1990;98:A230.
356. Doppman JL, Shawker TH, Miller DC. Localization of islet cell tumors. *Med Clin North Am* 1989;18:793–804.
357. Norton JA, Jensen RT. Unresolved issues in the management of patients with zollinger-ellison syndrome. *World J Surg* 1991;15:151–159.
358. Jensen RT, Gardner JD, Raufman J-P. Zollinger-Ellison syndrome: current concepts and management. *Ann Intern Med* 1983;98:59–75.
359. Wank SA, Doppman JL, Miller DL. Prospective study of the ability of computerized axial tomography to localize gastrinomas in patients with Zollinger-Ellison syndrome. *Gastroenterology* 1987;92:905–912.
360. Maton PN, Miller DL, Doppman JL. The role of selective angiography in the management of patients with Zollinger-Ellison syndrome. *Gastroenterology* 1987;92:913–919.

361. Eberle F, Grun R. Multiple endocrine neoplasia, type 1 (MEN1). *Ergebnisse Interen Med Kinderheilk* 1981;46:75–150.

362. Boden G. Glucagonomas and insulinomas. *Gastroenterol Clin North Am* 1989;18:831–845.

363. Wolfe MM, Jensen RT. Zollinger-Ellison syndrome. *N Engl J Med* 1987;317:1200–1209.

364. Norton JA, Doppman JL, Collen MJ. Prospective study of gastrinoma localization and resection in patients with Zollinger-Ellison syndrome. *Ann Surg* 1986;204:468–479.

365. London JF, Shawker TH, Doppman JL. Prospective assessment of abdominal ultrasound in patients with Zollinger-Ellison syndrome. *Radiology* 1991;178:763–767.

366. Shawker TH, Doppman JL, Dunnick NR, McCarthy DM. Ultrasound investigation of pancreatic islet cell tumors. *J Ultrasound Med* 1982;1:193–200.

367. Frucht H, Doppman JL, Norton JA. Gastrinomas: comparison of MR imaging with CT, angiography and ultrasound. *Radiology* 1989;171:713–717.

368. Pisegna JR, Doppman JL, Norton JA, Metz DC, Jensen RT. Prospective assessment of MR imaging in patients with Zollinger-Ellison syndrome. *Dig Dis Sci* (in press).

369. Barton JC, Hirschowitz BI, Maton PN, Jensen RT. Bone metastases in malignant gastrinoma. *Gastroenterology* 1986;91:915–925.

370. Norton JA, Shawker TH, Doppman JL. Localization and surgical treatment of occult insulinomas. *Ann Surg* 1990;212:615–620.

371. Krudy AG, Doppman JL, Jensen RT. Localization of islet cell tumors by dynamic CT: comparison with plain CT, arteriography, sonography, and venous sampling. *Am J Radiol* 1982;143:585–590.

372. Roche A, Raisonnier A, Gillon-Savouret MC. Pancreatic venous sampling and arteriography in localizing insulinomas and gastrinomas: procedure and results in 55 cases. *Radiology* 1982;145:621–627.

373. Pipeleers-Marichial M, Somers G, Willems G. Gastrinomas in the duodenum of patients with multiple endocrine neoplasia type 1 and the Zollinger-Ellison syndrome. *N Engl J Med* 1990;322:723–727.

374. Krenning EP, Breenan WAP, Kooij PP. Localization of endocrine-related tumors with radioiodinated analogues of somatostatin. *Lancet* 1989;1:242–244.

375. Doppman JL, Brennan MF, Dunnick NR. The role of pancreatic venous sampling in the localization of occult insulinoma. *Radiology* 1981;138:557–562.

376. Kingham J, Dick R, Bloom SR. VIPoma: localization by transhepatic portal venous sampling. *Br Med J* 1978;2:1682–1683.

377. Norton JA, Cromack DT, Shawker TH. Intraoperative ultrasonographic localization of islet cell tumors: a prospective comparison to palpation. *Ann Surg* 1988;207:160–168.

378. Frucht H, Norton JA, London JF. Detection of duodenal gastrinomas by operative endoscopic transillumination: a prospective study. *Gastroenterology* 1990;99:1622–1627.

379. Miller DL, Doppman JL, Metz DC, Matson PN, Jensen RT. Zollinger-Ellison syndrome: techniques, results and complications of portal venous sampling. *Radiology* 1992;182:235–241.

380. Croughs RJM, Hulsmans HAM, Israel DE, Hackeng WHL, Schopman W. Glucagonoma as part of the polyglandular adenoma syndrome. *Am J Med* 1972;52:690–698.

381. Stabile BE, Morrow DJ, Passaro E Jr: The gastrinoma triangle: operative implications. *Am J Surg* 1984;147:25–32.

382. Rosch T, Lightdale CJ, Botet JF. Localization of pancreatic endocrine tumors by endoscopic ultrasonography. *Endocrinology* 1992;326:1721–1726.

383. Doppman JL, Miller DL, Chang R. Gastrinomas: localization by means of selective intraarterial injection of secretin. *Radiology* 1990;174:25–29.

384. Thom AK, Norton JA, Doppman JL, Miller DL, Chang R, Jensen RT. Prospective study of the use of intraarterial secretin injection and portal venous sampling to localize duodenal gastrinomas. *Surgery* 1992;112:1002–1009.

385. Doppman JL, Miller DL, Chang R. Insulinomas: localization with selective intraarterial injection of calcium. *Radiology* 1991;178:237–241.

386. Reubi JC, Kvols LK, Nagorney DM. Detection of somatostatin receptor in surgical percutaneous needle biopsy samples of carcinoid and islet cell carcinomas. *Cancer Res* 1990;50:5969–5977.

387. Sheppard BC, Norton JA, Doppman JL, Maton PN, Gardner JD, Jensen RT. Management of islet cell tumors in patients with multiple endocrine neoplasia: A prospective study. *Surgery* 1989;106:1108–1118.

388. Imamura M, Takashi MP, Isobe Y, Hattori Y, Satomura K, Tobe T. Curative resection of multiple gastrinomas aided by selective arterial secretin injection and intraoperative secreting test. *Ann Surg* 1989;210:710–715.

389. Thompson NW. Surgical treatment of the endocrine pancreas and Zollinger-Ellison syndrome in MEN-1 syndrome. *Henry Ford Hosp Med J* 1992;40:195–198.

390. Friesen SR, Kimmel JR, Tomita T. Pancreatic polypeptide as a screening marker for pancreatic polypeptide apudomas in multiple endocrinopathies. *Am J Surg* 1980;139:61–72.

391. Wermer P. Endocrine adenomatosis and peptic ulcer in a large kindred. *Am J Med* 1963;35:205–212.

392. Hedman I, Hansson G, Lundberg LM, Tisell LE. A clinical evaluation of radiation-induced hyperparathyroidism based on 148 surgically treated patients. *World J Surg* 1984;8:96–105.

393. Langstein HN, Norton JA, Chiang HCV. The utility of circulating levels of human pancreatic polypeptide as a marker of islet cell tumors. *Surgery* 1990;108:1109–1116.

394. Kloppel G, Heitz PU. Pancreatic endocrine tumors. *Pathol Res Pract* 1988;183:155–175.

395. Stacpoole PW. The glucagonoma syndrome: clinical features, diagnosis and treatment. *Endocrine Rev* 1981;2:347–361.

396. Norton JA, Sugerbaker DH, Doppman JL. Aggressive resection of metastatic disease in selected patients with malignant gastrinoma. *Ann Surg* 1986;203:352–359.

397. Von Schrenk T, Howard JM, Doppman JL. Prospective study of chemotherapy in patients with metastatic gastrinoma. *Gastroenterology* 1988;94:1326–1334.

398. Heitz PU, Kasper M, Polak JM, Kloppel G. Pancreatic endocrine tumors: immunocytochemical analysis of 125 tumors. *Hum Pathol* 1982;13:163–271.

399. Kvols LK, Buck M. Chemotherapy of the metastatic carcinoid and islet cell tumors: a review. *Am J Med* 1987;82:77–83.

400. Buchanan KD, O'Hare MMT, Russell CJF, Kennedy TL, Hadden DP. Factors involved in the responsiveness of gastrointestinal apudomas to streptozotocin. *Dig Dis Sci* 1986;31:551S.

401. Moertel CG, Lefkopoulo M, Lipsitz S, Hahn RG, Klaassen D. Streptozotocin-doxorubicin, streptozotocin-fluorouracil or chlorozotocin in the treatment of advanced islet-cell carcinoma. *N Engl J Med* 1992;326:563–565.

402. Moertel CG, Hanely JA, Johnson LA. Streptozotocin alone compared with streptozotocin plus fluorouracil in the treatment of advanced islet-cell carcinoma. *N Engl J Med* 1980;303:1189–1192.

403. Pisegna JR, Slimak GG, Doppman JL, et al. Use of alpha interferon in patients with metastatic gastrinoma. *Gastroenterology* 1991;100:A299.

404. Ajani JA, Levin B, Wallace S. Systemic and regional therapy of advanced islet cell tumors. *Gastroenterol Clin North Am* 1989;18:923–930.

405. Eriksson B, Oberg K, Alm G. Treatment of malignant endocrine pancreatic tumors with human leukocyte interferon. *Lancet* 1986;2:1307–1309.

406. Ajani JA, Kavanagh J, Patt Y. Roferon and doxorubium combination against advanced islet cell or carcinoid tumors. *Proc Am Assoc Cancer Res* 1989;30:293.

407. Wadler S, Wiernick PH. Clinical update on the role of fluorouracil and recombinant interferon alpha-2a in the treatment of colorectal carcinoma. *Semin Oncol* 1990;17(Suppl. 1):16–21.

408. Kemeny N, Younes A, Seiter K. Interferon alpha-2a and 5-

fluorouracil for advanced colorectal carcinoma. Assessment of activity and toxicity. *Cancer* 1990;66:2470–2475.

409. Redding TW, Schally AV. Inhibition on growth of pancreatic carcinomas in animal models by analogs of hypothalamic hormones. *Proc Natl Acad Sci USA* 1984;84:248–252.

410. Reubi JC. Somatostatin analogue inhibits chondoscarcoma and insulinoma tumor growth. *Acta Endocrinol* 1985;109:108–114.

411. Carrasco CH, Chuang VP, Wallace S. Apudoma metastatic to the liver: treatment by hepatic artery embolization. *Radiology* 1983;149:79–83.

412. Moertel CG, May GR, Martin JK. Sequential hepatic artery occlusion and chemotherapy for metastatic islet carcinoid tumor and islet cell carcinoma. *Proc Amer Soc Clin Oncol* 1985;4:80.

413. Valette PJ, Souquet JC. Pancreatic islet cell tumors metastatic to the liver: treatment by hepatic artery chemo-embolization. *Hormone Res* 1989;32:77–79.

414. Kahn CR, Levy AG, Gardner JD, Miller JV, Gorden P, Schein PS. Pancreatic cholera: beneficial effects of treatment with streptozotocin. *N Engl J Med* 1975;292:941–945.

415. Zollinger RM, Ellison EH, Fabri PJ, Johnson J, Sparks J, Carey LC. Primary peptic ulceration of the jejunum associated with islet cell tumors: twenty-five year appraisal. *Ann Surg* 1980;192:422–430.

416. Zollinger RM, Martin EW, Carey LC, Sparks J, Minton JP. Observations on the postoperative tumor growth behavior of certain islet cell tumors. *Ann Surg* 1976;184:525–530.

417. McFadden D, Jaffe BM. Surgical approaches to endocrine-producing tumors of the gastrointestinal tract. In: *Hormone producing tumors of the gastrointestinal tract.* Cohen S, Soloway RD, eds. New York: Churchill Livingstone, 1985;139–158.

418. Carty SE, Jensen RT, Norton JA. Prospective study of aggressive resection of metastatic pancreatic endocrine tumors. *Surgery* 1992;112:1024–1032.

419. Thompson NW, Lloyd RV, Nishiyama RH. MEN pancreas: a histological and immunohistochemical study. *World J Surg* 1984;8:561–574.

420. Rasbach DA, van Heerden JA, Telander RL, Grant CS, Carney A. Surgical management of hyperinsulinism in the multiple endocrine neoplasia type 1 syndrome. *Arch Surg* 1985;123:584–589.

421. Goode PN, Farndon JR, Anderson J, Johnston ID, Morte JA. Diazoxide in the management of patients with insulinoma. *World J Surg* 1896;10:586–592.

422. Maton PN, Gardner JD, Jensen RT. Use of long-acting somatostatin analog SMS 201-995 in patients with pancreatic islet cell tumors. *Dig Dis Sci* 1989;34:(Suppl. 3):28s–39s.

423. Lamberts SW, Pieters GF, Metselaar HJ, Ong GL, Tan HS, Reubi JC. Development of resistance to a long-acting somatostatin analogue during treatment of two patients with metastatic endocrine pancreatic tumors. *Acta Endocrinol* 1988;119:561–566.

424. Lems WF, Fisher HR, Hackeng WH, Naafs MA. Aggravation of hypoglycemia in insulinoma patients by the long-acting somatostatin analogue ocreotide (Sandostatin). *Acta Endocrinol* 1989;121:34–50.

425. Bradows RG, Campbell RG. Control of refractory fasting hypoglycemia in a patient with suspected insulinoma with diphenylhydantion. *J Clin Endocrinol Metab* 1974;38:159–161.

426. Imanaka S, Matsuda S, Ito K, Matsouka T, Okada Y. Medical treatment for inoperable insulinoma: clinical usefulness of depheylhydantiin and diltiazem. *Jpn J Clin Oncol* 1986;16:65–71.

427. Blum I, Rusecki Y, Doron M, Lahav M, Laron Z, Atsman A. Evidence for a therapeutic effect of dl-propranolol in benign and malignant insulinoma: report of three cases. *J Endocrinol Invest* 1983;6:41–45.

428. Warren WH, Faber P, Gould VE. Neuroendocrine tumors of the lung. *J Thorac Carciovasc Surg* 1989;98:321–332.

429. Pass HI, Doppman JL, Nieman L. Management of the ectopic ACTH syndrome due to thoracic carcinoids. *Ann Thorac Surg* 1990;50:52–57.

430. Creutzfeldt W, Bartsch HH, Jacubaschke U, Stockmann F. Treatment of gastrointestinal endocrine tumours with interferon-alpha and octreotide. *Acta Oncol* 1991;30:529–535.

431. Burke CW, Adams CBT, Esiri MM, Morris C, Bevan JS. Transsphenoidal surgery for Cushing's disease: does what is removed determine the endocrine outcome? *Clin Endocrinol* 1990;33:525–537.

432. Burch W. A survey of results with transsphenoidal surgery in Cushing's disease. *N Engl J Med* 1983;308:103–105.

433. Wilson CB, Dempsey LC. Transsphenoidal microsurgical removal of 250 pituitary adenomas. *J Neurosurg* 1978;48:13–22.

434. Sheline GE, Wara WM, Smith V. Therapeutic irradiation and brain injury. *Int J Radiat Oncol Biol Phys* 1980;6:1215–1228.

435. Howlett TA, Plowman PN, Wass JA, Rees LH, Jones AE, Besser GM. Megavoltage pituitary irradiation in the management of Cushing's disease and Nelson's syndrome: long-term follow-up. *Clin Endocrinol* 1989;31:309–323.

436. Eastman RC, Gorden P, Roth J. Conventional supervoltage irradiation is an effective treatment for acromegaly. *J Clin Endocrinol Metab* 1979;48:931–940.

437. Linfoot JA, Nakagawa JS, Wiedemann E. Heavy particle therapy: pituitary tumors. *Bull Los Angeles Neurol Soc* 1977;42:175–189.

438. Levy RP, Fabrikant JI, Frankel KA. Heavy-charged-particle radiosurgery of the pituitary gland: clinical results of 840 patients. *Stereotact Funct Neurosurg* 1991;57:22–35.

439. Lawrence JH, Tobias CA, Linfoot JA, Born JL, Chong CY. Heavy-particle therapy in acromegaly and Cushing disease. *J Am Med Assoc* 1976;235:2307–2310.

440. Verde G, Oppizzi G, Chiodini PG, Dallabonzana D, Luccarelli G, Liuzzi A. Effect of chronic bromocriptine administration on tumor size in patients with "nonsecreting" pituitary adenomas. *J Endocrinol Invest* 1985:8:113.

441. Koppelman MC, Jaffee MJ, Rieth KG. Hyperprolactinemia, amenorrhea and galactorrhea. A retrospective assessment of twenty-five cases. *Ann Intern Med* 1984;100:115–121.

442. Klibanski A, Greenspan S. Increase in bone mass after treatment of hyperprolactinemic amenorrhea. *N Engl J Med* 1986;315:542.

443. Corenblum B, Taylor PJ. Long-term follow-up of hyperprolactinemic women treated with bromocriptine. *Fertil Steril* 1983;40:596.

444. Molitch ME, Elton RL, Blackwell RE, Caldwell B. Bromocriptine as primary therapy for prolactin-secreting macroadenomas: results of a prospective multicenter study. *J Clin Endocrinol Metab* 1985;60:698–705.

445. Ciccarelli E, Miola C, Grottoli S, Avataneo T, Lancranjan I, Camanni F. Long term therapy of patients with macroprolactinoma using repeatable injectable bromocriptene. *J Clin Endocrinol Metab* 1993;76:484–488.

446. Randall RV, Laws ER Jr, Abboud CF, Ebersold MJ, Kao PC, Scheithauer BW. Transsphenoidal microsurgical treatment of prolactin-producing pituitary adenomas. *Mayo Clin Proc* 1983;58:108–121.

447. Nelson PB, Goodfman M, Maroon JC. Factors in predicting outcome from operation in patients with prolactin-secreting pituitary adenomas. *Neurosurgery* 1983;13:634–641.

448. Parl F, Cruz VE, Cobb CA. Late recurrence of surgically removed prolactinomas. *Cancer* 1986;57:2422–2426.

449. Balagura S, Derome P, Guiot G. Acromegaly: analysis of 132 cases treated surgically. *Neurosurgery* 1981;8:413–416.

450. Ross DA, Wilson CB. Results of transsphenoidal microsurgery for growth hormone-secreting pituitary adenoma in a series of 214 patients. *J Neurosurg* 1988;68:854–867.

451. Laws EJ. Surgical management of pituitary adenomas. *Curr Probl Cancer* 1984;8:1–26.

452. Wass JA, Thorner MO, Morris DV. Long-term treatment of acromegaly with bromocriptine. *Br Med J* 1977;1:875–878.

453. Oppizzi G, Liuzzi A, Chiodini PG. Dopaminergic treatment of acromegaly: different effects on hormone secretion and tumor size. *J Clin Endocrinol Metab* 1984:58:988–992.

454. Mehltretter G, Heinz S, Schopohl J, von Werder K, Muller OA. Long-term treatment with SMS 201-995 in resistant ac-

romegaly: effectiveness of high doses and continuous subcutaneous infusion. *Klin Wochenschr* 1991;69:83–90.

455. Mukada K, Uozumi T, Takechi A, Arita K. Effect of long-term treatment with somatostatin analogue (SMS 201-995) on pituitary tumor shrinkage in acromegaly—report of two cases. *Neurol Med Chir* 1992;32:215–219.

456. Barkan AL, Lloyd RV, Chandler WF. Preoperative treatment of acromegaly with long-acting somatostatin analog SMS 201-995: shrinkage of invasive pituitary macroadenomas and improved surgical remission rate. *J Clin Endocrinol Metab* 1988;67:227–228.

457. Melby JC. Therapy of Cushing disease: a consensus for pituitary microsurgery. *Ann Intern Med* 1988;109:445–446.

458. Friedman RB, Oldfield EH, Nieman LK. Repeat transsphenoidal surgery for Cushing's disease. *J Neurosurg* 1989; 71:520–527.

459. Orth DN, Liddle GW. Results of treatment in 108 patients with Cushing's syndrome. *N Engl J Med* 1971;285:243–247.

460. Jennings AS, Liddle GW, Orth DN. Results of treating childhood Cushing's disease with pituitary irradiation. *N Engl J Med* 644;297:957–962.

461. Schteingart DE, Tsao HS, Taylor, CI, McKenzie A, Victoria R, Therrien BA. Sustained remission of Cushing's disease with mitotane and pituitary irradiation. *Ann Intern Med* 1980;92:613–619.

462. Ross WM, Evered DC, Hunter P, Benaim M, Cook D, Hall R. Treatment of Cushing's disease with adrenal blocking drugs and megavoltage therapy to the pituitary. *Clin Radiol* 1979;30:149–153.

463. Yanovski J, Cutler GBJ. Cushing's disease: medical treatment. In: *Contemporary diagnosis and management of pituitary adenomas.* Cooper P, ed. Park Ridge, IL: American Association of Neurological Surgeons, 1991;125–138.

464. Sarkar R, Thompson NW, McLeod MK. The role of adrenalectomy in Cushing's syndrome. *Surgery* 1990;108:1079–1084.

465. Guthrie FJ, Ciric I, Hayashida S, Kerr WJ, Murphy ED. Pituitary Cushing's syndrome and Nelson's syndrome: diagnostic criteria, surgical therapy, and results. *Surg Neurol* 1981;16:316–323.

466. Wynne AG, Gharib H, Scheithauer BW, Davis DH, Freeman SL, Horvath E. Hyperthyroidism due to inappropriate secretion of thyrotropin in 10 patients. *Am J Med* 1992;92:15–24.

467. Gharib M, Boellner JR, Zinsmeister AR. Fine needle aspiration biopsy of the thyroid: the problem of suspicious cytologic findings. *Ann Intern Med* 1993;125:184.

468. Robbins J, Merino MJ, Boice JD Jr, et al. Thyroid cancer: a lethal endocrine neoplasm. *Ann Intern Med* 1991;115:133.

469. Ross NS, Aron DC. Hormonal evaluation of the patient with an incidentally discovered adrenal mass. *N Engl J Med* 1990;323:1401.

470. Friesen SR. The development of endocrinopathies in the prospective screening of two families with multiple endocrine adenopathy, type 1. *World J Surg* 1979;3:753–764.

471. Skogseid B, Eriksson B, Lundqvist G, et al. Multiple endocrine neoplasia type 1: A 10-year prospective screening study in four kindreds. *J Clin Endocrinol Metab* 1991; 73:281–287.

472. Marx SJ, Vinik AI, Santen RJ, Floyd JC Jr, Mills JL, Green J. Multiple endocrine neoplasia type I: assessment of laboratory tests to screen for the gene in a large kindred. *Medicine* 1986;65:226–241.

473. Antonarakis SE. Diagnosis of genetic disorders at the DNA level. *N Engl J Med* 1989;302:153–163.

474. McKusick VA, Francomano CA, Antonarakis SE. *Mendelian inheritance in man: Catalogs of autosomal dominant autosomal recessive, and X-linked phenotypes.* Baltimore: The Johns Hopkins University Press, 1992.

475. Chang JC, Kan YW. Antenatal diagnoses of sickle cell anaemia by direct analysis of the sickle mutation. *Lancet* 1981;2:1127–1129.

476. Thompson MW, McInnes RR, Willard HF. Genetics in medicine. In: Ott J. *Analysis of human genetic linkage.* Baltimore: Johns Hopkins University Press, 1991.

477. Janson M, Larsson C, Werellus B, et al. Detailed physical map of human chromosomal region 11q12–13 shows high melotic recombination rate around the MEN1 locus. *Proc Natl Acad Sci USA* 1991;88:10609–10613.

478. Larsson C, Shepherd J, Nakamura Y, et al. Predictive testing for multiple endocrine neoplasia type I using DNA polymorphisms. *J Clin Invest* 1992;89:1344–1349.

479. Bale BJ, Bale AE, Stewart K, et al. Linkage analysis of multiple endocrine neoplasia type 1 with INT2 and other markers on chromosome 11. *Genomics* 1989;4:320–322.

480. Nakamura Y, Larsson C, Julier C, et al. Localization of the genetic defect in multiple endocrine neoplasia type 1 within a small region of chromosome 11. *Am J Hum Genet* 1989;44:751–755.

481. Fujimori M, Wells SA, Nakamura Y: Fine-scale mapping of the gene responsible for multiple endocrine neoplasia type 1 (MEN1). *Am J Hum Genet* 1992;50:399–403.

The Parathyroids, edited by J.P. Bilezikian, M.A. Levine, and R. Marcus. Raven Press, Ltd., New York © 1994.

CHAPTER 38

Multiple Endocrine Neoplasia Type I

Pathology, Pathophysiology, Molecular Genetics, and Differential Diagnosis

Eitan Friedman, Catharina Larsson, Andrea Amorosi, Maria-Luisa Brandi, Allen E. Bale, David C. Metz, Robert T. Jensen, Monica C. Skarulis, Richard C. Eastman, Lynette Nieman, Jeffrey A. Norton, and Stephen J. Marx.

Multiple endocrine neoplasia type I (MEN-I) is a distinctive syndrome with neoplasia in the parathyroids, gastrointestinal (GI)–endocrine cells, anterior pituitary, and other tissues. We have reviewed its clinical-presentation and its treatment in the previous chapter. The disorder usually results from mutation of an un-identified gene on the long arm (band q12–13) of chromosome 11. This chapter explores several related topics, including how mutation at the *men1* locus can contribute to multiple neoplasms in certain target tissues.

E. Friedman, C. Larsson: Department of Clinical Genetics, Karolinska Hospital, S-10401 Stockholm, Sweden.

M. Brandi, A. Amorosi: Endocrine Section, Department of Clinical Physiopathology, University of Florence Medical School, 50139 Florence, Italy.

A. E. Bale: Department of Genetics, Yale University School of Medicine, New Haven, Connecticut 06510.

D. C. Metz: Department of Medicine, Division of Gastroenterology, Hospital of the University of Pennsylvania, University of Pennsylvania, Philadelphia, Pennsylvania 19104.

R. T. Jensen: Digestive Disease Branch, National Institute of Diabetes, Digestive, and Kidney Diseases, National Institutes of Health, Bethesda, Maryland 20892.

M. C. Skarulis: Division of Intramural Research, National Institute of Diabetes, Digestive, and Kidney Diseases, National Institutes of Health, Bethesda, Maryland 20892.

R. C. Eastman: Diabetes Branch, National Institute of Diabetes, Digestive, and Kidney Disease, National Institutes of Health, Bethesda, Maryland 20892.

L. Nieman: Developmental Endocrinology Branch, National Institute of Child Health and Human Development, National Institutes of Health, Bethesda, Maryland 20892.

J. A. Norton: Department of Surgery, Washington University School of Medicine, St. Louis, Missouri 63110.

S. J. Marx: Genetics and Endocrinology Section, National Institute of Diabetes, Digestive, and Kidney Diseases, National Institutes of Health, Bethesda, Maryland 20892.

REGULATORY CONTROL OF SECRETION AND PROLIFERATION IN PARATHYROID, PANCREATIC ISLET, AND ANTERIOR PITUITARY

Parathyroid Glands

Short-term studies with dispersed cells or tissue explants have yielded considerable information about mechanisms controlling secretion of parathyroid hormone (PTH) (1), confirming results of in vivo experiments. Ionized calcium is the central factor, controlling release of PTH (2). Also in vitro models have been particularly helpful in analyzing the significance of cAMP in parathyroid secretion and in identifying a series of agents previously unrecognized as stimulators or inhibitors of PTH secretion. Any agent that increases cellular cAMP content in parathyroid chief cells also causes enhanced release of PTH from the cells and vice versa.

The actions of calcium and eventually of other agents that control parathyroid cell function are not limited to the control of PTH release. They may regulate proliferation in the same direction, as shown for calcium in parathyroid explants in organ culture (3). Primary cultures have been proposed as a model to analyze parathyroid cell growth. Functional parathyroid cells have been maintained in culture as mixed cell types for short periods, but have replicated poorly and eventually became overgrown by fibroblasts (4,5). The traditional conditions of primary cultures may not be optimal to study the growth of parathyroid cells.

The development of a long-term culture system of bovine parathyroid (PT-b) cells in serum-free medium made it possible to demonstrate that proliferation of parathyroid cells was extremely sensitive to calcium ion (6). Conversely, long-term cultures of parathyroid cells showed reduced sensitivity to calcium in suppressing hormone secretion (6). These cells, however, could not be cloned and eventually became senescent.

With extensions of these methods, a clonal line of epithelial cells was cloned from rat hyperplastic parathyroid glands (7). This clonal parathyroid cell strain (PT-r) provided a single, uniform population for studies on control of parathyroid cell proliferation. Like the PT-b cells, PT-r cell growth was controlled by calcium, in that increasing concentrations of calcium caused a progressive decrease in the rate of thymidine incorporation and cell growth (7). Moreover, secretin, a known stimulator of PTH release in isolated parathyroid cells, induced both cAMP accumulation and hormone release from PT-r cells (7). The senescence phenomenon reported for bovine parathyroid cells in long-term culture did not apply to PT-r cells. Similarly, a clonal population of endothelial cells (BPE-1) derived from bovine parathyroid tissue is immortal (8). Like other endothelial cells, BPE-1 cells showed organ-specific characteristics (i.e., the ability to take up exogenously added PTH), suggesting a unique role of the endothelial compartment in the parathyroid tissue (8).

These cellular models have been useful for in vitro studies of cell-to-cell relationships among the endocrine component and the endothelial counterpart. Communications between epithelial and endothelial cells in endocrine glands are particularly interesting. In response to a trophic hormone or to a circulating factor (i.e., changes of blood calcium levels), target endocrine tissues typically undergo dose-dependent increases in weight; this represents a coordinated growth of both parenchyma and stroma, such as the capillary network. How angiogenesis is coordinated with growth of parenchymal cells in response to a trophic factor is uncertain. It may represent a direct effect of the trophic factor on endothelial cells. Alternatively, angiogenesis may be secondary to products released by stimulated parenchymal cells, as proposed for tumor growth. To test this hypothesis, we measured the effect of media conditioned by PT-r cells on

BPE-1 cells and vice versa. Each cell line released mitogenic factor(s) which activated the other cell type (9). Moreover, direct contacts between PT-r and BPE-1 cells resulted in morphological and functional changes. PT-r cells adhered to the endothelial monolayers, forming clusters or miniglands on top of them (9). Similar interactions between epithelial and endothelial cells may be instrumental for the in vivo regulation of metabolically active parathyroid tissue and for the embryonic development of what is termed the parathyroid *endocrine structure*.

From studies of primary cultures and clonal continuous cell lines of parathyroid cells, a number of factors have been proposed as endocrine, paracrine, and autocrine regulators of parathyroid cell function and proliferation. 1,25-Dihydroxyvitamin D appears to inhibit parathyroid cell proliferation independently of calcium (10–12). Moreover, there is evidence for an autocrine mechanism whereby hypocalcemia increases the production of acidic fibroblast growth factor as well as its membrane receptors in parathyroid cells (13). Pancreastatin, a presumed product of chromogranin A processing, inhibits parathyroid cell secretory activity (14); expression of chromogranin A mRNA is qualitatively and quantitatively normal in hyperplastic and adenomatous parathyroid tissues (15). Among the additional factors proposed as potential in vivo regulators of parathyroid cell metabolism are endothelin (16), atrial natriuretic peptide (17), PTH-related protein (18,19), and P-glycoprotein (20). However, no definitive answers on the physiological role of these factors in parathyroid cell regulation are available yet.

Endocrine Pancreas

The islets of Langerhans make up only 1–2% of the total cell mass of the pancreas in most adult mammals. Insulin is produced by the B cells (beta cells), glucagon by the A cells (α or α_2 cells), pancreatic polypeptide by the F cells (PP cells), and somatostatin by the D cells (α_1 cells). The use of collagenase to isolate islets was a major breakthrough in the study of the physiology and biochemistry of the endocrine pancreas (21). Systematic studies on the influence of culture conditions on mouse islet cell function and growth were also initiated (22). Great efforts have been made to develop chemically defined media where the serum supplement is minimized or even totally replaced by hormones and well-defined growth factors.

Recent work has identified the DNA-binding site for an as yet unidentified islet and specific differentiation-inducing transcription factors (23,24).

In defined culture conditions, glucose induced insulin release and synthesis. However, the islet consists of several other cell types which by hormonal, paracrine, and autocrine mechanisms may interact one to each other in modulating hormone release. Indeed, under standard conditions (i.e., 11 mmol glucose) glucagon secretion is suppressed, and insulin seems to be of importance for the glucose-dependent suppression of the glucagon secretion. Somatostatin, present in the D cells of the islets, is known to inhibit secretion of both insulin and glucagon. There is some controversy with regard to the mitogenic effect of high glucose on the islet cells. Whether such an effect is observed probably depends on the experimental conditions. Insulin itself may be required for a mitogenic effect of glucose, since insulin has been found to promote the development and maturation of the beta cells in culture (25). Moreover, diabetic serum appears to contain a mitogenic protein with an apparent molecular weight ~ 60–100 kDa (26). The influence of pituitary hormones on glucose homeostasis has been recognized for more than a century. Growth hormone directly stimulates insulin release and islet proliferation of fetal tissues (27). The influence of the adrenal gland on glucose homeostasis has been known for a long time. From in vitro studies it can be concluded that glucocorticoids, in a narrow concentration range, stimulate the function of the β cells, but, in contrast to growth hormone, glucocorticoids inhibit mitotic activity (27). Acute exposure of pancreatic islets to PTH stimulates insulin secretion independent of glucose concentration of the medium (28). These observations suggest that PTH may play a role in the acute stimulation of insulin secretion.

Although functioning islet cell cultures have been maintained for various periods of time, they have consisted of mixtures of cell types and have eventually been overgrown by fibroblasts. Clonal cell lines were established in 1980 from a rat islet cell tumor (29). These cell clones secrete insulin in response to glucose and other insulin secretagogues. Studies on tumor-derived clonal and subclonal cell lines support the conclusion that a single islet cell has the potential of differentiating into cells expressing at least three of the islet hormones (30). The significance of the intraislet interaction among different endocrine cell types must await further studies on clonal populations of the individual cell types. Indeed, chronic endogenous hypergastrinemia promotes proliferation and differentiation of islet cells and stimulates the secretory function of B cells and, to a lesser extent, of A cells, providing evidence for a trophic and secretagogue action of gastrin on the endocrine pancreas (31). A major challenge for future research is to find out whether the various peptide hormones produced in the pancreatic islets participate in the local intercellular communication network.

Anterior Pituitary

It is generally accepted that the control of anterior pituitary secretion and proliferation depends on hypothalamic hypophysiotropic hormones and hormones from peripheral endocrine glands. Pituitary cells differentiate from a common stem cell. Pit-1 is a transcription factor that regulates this differentiation as well as it modulates transcription of genes for pituitary hormones (32). Efforts of a number of investigators for several years have been directed to delineating paracrine interactions within the anterior pituitary. Although anatomical arrangements of cells suggest and would facilitate cell-to-cell interactions, this evidence by itself is insufficient to prove interactions among cells. During recent years, however, evidence has been growing that anterior pituitary cells control their functional activity through a local intercellular communication network. Many groups have examined the effects on secretion of isolating different types of cells and restoring possible interactions by permitting different fractions to reaggregate (33). As an example, signals transmitted from gonadotrophs (33) and corticotrophs profoundly affect the secretory activity of lactotrophs and/or somatotrophs.

Moreover, the system is complicated by the fact that several biologically active peptides, besides pituitary hormones, are synthesized in the anterior pituitary cells. Indeed, brain–gut peptides, opioid peptides, peptides regulating salt–water balance, activin and inhibin, growth factors, and cytokines have been demonstrated in intracellular compartments, including secretory granules, of anterior pituitary cells. Although a paracrine action seems evident for a few, the precise function of most of these peptides remains unknown.

The pituitary gland is a rich source of several substances with growth-promoting activities. Many of these are uncharacterized. Some of these factors can modulate endocrine function, but much less is known about their possible effects on the replication of anterior pituitary cells. Basic fibroblast growth factor (bFGF) was isolated and characterized from bovine pituitary tissue (34). Basic FGF has a mitogenic effect on primary cultures of rat pituitary cells and increases the sensitivity of both thyrotrophs and lactotrophs to the effects of TRH in normal rat pituitary cells (35). In addition, bFGF also induces endothelial cell proliferation and could therefore be involved in angiogenesis of pituitary tissue in normal and pathological conditions. Follicular or folliculostellate cells, a morphologically well-characterized and versatile population of pituitary cells, are a major source of bFGF (36). Interestingly, pituitary follicular cells also secrete interleukin-6 (37), vascular endothelial growth factor (38), and leukemia-inhibitory factor (39). All these factors could have a role in the process of tumor development in the pituitary.

PATHOLOGY OF TUMORS INCLUDING HYPERPLASIAS IN MULTIPLE ENDOCRINE NEOPLASIA TYPE I

Parathyroid Tumors

Parathyroid gland abnormalities in MEN-I are often classified as chief cell hyperplasia (40–42). This term denotes a multiple gland disorder. In fact, the whole parathyroid tissue appears to be involved, although in the majority of cases individual glands from a patient are not simultaneously affected to the same extent.

Macroscopically, considerable asymmetry in gland size is a consistent finding in MEN-I-associated parathyroid hyperplasia. An average ratio of 9.6 for the maximum/minimum volume has been estimated in a detailed analysis of size heterogeneity of the parathyroid glands in patients with MEN-I (43). Histologically, a distinct cytoarchitectural variability is characteristic of the parathyroid glands in MEN-I with primary hyperparathyroidism (Fig. 1) (44). Chief cells dominate, but different types (dark and clear, small and large cells) are identified; oxyphil cells and, occasionally, water-clear cells are also present. The parathyroid cells may be arranged in cords, sheets, acini, or follicles. Two basic growth patterns, nodular and diffuse, are recognized, but intermediate patterns may occur in some glands. Nodules are commonly multiple, and they vary considerably in size (Fig. 2A). They may be unencapsulated or surrounded by a delicate to thick fibrous layer (adenomatous nodules) (Fig. 2B). The cytological and architectural features are usually different in neighboring nodules. Foci of normal parathyroid tissue, recognizable by smaller

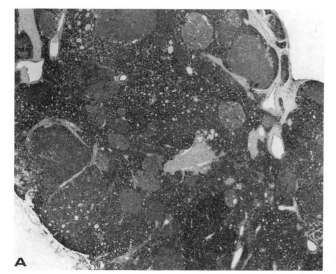

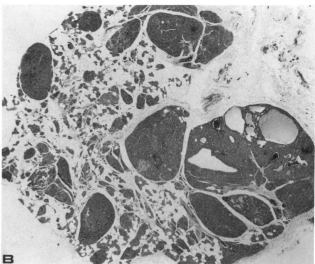

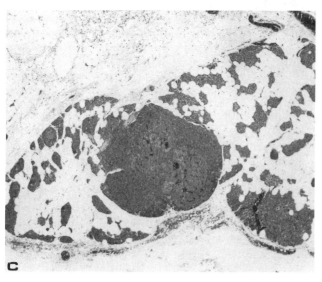

FIG. 1. Distinct pathological heterogeneity of three parathyroid glands from the same patient, suggesting progressive structural abnormalities. Hematoxylin-eosin. **A:** ×25; **B:** ×25; **C:** ×30.

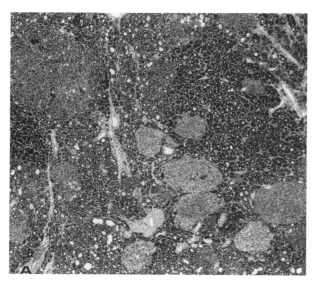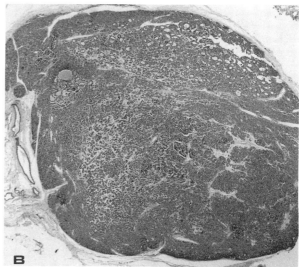

FIG. 2. Variable aspects of hyperplastic nodular parathyroid glands. **A:** Micronodules; **B:** adenomatous nodule. Hematoxylin-eosin. **A,** ×32; **B,** ×20.

cells, lobularity, and high adipose/parenchymal tissue ratio may be observed, either forming a rim around hyperplastic nodules or indistinctly merging with areas of diffuse hyperplasia. Markedly enlarged glands usually contain one or several large, encapsulated nodules. Slightly enlarged abnormal glands consist of small islands of chief cells separated by intervening areas containing abundant fat. An essentially diffuse hyperplasia may be observed in moderately enlarged glands. A single, histologically normal parathyroid gland in the context of a fully established hyperplasia of the remaining glands rarely occurs.

Parathyroid hormone immunoreactivity varies in intensity and distribution in different parathyroid glands and within the same gland (Fig. 3A) (44,45). Such a polymorphous staining pattern has been related to different stages of hormone synthesis, secretion, and storage by parathyroid cells. Chromogranin A (CgA) immunoreactivity shows a similar variability, with only a partial correlation to PTH staining on serial sections (Fig. 3B) (44–46).

The occurrence of parathyroid adenomas, or double adenomas, in MEN-I has not been reported until recently (47). However, taking into account the size heterogeneity and the cytoarchitectural polymorphism of the parathyroid glands, it seems likely that most cases originally diagnosed as adenomas actually represent adenomatous hyperplasia with asymmetric gland involvement (41).

Present difficulties in the pathological distinction between hyperplasia and adenoma are well known. A parathyroid nodule composed of a single cell type, lacking fat cells, lobular pattern, and continuity with the surrounding tissue could indeed represent a neoplastic growth (i.e., an adenoma) (48), but this cannot

definitively be ascertained on morphological bases in a context of generalized abnormalities of the parathyroid tissue. According to the current criteria, adenoma can reliably be diagnosed whenever there is a single abnormal parathyroid gland and the remaining glands are microscopically normal (42). Neither immunostaining for PTH, Chromogranin A, and parathyroid cell surface receptors involved in the regulation of hormone release, nor probing for PTH mRNA allows differentiation between hyperplasia and adenoma (44, 46,49,50). Uniform staining pattern with immunohistochemical markers, as well as concordance of PTH mRNA expression, have been reported in individual nodules from patients with non-MEN-1 parathyroid hyperplasia, and these have been cited as evidence of monoclonality (50,51).

In contrast to traditional histology, the study of clonality through molecular biology techniques has provided important information about the origin of parathyroid lesions in MEN-1. Allelic losses specific to chromosome 11 band q13 have been detected in the larger abnormal parathyroid glands, indicating that a monoclonal or oligoclonal outgrowth may develop after a phase of polyclonal proliferation (52). Unfortunately, no attempt has been made to characterize microscopically monoclonal vs. polyclonal "tumors." It will be of interest to prepare and to test DNA separately from single nodules or even from nondemarcated regions with a parathyroid "tumor" to analyze exactly the clonal composition of individual abnormal glands and to achieve reliable morphobiological correlations (52,53). It is conceivable that the wide spectrum of histological abnormalities of the parathyroid glands in MEN-1 represents different stages in the progression from hyperplasia to neoplasia under the cu-

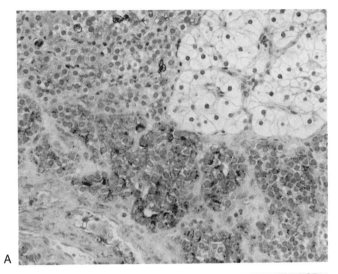

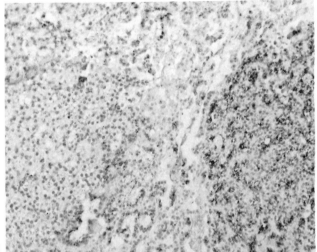

FIG. 3. Irregular distribution of PTH **(A)** and chromogranin **(B)** immunoreactivity in hyperplastic parathyroid tissue. Immunoperoxidase-hematoxylin. A, ×400; B, ×200.

mulative effects of intrinsic and extrinsic selective pressures on polyclonal cell populations (53,54). In some cases, the transition from hyperplasia to neoplasia could possibly correlate to a shift towards aneuploidy, recognizable via flow cytometric DNA analysis (55).

Tertiary hyperparathyroidism shares many functional and pathological features with MEN-I-associated hyperparathyroidism (56,57). Therefore, it provides an ideal system to investigate the development of clonal lesions in the context of a multicellular active growth. In our experience the progression of uremic hyperparathyroidism involves allelic losses on chromosome 11 in the larger parathyroid glands, but conventional histological analysis of glands harboring a monoclonal component fails to identify an unequivocal morphological association (58).

Pancreatic and Gastrointestinal Tumors

The characteristic pathological change in the pancreas of the MEN-I patient, referred to as *diffuse microadenomatosis,* consists of multiple nodular proliferations of endocrine cells ranging from 0.03 to 0.5 cm in maximum diameter (microadenomas), randomly distributed in the pancreatic gland (59–61). Histological features of the single lesion are those of an islet cell tumor (Fig. 4). The growth pattern is trabecular to solid. A newly formed stroma is present in variable amounts and some tumors have a distinct fibrous capsule. One or several endocrine tumors, showing the same histological patterns but larger than 0.5 cm, may also develop. Immunohistochemical investigations have demonstrated that the majority of pancreatic endocrine tumors (PETs) associated with MEN-I are composed of peptide hormone-producing cells and in a significant proportion contain multiple cell types (59–64). Most microadenomas appear to be almost composed exclusively of cell populations normally present in the pancreas (59–61,63). Intratumoral distribution of different cells is random and in no way reminiscent of the typical topographic distribution in the normal pancreatic islets, further supporting the neoplastic nature of these lesions. Tumors are classified according to the prevailing cell type. Glucagon cell and pancreatic polypeptide (PP) cell microadenomas predominate (Fig. 5A,B). Insulin cell microaden-

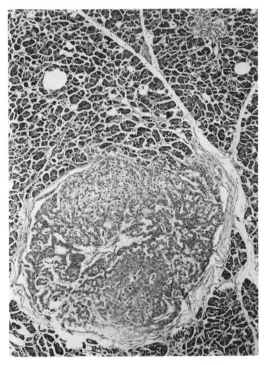

FIG. 4. Pancreatic microadenoma, with a distinct cytoarchitectural polymorphism. Hematoxylin-eosin. ×80.

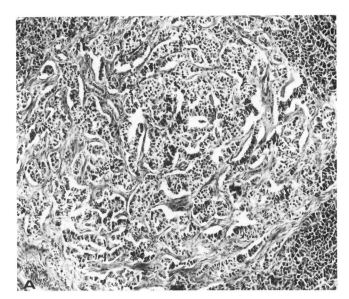

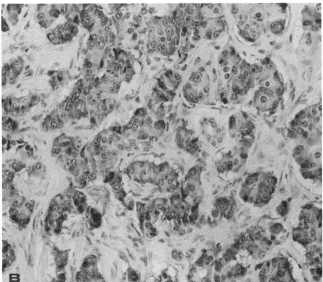

FIG. 5. A trabecular-to-solid pancreatic microadenoma containing PP immunoreactive cells. **A:** Hematoxylin-eosin. × 125. **B:** Immunoperoxidase, ×300.

omas are also frequent, but their number varies considerably from patient to patient. Somatostatin cell microadenomas seldom occur.

The development of hyperfunctional symptoms is usually associated with the presence of tumors larger than 0.5 cm (59,63). Ectopic cell types are more likely to be found in these lesions and may dominate the clinical picture (63,64). Functioning tumors are classified according to the hormone causing the clinically recognizable syndrome, although the responsible tumor frequently contains multiple cell types.

An overall low rate of metastases to regional lymph nodes and liver has been reported in MEN-I-associated PETs (59,62). Metastatic disease does not rule out long-term survival (47).

The Zollinger-Ellison syndrome (ZES) in MEN-I patients requires special considerations. Multiple gastrin-producing tumors in the pancreas have been considered responsible for the high serum gastrin levels and the related clinical symptoms. However, evidence that hypergastrinemia is in fact caused by pancreatic tumors has been provided in few cases. Recent immunohistochemical analyses have demonstrated that pancreatic gastrinomas are actually uncommon in patients with MEN-I and ZES (59–61,65). Conversely, single or more often multiple carcinoids, containing gastrin immunoreactive cells (Fig. 6), are usually found in the proximal duodenum (59,63,65–67). These observations indicate that duodenal rather than pancreatic gastrinomas are the main cause of ZES in MEN-I.

Duodenal gastrinomas appear as nodular or polypoid lesions arising in the deep part of the mucosa and expanding into the submucosa. The histological pattern is trabecular to solid. Immunohistochemical examination may reveal, in addition to gastrin-positive cells, focal reactivity for the glycoprotein hormone α subunit and a number of specific hormones/amines (more often somatostatin and serotonin) (65,67–69). Multiple tumor foci and hyperplasia of gastrin cells in the intervening nontumor mucosa are characteristic of duodenal gastrinomas associated with MEN-I (63,65). Small size (often <0.6 cm) is typical of duodenal carcinoids, either sporadic or MEN-I associated (65–72).

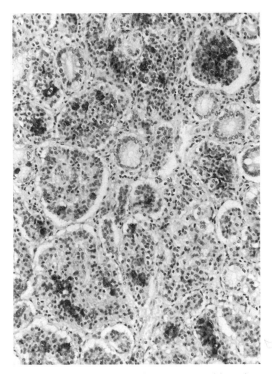

FIG. 6. Duodenal gastrinoma. Immunoperoxidase-hematoxylin. ×250.

The smallest lesions, encountered in MEN-I, may be overlooked despite a careful clinical and pathological examination. Because even small tumors appear to be potentially malignant, it has been suggested that gastrinoma occasionally found in peripancreatic lymph nodes may actually represent metastasis from a missed duodenal carcinoid rather than primary ectopic tumors (65,66).

The malignancy rate of MEN-I-associated gastrinoma is similar to that of sporadic gastrinoma (70). Hepatic metastases are generally regarded as the most important marker of a clinically malignant disease, while patients with gastrinoma confined to lymph nodes uncommonly follow a malignant clinical course.

At present it is unclear whether MEN-I appreciably influences survival in gastrinoma patients.

Gastric argyrophil carcinoids arising in the oxyntic mucosa have been reported in MEN-I patients with ZES (73,74). These tumors, usually multiple and small in size, have a microlobular–trabecular structure, and show silver staining technique, immunohistochemistry, and electron microscopy features of enterochromaffin-like (ECL) cell tumors (75). ECL-omas in ZES arise against a background of hypertrophic oxyntic mucosa, with a pronounced increase in the parietal cell mass, and are associated with proliferative changes of mucosal argyrophil cells, encompassing the whole spectrum of hyperplasia through multiple intramu-

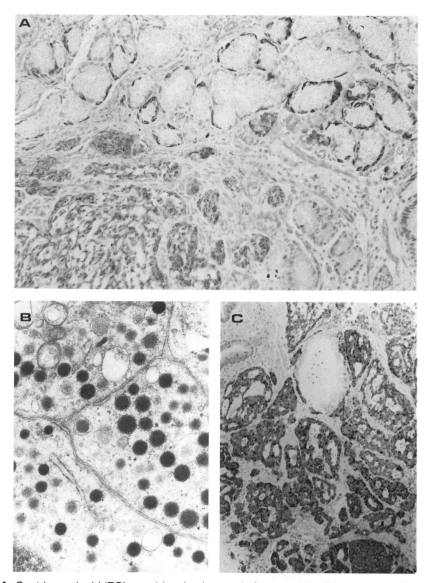

FIG. 7. A: Gastric carcinoid (ECL-oma) in a background of argyrophil cell hyperplasia. Grimelius silver. ×200. **B:** Ultrastructural appearance of nonvacuolated ECL-cell granules. Uranyl-lead. ×17,000. **C:** Diffuse immunostaining for chromogranin A of the tumor cells. Immunoperoxidase-hematoxylin. ×125.

cosal microcarcinoids (a condition referred to as *carcinoidosis*) to deeply invasive macroscopic tumors (76). Since ECL cells are sensitive to the trophic stimulus of gastrin (75), a relationship has been postulated between hypergastrinemia and the development of ECL cell tumors in ZES. Ultrastructural morphometry of the oxyntic mucosa in ZES has demonstrated a selective increase in number and size of ECL cells, while the other endocrine cell types are not affected (77). Moreover, the ECL cells may show ultrastructural features typical of ECL-omas, possibly reflecting preneoplastic changes in a presumptive hyperplasia–neoplasia sequence (77). However, the prevalence of ECL cell tumors in ZES patients is very low. Most cases so far reported have been observed in MEN-I patients, suggesting that genetic abnormalities play a major role in the genesis of these tumors. Carcinoid tumors of the stomach may occasionally occur in MEN-I patients without ZES (75,76). We have observed a case of ECL cell carcinoidosis associated with chronic fundic gastritis and hypergastrinemia of antral origin in an MEN-I patient (Fig. 7A–C). The malignant potential of gastric carcinoids is generally regarded as low (75,76). Tumors arising in the nonatrophic oxyntic mucosa seem to carry a less favorable prognosis than those associated with chronic atrophic gastritis type A. Jejunal and ileal carcinoids have also been reported in MEN-I patients (78). Clinicopathological and immunohistochemical features do not differ from those of corresponding sporadic tumors.

Pituitary Tumors

Adenoma is the most common pituitary lesion in MEN-I (79). Clinicopathological aspects of these tumors, such as distribution by patient age and sex, tumor size, and local invasion, are similar to those of sporadic adenomas (80). Although multiple tumors occur (80,81), multiplicity does not appear to be an impressive feature of MEN-I-associated pituitary adenomas. The prevalence of hormone hypersecretion is higher in MEN-I-associated than in sporadic tumor of the pituitary (80). A wide range of functional differentiation can be revealed by immunohistochemical investigations (79,80). A higher prevalence rate of growth hormone (GH)-producing adenomas (either mono- or plurihormonal), and a moderate increase of prolactin (PRL) cell adenomas have been reported in comparison with non-MEN-I pituitary tumors. Prolactinomas are the most common category (Fig. 8A,B), whereas adrenocorticotrophic hormone (ACTH)-producing adenomas are rare. MEN-I-associated adenomas represent a consistent subset of pituitary tumors engaged in the production of multiple hormones (82). The most frequently occurring variant produces GH, PRL, and glycoprotein hormones.

More recent application of a classification scheme of pituitary tumor function based on immunohistochemical, electron microscopy, and mRNA characteristics revealed that tumors previously considered nonfunctional expressed glycoprotein hormones and that more than one hormone, often of different classes, may be made within a single tumor, and often within a single cell (83–85).

Clinicopathological aspects of pituitary hyperplasia are still controversial (86). Hyperplasia of GH cells or ACTH cells, induced by ectopic gonadotropin hormone-releasing hormone (GHRH) (70,87–89) or corticotropin-releasing hormone (CRH) (80) production, has been reported in patients with MEN-I. However, in most of these cases pituitary tissue was not available for morphological evaluation. Moreover, the development of an adenomatous lesion, presumptively in a background of hyperplasia, has been suggested in a patient with a pancreatic GHRH-producing tumor (71), but histological confirmation is lacking.

In recent years, attention has been focused on a nonendocrine cell population, the so-called folliculostellate cells (Fig. 9). Their origin and functional role

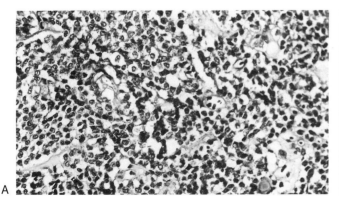
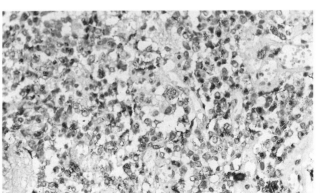

FIG. 8. Pituitary adenoma containing prolactin-positive cells. **A:** Hematoxylin-eosin. ×250. **B:** Immunoperoxidase-hematoxylin. ×250.

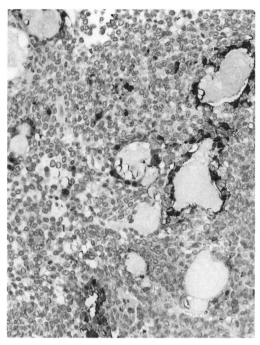

FIG. 9. Same case shown in Fig. 8. S100 reactivity of pituitary folliculostellate cells. Immunoperoxidase-hematoxylin. ×250.

in normal and adenomatous pituitary tissue are under active investigation (90,91). Production of a vascular endothelial growth factor (VEGF) has been reported only quite recently (92).

Other Tumors

Adrenocortical lesions are not uncommon in MEN-I, although they are only rarely functional (93). Adrenal involvement is frequently bilateral. Histologically diffuse and nodular cortical hyperplasia and adenomas are usually found. Adrenocortical carcinomas have also been reported. It has been suggested that in most instances pituitary-independent adrenocortical proliferations may be secondary lesions, possibly related to concurrent pancreatic endocrine tumors.

A variety of thyroid lesions have been observed in MEN-I, including Hashimoto's thyroiditis, nodular hyperplasia, follicular cell adenomas, and carcinomas. Bronchial and thymic carcinoids have also been reported in MEN-I patients (94). No histological differences from sporadic tumors are known. Subcutaneous and visceral lipomas are the only nonendocrine tumors found with some frequency in MEN-I patients (47). No features distinguish MEN-I-associated from sporadic lipoma.

EARLY THEORIES CONCERNING MULTIPLE ENDOCRINE NEOPLASIA TYPE I

The most widely accepted theory seems still to be that of Wermer (95), who proposed abnormal growth as a direct effect of the abnormal gene in the cells of the different affected tissues. A different hypothesis for the etiology of MEN-I syndrome grew out of the "neural crest" hypothesis, in that tumors of multiple endocrine organs could be the result of a genetic defect of the neural crest tissue. However, parathyroid tissue is not derived from the neuroectoderm. Therefore, this hypothesis is untenable for MEN-I.

A genetic transmission of a multipotential islet cell neoplasm capable of secreting glucagon as well as insulin and gastrin was proposed by Vance et al. (96). Hyperplasia of the primordial cell of the islets of Langerhans, so-called *nesidioblastosis* (97), would constitute the genetic defect, and changes in other endocrine glands would evolve as a consequence of islet cell hormone excess. No islet hormone has been identified with the potential to cause extrapancreatic effects.

Speculations have also arisen that hormonal, metabolic, and autoimmune influences have a role in promoting growth in several affected organs in the MEN-I syndrome. This theory is based on the assumption that a chronic and excessive stimulation of hormonal release would cause proliferative changes in the other glands under consideration. As an example one may cite that hypercalcemia, the first abnormality that can be observed in MEN-I, could play a major role in the development of hypergastrinemia (98). In addition, PTH stimulates the release of gastrin (99). Several lines of evidence have also suggested that gastrointestinal hormones may be important in calcium homeostasis. Indeed, secretin stimulates parathyroid cell function both in vitro and in vivo (100). Glucagon tends to decrease serum calcium and leads to parathyroid hyperplasia in rabbits after prolonged administration (101). Metabolic alkalosis, which can frequently be observed in Zollinger-Ellison syndrome, results in decreased ionized calcium and increased circulating PTH (102). GH and PRL are both believed to influence mineral metabolism in a variety of animal species, including man (103–105). In vitro data support a major role for PRL in the genesis of the hypercalcemia in rats bearing secreting pituitary tumors (106). Physiologic doses of insulin stimulate PRL expression in normal rat parathyroid cells (107). Moreover, insulin acts as a growth factor in bovine parathyroid cell cultures (6). The actual role of all these humoral factors in promoting hyperplasia and tumor growth in MEN-I syndrome is not yet understood but is currently not believed to be important.

MULTIPLE ENDOCRINE NEOPLASIA TYPE I GROWTH FACTOR AND FIBROBLAST GROWTH FACTOR FAMILY

Properties

Long-term cultures of bovine parathyroid (PT-b) cells allowed detection of a parathyroid growth factor in MEN-I plasma (6–8,108). The cloning of a pure cell line of bovine parathyroid endothelial (BPE-1) cells (8) led to recognition that all or portions of the circulating parathyroid growth factor in MEN-I plasma is acting on the endothelial component of the parathyroids (109). More recently, the establishment of a continuous clonal cell line of human endothelial (HPE) cells from an MEN-I parathyroid tumor further supported these observations (MLB, unpublished observations) Conversely, cloned rat parathyroid epithelial cells (PT-r) did not recognize the MEN-I mitogen (110). The discovery that the endothelium represented the target of the mitogenic effect of the MEN-I plasma suggested similarities between the MEN-I growth factor and the fibroblast growth factor (FGF) family of mitogens. This protein family has fewer than ten members; all are potent mitogens, and some can be oncogenic (111). The members of this family are characterized by homology throughout their amino acid sequence and by the ability to bind to immobilized heparin. Several of these growth factors also stimulate proliferation of endothelial cells. Distinct functions, besides fibroblast and endothelial cell proliferation, are now recognized as typical of some members of this family of molecules.

Similarities exist between the MEN-I mitogen and basic FGF (bFGF), a member of the FGF family of mitogens, which has been isolated from a variety of normal tissues, including the pituitary gland (83). The increased bFGF-like activity in MEN-I plasma had an apparent MW of ~110 kDa, which after treatment with 7 M urea was reduced to 14–16 kDa, a molecular size very similar to that of bFGF (109). A property useful in characterization of the MEN-I mitogen was its high affinity for immobilized heparin (109). Moreover, highly specific antibodies for the amino terminus of bFGF also recognized the MEN-I growth factor, as demonstrated by bioassay and immunoradiometric analyses (109). Despite the presence of abundant cellular stores, the amino acid sequence of bFGF lacks a conventional signal sequence, and bFGF has not been found in normal plasma (84). The MEN-I growth factor appears in the circulation, so, if it is a form of bFGF, a mechanism must exist accounting for its release from cells.

Recently, evidence for a plasma mitogenic protein has been demonstrated in patients affected by MEN-I syndrome (85). This mitogen appears to be active in a rat insulinoma cell line. The relationship between this islet-cell growth factor and the bFGF-like material active on parathyroid endothelial cells remains to be determined.

Tissue Origin(s)

Increased levels of FGF-like activity have been found in urine of patients with bladder and kidney cancer (112), and some tumor cells appear to release considerable amounts of bFGF-like substances into their culture medium (113). Thus it is possible that in MEN-I syndrome the increased levels of circulating bFGF-like activity reflect systemic release of bFGF-like substances from one or more affected endocrine glands in MEN-I.

The natural history of the disease suggested that hyperparathyroidism could be a prerequisite for the other types of endocrine neoplasms in MEN-I syndrome. However, the possibility that the high circulating MEN-I mitogenic activity was an autocrine product from the parathyroid gland was excluded, since conditioned medium from primary cultures of MEN-I parathyroid cells did not show any mitogenic effect on BPE-1 cells (108). In addition, no differences were found between mitogenic activity in peripheral blood and in venous effluents from parathyroid glands. Finally, high parathyroid mitogenic activity persisted after total parathyroidectomy (108).

Pancreatic tumors are another potential site for release of this growth activity. Studies on venous effluents and on pancreatic endocrine cells in culture are too limited to allow conclusions.

The high concentration of bFGF in the pituitary gland (83), together with the finding that bFGF-like immunoreactivity was increased in the plasma of MEN-I patients with untreated pituitary tumors (114), implies that pituitary tumors are one likely source of circulating bFGF immunoreactivity in MEN-I syndrome. Recent studies also showed that conditioned media of pituitary cells cultured from MEN-I prolactinomas were mitogenic for bovine and human parathyroid cells (M.L.B., unpublished observations). In addition, immunohistochemical staining for S100 protein (115) gave evidence that prolactinoma tissues associated with the MEN-I syndrome (Fig. 9) are characterized by the presence of follicular cells (M.L.B., A.A., unpublished observations), the main cellular source of bFGF in the pituitary (36).

Possible Functional Roles in Multiple Endocrine Neoplasia Type I

The idea that new vessels are necessary for tumor growth originated in the early 1960s (116) from an experiment in which tumors were implanted in isolated perfused organs, where capillary blood vessel proliferation did not occur. The tumors failed to vascularize and could not enlarge beyond a few millimeters. These results led to the hypothesis that "tumor growth" is dependent on angiogenesis. This hypothesis proposed a role for new capillary blood vessels in every further increase in tumor mass only once tumor has occurred. However, angiogenesis could also represent the first step in the induction of parenchymal proliferation in normal and pathological conditions. Indeed, immediately after fertilization, vessels form, and conditions favoring the growth of endothelium also promote proliferation of surrounding tissues.

Studies on the histogenesis of human parathyroid glands indicate that embryological vascularization of the parathyroid gland is followed by a period of active hyperplasia, marked increase in cell number and a consequent increase in gland size. Hyperplastic goiter is characterized by follicular cell hypertrophy and hyperplasia, but also by extensive enlargement of the endothelial cells, which start to proliferate earlier than follicular cells (117). We might, therefore, speculate that in MEN-I a bFGF-like growth factor with specificity for parathyroid is released into the circulation and acts in an endocrine fashion on parathyroid endothelial cell proliferation. It is even more speculative that endothelial cells from the other endocrine tissues affected in MEN-I syndrome could also represent targets of the MEN-I mitogen. Development of endothelial cell in vitro culture models from other districts, such as endocrine pancreas and anterior pituitary gland, could help to explore this possibility.

To analyze possible paracrine functions of the MEN-I mitogen on parathyroid tissue, pure parathyroid epithelial (PT-r) and endothelial (BPE-1) cells were cocultured in two separate wells and exposed thereby to the mitogenic activity of the MEN-I plasma; MEN-I plasma induced the production of paracrine soluble factor(s), which acted in turn on BPE-1 cells, greatly potentiating the mitogenic action of the MEN-I mitogen (118). These data may explain why the MEN-I mitogen stimulated the mixed long-term culture of parathyroid (PT-b) cells with a higher potency than pure parathyroid endothelial (BPE-1) cells (110).

Heparin-purified mitogenic activity from MEN-I plasma also influenced differentiation of BPE-1 cells, with induction of migratory responses and of collagen and glycosoaminoglycan synthesis (110). These observations suggest that, like the other members of the FGF family of mitogens, the MEN-I growth factor is implicated in nonmitogenic effects in target tissues. The possibility that these in vitro effects are also retained in vivo is of particular importance, because the differentiated response of endothelial cells is one of

the basic mechanisms that underlie the process of neovascularization.

The finding that the MEN-I growth factor acts as a potent mitogen on parathyroid endothelial cells led to the evaluation of the vascularization of MEN-I parathyroid tissue. Ultrastructural histomorphometric studies showed that proliferation of parathyroid epithelial cells in MEN-I patients is accompanied by parallel increase in the associated endothelial component that does not occur in patients with secondary hyperparathyroidism (119). These results provide the first evidence for an in vivo role of the MEN-I mitogenic factor in structural changes of parathyroid tissue.

Both pathological and molecular genetic studies suggest the possibility that final tumor formation in parathyroids is preceded by a stage of hyperplasia. Indeed, the monoclonality of large parathyroid tumors in MEN-I syndrome (120) need not reflect a clonal growth at early stages of tumor development but could reflect the cumulative effect of intrinsic and extrinsic pressures on polyclonal populations during active growth. Therefore, initial proliferation of parathyroid tissue could be polyclonal in MEN-I syndrome, and the bFGF-like mitogen could have a pathogenetic role in this first phase (Fig. 10). This has been supported by the finding that clonality in MEN-I is characteristic of large but not small parathyroid tumors (121). The MEN-I mitogen might also influence a late stage of progression of parathyroid tumors (i.e., loss of DNA alleles from chromosome 11 region q13) (Fig. 10). If, indeed, the MEN-I growth factor had a pathogenetic role in parathyroid tumor development, an early expression of the mitogenic activity should be expected. Earlier studies contributed to characterize both the age dependence and the relation to endocrine

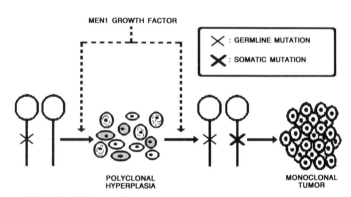

FIG. 10. Schematic representation of the speculative roles for the MEN-I growth factor in the development of parathyroid tumors. The first hit, carried as a germline mutation, could itself predispose the parathyroid tissue to hyperplastic growth, but the MEN-I growth factor may also have a pathogenetic role in this process. Alternatively, the factor could promote emergence of the monoclonal tumor whether or not a hyperplastic stage preceeds this.

indices of the circulating MEN-I mitogen in affected and unaffected subjects from a large kindred (122). The high plasma mitogenic activity in this kindred may be the direct cause of hyperfunction of the parathyroids, without a relation to hyperfunction of the pancreatic islets and anterior pituitary (122). Moreover, plasma mitogenic activity was higher in members expressing the *men1* gene than in their unaffected first-, second-, third-, or fourth-degree relatives (122). The lack of age dependence and the high values in MEN-I gene carriers suggested that the mitogenic activity is elevated in some gene carriers very early in life, before expression of endocrine hyperfunction (122). More recently, the availability of a premorbid genetic test made it possible to evaluate asymptomatic young (before age 15 years) MEN-I gene carriers from different kindreds for circulating mitogenic activity and to compare the data to those from age-matched gene non-carriers. The mitogenic activity evaluated using a clonal cell line of human parathyroid endothelial (HPE) cells is higher in the gene carriers than in the gene non-carriers (Fig. 11). These results support an early pathogenetic role of the MEN-I mitogen in parathyroid tumor development.

Possible Diagnostic and Therapeutic Applications

The use of the MEN-I growth factor measurement in the diagnosis and follow-up of the disease is limited by the intrinsic variability of the bioassay (108). Indeed, a great deal of overlap exists between normal values and results obtained in MEN-I patients (108). The use of an immunoradiometric method for the evaluation of circulating bFGF-like reactivity in MEN-I patients (114) would possibly represent a diagnostic advance. Certainly, the fact that bFGF-like immunoreactivity falls after successful treatment for pituitary tumors in MEN-I syndrome suggests that this may be a particularly useful marker for diagnosis and follow-up of pituitary adenomas, including the "hormonally silent" macroadenomas most common in MEN-I syndrome (112).

An emerging concept in tumor angiogenesis is that the switch to the angiogenic phenotype is the outcome of a balance between angiogenic stimulators and angiogenic inhibitors. Angiogenic factors have now been identified and isolated from a variety of normal tissues. An example of an angiogenic inhibitor at the tissue level is found in cartilage. In the circulation, angiostatic steroids have been discovered and recognized to be active in vivo. These mechanisms also serve as targets for antiangiogenic therapy. Could the growth of tumors in MEN-I syndrome be suppressed by specific inhibitors of capillary growth? Indeed, the use of systemic blockers of MEN-I growth factor is a potential therapeutic strategy for this disorder.

INTRINSIC PROCESSES IN MULTIPLE ENDOCRINE NEOPLASIA TYPE I

Chromosomal Instability

The term *chromosomal breakage syndrome* has been applied to a number of autosomal recessive disorders that predispose to various malignancies. Such chromosomal instability was first described in Bloom syndrome, then in Fanconi anemia, ataxia telangiectasia, and xeroderma pigmentosum (123–127). The underlying defect in several has been localized to a DNA repair enzyme. In 1983 similar findings were reported for MEN-I (128). Cultured lymphocytes from nine patients representing six MEN-I families showed an increased frequency of gaps and chromatid-type abnormalities but a normal range of sister chromatid exchanges. Lymphocytes from several MEN-I patients have also shown an increased frequence of chromosomal breakage (129). Recently, Scappaticci and coworkers (130) showed that cultured lymphocytes from three MEN-I patients had a high rate of chromosomal instability, which consisted of numerical as well as structural abnormalities, such as dicentric chromosomes, ring chromosomes, acentric fragments, and double minutes. In addition, fibroblasts from the same patients showed increased frequencies of chromosome breaks and hyperploidy (130). Though more than 60 chromosomally aberrant cells were analyzed in this

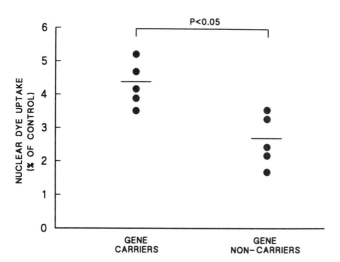

FIG. 11. Plasma mitogenic activity on human parathyroid endothelial cells in asymptomatic age-matched (within age 15 years) MEN-I offspring from five different kindreds grouped as gene carriers and gene non-carriers was determined by assessing genes tightly linked to MEN-I in each patient's family. The mitogenic activity was evaluated by a microfluorimetric assay as previously described (5).

study, no rearrangements were found that involved chromosome 11, despite evidence that the MEN-I gene is on chromosome 11 and undergoes inactivation by mutation in tumor precursor cells.

Activation of an Oncogene

Oncogenes, initially identified as transforming components of retroviruses, have been associated with tumor formation in several animal and human disorders (131–133). The viral genes with neoplastic transforming properties, viral oncogenes (v-onc genes), correspond to very closely related genes in vertebrates, protooncogenes (c-onc genes). The protooncogenes are involved in key regulatory functions in cell proliferation and differentiation. They are classified according to their subcellular localization and biochemical function. Some are found in the cell nucleus and may be recognized as transcription factors, while others are found outside the cell-surface, bound to a membrane receptor, i.e., growth factors. As a result of specific genetic alteration(s), they become capable of transforming the cell. The transforming capabilities of oncogenes are mediated by a "gain of function" either via overexpression of the normal, nonmutated gene product or via expression of an aberrant, inappropriately active protein. The underlying mutation may be an amplification, translocation, deletion, or point mutation of the gene.

Since only one of the two copies of the gene has to be activated to transform a cell, these genes act dominantly at the tissue level. Consequently, it is unlikely that this model will explain the type of genetic alteration that is inherited as an autosomal dominant predisposition to develop tumors stochastically in MEN-I.

Two different observations are, however, compatible with a gain of a functional mutation in nonneoplastic tissues from MEN-I patients. Brandi et al. (108) described in plasma from MEN-I patients factor(s) that were mitogenic on normal parathyroid cells. The recent finding of double minutes in lymphocyte cultures from MEN-I patients could reflect a dominant or gain of function type of underlying mechanism (130), considering that in malignancies the cytogenetic phenomenon of double minutes is usually associated with amplification of cellular oncogenes.

Although illegitimate expression of an oncogene is unlikely to account for the inherited mutation in MEN-I, it may still be operative in tumor development. The activating G protein gene, $G_{s\alpha}$, can show an activating mutation as gsp in a subset of growth hormone (GH)-secreting pituitary tumors (usually sporadic) with constitutive activation of adenylyl cyclase and GH hypersecretion (134,135); cAMP synthesis thus becomes autonomous. The cAMP is an intracellular second messenger for several trophic hormones and has the ability to stimulate growth in many cell types. It would not be surprising if the same direct oncogene contributed to tumor development in some GH-producing tumors in MEN-I.

DNA transfection experiments performed in NIH-3T3 cells determined the presence of transforming DNA sequences in prolactinomas (136). By ALU-PCR, the transforming DNA was shown to contain the human *hst1* gene, and expression of *hst1* mRNA in prolactinomas suggested that this growth factor gene may be associated with pituitary tumorigenesis. On the other hand, it is also possible that a gene (such as *pradl*) closely linked to *hst1* is the actual transforming gene rather than *hst1* itself.

Several tumor forms, e.g., breast cancer, have amplification of the 11q13 region resulting in expression of several putative oncogenes. In addition to *hst1*, this may also involve D11S287 (137). This marker was originally identified in a sporadic parathyroid adenoma in which a clonal chromosomal inversion placed the noncoding first exon of the *PTH* gene on 11p adjacent to a then unknown single copy DNA segment (*pradl*) that normally resides on 11q13 (see the chapter by Arnold; 138). Thus abnormal overexpression of *pradl* can be due to the influence of regulatory elements of the *PTH* gene. This type of rearrangement has been found in a small proportion of parathyroid adenomas, implicating *pradl* in only a subpopulation of the tumors (133,138,139). The normal *pradl* gene was shown to encode a member of the cyclin gene family of proteins believed to have central roles in control of the cell cycle. Southern blot analysis of 31 parathyroid tumors from MEN-I patients did not reveal any gene rearrangements with *pradl* (E.F., unpublished observations).

Inactivation of a Growth Suppressor Gene

The first experimental evidence for tumor suppressor genes came from studies of somatic cell hybrids, when it was shown that malignancy could be suppressed by the fusion of malignant and nonmalignant cells (140). The idea that some heritable tumors result from mutation causing a cell to become homozygous for a cancer-causing gene was proposed by de Mars (141), and 1 year later Alfred Knudson (142) introduced the two-mutation model of tumorigenesis. This model was first suggested and proven for retinoblastoma, which has since served as a prototype for identification of similar mechanisms in others types of tumors. The theory proposes that the inherited defective gene would make the individual a heterozygous carrier predisposed to tumor development. The tumor develops when a second mutational event has occurred, in a single susceptible cell so that the remaining "normal" gene or gene function is eliminated. Several types of second mutational events are possible, e.g., loss of one copy of a chromosome, somatic recombination, chromosomal deletion, or point mutation. Since the tumors grow after complete elimination of the normal function, these genes are called *tumor suppressor genes*. The synonym *recessive cancer genes* refers to the fact that at the cellular level the action is recessive, although the trait of tumor susceptibility is dominantly transmitted.

Approximately eight tumor suppressor genes that contribute to human neoplasia have been cloned (Table 1). It is noteworthy that, as with direct-acting oncogenes, their normal encoded products function in diverse cell compartments and in diverse manners. Their most important common feature is that the normal function of each in some manner involves growth suppression. Most of the cloned human tumor suppressor genes can contribute to either sporadic or hereditary neoplasia. Some of the tumor suppressor genes also cause developmental defects (e.g., Denys

TABLE 1. *Cloned human tumor-suppressor genes[a]*

Symbol	Chromos	Associated tumors and dystrophies	Normal cell compartment and functions of encoded protein	Inherited syndrome
nf2	22q	Acoustic neuroma, meningioma	Possible plasma membrane protein for cell-to-cell attachment	Neurofibromatosis type 2 (central neurofibromatosis)
dcc	18q	Colon polyps, colon adenocarcinoma	Possible fibronectin-like plasma membrane protein for cell-to-cell attachment (N-CAM homolog)	None proven
nf1	17q	Neurofibroma, glioma, pheochromocytoma, plexiform neuroma, cafè-au-lait spots	Cytoplasmic GTPase activating protein (GAP) homolog; might activate *ras* or other small G protein pathway	Neurofibromatosis type 1 (Von Recklinghausen's neurofibromatosis)
apc	5q	Colon polyps, colon adenocarcinoma, jaw cysts, cutaneous desmoids	Potential to form coiled coil suggests interaction with other protein(s) located in cytoplasm	Familial adenomatous polyposis, including Gardner's syndrome
p53	17p	Colon polyps, colon cancer, endometrial cancer, breast cancer, ovarian cancer, leukemia, lung cancer, bladder cancer, adrenal cancer, esophageal cancer, soft tissue sarcoma, other cancers	Nuclear phosphoprotein; probable transcription factor; it can bind to DNA recognition elements but normal target gene(s) not established; cell cycle checkpoint regulation	Li-Fraumeni (cancer family syndrome), familial soft tissue sarcoma
rb1	13q	Retinoblastoma, sarcoma; small cell lung cancer, lung adenocarcinoma, bladder cancer	Nuclear phosphoprotein; reversibly binds several classes of transcription factors; cell cycle regulation	Retinoblastoma
wt1	11p	Wilms tumor, rhabdomyosarcoma; as part of contiguous gene inactivation contributes to Beckwith-Weideman syndrome (hemihypertrophy, omphalocele, macroglossia, hypoglycemia Wilms tumor); Denys Drash syndrome (partial gonadal dysgenesis and gonadoblastoma, infantile nephropathy, Wilms tumor) from dominant negative mutation	Nuclear protein; probable transcription factor based on Cys2-His2 zinc finger domains	Wilms tumor; as contiguous gene inactivation can be associated with aniridia, genitourinary anomalies, and mental retardation (WAGR); Denys Drash syndrome

[a]The gene for von Hipple Lindau syndrome has been cloned (143).

Drash syndrome from *wt1*) (Table 1), apparently as a direct expression of the heterozygous germline mutation; some can be associated with developmental defects when the germline mutation is a deletion or inactivation of that gene plus contiguous genes (e.g., WAGR syndrome from *wt1* plus "aniridia gene" and perhaps other genes) (Table 1).

The two mutation model for tumorigenesis implies that it would be possible to determine which chromosome the gene for the heritable form of a neoplasia is situated on, simply by detecting chromosomal rearrangements which might reflect the "second mutational event." Such information may be available from karyotypes of cultured tumor cells or by genotypic comparison of constitutional and primary tumor tissue. The latter type of analysis involves detection of allele losses by the use of restriction fragment length polymorphism (RFLP) markers.

Localization of tumor-predisposing genes has in some cases, e.g., retinoblastoma and familial polyposis coli, been facilitated by the finding of constitutional chromosomal aberrations. Another possibility to localize the gene would be to test randomly chosen polymorphic markers from all chromosomes for genetic linkage to the disease. Cytogenetic analyses of *men1* patients have not revealed any constitutional chromosomal abnormalities that could indicate the localization of the *men1* gene. Neither could the hormones that are principally affected be regarded as candidate genes, since they are located on different chromosomes. However, if *men1* associated tumors result from unmasking of a recessive mutation according to the two-mutation model, chromosomal rearrangements in such tumors might indicate which chromosome the MEN-I gene is situated on. Therefore, constitutional and tumor genotypes were compared at different RFLP loci in two brothers with neuroendocrine pancreatic tumors, who had inherited the disease from their mother. Markers on 17 chromosomes showed retained constitutional genotypes, but both tumors had lost one of the constitutional alleles at all informative loci on chromosome 11 (144).

The significance of these findings was further supported when the parental origin of the lost chromosome was determined. In both cases the lost alleles were those of the unaffected father. These findings fit the hypothesis that the tumors had grown after elimination of the normal allele at the MEN-I locus, and the MEN-I gene would hence be a tumor suppressor gene located on chromosome 11. Subsequently, linkage of MEN-I to different RFLP markers on chromosome 11 was tested in four Swedish families. In these families, MEN-I was unlinked to the insulin locus (at 11p15) and apolipoprotein A1 (at 11q23). However, when markers closer to the centromeric part of the long arm were analyzed, results in favor of linkage were obtained. In

three informative families, MEN-I was closely linked to the skeletal muscle glycogen phosphorylase *(pygm)* locus at 11q13. No meiotic recombinants were detected with this marker, and the maximum LOD score was 4.37; i.e., the odds in favor of close linkage were $10^{4.37}$:1. The localization of MEN-I to 11q13 was then confirmed in four additional families (145,146). Based on the finding of bFGF-like substance circulating in plasma of MEN-I patients (108), a bFGF-related gene known to be localized at 11q13 was used as a marker. This gene locus, *int2*, was closely linked to MEN-I in all four families. Taken together, these findings strongly suggested that the MEN-I gene is on 11q13 and is a tumor suppressor gene, whose inactivation is involved in tumor development in MEN-I. Alternatively, the predisposing genetic defect in MEN-I could be a dominantly acting mutation, with loss of heterozygosity (LOH) serving to inactivate one or both copies of other loci on chromosome 11, which would also, in this setting, selectively involve the chromosome derived from the unaffected parent. However, several observations make this latter model unlikely.

Loss of heterozygosity involving the 11q13 region is seen in the majority of parathyroid and pancreatic tumors from MEN-I patients (146–151). Deletion mapping studies of familial parathyroid pancreatic tumors have revealed three regions with allele losses, two in addition to the *men1* locus on 11q13 itself: a region telomeric on 11q and one on 11p (147,148,151). They were separated by the *pga* locus (centromeric of the *men1* locus) and the D11S146–*int2* region (telomeric) that showed the tendency to be maintained. One particular pancreatic tumor showed LOH for all three regions and retained heterozygosity at *pga* and D11S146, and at each locus the allele derived from the unaffected parent was eliminated (C. Larsson, unpublished). Analysis of three cases of familial parathyroid tumors (146,148) revealed allelic deletions involving the chromosome carrying the normal *men1* allele, in agreement with the two-mutation model.

Loss of the wild-type chromosome has been found in four pancreatic tumors from three different patients (144,152). Two pancreatic tumors from two brothers with MEN-I both showed loss of the chromosome 11 alleles derived from the unaffected parent (144). DNA from microadenomatous "hyperplastic" pancreatic tissue of one of the brothers was also studied. This tissue was classified histopathologically as benign "hyperplasia" and showed the same type of chromosomal rearrangement as the malignant insulinoma (144). This is compatible with 11q13 deletions being primary events in tumor development, so the secondary mutational events involved in tumor progression would still need to be identified.

The MEN-I pituitary lesions are mostly prolactinomas, which are rarely operated on, and studies of

LOH in pituitary tumors have only in two cases involved familial tumors (148,153). One of these showed LOH at 11q13, and in this case combined tumor and pedigree analysis confirmed elimination of the wild-type allele (153).

MEN-I patients mainly develop neoplasias of the parathyroid glands, the neuroendocrine pancreas and duodenum, and the anterior pituitary gland, and autopsy findings suggest that with increasing age, all three tissues will be affected (154,155). In addition, however, MEN-I patients also develop tumors in other organs more frequently than in the general population. Examples of such lesions are adrenocortical tumors, carcinoid tumors, and lipomas. These associated tumors may reflect a pleiotropic effect of the underlying inherited MEN-I mutation but may also occur secondary to the MEN-I-phenotype. Most common of these associated tumors are benign enlargement of the adrenal cortex, which has been found in about one-third of MEN-I necropsy cases (156,157). As for the pituitary tumors, they are rarely operated on; thus, a genetic analysis of such tumors must rely on a small number of cases. Biochemical evaluation of 12 such individuals failed to demonstrate any disturbances in the hypothalamic–pituitary–adrenal axis (93). Benign adrenal enlargements from five of these MEN-I patients showed retained genotypes for markers flanking the *men1* region, in agreement with results from analysis of eight sporadic adrenocortical adenomas (158). However, one case of MEN-I-associated adrenocortical carcinoma displayed a complete loss of the normal chromosome 11 (93). There are several feasible explanations for the lack of 11q13 deletions in the benign adrenocortical tumors. A conclusive answer, however, will require cloning and analysis of the *men1* gene.

men1 Gene in Sporadic Neoplasms

Accumulating evidence has suggested a two-hit mechanism of tumor development in MEN-I. By analogy with findings in retinoblastoma, some sporadic counterparts of MEN-I-associated tumors are therefore expected to occur by inactivation of the *men1* gene. Hence the sporadic tumor forms would also show allelic losses for the 11q13 region.

In sporadic parathyroid "adenomas" and "hyperplasias," LOH for chromosome 11 markers is a less frequent finding than in those from MEN-I patients (146–149,151); LOH at 11q13 is seen in the majority of familial parathyroid tumors. This is present in approximately one-third of sporadic tumors. The situation for familial and sporadic pancreatic tumors is similar (93,144,150,159). It is possible that these differences reflect a heterogeneity within the group of sporadic tumors. On the other hand, LOH can be detected only

if it is present in a large proportion of the tumor cells. In sporadic tumors, this is only the case when all tumor cells originate from a single cell; i.e., the tumor is monoclonal.

The questions of clonality in primary hyperparathyroidism have been tested by different methods, including X inactivation analysis in females. In females who are heterozygous for an HPRT "marker on the X chromosome," subsequent digestion with the methylation-sensitive restriction enzyme HpaII will result in elimination of one of the constitutional bands if the tumor is monoclonal. The majority of "adenomas" had the DNA hybridization pattern of monoclonality, while that was not the case for any of the "hyperplasias" tested (156). These results are partly supported by the findings of tumor-specific LOH in a considerable proportion of "adenomas," as discussed above. However, in familial tumors, such losses do not necessary reflect a monoclonal origin of the tumor. Since these losses serve to eliminate the wild-type allele at the disease locus, polyclonal and monoclonal tumors may give similar patterns of allele losses for chromosome 11 markers, particularly those near the disease locus.

Studies of LOH in sporadic pituitary tumors have revealed 11q13 deletions in a total of only three cases (148,161). Another recent series showed LOH in four of twelve sporadic somato tropinomas (162). For many of these cases, the losses were partial; the hybridization signal for one of the alleles was reduced to ~50%. This can be due to either an admixture of normal cells or a subclonal secondary event during tumor progression. The latter explanation is most likely, since the vast majority of sporadic pituitary adenomas have been shown to be monoclonal (163,164). The observation of relatively few allele losses on chromosome 11 in pituitary adenomas suggests a difference in pathogenesis compared to the pancreatic and parathyroid lesions, but several explanations are feasible. The pathogenesis of sporadic pituitary adenomas may involve mutational events at the *men1* locus that could not be detected with the method applied, or the pituitary lesions might not reflect mutational events of this gene. One might also speculate that sporadic pituitary adenomas differ pathogenetically from MEN-I-associated lesions.

Efforts To Find the *men1* Gene

Regardless of which strategy has been chosen to isolate the *men1* gene, restriction of the putative gene containing region is a useful start. If the region can be restricted to no more than one or a few million base pairs, it can be cloned and screened for sequences expressed in the affected tissues, i.e., positional cloning.

The region of chromosome 11 harboring the *men1* locus was first defined by seven anchor markers, for which the relative order and genetic distance was determined in reference families (165,166). The loci covered approximately 12 cM, and, for markers at both ends of this region (D11S288 and *int2*), meiotic crossovers were detected (165). As a next step, cosmid clones were isolated from this region, through isolation of human specific clones from somatic cell hybrids (167,168). Then, a total of >50 DNA markers were mapped within this region by hybridization to a panel of radiation-reduced somatic cell hybrids. This panel was designed to carry different parts of the 11q11–13 region on a hamster background, and based on the hybridization pattern the markers were divided into nine groups (162). Such sublocalization provides a starting point for more precise mapping using pulse field gel electrophoresis (PFGE) (169–171), genetic linkage mapping (172,173), and isolation of candidate genes from VAC libraries (174).

For some of the clones new polymorphisms were identified (161,162,167) and used to identify and outline meiotic crossovers in MEN-I families (162,166, 168). As illustrated, multiple recombinants have been detected for D11S288 and in a few cases also for PGA on the centromeric side (Fig. 12). Several meiotic

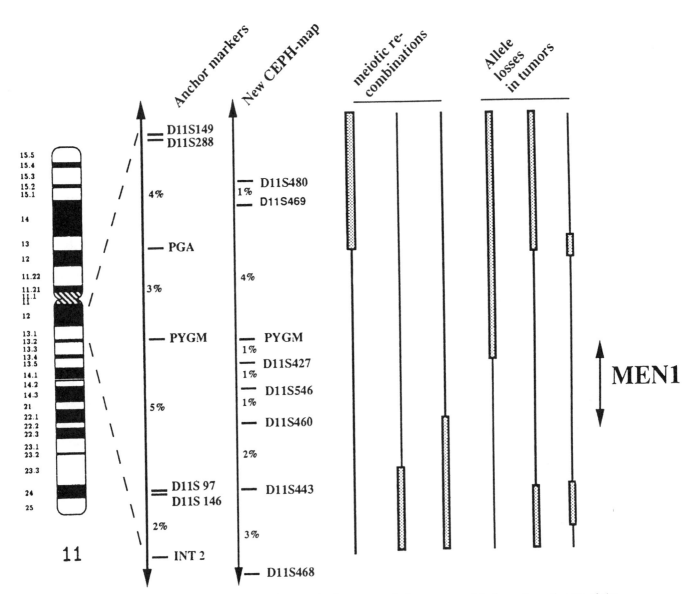

FIG. 12. Mapping of the *men1* region on the long arm of chromosome 11. An enlarged map of the 11q11–13 region shows the genetic order of anchor markers as well as newly isolated cosmid clones mapped in reference families (165,168,176). *Stippled boxes* indicates regions excluded to harbor the *men1* gene as determined by analysis of melotic recombinational events as well as deletion mapping of tumors.

crossovers have also been detected for *int2,* D11S146 and D11S97 on the telomeric side (150,165,168,176). On the other hand, despite extensive family studies, no meiotic recombinants have so far been detected with *pygm* (144,146,165,168,172–176). Taken together, these observations clearly located the *men1* gene between *pga* and D11S97.

Further restriction of the gene-containing region was based on the identification of a deletion telomeric of *pygm* in a parathyroid tumor from an MEN-I patient (148). Similarly, one meiotic recombinant detected for D11S807 (168) and one for D11S460 (172) further moved the telomeric border. *pygm* and D11S460 are located within 3% recombination distance, and their physical distance as determined by PFGE analysis is <2 Mb (171,172).

How the Gene May Be Exploited After Its Discovery

When the *men1* gene is cloned, several basic biological questions can be easily approached. In addition, presymptomatic diagnosis may be based on very reliable methods of mutation detection, and possible relationships between MEN-I-families may be determined. Another aspect is the correlation between genotype and phenotype. Within each affected family, all phenotypic stigmata of MEN-I are usually represented, but at varying frequencies in different families. Why some families for example exhibit mainly pituitary tumors may perhaps be explained by the nature and location of the segregating mutation. The extent and level of the involvement of the MEN-I gene in tumorigenesis of sporadic parathyroid, pituitary, and pancreatic–duodenal tumors might also be clarified.

If the *men-I* gene is a tumor-suppressor gene, its expression is expected to be altered or lost in the tumors. Furthermore, introduction of a cloned *men1*-gene into a tumor cell line should result in reversion of the neoplastic phenotype. Similarly, knockout experiments using transgenic animals should result in the occurrence of multiple endocrine tumors. This could be studied in species that spontaneously develop the MEN-I phenotype in low frequencies, i.e., functioning parathyroid, endocrine pancreatic–duodenal, and anterior pituitary tumors. However, no such animal model has been identified so far. Animal models could allow research into treatment options that would be difficult to study in humans, such as the effect of early parathyroidectomy on late development of gastrointestinal neoplasms.

Animal Models of Multiple Endocrine Neoplasia Type I

Sporadic prolactin-producing pituitary tumors associated with parathyroid "hyperplasia" and hyper-

calcemia but without pancreatic involvement have been found occasionally in dogs (54). Spontaneously occurring pituitary nodules consisting mainly of prolactin-producing cells have been found in aging Long-Evans rats (177). These animals also showed diffuse and nodular "hyperplasia" of the parathyroids, the thyroid, and the adrenal medulla. Thus this would rather be a model of mixed MEN-I and -II syndrome. Nonfunctioning parathyroid and thyroid tumors can be induced in rats by irradiation, and, if irradiation is given in combination with 3-methylcholantrene, pancreatic islet cell tumors may also develop (178,179).

Foreign DNA may be introduced into the germline of mammals by injecting the DNA directly into the pronucleus of fertilized eggs and then transferring the eggs to foster mothers so that development can continue. The resulting transgenic animals generally carry one or more copies of the foreign DNA integrated into one of their chromosomes. By fusing regulatory regions from genes that are known to be expressed in a tissue-specific manner to transforming genes, it is possible to direct expression of the transforming genes to specific cell types, thereby producing lines of mice that develop tumors only in specific organs. SV-40 large T antigen is oncogenic in transgenic mice, and, for example, when it is introduced in combination with the rat insulin gene promoter, endocrine pancreatic tumors develop (180). When T antigen is coupled to elastase, exocrine pancreatic tumors develop (181).

Endocrine pancreatic and pituitary tumors were found to develop in mice transgenic for vasopressin–SV40 hybrid (182). In contrast, when the SV40 large T antigen was placed under the control of a major histocompatibility complex class I gene enhancer, the resulting transgenic mice developed a variety of different tumors, including choroid plexus papillomas, lymphoid hyperplasia, and multiple endocrine neoplasias (183). The endocrine neoplasias were found to develop later in life; involved the pancreas, pituitary, thyroid adrenals, and testes; and rapidly progressed toward malignant growth (183).

The background of the transgene is such that it can modulate tumor formation. This is illustrated by recent observations from transgenic mice carrying the *c-mos* protooncogene (184). The majority of the mice were found to develop pheochromocytomas and C-cell thyroid neoplasms, as in MEN-IIa. When the transgenic mice that initially did not develop the MEN-IIa phenotype were crossed with C3H mice, the progeny were instead found to develop an MEN-I phenotype with pancreatic islet cell "hyperplasia" and pituitary adenomas (185). Therefore, this would be a good model to study phenotypic penetrance in MEN-I.

DIAGNOSIS AND COUNSELING

Incidence

The incidence of MEN-I in the general population remains unknown as prospective, long-term, population-based studies are lacking. Published reports, based on findings during randomly performed autopsies, estimate a prevalence of 0.25% (186,187). Other estimates, based on published reports in the literature, assume a prevalence in the range of 0.02–0.175 per thousand (188). Cancer registry data from Holland (population 15 million) estimate ~25 families with MEN-I (189), and ~16 families with 100 affected individuals are known in Sweden (population 8,000,000) (190,191). Since the disease manifests itself as hyperfunction of the parathyroids, the neuroendocrine pancreas, and the anterior pituitary, estimates of its occurrence have been made in unselected patient populations presenting with hyperparathyroidism, endocrine pancreatic hypersecretion syndromes, and pituitary tumors. Estimated figures for the prevalence of MEN-I patients among patients with primary hyperparathyroidism (HPT); (the most common endocrine anomaly in MEN-I) range from 1% to 18% (192). In a retrospective study of 119 patients with primary HPT, an overall incidence of MEN-I of 17.5% was reported, with a higher incidence (43%) in patients with more than one gland affected (193). Jackson and coworkers (194) identified three individuals with familial MEN-I among 91 consecutive patients who underwent neck exploration for primary HPT. Fifteen of 147 patients with hyperparathyroidism (10%) have evidence of coexisting pituitary adenoma (195). In contrast, not even a single case of MEN-I was detected in a prospective study with screening of many biochemical markers or among 63 consecutive patients with primary HPT (196). The cause for differing rates of MEN-I within groups with primary HPT is unknown but may be related to patient selection bias or to methods of screening in the patients and their relatives.

Neuroendocrine pancreatic tumors, particularly gastrinomas, are frequently expressed clinically in MEN-I (197). An early report by Kumerrelle and associates (197) states that only 12 of 282 patients with endocrine pancreatic tumors have associated MEN-I. In a Danish survey the prevalence of MEN-I was 38% (14/26) in individuals with the Zollinger-Ellison (ZE) syndrome (198). In a retrospective study of 90 patients treated surgically for ZE, 15 (16%) displayed other features of MEN-I (199). In a review from Ireland covering 16 years with 2.6–9.7 new pancreatic endocrine tumors diagnosed per year, one-third of gastrinomas and insulinomas were reported to be in the context of MEN-I, and the annual incidence of newly diagnosed MEN-I in this patient population was 0.05 per 100,000 (200).

The prevalence of pituitary involvement in MEN-I in various series ranges from 16% to 65%. In a prospective study of 176 patients with anterior pituitary adenoma, seven index cases of MEN-I were diagnosed (120), and 41 of 1500 consecutive pituitary adenomas (2.7%) were encountered in the context of MEN-I (201). In contrast, no patient with MEN-I features was diagnosed among 79 consecutive patients with pituitary neoplasm (201). This may be explained by the low frequency of prolactinoma (the most common pituitary tumor in MEN-I) in the latter study.

The Sporadic Case

The distinction between the familial form of MEN-I and the sporadic form is difficult, or virtually impossible to make in some cases. Only after the *men1* gene has been cloned and sequenced will it be possible to make a clear distinction between these two patient populations. Some cases of new mutation may be mosaics and, therefore, may not show that mutation clearly in all tissues. In the familial cases, a germline mutation that cosegregates with the disease gene will be found, whereas, in the sporadic cases, gene alterations (e.g., point mutations) will be found in a somatic, tumor-specific manner but not in the germline (unless there is a newly acquired germline mutation).

There are several factors that may account for the reported sporadic cases of MEN-I. First, it may reflect incomplete family evaluation, incomplete gene penetrance, or young age of the other family members. Second, the possibility of two unrelated, coincidental endocrine anomalies should be borne in mind. Third, there may be newly acquired germline mutations in the *men1* gene, similar to what has been described for other familial diseases for which the genes have been cloned, sequenced, and shown to act as tumor suppressor genes, like the presumed *men1* gene [include the neurofibromatosis type 1 gene (202), the familial adenomatous polyposis gene (203), and the retinoblastoma gene (204)]. Since it is not known at present how large the *men1* gene is, it is virtually impossible to assess the proportion with newly acquired mutations in the MEN-I patient population. Finally, some endocrine tumors secrete factors that stimulate growth in a paracrine or true endocrine fashion. Thus carcinoid tumors have been shown to secrete ACTH (205), which may account for the adrenal hyperplasia seen in some MEN-I patients; pancreatic endocrine tumors rarely secrete GH-releasing factor, which may cause pituitary hyperplasia (206,207). The relative proportion of tumors displaying this presumed paracrine/endocrine activity is unknown. However, this could imply that some of the MEN-I-associated tumors are polyclonal and not mono- or oligooclonal, as has been shown for the parathyroid and pancreatic tumors (121,208).

Differential Diagnosis

Multiple Sporadic Tumors

A combination of more than one endocrine tumor in the same patient, by definition, constitutes multiple endocrine neoplasia (see above). Many unusual tumors and dysplastic processes have coexisted with primary hyperparathyroidism in sporadic cases (51). These associations, invariably based on single case reports, prompted some authors to suggest the existence of variants or subtypes of the known MEN syndromes. However, it is not clear whether this is justified (209). As was mentioned above, some of these reports may represent simultaneous expression of common disorders, primary hyperparathyroidism and another less common disorder; incomplete gene penetrance; inadequate familial screening; or newly acquired germline mutation within the *men1* gene.

Several reports, based on retrospective surgical surveys, have made a case for the high frequency of coexisting parathyroid adenoma and nonmedullary thyroid carcinoma (210,211). In their review of published reports, Simpson and Moss (211) state that ~4% of patients with thyroid carcinoma have coexisting parathyroid tumor. This association could be explained by a coincidence, a common external environmental factor (such as irradiation; see below), the "goitrogenic" effect of hypercalcemia, or a common genetic abnormality, such as mutation in the *men1* gene. Interestingly, allelic losses involving the long arm of chromosome 11, and including the *men1* gene locus, were found in several follicular thyroid neoplasms (212). This may be indirect evidence that the *men1* gene is also involved in thyroid tumorigenesis and that the above-mentioned association is truly a genetic one.

Several endocrine syndromes have infrequently been described to accompany sporadic pancreatic endocrine tumors: Cushing's syndrome (caused by ACTH secretion) (213), atypical carcinoid tumor syndrome (serotonin) (214), and acromegaly (GHRH or GH) (206). The frequency of Cushing's syndrome associated with nonfamilial ZE syndrome in one large prospective study was 5% (3/59) (215), and, invariably, the pancreatic tumor was malignant (216). In some cases, the appropriate causative hormones have been shown to be ectopically produced by the pancreatic islet cell tumor.

Single, sporadic cases documented the concurrence of prolactinoma with adrenal aldosteronoma, gastric schwannoma, and colonic polyps (217), unilateral aldosteronoma (218), and neck paraganglioma (219,220). Acromegaly, which occurs much less frequently than prolactinoma, has been associated with a statistically significantly increased incidence of benign and malignant tumors, most notably thyroid carcinomas, nodules, and goiters (221). The underlying mechanism(s) of this increase is unknown, but the authors suggested an effect of the GH or its active metabolite, IGF-I, on the target tissues. In addition, the association of acromegaly or nonsecreting pituitary tumors with sporadic pheochromocytoma has been described in a few cases (222). In two cases, these tumors were accompanied by hyperparathyroidism. Schimke (209), reviewing all published data on this association, concluded that current evidence does not support a syndromal relationship between pituitary adenoma and pheochromocytoma. A single case report documented the coexistence of acromegaly and a unilateral adrenal adenoma (223). The association of bilateral, pituitary-dependent, adrenal hyperplasia and unilateral adrenal adenoma with thyroid nodules has been reported infrequently (224) in females only, and this suggested yet another variant of MEN syndromes. It was not clear, however, whether these represented familial or sporadic cases.

About 4% of all carcinoids have been associated with other endocrine tumors (94). For the most part, these are encountered in the setting of familial MEN-I. However, a few reports document the nonfamilial association between carcinoid tumors and medullary thyroid carcinoma (94) and several cases with associated pheochromocytoma (225). This latter association is intriguing, since duodenal carcinoid tumor and pheochromocytoma both occur with an increased frequency in neurofibromatosis type 1 (see below). Carcinoid tumors can secrete ectopic peptide hormones such as GHRH, that may in turn result in secondary endocrine syndromes. Thus interpreting data from patients with carcinoid tumors with associated endocrine tumors and deciding whether these represent separate, distinct tumor entities or are casually related may be difficult.

Neck Irradiation and Tumorigenesis

Radiation was a commonly used therapeutic modality in the 1930s through the mid-1950s for benign conditions such as facial acne and tinea capitis (226). When the association between external irradiation of the head and neck and subsequent development of benign and malignant tumors in the irradiated region became apparent, these uses of irradiation were discontinued (227,228). Since the original report in 1975 of hyperparathyroidism in a previously irradiated patient (229), numerous studies have documented this association (230–235). Prior radiation has occurred in 14–30% of patients with primary HPT (230,231,236), and the prevalence of primary HPT in patients with a history of irradiation is estimated at 4–11% (237) compared to an incidence of <0.4% in the general population (238). Hyperparathyroidism occurs after a mean time of several decades (32–47 years) following the radiation (232,234) and was noted with both high exposure (239) and low dose irradiation (such as in atomic bomb survivors) (235). Clinically, there are no apparent differences with regard to age at diagnosis, male to female ratio, calcium levels, or uni- vs. polyglandular involvement in the irradiated group of patients compared with the nonirradiated patients. In some studies, the irradiated patients seemed to have a higher proportion of asymptomatic presentation, and in all reports there is clearly a high proportion of cooccurring thyroid neoplasms ranging from 30% to 84% of patients with primary HPT (232,236,240–241). These epidemiological data clearly demonstrate the association of previous X-ray irradiation with the development of parathyroid tumors. Furthermore, in several studies (235,242), hyperparathyroidism seemed to occur more frequently in patients who received higher doses, suggesting a causal effect of irradiation in parathyroid tumor development. In animals irradiated with X-rays, it was also possible to induce parathyroid tumors, further supporting the causal role of irradiation in parathyroid tumor development.

The role of radioactive iodine in parathyroid tumorigenesis is less clear. Despite the detection of a high proportion of parathyroid tumors in rats exposed to ^{131}I (243), and the detection of an increased incidence of parathyroid tumors in patients previously exposed to ^{131}I (244), this could not be demonstrated in all studies (245). Another difficulty in interpreting the data linking ^{131}I to hyperparathyroidism is the fact that the underlying reason for the radioiodine treatment may have been a neoplastic process affecting the thyroids. Thus a "cancer susceptibility gene," unrelated to the ^{131}I treatment, may be operative in parathyroid tumor development in this patient population. Whatever the role of previous X-ray exposure or ^{131}I treatment may be in development of head and neck tumors, it is clear that patients who have undergone these types of irradiation should be monitored closely, clinically and biochemically, for the possible development of parathyroid and thyroid neoplasia. Jackson has suggested that neck radiation could contribute to development of parathyroid tumors in patients with susceptibility such as in MEN-I. He recommended minimizing exposure to radiation for dental and other procedures in these subjects (246).

Multiple Endocrine Tumor Different From Those in Multiple Endocrine Neoplasia Type I or II

Carney Syndrome

An unusual complex of myxomas (cardiac, cutaneous, and breast), pigmented skin lesions, and endocrine overactivity was first described by Schweitzer-Cagiaut and coworkers (247) and was best delineated by Carney et al. (248). The endocrine components of this syndrome include pigmented bilateral adrenal autonomous lesions (though not all patients clinically have Cushing's syndrome), acromegaly due to pituitary adenoma, and bilateral Sertoli or Leydig cell tumors of the testes that may result in precocious puberty (249). A pheochromocytoma (250) and a prolactin- and ACTH-secreting pituitary adenoma (251) have also been described in affected patients. A heritable form of the syndrome appears to follow autosomal dominant transmission (249). The precise genetic lesion is unknown, and suggestions about a role for circulating antibodies stimulating adrenal hyperplasia have been made (252). To date, there are no reported genetic linkage analyses in this syndrome, nor have any genetic abnormalities been reported in the associated tumors. Interestingly, sporadic tumors in two of the tissues that are commonly affected in this syndrome complex, namely, pituitary and adrenal, have shown tumor-specific mutations in the alpha subunits of two GTP-binding proteins (G proteins): Gs in pituitary GH-secreting tumors and Gi2 in adrenal tumors. Mutations in the Gsα gene have been documented in affected tissues from patients with the McCune-Albright syndrome (see below).

McCune-Albright Syndrome

This syndrome is characterized by polyostotic fibrous dysplasia, café-au-lait pigmentation of the skin, and a host of endocrinopathies: sexual precocity, hyperthyroidism, gigantism with GH-secreting pituitary adenomas, and autonomous adrenal hyperplasia (253, 254). Because of the sporadic occurrence of the syndrome and the pattern of skin pigmentation, it has been suggested that the underlying defect may be a somatic mutation affecting several tissues early in embryonic development, resulting in a mosaic tissue composition (255). The endocrine glands commonly affected in this syndrome are all autonomous (254). As was mentioned above, activating mutations in the Gsα gene have been found in a large proportion of solitary GH-secreting tumors (256) and in some thyroid tumors (257). Furthermore, these so-called *gsp* mutations are biochemically characterized by a decrease in the intrinsic GTPase activity of the Gsα subunit, with resultant constitutive activation of adenylyl cyclase and intracellular accumulation of cAMP (259). Thus it seemed logical to search for abnormalities in the signal transduction pathway that controls the production of cAMP. Indeed, Weinstein and coworkers (255) have demonstrated somatic *gsp*-activating mutations in a mosaic distribution pattern in all affected endocrine tissues as well as in some clinically unaffected tissues in McCune-Albright syndrome. Similar *gsp* mutations have been documented in skin and bone lesions (258). Although direct biochemical evidence of increased cAMP levels in affected tissues is lacking, the current data are highly suggestive of a pathogenetic role for *gsp* mutations in the McCune-Albright syndrome.

Pheochromocytoma and Islet Cell Tumors

The concurrence of pheochromocytoma and islet cell tumors has been documented in sporadic and familial cases (260,261). In the familial cases, the syndrome follows an autosomal dominant inheritance pattern with variable expression, whereas, in the sporadic cases, there is a predominance of females, and in the majority of the cases there was a history of pheochromocytoma or the von Hippel-Lindau disease in another family member. The pancreatic islet cell tumors occurring as part of this complex are often multicentric and clinically nonfunctional. Single case reports document coexisting unilateral pheochromocytoma with multiple pancreatic gastrinoma and a single parathyroid adenoma and adrenal adenomas (255) and the combination of islet cell tumors with extraadrenal paragangliomas (263). These may, in fact, represent "mixed" MEN syndromes (see below). Pheochromocytoma and islet cell tumors occur together or separately as part of the von-Hippel Lindau (VHL) syndrome (264). Furthermore, Hull and coworkers reported two sibs within a family with VHL, who both had pheochromocytoma and islet cell adenoma. Thus, before accepting the association of pheochromocytoma-islet cell tumor as a distinct, novel MEN syndrome, VHL should be excluded. This can be accomplished by direct analysis of the *vhl* gene or by performing linkage analyses in the familial cases to establish linkage to 3p markers that were linked to the VHL gene or by searching for allelic losses of material from the same chromosomal region in the appropriate tumors from the sporadic cases (see below).

Von Hippel-Lindau Disease

This rare, autosomally dominant inherited disorder is characterized by hemangioblastomas of the central nervous system, retinal angiomatosis, renal cell carcinoma, visceral cysts, and pheochromocytoma (264). In addition to pheochromocytoma, pancreatic islet cell tumors are observed (265,266) and were noted in six of 35 (17%) affected patients (266). The pancreatic tumors in VHL are usually nonfunctional and asymptomatic. Other endocrine abnormalities in VHL, all in the form of single case reports, include metastatic carcinoid tumor, carotid body tumor, pituitary adenoma (prolactinoma), and medullary thyroid carcinoma (264). The VHL disease gene has been localized by linkage analysis to chromosome 3p (267) and presumably acts as a tumor suppressor gene, as inferred from the frequent allelic loss of 3p markers in renal cell carcinoma from patients with VHL. The *vhl* gene has been cloned and found to encode a unique protein (143).

Neurofibromatosis Type 1

Neurofibromatosis type 1 is an inherited autosomal dominant disorder characterized by abnormalities in tissues, many of which are derived from the neural crest: cafè-au-lait spots, benign neurofibromas, mental retardation, Lisch nodules of the iris, and an increased risk of benign and malignant tumors of the nervous system (268). The disease gene, localized to the long arm of chromosome 17, has been cloned and sequenced (269), and the gene product (neurofibromin) has been shown to possess a GTPase activating protein (GAP)-like domain that is active in the down regulation of the active, GTP-bound *ras* gene product (270,271). Furthermore, tumor-specific mutations that inhibit the GTPase activity of *nf1* gene product have been shown in a few sporadic human tumors (272). The endocrine tumors that have been associated with NF1 include pheochromocytoma, which probably affects <1% of patients with NF1 (273), duodenal somatostatin-containing carcinoid tumors (with distinct histological features) (274), and sporadic case reports documenting NF1 in association with medullary and nonmedullary thyroid carcinomas (275,276), adrenocortical adenomas (277,278), and multiple paragangliomatosis (277). Parathyroid tumors in NF1 patients, usually single adenomas, had been reported in 11 patients by 1990 (279). A single case report described, in a probable MEN-I patient, the association of hyperparathyroidism, islet cell tumor, and mediastinal neurofibrosarcoma (280). The association between parathyroid tumors and NF1 may be totally coincidental. It would be interesting, however, to test these particular parathyroid tumors for allelic losses from 11q13 (the MEN-I gene locus) as well as to screen for somatic point mutations of the *nf1* gene.

Familial Syndromes Affecting Only One Endocrine Organ

Familial Hyperparathyroidism. More than 30 kindreds, mostly small, were reported to display primary hyperparathyroidism only (familial isolated hyperparathyroidism; FIHP), with no evidence of other associated endocrinopathies to suggest MEN (281). In most cases, the inheritance is autosomal dominant, but a single kindred with autosomal recessive transmission has been reported (282). Histopathologically, uni- or polyglandular adenoma or hyperplasia occur at a similar frequency, and in five families the histopathological diagnosis of parathyroid carcinoma was made in some family members. The unique cooccurrence of familial hyperparathyroidism and parathyroid cysts with ossifying fibromas of the jaw, in association with familial hypocalciuric hypercalcemia (FHH) has been reported by Mallette and coworkers (283). Some families reported initially to have FIHP were subsequently reclassified as having MEN-I (284). However, in others, linkage to the MEN-I locus has been excluded. Clinically, there are important distinctions between the two disease entities; hypercalcemia in FIHP tends to occur during adolescence, i.e., earlier then in MEN-I, and there is an apparent increased incidence of parathyroid carcinoma, a rare tumor reported in ~15% FIHP families (285–288), whereas it was reported only once with MEN-I (289), a more prevalent disease. Linkage analysis in one FIHP family clearly indicate that it is not linked to the MEN-I, the MEN-II, or the PTH gene loci and that in the parathyroid tumors examined there are no chromosome 11 allelic losses (290). The possibility of disease heterogeneity, with some families showing linkage to any of the MEN loci, should be considered. Furthermore, linkage to the FHH gene locus, recently localized to 3q (291), should be examined.

Familial Pancreatic Islet Cell Tumors. There are only two reports of a familial occurrence of isolated insulinoma without associated endocrinopathies (292, 293). In both families, a father and daughter were affected, and, in both parents, the tumors recurred after a long euglycemic period of up to 15 years. The tumors were diagnosed early in childhood in one family (292), and an association with diabetes mellitus was noted. The paucity of reports of this association speaks for itself, but it seems distinct clinically, and perhaps genetically, from any known MEN syndrome.

Familial Acromegaly. A few reports suggest familial isolated acromegaly as a distinct entity (294–299). The majority of the cases were diagnosed in the second or third decade of life, and, in the few cases examined, the tumors had some unique histological features (298). The mode of transmission is presumed to be autosomal dominant with variable penetrance. Obviously, in no case were there signs of either the McCune-Albright or the Carney syndrome, but the extent to which MEN-I was excluded is unclear from the reports. However, the early age at diagnosis and the infrequent occurrence of acromegaly in MEN-I make it likely that familial acromegaly is a separate entity. To date, no genetic abnormalities have been reported in these tumors.

The so-called prolactinoma variant of MEN-I deserves to be mentioned. Five families, including four from Newfoundland, Canada, show a unique pattern of MEN-I with a high prevalence of hyperparathyroidism and prolactinomas, with only one case among 42 gene carriers displaying associated gastrinoma (300,301). In the Canadian families, linkage has been shown to 11q13 (Green J et al. unpublished), similar to the "regular" variant of MEN-I (302), clearly demonstrating that this variant is part of MEN-I and not a unique entity.

Familial Carcinoid Tumors. Carcinoid tumors are considered an integral part of MEN-I (209). In addition, the association of carcinoid tumors with medullary thyroid carcinoma (303) and pheochromocytoma (303), both predominant features of MEN-II, has been reported occasionally. Rarely, carcinoid tumors have shown familial clustering (304–308). The mode of inheritance seems to be autosomal dominant (308), and the tumors were located either at the terminal ileum or at the appendix (five families) or were duodenal (one family). This latter location is rare in sporadic carcinoid tumors but appears to be the most common site for carcinoid tumors associated with NF1 (309). Any relationship between this rare syndrome and the known MEN syndromes or NF1 remains to be determined.

Familial Adrenal Hyperfunction. Adrenocortical neoplasms have been documented in several families, and these have been attributed to selective antibodies. Involvement of the adrenal cortex has been reported in a considerable proportion of patients with MEN-I (36–41%) (310,311). In the majority of cases, the lesions are bilateral, hyperplastic, and non-functional. Furthermore, only in rare cases of an aldosteronoma (312) or carcinoma (311) have allelic losses encompassing the *men1* locus been documented. Thus, despite its being a part of the MEN-I tumor complex, the majority of adrenal lesions in this context appear to develop via a different mechanism from parathyroid, pancreatic, or pituitary tumors. Familial clustering of functional adrenocortical tumors has been encountered in the Li-Fraumeni syndrome, and inactivating mutations in the *p53* gene (located on the short arm of chromosome 17) have been documented in these familial cases in germline DNA (313). Interestingly, the one adrenocortical carcinoma from an MEN-I patient that was analyzed for allelic losses does display allelic loss that includes 17p (311). It would be interesting to explore potential interactions between the still elusive *men1* gene and the *p53* gene, both tumor-suppressor genes. To date, no somatic mutations within the *p53* gene have been reported in islet cell or pituitary tumors (314).

Mixed Multiple Endocrine Neoplasia Syndromes

A few cases with disease manifestations or organ involvement that overlap the MEN-I and MEN-II syndromes have been published (Table 2). These reports prompted speculation that the known MEN syndromes are not pure entities and that reclassification is needed. All the reported cases represent either a sporadic occurrence of a tumor considered part of a specific MEN syndrome in a familial setting of another MEN syndrome (Table 2) or sporadic, nonfamilial cooccurrence of an "overlap" tumor constellation in a single patient. Some nonfamilial cases show features of MEN-I plus pheochromocytoma (328,329) or MEN-I plus chemodectoma (330,331). It is clear that the MEN-I and MEN-II genes are located on different chromosomes and presumably encode for different gene products. It is possible that these reported over-

TABLE 2. *Overlap syndromes in multiple endocrine neoplasia[a]*

MEN-1-related	REF	MEN2A- MEN2B-related	Fa./Sp. Age/Sex	Other findings
Cushing's syndrome (Source?) Hyperparathyroidism	(315)	Pheochromocytoma MTC	Fa.	
Parathyroid hyperplasia Acromegaly	(316)	Paragalgliomas, extraadrenal, multiple	Fa(?) 19/F	Pigmentary abnormalities; retinal anomalies NF1?
Duodenal carcinoid tumors Adrenal cortical adenoma		Pheochromocytoma; left adrenal + 2 paraaortic Ganglioneuroma	? 13/F	NF1?
Pituitary adenoma Basophils		Pheochromocytoma, Bilateral; MTC	? 43/F	
Intestinal carcinoid, metastatic	(317)	"Benign C-cell adenoma" of the thyroid	? 47/F	
Pancreatic islet cell Glucagonoma (?)	(318)	MTC	Fa.	No symptoms
Gastrinoma (?)	(319)	MTC	Sp. 28/M	Source of hypergastrinemia not found
Islet cell tumor (hormone?)	(320)	Pheochromocytoma	Sp. 31/F	
Pituitary tumor (hormone?)		Pheochromocytoma	Sp. ?/F	
Gastrinoma, multiple; adrenocortical adenoma	(321)	Pheochromocytoma Parathyroid hyperplasia	Sp. 36/F	
Granular cell pituitary tumor		MTC parathyroid hyperplasia (in the father)	Fa 36/F	
Hyperprolactinemia	(322)	Undefined thyroid disease		
Parathyroid Adenoma		Marfanoid habitus	Sp(?) 31/F	Optic atrophy Mental retardation
Prolactinoma	(323)			Mitral valve prolapse
Prolactinoma	(324)	MTC, bilateral Pheochromocytoma Parathyroid adenoma, single	Fa (MTC) 26/M	
Pancreatic polypeptide hypersecretion		MTC		
Microadenosis and nesidioblastosis	(325)			
Pancreatic gastrinoma, solitary	(326)	MTC; Pheochromocytoma, bilateral	Fa 36/M	Extra adrenal Cushing's syndrome
Prolactinoma	(327)	Ganglioneuroma, extra adrenal	Sp. 34/F	

[a]One patient with MTC from a family with MEN-I and hyperparathyroidism has been reported by Eberle MTC denotes medullary thyroid carcinoma; Sp., sporadic; Fa, familial; F, female; M, male.
*Fa.Sp., familial/sporadic

lap syndromes do represent a coincidence. Alternatively, there may be a direct interaction (in the form of either protein–protein interaction or transcriptional regulation) or sharing of a common biochemical pathway between the gene products, a pathway that is operative and crucial in the tumor development cascade of these particular tumors. Obviously, this can be answered with a degree of confidence only following the cloning of the appropriate genes.

Familial Hypocalciuric Hypercalcemia

The hereditary disorder most frequently requiring differentiation from MEN-I is familial hypocalciuric (or familial benign) hypercalcemia (FHH) (see the chapter by Heath; 332,333). The *fhh* gene (also called *hhc* gene) is on the long arm of chromosome 3 (291), widely separated from the *men1* gene on chromosome 11. FHH is an autosomal dominant disorder, showing life-long and stable hypercalcemia. The population prevalence of FHH kindreds is approximately the same as that of MEN-I kindreds (S.J.M., unpublished observations). Because of its clinical similarities and its incidence similarities to MEN-I, FHH can present a diagnostic challenge when a small kindred shows asymptomatic hypercalcemia in several members. The pathophysiology of FHH is believed to be quite different from that of MEN-I; MEN-I is principally an excessive proliferation in certain tissue groups; FHH is probably a defect in calcium recognition or transport at the level of the parathyroid gland, kidneys, and perhaps other tissues. The following description of FHH emphasizes those features that help to distinguish MEN-I from FHH (Table 2 in the chapter by Metz et al.).

Hypercalcemia onset age: Hypercalcemia in FHH is expressed within the first week of life (307), and the degree of hypercalcemia changes little throughout life. Since hypercalcemia is rare before age 15 years in MEN-I, hypercalcemia in a young child is an extremely useful differentiating feature.

Calcium in urine: Urinary calcium excretion follows a normal distribution in FHH; thus occasional hypercalciuria can occur, but this is the rare exception (335). Because urinary calcium is partly dependent on glomerular filtration rate (GFR), expression of urinary calcium corrected for GFR leads to the most useful diagnostic index. The most widely used index is the renal calcium clearance divided by the creatinine clearance; this clearance ratio is <0.01 in ~90% of FHH cases and >0.01 in ~90% of cases of primary hyperparathyroidism (either sporadic or from MEN-I). This index should be used only in hypercalcemic cases.

Serum magnesium: On average, serum magnesium is significantly higher in FHH than in MEN-I (336), but this is rarely helpful in individual cases.

Parathyroid hormone in serum: Typical PTH levels are normal in FHH, though 10–15% of cases show elevated PTH levels (337) even with immunoradiometric assays for intact PTH (338); thus hypercalcemia with nonsuppressed PTH levels in the middle to low portion of the normal range favors a diagnosis of FHH.

Outcome of parathyroid surgery: Unsuccessful parathyroidectomy is a feature common to FHH and MEN-I. While subtotal parathyroidectomy by an experienced surgeon can be at least temporarily successful in up to 95% of MEN-I cases, the outcome in FHH is almost always persistent hypercalcemia unless the patient becomes hypoparathyroid. The reasons for persistent hypercalcemia differ in the two disorders. The parathyroid glands in FHH generally appear normal, with evidence of only mild hyperplasia on close inspection. The increased calcium set point for PTH secretion by each cell and not the secretory cell mass is critical in FHH. A small parathyroid remnant is sufficient to regenerate immediately the preoperative state of hypercalcemia. In MEN-I, the typical finding is multiple adenomas; when surgery is unsuccessful, this reflects failure to remove one or more substantial masses of parathyroid tissue.

REFERENCES

1. Brown EM, Hurwitz S, Aurbach GD. Preparation of viable isolated bovine parathyroid cells. *Endocrinology* 1976;99: 1582–1588.
2. Brown EM. Calcium hemostasis. This volume.
3. Raisz LG. Regulation by calcium of parathyroid growth and secretion in vitro. *Nature* 1963;197:1115–1116.
4. Leboff MS, Rennke HG, Brown EM. Abnormal regulation of parathyroid cell secretion and proliferation in primary cultures of bovine parathyroid cells. *Endocrinology* 1983;113: 277–284.
5. MacGregor RR, Sarras MP Jr, Houle A, Cohn DV. Primary monolayer cell culture of bovine parathyroids: effects of calcium, isoproterenol and growth factors. *Mol Endocrinol* 1983;30:313–328.
6. Brandi ML, Fitzpatrick LA, Coon HG, Aurbach GD. Bovine parathyroid cells: cultures maintained for more than 140 population doublings. *Proc Natl Acad Sci USA* 1986;83: 1709–1713.
7. Sakaguchi K, Santora A, Zimering M, Curcio F, Aurbach GD, Brandi ML. Functional epithelial cell line cloned from rat parathyroid glands. *Proc Natl Acad Sci USA* 1987; 84:3269–3273.
8. Brandi ML, Ornberg R, Sakaguchi K, Curcio F, Fattorossi A, Lelkes P, Matsui T, Zimering M, Aurbach GD. Establishment and characterization of a clonal line of parathyroid endothelial cells. *FASEB J* 1990;4:3152.
9. Brandi ML. Cellular models for the analysis of paracrine communications in parathyroid tissue. *J Endocrinol Invest* 1993;16:303–314.
10. Kremer R, Bolivar I, Goltzman D, Hendy GN. Influence of calcium and 1,25-dihydroxycholecalciferol on proliferation

and proto-oncogene expression in primary cultures of bovine parathyroid cells. *Endocrinology* 1989;125:935–941.

11. Szabo A, Merke J, Beier E, Mall G, Ritz E. 1,25-(OH)$_2$ vitamin D$_3$ inhibits parathyroid cell proliferation in experimental uremia. *Kidney Int* 1989;35:1049–1056.

12. Ishimi Y, Russell J, Sherwood LM. Regulation by calcium and 1,25-(OH) 2D3 of cell proliferation and function of bovine parathyroid cells in culture. *J Bone Min Res* 1990;5:755–760.

13. Sakaguchi K. Autocrine and paracrine functions of parathyroid tissue. This volume.

14. Fasciotto BH, Borr SU, DeFranco DJ, Levine MA, Cohn DV. Pancreastatin, a presumed product of chromogranin-A (secretory protein-I) processing, inhibits secretion from porcine parathyroid cells in culture. *Endocrinology* 1989;125:1617–1622.

15. Levine MA, Dempsey MA, Helman LJ, Ahn TG. Expression of chromogranin-A messenger ribonucleic acid in parathyroid tissue from patients with primary hyperparathyroidism. *J Clin Endocrinol Metab* 1990;70:1668–1673.

16. Fujii Y, Moreira JE, Orlando C, et al. Endothelin as an autocrine factor in the regulation of parathyroid cells. *Proc Natl Acad Sci USA* 1991;88:4235–4239.

17. De Feo ML, Bartolini O, Orlando C, et al. Natriuretic peptide receptors regulate endothelin synthesis and release from parathyroid cells. *Proc Natl Acad Sci USA* 1991;88:6496–6500.

18. Ikeda K, Weir E, Mangin M, et al. Expression of messenger ribonucleic acids encoding a parathyroid hormone-like peptide in normal human and animal tissues with abnormal expression in human parathyroid adenomas. *Mol Endocrinol* 1988;2:1230–1236.

19. Ikeda K, Weir EC, Sakaguchi K, et al. Clonal rat parathyroid cell line expresses a parathyroid hormone-related peptide but not parathyroid hormone itself. *Biochem Biophys Res Commun* 1989;162:108–115.

20. Bani D, Axiotis C, Bianchi S, Pioli P, Tanini A, Brandi ML. Expression and calcium modulation of P-glycoprotein in parathyroid tissue. *Bone Mineral* 1992;17:S96.

21. Moskalewski S. Isolation and culture of the islets of Langerhans of the guinea pig. *Gen Comp Endocrinol* 1965;5:342–353.

22. Andersson A, Hellerstrom C. Metabolic characteristics of isolated pancreatic islets in tissue culture. *Diabetes* 1972;21:546–554.

23. Knepel W, Vallejo M, Chafitz JA, Habener JF. The pancreatic islet-specific glucagon G3 transcription factors recognize control elements in the rat somatostatin and insulin-I genes. *Mol Endocrinol* 1991;5:1457–1466.

24. Kruse F, Rose SD, Swift GH, Hammer RE, MacDonald RJ. An endocrine-specific element is an integral component of an exocrine-specific pancreatic enhancer. *Genes & Devel* 1993;7:774–776.

25. Rabinovitch A, Quigley C, Russell T, Patel Y, Mintz DH. Insulin and multiplication stimulating activity (an insulin-like growth factor) stimulate islet beta-cell replication in neonatal rat pancreatic monolayer cultures. *Diabetes* 1982;31:160–164.

26. Nielsen JH, Ezban M, Lernmark A. Presence of a factor in diabetic serum stimulating insulin release from mouse pancreatic islets in organ culture (abstract). *Acta Endocrinol* 1983;106:43.

27. Nielsen JH. Growth and function of the pancreatic beta cell in vitro. *Acta Endocrinol* 1985;105:1–40.

28. Fadda GZ, Akmal M, Lipson LG, Massry SG. Direct effect of parathyroid hormone on insulin secretion from pancreatic islets. *Am J Physiol* 1990;258:E975–E984.

29. Gazdar AF, Chick WL, Oie HK, et al. Continuous, clonal, insulin- and somatostatin-secreting cell lines established from a transplantable rat islet cell tumor. *Proc Natl Acad Sci USA* 1980;77:3519–3523.

30. Philippe J, Chick WL, Habener JF. Multipotential phenotypic expression of genes encoding peptide hormones in rat insulinoma cell lines. *J Clin Invest* 1987;79:351–358.

31. Bani Sacchi T, Bani D, Biliotti G. Nesidioblastosis and islet

cell changes related to endogenous hypergastrinemia. *Virchows Arch Cell Pathol* 1985;48:261–276.

32. Ingraham HA, Albert VR, Chen RP et al. A family of POU-domain and Pit-1 tissue-specific transcription factors in pituitary and neuroendocrine development. *Ann Rev Physiol* 1990;52:773–791.

33. Denef C, Andries M. Evidence for paracrine interaction between gonadotrophs and lactotrophs in pituitary cell aggregates. *Endocrinology* 1983;112:813–822.

34. Bholen P, Baird A, Esch F, Ling N. Isolation and partial molecular characterization of pituitary fibroblast growth factor. *Proc Natl Acad Sci USA* 1984;81:5364–5368.

35. Baird A, Mormede P, Ying S-Y, et al. A nonmitogenic pituitary function of fibroblast growth factor: regulation of thyrotropin and prolactin secretion. *Proc Natl Acad Sci USA* 1985;82:5545–5549.

36. Ferrara N, Schweigerer L, Neufeld G, Mitchell R, Gospodarowicz D. Pituitary follicular cells produce basic fibroblast growth factor. *Proc Acad Sci USA* 1987;84:5773–5777.

37. Vankelecom H, Carmeliet P, Van Damme J, Billiau A, Denef C. Production of interleukin-6 by folliculo-stellate cells of the anterior pituitary gland in histiotypic cell aggregate culture system. *Neuroendocrinology* 1989;49:102–106.

38. Ferrara N, Henzel WJ. Pituitary follicular cells secrete a novel heparin-binding growth factor specific for vascular endothelial cells. *Biochem Biophys Res Commun* 1989;161:851–858.

39. Ferrara N, Winer J, Henzel WJ. Pituitary follicular cells secrete an inhibitor of aortic endothelial cell growth: identification as leukemia inhibitory factor. *Proc Natl Acad Sci USA* 1992;89:698–702.

40. Castleman B, Roth SI. Tumors of the parathyroid glands. In: *Atlas of tumor pathology*. Hartman WH, ed. Washington, DC: Armed Forces Institute of Pathology, 1978.

41. LiVolsi VA. The thyroid and parathyroid. *Diagnostic Surgical Pathology*. Raven Press: New York. 1989;395–433.

42. Rosai J. Parathyroid glands. In: Rosai J. ed. *Ackerman's surgical pathology*. 7th ed. St. Louis: Mosby, 1989;449–466.

43. Marx SJ, Menczel J, Campbell G, Aurbach GD, Spiegel AM, Norton JA. Heterogeneous size of the parathyroid glands in familial multiple endocrine neoplasia type 1. *Clin Endocrinol* 1991;35:521–526.

44. Harach HR, Jasani B. Parathyroid hyperplasia in multiple endocrine neoplasia type 1: a pathological and immunohistochemical reappraisal. *Histopathology* 1992;20:305–313.

45. Pesce C, Tobia F, Carli F, Antoniotti GV. The sites of hormone storage in normal and diseased parathyroid glands: a silver impregnation and immunohistochemical study. *Histopathology* 1989;15:157–166.

46. Schmid KW, Hittmair A, Ladurner D, Sandbichler P, Gasser R, Totsch M. Chromogranin A and B in parathyroid tissue of cases of primary hyperparathyroidism: an immunohistochemical study. *Virchows Arch (Pathol Anat)* 1991;418:295–299.

47. Samaan NA, Ovais S, Ordonez NG, Choksi UA, Selvin RV, Hickey RC. Multiple endocrine syndrome type 1. Clinical laboratory findings, and management in five families. *Cancer* 1989;64:741–752.

48. Ghandur-Mnaymneh L, Kimura N. The parathyroid adenoma: a histopathologic definition with a study of 172 cases of primary hyperparathyroidism. *Am J Pathol* 1984;115:70–83.

49. Juhlin C, Rastad J, Klareskog L, Grimelius L, Akerstrom G. Parathyroid histology and cytology with monoclonal antibodies recognizing a calcium sensor of parathyroid cells. *Am J Pathol* 1989;135:321–328.

50. Kendall CH, Roberts PA, Pringle JH, Lauder I. The expression of parathyroid hormone messenger RNA in normal and abnormal parathyroid tissue. *J Pathol* 1991;165:111–118.

51. Oks T, Yoshioka T, Shrestha GR. Immunohistochemical study of nodular hyperplastic parathyroid glands in patients with secondary hyperparathyroidism. *Virchows Arch (Pathol Anat)* 1988;413:53–60.

52. Friedman E, Sakaguchi K, Bale AE, et al. Clonality of para-

thyroid tumors in familial multiple endocrine neoplasia type 1. *N Engl J Med* 1989;321:213–218.

53. Amorosi A, Cicchi P, Tonelli F. Multiple endocrine type 1: a model for the analysis of tumor clonality and its biological significance. In: Brandi ML, White R, eds. *Hereditary tumors*. New York: Raven Press, 1991.

54. Brandi ML, Marx SJ, Aurbach GD, Fitzpatrick LA. Familial multiple endocrine neoplasia type I: A new look at pathophysiology. *Endocrine Rev* 1987;8:391–405.

55. Obara T, Fujimoto Y, Kanaji Y. Flow cytometric DNA analysis of tumors. *Cancer* 1990;66:1555–1562.

56. Krause MW, Hedinger C. Pathologic study of parathyroid glands in tertiary hyperparathyroidism. *Hum Pathol* 1985; 16:772–784.

57. Harach HR, Jasani B. Parathyroid hyperplasia in tertiary hyperparathyroidism: a pathological and immunohistochemical reappraisal. *Histopathology* 1992;21:513–519.

58. Falchetti A, Bale AE, Amorosi A. Progression of uremic hyperparathyroidism involves allelic loss on chromosome 11. *J Clin Endocrinol Metab* 76:139–144.

59. Kloppel G, Willener S, Stamm B, Hacki WH, Heitz PU. Pancreatic lesions and hormonal profile of pancreatic tumors in multiple endocrine neoplasia type 1. An immunocytochemical study of nine patients. *Cancer* 1986;57:1824–1832.

60. Bordi C, De Vita O, Pilato EP, et al. Multiple islet cell tumors with predominance of glucagon-production cells and ulcer disease. *Am J Clin Pathol* 1987;88:153–161.

61. Pilato FP, A'dda T, Banchini E, Bordi C. Nonrandom expression of polypeptide hormones in pancreatic endocrine tumors. An immunohistochemical study in a case of multiple islet cell neoplasia. *Cancer* 1988;61:1815–1980.

62. Thompson NW, Lloyd RV, Nishiyama RH. MEN pancreas: a histological and immunohistochemical study. *World J Surg* 1984;8:561–574.

63. Solcia E, Capella C, Fiocca R, Cornaggia M, Bosi F. The gastroenteropancreatic endocrine system, and related tumors. *Gastroenterol Clin North Am* 1989;18:671–693.

64. Mukai K, Greider MH, Grotting JC, Rosai J. Retrospective study of 77 pancreatic endocrine tumors using the immunoperoxidase method. *Am J Surg Pathol* 1982;6:387–399.

65. Pipeleers-Marichal M, Somers G, Willems G. Gastrinomas in the duodenums of patients with multiple endocrine neoplasia type 1 and the Zollinger-Ellison syndrome. *N Engl J Med* 1990;322:723–727.

66. Donow C, Pipeleers-Marichal M, Schroder S, Stamm B, Heitz PU, Kloppel G. Surgical pathology of gastrinoma. Site, size, multicentricity, association with multiple endocrine neoplasia type 1, and malignancy. *Cancer* 1991;68: 1329–1334.

67. Stamm B, Hedinger CE, Saremaslani P. Duodenal and ampullary carcinoid tumors. A report of 12 cases with pathological characteristics, polypeptide content and relation to the MEN 1 syndrome and von Recklinghausen's disease (neurofibromatosis). *Virchows Arch (Pathol Anat)* 1986;408: 475–489.

68. Capella C, Riva C, Rindi G, Usellini L, Chiaravalli A, Solcia E. Endocrine tumors of the duodenum and upper jejunum. A study of 33 cases with clinicopathological characteristics and hormone content. *Hepatogastroenterology* 1990;37:247–252.

69. Birke AP, Federspiel BH, Sobin LH, Shekitka KM, Helwig EB. Carcinoids of the duodenum. A histologic and immunohistochemical study of 65 tumors. *Am J Surg Pathol* 1989;13:828–837.

70. Asa SL, Singer W, Kovacs K. Pancreatic endocrine tumour producing growth hormone-releasing hormone associated with multiple endocrine neoplasia type 1 syndrome. *Acta Endocrinol* 1987;115:331–337.

71. Sano T, Yamasaki R, Saito H. Growth hormone releasing hormone (GHRH)-secreting pancreatic tumor in a patient with multiple endocrine neoplasia type 1. *Am J Surg Pathol* 1987;11:810–819.

72. Solcia E, Capella C, Fiocaca R, Rindi G, Rosai J. Gastric argyrophil carcinoidosis in patients with Zollinger-Ellison

syndrome due to type 1 multiple endocrine neoplasia. A newly recognized association. *Am J Surg Pathol* 1990;14: 503–513.

73. Creutzfeldt W. The achlorhydria-carcinoid sequence: role of gastrin. *Digestion* 1988;39:61–79.

74. Mignon M, Lehy T, Bonnefond A, Ruszniewski P, Labeille D, Bonfils S. Development of gastric argyrophil carcinoid tumors in a case of Zollinger-Ellison syndrome with primary hyperparathyroidism during long-term antisecretory treatment. *Cancer* 1987;59:1959–1962.

75. Bordi C, D'Adda T, Pilato FP, Ferrari C. Carcinoid (ECL cell) tumor of the oxyntic mucosa of the stomach: a hormone-dependent neoplasm? In: *Progress in surgical pathology*. Fenoglic-Preiser CM, Wolff M, Rilke F, eds. Berlin: Springer-Verlag, 1988;177–195.

76. Solcia E, Bordi C, Cruetzfeldt W. Histopathologic classification of nonantral gastric endocrine growths in man. *Digestion* 1988;41:185–200.

77. D'Adda T, Corleto V, Pilato FP. Quantitative ultrastructure of endocrine cells of oxyntic mucosa in Zollinger-Ellison syndrome. *Gastroenterology* 1990;99:17–26.

78. Dayal Y. Neuroendocrine cells and their proliferative lesions. In: *Pathology of the colon, small intestine, and anus*. Norris HT, ed. New York: Churchill Livingstone, 1991;305–366.

79. Kovacs K, Horvath E. *Atlas of tumor pathology*. Washington, DC: Armed Forces, Institute of Pathology, 1986.

80. Scheithauer BW, Laws ER Jr, Kovacs K, Horvath E, Randall RV, Carney JA. Pituitary adenomas of the multiple endocrine neoplasia type 1 syndrome. *Semin Diagn Pathol* 1987;4:205–211.

81. Hershon KS, Kelly WA, Shaw CM, Schwartz R, Bierman EL. Prolactinomas as part of the multiple endocrine neoplastic syndrome Type 1. *Am J Med* 1983;74:713–720.

82. Scheithauer BW, Horvath E, Kovacs K. Plurihormonal pituitary adenomas. *Semin Diagn Pathol* 1986;8:69–82.

83. Gospodarowicz D, Cheng J, Lui GM, Baird A, Bohlen P. Isolation of brain fibroblast growth factor by heparin-sepharose affinity chromatography: identity with pituitary fibroblast growth factor. *Proc Natl Acad Sci USA* 1984; 81:6963–6967.

84. Gauthier T, Maftouh M, Picard C. Rapid enzymatic degradation of (125-I) (Tyr 10) FGF (1–10) by serum in vitro and involvement in the determination of circulating FGF by RIA. *Biochem Biophys Res Commun* 1987;145:775–781.

85. McLeod MK, Tutera AM, Vinik AI. Evidence for a plasma mitogenic glycoprotein in patients with multiple endocrine neoplasia type 1. *Clin Res* 1989;37:934A.

86. Horvath E. Pituitary hyperplasia. *Pathol Res Pract* 1988; 183:623–625.

87. Ramsay JA, Kovacs K, Asa SL, Pike MJ, Thorner MO. Reversible sellar enlargement due to growth hormone-releasing hormone production by pancreatic endocrine tumors in an acromegalic patient with multiple endocrine neoplasia type 1 syndrome. *Cancer* 1988;62:445–450.

88. Berger G, Tronillas J, Bloch B. Multihormonal carcinoid tumor of the pancreas. *Cancer* 1984;54:1097–2108.

89. Ch'ng JLC, Christofides ND, Kraenzlin M. Growth hormone secretion dynamics in a patient with ectopic growth hormone-releasing factor production. *Am J Med* 1985;79: 135–138.

90. Tachibana O, Yamashima T. Immunochistochemical study of folliculostellate cells in human pituitary adenomas. *Acta Neuropathol* 1988;76:458–464.

91. Sbarbati A, Fakhreddine A, Zancanaro C, Bontempini L, Cinti S. Ultrastructural morphology of folliculo-stellate cells in human pituitary adenomas. *Ultrastruct Pathol* 1991;15: 241–242.

92. Ferrara N, Henzel WJ. Pituitary follicular cells secrete a novel heparin-binding growth factor specific for vascular endothelial cells. *Biochem Biophys Res Commun* 1989;161: 851–858.

93. Skogseid B, Larsson C, Lindgran PG, et al. Clinical and genetic features of adrenocortical lesions in multiple endo-

crine neoplasia type 1. *J Clin Endocrinol Metab* 1992;75:76–81.

94. Duh Q-Y, Hybarger CP, Geist R, et al. Carcinoids associated with multiple endocrine neoplasia syndromes. *Am J Surg* 1987;154:142–148.

95. Wermer P. Genetic aspects of adenomatosis of endocrine glands. *Am J Med* 1954;16:363–371.

96. Vance JE, Kitabchi AE, Buchanan KD, Stoli RW, Hollander D, Wood FC Jr. Hypersecretion of insulin, glucagon and gastrin in a kindred with multiple adenomatosis. *Diabetes* 1968;17:299–305.

97. Laidlaw GF. Nesidioblastoma, the islet tumor of the pancreas. *Am J Pathol* 1938;14:125–134.

98. Trudeau WL, McGuigan JE. Effects of calcium on serum gastrin levels in the Zollinger-Ellison syndrome. *N Engl J Med* 1969;281:862–866.

99. Cooper CW, Bolman RM, Linehan WM, Wells SA Jr. Interrelationships between calcium, calcemic hormones and gastrointestinal hormones. *Rec Progr Hormone Res* 1978;34:259–283.

100. Windeck R, Brown EM, Gardner DG, Aurbach GD. Effect of gastrointestinal hormones on isolated bovine parathyroid cells. *Endocrinology* 1978;103:2020–2026.

101. Paloyan E, Lawrence AM, Ernst K, et al. Inter-relationships between parathyroids and islets of Langerhans. *Fed Proc* 1966;25:495–502.

102. Jaffe BM, Peskin GW, Kaplan EL. Serum levels of the parathyroid hormone in the Zollinger-Ellison syndrome. *Surgery* 1973;74:621–625.

103. Finkelstein JD, Schacter D. Active transport of calcium by intestine: effects of hypophysectomy and growth hormone. *Am J Physiol* 1962;203:873–880.

104. Magliola L, Forte LR. Prolactin stimulation of parathyroid hormone secretion in bovine parathyroid cells. *Am J Physiol* 1984;247:E675–E680.

105. Lancer SR, Bowser EN, Haris GK, Williams GA. The effect of growth hormone on parathyroid function in rats. *Endocrinology* 1976;98:1289–1293.

106. Carlson HE, Lamberts SWJ, Brichman AS, Deftos LJ, Horst RL, Forte LR. Hypercalcemia in rats bearing growth hormone- and prolactin-secreting transplantable pituitary tumors. *Endocrinology* 1985;117:1602–1607.

107. Prager D, Yamashita S, Melmed S. Insulin regulates prolactin secretion and messenger ribonucleic acid levels in pituitary cells. *Endocrinology* 1988;122:2946–2952.

108. Brandi ML, Auerbach GD, Fitzpatrick LA. Parathyroid mitogenic activity in plasma from patients with familial multiple endocrine neoplasia type-1. *N Engl J Med* 1986;314:1287–1293.

109. Zimering MB, Brandi ML, DeGrange DA, et al. Circulating fibroblast growth factor-like substance in familial multiple endocrine neoplasia type 1. *J Clin Endocrinol Metab* 1990;70:149–154.

110. Brandi ML, Zimering MB, Marx SJ, et al. Multiple endocrine neoplasia type I: role of a circulating growth factor in parathyroid cell hyperplasia. In: *Clinical disorders of bone and mineral metabolism.* Kleerekoper M, Krane SM, eds. New York: Mary Ann Liebert, 1989;323–328.

111. Brem H, Klagsbrun M. The role of fibroblast growth factors and related oncogenes in tumor growth. *Cancer Treat Res* 1992;63:211–231.

112. Chodak GW, Hospelhorn Y, Judge SM, Mayforth R, Koeppen H, Sasse J. Increased levels of fibroblast growth factor-like activity in urine from patients with bladder or kidney cancer. *Cancer Res* 1988;48:2083–2088.

113. Sato Y, Murphy PR, Sato R, Friesen HG. Fibroblast growth factor release by bovine endothelial cells and human astrocytoma cells in culture is density dependent. *Mol Endocrinol* 1989;3:744–748.

114. Zimering MB, Katsumata N, Sato Y, et al. Increased basic fibroblast growth factor in plasma from multiple endocrine neoplasia type 1: relation to pituitary tumors. *J Clin Endocrinol Metab* 1993;76:1182–1187.

115. Nakajima T, Yamaguchi H, Takahashi K. S100 protein in fol-

liculostellate cells of the rat pituitary anterior lobe. *Brain Res* 1980;191:523–531.

116. Folkman J, Long D, Becker F. Growth and metastasis of tumor in organ culture. *Cancer* 1963;16:453–467.

117. Wollman SH, Herveg JP, Ziligs JD, Ericson LE. Blood capillary enlargement during the development of thyroid hyperplasia in the rat. *Endocrinology* 1978;103:2306–2314.

118. Brandi ML. A novel endothelial cell growth factor circulates in familial multiple endocrine neoplasia type 1. *Nucl Med Biol* 1990;17:639–643.

119. D'Adda T, Amorosi A, Bussolati G, Brandi ML, Bordi C. Quantitative differences in parathyroid endothelial component between MEN-1 syndrome and secondary hyperparathyroidism. *Pathologia* 1992;325:76–77.

120. Schaaf L, Gerschner M, Geissler W, Eckert B, Seif FJ, Usadel KH. The importance of multiple endocrine neoplasia syndromes in differential diagnosis. *Klin Wochenschr* 1990;68:669–672.

121. Friedman E, DeMarco L, Gejman PV, et al. Allelic loss from chromosome 11 in parathyroid tumors. *Cancer Res* 1992;525:6804–6810.

122. Marx SJ, Sakaguchi K, Green J III, Aurbach GD, Brandi ML. Mitogenic activity on parathyroid cells in plasma from members of a large kindred with multiple endocrine neoplasia type I. *J Clin Endocrinol Metab* 1988;67:149–153.

123. German J, Archibald R, Bloom D. Chromosomal breakage in a rare and probably genetically determined syndrome of man. *Science* 1965;148:506–507.

124. Bloom GE, Warner S, Gerard PS, Diamond LK. Chromosome abnormalities in constitutional aplastic anemia. *N Engl J Med* 1966;274:8–14.

125. Hecht F, Koler RD, Rigas DA, et al. Leukemia and lymphocytes in ataxia teleanglectasia. *Lancet* 1966;2:1193.

126. Cleaver JE. Defective repair replication of DNA in xeroderma pigmentosum. *Nature* 1968;218:652–656.

127. Hecht F, Kaiser McCaw B. In: *Genetics of human cancer.* Muvihill JJ, Miller RW, Fraumuni Jr, eds. New York: Raven Press, 1977;105–123.

128. Gustavsson KH, Jansson R, Oberg K. Chromosomal breakage in multiple endocrine adenomatosis (type I and II). *Clin Genet* 1983;23:143–149.

129. Benson L, Gustavson K-H, Rastad J, Akerstrom G, Oberg K, Ljunghall S. Cytogenetical investigations in patient with primary hyperparathyroidism and multiple endocrine neoplasia type 1. *Hereditas* 1988;108:227–229.

130. Scappaticci S, Maraschio P, Del Ciotto N, Fossati GS, Zonta A, Fraccarp M. Chromosome abnormalities in lymphocytes and fibroblasts of subjects with multiple endocrine neoplasia type 1. *Cancer Genet Cytogenet* 1991;52:85–92.

131. Bishop JM. The molecular genetics of cancer. *Science* 1987;235:305–311.

132. Bishop JM. Molecular themes in oncogenesis. *Cell* 1991;64:235–248.

133. Arnold A. Molecular basis of primary hyperparathyroidism. This volume.

134. Landis CA, Master SB, Spada A, Pace AM, Bourne HR, Vallar L. GTPase inhibiting mutations activate the a chain of Gs and stimulate adenylyl cyclase in human pituitary tumours. *Nature* 1989;340:692–696.

135. Lyons J, Landis CA, Harsh G, et al. Two G protein oncogenes in human endocrine tumors. *Science* 1990;249:655–659.

136. Gonsky R, Herman V, Melmed S, Fagin J. Transforming DNA sequences present in human prolactin-secreting pituitary tumors. *Mol Endocrinol* 1991;5:1687–1695.

137. Lammie GA, Fanti V, Smith R, et al. D11S287, a putative oncogene on chromosome 11q13, is amplified and expressed in squamous cell and mammary carcinomas and linked to BCL-1. *Oncogene* 1991;6:439–444.

138. Arnold A, Kim HG, Gaz RD, et al. Molecular cloning and chromosomal mapping of DNA rearranged with the parathyroid hormone gene in a parathyroid adenoma. *J Clin Invest* 1989;83:2034–2040.

139. Friedman E, Bale AE, Marx SJ, et al. Genetic abnormalities

in sporadic parathyroid adenomas. *J Clin Endocrinol Metab* 1990;71:293–297.

140. Harris H. Suppression of malignancy by cell fusion. *Nature* 1969;223:363–368.

141. de Mars R. Discussion. In: *23rd Annual Symposium of Fundamental Cancer Research, 1969.* Baltimore: Williams & Wilkins, 1969, 105.

142. Knudson AG. Mutation and cancer: statistical study of retinoblastoma. *Proc Natl Acad Sci USA* 1971;68:820–823.

143. Latif F, Tory K, Gnara J et al. Identification of the von-Hipple–Lindau disease tumor suppressor gene. *Science* 1993; 260:1317–1320.

144. Larsson C, Skogseid B, Oberg K, Nakamura Y, Nordenskjold M. Multiple endocrine neoplasia type 1 gene maps to chromosome 11 and is lost in insulinoma. *Nature* 1988; 332:85–87.

145. Bale SJ, Bale AE, Stewart K, et al. Linkage analysis of Multiple Endocrine Neoplasia Type 1 with INT2 and other markers on chromosome 11. *Genomics* 1989;4:320–322.

146. Thakker RV, Bouloux P, Wooding C, et al. Association of parathyroid tumors in multiple endocrine neoplasia type 1 with loss of alleles on chromosome 11. *N Engl J Med* 1989;321:218–224.

147. Friedman E, Sakaguchi K, Bale AE, et al. Clonality of parathyroid tumors in familial multiple endocrine neoplasia type 1. *N Engl J Med* 1989;321:213–218.

148. Bystrom C, Larsson C, Blomberg C, et al. Localization of the MEN 1 gene to a small region within chromosome 11q13 by deletion mapping in tumors. *Proc Natl Acad Sci USA* 1990;87:1968–1972.

149. Radford DM, Ashley SM, Wells SA, Gerhard DS. Loss of heterozygosity of markers on chromosome 11 in tumors from patients with multiple endocrine neoplasia syndrome type 1. *Cancer Res* 1990;50:6529–6533.

150. Bale AE, Norton JA, Wong EL, et al. Allelic loss on chromosome 11 in hereditary and sporadic tumors related to familial multiple endocrine neoplasia type 1. *Cancer Res* 1991;51:1154–1157.

151. Friedman E, DeMarco L, Gejman PV, et al. Allelic loss from chromosome 11 in parathyroid tumors. *Cancer Res* 1992;52: 6804–6809.

152. Yoshimoto K, Lizuka M, Iwahana H, et al. Loss of the same alleles of HRAS 1 and D11S151 in two independent pancreatic cancers from a patient with multiple endocrine neoplasia type 1. *Cancer Res* 1989;49:2716–2721.

153. Yoshimoto K, Iwahana H, Kobo K, Saito S, Itakura M. Allele loss on chromosome 11 in a pituitary tumor from a patient with multiple endocrine neoplasia type 1. *Cancer Res* 1991;82:886–889.

154. Majewski JT, Wilson SD. The MEN-I syndrome: an all or none phenomenon? *Surgery* 1979;86:475–484.

155. Larsson C, Nordenskjold M. Multiple endocrine neoplasia. *Cancer Surv* 1990;9:703–723.

156. Ballard HS, Frame B, Hartsock RJ. Familial multiple endocrine adenoma–peptic ulcer complex. *Medicine* 1964;43: 481–516.

157. Croisier JC, Azerad E, Lubetzki J. L'adenomatse polyendocrinienne. A propos d'une observation peronelle et revenue de la litterature. *Semin Hop Paris* 1971;47:494–525.

158. Yano T, Linehan M, Anglard P, et al. Genetic changes in human adreno-cortical carcinomas. *JNCI* 1989;81:518–523.

159. Sawicki MP, Wan Y-J Y, Johnson CL, Berenson J, Gatti R, Passaro E. Loss of heterozygosity on chromosome 11 in sporadic gastrinomas. *Hum Genet* 1992;89:445–449.

160. Arnold A, Staunton CE, Kim HG, Gaz RD, Kronenberg HM. Monoclonality and abnormal parathyroid hormone genes in parathyroid adenomas. *N Engl J Med* 1983;318:658–662.

161. Herman V, Drazin NZ, Gonsky R, Melmed S. Molecular screening of pituitary adenomas for gene mutations and rearrangements. *J Clin Endocrinol Metab* 1993;77:50–55.

162. Thakker RV, Pook MA, Wooding C, et al. Association of somatotrophinomas with loss of alleles of chromosome 11 and with gsp mutations. *J Clin Invest* 1993;91:2815–2821.

163. Herman V, Fagin J, Gonsky R, Kovacs K, Melmed S. Clonal

origins of pituitary adenomas. *J Clin Endocrinol Metab* 1990;71:1427–1433.

164. Alexander JM, Biller BMK, Kikkal H, Zervas NT, Arnold A, Klibanski A. Clinically nonfunctioning pituitary tumors are monoclonal in origin. *J Clin Invest* 1990;86:336–340.

165. Nakamura Y, Larsson C, Julier C, et al. Localization of the genetic defect in multiple endocrine neoplasia type 1 within a small region of chromosome 11. *Am J Hum Genet* 1989;44:751–755.

166. Julier C, Nakamura Y, Lathrop M, et al. A detailed genetic map of the long arm of chromosome 11. *Genomics* 1990; 7:335–345.

167. Tokino T, Takahashi E, Mori M, et al. Isolation and mapping of 62 new RFLP markers on human chromosome 11. *Am J Hum Genet* 1991;48:258–268.

168. Larsson C, Weber G, Kvanta E, et al. Isolation and mapping of polymorphic cosmid clones used for sublocalization of the multiple endocrine neoplasia type 1 (MEN1) locus. *Hum Genet* 1992;89:187–193.

169. Janson M, Larsson C, Werelius B. Detailed physical map of human chromosomal region 11g12–13 shows high meiotic recombination rate around the MEN1 locus. *Proc Natl Acad Sci USA* 1991;88:10609–10613.

170. Szepetowski P, Simon M-P, Grosgeorge J, et al. Localization of 11q13 loci with respect to regional chromosomal breakpoints. *Genomics* 1992;12:738–744.

171. Tanigami A, Tokino T, Takita K-I, Takaguchi S, Nakamura Y. A 14 Mb physical map of the region at chromosome 11q13 harboring the MEN1 locus and the tumor amplicon region. *Genomics* 1992;13:16–20.

172. Fujimori M, Wells SA, Nakamura Y. Fine-scale mapping of the gene responsible for multiple endocrine neoplasia type 1 (MEN1). *Am J Hum Genet* 1992;50:399–403.

173. Litt M, Kramer P, Hauge XT, et al. A microsatellite-based index map of human chromosome 11. *Hum Molec Gen* 1993;2:909–913.

174. Qin S, Zhang J, Isaacs CN, et al. A chromosome 11 YAC library. *Genomics* 1993;16:580–585.

175. Iwasaki H, Stewart PW, Dilley WG, et al. A minisatellite and microsatellite polymorphism within 1.5 kb at the human muscle glycogen phosphorylase (PYGM) locus can be amplified by PCR and have combined informativeness of PIC 0.95. *Genomics* 1992;13:7–15.

176. Larsson C, Shepherd J, Nakamura Y, et al. Predictive testing for multiple endocrine neoplasia type 1 using DNA polymorphisms. *J Clin Invest* 1992;89:1344–1349.

177. Lee AK, DeLellis RA, Blount M, Nunemacher G, Wolfe HJ. Pituitary proliferative lesions in aging male Long-Evans rats. A model of mixed multiple endocrine neoplasia syndrome. *Lab Invest* 1982;47:595.

178. Fjalling M, Hansson G, Hedman J, Ragnhult I, Tissell LE. Radiation-induced parathyroid adenomas and thyroid tumors in rats. *Acta Pathol Microbiol Scand* 1981;89:425.

179. Boschetti A, Moloey WC. Observations on pancreatic islet cell and other radiation-induced tumors in the rat. *Lab Invest* 1966;15:565.

180. Hanahan D. Heritable formation of pancreatic B-cell tumors in transgenic mix expressing recombinant insulin/simian virus 40 oncogenes. *Nature* 1985;319:115–122.

181. Ornitz DM, Hammer RE, Messing A, Palmiter RD, Brinster RL. Pancreatic neoplasia induced by SV40 T-antigen expression in acinar cells of transgenic mice. *Science* 1987;238: 188–193.

182. Murphy D, Bishop A, Rindi G, et al. Mice transgenic for a vasopressin-SV40 hybrid oncogene develop tumors of the endocrine pancreas and the anterior pituitary. *Am J Pathol* 1987;129:552–566.

183. Reynolds RK, Hoekzema GS, Vogel J, Hinrichs SH, Jay G. Multiple endocrine neoplasia induced by the promiscuous expression of a viral oncogene. *Proc Natl Acad Sci USA* 1988;85:3135–3139.

184. Schulz N, Propst F, Linncila RI, Rosenberg M, Vande Woude GF. C-mos transgenic mice exhibit background dependent patterns of neoplasia relevant to multiple endocrine neoplasia. *Proc Am Assoc Cancer Res* 1992;33:376.

185. Schulz N, Propst F, Linnoila RI, Rosenberg M, Vande Woude GF. c-Mos transgenic mice exhibit background dependent patterns of neoplasia relevant to humn multiple endocrine neoplasia. *Proc Am Assoc Canc Res* 1992;33:376 (abstr).

186. Lipps CJM, Vassen HFA, Lamers CBWH, Berdjis CC. Polyglandular syndrome: II. Multiple endocrine adenomas in man. A report of 5 cases and a review of the literature. *Oncologia* 1962;15:288–311.

187. Lips CJM, Vassen HFA, Lamers CBHW. Multiple endocrine neoplasia syndromes. *CRC Crit Rev Oncol Hematol* 1984; 2:117–184.

188. Eberle F, Grun R. Multiple endocrine neoplasia, type I (MEN1). *Ergebnisse Interen Med Kinderheilk* 1981;46:759–149.

189. Vassen HFA, Griffioen G, Lips CJM, Struyvenberg A, van Slooten EA. Screening for families predisposed to cancer development in the Netherlands. *Anticancer Res* 1990;10: 555–564.

190. Oberg K, Skogseid B, Eriksson B. Multiple endocrine neoplasia type 1 (MEN-1): clinical, biochemical and genetical investigations. *Acta Oncol* 1989;28:383–387.

191. Betts JB, O'Malley BP, Rosenthal FD. Hyperparathyroidism: a prerequisite for Zollinger-Ellison syndrome in multiple endocrine adenomatosis type 1. *Q J Med* 1980;193:69–76.

192. Brandi ML, Marx SJ, Aurbach GD, Fitzpatrick LA. Familial multiple endocrine neoplasia type I: A new look at pathophysiology. *Endocrine Rev* 1987;8:391–405.

193. Boye JH, Cooke TJC, Gilbert JJM, Sweeny EC, Taylor S. Occurrence of other endocrine tumors in primary hyperparathyroidism. *Lancet* 1975;2:781–784.

194. Jackson CE, Frame B, Block MA. Prevalence of endocrine neoplasia syndromes in genetic studies of parathyroid tumors. *Progr Cancer Res Ther* 1977;3:205–208.

195. Wajngot A, Werner S, Granberg PO, Lindvall N. Occurrence of pituitary adenomas and other neoplastic diseases in primary hyperparathyroidism. *Surg Gynecol Obstet* 1980;151: 401–403.

196. Muhr C, Ljunghall S, Akstrom G, et al. Screening for multiple endocrine neoplasia syndrome (type 1) in patients with primary hyperparathyroidism. *Clin Endocrinol* 1984;20:153–162.

197. Eberle F, Grun R. Multiple endocrine neoplasia, type I (MEN1). *Ergebnisse Inneren Med Kinderheilk* 1981;46:75–149.

198. Bardram L, Stage JG. Frequency of endocrine disorders in patients with the Zollinger-Ellison syndrome. A collective surgical experience. *Scand J Gastroenterol* 1985;20:233–238.

199. Farley DR, van Heerden JA, Grant CS, Miller LJ, Ilstrup DM. The Zollinger-Ellison syndrome. A collective surgical experience. *Ann Surg* 1992;215:561–569.

200. Watson RGP, Johnston CF, O'Hare MMT, et al. The frequency of gastrointestinal endocrine tumors in a well defined population-Northern Ireland. *Q J Med* 1985;72:647–657.

201. Scheithauer BW, Laws ER Jr, Kovacs K, Horvath E, Randall RV, Carney JA. Pituitary adenomas of the multiple endocrine neoplasia type I syndrome. *Semin Diagn Pathol* 1987;4:205–211.

202. Cawthon RM, Weiss R, Xu C, et al. A major segment of the neurofibromatosis type 1 gene: cDNA sequence, genomic structure, and point mutations. *Cell* 1990;62:193–201.

203. Nishisho I, Nakamura Y, Miyoshi Y, et al. Mutations of chromosome 5q21 genes in FAP and colorectal cancer patients. *Science* 1991;253:665–669.

204. Dunne MJ, Philips RA, Becker AJ, Gallie BL. Identification of germline and somatic mutations affecting the retinoblastoma gene. *Science* 1988;241:1797–1800.

205. Leveston SA, McKeel DW, Buckley PJ, et al. Acromegaly and Cushing's syndrome associated with a foregut carcinoid tumor. *J Clin Endocrinol* 1981;53:632–639.

206. Melmed S, Ezrin C, Kovacs K, Goodman RS, Frohman LA. Acromegaly due to secretion of growth hormone by an ec-topic pancreatic islet-cell tumor. *N Engl J Med* 1986;312:9–17.

207. McCarthy DM, Peikin SR, Lopatin RN. Hyperparathyroidism: a reversible cause of cimetidine-resistant gastric hypersecretion. *Br Med J* 1979;1:765–766.

208. Baystrom C, Larsson C, Blomberg C, et al. Localization of the gene for multiple endocrine neoplasia type 1 to a small region within chromosome 11q13 by deletion mapping in tumor tissue. *Proc Natl Acad Sci USA* 1990;87:1968–1972.

209. Schimke RN. Multiple endocrine neoplasia: how many syndromes? *Am J Med Genet* 1990;37:375–383.

210. Calcatera TC, Paglia D. The coexistence of parathyroid adenoma and thyroid carcinoma. *Laryngoscope* 1979;89:1166–1169.

211. Simpson RJ, Moss J Jr. Parathyroid adenoma and nonmedullary thyroid carcinoma association. *Otolaryngol Head Neck Surg* 1989;101:584–587.

212. Matsuo K, Tang SH, Fagin JA. Allelotype on human thyroid tumors: loss of chromosome 11q13 sequences in follicular neoplasms. *Mol Endocr* 1991;5:1873–1879.

213. Melmed S, Yamashita S, Kovacs K, Ong J, Rosenblatt S, Braunstein G. Cushing's syndrome due to ectopic proopiomelanocortin gene expression by islet cell carcinoma of the pancreas. *Cancer* 1987;595:772–778.

214. Wilander E, El-Salhy M, Willen R, Grimelius L. Immunocytochemistry and electron microscopy of an argentaffin endocrine tumor of the pancreas. *Virchows Arch Pathol Anat* 1981;292:263–269.

215. Maton PN, Gardner JD, Jensen RT. Cushing's syndrome in patients with the Zollinger Ellison syndrome. *N Engl J Med* 1986;315:1–5.

216. Klöppel G, Heitz PU. Pancreatic endocrine tumors. *Pathol Res Pract* 1988;183:155–168.

217. Doumith R, Gennes JL, Cabane JP, Zygelman N. Pituitary prolactinoma, adrenal aldosterone producing adenoma, gastric schwannoma and clonic polyadenomas: a possible variant of multiple endocrine neoplasia (MEN) type I. *Acta Endocrinol* 1982;100:189–195.

218. Holland OB, Gomez-Sanchez CE, Kem DC, Weiberger MH, Kramer NJ, Higgins JR. Evidence against prolactin stimulation of aldosterone in normal subjects and in patients with primary hyperaldosteronism, including a patient with primary hyperaldosteronism and prolactin producing pituitary macroadenoma. *J Clin Endocrinol Metab* 1977;45:1064–1076.

219. Blumenkopf B, Boekelheide K. Neck paraganglioma with a pituitary adenoma. Case report. *J Neurosurg* 1982;57:426–429.

220. Nelson DR, Stachura ME, Dunlap DB. Case report: Illeal carcinoid tumor complicated by retroperitoneal fibrosis and prolactinoma. *Am J Med Sci* 1988;296:129–133.

221. Barzilay J, Heatley GJ, Cushing GW. Benign and malignant tumors in patients with acromegaly. *Arch Intern Med* 1991;151:1629–1632.

222. Anderson RJ, Lufkin EG, Sizemore SW, Carney JA, Sheps SG, Silliman YE. Acromegaly and pituitary adenoma with pheochromocytoma: a variant of multiple endocrine neoplasia. *Clin Endocrinol* 1981;14:605–612.

223. Watanobe H, Kudo K, Okushima T, Nakazono M, Kudo M, Takebe K. Coexisting acromegaly and a unilateral cortisol producing adrenal adenoma: a possible variant of multiple endocrine neoplasia type I. *J Endocrinol Invest* 1992;15:297–301.

224. Semple CG, Thompson JA. Cushing's syndrome and autonomous thyroid nodules, a variant of multiple endocrine neoplasia? *Acta Endocrinol* 1986;113:463–464.

225. Morris JA, Tymms DJ. Oat cell carcinoma, pheochromocytoma and carcinoid tumors—Multiple APUD neoplasia—A case report. *J Pathol* 1980;131:107–115.

226. Cohen J, Gierlowski TC, Schneider AB. A prospective study of hyperparathyroidism in individuals exposed to radiation in childhood. *JAMA* 1990;264:581–584.

227. Modan B, Baidatz D, Mart H, Steinitz R, Levin SG. Radiation-induced head and neck tumors. *Lancet* 1975;1:277–279.

228. Schneider AB, Shore-Freedman E, Weinstein RA. Radia-

tion-induced thyroid and other head and neck tumors: Occurrence of multiple tumors and analysis of risk factors. *J Clin Endocrinol* 1986;63:107–112.

229. Rosen IB, Strawbridge HG, Bain J. A case hyperparathyroidism associated with radiation of the head and neck area. *Cancer* 1975;36:1111–1114.

230. Tisell LE, Carlsson S, Lindberg S, Ragnhult I. Autonomous hyperparathyroidism. A possible late complication of neck radiotherapy. *Acta Chir Scand* 1976;142:889–904.

231. Christensson T. Hyperparathyroidism and radiation therapy. *Ann Intern Med* 1978;89:216–217.

232. Hedman I, Hansson G, Lundberg LM, Tisell LE. A clinical evaluation of radiation-induced hyperparathyroidism based on 148 surgically treated patients. *World J Surg* 1984;8:96–105.

233. Schneider AB, Shore-Freedman E, Weinstein RA. Radiation-induced thyroid and other head and neck tumors: occurrence of multiple tumors and analysis of risk factors. *J Clin Endocrinol Metab* 1986;63:107–112.

234. Christmas TJ, Chapple CR, Noble JG, Milroy EJG, Cowie AGA. Hyperparathyroidism after neck irradiation. *Br J Surg* 1988;75:873–874.

235. Fujiwara S, Spoto R, Ezaki HAB, et al. Hyperparathyroidism among atomic bomb survivors in Hiroshima. *Radiat Res* 1992;130:372–378.

236. Printz RA, Paloyan E, Lawrence AM, Pickleman JR, Braithwaite S, Brooks MH. Radiation-associated hyperparathyroidism: a new syndrome? *Surgery* 1977;82:276–302.

237. Tisell LE, Hansson G, Lindberg S, Ragnhult I. Hyperparathyroidism in persons treated with X-rays for tuberculosis cervical adenitis. *Cancer* 1977;40:846–854.

238. Heath H III, Hodgson S, Kennedy A. Primary hyperparathyroidism: incidence, morbidity, and potential economic impact in a community. *N Engl J Med* 1980;302:189–193.

239. Cohen H, Gieglowski TC, Schneider AB. A prospective study of hyperparathyroidism in individuals exposed to radiation in childhood. *JAMA* 1990;264:581–584.

240. Katz A, Braunstein GD: Clinical, biochemical and pathologic features of radiation-associated hyperparathyroidism. *Arch Intern Med* 1983;143:79–82.

241. DeJong SA, Demter JG, Jarosz H, Lawrence AM, Paloyan E. Thyroid carcinoma and hyperparathyroidism after radiation therapy for adolescent acne vulgaris. *Surgery* 1991;110:691–695.

242. Tisell LE, Carlsson S, Fjalling M, Hansson G, Lindberg S, Lundberg LM. Hyperparathyroidism subsequent to head and neck irradiation. Risk factors. *Cancer* 1985;56:1529–1533.

243. Triggs SM, Williams ED. Irradiation of the thyroid as a cause of parathyroid adenoma. *Lancet* 1977;1:593–594.

244. Bondeson AG, Bondeson L, Thompson NW. Hyperparathyroidism after treatment with radioactive iodine: not only a coincidence? *Surgery* 1989;106:1025–1027.

245. Fjalling M, Dackenberg A, Hedman I, Tisell LE. An evaluation developing hyperparathyroidism after 12qI treatment for thyrotoxicosis. *Acta Chir Scand* 1983;149:681–686.

246. Jackson CE. Limiting subsequent mutagenic events in carriers of hereditary tumor genes. *Am J Hum Genet* 1992;50:1350–1351.

247. Schweitzer-Cagianut M, Froesch ER, Hedinger C. Familial Cushing's syndrome with primary adrenocortical microadenomatosis (primary adrenocortical nodular dysplasia). *Acta Endocrinol* 1980;94:529–535.

248. Carney JA, Gordon H, Carpenter PC, Shenoy BV, Go VLW. The complex of myxomas, spotty pigmentation and endocrine overactivity. *Medicine* 1985;64:270–283.

249. Carney JA, Hruska LS, Beauchamp GD, Gordon H. Dominant inheritance of the complex of Myxomas, spotty pigmentation and endocrine overactivity. *Mayo Clin Proc* 1986;61:165–172.

250. Vidaillet HJ Jr, Seward JB, Fyke FE III, Su WPD, Tajik AJ. Syndrome Myxoma: a subset of patients with cardiac myxoma associated with pigmented skin lesions and peripheral and endocrine neoplasms. *Br Heart J* 1987;57:247–255.

251. Handley J, Carson D, Walsh M, Thornton C, Hadden D, Bigham EA. Multiple lentigines, myxoid tumors and endocrine overactivity: four cases of Carney's complex. *Br J Dermatol* 1992;126:367–371.

252. Duh Q-Y, Kawasaki E, Bourne HR, McCormick F. Two G protein oncogenes in human endocrine tumors. *Science* 1990;249:635–639.

253. Albright F, Butler AM, Hampton AO, Smith P. Syndrome characterized by osteitis fibrosis desseminata, areas of pigmentation and endocrine dysfunction, with precocious puberty in females: report of five cases. *N Engl J Med* 1937;216:727–746.

254. Mauras N, Blizzard RM. The McCune-Albright syndrome. *Acta Endocrinol* 1986;279(Suppl.):207–217.

255. Weinstein LS, Shenker A, Gegman PV, Merino MJ, Friedman E, Spiegel AM. Activating mutations of the stimulatory G protein in the McCune-Albright syndrome. *N Engl J Med* 1991;325:1688–1695.

256. Lyons J, Landis CA, Harsh G, et al. Two G protein oncogenes in human endocrine tumors. *Science* 1990;249:635–639.

257. Suarez HG, du-Villard JA, Caillou B, Schlumberger M, Parmentier C, Monier M. Gsp mutations in human thyroid tumors. *Oncogene* 1991;6:677–697.

258. Schwindinger WF, Francomano CA, Levine MA. Identification of a mutation in the gene encoding the α subunit of the stimulatory G protein of adenylyl cyclase in McCune-Albright syndrome. *Proc Natl Acad Sci* 1992;89:5152–5156.

259. Landis CA, Masters SB, Spada A, Pace AM, Bourne HR, Vallar L. GTPase inhibiting mutations activate the subunit of Gs and stimulate adenylyl cyclase in human pituitary tumors. *Nature* 1989;340:692–696.

260. Zeller JR, Kauffman M, Komorowski RA, Itskovitz HD. Bilateral pheochromocytoma and islet cell adenoma of the pancreas. *Arch Surg* 1982;117:827–830.

261. Carney JA, Go VLW, Gordon H, Northcutt RC, Pearse AGE, Sheps SG. Familial pheochromocytoma and islet cell tumor of the pancreas. *Am J Med* 1980;68:515–521.

262. Alberts WM, McMeekin JO, George JM. Multiple endocrine neoplasia syndromes. *J Am Med Assoc* 1980;244:1235–1277.

263. Hashomoto K, Suemaru S, Hattori T, et al. Multiple endocrine neoplasia with Cushing's syndrome due to paragaglioma producing Corticotropin-releasing factor and adrenocorticotropin. *Acta Endocrinol* 1986;113:189–195.

264. Neumann HPH. Basic criteria for clinical diagnosis and genetic counseling in von-Hippel Lindau syndrome. *J Vasc Dis* 1987;16:220–226.

265. Griffiths DFR, Williams GT, Williams ED. Duodenal carcinoid tumours, phaeochromocytoma and neurofibromatosis: islet cell tumor, phaeochromocytoma and the von Hippel-Lindau complex: two distinctive neuroendocrine syndromes. *Q J Med* 1987;245:769–782.

266. Binkovitz LA, Johnson CD, Stephens DH. Islet cell tumors in von Hippel-Lindau diseases: increased prevalence and relationship to the multiple endocrine neoplasias. *AJR* 1990;155:501–505.

267. Seizinger BR, Rouleau GA, Ozelius LJ, et al. Von Hippel-Lindau disease maps to the region of chromosome 3 associated with renal cell carcinoma. *Nature* 1988;332:268–269.

268. Riccardi VM, Eichner JE. *Neurofibromatosis: phenotype, natural history, and pathogenesis.* Baltimore: Johns Hopkins University Press, 1986.

269. Cawthon RM, Weiss R, Xu C, et al. A major segment of the neurofibromatosis type 1 gene: cDNA sequence, genomic structure, and point mutations. *Cell* 1990;62:193–201.

270. Ballester R, Marchuk Boguski M, Saulino A, Letcher R, Wigler M, Collins F. The NF1 locus encodes a protein functionally related to mammalian GAP and yeast IRA proteins. *Cell* 1990;63:857–859.

271. Xu G, O'Connel P, Viskochill D, et al. The neurofibromatosis type 1 gene encodes a protein related to GAP. *Cell* 1990;62:599–608.

272. Li C-Y, Bollag G, Clark R, et al. Somatic mutations in the Neurofibromatosis 1 gene in human tumors. *Cell* 1992;69: 275–281.

273. Samuelsson B, Azelsson R. Neurofibromatosis: a clinical genetic study of 96 cases in Gothenburg, Sweden. *Acta Derm Venereol* 1981;95:67–71.

274. Swinburn BA, Yeong ML, Lane MR, Nicholson GI, Holdaway IM. Neurofibromatosis associated with somatostatinoma: a report of two patients. *Clin Endocrinol* 1988;28:353–359.

275. Brasfield RO, Das-Gupta TK. Von Recklinhausen disease: a clinicopathological study. *Ann Surg* 1972;175:86–104.

276. Nakamura H, Koga M, Sato B, Noma K, Morimoto Y, Kashimoto S. Von Recklinhausen's disease with pheochromocytoma and non medullary thyroid cancer. *Ann Intern Med* 1986;105:796–797.

277. Sartori P, Symons JC, Taylor NF, Grant OB. Adrenal cortical adenoma in a 13 year old girl with neurofibromatosis. *Acta Paediatr Scand* 1989;78:476–478.

278. DeAngelis LM, Kelleher MB, Kalmon DP, Fetell MR. Multiple paragangliomatosis in neurofibromatosis: a new neuroendocrine neoplasia. *Neurology* 1987;37:129–133.

279. Weinstein RS, Harris RL. Hypercalcemic hyperparathyroidism and hypophosphatemic osteomalacia complicating neurofibromatosis. *Calcif Tissue Int* 1990;46:261–366.

280. Aach R, Kissane J. Multiple endocrine adenomatoses. *Am J Med* 1969;47:608–618.

281. Goldsmith RE, Sizemore GW, Chen I, Zalme E, Altemeier WA. Familial hyperparathyroidism. Description of a large kindred with physiologic observations and a review of the literature. *Ann Intern Med* 1976;84:36–43.

282. Law WM Jr, Hodgson S, Heath H III. Autosomal recessive inheritance of familial hyperparathyroidism. *N Engl J Med* 1983;309:650–653.

283. Mallette LE, Malini S, Rappaport MP, Kirkland JL. Familial adenomatosis. *Ann Intern Med* 1987;107:54–60.

284. Jung RT, Davie M, Grant AM, Jenkins D, Chalmers TM. Multiple endocrine adenomatosis (type I) and familial hyperparathyroidism. *Postgrad Med J* 1978;54:92–94.

285. Frayha RA, Nassar VH, Dagher F, Salti IS. Familial parathyroid carcinoma. *J Med Lib* 1972;25:299–309.

286. Leborgne J, le Neel JC, Buzelin G, Malvy P. Cancer familial des parathyroides. *J Chir Paris* 1975;109:315–326.

287. Dinnen JS, Greenwood RH, Jones JH, Walker DA, Williams ED. Parathyroid carcinoma in familial hyperparathyroidism. *J Clin Pathol* 1977;30:966–975.

288. Streeten EA, Weinstein LS, Norton JA. Studies in a kindred with parathyroid carcinoma. *J Clin Endocrinol Metab* 1992; 75:362–366.

289. Mallette LE, Bilezikian JP, Ketcham AS, Aurbach GD. Parathyroid carcinoma in familial hyperparathyroidism. *Am J Med* 1974;57:642–648.

290. Wassif SW, Moniz C, Friedman E, et al. Familial isolated hyperparathyroidism: a distinct genetic entity with an increased risk of parathyroid cancer. *J Clin Endocrinol Metab* 1993 (in press).

291. Chou Y-HW, Brown EM, Levi T, et al. The gene responsible for familial hypocalciuric hypercalcemia maps to chromosome 3q in four unrelated families. *Nature Genet* 1992; 1:295–300.

292. Tragl KH, Mayr WR. Familial islet cell adenomatosis. *Lancet* 1977;2:426–428.

293. Maioli M, Ciccarese M, Pacifico A, et al. Familial insulinoma description of two cases. *Acta Diabetol* 1992;29:38–40.

294. Kinnamon JEC. Heredity and symptoms in acromegaly. *Acta Otolaryngol* 1976;82:230–233.

295. Kurisaka M, Takei Y, Tsubokawa T, Motiyasu N. Growth hormone-secreting pituitary adenoma in uniovular twin brothers: case report. *Neurosurgery* 1981;8:226–230.

296. Jones MK, Evans PJ, Jopnes IR, Thomas JP. Familial acromegaly. *Clin Endocrinol* 1984;20:355–358.

297. Abbassioun K, Fatourechi V, Amirjamshidi A, Meibodi NA. Familial acromegaly with pituitary adenoma. Report of three accepted siblings. *J Neurosurg* 1986;64:510–512.

298. Pestell RG, Alford FP, Best JD. Familial acromegaly. *Acta Endocrinol* 1989;121:286–289.

299. McCarthy MI, Noonan K, Wass JAH, Monson JP, Familial acromegaly: studies in three families. *Clin Endocrinol* 1990;32: 719–728.

300. Farid NR, Buehler S, Russell NA, Maroun FB, Allerdice P, Smyth HS. Prolactinomas in familial multiple endocrine neoplasia syndrome type 1. *Am J Med* 1980;69:874–880.

301. Bear JC, Brione-Urbina R, Fahey JF, Farid NR. Variant multiple endocrine neoplasia I (MEN I-Burin): further studies and non-linkage to HLA. *Hum Hered* 1985;35:15–20.

302. Bale SJ, Bale AE, Stewart K, et al. Linkage analysis of multiple endocrine neoplasia type 1 with int-2 and other markers on chromosome 11. *Genomics* 1989;4:320–322.

303. Duh Q-Y. Carcinoids associated with multiple endocrine neoplasia syndromes. *Am J Surg* 1987;154:142–148.

304. Eschbach JW, Rinaldo JA. Metastatic carcinoid: a familial occurrence. *Ann Intern Med* 1962;57:647–650.

305. Anderson RE. A familial instance of appendiceal carcinoid tumors. *Am J Surg* 1966;111:738–740.

306. Moertel CG, Dockerty MB. Familial occurrence of metastizing carcinoid tumors. *Ann Intern Med* 1973;78:389–390.

307. Wale RJ, William JA, Veeley AH. Familial occurrence in carcinoid tumors. *Aust NZ J Surg* 1983;53:325–328.

308. Yeatman TJ, Sharp JV, Kimura AK. Can suceptibility to carcinoid tumors be inherited? *Cancer* 1989;63:390–393.

309. Swinborn PA, Yeong ML, Lane MR, Nicholson GI, Holdaway IM. Neurofibromatosis associated with somatostatinoma: Report of two patients. *Clin Endocrinol* 1988;28:353–359.

310. Eberle F, Grun R. Multiple endocrine neoplasia, type I (MENI). *Ergebnisse Inneren Med Kinderhelk* 1981;46:76–149.

311. Skogseid B, Larsson C, Lindgren PG, et al. Clinical and genetic features of adrenocortical lesions in multiple endocrine neoplasia type 1. *J Clin Endocrinol Metab* 1992;75: 76–81.

312. Beckers A, Abs R, Willems PJ, et al. Aldosterone-secreting adrenal adenoma as part of multiple endocrine neoplasia type 1 (MENI): loss of heterozygosity for polymorphic chromosome 11 deoxynucleic acid markers, including the MEN1 locus. *J Clin Endocrinol* 1992;75:564–570.

313. Sameshima Y, Tsunematsu Y, Watanabe S, et al. Detection of novel germ-line p53 mutations in diverse-cancer-prone families identified by selecting patients with childhood adrenocortical carcinoma. *JNCI* 1992;84:703–707.

314. de Fromentel CC, Sousi T. TP53 tumor suppressor gene: a model for investigating human mutagenesis. *Genes Chrom Cancer* 1992;4:1–15.

315. Steiner AL, Goodman AD, Powers SR. A study of a kindred with pheochromocytoma, medullary thyroid carcinoma, hyperparathyroidism and Cushing's disease: Multiple endocrine neoplasia type 2. *Medicine*. l968;47:371–409.

316. Farhi F, Dikman SH, Lawson W, Cobin RH, Zak FG. Paragangliomatosis associated with multiple endocrine adenomas. *Arch Pathol Lab Med* 1976;100:495–498.

317. Hansen OP, Hansen M, Hansen HH, Rose B. Multiple endocrine adenomatosis of the mixed type. *Acta Med Scand* 1976;200:327–331.

318. Boden G, Owen OE. Familial hyperglucagonemia. An autosomal dominant disorder. *N Engl J Med* 1977;296:534–538.

319. Cameron D, Spiro HM, Landsberg L. Zollinger Ellison syndrome with multiple endocrine adenomatosis type II. *N Engl J Med* 1978;299:152–153.

320. Janson KL, Roberts JA, Vareia M. Multiple endocrine adenomatosis. In support of the common origin theories. *J Urol* 1978;119:161–165.

321. Alberts MW, McMeekin JO, George JM. Mixed multiple endocrine neoplasia syndromes. *JAMA* 1980;244;1236–1237.

322. Cusick JF, Ho K-C, Hagen TC, Kun LE: Granular-cell pituicytoma associated with multiple endocrine neoplasia type 2. *J Neurosurg* 1982;56:594–596.

323. Manning GS, Stevens KA, Stock JL. Multiple endocrine neoplasia, type I. Association with marfanoid habitus, optic

atrophy, and other abnormalities. *Arch Intern Med* 1983; 143:2315–2316.

324. Bertnard J-H, Ritz P, Reznik Y, Grollier G, Potier J-C, Evrad C, Mahoudeau JA. Sipple's syndrome associated with a large prolactinoma. *Clin Endocrinol* 1987;27:607–614.

325. Jerkins TW, Sacks HS, O'Dorisio TM, Tuttle S, Solomon SS. Medullary carcinoma of the thyroid, pancreatic nesidioblastosis and microadenosis, and pancreatic polypepetide hypersecretion: a new association and clinical and hormonal response to a long-acting somatostatin analog. *J Clin Endocrinol Metab* 1987;64:1313–1319.

326. Maton PN, Norton JA, Nieman LK, Doppman JL, Jensen RT. Multiple endocrine neoplasia type II with Zollinger Ellison syndrome caused by a solitary pancreatic gastrinoma. *JAMA* 1989;262:535–537.

327. Reschini E, Catania A, Airaghi L, Manfredi MG, Crosignani PG. Scintigraphic study of extra-adrenal ganglioneuroma in a patient with overlap between multiple endocrine neoplasia types 1 and 2. *Clin Nucl Med* 1992;17:573–576.

328. Cohen N, Modal D, Pik A, Golik A, Weissgarten J, Segal M. Coexistence of sporadic multiple endocrine neoplasia and scapular ectopic braest: coincidence or biologically associated? *Arch Intern Med* 1986;146:1822–1823.

329. Jansson S, Tieseli L-E, Hansson G. Morphology of the adrenal medulla indicating multiple neuroectodetermal abnormalities in pheochromocytoma patients. *Acta Med Austriaca* 1988;15:99–100.

330. Palmer FJ, Sawyer TM. Hyperparathyroidism, chemodectoma, thymoma, and myasthenia gravis. *Arch Intern Med* 1978;138:1402–1403.

331. Steely WM, Davies RS, Brigham RA. Carotid body tumor and hyperparathyroidism. A case report and review of the literature. *Am Surg* 1987;53:337–338.

332. Marx SJ. Familial hypocalciuric hypercalcemia. In: *Primer on metabolic bone diseases and disorders of mineral metabolism*. Favus MR, ed. Richmond, VA: William Byrd Press, 1990:113–115.

333. Heath DA. Familial hypocalciuric hypercalcemia. This volume.

334. Orwoll E, Silbert J, McClung M. Asymptomatic neonatal familial hypercalcemia. *Pediatrics* 1982;69:109–111.

335. Marx SJ, Attie MF, Levine MA, Spiegel AM, Downs RW Jr, Lasker RD. The hypocalciuric or benign variant of familial hypercalcemia: clinical and biochemical features in fifteen kindreds. *Medicine* 1981;60:397–412.

336. Marx SJ, Spiegel AM, Brown EM, et al. Divalent cation metabolism. Familial hypocalciuric hypercalcemia versus typical primary hyperparathyroidism. *Am J Med* 1978;65:235–242.

337. Marx SJ, Spiegel AM, Brown EM, et al. Circulating parathyroid hormone activity: familial hypocalciuric hypercalcemia versus typical primary hyperparathyroidism. *J Clin Endocrinol Metab* 1978;47:1190–1197.

338. Firek AF, Kao PC, Heath H III. Plasma intact parathyroid hormone (PTH) and PTH-related peptide in familial benign hypercalcemia: greater responsiveness to endogenous PTH than in primary hyperparathyroidism. *J Clin Endocrinol Metab* 1991;72:541–546.

The Parathyroids, edited by J.P. Bilezikian,
M.A. Levine, and R. Marcus. Raven Press. Ltd.,
New York © 1994.

CHAPTER 39

Multiple Endocrine Neoplasia Type II

Robert F. Gagel

Multiple endocrine neoplasia type II (MEN-II) is an autosomal dominant multiglandular syndrome, which includes a diverse group of clinical manifestations unified by the fact that the involved cell types derive from the neural crest. The association of thyroid carcinoma and pheochromocytoma was first noted 30 years ago (1), although it is clear that some variants of the syndrome were described at least 50 years earlier (2). The components of the syndrome that have attracted the most attention are medullary thyroid carcinoma (MTC), pheochromocytoma, and hyperparathyroidism. Other features of variant syndromes include mucosal and alimentary neuromas, skeletal abnormalities, a rare cutaneous form of amyloidosis, and Hirschsprung's disease. It is difficult to understand this diverse group of manifestations, all of which have been linked to a single genetic locus, unless one accepts the hypothesis that they represent a defect in the normal differentiation of neural crest tissue. In this context, identification of the genes responsible for MEN-II may be important not only for defining a mechanism for an interesting model of endocrine neoplasia but also to provide a target for understanding dermal, gastrointestinal, and skeletal development.

This chapter attempts to integrate a rapidly evolving literature regarding the molecular abnormalities in MEN-II with recently developed concepts regarding neural crest development. No attempt is made to discuss the management of clinical manifestations of MEN-II, since adequate reviews have been published elsewhere (3–6); however, the impact of identifying specific molecular defects on clinical management is discussed briefly.

BRIEF HISTORY OF THE MULTIPLE ENDOCRINE NEOPLASIA TYPE II SYNDROMES

An association between thyroid carcinoma and pheochromocytoma was first described by Sipple in 1961 (1), although an understanding of its heritable components and distinction from multiple endocrine neoplasia type I (MEN-I) emerged over the subsequent decade (7). Despite the fact that the MEN-II syndrome has only recently been categorized, there is unequivocal evidence based on genealogical studies of affected kindreds that the gene existed in the eighteenth century or earlier (8). Williams and his coworkers (9) are generally credited with the rediscovery of the mucosal neuroma syndrome (MEN-IIb) first described by Froboese (2) and the recognition that this was associated with MTC and pheochromocytoma. Additional variants of MEN-II include familial medullary thyroid carcinoma (FMTC) with no other manifestations of MEN-II (10), MEN-IIa in association with cutaneous lichen amyloidosis (11,12), and MEN-IIa in association with Hirschsprung's disease (13) (Table 1).

MULTIPLE ENDOCRINE NEOPLASIA TYPE IIa

The term *Sipple's syndrome* is most correctly applied to the association of MTC, pheochromocytoma, and parathyroid neoplasia (14), now known as MEN-IIa (Table 1). During the first decade after Sipple's report, the three major components of the syndrome were characterized (7,15). The convergence of several observations led to the use of provocative tests for calcitonin in the diagnosis of early MTC. These observations include the identification and sequencing of the calcitonin (CT) peptide (16,17), recognition of the C cell (thyroid parafollicular cell) as the transformed cell type in MTC along with the observation that it

R. F. Gagel: Section of Endocrinology, M.D. Anderson Cancer Center, Houston, Texas 77030.

TABLE 1. *Classification of multiple endocrine neoplasia type 2 (MEN-II)*

MEN IIa
  Medullary thyroid carcinoma
  Pheochromocytoma
  Parathyroid neoplasia
Variants of MEN-IIa
  Familial medullary thyroid carcinoma only (FMTC)
  MEN 2A in association with Hirschsprung's disease
  MEN 2A in association with cutaneous lichen amyloidosis
MEN IIb
  Medullary thyroid carcinoma
  Pheochromocytoma
  Mucosal and alimentary tract ganglioneuromatosis
  Marfanoid features
  Absence of parathyroid neoplasia

produced CT (18), the development of radioimmunoassays for CT (19,20), and the finding that either a provocative calcium or pentagastrin test could be used to stimulate CT release (21–24). Use of provocative tests led to the identification of subclinical C-cell hyperplasia, a histologic lesion thought to represent a premalignant form of MTC (25) and to the systematic screening of families to detect these abnormalities (3,26,27). In parallel studies, hyperplasia of the adrenal medulla was identified as a precursor lesion (26,28,29). Implementation of prospective screening studies over the next 2 decades resulted in the routine identification of MTC and pheochromocytoma at early stages in their development and has led to the belief

that death related to either of these manifestations can be prevented by timely surgical intervention (3,30). In 1987, genetic linkage of MEN-IIa to a centromeric locus on chromosome 10 (31,32) abruptly shifted the focus of investigation for this syndrome and has led to an intense search for the predisposing gene, a quest that has recently culminated in the identification of point mutations of the *ret* protooncogene in MEN-IIa.

NATURAL HISTORY OF THE THREE NEOPLASTIC MANIFESTATIONS OF MULTIPLE ENDOCRINE NEOPLASIA TYPE II

C-Cell Hyperplasia and Medullary Thyroid Carcinoma

The parafollicular cells are distributed within the thyroid gland in a characteristic pattern (Fig. 1A). In each lobe, their greatest concentration occurs in the central upper portion, where the upper one-third and lower two-thirds intersect. Transformation of the C cell is thought to be a random, clonal event (33), and it is therefore not surprising that most examples of hereditary MTC develop in this anatomic location in contrast to the more random location of sporadic MTC (Fig. 1). Hyperplasia of the C cells is the earliest abnormality observed in hereditary MTC. This lesion most commonly develops in childhood in MEN-IIa (3,8,30), although its occurrence in adults (34) suggests random acquisition of genetic events, leading to transformation or the presence of modifier genes, which al-

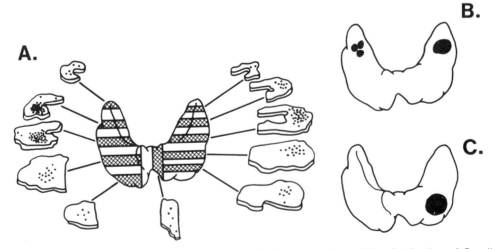

FIG. 1. Distribution of C cells in the thyroid gland. **A:** Reconstruction of the distribution of C cells in the thyroid gland. The greatest concentration of C cells occurs at the junction of the upper one-half and lower two-thirds of the gland. This distribution explains the characteristic location of hereditary medullary thyroid carcinoma. (Modified from Wolfe HJ, Voelkel EF, Tashjian AH Jr. Distribution of calcitonin containing cells in the normal adult human thyroid gland: a correlation of morphology with peptide content. *J Clin Endocrinol Metab* 1974;38:688–694.) **B:** Hereditary medullary thyroid carcinoma is almost always bilateral, although the extent of involvement may not be equal. **C:** Sporadic medullary thyroid carcinoma is most commonly a unilateral process that may develop at any location within the thyroid gland.

ter the onset of transformation. Histological progression of the lesion is evidenced by the development of nodular hyperplasia, which gives the appearance of C cells filling the thyroid follicle but actually represents displacement of the thyroid follicle by cells lying in a parafollicular location (Fig. 2A). Continued growth (or a transforming event) leads to the development of microscopic carcinoma (Fig. 2B). It is not clear at what point along this pathway metastasis occurs, although metastatic disease has been found in a few individuals with microscopic carcinoma in the thyroid (35,36). It is common to find separate lesions within the thyroid gland at different developmental points along the pathway from normal to carcinoma. Metastasis to central lymph nodes of the neck occurs commonly in patients with carcinoma detectable by the human eye. The fact that 25% of patients with lymph node metastasis without evidence of other metastatic disease can be cured by lymph node dissection of the neck suggests that spread to local lymph nodes occurs first, with dissemination occurring later on.

A considerable literature has developed regarding secretory or nonsecretory proteins produced by MTC, collectively categorized as tumor markers. Genes that are normally expressed by the C cell include CT, somatostatin, chromogrannin A, and DOPA decarboxylase (6,37–42). Their expression by MTC cells is normal, although the level of expression and subsequent processing events may be altered in the transformed C cell (43,44). Less is known about the expression of carcinoembryonic antigen, insulin-like growth factors

(IGF)-I and -II, fibroblast growth factor, and their receptors, although the suggestion has been made that IGF-I may be a growth factor for MTC (45). There is abundant evidence that one or more variants of the somatostatin receptor are expressed in normal or transformed C cells (46–48), although it is not clear at present which of the five cloned variants is expressed in the C cell. The utilization of each of these expressed genes for diagnostic or therapeutic purposes has been explored. Several, including CT, carcinoembryonic antigen, and somatostatin, have been useful for diagnostic purposes, although a unique cell surface or structural protein other than carcinoembryonic antigen has not been found.

Fully expressed MTC is characteristically multifocal. Each tumor appears as a whitish-yellow circumscribed lesion against a background of thyroid tissue. The characteristic histologic features of the tumor include a nested endocrine-type appearance or sheets of cells interspersed with amyloid; the amyloid is derived at least in part from calcitonin gene products (49).

Adrenal Medullary Hyperplasia and Pheochromocytoma

Pheochromocytomas occur in >50% of affected individuals. They are bilateral in approximately one-half of those affected. It is reasonable to believe that adrenal medullary abnormalities of a lesser degree (adrenal medullary hyperplasia) occur in a higher per-

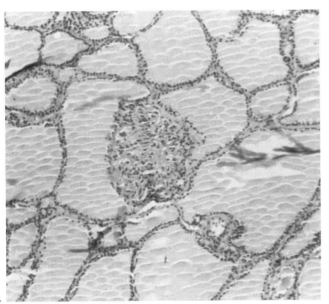
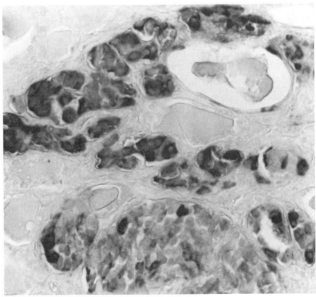

A   B

FIG. 2. Progression of histological changes in hereditary medullary thyroid carcinoma. **A:** Nodular hyperplasia with displacement of a thyroid follicle by parafollicular cells. ×100. (Reprinted from ref. 4 with permission.) **B:** Microscopic medullary thyroid carcinoma, which stains positive for calcitonin by immunohistochemical staining. ×400. (Reprinted from ref. 12 with permission.)

centage of patients and develop in parallel with hyperplastic events affecting the C cell.

Several features differentiate pheochromocytomas associated with MEN-II from sporadic pheochromocytoma. The most characteristic is the type of catecholamine produced. Almost all pheochromocytomas associated with MEN-II develop in the adrenal medulla and express the enzyme phenylethanolamine-N-methyltransferase, the enzyme that catalyzes the methylation of norepinephrine to epinephrine. Studies from multiple kindreds have demonstrated an increase in the relative production of epinephrine in MEN-II-associated pheochromocytomas. The first abnormality observed in an MEN-II gene carrier is an absolute increase in the 24 hr urine or an exercise-induced plasma epinephrine concentration (26,30,50,51). Palpitations, nervousness, jitteriness, and absence of hypertension, the earliest clinical signs and symptoms in MEN-II patients who are subsequently documented to have adrenal medullary hyperplasia or pheochromocytoma, are thought to relate directly to increased epinephrine production. In patients whose adrenal medullary abnormalities remain undetected, there may be a subsequent development of clinical features more characteristically associated with pheochromocytoma, including hypertension. A second characteristic feature is the invariable location of the pheochromocytoma in the adrenal medulla. The few examples of extraadrenal pheochromocytoma in this syndrome are thought to have arisen from adrenal rest tissue or to represent recurrence of a pheochromocytoma in the anatomic region of the adrenal gland (52,53).

Parathyroid Abnormalities

It has been difficult to study the natural history of hyperparathyroidism in MEN-II because of its low incidence (5–20%) and the frequent late onset of its clinical features. Nonetheless, several interesting points have emerged. First, there appears to be a familial predisposition to hyperparathyroidism. In some kindreds, hyperparathyroidism is found rarely, whereas, in others, it occurs frequently and at an early age. A second observation, made in several families, is the lack of hyperparathyroidism in gene carriers who were thyroidectomized for early C-cell abnormalities, despite follow-up periods of >15 years (30,54). Whether this observation has pathophysiologic significance or results from the inevitable loss of parathyroid tissue during total thyroidectomy is not clear. One hypothesis to explain the observation is the production of a growth factor by thyroid tissue that has effects on the adjacent parathyroid tissue, a mechanism analogous to the growth factor postulated for development of hyper-

parathyroidism in MEN-I (see chapters by Friedman et al.) (55–58).

The clinical syndrome of hyperparathyroidism does not appear to differ from that observed with sporadic hyperparathyroidism. Hypercalcemia and nephrolithiasis are the most common presenting manifestations found in MEN-II patients. Pheochromocytoma, possibly related to production of parathyroid hormone-related protein, may rarely cause hypercalcemia and should be excluded prior to surgery (30).

Hyperplasia of multiple parathyroid glands is the most common abnormality found in hyperparathyroidism associated with MEN-II, although many reports emphasize the occurrence of multiple parathyroid adenomas in individuals who present with the fully developed MEN-II syndrome, generally after the age of 35 years (3,19,59).

Familial Medullary Thyroid Carcinoma

In ~10–15% of MTC families, hereditary MTC occurs without other manifestations of MEN-IIa (FMTC) (10). The pattern of inheritance and clinical features in this variant do not differ from those found in MEN-IIa except that the MTC tends to occur later and is clinically less aggressive. Categorization of a family with the diagnosis of FMTC should be made only after a careful examination of the clinical spectrum of the disease in several generations of family members. The penetrance of pheochromocytoma and parathyroid disease in MEN-IIa is 50% or less, and categorization of a small family with the diagnosis of FMTC may result in inadequate screening for pheochromocytoma. There is a belief by some individuals that FMTC is late-onset MEN-IIa resulting in a lower penetrance rate for pheochromocytoma.

Hirschsprung's Disease in Association With Multiple Endocrine Neoplasia Type IIa

A small number of families have been described among whom classical Hirschsprung's disease has been observed in association with MEN-IIa (13). In contrast to MEN-IIb, where ganglioneuromatosis is generally found throughout the entire gastrointestinal tract, in the MEN-IIa/Hirschsprung's disease variant, aganglioneuromatosis may be found throughout the colon or in smaller intestinal segments. The gastrointestinal features of Hirschsprung's disease and those associated with MEN-IIb include megacolon, obstruction, and colonic atony. Clinical differentiation between Hirschsprung's/MEN-IIa and MEN-IIb based solely on gastrointestinal symptomatology may be difficult.

Multiple Endocrine Neoplasia Type IIa With Cutaneous Lichen Amyloidosis

In 10 to 12 kindreds, a pruritic skin lesion located over the upper back (dermatomes C6–T5) has been associated with MEN-IIa (Fig. 3) (11). The skin lesions may be unilateral or bilateral, and clinical features of MEN-IIa in these families do not differ in any other recognizable way from the more common MEN-IIa (60–63). Patients with this variant describe intermittent periods of intense pruritus, during which they scratch the upper back. These symptoms begin in early childhood in some families and may precede the development of MTC. In other kindreds, the skin lesion develops later. Biopsy of more advanced forms of this lesion has demonstrated typical findings of cutaneous lichen amyloidosis (12), whereas amyloid is infrequently found in early skin lesions (11,62,64). Several explanations have been considered to explain the presence of amyloid. One possibility, that the amyloid consists of CT gene products, has been excluded experimentally (12,65,66). Immunohistochemical studies indicate the amyloid consists of keratin, analogous to more common varieties of hereditary or sporadic cutaneous lichen amyloidosis (67). The combination of a dermatome-like distribution for the skin lesion (Fig. 3) and a clinical history of intense pruritus preceding the development of the skin lesion suggests to some that the primary abnormality is a neurologic disorder leading to pruritus and that the skin lesion and amyloid deposition are secondary to chronic irritation similar to that observed in notalgia parathetica, a localized

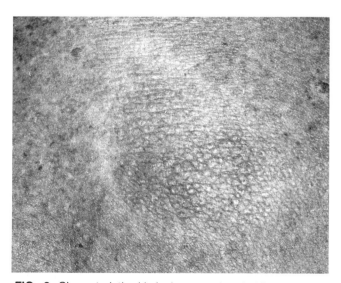

FIG. 3. Characteristic skin lesion associated with cutaneous lichen amyloidosis associated with MEN-IIa. The lesion has been found unilaterally or bilaterally over the upper back in all individuals affected with this variant.

form of cutaneous pruritus (68). One hypothesis put forward to explain the clinical findings is a disorder of neural crest differentiation, leading to increased sensory neuronal activity. Electromyographic studies of the paraspinal musculature has demonstrated a nonspecific abnormality between the T1 and T6 dermatomes in one of four patients (69). There have been no histologic studies of sensory nerves or dorsal root ganglia in the spinal cord of affected patients. Nonetheless, a defect in segmental neural crest differentiation is one hypothesis that links the diverse clinical features of MTC, pheochromocytoma, and a dermatome-specific skin lesion.

MULTIPLE ENDOCRINE NEOPLASIA TYPE IIb

The association of MTC, pheochromcytoma, mucosal ganglioneuromatosis, skeletal abnormalities suggestive of Marfan syndrome, and the absence of hyperparathyroidism has been categorized as multiple endocrine neoplasia type IIb. The most striking characteristic of this syndrome is the presence of mucosal neuromas, which occur on the tip of the tongue, on the conjunctival surface of the eyelids, and throughout the gastrointestinal tract. The most common presenting manifestations in children in whom the distinctive clinical phenotype is not recognized are related to the gastrointestinal manifestations of neuronal dysplasia. These include diarrhea, intestinal obstruction, megacolon, and crampy abdominal pain (70). The Marfanoid features include an altered upper/lower body ratio, long limbs, pectus abnormalities, arachnodactyly, hyperextensibility of joints, and epiphyseal abnormalities (9,71,72). Other manifestations of Marfan syndrome are rare, although the author is aware of one patient with aortic dissection and another with a dysfunctional mitral valve.

The penetrance of MTC in MEN-IIb approaches 100% and is evident at an early age. Metastastatic disease has been found in the first year of life and is uniformly present in patients diagnosed after the age of 10 years. If the disease is not diagnosed prior to development of metastasis, the tumor pursues a virulent course in ~50% of patients. Greater long-term experience with MEN-IIb indicates that the prognosis is not uniformly poor (73,74), and a number of multigenerational families have been identified (75). Pheochromocytomas are eventually found in ~50% of affected individuals and do not differ substantially from those found in MEN-IIa. Hyperparathyroidism occurs rarely (76), and, of interest, cutaneous lichen amyloidosis has not been described. The author has seen or is aware of examples of MEN-IIb in which some of the characteristic manifestations are absent (Table 2). It is possible that these unusual cases represent variable

TABLE 2. *Variants of multiple endocrine neoplasia type IIb*

MTC	Pheochromocytoma	Parathyroid neoplasia	Ganglioneuromatosis	Marfanoid features
+	+	−	+	+
+	−	−	+	+
+	+	−	−	+
−	−	−	+	+

penetrance of a common genetic defect or are examples of a unique genetic abnormality at the MEN-II locus or elsewhere. One example in the literature, a mother with fully developed MEN-IIb and two children with MTC, only one of whom had the ganglioneuromatosis phenotype, suggests that penetrance in the MEN-IIb can be variable (77).

There is considerable evidence that each of the tissue types involved in MEN-IIb is derived from the neural crest. The derivation of the C cells, adrenal medulla, and enteric nervous system from neural crest anlage is well established. The Marfanoid features are more difficult to understand, although considerable evidence suggests that cartilage and bone are derived from neural crest tissue.

MAPPING THE MEN-II LOCUS

The identification of frequent DNA polymorphism in the human genome and the revival of genetic linkage techniques based on these polymorphisms in the early 1980s led to the application of these techniques to study MEN-II, an ideal example because of the availability of large, well-defined families. Initial progress was disappointing and was hampered considerably by the lack of evenly spaced markers across the human genome. Nonetheless, linkage was established to a centromeric locus on chromosome 10 in 1987 (31,32). Subsequent efforts have led to the linkage of each of the major variants of MEN-II to this same centromeric locus (75,78–80). Efforts to narrow further the region containing the *MEN-II* gene(s) were slowed by a low recombination rate in this region (81). Through a combination of physical mapping and identification of a few key recombinants, the region containing the *MEN-II* gene has been narrowed to a 0.5 megabase (500,000 bases) sequence on proximal chromosome 10q (10q11–12) between D10S141 and D10S94 (Fig. 4). The genomic DNA for this entire region has been cloned into large vectors (82–84).

Of considerable potential importance is the inclusion of *ret*, a protooncogene, in the region flanked by D10S141 and D10S94, which contains the *MEN-II* gene(s) (Fig. 4). The *ret* protooncogene is a receptor similar to those for nerve growth factor (*trk* oncogene)

or fibroblast growth factor (Fig. 5). A characteristic feature of this class of receptor, which also includes the insulin, epidermal growth factor, and platelet-derived growth factor receptors, is a tyrosine kinase domain that autophosphorylates the cytoplasmic portion of the receptor. Several cDNAs for the *ret* protooncogene have been isolated (85,86). These cDNAs encode a protein with a single transmembrane domain and an intracellular tyrosine kinase (Fig. 6). A prominent feature is the presence of a cysteine-rich region immediately adjacent to the transmembrane section. The presence of several different variants of the cDNA is most readily explained by 5′ and 3′ alternative RNA processing events, which create at least five different mRNAs. The functional significance of the alternative RNA processing is unclear (87).

The tyrosine kinase class of receptors to which *ret* belongs has most commonly been linked to growth factor function. Activation of this type of receptor results

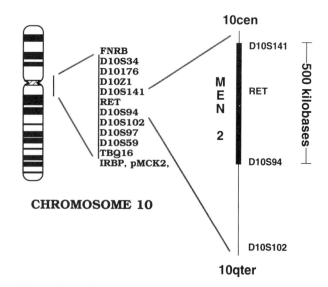

FIG. 4. Genetic and physical map of the centromeric chromosome 10 *MEN-II* locus. The genetic markers shown define the centromeric chromosome 10 locus for *MEN-II*. The *MEN-IIa* gene is located in a 0.5 megabase region on proximal chromosome 10q flanked by D10S94 and D10S141 and includes the *ret* protooncogene.

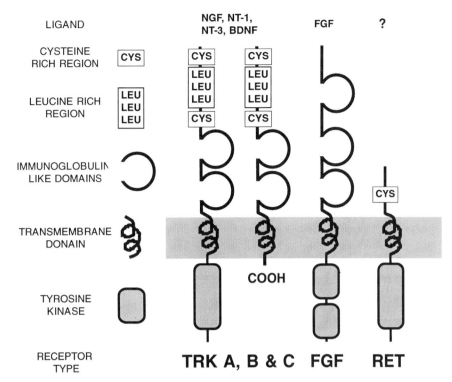

FIG. 5. Tyrosine kinases involved in neural crest differentiation. Schematic diagram of several of the tyrosine kinase receptor types involved in differentiation of neural crest tissue. Abbreviations: TRK A, B, and C, the tropomyosin kinase receptor; FGF, the receptor for fibroblast growth factor; RET, *ret* protooncogene; NGF, nerve growth factor; NT-1 and NT-3, neurotropins 1 and 3; and FGF, fibroblast growth factor.

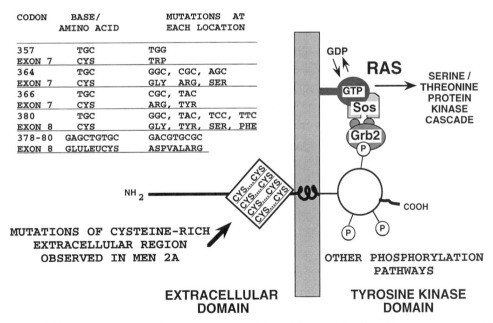

FIG. 6. Mutations of the *ret* protooncogene associated with MEN-IIa. Mutation of specific codons, which change a cysteine to another amino acid at codons 357, 364, 366, and 380 in exons 7 or 8, are found in the germlines of individuals who carry a mutant copy of the *MEN-II* gene. The *ret* receptor is thought to function in a manner analogous to other tyrosine kinase receptors by activation of *ras*, as outlined in the text. It is likely that *ret* activation will also be linked to other protein kinase pathways. Abbreviations are given in the text.

in autophosphorylation and configurational changes in the cytoplasmic portion of the receptor (Fig. 6), which cause association of GTP with *ras,* resulting in its activation. Recently the protein factors that mediate the link between the receptor and *ras* have been identified and include a class of proteins (of which Grb2 is the most well known) containing *src* homology domains that bind tyrosine phosphoproteins. The Grb2 protein associates with another protein (Sos) that links to *ras,* thereby activating *ras* and transmitting the signal from the activated receptor to serine/threonine protein kinases downstream (88,89). It seems likely that phosphorylated tyrosine residues also activate other phosphorylation pathways (Fig. 6).

A ligand for *ret* has not been identified, but the transforming capability of *ret* (the *ret* oncogene) in neoplasia has been confirmed for several neoplastic processes. One clearly defined example in which *ret* has been shown to have transforming activity is the most common malignant thyroid carcinoma, papillary thyroid carcinoma (90–94). Transformation of NIH 3T3 cells by DNA derived from papillary thyroid carcinoma led to the identification of the papillary thyroid carcinoma oncogene (PTC), a rearranged form of *ret* in which the expression of the cytoplasmic tyrosine kinase portion of *ret* is driven by the promoter from another gene (H4) as a result of a chromosome 10 rearrangement (most commonly an inversion) (95–98). The PTC oncogene is found in 20–35% of papillary thyroid carcinomas and is thought to be important in the development or progression of this tumor. Other rearrangements of the *ret* protooncogene have been described in nonthyroid tumors (87,99,100). In each of these cases, expression of the rearranged protooncogene is driven by promoter sequences thought to be constitutively expressed in the cell type and does not represent normal functioning of the receptor.

There is evidence of enhanced expression of the *ret* protooncogene in hereditary and sporadic MTCs and pheochromocytomas derived from MEN-II patients, an observation first made by Santoro et al. (101). These results were confirmed by Miya et al. (102), who demonstrated high levels of expression in 12 of 12 MTCs and six of eight pheochromocytomas, whereas there was no expression of *ret* in adjacent follicular cells. Moreover, these authors demonstrated mRNA sizes of 7.0, 6.0, 4.5, and 3.9 kilobases, consistent with a normally expressed and alternatively processed *ret* mRNA. Examination of a single tumor for rearrangement of *ret* demonstrated no abnormalities. What is less clear from results described to date is whether the *ret* protooncogene is expressed in normal thyroid C cells or adrenal medulla, although studies suggest a low level of expression in normal adrenal medulla (102).

Mutation of the *ret* Protooncogene in Multiple Endocrine Neoplasia Type-IIa

Studies by two groups of investigators have identified mutations in the *ret* protooncogene in MEN-IIa (103,104). These point mutations have been identified within a cysteine-rich extracellular region of the *ret* protooncogene (Fig. 6). In each mutation identified to date, there is the conversion of a cysteine to another amino acid at codon 357, 364, 366, or 380 [codon number derived from Takahashi et al. (85)]. A mutation seen in several cases involves codons 378–380 and results in a three-amino-acid change, including a mutation of the cysteine. Although these are exciting findings, additional studies will be required to demonstrate a causal relationship between the mutations and oncogenesis. Preliminary studies suggest that these mutations are not present in all cases of MEN-IIa, and there is currently no information regarding these mutations in MEN-IIb or other MEN-II variants.

The point mutations of *ret* are thought constitutively to activate the *ret* receptor. The only fact available to support this hypothesis is the expression of the *ret* protooncogene in tumor types derived from MEN-IIa and a precedent for this type of mutation in other tyrosine kinase receptors (105,106). The *ret* protooncogene promoter sequence is expressed in MTC cells, but there is no evidence to suggest an abnormality of the promoter region contributes to expression of the *ret* protooncogene in MTC or pheochromocytoma (107).

Whether abnormalities of *ret* will be identified in MEN-IIb and the other variants of MEN-IIa remains to be seen. There could be as many as ten to 20 genes in the 0.5 million base region encompassing the *MEN-II* locus, raising the possibility that other genes are involved as a result of small deletions or rearrangements in the region. One other newly described gene derived from the D10S94 locus encodes a cyclin type protein, although no abnormality of this gene has been described (108).

Is the *MEN-II* Gene an Important Regulator of Neural Crest Differentiation?

Multiple endocrine neoplasia is a syndrome in which each of the affected tissues could plausibly trace its derivation to the neural crest. C cells of the thyroid, adrenal medullary cells, parathyroid cells, neuromas in MEN-IIb, cartilaginous tissue leading to Marfanoid features, and neuronal dysplasia associated with Hirschsprung's disease involve cell types that originate in the neural crest. There is strong suspicion that the likely sensory defect associated with cutaneous lichen amyloidosis has its origins in neural crest tissue, although definitive proof is not available. It seems reasonable to hypothesize that the *MEN-II* gene may play an important role in neural crest cell differentiation or migration and that a defect in this gene could lead to abnormal development or aberrant growth of one or more cell types and eventually to the neoplastic and nonneoplastic manifestations associated with MEN-II.

The neural crest is a band of cells located between the neural tube and the developing epidermal ectoderm. Pluripotential cells from this structure give rise to diverse cell and tissue types (109). As a beginning, it may be instructive to sketch the development of neural crest tissue in broad strokes to provide a framework for subsequent discussion of individual cell types and relevant information relating to their development. It is important to recognize that what follows is an overview of very complex events and is focused on those elements of direct relevance to MEN-II. The field is evolving rapidly, and there is very little at present that can be accepted as established.

There is evidence showing that rostral-to-caudal segmentation of mammalian species is directed by a series of genes closely related to the *Hox* family of genes, which direct segmentation of *Drosophila melanogaster*. Studies in mammalian species indicate that these genes are conserved and are likely to play a similar role in higher organisms. Targeted recombination of these genes in mice results in defective rostral-to-caudal segmentation and provides evidence for a similar role in mammalian species (110,111).

Neural crest development proceeds within the overall context of segmentation provided by the *Hox* genes but has several unique characteristics. The neural crest coalesces around the neural tube during development (Figs. 7, 8). Cells migrate from the neural crest in clearly defined patterns (Figs. 7, 8) to form a variety of tissues. Migration of cells occurs in rostral-to-caudal and dorsal-to-ventral directions. These migratory patterns are observed most commonly within specific segments, defined as somites (Fig. 8B). Within these recurring units there is a pattern of organization. For example, the neural crest cells destined to become the dorsal root ganglion migrate in a dorsal-to-ventral direction within the most rostral portion of each somite (Fig. 8B), a concept explained most clearly in a review by Bronner-Fraser (112).

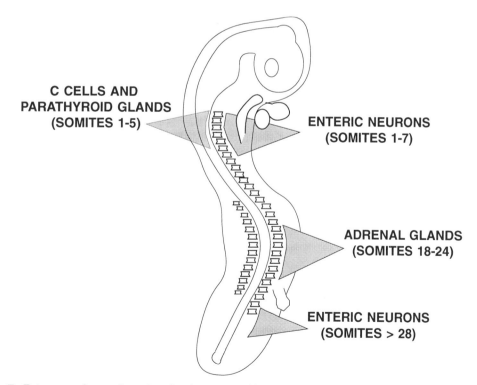

FIG. 7. Fate map of neural crest as it relates to multiple endocrine neoplasia type II. Section of chick embryo showing the origin of neural crest cells for the C cell, parathyroid glands, enteric neurons, and adrenal medulla.

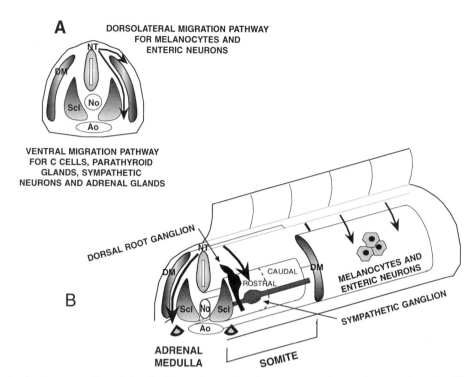

FIG. 8. A: Cross-section of developing embryo, showing patterns of neural crest migration. The pluripotential neural crest cells can either migrate in a ventral direction to form precursors for the sympathetic nervous system, adrenal medulla, C cells, or parathyroid glands or laterally to develop into melanocytes or enteric neurons. Scl, sclerotome; No, notochord; Ao, aorta; DM, dermatomyotome; NT, neural tube. **B:** Impact of somite organization on neural crest migration patterns. The neural crest migration is tighly regulated, resulting in a segmental pattern of migration within the confines of a particular somite. There is a specific organization of sympathetic neurons and other neural crest-derived structures within this organizational pattern. Scl, sclerotome; No, notochord; Ao, aorta; DM, dermatomyotome; NT, neural tube. (Modified from ref. 112.)

WHAT DETERMINES THE FATE OF NEURAL CREST CELLS?

The migration and differentiated functions of neural crest cells are shaped by several different factors. Expression of the *Hox* genes leads to segmentation of the embryo, an effect thought to be mediated by a transcription cascade. Although few specific details regarding regulation of this cascade are known, at least four general categories of factors have been implicated in subsequent development of the pluripotential cells of the neural crest within a particular segment. The first is the expression of neurotropins, which include but are not limited to basic fibroblast growth factor (bFGF), nerve growth factor (NGF), at least five neurotrophins (NTs-1–5), and brain-derived neurotrophic factor (BDNF). These factors interact with tyrosine kinase receptors, which form the second category and include the FGF receptor, the *trk* family of receptors (receptors for NGF and NT-1) (113) and several other tyrosine kinase receptors (Fig. 5) (114). Third, a group of glycoproteins, including laminin, fibronectin, and tenascin, are known to be important determinants of migration (115). These glycoproteins are produced along migration pathways and interact with specific receptors on the cell surface of the migrating neural crest derivative. Within this class there are positively acting glycoproteins, which serve a trophic function to guide migration along a particular pathway. It is likely that inhibitory factors will also be described, such as a factor that deflects ventrally migrating cells from the notochord (112). Finally, a class of helix–loop–helix transcription factors appears to be involved in cell differentiation and cell-specific expression of genes. This group of transcription factors includes Myo D (116,117), a transcription factor with dual roles of differentiation and cell-specific gene expression in muscle, and the mammalian homolog of *Drosophila* achaete-scute, mASH-1 (118). There is evolving evidence that this class of proteins is likely to be important for cell-specific expression of a variety of peptides produced by neuroendocrine cells, including CT, insulin, glucagon, and others. The following is an attempt to define the specific neural crest derivation of cell types involved in MEN-II, to provide insight regarding their developmental patterns, and to suggest points at which growth and differentiation may be affected in MEN-II. Although it is premature to draw firm conclusions, it seems likely that the *MEN-II* gene defect(s) will have an impact on this developmental process.

MIGRATORY PATHWAYS OF NEURAL CREST CELLS INVOLVED IN MULTIPLE ENDOCRINE NEOPLASIA TYPE II

Derivation of the C Cell

The migration of the C- or CT-producing cell type was among the first of the endocrine neural crest cells to be documented. Studies by Le Douarin and colleagues (119,120), performed by grafting of neural crest cells derived from quail with a distinctive nuclear structure, demonstrated unequivocally that C cells are derived from neural crest and migrate in a ventral direction to their ultimate resting place in the ultimobranchial body in birds (or the thyroid gland in mammals; Fig. 7). Despite these early observations, there is little information about molecular signals that cause differentiation or direct migration.

Derivation and Differentiation of the Adrenal Medulla

The neural crest cells destined to become the adrenal medulla are derived from somites 18–24 (Fig. 7) (121). These pluripotential neural crest cells migrate in a ventral direction (Fig. 8A, B) to form the progenitor cells for either the sympathetic nervous system or the adrenal medulla (112). What determines a ventral route of migration of neural crest cells has not been determined with certainty, although it seems clear that a series of molecular processes, which include growth factor and glycoprotein expression and expression of their receptors, constitute primary signals. Basic fibroblast growth factor (bFGF) causes the cell to differentiate to a neuronal phenotype. This includes the development of neuritic processes and the expression of *trk*A receptors for and a dependence on the presence of nerve growth factor (NGF). Expression of NGF further reinforces the neuronal phenotype and commits the cell to a sympathetic phenotype (122). Development of the neuronal phenotype can be suppressed by high concentrations of glucocorticoid present in the developing adrenal gland. Glucocorticoids have been shown experimentally to prevent the NGF-induced differentiation toward a sympathetic neuronal phenotype. This effect is thought to be mediated by positive or negative effects of glucocorticoid on transcription. For example, phenylethanolamine-N-methyl transferase, the enzyme responsible for methylation of

norepinephrine to produce epinephrine is induced by glucocorticoid. Transcription of other genes expressed preferentially by neurons, including peripherin, SCG10, and GAP 43, is inhibited (reviewed in 122).

A ROLE FOR THE *ret* PROTOONCOGENE IN NEURAL CREST DIFFERENTIATION?

Evidence for a role of the *ret* protooncogene in neural crest differentiation is fragmentary at present, but there is clear evidence of *ret* protooncogene expression in neural crest-derived tissue. Several studies have demonstrated normal expression of *ret* protooncogene in tissue derived from the neural crest, including normal mouse (86) and rat spinal cord and testis (85). In addition, *ret* protooncogene expression has been consistently observed in mouse and rat neuroblastoma cell lines and tumors as well as monocytic (THP-1) and promyelocytic (HL-60) cell lines (123). The identification of a cadherin-like sequence in the extracellular region of the *ret* protooncogene (86) has suggested that *ret* may function as a cell adhesion molecule in a manner analogous to the interaction between *boss* and *sevenless* in the formation of the retina in *D. melanogaster* (124,125).

Evidence that expression of the *ret* oncogene (the rearranged form of the *ret* protooncogene) can affect melanocytes, a neural crest-derived cell type, is provided by experiments in which overexpression of the *ret* oncogene in several transgenic animal lines driven by a mouse metallothionein promoter caused melanocyte hyperplasia and tumor formation (123,126–129). It is generally accepted that melanocytes are derived from the neural crest but pursue a migratory pathway very different from that observed for any of the cell types involved in MEN-II (Fig. 8B). Despite these intriguing fragments of information, it is probably premature to suggest a specific role for the *ret* protooncogene in neural crest differentiation.

IS THERE A ROLE FOR THE HELIX–LOOP–HELIX TRANSCRIPTION FACTORS IN THE DEVELOPMENT OF THE NEURAL CREST AND MULTIPLE ENDOCRINE NEOPLASIA TYPE II?

The helix–loop–helix (HLH) class of transcription factors have a dual role, that of promoting cell-specific expression of specific genes and a secondary role in differentiation of a specialized cell type. The most straightforward example of this phenomenon is the *achaete-scute* HLH transcription factor necessary for development of the peripheral nervous system in *Drosophila melanogaster* (130). These factors are relevant to MEN-II in that cell-specific expression of several genes coding for secretory peptides produced by neuroendocrine cells, most notably CT but including insulin and glucagon, are regulated by members of this family (131,132). In MTC there appears to be a direct correlation between the differentiation state of the cell and *CT* gene expression, with low levels of *CT* gene expression in poorly differentiated tumors (133–135). Furthermore, treatment of MTC cell lines with retinoic acid or other agents that slow growth and cause differentiation results in enhanced expression of calcitonin (134–136). Recently mammalian homologs of the *achaete-scute* gene have been cloned in rats (*mASH-1*) and human subjects (*hASH-1*) (137,138). *hASH-1* is expressed in human MTC cells, although its function there has not been clarified (138). Another HLH protein, Myo D, performs dual roles in muscle differentiation and cell-specific expression of muscle creatine kinase (117). At this point there is no known example of an HLH protein causing transformation of a cell type, although there is the belief that it may augment transformation caused by other transcription factors (e.g., *myc*) by the formation of heterodimers that facilitate transcriptional effects.

DERIVATION AND DIFFERENTIATION OF NEURONS AND NEUROENDOCRINE CELLS OF THE ENTERIC ENDOCRINE SYSTEM

Neural crest cells that migrate to the gastrointestinal tract are not primarily involved in the endocrine malignancy of MEN-II, but the presence of enteric neuronal dysplasia in both MEN-IIa and -IIb indicates that the causative gene(s) is involved in neuronal differentiation and/or migration of neural crest tissue. Because of the striking phenotypes associated with either MEN-IIa associated with Hirschsprung's disease or enteric ganglioneuromatosis associated with MEN-IIb, it may be useful to review the evidence for the *MEN-II* gene locus being involved in its development and outline what is currently known about enteric neuronal development.

The most compelling evidence pointing to a relationship between enteric neuronal development and the *MEN-II* locus was the identification of a child with Hirschsprung's disease and a centromeric chromosome 10 deletion (q11.2–q21.2) (139). Studies in this child failed to demonstrate MTC. Subsequent investigation led to the linkage of a form of familial Hirschsprung's disease without MEN-IIa to the MEN-II locus at centromeric chromosome 10 (140), further strengthening the relationship between some forms of Hirschsprung's disease and the *MEN-II* locus.

The enteric neuronal/endocrine system is derived from vagal (somites 1–7) and caudal somites (distal to somite 28) of the developing embryo (Figs. 7, 8B). There is some evidence that enteric neurons are derived from the same type of pluripotential cells that develop into the sympathetic and chromaffin precursors, a point of some importance in searching for a link between the enteric neuronal manifestations and C-cell/chromaffin manifestations of MEN-II. It is not clear what factors cause divergence of cells destined to be sympathoadrenal from those that will become enteric neurons, but there is evolving evidence that the type of *trk* receptor expressed by the cell may be important. Cells that evolve along a sympathoadrenal pathway express the *trk* A gp 140 receptor, which binds NGF with high affinity. In contrast, enteric neuroendocrine cells express the *trk* C receptor (Fig. 5), which binds NT-1 with high affinity and binds NGF or BDNF poorly (reviewed in 115). These factors lead to differentiation to the serotoninergic (instead of catecholaminergic) phenotype seen in gut neuronal/endocrine cells and the expression of a group of peptides that include vasoactive intestinal peptide (VIP), calcitonin gene-related peptide (CGRP), and substance P.

Another factor important in the development of the enteric nervous system is the expression of laminin and its receptor. Laminin is a glycoprotein of ~850 kd composed of three peptide chains. It is a prominent component of basement membranes, but is transiently expressed elsewhere. For example, laminin expression has been demonstrated along certain axonal tracts in the central (141) or peripheral (142) nervous system at a moment in development when axons pass through the area. It is the local expression of laminin combined with the expression of a 110 kDa laminin-binding protein on the migrating neuron that appears to direct migration of the pluripotential neural crest cell and in some cases to alter its phenotype. For example, in the gastrointestinal tract, the 110 kDa laminin-binding protein is not expressed by migrating neural crest-derived cells until they reach the gut, and at this point it appears to stimulate the development of a neuronal phenotype (reviewed in 115).

The observations related to laminin or a similar protein may be of direct relevance for development of neuronal manifestations of MEN-IIb and Hirschsprung's disease. Both are conditions in which there is disordered migration or differentiation of enteric neurons. One model of Hirschsprung's disease is the *ls/ls* mouse, in which the terminal segment of the gut is devoid of neuronal innervation, analogous to Hirschsprung's disease (143). There is compelling evidence that in this model system neural crest cells cannot migrate into the affected regions because of an accumulation of laminin and several other glycoproteins in the bowel wall, presumably preventing migration (144).

DERIVATION OF PARATHYROID CELLS

There is considerable evidence that the parathyroid glands are derived from cranial somites of the neural crest, which develop into mesoectoderm and contribute to the development of the third, fourth, and sixth branchial arches (145,146). Most of the information regarding migration and differentiation has been surmised from a series of experiments in which neural crest cells have been labeled and their migration determined (109) or by the identification of congenital abnormalities in which abnormalities of the parathyroid glands are associated with abnormalities of the great vessels or of immune function (Di George syndrome) (146,147). There is little information about specific molecular events that form the parathyroid glands and how a defect in the *ret* protooncogene might affect this development. At this point, any attempt to implicate *ret* in the development of parathyroid hyperplasia associated with MEN-IIa would be conjectural, although it seems likely that studies of *ret* function in parathyroid disease will be forthcoming.

CAN THE MARFANOID FEATURES OF MULTIPLE ENDOCRINE NEOPLASIA TYPE II BE RELATED TO NEURAL CREST DERIVATION?

One of the puzzling features of MEN-II has been the inclusion of Marfanoid features in the MEN-IIb variant (Table 2). Marfan syndrome has been associated with a defect in the fibrillin gene, located on chromosome 15 (148). One explanation for the developmental abnormalities in MEN-IIb lies in the neural crest origin of cartilage (121,149). It is known that pluripotential neural crest precursors form cartilaginous precursors. However, almost nothing is known about the signalling events that cause differentiation of the stem cell into a cell type terminally differentiated to produce collagen and other cartilaginous proteins. Several hypotheses could be advanced to explain the developmental abnormalities in MEN-IIb. The first is that the *ret* protooncogene is important for the development of the bony skeleton. A second hypothesis that could be advanced is that the defect in MEN-IIb is not restricted to the *ret* protooncogene and that a small deletion involves *ret* and a second gene important in cartilage development. Finally, it is possible that the peripheral nervous system, known to be abnormal in MEN-IIb, has a direct effect on skeletal development. All these possibilities will be directly testable in the near future and will undoubtedly add to current information about how Marfanoid features associated with MEN-IIb develop as well as to an understanding of skeletal development in general.

OTHER GENETIC ABNORMALITIES IN HEREDITARY OR SPORADIC TUMORS OF THE TYPE ASSOCIATED WITH MULTIPLE ENDOCRINE NEOPLASIA TYPE II

Multistep Model of Carcinogenesis

There is general agreement that the primary defect in MEN-II is an abnormality located at a centromeric chromosome 10 locus involving the *ret* protooncogene or other closely related genes. The consistent finding of abnormalities at other chromosomal loci, however, has suggested to most investigators that a single genetic abnormality is inadequate for transformation, and it is likely that mutational events at one or more of the loci mentioned below contribute to the transformed phenotype. The identification of the predisposition gene(s) at centromeric chromosome 10 will result in a refocusing of efforts to include these other loci and to define the causative genes.

Chromosome 1

A high percentage of MEN-II-associated tumors have a loss of heterozygosity on chromosome 1p (150). Mapping studies have further defined the region between D1S15 and D1Z22 (151). There is also evidence of a loss of heterozygosity in sporadic pheochromocytoma on 1p (152).

Chromosome 3

Studies by Taylor et al. (153) document frequent abnormalities of chromosome 3p in human and rat MTC cell lines. In addition, studies by Khosla et al. (152) in MTC and pheochromocytoma document loss of alleles on chromosome 3. Of interest is the recent identification of the predisposing tumor suppressor gene for Von Hippel-Lindau disease on chromosome 3p (154).

Chromosome 22

Reports from several sources provide evidence of a loss of heterozygosity on chromosome 22. Takai et al. (155) have reported a loss of heterozygosity in one of nine MTCs and two of five pheochromocytomas taken from MEN-II patients. Taylor et al. (153) have characterized two human and three rat MTC cell lines and found evidence for chromosome 22 abnormalities in all these cell lines. Finally, Khosla and coworkers (152) have demonstrated evidence for loss of alleles from chromosome 22q in 31% of pheochromocytomas.

HOW WILL MOLECULAR INFORMATION IMPACT ON THE MANAGEMENT OF PATIENTS WITH MULTIPLE ENDOCRINE NEOPLASIA TYPE 2?

The identification of specific molecular abnormalities of the *ret* protooncogene will have several immediate effects. It will be possible to identify gene carriers and to exclude unaffected individuals with 100% certainty by straightforward molecular techniques in families among whom a specific *ret* mutation has been identified. There is currently debate about what action should be taken in the event that a child carries a specific mutation of the *ret* gene. The author believes that thyroidectomy should be performed prior to age 4 years in children with a positive genetic test result. This recommendation is based on several observations. First, 90% of gene carriers will eventually develop MTC. Second, metastatic disease has been observed in children as young as 6 years of age (35,36). Third, early thyroidectomy eliminates the need for repetitive pentagastrin testing, a procedure families and physicians find unpleasant. Although the risks associated with surgery (hypoparathyroidism and recurrent laryngeal nerve damage) are real, the author has found no compelling evidence that the likelihood of these events is greater when surgery is performed at an early age by a competent surgeon. It seems unlikely that genetic testing will have any impact on the diagnosis and management of pheochromocytomas or hyperparathyroidism in this syndrome, since both are generally diagnosed and treated after identification of the thyroid lesion. Screening and management approaches for these manifestations have been outlined elsewhere (4).

Finally, the identification of specific mutations will permit the use of preimplantation screening techniques, making it possible for parents to eliminate the gene in their progeny by implantation of only nonaffected embryos (156). The techniques for this approach are evolving rapidly, although ethical considerations must be addressed by physicians and affected families.

Another important application of the identification of specific mutations will be to address the question of whether a patient with apparent sporadic MTC is, in fact, an *MEN-II* gene carrier. Since all forms of MEN-II have been linked to the same genetic locus, a compendium of genetic abnormalities of *ret* or other closely related genes will make it possible to exclude hereditary disease with a high degree of certainty.

In conclusion, the identification of a molecular defect in MEN-II will be a watershed event in the management of this interesting genetic syndrome. New questions will be asked and new directions plotted in our search for understanding of these interesting genetic syndromes.

REFERENCES

1. Sipple JH. The association of pheochromocytoma with carcinoma of the thyroid gland. *Am J Med* 1961;31:163–166.
2. Froboese C. Das aus markhaltigen Nervenfasern bestehende, ganglien-zelenlose, echte neurom in rankenform. Zugleich ein beitrag zu den nervosen geschwulsten der zunge und des augenlides. *Virchows Arch Pathol Anat* 1923;240:312–327.
3. Cance WG, Wells SA Jr. Multiple endocrine neoplasia type IIa. *Curr Probl Surg* 1985;22:1–56.
4. Gagel RF. Multiple endocrine neoplasia. In: Wilson JD and Foster DW, eds. *Williams textbook of endocrinology.* Philadelphia: WB Saunders, 1992;1537–1553.
5. Gagel RF, Robinson ML, Alford BR, Donovan DT. Medullary thyroid carcinoma: recent progress. *J Clin Endocrinol Metab* 1993;76:809–814.
6. de Bustros AC, Baylin SB. Medullary carcinoma of the thyroid. In: Braverman L and Utiger RD, eds. *The thyroid.* Philadelphia: JB Lippincott, 1993;1166–1183.
7. Steiner AL, Goodman AD, Powers SR. Study of a kindred with pheochromocytoma, medullary carcinoma, hyperparathyroidism and Cushing's disease: multiple endocrine neoplasia, type 2. *Medicine* 1968;47:371–409.
8. Telenius-Berg M, Berg B, Hamberger B, et al. Impact of screening on prognosis in the multiple endocrine neoplasia type 2 syndromes: natural history and treatment results in 105 patients. *Henry Ford Hosp Med J* 1984;32:225–231.
9. Williams ED, Pollock DJ. Multiple mucosal neuromata with endocrine tumours: a syndrome allied to Von Recklinghausen's disease. *J Pathol Bacteriol* 1966;91:71–80.
10. Farndon JR, Leight GS, Dilley WG, et al. Familial medullary thyroid carcinoma without associated endocrinopathies: a distinct clinical entity. *Br J Surg* 1986;73:278–281.
11. Nunziata V, Giannattasio R, di Giovanni G, D'Armiento MR, Mancini M. Hereditary localized pruritus in affected members of a kindred with multiple endocrine neoplasia type 2A (Sipple's syndrome). *Clin Endocrinol* 1989;30:57–63.
12. Gagel RF, Levy ML, Donovan DT, Alford BR, Wheeler T, Tschen JA. Multiple endocrine neoplasia type 2a associated with cutaneous lichen amyloidosis. *Ann Intern Med* 1989;111:802–806.
13. Verdy M, Weber AM, Roy CC, Morin CL, Cadotte M, Brochu P. Hirschsprung's disease in a family with multiple endocrine neoplasia type 2. *J Pediatr Gastroenterol Nutr* 1982;1:603–607.
14. Sipple JH. Multiple endocrine neoplasia type 2 syndromes: historical perspectives. *Henry Ford Hosp Med J* 1984;32:219–221.
15. Schimke RN, Hartmann WH. Familial amyloid-producing medullary thyroid carcinoma and pheochromocytoma: a distinct genetic entity. *Ann Intern Med* 1965;63:1027–1039.
16. Copp DH, Davidson AGF, Cheney BA. Evidence for a new parathyroid hormone which lowers blood calcium. *Proc Can Fed Biol Soc* 1961;4:17.
17. Hirsch PF, Gauthier GF, Munson PL. Thyroid hypocalcemic principle and recurrent laryngeal nerve injury as factors affecting the response to parathyroidectomy in rats. *Endocrinology* 1963;73:244–252.
18. Williams ED. Histogenesis of medullary carcinoma of the thyroid. *J Clin Pathol* 1966;19:114–118.
19. Melvin KEW, Tashjian AH Jr, Miller HH. Studies in familial (medullary) thyroid carcinoma. *Rec Progr Hormone Res* 1972;28:399–470.
20. Deftos LJ, Lee MR, Potts JT Jr. A radioimmunoassay for thyrocalcitonin. *Proc Natl Acad Sci USA* 1968;60:293–299.
21. Cooper CW, Deftos LJ, Potts JT Jr. Direct measurement of in vivo secretion of pig thyrocalcitonin by radioimmunoassay. *Endocrinology* 1971;88:747–754.
22. Hennessey JF, Gray TK, Cooper CW, Ontjes DA. Stimulation of thyrocalcitonin secretion by pentagastrin and calcium in 2 patients with medullary thyroid carcinoma of the thyroid. *J Clin Endocrinol Metab* 1973;36:200–203.

23. Hennessey JF, Wells SA, Ontjes DA, Cooper CW. A comparison of pentagastrin injections and calcium infusion as provacative agents for the detection of medullary carcinoma of the thyroid. *J Clin Endocrinol Metab* 1974;39: 487.

24. Melvin KEW, Miller HH, Tashjian AH Jr. Early diagnosis of medullary carcinoma of the thyroid gland by means of calcitonin assay. *N Engl J Med* 1971;285:1115–1120.

25. Wolfe HJ, Melvin KEW, Cervi-Skinner SJ, et al. C-cell hyperplasia preceding medullary thyroid carcinoma. *N Engl J Med* 1973;289:437–441.

26. Gagel RF, Melvin KE, Tashjian AH Jr, et al. Natural history of the familial medullary thyroid carcinoma-pheochromocytoma syndrome and the identification of preneoplastic stages by screening studies: a five-year report. *Trans Assoc Am Physicians* 1975;88:177–191.

27. Graze K, Spiler IJ, Tashjian AH Jr, et al. Natural history of familial medullary thyroid carcinoma: effect of a program for early diagnosis. *N Engl J Med* 1978;299:980–985.

28. Carney JA, Sizemore GW, Tyce GM. Bilateral adrenal medullary hyperplasia in multiple endocrine neoplasia, type 2: the precursor of bilateral pheochromocytoma. *Mayo Clin Proc* 1975;50:3–10.

29. DeLellis RA, Wolfe HJ, Gagel RF, et al. Adrenal medullary hyperplasia. A morphometric analysis in patients with familial medullary thyroid carcinoma. *Am J Pathol* 1976;83: 177–196.

30. Gagel RF, Tashjian AH Jr, Cummings T, et al. The clinical outcome of prospective screening for multiple endocrine neoplasia type 2a. An 18-year experience. *N Engl J Med* 1988;318:478–484.

31. Simpson NE, Kidd KK, Goodfellow PJ, et al. Assignment of multiple endocrine neoplasia type 2A to chromosome 10 by linkage. *Nature* 1987;328:528–530.

32. Mathew CG, Chin KS, Easton DF, et al. A linked genetic marker for multiple endocrine neoplasia type 2A on chromosome 10. *Nature* 1987;328:527–528.

33. Baylin SB, Gann DS, Hsu SH. Clonal origin of inherited medullary thyroid carcinoma and pheochromocytoma. *Science* 1976;193:321–323.

34. Gagel RF, Jackson CE, Block MA, et al. Age-related probability of development of hereditary medullary thyroid carcinoma. *J Pediatr* 1982;101:941–946.

35. Graham SM, Genel M, Touloukian RJ, Barwick KW, Gertner JM, Torony C. Provocative testing for occult medullary carcinoma of the thyroid: findings in seven children with multiple endocrine neoplasia type IIa. *J Pediatr Surg* 1987;22:501–503.

36. Telander RL, Zimmerman D, van Heerden JA, Sizemore GW. Results of early thyroidectomy for medullary thyroid carcinoma in children with multiple endocrine neoplasia type 2. *J Pediatr Surg* 1986;21:1190–1194.

37. Baylin SB, Beaven MA, Keiser HR, et al. Serum histaminase and calcitonin levels in medullary carcinoma of the thyroid. *Lancet* 1972;1:455–458.

38. Baylin SB, Beaven MA, Buja LM, et al. Histaminase activity: a biochemical marker for medullary carcinoma of the thyroid. *Am J Med* 1972;53:723–733.

39. Baylin SB, Mendelsohn G, Weisburger WR, et al. Levels of histaminase and L-dopa decarboxylase activity in the transition from C-cell hyperplasia to familial medullary thyroid carcinoma. *Cancer* 1979;44:1315–1321.

40. Baylin SB, Jackson RD, Goodwin G, Gazdar AF. Neuroendocrine-related biochemistry in the spectrum of human lung cancers. *Exp Lung Res* 1982;3:209–223.

41. Gagel R. Tumor markers of medullary thyroid carcinoma. In: Fishman W, ed. *Oncodevelopmental markers: Biologic, diagnostic and monitoring aspects*. New York: Academic Press, 1983;222–239.

42. Gagel RF, Palmer WN, Leonhart K, Chan L, Leong SS. Somatostatin production by a human medullary thyroid carcinoma cell line. *Endocrinology* 1986;118:1643–1651.

43. Cote GJ, Gagel RF. Dexamethasone differentially affects the levels of calcitonin and calcitonin gene-related peptide mRNAs expressed in a human medullary thyroid carcinoma cell line. *J Biol Chem* 1986;261:15524–15528.

44. Nelkin BD, Chen KY, de BA, Roos BA, Baylin SB. Changes in calcitonin gene RNA processing during growth of a human medullary thyroid carcinoma cell line. *Cancer Res* 1989.

45. Yang KP, Samaan NA, Liang Y, Castillo SG. Role of insulin-like growth factor-1 in the autocrine regulation of cell growth in TT human medullary thyroid carcinoma cells. *Henry Ford Hosp J* 1992;40:293–295.

46. Lamberts SW, Hofland LJ, van Koetsveld PM, et al. Parallel in vivo and in vitro detection of functional somatostatin receptors in human endocrine pancreatic tumors: consequences with regard to diagnosis, localization, and therapy. *J Clin Endocrinol Metab* 1990;71:566–574.

47. Reubi JC, Chayvialle JA, Franc B, Cohen R, Calmettes C, Modigliani E. Somatostatin receptors and somatostatin content in medullary thyroid carcinomas. *Lab Invest* 1991;64: 567–573.

48. Lamberts SW, Bakker WH, Reubi JC, Krenning EP. Somatostatin-receptor imaging in the localization of endocrine tumors. *N Engl J Med* 1990;323:1246–1249.

49. Livolsi VA. *Surgical pathology of the thyroid*. Philadelphia: WB Saunders, 1990.

50. Telenius-Berg M, Adolfsson L, Berg B, et al. Catecholamine release after physical exercise. A new provocative test for early diagnosis of pheochromocytoma in multiple endocrine neoplasia type 2. *Acta Med Scand* 1987;222:351–359.

51. Miyauchi A, Masuo K, Ogihara T, et al. Urinary epinephrine and norepinephrine excretion in patients with medullary thyroid carcinoma and their relatives. *Nippon Naibunpi Gakkai Zasshi* 1982;58:1505–1516.

52. Lips CJ, Minder WH, Leo JR, Alleman A, Hackeng WH. Evidence of multicentric origin of the multiple endocrine neoplasia syndrome type 2a (Sipple's syndrome) in a large family in The Netherlands. Diagnostic and therapeutic implications. *Am J Med* 1978;64:569–578.

53. Lips KJ, Van der Sluys Veer J, Struyvenberg A, et al. Bilateral occurrence of pheochromocytoma in patients with the multiple endocrine neoplasia syndrome type 2A (Sipple's syndrome). *Am J Med* 1981;70:1051–1060.

54. Bone HG, Deftos LJ, Snyder WH, Pak CYC. Mineral metabolic effects of thyroidectomy and long-term outcomes in a family with MEN 2A. *Henry Ford Hosp J* 1992;40:258–260.

55. Brandi ML, Aurbach GD, Fitzpatrick LA, et al. Parathyroid mitogenic activity in plasma from patients with familial multiple endocrine neoplasia type 1. *N Engl J Med* 1986;314: 1287–1293.

56. Marx SJ, Sakaguchi K, Green J III, Aurbach GD, Brandi ML. Mitogenic activity on parathyroid cells in plasma from members of a large kindred with multiple endocrine neoplasia type 1. *J Clin Endocrinol Metab* 1988;67:149–153.

57. Brandi ML, Zimering MB, Marx SJ, DeGrange D, Goldsmith P, Sakaguchi K, Aurbach GD. Multiple endocrine neoplasia type 1: Role of a circulating growth factor in parathyroid hyperplasia. In: Kleerekoper M and Krane S, eds. *Clinical disorders of bone and mineral metabolism*, New York: Mary Ann Liebert, 1989.

58. Brandi ML. A novel endothelial cell growth factor circulates in familial multiple endocrine neoplasia type 1. *Int J Rad Appl Instrum* 1990;17:639–643.

59. Keiser HR, Beaven MA, Doppman J, et al. Sipple's syndrome: medullary thyroid carcinoma, pheochromocytoma, and parathyroid disease. *Ann Intern Med* 1973;78:561–579.

60. Kousseff BG, Espinoza C, Zamore GA. Sipple syndrome with lichen amyloidosis as a paracrinopathy: pleiotropy, heterogeneity, or a contiguous gene? *J Am Acad Dermatol* 1991;25:651–657.

61. Robinson MF, Furst EJ, Nunziata V, et al. Characterization of the clinical features of five families with hereditary primary cutaneous lichen amyloidosis and multiple endocrine neoplasia type 2. *Hy Ford Hosp J* 1992;40:249–252.

62. Chabre O, Labat-Moleur F, Berthod F, et al. Cutaneous lesion associated with multiple endocrine neoplasia type 2A—an early clinical marker. *Presse Med* 1992;21:299–303.

63. Ferrer JP, Halperin I, Conget JI, et al. Primary localized cutaneous amyloidosis and familial medullary thyroid carcinoma. *Clin Endocrinol* 1991;34:435–439.

64. Ferrer JP, Halperin I, Palou J. Cutaneous lichen amyloidosis and familial medullary thyroid carcinoma [letter]. *Ann Intern Med* 1990;112:551–552.

65. Conri C, Ducloux G, Lagueny A, Kerrer M, Vital C. Polyneuropathy in type I multiple endocrine syndrome. *Presse Med* 1990;19:247–250.

66. Nunziata V, di Giovanni G, Lettera AM, D'Armiento M, Mancini M. Cutaneous lichen amyloidosis associated with multiple endocrine neoplasia type 2A. *Henry Ford Hosp J* 1989;37:144–146.

67. Yoneda K, Watanabe H, Yanagihara M, Mori S. Immunohistochemical staining properties of amyloids with anti-keratin antibodies using formalin-fixed, paraffin-embedded sections. *J Cutaneous Pathol* 1989;16:133–136.

68. Chabre O, Labat F, Pinel N, Berthod F, Tarel V, Bachelot I. Cutaneous lesion associated with multiple endocrine neoplasia type 2A: lichen amyloidosis or notalgia paresthetica. *Henry Ford Hosp J* 1992;40:245–248.

69. Robinson MF, Furst EJ, Nunziata V, et al. The multiple endocrine neoplasia type 2/cutaneous lichen amyloidosis syndrome-clinical features of a new variant. *Calcium Reg Bone Metab* (in press).

70. Carney JA, Go VL, Sizemore GW, Hayles AB. Alimentary-tract ganglioneuromatosis. A major component of the syndrome of multiple endocrine neoplasia, type 2b. *N Engl J Med* 1976;295:1287–1291.

71. Carney JA, Sizemore GW, Hayles AB. Multiple endocrine neoplasia, type 2b. *Pathobiol Annu* 1978;8:105–153.

72. Carney JA, Bianco AJJ, Sizemore GW, Hayles AB. Multiple endocrine neoplasia with skeletal manifestations. *J Bone Joint Surg [Am]* 1981;63:405–410.

73. Vasen HFA, van der Feltz M, Raue F, et al. The natural course of multiple endocrine neoplasia type IIb: a study of 18 cases. *Arch Intern Med* 1992;152:1250–1252.

74. Sizemore GW, Carney JA, Gharib H, Capen CC. Multiple endocrine neoplasia type 2B: eighteen-year follow-up of a four-generation family. *Henry Ford Hosp J* 1992;40:236–244.

75. Norum RA, Lafreniere RG, ONeal LW, et al. Linkage of the multiple endocrine neoplasia type 2B gene (MEN2B) to chromosome 10 markers linked to MEN2A. *Genomics* 1990;8:313–317.

76. Carney JA, Roth SI, Heath H III, Sizemore GW, Hayles AB. The parathyroid glands in multiple endocrine neoplasia type 2b. *Am J Pathol* 1980;99:387–398.

77. Sciubba JJ, DAmico E, Attie JN. The occurrence of multiple endocrine neoplasia type IIb, in two children of an affected mother. *J Oral Pathol* 1987;16:310–316.

78. Narod SA, Lavoue MF, Morgan K, et al. Genetic analysis of 24 French families with multiple endocrine neoplasia type 2A. *Am J Hum Genet* 1992;51:469–477.

79. Lairmore TC, Howe JR, Korte JA, et al. Familial medullary thyroid carcinoma and multiple endocrine neoplasia type 2B map to the same region of chromosome 10 as multiple endocrine neoplasia type 2A. *Genomics* 1991;9:181–192.

80. Robinson MF, Furst EJ, Nunziata V, et al. The multiple endocrine neoplasia type 2/cutaneous lichen amyloidosis syndrome is linked to the MEN 2 locus. Paper presented at *the Fourth International Workshop on Multiple Endocrine Neoplasia*, 1991.

81. Simpson NE. The exploration of the locus or loci for the syndromes associated with medullary thyroid cancer (MTC) on chromosome 10. In: Brandi and White R, eds. *Hereditary tumors*. New York: Raven Press, 1991;55–67.

82. Lairmore TC, Dou S, Howe JR, et al. A 1.5-megabase yeast artificial chromosome contig from human chromosome 10q11.2 connecting three genetic loci (RET, D10S94, and D10S102) closely linked to the MEN2A locus. *Proc Natl Acad Sci USA* 1993;90:492–496.

83. Gardner E, Papi L, Easton DF, et al. Genetic linkage studies map the multiple endocrine neoplasia type 2 loci to a small interval on chromosome 10q11.2. *Hum Mol Genet* 1993;2:241–246.

84. Mole SE, Mulligan LM, Healey CS, Ponder BAJ, Tunnacliffe A. Localisation of the gene for multiple endocrine neoplasia type 2A to a 480 kb region in chromosome band 10q11.2. *Hum Mol Genet* 1993;2:247–252.

85. Takahashi M, Buma Y, Iwamoto T, Inaguma Y, Ikeda H, Hiai H. Cloning and expression of the ret proto-oncogene encoding a tyrosine kinase with two potential transmembrane domains. *Oncogene* 1988;3:571–578.

86. Iwamoto T, Taniguchi M, Asai N, Ohkusu K, Nakashima I, Takahashi M. cDNA cloning of mouse ret proto-oncogene and its sequence similarity to the cadherin superfamily. *Oncogene* 1993;8:1087–1091.

87. Tahira T, Ishizaka Y, Itoh F, Sugimura T, Nagao M. Characterization of ret proto-oncogene mRNAs encoding two isoforms of the protein product in a human neuroblastoma cell line. *Oncogene* 1990;5:97–102.

88. Rozakis-Adcock M, Fernley R, Wade J, Pawson T, Bowtell D. The SH2 and SH3 domains of mammalian Grb2 couple the EGF receptor to the Ras activator mSos1. *Nature* 1993;363:83–85.

89. Egan SE, Giddings BW, Brooks MW, Buday L, Sizeland AM, Weinberg RA. Association of Sos Ras exchange protein with Grb2 is implicated in tyrosine kinase signal transduction and transformation. *Nature* 1993;363:45–51.

90. Zajac JD, Penschow J, Mason T, Tregear C, Coghlan J, Martin TJ. Identification of calcitonin and calcitonin gene-related peptide messenger ribonucleic acid in medullary thyroid carcinomas by hybridization histochemistry. *J Clin Endocrinol Metab* 1986;62:1037–1043.

91. Zaniewski M, Jordan PH Jr, Yip B, Thornby JI, Mallette LE. Serum gastrin level is increased by chronic hypercalcemia of parathyroid or nonparathyroid origin. *Arch Intern Med* 1986;146:478–482.

92. Tortella BJ, Matthews JB, Antonioli DA, Dvorak AM, Silen W. Gastric autonomic nerve (GAN) tumor and extra-adrenal paraganglioma in Carney's triad. A common origin. *Ann Surg* 1987;205:221–225.

93. Mannelli M, Maggi M, DeFeo ML, et al. Opioid modulation of normal and pathological human chromaffin tissue. *J Clin Endocrinol Metab* 1986;62:577–582.

94. Hadden DR, OReilly F, Kennedy L, Russell C. Multiple endocrine neoplasia type 2A: a Northern Ireland and Australian family. *Henry Ford Hosp Med J* 1987;35:107–109.

95. Grieco M, Santoro M, Berlingieri MT, et al. PTC is a novel rearranged form of the ret proto-oncogene and is frequently detected in vivo in human thyroid papillary carcinomas. *Cell* 1990;60:557–563.

96. Bongarzone I, Pierotti MA, Monzini N, et al. High frequency of activation of tyrosine kinase oncogenes in human papillary thyroid carcinoma. *Oncogene* 1989;4:1457–1462.

97. Donghi R, Sozzi G, Pierotti MA, et al. The oncogene associated with human papillary thyroid carcinoma (PTC) is assigned to chromosome 10 q11–q12 in the same region as multiple endocrine neoplasia type 2A (MEN2A). *Oncogene* 1989;4:521–523.

98. Pierotti MA, Santoro M, Jenkins RB, et al. Characterization of an inversion on the long arm of chromosome 10 juxtaposing D10S170 and RET and creating the oncogenic sequence RET/PTC. *Proc Natl Acad Sci USA* 1992;89:1616–1620.

99. Ishizaka Y, Ochiai M, Tahira T, Sugimura T, Nagao M. Activation of the ret-II oncogene without a sequence encoding a transmembrane domain and transforming activity of two ret-II oncogene products differing in carboxy-termini due to alternative splicing [published erratum appears in *Oncogene* 1989;4:1415]. *Oncogene* 1989;4:789–794.

100. Kunieda T, Matsui M, Nomura N, Ishizaki R. Cloning of an activated human ret gene with a novel 5′ sequence fused by DNA rearrangement. *Gene* 1991;107:323–328.

101. Santoro M, Rosati R, Grieco M, et al. The ret proto-oncogene is consistently expressed in human pheochromocytomas and thyroid medullary carcinomas. *Oncogene* 1990;5:1595–1598.

102. Miya A, Yamamoto M, Morimoto H, et al. Expression of the ret proto-oncogene in human medullary thyroid carcinomas

and pheochromocytomas of MEN 2A. *Henry Ford Hosp Med J* 1992;40:215–219.

103. Donis-Keller H, Shenshen D, Chi D, et al. Mutations in the RET proto-oncogene are associated with MEN2A and FMTC. *Hum Mol Genet* 1993;2:851–856.

104. Mulligan LM, Kwok JBJ, Healey CS, et al. Germline mutations of the RET proto-oncogene in multiple endocrine neoplasia type 2A (MEN 2A). *Nature* 1993;363:458–460.

105. Coulier F, Kumar R, Ernst M, Klein R, Martin-Zanca D, Barbacid M. Human trk oncogenes activated by point mutation, in-frame deletion, and duplication of the tyrosine kinase domain. *Mol Cel Biol* 1990;10:4202–4210.

106. Roussel MF, Downing JR, Rettenmier CW, Sherr CJ. A point mutation in the extracellular domain of the human CSF-1 receptor (c-fms oncogene product) activates its transforming potential. *Cell* 1988;55:979–988.

107. Itoh F, Ishizaka Y, Tahira T, et al. Identification and analysis of the ret proto-oncogene promoter region in neuroblastoma cell lines and medullary thyroid carcinomas from MEN2A patients. *Oncogene* 1992;7:1201–1206.

108. McDonald H, Smailus D, Jenkins H, Adams K, Simpson NE, Goodfellow PJ. Identification and characterization of a gene at D10S94 in the MEN2A region. *Genomics* 1992;13:344–348.

109. Le Douarin N. *The neural crest*. Cambridge: Cambridge University Press, 1982.

110. Chisaka O, Capecchi MR. Regionally restricted developmental defects resulting from targeted disruption of the mouse homeobox gene hox-1.5. *Nature* 1991;350:473–479.

111. Chisaka O, Musci TS, Capecchi MR. Developmental defects of the cranial nerves and hindbrain resulting from targeted disruption of the mouse homeobox gene Hox-1.6. *Nature* 1992;355:516–520.

112. Bronner-Fraser M. Environmental influences on neural crest cell migration. *J Neurobiol* 1993;24:233–247.

113. Ragsdale C, Woodgett J. *trk*ing neurotrophic receptors. *Nature* 1991;350:660–661.

114. Barbacid M. The *Trk* family of neurotropin receptors: molecular characterization and oncogenic activation in human tumors. In: Levine AJ and Schmidek HH, eds. *Molecular genetics of nervous system tumors*. New York: Wiley-Liss, 1993;123–136.

115. Gershon MD, Chalazonitis A, Rothman TP. From neural crest to bowel: development of the enteric nervous system. *J Neurobiol* 1993;24:199–214.

116. Sassoon D, Lyons G, Wright WE, et al. Expression of two myogenic regulatory factors myogenin and MyoD1 during mouse embryogenesis. *Nature* 1989;341:303–307.

117. Lassar AB, Buskin JN, Lockshon D, Davis RL, Alpone S, Hauschka SD, Weintraub H. Myo D is a sequence specific DNA binding protein requiring a region of myc homology to bind to the murine creatine kinase enhancer. *Cell* 1989;58:823–831.

118. Johnson JE, Birren SJ, Anderson DJ. Two rat homologues of Drosophila achaete-scute specifically expressed in neuronal precursors. *Nature* 1990;346:858–861.

119. Le Douarin N, Le Lievre C. Demonstration de l'origine neurales des cellules a calcitonine du corps ultimobranchial chez l'embryon de poulet. *CR Acad Sci* 1970;270:2857–2860.

120. Le Douarin NM. Cell line segregation during peripheral nervous system ontogeny. *Science* 1986;231:1515–1522.

121. Le Douarin NM, Dupin E. Cell lineage analysis in neural crest ontogeny. *J Neurobiol* 1993;24:146–161.

122. Anderson DJ. Cell fate determination in the peripheral nervous system: the sympathoadrenal progenitor. *J Neurobiol* 1993;24:185–214.

123. Takahashi M, Cooper GM. ret Transforming gene encodes a fusion protein homologous to tyrosine kinases. *Mol Cell Biol* 1987;7:1378–1385.

124. Tomlinson A, Bowtell DDL, Hafen E, Rubin GM. Localization of the *sevenless* protein, a putative receptor for positional information, in the eye imaginal disc of *Drosophila*. *Cell* 1987;51:143–150.

125. Basler K, Christen B, Hafen E. Ligand-independent activation of the sevenless receptor tyrosine kinase changes the fate of cells in the developing *Drosophila* eye. *Cell* 1991;64:728–739.

126. Taniguchi M, Iwamoto T, Nakashima I, et al. Establishment and characterization of a malignant melanocytic tumor cell line expressing the ret oncogene. *Oncogene* 1992;7:1491–1496.

127. Iwamoto T, Takahashi M, Ohbayashi M, Nakashima I. The ret oncogene can induce melanogenesis and melanocyte development in Wv/Wv mice. *Exp Cell Res* 1992;200:410–415.

128. Iwamoto T, Takahashi M, Ito M, et al. Aberrant melanogenesis and melanocytic tumour development in transgenic mice that carry a metallothionein/ret fusion gene. *EMBO J* 1991;10:3167–3175.

129. Takahashi M, Iwamoto T, Nakashima I. Proliferation and neoplastic transformation of pigment cells in metallothionein/ret transgenic mice. *Pigment Cell Res* 1992;5:344–347.

130. Ghysen A, Dambly-Chaudiere C. From DNA to form: the *achaete-scute* complex. *Genes Dev* 1988;2:495–501.

131. de Bustros A, Lee RY, Compton D, Tsong TY, Baylin SB, Nelkin BD. Differential utilization of calcitonin gene regulatory DNA sequences in cultured lines of medullary thyroid carcinoma and small-cell lung carcinoma. *Mol Cell Biol* 1990;10:1773–1778.

132. Peleg S, Abruzzese RV, Cote GJ, Gagel RF. Transcription of the human calcitonin gene is mediated by a C cell-specific enhancer containing E-box-like elements. *Mol Endocrinol* 1990;4:1750–1757.

133. Ruppert JM, Eggleston JC, de Bustros A, Baylin SB. Disseminated calcitonin-poor medullary thyroid carcinoma in a patient with calcitonin-rich primary tumor. *Am J Surg Pathol* 1986;10:513–518.

134. Nakagawa T, Mabry M, de Bustros A, Ihle JN, Nelkin BD, Baylin SB. Introduction of v-Ha-ras oncogene induces differentiation of cultured human medullary thyroid carcinoma cells. *Proc Natl Acad Sci USA* 1987;84:5923–5927.

135. Nakagawa T, Nelkin BD, Baylin SB, de Bustros A. Transcriptional and posttranscriptional modulation of calcitonin gene expression by sodium n-butyrate in cultured human medullary thyroid carcinoma. *Cancer Res* 1988;48:2096–2100.

136. Nelkin BD, Borges M, Mabry M, Baylin SB. Transcription factor levels in medullary thyroid carcinoma cells differentiated by Harvey ras oncogene: c-jun is increased. *Biochem Biophys Res Commun* 1990;170:140–146.

137. Ball DW, Diamond L, Borges M, Baylin SB, Nelkin BD. A basic helix–loop–helix protein enhances human calcitonin gene expression. *Program of the 75th Annual Meeting of the Endocrine Society, Las Vegas, NV, June 9–12, 1993, abstract 1260,* 1993.

138. Lo LC, Johnson JE, Wuenschell CW, Saito T, Anderson DJ. Mammalian achaete-scute homolog 1 is transiently expressed by spatially restricted subsets of early neuroepithelial and neural crest cells. *Genes Dev* 1991;5:1524–1537.

139. Martucciello EA. Chromosome 10 deletion in Hirschsprung's disease. *Pediatr Surg Int* 1992;7:308–310.

140. Yin L, Ceccherini I, Hofstra MW, et al. Linkage studies in two swiss pedigrees and physical mapping assign a recently localized Hirschsprung's gene to the interval between RBP3 and a breakpoint in 10q11.2 (abstract). *Proceedings of a Workshop on Hirschsprung's Disease* (in press).

141. Cohen J, Burke JF, McKinlay C. The role of laminin and the laminin/fibronectin receptor complex in the outgrowth of retinal ganglion cell axons. *Dev Biol* 1987;122:407–418.

142. Rogers SL, Edson KJ, Letourneau PC. Distribution of laminin in the developing peripheral nervous system of the chick. *Dev Biol* 1986;113:429–435.

143. Lane PW. Association of megacolon with two recessive spotting genes in the mouse. *J Hered* 1966;57:29–31.

144. Payette RF, Tennyson VM, Pomeranz HD, Pham TD, Rothman TP, Gershon MD. Accumulation of components of basal laminae: association with the failure of neural crest cells to colonize the presumptive aganglionic bowel of *ls/ls* mutant mice. *Dev Biol* 1988;125:341–360.

145. Merida-Velasco JA. Experimental study of the origin of the parathyroid glands. *Acta Anat* 1991;141:163–169.

146. Le Lievre CS, Le Douaarin NM. Mesenchymal derivatives of the neural crest: analysis of chimaeric quail and chick embryos. *J Embryol* 1975;34:125–154.

147. Couly G, Lagrue A, Griscelli C. Di George syndrome, exemplary rhomboencephalic neurocristopathy. *Rev Stomatol Chir Maxillofac* 1983;84:103–108.

148. Kainulainen K, Pulkkinen L, Savolainen A, Kaitila I, Peltonen L. Location on chromosome 15 of the gene defect causing Marfan syndrome. *N Engl J Med* 1990;323:935–939.

149. Couly GF, Coltey PM, Le Douarin NM. The triple origin of the skull in higher vertebrates: a study in quail-chick chimeras. *Development* 1993;117:409–429.

150. Mathew CG, Smith BA, Thorpe K, et al. Deletion of genes on chromosome 1 in endocrine neoplasia. *Nature* 1987;328:524–526.

151. Moley JF, Brother MB, Fong CT, et al. Consistent association of 1p loss of heterozygosity with pheochromocytomas from patients with multiple endocrine neoplasia type 2 syndromes. *Cancer Res* 1992;52:770–774.

152. Khosla S, Patel VM, Hay ID, et al. Loss of heterozygosity suggests multiple genetic alterations in pheochromocytomas and medullary thyroid carcinomas. *J Clin Invest* 1991;87:1691–1699.

153. Taylor LD, Elder FB, Knuth A, Gagel RF. Cytogenetic characterization of two human and three rat medullary thyroid carcinoma cell lines (abstract). *Henry Ford Hosp Med J* 1989;37:207.

154. Latif F, Kalman T, Gnarra J, et al. Identification of the von Hippel-Lindau disease tumor suppressor gene. *Science* 1993;260:1317–1320.

155. Takai S, Tateishi H, Nishisho I, et al. Loss of genes on chromosome 22 in medullary thyroid carcinoma and pheochromocytoma. *Jpn J Cancer Res* 1987;78:894–898.

156. Handyside AH, Lesko JG, Winston RM, Hughes MR. Birth of a normal girl after in vitro fertilization and preimplantation diagnostic testing for cystic fibrosis. *N Engl J Med* 1992;32:905–909.

The Parathyroids, edited by J.P. Bilezikian, M.A. Levine, and R. Marcus. Raven Press, Ltd., New York © 1994.

CHAPTER 40

Familial Hypocalciuric Hypercalcemia

David A. Heath

In 1966 Jackson and Boonstra (1) described a patient with hypercalcemia who on neck exploration was found to have hyperplasia of all four parathyroid glands. Following removal of three and one-half glands, the serum calcium fell, but not to normal. Subsequent investigations of the family revealed 17 other hypercalcemic individuals in three generations, with an inheritance pattern suggestive of an autosomal dominant disorder. Two subjects underwent neck surgery at which four gland hyperplasia was found; following the removal of two and three and one-half glands, their serum calcium levels remained elevated. Serum parathyroid hormone (PTH) concentrations were normal in eight of nine patients and were questionably elevated in the ninth. None of the patients had any symptoms or complications of hyperparathyroidism. The authors suggested that this might be a new inherited condition to be distinguished from familial hyperparathyroidism.

In 1972 Foley et al. (2) described a condition which they termed *familial benign hypercalcemia* (FBH). The proband was a 5-year-old boy who presented with headaches and was found to be hypercalcemic. Exploration of the neck and anterior mediastinum led to the removal of three normal parathyroid glands; the fourth was not removed. Surgery did not correct the hypercalcemia. Eleven hypercalcemic individuals were then discovered in four generations of the family, all of whom were asymptomatic. Other studies revealed the proband to have persistent hypocalciuria, and the PTH concentrations in the hypercalcemic family members were all within the normal range. The authors stressed the apparently benign nature of the condition and wondered whether hypocalciuria might be a characteristic hallmark. They also suggested that a primary excess of PTH secretion was an unlikely explanation for the

disorder suggesting rather that an altered parathyroid calcium set point was a more likely explanation.

In 1977 Marx and his colleagues (3) published the first of a series of articles from the National Institutes of Health delineating the condition they called *familial hypocalciuric hypercalcemia* (FHH). In this article, the authors specifically investigated the families of index patients with hypercalcemia who had been found to have primary parathyroid hyperplasia on neck surgery. In investigating 25 index patients, they discovered other hypercalcemic family members in 13 cases. Two index patients were part of large kindreds with FHH, four were members of families with multiple endocrine neoplasia type I (MEN-I), and seven kindreds were too small to allow definite classification. The authors reported FHH to be a condition distinct from MEN-I, with a better prognosis but a poor response to parathyroidectomy. This poor response to parathyroidectomy meant that, even after extensive parathyroid surgery, normocalcemia was rare and persistent hypercalcemia common. In reviewing 67 cases referred to the National Institutes of Health (NIH) because of failed parathyroid surgery, Marx et al. (4) subsequently showed that six were index cases of new FHH families. In fact it is likely that virtually all cases of FHH or FBH diagnosed prior to the late 1970s had initially been erroneously diagnosed as primary hyperparathyroidism and patients had undergone an unsuccessful parathyroidectomy.

By 1981 the NIH group had studied in detail 15 kindreds with FHH. Their studies (5) confirmed the benign nature of the condition, which had an autosomal dominant inheritance pattern with nearly 100% penetrance. They identified a number of mild symptoms that they thought were more common in FHH and two possible rare but serious complications, acute pancreatitis and severe neonatal hyperparathyroidism.

Also in 1981 Jackson and Kleerekoper (6) restudied the family reported in 1966 by Jackson and Boonstra

D. A. Heath: Department of Medicine, Selly Oak Hospital, Birmingham B15 2TH United Kingdom.

(1) and confirmed the presence of FHH, thus making this the first well documented family. In addition to the large series studied at the NIH, investigators at the Mayo Clinic began to collect a series of families and in 1985 reported 125 cases of FBH among 21 families (7). By 1989, an additional ten new families with >30 more affected individuals had been discovered (8). The studies from the Mayo Clinic confirmed the previous clinical observations made at the NIH. The two groups have continued to use two different terms (FBH and FHH) for what is clearly the same condition. Neither term is completely satisfactory. Although the condition is usually benign, there are very rare serious complications, and, while hypocalciuria is usual, it is not invariable. The author's preferred term is *familial benign hypercalcemia* but in the remainder of this chapter the term *familial hypocalciuric hypercalcemia* is used in deference to Dr. Gerald Aurbach, whose group introduced this name.

PRESENTATION

Until the introduction of multichannel autoanalyzers in the late 1960s, serum calcium measurements were not routinely performed and were restricted to patients suffering from bone diseases and renal problems, especially renal stones. As a result, primary hyperparathyroidism was discovered most commonly among those with skeletal and renal complications. With the advent of the autoanalyzer, serum calcium measurements became a routine laboratory test, leading to the discovery of many patients with primary hyperparathyroidism who had no overt complications of the disease (9). When hyperparathyroidism was thought to be commonly complicated by bone disease and renal stones, it was reasonable to recommend the only effective cure of the condition—parathyroidectomy—for all patients with the disease. The recognition of mild or asymptomatic cases of hyperparathyroidism initially was associated with the view that complications were likely to develop in the future and that treatment of the condition in its asymptomatic phase was to be recommended. This was the background leading to the recognition of FHH. Initial cases were misdiagnosed as primary hyperparathyroidism and referred for parathyroidectomy, which was invariably unsuccessful. Because the majority of patients with renal stones, peptic ulcer, pancreatitis, and so on, do not have primary hyperparathyroidism, it was inevitable that occasional patients with FHH would be reported to have complications associated with primary hyperparathyroidism. However, it is rather the fact that patients with FHH have few if any symptoms. In the initial review of families seen at the NIH, it was reported that fatigue, weakness, mental problems, headaches, arthralgia, polydipsia, and polyuria were more common

in FHH (5). Subsequent studies have not confirmed this. Menko et al. (10) found that these symptoms were no more common in affected patients than in a control group. Law and Heath (7) found that these symptoms were more common in the proband but not in affected members discovered by screening. Our own studies in a very large family with over 50 affected members have also failed to identify any symptoms that are more common in affected family members (11). Other reports of families with multiple affected members also stress that symptoms of hypercalcemia are no more common in the hypercalcemic than in the normocalcemic family members (12–14). The cardinal feature of FHH is therefore asymptomatic hypercalcemia.

Associated diseases are also uncommon in FHH. In the NIH series (5) adult-onset diabetes mellitus, symptomatic thyroid disease, cardiovascular disease, and pulmonary disease were observed in three or more hypercalcemic subjects. However, there was insufficient evidence to implicate FHH in any of these disorders. There was a 36% prevalence of articular chondrocalcinosis in hypercalcemic members over the age of 47 years, which is higher than that in previous reports of healthy subjects aged 60–80 years (15). Pancreatitis was noted in three hypercalcemic members, and several neonates in one family suffered severe primary hyperparathyroidism. The association of FHH with these last two conditions is considered in detail below.

In the studies of Law and Heath (7), 27 medical problems were sought in affected and unaffected family members. In index cases arthritis, gallstones, and arterial hypertension were significantly more common in affected members. However, in those cases found by family screening, only gallstones were more frequent in hypercalcemic members. In the four families studied by Toss et al. (14), several affected individuals had diabetes and pituitary insufficiency, and there were isolated cases of hypertension and nephrolithiasis, but no condition occurred significantly more frequently than would be expected by chance. Auwerx et al. (12) reported a family with FHH among whom there was an associated interstitial lung disease and disturbed host defense mechanisms expressed as granulocyte dysfunction.

PANCREATITIS AND FAMILIAL HYPOCALCIURIC HYPERCALCEMIA

Marx et al. (5) noted pancreatitis in three hypercalcemic family members from 15 separate families with over 121 affected subjects. Davies et al. (16) reported three patients with pancreatitis among the four families with 17 affected members. Other cases of pancreatitis in patients with FHH have been reported by Doumith et al. (17), Damoiseaux et al. (18), Stuckey et al. (19), and Toss et al. (13). Although other large kindreds have been studied among whom no examples of pancreatitis were identified, especially the 155 cases from 31 families studied at the Mayo Clinic (8), it is now accepted by some that pancreatitis is a definite but rare complication of FHH (20,21). Many cases of pancreatitis were recurrent and life threatening, leading to the unusual recommendations of total parathyroidectomy when this rare complication presents in this way (21). Stuckey et al. (22) reviewed the ten reported cases of pancreatitis occurring in patients with FHH. The authors were able to identify other possible causes of pancreatitis, such as alcoholism and gallstones, in seven cases; in one case no additional history was available, and in only two cases were no other etiological factors present. This result led the authors to conclude that a causal link between the two conditions was actually unlikely. An additional factor that argues against an association is that most if not all the cases of pancreatitis reported with FHH occurred in the index patient. Pancreatitis virtually always initiates the measurement of the serum calcium, which can lead to the false association of pancreatitis with a condition that otherwise appears to be asymptomatic. It therefore appears likely that the previously reported association between pancreatitis and FHH is a chance association and that hypercalcemia plays no etiological part in the pancreatic disorder. If this conclusion is accepted, then the previous advice to consider total parathyroidectomy (20) in such patients should be reconsidered, especially in light of the fact that normocalcemia is rarely achieved (13).

NEONATAL HYPERPARATHYROIDISM AND FAMILIAL HYPOCALCIURIC HYPERCALCEMIA

In the NIH review of their 15 families with FHH it was noted that three patients from two families had had severe primary hyperparathyroidism in the neonatal period associated with hypotonia, respiratory distress, and skeletal undermineralization (5). The following year, a detailed report of four cases from three families appeared (23). Primary hyperparathyroidism is a very rare condition in childhood and appears to be different in very young children from the case in older children. In 1967, Muhlethaler et al. (24) noted that, in all reported cases of neonatal hyperparathyroidism, multiglandular parathyroid hyperplasia was present rather than a single parathyroid adenoma. Rajasuriya et al. (25) reviewed 11 cases of parathyroid adenomata in childhood. The youngest reported patient was aged 7 years, with the rest ranging in age between 10 and 17 years. Neonatal primary hyperparathyroidism can be defined in children under age 6 months who have symptomatic hypercalcemia with hyperparathyroid bone disease. At least 49 cases have been reported (23,24,26–65). In 41 cases in which parathyroid tissue was removed either at surgery or postmortem, multi-

ple parathyroid glands were affected by parathyroid hyperplasia. Not one case of a parathyroid adenoma was noted.

Initial reports of siblings with neonatal hyperparathyroidism (24,32,37) raised the possibility that the condition could be inherited as an autosomal recessive condition; the parents of at least two of the families were reported to have a normal total serum calcium, whereas, in the other report, the parents' calcium was unknown (32). In 1977 Spiegel et al. (44) reported a case previously published by Garcia-Banniel et al. (40) in which the hypercalcemia was clearly inherited in an autosomal dominant manner. At the time, the family was also thought to have familial hyperparathyroidism, although this diagnosis was revised later to FHH (23). It now seems likely that, in the neonate with hypercalcemia, the familial syndrome will be FHH rather than familial hyperparathyroidism. If the condition is inherited as an autosomal dominant condition with high penetrance, then one of the parents should be hypercalcemic. In the 41 reported families, both parents have been tested in 23 cases, and in 15 at least one parent was found to be hypercalcemic, and in three instances, both parents were abnormal (23,55,56). Other studies since 1982 place the estimate of cases of neonatal hyperparathyroidism in families with FHH at closer to 75%. It is clear that neonatal primary hyperparathyroidism is a real but rare complication of FHH, perhaps the only one. In that the reported cases of neonatal hyperparathyroidism appear to be similar whether they occur within the setting of FHH or not, the clinical features of neonatal hyperparathyroidism discussed herein are taken from all the 49 reported cases.

With few exceptions, symptoms and signs are noted either at birth or within the first week of life. These commonly include failure to thrive, anorexia, constipation, hypotonia, and respiratory distress. Physical examination usually reveals prominent hypotonia. A number of children have been described with a very narrow or deformed chest (23,43–46,48,50,51). Craniotabes has been found in three (23,43,54). Other congenital abnormalities include dysmorphic facial features (31,36,48,65) and anovaginal and rectovaginal fistulas (40,41). Skeletal radiographs have shown striking demineralization, fractured ribs and long bones, subperiosteal erosions especially of the long bones, and widening of the metaphyses. The changes of rickets are occasionally present as well (48).

Hypercalcemia is found in all cases, often to an extreme degree. The highest reported serum calcium concentration appears to be 30.8 mg/dl (7.7 mmol/liter (35). The hypercalcemia has been elevated, with one exception (65), when first measured, often rising to extremely high levels in subsequent days or weeks. Early reported cases that were managed conservatively had a very high mortality, whereas patients who underwent emergency parathyroidectomy had a much better prognosis. Surgery was withheld in some babies thought to be too ill for surgery. Table 1 compares the degree of hypercalcemia and the outcome of medical and surgical treatment in cases reported before and after 1982. It can be seen that prior to 1982 the average highest serum calcium was 19.8 mg/100 ml (4.95 mmol/liter). There was no difference between the calcium levels of survivors compared to that in those who died. The patients who underwent parathyroidectomy had a very much better outcome. Since 1982, the degree of hypercalcemia has been significantly lower. There are probably a number of reasons for this, more accurate measurements of calcium, better methods for controlling hypercalcemia medically, and employing surgery at an earlier stage. The most dramatic change is that patients managed conservatively have had an excellent outcome. Of the 24 infants reported since 1982, only two have died, both following surgery (23,57). In one of these cases (23) the surgery was performed in the 1950s, so that, for cases actually managed in the past 10–15 years, the prognosis has been very good. The patients managed medically had a significantly milder degree of hypercalcemia.

The response to parathyroidectomy was similar in most of the reported cases in that, unless the infant was rendered permanently hypoparathyroid, the serum calcium concentration usually fell only transiently before rising again. Even when four parathyroid glands were found and removed, the hypercalcemia was not always cured.

The clinical state of the child has often improved dramatically after surgery, and there has usually been a rapid healing of the profound radiological changes even when the hypercalcemia was not cured. Similar radiological healing has been seen in patients managed conservatively (62,63,65), suggesting that the healing process, at least in part, occurs in the natural evolution of the condition.

In family studies of FHH, groups of children at all ages exhibit the expected number of hypercalcemic cases for a dominantly inherited condition. Children born to affected parents have been shown to be hypercalcemic within 2 hr of birth, suggesting that hypercalcemia is expressed at least from birth. Among the families studied, there appears to be no obvious increase in neonatal mortality. This means that the vast majority of affected neonates have no obvious clinical expression of the disorder in early life, and thus it does not require treatment. Whether such asymptomatic cases have radiological or histological evidence of parathyroid bone disease that spontaneously heals is not known, and it would be hard on ethical grounds to justify investigation of such cases.

Why severe symptomatic disease occurs in a small minority of cases is currently unclear. One obvious possibility is that these cases represent homozygous forms of the disease. Marx and his colleagues (66) have restudied a family previously reported by Hillman et al. (32), among whom two children had severe neonatal hyperparathyroidism and the consanguineous parents had normal total serum calcium concentrations. The new studies demonstrated that multiple family members had very mild and sometimes intermittent hypercalcemia and that the parents of the affected children, while still having normal total serum calcium levels, showed mild but definite elevations in ionized calcium activity together with hypocalciuria. It is very tempting to conclude that presumed heterozygotes in this family had mild hypercalcemia and that probable homozygotes, the affected neonates, had severe hypercalcemia. The other implication of this family study is that normal total serum calcium concentrations in the parents do not exclude FHH. Hence some or all of the previously reported families among whom the parents were normocalcemic could have had the inherited condition.

Among the families so far reported, consanguineous parents are known in six instances (32,35,56,59–61). In these cases, both parents are known to be affected or hypercalcemic in only two (32,61) or three (56). In one additional family, the parents were not known to be

TABLE 1. *Hypercalcemic severity and outcome in reported cases of familial hypocalciuric hypercalcemia*

	Pre-1982		1982 and after	
	mg/100 ml	mmol/liter	mg/100 ml	mmol/liter
Serum calcium[a]	19.8	4.95	14.6	3.65
In survivors	19.7	4.93	14.7	3.68
In nonsurvivors	20.0	5.00	14.0	3.50
Surgical management	20.9	5.23	15.6	3.90
Conservative management	17.9	4.48	12.7	3.18
Survival				
Surgical management (%)	73.3		88	
Conservative management (%)	12.5		100	

[a]Highest total serum calcium reported in the publication.

consanguineous but both were hypercalcemic (55). The father was shown to have FHH, but the mother was assumed (but not proved) to have primary hyperparathyroidism.

Marx et al. (23) put forward other possible explanations. One is that, if the expectant mother is normocalcemic and the fetus hypercalcemic, the tendency of the normal fetus to have a serum calcium level higher than that of the mother could be exaggerated, causing severe hypercalcemia in the fetus. Such a hypothesis would predict a preponderance of normocalcemic mothers and hypercalcemic fathers in affected families, but this does not appear to be the case. A third possible explanation is that severe neonatal hyperparathyroidism is one end of a clinical spectrum in the same way that severe clinical bone disease is a rare but recognized complication of primary hyperparathyroidism in adults.

There is definite evidence of a hyperparathyroid state in these neonates. The parathyroid glands are very much larger than normal for an infant, often described as being ten times normal size. Histology shows chief cell or water-clear cell hyperplasia. When it has been measured, the serum PTH concentration has been clearly elevated (23,44,46,50–58,60,61, 63,64), except in one case when it was within the normal range (65). In addition radiological and histological evidence of hyperparathyroidism has been seen. These findings are in contradistinction to those in the typical case of FHH, where unequivocal evidence of hyperparathyroidism is usually absent.

MANAGEMENT OF NEONATAL HYPERPARATHYROIDISM

The diagnosis of neonatal hyperparathyroidism with significant and often worsening hypercalcemia, increased serum PTH, and marked skeletal demineralization, with subperiosteal erosions of the long bones, would appear to be specific and is unlikely to be confused with the other rare conditions causing hypercalcemia in neonates. In view of the excellent results of conservative management in recent years, this form of management is to be recommended initially. Provided the baby's condition is satisfactory, parathyroid surgery should be avoided. If, despite adequate rehydration, the hypercalcemia worsens and is associated with clinical deterioration, neck exploration is necessary. Wherever possible, these children should be managed in special pediatric centers. If surgery is required, total parathyroidectomy with autotransplantation of part of one gland would appear to be the best operation. If facilities are available, cryopreservation of some of the parathyroid tissue is advantageous for later use if the initial operation leads to permanent hypoparathyroidism (60).

MANAGEMENT OF PREGNANCY IN FAMILIAL HYPOCALCIURIC HYPERCALCEMIA

Neonatal hyperparathyroidism appears to be a very rare complication in FHH, so affected family members can be reassured that the condition is unlikely to affect adversely the outcome of pregnancy. It is wise nevertheless to alert the obstetrician of the remote possibility of severe hypercalcemia in the neonatal period.

Apnea has been described in seven hypercalcemic children, due to idiopathic infantile hypercalcemia in six cases and to FHH in one (67). Late-presenting hypocalcemia, due possibly to transient hypoparathyroidism, was described in an infant born to a mother with FHH (68).

SELF-LIMITING NEONATAL HYPERPARATHYROIDISM

A single family has been reported with self-limiting neonatal hyperparathyroidism associated with persistent hypercalciuria, renal tubular acidosis, and nephrocalcinosis (69). Three siblings were affected, and all evidence of hypercalcemia disappeared within 2 years, although the other conditions continued to be manifest. Both parents had normal serum calcium concentrations, so autosomal recessive inheritance was suggested. Because these cases differ in many respects from all other reported cases of neonatal hyperparathyroidism, it is best at present to consider these patients to have a separate condition.

BIOCHEMICAL CHANGES IN FAMILIAL HYPOCALCIURIC HYPERCALCEMIA

Serum Calcium

Hypercalcemia is an important feature of FHH. The increase in total serum calcium is not due to any detectable abnormality of serum proteins, and the ultrafiltrable and ionized calcium levels are increased proportionally to the total calcium (2,70). In mild cases the total serum calcium may be within the normal range some or all of the time, while the ionized calcium activity is slightly elevated (66). All current evidence suggests that hypercalcemia is present from birth. It is the early occurrence of hypercalcemia that is one of the cardinal differentiating points between FHH and familial hyperparathyroidism. Hypercalcemia persists throughout life and, with the exception of the severe neonatal hypercalcemia, is usually mild and constant. Two studies have shown that the mean serum calcium level in affected children is higher than in affected adults (8,10), but in unaffected members the mean serum calcium concentration was also higher in children than in adults (10). Apart from the severe neonatal hypercalcemia, the highest serum calcium level reported in the literature in FHH is 14.6 mg/100 ml, or 3.65 mmol/liter. The vast majority of patients, however, have a serum calcium <12.0 mg/dl, or 3 mmol/liter. Some evidence suggests a clustering of serum calcium values in different families (5,71). One report of a family with six affected hypercalcemic members also noted four hypocalcemic subjects (72). Either the hypocalcemia noted was within the limits seen in a normal population or a trait for low calcium is inherited in families. These points were specifically examined by Rajala and Heath (71) in the families studied at the Mayo Clinic. The authors found five hypocalcemic FHH family members, but this was of a sporadic, nongenetic origin. They confirmed that the hypercalcemia in FHH is not an extreme of the normal distribution but a clear disturbance of calcium metabolism, with its own distribution around a supranormal mean serum calcium concentration.

Serum Phosphorus

Serum phosphorus values are reduced compared to normal and are similar to values seen in primary hyperparathyroidism (2,7,10,13,70).

Serum Electrolytes

Serum sodium, potassium, chloride, and bicarbonate levels are all within the normal range, although Menko et al. (10) found the mean serum sodium concentration to be lower in young patients than in controls. Serum chloride is higher in adult patients than in controls (10,70), suggesting a mild hyperchloremic acidosis, which is also commonly seen in primary hyperparathyroidism.

Serum Magnesium

Studies have shown that the serum magnesium concentration is consistently higher in FHH than in controls or in patients with primary hyperparathyroidism (7,10,13,70). In FHH patients the values tend to cluster towards or just above the upper limit of normal, whereas, in primary hyperparathyroidism, they tend to be in the lower one-half of the normal range. The change in magnesium persists after controlling for age, sex, and renal function (70). In FHH there is a positive correlation between serum calcium and magnesium, whereas in primary hyperparathyroidism the relationship is negative (70). Despite these differences in serum magnesium in the two hypercalcemic conditions, there is considerable overlap between them, so magnesium measurements in the individual patient will not differentiate between the two conditions.

Glomerular Filtration Rate

Glomerular filtration rate (GFR) in FHH is similar to that in controls (5,10,73) and shows a mild age-related decline similar to that seen in normal subjects (5).

Serum Citrate

In the early studies of Foley et al. (2), adult patients had a tendency toward increased serum citrate concentrations compared to normals and unaffected family members.

MEASUREMENTS OF RENAL FUNCTION

Renal Calcium Handling

Since the early description of FHH in 1972 by Foley et al. (2), hypocalciuria has been a well recognized feature of the disorder. The NIH group identified it as being a cardinal feature, which helped to differentiate it from familial primary hyperparathyroidism (5). Although 24 hr urine calcium excretion is typically low in FHH, there is marked overlap with the values seen in typical primary hyperparathyroidism. This overlap is reduced if the urine calcium excretion is related to creatinine clearance and is further reduced if the calcium excretion is expressed as a ratio of calcium clearance to creatinine clearance (5). Marx and his colleagues (5) studied 40 patients with FHH from 15 kindreds and compared the calcium excretion to that seen in 90 typical cases of primary hyperparathyroidism. The lowest 24 hr calcium excretion seen in hyperparathyroidism was 3 mEq, and 35% of the patients with FHH had a lower value. The highest 24 hr calcium excretion seen in FHH was 20 mEq, and 36% of the hyperparathyroid patients had a higher value. Excretion between 3 and 20 mEq was therefore an overlap area, within which 65% of the FHH patients fell. With calcium clearance/creatinine clearance ratios, no hyperparathyroid patient had a value <0.0057, while 45% of the FHH patients had ratios below this value. All but one hyperparathyroid patient had a ratio >0.01, while 80% of the FHH patients had lower values. Thus while a calcium clearance/creatinine clearance ratio <0.01 is very suggestive of FHH, 20% of patients will have a value above this, and occasionally patients with hyperparathyroidism have a value below it. Broadly similar findings were found by the Mayo Clinic group (8). Other methods of expressing renal calcium handling, such as theoretical tubular maximum for calcium reabsorption or fractional excretion of calcium, do not offer any advantages (74).

Although hypocalciuria is a major feature of FHH, hypercalciuria can also occur. Pasieka et al. (75) described a family with four hypercalcemic members. Two of the patients showed all the biochemical features of FHH, including high-normal magnesium, low 24 hr urine calcium excretion, and calcium clearance/creatinine clearance ratios <0.007. Two other members, including the index case, had similar results apart from frank hypercalciuria and high calcium/creatinine clearance ratios. The index case underwent an unsuccessful neck exploration, and parathyroid histology was typical of FHH.

Kristiansen et al. (76), studying ten patients in one family, found the 24 hr urine calcium excretion and the calcium clearance/creatinine clearance to be considerably higher than the values found by many other workers. This again suggests that renal calcium handling measurements can vary substantially both between members within one family and among families.

The occurrence of hypocalciuria in the presence of hypercalcemia indicates increased renal calcium reabsorption. The site of this increase appears to be exclusively the proximal renal tubule rather than the distal tubule (73). Enhanced proximal tubule calcium reabsorption is independent of PTH action; it persists even in those patients with FHH rendered hypoparathyroid by total parathyroidectomy (77,78).

Renal Phosphate Handling

The tubular maximal reabsorption rate per liter glomerular filtrate is lower in FHH than in normal controls but is higher than that in primary hyperparathyroidism (10,76,79). The higher the serum calcium in FHH, the lower the phosphate reabsorption. Marked overlap occurs in the values seen in FHH and primary hyperparathyroidism.

Renal Magnesium Handling

As with renal calcium handling, there is a relative hypomagnesuria, with an increased renal tubular reabsorption of magnesium (76).

Renal Concentrating Ability

Despite life-long hypercalcemia, renal concentrating ability is normally maintained, while it is occasionally impaired in primary hyperparathyroidism (80).

PARATHYROID FUNCTION IN FAMILIAL HYPOCALCIURIC HYPERCALCEMIA

Parathyroid Glands

In many of the studies of patients with FHH who have undergone parathyroid surgery, the parathyroid glands have been described as being enlarged and hyperplastic. In the first systematic analysis of parathyroid histology with glands removed from eight different kindreds, parathyroid hyperplasia was said to be present in 13 of 38 patients with increased parathyroid parenchymal area (81). A contrary view has been expressed by the Mayo Clinic group. Using high-resolution ultrasonography, they found no evidence of parathyroid gland enlargement (82). Among glands removed from patients with FHH, 83% had gland weights within the normal range, and the relative parenchymal area was slightly less than in control glands (83). The suggestion is that, when the glands are of greater than normal weight, the excess is due to an increased number of fat cells.

Although there is debate regarding whether there is increased parathyroid cell mass in FHH, even if there is, it seems unlikely that the hypercalcemia could be due simply to increased functioning parathyroid tissue. This is in contradistinction to the obvious increased parathyroid mass in neonatal hyperparathyroidism complicating rare cases of FHH (see above).

Serum Parathyroid Hormone Concentrations

Over the 20 years during which FHH emerged as a clinical entity, the methodology and performance of PTH assays have improved markedly. Early assays were unable to measure PTH concentrations in the majority of normal subjects and found elevated PTH values in only a proportion of cases of proven primary hyperparathyroidism. Nonspecific interference in the assay also led to elevated PTH concentrations being found in some cases of non-PTH-mediated hypercalcemia. Currently, with the new generation of two-site immunoradiometric assays, virtually all normal subjects have detectable "intact" PTH concentrations, and high-normal or clearly elevated PTH values are found in virtually all cases of primary hyperparathyroidism (see the chapter "Clinical Presentation of Primary Hyperparathyroidism," by Bilezikian et al.). It is not surprising therefore that early reports of PTH concentrations in FHH were variable. In seven of 32 patients studied initially at the NIH, PTH concentrations were above normal (5). Paterson and Gunn (84) found normal concentrations in ten affected patients, as did Menko et al. (10). Hunter Heath reviewed the various assays used in the Mayo Clinic studies and reported that, with all assays, the majority of patients had normal values. However, with these same assays, and even now with the new two-site assays, a few patients with FHH have slightly elevated values (8). The concentration of PTH, however, tends to be significantly lower than that seen in typical primary hyperparathyroidism. Gunn and Wallace (85), using a two-site "intact" PTH assay, found normal PTH concentrations in 20 subjects with FHH from four different families, but 14% of their primary hyperparathyroidism patients had similar, normal values (85). Serum PTH increases with age; the values in 60-year-old patients were on average three times higher than those in 20-year-old patients. A similar observation was made by McMurtry et al. (86), who studied a family with 19 affected members. Serum PTH measured via three different immunoassays increased with age and became supranormal by age ~30 years. Thus in older patients it became more difficult to distinguish between FHH and primary hyperparathyroidism. Even the finding of normal PTH concentrations in the presence of hypercalcemia can be considered abnormal, and such inappropriately normal values led to many patients being diagnosed mistakenly as having primary hyperparathyroidism. One explanation for such a discrepancy is that the parathyroid cells have an abnormally high calcium set point, secreting normal amounts of PTH at calcium concentrations that normally suppress secretion. This is discussed below under Pathophysiology.

URINARY CYCLIC ADENOSINE MONOPHOSPHATE EXCRETION

Urinary cyclic adenosine monophosphate (cAMP) excretion is an indicator of circulating PTH activity and is increased in primary hyperparathyroidism (87). Studies of 23 subjects with FHH showed normal nephrogenous cAMP excretion (79). Law and Heath (7) found urinary cAMP excretion to be identical in affected and unaffected family members. Although occasional patients have been reported to have increased cAMP excretion, the consensus is that it is usually normal and consistent with typically normal serum PTH concentrations. This also suggests that there is unlikely to be a circulating non-PTH substance that mimics the action of PTH.

BONE CHANGES IN FAMILIAL HYPOCALCIURIC HYPERCALCEMIA

Definite evidence of parathyroid bone disease is seen in babies with neonatal primary hyperparathyroidism complicating FHH. Excepting this complication, there is no clinical evidence of bone disease in FHH. However, subtle changes in bone structure and mass could easily be missed. Menko et al. (10) noted a small, nonsignificant increase in urinary hydroxyproline in their affected family members. Kristiansen et al. (88), however, found a significantly increased hydroxyproline/creatinine ratio, which could indicate increased bone breakdown. Measurements of bone density with various techniques have shown normal values and no evidence of any increased fracture risk (7,88,89). This suggests either that bone metabolism is normal in FHH or that any tendency to increase bone resorption is matched by an increase in bone formation.

A recent paper by McMurtry et al. (86) reported the occurrence of four family members with radiological evidence of osteomalacia. Three of the five affected members who were over 40 years of age appeared to have osteomalacia, and a bone biopsy performed in one showed histological changes compatible with this diagnosis. Clearly, further observations are required in patients with FHH, especially in those over the age of 40 years, to see whether these changes are found in other families.

RESPONSE TO PARATHYROIDECTOMY

One of the features of FHH that led to its recognition was the poor results of parathyroidectomy in curing the hypercalcemia. Among 27 patients who underwent between one and four neck explorations, only two patients became permanently normocalcemic; 21 remained hypercalcemic (six after three or four operations), and five were rendered permanently hypoparathyroid (5). This dismal result of surgery has been seen in all reports on FHH. As a result, one of the main reasons for making a definite diagnosis of FHH is to prevent unnecessary neck exploration.

PATHOPHYSIOLOGY

Most of the observations on the pathophysiology of FHH have centered on the role of the parathyroid glands. As was reviewed above, although there is some evidence of increased parathyroid parenchymal cell mass and/or PTH hypersecretion, most of the evidence does not support this. Consequently, efforts have concentrated on studying the mechanism of PTH secretion to see if the physiological control differs from that of normal parathyroid glands. By definition, a normal PTH concentration in the presence of an increased ionized serum calcium indicates that the parathyroid gland calcium set point is higher in FHH than in normal individuals. This higher set point appears to function otherwise normally, in that calcium infusions suppress serum PTH concentrations normally in FHH (2,7,79,90,91). Infusions of EDTA to lower serum calcium cause a normal PTH response (90). Comparisons of patients with FHH and primary hyperparathyroidism confirm that the functional parathyroid abnormality in FHH is a simple set point error, whereas in hyperparathyroidism it is a combination of a set point error with a varying degree of calcium-nonsuppressible PTH secretion (92). A single abnormality in the parathyroid glands would be unlikely to cause all the features of FHH. Specifically, repeated neck explorations should cause hypoparathyroidism just as frequently in FHH as in normal subjects and in hyperparathyroidism due to four-gland hyperplasia. This does not seem to be the case; persistent hypercalcemia is the most likely outcome. Peripheral responses to PTH have been studied, and there is some evidence of a greater responsiveness to both exogenous and endogenous PTH in FHH (8,93), but this could not be demonstrated in dermal fibroblasts (94).

In addition to a parathyroid cell abnormality, there is abundant evidence of renal tubular dysfunction. Relative to normal subjects and patients with primary hyperparathyroidism, patients with FHH have an increased tubular reabsorption of both calcium and magnesium. The change in calcium handling is specific to the proximal tubule (73) and is independent of PTH (77,78). If the parathyroid cell and renal tubule respond differently, there could be a widespread cellular abnormality of calcium sensing and/or transport. Initial support for this hypothesis came from studies indicating that active calcium efflux from erythrocytes of patients with FHH was higher than normal (95). The same group later showed an increased erythrocyte membrane calcium pump activity in FHH (96), but more recent studies have not confirmed this finding (97). To date, no definite abnormality of vitamin D metabolism (8), calcitonin (91), or PTH-related protein (93) has been described. In summary, the overwhelming evidence suggests that there is at least an abnormality of the parathyroid gland calcium "set point" and an abnormality of renal tubular function in FHH, although the molecular basis of such abnormalities remains obscure.

GENETICS OF FAMILIAL HYPOCALCIURIC HYPERCALCEMIA

With very few exceptions, an autosomal dominant inheritance with virtually complete penetrance has been the feature of all reported cases. Within reported families, "skip" generations have been extremely rare, although normal total serum calcium and elevated ionized calcium occasionally give this impression (66). New mutations seem to be extremely uncommon, but this may be due in part to the difficulty of diagnosing the condition in the absence of an affected parent or relative. An initial report suggested linkage of the trait to the HLA haplotype A11, BW55 CW3 DR4 (55), but subsequent reports have failed to confirm this (98–100). There was no evidence of linkage to the *PTH* gene (101), nor was there linkage with a series of candidate genes related to calcium metabolism (102). More recently, studies in 114 individuals in four unrelated families have mapped FHH to chromosome 3q, with a lod score of 20.67 (103). Studies in a series of

other families have not shown such linkage (Thakker and Heath, unpublished observations). At present it is not possible to be certain of the genetic defect in FHH, but there is no doubt that its ultimate identification will greatly enhance our understanding of calcium metabolism and aid in the diagnosis of this fascinating condition.

IDENTIFICATION AND MANAGEMENT OF FAMILIAL HYPOCALCIURIC HYPERCALCEMIA

Once it is recognized that FHH is occurring within a family, it becomes easy to make the correct diagnosis in additional family members who are found to be hypercalcemic. Occasionally it is difficult to differentiate between MEN-I and familial hyperparathyroidism. The recognition of disease due to pancreatic or pituitary tumor within other family members will obviously help to make the diagnosis of MEN-I. The best discriminating point is the identification of hypercalcemia in young children, which is to be expected in FHH but is extremely rare in the other two conditions. Marx et al. (5) in reviewing this point could find only two reported families among whom hypercalcemia was found in those under the age of 10 years in MEN-I and familial hyperparathyroidism. The challenge is to diagnose FHH in a new index case. The importance of this depends on the policy used to manage asymptomatic primary hyperparathyroidism. If all cases of asymptomatic primary hyperparathyroidism are referred for surgery, then it becomes imperative to differentiate this condition from FHH to avoid unnecessary surgery. Many centers are now prepared to consider conservative treatment for older patients with asymptomatic primary hyperparathyroidism but continue to recommend surgical treatment for younger patients (104). Basically, in any asymptomatic patient with presumed hyperparathyroidism, FHH should be excluded before surgery. The author's practice has been to recommend parathyroidectomy for all patients with presumed hyperparathyroidism who are under age 40 years. Prior to routinely evaluating our patients for FHH, two of 24 patients under age 40 years referred for parathyroidectomy had failed surgery and a revised diagnosis of FHH (11). Since that time, family screening of asymptomatic young patients has prevented such mistakes and has identified several new families with FHH. At a minimum, it seems essential to measure total serum calcium in both parents if they are alive. A completely normal total serum calcium in both parents would make the diagnosis of FHH unlikely, but care should be taken with serum calcium values in the upper part of the normal range (66). When both parents are unavailable for study, values of urinary calcium clearance/creatinine clearance <0.01

and low-normal serum PTH concentrations and high-normal serum magnesium values should suggest the possibility of FHH. Unfortunately, at present, no single test or series of tests unequivocally establishes the diagnosis of FHH. It remains a condition that has to be suspected, and, if the physician is in doubt, parathyroidectomy should be delayed. Elucidation of the genetic defect may well lead to more specific diagnostic tests.

Once FHH has been diagnosed, the patient should be reassured of its benign nature, and parathyroidectomy should be avoided. When appropriate, it is reasonable to advise patients that pregnancy carries minimal risks of complications. Further studies, however, are required to ensure that the disorder, especially in older life, does not carry appreciable risks of skeletal disease (86).

REFERENCES

1. Jackson CE, Boonstra CE. Hereditary hypercalcemia and parathyroid hyperplasia without definite hyperparathyroidism. *J Lab Clin Med* 1966;68:883.
2. Foley TP Jr, Harrison HC, Arnaud CD, Harrison HE. Familial benign hypercalcaemia. *J Pediatr* 1972;82:1060–1067.
3. Marx SJ, Spiegel AM, Brown EM, Aurbach GD. Family studies in patients with primary parathyroid hyperplasia. *Am J Med* 1977;62:698–706.
4. Marx SJ, Stock JL, Attie MG, et al. Familial hypocalciuric hypercalcemia: Recognisation among patients referred after unsuccessful parathyroid exploration. *Ann Intern Med* 1980;92:351–356.
5. Marx SJ, Attie MF, Levine MA, Spiegel AM, Downs RW Jr, Lasker RD. The hypocalciuric or benign variant of familial hypercalcemia: clinical and biochemical features in fifteen kindreds. *Medicine* 1981;60:397–412.
6. Jackson CE, Kleerekoper M. Hereditary hypocalciuric hypercalcemia is benign in 15 year follow up. *Clin Res* 1981;29:409A (abstract).
7. Law WM Jr, Heath H III. Familial benign hypercalcemia (Hypocalciuric hypercalcemia). Clinical and pathogenetic studies in 21 families. *Ann Intern Med* 1985;102:511–519.
8. Heath H III. Familial benign (hypocalciuric) hypercalcemia. *Endocrinol Metab Clin North Am* 1989;18:723–740.
9. Mundy GR, Cove DH, Fisken R, Heath DA, Somers S. Primary hyperparathyroidism: changes in the pattern of clinical presentation. *Lancet* 1980;1:1317–1320.
10. Menko FH, Bijvoet OLM, Fronen JLHH, et al. Familial benign hypercalcemia: study of a large family. *Q J Med* 1983;206:120–140.
11. Heath DA. Familial benign hypercalcemia. *Trends Endocrinol Metab* 1989;1:6–9.
12. Auwerx J, Demedts M, Bouillon R, Ceuppens JL, Desmet J. Co-existence of idiopathic pulmonary fibrosis and hypocalciuric hypercalcemia in a family: a cross sectional study. *Eur J Clin Invest* 1985;15:6–14.
13. Lyons TJ, Crookes PF, Postlethwaite W, Sheridan B, Brown RC, Atkinson AB. Familial hypocalciuric hypercalcemia as a differential diagnosis of hyperparathyroidism: studies in a large kindred and a review of surgical experience in the condition. *Br J Surg* 1986;73:188–192.
14. Toss G, Arnqvist H, Larsson L, Nilsson O. Familial hypocalciuric hypercalcemia: a study of four kindreds. *J Intern Med* 1989;225:201–206.
15. McCarty DJ, ed. *Calcium pyrophosphate deposition disease (pseudogout; articular chondrocalcinosis) in arthritis and allied conditions*, 9th ed. Philadelphia: Lea and Febiger, 1979;1276.
16. Davies M, Klimiuk PS, Adams PH, Laub GA, Large DM, Anderson DC. Familial hypocalciuric hypercalcemia and acute pancreatitis. *Br Med J* 1981;282:1023–1025.
17. Doumith R, Ulmann A, Biclet P, Rieu M, Dubost CI. Syndrome d'hypercalcemie-hypocalciurie: une cause meconnue d'hypercalcemie. *Nouv Presse Med* 1980;16:1157–1159.
18. Damoiseux P, Tafforeau M, Henkinbrant A. Episode unique de pancreatite aigue revelant une hypercalcemie hypocalciurique familiale. *Acta Clin Belg* 1985;40:247–250.
19. Stuckey BGA, Kent GN, Gutteridge DH, Pullan PT, Price RI, Bhagat C. Fasting calcium excretion and parathyroid hormone together distinguish familial hypocalciuric hypercalcemia from primary hyperparathyroidism. *Clin Endocrinol* 1987;27:525–534.
20. Leading article. Familial hypocalciuric hypercalcemia. *Lancet* 1982;1:488–489.
21. Auwerx J, Brunzell J, Bouillon R, Demedts M. Familial hypocalciuric hypercalcemia—familial benign hypercalcemia: a review. *Postgrad Med J* 1987;63:835–840.
22. Stuckey BGA, Kent GN, Gutteridge DH, Reed WD. Familial hypocalciuric hypercalcemia and pancreatitis: no causal link proven. *Aust NZ J Med* 1990;20:718–719.
23. Marx J, Attie MF, Spiegel AM, Levine MA, Laser RD, Fox M. An association between neonatal severe primary hyperparathyroidism and familial hypocalciuric hypercalcemia in three kindreds. *N Engl J Med* 1982;306:257–264.
24. Muhlethaler JP, Scharer K, Antener I. Akuter hyperparathyeoidismus bei primarer Nebenschilddrusen hyperplasie. *Helv Paediatr Acta* 1967;22:529–557.
25. Rajasuriya K, Peiris OA, Ratnaike VT, de Fonseka CP. Parathyroid adenomas in childhood. *Am J Dis Child* 1964;107:442–449.
26. Landon JF. Parathyroidectomy in generalised osteitis fibrosa cystica. *J Pediatr* 1932;1:544.
27. Anspach WE, Clifton WM. Hyperparathyroidism in children. Report of two cases. *Am J Dis Child* 1939;58:540–557.
28. Pratt EL, Geren BB, Neuhauser EBD. Hypercalcemia and idiopathic hyperplasia of the parathyroid glands in an infant. *J Pediatr* 1947;30:388–399.
29. Philips RN. Primary diffuse parathyroid hyperplasia in an infant of four months. *Pediatrics* 1948;2:428–434.
30. Roget J, Beaudoing A, Bernard, Jobert. Un cas d'hyperparathyroidie primitive chez un enfant de 30 mois. *Pediatrie* 1959;14:21–34.
31. Randall C, Lauchlan SC. Parathyroid hyperplasia in an infant. *Am J Dis Child* 1963;105:364–367.
32. Hillman DA, Scriver CR, Pedvis S, Shragovitch I. Neonatal familial primary hyperparathyroidism. *N Engl J Med* 1964;270:483–490.
33. Fretheim B, Gardborg O. Primary hyperparathyroidism in an infant. Report of a case. *Acta Chir Scand* 1965;129:557–566.
34. Farriaux JP, Maillard E, Tahon A, du Bois R, Dupont A, Fontaine G. Etude d'une nouvelle observation d'hyperparathyroidie primitive par hyperplasie chez une enfant de une mois. *Ann Pediatr* 1968;15:716–723.
35. Corbeel L, Casaer P, Malvaux P, Lormans J, Bourgeois N. Hyperparathyroidie congenitale. *Arch Fr Pediatr* 1968;25:879–891.
36. DuBois R, Farriaux JP, Maillard E, Maillard JP. Hyperparathyroidisime primitif chez un nouveau-ne. *Ann Radiol* 1969;12:407–412.
37. Goldbloom RB, Gillis DA, Prasad M. Hereditary parathyroid hyperplasia. A surgical emergency of early infancy. *Pediatrics* 1972;49:514–523.
38. Bradford WD, Wilson JW, Gaede JT. Primary neonatal hyperparathyroidism—an unusual cause of failure to thrive. *Am J Clin Pathol* 1973;59:267–275.
39. Grantmyre EB. Roentgenographic features of "primary" hyperparathyroidism in infancy. *J Can Assoc Radiol* 1973;24:257–260.
40. Garcia-Banniel R, Kutchemeshgi A, Brandes D. Hereditary hyperparathyroidism. The fine structure of the parathyroid gland. *Arch Pathol* 1974;97:399–403.
41. Nguyen VC, Sennot WM, Knox GS. Neonatal hyperparathyroidism. *Radiology* 1974;112:175–176.

42. Rhone DP. Primary neonatal hyperparathyroidism. Report of a case and review of the literature. *Am J Clin Pathol* 1975;64:488–499.

43. Proesmans W, Dhondt F, Logghe N. Congenital hyperparathyroidism. Case report and review of the literature. *Acta Paediatr Belg* 1977;30:45–52.

44. Spiegel AM, Harrison HE, Marx SJ, Brown EM, Aurbach GD. Neonatal primary hyperparathyroidism with autosomal dominant inheritance. *J Pediatr* 1977;90:269–272.

45. Thompson NW, Carpenter LC, Kessler DL, Nishiyama RH. Hereditary neonatal hyperparathyroidism. *Arch Surg* 1978; 113:100–103.

46. Matsuo M, Okita K, Takemine H, Fujita T. Neonatal primary hyperparathyroidism in familial hypocalciuric hypercalcemia. *Am J Dis Child* 1982;136:728–731.

47. Eichenbrenner TJ. Asymptomatic neonatal familial hypercalcemia. *Pediatrics* 1982;70:154.

48. Eftekhari F, Yousefzadeh DK. Primary infantile hyperparathyroidism: clinical, laboratory and radiographic features in 21 cases. *Skel Radiol* 1982;8:201–208.

49. Orwoll E, Silbert J, McChing M. Asymptomatic neonatal familial hypercalcemia. *Pediatrics* 1982;69:109–111.

50. Fujita T, Watanabe N, Fukase M et al. Familial hypocalciuric hypercalcemia involving four members of a kindred including a girl with severe neonatal primary hyperparathyroidism. *Mineral Electrolyte Metab* 1983;9:51–54.

51. Gaudelus J, Dandine M, Nathanson M, Perelman R, Hassan M. Rib cage deformity in neonatal hyperparathyroidism. *Am J Dis Child* 1983;137:408–409.

52. Lillquist K, Illum N, Brock Jacobsen B, Lockwood K. Primary hyperparathyroidism in infancy associated with familial hypocalciuric hypercalcemia. *Acta Pediatr Scand* 1983; 72:625–629.

53. Dezateux CA, Hyde JC, Hoey HMCV, et al. Neonatal hyperparathyroidism. *Eur J Pediatr* 1984;142:135–136.

54. Ch'ing JLC, Kaiser A, Lynn J, Joplin GF. Post parathyroidectomy restoration of normal calcium homeostasis in neonatal primary hyperparathyroidism. *Acta Endocrinol* 1984; 105:350–353.

55. Sopwith AM, Burns C, Grant DB, Taylor GW, Wolf E, Besser GM. Familial hypocalciuric hypercalcemia: association with neonatal primary hyperparathyroidism and possible linkage with HLA haplotype. *Clin Endocrinol* 1984;21:57–64.

56. Steinmann B, Griehm HE, Rao VH, Kind HP, Prader A. Neonatal severe hyperparathyroidism and alkaptonuria in a boy born to related parents with familial hypocalciuric hypercalcemia. *Helv Paediatr Acta* 1984;39:171–186.

57. Just J, Schmitt AM, Tournier G, Grumer M, Costil J, Couvreur J. L'hyperparathyroidie primitive neonatale chez deux jumelles dizygotes. Importance de la parathyroidectomie en urgence. *Ann Pediatr* 1986;33:217–220.

58. Ross AJ III, Cooper A, Attie M, Bishop HC. Primary hyperparathyroidism in infancy. *J Pediatr Surg* 1986;6:493–499.

59. Anast CS. Neonatal disorders of mineral homeostasis. In: Frame B, Potts JT Jr, eds. *Clinical disorders of bone and mineral metabolism.* Amsterdam: Excerpta Medica 1983;422–426.

60. Lutz P, Kane O, Pfersdorff A, Seiller F, Sauvage P, Levy JM. Neonatal primary hyperparathyroidism. Total parathyroidectomy with autotransplantation of cryopreserved parathyroid tissue. *Acta Paediatr Scand* 1986;75:179–182.

61. Cooper L, Wertheimer J, Levey R, et al. Severe primary hyperparathyroidism in a neonate with two hypercalcemic parents: management with parathyroidectomy and heterotopic autotransplantation. *Pediatrics* 1986;78:263–268.

62. Page LA, Haddow JE. Self limited neonatal hyperparathyroidism in familial hypocalciuric hypercalcemia. *J Pediatr* 1987;111:261–264.

63. Harris SS, D'Ercole AJ. Neonatal hyperparathyroidism: the natural course in the absence of surgical intervention. *Pediatrics* 1989;83:53–56.

64. Fujimoto Y, Hazama H, Oku K. Severe primary hyperpara-

thyroidism in a neonate having a parent with hypercalcemia: treatment by total parathyroidectomy and simultaneous heterotopic autotransplantation. *Surgery* 1990;108:933–938.

65. Pomeranz A, Wolach B, Raz A, Ben Ari Y. Neonatal hyperparathyroidism. Conservative treatment with intravenous and oral rehydration solutions. *Child Nephrol Urol* 1992; 12:55–58.

66. Marx SJ, Fraser D, Rapoport A. Familial hypocalciuric hypercalcemia. Mild expression of the gene in heterozygotes and severe expression in homozygotes. *Am J Med* 1985; 78:15–22.

67. Kooh S-W, Binet A. Hypercalcemia in infants presenting with apnea. *Can Med Assoc J* 1990;143:509–512.

68. Powell BR, Buist NRM. Late presenting, prolonged hypocalcemia in an infant of a women with hypocalciuric hypercalcemia. *Clin Pediatr* 1990;29:241–243.

69. Nishiyama S, Tomoeda S, Inoue F, Ohta T, Matsuda I. Self limiting neonatal familial hyperparathyroidism associated with hypercalciura and renal tubular acidosis in three siblings. *Pediatrics* 1990;86:421–427.

70. Marx SJ, Spiegel AM, Brown EM, Koehler JO, Gardner DG, Brennan MF, Aurbach GD. Divalent cation metabolism. Familial hypocalciuric hypercalcemia versus typical primary hyperparathyroidism. *Am J Med* 1978;65:235–242.

71. Rajala MM, Heath H III. Distribution of serum calcium values in patients with familial benign hypercalcemia (hypocalciuric hypercalcemia): evidence for a discrete genetic defect. *J Clin Endocrinol Metab* 1986;65:1039–1041.

72. Bannister P, Sheridan P, Dibble J, Payne RB. Benign hypercalcemia and "benign hypocalcemia" in the same family. *Ann Intern Med* 1986;105:217–219.

73. Kristiansen JH, Brochner-Mortensen J, Pederson KO. Renal tubular reabsorption of calcium in familial hypocalciuric hypercalcemia. *Acta Endocrinol* 1986;112:541–546.

74. Kent GN, Bhagat CI, Garcia-Webb P, Gutteridge DH. Tubular maximum for calcium reabsorption: lack of diagnostic usefulness in primary hyperparathyroidism and familial hypocalciuric hypercalcemia. *Clin Chim Acta* 1987;166:155–161.

75. Pasieka JL, Anderson MA, Hanley DA. Familial benign hypercalcemia: hypercalciuria and hypocalciuria in affected members of a small kindred. *Clin Endocrinol* 1990;33:429–433.

76. Kristiansen JH, Brochner-Mortensen J, Pederson KO. Familial hypocalciuric hypercalcemia I. Renal handling of calcium, magnesium and phosphate. *Clin Endocrinol* 1985;22:113–116.

77. Attie MF, Gill JR Jr, Stock JL, et al. Urinary calcium excretion in familial hypocalciuric hypercalcemia. Persistence of relative hypocalciuria after induction of hypoparathyroidism. *J Clin Invest* 1983;72:667–676.

78. Davies M, Adams PH, Lumb GA, Berry JL, Loveridge N. Familial hypocalciuric hypercalcemia: evidence for continued enhanced renal tubular reabsorption of calcium following total parathyroidectomy. *Acta Endocrinol* 1984;106:499–504.

79. Marx SJ, Speigel AM, Brown EM, et al. Circulating parathyroid hormone activity: familial hypocalciuric hypercalcemia versus typical primary hyperparathyroidism. *J Clin Endocrinol Metab* 1978;47:1190–1197.

80. Marx SJ, Attie MF, Stock JL, Spiegel AM, Levine MA. Maximal urine-concentrating ability: familial hypocalciuric hypercalcemia versus typical primary hyperparathyroidism. *J Clin Endocrinol Metab* 1981;52:736–740.

81. Thorgeirsson V, Costa J, Marx SJ. The parathyroid glands in familial hypocalciuric hypercalcemia. *Hum Pathol* 1982; 12:229–237.

82. Law WM Jr, James EM, Charboneau JW, Purnell DC, Heath H III. High-resolution parathyroid ultrasonography in familial benign hypercalcemia (familial hypocalciuric hypercalcemia). *Mayo Clin Proc* 1984;59:153–155.

83. Law WM Jr, Carney JA, Heath H III. Parathyroid glands in familial benign hypercalcemia (familial hypocalciuric hypercalcemia). *Am J Med* 1984;76:1021–1026.

84. Paterson CR, Gunn A. Familial benign hypercalcemia. *Lancet* 1981;2:61–63.

85. Gunn IR, Wallace JR. Urine calcium and serum ionised calcium, total calcium and parathyroid hormone concentrations in the diagnosis of primary hyperparathyroidism and familial benign hypercalcemia. *Ann Clin Biochem* 1992;29:52–58.

86. McMurtry CT, Schranck FW, Walkenhorst DA, et al. Significant developmental elevation in serum parathyroid hormone levels in a large kindred with familial benign (hypocalciuric) hypercalcemia. *Am J Med* 1992;93:247–258.

87. Broadus AE, Mahaffey JE, Bartter FC, Neer RM. Nephrogenous cyclic adenosine monophosphate as a parathyroid function test. *J Clin Invest* 1977;60:771–783.

88. Kristiansen JH, Rodbro P, Christiansen C, Johansen J, Jensen JT. Familial hypocalciuric hypercalcemia III: bone mineral metabolism. *Clin Endocrinol* 1987;26:713–716.

89. Abugassa S, Nordenstrom J, Jarhult J. Bone mineral density in patients with familial hypocalciuric hypercalcemia (FHH). *Eur J Surg* 1992;158:397–402.

90. Auwerx J, Demedts M, Bouillon R. Altered parathyroid set point to calcium in familial hypocalciuric hypercalcemia. *Acta Endocrinol* 1984;106:215–218.

91. Rajala MM, Klee GG, Heath H III. Calcium regulation of parathyroid and C cell function in familial benign hypercalcemia. *J Bone Mineral Res* 1991;6:117–124.

92. Khosla S, Ebeling PR, Firek AF, Burritt MM, Kao PC, Heath H III. Calcium infusion suggests a "set point" abnormality of parathyroid gland function in familial benign hypercalcemia and more complex disturbances in primary hyperparathyroidism. *J Clin Endocrinol Metab* 1993;76:715–720.

93. Firek AF, Kao PC, Heath H III. Plasma intact parathyroid hormone (PTH) and PTH-related peptide in familial benign hypercalcemia: greater responsiveness to endogenous PTH than in primary hyperparathyroidism. *J Clin Endocrinol Metab* 1991;72:541–546.

94. Firek AF, Carter WB, Heath H III. Cyclic adenosine 3′,5′-monophosphate responses to parathyroid hormone, prostaglandin E_2 and isoproterenol in dermal fibroblasts from patients with familial benign hypercalcemia. *J Clin Endocrinol Metab* 1991;73:203–206.

95. Hoare SF, Paterson CR. Familial benign hypercalcemia: a possible abnormality in calcium transport by erythrocytes. *Eur J Clin Invest* 1984;14:428–430.

96. Mole PA, Paterson CR. Calcium ATPase activity in erythrocyte ghosts from patients with familial benign hypercalcemia. *Scand J Clin Lab Invest* 1985;45:349–353.

97. Donahue HJ, Penniston JT, Heath H III. Kinetics of erythrocyte plasma membrane (Ca^{2+}, Mg^{2+}) ATPase in familial benign hypercalcemia. *J Clin Endocrinol Metab* 1989;68:893–898.

98. Paterson CR, Leheny W, O'Sullivan AF. HLA antigens and familial benign hypercalcemia. *Clin Endocrinol* 1985;85:111–113.

99. Kowalska G, Peacock C, Davies M, Dyer P. Absence of linkage between familial hypocalciuric hypercalcemia and the major histocompatibility system. *Tissue Antigens* 1987;30:91–95.

100. Menko FH, Bijvoet OLM, Khan PM, et al. Familial benign hypercalcemia (FBH) linkage in a large Dutch family. *Hum Genet* 1984;67:452–454.

101. Almarhoos GM, Docherty K, Fletcher JA, Webb T, Heath DA. Studies of the parathyroid hormone gene in normal subjects and in subjects with primary hyperparathyroidism and familial benign hypercalcemia. *J Endocrinol* 1987;115:183–186.

102. Heath H III, Leppert MF, Lifton RP, et al. Genetic linkage analysis in familial benign hypercalcemia using a candidate gene strategy. I. Studies in four families. *J Clin Endocrinol Metab* 1992;75:846–851.

103. Chou Y-HW, Brown EM, Levi T, et al. The gene responsible for familial hypocalciuric hypercalcemia maps to chromosome 3q in four unrelated families. *Nature Genet* 1992;1:295–300.

104. Heath DA, Heath EM. Conservative management of primary hyperparathyroidism. *J Bone Mineral Res* 1991;6 (Suppl. 2);117–124.

The Parathyroids, edited by J.P. Bilezikian, M.A. Levine, and R. Marcus. Raven Press, Ltd., New York © 1994.

CHAPTER 41

The Parathyroids in Renal Disease

Pathophysiology

Kevin J. Martin and Eduardo Slatopolsky

The association between renal failure, bone disease, and hyperplasia of the parathyroid glands has been recognized for more than 50 years (1–4). Since that time, considerable effort has been devoted to the elucidation of the pathogenesis of secondary hyperparathyroidism. The elucidation of the factors involved in the initiation and the maintenance of the state of disordered parathyroid hormone (PTH) secretion can form the basis of a rational approach to the treatment of this important and common complication of renal insufficiency.

Hyperplasia of the parathyroid glands and elevated levels of PTH in blood are among the earliest alterations of mineral metabolism seen in patients with decreased renal function. Elevated levels of PTH have been reported in patients with only mild decreases in renal function (5,6). Additional evidence of parathyroid overactivity was provided by the observation that patients with decreased renal function exhibit a greater than normal increase in serum PTH in response to hypocalcemia (7).

While under normal circumstances the principal determinant of PTH secretion is the concentration of ionized calcium in blood, in the presence of renal insufficiency there is a constellation of factors that contribute to alter the regulation of the secretion of PTH. The main factors involved in the pathogenesis of hy-

perparathyroidism in chronic renal disease are illustrated in Fig. 1 and include (a) phosphorus retention, (b) decreased levels of calcitriol, (c) abnormal parathyroid gland function, (d) hypocalcemia, and (e) skeletal resistance to the calcemic action of PTH. While these abnormalities are considered below separately, it should be emphasized that all these factors are closely interrelated, and some may predominate at different stages of renal insufficiency under a variety of clinical circumstances.

ROLE OF PHOSPHATE RETENTION

The importance of phosphate retention as a factor in the pathogenesis of the secondary hyperparathyroidism of renal insufficiency has been emphasized by Slatopolsky and colleagues (8–10). It was originally proposed that a transient small increase in serum phosphorus would occur early in the course of renal insufficiency as a consequence of decreased ability of the failing kidney to excrete phosphorus (8,9). This transient episode of hyperphosphatemia would result in a small decrease in the levels of ionized calcium in blood, which would consequently result in an increase in PTH secretion to restore the serum calcium to normal. The increased levels of PTH would decrease phosphorus reabsorption by the proximal tubule of the kidney and, thus, cause phosphaturia and restore the elevated serum phosphorus to normal. This new steady state would be maintained at the expense of higher circulating levels of PTH. Support for a role of phosphorus in the genesis of hyperparathyroidism is

K.J. Martin: Division of Nephrology, St. Louis University Medical Center, St. Louis, Missouri 63110.

E. Slatopolsky: Department of Internal Medicine, Renal Division, Washington University Medical Center at Barnes Hospital, St. Louis, Missouri 63110.

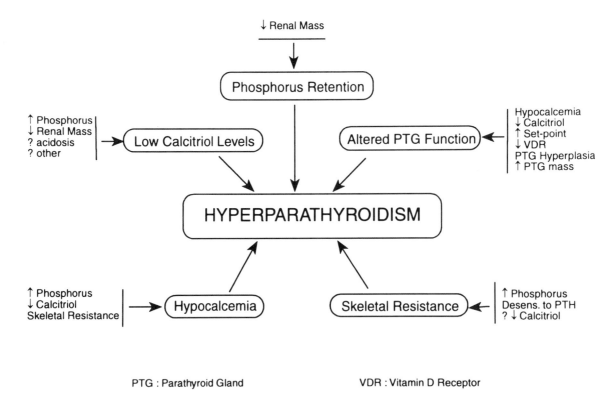

↓ Renal Mass

Phosphorus Retention

↑ Phosphorus
↓ Renal Mass
? acidosis
? other

→ Low Calcitriol Levels

Altered PTG Function ←

Hypocalcemia
↓ Calcitriol
↑ Set-point
↓ VDR
PTG Hyperplasia
↑ PTG mass

HYPERPARATHYROIDISM

↑ Phosphorus
↓ Calcitriol
Skeletal Resistance

→ Hypocalcemia

Skeletal Resistance ←

↑ Phosphorus
Desens. to PTH
? ↓ Calcitriol

PTG : Parathyroid Gland   VDR : Vitamin D Receptor

FIG. 1. Schematic diagram of the factors involved in the pathogenesis of hyperparathyroidism in renal insufficiency.

provided by the observation that a diet high in phosphorus results in parathyroid hyperplasia (11,12). More compelling are the studies of Slatopolsky et al. (13), who demonstrated that restriction of dietary phosphate in proportion to the decrease in glomerular filtration rate (GFR) (thereby negating the initial stimulus for series of events outlined above to increase the secretion of PTH) was successful in preventing the development of hyperparathyroidism in dogs with renal insufficiency (13). Subsequent studies by Llach and Massry (14) confirmed these findings in human subjects.

There is general agreement that phosphorus retention plays an important role in the genesis of the hyperparathyroidism of renal insufficiency. However, the mechanism by which this effect occurs is complex and is somewhat controversial. The mechanisms that have been considered are (a) phosphorus-induced hypocalcemia, (b) phosphorus-induced decrease in the levels of calcitriol, and (c) other unknown factors. Again, it is important to point out that these mechanisms are closely interrelated and are not mutually exclusive.

Phosphorus Retention and Hypocalcemia

That a rise in serum phosphorus can evoke an increase in PTH secretion was shown by Reiss et al.

(15), who demonstrated that an oral phosphorus load led to an increase in serum phosphorus, a fall in ionized calcium, and an increased level of PTH in normal human subjects. Whether this sequence of events occurs in early renal failure has been questioned, because fasting or even postprandial levels of serum phosphorus are not consistently elevated in early renal insufficiency (16,17). In fact, low levels of serum phosphorus are not uncommon. Furthermore, in early renal failure, although a trend towards a decrease in the levels of plasma ionized calcium has been demonstrated by Llach and Massry (18), hypocalcemia is not demonstrable in all patients. Portale et al. (16) also examined the possibility that intermittent hypocalcemia may occur after phosphate loading and again could not demonstrate hypocalcemia despite careful monitoring of the serum ionized calcium concentration. Thus it appears that the mechanism of the effect of phosphate retention may not be exerted exclusively through the induction of hypocalcemia. This concept was further tested directly by Lopez-Hilker et al. (19); hypocalcemia was prevented in dogs after the induction of uremia by the administration of a high-calcium diet. In these animals, which actually developed a mild increase in the serum calcium concentrations, increased levels of immunoreactive PTH nonetheless occurred. These studies clearly demonstrated that hypocalcemia is not essential for the development of secondary hyperparathyroidism in chronic renal failure.

These observations illustrate that other factors should be considered to explain the effects of phosphorus retention in the pathogenesis of secondary hyperparathyroidism.

Phosphorus Retention and Calcitriol

Since phosphorus plays a major role in the regulation of the production rate of 1,25-dihydroxyvitamin D (calcitriol) by altering the activity of the enzyme 1α-hydroxylase (20), it is possible that phosphorus retention leads directly to a decrease in the production of calcitriol. Conversely, the beneficial effects of phosphorus restriction on ameliorating the development or in decreasing established hyperparathyroidism could be explained by an increase in the levels of calcitriol. Evidence has been presented in support of a role of calcitriol deficiency in the studies of Lopez-Hilker et al. (19), in which the administration of calcitriol immediately after the induction of renal insufficiency was successful in preventing the development of hyperparathyroidism.

Other Mechanisms of the Effect of Phosphorus Retention

Although attention has focused primarily on the effects of phosphorus to alter serum levels of calcium and/or calcitriol, there is some evidence that other factors are involved. The mechanism of the phosphorus effect was studied in detail by Lopez-Hilker et al. (21) in chronically uremic dogs with severe hyperparathyroidism, in which dietary phosphorus was restricted in a progressive fashion. Simultaneously, dietary calcium was adjusted to maintain serum ionized calcium levels. Calcitriol concentrations remained low and did not change despite lowering of dietary phosphorus, which would have been expected to lead to an increase in calcitriol levels. Presumably, the production rate of calcitriol did not increase because total renal mass, reflecting 1α-hydroxylase activity, was reduced. As is shown in Fig. 2, under these circumstances, with no change in the levels of ionized calcium or calcitriol, the decrease in serum phosphorus was associated with a remarkable decrease in the levels of PTH as measured by an active-fragment, amino-terminal assay. These data raise the intriguing possibility that dietary phosphorus directly or indirectly affects the secretion of PTH. To date, however, when the levels of ionized calcium are carefully controlled, it has not been possible to show a direct effect of phosphorus on PTH secretion in vitro.

ROLE OF DECREASED SYNTHESIS OF CALCITRIOL

Since the kidney is the major site for the production of calcitriol, it follows that a decrease in renal mass as renal disease progresses may lead to a decrease in the ability of the diseased kidney to produce this important metabolite of vitamin D. The consequences of calcitriol deficiency on mineral metabolism contribute importantly to the development of secondary hyperparathyroidism. Substantial evidence has been presented in support of the role of abnormal vitamin D metabolism in the pathogenesis of hyperparathyroidism in renal insufficiency. In general, adults with

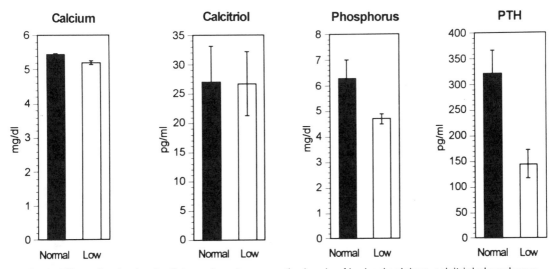

FIG. 2. Effect of reduction in dietary phosphorus on the levels of ionized calcium, calcitriol phosphorus, and amino-terminal PTH in dogs with chronic renal failure. *Solid bars* show the data on a diet of 1.6% calcium and 0.95% phosphorus. *Open bars* show the effect of changing the diet to 0.6% phosphorus and simultaneously lowering dietary calcium to 0.6% to prevent hypercalcemia. Data are mean ± SEM from studies in five animals. (Modified from ref. 21 with permission.)

chronic renal insufficiency have levels of calcitriol in the normal range until GFR falls to <50 ml/min (22–25). Some investigators, however, have found lower plasma levels of calcitriol, with creatinine clearances between 50 and 80 ml/min (26). Although blood levels of calcitriol may be normal, it is important to point out that these values still may be inappropriately low in view of the fact that levels of PTH are already elevated at this stage of renal insufficiency. The stimulus to raise calcitriol levels above normal is thus present. It is possible that, in this situation, phosphate retention is counteracting the stimulating actions of PTH on calcitriol production. An additional consideration is that the development of metabolic acidosis with renal failure decreases the levels of calcitriol. This issue is somewhat controversial, since acidosis has been reported to decrease, to increase, or not to change levels of calcitriol (27–31). Recent evidence suggests that the critical determinant of the changes in calcitriol during metabolic acidosis might be the effects of acidosis on phosphorus homeostasis (32). It is also possible that other factors that accumulate in plasma as a consequence of decreased GFR could potentially inhibit 1α-hydroxylase activity in the kidney (33). Such factors may be more relevant in advanced renal insufficiency. As renal disease advances and renal mass becomes limiting, the levels of calcitriol unquestionably fall, and this becomes a major factor in the genesis of hyperparathyroidism. Decreases in the level of calcitriol may lead to impaired intestinal calcium absorption, to hypocalcemia, and, importantly, to abnormal function of the parathyroid glands.

ROLE OF ALTERED PARATHYROID FUNCTION

Although many factors may lead to the development of hypocalcemia during the course of renal insufficiency and, thus, to increased secretion of PTH, evidence has accumulated that there may be an intrinsic abnormality that develops at the level of the parathyroid gland that leads to disordered calcium-regulated PTH secretion. It has been shown that the enzyme adenylyl cyclase in parathyroid cell membranes prepared from hyperplastic parathyroid glands is less susceptible to inhibition by calcium than that of membranes prepared from normal parathyroid tissue (34). Subsequent studies revealed that this difference could also be demonstrated for calcium-regulated PTH secretion in vitro (35,36). These data demonstrated that the set point for calcium was elevated in hyperplastic parathyroid glands; that is, a higher calcium concentration was required to decrease PTH secretion by 50%. These data thus suggested an intrinsic abnormality in calcium-regulated PTH secretion.

Current evidence increasingly implicates calcitriol as a major factor in the direct regulation of PTH secre-

tion. The finding of cytoplasmic and nuclear binding components for calcitriol in chick parathyroid glands by Brumbaugh et al. (37) first demonstrated that the parathyroid glands may be an important target tissue for calcitriol. These observations were followed by the demonstration that calcitriol decreased PTH secretion in vitro (38). Despite the controversial nature of the initial reports (39), it was subsequently demonstrated by Cantley et al. (40) with more prolonged experimental protocols that calcitriol clearly suppresses PTH secretion. This observation was confirmed by others (41) and was further detailed by Silver et al. (42) and Russell et al. (43), who demonstrated that the effect of calcitriol was at the level of transcription of PTH gene itself. These data were subsequently confirmed in studies in vivo by Silver et al. (44). Okazaki et al. (45) have extended these observations and identified a region in the 5′-flanking region of the PTH gene that appears to mediate the inhibition of PTH gene transcription by calcitriol. These studies clearly show that calcitriol has a direct effect on the synthesis and secretion of PTH.

The mechanisms by which low levels of calcitriol may alter PTH secretion are illustrated diagrammatically in Fig. 3. In addition to the indirect effect of low levels of calcitriol of increasing PTH secretion by leading to hypocalcemia as a consequence of impaired intestinal absorption of calcium and the direct effect of calcitriol on the transcription of the PTH gene, there are additional direct effects of low levels of calcitriol on the parathyroid cell indicating that the effects of calcitriol on parathyroid function may be even more complex. Observations by Korkor (46) have indicated that the number of receptors for calcitriol in parathyroid glands appears to be reduced in patients with chronic renal failure compared to either patients undergoing renal transplantation or patients with pri-

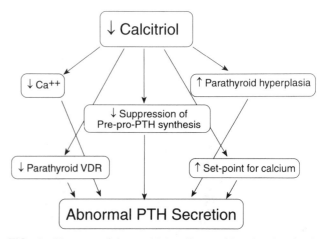

FIG. 3. Diagram of the multiple effects of low levels of calcitriol on the parathyroid gland that may lead to abnormal regulation of the secretion of parathyroid hormone.

mary hyperparathyroidism. These observations suggest that a decrease in parathyroid vitamin D receptor number may contribute to the pathogenesis of hyperparathyroidism by reducing the ability of calcitriol to inhibit PTH secretion on this basis. Similar observations have been made by Merke et al. (47) and Brown et al. (48), who also found a decreased number of calcitriol receptors in the parathyroid glands from uremic rats and dogs, respectively. Further studies by Naveh-Many et al. (49) have shown that the administration of calcitriol led to a dose-dependent increase in the number of vitamin D receptors in the parathyroid glands of normal rats. These data are all consistent with the view that calcitriol may regulate its own receptor number in the parathyroid cell. An additional effect of calcitriol on parathyroid function is suggested by the studies of Kremer et al. (50), who showed that exposure of quiescent bovine parathyroid cells in culture to serum or serum substitute results in an increase in tritiated thymidine incorporation, followed by an increase in cell number. These changes were preceded by an increase in *c-myc* and *c-fos* protooncogene mRNA levels. Alterations in medium calcium concentration have no effect on the growth rate of quiescent parathyroid cells. However, calcitriol, when added with serum or serum substitute, blocked the increase in *c-myc* mRNA levels, and the expected increase in parathyroid cell number failed to occur. These results indicated that calcitriol may directly modulate parathyroid cell proliferation by altering the expression of specific replication-associated oncogenes. Thus, if cal-

citriol is also an important growth regulator of parathyroid cells, as is suggested by the data, low levels of calcitriol may allow parathyroid cells to proliferate. Conversely, the administration of calcitriol may suppress proliferation of parathyroid cells.

The observation that calcitriol directly effects parathyroid function was investigated in clinical studies by Slatopolsky et al. (51), who showed that the intravenous administration of calcitriol to patients with end-stage renal disease maintained on chronic hemodialysis resulted in substantial suppression of PTH levels (Fig. 4). Although serum calcium levels gradually rose during the treatment with calcitriol, it appeared that the levels of PTH in serum began to decrease prior to the elevation in serum calcium. Because observations in vitro in parathyroid cells obtained from hyperplastic parathyroid glands from uremic patients indicated that the set point for calcium-regulated PTH secretion was shifted to the right, Delmez et al. (52) performed studies to determine if changes in calcitriol levels might affect the set point for calcium-regulated PTH secretion. The set point for calcium-regulated PTH secretion was determined by altering the levels of serum calcium during hemodialysis treatment. After baseline studies, the patients received calcitriol parenterally for a period of 2 weeks, and the set point for calcium regulated PTH secretion was again determined. Following the treatment with calcitriol, the set point for calcium was returned toward normal (Fig. 5). The finding that administration of calcitriol appears to result in a downward and leftward shift in the curve relating PTH

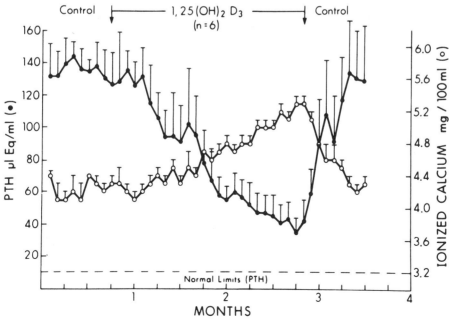

FIG. 4. Effect of intravenous calcitriol on the levels of PTH and ionized calcium in patients on hemodialysis. (Reprinted from ref. 51 with permission.)

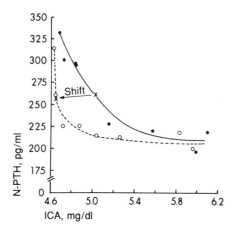

FIG. 5. Effects of treatment with calcitriol for a period of 2 weeks on the relationship between PTH levels and serum ionized calcium (ICA). ●, Baseline; ○, after 2 weeks. The set point for calcium was reduced by the administration of calcitriol. (Reprinted from ref. 52 with permission.)

secretion to serum calcium has also been made by Dunlay et al. (53).

In summary (Fig. 3), the effects of calcitriol on parathyroid gland function are complex and may occur at many levels. Calcitriol deficiency may lead to hypocalcemia principally by decreasing intestinal calcium absorption. Low levels of calcitriol may also play a role in initiating parathyroid cell hyperplasia by its effect on the regulation of parathyroid cell growth. Low levels of calcitriol have a profound effect on preproPTH synthesis by a direct effect on the regulation of PTH gene transcription. Evidence has also been presented that low levels of calcitriol may decrease the expression of vitamin D receptor in parathyroid tissue and consequently may influence the responsivity of the parathyroid gland to changes in calcitriol. Decreased levels of calcitriol may also play a role in the regulation of the set point for calcium-regulated PTH secretion. These abnormalities in parathyroid gland function as a consequence of decreased levels of calcitriol may contribute to the generation and maintenance of hyperparathyroidism in the course of renal insufficiency and provide the basis for the therapeutic effects of calcitriol in the treatment of hyperparathyroidism in uremia.

ROLE OF HYPOCALCEMIA

Hypocalcemia is not uncommon during the course of renal insufficiency. The potential mechanisms for the development of hypocalcemia are several. The retention of phosphorus leading to hyperphosphatemia may result in the formation of complexes with calcium. Hypocalcemia may occur as a result of deposi-

tion of these complexes in soft tissue and/or bone. Since a major action of calcitriol is to regulate intestinal absorption of calcium, it follows that, as levels of calcitriol decline with progressive renal disease, the intestinal absorption of calcium also falls. Decreased intestinal absorption of calcium may contribute to the development of hypocalcemia, which in turn would provide a stimulus for increased PTH secretion. Studies of the measurement of intestinal calcium absorption at various levels of renal function have revealed results similar to the relationship between calcitriol and renal function and reflect the major role of calcitriol in the regulation of intestinal calcium absorption. An additional cause of hypocalcemia is that of skeletal resistance to the calcemic actions of PTH (see below).

SKELETAL RESISTANCE TO PARATHYROID HORMONE

Resistance of the skeleton to the hypercalcemic action of PTH is another potential cause of hypocalcemia and hyperparathyroidism in patients with renal insufficiency. It has been demonstrated that the increase in serum calcium in response to infusion of PTH is significantly less in hypocalcemic patients with renal failure than in normal subjects (54,55). Additional observations have indicated that recovery from induced hypocalcemia in patients with mild renal insufficiency is delayed compared to results from normal subjects, despite a greater augmentation of PTH levels in those with renal insufficiency. These findings could be interpreted to indicate that the skeleton is resistant to the calcemic actions of PTH (56). In experimental acute renal failure, it has been shown that treatment with calcitriol results in the partial correction of the blunted calcemic response to PTH (56,57). Further observations in rats have shown that hyperphosphatemia may play an important role in skeletal resistance (58,59). In studies in isolated, perfused bone, it has been shown that there is a blunted release of cyclic adenosine monophosphate (cAMP) in response to PTH. However, if parathyroidectomy is performed prior to the perfusion of isolated bone, the cAMP response to PTH is restored to normal (60,61). These studies indicate the possibility that desensitization or downregulation of the PTH receptor–adenylyl cyclase system in bone as a result of endogenous high levels of PTH leads to a resistance to further infusions of PTH. Further in vivo studies by Galceran (62) have demonstrated that parathyroidectomy prior to the study of the calcemic response to PTH results in a normalization of the response, while, when parathyroid glands were intact in the animal, a blunted response to PTH was observed. These observations provide further support for the concept of desensitization of the PTH receptor–effector mechanisms and minimize a direct role for calcitriol, since the levels of calcitriol remain low in both groups of animals. Similar results were obtained in uremic rats by Rodriguez et al. (63). An additional mechanism for skeletal resistance has been suggested from studies in organ culture in which high levels of medium phosphorus result in blunted release of calcium on bone in response to PTH (64). These abnormalities at the level of bone can, therefore, contribute to the pathogenesis of hyperparathyroidism in uremia.

EFFECT OF ALUMINUM ON PARATHYROID FUNCTION

As is discussed above, central to the control of hyperparathyroidism is the control of serum phosphorus. This was initially accomplished by the use of aluminum-containing antacids to bind dietary phosphorus and prevent its absorption. While it was believed that such treatment was safe and had been shown to be effective, following the demonstration of aluminum toxicity in patients with end-stage renal disease as result of high aluminum content of the dialysis water (65), the issue of aluminum accumulation as a result of the ingestion of aluminum-containing antacids was reevaluated. It has now been realized that aluminum can, indeed, accumulate in the bodies of patients with end-stage renal disease as a result of antacid ingestion (66) and can result in significant toxicity (67). Characteristics of the syndrome of aluminum toxicity are related mainly to the skeleton and include bone pain; easy fracturability; hypercalcemia, especially if vitamin D analogs are administered; relatively low levels of PTH in serum; and a characteristic appearance by bone biopsy (see the chapter by Coburn and Salusky). Special staining of the bone biopsy may show aluminum deposition in bone, often localized at the mineralization front (68). The low levels of PTH in blood can be explained by the observation that aluminum can accumulate in the parathyroid gland (69). Furthermore, it has been shown that aluminum may directly decrease PTH secretion in vitro, as is shown in Fig. 6 (70). Since it has been shown that cessation of aluminum ingestion is associated with a gradual reduction in the levels of plasma aluminum in patients with end-stage renal disease, it is now recommended that aluminum-containing antacids should be avoided if possible, that aluminum levels be carefully monitored, and that phosphate binding be achieved with calcium salts.

SUMMARY

The pathogenesis of hyperparathyroidism in chronic renal disease is multifactorial. The major factors involved are the retention of phosphorus and the decreased levels of calcitriol, which set in motion a series of events resulting in a state of disordered calcium-regulated PTH secretion. While each of these factors may contribute to the development of hyperparathyroidism in a variety of ways, the relative role of each of these mechanisms in the development of hyperparathyroidism may vary from patient to patient. It may also vary as a result of the particular nature of the renal disease (tubulointerstitial or glomerular/vascular); overall vitamin D status of the patient; and individual dietary habits with respect to the intake of calcium, phosphorus, and protein. The elucidation of the pathogenetic factors involved in the genesis of secondary hyperparathyroidism in renal failure provides the basis for a rational therapeutic approach to its treatment.

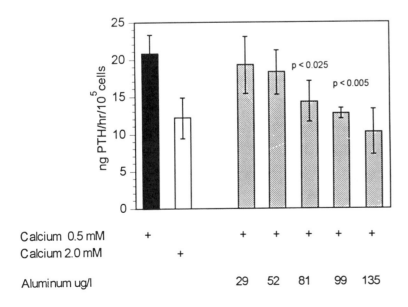

FIG. 6. Effect of aluminum on the secretion of parathyroid hormone in dispersed bovine parathyroid cells in vitro. *Solid bar,* 0.5 mM calcium; *open bar,* 2.0 mM calcium; *shaded bars,* 0.5 mM calcium plus aluminum. The aluminum concentrations represent the measured levels of free aluminum in the medium. (Reprinted from ref. 70 with permission.)

ACKNOWLEDGMENTS

The authors thank Emma Williams for secretarial assistance. This work was supported in part by grants DK09976 and AR39561 from the National Institutes of Health.

REFERENCES

1. Albright F, Drake TG, Sulkowitch HW. Renal osteitis fibrosa cystica: report of case with discussion of metabolic aspects. *Johns Hopkins Med J* 1937;60:377.
2. Follis RH Jr, Jackson DA. Renal osteomalacia and osteitis fibrosa in adults. *Johns Hopkins Med J* 1943;72:232.
3. Pappenheimer AM. Effect of an experimental reduction of kidney substance upon parathyroid glands and skeletal tissue. *J Exp Med* 1936;64:965.
4. Pappenheimer AM, Wilens SL. Enlargement of the parathyroid glands in renal disease. *Am J Pathol* 1935;11:73.
5. Reiss E, Canterbury JM, Bilinsky RT. Measurement of serum parathyroid hormone in renal insufficiency. *Trans Assoc Am Physicians* 1968;81:104.
6. Arnaud CD. Hyperparathyroidism and renal failure. *Kidney Int* 1973;4:89.
7. Llach F, Massry SG, Singer FR, Kurokawa K, Kaye JM, Coburn JW. Skeletal resistance of endogenous parathyroid hormone in patients with early renal failure: a possible cause of secondary hyperparathyroidism. *J Clin Endocrinol Metab* 1975;41:333–345.
8. Slatopolsky E, Caglar S, Pennell JP, et al. On the pathogenesis of hyperparathyroidism in chronic experimental insufficiency in the dog. *J Clin Invest* 1971;50:492–499.
9. Slatopolsky E, Caglar S, Gradowska L, Canterbury J, Reiss E, Bricker NS. On the prevention of secondary hyperparathyroidism in experimental chronic renal disease using "proportional reduction" of dietary phosphorus intake. *Kidney Int* 1972;2:147–151.
10. Slatopolsky E, Bricker NS. The role of phosphorus restriction in the prevention of secondary hyperparathyroidism in chronic renal disease. *Kidney Int* 1973;4:141.
11. LaFlame FG, Jowsey J. Bone and soft tissue changes with oral phosphate supplements. *J Clin Invest* 1972;51:2834.
12. Jowsey J, Reiss E, Canterbury JM. Long-term effects of high phosphate intake on parathyroid hormone levels and bone metabolism. *Acta Orthop Scand* 1974;45:801.
13. Rutherford WE, Bordier P, Marie P, et al. Phosphate control and 25-hydroxycholecalciferol administration in preventing experimental renal osteodystrophy in the dog. *J Clin Invest* 1977;60:332–341.
14. Llach F, Massry SG. On the mechanism of the prevention of secondary hyperparathyroidism in moderate renal insufficiency. *J Clin Endocrinol Metab* 1985;61:601.
15. Reiss E, Canterbury MJ, Bercovitz MA, Kaplan EL. The role of phosphate in the secretion of parathyroid hormone in man. *J Clin Invest* 1970;49:2146.
16. Portale AA, Booth BE, Halloran BP, Morris RC Jr. Effect of dietary phosphorus on circulating concentrations of 1,25-dihydroxyvitamin D_3 and immunoreactive parathyroid hormone in children with moderate renal insufficiency. *J Clin Invest* 1984;73:1580–1589.
17. Wilson L, Felsenfeld A, Drezner MK, Llach F. Altered divalent ion metabolism in early renal failure: Role of 1,25(OH)₂D. *Kidney Int* 1985;17:565–573.
18. Llach F, Massry SG. On the mechanisms of secondary hyperparathyroidism in moderate renal insufficiency. *J Clin Endocrinol Metab* 1985;61:601–606.
19. Lopez-Hilker S, Galceran T, Chan Y, Rapp N, Martin KJ, Slatopolsky E. Hypocalcemia may not be essential for the development of secondary hyperparathyroidism in chronic renal failure. *J Clin Invest* 1986;78:1097–1102.
20. Tanaka Y, DeLuca HF. The control of 25-hydroxyvitamin D metabolism by inorganic phosphorus. *Arch Biochem Biophys* 1973;159:566.
21. Lopez-Hilker S, Dusso AS, Rapp NS, Martin KJ, Slatopolsky E. Phosphorus restriction reverses hyperparathyroidism in uremia independent of changes in calcium and calcitriol. *Am J Physiol* 1990;259:F432–F437.
22. Mason RS, Lissner D, Wilkinson M, Posen S. Vitamin D metabolites and their relationship to azotemic osteodystrophy. *Clin Endocrinol* 1980;13:375.
23. Christiansen C, Christensen MS, Melsen F, Ridbro P, DeLuca HF. Mineral metabolism in chronic renal failure with special reference to serum concentrations of 1,25(OH)₂D and 24,25(OH)₂D. *Clin Nephrol* 1981;15:18–22.
24. Juttmann JR, Buurman CJ, DeKam E, et al. Serum concentrations of metabolites of vitamin D in patients with chronic renal failure (CRF). Consequences for the treatment with 1-α-hydroxy-derivatives. *Clin Endocrinol* 1981;14:225.
25. Tessitore N, Lund B, Lund B, et al. Vitamin D metabolites in patients with early renal failure: effects of dietary phosphate restriction and calcium supplementation. *Kidney Int* 1981;20:303.
26. Wilson L, Felsenfeld A, Drezner MK, Llach F. Altered divalent ion metabolism in early renal failure: Role of 1,25(OH)₂D. *Kidney Int* 1985;27:565.
27. Gafter U, Kraut JA, Lee DBN, et al. Effect of metabolic acidosis on interstitial absorption of calcium and phosphorus. *Am J Physiol* 1980;239:G480–G484.
28. Bushinsky DA, Favus AMJ, Schneider AB, Sen PK, Sherwood LM, Coe FL. Effects of metabolic acidosis on PTH and 1,25(OH)₂D₃ response to low calcium diet. *Am J Physiol* 1982;243:F570–F575.
29. Kraut JA, Gordon EM, Ransom JC, et al. Effect of chronic metabolic acidosis on vitamin D metabolism in humans. *Kidney Int* 1983;24:644–648.
30. Bushinsky DA, Riera GS, Favus MJ, Coe FL. Response of serum 1,25(OH)₂D₃ to variation of ionized calcium during chronic acidosis. *Am J Physiol* 1985;249:F361–F365.
31. Langman CB, Bushinsky DA, Favus MJ, Coe FL. Ca and P regulation of 1,25(OH)₂D₃ synthesis by vitamin D-replete rat tubules during acidosis. *Am J Physiol* 1986;251:F911–F918.
32. Krapf R, Vetsch R, Vetsch W, Hulter HN. Chronic metabolic acidosis increases the serum concentration in 1,25-dihydroxyvitamin D in humans by stimulating its production rate. *J Clin Invest* 1992;90:2456–2463.
33. Hsu CH, Patel S. Uremic plasma contains factors inhibiting 1-α-hydroxylase activity. *J Am Soc Nephrol* 1991;3:947–952.
34. Bellorin-Font E, Martin KJ, Freitag JJ, et al. Altered adenylate cyclase kinetics in hyperfunctioning human parathyroid glands. Comparison with normal human and bovine parathyroid tissue. *J Clin Endocrinol Metab* 1981;52:499–507.
35. Brown EM, Brennan MF, Hurwitz S, et al. Dispersed cells prepared from human parathyroid glands. Distinct calcium sensitivity of adenomas vs. primary hyperplasia. *J Clin Endocrinol Metab* 1978;46:267–275.
36. Brown EM, Wilkson RE, Eastman RC, Pallotta J, Marynick SP. Abnormal regulation of parathyroid hormone release by calcium in secondary hyperparathyroidism due to chronic renal failure. *J Clin Endocrinol Metab* 1982;54:172–179.
37. Brumbaugh PF, Hughes MR, Haussler MR. Cytoplasmic and nuclear binding components for 1 alpha, 25-dihydroxyvitamin D₃ in chick parathyroid glands. *Proc Natl Acad Sci USA* 1975;72:4871–4875.
38. Chertow BS, Baylink DJ, Wergedal JE, Su MHH, Norman AW. Decrease in serum immunoreactive parathyroid hormone in rats in a parathyroid hormone section in vitro by 1,25-dihydroxycholecalciferol. *J Clin Invest* 1975;56:668–678.
39. Golden P, Greenwalt A, Martin K, et al. Lack of direct effect of 1,25-dihydroxycholecalciferol on parathyroid hormone secretion by normal bovine parathyroid glands. *Endocrinology* 1980;107:602–607.
40. Cantley LK, Russell J, Lettieri D, Sherwood LM. 1,25-Dihydroxyvitamin D₃ suppresses PTH secretion from bovine

parathyroid cells in tissue culture. *Endocrinology* 1985; 227:2114–2119.

41. Chan YL, McKay C, Dye E, Slatopolsky E. The effect of 1,25-dihydroxycholecalciferol on parathyroid hormone section by monolayer cultures of bovine parathyroid cells. *Calcif Tissue Int* 1986;38:27–32.

42. Silver J, Russell J, Sherwood LM. Regulation of vitamin D metabolites of messenger RNA for pre-proparathyroid hormone in isolated bovine parathyroid cells. *Proc Natl Acad Sci USA* 1985;82:4270–4273.

43. Russell J, Lettieri D, Sherwood LM. Suppression by 1,25(OH)$_2$D$_3$ of transcription of the parathyroid hormone gene. *Endocrinology* 1986;119:2864–2866.

44. Silver J, Naveh-Many T, Mayer H, Schmeizer HJ, Popovtzer MM. Regulation by vitamin D metabolites of parathyroid gene transcription in vitro in the rat. *J Clin Invest* 1986; 78:1296–1301.

45. Okazaki T, Igarashi T, Kronenberg HM. 5′-Flanking region of the parathyroid hormone gene mediates negative regulation by 1,25(OH)$_2$D$_3$. *J Biol Chem* 1988;263:2203–2208.

46. Korkor AB. Reduced binding of [^{3}H]1,25-dihydroxyvitamin D$_3$ in the parathyroid glands of patients with renal failure. *N Engl J Med* 1987;316:1573–1577.

47. Merke J, Hugel U, Zlotkowski A, et al. Diminished parathyroid 1,25(OH)$_2$D$_3$ receptors in experimental uremia. *Kidney Int* 1987;32:350–353.

48. Brown AJ, Dusso A, Lopez-Hilker S, Lewis-Finch J, Grooms P, Slatopolsky E. 1,25(OH)$_2$D receptors are decreased in parathyroid glands from chronically uremic dogs. *Kidney Int* 1989;35:19–23.

49. Naveh-Many T, Marx R, Keshet E, Pike JW, Silver J. Regulation of 1,25-dihydroxyvitamin D$_3$ in the parathyroid in vivo. *J Clin Invest* 1990;86:1968–1975.

50. Kremer R, Bolivar I, Goltzman D, Hendy GN. Influence of calcium and 1,25-dihydroxycholecalciferol on proliferation and proto-oncogene expression in primary cultures of bovine parathyroid cells. *Endocrinology* 1989;125:935–941.

51. Slatopolsky E, Weerts C, Thielan J, Horst R, Harter H, Martin KJ. Marked suppression of secondary hyperparathyroidism by intravenous administration of 1,25-dihydroxycholecalciferol in uremic patients. *J Clin Invest* 1984;74:2136–2143.

52. Delmez AJ, Tindira C, Grooms P, Dusso A, Windus DW, Slatopolsky E. Parathyroid hormone suppression by intravenous 1,25-dihydroxyvitamin D: a role for increased sensitivity to calcium. *J Clin Invest* 1989;83:1349–1355.

53. Dunlay R, Rodriguez M, Felsenfeld AJ, Llach F. Direct inhibitory effect of calcitriol on parathyroid function (sigmoidal curve) in dialysis. *Kidney Int* 1989;36:1093–1098.

54. Evanson JM. The response to the infusion of parathyroid extract in hypocalcemia states. *Clin Sci* 1966;31:63.

55. Massry SG, Coburn JW Lee DBM, et al. Skeletal resistance to parathyroid hormone in renal failure: study in 105 human subjects. *Ann Intern Med* 1973;78:357.

56. Somerville PJ, Kaye M. Resistance to parathyroid hormone in renal failure: role of vitamin D metabolites. *Kidney Int* 1978;14:245–254.

57. Massry SG, Stein R, Garty J, et al. Skeletal resistance to the calcemic action of parathyroid hormone in uremia: role of 1,25(OH)$_2$D$_3$. *Kidney Int* 1976;9:467–474.

58. Somerville PJ, Kaye M. Evidence that resistance to the calcemic action of parathyroid hormone in rats with actue uremia is caused by phosphate retention. *Kidney Int* 1979; 16:552–560.

59. Rodriguez M, Martin-Malo A, Martinez ME, Torres A, Felsenfeld AJ, Llach F. Calcemic response to parathyroid hormone in renal failure: role of phosphorus and its effect on calcitriol. *Kidney Int* 1991;40:1055–1062.

60. Olgaard K, Schwartz J, Finco D, et al. Extraction of parathyroid hormone and release of cyclic-AMP by isolated perfused bones obtained from dogs with acute uremia. *Endocrinology* 1982;111:1678–1682.

61. Olgaard K, Arbelaez M, Schwartz J, Klahr S, Slatopolsky E. Abnormal skeletal response to parathyroid hormone in dogs with chronic uremia. Skeletal cyclic-AMP response to PTH in chronic uremia. *Calcif Tissue Int* 1982;34:403–407.

62. Galceran T, Martin KJ, Morrissey JJ, Slatopolsky E. Role of 1,25-dihydroxyvitamin D on the skeletal resistance to parathyroid hormone. *Kidney Int* 1987;32:801–807.

63. Rodriguez M, Felsenfeld AJ, Llach F. Calcemic response to parathyroid hormone in renal failure: role of calcitriol and the effect of parathyroidectomy. *Kidney Int* 1991;40:1063–1068.

64. Raisz LG, Niemann I: Effect of phosphate, calcium and magnesium on bone resorption and hormonal responses in tissue culture. *Endocrinology* 1969;85:446–452.

65. Platts MM, Goode GC, Hislup JS. Composition of the domestic water supply and the incidence of fractures and encephalopathy in patients on home dialysis. *Br Med J* 1977; 2:657–660.

66. Kaehny W, Hegg A, Alfrey A. Gastrointestinal absorption of aluminum from aluminum containing antacids. *N Engl J Med* 1977;296:1389–1390.

67. Ott SM, Maloney NA, Coburn JW, Alfrey AC, Sherrard DJ. The prevalence of bone aluminum deposition in renal osteodystrophy and its relation to the response to calcitriol therapy. *N Engl J Med* 1982;307:709–713.

68. Sherrard DJ, Andress DL. Aluminum-related osteodystrophy. *Adv Intern Med* 1989;34:307–324.

69. Cann C, Prussin S, Gordon G. Aluminum uptake by the parathyroid glands. *J Clin Endocrinol Metab* 1979;49:543–545.

70. Morrissey J, Slatopolsky E. The effect of aluminum on parathyroid hormone secretion. *Kidney Int* 1986;29:S41–S44.

The Parathyroids, edited by J.P. Bilezikian,
M.A. Levine, and R. Marcus. Raven Press, Ltd.,
New York © 1994.

CHAPTER 42

Hyperparathyroidism in Renal Failure

Clinical Features, Diagnosis, and Management

Jack W. Coburn and Isidro B. Salusky

The prevention and management of secondary hyper-parathyroidism are major challenges to physicians who care for patients with renal failure, particularly insofar as the lives of these patients are extended with improved conservative management and various modes of dialysis. The development of secondary hyperparathyroidism is ubiquitous in patients with advanced renal failure (1), and it was once believed that its occurrence was almost inevitable as renal function decreased (2). However, the recent findings in a cross-sectional study of bone biopsies from 249 Canadian dialysis patients suggest that there is major change in the distribution of the types of bone diseases encountered during the last 3–4 years in dialysis patients compared to the distribution 10–15 years ago (3).

This chapter considers the types of bone disorders that occur in uremia, the various syndromes and clinical features encountered, the methods for recognition and diagnosis of these disorders, and the clinical management of uremic secondary hyperparathyroidism. Pathophysiological mechanisms are covered in the previous chapter by Martin and Slatopolsky. It must be emphasized that the diagnosis of secondary hyperparathyroidism differs from the recognition of primary hyperparathyroidism. Thus there is a qualitative difference between patients with primary hyperparathyroidism compared to normal individuals, while there is a continuum in renal insufficiency, with the condition varying from profound secondary hyperparathyroidism to "mild" disease and even to subnormal bone

turnover, the latter condition arising, in part, from "oversuppressed" parathyroid glands.

CLASSIFICATION OF RENAL BONE DISEASES

The renal bone diseases are classified based on bone biopsy features, including the bone formation rate as measured with double tetracycline labelling and the surface staining with aluminum. The disorders can be divided, from a pathogenic standpoint, into a broad group with normal or increased bone turnover, compared to those with a subnormal rate of bone turnover. The groups with normal/high turnover include: (a) osteitis fibrosa, (b) "mild" hyperparathyroid disease, and (c) mixed bone disease patients.

The other major type of disorder includes patients with low rates of bone turnover. These include (d) osteomalacia and (e) "aplastic" bone. Nearly all *symptomatic* renal patients with these types of lesions have aluminum-related bone disease, as identified by significant surface stainable aluminum (4). The differentiation between osteomalacia and "aplastic" bone is determined by the presence of widened or increased osteoid in the former. There is a newly recognized condition of "idiopathic" low bone turnover, also termed *aplastic* bone or *adynamic* bone, which lacks significant aluminum staining. Mixed bone disease exhibits markedly increased osteoid plus peritrabecular fibrosis, features of both osteitis fibrosa and osteomalacia.

MANIFESTATIONS AND SYNDROMES OBSERVED

The symptoms and signs of severe secondary hyperparathyroidism and the other forms of renal osteodys-

J. W. Coburn, I. B. Salusky: Departments of Medicine and Pediatrics, UCLA School of Medicine; and Nephrology Section, West Los Angeles Veterans Affairs Medical Center, Los Angeles, California 90073.

trophy are usually nonspecific, and the laboratory and radiographic abnormalities generally antedate the appearance of any clinical manifestations. It must be emphasized that most renal patients with immunoreactive parathyroid hormone (iPTH) levels and bone biopsies that show severe osteitis fibrosa have no symptoms that can be clearly attributed to overactivity of the parathyroid glands. Some specific symptoms and certain syndrome complexes occur in dialysis patients; these are described below.

Bone and/or Joint Pain

Bone pain is a common manifestation of severe bone disease in patients with advanced renal failure. It is usually insidious in appearance and is often aggravated by weight bearing or a change in posture. Physical findings are often absent. Pain is most common in the lower back, hips, and legs, but it may occur in the peripheral skeleton. Deep, generalized bone pain is more common and often much worse in patients with aluminum-related bone disease than in those with osteitis fibrosa; the pain is perceived by the patient as being more deeply seated than in joints or muscles (5–7).

On rare occasions, acute, severe, localized bone pain can develop in patients with marked secondary hyperparathyroidism. The sudden appearance of pain around the knee, ankle, or heel can suggest an acute arthritis; such pain is usually not relieved by massage or local heat. Radiographs may or may not show localized subperiosteal erosions; a bone scan may show increased uptake in an area corresponding to the symptoms. The disappearance of the pain after the PTH is lowered via calcitriol therapy or following parathyroidectomy is the feature indicating that the pain arose from secondary hyperparathyroidism.

Acute periarthritis that is associated with periarticular calcium deposition and crystals characteristic of hydroxypapatite (8) was not uncommon in the past in dialysis patients with marked hyperphosphatemia and a significantly elevated Ca X P product in serum (Ca X P product >75 for prolonged periods). This condition is manifested by acute pain, redness, and swelling, leading to a suspicion of gout or pseudogout. The discomfort often responds to therapy with nonsteroidal antiinflammatory drugs, and it usually disappears completely after parathyroidectomy (8,9). This problem is almost never seen in dialysis patients with reasonable control of serum phosphorus levels.

In long-term dialysis patients, severe arthralgias develop in association with the disposition of a unique amyloid made up of β_2-microglobulin; this type of amyloid is characteristically deposited in articular and periarticular structures (10). The pain about the joint may be asymmetrical, and the joints most commonly affected are the shoulders, knees, wrists, and small joints of the hand. The symptoms are typically worse at night or after a period of inactivity, and the pain is reduced or relieved by moving about (11,12). The presence of such pain in association with thin-walled bone cysts, which are erroneously described as brown tumors, may lead to an erroneous diagnosis of secondary hyperparathyroidism. Other syndromes associated with dialysis amyloidosis are described below.

Proximal Myopathy

Muscle weakness can be marked in patients with advanced renal failure. Symptoms appear so gradually that they are often ignored until the patient is limited to crutches or a wheelchair. The gait is commonly abnormal, so that the patient waddles from side to side with a typical "penguin gait." Patients note difficulty in climbing stairs or rising from a low chair, and they can have difficulty in holding their arms elevated to comb their hair. This proximal muscle weakness resembles that observed with nutritional vitamin D deficiency and that reported in primary hyperparathyroidism. Plasma levels of muscle enzymes are usually normal, and electromyographic changes are nonspecific.

The pathogenesis of such myopathy is not known; the mechanisms implicated include secondary hyperparathyroidism (13), phosphate depletion (14), abnormal vitamin D metabolism (15), and aluminum intoxication (16). Improvement in the gait posture has been observed in azotemic children after treatment with 1,25-dihydroxyvitamin D_3 [1,25-$(OH)_2D_3$] (17), and muscle weakness can improve rapidly after this treatment in affected adults (18). Improvement in proximal muscular strength has occurred after treatment with 25-hydroxyvitamin D_3 [25-$(OH)D_3$], following subtotal parathyroidectomy, after successful renal transplantation, and after chelation therapy of aluminum toxicity using desferrioxamine (16). The favorable response of some uremic patients to treatment with 25-$(OH)D_3$ or 1,25-$(OH)_2D_3$ suggests that a therapeutic trial with an active vitamin D sterol is warranted in uremic patients with myopathy. The presence of aluminum intoxication or severe secondary hyperparathyroidism must be excluded.

Pruritus

Severe itching, a common symptom in patients with advanced renal failure, sometimes improves or disappears when regular dialysis is initiated. Pruritus is particularly common in dialysis patients with severe or overt secondary hyperparathyroidism; moreover, this symptom often improves substantially or even vanishes within a few days after total or subtotal parathyroidectomy (19). The mechanism whereby secondary hyperparathyroidism leads to pruritus is unclear. Unfortunately, this symptom is not at all specific, and many dialysis patients have troublesome pruritus but lack significant secondary hyperparathyroidism. Parathyroid surgery should never be done for pruritus unless there is objective evidence of secondary hyperparathyroidism (see below under Diagnosis of Secondary Hyperparathyroidism).

Spontaneous Tendon Rupture

Spontaneous tendon rupture occurs in patients with advanced renal failure, and this occurrence is almost always associated with evidence of marked secondary hyperparathyroidism (20). The mechanism for tendon rupture is uncertain; it has been postulated to arise due to alterations in collagen metabolism affecting the structure of tendons (21,22) or secondary to microfractures in bone at the site of the tendon insertion (23). When a patient with end-stage renal disease (ESRD) has a tendon rupture, there should be a careful search for features of secondary hyperparathyroidism, and aggressive therapy should be directed to correct the overactive parathyroid glands.

Deformities of Bone

Bone deformities are particularly common in uremic patients with severe aluminum toxicity, but they can also occur as a consequence of secondary hyperparathyroidism. Bone deformities are common in children with renal failure and secondary hyperparathyroidism, almost certainly related to the high rates of bone growth, modeling, and remodeling that exist in the immature skeleton; both the axial and the appendicular skeletons are involved in children. In adults, bony deformities arise due to fractures or to remodeling, with the axial skeleton most commonly affected (24). Thus rib deformities and kyphoscoliosis commonly produce a "funnel chest" abnormality. Enlargement of the distal tufts of the fingers due to osteitis fibrosa produces an appearance that is appropriately termed *pseudoclubbing* (25). In children <10 years of age, bowing of long bones, genu valgum, and ulnar deviation of the wrist are frequent. Slipped epiphyses occur most commonly in the preadolescent period and are particularly common in patients with long-standing congenital renal disease (24). The radiographic features of a "rickets-like" lesion observed in uremic children has histologic features of osteitis fibrosa and secondary hyperparathyroidism rather than vitamin D deficiency or osteomalacia (26).

Calciphylaxis

This is an unusual syndrome that occasionally develops in patients with advanced renal failure, those treated with regular dialysis, and those with functioning kidney transplants; it is characterized by spontaneous ischemic necrosis of the skin, muscles, and/or subcutaneous fat (27). The pathogenesis of this syndrome is unknown. Extensive medial calcification of the arteries is present, but such calcification commonly exists without causing gangrene or ulcerations; thus it is not certain that the vascular calcification, per se, is the cause of the ischemic necrosis. Most patients with this syndrome have a history of marked hyperphosphatemia and severe secondary hyperparathyroidism. A significant percentage of such patients have shown clinical improvement within a few days after parathyroidectomy (27). In some patients (28) and in an animal model of this syndrome (29), glucocorticoid therapy may predispose to the development of the lesion.

Patients with calciphylaxis often die from secondary infection. Because of this poor prognosis, urgent parathyroidectomy is often recommended in patients with secondary hyperparathyroidism. Patients with diabetes mellitus and renal failure also develop ischemic lesions, medial vascular calcification, and a similar clinical picture. However, the lesions observed in diabetic patients rarely improve following parathyroidectomy, and parathyroid surgery should be reserved for patients with definite evidence of overt secondary hyperparathyroidism.

Growth Retardation

Delayed growth is common in children with chronic renal failure. Chronic acidosis, malnutrition, secondary hyperparathyroidism, and low levels of somatomedin are factors suggested to cause this complex problem (30–32). The correction of certain of these abnormalities has been associated with improved growth velocity; however, this does not occur in all cases. Improved or even catch-up growth has been observed in a few children following treatment with calcitriol (33); however, the number of patients studied was small, and subsequent reports have not confirmed the original findings (34). Recombinant growth hormone has been introduced for the management of the growth retardation found in uremic children, and initial reports demonstrated increased growth velocity, particularly in prepubertal patients with stable renal insufficiency (35). The long-term results and potential side effects of such intervention require further evaluation.

Dialysis Amyloidosis

Dialysis-related amyloidosis can lead to certain clinical syndromes that resemble secondary hyperparathyroidism or other types of renal osteodystrophy; moreover, such amyloidosis often exists concurrently with one of the metabolic bone conditions. Dialysis amyloidosis arises from the deposition in bone and periarticular structures of a specific type of amyloid made up of β_2-microglobulin (36). The frequency of its clinical presentation increases substantially in patients treated with regular dialysis for >5–10 years, and it is much more common in patients who start dialysis after age 50 years (37). The blood levels of β_2-microglobulin are strikingly elevated in all patients with ESRD because of failure of the normal renal catabolism of this normal plasma constituent.

The clinical manifestations can include: 1) carpal tunnel syndrome, which is the most common feature; 2) destructive or erosive arthropathy involving the large and medium-sized joints, with shoulder, knee, hip or back pain the most common manifestations; 3) spondyloarthropathy, most commonly affecting the cervical spine; 4) subchondral, thin-walled cysts of bone, most commonly affecting the carpal bones, humoral and femoral heads, distal radius, acetabulum, and tibial plateau (Fig. 1); 5) local tendinitis, particularly of the hand; and 6) joint effusions and tendon sheath cysts. The involvement of the tendons of the hand can cause trigger fingers, swan-neck deformities, and camptodactly. The subchondral cysts probably represent amyloidomas infiltrating the cavity of the bone at a site of a tendon insertion. They are at times confused with brown tumors of secondary hyperparathyroidism. However, their location and multiple occurrence differs from brown tumors, which are usually solitary and occur most commonly in the rib or mandible (38). Nonetheless, one must consider this syndrome as a potential cause of musculoskeletal and periarticular symptoms that are encountered in a long-term dialysis patient. One pitfall to avoid is to recommend parathyroid surgery for a dialysis patient whose musculoskeletal symptoms do not improve after lowering of PTH levels with calcitriol therapy; the symptoms may be due to dialysis-related amyloidosis. A specific diagnosis of the latter can be made from the biopsy demonstration of amyloid made up of β_2-microglobulin. However, invasive procedures are rarely indicated to establish the diagnosis, which can generally be made from the clinical presentation (38), the finding of multiple thin-walled cysts on skeletal radiographs, and/or the demonstration of thickened shoulder tendons by ultrasound examination of the shoulders (39). The management of this syndrome is largely unsatisfactory. Successful renal transplantation leads to rapid normalization of plasma levels of β_2-microglobulin, the symptoms often disappear (40), and there may be no further progression of the bony cysts on subsequent radiographs (41); however, the histologic features of amyloid may persist (42).

Destructive Spondyloarthropathy

The frequency of reports suggests that destructive spondyloarthropathy is more common in patients with uremia, particularly those undergoing hemodialysis (43). The cervical spine may be more commonly involved. The underlying pathogenic mechanisms include secondary hyperparathyroidism [both with (44) and without brown tumors (45)], dialysis amyloidosis (41,46), and microcrystalline deposits (hydroxy apatite) (43); in yet other cases, no etiologic diagnosis has been established (personal observations). In many patients the manifestations are merely radiographic, but in others spinal cord compression with severe neurologic sequelae follows. The prognosis for such patients, particularly those who are symptomatic, has not been good (47), although neurologic improvement has been reported following spinal cord decompression and parathyroidectomy (45). The finding of this clinical syndrome in a dialysis patient should lead to a search for both secondary hyperparathyroidism and dialysis amyloidosis.

Low Turnover Bone Without Aluminum: Idiopathic Aplastic or Adynamic Bone

This condition, which is defined above, is a histologic diagnosis from bone biopsy. It is included because it may be related to "oversuppressed" PTH levels and because its presence may impact on the maneuvers used to prevent and treat renal bone disease. Several reports have noted the finding of "aplastic" or "adynamic" bone without aluminum staining in

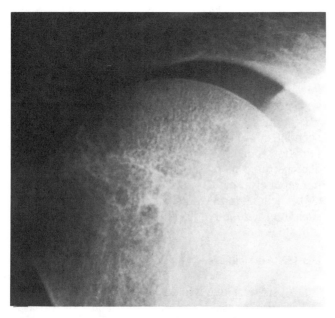

FIG. 1. Thin-walled cysts characteristic of dialysis amyloidosis in the proximal humerus of a long-term dialysis patient.

dialysis patients (37,48–53). They were identified not because of symptoms or biochemical features but because bone biopsies were done in cross-sectional studies of dialysis patients. This lesion has occurred in both children (48) and adults (49,50,52,53). The percentage of patients with this lesion has varied from 10% (48) to 31% (52) and to as high as 48% (53) among those treated with continuous ambulatory peritoneal dialysis (CAPD), and it has been seen in up to 17% of hemodialysis patients (53). The patients with this "idiopathic" aplastic bone do not have fractures, bone pain, or muscle weakness with any higher frequency than patients with only "mild" hyperparathyroidism. They may be more prone to development of hypercalcemia with intake of the calcium-containing phosphate binders (37,52,53) and during calcitriol therapy (54). One would expect such patients to be more susceptible to aluminum toxicity if they were given aluminum gels (55,56).

The factors associated with the occurrence of this disorder include 1) the ingestion of large doses of calcium carbonate/calcium acetate as phosphate binders, 2) the use of continuous ambulatory peritoneal dialysis as the dialysis modality; 3) the presence of diabetes mellitus, and 4) the use of dialysate calcium concentrations of 3.0–3.5 mEq/liter. Serum iPTH levels (intact) have ranged from normal to 1.5 times the upper normal limit (49,51–53). Another factor that may predispose to this lesion is therapy with calcitriol, particularly when serum PTH levels are not significantly elevated (54). There has been no difference between iPTH levels in patients with the idiopathic disorder compared to those with the low turnover state and significant aluminum staining (37,52), and the dynamics of parathyroid function during acute hypocalcemia and hypercalcemia did not differ (37). On the theory that PTH levels were "oversuppressed" by the flux of calcium from dialysate, Hercz et al. (57) lowered the calcium concentration in peritoneal dialysate from 3.5 to 2.0 mEq/liter for several months; this was followed by a fourfold rise in the mean intact (IRMA) PTH from 38 to 139 pg/ml, indicating that the "high" dialysate calcium contributes to the "suppressed" PTH levels. Whether this "disorder" will lead to overt clinical problems is presently unknown, and long-term observations are needed to identify whether such patients may be at greater risk of developing symptoms or other bone pathology with longer follow-up. Until more is known about the natural history of this condition, it would seem prudent that iPTH levels in dialysis patients should be maintained at >1.5-fold the upper normal limits (see below).

DIAGNOSIS OF THE RENAL BONE DISEASES

Because more than one pathologic process is involved in producing the "renal bone diseases," it is important to identify the type of disorder and its cause. Serum levels of iPTH were initially believed to hold the key to recognizing secondary hyperparathyroidism in patients with renal failure. However, the heterogeneity of iPTH and its fragments in the plasma (58) and the fact that renal failure, per se, leads to retention of certain PTH fragments (59) have led to difficulty with the interpretation of a given iPTH value in recognizing significant or overt secondary hyperparathyroidism. Several studies have reported correlations between serum iPTH levels and various histologic features of secondary hyperparathyroidism observed on bone biopsy (48,60–63), but most do not provide information on the sensitivity and specificity of an iPTH level for a diagnosis. Aluminum toxicity, which causes bone disease by a different process and requires totally different management (56), must be distinguished from secondary hyperparathyroidism. Three questions that must be answered are 1) does the patient have significant secondary hyperparathyroidism? 2) is aluminum toxicity present? and 3) does the patient have features consistent with low bone turnover without aluminum? This chapter considers the procedures and laboratory tests that can assist in the diagnosis of the specific type of renal bone disease present. Clinicians also encounter many dialysis patients with musculoskeletal symptoms that arise from dialysis amyloidosis (38); the diagnosis of this disorder is generally based on clinical features, radiographs, and ultrasonography; there are no laboratory tests that aid in the recognition of this problem. Except for a brief description of its clinical features, this condition is beyond the scope of this review.

Bone Biopsy

The evaluation of bone histology provides 1) a diagnosis of the specific type of renal bone disease present, 2) a method for understanding the pathophysiology of renal bone disease, and 3) a guide to its proper management. Currently, bone biopsy procedures can be done on an outpatient basis with minimal morbidity in both adult and pediatric patients (48,64,65). Double tetracycline labeling combined with quantitative histomorphometry permits evaluation of bone formation rate and is the method to identify defective mineralization (5,66). For this, tetracycline is given on two occasions, separated by a specific time interval, usually 10–17 days. The width of separation of the two fluorescent bands of tetracycline observed on the biopsy and the length of bone surface showing such labels permit calculation of the bone formation rate (BFR); the finding of subnormal bone turnover is critical in identifying certain disorders of bone.

The disorders with normal/high turnover include osteitis fibrosa and mild hyperparathyroidism. The bone in osteitis fibrosa shows increased bone turnover, with increased numbers of osteoblasts and osteoclast and variable degrees of peritrabecular fibrosis. Such bone shows increased amounts of woven osteoid, with a haphazard arrangement of collagen fibers, in contrast to the usual lamellar pattern of osteoid in normal bone. Mild hyperparathyroidism has normal or increased formation, but there is minimal or no peritrabecular fibrosis. With these lesions, the major pathogenic factor is increased levels of PTH.

The other major category of alteration in uremic bone is the state of low bone turnover, with either 1) osteomalacia or 2) a state of reduced bone formation without osteomalacia. Osteomalacia is characterized by the presence of wide osteoid seams, increased numbers of osteoid lamellae, increased trabecular surface covered with osteoid, and diminished rate of bone formation, as assessed by double tetracycline labeling. Peritrabecular fibrosis is absent or minimal (67). Biopsies that show normal osteoid volume, the absence of fibrosis, and yet a reduced bone formation rate, as measured via double tetracycline label, are classified as "aplastic" or "adynamic" bone lesion (4,67). Patients with >25% surface staining with aluminum along the bone surfaces and a paucity of osteoblasts and osteoclast often present all the clinical features of aluminum-related bone disease (5). Patients with the aplastic or adynamic lesion but without significant surface-stainable aluminum are believed to represent a different process, which is reviewed above.

When osteitis fibrosa co-exists with osteomalacia, the pattern is called a *mixed* lesion (5). Mixed lesions, as observed in the past, were often associated with significant hypocalcemia and elevated serum PTH levels; the disorder responded readily to calcitriol therapy (67). Such a lesion is more commonly seen as a transition from osteitis fibrosa to aluminum-related bone disease or the reverse (3). The reader is referred elsewhere for a more complete description of bone histology and histomorphologic findings in the renal bone diseases (68,69).

Serum Calcium, Phosphorus, and Alkaline Phosphatase

The measurement of serum calcium and phosphorus levels in a large number of ESRD patients often reveals differences between groups with different types of bone disease (55,70); however, these levels are of little value to separate individual patients. Significant hypercalcemia is not uncommon in patients with osteitis fibrosa (55,70) or aluminum-related bone disease (55,70); it may be more common in those with the low turnover bone condition without aluminum ("aplastic" or "adynamic" bone) (71). The measurement of ionized calcium increases the sensitivity to recognize hy-

percalcemia, particularly in patients undergoing peritoneal dialysis (72), since their serum albumin levels are often below normal and are generally lower than those observed in hemodialysis patients (63). Serum phosphorus levels are commonly higher in a group of patients with osteitis fibrosa than in those with aluminum bone disease (70), but serum phosphorus levels are not discriminating in individual patients.

The serum alkaline phosphatase levels are commonly elevated in patients with osteitis fibrosa; normal levels are also common, however. A slow progressive rise of alkaline phosphatase, even within the normal range (73), may indicate worsening secondary hyperparathyroidism. This is because the bone isoenzyme of alkaline phosphatase represents a small fraction of total of alkaline phosphatase. Thus the bone isoenzyme of alkaline phosphatase was above normal in 30% of dialysis patients who had normal total alkaline phosphatase levels (74). Patients with severe aluminum-related osteomalacia that arose from aluminum-contaminated dialysate were reported to have normal total alkaline phosphatase levels (75), while other patients with a similar disorder that developed slowly from the ingestion of aluminum gels often had elevated levels (55). From this, one could conclude that alkaline phosphatase levels are not as specific for separation of osteitis fibrosa from osteomalacia as was once believed. The serial evaluation of alkaline phosphatase levels is of value, however, in following the course of a dialysis patient both over a period of many months and also during specific therapy, e.g., with calcitriol.

Parathyroid Hormone Assays

One major goal of internists and endocrinologists who use an immunoassay for PTH is the differential diagnosis of hypercalcemia, separating primary hyperparathyroidism from other causes. The interpretation of results in patients with renal insufficiency is more complex. The heterogeneity of iPTH (58) and the major role of the kidney in clearing certain immunoreactive fragments of PTH from the blood (76) create problems in interpreting PTH assays in patients with renal insufficiency. The retention of carboxyl (C)-terminal fragments and particularly the midmolecule (MM) or midregion of the C-terminal fragment of PTH in uremic patients (59) causes the levels to be markedly elevated above normal in almost all uremic patients (60), independent of whether secondary hyperparathyroidism is present. Thus the "normal" range cannot be used to interpret the results of these PTH assays. Moreover, the results from certain commercial laboratories are reported in charts in a way that either excludes patients with renal failure or assumes that all patients with renal failure have secondary hyperparathyroidism (77).

For the diagnosis of clinically significant or "overt" secondary hyperparathyroidism from serum iPTH levels in patients with renal failure, it is important to have data on specific iPTH results in relation to the features observed on bone biopsy in a large population of uremic patients. It is well known that "skeletal resistance" to the calcemic action of PTH exists in patients with renal failure (78), and there is evidence that the levels of the intact PTH must be substantially above the normal range before the skeletal features of hyperparathyroidism are present in dialysis patients (79). The clinician who evaluates a dialysis patient must ask, "Is this PTH level high enough to cause osteitis fibrosa and/or to produce the clinical symptoms of secondary hyperparathyroidism (e.g., proximal myopathy, hypercalcemia, etc.)?"

Despite some of the limitations noted above, good correlations have been reported between the results of both midregion C-terminal PTH assays (48,60,80) and C-terminal PTH assays (80–82) in comparison to several histologic features of osteitis fibrosa in biopsies of hemodialysis patients; thus correlation coefficients ranging between 0.62 (60), 0.59 (83), and 0.56 (80) have been reported. A study using the MM PTH assay in children and adolescent patients being treated with peritoneal dialysis showed little ability to separate the different types of bone diseases (48). This is almost certainly due to the removal of greater quantities of the PTH fragments by peritoneal dialysis compared to minimal removal of intact PTH (84) and to the very short circulating half-life of the intact PTH molecule compared to the very long half-life of the C-terminal fragments. Certain reports failed to observe significant correlations between histologic features of secondary hyperparathyroidism and results of a C-terminal assay for PTH (62); whether this is due to differences in the antiserum used for the PTH assay or differences in the patient population is uncertain.

With several of the PTH assays that have been used commercially, the units used to measure iPTH levels and details regarding the antiserum used often were not provided, and a report might not distinguish between a C-terminal assay or a midregion assay. Also, the normal ranges were highly variable even with assays that were called "C-terminal" or "N-terminal" assays (77). Therefore, it was very difficult to interpret the meaning of a given iPTH level in a patient with renal failure; also, few commercially available PTH methods provide information about results of PTH levels with different types of bone disease observed in patients with renal failure. It was often difficult or even impossible to compare the results from two different laboratories (77). For this reason, nephrologists have been forced to use their own experience in recognizing a specific PTH level that indicates the presence of significant secondary hyperparathyroidism.

With the in vitro synthesis of specific fragments of the PTH molecule and use of these fragments to generate antisera, the assays for PTH have been more consistent and predictable. Several studies have used antisera prepared in this manner and directed specifically toward the amino or N terminus of the PTH molecule (61,62,83,85), the biologically active region of the molecule. Because the N-terminal fragment of PTH can almost never be detected in plasma, such an assay reflects the "intact" hormone. Voigts et al. (62) and Andress et al. (83) found slightly better correlations with histologic features of hyperparathyroidism on bone biopsies of dialysis patients utilizing the N-terminal PTH assay in comparison to results with the C-terminal or midregion assays. The specific relationships between various PTH assays and the various histomorphometric features on bone biopsy of dialysis patients are reviewed in detail elsewhere (86).

The development of sensitive immunoradiometric assays or chemiluminescence assays for the intact PTH-(1–84) that employ two populations of region-specific antibodies represents a significant advance. Such assays utilize saturation kinetics rather than competitive binding and have many technical advantages over a conventional radioimmunoassay (see the chapter by Nussbaum and Potts) (87). Also, the results from the two-site assays for the "intact" PTH peptide, utilizing either an immunoradiometric assay (IRMA) (87) or a chemiluminescence assay (88), reveal remarkably similar ranges of normal from one commercial laboratory to another (87); their ability to separate patients with primary hyperparathyroidism is good and is very similar from one assay to another (87). In a comparison of the IRMA and a two-site immunochemiluminescent assay in 104 dialysis patients, Morita et al. (89) found very good correlation ($r = 0.93$). Also, the results of several studies that utilized these intact PTH assays in relation to the bone biopsy features of dialysis patients (63,80,90) show reasonably good separation of one type of disorder from another; moreover, there are similarities from one report to another. Such assays may become the "gold standard" in the future.

With the measurement of serum iPTH levels, it is important to know whether the patient is in a "steady state." In ESRD, most PTH levels are obtained just prior to dialysis. However, the PTH levels can change during dialysis, depending on the assay used and the calcium level in the dialysate. Thus the intact PTH levels showed a substantial fall during the dialysis procedure as the serum calcium rose slightly; at the same time, there was no significant change in the MM PTH (63,89). Another study of dialysis patients with profound secondary hyperparathyroidism receiving long-term therapy with intravenous calcitriol (91) disclosed no significant reduction in MM PTH compared to a significant fall in N-terminal PTH, even though the bone biopsies improved significantly. Thus the slow turnover of MM PTH may not permit the recognition of a significant change during treatment; also, the intact PTH is the ideal assay for acute physiologic studies. Solal et al. (80) used three different PTH assays, "intact" PTH using an IRMA assay, midregion PTH assay, and carboxyl-terminal PTH assay, in 24 dialysis patients who had never received aluminum gels and whose dialysate aluminum levels were very low. The intact PTH showed the best correlation with bone formation rate (BFR) (r = 0.63) and provided the best separation between groups. Patients with "severe" hyperparathyroidism (increased resorption and high BFR) had intact PTH levels that were 1.2–5 times the upper limit of normal. In separating this group with hyperparathyroidism from a small group of patients with subnormal bone formation rate but no aluminum staining (adynamic or aplastic bone), the intact PTH had a sensitivity of 100% and a specificity of ~70%. Quarles et al. (79) reported the relationship between intact PTH using an IRMA and bone biopsy features of secondary hyperparathyroidism in 39 dialysis patients, although data from the biopsies from 17 additional patients with a low BFR, aluminum staining, or both features were excluded from the analysis. The correlation between the intact PTH assay and BFR was high over a very wide range of iPTH levels (r = 0.84), and linear regression analysis was used to evaluate the relation between iPTH and various histologic indices of secondary hyperparathyroidism. In those with an average PTH 2.6 times the upper limit of normal, the BFR was above normal and there was minimal fibrosis; woven osteoid was present when the mean PTH level exceeded the normal limit by 3.2-fold. Histological findings of severe hyperparathyroidism were invariable when the levels averaged 7.5 times normal. At the other extreme, the patients with PTH levels averaging 1.5-fold the upper normal limit had normal bone formation and resorption surfaces and lacked both peritrabecular fibrosis and woven bone. The results were not reported in a way that indicates the sensitivity or specificity of the PTH assay for the identification of secondary hyperparathyroidism.

Segre et al. (90) and Sherrard et al. (3) have summarized the results IRMA of intact PTH in relation to histologic findings on bone biopsy in 259 ESRD patients from Toronto; these results are shown in Fig. 2. In those with a PTH level >7.7-fold the upper limit of normal (500 pg/ml), there was 100% specificity for identification of severe osteitis fibrosa, but the sensitivity was only 46%. In those with PTH lowered to 4.6-fold the upper normal value (300 pg/ml), the sensitivity was 85% and the false-positive rate was 5%. Finally, at a PTH value below 3.1-fold normal (200 pg/ml), 99% of those with severe osteitis fibrosa were excluded.

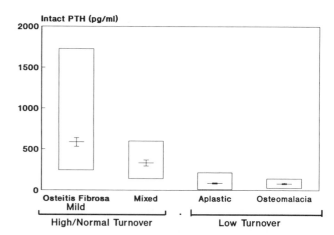

FIG. 2. Intact PTH levels (IRMA) in 259 dialysis patients from Toronto with iliac crest bone biopsies and classification of the type of bone disease. The entire ranges of PTH and mean values ± SEM for each group are given. The numbers of patients with each of the disorders are: osteitis fibrosa and mild, 112; mixed, 18; aplastic, 128; and osteomalacia, 11. (Modified from refs. 3 and 90 with permission.)

Considerations Regarding Aluminum-Related Bone Disease

A lengthy description of aluminum-related bone disease is beyond the scope of this chapter. However, the distinction between hyperparathyroidism and aluminum-related bone disease is not always simple, and there are several reasons why the methods used to make a diagnosis of aluminum toxicity or aluminum loading are included. For example, an aluminum-loaded patient with osteitis fibrosa will often convert to symptomatic aluminum-related bone disease after parathyroidectomy. It is more difficult to treat aluminum-related bone disease after parathyroidectomy when serum PTH levels remain very low (92); thus it is generally recommended that the aluminum overload be treated before parathyroidectomy is performed in patients who have aluminum overload combined with severe secondary hyperparathyroidism (16,68).

Patients with aluminum-related bone disease who undergo parathyroidectomy often become worse, sometimes markedly so (93), and so the correct diagnosis is important. Sherrard et al. (94) coined the term, *pseudohyperparathyroidism*, to describe patients with bone pain, fractures, variable degrees of hypercalcemia, elevated PTH levels (usually with a C-terminal or MM assay), and skeletal radiographs that show subperiosteal erosions. Parathyroidectomy usually led to worsening of the symptoms, and bone biopsies disclosed features of aluminum-related bone disease. The radiographic finding of erosions represents earlier osteoclastic erosions that had not "healed" or mineralized but were filled with unmineralized osteoid as a consequence of the superimposed aluminum loading.

Because of the tendency for substantial worsening after parathyroidectomy (93,95–97), aluminum toxicity should be excluded as a possible diagnosis before parathyroid surgery is undertaken (94). This matter is much less of a problem now that fewer and fewer dialysis patients are receiving aluminum gels for control of hyperphosphatemia. The "gold standard" for recognizing aluminum-related bone disease is a bone biopsy, which must be seriously considered in a patient who has ingested large doses of aluminum gels in the past. The value of plasma aluminum, the change in plasma aluminum after desferrioxamine, and the serum iPTH level are briefly considered below.

PTH levels are lower in patients with aluminum toxicity than in a usual dialysis population (55,70), and such levels are of value in identification of these patients. Among a study of 40 patients with severe aluminum toxicity referred for therapy with desferrioxamine, Norris et al. (55) found the MM iPTH to average 10.8-fold the upper limit of normal compared to a mean value of 120-fold normal in 21 patients with symptomatic osteitis fibrosa. Overlap existed, however, and 20% of those with aluminum toxicity had MM iPTH values >190 μlEq/ml (normal 2–9 μlEq/ml), the lowest value observed in the patients with severe osteitis fibrosa.

Plasma aluminum levels are believed to represent evidence of recent exposure to aluminum rather than evidence of aluminum toxicity (98), and the levels will fall over 2–4 months in an aluminum-loaded dialysis patient after all exposure to aluminum has been withdrawn (99). There is considerable controversy regarding the value of plasma aluminum (100–103). Nonetheless, the monitoring of these levels in dialysis patients is of value when patients do become exposed (104). If plasma aluminum levels are high (>100 μg/liter), there is a possibility that aluminum loading and toxicity may be present; if they are very high (>200–300 μg/liter), the risk of toxicity becomes greater. On the other hand, if the plasma levels are below 30–40 μg/liter, aluminum toxicity is far less likely unless such a patient has been totally withdrawn from aluminum exposure for 6–8 months or longer. For this reason, the desferrioxamine infusion has been suggested for detecting aluminum loading (105); its sensitivity is not very high, however (106).

A combination of the iPTH level combined with the increment in serum aluminum after a desferrioxamine infusion has been suggested as a useful method. With use of the IRMA intact PTH assay, Pei et al. (107) used a "cut-off" intact PTH level <3.1-fold the upper normal value (200 pg/ml) combined with an increment in plasma aluminum after a desferrioxamine infusion to identify dialysis patients with aluminum-related bone disease among 259 Canadian dialysis patients who underwent biopsies. The combination of intact PTH

<200 pg/ml and an increment in plasma aluminum after DFO of ≥150 μg/liter provided the best positive predictive value (≥95%) in both peritoneal dialysis and hemodialysis patients (107); however, the sensitivity was only 35–45%. The authors evaluated "cut-off" increments in plasma aluminum of ≥100 μg/liter and ≥50 μg/liter combined with the same limit for PTH level. There was a modest reduction in positive predictive value, but the sensitivity rose substantially. Pei et al. noted that the sensitivity of these methods, as indicated by a change in false-negative rates, was substantially lower in patients who had had aluminum gels withdrawn for >6 months compared to patients still ingesting aluminum gels. They considered the usefulness of these tests under circumstances when the prevalence of aluminum loading becomes lower, as would occur with decreased use of aluminum gels (108); under such circumstances, a bone biopsy would much more likely be required. These authors suggest that these evaluations, done at various intervals, would be of most value in dialysis patients who continue to require aluminum gels for the control of serum phosphorus. From our experience, it seems likely that monitoring serum aluminum per se is also useful; as long as serum aluminum levels remain <30–40 μg/liter, it is unlikely that such a patient could develop aluminum loading and toxicity de novo. If the levels rise progressively in a patient, there should be concern about aluminum loading, and the clinician should explore the possibility of aluminum loading from a new source, either the breakdown of a water-treatment system or markedly augmented aluminum absorption due to the ingestion of citrate (109).

Other Biochemical Tests

Several other biochemical tests have been utilized in uremic patients to identify the degree of activity of bone disease; these include osteocalcin or bone Gla protein (BGP) and insulin-like growth factor-I (IGF-I). In two studies that reported levels of both iPTH and osteocalcin (61,82), the correlations between bone histologic features and either iPTH levels or osteocalcin levels were quite similar. The osteocalcin levels of all uremic patients exceeded normal, most likely due to renal retention of this peptide in a manner similar to that in the MM PTH assay. Another report showed similar correlations between bone formation rate and osteoclast number and either PTH levels or levels of IGF-I (110). However, the lack of general availability of these determinations limits their clinical usefulness.

When persistent and unexplained hypercalcemia develops in a patient with renal failure, the measurement of serum calcitriol [1,25-$(OH)_2D_3$] may aid in identification of a granulomatous process, such as sarcoidosis

(111) or tuberculosis (112), as a cause of extrarenal generation of the active vitamin D sterol. Under usual circumstances, the serum calcitriol levels are either undetectable or below the normal range in patients with ESRD; thus the finding of a value that is in the upper range of normal or higher would suggest the existence of such a problem.

Radiological Evaluation of Secondary Hyperparathyroidism

Radiographic Features

Subperiosteal erosions are the most consistent radiographic feature of secondary hyperparathyroidism (5,24,113). The degree of subperiosteal erosions can correlate with serum PTH and alkaline phosphatase levels, but radiographs are quite insensitive and can be normal in patients with histological features of marked osteitis fibrosa on bone biopsy (60). Among pediatric patients, metaphyseal changes (i.e., growth zone lesions that are termed *rickets-like lesions*) are common (24,26).

Radiographic features of secondary hyperparathyroidism are best detected by hand radiographs, with several techniques used to enhance their sensitivity. Meema et al. (114) use fine-grain films and then magnify them six- to sevenfold with a hand lens. Direct magnification X-rays can also be employed (115). Subperiosteal erosions occur as well in the distal ends of clavicles, at the surface of the ischium and pubis, at the sacroiliac joints, and at the junction of the metaphysis and diaphysis of long bones (113,116).

Subperiosteal erosions can also be observed in patients with aluminum-related bone disease (117), so they are not always specific. This occurrence represents the residual manifestations of previous secondary hyperparathyroidism with osteitis fibrosa, as was noted above. Aluminum toxicity prevents remineralization of bone and prevents normalization of the radiograph when secondary hyperparathyroidism is replaced by aluminum loading (117); the term *pseudohyperparathyroidism* has been used to describe such patients (94). The radiographic abnormalities of the skull in secondary hyperparathyroidism (116) can include (a) a diffuse "ground glass" appearance, (b) a generalized mottled or granular appearance, (c) focal radiolucencies, and (d) focal sclerosis.

Among children with renal failure, abnormalities of the growth zone are common. The radiographic changes arising from secondary hyperparathyroidism resemble true rachitic abnormalities. Mehls (118) demonstrated that the histological features of these epiphyseal lesions in uremic children are those of osteitis fibrosa and noted radiographic features that are distinct from those of rickets due to vitamin D deficiency.

Brown tumors do develop in renal patients with secondary hyperparathyroidism, but their occurrence is unusual, even in patients with bone biopsy findings of severe osteitis fibrosa. They are most commonly seen in the jaw or ribs, and they are generally single. The radiographic features of dialysis amyloidosis, noted above, can be misinterpreted as brown tumors. Indeed, serial skeletal radiographs are presently of the most value in both detecting the appearance and following the progress of the cystic lesions of dialysis amyloidosis.

Bone Scintiscan

The scintiscan of bone, using technetium-99-labeled diphosphonate, will detect osteitis fibrosa, and this procedure can be used to estimate the severity of skeletal disease in patients with advanced renal failure (119); also, the response to a specific treatment can be followed by serial bone scans (120). In one study, the scintiscan were abnormal in 13 of 14 dialysis patients, with symmetrically increased uptake over the skull, mandible, sternum, shoulders, vertebrae, and distal aspects of the femur and tibia. This symmetrically increased uptake of the diphosphonate by the axial skeleton and around the epiphyseal areas of the long bones leads to a feature that has been termed the *super scan*. In contrast to this finding, there is generally a diffuse reduction of the uptake in renal patients with aluminum-related bone disease and osteomalacia (121,122). Karsenty et al. (120) were able to differentiate between patients with osteitis fibrosa and those with osteomalacia from aluminum intoxication by the uptake on bone scan. However, patients with mixed lesions on biopsy could not be identified. Hodson et al. (123) concluded from their results that bone scans did not provide enough useful information on either the type or the severity of renal osteodystrophy in their comparison of scintiscan and results on bone biopsy.

The bone scintiscan will also detect nondisplaced fractures (pseudofractures) in the ribs and elsewhere in patients with osteomalacia (24); it is also useful to detect ectopic calcification. Thus the bone scan is a noninvasive diagnostic method that can establish the severity or type of bone disease in some but not all patients. A bone biopsy is still required, however, to establish the specific type of renal bone disease in many cases.

TREATMENT OF SECONDARY HYPERPARATHYROIDISM

For the prevention and management of secondary hyperparathyroidism arising with renal failure, the specific goals are (a) to maintain the blood levels of calcium and phosphorus as near to normal as possible,

(b) to prevent hyperplasia of the parathyroid glands and to suppress PTH secretion appropriately if secondary hyperparathyroidism is already present, and (c) to avoid the development of extraskeletal calcification. In addition, it is important to prevent or minimize other disorders affecting bone that can develop in advanced renal failure, namely, aluminum toxicity and the idiopathic aplastic or adynamic bone disorder.

Modification of Dietary Phosphorus and Calcium

A major therapeutic goal is to avoid phosphate retention and hyperphosphatemia in renal failure. As is noted in the chapter by Martin and Slatopolsky, phosphate retention is a major factor leading to the development of secondary hyperparathyroidism in renal patients. Thus, in human subjects with mild to moderate renal failure, a reduction in dietary phosphorus was associated with reductions in serum PTH values and improvement in the calcemic response to parathyroid hormone (124,125); moreover, in advanced renal failure, the degree of hyperphosphatemia correlates with the degree of secondary hyperparathyroidism (126), and marked hyperphosphatemia can block the effect of calcitriol of suppressing serum iPTH levels (127).

Dietary phosphorus is derived primarily from meat and dairy products, and phosphorus intake commonly ranges from 1.0 to 1.8 g/day in adults in the United States and Western Europe. To prevent hyperphosphatemia, the dietary intake of phosphorus should be reduced to <1,000 mg/day by sharply restricting the intake of dairy products in patients with moderate to advanced renal failure. There is growing evidence that dietary protein restriction can slow the usual progressive nature of most chronic renal diseases (128), and such a low-protein diet contains less phosphate. In patients with ESRD, one relies on the dialysis procedure to remove a substantial amount of phosphate (129); however, the excess phosphate that accumulates during the interval between two dialysis treatments has a space of distribution well beyond the extracellular fluid. Because of the slow movement of such phosphate into the extracellular fluid, the serum phosphorus levels fall very rapidly during the first 30–60 min of a hemodialysis procedure; subsequently, there is a very small gradient for phosphate diffusion from the blood into the dialysis fluid, limiting the net amount of phosphate that is removed by dialysis (130). The ingestion of a highly phosphate-restricted diet (e.g., <600 mg/day) would be very useful; however, such a diet is highly unpalatable, particularly to patients who are accustomed to the typical high-protein diet consumed in North America (131). Therefore, a reasonable "target" for dietary phosphate is 800–900 mg/day in patients with ESRD. With such a diet, phosphate-binding agents must be given to most dialysis patients to prevent the development of hyperphosphatemia, and such

phosphate-binding agents are indicated in most predialysis patients with advanced renal failure and creatinine clearances <15–20 ml/min. If the dietary intake of phosphate increases, the required dosages of phosphate binders become very large, so attention must be paid to both dietary phosphate restriction and phosphate binders (Fig. 3).

There is a recommendation that the calcium intake should be augmented in patients with advanced renal failure. This is done by adding calcium salts, usually calcium acetate or calcium carbonate. There are two reasons for this. First, calcium salts, either calcium carbonate or calcium acetate, are safe and effective for the intestinal binding of ingested phosphate in patients with ESRD (132–134), and, second, calcium supplements are indicated because calcium absorption is impaired in uremia and because the calcium intake is suboptimal in most patients with ESRD (135). Because of the importance of reducing the intake of dairy products to limit the phosphate intake, the amount of calcium in the diet is often as low as 400–700 mg/day in patients with renal failure (135). Furthermore, studies of net intestinal calcium absorption in uremic patients indicate that a neutral or positive calcium balance is commonly achieved when the dietary calcium is increased >1.5 g/day with calcium carbonate, calcium citrate, or calcium lactate (136,137).

Long-term treatment with large doses of calcium supplements has been shown to reduce the incidence of (a) the erosive skeletal lesions of secondary hyperparathyroidism, (b) fractures, and (c) the prevalence of extraskeletal calcification (137a). The calcium salts, calcium carbonate (99,133,134,138) and calcium acetate (139), are presently the safest and most widely used phosphate-binding agents. It is generally safe to give calcium carbonate or calcium acetate as the initial phosphate binder, and the serum phosphorus usually

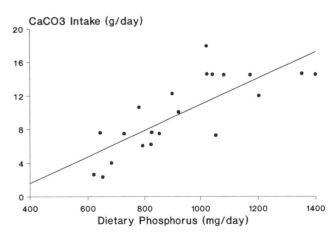

FIG. 3. Relation between total daily dose of calcium carbonate and dietary phosphate intake in 21 compliant patients who exhibited good control of their serum phosphate levels. (Modified from ref. 141 with permission.)

falls over a period of 2–4 weeks after therapy with calcium salts is initiated, long before the serum calcium rises. Patients who receive such calcium supplements, particularly when they are also receiving vitamin D sterols, should have their serum calcium levels monitored every 2–3 weeks to detect the development of hypercalcemia. Mild hypercalcemia (11.0–12.0 mg/dl) is usually associated with no symptoms (140); however, attention should be paid to the appearance of pruritus (19); also, nausea, anorexia, vomiting, mental confusion, and lethargy can occur when serum calcium levels are high; occasionally, ESRD patients will develop such symptoms insidiously and with serum calcium levels no higher than 11.5–12.5 mg/dl.

The calcium salts should be given somewhat more cautiously when the serum calcium levels are in the upper range of normal and when the serum phosphorus levels are >7.5–8.0 mg/dl. Under such circumstances, there is a substantial risk of hypercalcemia with a rise in the Ca X P product, which can predispose to extraskeletal calcification. Under such circumstances, it is wise to reduce the dialysate calcium from a usual value of 3.0–3.5 mEq/liter to 2.5 mEq/liter to reduce the risk of hypercalcemia (134,141–144).

Phosphate-Binding Agents

Because dietary phosphate restriction alone cannot control the hyperphosphatemia that exists in almost every patient undergoing regular dialysis, the intake of phosphate-binding agents has become standard. The aluminum-containing gels, aluminum hydroxide and aluminum carbonate, were the agents used in the past to reduce phosphate absorption and to control the serum phosphorus levels in patients with advanced renal failure and in those undergoing hemodialysis (145). However, it was recognized that the ingestion of aluminum-containing gels is a major risk factor for the development of aluminum intoxication, particularly that causing osteomalacia and other symptomatic "low turnover" disorders of bone (146–150). Kaehny et al. (151) and Recker et al. (152) found that small amounts of aluminum were absorbed and excreted in the urine following the ingestion of large doses of aluminum-containing gels by normal men. When aluminum is absorbed by patients with renal failure, it cannot be excreted, and it accumulates in the body. Thus both dialysis encephalopathy and aluminum-related bone disease have been reported prior to the initiation of dialysis in azotemic adults and children who were ingesting aluminum gels (146–150). It was shown that plasma aluminum levels correlated with the amount of oral aluminum intake from the phosphate-binding agents (153). Such observations implied a role of aluminum absorption from the gastrointestinal tract as a source of aluminum loading and toxicity. The

observations that plasma aluminum levels fall strikingly (99,108,140) and that aluminum-related bone disease will reverse after the total withdrawal of aluminum gels (108) provide proof that the oral intake of aluminum gels can be responsible for aluminum intoxication.

Guidelines for "safe" doses of aluminum hydroxide have been developed, and the safe maximum dose was considered to be 30 mg/kg/day for children (154) and 4–6 tablets/day for adult patients treated with hemodialysis (155). However, when this recommended dose was prospectively evaluated in pediatric dialysis patients, there was a progressive increase in the body burden of aluminum as judged by increments in plasma aluminum levels (Fig. 4), increases in plasma aluminum levels after a desferrioxamine infusion test, and by histologic evidence of aluminum deposition in bone (156). Indeed, one patient developed bone biopsy evidence of aluminum-related bone disease after only 12 months of therapy with a "recommended dose" of aluminum hydroxide (156). Thus aluminum-containing drugs should be avoided in the vast majority of patients with renal failure. In 5–10% of dialysis patients, aluminum gels are still required to control hyperphosphatemia; under such situations, the gels can be combined with the calcium salts, with the "recommended dosages" of aluminum gels not exceeded in such cases.

In patients receiving aluminum gels, there should be caution concerning the intake of medications that will augment aluminum absorption. Among the factors that enhance aluminum absorption, the most potent is citrate, as citric acid or a salt (157). The simultaneous ingestion of citrate with an aluminum-containing gel

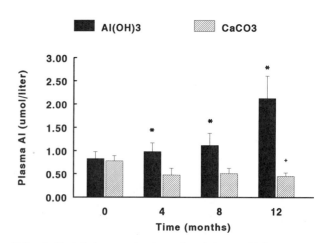

FIG. 4. Serial plasma aluminum levels in 17 children treated with CCPD and receiving either aluminum hydroxide (n = 7; *solid bars*) or calcium carbonate (n = 10; *hatched bars*) as phosphate binders. *Asterisks* indicate a significant change from baseline values ($P < 0.05$). (Reprinted from ref. 156 with permission.)

will markedly augment aluminum absorption, e.g., will produce a 20-fold or greater increase (158). Fatal cases of acute aluminum toxicity have occurred in patients with advanced renal insufficiency (159,160) due to the simultaneous intake of aluminum hydroxide for hyperphosphatemia and the prescription of Shohl's solution or Bicitra for metabolic acidosis. Other sources of citrate should be avoided with advanced renal failure as well. Thus calcium citrate is an effective phosphate-binding agent (161), but calcium citrate should be avoided because of the potential risk for aluminum intoxication if aluminum gels are coincidentally ingested (157,158). Another drug, Alka Seltzer, which is often ingested by patients with dyspepsia, contains citric acid and has produced aluminum toxicity in a dialysis patient (162).

Calcium carbonate has proved effective as the sole phosphate-binding agent in at least 80–90% of adult and pediatric dialysis patients (Fig. 5). Hypercalcemia is the major side effect, either with or without simultaneous vitamin D therapy (99,133,140,141,144). Calcium carbonate should be ingested together with a meal, both to maximize its phosphate-binding efficiency and to minimize the absorption of calcium (163). The required dosage of calcium carbonate varies from patient to patient, but the initial doses have averaged 4–7 g/day. In individual patients, the dose is adjusted empirically according to the levels of serum phosphorus (99,133,138,140).

Theoretical calculations, using a well-defined equilibrium constant, suggested that calcium acetate was effective as a phosphate binder (164). In vitro studies of phosphate-binding capacity demonstrated that calcium acetate was more potent than calcium carbonate

or calcium citrate based on the calcium content of each calcium salt (164,165). Because of this, the total calcium load could theoretically be lowered with less potential risk of hypercalcemia. However, calcium carbonate is 40% calcium by weight, compared to 25% for calcium acetate; thus the number and size of the pills required do not differ greatly between the two compounds. Also, there are pharmaceutical advantages of calcium carbonate, with several forms available (e.g., capsules, a powder, and flavored "chewable" tablets), compared to a single form and dose for calcium acetate. Also, if the coating of the tablet is dissolved, calcium acetate has an unpleasant taste, and the latter is more costly than calcium carbonate. When the efficacy and side effects of calcium acetate and calcium carbonate were compared in hemodialysis patients, neither Cunningham et al. (166) nor Delmez et al. (133) were able to identify a major advantage of calcium acetate compared to calcium carbonate; on the other hand, Ring et al. (167) reported that calcium acetate use was associated with slightly lower serum phosphorus levels than calcium carbonate in a double-blind, crossover study. One caution about the use of calcium carbonate is the necessity of employing a preparation that has the proper solubility, or calcium carbonate may be totally ineffective (168).

Hypercalcemia is the major side effect associated with the long-term use of the calcium salts, either with or without concomitant vitamin D therapy (99, 133,140,141,144). The use of dialysate solutions with the calcium concentration reduced to 2.5 mEq/liter has been very useful in patients treated with hemodialysis (144). When calcium carbonate was given as the sole phosphate binder in adult continuous ambulatory peritoneal dialysis (CAPD) patients who used dialysate with 3.5 mEq/liter calcium, the "standard" peritoneal dialysate calcium concentration for several years, hypercalcemia occurred in as many as 44% of patients, and many required the addition of aluminum gels (166). A controlled comparison of groups of patients who utilized dialysate with either 2.5 or 3.5 mEq/liter calcium concentrations has shown equal control of serum phosphorus levels, but there was no need to add aluminum hydroxide in the patients using the lower dialysate calcium dose (166). It is likely that the use of a dialysate calcium concentration of 2.5 mEq/liter will become standard in many dialysis units, particularly for adults ingesting large doses of calcium-containing, phosphate-binding agents (141,144,169), and there is growing evidence that this should be true for patients treated with peritoneal dialysis as well (169).

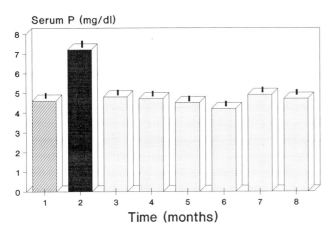

FIG. 5. Serum phosphorus levels in ten hemodialysis patients converted from aluminum hydroxide (*hatched column*) to calcium carbonate (*stippled columns*), with 3 weeks in between when no phosphate-binder was ingested (*solid column*). Data are mean ± SE. (Modified from ref. 99 with permission.)

Active Vitamin D Sterols

Despite dietary phosphate restriction, the intake of phosphate-binding agents, the use of an appropriate level of calcium in dialysate, and an adequate intake of calcium, a significant number of uremic patients develop progressive osteitis fibrosa. Appropriate therapy with an active vitamin D sterol can halt or retard the progression of the bone disease in patients with overt secondary hyperparathyroidism. The uses of vitamin D_3 or D_2 in pharmacologic doses (1), dihydrotachysterol (170), 25-hydroxyvitamin D_3 (calcifediol) (171,172), 1α-hydroxyvitamin D_3 (173,174), or 1,25-$(OH)_2D_3$ (calcitriol) (18,175–177) have all been associated with improved symptoms and correction of certain biochemical and radiological features of secondary hyperparathyroidism. No controlled studies have yet compared the effectiveness of the different vitamin D sterols.

Certain data suggest that vitamin D_2 or D_3 can produce more normal mineralization of bone than calcium carbonate (178). In doses of 50,000–200,000 IU/day, vitamin D_2 can improve secondary hyperparathyroidism in uremic patients (1). The use of vitamin D itself, however, can be accompanied by hypercalcemia that persists for weeks after the drug is stopped.

Calcifediol has also been employed in the management of renal osteodystrophy. Considerable data exist to indicate that both adult and pediatric renal patients respond favorably to this sterol in doses of 25–100 μg/day (171,172). The results from a six-center study of therapy with 25-$(OH)_2D_3$ in dialysis patients demonstrated a reversal of bone pain and tenderness, a fall in the serum alkaline phosphatase activity, and a decrease in the extent of osteitis fibrosa.

Several clinical trials have documented the efficacy of 1,25-$(OH)_2D_3$ for the treatment of patients with symptomatic renal osteodystrophy (18,33,175–177, 179). The results of these studies can be summarized as follows. With regard to symptoms and signs, there has been a decrease in bone pain, improvement in proximal muscle weakness, and improvement in postural gait. An increase in growth velocity of uremic children was shown in patients with very severe secondary hyperparathyroidism (33); other groups failed to confirm significant improvement in height velocity in children, although plasma alkaline phosphatase levels and serum PTH levels fell toward normal (175). Studies of bone histology have demonstrated improved osteitis fibrosa (176,180,181). An example of the biochemical response to therapy with calcitriol is shown in Fig. 6.

The doses of oral 1,25-$(OH)_2D_3$ used in these trials have ranged from 0.25 to 1.5 μg/day. The major side effect was the appearance of hypercalcemia. The increments in serum calcium levels were sometimes rapid and marked, and they were more common in two situations: (a) after many weeks or months of treatment in patients with osteitis fibrosa who had experienced a favorable response to therapy and (b) after only a few weeks of calcitriol treatment in patients receiving relatively low doses and with no clinical re-

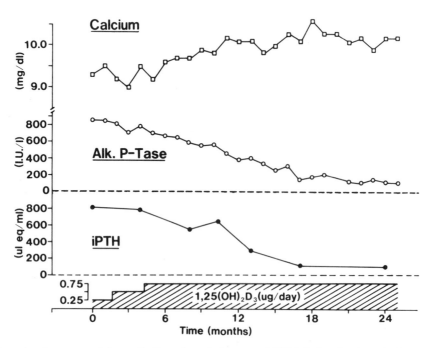

FIG. 6. Levels of serum calcium, alkaline phosphatase, and PTH during treatment of secondary hyperparathyroidism with daily oral calcitriol. (Reprinted from Coburn JW, Norris KC: A CPC series. In *Cases in metabolic bone disease.* Vol 1. Zackson DA, ed. New York: Rogosin Institute, Medical Projects Inc., 1985;1, with permission.)

sponse to treatment. In the latter group, who developed hypercalcemia while receiving calcitriol in dosages of 0.25–0.5 μg/day, aluminum-related bone disease should be suspected (181). In patients with secondary hyperparathyroidism, the development of hypercalcemia can often be anticipated by a fall in serum alkaline phosphatase into or toward the normal range. Thus the response to treatment with 1,25-$(OH)_2D_3$ may suggest the type of renal bone disease that is present (66,181). Increments in serum phosphorus or a greater requirement for a phosphate-binding agent are also observed, probably due to the action of 1,25-$(OH)_2D_3$ of augmenting intestinal phosphate absorption as well as that of calcium (Fig. 7).

1α-Hydroxyvitamin D_3, or alfacalcidol, is the active vitamin D sterol that has been widely used for the management of ESRD patients in Europe, Canada, and Japan (174,182). This sterol undergoes hepatic 25-hydroxylation to 1,25-$(OH)_2D_3$; its effects are very similar to those of 1,25-$(OH)_2D_3$. The required dosage is generally 50–75% higher. Patients who receive anticonvulsant therapy concomitantly may fail to respond, perhaps due to impaired hepatic 25-hydroxylation (183).

Another vitamin D sterol that has been investigated is 24,25-dihydroxyvitamin D_3 [24,25-$(OH)_2D_3$]. Short-term studies in patients with nutritional vitamin D deficiency suggest that 24,25-$(OH)_2D_3$ has effects different from those of 1,25-$(OH)_2D_3$ (178,184). Serum calcium levels fell slightly and alkaline phosphatase levels increased in dialysis patients given 24,25-$(OH)_2D_3$ (185), and some uremic patients with aluminum-related bone disease have shown improved min-

eralization following treatment with 24,25-$(OH)_2D_3$ and 1,25-$(OH)_2D_3$ (185a). Further studies are needed to clarify the actions of 24,25-$(OH)_2D_3$ compared to other vitamin D sterols.

Analogs of Calcitriol

The recent development of analogs of 1,25-$(OH)_2D_3$ with low calcemic activity have raised the possibility of their therapeutic utility (186). Brown et al. (187) demonstrated that oxacalcitriol (OCT) suppressed PTH secretion in primary cultures of bovine parathyroid cells in a dose-dependent manner, similar to the effect of 1,25-$(OH)_2D_3$. In dogs with chronic renal failure, OCT suppressed PTH levels, with no change in serum calcium level. It is important that such observations be confirmed in further studies carried out for longer periods of time; the availability of a vitamin D sterol, such as OCT, that may reduce PTH secretion without causing hypercalcemia, may be an important adjunct to the therapy available. Further trials in humans with secondary hyperparathyroidism are also needed to test the efficacy of this analog of vitamin D (186).

Intravenous Calcitriol and "Pulse" Oral Dosing

A major advance in the therapeutic approach with vitamin D sterols has been the introduction of parenteral calcitriol and pulse-dose oral therapy. Slatopolsky et al. (188) first reported the marked effect of intravenous 1,25-$(OH)_2D_3$ of suppressing the serum PTH levels in hemodialysis patients. These studies showed a suppression of PTH that was significantly greater than that observed with calcium carbonate and was more marked than that previously observed with the daily oral administration of 1,25-$(OH)_2D_3$. Moreover, there was a 20% inhibition of PTH release before serum ionized calcium rose (as is shown in Fig. 4 in the chapter by Martin and Slatopolsky). This effect of 1,25-$(OH)_2D_3$ is probably due to the action of calcitriol in suppressing the synthesis of mRNA for prepro-PTH by the parathyroid cells (189,190). Slatopolsky et al. (188) postulated that the higher blood levels of calcitriol after intravenous administration may allow a direct effect on the parathyroid glands and bypass part of the effect of augmenting intestinal calcium absorption.

Since the initial use of intravenous calcitriol, other reports have documented that calcitriol, given intravenously two or three times weekly at the time of regular dialysis, was effective in reversing features of uremic secondary hyperparathyroidism (91,126,191–195). Andress et al. (91) ave intravenous calcitriol for 1 year or longer in thrice weekly doses of 1.0–2.5 μg/

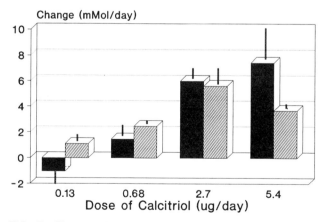

FIG. 7. Changes in net absorption of calcium (*solid bars*) and phosphorus (*hatched bars*) in patients with advanced renal failure during therapy with either calcitriol or 1α-$(OH)_2D_3$ as determined from metabolic balance studies of 14–28 days' duration. The data with the two sterols are combined because of trivial differences between the two sterols. Data are mean ± SE. (Modified from ref. 218 with permission.)

dialysis to 12 hemodialysis patients with severe secondary hyperparathyroidism; all had previously received daily oral calcitriol, but the dose was limited by hypercalcemia. Bone biopsies, carried out before and after 12 months of therapy, showed substantial improvement in bone formation rate, osteoblastic osteoid, and magnitude of peritrabecular fibrosis (Fig. 8); there was also a substantial reduction in amino-terminal PTH and in alkaline phosphatase; MM PTH

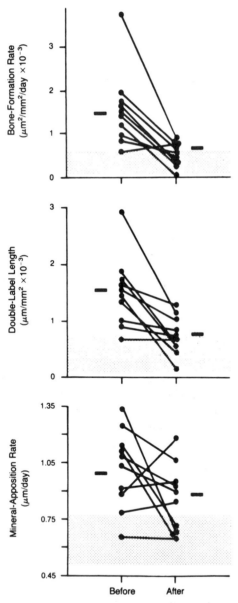

FIG. 8. Changes in bone formation rate, double tetracycline label length, and mineral apposition rate in ten patients with severe osteitis fibrosa. The values are from bone biopsies obtained before and after 11 months of therapy with intravenous calcitriol. The *horizontal line* indicates the mean, and the normal range is indicated by the *shaded area*. (Reprinted from ref. 91 with permission.)

changed less significantly, perhaps related to therapy being interrupted periodically. Hamdy et al. (196) noted a 5–7% *decrease* in serum calcium level from the fourth to eighth weeks of intravenous calcitriol therapy in patients with severe hyperparathyroidism and mild hypercalcemia prior to the treatment; moreover, the fall in serum calcium occurred as MM PTH was also lower. These observations and the study of Dunlay et al. (191) and Delmez et al. (197) suggest that calcitriol may make the gland more susceptible to suppression by calcium.

In these studies of intravenous calcitriol, the degree of hyperparathyroidism has varied substantially from very mild (188) to very marked (91). Also, the doses have varied substantially from study to study. The average dose of 0.87 μg/dialysis was used in a large multicenter study from Italy that included 76 patients (194); yet another study increased the average dose to as high as 7.0 μg per dialysis (195). Sprague and Moe (192) titrated the dose up from 0.50 μg per dialysis based on iPTH, serum calcium and phosphorus to an average maximum dose of 0.97 μg. They also noted a need for higher doses in patients with the highest PTH levels. A tendency to rising serum phosphorus levels was common (128,193–195), and the development of marked hyperphosphatemia due to noncompliance with phosphate-binding agents was associated with a rise in serum iPTH despite the continued administration of calcitriol and a continued slight increase in ionized calcium level (128).

During this same period, other reports have shown substantial suppression of serum iPTH levels following the administration of large oral doses of calcitriol given twice weekly. Thus the "pulse" oral doses of calcitriol, 3.0–5.0 μg given twice weekly (198–200), led to reductions in serum iPTH over a period of 4–8 weeks without any change in serum calcium or with only a slight increment. A comparison of serum calcitriol levels after a single oral dose vs. an intravenous dose in the same patients revealed serum levels that exceeded the normal range for a period up to 24 hr by both routes (201). Over the first 3 hr after dosing, the blood levels were higher after the intravenous dose than after the oral dose, but they were no different thereafter. The overall area under the curve after intravenous calcitriol was 62% greater than that after oral dosing (Fig. 9). Fukagawa et al. (198) demonstrated the intermittent "pulse" oral calcitriol, in doses of 4.0 μg twice weekly, lowered the PTH levels (Fig. 10) and also reduced the size of the parathyroid glands by ~41% as measured via ultrasound in hemodialysis patients with hyperparathyroidism (198). Tsukamoto et al. (199) studied 19 long-term hemodialysis patients who had previously received calcitriol or alphacalcidol for 4 years, with the dose limited by hypercalcemia. With "pulse dose," 4.0 μg twice weekly,

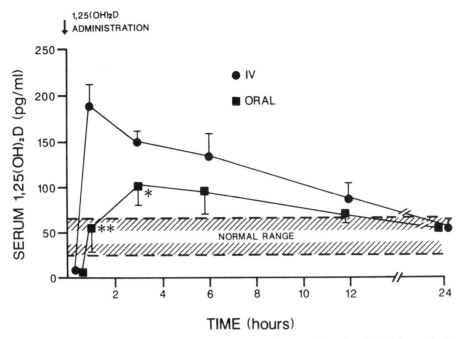

FIG. 9. Serum levels of 1,25-(OH)$_2$D in six adolescent patients undergoing CAPD for end-stage renal disease. On two separate occasions, separated by 1 month, the patients received single doses of both oral and intravenous calcitriol, 4.0 μg/70 kg body weight. The values are shown as mean ± SE; the values differ with the two routes of administration: *P < 0.05, **P < 0.01. (Modified from ref. 201 with permission.)

PTH was lowered by 52–59% in 16 patients treated for 6 months; three other patients discontinued the "pulse" treatment because of hypercalcemia. Similar reductions in serum iPTH levels after pulse oral doses of calcitriol in patients undergoing CAPD have been reported by Martin et al. (200). The question of whether pulse dose calcitriol can lead to regression of

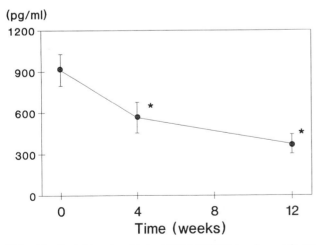

FIG. 10. Serial levels of intact PTH (IRMA) in nine patients with severe secondary hyperparathyroidism who received oral calcitriol, 4.0 μg twice weekly. Over this period, the mean serum calcium increased from 10.0 ± 0.16 to 10.92 ± 0.28 mg/dl. (Modified from ref. 198 with permission.)

the hyperplastic glands, as suggested by Fukagawa et al. (198), is not entirely certain. Most studies have shown a rather rapid return of serum iPTH levels to pretreatment levels within a short time after the calcitriol has been discontinued, an observation suggesting little regression in gland size (Fig. 11).

There are also reports documenting the effectiveness of intermittent intravenous doses of 1α-hydroxy-vitamin D$_3$ in lowering serum iPTH levels (202–204); it almost certainly does this by increasing the serum concentration of 1,25-(OH)$_2$D$_3$. There have been no studies of 1,25-(OH)$_2$D$_3$, given either in pulsed oral doses or intravenously, and 1α-hydroxyvitamin D$_3$ that permit a comparison of the relative effectiveness of the two sterols.

From the observations that have been reported, it is not certain whether the intravenous route for calcitriol is superior to intermittent "pulse" oral doses of the sterol for the management of secondary hyperparathyroidism in patients with chronic renal failure. Regardless of the route of calcitriol administration, the data suggest that the use of intermittent or "pulse" therapy with calcitriol may have advantages over daily dosing in the control of iPTH levels in these patients. It seems likely that "supranormal" plasma levels of calcitriol may have effects on the parathyroid glands that are not achieved with normal levels. It is of interest that such "supranormal" plasma levels of 1,25-(OH)$_2$D are observed during the recovery period as patients with nu-

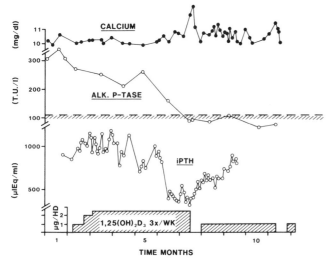

FIG. 11. Serial changes in serum calcium, alkaline phosphatase, and serum MM PTH (midregion; normal <9 μIEq/ml) in a dialysis patient with severe, symptomatic secondary hyperparathyroidism during treatment with intravenous calcitriol with each dialysis. Serum iPTH decreased by 45% before the patient became hypercalcemic, and the calcitriol was discontinued briefly. Later, as calcitriol was resumed at a lower dose, serum iPTH levels rose almost to the pretreatment levels, but the alkaline phosphatase levels continued to fall. (Reprinted from ref. 219 with permission.)

tritional vitamin D deficiency are given moderate doses of vitamin D (205); this observation suggests that the "recovery" from the secondary hyperparathyroidism may involve serum calcitriol levels that exceed the normal range.

Summary of Calcitriol in ESRD: A Current View

There have been several changes in the evaluation and management of patients with ESRD that affect the use of calcitriol and other vitamin D sterols in uremic patients. These include (a) the substantial effectiveness of "pulse" calcitriol in suppressing serum iPTH levels; (b) the widespread use of calcium salts rather than aluminum gels as phosphate in most ESRD patients, resulting in substantially higher calcium intake; (c) the use of dialysate calcium levels that do not raise the total or ionized calcium levels, thereby giving greater safety with use of calcium salts, and perhaps calcitriol as well; (d) the recognition of the syndrome of idiopathic low bone turnover, which arises in part from "oversuppression" of PTH; and (e) the use of intact PTH measurements, with their close correlations with the histologic types of renal bone disease; this may permit better prediction of the renal bone disease present and the treatment needed in these patients. On the basis of these changes, it seems reasonable that intact PTH levels will be used as guides to therapy

with calcitriol and other active vitamin D sterols, particularly in adults. (a) With intact PTH levels more than six- to eightfold greater than normal, calcitriol therapy should almost always be initiated. (b) With intact PTH levels of three to six times normal, therapy might be considered, particularly if serial levels of PTH are showing an increase. (c) With intact PTH levels between one and one-half and three times normal, calcitriol is not indicated in that it might lower PTH levels further, with a risk of inducing a "low-turnover" state. (d) With intact PTH levels within the normal range or up to 1.5-fold greater than normal, there is a strong likelihood that such a patient has the condition with subnormal bone turnover, and there is no reason to add calcitriol; indeed, such a patient's dialysate calcium should be lowered to 2.5 mEq/liter. The levels of serum calcium and the phosphorus levels would be used primarily to avoid toxicity with calcitriol rather than being an indication for such treatment. With the midregion PTH levels, there may also be guidelines; with an MM PTH below 15-fold of normal, hyperparathyroid bone disease is usually not present, while the bone usually exhibits hyperparathyroidism when the value is 15–20-fold of normal (206).

When therapy with calcitriol is initiated, a "pulse" dose regimen would seem appropriate, with the dose of 1.0–2.0 μg given two or three times weekly as long as serum calcium and phosphorus levels are well controlled. If hyperphosphatemia is marked (>7.0–7.5 mg/dl), the dose of phosphate binder should be increased and calcitriol treatment postponed until the phosphorus level falls. If serum calcium is more than mildly increased (>11.0–11.5 mg/dl), the dialysate calcium should be lowered to 2.5 mEq/liter before calcitriol is given. Serum iPTH levels should be followed at intervals of 2–3 months; if the iPTH level falls to below four- to fivefold of normal, the dose should be reduced substantially. On the other hand, if serum iPTH does not fall, the dosage of calcitriol may be increased as long as serum calcium and phosphorus are adequately controlled.

Calcitriol in "Early" and Predialysis Renal Failure

Since reductions in calcitriol synthesis by the kidney are important in the pathogenesis of secondary hyperparathyroidism in renal failure, and since some patients have already developed significant hyperparathyroidism by the time they enter upon dialysis, one can raise the question "should calcitriol therapy be given in the predialysis phase of renal failure?" Several well controlled studies have been done with daily calcitriol administration (207–209); the results are in general agreement, and these data are reviewed in detail elsewhere (210,211). From some of the very early reports, there has been concern that the 1α-hydroxylated vitamin D sterols may accelerate the rate of progression of renal disease in such patients (212,213). However, when either 1,25-(OH)$_2$D$_3$ or 1α-hydroxyvitamin D$_3$ has been given in daily doses of 0.25–0.50 μg, the occurrence of hypercalcemia, hyperphosphatemia, or any impairment of renal function has been very rare (210,211). There is some evidence that calcitriol impairs creatinine secretion by the renal tubule, accounting for the reversible change in serum creatinine and creatinine clearance reported in some studies with calcitriol therapy at doses of 0.50 μg/day or higher (214). With daily doses that rarely exceeded 0.25 μg/day, calcitriol therapy reversed secondary hyperparathyroidism, as judged from both biochemical findings and the histologic features found on bone biopsy (207–209). Such therapy may be particularly valuable in patients, such as children and those with very slowly progressive tubulointerstitial renal disease, who are at high risk of developing progressive secondary hyperparathyroidism as their renal disease slowly worsens (215).

Parathyroidectomy

Certain laboratory and clinical features of severe secondary hyperparathyroidism indicate the necessity for parathyroidectomy. The presence of hyperplasia and/or hypertrophy of the parathyroid glands should be documented by the finding of very high levels of serum PTH and the presence of osteitis fibrosa on bone biopsy. When this is the case, the indications for parathyroid surgery include (a) persistent hypercalcemia (serum calcium levels 11.5–12.0 mg/dl), particularly when the hypercalcemia is symptomatic; (b) intractable and severe pruritus that fails to respond to dialysis or other medical treatment; (c) progressive extraskeletal calcification when the Ca X P product in serum exceeds 75–80 mg/dl despite appropriate phosphate restriction; (d) severe skeletal pain, fractures, skeletal deformities or tendon rupture; and (e) the syndrome of calciphylaxis. When the patient does not have (a) significant hypercalcemia or (b) hyperphosphatemia that is refractory to management or (c) progressive calciphylaxis, a therapeutic trial with intravenous or pulse oral calcitriol may certainly be indicated prior to resorting to parathyroidectomy.

Persistent hypercalcemia can occur in patients with aluminum-related bone disease (55,181,211), and aluminum toxicity must be excluded prior to parathyroid surgery. Other causes of hypercalcemia, such as sarcoidosis, malignancy-related hypercalcemia, intake of calcium supplements, and presence of adynamic/aplastic bone lesion not related to aluminum, should also be considered (69).

When a decision to perform parathyroid surgery has been made, it is essential to avoid a marked postoperative fall in serum calcium levels due to the "hungry bone" syndrome. Because of the severity of the bone disease, this hypocalcemia is often more marked and more prolonged than that following parathyroidectomy for primary hyperparathyroidism. Renal patients should receive oral calcitriol, 0.5–1.0 μg, or intravenous calcitriol, 1.5–2.0 μg per hemodialysis treatment, for 2–6 days before the parathyroid surgery to stimulate intestinal calcium absorption during the postoperative period and to maximize the effectiveness of oral calcium salts. Following surgery, serum calcium and potassium levels should be monitored every 8–12 hr, and serum phosphorus and magnesium should be measured daily. By 24–36 hr after surgery, marked hypocalcemia, with serum calcium falling to levels below 6–7 mg/dl, may be seen; this can be associated with serious symptoms, including major convulsive seizures that can cause fractures and tendon avulsion. Such seizures may occur within 2–3 days up to 3–4 weeks after the surgery. For uncertain reasons, these seizures most commonly occur during the last 1–2 hr of a hemodialysis procedure. To reduce the risk of this serious problem, an infusion containing calcium gluconate should be initiated when the serum calcium falls below 7.5–8.0 mg/dl; enough ampules of calcium gluconate (calcium content ~110 mg/10 ml ampule) should be added to an intravenous infusion to provide 100 mg calcium ion per 1 hr, and the infusion should be continued for 8–12 hr or longer if serum calcium does not rise. During this infusion, the serum calcium should be measured every 4–6 hr; if the serum calcium continues to fall, the infusion of calcium should be increased to deliver 200 mg calcium per 1 hr. Recommended doses of infused calcium have also been based on the degree of preoperative elevation of serum alkaline phosphatase (216) or the weight of the parathyroid glands removed at surgery (217). Oral calcium carbonate, in doses that provide up to 2–3 g of ionic calcium and given five or six times daily, should be used; oral calcitriol in doses of 1.0–2.0 μg/day or higher should be added if the hypocalcemia persists. The length of time for which intravenous calcium is required varies greatly: Most patients require it for only 2 or 3 days, but severe hypocalcemia can persist for several weeks or months, and a "permanent" central catheter may be required for the daily home infusions of 800–1,000 mg calcium ion. When the serum calcium begins to rise toward normal, intravenous calcium can be discontinued, the calcitriol treatment can be reduced or stopped, and the dosage of oral calcium salts can be reduced and then adjusted to control hyperphosphatemia.

Serum phosphorus levels often fall to normal or even subnormal levels postoperatively; any phosphate treatment will markedly aggravate the hypocalcemia, and patients should not receive phosphate unless the serum phosphorus falls to very low levels, e.g., below 1.5–2.0 mg/dl. Serum phosphorus levels are ideally maintained between 2.5 and 4.0 mg/dl to avoid a risk of aggravating the hypocalcemia. Calcium carbonate or calcium acetate should be the phosphate-binding agent of choice, and $Al(OH)_3$ should be avoided after surgery unless it is absolutely necessary because of the increased susceptibility to aluminum toxicity after parathyroidectomy (93,97).

ACKNOWLEDGMENTS

This work was supported by U.S. PHS grants DK-35423 and RR-00865 and by research funds from the U.S. Department of Veterans Affairs.

REFERENCES

1. Dent CE, Harper CN, Philpot G. Treatment of renal glomerular osteodystrophy. *Q J Med* 1961;30:1–31.
2. Slatopolsky E, Bricker NS. The role of phosphorus restriction in the prevention of secondary hyperparathyroidism in renal disease. *Kidney Int* 1973;4:141–148.
3. Sherrard DJ, Hercz G, Pei Y, et al. The spectrum of bone disease in end-stage renal failure—An evolving disorder. *Kidney Int* 1993;43:435–436.
4. Andress DL, Maloney NA, Coburn JW, Endres DB, Sherrard DJ. Osteomalacia and aplastic bone disease in aluminum-related osteodystrophy. *J Clin Endocrinol Metab* 1987; 65:11–16.
5. Sherrard DJ. Renal osteodystrophy. *Semin Nephrol* 1986;6: 56–67.
6. Coburn JW, Henry DA. Renal osteodystrophy. *Adv Intern Med* 1984;30:387–424.
7. Nebeker HG, Coburn JW. Aluminum and renal osteodystrophy. *Annu Rev Med* 1986;37:79–95.
8. Mirahmadi KS, Coburn JW, Bluestone R. Calcific periarthritis and hemodialysis. *J Am Med Assoc* 1973;223:548–549.
9. Llach F, Pederson JA. Acute joint syndrome and maintenance hemodialysis. *Proc Clin Dialysis Transplant Forum* 1979;9:17–23.
10. Noel LH, Zingraff J, Bardin T, Atienza C, Kuntz D, Drueke T. Tissue distribution of dialysis amyloidosis. *Clin Nephrol* 1987;27:175–178.
11. Kleinman KS, Coburn JW. Amyloid syndromes associated with hemodialysis. *Kidney Int* 1989;35:567–575.
12. Hampl H, Lobeck H, Bartel-Schwarze S, Stein H, Eulitz M, Linke RP. Clinical, morphologic, biochemical, and immunohistochemical aspects of dialysis-associated amyloidosis. *ASAIO Trans* 1987;33:250–259.
13. Malette LE, Patten BM, Engel WK. Neuromuscular disease in secondary hyperparathyroidism. *Ann Intern Med* 1975;82: 474–483.
14. Baker LRI, Ackrill P, Cattell WR, Stamp TCB, Watson L. Iatrogenic osteomalacia and myopathy due to phosphate depletion. *Br Med J* 1974;3:150–152.
15. Smith R, Stern G. Myopathy, osteomalacia and hyperparathyroidism. *Brain* 1967;90:593–602.
16. Coburn JW, Nebeker HG, Hercz G, et al. Role of aluminum accumulation in the pathogenesis of renal osteodystrophy. In: Robinson RR, ed. *Nephrology,* Vol. II. New York: Springer-Verlag, 1984;1383–1395.
17. Kanis JA, Cundy T, Earnshaw M, et al. Treatment of renal bone disease with 1α-hydroxylated derivatives of vitamin

D_3: clinical, biochemical, radiographic and histological responses. *Q J Med* 1979;48:289–322.
18. Brickman AS, Sherrard DJ, Jowsey J, et al. 1,25-Dihydroxycholecalciferol: effect of skeletal lesions and plasma parathyroid hormone levels in uremic osteodystrophy. *Arch Intern Med* 1974;134:883–888.
19. Massry SG, Popovtzer MM, Coburn JW, Makoff DL, Maxwell MH, Kleeman CR. Intractable pruritus as manifestation of 2° hyperparathyroidism in uremia. Disappearance of itching following subtotal parathyroidectomy. *N Engl J Med* 1969;279:697–700.
20. Lotem M, Bernheim J, Conforty B. Spontaneous rupture of tendons: a complication of hemodialyzed patients treated for renal failure. *Nephron* 1978;21:201–208.
21. Avioli L. Collagen metabolism, uremia and bone. *Kidney Int* 1973;4:105–113.
22. Cirincione RJ, Baker BE. Tendon rupture with secondary hyperparathyroidism. *J Bone Joint Surg* 1975;57A:852–857.
23. Ryuzaki M, Konishi K, Kasuga A, et al. Spontaneous rupture of the quadriceps tendon in patients on maintenance hemodialysis—report of three cases with clinicopathological observations. *Clin Nephrol* 1989;32:144–148.
24. Wright RS, Mehls O, Ritz E, Coburn JW. Musculoskeletal manifestations of chronic renal failure, dialysis and transplantation. In: Bacon P, Hadler N, eds. *Renal manifestations in rheumatic disease*. London: Butterworth, 1982;352.
25. Eastwood JB, Bordier PJ, De Wardener HE. Some biochemical histological, radiological and clinical features of renal osteodystrophy. *Kidney Int* 1973;4:128–140.
26. Mehls O, Ritz E, Krempien B, et al. Slipped epiphysis in renal osteodystrophy. *Arch Dis Child* 1975;50:545–554.
27. Gipstein RM, Coburn JW, Adams JA, et al. Calciphylaxis in man. *Arch Intern Med* 1976;136:1273–1280.
28. Massry SG, Gordon A, Coburn JW, et al. Vascular calcification and peripheral necrosis in a renal transplant recipient: reversal of lesions following subtotal parathyroidectomy. *Am J Med* 1970;49:416–422.
29. Selye H. *Calciphylaxis*. Chicago: University of Chicago Press, 1962.
30. McSherry E, Morris RC. Attainment and maintenance of normal growth status with alkali therapy in infants and children with classic renal tubular acidosis (RTA). *J Clin Invest* 1978;61:509–527.
31. Stickler GB, Bergen BJ. A review: short stature in renal disease. *Pediatr Res* 1973;7:978–982.
32. Simmons JM, Wilson CJ, Potter DE, Holliday MA. Relation of caloric deficiency to growth failure in children on hemodialysis and the growth response to caloric supplementation. *N Engl J Med* 1971;285:653–656.
33. Chesney RW, Moorthy AV, Eisman JA, Tax DK, Mazess RB, Deluca HF. Increased growth after long-term oral 1,25-vitamin D_3 in childhood renal osteodystrophy. *N Engl J Med* 1978;298:238–242.
34. Bulla M, Delling G, Offerman G, et al. Renal bone disorders in children: Therapy with vitamin D_3 and 1,25 dihydroxycholecalciferol. In: Norman AW, Schaefer K, V. Herrath D, et al., eds. *Vitamin D: basic research and its clinical application*. Berlin: de Gruyter, 1979, p. 853.
35. Tonshoff B, Mehls O, Heinrich U, Blum WF, Ranke MB, Schauer A. Growth-stimulating effect of recombinant human growth hormone in child with end-stage renal disease. *J Pediatr* 1990;116:561–566.
36. Bardin T, Kuntz D, Zingraff J, Voisin MC, Zelmar A, Lansaman J. Synovial amyloidosis in patients undergoing long-term hemodialysis. *Arthritis Rheum* 1985;28:1052–1058.
37. Felsenfeld AJ, Rodriguez M, Dunlay R, Llach F. A comparison of parathyroid-gland function in haemodialysis patients with different forms of renal osteodystrophy. *Nephrol Dialysis Transplant* 1991;6:244–251.
38. Koch KM. Dialysis-related amyloidosis. *Kidney Int* 1992;41: 1416–1429.
39. McMahon LP, Radford J, Dawborn JK. Shoulder ultrasound in dialysis related amyloidosis. *Clin Nephrol* 1991;35:227–232.
40. Hutchinson AJ, Freemont AJ, Lumb GA, Gokal R. Renal

osteodystrophy in CAPD. In: Khanna R, Nolph KD, Prowant BF, Twardowski ZJ, Oreopoulos DG, eds. *Advances in peritoneal dialysis.* Toronto: University of Toronto Press, 1991;237.

41. Bindi P, Chanard J. Destructive spondyloarthropathy in dialysis patients: an overview. *Nephron* 1990;55:104–109.

42. Nelson SR, Sharpstone P, Kingswood JC. Does dialysis-associated amyloidosis resolve after transplantation? *Nephrol Dialysis Transplant* 1993;8:369–370.

43. Kuntz D, Naveau B, Bardin T, Drueke T, Treves R, Dryll A. Destructive spondylarthropathy in hemodialyzed patients. *Arthritis Rheum* 1984;27:369–375.

44. Bohlman ME, Kim YC, Eagan J, Spees EK. Brown tumor in secondary hyperparathyroidism causing acute paraplegia. *Am J Med* 1986;81:545–547.

45. DeForges-Lasseur C, Combe C, Cernier A, Vital JM, Aparicio M. Destructive spondyloarthropathy presenting with progressive paraplegia in a dialysis patient. Recovery after surgical spinal cord decompression and parathyroidectomy. *Nephrol Dialysis Transplant* 1993;8:180–184.

46. Sebert JL, Fardellone P, Marie A, et al. Destructive spondyloarthropathy in hemodialyzed patients: possible role of amyloidosis. *Arthritis Rheum* 1986;29:301–302.

47. Allard JC, Artze ME, Porter G, Ghandur-Mnaymned L, De Velasco R, Perez GO. Fatal destructive spondyloarthropathy in two patients on long-term dialysis. *Am J Kidney Dis* 1992;19:81–85.

48. Salusky IB, Coburn JW, Brill J, et al. Bone disease in pediatric patients undergoing dialysis with CAPD or CCPD. *Kidney Int* 1988;33:975–982.

49. Moriniere P, Cohen-Solal M, Belbrik S, et al. Disappearance of aluminic bone disease in a long term asymptomatic dialysis population restricting Al(OH)₃ intake: emergence of an idiopathic adynamic bone disease not related to aluminum. *Nephron* 1989;53:93–101.

50. Hercz G, Goodman WG, Pei Y, Segre GV, Coburn JW, Sherrard DJ. Low turnover bone disease without aluminum in dialysis patients (abstract). *Kidney Int* 1989;35:378.

51. Hercz G, Pei Y, Manuel A, et al. Aplastic osteodystrophy without aluminum in dialysis patients (abstract). *Kidney Int* 1990;37:449.

52. Hutchison AJ, Whitehouse RW, Boulton HF, et al. Characteristics and natural history of adynamic bone in CAPD (abstract). *Nephrol Dialysis Transplant* 1992;7:759–760.

53. Hercz G, Pei Y, Greenwood C, et al. Low turnover osteodystrophy without aluminum: the role of "suppressed" parathyroid function. *Kidney Int* 1993;44:860–866.

54. Goodman WG, Ramirez JA, Gales G, Segre GV, Salusky IB. Skeletal response to one year of intermittent calcitriol therapy in dialyzed children (abstract). *J Am Soc Nephrol* 1992;3:672.

55. Norris KC, Crooks PW, Nebeker HG, et al. Clinical and laboratory features of aluminum-related bone disease: differences between sporadic and "epidemic" forms of the syndrome. *Am J Kidney Dis* 1985;6:342–347.

56. Coburn JW, Norris KC, Nebeker HG. Osteomalacia and bone disease arising from aluminum. *Semin Nephrol* 1986;6:68–89.

57. Hercz G, Pei Y, Manuel A, et al. Aplastic osteodystrophy: Role of suppressed parathyroid hormone levels (abstract). *Abstract Book XIth Int Congr Nephrol* 1990;402A.

58. Berson SA, Yalow RS. Immunochemical heterogeneity of parathyroid hormone in plasma. *J Clin Endocrinol Metab* 1968;28:1037–1047.

59. Martin KJ, Hruska KA, Freitag JJ, Klahr S, Slatopolsky E. The peripheral metabolism of parathyroid hormone. *N Engl J Med* 1979;301:1092–1098.

60. Hruska KA, Teitelbaum SL, Kopelman R, et al. The predictability of the histological features of uremic bone disease by non-invasive techniques. *Metab Bone Dis Rel Res* 1978; 1:39–44.

61. Malluche HH, Faugere MC, Fanti P, Price PA. Plasma levels of bone Gla-protein reflect bone formation in patients on chronic maintenance hemodialysis. *Kidney Int* 1984;26:869–874.

62. Voigts A, Felsenfeld AJ, Andress D, Llach F. Parathyroid hormone and bone histology: response to hypocalcemia in osteitis fibrosa. *Kidney Int* 1984;25:445–454.

63. Blind E, Schmidt-Gayk H, Scharla S, et al. Two-site assay of intact parathyroid hormone in the investigation of primary hyperparathyroidism and other disorders of calcium metabolism compared with a midregion assay. *J Clin Endocrinol Metab* 1988;67:353–360.

64. Hodgson SF. Skeletal remodeling and renal osteodystrophy. *Semin Nephrol* 1986;6:42–55.

65. Norris KC, Goodman WG, Howard N, Nugent ME, Coburn JW. The iliac crest bone biopsy for the diagnosis of aluminum toxicity and a guide to the use of deferoxamine. *Semin Nephrol* 1986;6(Suppl 1):27–34.

66. Ott SM, Maloney NA, Coburn JW, Alfrey AC, Sherrard DJ. The prevalence of bone aluminum deposition in renal osteodystrophy and its relation to the response to calcitriol therapy. *N Engl J Med* 1982;307:709–713.

67. Sherrard DJ, Ott SM, Maloney NA, Andress DL, Coburn JW. Uremic osteodystrophy: classification, cause and treatment. In: Frame B, Potts JT Jr, eds. *Clinical disorders of bone and mineral metabolism.* Amsterdam: Excerpta Medica, 1984;254.

68. Andress DL, Sherrard DJ. The osteodystrophy of chronic renal failure. In: Schrier RW, Gottschalk CW, eds. *Diseases of the Kidney, 5th ed.* Boston: Little, Brown, & Co., 1993;2759.

69. Malluche H, Faugere M-C: Renal bone disease 1990: an unmet challenge for the nephrologist. *Kidney Int* 1990;38:193–211.

70. Hodsman AB, Sherrard DJ, Alfrey AC, et al. Bone aluminum and histomorphometric features of renal osteodystrophy. *J Clin Endocrinol Metab* 1982;54:539–546.

71. Hutchison AJ, Freemont AJJ, Boulton HF, Gokal R. Low-calcium dialysis fluid and oral calcium carbonate in CAPD: a method for controlling hyperphosphatemia whilst minimizing aluminum exposure and hypercalcaemia. *Nephrol Dialysis Transplant* 1992;7:1219–1225.

72. Morton AR, Hercz G. Hypercalcemia in dialysis patients: comparison of diagnostic methods. *Dialysis Transplant* 1991; 20:661–667.

73. Mirahmadi KS, Duffy BS, Shinaberger JH, Jowsey J, Massry SG, Coburn JW. A controlled evaluation of clinical and metabolic effects of dialysate calcium levels during regular hemodialysis. *Trans ASAIO* 1971;17:118–124.

74. Tibi L, Chhabra SC, Sweeting VM, Winney RJ, Smith AF. Multiple forms of alkaline phosphatase in plasma of hemodialysis patients. *Clin Chem* 1991;37:815–820.

75. Alvarez-Ude F, Feest TG, Ward MK, et al. Hemodialysis bone disease: correlation between clinical, histologic and other findings. *Kidney Int* 1978;14:68–73.

76. Brickman AS, Coburn JW, Norman AW. Action of 1,25-dihydroxycholecalciferol, a potent kidney-produced metabolite of vitamin D₃ in uremic man. *N Engl J Med* 1972; 287:891–895.

77. Nebeker HG, Coburn JW. Parathyroid hormone and chronic renal failure. *AACC ENDO* 1985;3:1–9.

78. Massry SG, Coburn JW, Lee DBN, Jowsey J, Kleeman CR. Skeletal resistance to parathyroid hormone in renal failure. *Ann Intern Med* 1973;78:357–364.

79. Quarles LD, Lobaugh B, Murphy G. Intact parathyroid hormone overestimates the presence and severity of parathyroid-mediated osseous abnormalities in uremia. *J Clin Endocrinol Metab* 1992;75:145–150.

80. Solal MC, Sebert JL, Boudailliez B, et al. Comparison of intact, midregion, and carboxy terminal assays of parathyroid hormone for the diagnosis of bone disease in hemodialyzed patients. *J Clin Endocrinol Metab* 1991;73:516–524.

81. Chan YL, Furlong TJ, Cornish CJ, Posen S. Dialysis osteodystrophy. A study involving 94 patients. *Medicine* 1985;64: 296–309.

82. Charhon SA, Delmas PD, Malaval L, et al. Serum bone Gla-protein in renal osteodystrophy: comparison with bone histomorphometry. *J Clin Endocrinol Metab* 1986;63:892–897.

83. Andress DL, Endres DB, Maloney NA, Kopp JB, Coburn

JW, Sherrard DJ. Comparison of parathyroid hormone assays with bone histomorphometry in renal osteodystrophy. *J Clin Endocrinol* 1986;63:1163–1169.

84. Hruska KA, Kopelman R, Rutherford WE, Klahr S, Slatopolsky E. Metabolism of immunoreactive parathyroid hormone in the dog. *J Clin Invest* 1975;56:39–48.

85. Piraino B, Chen T, Cooperstein L, Segre G, Puschett J. Fractures and vertebral bone mineral density in patients with renal osteodystrophy. *Clin Nephrol* 1988;30:57–62.

86. Felsenfeld AJ. The diagnosis of secondary hyperparathyroidism. *Nephrologia* (in press).

87. Nussbaum SR, Potts JT Jr. Immunoassays for parathyroid hormone 1–84 in the diagnosis of hyperparathyroidism. *J Bone Mineral Res* 1991;6(Suppl. 2):S43–S50.

88. Brown RC, Aston JP, Weeks I, Woodhead S. Circulating intact parathyroid hormone measured by a two-site immunochemiluminometric assay. *J Clin Endocrinol Metab* 1987;65:407–414.

89. Morita A, Tabata T, Koyama H, et al. A two-site immunochemiluminometric assay for intact parathyroid hormone and its clinical utility in hemodialysis patients. *Clin Nephrol* 1992;38:154–157.

90. Segre GV, Sherrard DJ, Carlton EI. *Use of the PTH (IRMA) assay in patients with impaired renal function and renal osteodystrophy.* San Juan Capistrano, CA: Nichols Institute, 1990;1.

91. Andress DL, Norris KC, Coburn JW, Slatopolsky EA, Sherrard DJ. Intravenous calcitriol in the treatment of refractory osteitis fibrosa of chronic renal failure. *N Engl J Med* 1989;321:274–279.

92. Andress DL, Nebeker HG, Ott SM, et al. Bone histologic response to deferoxamine in aluminum-related bone disease. *Kidney Int* 1987;1:1344–1350.

93. Andress DL, Ott SM, Maloney NA, Sherrard DJ. Effect of parathyroidectomy on bone aluminum accumulation in chronic renal failure. *N Engl J Med* 1985;312:468–473.

94. Sherrard DJ, Ott SM, Andress DL. Pseudohyperparathyroidism. A syndrome associated with aluminum intoxication in patients with renal failure. *Am J Med* 1985;79:127–130.

95. Campistrus De Gencarelli N, Cournot-Witmer G, Zingraff J, Drueke T. The role of parathyroid function and parathyroidectomy in the outcome of aluminum-related dialysis encephalopathy. *Nephrol Dialysis Transplant* 1986;1:192–198.

96. Charhon SA, Berland YF, Olmer MJ, Delawari E, Traeger J, Meunier PJ. Effects of parathyroidectomy on bone formation and mineralization in hemodialyzed patients. *Kidney Int* 1985;27:426–435.

97. De Vernejoul M-C, Marchais S, London G, Morieux C, Bielakoff J, Miravet L. Increased bone aluminum deposition after subtotal parathyroidectomy in dialyzed patients. *Kidney Int* 1985;27:785–791.

98. Alfrey AC, Hegg A, Craswell P. Metabolism and toxicity of aluminum in renal failure. *Am J Clin Nutr* 1980;33:1509–1516.

99. Hercz G, Kraut JA, Andress DL, et al. Use of calcium carbonate as a phosphate binder in dialysis patients. *Mineral Electrolyte Metab* 1986;12:314–319.

100. Von Herrath D, Asmus G, Pauls A, Delling G, Schaefer K. Renal osteodystrophy in asymptomatic hemodialysis patients: evidence of a sex-dependent distribution and predictive value of serum aluminum measurements. *Am J Kidney Dis* 1986;8:430–435.

101. Hodsman AB, Hood SA, Brown P, Cordy PE. Do serum aluminum levels reflect underlying skeletal aluminum accumulation and bone histology before or after chelation by deferoxamine? *J Lab Clin Med* 1985;106:674–681.

102. De Vernejoul MC, Marchais S, London G, et al. Deferoxamine test and bone disease in dialysis patients with mild aluminum accumulation. *Am J Kidney Dis* 1989;14:124–130.

103. Hodsman AB, Steer BM. Serum aluminum levels as a reflection of renal osteodystrophy status and bone surface aluminum staining. *J Am Soc Nephrol* 1992;2:1318–1327.

104. De Broe ME, D'Haese PC, Couttenye M-M, Van Landeghem GF, Lamberts LV. New insights and strategies in the diagnosis and treatment of aluminum overload in dialysis patients. *Nephrol Dialysis Transplant* 1993;8(Suppl. 1):47–50.

105. Milliner DS, Nebeker HG, Ott SM, et al. Use of the deferoxamine infusion test in the diagnosis of aluminum-related osteodystrophy. *Ann Intern Med* 1984;101:775–779.

106. Malluche HH, Smith AJ, Abreo K, Faugere MC. The use of deferoxamine in the management of aluminum accumulation in bone in patients with renal failure. *N Engl J Med* 1984;311:140–144.

107. Pei Y, Hercz G, Greenwood C, et al. Non-invasive prediction of aluminum bone disease in hemo- and peritoneal dialysis patients. *Kidney Int* 1992;41:1374–1382.

108. Hercz G, Andress DL, Norris KC, et al. Improved bone formation in dialysis patients after substitution of calcium carbonate for aluminum gels. *Trans Assoc Am Physicians* 1987;100:139–145.

109. Podenphant J, Heaf JG, Joffe P. Metabolic bone disease and aluminum contamination in 38 uremic patients. A bone histomorphometric study. *Acta Pathol Microbiol Immunol Scand* 1986;94:1–6.

110. Andress DL, Pandian MR, Endres DB, Kopp JB. Plasma insulin-like growth factors and bone formation in uremic hyperparathyroidism. *Kidney Int* 1989;36:471–477.

111. Barbour GL, Coburn JW, Slatopolsky E, Norman AW, Horst RL. Hypercalcemia in an anephric patient with sarcoidosis, evidence for extrarenal generation of 1,25 dihydroxyvitamin D. *N Engl J Med* 1981;305:440–446.

112. Felsenfeld AJ, Drezner MK, Llach F. Hypercalcemia and elevated calcitriol in a maintenance dialysis patient with tuberculosis. *Arch Intern Med* 1986;146:1941–1944.

113. Dent CE, Hodson CJ. Radiological changes associated with certain metabolic bone diseases. *Br J Radiol* 1954;27:605–608.

114. Meema HE, Rabinovich S, Meema S, Lloyd GJ, Oreopoulos DG. Improved radiological diagnosis of azotemic osteodystrophy. *Radiology* 1972;102:1–10.

115. Meema HE, Meema S. Microradioscopic quantitation of periosteal resorption in secondary hyperparathyroidism of chronic renal failure. *Clin Orthop* 1978;130:297.

116. Parfitt AM. Clinical and radiographic manifestations of renal osteodystrophy. In: David DS, ed. *Calcium metabolism in renal failure and nephrolithiasis.* New York: John Wiley & Sons, 1977;150.

117. Shimada H, Nakamura M, Marumo F. Influence of aluminum on the effect of 1-alpha-(OH)D₃ on renal osteodystrophy. *Nephron* 1983;35:163–170.

118. Mehls O. Renal osteodystrophy in children: etology and clinical aspects. In: Fine RN, Gruskin AB, eds. *Endstage renal disease in children.* Philadelphia: W.B. Saunders, 1984;227–250.

119. Olgaard K, Heerfordt J, Madsen S. Scintographic skeletal changes in uremic patients on regular hemodialysis. *Nephron* 1976;17:325–334.

120. Karsenty G, Vigneron N, Jorgetti V, et al. Value of the 99-mTc-methylene diphosphonate bone scan in renal osteodystrophy. *Kidney Int* 1986;29:1058–1065.

121. Vanherweghem J-L, Schoutens A, Bergman P, et al. Usefulness of 99mTc-pyrophosphate bone scintography in aluminum bone disease. *Trace Elements Med* 1984;1:80–83.

122. Botella J, Gallego JL, Fernandez-Fernandez J, et al. The bone scan in patients with aluminum-associated bone disease. *Proc EDTA-ERA* 1985;21:403–409.

123. Hodson EM, Howman-Gilles RB, Evans RB, et al. The diagnosis of renal osteodystrophy: A comparison of technitium⁹⁹ pyrophosphate bone scintography with other techniques. *Clin Nephrol* 1981;16:24–28.

124. Llach F, Massry SG. On the mechanism of secondary hyperparathyroidism in moderate renal insufficiency. *J Clin Endocrinol Metab* 1985;61:601–606.

125. Portale AA, Booth BE, Halloran BP, Morris RC Jr. Effect of dietary phosphorus on circulating concentrations of 1,25-dihydroxyvitamin D and immunoreactive parathyroid hormone in children with moderate renal insufficiency. *J Clin Invest* 1984;73:1580–1589.

126. Fournier AE, Arnaud CD, Johnson WJ. Etiology of hyperparathyroidism and bone disease during chronic hemodialysis. II. Factors affecting serum immunoreactive parathyroid hormone. *J Clin Invest* 1971;50:599.

127. Rodriguez M, Felsenfeld AJ, Williams C, Pederson JA, Llach F. The effect of long-term calcitriol administration on parathyroid function in hemodialysis patients. *J Am Soc Nephrol* 1991;2:1014–1020.

128. Maschio G, Oldrizzi L, Tessitore N, et al. Effects of dietary and protein restriction on the progression of early renal failure. *Kidney Int* 1982;22:597–607.

129. Kaye M, Turner M, Ardila M, Wiegmann T, Hodsman A. Aluminum and phosphate. *Kidney Int* 1988;24(Suppl.):S172–S174.

130. Hercz G, Coburn JW. Prevention of phosphate retention and hyperphosphatemia in uremia. *Kidney Int* 1987;32(Suppl. 22):S215–S220.

131. Kopple JD, Coburn JW. Metabolic studies of low protein diets in uremia. II. Calcium, phosphorus and magnesium. *Medicine* 1973;52:597.

132. Coburn JW, Salusky IB. Control of serum phosphorus in uremia. *N Engl J Med* 1989;320:1140–1142.

133. Slatopolsky E, Weerts C, Lopez-Hilker S, et al. Calcium carbonate is an effective phosphate binder in patients with chronic renal failure undergoing dialysis. *N Engl J Med* 1986;315:157–161.

134. Delmez JA, Tindira CA, Windus DW, et al. Calcium acetate as a phosphorus binder in hemodialysis patients. *J Am Soc Nephrol* 1992;3:96–102.

135. Coburn JW, Hartenbower DL, Massry SG. Intestinal absorption of calcium and the effect of renal insufficiency. *Kidney Int* 1973;4:96–103.

136. Clarkson EM, McDonald SJ, De Wardener HE. The effect of a high intake of calcium carbonate in normal subjects and patients with chronic renal failure. *Clin Sci* 1966;30:425–438.

137. Clarkson EM, Eastwood JB, Koutsaimanis K, De Wardener H. Net intestinal absorption of calcium in patients with chronic renal failure. *Kidney Int* 1973;3:258.

137a. Meyrier A, Marsac J, Richet G. The influence of a high calcium carbonate intake on bone disease in patients undergoing hemodialysis. *Kidney Int* 1973;4:146–153.

138. Fournier A, Moriniere PH, Sebert JL, et al. Calcium carbonate, an aluminum-free agent for control of hyperphosphatemia, hypocalcemia and hyperparathyroidism in uremia. *Kidney Int* 1986;29(Suppl. 18):S115–S119.

139. Emmett M, Sirmon MD, Kirkpatrick WG, Nolan CR, Schmitt GW, Cleveland MVB. Calcium acetate control of serum phosphorus in hemodialysis patients. *Am J Kidney Dis* 1991;17:544–550.

140. Salusky IB, Coburn JW, Foley J, Nelson P, Fine RN. Effects of oral calcium carbonate on control of serum phosphorus and changes in plasma aluminum levels after discontinuation of aluminium-containing gels in children receiving dialysis. *J Pediatr* 1986;108:767–770.

141. Slatopolsky E, Weerts C, Norwood K, et al. Long-term effects of calcium carbonate and 2.5 mEq/liter calcium dialysate on mineral metabolism. *Kidney Int* 1989;36:897–903.

142. MacTier RA, Van Stone J, Cox A, Van Stone M, Twardowski Z. Calcium carbonate is an effective phosphate binder when dialysate calcium concentration is adjusted to control hypercalcemia. *Clin Nephrol* 1987;28:222–226.

143. Sawyer N, Noonan K, Altmann P, Marsh F, Cunningham J. High dose calcium carbonate with stepwise reduction in dialysate calcium concentration: Effective phosphate control and aluminum avoidance in haemodialysis patients. *Nephrol Dialysis Transplant* 1988;3:1–5.

144. Oettinger CW, Oliver JC, Macon EJ. The effects of calcium carbonate as the sole phosphate binder in combination with low calcium dialysate and calcitriol therapy in chronic dialysis patients. *J Am Soc Nephrol* 1992;3:995–1001.

145. Coburn JW, Slatopolsky E. Vitamin D, parathyroid hormone, and renal osteodystrophy. In: Brenner BM, Rector FC Jr, eds. *The Kidney*, 3rd ed. Philadelphia: WB Saunders, 1986;1657.

146. Felsenfeld AJ, Gutman RA, Llach F, Harrelson JM. Osteomalacia in chronic renal failure: a syndrome previously reported only with maintenance dialysis. *Am J Nephrol* 1982;2:147–154.

147. Griswold WR, Reznik V, Mendoza SA, Trauner D, Alfrey AC. Accumulation of aluminum in a nondialyzed uremic child receiving aluminum hydroxide. *Pediatrics* 1983;71:56–58.

148. Nathan E, Pederson SE. Dialysis encephalopathy in a non-dialysed uremic boy treated with aluminum hydroxide orally. *Acta Paediatr Scand* 1980;69:793–796.

149. Kaye M. Oral aluminum toxicity in a non-dialyzed patient with renal failure. *Clin Nephrol* 1983;20:208–211.

150. Andreoli SP, Bergstein JM, Sherrard DJ. Aluminum intoxication from aluminum-containing phosphate binders in children with azotemia not undergoing dialysis. *N Engl J Med* 1984;310:1079–1084.

151. Kaehny WD, Hegg P, Alfrey AC. Gastrointestinal absorption of aluminum from aluminum-containing antacids. *N Engl J Med* 1977;296:1389–1390.

152. Recker RR, Blotchky AJ, Leffler JA, Rack EP. Evidence for aluminum absorption from the gastrointestinal tract and bone deposition by aluminum carbonate ingestion with normal renal function. *J Lab Clin Med* 1977;90:810–815.

153. Salusky IB, Coburn JW, Paunier L, Sherrard DJ, Fine RN. Role of aluminum hydroxide in raising serum aluminum levels in children undergoing continuous ambulatory peritoneal dialysis. *J Pediatr* 1984;105:717–720.

154. Sedman AB, Miller NL, Warady BA, Lum GM, Alfrey AC. Aluminum loading in children with chronic renal failure. *Kidney Int* 1984;26:201–204.

155. Winney RJ, Cowie JF, Robson JS. The role of plasma aluminum in the detection and prevention of aluminum toxicity. *Kidney Int* 1986;29(Suppl. 18):S91–S95.

156. Salusky IB, Foley J, Nelson P, Goodman WG. Aluminum accumulation from recommended doses of aluminum hydroxide in dialyzed children. *N Engl J Med* 1991;324:527–531.

157. Molitoris BA, Froment DH, MacKenzie TA, Huffer WH, Alfrey AC. Citrate: a major factor in the toxicity of orally administered aluminum compounds. *Kidney Int* 1989;36:949–953.

158. Coburn JW, Mischel MG, Goodman WG, Salusky IB. Calcium citrate markedly enhances aluminum absorption from aluminum hydroxide. *Am J Kidney Dis* 1991;17:708–711.

159. Bakir AA, Hryhorczuk DO, Berman E, Dunea G. Acute fatal hyperaluminemic encephalopathy in undialyzed and recently dialyzed uremic patients. *Trans Am Soc Artif Intern Organs* 1986;32:171–176.

160. Kirschbaum BB, Schoolwerth AC. Acute aluminum toxicity associated with oral citrate and aluminum-containing antacids. *Am J Med Sci* 1989;297:9–11.

161. Cushner HM, Copley JB, Lindberg JS, Foulks CJ. Calcium citrate, a nonaluminum-containing phosphate-binding agent for treatment of CRF. *Kidney Int* 1988;33:95–99.

162. Sherrard DJ. Aluminum, much ado about something. *N Engl J Med* 1991;324:558–559.

163. Schiller LR, Santa Ana CA, Sheikh MS, Emmett M, Fordtran JS. Effect of the time of administration of calcium acetate on phosphorus binding. *N Engl J Med* 1989;320:1110–1113.

164. Sheikh MS, Maguire JA, Emmett M, et al. Reduction of dietary phosphorus absorption by phosphorus binders: a theoretical, in vitro, and in vivo study. *J Clin Invest* 1989;83:66–73.

165. Mai ML, Emmett M, Sheikh MS, Santa Ana CA, Schiller L, Fordtran JS. Calcium acetate, an effective phosphorus binder in patients with renal failure. *Kidney Int* 1989;36:690–695.

166. Cunningham J, Beer J, Coldwell RD, Noonan K, Sawyer N, Makin HLJ. Dialysate calcium reduction in CAPD patients treated with calcium carbonate and alphacalcidol. *Nephrol Dialysis Transplant* 1992;7:63–68.

167. Ring T, Nielsen C, Paulin Anderson S, Behrnes JK, Sodemann B, Kornerup HJ. Calcium acetate versus calcium carbonate as phosphorus binders in patients on chronic haemodialysis: a controlled study. *Nephrol Dialysis Transplant* 1993;8:341–346.

168. Kobrin SM, Goldstein SJ, Shangraw RF, Raja RM. Variable efficacy of calcium carbonate tablets. *Am J Kidney Dis* 1989;14:461–465.

169. Coburn JW. Mineral metabolism and renal bone disease: effects of CAPD versus hemodialysis. *Kidney Int* 1993;43 (Suppl. 40):S92–S100.

170. Kaye M, Chatterjee G, Cohen GF. Arrest of hyperparathyroid bone disease with dihydrotachysterol in patients undergoing chronic hemodialysis. *Ann Intern Med* 1970;73: 225–233.

171. Witmer G, Margolis A, Fontaine O, et al. Effects of 25-hydroxycholecalciferol on bone lesions of children with terminal renal failure. *Kidney Int* 1976;10:395–408.

172. Recker R, Schoenfeld P, Letteri J, Slatopolsky E, Goldsmith R, Brickman AS. The efficacy of calcifediol in renal osteodystrophy. *Arch Intern Med* 1978;138:857.

173. Peacock M, Heyburn P, Aaron J, Taylor GA, Brown WB, Speed R. Osteomalacia: treated with 1 hydroxy or 1,25 dihydroxy vitamin D. In: Norman AW, Schaefer K, V. Herrath D, et al., eds. *Vitamin D: basic research and its clinical application*. Berlin: de Gruyter, 1979;1177.

174. Peacock M. The clinical uses of 1 α-Hydroxyvitamin D$_3$. *Clin Endocrinol.* 1977;7:15–2465 (suppl).

175. Salusky IB, Fine RN, Kangarloo H, et al. "High-dose" calcitriol for control of renal osteodystrophy in children on CAPD. *Kidney Int* 1987;32:89–95.

176. Baker LRI, Abrams SML, Roe CJ, et al. Early therapy of renal bone disease with calcitriol: a prospective double-blind study. *Kidney Int* 1989;36(Suppl. 27):S140–S142.

177. Baker LR, Muir JW, Sharman VL, et al. Controlled trial of calcitriol in hemodialysis patients. *Clin Nephrol* 1986;26: 185–191.

178. Bordier P, Rasmussen H, Marie P, Miravet L, Gueris J, Ryckwaert A. Vitamin D metabolites and bone mineralization in man. *J Clin Endocrinol Metab* 1976;46:284–294.

179. Berl T, Berns AS, Huffer WE, et al. 1,25-Dihydroxycholecalciferol effects in chronic dialysis. A double-blind controlled study. *Ann Intern Med* 1978;88:774–780.

180. Sherrard DJ, Coburn JW, Brickman AS, Singer FR, Maloney N. Skeletal response to treatment with 1,25-dihydroxyvitamin D in renal failure. *Contrib Nephrol* 1980;18:92–97.

181. Coburn JW, Brickman AS, Sherrard DJ, et al. Use of 1,25(OH)$_2$-vitamin D$_3$ to separate "types" of renal osteodystrophy. *Proc EDTA* 1977;14:442–450.

182. Tougaard L, Sorensen E, Brochner-Mortensen J, Christensen MS, Rodbro P, Sorenson AWS. Controlled trial of 1α-hydroxycholecalciferol in chronic renal failure. *Lancet* 1976; 1:1044–1047.

183. Pierides AM, Kerr DNS, Ellis HA. 1α-Hydroxycholecalciferol in hemodialysis renal osteodystrophy. Adverse effects of anticonvulsant therapy. *Clin Nephrol* 1976;5:189–192.

184. Voigts AL, Felsenfeld AJ, Llach F. The effects of calciferol and its metabolites on patients with chronic renal failure. II. Calcitriol, 1 alpha-hydroxyvitamin D$_3$, and 24,25-dihydroxyvitamin D$_3$. *Arch Intern Med* 1983;143:1205–1211.

185a.Hodsman AB, Wong EGC, Sherrad DJ, et al. Preliminary trials with 24,25-dihydroxyvitamin D$_3$ in dialysis osteomalacia. *Am J Med* 1983;74:407–414.

185. Llach F, Brickman AS, Singer FR, Coburn JW. 24,25-Dihydroxycholecalciferol, a vitamin D sterol with qualitatively unique effects in uremic man. *Metab Bone Dis Rel Res* 1979;2:11–15.

186. Brown AJ, Ritter CR, Finch JL, et al. The noncalcemic analogue of vitamin D, 22-oxacalcitriol, suppresses parathyroid hormone synthesis and secretion. *J Clin Invest* 1989; 84:728–732.

187. Brown AJ, Finch JL, Lopez-Hilker S, et al. New active analogues of vitamin D with low calcemic activity. *Kidney Int* 1990;29(Suppl. 29):S22–S27.

188. Slatopolsky E, Weerts C, Thielan J, Horst RL, Harter H, Martin KJ. Marked suppression of secondary hyperparathyroidism by intravenous administration of 1,25-dihydroxycholecalciferol in uremic patients. *J Clin Invest* 1984;74: 2136–2143.

189. Silver J, Naveh-Many T, Mayer H, Schmelzer HJ, Popvtzer MM: Regulation by vitamin D metabolites of parathyroid hormone gene transcription in vivo in the rat. *J Clin Invest* 1986;78:1296–1301.

190. Russell J, Lettieri D, Sherwood LM. Suppression by 1,25(OH)$_2$D$_3$ of transcription of the parathyroid hormone gene. *Endocrinology* 1986;119:2864–2866.

191. Dunlay R, Rodriguez M, Felsenfeld AJ, Llach F. Direct inhibitory effect of calcitriol on parathyroid function (sigmoidal curve) in dialysis. *Kidney Int* 1989;36:1093–1098.

192. Sprague SM. Safety and efficacy of long-term treatment of secondary hyperparathyroidism by low-dose intravenous calcitriol. *Am J Kidney Dis* 1992;19:532–539.

193. Malberti F, Surian M, Cosci P. Effect of chronic intravenous calcitriol on parathyroid function and set point of calcium in dialysis patients with refractory secondary hyperparathyroidism. *Nephrol Dialysis Transplant* 1992;7:822–828.

194. Gallieni M, Brancaccio D, Padovese P, et al. Low-dose intravenous calcitriol treatment of secondary hyperparathyroidism in hemodialysis patients. *Kidney Int* 1992;42:1191–1198.

195. Dressler R, Laut J, Lynn RI, Ginsberg N. Intravenous calcitriol for secondary hyperparathyroidism in patients with and-stage renal disease. In: Llach F, ed. *Renal osteodystrophy*. London: Oxford Press (in press).

196. Hamdy NAT, Brown CB, Kanis JA. Intravenous calcitriol lowers serum calcium concentrations in uraemic patients with severe hyperparathyroidism and hypercalcaemia. *Nephrol Dialysis Transplant* 1989;4:545–548.

197. Delmez JA, Tindira C, Grooms P, Dusso A, Windus DW, Slatopolsky E. Parathyroid hormone suppression by intravenous 1,25-dihydroxyvitamin D. A role for increased sensitivity to calcium. *J Clin Invest* 1989;83:1349–1355.

198. Fukagawa M, Orazaki R, Takano K, et al. Regression of parathyroid hyperplasia by calcitriol-pulse therapy in patients on long-term dialysis. *N Engl J Med* 1990;323:421–422.

199. Tsukamoto Y, Nomura M, Takahashi Y, et al. The "oral 1,25-dihydroxyvitamin D$_3$ pulse therapy" in hemodialysis patients with severe secondary hyperparathyroidism. *Nephron* 1991;57:23–28.

200. Martin KJ, Bullal HS, Domoto DT, Blalock S, Weindel M. Pulse oral calcitriol for the treatment of hyperparathyroidism in patients on continuous ambulatory peritoneal dialysis: preliminary observations. *Am J Kidney Dis* 1992;19: 540–545.

201. Salusky IB, Goodman WG, Horst R, et al. Pharmacokinetics of calcitriol in CAPD/CCPD patients. *Am J Kidney Dis* 1990;16:126–132.

202. Lind L, Wengle B, Wide L, Wrege U, Ljunghall S. Suppression of serum parathyroid hormone levels by intravenous alphacalcidol in uremic patients on maintenance hemodialysis: a pilot study. *Nephron* 1988;48:296–299.

203. Brandi L, Daugaard H, Tvedegaard E, Storm T, Olgaard K. Effect of intravenous 1-alpha-hydroxyvitamin D$_3$ on secondary hyperparathyroidism in chronic uremic patients on maintenance hemodialysis. *Nephron* 1989;53:194–200.

204. Ljunghall S, Althoff P, Fellström B, et al. Effects on serum parathyroid hormone of intravenous treatment with alphacalcidol in patients on chronic hemodialysis. *Nephron* 1990; 55:380–385.

205. Papapoulos SE, Fraher LJ, Clemens TL, Gleed J, O'Riordan JLH. Metabolites of vitamin D in human vitamin-D deficiency: effect of vitamin D$_3$ or 1,25-dihydroxy-cholecalciferol. *Lancet* 1980;2:612–615.

206. Coburn JW, Slatopolsky E. Vitamin D, parathyroid hormone, and the renal osteodystrophies. In: Brenner BM, Rector FC Jr, eds. *The Kidney*. Philadelphia: WB Saunders, 1991;2036.

207. Massry SG. Assessment of 1,25(OH)$_2$D$_3$ in the correction and prevention of renal osteodystrophy in patients with mild to moderate renal failure. In: Norman AW, Schaefer K, Grigoleit H-G, V. Herrath D, eds. *Vitamin D: a chemical, biochemical and clinical update*. Berlin: de Gruyter, 1985; 935.

208. Nordal KP, Dahl E. Low dose calcitriol versus placebo in patients with predialysis chronic renal failure. *J Clin Endocrinol Metab* 1988;67:929–936.

209. Baker LRI, Abrams SML, Roe CJ, et al. 1,25(OH)$_2$D$_3$ in

moderate renal failure: a prospective double-blind trial. *Kidney Int* 1989;35:661–669.

210. Goodman WG, Coburn JW: Calcitriol in "early" and predialysis renal failure: what are the risks and benefits: In: Norman AW, Bouillon R, Thomasset M, eds. *Vitamin D: gene regulation, structure-function analysis, and clinical application.* Berlin: de Gruyter, 1991;849.

211. Goodman WG, Coburn JW. The use of 1,25-dihydroxyvitamin D₃ in early renal failure. *Annu Rev Med* 1992;43:227–237.

212. Nielsen HE, Romer FK, Melsen F, Christensen MS, Hansen HE. 1α-Hydroxylated vitamin D₃ treatment of non-dialyzed patients with chronic renal failure. Effects on bone, mineral metabolism and kidney function. *Clin Nephrol* 1980;13:103–108.

213. Christiansen C, Rodbro P, Christensen MS, Hartnack B. Is 1,25-dihydroxy-cholecalciferol harmful to renal function in patients with chronic renal failure? *Clin Endocrinol* 1981; 15:229–236.

214. Bertoli M, Luisetto G, Ruffatti A, Urso M, Romagnoli G. Renal function during calcitriol therapy in chronic renal failure. *Clin Nephrol* 1990;33:98–102.

215. Cundy T, Hand DJ, Oliver DO, Woods CG, Wright FW, Kanis JA. Who gets renal bone disease before beginning dialysis? *Br Med J* 1985;290:271–275.

216. Dawborn JK, Brown DJ, Douglas MC, et al. Parathyroidectomy in chronic renal failure. *Nephron* 1983;33:100–105.

217. Sherrard DJ. Renal osteodystrophy. In: Henrich WJ, ed. *The principle and practice of dialysis.* Baltimore: Williams & Wilkins (in press).

218. Brickman AS, Hartenbower DL, Norman AW, Coburn JW. Actions of 1α-hydroxy- and 1,25-dihydroxyvitamin D₃ on mineral metabolism in man. I. Effects on net absorption of phosphorus. *Am J Clin Nutr* 1977;30:1064–1070.

219. Coburn JW. Use of oral and parenteral calcitriol in the treatment of renal osteodystrophy. *Kidney Int* 1990;38(Suppl. 29):S54–S61.

The Parathyroids, edited by J.P. Bilezikian,
M.A. Levine, and R. Marcus. Raven Press, Ltd.,
New York © 1994.

CHAPTER 43

Hypoparathyroid States in the Differential Diagnosis of Hypocalcemia

Louis M. Sherwood and Arthur C. Santora II

Hypocalcemia may present as an asymptomatic condition detected on routine screening or as a life-threatening medical emergency. While the latter, particularly if related to acute illness, is relatively straightforward to control, treatment of chronic hypocalcemia represents a significant therapeutic challenge. Advances in our knowledge of the physiology, biochemistry, and molecular biology and genetics of the calcium-regulating hormones, particularly parathyroid hormone (PTH) and the active form of vitamin D_3 [1,25-$(OH)_2D_3$], have helped us to understand the interplay of pathogenetic factors in hypocalcemia and to develop a rational basis for the therapy of this clinical condition.

Calcium plays a critical role in maintaining normal physiologic processes, and, in order to prevent hypocalcemia, rapid response systems of homeostasis have developed during vertebrate evolution. This is particularly relevant when animals left the sea, which is rich in calcium, and developed a base on land (1). The skeleton developed, at least in part, to create stable stores of calcium and other ions, that could compensate for wide variations in oral intake. In fresh water, which was deficient in calcium, calcium storage organs developed as primitive precursors to mammalian bone. In sea water, which was high in calcium, no such structures developed. Calcitonin (a peptide hormone derived from the ultimobranchial bodies) presumably developed to prevent the high calcium concentrations in sea water from overwhelming the organism (al-

though this still remains a working hypothesis). Our understanding of the calcium-regulating mechanisms in fish, which include the pituitary and Stannius corpuscles, is incomplete. In amphibious animals, paravertebral lime sacs as well as bone serve as calcium reservoirs, and the first appearance of the parathyroid gland occurs. Highly sophisticated mechanisms for regulating calcium have evolved in chickens and other birds because of large calcium fluxes, particularly during the formation of the eggshell. During evolution, mammals developed a tightly regulated mineral homeostatic system, including the hormones, PTH, and 1,25-$(OH)_2D_3$, that regulate the activity of targets in the skeleton, kidney, and gastrointestinal tract. Calcitonin, while perhaps an important hormone in fetal development and in the neonate, is relegated to a more vestigial role in evolution and in adult calcium homeostatis.

Important adaptive mechanisms are activated during decreases in dietary calcium intake and constitute a first defense against hypocalcemia (2). These include an increase in PTH secretion and an increase in the formation of 1,25-$(OH)_2D_3$. Together, these hormones increase movement of calcium into the plasma by way of enhanced gastrointestinal absorption of calcium, stimulation of calcium release from the skeleton, and enhanced renal tubular reabsorption of calcium. During chronic hypocalcemia the parathyroid glands undergo marked adaptive changes, not only in terms of hormone secretion but also in terms of hypertrophy and hyperplasia. Some of the cellular and subcellular mechanisms for these changes, have been identified, but others remain a mystery. It has now been well established that 1,25-$(OH)_2D_3$ feeds back on the parathyroid gland, exerting a negative regulation of PTH synthesis and ultimately PTH secretion (2). The details of calcium homeostasis and the role of the various hormones are described in detail in the chapter by Brown and will not be reviewed further here.

L. M. Sherwood: Medical and Scientific Affairs, U.S. Human Health, Merck and Company, West Point, Pennsylvania 19486; Department of Medicine, Albert Einstein College of Medicine, Bronx, New York 10461.

A. C. Santora II: Department Endocrine and Metabolism Clinical Research, Merck Research Laboratories, Rahway, New Jersey 07065.

Hypocalcemia was first recognized as a clinical problem when calcium measurements became available earlier in this century. In the late 1800s, with thyroidectomy for goiter becoming a commonly performed procedure, inadvertent removal of the parathyroid glands became a frequent complication of the operation. Some of these patients had latent or overt tetany or seizures, and the importance of the parathyroids in calcium homeostasis was recognized (3). It was actually in the 1800s that Richard Owen, a British biologist, first recognized the parathyroid gland as a discreet structure in the Indian rhinoceros. In 1880, the Swedish anatomist Ivar Sandström first identified the parathyroid glands in man, calling them "glandulae parathyroideae," to emphasize their location near the thyroid gland.

EPIDEMIOLOGY AND PREVALENCE OF HYPOCALCEMIA

The routine availability of calcium measurements and the frequent performance of laboratory testing have increased the rate of detection of asymptomatic or minimally symptomatic patients with hypocalcemia (3). As a result, more adults with hypocalcemia due to parathyroid-deficient states have been identified. At the same time, however, hypoparathyroidism and its variants remain fairly uncommon. On the other hand, hypocalcemia is now recognized as a frequent concomitant of severe illness and is particularly common in critical care units and in emergency room situations. In these states, hypoalbuminemia, hypomagnesemia, alkalosis, and other factors contribute to the enhanced incidence of this presentation. Surveys of a hospital population present a somewhat skewed distribution; patients being hospitalized tend to be acutely ill. Moreover, the growth in critical care units has increased the apparent prevalence of hypocalcemia in the hospitalized population. In a recent study of cancer patients, hypocalcemia and hypomagnesemia were present in 13.4% and 17.1%, respectively, of a group of 82 hospitalized cancer patients, 61% of whom were in the terminal phase of their disease (4). Furthermore, in a group of patients admitted to a medical intensive care unit, Desai et al. (5) found that 70% of patients had decreased levels of both total and ionized calcium, and known causes of hypocalcemia could be identified in 45%. These causes included hypomagnesemia, renal insufficiency, and acute pancreatitis. Serum albumin was correlated directly with ionized calcium levels, and there was a strong association between sepsis and hypocalcemia. In another retrospective analysis, Chernow et al. (6) found that 64% of critical care patients were hypocalcemic (total calcium <8.5 mg/dl), with albumin concentrations that were <3.5 g/dl in 70% of the patients. In addition, 32% of the patients

were alkalotic. Those patients with gastrointestinal bleeding and intraabdominal surgery were more likely to have a low serum calcium, whereas cardiac and neurosurgical patients generally had a normal serum calcium. A greater mortality rate was found in hypocalcemic patients. Rapid measurement of ionized calcium can be very useful in many ICU patients because alterations in both arterial pH and serum albumin make predictions of the ionized calcium concentration unreliable when they are based on nomograms or calculations referenced to total serum calcium and protein concentrations. Renal failure, blood transfusions, sepsis, low albumin, and hypomagnesemia are predisposing factors. In addition, hypocalcemia has been frequently found in pediatric intensive care units, particularly in prenatal infants. Mimouni et al. (7) studied retrospectively 13,462 infants born at the University of Cincinnati Hospital. Serum calcium was measured routinely in infants with low birth weight (<2,500 g) and at 24 hr in infants with preterm delivery, neonatal asphyxia, and diabetic mothers. After excluding neonates with diabetic mothers and those with major congenital abnormalities, low serum calcium was found to be associated with low gestational age, low Apgar score, and a caucasian ethnic background. The fetus is normally exposed to high calcium concentrations in utero, and transient hypocalcemia is not uncommon in the immediate postpartum period, particularly in infants who have any of the risk factors described above. Neonatal hypocalcemia may reflect deficient parathyroid function or immature tubular renal function. Thus neonatal hypocalcemia is found more commonly today because of an increased number of infants who are preterm as well as the expansion of neonatal intensive care units. In addition, routine screening of calcium has identified infants with minimal or no symptoms of hypocalcemia. Functional disturbances in albumin or magnesium have become important pathogenetic factors in hypocalcemia and must be considered in the hypocalcemic patient.

ETIOLOGY OF HYPOCALCEMIA

Parathyroid Causes of Hypocalcemia

Hypoparathyroidism, while relatively uncommon, usually presents as a postoperative metabolic disturbance and rarely as a genetic or sporadic disorder (3) (see Tables 1, 2). Total thyroidectomy, radical neck dissection, or repeated operations for primary hyperparathyroidism (particularly due to hyperplasia of the glands) are the most common surgical causes of hypoparathyroidism (1). With good surgical technique, the incidence of hypoparathyroidism is 1–2%, although some series have reported much higher numbers (8,9). While prolonged hypocalcemia after neck

TABLE 1. *Hypoparathyroid etiologies of hypocalcemia*

Agenesis or dysgenesis
  Isolated
  DiGeorge syndrome
Parathyroid ablation
  Surgical excision
  Neoplastic invasion or granulomatous infiltration
Parathyroid degeneration
  Autoimmune
    Isolated
    Polyglandular
  Systemic disease
    Hemochromatosis
    Wilson's disease
    Thalassemia
  Radiation
Deficient parathyroid hormone secretion
  Genetic
    Abnormal protein synthesis
    Secretion
  Hypomagnesemia/hypermagnesemia
  Neonatal hypocalcemia

TABLE 2. *Nonparathyroid hypocalcemia with increased parathyroid hormone secretion*

Parathyroid hormone resistance
  Bioinactive parathyroid hormone
  Pseudohypoparathyroidism
Calcium sequestration
  Rhabdomyolysis
  Chemotherapy
    Tumor lysis syndrome
  Acute pancreatitis
  "Hungry bones"
    Postparathyroidectomy
    Paget's disease after treatment
    Healing osteomalacia/rickets
    Post-hyperthyroidism
  Osteoblastic malignancy
    Metastatic prostate and breast carcinoma
Renal insufficiency
Vitamin D disorders
  Nutritional vitamin D deficiency
  Vitamin D–dependent/resistant rickets
Gastrointestinal disease
  Malabsorption
Drugs
  Calcium chelators
    Citrated blood transfusions
    Phosphate
  Inhibitors of bone resorption
    Bisphosphonates
    Calcitonin
    Gallium nitrate
    Plicamycin
  Vitamin D metabolism
    Anticonvulsants:
      Phenytoin and phenobarbital
    Ketoconazole
Multifactorial
  Critical illness

surgery can indicate permanent hypoparathyroidism, transient hypocalcemia is usually reversible and is typically due to edema or hemorrhage into the parathyroids, "hungry bone syndrome" in patients with severe hyperparathyroidism or hyperthyroidism, or postoperative hypomagnesemia (see the chapter by Nussbaum and Potts). It is advisable to avoid surgical maneuvers that may lead to the development of hypoparathyroidism, as it is challenging to treat hypocalcemia chronically. It is now possible to transplant parathyroid tissue at the time of parathyroidectomy (particularly in patients with primary hyperplasia of the glands) into the brachioradialis or sternocleidomastoid muscle or to cryopreserve tissue in dimethylsulfoxide (DMSO) for later transplantation if necessary (10). (See the chapter by O'Riordan.)

In addition to surgical excision of damage to the parathyroids, neoplastic invasion or granulomatous infiltration of the parathyroids may cause hypoparathyroidism, but these disorders are relatively uncommon. They could be associated with lymphomas or other neoplasms in the neck. More likely is hypocalcemia that results from mantle irradiation of patients with Hodgkin's disease and other lymphomas. Likewise, systemic disorders in which iron, such as primary or secondary (e.g., multiple transfusions for thalassemia major) hemochromatosis (see Table 1), or copper, such as Wilson's disease, may be associated with decreased parathyroid function or reserve due to metal in deposits in the lesser.

Idiopathic hypoparathyroidism is much less common. Serum levels of PTH are undetectable or very low in patients who lack parathyroid tissue or who have hypoplastic parathyroid glands. The parathyroid glands are derived from the third and fourth branchial pouches and thus development may vary in different congenital disorders. The apparent incidence of idiopathic hypoparathyroidism has increased with the routine measurement of plasma calcium. In early childhood, developmental abnormalities of both the third and the fourth branchial pouches (DiGeorge syndrome) lead to both hypoparathyroidism and cellular immune deficiency because of the common derivation of the parathyroids and thymus. More commonly, idiopathic hypoparathyroidism may occur in early childhood (6–10 years) and can be associated with other endocrine autoimmune deficiency states such as diabetes, gonadal dysfunction, decreased adrenal function, and moniliasis (see the chapter by Whyte). Antibodies to various involved endocrine tissues have often been found. A genetic etiology has been suggested through sex-linked recessive or autosomal dominant transmission in some, but the familial cases are primarily those that present in childhood. Adults with late onset hypoparathyroidism are much more likely to have a sporadic, limited autoimmune disorder (3).

The pathway for parathyroid hormone synthesis and its regulation has been well characterized (see the chapter by Kronenberg et al.). Parathyroid hormone is synthesized as a 115-amino acid precursor protein, prepro-PTH, the "pre" signal sequence being necessary to transport the nascent peptide across the endoplasmic reticulum. The pro PTH hormone is transported to the Golgi region of the cell and packaged in secretory granules. The prohormone contains a highly basic hexapeptide sequence, whose functional importance is not known. The prohormone is quantitatively converted to the mature 84 residue PTH in the secretory granule, and pro-PTH is not secreted from the gland either during stimulation of the glands by hypocalcemia or in gland abnormalities such as parathyroid-adenoma or carcinoma. While the production of an abnormal PTH or PTH inhibitor has been suggested (pseudoidiopathic hypoparathyroidism) (11), more recent data do not support the existence of such a mutant molecule (12). It is certainly possible, however, based on other proteins, to speculate that there are occasional mutations in the PTH molecule, leading to decreased or absent function. Other molecular abnormalities, however, in the regulation and processing of the PTH gene product have been described (see the chapter by Thakker). Much more common is hypomagnesemia (see below), which leads to functional abnormalities in PTH secretion (13,14). PTH synthesis is not decreased in the presence of magnesium deficiency, but hypomagnesemia (often found in acute alcoholism, parenteral nutrition, excessive vomiting, malabsorption, excessive diuretic use, etc.) may be associated with decreased secretion of PTH, leading to hypocalcemia (see the chapter by Rude). Under such circumstances, administration of intravenous calcium alone will not solve the problem, and administration of magnesium will be necessary to restore a fully functional parathyroid gland. In addition to the effect of hypomagnesemia on PTH secretion, where the mechanism is not known (possibly the effect of hypomagnesemia on cAMP signal transduction), hypomagnesemia may also be associated with resistance to PTH effect both in the skeleton and in the kidney. Again, effects of low magnesium on the cAMP signal transduction process are theoretically possible, but this has not been documented (13).

Neonatal hypocalcemia may occur during either the early or the late neonatal period and is commonly associated with prematurity (15). Deficient maturation of the parathyroid gland or renal tubule may be an important component in some infants, whereas magnesium deficiency may be associated with hypocalcemia in other infants.

Occasionally functional hypoparathyroidism occurs in infants born to mothers with primary hyperparathyroidism. Hypercalcemia in the mother is associated with enhanced transport of ionized calcium across the placenta, and the persistent hypercalcemia in the fetus causes transient suppression of its parathyroid glands, leading to hypocalcemia after birth. This is an exaggeration of the hypercalcemia that is usually present in the newborn infant and that leads to transient hypocalcemia at 24 hr of age.

Nonparathyroid Causes of Hypocalcemia Associated With Increased Parathyroid Hormone Secretion

Nutritional causes of hypocalcemia are common (16). Approximately 15–30% of an average dietary intake of 1,000 mg calcium is absorbed from the gastrointestinal tract and excreted in the urine. The actual flux in the gastrointestinal tract is much greater, as intestinal and pancreatic secretions release an additional 200–400 mg calcium into the gut, all of which is reabsorbed (endogenous calcium reabsorption) (see the chapter by Brown). In the presence of gastrointestinal disorders such as malabsorption, short bowel syndrome, or chronic pancreatitis, significant amounts of calcium can be lost in the stool. In chronic pancreatitis, deficiency of pancreatic enzymes such as lipase leads to decreased absorption of fat-soluble vitamins (particularly vitamin D), contributing to the low calcium absorption and hypocalcemia. Decreased albumin may also be associated with hypocalcemia. In acute pancreatitis, there may be complexes of calcium and free fatty acids or calcium soaps deposited in the hemorrhagic and damaged pancreas and surrounding retroperitoneal fat. If, however, magnesium deficiency also complicates the acute pancreatitis (which is common in patients with alcoholism), decreased PTH secretion rather than increased secretion would be expected.

Abnormalities in vitamin D may be associated with hypocalcemia and may be due to vitamin D deficiency, inherited or acquired disorders of metabolism, as well as resistance to vitamin D action (16). While vitamin D deficiency is quite uncommon in the United States (because of vitamin D supplementation of dairy products), it is common in developing countries. Vitamin D deficiency may be found in the United States in breast-fed infants who are black and receive no vitamin D as well as in older individuals who have limited exposure to ultraviolet light or whose diets are very deficient. In patients with sprue, inflammatory bowel disease, or chronic pancreatitis, poor absorption of vitamin D leads to hypocalcemia and may be associated with osteomalacia and rickets. PTH secretion is increased due to the hypocalcemia, and severe parathyroid hyperplasia may result. Patients with biliary cirrhosis or cholestatic liver disease may also have problems with decreased 25 hydroxylation and/or malabsorption of vitamin D. Those patients who take anticonvulsants such as phenytoin or phenobarbital have increased activity of microsomal hydroxylases in the liver, and consequent accelerated metabolism of vitamin D can lead to functional vitamin D deficiency.

A genetic disorder of vitamin D metabolism (vitamin D-dependent rickets type I; VDDRI) is a very rare autosomal recessive disorder characterized by deficient 1α-hydroxylase activity and decreased conversion of $25\text{-}(OH)D_3$ to $1,25\text{-}(OH)_2D_3$ (17). These individuals have low levels of $1,25\text{-}(OH)_2D_3$, which can be corrected by administration of the appropriate vitamin D metabolite. In contrast, individuals with VDDR type II have striking elevations of circulating $1,25\text{-}(OH)_2D_3$ because of resistance in their target tissues to the action of the vitamin. Some of these individuals have complete or partial alopecia, and different types of defects have been found in the target tissues in relation to the steps of steroid hormone uptake and activation. Unique genetic mutations in the zing finger region of the vitamin D receptor protein have been identified in some affected subjects (18).

Renal disease is one of the most common causes of hypocalcemia and has a complex pathogenesis (2), including hyperphosphatemia due to decreased nephron function and decreased synthesis of $1,25\text{-}(OH)_2D_3$ by the diseased kidney (see the chapters by Martin and Slatopolsky and Coburn and Salusky). Hypertrophy and marked hyperplasia of the parathyroid glands may result, particularly in patients with long-standing disease or in those who have not been treated appropriately with high-calcium dialysis or calcium and active vitamin D supplements. Osteitis fibrosa cystica (the classical form of hyperparathyroid bone disease) may be seen in some patients with severe secondary hyperparathyroidism, but a spectrum of bone disease varying from osteomalacia to osteitis fibrosa cystica is typically seen in patients with chronic renal dysfunction. The low levels of $1,25\text{-}(OH)_2D_3$ lead to overexpression of the PTH gene and increased release of hormone, and may be an important factor that contributes to development of parathyroid hyperplasia. In addition, the chronically low levels of calcium lead to enhanced synthesis and secretion of PTH from individual cells. Parathyroid hyperplasia may be so severe that, in some patients, hypercalcemia and hypophosphatemia (the classical biochemical hallmarks of primary hyperparathyroidism) may appear after restoration of renal function with a renal transplant. In some patients, subtotal parathyroidectomy may actually be necessary, but recent studies (2,19) show that administration of large amounts of active metabolites of vitamin D may

prevent or reverse parathyroid hypersecretion and hyperplasia (see the chapter by Coburn and Salusky).

Hyperphosphatemia may be associated with either oral or parenteral phosphate administration, lysis of tumors with chemotherapy, or rhabdomyolysis associated with acute renal failure (where large amounts of phosphate are released into the circulation) and can be associated with marked hypocalcemia. Hyperphosphatemia can produce hypocalcemia by exceeding the Ca × P physicochemical solubility product, and inducing metastatic calcifications, and by inhibiting synthesis of $1,25\text{-}(OH)_2D$. Rhabdomyolysis can be caused by muscle trauma or alcohol or drug abuse and typically is associated with hypocalcemia in the early phase, when the patient is oliguric; it is associated with hypercalcemia in the polyuric phase (20). While oral and parenteral phosphates have been used to treat hypercalcemia, with the advent of new approaches such as calcitonin and bisphosphonates, phosphate administration is much less common.

Osteoblastic metastases, frequently found in prostate cancer and occasionally in metastatic breast cancer, may be associated with hypocalcemia and hypophosphatemia due to uptake of calcium and phosphate ions into the skeleton (16). Likewise, in the "hungry bone syndrome," which can occur postoperatively in patients with severe hyperparathyroidism or with treatment of Paget's disease, continuous uptake of calcium and phosphate may occur for days, weeks, or even months.

Finally, resistance to the effects of PTH either due to hereditary disorders such as pseudohypoparathyroidism (see the chapter by Levine et al.) or magnesium deficiency (see the chapter by Rude) may cause hypocalcemia. The details of the various genetic forms of pseudohypoparathyroidism are well described in the chapter by Levine et al. and are not reviewed here. With variable resistance at the level of bone and/or kidney, these individuals have high levels of circulating PTH, but the hormone does not activate its target sites, leading to hypocalcemia and hyperphosphatemia. The resulting hypocalcemia leads to a stimulation of further PTH secretion, and the low levels of $1,25\text{-}(OH)_2D_3$ (resulting from hyperphosphatemia) cause a further increase in PTH synthesis and secretion, as well as parathyroid hyperplasia. A variety of associated phenotypic manifestations make up the clinical syndrome (1).

DIFFERENTIAL DIAGNOSIS

The differential diagnosis of hypocalcemia is relatively straightforward when one has access to a reliable PTH assay (see the chapter by Nussbaum and Potts). Initial findings of hypocalcemia in a patient should be confirmed by repeat determinations, and associated biochemical causes such as hypoalbuminemia and hypomagnesemia should be sought. In some circumstances, such as treatment of the complicated patient in the intensive care unit, it may be necessary to resort to ionized calcium measurement (using a calcium-sensitive electrode) because of the complexity of associated factors such as low albumin, low serum magnesium, and increased or decreased pH. In the nonacute situation, it is essential to determine whether an individual with hypocalcemia has increased or decreased circulating PTH. The history related to the various disorders given in Tables 1 and 2 can be useful in trying to assess etiology. Now that the assay for PTH has been markedly enhanced and made reliable through the immunometric method (21), differential diagnosis is relatively straightforward. More subtle differentiation of the different types of pseudohypoparathyroidism is described in the chapter by Levine et al. but differentiating the hypoparathyroid from the hyperparathyroid state in hypocalcemia is the critical differential diagnostic point. In the chapter to follow, hypoparathyroidism will be covered in greater detail with respect to etiology, molecular basis, and management.

REFERENCES

1. Schneider A, Sherwood LM. Pathogenesis and management of hypoparathyroidism and other hypocalcemic disorders. *Metabolism* 1975;24:871–898.
2. Feinfeld D, Sherwood LM. Parathyroid hormone and 1,25-(OH)₂D₃ in chronic renal failure. *Kidney Int* 1988;33:1049–1058.
3. Sherwood LM. Hypoparathyroidism. In: Favus M, ed. *Primer on metabolic bone diseases and disorders of mineral metabolism* 2nd ed. Raven Press: New York, 1993;2:191–193.
4. Derasmo AU, Celi FS, Acc M, Ministola S, Aliberti G, Mazuroli GF. Hypocalcemia and hypomagnesemia in cancer patients. *Biomed Pharmacol* 1991;45:315–317.
5. Desai TK, Carlson RW, Geheb MA. Prevalence and clinical implication of hypocalcemia in acutely ill patients in the medical intensive care setting. *Am J Med* 1988;84:209–214.
6. Chernow B, Zaloga G, McFadden E, et al. Hypocalcemia in critically ill patients. *Crit Care Med* 1982;10:848–851.
7. Mimouni CP, Loughead JL, Tsang RC. A case control of hypocalcemia in high risk neonates: racial but no seasonal differences. *J Am Coll Nutr* 1991;10:196–199.
8. Parfitt AM. The incidence of hypoparathyroid-tetany after thyroid operations: Relationship to age, extent of resection and surgical experience. *Med J Aust* 1971;1:1103–1107.
9. Laitinen O. Hypocalcemia after thyroidectomy. *Lancet* 1976;2:859–860.
10. Wells SA, Gunnells JC, Gutman RA, Shelburne D, Schneider AB, Sherwood LM. The successful transplantation of frozen parathyroid tissue in man. *Surgery* 1977;81:86–90.
11. Nusynowitz ML, Klein MH. Pseudoidiopathic hypoparathyroidism with ineffective parathyroid hormone. *Am J Med* 1973;55:667–686.
12. Ahn TG, Antonarakis SE, Kronenberg HM, Igaraskhi T, Levine MA. Hypoparathyroidism: a molecular genetic analysis of 8 families with 23 affected persons. *Medicine* 1986;65:73–81.
13. Leicht E, Biro G. Mechanisms of hypocalcemia in the clinical form of severe magnesium deficit in the human. *Magnesium Res* 1992;5:37–44.
14. Takatsuki K, Hanley DA, Schneider AB, Sherwood LM. The effects of magnesium ion on parathyroid hormone secretion in vitro. *Calcif Tissue Int* 1980;32:201–206.
15. Carpenter TO. Neonatal hypocalcemia. In: *Primer on metabolic bone diseases and disorders of mineral metabolism* 2nd ed. Favus MJ, ed. New York: Raven Press, 1993;2:207–209.
16. Porat A, Sherwood LM, eds. *Disorders of mineral homeostasis and bone.* New York: John Wiley and Sons, 1986;377–426.
17. Insogna K. Hypocalcemia due to vitamin D disorders. In: Favus MJ, ed. *Primer on the metabolic bone diseases and disorders of mineral metabolism* 2nd ed. New York: Raven Press, 1993;2:203–204.
18. Hughes M, Malloy P, Kieback D, Kestersen R, Pike J, Feldman D, O'Malley B. Point mutation in the human vitamin D receptor gene associated with hypocalcemic rickets. *Science* 1988;242:1702–1705.
19. Delmez JA, Dougan CS, Gearing BK, et al. The effects of intraperitoneal calcitriol on calcium and parathyroid hormone. *Kidney Int* 1987;31:795–799.
20. Llach F, Felsenfeld D, Haussler M. The pathophysiology of altered calcium metabolism in rhabdomyolysis-induced acute renal failure. *N Engl J Med* 1981;305:117–123.
21. Nussbaum SR, Sahradnik RJ, Lavigne JR, et al. Highly sensitive two-site immunoradiometric assay of parathyrin and its clinical utility in evaluating patients with hypercalcemia. *Clin Chem* 1988;33:1364–1367.

The Parathyroids, edited by J.P. Bilezikian,
M.A. Levine, and R. Marcus. Raven Press, Ltd.,
New York © 1994.

CHAPTER 44

Autoimmune Aspects of Hypoparathyroidism

Michael P. Whyte

Hypoparathyroidism may be transient or permanent; there are a considerable number of etiologies for each type. The many different causes of hypoparathyroidism are covered in the preceeding chapter by Sherwood and Santora.

Among the genetic defects that can result in hypoparathyroidism, some are inherited as an autosomal recessive, X-linked recessive, or autosomal dominant traits. Most cases, however, are developmental and occur sporadically. Some heritable forms of hypoparathyroidism have been linked to specific chromosomal loci, and mutations within the preproPTH gene have been identified (see the chapter by Thakker).

One of the incompletely understood heritable forms of hypoparathyroidism occurs within the context of a complex syndrome characterized by hypofunction of several endocrine glands. This polyglandular deficiency syndrome evolves during childhood and is transmitted as an autosomal recessive trait (1). In addition to hypoparathyroidism, the other major clinical components are adrenal insufficiency and chronic mucocutaneous candidiasis (moniliasis). Although the gene defect(s) is unknown, and indeed the chromosome locus has yet to be identified, the pathogenesis appears to involve autoimmune destruction of endocrine tissues. Several hundred patients with this syndrome have been described. Defective cell-mediated immunity occurs in the DiGeorge anomaly (III–IV brachial pouch dysembryogenesis), but the immune dysfunction is not related to the pathogenesis of the associated hypoparathyroidism (2,3). However, other less well-characterized syndromes suggest additional forms of hypoparathyroidism in which autoimmu-

nity is a pathogenetic factor (4–9). This chapter reviews the autoimmune aspects of idiopathic hypoparathyroidism.

HISTORY

Many years ago, pituitary failure was thought to be the sole basis for hypofunction of multiple endocrine glands in one subject. In 1908, however, Claude and Gougerot (10) discovered an additional potential pathogenesis, which they reported as infiltration of lymphocytes together with fibrosis of several endocrine tissues of individual patients. They coined the term *pluriglandular endocrine atrophy* (10). Four years later, Falta (11) suggested that a more mild form of the syndrome could be associated with partial glandular atrophy. This mechanism was first documented as the basis for failure of multiple endocrine glands in 1926, when Schmidt described two patients in whom there was adrenal insufficiency as well as thyroid hypofunction due to chronic lymphocytic thyroiditis (12).

Additional descriptions of multiple endocrine deficiencies in association with other unusual disorders then began to gradually appear in the medical literature. In 1929, Thorpe and Handley (13) published the first report of a child with both hypoparathyroidism and oral candidiasis. In 1943, reports of familial cases of idiopathic hypoparathyroidism with Addison's disease (14) and with moniliasis (15) appeared. Three years afterwards, adrenal insufficiency became the first endocrinopathy recognized to be pathogenetically associated with idiopathic hypoparathyroidism (16). In 1955, Craig and associates (17) emphasized the familial occurrence of chronic candidiasis with hypoparathyroidism or nontuberculous Addison's disease. One year later, Whitaker and coworkers (18) called attention to a syndrome of "familial juvenile hypoadrenocorticism, hypoparathyroidism, and superficial moniliasis."

M. P. Whyte: Metabolic Research Unit, Shriners Hospital for Crippled Children; Division of Bone and Mineral Diseases, The Jewish Hospital of St. Louis; and Departments of Medicine and Pediatrics, Division of Endocrinology and Metabolism, Washington University School of Medicine, St. Louis, Missouri 63110.

Insight concerning the pathogenesis of these unusual conditions came in 1956 with the discovery by Roitt and coworkers (19) of thyroglobulin autoantibodies in the serum of patients with lymphocytic (Hashimoto's) thyroiditis. These investigators proposed that organ-specific antibodies might be a cause of endocrine atrophy (19). In 1957 and 1962, respectively, Anderson et al. (20) and Blizzard et al. (21) suggested that autoantibodies could account for some cases of nontuberculous Addison's disease.

During the early 1960s the overall clinical picture of this disorder involving hypoparathyroidism, Addison's disease, and candidiasis came into clearer focus. In 1962, Gass (22) identified the syndrome of "keratoconjunctivitis, superficial moniliasis, idiopathic hypoparathyroidism, and Addison's disease." In 1963, Kunin and colleagues (23) noted the frequent association of moniliasis, steatorrhea, macrocytic anemia, and posthepatitic cirrhosis with hypoparathyroidism and Addison's disease. In 1966, recognizing that approximately one-third of individuals affected by these combined endocrine deficiencies had moniliasis as well, Taitz and coworkers (24) proposed the acronym "HAM" (hypoparathyroid–Addison's–monilia) to describe this syndrome. By 1972 (25), eight patients with the complete syndrome triad had been reported (14,15,17,18,26–28).

Further progress in defining this disorder and elucidating its pathogenesis was made during the early 1980s. In a series of papers published in 1980 and 1981, Neufeld and colleagues (29–31) characterized a group of conditions they called *polyglandular autoimmune (PGA) disease.* Three principal clinical forms, types I, II, and III, and possibly an additional type, type IV, were delineated. As summarized in Table 1, PGA disease type I includes hypoparathyroidism, adrenocortical insufficiency, and/or chronic mucocutaneous candidiasis that appear during childhood. PGA type I may also be complicated by insulin-dependent diabetes mellitus, primary hypogonadism, autoimmune thyroid disease, pernicious anemia, chronic active hepatitis, steatorrhea with malabsorption, alopecia, and/or vitiligo (see below) (31). PGA disease type II is *not associated with hypoparathyroidism,* but does include adrenocortical insufficiency, autoimmune thyroid disease, and/or insulin-requiring diabetes mellitus (31,32). Onset is usually during adulthood, and women are more commonly affected than men (30). PGA disease type III involves associations of autoimmune thyroid disease with (a) insulin-dependent diabetes mellitus, (b) pernicious anemia, or (c) vitiligo and/or alopecia, and/or additional organ-specific autoimmune diseases (e.g., hepatic dysfunction) (31). Finally, Neufeld and Blizzard (31) have defined PGA disease type IV as a disorder characterized by the presence of two or more organ-specific autoimmune diseases that do not fall

TABLE 1. *Classification of polyglandular autoimmune disease[a]*

Type	Features
I	Candidiasis, hypoparathyroidism, Addison's disease, and two or three of the following: Insulin-dependent diabetes mellitus, primary hypogonadism, autoimmune thyroid disease, pernicious anemia, chronic active hepatitis, steatorrhea (malabsorption), alopecia (totalis or areata), and vitiligo[b]
II	Addison's disease + thyroid autoimmune disease and/or insulin-dependent diabetes mellitus
IIIA	Thyroid autoimmune disease + insulin-dependent diabetes mellitus
IIIB	Thyroid autoimmune disease + pernicious anemia
IIIC	Thyroid autoimmune disease + vitiligo and/or alopecia and/or other organ-specific autoimmune disease
IV	Two or more organ-specific autoimmune diseases not falling into types I, II, or III

[a]From ref. 31 with permission.
[b]Adapted from ref. 30.

into types I, II, or III. In addition, Neufeld and colleagues (30) found a 20% incidence of *antiparathyroid* antibodies in patients with isolated Addison's disease. This and subsequent advances in our knowledge concerning the pathogenesis of PGA disease type I are discussed below (see under Pathogenesis).

Several other nosological designations have been used to describe PGA disease type I. As was noted above, in 1956 it was called *familial juvenile hypoadrenocorticism, hypoparathyroidism and superficial moniliasis* (18) and in 1966 "HAM" syndrome (24). The terms *MEDAC syndrome* (multiple endocrine deficiency, autoimmune candidiasis), *type I polyendocrine autoimmune disease,* and *APECS* (autoimmune polyendocrine-candidiasis syndrome) were introduced later (33).

More recently the association of idiopathic hypoparathyroidism with yet other disorders has also been hypothesized to have an autoimmune basis. Hypoparathyroidism (and occasionally additional endocrine disturbances such as hypothyroidism and diabetes mellitus) can occur in patients with Kearns-Sayre syndrome (oculocraniosomatic neuromuscular disease with mitochondrial myopathy) (6). In one patient, hypoparathyroidism occurred with Down's syndrome and autoimmune hyperthyroidism (4). Primary hypoparathyroidism has accompanied acute interstitial nephritis and uveitis (5). An elderly man with hypoparathyroidism, and probably incidental Paget's disease of bone, had parathyroid glands that showed severe lipomatosis and a diffuse lymphocytic infiltration with atrophy of the endocrine cells (8). An elderly woman with postsurgical hypoparathyroidism had spuriously elevated serum levels of iPTH in a radioimmunoassay that used antiserum specific for the C-terminal region of human PTH-(65–69). She appeared to have an IgG that was cross reactive with the assay antiserum (7). Another aged patient with acquired hypoparathyroidism had detectable serum levels of PTH owing to the presence of antiidiotypic PTH autoantibodies (9). Finally, in other disorders believed to have an autoimmune basis, hypoparathyroidism can apparently result from fibrosis of the parathyroid glands themselves [e.g., progressive systemic sclerosis (34) and Riedel's thyroiditis (35)].

CLINICAL FEATURES

Patients with PGA disease type I have an especially interesting form of "idiopathic hypoparathyroidism." The considerable number of associated conditions, however, diversifies the clinical presentation of PGA disease and results in important diagnostic and therapeutic challenges (25,33).

The incidence of autoimmune diseases increases significantly with age. Children and adolescents with an autoimmune disorder, however, also frequently have other conditions. In early infancy and childhood, the most common association of endocrine and nonendocrine autoimmune disease involves candidiasis, hypoparathyroidism, and/or adrenal insufficiency. In fact, these disorders occur together primarily in young patients. Syndromes with polyglandular associations are possibly more prevalent than autoimmune disorders in which a single tissue is affected.

Most cases of PGA disease type I have been familial. Genetic analyses of affected families have indicated an autosomal recessive pattern of inheritance (1,36,37). Consanguinity has been recorded (36,38). The age of onset does not differ between the familial and sporadic cases.

PGA disease type I occurs about equally in both sexes (36). The average age of onset of symptoms is ~8 years. A few individuals have apparently developed the condition after 10 years of age (30,39). The clinical onset of the three major components of PGA type I is typically chronic mucocutaneous candidiasis, hypoparathyroidism, and then Addison's disease. In one review, these disorders occurred, on average, at 5, 9, and 14 years of age, respectively (33).

Of interest, within a family, one affected patient may have candidiasis, hypoparathyroidism, and adrenal insufficiency, whereas other affected siblings may develop only one or two of these conditions (18,36,40). Hypoparathyroidism or Addison's disease may appear to occur independently within a sibship (37). Because

hypoparathyroidism almost invariably precedes the onset of Addison's disease, very few individuals who have isolated Addison's disease will later develop hypoparathyroidism (30,36).

As is detailed below, many children who have two or all three of these interrelated disorders will also have other "atrophic" problems, including pernicious anemia, alopecia, premature ovarian failure, diabetes mellitus, vitiligo, and autoimmune thyroid disease (30,33). Autoimmune thyroiditis is indistinguishable from the isolated illness (41). In 1966, Blizzard and coworkers (42) described 32 patients with idiopathic hypoparathyroidism who had one or more of the following associated conditions: moniliasis (66%), Addison's disease (56%), pernicious anemia (22%), thyroid disease (19%), alopecia totalis (13%), premature menopause before age 25 years (6%), and juvenile cirrhosis (6%). Review of a large series of patients in 1969 by Fanconi (43) disclosed that moniliasis occurred in 72% (mean age of 3 years), Addison's disease in 58% (mean age of 11 years), steatorrhea in 26% (mean age of 8 years), and pernicious anemia in 9% (mean age of 16.5 years). Complete PGA disease type I affected 32%, whereas hypoparathyroidism occurred with only moniliasis in 40% and with only Addison's disease in 28% of the study population.

Candidiasis

Chronic mucocutaneous candidiasis is a common feature of a variety of conditions (44). These include disorders with morphologic abnormalities of the thymus and thymus-dependent tissues that lead to profound deficiencies of cell-mediated immunity (e.g., DiGeorge anomaly) and those associated with both defective cellular and humoral immunity (e.g., Swiss-type agammaglobulinemia and thymic dysplasia). In fact, it is best to consider chronic mucocutaneous candidiasis as a secondary manifestation of an underlying disorder rather than as a primary disease (44). Hypoparathyroidism is most commonly accompanied by chronic mucocutaneous candidiasis, but Addison's disease is also frequently associated (45).

Infection with *Candida albicans* occurs in ~14% of all patients with idiopathic hypoparathyroidism. Candidiasis is usually the initial clinical manifestation of PGA disease type I and typically appears first in early childhood. It develops for 1–4 years before there is overt evidence of endocrine disease (23). Hypoparathyroidism typically precedes the development of adrenal insufficiency (15), and the reverse order of presentation seldom, if ever, occurs (40). Candidiasis develops even before hypocalcemia is detected (27). It is more apt to occur in patients who also have adrenocorticoid insufficiency or pernicious anemia.

Monilial lesions may be limited in distribution but occasionally involve almost the entire body. When present, mucocutaneous candidiasis invariably affects the oral cavity. Oral lesions are diffuse and commonly cause perlèche (cracks at the corners of the mouth) and lip fissures. The next most commonly involved site is the fingernails; the toenails are only occasionally infected. The entire width of the nail plate is affected, and the nails become thickened and dystrophic. There may be associated paronychia. Affected nails are typically pitted and friable, features that may be mistakenly attributed to hypocalcemia per se (15). The vagina can also be infected. Rarely, the skin of the hands and feet becomes hyperkeratotic and disfigured (Fig. 1) (46). Patients with chronic mucocutaneous candidiasis are predisposed to other cutaneous infections (44).

Obviously, it is important to be aware of the association between hypoparathyroidism and candidiasis, although the basis for this relationship is unknown (see below). Many individuals with chronic mucocutaneous candidiasis will later manifest endocrine dysfunction, but such patients are clinically indistinguishable from those subjects who will not develop these problems (44,45). By contrast, *systemic* candidiasis is rare and occurs only if there is another predisposing factor that impairs immune defense mechanisms (e.g., diabetes mellitus).

Idiopathic Hypoparathyroidism

Idiopathic hypoparathyroidism *without* Addison's disease and/or candidiasis typically presents between 6 months and 20 years of age (22), as does hypoparathyroidism associated *with* Addison's disease and/or mucocutaneous candidiasis. Symptoms of hypoparathyroidism begin, on average, ~4 years *after* candidiasis is noted, with a mean age of onset from 6 years (see 87) to 9 years (33), depending upon the reported series. Importantly, hypoparathyroidism almost invariably *precedes* the onset of Addison's disease (30,36).

Hypoparathyroidism in patients with PGA type I does not appear to differ clinically or biochemically from isolated idiopathic hypoparathyroidism. As in other causes of hypoparathyroidism, high serum levels of creatine kinase can occur in affected children during episodes of hypocalcemia (47).

Addison's Disease

By 1974, idiopathic and tuberculosis-related Addison's disease were recognized to be distinct entities (48). In contradistinction to Addison's disease due to tuberculosis, ~14% of patients with *idiopathic* Addison's disease had two or more additional conditions, e.g., diabetes mellitus, thyroid disorders, pernicious anemia, or gonadal insufficiency (48).

Autoimmune Addison's disease is a component of both PGA disease types I and II (Table 1), but each type has a different mean age-of-onset, apparent genetic basis, and pathogenesis (30).

Addison's disease may occasionally occur before the onset of hypoparathyroidism (30,46), but it never appears prior to development of moniliasis. Addison's disease is noted on average 5 years after onset of hypoparathyroidism, at a mean age of 14 years (33).

If unrecognized and untreated (see below), Addison's disease may be fatal (16). Rarely, selective involvement of the adrenal cortex may limit destruction to the zona glomerulosa, with development of isolated hypoaldosteronism (49). Addison's disease is associated with an unusually high mortality rate, perhaps in part because of the early age of onset, difficulty in treating hypoadrenalism, and additional clinical problems (27,50). It is important to recognize that *untreated* Addison's disease can mask the diagnosis of hypoparathyroidism (see below).

Other Endocrine Disease

Other endocrinopathies that may occur in conjunction with hypoparathyroidism in PGA disease type I include insulin-dependent diabetes mellitus, Hashimoto's thyroiditis (38,41,51), hypothyroidism (52), and ovarian failure (53–57). Several patients have developed severe, multiple endocrine gland hypofunction, in some cases involving the parathyroids, adrenals, thyroid, and ovaries in succession (nevertheless, moniliasis was the first manifestation) (38,53). The pituitary gland has not been directly affected, although hypopituitarism due to a pituitary tumor has been reported (58).

Ovarian failure associated with antiovarian antibodies has been well documented in PGA disease type I (53). In cases of primary amenorrhea, ovarian histopathology may resemble gonadal dysgenesis (38). Otherwise, menses are typically regular until there is sudden secondary amenorrhea and premature menopause. Fertility can be present in early adulthood (61). As in other forms of primary gonadal failure, serum levels of follicle-stimulating hormone (FSH) are elevated to a greater extent than those of luteinizing hormone (LH).

Nonendocrine Diseases

Nonendocrine problems other than candidiasis occur not infrequently in PGA disease type I. Pernicious anemia is the most common (25,26,38,39,50,56,59,60) and usually occurs 5–10 years after onset of hypoparathyroidism (25) but occasionally first manifests during

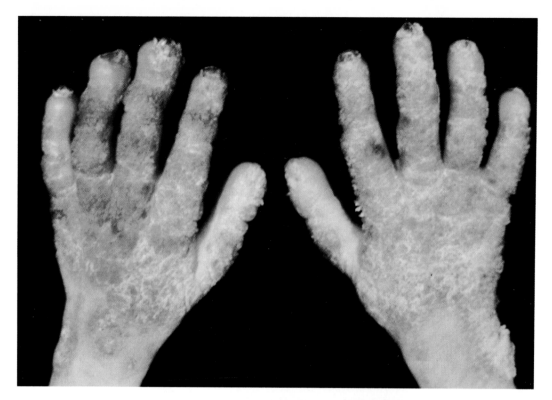

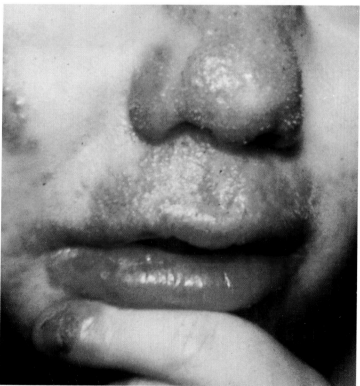

FIG. 1. This white boy with PGA disease type I illustrates the most severe expression of the associated mucocutaneous moniliasis, i.e., striking hyperkeratosis from infection of the skin of the hands (**top**) and face (**bottom**) in addition to involvement of the oropharynx and nails with *Candida albicans.*

adult life (39). Despite its early onset, the pernicious anemia is the "adult type," which is otherwise unusual before age 20 years (25). There is acquired gastric atrophy, with loss of all secretory components. Usually, antibodies to parietal cells and intrinsic factor are present in serum. This is in contrast to the "juvenile type" of pernicious anemia that is characterized by selective deficiency of intrinsic factor in the absence of antibodies.

Distinction should be made between cases of true pernicious anemia, in which intrinsic factor is deficient, and those cases in which impaired vitamin B_{12} absorption results from steatorrhea or nonspecific changes in the gastric mucosa (such as gastritis or achlorhydria secondary to chronic hypocalcemia). Ikkala and colleagues (60) in 1964 showed that these latter changes may also occur in cases of postoperative hypoparathyroidism. Indeed, in other types of hypoparathyroidism, successful treatment of the hypocalcemia occasionally leads to improved absorption of fat or vitamin B_{12}.

Corneal changes in a patient with idiopathic hypoparathyroidism were first described in 1929 (61). Early on, phlyctenular keratoconjunctivitis seemed to be one of the less frequently occurring conditions associated with PGA disease type I (15,16,62). In 1962, a review by Pohjola indicated the prevalence to be 10% (63). That same year, however, Gass (22) reported 12 cases of keratoconjunctivitis, all of whom had associated moniliasis and/or endocrinopathies. We now recognize that keratoconjunctivitis occurs in as many as 50% of patients with PGA disease type I (22). In fact, keratonconjunctivitis is one of the earliest presenting manifestations (22). In most patients the symptoms are often chronic, recurrent, and disabling. The symptoms can also be minimal. However, there may also be long periods of remission (22). In mild cases, slight redness of the eyes, photophobia, and blepharospasm can occur. Intense photophobia and excessive lacrimation occur during the acute phase of the keratitis (16,40,62). In severe cases, there is ulceration, scarring, and vascularization that can opacify the cornea and impair vision (22). Conjunctival biopsy specimens may disclose a heavy subepithelial infiltration of lymphocytes and plasma cells (64). There is also a bilateral superficial keratitis with corneal vascularization (62,65,66). Keratoconjunctivitis has been postulated to be a hypersensitivity response to the candidiasis rather than an independent component of the syndrome. However, this complication has occurred in the absence of clinical evidence of *Candida* infection (22). Wagman and coworkers (64), in a 1987 review of 16 cases of PGA disease type I, identified four children with bilateral, self-limited keratitis that began between 2 and 9 years of age (64). It preceded the onset of endocrinopathy in two of these patients and caused some impairment of vision. The authors concluded that the keratitis was not caused by the hypoparathyroidism or candidiasis.

Others have noted that keratitis may improve when serum calcium levels are well controlled (62).

Other reported ocular abnormalities include strabismus, loss of eyebrows and eyelashes, recurrent blepharitis, keratic precipitates, retinitis pigmentosa, exotropia, pseudoptosis, cataracts, and papilledema (62,64). The cataracts and papilledema are probably related to the hypocalcemia and hyperphosphatemia of hypoparathyroidism (64).

Patients with idiopathic hypoparathyroidism have ectodermal problems that include dry, rough skin (16); coarse and brittle hair; and lusterless, somewhat hypoplastic, distally split nails (16,51,61,67). Alopecia totalis is another frequently mentioned complication (16,42,45,51,57). There can also be alopecia areata (15,16,28,51,57,61), piebaldism (61), or vitiligo (51,59). Alopecia manifests in about 30% of affected individuals and may include loss of eyebrows and eyelashes (62). There may be dental abnormalities (16,28), including partial anodontia, enamel hypoplasia, and delayed eruption (40,50,62,68). Dental dysplasia may occur before or in the absence of hypocalcemia. There may also be darkly pigmented skin (16,28) with hyperkeratosis (15). Pigmented nevi have been described (18). A patient with prominent ectodermal dysplasia has been reported (67). Occasionally, there is cutaneous infection with other fungi, such as *Trichophyton rubrum* (57,61). Recurrent staphylococcal infections of the skin are also common (44).

Intracranial calcification (16,50,67) may be present, and some affected individuals can be mentally deficient (50). Papilledema can occur from raised intracranial pressure (15,16).

Patients may be troubled by a variety of intraabdominal disorders. Hepatitis that can progress to cirrhosis of the liver is well established (17,18). Indeed, it has been speculated that the hypoparathyroidism and Addison's disease could be sequellae (23). Chronic active hepatitis (40), "juvenile cirrhosis" (42), posthepatitic cirrhosis (18,22,23,68), pancreatic cystic fibrosis or mucoviscidosis (50,59), and steatorrhea (40,56, 59,69,70) have been described. Steatorrhea can lead to overt malabsorption (55,56). There may be predisposition to severe bouts of measles, viral hepatitis, and encephalomyelitis (61).

PATHOGENESIS

DiGeorge syndrome has clinical characteristics similar to those of PGA disease type I (i.e., hypoparathyroidism and candidiasis), but this syndrome results from developmental defects in the parathyroid glands and thymus. The absence of a thymus leads to diminished T-lymphocyte function, which appears to explain the predisposition to candidiasis (3). The pathogenesis of PGA disease type I is less clear-cut. It is apparent that the basis is a genetic defect(s); the syndrome is inherited in an autosomal recessive pat(1). Nevertheless, the molecular basis is not yet characterized and the gene locus has not been identified. As is reviewed below, the possibility that endocrine dysfunction in PGA disease type I is pathogenetically related to the associated candidiasis has led to exploration of an autoimmune pathogenesis. It is alsoconceivable that autoimmunity accounts for the development of idiopathic hypoparathyroidism in several other syndromes as well (4–9). By contrast, in 1961, Morse and coworkers (71) postulated inheritance of a gastrointestinal defect that impaired absorption of a factor necessary for parathyroid and adrenal function. Also, in 1963, Kunin and colleagues (23) reviewed cases in which posthepatitic cirrhosis was documented, and raised the possibility of a viral etiology that could present with hepatitis.

Until the 1970s it was hypothesized that candidiasis could cause the hypoparathyroidism and other endocrine dysfunction of PGA disease type I (71–73). However, autopsy studies have never shown invasion of the viscera or of the parathyroid glands by *Candida albicans* (18,38,59). As an alternative to direct infection by *Candida*, in 1966, Sjöberg (56) and in 1970 Windorfer (74) postulated that the fungus elaborated a toxin that affects the endocrine glands. Indeed, in 1971, it was proposed that documentation of such a causal relationship between the candidiasis and the endocrinopathies would provide a rationale for amputation of the ends of the fingers because of the high mortality rate from the Addison's disease (75). However, such a toxin has not been demonstrated, and candidiasis does not appear to cause the other defects (45).

Whitaker and colleagues (18) proposed that the candidiasis was secondary to the other dystrophic lesions of the skin, mucosa, and nails caused by hypoparathyroidism. This hypothesis seems unlikely, however, in that candidiasis precedes the onset of idiopathic hypoparathyroidism by an average of 5 years. Moreover, the dystrophic ectodermal changes improve when hypocalcemia is corrected, whereas the fungal disease usually does not (15).

In 1966, Sjöberg (56) found high serum titers of antibodies against *Candida albicans* in three patients. In normal individuals, it had been reported that there is a potent, heat-stable inhibitory factor(s) in serum that prevents the growth of *Candida albicans* (76), which is deficient in patients with chronic moniliasis (77). However, in 1967, Esterly and coworkers (78) showed that the presence or absence of this inhibitory factor was not a determining factor for the fungal disease.

An autoimmune pathogenesis for PGA disease type I was initially suspected from histopathologic and serologic studies of patients (48). Early autopsy investigations initially disclosed fibrous and lymphocytic infiltration of endocrine glands that replaced normal tissue and presumably caused gradual destruction of epithelial cells (61). Absence, fatty replacement, atrophy with atypical cells, and various degrees of lymphocytic infiltration of the parathyroid glands was documented at autopsy (22). Remnants (17,38) as well as absence of parathyroid tissue (16,18,79) were observed, suggesting that the parathyroid lesion was an acquired atrophy rather than developmental aplasia or hypoplasia (18). The adrenal cortex also appeared atrophic and was replaced by dense fibrous connective tissue that was infiltrated by lymphocytes (16,22).

The role of autoimmunity in PGA disease type I became well established by the 1960s. The notion that autoantibodies could cause disease of the *parathyroid glands* was given great impetus in 1966 by Blizzard, Chee, and Davis (42), who used both normal and pathological human parathyroid tissue to demonstrate *antiparathyroid* antibodies in the sera of 38% of patients with idiopathic hypoparathyroidism, 26% with Addison's disease, 12% with Hashimoto's thyroiditis, and 6% of normal controls. These autoantibodies appeared to be parathyroid-specific, since they were neutralized by exposure to parathyroid tissue alone. The antigen was detected in some, but not all, parathyroid adenomas. However, these investigations were hindered by limited availability of normal parathyroid tissue. Therefore, it was not possible to learn as much about the incidence, characteristics, and significance of parathyroid autoantibodies as had been learned about antibodies against other endocrine tissues (42). In this patient population with idiopathic hypoparathyroidism, the authors also detected antiadrenal antibodies in 10% and antigastric parietal cell antibodies in 7%, representing mostly children (42). The antibodies did not react with *Candida albicans*. Moreover, a 20% incidence of antiparathyroid antibodies has been reported in patients with isolated idiopathic adrenocortical insufficiency (30).

In 1967, Wuepper and Fudenberg (40) identified immunologic abnormalities in family members of patients with hypoparathyroidism and speculated that the autoimmune pathogenesis was probably genetic. Their patient showed delayed hypersensitivity to *Candida* (positive skin test), but lacked an anti-*Candida* factor found in normal serum (40). The following year, Blizzard and Gibbs (45) found that 40% of 44 patients with mucocutaneous moniliasis had an associated disease with a presumed autoimmune basis and that most of these subjects had antibodies that were reactive with endocrine glands or stomach. The presence of such antibodies was believed to reflect focal or generalized lymphocytic infiltration and at least subclinical involvement of the various tissues. A causal relationship between the candidiasis and the endocrinopathies was not established, however (45). There was no cross-antigenicity between *Candida albicans* and adrenal or thyroid tissue (80). In 1969, Irvine and Scarth (81) found IgG antibodies against parathyroid oxyphil cells in only one of nine patients with idiopathic hypoparathyroidism (81), but patients with "autoimmune" hypoparathyroidism were not tested. That same year, Spinner and coworkers (82) studied parents and siblings for antibodies to endocrine and gastric tissue and found additional evidence to support their genetic/clinical classification of individuals with hypoparathyroidism and/or Addison's disease (36).

Beginning in the 1960s, several groups of investigators were able to show lymphocytic infiltration and even atrophy of parathyroid glands in animals that were immunized with parathyroid tissue (83,84). In 1968, Lupulescu and coworkers (85) produced lymphocytic and plasma cell infiltration and atrophy of the parathyroid glands in dogs that had been immunized with extracts of allogeneic parathyroid tissue. Moreover, similar changes were noted in adrenal cortex as well. In 1974, passive immunization of rats with antiserum against rat parathyroid tissue was observed to cause marked immunoparathyroiditis, but hypoparathyroidism did not ensue (86).

The immunologic aspects of PGA disease type I are at best confusing. There is little correlation between the presence of antibodies and clinical manifestations even among members of a single kindred. The occurrence of antibodies in affected individuals, however, may be a harbinger of eventual endocrine deficiency, but the significance of antibodies found in apparently normal family members is unclear.

In 1971, Kirkpatrick and coworkers (44) and Block and colleagues (88) summarized evidence for various abnormalities in cell-mediated immunity in PGA disease type I. A woman with hypoparathyroidism, moniliasis, Addison's disease, and primary ovarian failure was described who lacked a delayed hypersensitivity response in vivo to *Candida albicans*, although there was evidence of immune cellular activity in vitro (88). That same year, Levy et al. (89) reported impaired cellular immunity in a 17-year-old man with chronic mucocutaneous moniliasis, Addison's disease, pernicious anemia, and gastrointestinal malabsorption in whom thrush cleared after transplantation of fetal thymus tissue. In a preliminary report in 1974, Rao and coworkers (87) noted that cell-mediated immunity to *Candida albicans* could be impaired in idiopathic hypoparathyroidism. In 1975, patients with PGA type I and hypoparathyroidism were shown to have abnormalities of T-cell function (91). PGA disease type I was postulated to reflect a defect in T-lymphocyte action. In 1979, abnormal suppressor T-lymphocyte function, low circulating levels of IgA, and deficient cell-mediated immunity to *Candida albicans* were reported (92,93). By that time, however, autoantibodies had

been described to endocrine glands, intrinsic factor, and the parietal cells of the stomach.

In the late 1970s, evidence was reported suggesting that the group of disorders called *polyglandular failure syndrome* was HLA-B8-associated (94,95). Thus, immunologic dysfunction involving genes on chromosome 6 could be a factor in the pathogenesis (94,95). However, other studies of HLA type have shown no consistent haplotypes in PGA disease type I (30,92,96), although type II is indeed associated with HLA-B8 (DW3) (30,94,95).

In 1969, Hermans and coworkers (61) suggested that viral infection, in a genetically predisposed individual, might play a pathogenetic role in PGA disease type I and that "immunologic deficiencies, especially those related to delayed hypersensitivity, appear to be of importance in the development of chronic mucocutaneous candidiasis." In 1983, Haspel and coworkers (97) reported that mice infected with retrovirus type I can develop an autoimmune polyendocrine disease in which autoantibodies are organ specific.

In 1977, Swana and coworkers (90) reported that reactivity against human parathyroid tissue in patients with hypoparathyroidism was due to an anti-human mitochondrial autoantibody (90). Yet, in 1981, Doniach and Bottazzo (98) noted that organ-specific parathyroid autoantibodies occur rarely in patients with autoimmune polyendocrinopathy and/or hypoparathyroidism. Subsequently, in 1985, Betterle and coworkers (99) described an IgG-class antihuman mitochondrial antibody that reacted with a 46 kDa mitochondrial membrane protein in 31% of patients with PGA disease type I that was not specific for parathyroid tissue. Indeed, antibodies could appear before endocrine dysfunction (100). In 1986, Posillico and coworkers (101) described three patients with idiopathic hypoparathyroidism in whom sera contained autoantibodies that inhibited secretion of PTH from dispersed human parathyroid cells. These antibodies were reactive with epitopes on the extracellular surface of the parathyroid cell and were postulated to interfere with signal recognition/transduction mechanisms for calcium-regulated PTH secretion (101).

In 1986, Brandi and coworkers (102) adapted a ^{51}Cr-release assay to cultured bovine parathyroid cells and showed that complement-dependent cytotoxic antibodies were present in sera from seven patients with autoimmune hypoparathyroidism. Cytotoxic antibodies were not present in 15 normal subjects or 41 patients with other diverse conditions associated with immune dysfunction (102). Adsorption of the sera with parathyroid or adrenal tissue caused a marked decrease in this effect. These investigators suggested that the technique could help to characterize further the nature of the tissue cell-specific, species-nonspecific antibodies in autoimmune hypoparathyroidism and perhaps identify the involved antigen(s) (102).

In 1988, Fattorossi and coworkers (103) extended this group's work and used fluorescence flow cytometry and tissue immunohistology to show IgM in patient sera that reacted with cultured *endothelial* cell membranes and tissue sections from bovine parathyroid glands. The antibody was not, however, completely species or organ specific; for example, it also reacted with human endothelial cells from adrenal tissue. Two major proteins of 130 and 200 kDa molecular weight were associated with the parathyroid endothelial membranes and could be the major target of the antibody. The significance of the antiendothelial IgM antibodies required further study, but an interesting postulate is that these immunoglobulins disturb an important physiologic relationship between endocrine and endothelial cells (103). Of interest, mice with autoimmune polyendocrine disease also have antibodies of the IgM class.

In 1992, Wortsman and coworkers (104) found generalized T-cell activation to be a novel feature of *adult*-onset idiopathic hypoparathyroidism. This observation suggested that an immune disturbance, possibly related to autoimmunity, could cause this type of hypoparathyroidism as well (104).

Although the pathogenesis of the chronic bilateral keratoconjunctivitis in PGA disease type I is unclear, hypoparathyroidism appears not to be the cause; this eye problem is not a feature of other types of hypoparathyroidism and can occur without hypoparathyroidism (64). Although hypothesized to be an allergic reaction to *Candida albicans* protein (22), for similar reasons phlyctenular keratitis is unlikely to reflect hypersensitivity to candidiasis (64). Laboratory studies have not confirmed an autoimmune basis for the keratitis (64).

The steatorrhea of patients with idiopathic hypoparathyroidism has been explained as an independent event, a direct effect of the hypoparathyroidism and hypocalcemia, a complication of intestinal candidiasis (71,86,105–107), or a result of abnormal liver function (23,108).

TREATMENT

For children with hypoparathyroidism or Addison's disease, the possibility that they may develop the full-blown PGA syndrome must be kept in mind. Of critical importance, one must recognize that Addison's disease can mask the presence of hypoparathyroidism (79), and glucocorticoid therapy alone may have a fatal outcome (16–18,28,109). Serum calcium concentration rises in adrenocortical insufficiency and could suddenly decrease after the introduction of corticosteroid

therapy because of diminished gastrointestinal absorption and increased renal excretion of calcium (18). Similarly, the introduction of estrogen-replacement therapy for ovarian failure can also diminish serum calcium levels (56). Patients with these two diseases are, therefore, more likely to show considerable fluctuations of serum calcium concentrations, and require especially careful regulation of doses of vitamin D sterols, etc. (28).

Absense of intrinsic factor production by gastric mucosa can cause pernicious anemia. The treatment is vitamin B_{12}, as in any other form of intrinsic factor deficiency. Steatorrhea, as was mentioned above, is also a known complication of autoimmune hypoparathyroidism. Patients with hypocalcemia, steatorrhea, and megaloblastic anemia have on occasion mistakenly been thought to have folate deficiency. When steatorrhea is severe, with its potential for vitamin D malabsorption, etc., hypoparathyroidism can be very difficult to treat. It may be necessary to give calcium intravenously for a period of time (55). A diet enriched with medium-chain triglycerides has been reported to be helpful, perhaps by decreasing calcium loss due to saponification (55).

Of interest, a 10-year-old girl with PGA type I who developed pure red cell aplasia resistant to conventional therapy showed hematologic remission after intramuscular injections of gammaglobulin (110). The authors of this report suggested an idiotype–antiidiotype interaction in which specific suppression by antiidiotype antibodies caused correction of the hematologic disease (110).

Patients with features of PGA disease type I must be screened regularly for the associated abnormalities (30). Healthy siblings should be tested during at least the first decade of life (111). Since ~13% will develop chronic active hepatitis, they should be monitored regularly with liver function tests and assays for smooth muscle and mitochondrial antibodies (30).

Hypoparathyroidism

Management of hypoparathyroidism in patients with PGA type I is essentially the same as that outlined in the chapter by O'Riordan on the treatment of idiopathic hypoparathyroidism per se. However, it is important to recognize that PGA disease type I is a much more complex disorder than isolated idiopathic hypoparathyroidism, and therefore the many potentially interacting medical problems will likely complicate such therapy. For example, in a child with candidiasis and hypoparathyroidism, there appeared to be defective 25-hydroxylation of vitamin D sterols from concomitant giant cell hepatitis and severe cirrhosis. Thus 1,25-dihydroxyvitamin D was considered to be the prudent form of vitamin D therapy to use in this circumstance (112). Steatorrhea would also affect the type of vitamin D that would be most efficacious. As discussed below, the presence or absence of Addison's disease is an especially important factor to consider in therapy.

Addison's Disease

Among the major confounding issues to consider when treating hypoparathyroidism in patients with PGA disease type I is Addison's disease. Prior to the 1950s, adrenocortical insufficiency was a fatal disorder, and >80% of affected patients were dead within 2 years of diagnosis (61). In a report published in 1969, one-third of patients had succumbed to this complication (43). Now, conventional replacement therapy of Addison's disease with glucocorticoids and mineralocorticoids enables long-term survival.

Addison's disease and its treatment have significant impact on the manifestations of hypoparathyroidism. When hypoadrenalism supervenes, the clinical and biochemical expression of associated hypoparathyroidism can diminish considerably but rapidly returns after glucocorticoid replacement therapy is begun (28). Presumably the glucocorticoids abruptly lower blood calcium levels by decreasing dietary absorption of calcium and by enhancing renal excretion as glomerular filtration rate is increased. Accordingly, particular care must be paid to exclude hypoparathyroidism when glucocorticoid therapy is started for Addison's disease. Similarly, if hypocalcemia is already present, it may be rapidly and severely exacerbated. An example of this situation is case 2 described in 1961 by Morse and colleagues (50). They encountered an 11-year-old child with hypoparathyroidism manifested by a serum calcium level of 5.5 mg/dl. Hypocalcemia was "corrected" to 10.3 mg/dl with the onset of Addison's disease. When glucocorticoid replacement treatment (without additional vitamin D therapy) was initiated, the serum calcium level abruptly fell to 4.7 mg/dl. Similar clinical scenarios have been described by Leonard (16), Leifer and Hollander (113), Papadatos and Klein (28), and Quichaud and colleagues (114). Conversely, in 1964, Kenny and Holliday (41) reported that the onset of Addison's disease in a patient who was successfully treated for hypoparathyroidism was followed by marked hypercalcemia of 14.5 mg/dl.

Candidiasis

The ectodermal changes that result from hypoparathyroidism per se (including brittleness of nails), will respond to successful treatment of the mineral distur-

bances. However, the superficial candidiasis often will not (15). Intractable candidiasis involving mucous membranes, skin, and nails is one of the most perplexing and frustrating problems associated with autoimmune hypoparathyroidism. The candidiasis once established may be difficult to eradicate even when serum calcium concentrations are maintained in the normal range.

Long-term therapy with ketoconazole is now considered to be the treatment of choice for chronic mucocutaneous candidiasis (115). Ketoconazole, 200–400 mg/day orally, is a very effective treatment for extensive and resistant mucocutaneous candidiasis (116,117). Mycostatin applied topically as well as administered orally (to reduce intestinal colonization) may prevent spread of the fungal lesions but will rarely eradicate infection. Local hypochlorite treatment has been suggested, since candidiasis of skin and nails is improved in patients who swim frequently in chlorinated pools. Infected nails have been avulsed, but recurrence during nail regrowth will occur unless the candidiasis is controlled elsewhere (44).

Although treatment in the past was often discouraging, success was reported for a significant number of patients who received transfer factor and amphotericin B. Transfer factor was prepared from lymphocytes of normal individuals immunized to *Candida albicans*. Kirkpatrick and Greenberg (118), however, studied 19 patients with chronic mucocutaneous candidiasis, the majority of whom had abnormalities in cell-mediated immunity. All had normal numbers of circulating T and B lymphocytes and normal lymphocyte responses to phytohemagglutinin and concanavalin A. Nevertheless, most had negative skin tests for *Candida albicans*. In that study, transfer factor administered for several months (with only local treatment with antifungal agents) was ineffective. Amphotericin B alone given intravenously, however, induced remissions in most of the patients (44). However, complete and lasting eradication of all clinical evidence of the disease proved to be an elusive goal. Face and scalp lesions cleared most readily and relapsed least frequently. Thrush often reoccurred and remained the most symptomatic lesion (44).

Additional Disorders

Medical therapy of keratoconjunctivitis may include corticosteroid eye drops; surgical treatment involves keratectomy or corneal transplant (62,64). Wagman and colleagues (64) recommend medical management of the corneal disease without surgical intervention. The active phase is helped by topical antibiotic/corticosteroid medication; systemic corticosteroids or immunosuppression were not required (64). Of importance, the authors noted that there appears to be a transition from an active to a quiescent phase ~10 years after the onset. Interestingly, cimetidine has also been reported to have some efficacy, perhaps acting as an immunomodulator (119).

ACKNOWLEDGMENTS

This work was supported by grant 15958 from the Shriners Hospitals for Crippled Children. The author is grateful to Frances Wilson for her expert secretarial assistance.

REFERENCES

1. McKusick VA. *Mendelian Inheritance In Man: Catalogs of Autosomal Dominant, Autosomal Recessive, and X-Linked Phenotypes.* 10th ed. Baltimore: The Johns Hopkins University Press, 1992.
2. Greenberg F, Valdes C, Rosenblatt HM, Kirkland JL, Ledbetter DH. Hypoparathyroidism and T cell immune defect in a patient with 10p deletion syndrome. *J Pediatr* 1986;109:489–492.
3. Hong R. The DiGeorge anomaly. *Immunodeficiency Rev* 1991;3:1–14.
4. Blumberg D, AvRuskin T. Down's syndrome, autoimmune hyperthyroidism, and hypoparathyroidism: a unique triad (letter). *AJDC* 1987;141:1149.
5. Catalano C, Harris PE, Enia G, Postorino M, Martorano C, Maggiore Q. Acute interstitial nephritis associated with uveitis and primary hypoparathyroidism. *Am J Kidney Dis* 1989;14:317–318.
6. Scully RE, Mark EJ, McNeely WF, McNeely BU. Case records of the Massachusetts General Hospital. *N Engl J Med* 1987;317:493–501.
7. Kasono K, Sato K, Suzuki T, et al. Falsely elevated serum parathyroid hormone levels due to immunoglobulin G in a patient with idiopathic hypoparathyroidism. *J Clin Endocrinol Metab* 1991;72:217–222.
8. Van de Casseye M, Gepts W. Primary (autoimmune?) parathyroiditis. *Virchows Arch Abt A Pathol Anat* 1973;361:257–261.
9. McElduff A, Lackmann M, Wilkinson M. Antidiotypic PTH antibodies as a cause of elevated immunoreactive parathyroid hormone in idiopathic hypoparathyroidism, a second case: another manifestation of autoimmune endocrine disease? *Calcif Tissue Int* 1992;51:121–126.
10. Claude M, Gougerot H. Insuffisance pluriglandulaire endocrinienne. *J Physiol Pathol Gen* 1908;10:469–480.
11. Falta W. Spateunuchoidismus und multiple Blutdrusen-sklerose. II. Die multiple Blut drusensklerose. *Klin Wochenschr* 1912;49:1477–1481.
12. Schmidt MB. Eine biglanduläre erkrankung (Nebennieren und Schilddrüsse) be: morbus Addisonii. *Verh Deutsch Pathol Ges* 1926;21:212–221.
13. Thorpe E, Handley H. Chronic tetany and chronic mycelial stomatitis in a child aged four and one-half years. *Am J Dis Child* 1929;38:328–338.
14. Talbot NB, Butler AM, MacLachlan EA. Effect of testosterone and allied compounds on mineral, nitrogen, and carbohydrate metabolism of a girl with Addison's disease. *J Clin Invest* 1943;22:583–593.
15. Sutphin A, Albright F, McCune DJ. Five cases (three in siblings) of idiopathic hypoparathyroidism associated with moniliasis. *J Clin Endocrinol Metab* 1943;3:625–634.
16. Leonard MF. Chronic idiopathic hypoparathyroidism with superimposed Addison's disease in a child. *J Clin Endocrinol Metab* 1946;6:493–506.
17. Craig JM, Schiff LH, Boone JE. Chronic moniliasis associated with Addison's disease. *Am J Dis Child* 1955;89:669–684.
18. Whitaker J, Landing BH, Esselborn VM, Williams RR. The syndrome of familial juvenile hypoadrenocorticism, hypoparathyroidism and superficial moniliasis. *J Clin Endocrinol Metab* 1956;16:1374–1387.
19. Roitt IM, Doniach D, Campbell PN, Hudson RV. Autoantibodies in Hashimoto's disease (lymphadenoid goitre). *Lancet* 1956;2:820–821.
20. Anderson JR, Goudie RB, Gray KG, Timbury GC: Auto-antibodies in Addison's disease. *Lancet* 1957;1:1123–1124.
21. Blizzard RM, Chandler RW, Kyle MA, Hung W. Adrenal antibodies in Addison's disease. *Lancet* 1962;2:901–905.
22. Gass JDM. The syndrome of keratoconjunctivitis, superficial moniliasis, idiopathic hypoparathyroidism and Addison's disease. *Am J Ophthalmol* 1962;54:660–674.
23. Kunin AS, MacKay BR, Burns SL, Halberstam MJ. The syndrome of hypoparathyroidism and adrenocortical insufficiency, a possible sequel of hepatitis. *Am J Med* 1963;34:856–866.
24. Taitz LS, Zarate-Salvador C, Schwartz E. Congenital absence of the parathyroid and thymus glands in an infant (III and IV pharyngeal pouch syndrome). *Pediatrics* 1966;38:412–418.
25. Olin R, Poindexter MH. Familial idiopathic hypoparathyroidism: with superficial moniliasis, pernicious anemia and Addison's disease. *Minn Med* 1972;55:701–704.
26. Hung W, Migeon CJ, Parrott RH. Possible autoimmune basis for Addison's disease in three siblings—one with idiopathic hypoparathyroidism, pernicious anemia and superficial moniliasis. *N Engl J Med* 1963;269:658–663.
27. Castleman B, Towne VW: Case records of the Massachusetts General Hospital. *N Engl J Med* 1954;251:442–448.
28. Papadatos C, Klein R. Addison's disease in a boy with hypoparathyroidism. *J Clin Endocrinol Metab* 1954;14:653–660.
29. Neufeld M, MacLaren N, Blizzard RM: Autoimmune polyglandular syndromes. *Pediatr Ann* 1980;9:154–162.
30. Neufeld M, MacLaren NK, Blizzard RM. Two types of autoimmune Addison's disease associated with different polyglandular autoimmune (PGA) syndromes. *Medicine* 1981;60:355–362.
31. Neufeld M, Blizzard RM: Polyglandular autoimmune disease. In: Pinchera A, Doniach D, Fenzi GF, et al., eds. *Symposium on autoimmune aspects of endocrine disorders.* New York: Academic Press, 1980;357–365.
32. Lechuga-Gomez EE, Meyerson J, Bigazzi PE, Walfish PG. Polyglandular autoimmune syndrome type II. *Can Med Assoc J* 1988;138:632–634.
33. Parfitt AM: Surgical, idiopathic, and other varieties of parathyroid hormone-deficient hypoparathyroidism. In: DeGroot LJ, Cahill GF Jr, Odell WD, et al., eds. *Endocrinology,* vol 2. New York: Grune & Stratton, 1979;755–768.
34. Sentochnik DE, Hoffman GS: Hypoparathyroidism due to progressive systemic sclerosis. *J Rheumatol* 1988;15:711–713.
35. Best TB, Munro RE, Burwell S, Volpé R. Riedel's thyroiditis associated with Hashimoto's thyroiditis, hypoparathyroidism, and retroperitoneal fibrosis. *J Endocrinol Invest* 1991;14:767–772.
36. Spinner MW, Blizzard RM, Childs B. Clinical and genetic heterogeneity in idiopathic Addison's disease and hypoparathyroidism. *J Clin Endocrinol Metab* 1968;28:795–804.
37. Hooper MJ, Carter JN, Stiel JN. Idiopathic hypoparathyroidism and idiopathic hypoadrenalism occurring separately in two siblings. *Med J Aust* 1973;1:990–993.
38. Drury MI, Keelan DM, Timoney FJ, Irvine WJ. Juvenile familial endocrinopathy. *Clin Exp Immunol* 1970;7:125–132.
39. Comin DB, Hines JD, Wieland RG. Coexistent pernicious anemia and idiopathic hypoparathyroidism in a woman. *J Am Med Assoc* 1969;207:1147–1149.
40. Wuepper KD, Fudenberg HH. Moniliasis, "autoimmune" polyendocrinopathy, and immunologic family study. *Clin Exp Immunol* 1967;2:71–82.

41. Kenny FM, Holliday MA. Hypoparathyroidism, moniliasis, Addison's and Hashimoto's disease. *N Engl J Med* 1964; 271:708–713.
42. Blizzard RM, Chee D, Davis W. The incidence of parathyroid and other antibodies in the sera of patients with idiopathic hypoparathyroidism. *Clin Exp Immunol* 1966;1:119–128.
43. Fanconi A. Hypoparathyreoidismus im Kindesalter. *Ergeb Inn Med Kinderheik* 1969;28:54–119.
44. Kirkpatrick CH, Rich RR, Bennett JE. Chronic mucocutaneous candidiasis: model-building in cellular immunity. *Ann Intern Med* 1971;74:955–978.
45. Blizzard RM, Gibbs JH. Candidiasis: studies pertaining to its association with endocrinopathies and pernicious anemia. *Pediatrics* 1968;42:231–237.
46. Lehner T. Classification and clinicopathological features of Candida infections in the mouth. In: *Symposium on* Candida *Infections*. Winner HI, Hurley R, eds. Edinburg: E & S Livingstone, 1966;119.
47. Battistella PA, Pozzan GB, Rigon F, Zancan L, Zacchello F. Autoimmune hypoparathyroidism and hyper-CK-emia (letter). *Brain Dev* 1991;13:61.
48. Nerup J: Addison's disease—a review of some clinical, pathological and immunological features. *Danish Med Bull* 1974; 21:201–217.
49. Marieb NJ, Melby JC, Lyall SS. Isolated hypoaldosteronism associated with idiopathic hypoparathyroidism. *Arch Intern Med* 1974;134:424–429.
50. Morse WI, Cochrane WA, Landrigan PL. Familial hypoparathyroidism with pernicious anemia, steatorrhea and adrenocortical insufficiency. *N Engl J Med* 1961;264:1021–1026.
51. Fields JP, Fragola L, Hadley TP. Hypoparathyroidism, candidiasis, alopecia and vitiligo. *Arch Dermatol* 1971;103:687–689.
52. Presley SJ, Paul JT. Idiopathic hypoparathyroidism. Report of a case. *Ill Med J* 1960;118:298–300.
53. Vazquez AM, Kenny FM. Ovarian failure and antiovarian antibodies in association with hypoparathyroidism, moniliasis, and Addison's and Hashimoto's diseases. *Obstet Gynecol* 1973;41:414–418.
54. Golonka JE, Goodman AD. Coexistence of primary ovarian insufficiency, primary adrenocortical insufficiency and idiopathic hypoparathyroidism. *J Clin Endocrinol Metab* 1968; 28:79–82.
55. Lorenz R, Burr IM. Idiopathic hypoparathyroidism and steatorrhea: a new aid in management. *J Pediatr* 1974;85:522–525.
56. Sjöberg K-H. Moniliasis—an internal disease?: three cases of idiopathic hypoparathyroidism with moniliasis, steatorrhea, primary amenorrhea and pernicious anemia. *Acta Med Scand* 1966;179:157–166.
57. Kleerekoper M, Basten A, Penny R, Posen S. Idiopathic hypoparathyroidism with primary ovarian failure. *Arch Intern Med* 1974;134:944–947.
58. Muir A, MacLaren NK. Autoimmune diseases of the adrenal glands, parathyroid glands, gonads, and hypothalamic–pituitary axis. *Endocrinol Metab Clin North Am* 1991;20:619–44.
59. McMahon FG, Cookson DU, Kabler JD, Inhorn SL. Idiopathic hypoparathyroidism and idiopathic adrenal cortical insufficiency occurring with cystic fibrosis of the pancreas. *Ann Intern Med* 1959;51:371–384.
60. Ikkala E, Siurala M, Viranko M. Hypoparathyroidism and pernicious anemia. *Acta Med Scand* 1964;176:73–77.
61. Hermans PE, Ulrich JA, Markowitz H. Chronic mucocutaneous candidiasis as a surface expression of deep-seated abnormalities. Report of a syndrome of superficial candidiasis, absence of delayed hypersensitivity and aminoaciduria. *Am J Med* 1969;47:503–519.
62. Stieglitz LN, Kind HP, Kazdan JJ, Fraser D, Kooh SW. Keratitis with hypoparathyroidism. *Am J Ophthalmol* 1977;84: 467–472.
63. Pohjola S. Ocular manifestations of idiopathic hypoparathyroidism: case report and review of the literature. *Acta Ophthalmol* 1962;40:255–265.
64. Wagman RD, Kazdan JJ, Kooh SW, Fraser D. Keratitis associated with the multiple endocrine deficiency, autoimmune disease, and candidiasis syndrome. *Am J Ophthalmol* 1987;103:569–575.
65. Svane-Knudsen P. Severe secondary ocular changes in a patient suffering from idiopathic hypoparathyroidism and pernicious anemia. *Acta Ophthalmol* 1959;37:560–567.
66. Wagner R. The syndrome of chronic hypoparathyroidism, Addison's disease and superficial moniliasis. *Exp Med Surg* 1960;18:157–160.
67. Kalb RE, Grossman ME. Ectodermal defects and chronic mucocutaneous candidiasis in idiopathic hypoparathyroidism. *J Am Acad Dermatol* 1986;15:353–356.
68. Williams E, Wood C. The syndrome of hypoparathyroidism and steatorrhoea. *Arch Dis Child* 1959;302–306.
69. Jackson WPU. Steatorrhoea and hypoparathyroidism (letter). *Lancet* 1957;1:1086–1087.
70. Cochrane WA, Morse WI, Landrigan P. Familial hypoparathyroidism with pernicious anemia and adrenal insufficiency related to intestinal dysfunction. *Am J Dis Child* 1960;100: 544–545.
71. Morse WI, Cochrane WA, Landrigan PL. Familial hypoparathyroidism with pernicious anemia, steatorrhea and adrenocortical insufficiency. *N Engl J Med* 1961;264:1021.
72. Dobias B. Moniliasis in pediatrics. *J Dis Child* 1957;94:234–239.
73. Strom L, Winberg J. Idiopathic hypoparathyroidism. *Acta Pediatr* 1954;43:574–581.
74. Windorfer A. Kasuistischer beitrag zum syndrom moniliasis, hypoparathyreoidismus und morbus Addison. *Mschr Kinderheilk* 1970;118:103–105.
75. Jellinek. Discussion. In: Fields JP, Fragola L, Hadley TP. Hypoparathyroidism, candidiasis, alopecia, and vitiligo. *Arch Dermatol* 1971;103:687–689.
76. Roth FJ Jr, Boyd CC, Sagami S, Blank H. An evaluation of the fungistatic activity in serum. *J Invest Dermatol* 1959; 32:549–556.
77. Louria DB, Brayton RG. Substance in blood lethal for *Candida albicans*. *Nature* 1964;201:309.
78. Esterly NB, Brammer SR, Crounse RG. In vitro inhibition of candidal growth by human serum. *J Invest Dermatol* 1967;49:246–250.
79. McQuarrie I, Hansen AE, Zeigler MR. Studies on the convulsive mechanism in idiopathic hypoparathyroidism. *J Clin Endocrinol Metab* 1941;1:789–798.
80. Blizzard RM, Kyle M. Studies of the adrenal antigens and antibodies in Addison's disease. *J Clin Invest* 1962;42:1653–1660.
81. Irvine WJ, Scarth L. Antibody to the oxyphil cells of the human parathyroid in idiopathic hypoparathyroidism. *Clin Exp Immunol* 1969;4:505–510.
82. Spinner MW, Blizzard RM, Gibbs J, Abbey H, Childs B. Familial distributions of organ specific antibodies in the blood of patients with Addison's disease and hypoparathyroidism and their relatives. *Clin Exp Immunol* 1969;5:461–468.
83. Jankovic BD, Isvaneski M, Popeskovic L, Mitrovic K. Experimental allergic thyroiditis (and parathyroiditis) in neonatally thymectomized and bursectomized chickens. Participation of the thymus in development of disease. *Int Arch Allergy* 1965;26:18–33.
84. Lupulescu A, Pop A, Merculiev E, Neascu C, Heithmanek C. Experimental iso-immune hypothyroidism in rats. *Nature* 1965;206:415–416.
85. Lupulescu A, Potorac E, Pop A, et al. Experimental investigations on immunology of the parathyroid gland. *Immunology* 1968;14:475–482.
86. Clarkson B, Kowlessar OD, Horwith M, Sleisenger MH. Clinical and metabolic study of a patient with malabsorption and hypoparathyroidism. *Metabolism* 1960;9:1093–1106.
87. Rao KJ, Tomar RH, Moses AM. Cell mediated immunity in hypoparathyroidism (abstract). *Clin Res* 1974;22:704A.
88. Block MB, Pachman LM, Windhorst D, Goldfine ID. Immunological findings in familial juvenile endocrine deficiency syndrome associated with mucocutaneous candidiasis. *Am J Med Sci* 1971;261:213–218.
89. Levy RL, Huang S-W, Bach ML, et al. Thymic transplan-

tation in a case of chronic mucocutaneous candidiasis. *Lancet* 1971;2:898–900.

90. Swana GT, Swana MR, Bottazzo CF, Doniach D. A human specific mitochondrial antibody: its importance in the identification of organ-specific reactions. *Clin Exp Immunol* 1977;28:517–525.

91. Irvine WJ, Barnes EW. Addison's disease, ovarian failure, and hypoparathyroidism. *J Clin Endocrinol Metab* 1975;4:379–434.

92. Arulanantham K, Dwyer JM, Genel MD. Evidence for defective immunoregulation in the syndrome of familial candidiasis endocrinopathy. *N Engl J Med* 1979;300:164–168.

93. Wirfält A. Genetic heterogeneity in autoimmune polyglandular failure. *Acta Med Scand* 1981;210:7–13.

94. Eisenbarth G, Wilson P, Ward F, Lebovitz HE. HLA type and occurrence of disease in familial polyglandular failure. *N Engl J Med* 1978;298:92–94.

95. Eisenbarth GS, Wilson PW, Ward F, Buckley C, Lebovitz H. The polyglandular failure syndrome: disease inheritance, HLA type, and immune function: studies in patients and families. *Ann Intern Med* 1979;91:528–533.

96. Perlmutter M, Ellison RR, Norsa L, Krantrowitz AR. Idiopathic hypoparathyroidism and Addison's disease. *Am J Med* 1956;21:634–643.

97. Haspel MV, Onodera T, Prabhaker BS, Horita M, Suzuki H, Notkins AL. Viral-induced autoimmunity: monoclonal antibodies that react with endocrine tissues. *Science* 1983;220:304–306.

98. Doniach D, Bottazzo GF: Polyendocrine autoimmunity. In: EC Franklin, ed. *Clinical Immunology Update*, vol 2. New York: Elsevier, 1981;95–121.

99. Betterle C, Caretto A, Zeviani M, Pedini B, Salviati C. Demonstration and characterization of anti-human mitochondria autoantibodies in idiopathic hypoparathyroidism and in other conditions. *J Exp Immunol* 1985;62:353–360.

100. Burckhardt P. Idiopathic hypoparathyroidism and autoimmunity. *Hormone Res* 1982;16:304–307.

101. Posillico JT, Wortsman J, Srikanta S, Eisenbarth GS, Mallette LE, Brown EM. Parathyroid cell surface autoantibodies that inhibit parathyroid hormone secretion from dispersed human parathyroid cells. *J Bone Mineral Res* 1986;1:475–483.

102. Brandi M-L, Aurbach GD, Fattorossi A, Quarto R, Marx SJ, Fitzpatrick LA. Antibodies cytotoxic to bovine parathyroid cells in autoimmune hypoparathyroidism. *Proc Natl Acad Sci USA* 1986;83:8366–8369.

103. Fattorossi A, Aurbach GD, Sakaguchi K, et al. Anti-endothelial cell antibodies: Detection and characterization in sera from patients with autoimmune hypoparathyroidism. *Proc Natl Acad Sci USA* 1988;85:4015–4019.

104. Wortsman J, McConnachie P, Baker JR Jr, Mallette LE. T-lymphocyte activation in adult-onset idiopathic hypoparathyroidism. *Am J Med* 1992;92:352–356.

105. DiGeorge AM, Paschkis K. The syndrome of Addison's disease, hypoparathyroidism and superficial moniliasis. *Am J Dis Child* 1957;94:476–478.

106. Russell RI. Hypoparathyroidism and malabsorption. *Br Med J* 1967;3:781.

107. Snodgrass RW, Mellinhoff SM. Idiopathic hypoparathyroidism with small bowel x-ray features of sprue, without steatorrhea. *Am J Dig Dis* 1962;7:273–280.

108. Miettinen TA, Perheentupa J. Bile salt deficiency in fat malabsorption of hypoparathyroidism. *Scand J Clin Lab Invest* 1971;27(Suppl 116):36.

109. Jeffcoate WJ, Hosking DJ, Jones RM. Hypoparathyroidism and Addison's disease: a potentially lethal combination. *J R Soc Med* 1987;80:709–710.

110. Etzioni A, Atias D, Pollack S, et al. Complete recovery of pure red cell aplasia by intramuscular gammaglobulin therapy in a child with hypoparathyroidism. *Am J Hematol* 1986;22:409–414.

111. Daneman D, Kooh SW, Fraser D. Hypoparathyroidism and pseudohypoparathyroidism in childhood. *J Clin Endocrinol Metab* 1982;11:211–231.

112. Gustafsson J, Holmberg I, Hardell L-I, Foucard T: Hypoparathyroidism and liver disease—evidence for a vitamin D hydroxylation defect: a case report. *Acta Endocrinol* 1984;105:211–214.

113. Leifer E, Hollander W. Idiopathic hypoparathyroidism and chronic adrenal insufficiency: a case report. *J Clin Endocrinol Metab* 1953;13:1264–1269.

114. Quichaud J, Le Bozec R, Frison B, Galez A, Massy B, Blanchard J. Syndrome candidose–Hypoparathyroïdie insuffisance surrénale idiopathique chez un garçon de 10 ans: considérations nosologiques et étiopathogéniques. *Ann D'Endocrinol* 1969;30:682–695.

115. Tomeck KJ, Dijkstra JWE. Superficial fungal infections of the skin. In: *Conn's Current Therapy 1993*. RE Rakel, ed. Philadelphia: W.B. Saunders, 1993;792–794.

116. Petersen EA, Alling DW, Kirkpatrick CH. Treatment of chronic mucocutaneous candidiasis with ketoconazole: controlled clinical trial. *Ann Intern Med* 1980;93:791–795.

117. Horsburg CR Jr, Kirkpatrick CH. Long-term therapy of mucocutaneous candidiasis with ketoconazole: Experience with twenty-one patients. *Am J Med* 1983;74:23–29.

118. Kirkpatrick CH, Greenberg LE. In: *Immune Regulators In Transfer Factor*. Khan A, Kirkpatrick CH, Hill NO, eds. New York: Academic Press, 1979.

119. Jorizzo JL, Sams WM Jr, Jegasothy BV, Olansky AJ. Cimetidine as an immunomodulator: chronic mucocutaneous candidiasis as a model. *Ann Intern Med* 1980;92:192–195.

The Parathyroids, edited by J.P. Bilezikian,
M.A. Levine, and R. Marcus. Raven Press, Ltd.,
New York © 1994.

CHAPTER 45

Molecular Genetics of Hypoparathyroidism

Rajesh V. Thakker

In recent years, important advances in endocrinology have resulted from the application of the methods of molecular biology (1). Thus the molecular basis for mammalian sex development (2–4), for papillary thyroid cancers (5–8), for nephrogenic diabetes insipidus (9,10), and for Kallmann's syndrome (11,12) have been elucidated. In addition, some of the susceptibility genes involved in the development of hypertension (13), insulin-dependent diabetes mellitus (14–16), and noninsulin-dependent diabetes mellitus (17) have been identified. In these studies, the first important step towards elucidating the genetic abnormality and in subsequently characterizing the gene product, i.e., protein, was taken by the localization of the disease gene locus. This approach has been referred to as *reverse genetics* (18) or *positional cloning* (19), and the chromosomal localization of candidate genes (i.e., *gene mapping*) may be accomplished either by the cytogenetic detection of chromosomal abnormalities in affected individuals or by segregation studies in affected families using recombinant DNA genetic markers (20). Development of these techniques has made it possible to investigate the molecular basis of the hypoparathyroid disorders.

Hypoparathyroidism is an endocrine disorder in which hypocalcemia and hyperphosphatemia are the result of a deficiency in parathyroid hormone (PTH) secretion. There are a variety of causes (21) of hypoparathyroidism (Table 1), and the disorder may occur as part of a pluriglandular autoimmune disorder or as a complex congenital defect, such as in the DiGeorge syndrome or in association with other developmental anomalies involving dysmorphic features, nephropa-

thy, sensorineural deafness, lymphedema, and cortical thickening of tubular bones. In addition, hypoparathyroidism may develop as a solitary endocrinopathy and this form has been called *isolated* or *idiopathic hypoparathyroidism*. Familial occurrences of isolated hypoparathyroidism have been reported, and autosomal dominant (22,23), autosomal recessive (24,25), and X-linked recessive (26–28) inheritances have been established (29). The molecular genetic basis for each of these forms of hypoparathyroidism has been investigated either by examining the *PTH* gene, located (30) on the short arm of chromosome 11, band 11p15, for abnormalities or by pursuing positional cloning studies in which the chromosomal location of the mutant gene was first elucidated. Progress in these molecular genetic studies of the hypoparathyroid disorders is discussed in this chapter.

PTH GENE ABNORMALITIES IN ISOLATED HYPOPARATHYROIDISM

Deficiency of PTH, an 84-amino-acid polypeptide (31) encoded by a single gene located on 11p15 (30), is the hallmark of hypoparathyroidism. The *PTH* gene has been investigated for abnormalities in patients with autosomal familial isolated hypoparathyroidism (23,25,32). Families with autosomal hypoparathyroidism have been initially investigated for segregation of the disease and *PTH* gene polymorphisms, and families who showed cosegregation have been further investigated for DNA sequence abnormalities of the *PTH* gene. The identification of polymorphisms at the *PTH* locus together with the ability to amplify and determine the sequence of selected DNA segments by use of the polymerase chain reaction (PCR) has facilitated the investigation of these families for *PTH* gene abnormalities.

R. V. Thakker: MRC Molecular Medicine Group, Royal Postgraduate Medical School, Hammersmith Hospital, London W12 0NN, United Kingdom.

TABLE 1. *The hypoparathyroid disorders and their chromosomal localization*

Disorder	Inheritance	Chromosomal location
Isolated hypoparathyroidism	Autosomal dominant	11p15[a]
	Autosomal recessive	11p15[a]
	X-linked recessive	Xq26-q27
Associated complex congenital syndrome		
DiGeorge	Autosomal dominant	22q11
Kenney-Caffey	Autosomal dominant[b]	?[c]
Barakat	Autosomal recessive[b]	?[c]
Lymphedema	Autosomal recessive[b]	?[c]
Nephropathy, nerve deafness	Autosomal dominant	?[c]
	Autosomal recessive	?[c]
Dysmorphology, growth failure	Autosomal recessive[b]	?[c]
Pluriglandular autoimmune syndrome	Autosomal recessive	?[c]

[a]Mutation of PTH gene identified only in some families.
[b]Most likely inheritance shown.
[c]Location not known.

PTH Gene Polymorphisms

The *PTH* gene consists of three exons and 2 introns (Fig. 1). Exon 1, which is 85 base pairs (bp) in size, encodes an untranslated region: exon 2, which is 90 bp in size, encodes the initiation codon, signal peptide and part of the prohormone sequence; and exon 3, which is 612 bp in size, encodes the remainder of the prohormone sequence, the 84-amino-acid PTH peptide, and the 3'-untranslated region. Five polymorphisms of the *PTH* gene have been reported and two of these are associated with restriction fragment length polymorphisms (RFLPs) (33), another two are the result of point mutations (34), and one is due to a variation in the length of a microsatellite repetitive sequence in intron 1 (35). These polymorphisms are inherited in a Mendelian manner and are thus useful as genetic markers in family studies, and it is useful to consider these polymorphisms in greater detail.

Restriction Fragment Length Polymorphisms (RFLPs)

Restriction fragment length polymorphisms are the result of variations in the primary DNA sequence of individuals and may be due to single base changes, deletions, additions, or translocation. These changes in DNA sequence occur frequently (approximately once in every 250 base pairs), usually in the noncoding regions; do not affect gene function; and are often at a distance from the disease gene (36). Four such neutral mutations are known to be associated with polymorphisms of the *PTH* gene. Two of these point mutations, designated Mir1 and Mir2, which were due, respectively, to transition of an adenine (A) to guanine (G) residue in intron 1, and to a transversion of cytosine (C) to adenine (A) in exon 3, were revealed by altered migration of amplified prepro-PTH gene fragments through denaturing gels (34). The other two point mutations detected were associated with the

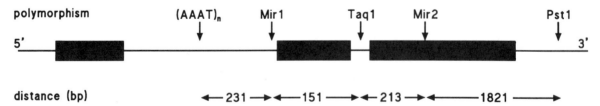

FIG. 1. Schematic representation of the PTH gene. The PTH gene consists of three exons and two introns, with the order 5'–exon 1–intron 1–exon 2–intron 2–exon 3–3' The three exons of the PTH gene are shown as *solid boxes* and the introns as *lines*. The polymorphic sites associated with the PTH gene are indicated. Two restriction fragment length polymorphisms RFLPs are associated with the PTH gene, and the TaqI polymorphic site is within intron 2 and the PstI polymorphic site is 1.7 kbp downstream in the 3' direction of the gene (33). Two internal polymorphic mutations (34) of the PTH gene designated Mir1 and Mir2 are located in intron 1 and exon 3, respectively, and the tetranucleotide (AAAT)ₙ polymorphism is in intron 1 (35). The distance between the tetranucleotide (AAAT)ₙ polymorphism and the polymorphic Mir1 mutation is 231 base pairs (bp), that between the Mir1 mutation and the Taq1 RFLP site is 152 bp, that between the TaqI RFLP site and the polymorphic Mir2 mutation is 212 bp, and that between the Mir2 mutation and the PstI RFLP site is 1821 bp. Linkage disequilibrium between the (AAAT)ₙ, TaqI, and PstI polymorphic sites has been established (35).

presence or absence of a cleavage site for a restriction enzyme (33). Restriction enzymes are derived from microorganisms and have been found to cleave DNA in a sequence-specific manner. For example, the enzyme HindIII, which originates from *Haemophilus influenzae,* will only cleave if the sequence AAGCTT is present, and then will cleave specifically (↓) between the two adenine (A) residues, i.e., A ↓ AGCTT. A DNA polymorphism such as a single base change in this sequence would result in loss of an enzyme cleavage site, and this would be revealed as an RFLP as follows (37).

A restriction enzyme is used to cleave human leukocyte DNA and the resulting DNA fragments are separated according to size by agarose gel electrophoresis, the smaller fragments migrating farthest away from the cathode. The DNA fragments are then transferred by passive capillary (Southern) blotting (38) to a nylon or nitrocellulose membrane. Digested fragments of single-stranded human DNA are thus immobilized according to size (i.e., fragment length) on the membrane, which is next hybridized with a single-stranded, radiolabelled DNA probe. The labelled DNA probe will anneal to any fragments that have a complementary sequence, and these restricted fragments of varying lengths are revealed by autoradiography. The exact number and size of restriction fragments will vary from individual to individual in relation to the number of recognition sites for the restriction enzyme, as shown in Fig. 2. In this example, the DNA sequence of individual 1 has three restriction en-

zyme cleavage sites, and, following digestion, fragments of two sizes will result. One fragment size will be 5 kilobases (kb) in length, and the other fragment size will be 10 kb in length. The labelled DNA probe will hybridize only to the 5 kb fragments, which contain a complementary sequence, and autoradiography will therefore only reveal one band, corresponding to the 5 kb fragment. However, in individual 2, there has been a loss of one restriction enzyme cleavage site, due to a change in the DNA sequence, and following digestion only restriction fragments of 15 kb in size will result. Therefore, a single 15 kb band is observed at autoradiography. The heterozygous individual who has one chromosome with three cleavage sites and another with two cleavage sites will reveal two restriction fragments at autoradiography, one at 15 kb and one at 5 kb. Alleles can be designated to these RFLPs; for example, individual 1, who has the smaller RFLP, is designated as having allele "aa"; individual 2, who has the larger RFLP is designated "AA"; and the heterozygous individual with both the large and smaller RFLPs is designated "Aa". Such RFLPs have been detected at the PTH locus by the two restriction endonucleases TaqI and PstI. The TaqI-derived RFLPs are 2.5 and 2.4 kb in size, and the PstI-derived RFLPs are 2.7 and 2.2 kb in size (33). These RFLPs and the polymorphic point mutations Mir1 and Mir2 are useful genetic markers for linkage studies; they are inherited in a mendelian manner, and their inheritance can be followed together with a disease in an affected family.

Microsatellite Polymorphisms

Many of the currently available DNA probes utilized to detect either RFLPs or variable numbers of tandem repeats (VNTRs) in minisatellite sequences by Southern blotting have limited application in that they are not highly polymorphic, and information from the marker locus will not be obtained for family studies. To gain maximal genetic information from limited numbers of families with rare clinical disorders, such as hypoparathyroidism, highly polymorphic genetic markers are required. PCR is useful in the detection of DNA sequence polymorphisms by revealing length variations in microsatellite tandem repeats (39), for example $(CA)_n$, where $n = 10–60$. In addition to tandem repeats in the sequence (CA), microsatellite tandem repeats consisting of $(AT)_n$, $(GA)_n$, $(ATT)_n$, $(ATTT)_n$, $(AAAT)_n$, and the hexanucleotide $[T(Pu)T(Pu)T(Pu)]_n$ have also been reported (35,39). These tandem repeats, which are highly polymorphic and are inherited in a Mendelian manner, are estimated to occur once in every 50–100 kilobase pairs (kbp). Thus, they represent a powerful approach to obtaining a detailed genetic map around a disease locus, for example, that for hypoparathyroidism. With this technique, oligonucle-

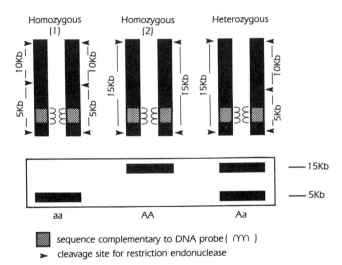

FIG. 2. Schematic representation of RFLPs resulting from variations in the number of restriction endonuclease sites. **Top:** a pair of chromosomal DNA segments from three individuals—two of whom are homozygous (1) and (2) and one of whom is heterozygous—for the polymorphisms. **Bottom:** the bands, i.e., RFLPs, revealed on autoradiography, and the upper 15 kb RFLP has been designated allele "A" and the lower 5 kb RFLP has been designated allele "a".

otide primers that flank the repeat are synthesized, and PCR is used to amplify the repeat sequence (Fig. 3). The smaller and larger fragment length polymorphisms in these repetitive sequences are detected by separation on a polyacrylamide sequencing gel or an agarose gel, respectively. The use of one such polymorphic tetranucleotide [(AAAT)$_n$] repetitive sequence from intron 1 of the *PTH* gene (35) is illustrated in Fig. 4.

Family Studies

PTH gene polymorphisms have been used in segregation studies of families affected with autosomal dominant and recessive forms of isolated hypoparathyroidism, and abnormalities of the *PTH* gene were excluded in 50% of the families by demonstrating recombination between the disease and the *PTH* gene (23,34,35,40). However, in families among whom cosegregation of hypoparathyroidism and the *PTH* locus was found, restriction endonuclease studies of DNA from affected individuals did not reveal an absence of the *PTH* gene or abnormal restriction patterns to suggest major structural rearrangements, deletions or insertions in the DNA of affected individuals (23,25,35,41). Detailed sequence analysis of the *PTH* gene was therefore undertaken, and the results from patients in four families, two with autosomal dominant (32,41) and two with autosomal recessive isolated hypoparathyroidism, have been reported (25,35).

Autosomal Dominant Isolated Hypoparathyroidism

DNA sequence analysis of the *PTH* gene from one patient with autosomal dominant isolated hypoparathyroidism has revealed a single base substitution (T→C) in exon 2 (32). This resulted in the substitution of arginine (CGT) for cysteine (TGT) in the amino acid signal peptide. A mutation involving the signal peptide is of importance in that signal sequences, which are present in the precursors of most secreted proteins, are required for correct processing of the protein through the cell's secretory pathway. This entails delivery of the protein to the outer membrane of the endoplasmic reticulum (ER), where the protein undergoes insertion and translocation, during which the signal peptide is cleaved of the protein. To facilitate this passage through the ER membrane, the signal peptide contains predominantly hydrophobic amino acids. However, the T→C mutation in the patient with hypoparathyroidism would result in the replacement of cysteine by arginine, a charged amino acid, in the midst of the hydrophobic core of the signal peptide, and this would impede the translocation of the prepro-PTH protein. The processing of this mutant prepro-

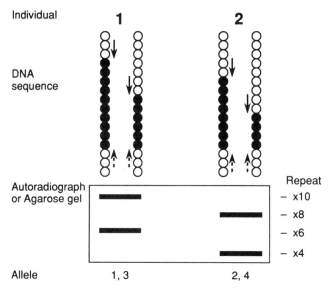

FIG. 3. Schematic representation of polymorphisms in microsatellite tandem repetitive DNA sequences, which may consist, for example, of the dinucleotide CA, or the trinucleotide ATT, or the tetranucleotide AAAT, or the hexanucleotide TATATG. Oligonucleotide primers (*arrows*) corresponding to the nonrepetitive sequences (*open circles*) on either side of the repetitive DNA sequence (*solid circles*) are synthesized and the polymerase chain reaction (PCR) is utilized to amplify the repeat in genomic DNA obtained from different individuals. The resulting PCR products are separated either by polyacrylamide gel or agarose gel electrophoresis, and the polymorphisms are revealed by autoradiography or by viewing of an ethidium bromide-stained agarose gel under ultraviolet light. Thus, of the pair of chromosomes from individual 1, one has ten repeats and the other has six repeats, whereas, of the pair of chromosomes from individual 2, one has eight repeats and the other has four repeats. Following PCR amplification and separation by gel electrophoresis, these variations in the length of the repeats will be revealed by the differences in the size of the bands, which have been designated alleles; for example, the larger band consisting of ten repeats is designated allele 1, and those consisting of eight, six, and four repeats are designated alleles 2, 3, and 4, respectively. These microsatellite tandem repetitive sequences, which are highly polymorphic, show Mendelian inheritance (Fig. 4) and can be used as genetic markers in family linkage studies. Such a polymorphic microsatellite consisting of the sequence (AAAT)$_n$ has been identified in intron 1 of the PTH gene (35). (Reprinted from ref. 1 with permission.)

PTH has been assessed (32) by in vitro translation studies using recombinant plasmids containing either the normal or the mutant form of prepro-PTH cDNA. The results of this study (32) revealed that RNA was transcribed from the cDNAs and that both normal and mutant PTH RNA were translated efficiently to the protein. However, the processing of the mutant prepro-PTH protein to the pro-PTH protein was greatly impaired, revealing the genetic and cellular basis of hypoparathyroidism in this patient.

The *PTH* gene sequence has also been investigated

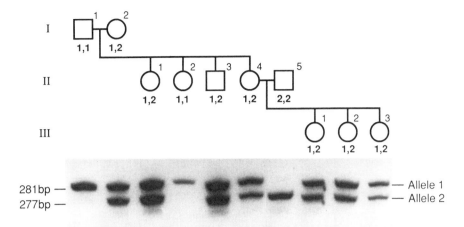

FIG. 4. Mendelian inheritance of the tetranucleotide (AAAT)$_n$ polymorphism associated with the PTH gene. The presence of the tandem repeat (AAAT)$_5$ was revealed by the 281 bp fragment (allele 1) and that of (AAAT)$_4$ was revealed by the 277 bp fragment (allele 2). An analysis of the inheritance of these alleles is shown for family 18/92, who are of northern European origin and are not affected with hypoparathyroidism. The family is drawn so that each individual appears above his or her alleles, and the genotype is indicated for each individual. The grandmother (I.2) is heterozygous (allele 1,2) and the grandfather (I.1) is homozygous (allele 1,1). An examination of their children and grandchildren reveals Mendelian inheritance of the alleles.

in another family among whom autosomal dominant hypoparathyroidism was associated with sensorineural deafness and renal dysplasia (41). The locations of the PTH gene and a gene encoding renal development, the Wilms' tumor gene, in 11p15 and 11p13, respectively, suggested this region as a candidate for genetic abnormalities in the family. A detailed analysis of the *PTH* gene revealed no abnormalities, and the results of this and other studies indicate that there is likely to be considerable genetic and molecular heterogeneity in autosomal dominant isolated hypoparathyroidism.

Autosomal Recessive Isolated Hypoparathyroidism

Autosomal recessive hypoparathyroidism has usually arisen in families with consanguineous marriages (25,35,42). Abnormalities in the *PTH* gene have been sought, and in one such family a donor splice site mutation at the exon 2–intron 2 boundary has been identified (25). This mutation involved a single base substitution (g→c) at position 1 of intron 1, and this altered the invariant gt dinucleotide of the 5' donor splice site (43) consensus sequence (gtaagt) (44) (Fig. 5). The mutation resulted in the creation of a DdeI restriction enzyme site (ctaag) which facilitated the detection of this donor splice mutation in other members of the family (Fig. 6). The donor splice site mutation of the *PTH* gene, which was found to segregate with hypoparathyroidism in this family, is of importance in that it would alter the consensus sequence (gtaagt), which is complementary to the sequence of the small

ribonucleoprotein (snRNP) designated U1 (45,46,47). The U1-snRNP is the 5' recognition component of the nuclear RNA splicing enzyme, which forms base pairs with the 5' and 3' ends of an intron so as to align these terminal regions for cutting and splicing. Thus an alteration of the complementary 5' donor splice site sequence of the intron will affect annealing of the U1–snRNP, and previous studies of β-thalassaemia have demonstrated that such mutations are associated with abnormalities of mRNA processing (48–50) in which there is either an accumulation of unspliced precursor mRNA, or retention of incompletely spliced precursors, or a complete absence of transcripts, or the appearance of aberrantly processed mRNA that resulted from the utilization of alternative normally occurring 5' splice sites or from the use of cryptic splice sites. In addition, in vitro studies utilizing the human adenovirus late transcription unit (51) and the rat preprotachykinin gene (52) have demonstrated that alterations at an internal exon–intron boundary result in the splicing out of the exon together with its adjacent introns. This form of abnormal splicing out of the exon has been referred to as *exon skipping*. These possibilities were investigated in the hypoparathyroid patient who had inherited a 5' donor splice size mutation (Fig. 6) of the *PTH* gene by a study of mRNA processing. However, *PTH* gene expression is usually limited to the parathyroid glands, which were not available from these patients. Thus a novel method that entailed the detection of *PTH* gene expression by PCR in cultured lymphocytes was utilized (Fig. 7).

The detection by PCR of a low level of transcription of a tissue-specific gene in cells that do not exhibit

770

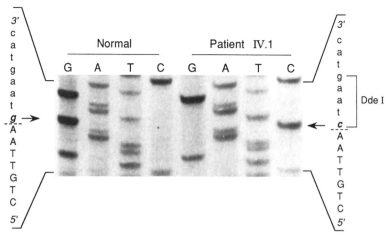

FIG. 5. Direct sequence analysis of genomic DNA amplified via PCR. The autoradiographs show the nucleotide sequences of the PTH exon 2–intron 2 boundary obtained from a normal individual and patient IV.1 (Fig. 6) who suffers from autosomal recessive idiopathic hypoparathyroidism. The exon sequence is indicated in uppercase letters, the intron sequence is indicated by lowercase letters, and the exon–intron boundary is shown (*dashed line*). At the first base of intron 2 (*arrow*), there is a guanine (g) residue in the DNA sequence of the normal individual. However, in patient IV.1, this g residue is absent and has been replaced by a cytosine (c) residue. Thus, there has been a single base substitution (g→c), and this has altered the normal consensus 5' donor splice site sequence (gtaagt). This mutation has resulted in the occurrence of a DdeI restriction enzyme site (c ↓ taag) in the DNA of the patient and this has facilitated the detection of this donor splice mutation in other members of the family (Fig. 6). The demonstration of a donor splice site mutation in the PTH gene of the patient indicates that hypoparathyroidism may be associated with an abnormality in PTH mRNA processing. (Reprinted from ref. 25 with permission.)

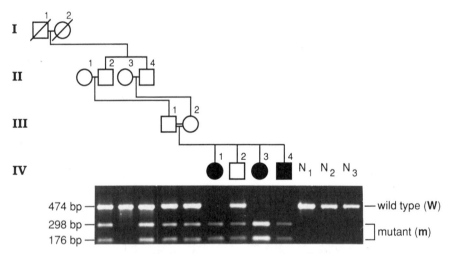

FIG. 6. DdeI restriction enzyme analysis in family A/89 detects a donor splice site mutation in the PTH gene. Family A/89, who are of Bangladeshi origin, are shown at *top,* with each individual appearing above his or her DNA fragments. Nine members from three generations of the family among whom the parents (III.1 and III.2) of the affected children (IV.1, IV.3, and IV.4) are consanguineous were investigated together with ten unrelated normal (N_n) Bangladeshi individuals. Genomic DNA was prepared using peripheral blood leukocytes from each individual, and the 474 bp PTH gene segment spanning the exon 2–intron 2 region was amplified by PCR. The PCR product was incubated with DdeI, and the samples were analyzed by electrophoresis on a 1.4% agarose gel stained with ethidium bromide to enable visualization of the DNA fragments, which are shown at *bottom.* The results from all ten normal individuals (results from N_1, N_2, and N_3 are shown) revealed that the 474 bp PCR product was not cleaved with DdeI, and this 474 bp fragment was designated the wild-type (W) allele. However, the presence of the DdeI site in the patients (IV.1, IV.3, and IV.4) was revealed as cleavage by DdeI resulted in two fragments of 298 bp and 176 bp, which were designated mutant (m) alleles. In the unaffected members (II.2, II.4, III.1, III.2, and IV.2) of the family, both the normal 474 bp fragment and the abnormal 298 bp and 176 bp fragments were detected, indicating heterozygosity. Thus the unrelated normal individuals are homozygous (WW) for the wild-type allele, the patients are homozygous (mm) for the mutant allele, and the unaffected family members are heterozygous (Wm). These results demonstrate that a g→c donor splice site mutation, which is detected by DdeI, in the PTH gene segregates with hypoparathyroidism. (Reprinted from ref. 25 with permission.)

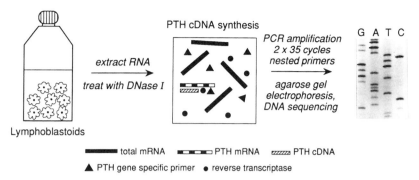

FIG. 7. Schematic representation for the detection of "illegitimate" or "nontissue-specific" transcription of the PTH gene via PCR. Epstein-Barr virus (EBV)-transformed lymphocytes were cultured, and total RNA was extracted and treated with Dnase I to remove any contaminating DNA. A specific first strand cDNA copy of the PTH mRNA sequence was made by using a PTH gene-specific oligonucleotide as a primer for the avian myeloblastosis virus (AMV) reverse transcriptase. The yield of the reverse transcribed PTH cDNA was increased by two rounds of PCR amplification, in which two pairs of nested primers were used to enhance the sensitivity and specificity of the amplification. On completion, the PCR amplification products were analyzed via agarose gel electrophoresis (Fig. 8) and by direct DNA sequencing (25). (Reprinted from ref. 53 with permission.)

physiological expression of the gene has been referred to as *non-tissue specific* or *ectopic*, or *illegitimate* transcription (54–56). For example, such non-tissue specific transcription of the Duchenne muscular dystrophy (DMD) gene encoding dystrophin, which is physiologically expressed only in muscle, has been observed to occur in fibroblasts, lymphoblastoid cells, HepG2 hepatoma cell lines, and peripheral blood lymphocytes (57,58). Additional studies have demonstrated that such ectopic transcription with correct splicing of the mRNA also occurs for other highly tissue-specific genes encoding clotting factor VIIIc, β-globin, anti-Müllerian hormone, and aldolase A (55). The extent of the non-tissue specific expression of these genes has been estimated (55–57) to be one molecule of correctly spliced mRNA per 1,000 cells, and the physiological relevance and mechanisms involved in this low level of ectopic transcription are not known. It has been postulated that the promoter regions of a tissue-specific gene may be activated by some of the ubiquitous transcriptional factors, such as TATA box factors, and CAAT box binding proteins, in the absence of the respective tissue-specific transcriptional factors (55). The binding of these ubiquitous transcriptional factors to their respective DNA elements would be facilitated by the chromatin disruption that occurs during DNA replication, and non-tissue specific transcription has been observed to be greater in actively proliferating lymphoblasts than in confluent fibroblasts (55). The demonstration of non-tissue specific transcription is of medical importance in that it permits the use of easily accessible cells (e.g., peripheral blood lymphocytes) for the detection of abnormalities in mRNA processing and thereby avoids the requirement for expressing tissue that may be obtained

only by biopsy. Advantage was taken of these methods to demonstrate abnormal processing of PTH mRNA in patients with autosomal recessive isolated hypoparathyroidism who were shown to have the donor splice site mutation in the *PTH* gene (25).

The non-tissue specific transcription of the *PTH* gene was demonstrated from cultured lymphocytes, as illustrated in Fig. 7. An analysis of the PTH cDNA obtained from normal and hypoparathyroid individuals (Fig. 8) revealed a mutant PTH cDNA from the hypoparathyroid patients, which was 90 bp smaller, a size that corresponded to that of exon 2. In addition, DNA sequence analysis of the wild-type or normal PTH cDNA sequence revealed a correctly spliced PTH cDNA with the order exon 1–exon 2–exon 3. However, DNA sequence analysis of the mutant PTH cDNA from the patient with autosomal recessive hypoparathyroidism demonstrated exon skipping, in which exon 2 was lost and exon 1 was spliced to exon 3. Thus, the donor splice site mutation, which is at the exon 2–intron 2 boundary, led to an abnormality of mRNA processing in which the other normally occurring 5' donor splice site at the exon 1–intron 1 boundary was utilized to splice exon 1 to exon 3. The resulting abnormal mRNA transcript did not contain exon 2, and thus lacked the initiation codon and the signal peptide sequence, which are required for the commencement of PTH mRNA translation (59) and for the translocation (60) of the prepro-PTH peptide, respectively. Thus these findings defined the molecular pathology of the *PTH* gene that causes autosomal recessive idiopathic hypoparathyroidism in this family. In addition, the ability to detect non-tissue specific expression of the *PTH* gene in cultured lymphocytes overcame the requirement for parathyroid tissue biop-

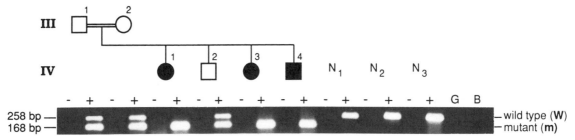

FIG. 8. Non-tissue specific transcription of the PTH gene revealed by detection of PTH cDNA in cultured lymphocytes. The ectopic transcription of the PTH gene in EBV-transformed lymphocytes was detected by PCR amplification of PTH cDNA (Fig. 7), which had been synthesised by addition (+) of the enzyme reverse transcriptase to extracts of RNA obtained from EBV-transformed lymphocytes of normal and affected individuals. The samples were analyzed via electrophoresis on a 1.5% agarose gel stained with ethidium bromide to enable visualization of the PTH cDNA fragments, which are shown at *bottom,* with the respective family member or control shown above. In ten normal individuals (N_1–N_3 shown), the PCR-amplified PTH cDNA was observed at the expected size of 258 bp. This product was not present when reverse transcriptase was omitted (−) from the reaction or when only genomic DNA (G) or a water blank (B) was used, demonstrating that this product is not due to amplification of a genomic sequence but is RNA specific. Thus non-tissue specific transcription of the PTH gene was demonstrated to occur in lymphocytes. In family A/89, the affected individuals (IV.1, IV.3, and IV.4) who were homozygous for the donor splice site mutation (Fig. 6) were found to differ from the normal individuals in having an abnormal PTH cDNA of 168 bp in size. Thus the mutant (m) PTH cDNA differed from the normal or wild-type (W) by 90 bp, which corresponds to the size of exon 2. The parents (III.1 and III.2) and the unaffected sibling (IV.2) who are heterozygous for the mutation (Fig. 6) have both the mutant and wild-type PTH cDNA. Thus the donor splice site mutation causing hypoparathyroidism in this family is associated with an abnormal PTH cDNA, which indicates an alteration in the processing of PTH mRNA. (Reprinted from ref. 25 with permission.)

sies. Use of this method will help to characterize further defects in the processing of PTH mRNA that may cause disorders of parathyroid activity.

The *PTH* gene sequence has been similarly investigated (35) in another consanguineous family with autosomal recessive hypoparathyroidism associated with renal insufficiency and developmental delay (42). Abnormalities of the *PTH* gene were not found, and other loci at which mutations may affect the embryological development, cell structure, or regulation of the parathyroids should be elucidated.

X-LINKED RECESSIVE HYPOPARATHYROIDISM

Isolated hypoparathyroidism has been reported to occur as an X-linked recessive disorder in two multi-generation kindreds (26,27) from Missouri. Only males were affected, and they suffered from infantile-onset epilepsy and hypocalcaemia, which was due to an isolated defect of parathyroid gland development (61). Linkage studies utilizing X-linked RFLPs in these families have localized (28) the mutant gene to the distal end of the long arm of the X chromosome to band Xq26–Xq27 by establishing linkage between hypoparathyroidism and an MspI-derived RFLP for the probe 4D.8, which defines the locus DXS98. An example of the inheritance of hypoparathyroidism and the RFLPs obtained with probe 4D.8 is shown in a por-

tion of one of the families (27) designated family W (Fig. 9). In this family, the two sons in generation IV are affected and have allele "a." Their mother, grandmother, and great grandmother are all carriers and are heterozygous allele "Aa," while their uncle in generation III is unaffected and has allele "A." These results indicate that the disease is segregating with the 8 kb allele "a," and the probability of linkage between hypoparathyroidism and the 4D.8 (DXS98) locus exceeded 6,500 to 1. It is useful to consider the results of this linkage analysis in greater detail.

Linkage Analysis

Restriction fragment length polymorphisms are inherited in a mendelian manner, and their inheritance can be followed together with a disease in an affected family. The consistent inheritance of an RFLP allele with the disease indicates that the two genetic loci are close together, i.e., are "linked." Genes that are far apart do not consistently cosegregate but show recombination because of the crossing over during meiosis. By studying recombination events in family studies, the distance between two genes and the probability that they are linked can be ascertained (62,63). The distance between two genes is expressed as the *recombination fraction* (θ), which is equal to the number of recombinants divided by the total number of offspring resulting from informative meioses within a

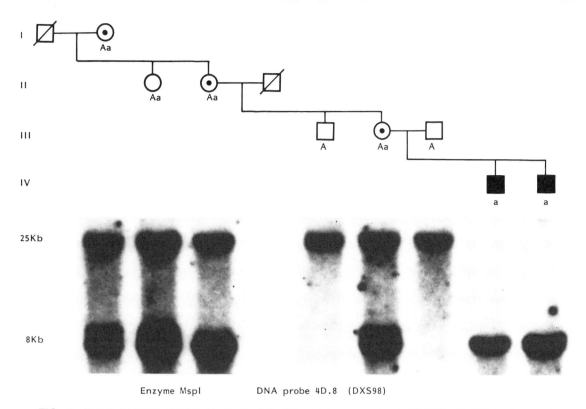

Enzyme MspI   DNA probe 4D.8   (DXS98)

FIG. 9. Autoradiograph obtained in eight of the 50 members from family W (27) with X-linked recessive hypoparathyroidism in which the X-linked probe 4D.8 has been hybridized to genomic DNA digested with the enzyme MspI to reveal RFLPs. The detection of RFLPs and the designation of alleles have been described earlier and illustrated in Fig. 2. The 25 kb allele is designated allele "A", and the 8 kb allele is designated allele "a". However, it is important to note that males have one X chromosome only and are thus hemizygous at this X-linked locus. The family tree is drawn so that each member appears above his or her RFLP pattern. Analysis reveals that the disease is segregating with the 8 kb allele (a). *Open squares,* normal male; *solid squares,* affected male; *open circle,* normal female; *circle with bullet,* carrier female.

family. The value of the recombination fraction (θ) can range from 0 to 0.5. A value of 0 indicates that the genes are very closely linked, while a value of 0.5 indicates that the genes are far apart and not linked. The probability that the two loci are *linked* at these distances is expressed as a "LOD" score, which is $\log_{10}$ of the odds ratio favoring linkage. The odds ratio favoring linkage is defined as the likelihood that two loci are *linked* at a specified recombination (θ) vs. the likelihood that the two loci are *not linked*. A LOD score of +3, which indicates a probability in favor of linkage of 1,000 to 1, establishes linkage between two loci, and a LOD score of -2, indicating a probability against linkage of 100 to 1, is taken to exclude linkage between two loci. LOD scores are usually evaluated over a range of recombination fractions (θ), allowing the genetic distance and the maximum (or peak) probability favoring linkage between two loci to be ascertained. A fuller description of linkage in families with inherited metabolic and endocrine disorders has been previously published (64).

Location of the X-Linked Recessive Hypoparathyroid Gene

The results from linkage analysis in family W (27), among whom isolated hypoparathyroidism had been inherited in an X-linked recessive manner over five generations, are shown in Fig. 10. A total of 50 members (four affected, seven carriers, and 39 unaffected) were studied with 17 X-linked genetic markers, of which 11 were informative. Linkage between hypoparathyroidism and the 4D.8 locus was established (28), with a peak LOD score of 3.82 ($\theta = 0.05$), indicating a probability in favor of linkage in excess of 6,500 to 1. All the other X-linked RFLP loci gave negative or low (i.e., <3) LOD scores, although many of these are also in the distal segment (Xq26–q27) of the long arm of the X chromosome. Thus the gene causing X-linked recessive hypoparathyroidism was mapped to the distal region of the long arm of the X chromosome, band Xq26–q27, where the DNA probe 4D.8 had been previously localized. An analysis of recom-

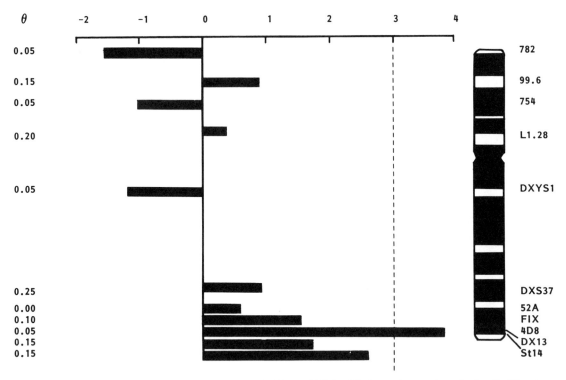

FIG. 10. Results of linkage analysis obtained with 11 X-linked informative probes in family W, who suffer from X-linked recessive hypoparathyroidism (27). The *bar* presents the peak LOD score between hypoparathyroidism and the genetic marker, whose position is shown on the X chromosome, while θ is the recombination fraction at which the peak LOD score was obtained. A significant peak LOD score, in excess of +3, established linkage between hypoparathyroidism and the locus 4D.8, thereby mapping the X-linked recessive hypoparathyroid gene to Xq26-q27.

bination events within this distal segment of the long arm of the X chromosome helped to localize further the hypoparathyroid locus (28). The pedigree shown in Fig. 11 includes 40 members (29 surviving and 11 deceased) in five generations from family W (27) with genetic marker data. The pedigree is informative for five X-linked RFLP loci, whose order in the region Xq25–Xq28 has been established as Xcen–DXS37–F9–DXS98–DXS52–DXS15–Xqter, and multipoint crosses exist. Individual IV.4 is a carrier mother who is heterozygous for F9, DXS98, DXS52, and DXS15, and the alleles she has inherited from her mother (III.2) and father (III.1) can be ascertained by examination of her mother's (III.2) and unaffected brother's (IV.1) genotypes. Her affected son, V.2, shows segregation of the disease with the alleles (N, a, 3, t), defined, respectively, by the polymorphic loci F9, DXS98, DXS52, and DXS15. Her other affected son, V.1, reveals segregation of the disease with the distal loci DXS98, DXS52, and DXS15 (alleles a, 3, t) but demonstrates recombination between hypoparathyroidism and the proximal locus F9 (allele n*). This observation locates hypoparathyroidism distal to the F9 locus. Analysis of the 11 children of individual II.4 further helps to localize the hypoparathyroid gene. The af-

fected male III.15 shows that, in this branch of the family, hypoparathyroidism is segregating with the alleles (E, a, 3, t). His carrier sister, III.12, is recombinant for hypoparathyroidism and the distal loci DXS52 and DXS15 and for the proximal locus DXS37 but nonrecombinant for DXS98. This observation locates hypoparathyroidism proximal to DXS52 and distal to DXS37. The combined observations of multipoint crossovers from III.12 and V.1 locate hypoparathyroidism distal to F9 and proximal to DXS52, i.e., in the vicinity of DXS98. Examination of the multipoint cross in the unaffected male III.6 locates hypoparathyroidism proximal to DXS98; this individual, who has inherited the alleles [a, 3, t] but has not inherited the disease, demonstrates recombination between hypoparathyroidism and the distal loci DXS98, DXS52, and DXS15 and indicates that the location of hypoparathyroidism is not in the chromosome segment distal to DXS98. Thus the combined observations from all the multipoint crosses suggest that hypoparathyroidism is located distal to F9 and proximal to DXS98. The likelihood of this location of hypoparathyroidism vs. the other possible locations of the disease within the fixed order Xcen–DXS37–F9–DXS98–DXS52–DXS15–Xqter was quantitatively assessed using the LINK-

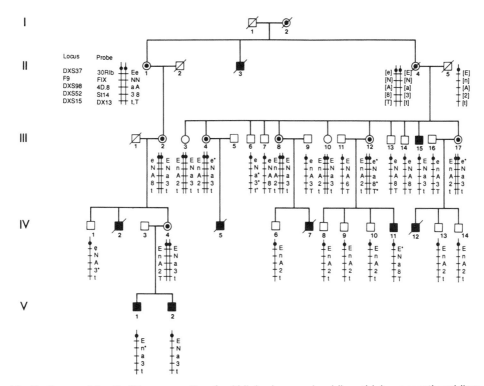

FIG. 11. Pedigree of family W, segregating for X-linked recessive idiopathichypoparathyroidism and distal long arm RFLP loci, whose respective alleles are indicated in parenthesis: DXS37 (Ee), F9 (Nn), DXS98 (Aa), DXS52 (2,3,6,8), and DXS15 (Tt). The loci are shown in the correct order but not the correct distances apart. Individuals are represented as unaffected male (*open squares,*) affected male (*solid squares*), unaffected female (*open circles*), and carrier female (*circles with bullet*). In some females the inheritance of paternal and maternal alleles can be ascertained, and for these females the paternal X chromosome is shown on the left. Recombinants between hypoparathyroidism and each allele are indicated by asterisks. Deduced genotypes are shown in brackets. Subject IV.4 is a carrier mother who is heterozygous for F9, DXS98, DXS52, and DXS15. Her affected son, V.1, is recombinant for hypoparathyroidism and the proximal locus F9 but nonrecombinant for DXS98, DXS52, and DXS15. Subject II.4 is a deceased carrier mother, whose genotype was deduced from her 11 children. Her carrier daughter, III.12, is recombinant for hypoparathyroidism and the distal loci DXS52 and DXS15 and for the proximal locus DXS37 but nonrecombinant for F9 and DXS98, whereas the unaffected son, III.6, is recombinant for hypoparathyroidism and the distal group of loci DXS98, DXS52, and DXS15 and nonrecombinant for the proximal locus DXS37. The minimal number of total recombinants in this pedigree is therefore obtained by locating the hypoparathyroid gene between F9 and DXS98. (Reprinted from ref. 28 with permission.)

MAP program (64), and a location of the hypoparathyroid gene between DXS98 and F9 was favored above all other locations [28]. The odds favoring the location of the hypoparathyroid gene proximal to DXS98 were 32 to 1, and those favoring a location distal to F9 were 17 to 1. More recent studies have further defined the genetic map around the hypoparathyroid gene, and a region of ~400 kb containing this mutant gene has been identified (65). The mapping of the X-linked idiopathic recessive hypoparathyroid gene to Xq26–Xq27 demonstrates that a mutation at a locus distant from the *PTH* gene, the location (30) of which is on the short arm of chromosome 11, is involved in altering parathyroid gland function. A possible role for this X-linked gene in parathyroid gland development is suggested by the neonatal or early-infantile onset of hy-

pocalcemic seizures in the two families. This suggests that the disorder may be due to parathyroid agenesis or hypoplasia, and a careful autopsy of a patient from one family has supported this (61). Thus the X-linked recessive idiopathic hypoparathyroid gene would appear to be important for the embryological development of the parathyroids and the situation may be analogous to that occurring in the DiGeorge syndrome. The precise mapping of the X-linked recessive idiopathic hypoparathyroid gene locus to Xq26–Xq27 represents an important step towards understanding this genetic component of parathyroid gland formation; it has identified the chromosomal segment the characterization of which will further elucidate the factors controlling parathyroid development and calcium homeostasis.

COMPLEX SYNDROMES ASSOCIATED WITH HYPOPARATHYROIDISM

Hypoparathyroidism may occur as part of a complex syndrome, which may be associated either with a congenital developmental anomaly or with an autoimmune syndrome.

Congenital Syndromes

Hypoparathyroidism has been reported to occur in association with the congenital development anomalies of the DiGeorge, the Kenney-Caffey, and the Barakat syndromes and also in syndromes associated with either lymphoedema, or renal dysplasia and deafness or with dysmorphic features and growth failure (Table 1). The inheritance of these congenital disorders, which has been reported in a few patients or a single family, has sometimes not been fully established. However, an autosomal dominant inheritance for the DiGeorge syndrome, which has been investigated by the methods of molecular genetics, is established.

DiGeorge Syndrome

Patients with the DiGeorge syndrome suffer from neonatal hypocalcemic seizures due to PTH deficiency and from severe infections resulting from an immunodeficiency due to thymic aplasia. The disorder arises from a congenital failure in the development of the derivatives of the third and fourth pharyngeal pouches, with resulting absence or hypoplasia of the parathyroids and thymus. In addition, deformities of the ear, nose, mouth, and aortic arch, as well as congenital heart defects may also occur. An autosomal dominant inheritance of DiGeorge syndrome has been observed (66), and an association between the syndrome and an unbalanced translocation and deletion involving 22q11 has also been reported [67,68]. Molecular genetic analysis utilizing in situ hybridization methods and deletion mapping studies have further defined this deletion (69–71). The DiGeorge syndrome deletion breakpoint was found to be proximal to the locus for the immunoglobulin λ polypeptide constant region but distal to the locus for the DNA probe D22S9, which was also found to be deleted in some patients (72). Analysis of the parental origin of the 22q11 unbalanced translocation revealed that imprinting does not play an important role in the pathogenesis of the DiGeorge syndrome (73). However, in some patients, deletion of another locus on chromosome 10p may also be involved in the DiGeorge syndrome (74,75). This mapping of the DiGeorge syndrome locus will help in characterizing the gene, which may resemble a homeobox gene as indicated by recent studies in the mouse (76).

The homeobox genes are a group of genes that specify the body plans of invertebrates, e.g., *Drosophila*, and in all likelihood vertebrates. In *Drosophila* these homeobox genes specify the identity of cells within each parasegment. The function of the corresponding genes in man and mouse is not known, but, as the order of these genes on the chromosomes of *Drosophila*, man, and mouse is the same, and because this gene order reflects the order of the anterior boundaries of gene expression along the anteroposterior body axis of the early embryos of all three species, it would appear that these homeobox genes are equally important in mammalian development. In man and mouse this set of 30 or more genes is known collectively as the *HOX* genes, and they are distributed in the genome in four separate linkage groups, which may have arisen during chordate evolution as the result of two duplications of chromosomal segments (77). The homeobox genes of *Drosophila* encode transcription factors that share a DNA binding motif, and these genes act as master switches directing the course of morphogenic development of each segment. As the human and mouse genes share similar homeobox sequences, the HOX proteins are thought to function also as transcriptional factors participating in the specification of regional information in the early mammalian embryo. In order to determine the genetic function of some of the *HOX* genes in the mouse, specific mutations have been induced by the use of gene targeting methods in embryo-derived stem (ES) cells. Disruption of the *hox 1.5* gene resulted in an abnormal phenotype, which resembled the DiGeorge syndrome (76). Mice that were homozygous for the mutation in *hox 1.5* died in the neonatal period and were found to be athymic and aparathyroid together with a wide range of throat abnormalities and a reduction in the mass of the thyroid and submaxillary tissue. In addition, these homozygous mice often suffered from defects of the heart and arteries as well as craniofacial abnormalities. Mice that were heterozygous were phenotypically normal. Thus the phenotype of the mice with homozygous mutations of the *hox 1.5* gene was very similar to the human DiGeorge syndrome, and this suggests that a *HOX* gene may be involved in the pathogenesis of the DiGeorge syndrome. However, the human syndrome is autosomal dominant, whereas the mouse syndrome is autosomal recessive, and the known location of the human *hox 1.5* gene to chromosome 7 makes it unlikely that the human *hox 1.5* gene is involved in the DiGeorge syndrome, which is associated with deletions and translocations of chromosome 22q11. It is important to note that most patients with the DiGeorge syndrome are karyotypically normal, and it is possible that the DiGeorge syndrome may result from mutations in separate genes. Additional studies of the human and mouse syndromes will help to elucidate this and a possible common developmental pathway.

Kenney-Caffey Syndrome

Hypoparathyroidism has been reported to occur in >50% of patients with the Kenney-Caffey syndrome, in which hypoparathyroidism is associated with short stature, osteosclerosis and cortical thickening of the long bones, delayed closure of the anterior fontanel, basal ganglia calcification, nanophthalmos, and hyperopia (78,79). Parathyroid tissue could not be found in a detailed postmortem examination of one patient (80), suggesting that hypoparathyroidism may be due to an embryological defect of parathyroid development. A molecular genetic analysis using *PTH* gene RFLP analysis revealed no abnormalities (81), and mutations at other loci, for example, in developmental genes, used to be investigated.

Additional Familial Syndromes

Single familial syndromes in which hypoparathyroidism is a component have been reported (Table 1). The inheritance of the disorder in some instances has been established, and molecular genetic analysis of the *PTH* gene has revealed no abnormalities. Thus an association of hypoparathyroidism, sensorineural deafness, and renal dysplasia has been observed in one British family, among whom an autosomal dominant inheritance of the disorder was established [41]. An analysis of the *PTH* gene in this family revealed no abnormalities. Autosomal recessive inheritance of hypoparathyroidism in association with renal insufficiency and developmental delay has been reported in one Asian family (42), and a similar analysis of the PTH gene revealed no abnormalities (35). The occurrence of hypoparathyroidism, nerve deafness, and a steroid-resistant nephrosis leading to renal failure, which has been referred to as the *Barakat syndrome* (82), has been reported in four brothers from one family, and an association of hypoparathyroidism with congenital lymphedema, nephropathy, mitral valve prolapse, and brachytelephalangy has been observed in two brothers from another family (83). Molecular genetic studies have not been reported from these two families. Recently, a novel syndrome in which hypoparathyroidism was associated with severe growth failure and dysmorphic features was reported in 12 patients from Saudi Arabia (84). Consanguinity was noted in 11 of the 12 patients' families, the majority of whom originated from the western province of Saudi Arabia. This syndrome is most likely to be inherited as an autosomal recessive disorder. Molecular genetic investigations of these disorders will help to identify additional genes that regulate the development of the parathyroid glands.

Pluriglandular Autoimmune Hypoparathyroidism

Hypoparathyroidism may occur in association with moniliasis and autoimmune Addison's disease, and the disorder has been referred to either as the autoimmune polyendocrinopathy–candidiasis–ectodermal dystrophy (APECED) syndrome or as the polyglandular autoimmune type 1 syndrome (85). Additional features of the syndrome include pernicious anaemia, hypothyroidism, and occasionally alopecia or vitiligo. A genetic analysis of 58 patients in 42 families indicated autosomal recessive inheritance of the disorder (86), which has a high incidence in Finland. In addition, the disorder has been reported to have a high incidence among Iranian Jews (87), though the occurrence of candidiasis was lower among the Iranian Jews. An association between hypoparathyroidism and the *HLA* loci, which are located on the short arm of chromosome 6 and which are associated with some autoimmune disorders, has not been established, and the molecular basis of hypoparathyroidism in this syndrome remains to be elucidated.

CONCLUSIONS

Recent advances in molecular biology and cytogenetics have made it possible to localize, clone, and characterize some of the genetic abnormalities that result in the hypoparathyroid disorders. Thus mutations of the gene encoding PTH have been demonstrated to be associated with some forms of autosomal dominant and autosomal recessive isolated hypoparathyroidism, and the detection of non-tissue specific transcription of the *PTH* gene in lymphocytes has enabled abnormalities in mRNA processing to be investigated. In addition, the locations for two genes that regulate the embryological development of the parathyroids have been identified. Thus the X-linked recessive hypoparathyroid gene has been mapped to Xq26–q27 and that for the DiGeorge syndrome has been mapped to 22q11. The identification of additional clinical developmental anomalies associated with hypoparathyroidism, together with the recent advances in molecular genetics, provides a unique opportunity to elucidate the pathogenesis of these disorders of calcium homeostasis.

ACKNOWLEDGMENTS

The author is grateful to the U. K. Medical Research Council (CMRC) for support, to D.B. Parkinson (MRC PhD student) for some of the illustrations, to

Dr. M.P. Whyte (St. Louis, MO) for his encouragement and support, and to Ms. Lesley Sargeant for typing the manuscript.

REFERENCES

1. Thakker RV. The molecular genetics of the multiple endocrine neoplasia syndromes. *Clin Endocrinol* 1993:38:1–14.
2. Sinclair AH, Berta P, Palmer MS, et al. A gene from the human sex-determining region encodes a protein with homology to a conserved DNA-binding motif. *Nature* 1990;346:240–244.
3. Gubbay J, Collignon J, Koopman P, et al. A gene mapping to the sex-determining region of the mouse Y chromosome is a member of a novel family of embryonically expressed genes. *Nature* 1990;346:245–250.
4. Koopman P, Gubbay J, Vivian N, Goodfellow P, Lovell-Badge R. Male development of chromosomally female mice transgenic for *Sry. Nature* 1991;351:117–121.
5. Grieco M, Santoro M, Berlingieri MT, et al. PTC is a novel rearranged form of the ret proto-oncogene and is frequently detected *in vivo* in human thyroid papillary carcinomas. *Cell* 1990;60:557–563.
6. Herrmann MA, Hay ID, Bartelt DH Jr, et al. Cytogenetic and molecular genetic studies of follicular and papillary thyroid cancers. *J Clin Invest* 1991;88:1596–1604.
7. Pierotti MA, Santoro M, Jenkins RB, et al. Characterization of an inversion on the long arm of chromosome 10 juxtaposing D10S170 and RET and creating the oncogenic sequence RET/PTC. *Proc Natl Acad Sci USA* 1992;89:1616–1620.
8. Sozzi G, Bongarzone I, Miozzo M, et al. Cytogenetic and molecular genetic characterization of papillary thyroid carcinomas. *Genes Chromosomes Cancer* 1992;5:212–218.
9. van den Ouweland AMW, Dreesen JCFM, Verdijk M, et al. Mutations in the vasopressin type 2 receptor gene *(AVPR2)* associated with nephrogenic diabetes insipidus. *Nature Genet* 1992;2:99–102.
10. Pan Y, Metzenberg A, Das S, Jing B, Gitschier J. Mutations in the V2 vasopressin receptor gene are associated with X-linked nephrogenic diabetes insipidus. *Nature Genet* 1992;2:103–106.
11. Franco B, Guioli S, Pragliola A, et al. A gene deleted in Kallmann's syndrome shares homology with neural cell adhesion and axonal path-finding molecules. *Nature* 1991;353:529–536.
12. Legouis R, Hardelin JP, Levilliers J, et al. The candidate gene for the X-linked Kallman syndrome encodes a protein related to adhesion molecules. *Cell* 1991;67:423–435.
13. Hilbert P, Lindpainter K, Beckmann JS, et al. Chromosomal mapping of two genetic loci associated with blood-pressure regulation in hereditary hypertensive rats. *Nature* 1991;353:521–529.
14. Todd JA, Aitman TJ, Cornall RJ, et al. Genetic analysis of autoimmune type 1 diabetes mellitus in mice. *Nature* 1991;351:542–547.
15. Cornall RJ, Prins J-B, Todd JA, et al. Type 1 diabetes in mice is linked to the interleukin-1 receptor and *Lsh/Ity/Bcg* genes on chromosome 1. *Nature* 1991;353:262–265.
16. Julier C, Hyer RN, Davies J, et al. Insulin-IGF2 region on chromosome 11p encodes a gene implicated in HLA-DR4-dependent diabetes susceptibility. *Nature* 1991;354:155–159.
17. Froguel P, Vaxillaire M, Sun F, et al. Close linkage of glucokinase locus on chromosome 7p to early-onset non-insulin-dependent diabetes mellitus. *Nature* 1992;356:162–164.
18. Ruddle FH. The William Allan Memorial Award Address: reverse genetics and beyond. *Am J Hum Genet* 1984;36:944–953.
19. Collins FS. Positional cloning: let's not call it reverse any more. *Nature Genet* 1992;1:3–6.
20. Thakker RV, Bouloux P, Wooding C, et al. Association of parathyroid tumors in multiple endocrine neoplasia type 1 with loss of alleles on chromosome 11. *N Engl J Med* 1989;321:218–224.
21. Thakker RV. Molecular genetics of mineral metabolic disorders. *J Inher Metab Dis* 1992;15:592–609.
22. Barr DGD, Prader A, Esper U, Rampini S, Marrian VJ, Forfar JO. Chronic hypoparathyroidism in two generations. *Helv Paediatr Acta* 1971;26:507–521.
23. Ahn TG, Antonarakis SE, Kronenberg HM, Igarashi T, Levine MA. Familial isolated hypoparathyroidism: a molecular genetic analysis of 8 families with 23 affected persons. *Medicine* 1986;65:73–81.
24. Bronsky D, Kiamlko RT, Waldstein SS. Familial idiopathic hypoparathyroidism. *J Clin Endocrinol Metab* 1968;28:61–65.
25. Parkinson DB, Thakker RV. A donor splice site mutation in the parathyroid hormone gene is associated with autosomal recessive hypoparathyroidism. *Nature Genet* 1992;1:149–152.
26. Peden VH. True idiopathic hypoparathyroidism as a sex-linked recessive trait. *Am J Hum Genet* 1960;12:323–337.
27. Whyte MP, Weldon VV. Idiopathic hypoparathyroidism presenting with seizures during infancy: X-linked recessive inheritance in a large Missouri kindred. *J Pediatr* 1981;99:608–611.
28. Thakker RV, Davies KE, Whyte MP, Wooding C, O'Riordan JLH. Mapping the gene causing X-linked recessive idiopathic hypoparathyroidism to Xq26-Xq27 by linkage studies. *J Clin Invest* 1990;86:40–45.
29. McKusick VA. *Mendelian inheritance in man.* Baltimore: John Hopkins University Press, 1988.
30. Naylor SL, Sakaguchi AY, Szoka P, et al. Human parathyroid hormone gene (PTH) is on short arm of chromosome 11. *Somat Cell Genet* 1983;9:609–616.
31. Keutmann HT, Sauer MM, Hendy GN, O'Riordan JLH, Potts JT Jr. Complete amino acid sequence of human parathyroid hormone. *Biochemistry* 1978;12:5723–5729.
32. Arnold A, Horst SA, Gardella TJ, Baba H, Levine MA, Kronenberg HM. Mutation of the signal peptide-encoding region of the preproparathyroid hormone gene in familial isolated hypoparathyroidism. *J Clin Invest* 1990;86:1084–1087.
33. Schmidtke J, Pape B, Krengel U, et al. Restriction fragment length polymorphisms at the human parathyroid hormone gene locus. *Hum Genet* 1984;67:428–431.
34. Miric A, Levine MA. Analysis of the preproPTH gene by denaturing gradient gel electrophoresis in familial isolated hypoparathyroidism. *J Clin Endocrinol Metab* 1992;74:509–516.
35. Parkinson DB, Shaw NJ, Himsworth RL, Thakker RV. Parathyroid hormone gene analysis in autosomal hypoparathyroidism using an intragenic tetranucleotide (AAAT)n polymorphism. *Hum Genet* 1993;91:281–284.
36. Cooper DN, Schmidtke J. DNA restriction fragment length polymorphisms and heterozygosity in the human genome. *Hum Genet* 1984;66:1–16.
37. Thakker RV, Ponder BAJ. Multiple endocrine neoplasia. In: Sheppard MC, ed. *Clinical endocrinology and metabolism,* Vol. 2, No. 4. London: Bailliere Tindall, 1988;1031–1067.
38. Southern EM. Detection of specific sequences among DNA fragments separated by gel electrophoresis. *J Mol Biol* 1975;98:503–517.
39. Weber JL, May PE. Abundant class of human DNA polymorphisms which can be typed using the polymorphisms which can be typed using the polymerase chain reaction. *Am J Hum Genet* 1989;44:388–396.
40. Schmidtke J, Kruse K, Pape B, Sippell G. Exclusion of close linkage between parathyroid hormone gene and a mutant gene locus causing idiopathic hypoparathyroidism. *J Med Genet* 1986;23:217–219.
41. Bilous RW, Murty G, Parkinson DB, et al. Autosomal dominant familial hypoparathyroidism, sensorineural deafness and renal dysplasia. *N Engl J Med* 1992;327:1069–1084.
42. Shaw NJ, Haigh D, Lealmann GT, Karbani G, Brocklebank JT, Dillon MJ. Autosomal recessive hypoparathyroidism with renal insufficiency and development delay. *Arch Dis Childhood* 1991;66:1191–1194.
43. Breathnach R, Benoist C, O'Hare K, Gannon F, Chambon P. Ovalbumin gene: evidence for a leader sequence in mRNA and DNA sequences at the exon-intron boundaries. *Proc Natl Acad Sci USA* 1978;75:4853–4857.
44. Mount SM. A catalogue of splice junction sequences. *Nucleic Acids Res* 1982;10:459–472.
45. Lewin B. Alternatives for splicing: recognizing the ends of introns. *Cell* 1980;22:324–326.

46. Lerner MR, Boyle JA, Mount SM, Wolin SL, Steitz JA. Are snRNPs involved in splicing? *Nature* 1980;283:220–224.
47. Rogers J, Wall R. A mechanism for RNA splicing. *Proc Natl Acad Sci USA* 1980;77:1877–1879.
48. Wieringa B, Meyer F, Reiser J, Weissmann C. Unusual splice sites revealed by mutagenic inactivation of an authentic splice site of the rabbit β-globin gene. *Nature* 1983;301:38–43.
49. Weatherall DJ, Clegg JB. Thalassemia revisited. *Cell* 1982; 29:7–9.
50. Treisman R, Proudfoot NJ, Shander M, Maniatis T. A single-base change at a splice site in a β-thalassaemic gene causes abnormal RNA splicing. *Cell* 1982;29:903–911.
51. Talerico M, Berget SM. Effect of 5' splice site mutations on splicing of the preceding intron. *Mol Cell Biol* 1990;10:6299–6305.
52. Kuo H-C, Nasim F-UH, Grabowski PJ. Control of alternative splicing by the differential binding of U1 small nuclear ribonucleoprotein particle. *Science* 1991;251:1045–1050.
53. Parkinson DB, Thakker RV. Illegitimate transcription of the parathyroid hormone gene in lymphocytes from normal and hypoparathyroid individuals. In: Cohn DV, Glorieux FH, Martin TJ, eds. *Calcium regulation and bone metabolism. Basic and clinical aspects.* London: Elsevier Science Publishers, 1992;41–45.
54. Sarkar G, Sommer SS. Access to a messenger RNA sequence or its protein product is not limited by tissue or species specificity. *Science* 1989;244:331–334.
55. Chelly J, Concordet J-P, Kaplan J-C, Kahn A. Illegitimate transcription: transcription of any gene in any cell type. *Proc Natl Acad Sci USA* 1989;86:2617–2621.
56. Berg L-P, Wieland K, Millar DS, et al. Detection of a novel point mutation causing haemophilia A by PCR/direct sequencing of ectopically-transcribed factor VIII mRNA. *Hum Genet* 1990;85:655–658.
57. Chelly J, Kaplan J-C, Maire P, Gautron S, Kahn A. Transcription of the dystrophin gene in human muscle and non-muscle tissues. *Nature* 1988;333:858–860.
58. Schloesser M, Slomski R, Wagner M, et al. Characterization of pathological dystrophin transcripts from the lymphocytes of a muscular dystrophy carrier. *Mol Biol Med* 1990;7:519–523.
59. Kozak M. The scanning model for translation: an update. *J Cell Biol* 1989;108:229–241.
60. Emr SD, Hall MN, Silhavy TJ. A mechanism of protein localisation: the signal hypothesis and bacteria. *J Cell Biol* 1980;86:701–711.
61. Whyte MP, Kim GS, Kosanovich M. Absence of parathyroid tissue in sex-linked recessive hypoparathyroidism. *J Pediatr* 1986;109:915.
62. Morton NE. Sequential tests for the detection of linkage. *Am J Hum Genet* 1955;7:277–318.
63. Ott J. Estimation of the recombination fraction in human pedigrees: efficient computation of the likelihood for human linkage studies. *Am J Hum Genet* 1974;26:588–597.
64. Thakker RV, O'Riordan JLH. Inherited forms of rickets and osteomalacia. In: Martin TJ, ed. *Clinical endocrinology and metabolism.* Vol. 2, No. 1, *Metabolic bone disease.* London: Balliere Tindall, 1988;157–191.
65. Thakker RV, Wooding C, Parkinson DB, Blake D, Whyte MP, Davies KE. Linkage analysis of three cloned DNA sequences, DXS294, CDR and DXS105, in X-linked recessive hypoparathyroid families. *Cytogenet Cell Genet* 1992;58:2087.
66. Rohn RD, Leffell MS, Leadem P, Johnson D, Rubio T, Emanuel BS. Familial third-fourth pharyngeal pouch syndrome with apparent autosomal dominant transmission. *J Pediatr* 1984;105:47–51.
67. de la Chapelle A, Herra R, Koivisto M, Aula P. A deletion in chromosome 22 can cause Di George syndrome. *Hum Genet* 1981;57:253–256.
68. Kelley RI, Zackai FH, Emmanuel BS, Kistenmacher M, Greenberg F, Punnett HH. The association of the Di George anomalad with partial monosomy of chromosome 22. *J Pediatr* 1982;101:197–200.
69. Cannizzaro LA, Emmanuel BS. In situ hybridisation and translocation breakpoint mapping. II Di George syndrome with partial monosomy of chromosome 22. *Cytogenet Cell Genet* 1985;39:179–183.
70. Fibison WJ, Budarf M, McDermid H, Greenberg F, Emanuel BS. Molecular studies of Di George syndrome. *Am J Hum Genet* 1990;46:888–895.
71. Scambler PJ, Carey AH, Wyse RKH, Roach S, Dumanski JP, Nordenskjold M, Williamson R. Microdeletions within 22q11 associated with sporadic and familial Di George syndrome. *Genomics* 1991;10:201–206.
72. Carey AH, Kelly D, Halford S, et al. Molecular genetic study of the frequency of monosomy 22q11 in DiGeorge syndrome. *Am J Hum Genet* 1992;51:964–970.
73. Driscoll DA, Budarf ML, Emanuel BS. A genetic etiology for DiGeorge syndrome: consistent deletions and microdeletions of 22q11. *Am J Hum Genet* 1992;50:924–933.
74. Monaco G, Pignata C, Rossi E, Mascellaro O, Cocozza S, Ciccimarra F. DiGeorge anomaly associated with 10p deletion. *Am J Med Genet* 1991;39:215–216.
75. Lai MMR, Scriven PN, Ball C, Berry AC. Simultaneous partial monosomy 10p and trisomy 5q in a case of hypoparathyroidism. *J Med Genet* 1992;29:586–588.
76. Chisaka O, Capecchi MR. Regionally restricted developmental defects resulting from targeted disruption of the mouse homeobox gene hox-1.5. *Nature* 1991;350:473–479.
77. Kappen C, Schughart K, Ruddle FH. Two steps in the evolution of *Antennapedia*-class vertebrate homeobox genes. *Proc Natl Acad Sci USA* 1989;86:5459–5463.
78. Fanconi S, Fischer JA, Wieland P, et al. Kenny syndrome: evidence for idiopathic hypoparathyroidism in two patients and for abnormal parathyroid hormone in one. *J Pediatr* 1986;109:469–475.
79. Franceschini P, Testa A, Bogetti G, et al. Kenny-Caffey syndrome in two sibs born to consanguineous parents: evidence for an autosomal recessive variant. *Am J Med Genet* 1992; 42:112–116.
80. Boynton JR, Pheasant TR, Johnson BL, Levin DB, Streeten BW. Ocular findings in Kenny's syndrome. *Arch Ophthalmol* 1979;97:896–900.
81. Bergada I, Schiffrin A, Abu Srair H, et al. Kenny syndrome: description of additional abnormalities and molecular studies. *Hum Genet* 1988;80:39–42.
82. Barakat AY, D'Albora JB, Martin MM, Jose PA. Familial nephrosis, nerve deafness, and hypoparathyroidism. *J Pediatr* 1977;91:61–64.
83. Dahlberg PJ, Borer WZ, Newcomer KL, Yutuc WR. Autosomal or X-linked recessive syndrome of congenital lymphedema, hypoparathyroidism, nephropathy, prolapsing mitral valve, and brachytelephalangy. *Am J Med Genet* 1983;16:99–104.
84. Sanjad SA, Sakati NA, Abu-Osba YK, Kaddoura R, Milner RD. A new syndrome of congenital hypoparathyroidism, severe growth failure, and dysmorphic features. *Arch Dis Child* 1991;66:193–196.
85. Ahonen P, Myllarniemi S, Sipila I, Perheentupa J. Clinical variation of autoimmune polyendocrinopathy-candidiasis-ectodermal dystrophy (APECED) in a series of 68 patients. *N Engl J Med* 1990;322:1829–1836.
86. Ahonen P. Autoimmune polyendocrinopathy-candidosis-ectodermal dystrophy (APECED): autosomal recessive inheritance. *Clin Genet* 1985;27:535–542.
87. Zlotogora J, Shapiro MS. Polyglandular autoimmune syndrome type 1 among Iranian Jews. *J Med Genet* 1992;29:824–826.

The Parathyroids, edited by J.P. Bilezikian,
M.A. Levine, and R. Marcus. Raven Press, Ltd.,
New York © 1994.

CHAPTER 46

Pseudohypoparathyroidism

Clinical, Biochemical, and Molecular Features

Michael A. Levine, William F. Schwindinger, Robert W. Downs, Jr., and
Arnold M. Moses

The term *pseudohypoparathyroidism* (PHP) describes a heterogeneous syndrome characterized by biochemical hypoparathyroidism (i.e., hypocalcemia and hyperphosphatemia), increased plasma levels of parathyroid hormone (PTH), and unresponsiveness of target tissues to the biological actions of PTH. Thus PHP differs substantially and fundamentally from true hypoparathyroidism, in which hypocalcemia is associated with low or undetectable levels of PTH and target tissue responsiveness.

In the initial, classical description of PHP, Fuller Albright and his associates (1) focused on the failure of patients with this syndrome to show either a calcemic or a phosphaturic response to administered parathyroid extract. These observations provided the basis for the hypothesis that biochemical hypoparathyroidism in PHP is due not to a deficiency of PTH but rather to resistance of the target organs, bone and kidney, to PTH.

PTH activates its target cells by binding to specific receptors located on the external surface of the cell plasma membrane. The recent cloning of cDNAs en-

coding an opossum kidney PTH receptor (2) and a rat bone PTH receptor (3) indicates that the PTH receptor is a member of the superfamily of receptors predicted to contain seven transmembrane spanning domains and that are coupled by G proteins to intracellular signal effector molecules (Fig. 1). Agonist binding to the cloned PTH receptor expressed in COS-7 cells leads to stimulation of adenylyl cyclase and phosphatidyl inositol turnover (3), implying that the PTH receptor can be linked to several different G proteins (e.g., Gs and a G protein linked to phospholipase C) to activate multiple second messengers, including cyclic adenosine monophosphate (cAMP) (4,5), inositol 1,4,5-trisphosphate, and diacylglycerol (DAG) (6,7), and cytosolic calcium (8–11) (see the chapter by Coleman et al.). The best characterized mediator of PTH action is cAMP, which rapidly activates protein kinase A (12). The relevant target proteins that are phosphorylated by protein kinase A and the precise mode(s) of action of these proteins remain uncharacterized, though proteins that activate genes responsive to cAMP and ion channel proteins are strong candidates. The intracellular accumulation of cAMP triggers a biochemical chain reaction that begins with phosphorylation of specific protein substrates by cAMP-activated protein kinase A and ultimately concludes with the physiologic response of the cell to agonist recognition (Fig. 2). In contrast to the well-recognized biologic effects of cAMP in PTH target tissues, the physiological importance of metabolites of phosphatidylinositol and intracellular calcium as PTH-induced second messengers has not yet been established.

In addition to the clinical and biochemical features of hypoparathyroidism, the patients described by Al-

M. A. Levine: Departments of Medicine and Pathology, The Johns Hopkins University School of Medicine, Baltimore, Maryland 21205.

W. F. Schwindinger: Department of Medicine, The Johns Hopkins University School of Medicine, Baltimore, Maryland 21205.

R. W. Downs: Department of Medicine, Medical College of Virginia, Virginia Commonwealth University, Richmond, Virginia 23298.

A. M. Moses: Department of Medicine, University Hospital, State University of New York, Syracuse, New York 13210.

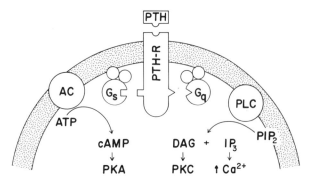

FIG. 1. Cell surface receptors for PTH are coupled to two classes of G proteins. Gs mediates stimulation of adenylyl cyclase (AC) and the production of cAMP, which in turn activates protein kinase A (PKA). Gq stimulates phospholipase C (PLC) to form the second messengers inositol-(1,4,5)-triphosphate (IP$_3$) and diacylglycerol (DAG) from membrane bound phosphatidylinositol-(4,5)-biphosphate; IP$_3$ increases intracellular calcium (Ca^{2+}), and DAG stimulates protein kinase C (PKC) activity. Each G protein consists of a unique α chain and a βγ dimer.

bright et al. exhibited a peculiar physical appearance, subsequently referred to as Albright's hereditary osteodystrophy (AHO), which is characterized by distinctive skeletal and developmental defects, which are described in detail below. The relationship between the biochemical abnormalities (hypocalcemia and hyperphosphatemia) and the unusual physical features of AHO could not be explained by Albright et al. or by anyone else. Indeed, in certain families, several af-

fected members may show both AHO and PTH resistance, whereas other family members, with so-called pseudopseudohypoparathyroidism (pseudo-PHP), may have AHO without evidence of hypocalcemia, PTH resistance, or any other dysfunction.

Recently, diagnostic classification of PHP has become even more complex with reports that clearly document individuals and families with PTH resistance and biochemical hypoparathyroidism but without any of the features of AHO (13). A classification of the many different forms of PHP is given in Table 1.

PATHOPHYSIOLOGY

Characterization of the molecular basis for PHP began with the observation that cAMP mediates many of the actions of PTH on kidney and bone and that administration of biologically active PTH to normal subjects leads to a significant increase in the urinary excretion of nephrogenous cAMP and phosphate (14). The PTH infusion test remains the most reliable test available for the diagnosis of PHP and allows distinction between the several variants of the syndrome (Fig. 2). Patients with PHP type I fail to show an appropriate increase in urinary excretion of both cAMP and phosphate (14), suggesting that an abnormality in the renal PTH receptor–adenylyl cyclase complex that produces cAMP is the basis for impaired PTH responsiveness. Subsequent studies by Bell et al. (15), in

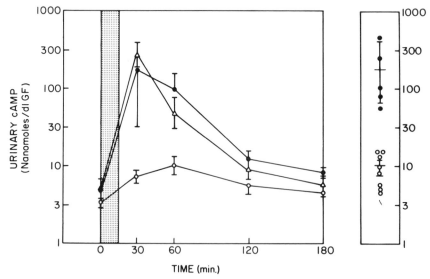

FIG. 2. Urinary cAMP excretion in response to an infusion of bovine parathyroid extract (300 USP units). The peak response in normal subjects (*open triangles*) as well as those with pseudo (*solid circles*) PHP is 50–100-fold times the basal level. Subjects with PHP type Ia (*open circles*) or PHP type Ib (not shown) show only a two- to fivefold increase. Urinary cAMP is expressed as nanomoles per 100 milliliters GF, U$_{cAMP}$ (nanomoles per 100 milliliters GF) = U$_{cAMP}$ (nanomoles/dl) × S$_{Cre}$ (mg/dL)/U$_{Cre}$ (mg/dL). (Reprinted from ref. 32 with permission.)

TABLE 1. *Salient features of the various forms of pseudohypoparathyroidism*

	PHP type Ia	PseudoPHP	PHP type Ib	PHP type Ic	PHP type II
Physical appearance	AHO; although physical findings may be subtle or (rarely) absent		Normal	AHO	Normal
Response to PTH					
Urine cAMP	Defective	Normal	Defective	Defective	Normal
Urine phosphorous	Defective	Normal	Defective	Defective	Defective
Serum calcium level	Low or (rarely) normal	Normal	Low	Low	Low
Hormone resistance	Generalized	Absent	Limited to PTH target tissues	Generalized	Limited to PTH target tissues
Gsα activity	Reduced		Normal	Normal	Normal
Inheritance	Autosomal dominant		Autosomal Dominant	Autosomal Dominant	Sporadic
Molecular defect	Mutations of the Gsα gene		PTH receptor (presumed)	Unknown; possibly adenylyl cyclase	Unknown; possibly cAMP target(s)

which administration of dibutyryl cAMP to patients with PHP type I produced a phosphaturic response, added further support for this theory and confirmed that the renal response mechanism to cAMP was intact. These studies indicate that proximal renal tubule cells fail to respond appropriately to PTH. In contrast, cells in other regions of the kidney appear to be responsive to PTH. Evidence in favor of at least partial responsiveness of the kidney to PTH comes from the observation that the degree of hypercalciuria in patients with PHP type I is less marked than in patients with hormonopenic hypoparathyroidism when the patients are compared after normalization of blood calcium levels in each group with high-dose vitamin D and oral calcium supplements (16,17). These results indicate that calcium reabsorption in the distal tubule is responsive to the high circulating levels of PTH in subjects with PHP type I and imply that other second messengers (e.g., cytosolic calcium or DAG) may mediate PTH action in these cells.

Subjects with another variant of the disorder, PHP type II, show a normal increase in urinary cAMP excretion to infused PTH but fail to demonstrate an appropriate phosphaturic response (18). Thus PHP type II results from a biochemical defect that is distal to the PTH-stimulated generation of cAMP. Although PHP type I is a rare disorder, PHP type II is even more uncommon.

Target organ resistance to PTH results in an inadequate flow of calcium into the extracellular fluid and deficient phosphate excretion by the kidney. Hypocalcemia results from impaired mobilization of calcium from bone, reduced intestinal absorption of calcium, and increased urinary calcium loss. Of the three defects, the diminished movement of calcium out of bone stores into the extracellular fluid probably plays the greatest role in producing hypocalcemia.

It has been generally assumed that bone cells in patients with PHP type I are innately resistant to PTH, but this remains unproven. In fact, cultured bone cells from a patient with PHP type I have been found to increase intracellular cAMP levels normally in response to PTH in vitro (19). That bone cells are unresponsive to PTH is inferred largely from the observation that these patients are hypocalcemic and that the plasma calcium level does not increase when PTH is administered. However, clinical, roentgenographic, or histologic evidence of increased bone turnover and demineralization (Fig. 3) is common in patients with PHP type I. One possible explanation for variable skeletal responsiveness to PTH is the existence of two distinct cellular systems in bone upon which PTH exerts action: the remodeling system and the mineral mobilization or homeostatic system. The bone remodeling system appears to be responsive to PTH in patients with PHP type I, whereas the homeostatic system appears to be nonresponsive. One explanation for this variability may reside in the lesser dependence of the remodeling system on normal 1,25-dihydroxyvitamin D [1,25-(OH)$_2$D] levels. Plasma levels of 1,25-(OH)$_2$D are reduced in hypocalcemic patients with PHP type I (20), and this could account for the concurrence of hypocalcemia and osteitis fibrosa cystica in these patients. Hypocalcemia leads to a compensatory overproduction of PTH, which may eventually overcome the 1,25-(OH)$_2$D dependency for remodeling but not for PTH-directed calcium mobilization.

A role of 1,25-(OH)$_2$D in modulating the responsiveness of the calcium homeostatic system to PTH is suggested by several observations. First, the calcemic response to PTH is deficient in patients with PHP type I or other hypocalcemic disorders in which plasma levels of 1,25-(OH)$_2$D are low. Moreover, normalization of the plasma calcium level by administration of phys-

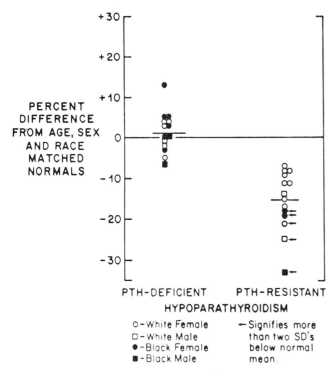

FIG. 3. Percentage difference in bone density in distal radius in patients with hypoparathyroidism and pseudohypoparathyroidism from age-, sex-, and race-matched normal controls. (Reprinted from ref. 72 with permission.)

iologic amounts of 1,25-$(OH)_2D$ or pharmacologic amounts of vitamin D restores calcemic responsiveness (21). Second, patients with PHP type I who have normal serum levels of calcium and 1,25-$(OH)_2D_3$ without vitamin D treatment (so-called normocalcemic PHP) show a normal calcemic response to administered PTH (21). These findings suggest that 1,25-$(OH)_2D$ deficiency is the basis for hypocalcemia and PTH unresponsiveness of the bone homeostatic mechanism in PHP type I and call into question the premise that bone cells are intrinsically resistant to the actions of PTH.

Subjects with PHP type I have increased serum levels of phosphate owing to the failure of PTH to promote phosphate clearance in the kidney. Hypocalcemia per se also contributes to the development of hyperphosphatemia, in that phosphate excretion is impaired by reduced levels of intracellular calcium. Accordingly, restoration of plasma calcium levels to normal by chronic high-dose vitamin D therapy has been noted to reverse the defective phosphaturic response in certain patients with PHP type I, although the urinary cAMP response to administered hormone remains markedly deficient (22). Therefore, persistence of a blunted urinary cAMP response to PTH in PHP type I patients in whom chronic vitamin D therapy is accompanied by normalization of plasma calcium lev-

els and restoration of a phosphaturic response need not imply, as has been at least suggested (22), a dissociation between cAMP production and phosphate clearance.

There are several important metabolic consequences of hyperphosphatemia. It is well recognized that high plasma phosphate levels can lower plasma calcium levels. This occurs both through increasing the rate of deposition of calcium from extracellular fluid into bone and extraossesous tissues and through decreasing the rate of resorption of calcium from bone. Furthermore, elevated plasma phosphate concentrations and increased levels of inorganic phosphorous in renal cells can reduce activity of renal 1α-hydroxylase and impair production of 1,25-$(OH)_2D$. This effect may be of significance equal to or greater than that of the defective renal cAMP response to PTH as a cause of deficient production of 1,25-$(OH)_2D$. It is therefore conceivable that reduced synthesis of 1,25-$(OH)_2D$ in PHP type I ultimately occurs as a consequence of two defects related to impaired PTH responsiveness: (a) decreased renal phosphate clearance resulting in elevated plasma phosphate levels, which inhibit activity of renal 1α-hydroxylase, and (b) decreased PTH activation of the enzyme.

The overall evidence suggests that the disturbances in calcium, phosphorous, and vitamin D metabolism in most patients with PHP type I result directly or indirectly from reduced responsiveness of both bone and kidney to PTH. Aggressive treatment with calcitriol [1,25-$(OH)_2D$] or other vitamin D analogs leads to improvement in intestinal calcium absorption and bone calcium mobilization, restoration of plasma calcium to normal, and reduction in circulating PTH levels. Thus, although PTH resistance appears to be the proximate biochemical defect, the major abnormalities in mineral metabolism found in patients with PHP type I can be explained largely on the basis of deficiency of circulating 1,25-$(OH)_2D$.

MOLECULAR BASIS OF PARATHYROID HORMONE RESISTANCE

Hormone action may be divided conceptually into prereceptor, receptor, and postreceptor events; defects at each of these steps have been proposed as the basis of hormone resistance in PHP (Fig. 1). A circulating inhibitor of PTH action has been proposed to explain PTH resistance as a prereceptor defect. In PHP type Ib, isolated PTH resistance likely is due to a mutation in the PTH receptor. Postreceptor defects are potentially the most diverse and yet are the best characterized. Patients with the most classical form of PHP, type Ia, are resistant to a variety of hormones that utilize cAMP as a second messenger, due presumably to decreased levels of Gsα, the G protein that couples cell surface receptors to adenylyl cyclase. Patients with PHP type Ic also show resistance to multiple hormones but have apparently normal Gsα activity. Hormone resistance in these subjects may be due to defects in other components of the signal transduction system that are not tissue specific, such as defects in adenylyl cyclase (23). Finally, patients with PHP type II have a normal urinary cAMP response to PTH but fail to generate a phosphaturic response. These subjects may have a defect in protein kinase A, in one of its substrates, or in another PTH signalling pathway (e.g., phospholipase C).

Prereceptor Defect

Several studies have reported an apparent dissociation between plasma levels of endogenous immunoreactive and bioactive PTH in subjects with PHP type I. Despite high circulating levels of immunoreactive PTH, the levels of bioactive PTH in many patients with PHP type I have been found to be within the normal range when measured with highly sensitive renal (24) and metatarsal (25) cytochemical bioassay systems. Furthermore, plasma from many of these patients has been shown to diminish the biological activity of exogenous PTH in these in vitro bioassays (26). Currently, the nature of this putative inhibitor or antagonist remains unknown. The observation that prolonged hypercalcemia can remove or reduce significantly the level of inhibitory activity in the plasma of patients with PHP has suggested that the parathyroid gland may be the source of the inhibitor. In addition, analysis of circulating PTH immunoactivity after fractionation of patient plasma by reversed-phase high-performance liquid chromatography has disclosed the presence of aberrant forms of immunoreactive PTH in many of these patients (27). Although it is conceivable that a PTH inhibitor causes PTH resistance in some patients with PHP, it is more likely that circulating antagonists of PTH action arise as a consequence of the sustained secondary hyperparathyroidism that results from the primary biochemical defect.

Receptor Defect: PHP Type Ib

Some subjects with PHP type I lack features of AHO. These patients typically show hormone resistance that is limited to target organs of PTH (Fig. 2) and have normal Gsα activity (Fig. 4) (28). This form of PHP has been termed *PHP type Ib*. Cultured fibroblasts from subjects with PHP type Ib show deficient cAMP responses to PTH but normal responses to other agonists (29). In some cases, this cellular defect

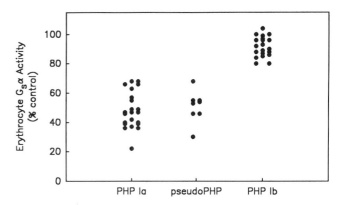

FIG. 4. Gsα activity of erythrocyte membranes. Gsα is quantified in complementation assays with S49 cyc⁻ membranes, which genetically lack Gsα but retain all other components necessary for hormone-response adenylyl cyclase activity. Activity was reduced ~50% in patients with AHO subjects with either PHP type Ia or pseudo-PHP but was normal in patients with PHP type Ib.

can apparently be reversed in vitro by treatment of the cultured fibroblasts with dexamethasone (30). Thus it seems likely that PTH resistance in subjects with PHP type Ib is due to a defect in the receptor for PTH. Although patients with PHP type Ib fail to show a nephrogenous cAMP response to PTH, they often manifest skeletal lesions similar to those that occur in patients with hyperparathyroidism (31). These observations have suggested that at least one intracellular signalling pathway coupled to the PTH receptor may be intact in patients with PHP type Ib.

The molecular basis for reduced PTH receptor activity in PHP type Ib has not been clearly defined. The PTH receptor can couple efficiently to two divergent signal transduction pathways (i.e., adenylyl cyclase and phospholipase C) (Fig. 1). Hence defects in the PTH receptor that uncouple the PTH receptor from adenylyl cyclase but leave intact the ability of the receptor to activate phospholipase C may explain the clinical observations noted above.

Postreceptor Defects: PHP Type Ia

Cell membranes from subjects with AHO have an ~50% reduction in Gs activity (Fig. 4) (32). Most patients with AHO have also been found to have a similar 50% reduction in levels of immunoreactive Gsα (33) and Gsα mRNA (34,35) (Fig. 5). Within a given family, patients may have these features alone, without hormone resistance (pseudo-PHP), or in association with multiple hormone resistance (PHP type Ia).

The observation that some patients with AHO have normal levels of Gsα mRNA first suggested that Gsα deficiency might result from a variety of different mu-

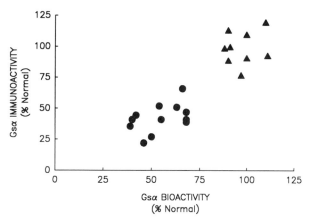

FIG. 5. Comparative analysis of cell membrane Gsα immunoactivity and bioactivity. Cell membranes from AHO patients with Gsα deficiency (*circles*) or normal phenotype with normal Gsα activity [PHP type Ib (*triangles*)] were analyzed. The relative level of immunoactive Gsα protein was determined by quantitative immunoblot analysis using an antisera generated against peptide sequences from exon 12. Results are expressed as a percentage of values obtained from a group of normal subjects. Gsα bioactivity (on the abscissa) was determined by a complementation assay based on the ability of detergent extracts of patient membranes to reconstitute an active adenylyl cyclase in membranes from the S49 cyc⁻ cell line, which genetically lacks Gsα. Gsα bioactivity is expressed as percentage mean activity of control membranes. (Modified from ref. 33 with permission.)

tations (35). The recent identification of heterozygous mutations in the gene encoding Gsα (*GNAS1*) provides confirmation that transmission of defects in the *GNAS1* gene accounts for AHO (Fig. 6). The *GNAS1* gene, located on chromosome 20q13.2→q13.3 (36), contains 13 exons and spans 20 kb (36). Alternative splicing accounts for the production of at least four distinct mRNA species. Inclusion of exon 3 results in the insertion of 15 codons into the mRNA, while use of an alternative splice site in exon 4 results in the insertion of a single additional codon into the mRNA. This gives rise to two Gsα proteins with apparent molecular weights of 45 kDa and two Gsα proteins with apparent molecular weights of 52 kDa (36,37). The alternatively spliced forms of Gsα are expressed in a tissue-specific distribution (38). Biochemical characterization of the short and long forms of Gsα has revealed subtle differences in the binding constant for guanosine diphosphate (GDP), the rate at which the forms are activated by agonist binding, efficiency of adenylyl cyclase stimulation, or the rate of guanosine triphosphate (GTP) hydrolysis. None of these differences appears to be physiologically relevant, however (39–41). Both long and short forms of Gsα can stimulate adenylyl cyclase and open calcium channels (40). Additional complexity in the processing of the *GNAS1* gene may derive from the use of an alternative upstream promoter to

produce a mRNA that has a novel exon spliced to exon 2 (42,43). The use of an alternative promoter provides the potential for greater tissue-specific and developmental regulation of Gsα expression. The deletion of exon 1, which encodes sequences important for GTP binding and interaction with βγ subunits, is predicted to affect dramatically the biological function of Gsα.

Distinct mutations in the *GNAS1* gene, including missense mutations (44–46), point mutations in sequences required for efficient splicing (47), and small deletions (45,47,48), have been found in each kindred studied, implying that new and independent mutations sustain this disorder in the population (Fig. 6). Most patients with AHO have genetic defects that impair the synthesis of Gsα protein and therefore have a Gsα deficiency. In other patients, mutations in the gene encoding Gsα lead to synthesis of dysfunctional proteins (Fig. 6). The first mutation in *GNAS1* that was identified in a patient with AHO altered the initiator ATG codon and led to synthesis of a Gsα protein that was truncated at the amino-terminal end (44). This protein presumably lacks the ability to interact with receptors or adenylyl cyclase. In other cases, missense mutations may selectively impair a specific function of Gsα. A point mutation in exon 13 of the Gsα gene that results in the replacement of Arg³⁸⁵ with His near the carboxy terminus of Gsα has recently been described in one patient with PHP type Ia (Fig. 6) (46). This mutation is located five amino acids upstream from a mutation in Gsα that was previously identified in the S49 murine lymphoma cell line *unc* (49,50). The *unc* mutation (Arg³⁸⁹→Pro) "uncouples" Gsα from cell-surface receptors (51). Similarly, expression studies of the Arg³⁸⁵→His mutation in Gsα indicate that this molecule is also unable to couple cell surface receptors to activation of adenylyl cyclase (52).

In AHO, inherited mutations in the gene encoding Gsα lead to diminished expression or reduced function of the Gsα protein. By contrast, postzygotic mutations that enhance the activity of the Gsα protein are responsible for the McCune-Albright syndrome (53,54). In this syndrome constitutive activation of Gsα leads to the clinical triad of café-au-lait pigmentation, polyostotic fibrous dysplasia, and autonomous hyperfunctioning of multiple endocrine glands. There is a satisfying symmetry in the realization that these two contrasting syndromes, both initially described by Fuller Albright, result from distinct mutations in the same gene.

Postreceptor Defects: PHP Type Ic

Resistance to multiple hormones has been described in several patients with AHO who do not have a demonstrable defect in Gs or Gi (28,55,56). These pa-

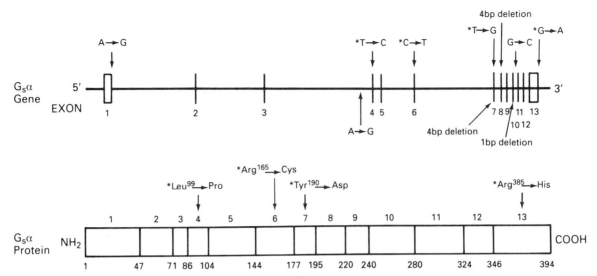

FIG. 6. The Gsα gene and protein. The *GNAS1* gene contains 13 exons (*boxes*) and 12 introns. The large form of the Gsα protein, containing exon 3, is shown below the gene structure. Unique mutations that have been identified in ten AHO kindreds are illustrated. A mutation in exon 1 eliminates the initiator ATG and results in the synthesis of Gsα protein that is truncated at the amino terminus (44). Small deletions in exon 7 (165), exon 8 (45), or exon 10 (47) result in frame shifts that prevent normal protein synthesis. Mutations in intron 3 and intron 10 (47) cause splicing abnormalities. Several missense mutations scattered throughout the molecule result in proteins with amino acid substitutions (45,46).

tients have PHP type Ic. The nature of the lesion in such patients is unclear, but it could be related to some other general component of the receptor–adenylyl cyclase system, such as the catalytic unit (23). Alternatively, these patients could have functional defects of Gs (or Gi) that are not apparent with the assays presently available. On the other hand, they may have a mutation in a more distal component of the signal transduction apparatus, such as the catalytic unit of adenylyl cyclase (Fig. 1) (23).

Postreceptor Defects: PHP Type II

PHP type II is a heterogeneous disorder without a clear genetic or familial basis. In these patients, renal resistance to PTH is manifested by a reduced phosphaturic response to administration of PTH, despite a normal increase in urinary cAMP excretion (18). A similar dissociation between the effects of PTH on generation of cAMP and tubular reabsorption of phosphate has been observed in patients with profound hypocalcemia due to vitamin D deficiency (57). These observations suggest that the PTH receptor–adenylyl cyclase complex functions normally to increase cAMP in response to PTH and are consistent with a model in which PTH resistance arises from an inability of intracellular cAMP to initiate the chain of metabolic events that results in the ultimate expression of PTH action. Although no supportive data are yet available, a defect in cAMP-dependent protein kinase A has been pro-

posed as the basis for this disorder (18). Alternatively, the defect in PHP type II may not reside in an inability to generate a physiological response to intracellular cAMP: a defect in another PTH-sensitive signal transduction pathway may explain the lack of a phosphaturic response. One candidate is the PTH-sensitive phospholipase C pathway that leads to increased concentrations of the intracellular second messengers inositol 1,4,5-trisphosphate and DAG (6,7) and cytosolic calcium (Fig. 1) (8–11).

In some patients with PHP type II, the phosphaturic response to PTH has been restored to normal after serum levels of calcium have been normalized by treatment with calcium infusion or vitamin D therapy (58). These results point to the importance of Ca^{2+} as an intracellular second messenger.

GENETICS

Genetic studies of AHO and other forms of PTH resistance have been hampered by incomplete clinical descriptions of affected patients and inadequate characterization of their biochemical defects. The inheritance of AHO has been controversial. X-linked (59), autosomal dominant (60), and autosomal recessive (61) inheritance of AHO have been proposed. However, the observation of father-to-son transmission of AHO with Gsα deficiency excludes an X-linked mode of inheritance (62). Moreover, the human gene for Gsα *(GNAS1)* has been mapped to chromosome 20 (63).

Thus autosomal dominant inheritance of AHO, including PHP type Ia and pseudo-PHP, is most consistent with the transmission of defects in the Gsα gene.

A striking feature of AHO is the occurrence of subjects with PHP type Ia and pseudo-PHP in the same family, who have identical mutations in the Gsα gene and show similarly reduced levels of Gsα. A comprehensive review of the inheritance of AHO indicates that pseudo-PHP and PHP type Ia do not occur in the same generation. Moreover, subjects with pseudo-PHP appear to have acquired the mutation from their fathers, while subjects with PHP type Ia appear to have acquired the mutation from their mothers (Schwindinger and Levine, unpublished). These observations suggest that parental imprinting may be important in determining the phenotype of subjects with AHO (64). Specifically, if the offspring receive the mutant allele from the father, they will develop pseudo-PHP, while, if they receive the same mutant allele from the mother, they will develop PHP type Ia.

The inheritance of other forms of PHP is less well characterized. Inheritance of PHP type Ib appears to be consistent with an autosomal dominant pattern. PHP type II is typically a sporadic disorder, although one case of familial PHP type II has been reported (65).

CLINICAL FEATURES

Hypocalcemia

The sine qua non of PHP is resistance to the biological effects of PTH, and the major symptoms of PHP are the consequence of reduced concentrations of ionized calcium in blood and extracellular fluid. Hypocalcemia leads to increased neuromuscular excitability, a condition termed *tetany*. Symptoms of tetany include carpopedal spasm, convulsions, paresthesias, muscle cramps, and stridor. Laryngeal spasm occurs most commonly in young children during episodes of severe hypocalcemia. Tetany is potentiated by hypomagnesemia and may be mimicked by hypokalemia. Hypocalcemia may also unmask a previously unsuspected seizure disorder or may greatly aggravate epilepsy. Clinical signs of the neuromuscular irritability associated with latent tetany include the Chvostek and Trousseau signs. Slightly positive reactions to the Chvostek sign may occur in 15% of normal adults. Importantly, both these signs can be absent even in patients with severe hypocalcemia. Although the clinical course of PHP is quite variable, the initial symptoms of neuromuscular irritability typically occur in subjects with PHP at approximately the eighth year of life. Hypocalcemia is not present from birth. A progressive decline in serum calcium and increasing levels of se-

rum phosphate, PTH, and 1,25-$(OH)_2D_3$ have been documented in one child as he advanced from 3 to 3.5 years of age (66). In most older children and in adults, the serum level of 1,25-$(OH)_2D_3$ is low and contributes to development of hypocalcemia (20). Some affected children show few symptoms of tetany, and the diagnosis of PHP is made only later in life. Moreover, some PHP patients may have normal levels of serum calcium without treatment (i.e., normocalcemic PHP) despite PTH resistance (21).

As in other forms of hypoparathyroidism, longstanding hypocalcemia and hyperphosphatemia may lead to soft tissue calcifications in patients with PHP. Posterior subcapsular cataracts develop frequently. Occasionally patients also have calcifications in the heart (67). In most patients, computerized tomography (CT) of the brain reveals calcification of the basal ganglion (68) and frontal lobes.

Skeletal Remodeling

Parathyroid hormone responsiveness of the skeleton appears to be variable in subjects with PHP. In contrast to the well-documented resistance of the kidney to PTH, there is less compelling evidence to support the notion that bone cells are resistant to PTH in PHP. There is a spectrum of bone disease in PHP: some subjects have apparently normal bone, while others have radiological or histological evidence of significant bone resorption (69). Patients with PHP type Ia typically show little or no evidence of diffuse skeletal involvement, while patients with PHP type Ib often demonstrate evidence of osteopenia or hyperparathyroid bone disease, including osteitis fibrosa cystica. Cultured bone cells from one patient with PHP type Ib and osteitis fibrosa cystica were shown to have normal adenylyl cyclase responsiveness to PTH in vitro (19).

Patients with PHP may develop additional abnormalities in bone metabolism, including osteomalacia (69), rickets (70), renal osteodystrophy (71), and osteopenia (72). These skeletal abnormalities result from excessive PTH or deficient 1,25-$(OH)_2D_3$.

Albright Hereditary Osteodystrophy and Developmental Defects

Subjects with AHO manifest a characteristic constellation of developmental defects that includes short stature, obesity, round face, shortening of the digits (brachydactyly), subcutaneous ossification, and dental hypoplasia (Fig. 7) (1,73). Considerable variability occurs in the clinical expression of these features even among affected members of a single family, and all these features are not present in every case (74).

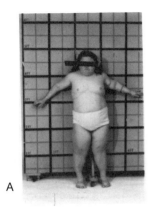
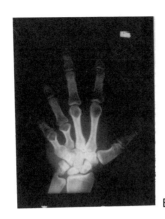
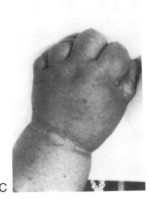
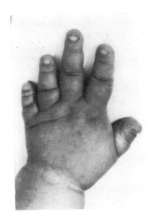

FIG. 7. Typical features of Albright hereditary osteodystrophy. **A:** A young woman with characteristic features of AHO; note the short stature, disproportionate shortening of the limbs, obesity, and round face. **B:** Radiograph of patient's hand showing marked shortening of fourth and fifth metacarpals. **C:** Archibald sign, with dimples in place of knuckles. **D:** Brachydactyly of the hand, note thumb sign and shortening of the fourth and fifth digits.

Although patients with AHO may be of normal height and weight, ~66% of children and ~80% of adults are below the 10th percentile for height. This reflects a disproportionate shortening of the limbs; arm span is less than height in the majority of patients. Obesity is a common feature of AHO, and approximately one-third of all patients with AHO are above the 90th percentile of weight for their age, despite their short stature (Fig. 7A) (75). Patients with AHO typically have a round face, a short neck, and a flattened nasal bridge. Numerous other abnormalities of the head and neck have also been noted. Ocular findings include hypertelorism, strabismus, nystagmus, unequal pupils, diplopia, microphthalmia, and a variety of abnormal findings on funduscopic examination that range from irregular pigmentation to optic atrophy and macular degeneration. Head circumference is above the 90th percentile in a significant minority of children

(75). Dental abnormalities are common in subjects with PHP and include dentin and enamel hypoplasia, short and blunted roots, and delayed or absent tooth eruption (76).

Brachydactyly is the most reliable sign for the diagnosis of AHO and may be symmetrical or asymmetrical and involve one or both hands or feet (Fig. 7C,D). Shortening of the distal phalanx of the thumb is the most common abnormality. This is apparent on physical examination as a thumb in which the ratio of the width of the nail to its length is increased ("Murder's thumb" or "potter's thumb"). Shortening of the metacarpals causes shortening of the digits, particularly the fourth and fifth digits. Shortening of the metacarpals may also be recognized on physical examination as dimpling over the knuckles of a clenched fist (Archibald sign). Often a definitive diagnosis requires careful examination of radiographs of the hands and feet (Fig. 7B). A specific pattern of shortening of the bones in the hand has been identified, in which the distal phalanx of the thumb and third through fifth metacarpals are the most severely shortened (77,78). This may be useful in distinguishing AHO from other unrelated syndromes in which brachydactyly occurs, such as familial brachydactyly, Turner's syndrome, and Klinefelter's syndrome (77).

In addition to brachydactyly, several other skeletal abnormalities are present in AHO. Numerous deformities of the long bones have been reported, including short ulna, bowed radius, deformed elbow or cubitus valgus, coxa vara, coxa valga, genu varum, and genu valgus deformities (75). The most common abnormalities of the skull are hyperostosis frontalis interna and a thickened calvarium. The skeletal abnormalities of AHO may not be apparent until a child is 5 years old (79). Bone age is advanced 2–3 years in the majority of patients (75). Spinal cord compression has also been reported in patients with AHO (80).

Patients with AHO develop heterotopic ossifications of the soft tissues or skin (osteoma cutis) that appear to be unrelated to abnormalities in serum calcium or phosphorus levels. Osteoma cutis is present in 25–50% of cases of AHO and is usually first noted in infancy or early childhood. Blue-tinged, stony-hard papular or nodular lesions that range from pinpoint size to 5 cm in diameter often occur at sites of minor trauma and may appear to be migratory on repeated examinations (81). Biopsy of these lesions reveals heterotopic ossification, with spicules of mineralizing osteoid and calcified cartilage.

Multiple Hormone Resistance

Although biochemical hypoparathyroidism is the most commonly recognized endocrine deficiency in

PHP, early clinical studies described additional hormonal abnormalities in patients with PHP type I, such as hypothyroidism (82,83) and hypogonadism (84). Consistent with these multiple endocrine defects, these patients have a deficiency in functional Gsα rather than a defect in a specific component of the adenylyl cyclase complex such as the receptor for PTH. Because available evidence suggests that Gsα is similar in all tissues, a ubiquitous deficiency of Gsα could be the basis for PTH resistance, the hallmark of PHP type Ia, and could explain the decreased responsiveness of diverse tissues (e.g., kidney, thyroid gland, gonads, and liver) to hormones that act via cAMP [e.g., PTH, thyroid-stimulating hormone (TSH), gonadotropins, and glucagon] (Fig. 8) (17,28,85).

Multiple hormone resistance occurs exclusively in patients with AHO. Furthermore, with rare exception, these patients show deficient Gsα activity (PHP type Ia).

Thyroid-Stimulating Hormone Resistance

Primary hypothyroidism occurs in most patients with PHP type Ia (28). Typically, patients lack a goiter or antithyroid antibodies and have an elevated serum TSH, with an exaggerated response to TRH. Serum levels of T_4 may be low or low-normal. Hypothyroidism may occur early in life prior to the development of hypocalcemia, and elevated serum levels of TSH are not uncommonly detected during perinatal screening (86–88). Unfortunately, early institution of thyroid hormone replacement does not seem to prevent the development of mental retardation (87).

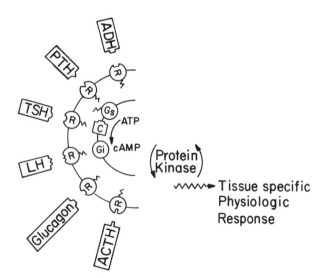

FIG. 8. Model of multihormone resistance in subjects with Gsα deficiency.

Gonadotropin Resistance

Hypogonadism is common in subjects with PHP type Ia. Women may have delayed puberty, oligomenorrhea, and infertility (28). Plasma gonadotropins may be elevated or normal, and some patients show an exaggerated serum gonadotropin response to gonadotropin-releasing hormone (GnRH) (84,89). Features of hypogonadism may be less obvious in men. Serum testosterone may be normal or reduced. Testes may show evidence of a maturation arrest or may fail to descend normally. Fertility appears to be decreased in men with PHP type Ia. Deficiency of prolactin secretion (basal and in response to secretagues such as TRH) has been reported in some patients with PHP type I by Carlson and his associates (90). In contrast, other investigators have found no evidence for reduced prolactin secretion (28). The role of cAMP in mediating prolactin secretion is controversial, and it is thought that cytosolic calcium may be the second messenger. Thus it is not clear that a deficiency of Gsα would impair prolactin secretion.

Miscellaneous Features

The incidence of hypertension appears to be increased among patients with PHP, and abnormal circadian variations of plasma renin, aldosterone, and catecholamines have been noted (91). Abnormal hormone responsiveness may occur in some tissues without obvious clinical sequelae. For example, the hepatic glucose response to glucagon is normal, although plasma cAMP concentrations fail to increase normally (28,92). In other tissues, significant hormone resistance does not occur despite the apparent reduction in Gsα. Diabetes insipidus is not a feature of AHO, and urine is concentrated normally in response to vasopressin in patients with PHP type Ia (93). Although there is a report of adrenal insufficiency in a single individual with PHP type Ia (94), hypoadrenalism is not a feature of PHP type Ia, and adrenal cortical responsiveness to adrenocorticotropic hormone (ACTH) is typically normal (28).

Neurological Abnormalities

A surprising variety of neurologic abnormalities have been described in patients with AHO. Mild-to-moderate mental retardation is common in patients with PHP type Ia. Farfel and Friedman (95) assessed intelligence in 25 patients with PHP type I whose Gsα activity had been determined. The authors suggested that mental deficiency was associated with PHP type Ia (Gsα deficiency) and that reduced cAMP levels in cortical tissue may have been related to the mental retardation. Factors contributing to the mental retardation may include hypothyroidism and hypocalcemia; however, efforts to control these have not prevented cognitive dysfunction in all patients, suggesting that Gsα deficiency may cause a primary abnormality of neurotransmitter signaling. Seizure disorders are also frequently reported. These may reflect atypical seizures due to hypocalcemia (cerebral tetany) or exacerbation of epileptic seizures. These seizures may occur prior to recognition of hypocalcemia (96,97). There have been reports of psychosis in patients with AHO (98). Patients with calcifications of the basal ganglia may rarely develop movement disorders (99).

Primary Sensory Abnormalities

Patients with PHP type Ia frequently manifest distinctive olfactory (100), gustatory (101), and auditory (102) abnormalities that are apparently unrelated to endocrine dysfunction [e.g., primary hypothyroidism must be properly treated, since defects in taste and smell occur in patients who are hypothyroid (103)]. The molecular basis of these neurosensory deficits has become more obscure with the discovery of unique G proteins for signal transduction in vision (104,105), olfaction (106), and taste (107).

Henkin (101) first reported disturbances in gustatory sensation in patients with PHP. He found that the thresholds for detection and recognition of sour and bitter taste were elevated above normal. Moreover, the olfactory thresholds for detection and recognition of all vapors tested were also elevated. Treatment with calcium, parathyroid extract, or both did not restore taste or olfaction to normal. However, modern biochemical means of classifying the types of PHP were not available, and the sophistication of sensory testing was very limited. In the mid-1980s, in vitro studies demonstrated an odorant-sensitive adenylyl cyclase in olfactory receptor cells from frog and rat (108,109). The olfactory G protein of isolated dendritic membranes from frog olfactory neuroepithelial cells was found to be similar to Gs proteins of endocrine cells (110). Shortly thereafter, patients with PHP type Ia were found to have impaired olfaction in comparison with patients with PHP who had normal Gsα activity (Fig. 9) (100). Olfaction was evaluated by a quantitative test, which required the patients to identify ten common odorants that were repeatedly presented in a random fashion. All five PHP type Ia patients demonstrated impaired olfaction compared with the seven PHP type Ib patients. One of the latter had a quantitative olfactory dysfunction in comparison with normal subjects, but even this patient scored much better on olfactory testing than any of the PHP type Ia pa-

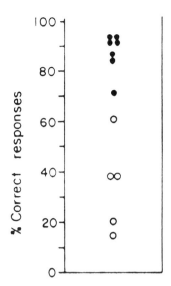

FIG. 9. Results of olfactory testing in patients with PHP type Ia (*open circles*) and patients with PHP type Ib (*solid circles*). (For details, see ref. 100.)

tients (100). The pattern of response from the PHP type Ia patients was consistent with what had previously been observed in patients with known absence of olfactory nerve input resulting from trauma or surgery (111). Adequate responses were limited to strong trigeminal stimulants (ammonia, isopropyl alcohol, acetic acid). Similar findings of decreased olfactory ability have been described in additional patients with PHP type Ia who have Gsα deficiency (112). These findings suggest that Gsα may have a role in odorant signal detection. More recent studies indicate that olfactory dysfunction does not occur in all AHO subjects with Gsα deficiency. Whereas olfactory disturbances are commonly observed in PHP type Ia subjects, who have evidence of defective signal transduction in other tissues (i.e., multiple hormone resistance), subjects with Gsα deficiency who do not have hormone resistance (i.e., pseudo-PHP) also do not manifest olfactory dysfunction (Fernandez, Levine, and Doty; unpublished observations).

It is not immediately obvious how a defect in Gsα can impair odorant signal detection (113). Olfactory neuroepithelial cells contain a unique G protein termed G_{olf} (106) and a specific form of adenylyl cyclase [type III (114)]. Perhaps Gsα deficiency impairs subsequent neurotransmission of the odorant signal generated by olfactory neuroepithelial cells.

Koch et al. (102) found that PHP type Ia patients with Gsα deficiency had symmetrical sensorineural hearing losses. The authors speculated that loss of the G protein–adenylyl cyclase complex causes progressive damage to cochlear hair cells induced by a disorder in the electrolyte composition of the inner ear fluids.

Alterations in visual function have been described in patients with PHP type Ia as well. Phototransduction in retinal rods and cones employs a signal transduction cascade that is homologous to the G protein-coupled adenylyl cyclase system. Light activation of the specialized receptor proteins rhodopsin and opsin that are expressed in rods and cones, respectively, is coupled to stimulation of cyclic guanosine monophosphate (GMP) phosphodiesterase by unique G proteins termed *transducins* (104,105). Although these G proteins share substantial similarity to Gs in subunit structure and mechanism of action, their expression is limited to retinal photoreceptor cells, and they subserve unique signalling functions. Rod and cone transducins are composed of distinct but highly homologous α chains and closely related βγ dimers. The important function of G proteins in phototransduction has stimulated interest in visual function in subjects with Gsα deficiency. Ellie et al. (115) reported a woman with PHP type Ia who had visual impairment and an abnormality of the electroretinogram that suggested a retinopathy involving mainly rods. Psychophysical studies in five patients with PHP type Ia demonstrated decreased rod photoreceptor adaptation (personal observation). This evidence for impaired rod function is based on the determination of visual recovery in the dark following a standard bleaching light stimulus. Decreased color discrimination and enhanced contrast sensitivity have also been observed in patients with PHP type Ia (116). The pathophysiological basis for these photoreceptor defects is unknown.

DIAGNOSIS OF PSEUDOHYPOPARATHYROIDISM

Clinical Evaluation

The diagnosis of PHP is generally suspected when a patient with symptoms or signs of biochemical hypoparathyroidism is found to have an elevated serum level of PTH. Occasionally, serum levels of PTH are "inappropriately" normal in subjects with PHP, owing to confounding hypomagnesemia (117) or other factors (118). The following clinical vignettes represent common presentations.

First, patients may have complained of paresthesias or may have had a convulsive seizure. The onset of symptoms may occur during times of "stress" on calcium homeostasis, such as during early pregnancy, during lactation, or during an episode of acute pancreatitis. Occasionally, patients with PHP do not develop symptoms until they are in their fifties (119). Second, a low serum calcium level may be reported after multichannel analysis of a blood specimen obtained as part of a routine examination. Third, PHP may be considered because of skeletal abnormalities, most often

a short metacarpal or other features of AHO. The fourth circumstance that dictates an evaluation for PHP is the screening of relatives of patients with known PHP. Other unusual presenting manifestations of PHP include neonatal hypothyroidism (86,87), unexplained cardiac failure (120), Parkinson's disease (121), and spinal cord compression (122).

The typical phenotype of AHO, including short stature, obesity, brachydactyly of hands and feet, and subcutaneous and cutaneous calcification, should raise suspicion of PHP type Ia or pseudo-PHP (Fig. 7). However, the presence of these developmental and skeletal abnormalities does not always indicate that the patient has AHO and Gsα deficiency. Features of AHO, particularly shortened metacarpals or metatarsals, may occur in normal subjects and in patients with hormone-deficient hypoparathyroidism (123–125), renal hypercalciuria (126), and primary hyperparathyroidism (127). Patients with a variety of skeletal anomalies may exhibit certain features of AHO. Developmental defects such as short stature, brachydactyly, or basal ganglion calcification are found in patients with Gardner's syndrome, Turner's syndrome, and the basal cell nevus syndrome. However, these disorders are genetically distinct from AHO, and affected patients have normal calcium and phosphorus metabolism and show a normal urinary cAMP response to PTH (128).

Basal ganglion calcification, as well as more extensive intracranial calcification, occurs often in patients with hypoparathyroidism, especially when CT scanning is employed (129,130). The calcification may be associated with symptoms such as Parkinson's disease. Unfortunately from a diagnostic viewpoint, this finding occurs in patients with hormone-deficient as well as hormone-resistant hypoparathyroidism and is therefore not helpful in differentiating between the two types of hypoparathyroidism (131).

The diagnosis of PHP can be made with reasonable certainty when there is hypocalcemia (ionized), hyperphosphatemia, elevated circulating levels of immunoreactive PTH, and normal renal function. A positive family history lends further support to the diagnosis. The presence of AHO and hypothyroidism and/or hypogonadism, resistant to their trophic hormones, supports the diagnosis of PHP type Ia (28). When most or all of these features are present, more sophisticated tests may not be necessary for the clinical diagnosis of PHP. Patients with PHP may spontaneously change from hypocalcemia to normocalcemia and vice versa, contributing to the confusion regarding possible transition between pseudo-PHP and PHP (21,132). The urinary response to PTH infusion (see below) will not change, however, regardless of the serum calcium level, and this remains the most reliable criteria to distinguish between these two variants.

Biochemical Tests

The biochemical hallmark of PHP is the failure of the target organs, bone and kidney, to respond adequately to PTH. Additional tests have been developed to identify subjects with PHP type Ia; these research tests, which are based on analysis of Gsα protein or the Gsα gene, are only rarely indicated under typical clinical circumstances. The classical tests of Ellsworth and Howard and of Chase, Melson, and Aurbach involved the administration of 200–300 USP units of bovine parathyroid extract (parathyroid injection, USP; Lilly) with the usual response parameters being urine cAMP (Fig. 3) and phosphate. The unavailability of this relatively crude PTH preparation has led to the development of tests in which synthetic human PTH-1–34 fragment (Parathar; teriparatide acetate; Rhone-Poulenc-Rorer) is infused. Normal subjects and patients with hormonopenic hypoparathyroidism usually display a ten- to 20-fold increase in urinary cAMP excretion, whereas patients with PHP type I (type Ia and type Ib), regardless of their serum calcium concentration, show a markedly blunted response. Thus this test can distinguish patients with so-called normocalcemic PHP (i.e., patients with PTH resistance who are able to maintain normal serum calcium levels without treatment) from subjects with pseudo-PHP (who will have a normal urinary cAMP response to PTH (Fig. 3) (14,32). Tests that measure the calcemic response to PTH are no longer used as a means of diagnosing PHP.

The definitive diagnosis of PHP at present depends on the demonstration of a deficient cAMP, 1,25-$(OH)_2D_3$, or phosphate response to an active preparation of PTH. Several diagnostic protocols have been described in which the response to an infusion of synthetic human PTH-1–34 peptide is used to differentiate among disorders of PTH responsiveness (133–135). The protocol recommended by the present authors involves the infusion of this PTH fragment, 200 units in an adult and 3 units/kg body weight (200 units maximum) in children over the age of 3 years, intravenously over 10 min (135,136). Test subjects should be in a fasting state, and active urine output should be initiated and maintained by the ingestion of 200 ml water per hour beginning 2 hr prior to the infusion of PTH and continuing through the study. A baseline urine collection should be made in a 60 min period preceding the PTH infusion. From time 0, urine should be collected in separate collections at the 0–30 min, 30–60 min, and 60–120 min periods. Blood samples should be obtained at time 0 and at 2 hr after the start of PTH infusion for measurement of serum creatinine and phosphorus concentrations. Urine samples should be analyzed for cAMP, phosphorus, and creatinine concentrations.

The preferred response parameter for urinary cAMP is nmol/100 ml (or per liter) glomerular filtrate (GF).

The cAMP response during the first 30 min from the start of PTH infusion differentiates patients with PHP type I from those with hypoparathyroidism and from normal subjects better than other parameters of cAMP metabolism (Fig. 10) (136). The mean increase in cAMP excretion in the first 30 min collection period was 6.3 nmol/liter GF, with individual values ranging from 0 to 20 nmol/liter GF. In patients with hypoparathyroidism, the increase was 1,512 nmol/liter GF, with the minimum being > 500 nmol/liter GF. In normal subjects the mean rise in cAMP was 937 nmol/liter GF, with a minimum increase of ~300 nmol/liter GF. The change in urinary cAMP/mg creatinine during the same 30 min period also discriminated well between patients with PHP and those with hypoparathyroidism or normal subjects (136). Several metabolic abnormalities such as hypo- and hypermagnesemia and metabolic acidosis may interfere with the renal generation and excretion of cAMP in response to PTH (137–140). These abnormalities should be corrected if possible but probably do not interfere with the interpretation of the test.

The response of plasma cAMP to PTH can be used to differentiate patients with type I PHP from normal subjects and patients with hypoparathyroidism (133,141). Patients with PHP type II can be expected to show normal responsiveness. This test offers few advantages over protocols that assess the urinary excretion of cAMP, in that changes in plasma cAMP in normal subjects and patients with hypoparathyroidism are much less dramatic than changes in urine cAMP, and urine must still be collected to assess the phosphaturic response to PTH. One reasonable indication

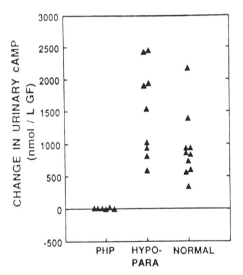

FIG. 10. Change in urinary cAMP excretion in response to PTH infusion in patients with pseudohypoparathyroidism or hypoparathyroidism and in normal subjects. (Reprinted from ref. 136 with permission.)

for measuring the plasma cAMP response to PTH is the evaluation of patients in whom proper collection of urine is not possible.

Calculation of the phosphaturic response to PTH as the percentage decrease in tubular maximum for phosphate reabsorption (percentage fall in TmP/GF) during the first 1 hr after infusion yielded the best separation between groups (Fig. 11) (136). However, the separation was also very good when the parameter was the fall in percentage tubular reabsorption of phosphorus (decrease in % TRP). A nomogram has been developed that facilitates calculation of TmPO/GF (142). TmP/GF is elevated in patients with PHP and hypoparathyroidism. Patients with hormone-deficient hypoparathyroidism have a steep fall in TmP/GF during the first 1 hr after the beginning of the infusion of PTH. This fall does not occur in patients with PHP. For further details, see references in Mallette and colleagues (135,136). In patients with PHP type II, the phosphaturic response to PTH is not changed despite at least a tenfold increase in cAMP excretion. Unfortunately, interpretation of the phosphaturic response to PTH is often complicated by random variations in phosphate clearance, and it is sometimes not possible to classify a phosphaturic response as normal or subnormal regardless of the criteria employed. More perplexing yet is the observation that biochemical findings that resemble PHP type II have been found in patients with various forms of vitamin D deficiency (57). In these patients, marked hypocalcemia is accompanied by hyperphosphatemia due presumably to an acquired dissociation between the amount of cAMP generated in the renal tubule and its effect on phosphate clearance.

The plasma 1,25-$(OH)_2D_3$ response to PTH has been used to differentiate between hormone-deficient and hormone-resistant hypoparathyroidism (134,143). In contrast to normal subjects and patients with hypoparathyroidism, patients with PHP had no significant increase in circulating levels of 1,25-$(OH)_2D_3$. This proposed test demonstrates nicely the difference in the pathophysiology between hypoparathyroidism and PHP. Its clinical relevance is probably limited to distinguishing type I from type II PHP, where the expected increase in the latter form of PHP might be a more reliable parameter than the phosphaturic response to PTH.

TREATMENT

Urgent treatment of acute or severe symptomatic hypocalcemia in patients with PHP (or other forms of hypoparathyroidism) is best accomplished with the infusion of calcium intravenously. Vitamin D is not required. The goal is alleviation of symptoms and prevention of laryngeal spasm and seizures. Hyperphosphatemia, alkalosis, and hypomagnesemia should be corrected. The serum calcium should be increased to the midnormal range. The desired serum calcium levels can usually be obtained by administering 1–3 g calcium gluconate (90–270 mg calcium, 10–30 ml 10% calcium gluconate) over a 10 min period and following this by administering up to 30–40 ml 10% solution (270–360 mg calcium) in 500 ml 5% dextrose in water over each subsequent 8 hr period. A 10% solution of calcium chloride is available for intravenous use, but it is very irritating to the veins. The serum calcium level should be measured at frequent intervals, and the amount of intravenous calcium should be adjusted accordingly. If patients are on digitalis therapy, electrocardiographic monitoring is advisable, because increasing serum calcium levels can predispose to digitalis toxicity. Oral calcium and vitamin D therapy should be started as soon as possible and gradually adjusted to replace the need for intravenous calcium (144).

The long-term treatment of hypocalcemia in patients with PHP involves the administration of oral calcium and vitamin D or analogs and the elimination of the metabolic abnormalities noted above. These patients are treated as are those with hormonopenic hypoparathyroidism, but with several distinctions as noted below. In addition, patients with PHP type Ia should be treated for their associated hypogonadism and hypothyroidism. Other differences are considered below.

The goal of chronic therapy is to normalize serum ionized calcium levels without inducing hypercalciuria

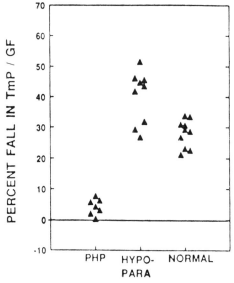

FIG. 11. Percent fall in TmP/GF from the baseline value in the first hour after infusion of PTH in patients with pseudohypoparathyroidism or hypoparathyroidism and in normal subjects. (Reprinted from ref. 136 with permission.)

and to suppress PTH levels to normal. Patients with hypoparathyroidism have increased urinary calcium excretion in relation to serum calcium and are therefore prone to hypercalciuria (145). By contrast, patients with PHP have significantly lower urinary calcium in relation to serum calcium (145,146) and can tolerate serum calcium levels that are within the normal range without developing hypercalciuria (16).

Once normocalcemia has been attained, attention should be directed toward suppression of PTH levels to normal. This is important in that elevated PTH levels in patients with PHP are frequently associated with increased bone remodeling. Hyperparathyroid bone disease, including osteitis fibrosa cystica (31,79,147) and cortical osteopenia (Fig. 3) (72), can occur in patients with PHP type I. These subjects may have elevated serum levels of alkaline phosphatase (147) and urine hydroxyproline (72). In this regard, calcitriol has an advantage over other vitamin D preparations, since it may inhibit PTH release directly (148) in addition to the indirect inhibition caused by elevating the serum calcium. Since thiazide diuretics effectively increase renal calcium reabsorption in patients with PHP (149), these agents along with a low-sodium diet can be utilized as an additional means of attaining higher serum calcium levels and better suppression of PTH without inducing hypercalciuria.

Oral calcium in the treatment of hypocalcemia in patients with PHP is usually administered in amounts ranging from 1 to 3 g calcium per day (including that contained in food) in divided doses. To ensure optimal absorption, oral calcium supplements should be taken with water or other fluids and with food in the stomach (150). Many considerations are involved in the selection of a calcium supplement. Chemically pure calcium salts are preferred, because bone meal and dolomite calcium may contain substantial amounts of lead (151). Calcium carbonate tablets are not properly dissolved or absorbed in patients with achlorhydria, including patients on H_2 blocker therapy (152,153). Some calcium carbonate tablets are relatively insoluble even in acid, so generic brands should be tested to determine if they dissolve during 30 min of vigorous stirring at room temperature in a glass of vinegar (150). Many house brands and private label brands of calcium carbonate do not dissolve in this test and are therefore considered to be biologically unavailable. The absorption of calcium from lactate and gluconate salts is less dependent on the acidity of the stomach contents. However, due to the low content of calcium in these salts (13% in lactate and 9% in gluconate), the bulk of the tablets is large and this often is not acceptable to patients. Calcium citrate is 21% calcium and is well absorbed even in the absence of stomach acidity (154). In the present authors' opinion, it is the best available means of supplying calcium to patients with PHP. For those who prefer a liquid calcium supplement, calcium glubionate is very palatable and contains 252 mg calcium/10 ml. Ten to thirty milliliters of a 10% calcium chloride solution (360–1,080 mg calcium) every 8 hr may be very effective in patients with achlorhydria (153). Hyperchloremic acidosis may occur, which can be prevented by giving one-half of the calcium as chloride and one-half as carbonate simultaneously (153).

Calcium phosphate salts should be avoided, and intake of dairy products should be limited in order to restrict phosphate intake. When phosphate intake is properly restricted, treatment with calcium and vitamin D usually decreases the elevated serum phosphate to a high-normal level because of a favorable balance between increased urinary phosphate excretion and decreased intestinal phosphate absorption. Occasionally, this balance is unfavorable and the serum phosphate is increased. This in turn interferes with normalization of serum calcium and predisposes to extraskeletal calcification.

All patients with PHP who are hypocalcemic require vitamin D or its analogs in addition to calcium. Calcitriol, the active form of vitamin D, is the most physiological treatment choice in patients with PHP. Patients with PHP require ~75% as much calcitriol to maintain normocalcemia as do patients with hypoparathyroidism (155). Almost all patients with PHP can be effectively treated with calcitriol in amounts ranging from 0.25 µg twice per day to 0.5 µg four times per day. Because of the expense of calcitriol and the need to administer the drug several times per day, other vitamin D choices may be preferred. PHP patients respond well to pharmacological doses of ergocalciferol and calcidiol. Ergocalciferol is the least expensive choice for vitamin D therapy and provides a long duration of action (with corresponding prolonged potential toxicity). Patients with PHP require lower doses of vitamin D than patients with hypoparathyroidism (155), an observation that reflects the response of bone and renal distal tubular cells to endogenous PTH (156).

Attention should be directed to a number of special situations. Because thiazide diuretics increase renal calcium reabsorption in patients with PHP (149), the inadvertent institution or discontinuation of these diuretics may increase or decrease, respectively, plasma calcium levels in patients who had been properly treated for hypocalcemia. Furosemide and similar diuretics may cause hypocalcemia in patients whose serum calcium had been normalized with calcium and vitamin D. The administration of glucocorticoids antagonizes the action of vitamin D (and its analogs) and may also precipitate hypocalcemia. The development of hypomagnesemia may also interfere with the effectiveness of treatment with calcium and vitamin D (157).

Estrogen therapy and pregnancy have particularly interesting effects on the maintenance of normocalcemia in patients with PHP. Estrogen therapy caused a consistent, dose-related, reversible reduction of serum calcium in two women with PHP type 1b who were not pregnant (158). This is similar to what occurs in women with hypoparathyroidism (159). In contrast, at the time of the menses, when estrogen levels are low, some well-treated hypoparathyroid women may develop symptomatic hypocalcemia, with the cause remaining unknown (160). The same phenomenon occurs occasionally in women with PHP (personal observation). The symptoms are relieved in 30–60 min by ingestion of 200–400 mg calcium.

Paradoxically, during the high-estrogen state of pregnancy, the two PHP type 1b patients of Zerwekh and Breslau (161) remained normocalcemic even without therapeutic amounts of calcium and vitamin D. During pregnancy, serum $1,25\text{-}(OH)_2D_3$ concentrations increased two- to threefold, while the PTH levels were nearly one-half of those present before pregnancy. After delivery, serum calcium and $1,25\text{-}(OH)_2D_3$ levels decreased and PTH rose (158). Since placental synthesis of $1,25\text{-}(OH)_2D$ is not compromised in patients with PHP (161), the placenta may have contributed to the maintenance of normocalcemia during pregnancy in these patients. In contrast, patients with hypoparathyroidism may require treatment with larger amounts of vitamin D and calcium in the latter one-half of pregnancy (162).

Patients with AHO may require specific treatment for unusual problems related to their developmental and skeletal abnormalities. Ectopic calcification occurs in ~30% of patients with AHO (75). This rarely causes a problem. However, at times, large extraskeletal osteomas occur (81). These may require surgical removal to relieve pressure symptoms. Surgery may also be required to relieve neurological symptoms caused by ossification of ligaments (163). Skeletal abnormalities such as deformed elbows, coxa valga and vara, and bowed tibia may require orthopedic evaluation and treatment. More commonly, treatment is directed at bone abnormalities in the feet. The symptoms are caused by deformities such as painful hyperkeratotic lesions beneath prominent metatarsal heads, bursitis of effected metatarsal phalangeal joints, dislocated toes that do not fit well into shoes, ulcerative lesions from malalignment, or pressure and exostoses (164). Measures that have been recommended to relieve pedal symptoms include reduction of hyperkeratotic lesions, padding of the plantar aspects of the feet to accommodate the lesions, soft orthotic devices that can be placed in shoes to cushion weight-bearing areas, custom-made molded shoes, and various medical and physical therapies to relieve acute capsulitis and bursitis (164).

CONCLUSIONS

The discovery and biochemical characterization of the components of the PTH receptor signal transduction pathway have facilitated development of molecular approaches to the investigation of the pathophysiology of PTH resistance. As with many other human disorders for which the disease gene has been identified, it is predicted that the ability to diagnose these disorders on a molecular level will extend the clinical spectrum of disease. This prediction has already been fulfilled in PHP type Ia, where identification of defects in the gene encoding $Gs\alpha$ permits categorization of patients into subgroups in which $Gs\alpha$ deficiency is accompanied by AHO and hormone resistance (i.e., PHP type Ia), AHO without hormone resistance (i.e., pseudo-PHP), and no clinical or biochemical manifestations. Future work must be directed towards identification of the basis for these differences in the biochemical and clinical expression of the $Gs\alpha$ mutation.

Investigation over the next several years should clarify the molecular defects that cause the other forms of PTH resistance so that all forms of PHP can be described on the basis of their pathophysiology. The insights gained from studies of these unusual patients will provide new information concerning the physiological regulation of PTH responsiveness in classical target tissues, such as bone and kidney, as well as in nonclassical targets.

ACKNOWLEDGMENTS

This work was supported in part by grants from the National Institutes of Health (DK 34281) and by The March of Dimes.

REFERENCES

1. Albright F, Burnett CH, Smith PH. Pseudohypoparathyroidism: an example of "Seabright-Bantam syndrome." *Endocrinology* 1942;30:922–932.
2. Juppner H, Abou Samra AB, Freeman M, et al. A G protein-linked receptor for parathyroid hormone and parathyroid hormone-related peptide. *Science* 1991;254:1024–1026.
3. Abou Samra AB, Juppner H, Force T, et al. Expression cloning of a common receptor for parathyroid hormone and parathyroid hormone-related peptide from rat osteoblast-like cells: a single receptor stimulates intracellular accumulation of both cAMP and inositol trisphosphates and increases intracellular free calcium. *Proc Natl Acad Sci USA* 1992;89:2732–2736.
4. Melson GL, Chase LR, Aurbach GD. Parathyroid hormone-sensitive adenyl cyclase in isolated renal tubules. *Endocrinology* 1970;86:511–518.
5. Chase LR, Fedak SA, Aurbach GD. Activation of skeletal adenyl cyclase by parathyroid hormone in vitro. *Endocrinology* 1969;84:761–768.
6. Civitelli R, Reid IR, Westbrook S, Avioli LV, Hruska KA. PTH elevates inositol polyphosphates and diacylglycerol in

a rat osteoblast-like cell line. *Am J Physiol* 1988;255:E660–E667.

7. Dunlay R, Hruska K. PTH receptor coupling to phospholipase C is an alternate pathway of signal transduction in bone and kidney. *Am J Physiol* 1990;258:F223–F231.

8. Gupta A, Martin KJ, Miyauchi A, Hruska KA. Regulation of cytosolic calcium by parathyroid hormone and oscillations of cytosolic calcium in fibroblasts from normal and pseudohypoparathyroid patients. *Endocrinology* 1991;128:2825–2836.

9. Civitelli R, Martin TJ, Fausto A, Gunsten SL, Hruska KA, Avioli LV. Parathyroid hormone-related peptide transiently increases cytosolic calcium in osteoblast-like cells: comparison with parathyroid hormone. *Endocrinology* 1989;125:1204–1210.

10. Reid IR, Civitelli R, Halstead LR, Avioli LV, Hruska KA. Parathyroid hormone acutely elevates intracellular calcium in osteoblastlike cells. *Am J Physiol* 1987;253:E45–E51.

11. Yamaguchi DT, Hahn TJ, Iida-Klein A, Kleeman CR, Muallem S. Parathyroid hormone-activated calcium channels in an osteoblast-like clonal osteosarcoma cell line. *J Biol Chem* 1987;262:7711–7718.

12. Bringhurst FR, Zajac JD, Daggett AS, Skurat RN, Kronenberg HM. Inhibition of parathyroid hormone responsiveness in clonal osteoblastic cells expressing a mutant form of 3′,5′-cyclic adenosine monophosphate-dependent protein kinase. *Mol Endocrinol* 1989;3:60–67.

13. Winter JSD, Hughes IA. Familial pseudohypoparathyroidism without somatic anomalies. *Can Med Assoc J* 1980;123:26–31.

14. Chase LR, Melson GL, Aurbach GD. Pseudohypoparathyroidism: defective excretion of 3′,5′-AMP in response to parathyroid hormone. *J Clin Invest* 1969;48:1832–1844.

15. Bell NH, Avery S, Sinha T, et al. Effects of dibutyryl cyclic adenosine 3′,5′-monophosphate and parathyroid extract on calcium and phosphorous metabolism in hypoparathyroidism and pseudohypoparathyroidism. *J Clin Invest* 1972;51:816.

16. Mizunashi K, Furukawa Y, Sohn HE, Miura R, Yumita S, Yoshinaga K. Heterogeneity of pseudohypoparathyroidism type I from the aspect of urinary excretion of calcium and serum levels of parathyroid hormone. *Calcif Tissue Int* 1990;46:227–232.

17. Shima M, Nose O, Shimizu K, Seino Y, Yabuuchi H, Saito T. Multiple associated endocrine abnormalities in a patient with pseudohypoparathyroidism type 1a. *Eur J Pediatr* 1988;147:536–538.

18. Drezner MK, Neelon FA, Lebovitz HE. Pseudohypoparathyroidism type II: a possible defect in the reception of the cyclic AMP signal. *N Engl J Med* 1973;280:1056–1060.

19. Murray TM, Rao LG, Wong MM, et al. Pseudohypoparathyroidism with osteitis fibrosa cystica: direct demonstration of skeletal responsiveness to parathyroid hormone in cells cultured from bone. *J Bone Mineral Res* 1993;8:83–91.

20. Drezner MK, Neelon FA, Haussler M, McPherson HT, Lebovitz HE. 1,25-Dihydroxycholecalciferol deficiency: the probable cause of hypocalcemia and metabolic bone disease in pseudohypoparathyroidism. *J Clin Endocrinol Metab* 1976;42:621–628.

21. Drezner MK, Haussler MR. Normocalcemic pseudohypoparathyroidism. *Am J Med* 1979;66:503–508.

22. Stogmann W, Fischer JA. Pseudohypoparathyroidism. Disappearance of the resistance to parathyroid extract during treatment with vitamin D. *Am J Med* 1975;59:140–144.

23. Barrett D, Breslau NA, Wax MB, Molinoff PB, Downs RW, Jr. New form of pseudohypoparathyroidism with abnormal catalytic adenylate cyclase. *Am J Physiol* 1989;257:E277–E283.

24. Nagant de Deuxchaisnes C, Fischer JA, Dambacher MA, et al. Dissociation of parathyroid hormone bioactivity and immunoreactivity in pseudohypoparathyroidism type I. *J Clin Endocrinol Metab* 1981;53:1105–1109.

25. Bradbeer JN, Dunham J, Fischer JA, Nagant de Deuxchaisnes C, Loveridge N. The metatarsal cytochemical bioassay of parathyroid hormone: validation, specificity, and application to the study of pseudohypoparathyroidism type I. *J Clin Endocrinol Metab* 1988;67:1237–1243.

26. Loveridge N, Fischer JA, Nagant de Deuxchaisnes C, et al. Inhibition of cytochemical bioactivity of parathyroid hormone by plasma in pseudohypoparathyroidism type I. *J Clin Endocrinol Metab* 1982;54:1274–1275.

27. Mitchell J, Goltzman D. Examination of circulating parathyroid hormone in pseudohypoparathyroidism. *J Clin Endocrinol Metab* 1985;61:328–334.

28. Levine MA, Downs RW Jr, Moses AM, et al. Resistance to multiple hormones in patients with pseudohypoparathyroidism. Association with deficient activity of guanine nucleotide regulatory protein. *Am J Med* 1983;74:545–556.

29. Silve C, Santora A, Breslau N, Moses A, Spiegel A. Selective resistance to parathyroid hormone in cultured skin fibroblasts from patients with pseudohypoparathyroidism type Ib. *J Clin Endocrinol Metab* 1986;62:640–644.

30. Silve C, Suarez F, el Hessni A, Loiseau A, Graulet AM, Gueris J. The resistance to parathyroid hormone of fibroblasts from some patients with type Ib pseudohypoparathyroidism is reversible with dexamethasone. *J Clin Endocrinol Metab* 1990;71:631–638.

31. Kidd GS, Schaaf M, Adler RA, Lassman MN, Wray HL. Skeletal responsiveness in pseudohypoparathyroidism: a spectrum of clinical disease. *Am J Med* 1980;68:772–781.

32. Levine MA, Jap TS, Mauseth RS, Downs RW, Spiegel AM. Activity of the stimulatory guanine nucleotide-binding protein is reduced in erythrocytes from patients with pseudohypoparathyroidism and pseudopseudohypoparathyroidism: biochemical, endocrine, and genetic analysis of Albright's hereditary osteodystrophy in six kindreds. *J Clin Endocrinol Metab* 1986;62:497–502.

33. Patten JL, Levine MA. Immunochemical analysis of the alpha-subunit of the stimulatory G-protein of adenylyl cyclase in patients with Albright's hereditary osteodystrophy. *J Clin Endocrinol Metab* 1990;71:1208–1214.

34. Carter A, Bardin C, Collins R, Simons C, Bray P, Spiegel A. Reduced expression of multiple forms of the alpha subunit of the stimulatory GTP-binding protein in pseudohypoparathyroidism type Ia. *Proc Natl Acad Sci USA* 1987;84:7266–7269.

35. Levine MA, Ahn TG, Klupt SF, et al. Genetic deficiency of the alpha subunit of the guanine nucleotide-binding protein Gs as the molecular basis for Albright hereditary osteodystrophy. *Proc Natl Acad Sci USA* 1988;85:617–621.

36. Kozasa T, Itoh H, Tsukamoto T, Kaziro Y. Isolation and characterization of the human Gs alpha gene. *Proc Natl Acad Sci USA* 1988;85:2081–2085.

37. Robishaw JD, Smigel MD, Gilman AG. Molecular basis for two forms of the G protein that stimulates adenylate cyclase. *J Biol Chem* 1986;261:9587–9590.

38. Granneman JG, Haverstick DM, Chaudhry A. Relationship between $G_S\alpha$ messenger ribonucleic acid splice variants and the molecular forms of Gss protein in rat brown adipose tissue. *Endocrinology* 1990;127:1596–1601.

39. Jones DT, Master SB, Bourne HR, Reed RR. Biochemical characterization of three stimulatory GTP-binding proteins. *J Biol Chem* 1990;265:2671–2676.

40. Mattera R, Graziano MP, Yatani A, et al. Splice variants of the alpha subunit of the G protein Gs activate both adenylyl cyclase and calcium channels. *Science* 1989;243:804–807.

41. Graziano MP, Freissmuth M, Gilman AG. Expression of Gs alpha in Escherichia coli. Purification and properties of two forms of the protein. *J Biol Chem* 1989;264:409–418.

42. Ishikawa Y, Bianchi C, Nadal-Ginard B, Homcy CJ. Alternative promoter and 5′ exon generate a novel G_s alpha mRNA. *J Biol Chem* 1990;265:8458–8462.

43. Swaroop A, Agarwal N, Gruen JR, Bick D, Weissman SM. Differential expression of novel Gsα signal transduction protein cDNA species. *Nucleic Acids Res* 1991;17:4725–4729.

44. Patten JL, Johns DR, Valle D, et al. Mutation in the gene encoding the stimulatory G protein of adenylate cyclase in

Albright's hereditary osteodystrophy. *N Engl J Med* 1990; 322:1412–1419.

45. Miric A, Vechio JD, Levine MA. Heterogeneous mutations in the gene encoding the alpha subunit of the stimulatory G protein of adenylyl cyclase in Albright hereditary osteodystrophy. *J Clin Endocrinol Metab* 1993;76:1560–1568.

46. Schwindinger WF, Miric A, Levine MA. Identification of a novel missense mutation in the gene encoding the alpha subunit of the stimulatory G protein of adenylyl cyclase in a subject with Albright hereditary osteodystrophy. *Program and Abstracts, 74th Annual Meeting of the Endocrine Society.* San Antonio, Texas, 1992;abstract 35.

47. Weinstein LS, Gejman PV, Friedman E, et al. Mutations of the Gs alpha-subunit gene in Albright hereditary osteodystrophy detected by denaturing gradient gel electrophoresis. *Proc Natl Acad Sci USA* 1990;87:8287–8290.

48. Weinstein LS, Gejman PV, de Mazancourt P, American N, Spiegel AM. A heterozygous 4-bp deletion mutation in the $G_s\alpha$ gene (GNAS1) in a patient with Albright hereditary osteodystrophy. *Genomics* 1992;13:1319–1321.

49. Loveridge N, Dean V, Goltzman D, Hendy GN. Bioactivity of parathyroid hormone and parathyroid hormone-like peptide: agonist and antagonist activities of amino-terminal fragments as assessed by the cytochemical bioassay and in situ biochemistry. *Endocrinology* 1991;128:1938–1946.

50. Rall T, Harris BA. Identification of the lesion in the stimulatory GTP-binding protein of the uncoupled S49 lymphoma. *FEBS Lett* 1987;224:365–371.

51. Sullivan KA, Miller RT, Masters SB, Beiderman B, Heideman W, Bourne HR. Identification of receptor contact site involved in receptor–G protein coupling. *Nature* 1987;330:758–760.

52. Schwindinger WF, Levine MA. A mutation that uncouples receptors from adenylyl cyclase in Albright hereditary osteodystrophy. *J Bone Miner Res* 1992;7:S114.

53. Weinstein LS, Shenker A, Gejman PV, Merino MJ, Friedman E, Spiegel AM. Activating mutations of the stimulatory G protein in the McCune-Albright syndrome. *N Engl J Med* 1991;325:1688–1695.

54. Schwindinger WF, Francomano CA, Levine MA. Identification of a mutation in the gene encoding the alpha subunit of the stimulatory G protein of adenylyl cyclase in McCune-Albright syndrome. *Proc Natl Acad Sci USA* 1992;89:5152–5156.

55. Farfel Z, Brothers VM, Brickman AS, Conte F, Neer R, Bourne HR. Pseudohypoparathyroidism: inheritance of deficient receptor-cyclase coupling activity. *Proc Natl Acad Sci USA* 1981;78:3098–3102.

56. Izraeli S, Metzker A, Horev G, Karmi D, Merlob P, Farfel Z. Albright hereditary osteodystrophy with hypothyroidism, normocalcemia, and normal Gs protein activity. *Am J Med* 1992;43:764–767.

57. Rao DS, Parfitt AM, Kleerekoper M, Pumo BS, Frame B. Dissociation between the effects of endogenous parathyroid hormone on adenosine 3′,5′-monophosphate generation and phosphate reabsorption in hypocalcemia due to vitamin D depletion: An acquired disorder resembling pseudohypoparathyroidism type II. *J Clin Endocrinol Metab* 1985;61:285–290.

58. Kruse K, Kracht U, Wohlfart K, Kruse U. Biochemical markers of bone turnover, intact serum parathyroid horn and renal calcium excretion in patients with pseudohypoparathyroidism and hypoparathyroidism before and during vitamin D treatment. *Eur J Pediatr* 1989;148:535–539.

59. Mann JB, Alterman S, Hills AG. Albright's hereditary osteodystrophy comprising pseudohypoparathyroidism and pseudo-pseudohypoparathyroidism with a report of two cases representing the complete syndrome occurring in successive generations. *Ann Intern Med* 1962;56:315–342.

60. Weinberg AG, Stone RT. Autosomal dominant inheritance in Albright's hereditary osteodystrophy. *J Pediatr* 1971;79:996–999.

61. Cedarbaum SD, Lippe BM. Probable autosomal recessive inheritance in a family with Albright's hereditary osteodys-

trophy and an evaluation of the genetics of the disorder. *Am J Hum Genet* 1973;25:638–645.

62. Van Dop C, Bourne HR, Neer RM. Father to son transmission of decreased Ns activity in pseudohypoparathyroidism type Ia. *J Clin Endocrinol Metab* 1984;59:825–828.

63. Levine MA, Modi WS, OBrien SJ. Mapping of the gene encoding the alpha subunit of the stimulatory G protein of adenylyl cyclase (GNAS1) to 20q13.2–q13.3 in human by in situ hybridization. *Genomics* 1991;11:478–479.

64. Davies SJ, Hughes HE. Imprinting in Albright's hereditary osteodystrophy. *J Med Genet* 1993;30:101–103.

65. Van Dop C. Pseudohypoparathyroidism: clinical and molecular aspects. *Semin Nephrol* 1989;9:168–178.

66. Tsang RC, Venkataraman P, Ho M, Steichen JJ, Whitsett J, Greer F. The development of pseudohypoparathyroidism. *Am J Dis Child* 1984;138:654–658.

67. Schuster V, Sandhage K. Intracardiac calcifications in a case of pseudohypoparathyroidism type Ia (PHP-Ia). *Pediatr Cardiol* 1992;13:237–239.

68. Illum F, Dupont E. Prevalences of CT-detected calcification in the basal ganglia in idiopathic hypoparathyroidism and pseudohypoparathyroidism. *Neuroradiology* 1985;27:32–37.

69. Burnstein MI, Sambasiva RK, Pettifor JM, Sochett E, Ellis BI, Frame B. Metabolic bone disease in pseudohypoparathyroidism: radiologic features. *Radiology* 1985;155:351–356.

70. Dabbaugh S, Chesney RW, Langer LO, DeLuca HF, Gilbert EF, DeWeerd JH, Jr. Renal-non-responsive, bone-responsive pseudohypoparathyroidism. A case with normal vitamin D metabolite levels and clinical features of rickets. *Am J Dis Child* 1984;138:1030–1033.

71. Hall FM, Segall-Blank M, Genant HK, Kolb FO, Hawes LE. Pseudohypoparathyroidism presenting as renal osteodystrophy. *Skel Radiol* 1981;6:43–46.

72. Breslau NA, Moses AM, Pak CYC. Evidence for bone remodeling but lack of calcium mobilization response to parathyroid hormone in pseudohypoparathyroidism. *J Clin Endocrinol Metab* 1983;57:638–644.

73. Albright F, Forbes AP, Henneman PH. Pseudopseudohypoparathyroidism. *Trans Assoc Am Physicians* 1952;65:337–350.

74. Faull CM, Welbury RR, Paul B, Kendall Taylor P. Pseudohypoparathyroidism: its phenotypic variability and associated disorders in a large family. *Q J Med* 1991;78:251–264.

75. Fitch N. Albright's hereditary osteodystrophy: a review. *Am J Med Genet* 1982;11:11–29.

76. Croft LK, Witkop CJ, Glas J-E. Pseudohypoparathyroidism. *Oral Surg Oral Med Oral Pathol* 1965;20:758–770.

77. Poznanski AK, Werder EA, Giedion A. The pattern of shortening of the bones of the hand in PHP and PPHP—a comparison with brachydactyly E, Turner syndrome, and acrodysostosis. *Radiol* 1977;123:707–718.

78. Graudal N, Galloe A, Christensen H, Olesen K. The pattern of shortened hand and foot bones in D- and E-brachydactyly and pseudohypoparathyroidism/pseudopseudohypoparathyroidism. *ROFO Fortschr Geb Rontgenstr Nuklearmed* 1988;148:460–462.

79. Steinbach HL, Rudhe U, Jonsson M, et al. Evolution of skeletal lesions in pseudohypoparathyroidism. *Radiology* 1965;85:670–676.

80. Alam SM, Kelly W. Spinal cord compression associated with pseudohypoparathyroidism. *J R Soc Med* 1990;83:50–51.

81. Prendiville JS, Lucky AW, Mallory SB, Mughal Z, Mimouni F, Langman CB. Osteoma cutis as a presenting sign of pseudohypoparathyroidism. *Pediatr Dermatol* 1992;9:11–18.

82. Marx SJ, Hershman JM, Aurbach GD. Thyroid dysfunction in pseudohypoparathyroidism. *J Clin Endocrinol Metab* 1971;33:822–828.

83. Werder EA, Illig R, Bernasconi S, Kind H, Prader A. Excessive thyrotropin-releasing hormone in pseudohypoparathyroidism. *Pediatr Res* 1975;9:12–16.

84. Wolfsdorf JI, Rosenfield RL, Fang VS, et al. Partial gonadotrophin-resistance in pseudohypoparathyroidism. *Acta Endocrinol* 1978;88:321–328.

85. Tsai KS, Chang CC, Wu DJ, Huang TS, Tsai IH, Chen FW.

Deficient erythrocyte membrane Gs alpha activity and resistance to trophic hormones of multiple endocrine organs in two cases of pseudohypoparathyroidism. *Taiwan I Hsueh Hui Tsa Chih* 1989;88:450–455.

86. Levine MA, Jap TS, Hung W. Infantile hypothyroidism in two sibs: an unusual presentation of pseudohypoparathyroidism type Ia. *J Pediatr* 1985;107:919–922.

87. Weisman Y, Golander A, Spiere Z, et al. Pseudohypoparathyroidism type Ia presenting as congenital hypothyroidism. *J Pediatr* 1985;107:413–415.

88. Yokoro S, Matsuo M, Ohtsuka T, Ohzeki T. Hyperthyrotropinemia in a neonate with normal thyroid hormone levels: the earliest diagnostic clue for pseudohypoparathyroidism. *Biol Neonate* 1990;58:69–72.

89. Downs RW Jr, Levine MA, Drezner MK, Burch WM Jr, Spiegel AM. Deficient adenylate cyclase regulatory protein in renal membranes from a patient with pseudohypoparathyroidism. *J Clin Invest* 1983;71:231–235.

90. Carlson HE, Brickman AS, Bottazzo CF. Prolactin deficiency in pseudohypoparathyroidism. *N Engl J Med* 1977; 296:140–144.

91. Brickman AS, Stern N, Sowers JR. Circadian variations of catecholamines and blood pressure in patients with pseudohypoparathyroidism and hypertension. *Chronobiologia* 1990;17:37–44.

92. Brickman AS, Carlson HE, Levin SR. Responses to glucagon infusion in pseudohypoparathyroidism. *J Clin Endocrinol Metab* 1986;63:1354–1360.

93. Moses AM, Weinstock RS, Levine MA, Breslau NA. Evidence for normal antidiuretic responses to endogenous and exogenous arginine vasopressin in patients with guanine nucleotide-binding stimulatory protein-deficient pseudohypoparathyroidism. *J Clin Endocrinol Metab* 1986;62:221–224.

94. Ridderskamp P, Schlaghecke R. Pseudohypoparathyroidism and adrenal cortex insufficiency. A case of multiple endocrinology due to peripheral hormone resistance. *Klin Wochenschr* 1990;68:927–931.

95. Farfel Z, Friedman E. Mental deficiency in pseudohypoparathyroidism type I is associated with Ns-protein deficiency. *Ann Intern Med* 1986;105:197–199.

96. Faig JC, Kalinyak J, Marcus R, Feldman D. Chronic atypical seizure disorder and cataracts due to delayed diagnosis of pseudohypoparathyroidism. *West J Med* 1992;157:64–65.

97. Bonadio WA. Hypocalcemia caused by pseudohypoparathyroidism presenting as convulsion. *Pediatr Emerg Care* 1989;5:22–23.

98. Furukawa T. Periodic psychosis associated with pseudopseudohypoparathyroidism. *J Nerv Ment Dis* 1991;179:637–638.

99. Klawans HL, Lupton M, Simon L. Calcification of the basal ganglia as a cause of levodopa-resistant parkinsonism. *Neurology* 1976;26:221–225.

100. Weinstock RS, Wright HN, Spiegel AM, Levine MA, Moses AM. Olfactory dysfunction in humans with deficient guanine nucleotide-binding protein. *Nature* 1986;322:635–636.

101. Henkin RI. Impairment of olfaction and of the tastes of sour and bitter in pseudohypoparathyroidism. *J Clin Endocrinol Metab* 1968;28:624.

102. Koch T, Lehnhardt E, Bottinger H, et al. Sensorineural hearing loss owing to deficient G proteins in patients with pseudohypoparathyroidism: results of a multicentre study. *Eur J Clin Invest* 1990;20:416–421.

103. McConnell RJ, Menendez CE, Smith FR, Henkin RI, Rivlin RS. Defects of taste and smell in patients with hypothyroidism. *Am J Med* 1975;59:354–364.

104. Lerea CL, Somers DE, Hurley JB, Klock IB, Bunt Milam AH. Identification of specific transducin alpha subunits in retinal rod and cone photoreceptors. *Science* 1986;234:77–80.

105. Lochrie MA, Hurley JB, Simon MI. Sequence of the alpha subunit of photoreceptor G protein: homologies between transducin, ras, and elongation factors. *Science* 1985;228: 96–99.

106. Jones DT, Reed RR. Golf: an olfactory neuron specific-G protein involved in odorant signal transduction. *Science* 1989;244:790–795.

107. McLaughlin SK, McKinnon PJ, Margolskee RF. Gustducin is a taste-cell specific G protein closely related to the tranducins. *Nature* 1992;357:563–568.

108. Sklar PB, Anholt RRH, Snyder SH. The odorant-sensitive adenylate cyclase of olfactory receptor cells. *J Biol Chem* 1986;261:15538–15543.

109. Pace U, Hanski E, Salomon Y, Lancet D. Odorant-sensitive adenylate cyclase may mediate olfactory reception. *Nature* 1985;316:255–258.

110. Pace U, Lancet D. Olfactory GTP-binding protein: signal-transducing polypeptide of vertebrate chemosensory neurons. *Proc Natl Acad Sci USA* 1986;83:4947–4951.

111. Wright HN, Weinstock RS, Spiegel AM, Levine MA, Moses AM. Guanine nucleotide-binding stimulatory protein. *Ann NY Acad Sci* 1987;510:719–722.

112. Ikeda K, Sakurada T, Sasaki Y, Takasaka T, Furukawa Y. Clinical investigation of olfactory and auditory function in type I pseudohypoparathyroidism: participation of adenylate cyclase system. *J Laryngol Otol* 1988;102:1111–1114.

113. Levy NS, Bakalyar HA, Reed RR. Signal transduction in olfactory neurons. *J Steroid Biochem Mol Biol* 1991;39:633–637.

114. Bakalyar HA, Reed RR. Identification of a specialized adenylyl cyclase that may mediate odorant detection. *Science* 1990;250:1403–1406.

115. Ellie E, Julien J, Ferrer X, Riss I, Durquety MC. Extensive cerebral calcification and retinal changes in pseudohypoparathyroidism. *J Neurol* 1989;236:432–434.

116. Jackowski MM, Hannon D, Sturr JF, Moses AM. Enhanced contrast sensitivity in patients with pseudohypoparathyroidism (abstract 1371). *Program of the Annual Meeting of ARVO* 1992;20:966.

117. Allen DB, Friedman AL, Greer FR, Chesney RW. Hypomagnesemia masking the appearance of elevated parathyroid hormone concentrations in familial pseudohypoparathyroidism. *Am J Med Genet* 1988;31:153–158.

118. Attanasio R, Curcio T, Giusti M, Monachesi M, Nalin R, Giordano G. Pseudohypoparathyroidism. A case report with low immunoreactive parathyroid hormone and multiple endocrine dysfunctions. *Minerva Endocrinol* 1986;11:267–273.

119. Hamilton DV. Familial pseudohypoparathyroidism presenting in adult life. *J R Soc Med* 1980;73:724–726.

120. Miano A, Casadel G, Biasini G. Cardiac failure in pseudohypoparathyroidism. *Helv Paediatr Acta* 1981;36:191–192.

121. Pearson DWM, Durward WF, Fogelman I, Boyle IT, Beastall G. Pseudohypoparathyroidism presenting as severe Parkinsonism. *Postgrad Med J* 1981;57:445–447.

122. Cavallo A, Meyer WJ III, Bodensteiner JB, Chesson AL. Spinal cord compression: an unusual manifestation of pseudohypoparathyroidism. *Am J Dis Child* 1980;134:706–707.

123. Moses AM, Rao KJ, Coulson R, Miller R. Parathyroid hormone deficiency with Albright's hereditary osteodystrophy. *J Clin Endocrinol Metab* 1974;39:496–500.

124. Isozaki O, Sato K, Tsushima T, Shizume K, Takamatsu J. A patient of short stature with idiopathic hypoparathyroidism, round face and metacarpal signs. *Endocrinol Jpn* 1984;31: 363–367.

125. Le Roith D, Burshell AC, Ilia R, Glick SM. Short metacarpal in a patient with idiopathic hypoparathyroidism. *Isr J Med Sci* 1979;15:460–461.

126. Moses AM, Notman DD. Albright's osteodystrophy in a patient with renal hypercalciuria. *J Clin Endocrinol Metab* 1979;49:794–797.

127. Sasaki H, Tsutsu N, Asano T, Yamamoto T, Kikuchi M, Okumura M. Co-existing primary hyperparathyroidism and Albright's hereditary osteodystrophy—an unusual association. *Postgrad Med J* 1985;61:153–155.

128. Aurbach GD, Marcus R, Winickoff RN, Epstein EH, Jr., Nigra TP. 3′,5′-cAMP in syndromes considered refractory to parathyroid hormone. *Metabolism* 1970;19:799–808.

129. Sachs C, Sjoberg HE, Ericson K. Basal ganglia calcifications on CT: relation to hypoparathyroidism. *Neurology* 1982;32:779–782.

130. Korn-Lubetzki I, Rubinger D, Siew F. Visualization of basal ganglion calcification by cranial computed tomography in

a patient with pseudohypoparathyroidism. *Isr J Med Sci* 1980;16:40–41.

131. Litvin Y, Rosler A, Bloom RA. Extensive cerebral calcification in hypoparathyroidism. *Neuroradiology* 1981;21:271.

132. Breslau NA, Notman D, Canterbury JM, Moses AM. Studies on the attainment of normocalcemia in patients with pseudohypoparathyroidism. *Am J Med* 1980;68:856–860.

133. Furlong TJ, Seshadri MS, Wilkinson MR, Cornish CJ, Luttrell B, Posen S. Clinical experiences with human parathyroid hormone 1–34. *Aust NZ J Med* 1986;16:794–798.

134. McElduff A, Lissner D, Wilkinson M, Cornish C, Posen S. A 6-hour human parathyroid hormone (1–34) infusion protocol: studies in normal and hypoparathyroid subjects. *Calcif Tissue Int* 1987;41:267–273.

135. Mallette LE. Synthetic human parathyroid hormone 1–34 fragment for diagnostic testing. *Ann Intern Med* 1988;109:800–804.

136. Mallette LE, Kirkland JL, Gagel RF, Law WM Jr, Health H III. Synthetic human parathyroid hormone-(1–34) for the study of pseudohypoparathyroidism. *J Clin Endocrinol Metab* 1988;67:964–972.

137. Rude RK, Oldham SB, Singer FR. Functional hypoparathyroidism and parathyroid hormone end-organ resistance in human magnesium deficiency. *Clin Endocrinol* 1976;5:209–224.

138. Slatopolsky E, Mercado A, Morrison A, Yates J, Klahr S. Inhibitory effects of hypomagnesemia on the renal action of parathyroid hormone. *J Clin Invest* 1976;58:1273–1279.

139. Beck N, Davis BB. Impaired renal response to parathyroid hormone in potassium depletion. *Am J Physiol* 1975;228:179–183.

140. Beck N, Kim HP, Kim KS. Effect of metabolic acidosis on renal action of parathyroid hormone. *Am J Physiol* 1975;228:1483–1488.

141. Sohn HE, Furukawa Y, Yumita S, Miura R, Unakami H, Yoshinaga K. Effect of synthetic 1–34 fragment of human parathyroid hormone on plasma adenosine 3′,5′-monophosphate (cAMP) concentrations and the diagnostic criteria based on the plasma cAMP response in Ellsworth-Howard test. *Endocrinol Jpn* 1984;31:33–40.

142. Walton RJ, Bijvoet OLM. Nomogram for derivation of renal threshold phosphate concentration. *Lancet* 1975;2:309–310.

143. Miura R, Yumita S, Yoshinaga K, Furukawa Y. Response of plasma 1,25-dihydroxyvitamin D in the human PTH (1–34) infusion test: an improved index for the diagnosis of idiopathic hypoparathyroidism and pseudohypoparathyroidism. *Calcif Tissue Int* 1990;46:309–313.

144. Lebowitz MR, Moses AM. Hypocalcemia. *Semin Nephrol* 1992;12:146–158.

145. Litvak J, Moldawer MP, Forbes AP, Henneman PH. Hypocalcemic hypercalciuria during vitamin D and dihydrotachysterol therapy of hypoparathyroidism. *J Clin Endocrinol Metab* 1958;18:246–252.

146. Yamamoto M, Takuwa Y, Masuko S, Ogata E. Effects of endogenous and exogenous parathyroid hormone on tubular reabsorption of calcium in pseudohypoparathyroidism. *J Clin Endocrinol Metab* 1988;66:618–625.

147. Kolb FO, Steinbach HL. Pseudohypoparathyroidism with secondary hyperparathyroidism and osteitis fibrosa. *J Clin Endocrinol Metab* 1962;22:59–64.

148. Slatopolsky E, Weerts C, Thielan J, Horst R, Harter H, Martin KJ. Marked suppression of secondary hyperparathyroidism by intravenous administration of 1,25-dihydroxycholecalciferol in uremia patients. *J Clin Invest* 1984;74:2136–2143.

149. Breslau N, Moses AM. Renal calcium reabsorption caused by bicarbonate and by chlorothiazide in patients with hormone resistant (pseudo) hypoparathyroidism. *J Clin Endocrinol Metab* 1978;46:389–395.

150. Shangraw RF. Factors to consider in the selection of a calcium supplement. *Public Health Rep Suppl* 1989;104:46–50.

151. Food and Drug Administration. Advice on limiting intake of bone meal. *FDA Drug Bull* 1982;12:5–6.

152. Recker RR. Calcium absorption and achlorhydria. *N Engl J Med* 1985;313:70–73.

153. Komindr S, Schmidt LW, Palmieri GMA. Case report: oral calcium chloride in hypoparathyroidism refractory to massive doses of calcium carbonate and vitamin D. *Am J Med Sci* 1989;296:182–184.

154. Harvey JA, Zobitz MM, Pak CYC. Dose dependency of calcium absorption: a comparison of calcium carbonate and calcium citrate. *J Bone Mineral Res* 1988;3:253–258.

155. Okano K, Furukawa Y, Morii H, Fujita T. Comparative efficacy of various vitamin D metabolites in the treatment of various types of hypoparathyroidism. *J Clin Endocrinol Metab* 1982;55:238–243.

156. Breslau NA. Pseudohypoparathyroidism: current concepts. *Am J Med Sci* 1989;298:130–140.

157. Rosler A, Rabinowitz D. Magnesium-induced reversal of vitamin D resistance in hypoparathyroidism. *Lancet* 1973;1:803–805.

158. Breslau NA, Zerwekh JE. Relationship of estrogen and pregnancy to calcium homeostasis in pseudohypoparathyroidism. *J Clin Endocrinol Metab* 1986;62:45–51.

159. Verbeelen D, Fuss M. Hypercalcemia induced by estrogen withdrawal in vitamin D-treated hypoparathyroidism. *Br Med J* 1979;1:522–523.

160. Mallette LE. Case report: hypoparathyroidism with menses-associated hypocalcemia. *Am J Med Sci* 1992;304:32–37.

161. Zerwekh JE, Breslau NA. Human placental production of 1 alpha,25-dihydroxyvitamin D3: biochemical characterization and production in normal subjects and patients with pseudohypoparathyroidism. *J Clin Endocrinol Metab* 1986;62:192–196.

162. Caplan RH, Beguin EA. Hypercalcemia in a calcitriol-treated hypoparathyroid woman during lactation. *Obstet Gynecol* 1990;76:485–489.

163. Firooznia H, Golimbu C, Rafii M. Progressive paraparesis in a woman with pseudohypoparathyroidism with ossification of the posterior longitudinal ligament from C4 to T5. *Skel Radiol* 1985;13:310–313.

164. Kalajian A. Pseudo-pseudohypoparathyroidism and its manifestations in the foot. *Arch Podiatr Med Foot Surg* 1978;5:9–12.

165. Rabbani SA, Kaiser SM, Henderson JE, et al. Synthesis and characterization of extended and deleted recombinant analogues of parathyroid hormone-(1–84): correlation of peptide structure with function. *Biochemistry* 1990;29:10080–10089.

The Parathyroids, edited by J.P. Bilezikian, M.A. Levine, and R. Marcus. Raven Press, Ltd., New York © 1994.

CHAPTER 47

Treatment of Hypoparathyroidism

J. L. H. O'Riordan

Since the realization that vitamin D could cause increased calcium absorption and hypercalcemia, the vitamin has been used in the treatment of hypoparathyroidism, whatever its origin. Relatively little is written about this treatment, and it remains more of an art than a science. For this reason, it is best practiced by those who see the condition frequently rather than by those who are unfamiliar with the problem. Inevitably in this situation much will depend on personal preference rather than universally accepted practice. The contents of this chapter reflect this situation; it illustrates the views and practices of the author.

Interestingly, there are wide variations in treatment regimes used in different parts of the world. To some extent this depends on the preparations of vitamin D, its analogs, and its metabolites that are available. In the United States and in the United Kingdom, vitamin D_2 (calciferol, ergocalciferol) and to a lesser extent vitamin D_3 (cholecalciferol) have been used rather commonly. Dihydrotachysterol (Tachyrol, AT10) has been used extensively in the United States and in mainland Europe and to some extent in the United Kingdom. 25-Hydroxycholecalciferol has been available in the United States, while 1α-hydroxycholecalciferol (Alfacalcidol, 1α-alfacalcidol) has been available in Europe but not in the United States. 1,25-Dihydroxycholecalciferol (calcitriol, Rocaltrol) has been available both in Europe and in the United States.

At this point, let me define several terms. When a particular form is being considered, it will be given its own name, but, when a general comment is being made, the term "vitamin D" is used and this will apply to any of the forms of the vitamin that were introduced above.

The advantage of using 1-hydroxylated forms of vi-

tamin D is that they act more quickly. The serum calcium can rise with their use, from 1.5 mmol/liter (6 mg/dl) up to 2.2 mmol/liter (8.8 mg/dl) in only a few days rather than the few weeks it would take if vitamin D_2 or vitamin D_3 had been administered. The 1-hydroxylated forms of vitamin D are also much more potent. While the maintenance dose of calcitriol might be 0.5 μg/day and that for 1α might be 1 μg/day, it might be necessary to give as much as 1–2 mg of vitamin D_2 or vitamin D_3 (40,000–80,000 units a day). Just as the action of 1-hydroxylated compounds develops more rapidly, so the effect of their excess disappears more quickly. Thus hypercalcemia can be reversed within a few days if calcitriol treatment is stopped but may take a few weeks or even months if vitamin D_2 or vitamin D_3 have been given. The longer duration of vitamin D_2 or vitamin D_3 is due to storage in body fat and slow release. In addition, 25-hydroxyergocalciferol and 25-hydroxycholecalciferol, the initial hydroxylated products of vitamin D_2 and vitamin D_3, respectively, circulate bound to a plasma carrier protein and so are less labile.

PREPARATIONS

Only the main preparations are considered here. It is a major undertaking to switch from one preparation to another, and this should not be done lightly. For example, a change from a long-acting preparation to a more quickly acting one should be phased in over a period of 1–2 months. Because the equivalence of the different preparations is not well defined, there is considerable room for confusion among physicians, pharmacists, and patients. Uncertainty about dosage equivalence is caused further by the availability of different strengths of preparations. For some preparations, the dose can be given in terms of weight (micrograms or milligrams) or in international unitage, and in

J. L. H. O'Riordan: Department of Metabolic Medicine, University College London, The Middlesex Hospital, London W1N 8AA United Kingdom.

such cases it is wise to cite both. For example, when 1.25 mg calciferol is given daily, it is wise to specify the dose as 50,000 units daily as well. Rather confusingly, in Britain, the descriptions "high-strength" and "strong" were also used for different preparations of vitamin D (the former referred to 10,000 units and the latter to 50,000 units). Such terms are undesirable. Whatever preparation is being used, it is best in discussions with the patient to be very precise, referring to the content and the color of the capsules. Patients should be encouraged to bring their capsules to show the physician and to be equally precise in describing their treatment. They should be warned to query any change in the appearance of their medication. In some centers, special preparations are available for particular purposes. These must be used with caution because of the problems of quality control and stability. In solutions, preservatives are needed. In a capsule containing high-quality arachis oil with antioxidants, they may be stable for 1 year, but reassay will be necessary to confirm this. Even commercial preparations made on a large scale can cause problems for reasons that are not always clear. Recently, in the United Kingdom, the supply of dihydrotachysterol has been discontinued and the supply of calciferol (ergocalciferol) has been interrupted temporarily. Some manufacturers allow "overage" to ensure that with prolonged storage there will still be a specified content in the preparation. This may mean that to allow greater "shelf-life" and still have, say, 1.25 mg calciferol, there may initially be 10–20% excess in a fresh batch. Since this is not generally known, and the presence of excess is not clear, errors may be caused unwittingly. Attention should be paid whenever an expiration date is given, of course. If a particular preparation is not available temporarily, it is better to change to another preparation containing the same form of vitamin D rather than restabilize the patient on a different compound. For example, if a pharmacy runs out of stock, it would be better to substitute 0.25 μg capsules of alfacalcidol in place of 1 μg capsules, and not to change to calcitriol, even though they are both 1-hydroxylated compounds.

MANAGEMENT

Long-Standing Hypoparathyroidism

Patients with long-standing hypoparathyroidism (be it due to idiopathic hypoparathyroidism, pseudohypoparathyroidism, or surgical hypoparathyroidism) can be considered together. It is likely that these patients on long-term therapy have been treated with vitamin D_2 or vitamin D_3 in doses of 1–3 mg or with dihydrotachysterol (0.2–1 mg/day). Long-term follow-up is necessary, with measurement of serum calcium every 3–4 months. The response to change in dosage will be slow, so any alteration to gain better control must be gradual. The adjustments will depend on the variety of sizes of tablet or capsule available. Since this variety is likely to be limited, it may be necessary to prescribe different doses on different days of the week or month. For example, a patient taking 1.25 mg calciferol/day might be given an extra tablet once per week; patients might take one tablet on odd days and two on even days to facilitate compliance. If hypercalcemia develops in a patient taking a long-acting preparation, treatment should be stopped until normocalcemia is restored. Assuming that the patient is not symptomatic and that renal function has not deteriorated because of vitamin D intoxication, nothing else will be needed. If the hypercalcemia is minimal (say, 2.6 mmol/liter, 10.4 mg/dl), it is reasonable merely to reduce the dose and to review the situation in several months if the disorder has previously been well controlled. If a serious episode of hypercalcemia has occurred and treatment has had to be stopped until normocalcemia is restored, a decision has to be made about whether to restart the patient on a smaller dose of the same preparation or to change to a newer, more rapidly acting form. In general, it would be much simpler to restart the patient on a lower dosage of the same preparation.

Newly Diagnosed Cases

It is reasonable to start these patients on a newer preparation such as calcitriol. If the patient has idiopathic hypoparathyroidism or pseudohypoparathyroidism, the hypocalcemia will probably have been long-standing, and it is better tolerated than it would be, for example, in a patient who has had thyroid surgery and inadvertently has been rendered hypoparathyroid. In the latter situation, hypocalcemia and tetany will develop within a few days, and, under such circumstances, intravenous calcium may be needed while other therapy is taking effect. In an adult it would be reasonable to start with 0.5 μg calcitriol twice daily or 1 μg alfacalcidol twice daily, monitoring serum calcium frequently, and changing the dose upward or downward as necessary. Changes in dosage can be made in general every 2–3 days. The maintenance dose of calcitriol is ~0.5 μg/day and that of alfacalcidol is ~1 μg/day, but at the start of treatment larger doses may be needed (up to 3 μg calcitriol/day, for example). It should be possible to stabilize the treatment regimen within 1 month.

A special situation is presented by the patient whose hypoparathyroidism was heralded by seizures. If the patient is to be treated with alfacalcidol, it should be remembered that this compound has to be 25-hydroxylated in the liver to be active. Antiseizure medications will inhibit this hydroxylation step. In these patients, therefore, a higher dose of alfacalcidol will be needed while the antiseizure medication is used. When the antiseizure medication is reduced, the dose of alfacalcidol also will have to be reduced. If the patient has a long-term seizure disorder and hypoparathyroidism has occurred separately, treatment for the seizures will have to be continued. Caution, however, is needed if any form of vitamin D apart from calcitriol is used, since metabolism to the active form is needed, and the dose required will change with any alteration in treatment of the seizure disorder.

Once treatment has been stabilized, serum calcium should be monitored every few months. Measurements of urine calcium are not essential. If they are taken, hypercalciuria will often be found. In the absence of renal stone formation, hypercalcemia per se is not worrisome. It is wise, however, to obtain a plain x-ray or ultrasound of the abdomen every few years to ensure that nephrocalcinosis or stone formation is not developing. It is sensible to check for occult kidney stones or nephrocalcinosis at the beginning of treatment to establish the baseline.

In a small proportion of patients (perhaps a few percent) control will not be satisfactory, and serum calcium will fluctuate wildly, being sometimes too high and sometimes too low, apparently with the same dose. The reason for this is generally not clear. Poor and variable compliance could be suspected. In part, the fluctuations may be attributed to variation in calcium intake, sometimes being high and at other times low. Strict dieting to reduce weight may also contribute to this. If a patient is on a rapidly acting form of vitamin D (e.g., calcitriol), it may be reasonable, in desperation because of rapid swings, to change to a longer acting preparation (e.g., vitamin D_2). It may also be sensible to try giving calcium supplements to provide high intake that will not be greatly affected by dietary variations. In this way, the speed of swings may be slowed, but it is unlikely that they will be eliminated. Motivation of the patient is important, and this has to be encouraged to obtain the best results of therapy.

Use of Calcium Supplements

It is possible to maintain patients very well on vitamin D, with calcium supplements. If hypercalcemia develops, it can be rapidly reversed by reducing the calcium intake, without changing the vitamin D intake (Bijvoet, personal communication). In general, however, it seems preferable to control the problem with a single substance, i.e., vitamin D or one of its derivatives. In acute hypocalcemia (after an inadvertent parathyroidectomy during thyroid surgery, for example), intravenous calcium may be needed intermittently to avoid tetany while long-term therapy is estab-

lished and stabilized. A special example of this occurs in patients undergoing radical surgery for pharyngeal or laryngeal neoplasms, since they are often very ill for long periods postoperatively, are not eating, and may become hypoalbuminemic. In this case, intravenous calcium will be needed until the patient can swallow satisfactorily, since vitamin D, even calcitriol, will have little benefit in the absence of a normal calcium intake.

Treatment of Patients After Surgery for Hyperparathyroidism

It is expected, after parathyroidectomy for hyperparathyroidism, that serum calcium will fall to normal within a few days, though this can sometimes take 7–10 days. Symptoms of hypocalcemia may develop postoperatively, even when the serum calcium is still elevated. Those symptoms do not require treatment. Transient hypocalcemia after neck exploration is quite common, and normocalcemia should be achieved, again within 1 week. Generally, it is reasonable to do no more in this situation, apart from giving oral calcium supplements if there are symptoms. It seems reasonable to delay more specific treatment if possible for 2–3 weeks, since, once vitamin D treatment is started, it is likely to be lifelong. It has been argued that a previously suppressed normal gland can be stimulated back to activity by permitting serum calcium to fall. The evidence for this, however, is not great.

If, preoperatively, there is hyperparathyroid bone disease (as witnessed on x-ray changes or raised alkaline phosphatase), then hypocalcemia is to be expected postoperatively. This is more likely to occur in patients with large tumors. In such patients, it is wise to start treatment as soon as serum calcium falls below normal (indicating the success of surgery). It has been suggested that preoperative treatment with alfacalcidol or calcitriol helps in postoperative control. This is difficult to prove. The so-called hungry bone disease that occurs after removal of parathyroids in patients with hyperparathyroid bone disease can cause severe, serious hypocalcemia and is resistant to treatment. High doses of calcitriol can be given, with large calcium supplements. The initial dose of calcitriol in this situation may reasonably be 1 μg twice per day, doubling this dose every 3–4 days as necessary, and increasing calcium supplements until control is achieved. This may require as much as 20 μg calcitriol/day, with 120 mM calcium per day, for example, as calcium lactate gluconate daily (this can be given as Sandocal 400 effervescent tablets each of which contains Ca^{++} 10 mM, 400 mg). Potentially, of course, this is a dangerous regime, and daily monitoring of serum calcium is necessary for a few weeks. As soon as normocalcemia is achieved, quite rapid reduction in dosage is necessary. In the longer term, high doses of calcitriol (4 μg/ day) may be needed for several months. Suddenly, when the bone disease is healed, the requirement for vitamin D and calcium will fall dramatically. The best way to anticipate this and to avoid hypercalcemia is to follow the alkaline phosphatase activity. The alkaline phosphatase level may take 6–9 months to fall to normal, but once it is normal there is a risk of hypercalcemia. Such patients can usually then be maintained on relatively small doses of calcitriol (say, 0.5–1 μg/day).

In patients in whom multiple operations have been performed to cure hyperparathyroidism and in whom several normal glands have previously been removed before the adenoma is found, it is likely that long-lasting hypoparathyroidism will ultimately result. This may, of course, be the result of initial surgery, as with patients with familial multiple endocrine neoplasia type I, because of the risk of recurrence if limited surgery is performed. In such cases, postoperatively treatment may start sooner than might otherwise be the case.

Management of Hypoparathyroidism in Pregnancy

Obviously it is desirable to maintain normocalcemia insofar as possible before, during, and after pregnancy, to avoid any adverse effects on the outcome. Patients can be reassured that this does not pose major problems, though particular care is needed in the third trimester and in the puerperium. The obstetrician and pediatrician should be made aware of the situation and appropriate supervision arranged. During the last 3 months of pregnancy, the dose of vitamin D (whatever form is used) may have to be reduced; this may be the result of the placenta having a 1α-hydroxylase enzyme capable of synthesizing 1,25-dihydroxyvitamin D_3. Serum calcium should therefore be measured monthly at that stage. After delivery, even in patients treated with calcitriol, there is again risk of hypercalcemia, probably the consequence of the effect of prolactin in stimulating 1α-hydroxylation. The dose of vitamin D therefore may have to be reduced. Breast feeding, with consequent temporary loss of calcium, is perfectly reasonable. For the first month after delivery, it is probably wise to measure serum calcium once per week.

CONCLUSIONS

It should be realized that vitamin D in all its forms can be a difficult drug to use and that treatment for hypoparathyroidism is necessary on a life-long basis. It is therefore necessary to inform the patient accordingly. Unpredictable changes in therapeutic requirements are the rule rather than the exception. Even after a period of several years with a stable dose, hypercalcemia and vitamin D intoxication may develop, so continued vigilance is required.

Continuity of care is important, though, inevitably in the lifetime of the patient, more than one physician is likely to be involved. With care, the problems of both low and high calcium can be avoided.

The Parathyroids, edited by J.P. Bilezikian,
M.A. Levine, and R. Marcus. Raven Press, Ltd.,
New York © 1994.

CHAPTER 48

Parathyroid Function and Responsiveness in Osteoporosis

Shonni J. Silverberg and John P. Bilezikian

As the incidence and prevalence of osteoporosis increases, with the attendant rise in economic and social costs, efforts to delineate the pathophysiologic basis of this disorder have intensified. Although estrogen deficiency characterizes the menopause in all women and is considered to be an important pathophysiologic feature, only 10–20% of postmenopausal women develop osteoporotic fractures within 20 years of cessation of menses (1). Despite some supporting data (2–4), most evidence argues against the hypothesis that postmenopausal women who develop osteoporosis are relatively more estrogen deficient than their counterparts who do not develop osteoporosis (5,6). Even studies that have noted a difference in sex steroid levels among those who develop osteoporosis have implicated additional factors in the pathogenesis of osteoporotic bone disease. Identifiable risk factors such as family history, racial and ethnic background, and peak bone mass achieved in young adulthood, as well as smoking, alcohol, and lack of physical exercise, are all believed to be important (7,8). In conjunction with estrogen deficiency, these other risk factors, knowledge of which is based on epidemiological studies, give a more satisfactory accounting of bone loss in the postmenopausal years. However, the epidemiological approach does not address mechanisms by which bone is lost. It is reasonable to consider the possibility that calcium-regulating hormones play a mechanistic role in the development of osteoporosis. For example, parathyroid function and responsiveness in osteoporosis have been a subject of active investigation in recent years. Vitamin D has also been implicated. This chapter reviews the evidence that the calcium-regulating hormones parathyroid hormone (PTH) and vitamin D play an important role in the pathophysiology of osteoporosis.

In osteoporosis, the normally tight balance between bone formation and bone resorption is lost. When this balance is at its most efficient, the amount of bone resorbed during the initial phase of bone remodeling is completely replaced by new bone formed in the subsequent stage of the remodeling sequence. With age, the efficiency of this process is reduced so that the amount of bone formed does not quite match the amount of bone lost. Over many years, this inefficiency leads to gradual loss of bone. It is this process of gradual bone loss in which PTH and vitamin D have been investigated as possible etiologic factors. For example, intestinal calcium absorption, a function dependent in part on vitamin D, has long been known to decrease with advancing age and may be reduced to a greater extent in osteoporotic subjects (9–11). A likely candidate to account for this age-related reduction in calcium absorption is the active metabolite of vitamin D, 1,25-dihydroxyvitamin D [$1,25(OH)_2D_3$].

Parathyroid hormone is also worthy of consideration as a potential causative agent in osteoporosis. The rationale for focusing on this hormone stems in part from its pivotal role in bone remodeling. Parathyroid hormone normally activates the remodeling cycle by indirectly stimulating the osteoclast through intercellular signals generated by its direct target cell, osteoblasts or osteoblast-like cells (12–14). When increased in pathologic states, PTH will induce excessive bone remodeling characterized by a rate of bone resorption that exceeds the rate of bone formation. Because of the inherent inefficiency of bone remodel-

S. J. Silverberg: Department of Medicine, Division of Endocrinology, College of Physicians and Surgeons, Columbia University, New York, New York 10032.

J. P. Bilezikian: Departments of Medicine and Pharmacology, College of Physicians and Surgeons, Columbia University, New York, New York 10032.

ing in adults, a higher remodeling rate is likely to lead to bone loss.

Another hypothesis rests on the idea that PTH in postmenopausal women becomes more catabolic for bone because of enhanced skeletal sensitivity (15). This catabolic action of PTH would surface in postmenopausal women because estrogens, which normally counteract the actions of parathyroid hormone, are reduced. Thus, for the same circulating level of PTH, postmenopausal women would become more sensitive than others to its actions.

Recognition that PTH is catabolic under pathologic conditions has tended to obscure its key physiologic role as an anabolic peptide for bone (see the chapters by Canalis et al. and by Marcus). This important physiologic effect under normal conditions has led to efforts to reveal abnormalities in PTH regulation in osteoporosis. Calvo et al. (16) suggested that differences between men and women in circadian variations in circulating PTH levels could contribute to the greater bone loss in women. These authors showed that women have a less vigorous rise in circulating PTH than men in response to mild hypocalcemia induced by overnight fasting. With blunted parathyroid responsiveness to this subtle hypocalcemic signal, the kidneys are less efficient in conserving calcium. Over years, such subtle differences in circadian responses of the parathyroid glands could contribute to a major loss of bone mass. This formulation is keyed to the notion that PTH is a major anabolic hormone for bone and that in postmenopausal women its overall availability to function in this capacity is reduced. The potential importance of the anabolic actions of PTH on skeletal metabolism is well illustrated in another disorder of mineral metabolism, primary hyperparathyroidism. In the mild presentation of the disease most commonly seen today, potential sites of postmenopausal bone loss, namely, the cancellous skeleton, are not affected (17). Rather, postmenopausal estrogen-deficient women with primary hyperparathyroidism show a preservation of cancellous bone as demonstrated by bone mineral densitometry and histomorphometric analysis of bone biopsies (see the chapter by Parisien et al.) (18–20).

Despite data suggesting a possible role for PTH in the development of osteoporosis, definitive answers remain elusive. Many studies have been flawed by the lack of an appropriate control group or by use of pharmacologic doses of PTH to assess physiologic responses. Improvements in assays for PTH have required reconsideration of older studies whose validity was limited by assay methodology. In addition, it has been necessary, but often is not possible, to distinguish between age-related changes in mineral metabolism that do not necessarily lead to osteoporosis and those that do.

PARATHYROID HORMONE AND 1,25-DIHYDROXYVITAMIN D LEVELS IN OSTEOPOROSIS

Advances in immunoassay techniques (see the chapter by Nausbaum and Potts) have aided in the characterization of basal and stimulated levels of PTH in osteoporosis. Basal levels of PTH clearly increased with age in most studies, as measured by both radioimmunoassay and bioassay (21–25). However, in postmenopausal osteoporosis, basal levels of PTH have been reported to be increased (5,21,26), normal (27,28), or decreased (5,11,29) relative to those in age-matched controls. No difference was reported between osteoporotic and normal women using the immunoradiometric assay for parathyroid hormone (IRMA) (4,30), while the even newer, more sensitive immunochemiluminometric assay has shown reduced basal PTH levels in osteoporotic patients (4,31). Several studies have identified a small subgroup of osteoporotic women, first identified by Jowsey and Riggs in 1973, who have increased PTH levels (5,21,26,32). If this is documented, this subset is unlikely to account for more than a small fraction of osteoporotic women.

The effect of advancing age on levels of 1,25-dihydroxyvitamin D [$1,25(OH)_2D_3$] is less controversial. There is a decrease in circulating levels of $1,25(OH)_2D_3$ in the elderly (11,22,29,33). Individuals with osteoporosis have $1,25(OH)_2D_3$ levels that are generally lower than those in age- and sex-matched normal individuals (11,34). This reduction is accompanied by a reduction in calcium absorption (11).

PATHOPHYSIOLOGIC IMPLICATIONS OF PARATHYROID HORMONE AND VITAMIN D IN OSTEOPOROSIS

It is likely that osteoporosis is not a single entity but instead a descriptive endpoint for a number of distinct pathogenetic pathways (35). With regard to parathyroid hormone, four different pathogenetic mechanisms leading to osteoporosis have been postulated (see Table 1).

TABLE 1. *Pathophysiology of osteoporosis: hypotheses*

Postulated primary mechanism	PTH change
1. Altered vitamin D metabolism	Increase
2. Altered skeletal sensitivity to PTH	Normal/decrease
3. Suppression of parathyroid gland	Decrease
4. Altered parathyroid gland responsiveness	Normal/decrease

For each hypothesis, the primary abnormality is placed at a different physiologic "level." In hypothesis 1, the abnormality in PTH activity is due to a primary disturbance in vitamin D metabolism. In hypothesis 2, the skeleton has become abnormally sensitive to PTH. In hypothesis 3, unidentified factor(s) lead to secondary suppression of a normally functioning parathyroid glands. In hypothesis 4, abnormalities in responsiveness of the parathyroid glands themselves are accountable for the development of osteoporosis.

Altered Vitamin D Metabolism

Decreased intestinal calcium among the elderly has been reported in studies of fractional calcium absorption and metabolic balance, with an even greater decrease in calcium absorption noted in osteoporotic subjects (9,11,36–38). Bone loss resulting from reduced calcium absorption could be due to a primary abnormality in vitamin D metabolism, with reduced levels of 1,25-dihydroxyvitamin D. The decrease in intestinal calcium absorption would lead to a subtle reduction in serum calcium concentration, which might not be detected. However, the hypocalcemic signal would induce a secondary increase in PTH. While most studies to test this hypothesis have implicated a defect in $1,25(OH)_2D_3$ production, a potential abnormality in metabolism of the precursor to $1,25(OH)_2D_3$, 25-hydroxyvitamin D, has not escaped notice. Villareal et al. (39) found that 9.1% of their population of midwestern U.S. women with postmenopausal osteoporosis had low (<38 nmol/liter; mean −2 SD of their normal population) 25-hydroxyvitamin D levels. In this group vertebral bone density correlated positively with levels of 25-hydroxyvitamin D and inversely with PTH levels, which were increased. Multivariate analysis demonstrated that the rise in PTH was best correlated with the decrease in bone density.

Early studies used pharmacologic doses of parathyroid extract to investigate whether decreased $1,25(OH)_2D_3$ levels in postmenopausal osteoporosis were due to a decrease in renal 1α-hydroxylase activity. A similar rise in $1,25(OH)_2D_3$ was observed in normal and osteoporotic individuals when high doses of PTH were administered. Although normal renal responsiveness could thus be demonstrated under these pharmacologic conditions, it remained possible that an abnormality existed in renal responsiveness to more physiologic levels of PTH (29,40). Subsequent studies suggested that the ability of kidney to generate $1,25(OH)_2D_3$ in response to PTH decreases with advancing age, with a further unexplained impairment in a group with age-related osteoporosis (33). However, the two older groups of subjects in this study, one with and one without osteoporosis, were not directly comparable be-

cause of differences in renal function. It remained possible that the differences observed between the two older groups of subjects were due primarily to differences in renal function and not to a particular abnormality in the osteoporotic group. Using more physiologic doses, Slovik et al. showed a blunted rise in $1,25(OH)_2D_3$ to PTH osteoporotic patients (41). Unfortunately, the control group in this study consisted of normal young individuals, making it impossible to know whether the observed abnormality in PTH responsiveness was due merely to advancing age or to the osteoporotic process itself.

In addition to impaired formation of $1,25(OH)_2D_3$, other factors that could contribute to altered $1,25(OH)_2D_3$ metabolism in osteoporosis include a decrease in $1,25(OH)_2D_3$ receptors in the small intestine (42,43). In 44 healthy women aged 20–87 years, a decrease in the concentration of duodenal $1,25(OH)_2D_3$ receptors was shown to be a function of age. Reduced calcitriol receptors could account for a reduction in gastrointestinal tract calcium absorption, offering an explanation for the PTH concentration.

A third mechanism to account for altered vitamin D metabolism in osteoporosis involves altered binding of $1,25(OH)_2D_3$ to its receptors (44) rather than a decrease in receptor number. Fourth, a postreceptor defect in $1,25(OH)_2D_3$ responsiveness may be proposed. Evidence for this possibility comes from a study of normal young women who had undergone oophorectomy (45). Six months after oophorectomy, a reduction in fractional calcium absorption and vertebral bone density was seen. Calcium absorption in response to $1,25(OH)_2D_3$ administration was blunted. The subnormal response, which could be prevented by estrogen replacement, was thought to be consistent with end-organ resistance to $1,25(OH)_2D_3$.

Altered Skeletal Sensitivity to Parathyroid Hormone

According to this hypothesis, originally proposed by Heaney in 1965, enhanced sensitivity to PTH in osteoporosis leads to greater bone resorption at any given level of circulating hormone (4,5,11,15,46). Early data from Riggs et al. (5) provided indirect support for this idea, with histologic evidence of increased bone resorption in the face of normal or low serum PTH immunoactivity. More recently, the same group published histomorphometric data supporting their earlier conclusions (4). Indices of bone remodeling were analyzed with regard to PTH levels by both immunoradiometric and immunochemiluminometric assays in normal and osteoporotic postmenopausal women. Measures of bone turnover, including bone resorption rate, bone formation rate, activation frequency, and rate of bone loss, all correlated with PTH levels in osteoporotic but not in normal individuals. For each pmol/liter increase in PTH, as measured in the immunochemiluminometric assay, there was greater activation frequency (1.3%/year), higher bone resorption rate (3.9%/year), and more cancellous bone loss (2.8%/year) in the women with postmenopausal osteoporosis.

These conclusions, however, were not supported by Tsai et al. (47) in a study employing pharmacologic doses of PTH to assess biochemical, rather than histologic, markers. Bovine PTH-(1–34) and 400 U/day was administered for 3 days to premenopausal and postmenopausal normal women and to women with postmenopausal osteoporosis. Although the osteoporotic women had evidence for increased bone turnover at baseline (higher urinary hydroxyproline levels than postmenopausal control subjects), the hormone-induced rise in both serum calcium concentration and urinary hydroxyproline was similar in all three groups. The authors concluded that these data speak against enhanced sensitivity to PTH in osteoporosis. Problems in this study, clearly noted by the authors, include a very high dose of PTH, the relative insensitivity of measured indices of increased resorption, and inadequate statistical power inherent in the study design.

Suppression of Parathyroid Gland Function

A third hypothesis implicating PTH in the pathophysiology of osteoporosis argues for a secondary suppression of parathyroid gland function. The hypothesis recognizes the importance of PTH action as anabolic for bone. This concept differs from the first two hypotheses in invoking a process that, independent of PTH, increases bone resorption and leads ultimately to osteoporosis. The increase in bone resorption leads to a subclinical rise in ionized calcium, with a compensatory suppression of PTH secretion. In this model, an associated decrease in intestinal calcium absorption would be a secondary phenomenon, due to lack of action of PTH to stimulate $1,25(OH)_2D_3$ formation. The list of agents potentially responsible for this suppression of PTH include interleukin-1, which has been reported to be produced at an enhanced rate by activated monocytes from postmenopausal osteoporotic women (48). In vitro interleukin-1 is a most potent stimulus to bone resorptive activity when assessed on a molar basis (49). Interleukin-6, another potent cytokine, has been implicated specifically in the enhanced bone resorption that occurs in conjunction with estrogen deficiency (50,51). Other local factors shown to stimulate bone resorption in vitro include lymphotoxin (52), tumor necrosis factor (52),

transforming growth factor (53,54), and certain prostaglandins (55–57).

Among recent studies supporting the concept of parathyroid suppression in osteoporosis, the work of Ebeling et al. (58) is noteworthy. These authors compared biochemical indices and bone markers in normal and osteoporotic women before and after calcium deprivation. At baseline, the osteoporotic cohort had lower PTH and higher osteocalcin and hydroxypyridinium collagen cross-link levels compared to normal women. After calcium deprivation, no difference was noted among the two groups in the decrement of serum calcium concentration or in the rise of PTH, $1,25(OH)_2D_3$, or hydroxypyridinium cross-link levels. The baseline data were interpreted to be consistent with a non-PTH-mediated increase in bone resorption, with a secondary suppression of PTH. The similar response to a hypocalcemic stimulus in both groups was considered to be evidence against any enhanced skeletal sensitivity to PTH or any change in parathyroid gland responsiveness.

Altered Parathyroid Gland Responsiveness

This hypothesis suggests that an abnormality in parathyroid gland responsiveness is important in the development of osteoporosis. Using oral phosphate administration as a hypocalcemic stimulus, Silverberg et al. (59) studied the effects of the ensuing mild hypocalcemia on PTH and calcitriol levels. Using a protocol of 5 days of oral phosphate administration, three groups were studied: postmenopausal healthy and osteoporotic women and young healthy individuals. Despite a similar increase in inorganic phosphorus concentration in response to the oral phosphate challenge, and a similar fall in serum calcium concentration among the groups, hormonal responses varied. Parathyroid hormone levels rose by a modest 43% in those with osteoporosis, a change similar to the 53% increase in young normal subjects. This modest response differed considerably from the more marked 2.5-fold rise in circulating parathyroid hormone seen in the older control group (see Fig. 1). Despite these markedly different responses, $1,25(OH)_2D_3$ levels were unchanged. In those with osteoporosis, whose response was modest and similar to that of young normal subjects, $1,25(OH)_2D_3$ levels fell by 50%. Normal older women thus appeared to require greater PTH reactivity than their younger counterparts to overcome the suppressive effects of phosphate on $1,25(OH)_2D_3$ formation. The data suggest that there is an age-related decline in the formation of $1,25(OH)_2D_3$ and that, as part of the normal aging process, postmenopausal women maintain their $1,25(OH)_2D_3$ levels only by mounting a more vigorous PTH response to hypocal-

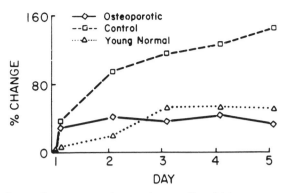

FIG. 1. Percentage change in parathyroid hormone after phosphate administration in osteoporotic and young and older normal subjects. (Reprinted from ref. 59 with permission.)

cemia than is required at a younger age. In osteoporosis, the age-appropriate rise in PTH responsiveness is not seen, suppressive effects of elevated phosphate prevail, and 1,25(OH)$_2$D$_3$ levels fall. The results support the concept of abnormal PTH responsiveness in osteoporosis, superimposed on a universal age-related decline in calcitriol production. This possibility is also consistent with suppression of parathyroid gland activity due to a nonparathyroid mechanism for activation of bone resorption (hypothesis 3).

Another assessment of parathyroid gland responsiveness to test this hypothesis avoided potential confounding effects of phosphorus on 1,25(OH)$_2$D$_3$ metabolism (30). Suppression of endogenous parathyroid hormone secretion was accomplished by infusing PTH-(1–34) at physiologic doses (0.55 U/kg/hr for 24 hr). Intact PTH-(1–84) was measured to assess endogenous hormone secretion. The extent of the response to PTH infusion, as reflected in both absolute and -fold increase in serum calcium and decrease in endogenous PTH, was indistinguishable among premenopausal and postmenopausal normal women as well as between untreated and estrogen-replaced postmenopausal women with osteoporosis. However, for any given increment in serum calcium concentration, osteoporotic individuals showed less suppression of endogenous PTH secretion compared to healthy women. Abnormal PTH suppressibility in osteoporotic subjects was not improved by estrogen-replacement therapy. Age, or the menopause itself, did not seem to affect the result. The authors concluded that skeletal sensitivity to PTH is not altered by aging or osteoporosis. Rather, in osteoporosis there is an alteration in parathyroid gland responsiveness, characterized by a change in the set point for hormone secretion. Parathyroid insensitivity to circulating calcium is consistent with the blunted stimulatory response to hypocalcemia reported by Silverberg et al. (59).

RELATIONSHIP OF PARATHYROID HORMONE TO CLASSIC DESIGNATIONS OF OSTEOPOROSIS

In 1947, Albright et al. (60) divided those with osteoporosis into two populations: a postmenopausal group and one with senile (age-related) osteoporosis. This concept was refined by Riggs and Melton (35), who suggested a different nomenclature, type I and type II osteoporosis. Because this nomenclature is in widespread use, these "types" are described here in an attempt to place them into the mechanistic framework outlined above.

Type I osteoporosis (postmenopausal osteoporosis) overwhelmingly affects women and develops within 15 years of menopause. Skeletal sites of primarily cancellous bone (the thoracic and lumbar vertebrae) are involved initially. Parathyroid hormone levels tend to be decreased in this group (Fig. 2). Suppressed PTH levels fit with hypothesis 3 (Table 1). Type II osteoporosis is the clinical endpoint of age-related bone loss. It is recognized later than type I, after age 70 years, and affects females more frequently than males. However, type II osteoporosis is seen in both women and men. Biochemically, this group is characterized by an increase in PTH concentration, generally thought to be a secondary response to decreased calcium absorption (Fig. 3) (21,61,62). From a mechanistic viewpoint, type II osteoporosis could be explained by hypothesis 1. Patients with postmenopausal (type I) disease have an abnormality of vitamin D metabolism, suggesting that the pathogenesis of this disorder may be even more complicated than the simple designation would suggest. Finally, Riggs et al. (63) have identified a subgroup of postmenopausal osteoporotic women with increased circulating PTH concentrations. This

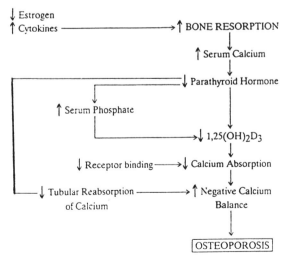

FIG. 2. Pathogenesis of type I (postmenopausal) osteoporosis. (Reprinted from ref. 1 with permission.)

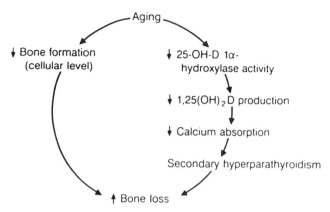

FIG. 3. Pathogenesis of type II (senile) osteoporosis. (Reprinted from ref. 42 with permission.)

subgroup has been designated at type III or Ia. Clinically, these individuals appear as with type I, with early development of vertebral fractures (in their 60s). Biochemically, however, their disease appears more similar to type II, with increased levels of PTH, decreased levels of $1,25(OH)_2D_3$, and reduced calcium absorption. While the type III or Ia group has not been well studied, their disease is thought to be related to a defect in $1,25(OH)_2D_3$ generation (hypothesis 1).

ESTROGEN AND PARATHYROID HORMONE

A full discussion of the interaction between estrogen and parathyroid hormone is beyond the scope of this chapter (see the chapters by Dawson-Hughes and Marcus). However, known relationships between estrogen and PTH are appropriately considered within the concepts of this chapter. Despite in vitro (64,65) evidence that estrogen plays a role in the control of PTH secretion, in vivo data are not supportive (66,67). No estrogen receptors have been identified yet in parathyroid glandular tissue (68). However, clinical observations support the idea of interactions between PTH and estrogen. Several considerations lead to this conclusion. Increased bone resorptive activity, a skeletal effect of PTH, emerges in the menopause when estrogen deficiency develops. Furthermore, the clinical disorder primary hyperparathyroidism is often unmasked by the menopause (18). In addition, use of estrogen in postmenopausal women with primary hyperparathyroidism is associated with a reduction in serum calcium levels (see the chapter by Stock and Marcus) (69,70). It has thus been postulated that estrogen is somehow antagonistic to PTH. It is believed by some that estrogen deficiency, in the menopause, potentiates PTH-mediated postmenopausal bone loss.

Current understanding of the interplay between estrogen deficiency and parathyroid function in either healthy or osteoporotic menopause remains limited.

Available information often comes mostly from studies describing the effects of estrogen repletion in the menopause. The relative contributions of estrogen loss and subsequent changes in PTH as altered mineral metabolism develops in the menopause can only be inferred. In addition, data obtained from normal postmenopausal women are not necessarily applicable to postmenopausal women with osteoporosis.

Early studies noted that the menopause was associated with a state of negative calcium balance (71). Decreased intestinal calcium absorption contributed to the negative balance. This abnormality was more pronounced in osteoporotic women than in normal women and could be reversed by estrogen-replacement therapy. Data from Gallagher et al. (72) suggested that estrogen treatment increased calcium absorption in postmenopausal osteoporosis by increasing PTH levels. The ensuing stimulation of renal 1α-hydroxylase activity due to PTH would lead to a rise in $1,25(OH)_2D_3$ and hence to the positive effect on the gastrointestinal tract.

More recent studies have led to a revision of this formulation. Estrogen deficiency does seem to be associated with a small decrement in total and ionized serum calcium, which can be reversed by replacement therapy. The reported effect of this mild hypocalcemia on PTH levels has been variable, with a decrease (66) or no change (67,73,74) in normal postmenopausal women and an increase (72,75) or no change (30,76) reported in osteoporotic individuals. Free as well as total $1,25(OH)_2D_3$ and vitamin D binding protein levels rise when normal postmenopausal women are given estrogen replacement (66,77,78). Recently, several studies have proposed that estrogen deficiency may alter the set point for PTH stimulation by circulating calcium. Estrogen replacement reportedly leads to a decrease in set point for PTH secretion in normal women, while, in osteoporotic women, blunted parathyroid gland sensitivity to circulating calcium was also found (30). In addition, estrogen treatment of the postmenopausal woman with osteoporosis leads to reduced bone resorptive (but not bone formative) activity in response to PTH administration (79).

SUMMARY

Although estrogen deficiency clearly plays a significant role in the development of postmenopausal osteoporosis, other factor(s) clearly contribute to the pathogenesis of this disorder. Evidence reviewed in this chapter implicates the parathyroid axis in the pathophysiologic abnormalities in osteoporosis. Several pathophysiologic mechanisms to explain possible relationships between PTH or parathyroid gland function and osteoporosis have been reviewed. Whether perturbations in PTH are a primary or a reactive mechanism remains unclear. Alterations at the level of the parathyroid glands are described in the hypothesis of modified parathyroid responsiveness leading to osteoporosis. Among the hypotheses that describe a secondary change in PTH are those based on alterations in $1,25(OH)_2D_3$ generation, enhanced skeletal sensitivity to the catabolic effects of PTH, and suppression of the parathyroids in the face of bone resorption driven by other agents. It is likely that several of these mechanisms will be found to be operative in this complex, yet common, disorder of skeletal metabolism.

REFERENCES

1. Riggs B, Melton L. Medical progress: involutional osteoporosis. N Engl J Med 1986;314:1676–1686.
2. Marshall D, Crilly R, Nordin B. Plasma androstenedione and estrone levels in normal and osteoporotic postmenopausal women. Br Med J 1977;2:1177–1179.
3. Crilly R, Cawood M, Marshall D, et al. Hormonal status in normal, osteoporotic and corticosteroid treated postmenopausal women. R Soc Med 1978;71:733–736.
4. Kotowicz M, Klee G, Kao P, et al. Relationship between serum intact PTH and bone remodeling in Type I osteoporosis: evidence that skeletal sensitivity is increased. Osteoporosis 1990;1:14–20.
5. Riggs B, Ryan R, Wahner H, et al. Serum concentration of estrogen, testosterone and gonadotropins in osteoporotic and nonosteoporotic postmenopausal women. J Clin Endocrinol Metab 1973;36:1097–1099.
6. Davidson B, Riggs B, Wahner H, Judd H. Endogenous cortisol and sex steroids in patients with osteoporotic spinal fractures. Obstet Gynecol 1983;61:275–278.
7. Lindsay RL, Cosman F. Primary osteoporosis. In: Coe FL, Favus MJ, eds. Disorders of bone and mineral metabolism. New York: Raven Press, 1992.
8. Aurbach GD, Marx SJ, Spiegel AM. Metabolic bone disease. In: Wilson JD, Foster DW, eds. Williams textbook of endocrinology. Philadelphia: WB Saunders, 1992.
9. Bullamore J, Gallagher J, Wilkinson R, Nordin B, Marshall D. Effect of age on calcium absorption. Lancet 1970;2:535–537.
10. Avioli L, McDonald J, Lee S. The influence of age on the intestinal absorption of 47 Ca in women and its relation to calcium absorption in postmenopausal osteoporosis. J Clin Invest 1965;44:1960.
11. Gallagher J, Riggs B, Eisman J, Hamstra A, Arnaud S, DeLuca H. Intestinal calcium absorption and serum vitamin D metabolites in normal subjects and osteoporotic patients. J Clin Invest 1979;66:729.
12. Chambers TJ, McSheehy PM, Thompson BM, Fuller K. The effect of calcium regulating hormones and prostaglandins on bone resorption by osteoclasts disaggregated from neonatal rabbit bones. Endocrinology 1985;116:234.
13. McSheehy PM, Chambers T. Osteoblast-like cells in the presence of parathyroid hormone release soluble factor that stimulates osteoclastic bone resorption. Endocrinology 1986;119:1654.
14. Perry HM, Skogen W, Chappel JC, Wilner GD, Kahn AJ, Teitelbaum SL. Conditioned medium from osteoblast-like cells mediate parathyroid hormone induced bone resorption. Calcif Tissue Int 1987;40:298.
15. Heaney R. A unified concept of osteoporosis. Am J Med 1965;39:377–380.
16. Calvo MS, Eastell R, Offord KP, Bergsalh EJ, Burritt MF. Circadian variation in ionized calcium and intact parathyroid hormone: evidence for sex differences in calcium homeostasis. J Clin Endocrinol Metab 1991;72:77–82.
17. Silverberg S, Shane E, de la Cruz L, et al. Skeletal disease in primary hyperparathyroidism. J Bone Mineral Res 1989;4:283–291.
18. Bilezikian J, Silverberg S, Shane E, Parisien M, Dempster D. Characterization and evaluation of asymptomatic primary hyperparathyroidism. J Bone Mineral Res 1991;6:585–589.
19. Parisien M, Silverberg S, Shane E, et al. The histomorphometry of bone in primary hyperparathyroidism: preservation of cancellous bone. J Clin Endocrinol Metab 1990;70:930–938.
20. Parisien M, Mellish R, Silverberg S, et al. Maintenance of cancellous bone connectivity in primary hyperparathyroidism: trabecular and strut analysis. J Bone Mineral Res 1992;7:913–920.
21. Gallagher J, Riggs B, Jerpbak C, Arnaud C. The effect of age on serum immunoreactive parathyroid hormone in normal and osteoporotic women. J Lab Clin Med 1980;95:373–385.
22. Epstein S, Bryce G, Hinman J, et al. The effect of age on bone mineral regulating hormones. Bone 1986;7:421–425.
23. Orwoll E, Meier D. Alterations in calcium, vitamin D and parathyroid hormone physiology in normal men with aging: relationship to the development of senile osteoporosis. J Clin Endocrinol Metab 1986;63:1262–1269.
24. Young G, Marcus R, Minkoff J, Kim L, Segre G. Age-related rise in parathyroid hormone in man: the use of intact and midmolecule antisera to distinguish hormone secretion from retention. J Bone Mineral Res 1987;2:366–367.
25. Forero M, Klein R, Nissenson R, et al. Effect of age on circulating immunoreactive and bioactive parathyroid hormone levels in women. J Bone Mineral Res 1987;2:363–366.
26. Teitelbaum S, Rosenberg E, Richardson C, Avioli L. Histologic studies of bone from normocalcemic postmenopausal women with increased circulating parathyroid hormone levels. J Clin Endocrinol Metab 1976;42:537–543.
27. Civitelli R, Agnusdei D, Nardi P, et al. Effect of one year treatment with estrogens on bone mass, intestinal calcium absorption, and 25-dihydroxyvitamin D 1-alpha hydroxylase reserve in postmenopausal osteoporosis. Calcif Tissue Int 1988;42:76–86.
28. Bouillon R, Geusens P, Dequeker J, DeMoor P. Parathyroid function in primary osteoporosis. Clin Sci 1979;578:167–171.
29. Sorenson O, Lumholtz B, Lund B, et al. Acute effects of parathyroid hormone on vitamin D metabolism in patients with the bone loss of aging. J Clin Endocrinol Metab 1981;54:1258–1261.
30. Cosman F, Shen V, Herrington B, Lindsay R. Response of the parathyroid gland to infusion of human parathyroid hormone-(1–34). J Clin Endocrinol Metab 1991;73:1345–1351.
31. Brown R, Atson J, Weeks I, Woodhead J. Circulating intact parathyroid hormone measured by immunochemiluminometric assay. J Clin Endocrinol Metab 1987;65:407–414.
32. Saphier P, Stamp T, Kelsey C, Loveridge N. PTH bioactivity in osteoporosis. Bone Mineral 1987;3:75–83.
33. Tsai K, Heath H, Kumar R, Riggs B. Impaired vitamin D metabolism with aging in women. J Clin Invest 1984;73:1668–1672.
34. Aloia JF, Cohn S, Vaswani A. Risk factors for postmenopausal osteoporosis. Am J Med 1985;78:95–100.
35. Riggs B, Melton L. Evidence for two distinct syndromes of involutional osteoporosis. Am J Med 1983;75:899–901.
36. Caniggia A, Gennari C, Bianchi V, Guideri R. Intestinal absorption of 47calcium in senile osteoporosis. Acta Med Scand 1963;173:613–617.
37. Szymendera J, Heaney R, Saville P. Intestinal calcium absorption: concurrent use of oral and intravenous tracers and calculation by the inverse convolution method. J Lab Clin Med 1972;79:570–578.
38. Kinney V, Tauxe W, Dearing W. Isotopic tracer studies of intestinal calcium absorption. J Lab Clin Med 1966;66:187–203.
39. Villareal D, Civitelli R, Chines A, Avioli L. Subclinical vitamin D deficiency in postmenopausal women with low vertebral bone mass. J Clin Endocrinol Metab 1991;72:628–634.
40. Riggs B, Hamstra A, DeLuca H. Assessment of 25-hydroxyvitamin D 1-alpha hydroxylase reserve in postmenopausal osteoporosis by administration of parathyroid extract. J Clin Endocrinol Metab 1981;53:833–835.
41. Slovik DM, Adams JS, Neer RM, Holick MF, Potts JT Jr.

Deficient production of 1,25-dihydroxyvitamin D in elderly osteoporotic patients. *N Engl J Med* 1981;305:372–374.

42. Gallagher J. The pathogenesis of osteoporosis. *Bone Mineral* 1990;9:215–227.

43. Ebeling P, Sandgren M, DiMango E, Lane A, DeLuca H, Riggs B. Evidence of an age-related decrease in intestinal responsiveness to vitamin D: relationship between serum 1,25-dihydroxyvitamin D and intestinal vitamin D receptor concentrations in normal women. *J Clin Endocrinol Metab* 1992;75:176–182.

44. Francis R, Peacock M, Taylor G, Storer J, Nordin B. Calcium malabsorption in elderly women with vertebral fractures: evidence for resistance to the action of vitamin D metabolites on the bowel. *Clin Sci* 1984;66:103–107.

45. Gennari C, Agnusdei D, Nardi P, Civitelli R. Estrogen preserves a normal intestinal responsiveness to 1,25-dihydroxyvitamin D in oophorectomized women. *J Clin Endocrinol Metab* 1990;71:1288–1293.

46. Jasani C, Nordin B, Smith D, Swanson I. Spinal osteoporosis and the menopause. *Proc R Soc Med* 1965;58:441–444.

47. Tsai K, Ebeling P, Riggs B. Bone responsiveness to parathyroid hormone in normal and osteoporotic postmenopausal women. *J Clin Endocrinol Metab* 1989;69:1024–1027.

48. Pacifici R, Rifas L, Teitelbaum S, et al. Spontaneous release of interleukin-1 from human blood monocytes reflects bone formation in idiopathic osteoporosis. *Proc Natl Acad Sci USA* 1987;84:4616–4620.

49. Gowen M, Mundy G. Actions of recombinant interleukin-1, interleukin-2 and interferon-gamma on bone resorption in vitro. *J Immunol* 1986;136:2478–2482.

50. Jilka R, Girasole G, Passeri G, et al. Increased osteoclast development after estrogen loss: mediation by interleukin-6. *Science* 1992;257:88–91.

51. Roodman GD. Interleukin-6: an osteotropic factor? *J Bone Mineral Res* 1992;7:475–478.

52. Bertolini D, Nedwin G, Bringman T, Smith D, Mundy G. Stimulation of bone resorption and inhibition of bone formation in vitro by human tumor necrosis factor. *Nature* 1986;319:516–518.

53. Tashjian A, Tice J, Sides K. Biological activities of prostaglandin analogues and metabolites on bone in organ culture. *Nature* 1977;266:645–647.

54. Raisz L, Simmons H, Sandberg A, Canalis E. Direct stimulation of bone resorption by epidermal growth factor. *Endocrinol* 1980;107:270–273.

55. Dietrich J, Goodson J, Raisz L. Stimulation of bone resorption by various prostaglandins in organ culture. *Prostaglandins* 1975;10:231–238.

56. Tashjian A, Levine L. Epidermal growth factor stimulates prostaglandin production and bone resorption in cultured mouse calvaria. *Biochem Biophys Res Commun* 1978;85:966–975.

57. Dewhirst F. 6-Keto-prostaglandin E1-stimulated bone resorption in organ culture. *Calcif Tissue Int* 1984;36:380–383.

58. Ebeling P, Jones J, Burritt M, et al. Skeletal responsiveness to endogenous parathyroid hormone in postmenopausal osteoporosis. *J Clin Endocrinol Metab* 1992;75:1033–1038.

59. Silverberg S, Shane E, de la Cruz L, Segre G, Clemens T, Bilezikian J. Abnormalities in parathyroid hormone secretion and 1,25-dihydroxyvitamin D_3 formation in women with osteoporosis. *N Engl J Med* 1989;320:277–281.

60. Albright F, Smith P, Richardson A. Postmenopausal osteoporosis. *J Am Med Assoc* 1941;116:2465–2474.

61. Wiske P, Epstein S, Bell N, Queener S, Edmondson J, Johnston CJ. Increases in immunoreactive parathyroid hormone with age. *N Engl J Med* 1979;300:1419–1421.

62. Marcus R, Madvig P, Young G. Age-related changes in parathyroid hormone and parathyroid hormone in normal humans. *J Clin Endocrinol Metab* 1984;58:223–230.

63. Riggs B, Gallagher J, DeLuca H, Edis A, Lambert P, Arnaud C. A syndrome of osteoporosis, increased serum immunoreactive parathyroid hormone, and inappropriately low serum 1,25-dihydroxyvitamin D. *Mayo Clin Proc* 1978;53:701–706.

64. Duarte B, Hargis G, Kukreja S. Effects of estradiol and progesterone on parathyroid hormone secretion from human parathyroid tissue. *J Clin Endocrinol Metab* 1988;66:584–587.

65. Greenberg C, Kukreja S, Bowser E, Hargis G, Henderson W, Williams G. Parathyroid hormone secretion: effect of estradiol and progesterone. *Metabolism* 1987;36:151–154.

66. Stock J, Coiderre J, Mallette L. Effects of a short course of estrogen on mineral metabolism in postmenopausal women. *J Clin Endocrinol Metab* 1985;61:595–600.

67. Selby P, Peacock M, Barkworth S, Brown W. Early effects of ethynyloestradiol and norethindrone treatment in postmenopausal women on bone resorption and calcium regulating hormones. *Clin Sci* 1985;69:265–271.

68. Prince R, Neer R, MacLaughlin D, Schiff I. Estrogen does not directly modulate parathyroid hormone secretion. *J Bone Mineral Res* 1989;4:S250.

69. Marcus R, Madvig P, Crim M, Pont A, Kosek J. Conjugated estrogens in the treatment of postmenopausal women with hyperparathyroidism. *Ann Intern Med* 1984;100:633–640.

70. Selby P, Peacock M. Ethinyl estradiol and norethindrone in the treatment of primary hyperparathyroidism in postmenopausal women. *N Engl J Med* 1986;314:1481–1485.

71. Heaney R, Recker R, Saville P. Menopausal changes in calcium balance performance. *J Lab Clin Med* 1978;92:953–963.

72. Gallagher J, Riggs B, DeLuca H. Effect of estrogen on calcium absorption and serum vitamin D metabolites in postmenopausal osteoporosis. *J Clin Endocrinol Metab* 1980;51:1359–1364.

73. Stevenson J, Abeyasekera G, Hillyard C, et al. Calcitonin and the calcium regulating hormones in postmenopausal osteoporosis. *Lancet* 1981;1:693–695.

74. Marshall R, Selby P, Chilvers D, Hodgkinson A. The effect of ethinyl estradiol on calcium and bone metabolism in peri- and postmenopausal women. *Hormone Metabol Res* 1984;16:1359–1364.

75. Riggs B, Ryan R, Wahner H, et al. Serum concentration of estrogen, testosterone and gonadotropins in osteoporotic and nonosteoporotic postmenopausal women. *J Clin Endocrinol Metab* 1973;36:1097–1099.

76. Boucher A, D'Amour P, Hamel L, et al. Estrogen replacement decreases the set point of parathyroid hormone stimulation by calcium in normal postmenopausal women. *J Clin Endocrinol Metab* 1989;68:831–836.

77. Marcus R, Villa M, Cheema M, Cheema C, Newhall K, Holloway L. Effects of conjugated estrogen on the calcitriol response to parathyroid hormone in postmenopausal women. *J Clin Endocrinol Metab* 1992;74:413–418.

78. Cheema C, Grant B, Marcus R. Effects of estrogen on circulating "free" and total 1,25-dihydroxyvitamin D and on the parathyroid-vitamin D axis. *J Clin Invest* 1989;83:537–542.

79. Cosman F, Shen V, Xie F, Seibel M, Ratcliffe A, Lindsay R. Estrogen protection against bone resorbing effects of parathyroid hormone infusion. *Ann Intern Med* 1993;118:337–343.

The Parathyroids, edited by J.P. Bilezikian,
M.A. Levine, and R. Marcus. Raven Press, Ltd.,
New York © 1994.

CHAPTER 49

Parathyroid Hormone and Growth Hormone in the Treatment of Osteoporosis

Robert Marcus

INTRODUCTION

Recent years have seen considerable progress in our understanding of the normal processes by which peak adult bone mass is acquired and maintained; the physical, nutritional, and hormonal factors that regulate bone mass throughout adult life (1–5); and the critical role of reproductive hormonal replacement for maintaining bone mass within the early years after menopause (6). For this same period, a number of therapeutic agents have been shown to minimize bone loss and to confer protection against osteoporotic fracture (6–8). Almost exclusively, these agents act to reduce the rate of bone resorption. Each shows significant positive effects on bone mass, and estrogen, in particular, exerts a profound influence on fracture risk (9), but none of these agents restores bone mineral of osteopenic patients to normal levels. To date, the goal of achieving major increases in bone mass remains an elusive and formidable research challenge. This chapter discusses two classical peptide hormones, parathyroid hormone (PTH) and growth hormone (GH), which have provoked considerable interest as potential osteotropic factors. For each hormone pertinent animal data as well as the results of studies in humans are reviewed. Because effective treatments require an understanding of factors that regulate bone mass and the mechanisms by which they operate, this chapter first summarizes the central role of bone remodeling in skeletal maintenance.

Remodeling is a continuous cycle of destruction and renewal that is carried out by individual, independent "bone remodeling units," illustrated in Fig. 1. Normally, 90% of bone surfaces are inactive, covered by a thin layer of lining cells. Remodeling is initiated by hormonal or physical signals that cause precursor cells in the marrow to cluster on the bone surface, where they fuse to become multinucleated osteoclasts and excavate a cavity into the bone. In cortical bone this appears as a resorption tunnel within a haversian canal. On trabecular surfaces it is a scalloped area called a Howship's lacuna. The resorption front leaves a cavity ~60 μm deep. The extent of deepest resorption appears as a thin cement line, a region of poorly organized collagen fibrils, as opposed to normal bone, which shows lamellar collagen deposition.

Coupled to resorption, bone formation ensues when local release of chemical mediators attracts preosteoblasts into the resorption cavity. These cells mature into osteoblasts that replace the missing bone by secreting new collagen and matrix constituents. Matrix production is initially rapid, the new osteoid seam approaching a thickness of 20 μm in 30 days. At that point, mineral deposition begins. Mineralization catches up to matrix deposition with time, and the new bone becomes fully mineralized. Resorption and formation are complete within 8–12 weeks, several additional weeks being required to complete mineralization.

If the remodeling cycle were completely efficient, bone would be neither lost nor gained. Each remodeling unit would be associated with complete replacement of the packet of bone that was initially lost. However, remodeling, like most biological processes, is not entirely efficient, so that a small bone deficit persists after completion of each cycle. The consequence of this inefficiency is age-related bone loss, a normal, predictable phenomenon, that begins shortly after ces-

R. Marcus: Department of Medicine, Stanford University School of Medicine, Stanford, California 94305; and Aging Study Unit, Veterans Affairs Medical Center, Palo Alto, California 94304.

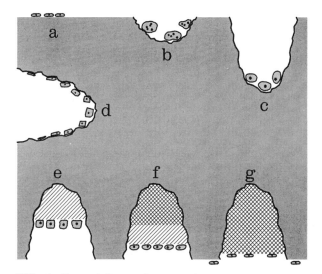

FIG. 1. Remodeling cycle: *a,* resting trabecular surface; *b,* multinucleated osteoclasts excavate a cavity of ~20 μm; *c,* completion of resorption to 60 μm by mononuclear phagocytes; *d,* recruitment of osteoblast precursors to the base of the resorption cavity; *e,* secretion of new matrix by osteoblasts; *f,* continued secretion of matrix, with initiation of calcification; and *g,* completion of mineralization of new matrix. Bone has returned to quiescent state, but a small deficit persists. (Reprinted from ref. 10 with permission.)

sation of linear growth. Alterations in remodeling activity represent the final pathway through which diverse stimuli, such as dietary or hormonal insufficiency, affect the rate of bone loss. Although it is not intuitively obvious, any stimulus that increases the rate of bone remodeling will increase the rate of bone loss. Moreover, a change in overall bone remodeling rate can reflect distinct perturbations in individual components of the remodeling cycle. These components include a change in the activation, or birth rate, of remodeling units; in the resorptive capacity of individual units; or in the vigor of bone formation. Even a small change in activation rate can exert a greater effect on overall bone loss than changes in remodeling balance within existing remodeling units. For a more detailed discussion of bone remodeling, the reader is referred to the review by Marcus (10).

Several points directly relevant to osteoporosis therapy can be inferred from this description. Resorption and formation are coupled, so drugs that act by decreasing either the activation of remodeling osteons or the formation of osteoclasts will eventually reduce overall bone formation rate. Furthermore, there is at any given time a transient deficit in bone mass, representing bone that was previously resorbed but has not yet been replaced. This so-called remodeling space (11) constricts if activation slows, and measured bone mass will rise until a new steady-state remodeling space has been achieved. This increase accounts for

the relatively modest rise in bone mass that occurs during the first months of antiresorptive therapy. By contrast, agents that activate remodeling will expand the remodeling space and decrease bone mass. It is important to realize that any agent that stimulates osteoblast proliferation or function may not increase bone mass in the early months of therapy if it simultaneously increases the remodeling space through a concurrent effect on activation of new remodeling units. Important questions must be addressed before a therapeutic role can be clarified for agents that initiate remodeling activity, including, as is discussed below, PTH and growth hormone. For example, both agents will be shown to be remodeling activators, and it may prove necessary to limit the degree of resorption to maximize gains in bone due to stimulation of formation. However, current information does not permit us to know whether the bone formation response is contingent on a fully expressed resorptive phase. If so, combination therapy might prove ineffective.

PARATHYROID HORMONE

The structural features and biological actions of PTH are reviewed in other chapters in this volume. The devastating skeletal consequences associated with sustained hypersecretion of PTH have been recognized for several decades, and comprehesive reviews of the skeletal actions of PTH have been published by Parfitt (12) and Wong (13). In accordance with predictions based on clinical experience, continuous infusion of PTH reliably decreases bone mass in animals, an effect that is due primarily to increased bone resorption as well as to osteoblast suppression. However, a sustained body of other data provides a rationale for considering PTH as an osteotropic agent when administered under appropriate circumstances. As early as the 1930s, Selye (14) and Shelling et al. (15) induced osteosclerosis in experimental animals following injection of parathyroid extract. Development of osteosclerosis with high doses of PTH has been confirmed more recently in other laboratories (16–18). Walker (16) demonstrated a profound age-dependent effect of daily PTH administration on metaphyseal trabeculae in rats. Initiation of treatment before birth resulted in substantial increases in matrix formation and obliteration of the medullary canal; if PTH was started 8 days postpartum, the increase in matrix was reduced by 50%, and treatment after 60 days of age had no effect. Parsons and colleagues (19) demonstrated that administration of PTH is rapidly followed by a shift of calcium from plasma into the skeleton and that low doses of PTH induced calcium retention in dogs (20). These results were attributed to an anabolic effect of PTH on bone.

Over the past decade, several laboratories have addressed this problem using synthetic human PTH-(1–34) in well-defined animal models. Hermann-Erlee et al. (21) showed that hPTH-(1–34) induces anabolic responses in embryonic rabbit bone in vitro. Tam et al. (22) stimulated bone apposition rate in parathyroidectomized rats with PTH. In that study the critical element was intermittent hormone administration. When PTH was given by continuous infusion, no increase in mineral apposition was observed. However, in a companion study in which these authors used a triple tetracycline-labeling method to measure bone apposition, dose-dependent increases were observed with either pulsatile or continuous infusion. Guiness-Hey and Hock (23) reported that treatment with PTH for 12 days increased trabecular, but not cortical, bone mass in weanling rats. In a second study using a similar protocol, they showed an increase in both trabecular and cortical bone and, in addition, showed disappearance of this effect after discontinuing hormone treatment (24).

Other laboratories have confirmed the fundamental observation that daily injections of hPTH-(1–34) at doses that maintain normal blood calcium concentrations promote bone mass (18,25,26) and whole-body calcium (27) in animals. Most recently, Ibbotson et al. (28) showed a striking increase in bone mineral content of the distal femur and trabecular bone volume of lumbar vertebrae of rats that had been oophorectomized for 1 year and then treated with daily injections of PTH for 14 days (Fig. 2).

To explore more fully the role of intermittent administration of PTH, Podbesek et al. (27) administered hPTH-(1–34) to mature greyhound dogs either by single daily subcutaneous injection or by continuous infusion. Daily injections of 50 µg hPTH-(1–34) led to peak circulating PTH concentrations of ~4 ng/ml. Elevated values were maintained for no more than 3 hr each day. Continuous infusions were given at a daily dose of 0.5 µg/kg, which maintained blood calcium in the normal range. Daily hPTH-(1–34) produced highly significant increases in the rate of bone formation as determined by ^{47}Ca kinetics, in plasma alkaline phosphatase activity, and in several parameters of bone formation as determined directly by histomorphometric analysis of iliac crest bone biopsies. After 4 months of hormone treatment, trabecular bone volume increased by 30%, and osteoid surfaces increased by 18%. Increased resorptive activity was also observed, as measured by resorption surfaces and osteoclast numbers. By contrast, calcium accretion and alkaline phosphatase activities in dogs treated by continuous infusion did not change over the course of this experiment. Technical difficulties limited the amount of biopsy material from the animals that received continuous infusions, but, in those from whom adequate paired biopsies were taken, no change in trabecular bone volume was observed, and resorption surfaces appeared to increase substantially. This study and an earlier report by Malluche et al. (29) suggest that continuous administration of hPTH-(1–34) does not increase iliac crest trabecular bone mass.

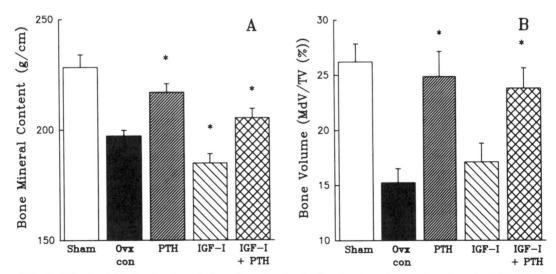

FIG. 2. Effects of 14 day treatment of oophorectomized (Ovex) rats on bone mineral content (BMC) of the distal femur (**A**) and mineralized bone volume (MBV), expressed as percentage of total bone tissue in lumbar vertebrae (**B**). Sham, intact animals; Ovx con, Ovex rats treated with no active drug; PTH, Ovex animals treated with hPTH-(1–34); IGF-I, Ovex rats treated with recombinant human IGF-I; IGF-I + PTH, Ovex rats treated with both hormones. Human PTH-(1–34) increased both the BMC and MBV of Ovex rats, whereas IGF-I did not increase either variable. (Reprinted from ref. 28 with permission.)

Clinical Studies

Encouraged by results in animals, workers in a few laboratories have undertaken to examine the effects of PTH on bone mass in patients with osteoporosis. Early forays into this area were carried out primarily by one group, using hPTH-(1–34) peptide prepared and standardized for clinical use. More recently, a commercial preparation of hPTH-(1–34) has been employed, as has a slightly larger peptide, hPTH-(1–38). Clinical studies with these peptides have been ongoing since the 1970s, but the results must still be considered preliminary, since conclusions from them are seriously hampered by the fact that most of the enrolled subjects are not representative of the general osteoporotic population, by lack of randomization, by poor standardization of subjects, and by the confounding effects of previous or concurrent therapy. Nevertheless, the results are of interest.

Reeve et al. (30) administered synthetic hPTH-(1–34) to four postmenopausal women with osteoporosis and monitored calcium balance, iliac crest biopsies, and ^{47}Ca kinetics over a period of 18 months. Bone mineral density of the distal femoral shaft was also monitored by single energy photon absorptiometry, but no measurement of trabecular bone was made. Calcium and phosphorus balances improved in three women, attended by a two- to threefold increase in estimates of bone accretion rate by tracer kinetics. Iliac crest bone biopsies showed a doubling of osteoid surfaces, with no change in resorption. Urinary hydroxyproline excretion did not change, confirming that bone resorption was not increased. Gross and net calcium absorption increased, with little change in urinary or endogenous fecal calcium excretion. Bone mineral density did not change in this experiment.

In a multicenter follow-up study, Reeve et al. (31) used hPTH(1–34) to treat 16 women and five men with osteoporosis. One hundred micrograms (~500 U) were administered per day by subcutaneous injection. Mineral balance, tracer kinetics, and iliac crest biopsy were carried out at baseline and at 6 months. In this study bone density of the midradius was assessed in 14 subjects, and femoral shaft density was monitored in eight subjects. Treatment produced no overall changes in plasma calcium concentration, but four individuals did show small increases. Biochemical markers of bone turnover rose, including serum alkaline phosphatase activity and urinary excretion of hydroxyproline, calcium, and phosphorus. There was no significant change in calcium balance, but a marginal increase in phosphorus balance was observed. Major increases were seen in bone formation rate and in trabecular osteoid surfaces. By bone biopsy, trabecular bone volume increased from 9.3% to 17.3% in nine of the ten subjects in whom material was adequate for

examination. By contrast, no significant changes were observed in bone mineral density at either of the monitored cortical sites. The authors concluded that the marked increases in trabecular bone could be attributed only partly to exchange with cortical bone. Furthermore, the authors suggested that lack of a therapeutic response in cortical bone reflected a failure of PTH to increase calcium absorption and balance, perhaps because the hormonal stimulus was insufficient to activate calcitriol production. Finally, they proposed that PTH-(1–34) might best be used in combination with an agent to limit bone resorption. In a study published soon thereafter, Hesp et al. (32) showed significant loss of cortical bone from the femoral shaft in osteoporotic subjects given PTH-(1–34) as monotherapy.

In a subsequent report, Reeve et al. (33) incorporated an antiresorptive drug into the treatment regimen. Human PTH(1–34) was administered for 1 year to 12 patients with vertebral osteoporosis. Nine subjects were also treated with estrogen, and three were treated with the anabolic steroid nandrolone. Estrogen was initiated 4 months into the treatment schedule, whereas the timing of nandrolone was variable. Bone mineral status was assessed by both computed tomography (CT) and dual photon absorptiometry (DPA) at entry and yearly for the 2 years of the protocol. Treatment with the parathyroid peptide produced a marked increase in trabecular bone mass, representing an increase of ~50% over baseline values. The authors estimated the effect of treatment on the *cortical* portion of vertebral bone by comparing the DPA results, which include both the trabecular and cortical elements of vertebrae, with results of CT, which is selective for trabecular bone. They concluded that vertebral *cortical* bone had not changed. Similarly, no increase in bone density of the forearm, a site of predominantly cortical bone, was observed. Supplementary results showed confirmation by bone biopsy of increased trabecular volume and improved calcium balance (34). Although it is encouraging that vertebral mineral increased substantially in the absence of a deleterious effect on appendicular (i.e., cortical) bone, failure to randomize the subjects and the lack of separate estrogen or nandrolone control groups limit interpretation of this study. As the authors themselves point out, "there is uncertainty whether hPTH-(1–34) provided sufficient additional benefit when added to long-term hormone replacement therapy." They concluded that a randomized, controlled trial is warranted.

A slightly different strategy was employed by Slovik et al. (35). These authors had reported previously (36) that elderly osteoporotic women were deficient in their production of calcitriol following a PTH challenge, so they elected to add exogenous calcitriol to the treatment regimen. Accordingly, they administered for 1 year a combination of daily hPTH-(1–34) (400–500 units), calcium, and 1,25(OH)$_2$D (calcitriol, 0.25 μg/day) to eight men with idiopathic osteoporosis. Bone mass was assessed at the lumbar spine by CT and at the radius by single photon abosrptiometry (Fig. 3). In all four patients in whom spine mineral was measured, large increases in trabecular bone density were observed, averaging a 198% increase over baseline. Four other patients either had completed the protocol before CT measurements became available or could not be evaluated because of vertebral fractures. Cortical bone density did not change. Calcium balance improved by 120 mg/day in four patients who were studied, and this was attended by an increase in calcium absorption. The authors proposed that combination therapy with calcitriol is essential to avoid cortical bone loss and to promote calcium retention. Because all subjects received both calcitriol and the PTH peptide, it is possible that some of the change in trabecular bone mass was due to calcitriol alone. This is not likely to be the case, however, since the modest dose of calcitriol that was used is well below that found to increase bone mass in other studies (8,37).

Hesch et al. (38) studied the effects of a slightly longer parathyroid peptide, hPTH-(1–38), in six men and two women with osteoporosis who were treated with four cycles of a complex regimen of 70 daily injections of PTH peptide interspersed with two separate 14 day periods with intranasal salmon calcitonin, 200 U/day. Vertebral mineral density, assessed by CT, increased over the 14 month study from 12% to 89% of initial bone mineral density (BMD), but forearm BMD showed no change. The stated rationale of this protocol was to administer PTH over the functional life span of the osteoblast and to give CT according to the life span of osteoclasts. In the absence of control groups treated with either hPTH-(1–38) or cyclical calcitonin alone, it is impossible to determine from this report what the contribution of calcitonin may have been to the results, and the relatively abstract theoretical rationale for this particular protocol cannot be evaluated.

Although the published experience to date does not permit firm statements regarding the therapeutic potential for PTH in osteoporosis, a few tentative conclusions seem justified. Administration of PTH peptide stimulates potentially important increases in trabecular, but not cortical, bone mass. Given alone, PTH may improve overall calcium balance in subjects who increase circulating calcitriol levels in response to the treatment. Otherwise, whole-body calcium balance may not improve, and trabecular bone mass may increase at the expense of cortical bone. Recent presentations at international meetings indicate that in a properly controlled trial the combination of PTH-(1–34) with estrogen produces dramatic results on axial bone mass and no deleterious effect on appendicular bone (J. Reeve, personal communication). One looks forward to the publication of these results and to the initiation of additional formal clinical trials.

GROWTH HORMONE

Pituitary growth hormone (GH) is a classical peptide hormone with profound effects on somatic growth and body composition. Circulating concentrations of GH decline with advancing age, as do GH secretion rates and pituitary GH responsiveness to a variety of provocative stimuli (39–42). These declines are accompanied by reduced levels of insulin-like growth factors (IGFs), the putative mediators of many of the actions of GH. Rudman (43) has called attention to the fact that changes in body composition associated with normal human aging are also characteristic of patients with GH deficiency. These changes include increased adiposity, reduced muscle mass and strength, and loss of bone mineral. Thus it seems reasonable to ask whether some age-related changes in body composition are directly related to relative GH deficiency and, further, whether GH therapy might have clinical utility in reversing them.

The major actions of GH on skeletal growth in children are well described and are not reviewed here. Less well defined are the skeletal actions of GH in adults. Although traditional models of GH action were predicated on an intermediary role for circulating IGFs, recent evidence indicates that GH directly stimulates IGF production in osteoblasts. GH activates

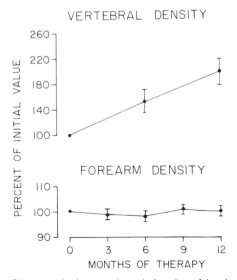

FIG. 3. Changes in bone mineral density of lumbar spine (n = 4) and forearm (n = 8) of patients treated for 1 year with hPTH-(1–34). (Reprinted from ref. 35 with permission.)

cell surface receptors in cultured osteoblast-like cells to increase IGF-I production (44–46). In murine osteoblasts, GH induces expression of the oncogenes *c-jun* and *c-fos* by a mechanism that involves activation of the protein kinase C transduction complex (47). In osteoblasts raised in serum-free medium, GH stimulates proliferation and increases the relative amount of newly synthesized type I collagen, an effect obliterated by anti-IGF-I immunoglobulin (48). There appears to be redundancy in the control of IGF-I production in osteoblasts, since PTH and estradiol also promote accumulation of this somatomedin. In vivo, both GH and IGF-I increase bone turnover.

In a classic experiment, Harris and Heaney (49) showed that administration of GH to adult dogs increased bone mass. More recently, recombinant human GH (rhGH) has been shown to maintain trabecular bone mass in primates rendered hypogonadal by a gonadotropin-releasing hormone analog (50). Such in vivo demonstrations, combined with an increasing volume of in vitro evidence, invite the conclusion that GH or IGF-I might have the potential to activate osteoblast proliferation and function to repair bone mineral deficits in osteoporosis.

Clinical Studies

Until recently, GH treatment other than of GH-deficient children was restricted by hormone supply. Limited experience with GH derived from human pituitaries gave interesting results, suggesting a possibly useful role for this hormone in man (51,52). Aloia et al. (52) described a 2-year intervention trial comparing the effect of GH followed by calcitonin to that of calcitonin alone in 14 osteoporotic women. GH and calcitonin increased whole-body bone mineral by 2.3% per year, whereas calcitonin alone produced no change. The effect of GH in this limited study seemed to be progressive, that is, without a plateau effect, which would have occurred if treatment merely condensed the remodeling space. No changes were seen by analysis of iliac crest bone biopsies in either group, but this could have been due to an insufficient number of subjects. Unfortunately, the authors did not report blood levels of IGF-I, so it was not possible to judge dose adequacy. Finally, concerns about the relationship between pituitary GH and the development of Jakob-Creutzfeld disease led to cessation of clinical trials with this agent (53).

With the availability of rhGH, therapy of adults has become feasible, albeit expensive. Our research group (54) reported the effects of 7 days of rhGH administration to 16 healthy men and women over 60 years of age. Recombinant human GH produced a brisk rise in circulating IGF-I, which was associated with striking increases in nitrogen and sodium retention and alterations in the parathyroid–vitamin D axis. Twenty-four hour urinary nitrogen and sodium excretion decreased by 38% and 50%, respectively, whereas urine calcium excretion markedly increased. Thus rhGH uncoupled the usual tight relationship between urinary sodium and calcium excretion. Significant increases were observed in circulating osteocalcin and in urinary hydroxyproline, suggesting that bone remodeling had been activated. In this regard, Brixen et al. (55) also showed that several daily injections of rhGH in young men initiated a prompt and very sustained elevation in circulating concentrations of osteocalcin.

The most widely publicized clinical trial of GH to date was reported by Rudman et al. (56). In a randomized, placebo-controlled intervention trial in 21 elderly men, rhGH (0.03 mg/kg three times per week) was given for 6 months and was found to produce significant increases in lean mass by ^{40}K analysis. Bone density was assessed via DPA at nine different sites. A 1.6% increase in lumbar spine mineral density was reported. The authors stated that "the effects of 6 months of hGH on lean body mass and adipose-tissue mass were equivalent in magnitude to the changes incurred during 10–20 years of aging." This statement has been extrapolated subsequently by the nonmedical community, especially the news media, to suggest that GH reverses aging.

Although the results of this experiment are provocative, several concerns must be raised. The ^{40}K data provide convincing evidence of a true increase in lean mass. However, with respect to the stated changes in adiposity, changes in skinfold thickness may have been confounded by fluid retention. The changes in bone mass were marginally significant at best and pose questions about analytical methodology, since bone mass was measured at nine different sites without adjustment for multiple comparisons.

We have recently completed a randomized, placebo-controlled 1 year intervention trial of rhGH (0.025 mg/kg/day) in 23 healthy elderly women. Eight women received rhGH as a daily injection, and 15 received daily placebo injections. Compared to the placebo group, the treated women showed significantly elevated circulating levels of IGF-I throughout the trial. Recombinant human GH stimulated a persistent increase in bone turnover. In the treatment group, sustained elevations were observed in circulating osteocalcin, type I procollagen peptide, and bone alkaline phosphatase as well as in urinary excretion of hydroxyproline. These changes associated with rhGH reverted to baseline values by 3 months after stopping treatment. Despite clear changes in markers of bone metabolism, no significant changes were observed in BMD at either the lumbar spine or the proximal femur. However, it is of interest that BMD at the femoral trochanter and

Ward's triangle decreased significantly in the placebo group. Thus, although rhGH did not increase bone mass, it may have been responsible for maintaining BMD at the hip. No significant changes in lean body mass or adiposity were observed by hydrostatic weighing, although an increase in lean mass was suggested by skinfold thickness.

With respect to safety, results of this trial were fairly reassuring. A transient increase in insulin resistance was observed several weeks after starting therapy, but this resolved by 6 weeks. No significant changes were observed at any time in blood pressure, lipoprotein concentrations, thyroid function tests, or fibrinogen levels. Thus, with respect to a panel of cardiovascular risk factors, rhGH appears to have been a safe intervention. It is important to note that the margin of safety may not be very large for rhGH. An attempt to treat older women with a twofold higher dose of rhGH led to intolerable fluid retention and symptoms of carpal tunnel compression in two cases.

Role of GH in Therapy of Osteoporosis

The osteotropic actions of GH suggest a rationale for considering this hormone to increase bone mass in patients with osteopenia. Unfortunately, neither the report of Rudman et al. (56) nor our own experience permits the conclusion that rhGH, *given as single daily monotherapy,* will offer meaningful increases in bone mass. Although a small rise in lumbar BMD (56) or maintenance of BMD at the hip may have occurred, several antiresorptive agents currently offer similar protection, and it would be hard to justify the use of an expensive, injectable protein hormone to achieve a similar result. Since the doses employed are close to maximally tolerated levels, it is unlikely that an upwards adjustment of dose will make the therapy more attractive. Nevertheless, the results do establish clearly that rhGH promptly induces a sustained increase in bone remodeling. Since bone remodeling is an inherently inefficient process, anything that activates remodeling should ultimately aggravate bone loss. Net acquisition of bone in response to GH would require a favorable alteration in the remodeling process, either by shortening the resorption phase or by increasing the osteoblastic response. Furthermore, Parfitt (57) has pointed out that, even if GH increases bone mass, it would be important to establish that the sites of new bone formation are in desired areas. For example, new bone formation around cranial foramina could have disastrous consequences.

These considerations temper the enthusiasm for GH as a therapy for osteoporosis. Any role for GH is likely to involve other agents, such as estrogen or other antiresorbers, in a complex treatment schedule. A number of questions must be addressed before such a role can be established. Should treatment be reserved for patients with low levels of IGF-I? What are the effects of rhGH on bone remodeling as defined by dynamic parameters of bone histomorphometry? Should GH be used cyclically in combination with an antiresorptive agent? Recombinant IGF-I is itself available for clinical studies. Some of the adverse metabolic effects of GH may be overcome with IGF-I, giving support to the idea that IGF-I might have therapeutic benefit. Potential adverse consequences of this agent, however, will require careful evaluation.

Finally, it should be remembered that GH, at least transiently, promotes nitrogen retention in adults. Since decreased muscle mass and strength contribute to the risk for falls, and therefore to the risk for hip fracture, a therapeutic role for rhGH might be found that is independent of bone mass per se. Although our own results did not confirm a persistent effect of rhGH on nitrogen balance, it is conceivable that GH may synergize with an exercise program to improve muscle mass and strength.

REFERENCES

1. Dequeker J, Nijs J, Verstraeten A, Geusens P, Gevers G. Genetic determinants of bone mineral content at the spine and radius: a twin study. *Bone* 1987;8:207–209.
2. Seeman E, Hopper JL, Bach LA, et al. Reduced bone mass in daughters of women with osteoporosis. *N Engl J Med* 1988;320:554–558.
3. Marcus R, Carter DR. The role of physical activity in bone mass regulation. *Adv Sports Med Fitness* 1988;1:63–82.
4. Marcus R. Calcium intake and skeletal integrity: is there a critical relationship? *J Nutr* 1987;117:631–635.
5. Longcope C, Baker RS, Hui SL, Johnston CC Jr. Androgen and estrogen dynamics in women with vertebral crush fractures. *Maturitas* 1985;6:309–318.
6. Lindsay R, Hart DM, Forrest C, Baird C. Prevention of spinal osteoporosis in oophorectomised women. *Lancet* 1980;2:1151–1154.
7. Watts NB, Harris ST, Genant HK, et al. Intermittent cyclical etidronate treatment of postmenopausal osteoporosis. *N Engl J Med* 1990;323:73–79.
8. Tilyard MW, Spears GFS, Thomson J, Dovey S. Treatment of postmenopausal osteoporosis with calcitriol or calcium. *N Engl J Med* 1992;326:357–362.
9. Weiss NS, Ure CL, Ballard JH, Williams AR, Daling JR. Decreased risk of fractures of the hip and lower forearm with postmenopausal use of estrogen. *N Engl J Med* 1980;303:1195–1198.
10. Marcus R. Normal and abnormal bone remodeling in man. *Annu Rev Med* 1987;38:129–141.
11. Jaworski ZFG. Parameters and indices of bone resorption. In: Meunier PJ, ed. *Bone histomorphometry, 2nd Int Workshop.* Paris: Armour Montague, 1976.
12. Parfitt AM. The actions of parathyroid hormone on bone: relation to bone remodeling and turnover, calcium homeostasis and metabolic bone disease. Part III of IV Parts: pTH and osteoblasts, the relationship between bone turnover and bone loss, and the state of the bones in primary hyperparathyroidism. *Metabolism* 1976;25:1033–1069.
13. Wong GL. Skeletal effects of parathyroid hormone. In: Peck WA, ed. *Bone and mineral research 4.* Amsterdam: Elsevier Science Publishers, 1986;103–129.

14. Selye H. On the stimulation of new bone formation with parathyroid extract and irradiated ergosterol. *Endocrinology* 1932; 16:547–558.

15. Shelling DH, Asher DE, Jackson DA. Calcium and phosphorus studies. VII: The effects of variations in dosage of parathormone and of calcium and phosphorus in the diet on the concentrations of calcium and inorganic phosphorus in the serum and on the histology and chemical composition of the bones of rats. *Bull Johns Hopkins Hosp* 1933;53:348–389.

16. Walker DG. The induction of osteopetrotic changes in hypophysectomized thyroparathyroidectomized and intact rats of various ages. *Endocrinology* 1971;89:1389–1406.

17. McGuire JL, Marks SL. The effects of parathyroid hormone on bone cell structure and function. *Clin Orthop* 1974; 100:392–405.

18. Kalu DN, Pennock J, Doyle FH, Foster GV. Parathyroid hormone and experimental osteosclerosis. *Lancet* 1970;1:1363–1366.

19. Parsons JA, Robinson CJ. Calcium shift into bone causing transient hypocalcemia after injection of parathyroid hormone. *Nature* 1971;230:581–582.

20. Parsons JA, Reit B. Chronic response of dogs to parathyroid hormone infusion. *Nature* 1974;250:254–257.

21. Hermann-Erlee MPM, Heersche JNM, Hekkelman JW, et al. Effects on bone in vitro of bovine parathyroid hormone and synthetic fragments representing residues 1–34, 2–34, and 3–34. *Endocrinol Res Commun* 1976;3:21.

22. Tam CS, Heersche JNM, Murray TM, Parsons JA. Parathyroid hormone stimulates the bone apposition rate independently of its resorptive action: differential effects of intermittent and continuous administration. *Endocrinology* 1982; 110:506–512.

23. Guiness-Hey M, Hock JM. Increased trabecular bone mass in rats treated with human synthetic parathyroid hormone. *Metab Bone Dis Rel Res* 1984;5:177–182.

24. Guiness-Hey M, Hock JM. Loss of the anabolic effect of parathyroid hormone on bone after discontinuation of hormone in rats. *Bone* 1989;10:447–452.

25. Hock JM, Gera I, Fonseca J, Raisz LG. Human parathyroid hormone (1–34) increases bone mass in ovariectomized and orchidectomized rats. *Endocrinology* 1988;122:2899–2904.

26. Hefti E, Trechsel U, Bonjour JP, Fleisch H, Schenk R. Increase of whole body calcium and skeletal mass in normal and osteoporotic adult rats treated with parathyroid hormone. *Clin Sci* 1982;62:389–392.

27. Podbesek R, Edouard C, Meunier PJ, et al. Effects of two treatment regimens with synthetic human parathyroid hormone fragments on bone formation and the tissue balance of trabecular bone in greyhounds. *Endocrinology* 1983;112:1000–1006.

28. Ibbotson KJ, Orcutt CM, D'Sousa SM, et al. Contrasting effects of parathyroid hormone and insulin-like growth factor I in an aged ovariectomized rat model of postmenopausal osteoporosis. *J Bone Mineral Res* 1992;7:425–432.

29. Malluche HH, Sherman D, Meyer W, Ritz E, Norman AW, Massry SG. Effects of long-term infusion of physiological doses of 1-34 PTH on bone. *Am J Physiol* 1982;242:197.

30. Reeve J, Williams D, Hesp R, et al. Anabolic effect of low doses of a fragment of human parathyroid hormone on the skeleton in postmenopausal osteoporosis. *Lancet* 1976;1:1035–1038.

31. Reeve J, Meunier PJ, Parsons JA, et al. Anabolic effect of human parathyroid hormone fragment (hPTH 1–34) therapy on trabecular bone in involutional osteoporosis: report of a multi-centre trial. *Br Med J* 1980;280:1340–1344.

32. Hesp R, Hulme P, Williams D, Reeve J. The relationship between changes in femoral bone density and calcium balance in patients with involutional osteoporosis treated with human parathyroid hormone fragment (hPTH 1–34). *Metab Bone Dis Rel Res* 1981;2:331–334.

33. Reeve J, Davies UM, Hesp R, McNally E, Katz D. Treatment of osteoporosis with human parathyroid peptide and observations on effect of sodium fluoride. *Br Med J* 1990;301:314–318.

34. Reeve J, Bradbeer JN, Arlot M, et al. hPTH 1–34 treatment of osteoporosis with added hormone replacement therapy: biochemical, kinetic and histological responses. *Osteoporosis Int* 1991;1:162–170.

35. Slovik DM, Rosenthal DI, Doppelt SH, et al. Restoration of spinal bone in osteoporotic men by treatment with human parathyroid hormone (1–34) and 1,25-dihydroxyvitamin D. *J Bone Mineral Res* 1986;1:377–381.

36. Slovik DM, Adams JS, Neer RM, Holick MF, Potts JT Jr. Deficient production of 1,25-dihydroxyvitamin D in elderly osteoporotic patients. *N Engl J Med* 1981;305:372–374.

37. Ott SM, Chesnut CH III. Calcitriol treatment is not effective in postmenopausal osteoporosis. *Ann Intern Med* 1989; 110:267–274.

38. Hesch R-D, Busch U, Prokop M, Delling G, Rittinghaus E-F. Increase of vertebral density by combination therapy with pulsatile 1–38hPTH and sequential addition of calcitonin nasal spray in osteoporotic patients. *Calcif Tissue Intl* 1989; 44:176–180.

39. Rudman D, Kutner MH, Rogers M, Lubin MF, Fleming GA, Baine RP. Impaired growth hormone secretion in the adult population. *J Clin Invest* 1981;67:1361–1369.

40. Ho KY, Evans WS, Blizzard RM, et al. Effects of sex and age on the 24-hour profile of growth hormone secretion in man: importance of endogenous concentrations. *J Clin Endocrinol Metab* 1987;64:51–58.

41. Franchimont P, Urbain-Choffray D, Lambelin P, Fontaine M-A, Frangin G, Reginster J-Y. Effects of repetitive administration of growth hormone-releasing hormone on growth hormone secretion, insulin-like growth factor I, and bone metabolism in postmenopausal women. *Acta Endocrinol* 1989;120:121–128.

42. Pyka G, Wiswell RA, Marcus R. Age-dependent effect of resistance exercise on growth hormone secretion in people. *J Clin Endocrinol Metab* 1992;75:404–407.

43. Rudman D. Growth hormone, body composition, and aging. *J Am Geriatr Soc* 1985;33:800–807.

44. Stracke H, Schultz A, Moeller D, Rossol S, Schatz H. Effect of growth hormone on osteoblasts and demonstration of somatomedin C/IGF-1 in bone organ culture. *Acta Endocrinol* 1984;107:16–24.

45. Chenu C, Valentin-Opran A, Chavassieux P, Saez S, Meunier PJ, Delmas PD. Insulin growth factor I hormonal regulation by growth hormone and by $1,25(OH)_2D_3$ and activity on human osteoblast-like cells in short-term cultures. *Bone* 1990; 11:81–86.

46. Barnard R, Ng KW, Martin TJ, Waters MJ. Growth hormone (GH) receptors in clonal osteoblast-like cells mediate a mitogenic response to GH. *Endocrinology* 1991;128:1459–1464.

47. Slootweg MC, de Groot RP, Herrmann-Erlee MPM, Koornneef I, Kruijer W, Kramer YM. Growth hormone induces expression of c-jun and jun B oncogenes and employs a protein kinase C signal transduction pathway for the induction of c-fos oncogene expression. *J Mol Endocrinol* 1991;6:179–188.

48. Ernst M, Froesch ER. Growth hormone dependent stimulation of osteoblast-like cells in serum-free cultures via local synthesis of insulin-like growth factor I. *Biochem Biophys Res Commun* 1988;151:142–147.

49. Harris WH, Heaney RP. Effect of growth hormone on skeletal mass in adult dogs. *Nature* 1969;273:403–404.

50. Mann DR, Rudman CG, Akinbami MA, Gould KG. Preservation of bone mass in hypogonadal female monkeys with recombinant human growth hormone administration. *J Clin Endocrinol Metab* 1992;74:1263–1269.

51. Aloia JF, Zanzi I, Ellis K, Jowsey J. Effects of growth hormone in osteoporosis. *J Clin Endocrinol Metab* 1976;43:992–999.

52. Aloia JF, Vaswani A, Kapoor A, Yeh JK, Cohn SH. Treatment of osteoporosis with calcitonin, with and without growth hormone. *Metabolism* 1985;34:124–129.

53. Brown P, Gajdusek DC, Gibbs CJ Jr, Asher DM. Potential

epidemic of Creutzfeld-Jakob disease from human growth hormone therapy. *N Engl J Med* 1985;313:728–731.

54. Marcus R, Butterfield G, Holloway L, et al. Effects of short-term administration of recombinant human growth hormone to elderly people. *J Clin Endocrinol Metab* 1990;70:519–527.

55. Brixen K, Nielsen HK, Mosekilde L, Flyvbjerg A. A short course of recombinant human growth hormone treatment stimulates osteoblasts and activates bone remodeling in normal human volunteers. *J Bone Mineral Res* 1900;5:609–618.

56. Rudman D, Feller AG, Nagraj HS, et al. Effects of human growth hormone in men over 60 years old. *N Engl J Med* 1990;323:1–6.

57. Parfitt AM. Growth hormone and adult bone remodeling. *Clin Endocrinol* 1991;35:467–470.

The Parathyroids, edited by J.P. Bilezikian,
M.A. Levine, and R. Marcus. Raven Press, Ltd.,
New York © 1994.

CHAPTER 50

Parathyroid Function in Paget's Disease of Bone

Ethel S. Siris and Robert E. Canfield

Paget's disease of bone is a localized disorder of bone remodelling, which may affect 3% of people over the age of 50 years in the United States. In this condition an increase in osteoclast-mediated bone resorption and a coupled, secondary increase in new bone formation at affected skeletal areas produce an alteration of bone architecture and a variety of signs and symptoms. The initiating lesion appears to reside in the osteoclasts at pagetic sites, cells that are increased in both size and number at foci of the disorder. Although the cause of the abnormality in both the morphology and the function of the osteoclasts is not known, it has been hypothesized that a paramyxovirus infection of these cells in a genetically susceptible host may lead to the remodelling abnormality that produces the characteristic mosaic of woven and lamellar bone (1,2).

The distortion of bone architecture may be appreciated on skeletal X-rays that demonstrate a thickening of the cortex, increased trabecular markings, expansion of the size of the bone, and variable degrees of gross bone deformity. This can be seen in Fig. 1. Depending on the number and the location of affected skeletal sites as well as the degree of the ongoing increases in bone turnover, the condition may produce no signs or symptoms or may cause a range of clinically significant problems. The latter may include bone pain; increased warmth over the bone (due to hypervascularity of actively remodeling pagetic bone); deformity (including an increase in skull size, bowing or enlargement of extremities, kyphosis, or spinal stenosis); secondary arthroses or arthritis; neurological complications such as spinal cord or nerve root compression, deafness in the setting of skull involvement, and rare cases of brainstem or cerebellar compression with or without hydrocephalus due to basilar invagination of the skull; traumatic or pathological fracture; and rare malignant degeneration and development of an osteogenic sarcoma.

Thus Paget's disease is not a metabolic bone disease as the term is currently defined. Nonaffected areas of the skeleton do not reveal increased numbers of enlarged and "supernucleated" osteoclasts; moreover, it is the impression of most investigators of this disease that, once the condition declares itself at specific locations, it is extremely uncommon for new sites to appear. Changes may progress within an affected site, but the disease does not appear to move across joint spaces or to emerge in new locations after its initial foci have been established.

It has generally been accepted that parathyroid hormone (PTH) plays no role in the etiology of Paget's disease. Nonetheless, it has become apparent in the past few years that levels of circulating PTH may have a role in the expression of the pagetic process and that some aspects of the treatment of the disorder should take these issues into account.

EFFECTS OF PARATHYROID HORMONE ON PAGETIC BONE

One of the first indications of the possible modulating role of PTH in Paget's disease came from work demonstrating an exquisite sensitivity of the large, hypernucleated pagetic osteoclasts to this hormone. Genuth and Klein (3) described a man with idiopathic

E. S. Siris: Department of Medicine, Division of Endocrinology, College of Physicians and Surgeons, Columbia University, New York, New York 10032.

R. E. Canfield: Department of Medicine, Irving Center for Clinical Research, College of Physicians and Surgeons, Columbia University, New York, New York 10032.

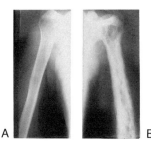

FIG. 1. Radiographs contrasting the appearance of a normal humerus (**A**) and a humerus with extensive changes due to Paget's disease (**B**). Note the irregular and thickened width of the cortex of the pagetic bone as well as the heterogeneous juxtaposition of sclerotic and lucent or lytic areas. The pagetic bone is also expanded in size due to the alterations in bone architecture. (Reprinted from ref. 2a with permission.)

hypoparathyroidism and active Paget's disease who had a greater than usual increase in urinary hydroxyproline excretion after an injection of parathyroid extract; a euparathyroid subject with Paget's disease described in the same study had an exaggerated hypercalcemic response to a similar injection. These data indicated both the possibility of active Paget's disease in the total absence of PTH and the increased stimulus to the already enhanced rate of bone resorption that occurs in Paget's disease when PTH is introduced.

PAGET'S DISEASE AND COEXISTENT PRIMARY HYPERPARATHYROIDISM

A second line of evidence supporting a modulating role of PTH comes from a series of case reports of patients with both Paget's disease and documented primary hyperparathyroidism in whom there was a marked reduction in the elevated levels of urinary hydroxyproline and serum alkaline phosphatase after the surgical removal of a parathyroid adenoma (4–8). In that PTH stimulates osteoclast-mediated bone resorption, it is not surprising that PTH excess would have a particularly profound effect at sites of Paget's disease. Specifically, one would expect a further increase above the intrinsically elevated rate of bone turnover, exacerbating the process. Elimination of the hormone excess would permit a restoration of a less marked increase in bone turnover, as the reported cases demonstrated.

The coexistence of single or multiple parathyroid adenomas in patients with Paget's disease has now been described on a number of occasions (4–21). In our own experience, we have had nine such patients, and we have also noted an improvement in the Paget's disease when the primary hyperparathyroidism was surgically cured. Posen (18), in describing his nine cases, wondered whether the coexistence of the two

disorders was a coincidence or whether there might be a linkage between them. An epidemiologic study performed by our group found that, among 864 patients with Paget's disease and 500 nonpagetic controls, adjusted for age and gender, there was a 5% prevalence of primary hyperparathyroidism self-reported by the Paget's disease cases compared with a 1% prevalence reported by the controls (22). This difference was significant at $P < 0.001$. Curiously, the same study found, when comparing calcium intake (determined by estimating milk intake) during ages 5–15 years, that the Paget's disease patients' intake was very much lower than that of the controls ($P < 0.0001$) (22). It is not known whether low calcium intake promotes a long-term stimulation of PTH secretion at higher levels or what modulating role this might play in the expression of Paget's disease, but if confirmed this would be a provocative concept.

PAGET'S DISEASE AND COEXISTENT SECONDARY HYPERPARATHYROIDISM

In addition to this as yet undefined relationship between Paget's disease and primary hyperparathyroidism, there is information regarding the presence of secondary hyperparathyroidism in some patients with Paget's disease. Early studies of levels of circulating PTH in patients with Paget's disease, performed as the first assays for the hormone were developed and utilizing very small numbers of patients, found these measurements to be within normal limits (23). More recently, however, several lines of evidence have suggested that a secondary increase in PTH concentrations may occur in Paget's disease, possibly in response to the relative lack of availability of calcium during periods of heightened calcium requirements for increased new bone formation. Several years ago, our group studied eight patients with very severe Paget's disease to follow the changes in calcium-related physiology after treatment with plicamycin (24). We were struck by the fact that baseline values for PTH, urinary cyclic adenosine monophosphate (cAMP) and $1,25(OH)_2D_3$ were near or slightly above the upper limit of normal in these normocalcemic patients who were experiencing very elevated levels of increased bone turnover from Paget's disease. At the same time, Meunier et al. (25) analyzed transiliac bone biopsies from 136 untreated patients with Paget's disease in Lyon, France, and found that nearly one-half of those whose biopsies were from a nonpagetic iliac crest site had evidence of increased bone remodelling, thought possibly to be due to an effect of excess PTH. Subsequently, Chapuy et al. (26) found an increase in PTH levels in 13 of 109 (12%) healthy, normocalcemic Paget's disease patients in Lyon; however, five of the 13 also had borderline or low values for 25-hydroxyvitamin D$_3$, which might have contributed to the increases in PTH. Harinck et al. (27) also called attention in a general way to the presence of secondary hyperparathyroidism in pagetic patients in The Netherlands.

To estimate the prevalence of secondary hyperparathyroidism in U.S. patients with Paget's disease, we measured serum PTH levels, using an N-terminal assay, in 39 consecutive patients who came to our General Clinical Research Center (28). These individuals had a wide range of pagetic involvement and activity, including serum alkaline phosphatase values of 57–2950 U/liter (mean 717 U/liter), with 30–100 U/liter being normal. All were ambulatory, otherwise healthy, and normocalcemic. In addition, all were shown to have normal serum concentrations of both 25-hydroxyvitamin D$_3$ and 1,25(OH)$_2$D$_3$. Thirty of the 39 either were untreated or had received no treatment for at least 6 months prior to the study; the remaining nine were on stable doses of long-term salmon calcitonin (in three) or had just completed 6 months of 400 mg/day of etidronate (in six). The results of the study revealed that seven of 39 patients (18%) had PTH levels that were above the upper limit of normal for the assay. As is shown in Fig. 2, these patients were among the most severely affected as indicated by the levels of the increases in both serum alkaline phosphatase and 24 hr urinary hydroxyproline:creatinine ratios.

A second interesting result from this study was revealed when we compared the relationships between PTH and the serum calcium levels, serum alkaline phosphatase levels, and urinary hydroxyproline:creatinine ratios for the entire group of 39 subjects.

Contrary to expectations, PTH values did not correlate with measurements of serum calcium ($r = -0.241$, $P = $ ns); however, there were significant correlations between parathyroid hormone and serum alkaline phosphatase ($r = 0.496$, $P < 0.001$) and PTH and urinary hydroxyproline:creatinine ratios ($r = 0.450$, $P < 0.011$).

We concluded from these data that a substantial subset of patients with Paget's disease, particularly those with the highest levels of pagetic biochemical indices of increased bone turnover, have evidence of absolute secondary hyperparathyroidism. Moreover, a "relative" secondary hyperparathyroidism, reflecting the degree of pagetic bone turnover, may exist in many patients. This relative increase, representing presumably higher levels of PTH than would be expected if the patient did not have Paget's disease, may reflect a homeostatic mechanism to maintain normocalcemia during phases of active new bone formation at sites of pagetic bone for which calcium demands may be great. As a consequence of absolute or relative increases in PTH, however, there is the potential for a greater stimulus to increased bone resorption and secondary new bone formation at these sites, possibly worsening the remodelling abnormality.

IS THERE A CONNECTION BETWEEN PRIMARY AND SECONDARY HYPERPARATHYROIDISM IN PAGET'S DISEASE?

The existence of a state in which there is an ongoing stimulus to parathyroid secretion leads one to speculate on whether there may in fact be a true increase in

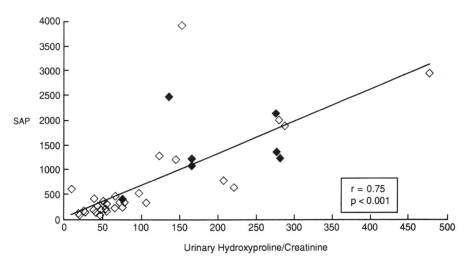

FIG. 2. Correlation between serum alkaline phosphatase (SAP) and 24 hr urinary hydroxyproline: creatinine ratios (mg/g) in 39 patients with Paget's disease in whom parathyroid hormone was measured. Seven of the patients had parathyroid hormone values above the upper limit of normal for the assay (solid diamonds). Of the seven, six were among the subjects with the highest pagetic indices. (Reprinted from ref. 28 with permission.)

the incidence of primary hyperparathyroidism in patients with Paget's disease as a consequence of the chronic overproduction of PTH by these glands. The fact that the reported cases harbored predominantly single (or multiple) adenomas rather than four-gland hyperplasia may argue against this hypothesis; however, it is also possible that the Paget's disease setting may offer a clue to the possible evolution of adenoma formation in the setting of prior hyperplasia; once an adenoma evolves and frank hypercalcemia emerges, the previously hyperplastic glands may regress. Indeed, one of our pagetic patients with primary hyperparathyroidism was a woman with extremely severe Paget's disease affecting the majority of her bones and associated with a serum alkaline phosphatase of 6,000 U/liter. When her neck was explored, a large adenoma was found and excised. Portions of the other glands were examined, and two of the three showed various degrees of hyperplasia. She remained eucalcemic after the surgery. Thus, although there is no clear evidence to prove either that there is an increased incidence of primary hyperparathyroidism in Paget's disease or that this is due to the increased prevalence of secondary hyperparathyroidism, the data acquired to date suggest that this is an area worthy of future research.

CALCIUM TREATMENT OF PAGET'S DISEASE

In terms of the well-documented presence of some degree of secondary hyperparathyroidism in Paget's disease, the question appropriately arises of whether supplemental oral calcium might play a therapeutic role in at least some patients. Evans (29) and colleagues in Australia described up to 30% decreases in pagetic indices when they treated patients with a combination of calcium supplements and thiazides, causing mild increases in serum calcium above normal, in uncontrolled studies. Such an effect might have been the result of either a decrease in PTH or an increase in endogenous calcitonin in response to the mild hypercalcemia or both.

Our group subsequently undertook an ongoing controlled study of oral calcium, 2.4 g/day in divided doses, taken as calcium citrate, vs. placebo for 24 weeks. Preliminary results from the first 24 patients (including 12 who received calcium and 12 who received placebo in the double-blind phase as well as five patients who subsequently received open-label calcium in an identical protocol after completing the placebo phase in the double-blind phase) are available (30). These data show that after 24 weeks the placebo patients had small and nonsignificant increases in mean serum alkaline phosphatase ($9\% \pm 0.3\%$; SEM) and mean hydroxyproline to creatinine ratios ($10\% \pm 0.2\%$; SEM), whereas the calcium-treated patients had

significant mean decreases in alkaline phosphatase ($13\% \pm 0.1\%$; SEM; $P < 0.001$) and hydroxyproline:creatinine ratios ($8\% \pm 0.2\%$; SEM; $P < 0.05$). The calcium and the placebo groups were significantly different from each other with respect to the changes in the indices over the 24 week study (serum alkaline phosphatase, $P < 0.01$; hydroxyproline:creatinine ratio, $P < 0.02$).

Although the average changes were small, it was interesting to note that the serum alkaline phosphatase fell by 18–34% in seven of 17 calcium-treated patients and none of 12 placebo patients; similarly, the urinary hydroxyproline:creatinine ratios decreased by 11–37% in nine of 17 calcium-treated patients and one of 12 placebo patients. Thus, while some of the calcium-treated patients had essentially no change in response to treatment, others had a biologically significant decrease in the indices of increased bone turnover. Moreover, PTH levels, which were increased above the upper limit of normal in five of the 24 patients at the start of the study, were unchanged in the placebo-treated patients at the end of 24 weeks but were decreased by a mean of 25% in the calcium-treated patients ($P < 0.001$). Levels of serum calcium and vitamin D metabolites were normal in all patients. Thus it may be that patients with active Paget's disease and secondary hyperparathyroidism do require added oral intake of calcium, an inexpensive and relatively benign treatment, as a part of their management.

SECONDARY HYPERPARATHYROIDISM IN PAGET'S DISEASE DURING TREATMENT WITH BISPHOSPHONATES

Added calcium is often required in the setting of mild hypocalcemia and secondary hyperparathyroidism that occurs during the course of treatment in some patients who receive the newer and more potent bisphosphonates. Although etidronate use does not pose this problem, these changes may be seen with pamidronate, clodronate, alendronate, risedronate, and aminohexane bisphosphonate (31). These agents rapidly decrease levels of increased bone resorption through effects on pagetic osteoclasts, quickly diminishing the release of calcium from bone. Since the previously well-coupled increased new bone formation lags behind in its reduction in response to these agents, new bone continues to be made, with a decrease in the availability of calcium previously provided through the ongoing increased bone resorption. Serum calcium levels typically fall, and there is a secondary increase in PTH, an effect that may last for several weeks. Here the issue is not one of the pagetic process being further stimulated by the increase in PTH; the capacity for bone resorption is effectively blocked by the potent bisphosphonate. Rather, the problem is one of some-times rather dramatic hypocalcemia (although more typically the decreases below the lower end of the normal range are modest and do not cause symptoms), which requires correction. One gram of elemental calcium per day, orally, has generally ameliorated this problem in our experience. With the eventual reduction in new bone formation at the pagetic sites in response to the bisphosphonate, the demand for added oral calcium diminishes, and both serum calcium and PTH return to the normal range in most patients.

SECONDARY HYPERPARATHYROIDISM DURING THE TREATMENT OF PAGET'S DISEASE WITH CALCITONIN OR PLICAMYCIN

The use of both salmon and human calcitonin and plicamycin is also associated with acute decreases in serum calcium and increases in PTH (24,32). The decreases in serum calcium are typically mild with the former, and they may be noted only if blood is drawn shortly after the dose is administered. Sustained secondary hyperparathyroidism does not occur with chronic administration of a calcitonin (32). Conversely, the very potent agent plicamycin can cause more striking transient decreases in serum calcium, producing a rapid rise in PTH and subsequent increase in serum $1,25(OH)_2D_3$ after an intravenous dose (24). Oral calcium supplements (along with a multivitamin providing adequate vitamin D), administered as required for the degree of hypocalcemia, are effective in correcting this problem during the course of treatment with plicamycin.

SUMMARY

The early evidence suggesting that PTH plays no significant role in the etiology of Paget's disease remains convincing. However, the more recent recognition of significant absolute or "relative" secondary hyperparathyroidism in many patients with Paget's disease is of interest in terms of its potential for driving the pagetic process beyond its intrinsically augmented state of increased bone turnover. The possibility that oral calcium supplements may be useful to restore calcium homeostasis while the disease is active is still being evaluated. The requirement to add oral calcium in the setting of overt hypocalcemia in the course of treatment with potent new bisphosphonates is determined by the clinical circumstances of each patient.

Finally, the interesting query of Posen et al. (18) on whether the coexistence of primary hyperparathyroidism and Paget's disease in the same patient is a clinical coincidence or is causally linked remains unanswered.

The question is especially intriguing in view of the data regarding secondary hyperparathyroidism in severe Paget's disease. Our epidemiological data suggest a possible increase in the prevalence of primary hyperparathyroidism in Paget's disease, but further study is needed. If this finding is borne out, it may provide some additional clues not about the etiology of Paget's disease but rather about the evolution, at least in some cases, or parathyroid adenomas.

ACKNOWLEDGMENTS

This work was supported by NIH grants FD-R 000762 and RR 00645.

REFERENCES

1. Mills BG, Singer FR. Critical evaluation of viral antigen data in Paget's disease of bone. *Clin Orthop* 1987;217:16–25.
2. Siris ES, Ottman R, Flaster E, Kelsey JL. Familial aggregation of Paget's disease of bone. *J Bone Mineral Res* 1991;6:495–500.
2a. Siris ES. Paget's disease of bone: In: Mazzaferri EL ed, *Advances in endocrinology and metabolism, vol. 4.* Mosby Yearbook, 1993;335–355.
3. Genuth SM, Klein L. Hypoparathyroidism and Paget's disease: the effect of parathyroid hormone administration. *J Clin Endocrinol Metab* 1972;35:693–699.
4. Gutman A, Parsons WB. Hyperparathyroidism simulating or associated with Paget's disease; with three illustrative cases. *Ann Intern Med* 1938;12:13–31.
5. Rosen H. Paget's disease complicated by hyperparathyroidism. *Bull Hosp Joint Dis* 1950;11:113–127.
6. Law WB. Hyperparathyroidism simulating Paget's disease. *Med J Aust* 1957;2:455–457.
7. Kontos HA, Kemp EV, Sharpe AR. Coexistence of Paget's disease and primary hyperparathyroidism. *Am Pract* 1962;13:620–624.
8. Bordier P, Rasmussen H, Dorfmann H. Effectiveness of parathyroid hormone, calcitonin and phosphate on bone cells in Paget's disease. *Am J Med* 1974;56:850–857.
9. Albright F, Aud JC, Bauer W. Hyperparathyroidism. *J Am Med Assoc* 1934;102:1276–1287.
10. Zimmerman SP. Hyperparathyroidism-simulating Paget's disease. *Ann Intern Med* 1949;30:675–681.
11. Rockney RE, Kleeman CR, Maxwell HM. Hyperparathyroidism in a patient with Paget's disease and carcinoma of the breast. *Arch Intern Med* 1959;104:797–801.
12. Kohn NN, Myerson RM. Hyperparathyroidism associated with Paget's disease. *Ann Intern Med* 1961;54:985–992.
13. Martin MM. Coexisting hyperparathyroidism and Paget's disease. *Arch Intern Med* 1964;114:482–486.
14. Hockaday TDR, Keynes WM, McKenzie JK. Catatonic stupor in an elderly woman with hyperparathyroidism. *Br Med J* 1966;1:85–87.
15. Frank M, deVries A, Nathan P, et al. Paget's disease of bone, hyperparathyroidism, gout and nephrolithiasis. *Harefuah* 1967;42:465–470.
16. Ben-Asuly S, Horne T, Goldschmidt Z, Eyal Z, Eliakim M, Chowers I. Coma due to hypercalcemia in a patient with Paget's disease and multiple parathyroid adenomata. *Am J Med Sci* 1975;269:267–275.
17. Lester E. Paget's disease and primary hyperparathyroidism. *Br Med J* 1978;1:1111–1112.
18. Posen S, Clifton-Bligh P, Wilkinson M. Paget's disease of bone and hyperparathyroidism: coincidence or causal relationship? *Calcif Tissue Res* 1978;26:107–109.

19. Gillespie WJ. Hypercalcemia in Paget's disease of bone. *Aust NZ J Surg* 1979;49:84–86.
20. Ooi TC, Spiro TP, Ibbertson HK. Coexisting Paget's disease of bone and hyperparathyroidism. *NZ Med J* 1980;91:134–136.
21. Avramides A, Leonidas J-R, Chen C-K, Nicastri A. Coexistence of Paget's disease and hyperparathyroidism. *NY State J Med* 1981;81:1660–1662.
22. Siris ES. Epidemiologic aspects of Paget's disease: family history and relationship to other medical conditions. *Semin Arthr Rheum* (Suppl: First International Paget's Disease Symposium, Manchester, England, 1992), in press.
23. Burckhardt PM, Singer FR, Potts JT. Parathyroid function in patients with Paget's disease treated with salmon calcitonin. *Clin Endocrinol* 1973;2:15–22.
24. Bilezikian JP, Canfield RE, Jacobs TP, et al. Response of 1-alpha, 25-dihydroxyvitamin D_3 to hypocalcemia in human subjects. *N Engl J Med* 1978;299:437.
25. Meunier PJ, Coindre JM, Edouard CM, Arlot ME. Bone histomorphometry in Paget's disease. *Arthr Rheum* 1980;23:1095–1103.
26. Chapuy MC, Zucchelli P, Meunier PJ. Parathyroid function in Paget's disease of bone. *Minerals Electrolyte Metab* 1981;6:112–118.
27. Harinck HI, Bijvoet OLM, Vellenga CJ, Blanksma HJ, Frijlink WB. Relation between signs and symptoms in Paget's disease of bone. *Q J Med* 1986;58:133–151.
28. Siris ES, Clemens TP, McMahon D, et al. Parathyroid function in Paget's disease of bone. *J Bone Mineral Res* 1989;4:75–79.
29. Evans RA. Treatment of Paget's disease of bone. *Med J Aust* 1983;1:159–163.
30. Siris E, Flaster E, Diamond B, Karmally W. Oral calcium in Paget's disease: a controlled trial. *J Bone Mineral Res* 1991;6:S191 (abstract).
31. Kanis JA. *Pathophysiology and treatment of Paget's disease of bone.* Durham, NC: Carolina Academic Press/Martin Dunitz, 1991;186–187.
32. Chapuy MC, David L, Meunier PJ. Parathyroid function during treatment with salmon calcitonin. *Horm Metab Res* 1980;12:486–487.

The Parathyroids, edited by J.P. Bilezikian,
M.A. Levine, and R. Marcus. Raven Press, Ltd.,
New York © 1994.

CHAPTER 51

Parathyroid Function in Magnesium Deficiency

Robert K. Rude

Magnesium (Mg) is one of the most plentiful elements on earth. In vertebrates it is the fourth most abundant cation and the second most abundant intracellular cation. Therefore, it is not surprising that Mg is involved in numerous biological processes and is essential for life (1). Mg was involved in early evolution as a means of harnessing energy from the sun. Chlorophyll is the Mg chelate of porphyrin. Through the process of photosynthesis, adenosine triphosphate (ATP) is formed, which provides energy for the synthesis of carbon dioxide and water into carbohydrate and oxygen. In animal cells, as well as in plant cells in the absence of the sun, stored chemical energy is utilized to maintain life. This chemical energy is released by Mg-dependent oxidative phosphorylation, in which ATP is again formed. Mg has evolved to become a required cofactor in literally hundreds of enzyme systems (1,2). Examples of the physiological role of Mg are shown in Table 1. Mg may be required for substrate formation. For example, all enzymes that utilize ATP do so as the metal chelate MgATP. Free Mg^{++} also acts as an allosteric activator of numerous enzyme systems as well as playing a role in ion currents and for membrane stabilization. Mg is therefore critical for a great number of cellular functions, including oxidative phosphorylation, glycolysis, DNA transcription, and protein synthesis.

MAGNESIUM METABOLISM

The normal adult total body Mg content is ~25 g, of which 50–60% resides in bone. One-third of skeletal

Mg is exchangeable, and this fraction may serve as a reservoir for maintaining a normal extracellular Mg concentration. Extracellular Mg accounts for ~1% of total body Mg. The normal serum Mg concentration is 0.71–0.91 mmol/liter (1.7–2.2 mg/dl). Approximately 70–75% of plasma Mg is ultrafilterable, of which the major portion is ionized. The remainder is protein bound, chiefly to albumin. The concentrations of Mg within cells is on the order of $1–3 \times 10^{-3}$ mol/liter, of which 0.5–5% is ionized or free (for reviews, see 1–3).

The kidney is the principal organ involved in Mg homeostasis (4). During Mg deprivation, the kidney avidly conserves Mg, and < 1 mEq is excreted in the urine per day. Conversely, when excess Mg is taken, it is rapidly excreted into the urine. The major sites of Mg reabsorption in the nephron are the proximal convoluted tubule (20–30%) and the thick ascending limb of Henle (65%) (4,5). The factor(s) that regulate renal Mg homeostasis are unknown. Parathyroid hormone (PTH), when given in large doses in man or other species, will decrease urinary Mg excretion. Patients with either primary hyperparathyroidism or hypoparathyroidism usually have normal serum Mg levels, however, suggesting that PTH is not an important physiological regulator of Mg homeostasis (6).

Intestinal Mg absorption is inversely proportional to the amount ingested. Under normal dietary conditions in healthy individuals, ~30–50% of ingested Mg is absorbed (2). Mg is absorbed along the entire intestinal tract, including the large and small bowel, but the sites of maximal Mg absorption appear to be the ilium and distal jejunum (7). There exist both a passive and an active transport system for Mg. A principal factor regulating intestinal Mg transport has not been described. Vitamin D and its metabolites 25-hydroxyvitamin D and $1,25(OH)_2D_3$ have been found in some studies to enhance intestinal Mg absorption but to a much lesser extent than they do calcium absorption (8,9).

R. K. Rude: Department of Medicine, University of Southern California, Los Angeles, California 90033.

TABLE 1. *Physiological role of magnesium*

Enzyme substrate (ATPMg, GTPMg)
   Kinase (hexokinase, creatine kinase, protein kinase)
   ATPase or GTPase (Na$^+$, K$^+$-ATPase, Ca^{++}-ATPase)
   Cyclases (adenylyl cyclase, guanylyl cyclase)
Direct enzyme activation
   Phosphofructokinase
   Creatine kinase
   5-Phosphoribosyl-pyrophosphate synthetase
   Adenylyl cyclase
   Phospholipase C
   Na$^+$, K$^+$-ATPase
Influence membrane properties
   Nerve conduction
   Calcium channel activity
   Potassium transport

TABLE 2. *Causes of magnesium deficiency*

Gastrointestinal disorders
   Prolonged nasogastric suction
   Malabsorption syndromes
   Extensive bowel resection
   Acute and chronic diarrhea
   Intestinal and biliary fistulas
   Protein-calorie malnutrition
   Acute hemorrhagic pancreatitis
   Primary hypomagnesemia (neonatal)
Renal loss
   Chronic parenteral fluid therapy
   Osmotic diuresis
      Glucose (diabetes mellitus)
      Mannitol
      Urea
   Hypercalcemia
   Alcohol
   Drugs
      Diuretics (furosemide, ethacrynic acid)
      Aminoglycosides
      Cisplatin
      Cyclosporin
      Amphotericin B
      Pentamidine
      Cardiac glycosides (possible)
   Metabolic acidosis (starvation, ketoacidosis, alcoholism)
   Renal diseases
      Chronic pyelonephritis, interstitial nephritis, and
         glomerulonephritis
      Diuretic phase of acute tubular necrosis
      Postobstructive nephropathy
      Renal tubual acidosis
      Postrenal transplantation
   Primary hypomagnesemia

MAGNESIUM DEFICIENCY

Magnesium deficiency is more prevalent than was previously appreciated. Approximately 10% of patients admitted to large city hospitals are hypomagnesemic (10). This incidence may increase to as high as 65% in a medical intensive care unit (11). Because Mg is ubiquitous in food, moderate to severe degrees of Mg depletion are most unusual in healthy individuals with a normal caloric intake. Clinically apparent hypomagnesemia and/or Mg deficiency is usually due to losses of Mg from either the gastrointestinal tract or the kidney. Causes of Mg deficiency are given in Table 2 (for reviews, see 1,2,12).

The Mg content of upper intestinal tract fluids is ~1 mEq/liter. Vomiting and nasogastric suction, therefore, may contribute to Mg depletion. The Mg content of diarrheal fluids and fistulous drainage are much higher (up to 15 mEq/liter). Consequently, Mg depletion is common in acute and chronic diarrhea, regional enteritis, ulcerative colitis, and intestinal and biliary fistulas.

Malabsorption syndrome due to nontropical sprue, radiation injury resulting from therapy for disorders such as Whipple's disease and carcinoma of the cervix, and intestinal lymphangiectasia may result in Mg deficiency, presumably due to intestinal mucosal damage. Steatorrhoea may also cause or contribute to Mg malabsorption through formation of nonabsorbable magnesium-lipid salts. Resection or bypass of the small bowel, particularly the ileum, for obesity, enteritis, or vascular infarction, also often results in Mg deficiency.

Excessive excretion of Mg into the urine underlies the basis of Mg depletion in many patients. Proximal tubular Mg reabsorption is proportional to tubular fluid flow and sodium reabsorption. Therefore, chronic parenteral fluid therapy, particularly with so-dium-containing fluids, and volume expansion states, such as primary aldosteronism, may result in Mg deficiency. Similarly, osmotic diuresis due to glucosuria (diabetes mellitus) (13), mannitol, and urea will result in urinary Mg wasting. Hypercalcemia has been shown to decrease renal Mg reabsorption and is probably the mechanism of renal Mg wasting and the tendency toward hypomagnesemia in most hypercalcemic states.

Certain drugs are becoming recognized as common causes of renal Mg wasting and Mg depletion. Diuretics acting at the loop of Henle (e.g., furosemide, bumetamide, and ethacrynic acid) have been shown by micropuncture studies and clinical studies to result in marked Mg wasting. The effect of thiazide diuretics is controversial, some studies demonstrating an Mg wasting effect, while others do not. The commonly used aminoglycosides have been shown to cause a reversible renal lesion, which results in hypermagnesuria and hypomagnesemia (14). Similarly, amphotericin B therapy has been reported to result in renal Mg wasting. Cisplatin is a chemotherapeutic agent used in the treatment of epithelial neoplasms. Renal Mg wasting resulting in hypomagnesemia has been reported in up to 100% of patients receiving this agent. Cyclosporin is an immunosuppressive agent that also results in nephrotoxicity and renal Mg wasting. Recently pentamidine has been reported to result in renal Mg loss in patients with acquired immunodeficiency syndrome (AIDS) (15). A rising blood alcohol level has been associated with renal Mg wasting and is one factor contributing to Mg deficiency in chronic alcoholism. Metabolic acidosis due to diabetic ketoacidosis, starvation, or alcoholism also causes renal Mg wasting.

Some renal tubular, glomerular, or interstitial diseases have been associated with renal Mg wasting. There may be other accompanying tubular abnormalities, and reduced glomerular filtration rate (GFR) may or may not be present.

Diabetes mellitus is probably the most common disorder associated with Mg deficiency (13). The incidence of hypomagnesemia in diabetes mellitus has been reported to vary from 25% to 39% (2). The serum Mg concentration correlates inversely with the serum glucose concentration and the degree of glucosuria. The Mg depletion is probably mostly due to the glucosuria (osmotic diuresis). Patients with ketoacidosis may also waste Mg into the urine during the acidosis per se. Hypomagnesemia can be found in association with a number of other endocrine disorders, as listed in Table 3. The mechanism leading to the hypomagnesemia most frequently involves urinary Mg wasting. Phosphate depletion has been shown experimentally in humans and rats to result in urinary Mg wasting and hypomagnesemia (16). Excessive urinary Mg wasting and hypomagnesemia can be seen in severe primary hyperparathyroidism, treated hypoparathyroidism, and thyrotoxicosis; the urinary losses may be due to the hypercalcemia and/or hypercalciuria occurring in these states (2). The hypomagnesemia that may be seen in primary hyperaldosteronism has been related to plasma volume expansion and subsequent renal Mg wasting. Hypomagnesemia may also accompany the hungry bone syndrome, a phase of rapid bone mineral

accretion in subjects with overt skeletal disease who undergo successful parathyroidectomy.

MANIFESTATIONS OF MAGNESIUM DEFICIENCY

Since Mg deficiency is usually secondary to another disease process or to a therapeutic agent, the features of the primary disease process may complicate or mask Mg deficiency. A high index of suspicion is therefore warranted.

Frequent manifestations of moderate to severe Mg deficiency are given in Table 4 (for reviews, see 1,2,12). Neuromuscular hyperexcitability is often the presenting complaint. Latent tetany, as elicited by a positive Chvostek's and Trousseau's sign, or spontaneous carpal–pedal spasm may be present. Frank generalized seizures may also occur. While hypocalcemia may contribute to the neurological signs, hypomagnesemia without hypocalcemia has been reported to result in neuromuscular hyperexcitability (17). Other signs may include vertigo, ataxia, nystagmus, and athetoid and choreiform movements as well as muscular tremor, fasciculation, wasting, and weakness.

Electrocardiographic abnormalities of Mg deficiency in man include prolonged P-R interval and Q-T interval. Mg deficiency may also result in arrhythmias. Supraventricular arrhythmias, including premature atrial complexes, atrial tachycardia, atrial fibrillation,

TABLE 3. Endocrine and metabolic disorders associated with magnesium deficiency

Diabetes mellitus
Phosphate depletion
Primary hyperparathyroidism
Hypoparathyroidism
Hyperthyroidism
Primary aldosteronism
Hungry bone syndrome
Excessive lactation
Bartter's syndrome

TABLE 4. Manifestations of moderate to severe magnesium deficiency

Neuromuscular
  Positive Chvostek's and Trousseau's signs
  Spontaneous carpal–pedal spasm
  Seizures
  Vertigo, ataxia, nystagmus, athetoid, chlorioform movements
  Muscular weakness, tremor, fasciculation, wasting
  Psychiatric: depression, psychosis
Cardiac arrhythmia
  EKG: prolonged P-R interval and Q-T intervals, U waves
  Atrial tachycardia, premature contractions, fibrillation
  Junctional arrhythmias
  Ventricular premature contractions, tachycardia, fibrillation
  Sensitivity to digitalis intoxication
  Torsades de pointes
Biochemical
  Hypokalemia
    Renal potassium wasting
    Decreased intracellular potassium
  Hypocalcemia
    Impaired PTH secretion
    Renal and skeletal resistance to PTH
    Resistance to vitamin D

and junctional arrhythmias, have been described (18). Ventricular premature complexes, ventricular tachycardia, and ventricular fibrillation are more serious complications (19).

A common laboratory feature of Mg deficiency is hypokalemia. During Mg deficiency there is loss of potassium from the cell, with intracellular potassium depletion as well as an inability of the kidney to conserve potassium. Attempts to replete the potassium deficit with potassium therapy alone are not successful without simultaneous Mg therapy (20,21). This biochemical feature may be a contributing cause of the electrocardiologic findings and cardiac arrhythmias discussed above.

Soon after the observation that Mg deficiency may cause neuromuscular hyperexcitability, it was noted that hypocalcemia was also a common finding in moderate to severe Mg deficiency (22). Correction of the hypocalcemia was possible only with Mg therapy. The relationship of Mg with mineral homeostasis in normal physiology as well as in the pathophysiological events leading to hypocalcemia soon followed.

EFFECT OF MAGNESIUM ON PARATHYROID HORMONE SECRETION

Calcium is considered to be the major regulator of PTH secretion. A number of in vitro and in vivo studies, however, have demonstrated that Mg can modulate PTH secretion in a manner similar to calcium. Perfusion of isolated parathyroid glands of goats and sheep with varying concentrations of Mg showed that acute elevations of Mg inhibited PTH secretion, while acute reductions stimulated PTH secretion, as shown in Fig. 1 (23). These findings were later confirmed in studies of bovine and rat parathyroid glands in vitro, in which an increase in media Mg concentration inhibited release of PTH, while low media Mg stimulated PTH release (24,25). Recent studies have also demonstrated that hypermagnesemia will inhibit PTH secretion in humans (26–28). It became apparent that Mg could be a physiologic regulator of PTH secretion. Early investigations suggested that Mg was equipotent to calcium in its effect on parathyroid gland function (24); however, more recent studies demonstrated that Mg has ~30–50% the effect of calcium in either stimulating or inhibiting PTH secretion (27–31). The recent finding in humans that a 5% (0.03 mM) decrease in serum ultrafilterable Mg did not result in any detectable change in intact serum PTH concentration while a 5.5% (.07mM) decrease in ionized calcium resulted in a 400% increase in serum PTH supports this concept (28).

The mechanism by which Mg alters parathyroid function is unclear but is probably different from that

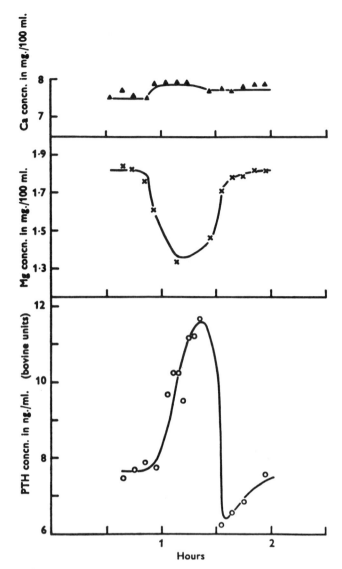

FIG. 1. Increase in parathyroid hormone secretion by hypomagnesemic perfusion of a surgically isolated parathyroid gland in an anesthetized goat. Effect of changes in plasma magnesium concentration in the perfusing blood on PTH concentration in the parathyroid venous plasma is shown. The plasma concentration of ionized calcium was raised from 5.0 mg/dl to 5.2 mg/dl during the perfusion. (Reprinted from ref. 23 with permission.)

of calcium in that the inhibitory effects of Mg on PTH secretion may vary dependent on the extracellular calcium concentration (32). At physiological calcium and Mg concentrations, these divalent cations were found to be relatively equipotent in inhibiting PTH secretion from dispersed bovine parathyroid cells (32). At a low calcium concentration (0.5 mM), however, a threefold greater Mg concentration was required for similar PTH inhibition. Altering the Mg concentration did not diminish the ability of calcium to inhibit PTH secretion. Differences have also been noted in the effect of Mg and calcium on the biosynthesis of PTH in vitro. Changes in calcium over the range 0–3.0 mM resulted in increased PTH synthesis as assessed by amino acid incorporation (33–35) or DNA synthesis (35), whereas changes in Mg over the range 0–1.7 mM had no effect. It is probable, therefore, that calcium and Mg affect PTH secretion by independent but complementary mechanisms. Nevertheless, it is apparent that acute changes in the serum Mg concentration may modulate PTH secretion and should be considered in the evaluation of the determination of serum PTH concentrations.

EFFECT OF MAGNESIUM DEFICIENCY ON PARATHYROID GLAND FUNCTION

While acute changes in the extracellular Mg concentrations will influence PTH secretion qualitatively similarly to calcium, it is clear that Mg deficiency markedly perturbs mineral homeostasis (22). Hypocalcemia is a prominent manifestation of Mg deficiency in man (22). This has been found to be true in most species, including monkey, cow, sheep, pig, dog, chick, guinea pig, and mouse (1,36). The rat, however, will develop hypercalcemia when Mg depleted and maintained on a normal-calcium diet (36–38). On a low-calcium diet, however, the rat will become hypocalcemic (36). In humans, Mg deficiency must become moderate to severe before symptomatic hypocalcemia develops. A positive correlation has been found between serum Mg and calcium concentrations in hypocalcemic hypomagnesemic patients (22). Mg therapy alone will restore serum calcium concentrations to normal in such patients within days (22). Calcium and/or vitamin D therapy will not correct the hypocalcemia (2,22). Even mild degrees of Mg depletion, however, may result in a significant fall in the serum calcium concentration, as was recently demonstrated in experimental human Mg depletion (39).

One major factor resulting in the fall in the serum calcium is impaired parathyroid gland function. Low Mg in the media of bovine or rat parathyroid cell cultures impairs PTH release in response to a low media calcium concentration (40,41). Determinations of serum PTH concentrations in hypocalcemic hypomagnesemic patients have given heterogenous results, as is shown in Fig. 2. The majority of patients have low or normal serum PTH levels (22,42–47). Normal serum PTH concentrations are thought to be inappropriately low in the presence of hypocalcemia. Therefore, a state of hypoparathyroidism exists in most hypocalcemic Mg-deficient patients. Some patients, however, have elevated levels of PTH in the serum (22,46,47). The administration of Mg will result in an immediate rise in the serum PTH concentration regardless of the

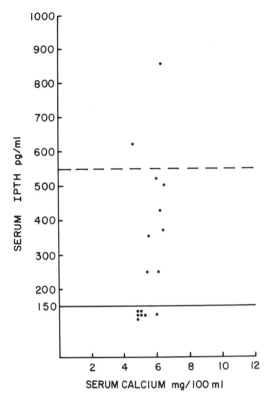

FIG. 2. Correlation of the serum PTH concentration with the serum calcium concentration in hypocalcemic hypomagnesemic patients. The *dashed line* denotes the upper limit of normal and the *solid line* represents the level of detectability of the serum PTH concentration. (Reprinted from ref. 22 with permission.)

basal PTH level (22,42,46,47). As is shown in Fig. 3, 10 mEq Mg administered intravenously over 1 min caused an immediate marked rise in the serum PTH in patients with either low, normal, or elevated basal serum PTH concentrations. This is distinctly different from the effect of an Mg injection in normal subjects, in whom, as was discussed above, Mg will cause an inhibition of PTH secretion (39). The ability of Mg to stimulate the rise in PTH appears to be specific for Mg depletion; Mg injection does not result in an increase in PTH in primary or secondary hyperparathyroidism (46). The serum PTH concentration will gradually fall to normal within several days of therapy as the serum calcium concentration normalizes (22,42,45,46,47), as is shown in Fig. 4. The impairment in PTH secretion appears to occur early in Mg depletion. Normal human subjects experimentally placed on a low-Mg diet for only 3 weeks showed similar, but not as marked, changes in the serum PTH levels (39). In this study there was a fall in both serum calcium and PTH concentrations in 20 of 26 subjects at the end of a 3 week dietary Mg-deprivation period. The administration of intravenous Mg at the end of the Mg-depletion period

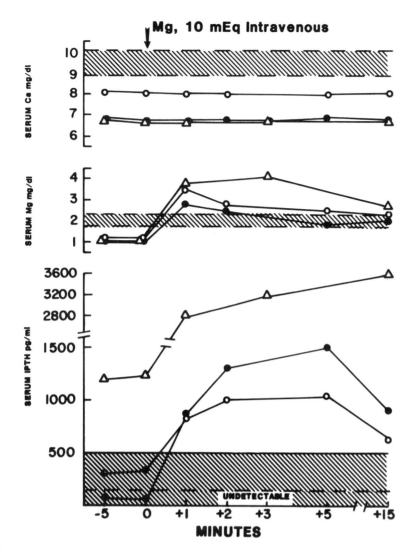

FIG. 3. Effect of an intravenous injection of 10 mEq Mg on the serum concentrations of calcium, magnesium, and immunoreactive parathyroid hormone (IPTH) in hypocalcemic magnesium-deficient patients with undetectable (●), normal (○), or elevated (△) levels of IPTH. Shaded areas represent the range of normal of each assay. The *broken line* for IPTH assay represents the level of detectability. The magnesium injection resulted in a marked rise in PTH secretion within 1 min in all three patients. (Reprinted from ref. 115 with permission.)

resulted in a significant rise in the serum PTH concentration, whereas a similar Mg injection suppressed PTH secretion prior to the low-Mg diet. In this study, as with hypocalcemia hypomagnesemic patients, some subjects had elevations in the serum PTH concentration. The heterogeneous serum PTH values may be explained based on the severity of Mg depletion. As hypomagnesemia develops, the parathyroid gland will react normally with an increase in PTH secretion. As intracellular Mg depletion develops, however, the ability of the parathyroid to secrete PTH is impaired resulting in a fall in the serum PTH levels, and subsequently a fall in the serum calcium concentration. This concept is supported by the observation that the change in serum PTH in experimental human Mg depletion is positively correlated with the fall in red blood cell intracellular free Mg^{++} (39). A slight fall in red blood cell Mg^{++} resulted in a increase in PTH. However, a greater decrease in red blood cell Mg^{++}

correlated with a progressive fall in serum PTH concentrations.

It is conceivable that PTH synthesis and/or PTH secretion may be affected given the wide requirement of Mg for energy generation and protein synthesis. The immediate rise in PTH following the administration of intravenous magnesium to Mg-deficient patients strongly suggests that the defect is in secretion, because biosynthesis of PTH is estimated to take ~45 min in vitro (33).

EFFECT OF MAGNESIUM DEFICIENCY ON PARATHYROID HORMONE ACTION

The above discussion strongly supports the notion that impairment in the secretion of PTH in Mg deficiency is a major contributing factor in the hypocalcemia. However, the presence of normal or elevated

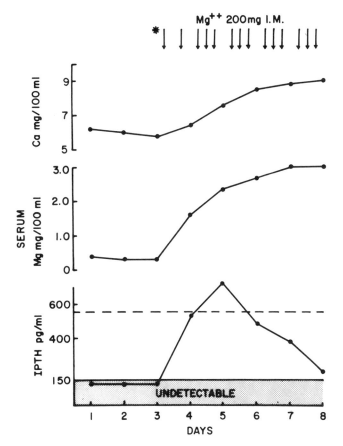

FIG. 4. Changes in the serum calcium, magnesium, and PTH concentrations during 5 days of magnesium therapy. The *dashed line* indicates the upper limit of normal for serum PTH. *Arrows* indicate times of intramuscular injection of 200 mg magnesium. *Asterisk* indicates an initial intravenous injection of 300 mg magnesium. (Reprinted from ref. 22 with permission.)

serum concentrations of PTH in the face of hypocalcemia (22,46,47) suggests that there may also be end-organ resistance to PTH action, such as exists in pseudohypoparathyroidism. In hypocalcemic Mg-deficient patients treated with Mg, the serum calcium concentration does not rise appreciably within the first 24 hr despite elevated serum PTH concentrations, as is illustrated in Fig. 4 (22,47). This also suggests skeletal resistance to PTH, since exogenous PTH administered to hypoparathyroid patients causes a rise in the serum calcium within 24 hr (48). A number of clinical studies have been reported in which exogenous PTH was administered to hypocalcemic Mg-deficient patients, demonstrating that PTH had little effect in raising the serum calcium concentration (22,49–52). In one such study, represented in Fig. 5, parathyroid extract did not result in an elevation in the serum calcium concentration or urinary hydroxyproline excretion in hypocalcemic hypomagnesemic patients (49). Following Mg repletion, however, a clear response to PTH was observed. PTH has also been shown to have a reduced calcemic effect in Mg-deficient dogs, chicks, and rats (53–57). The ability of PTH to resorb bone in vitro is also greatly diminished in the presence of low media Mg (58). In one in vivo study of isolated, perfused dog femur, the ability of PTH to simulate an increase in the venous cAMP was impaired during perfusion with low-Mg fluid, suggesting skeletal PTH resistance (59). Not all human studies have shown skeletal resistance to PTH, however (60–63). It appears likely that skeletal PTH resistance may be observed in patients with more severe degrees of Mg depletion. In human studies, a normal calcemic response to PTH was demonstrated in subjects who had been on recent Mg therapy

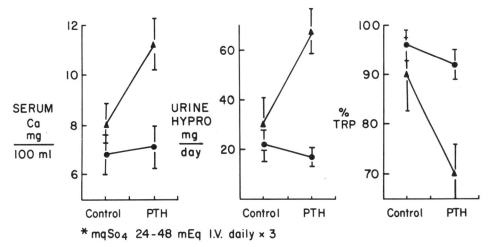

FIG. 5. Mean and standard deviations of serum calcium concentration and urinary hydroxyproline and phosphate excretion in hypocalcemic magnesium-deficient patients before (●) and after (▲) 3 days of parenteral magnesium therapy. (Reprinted from ref. 49 with permission.)

(60–63). Patients who have been found to be resistant to PTH have, in general, not had prior Mg administration (22,49–52). Consistent with this notion is that, in the Mg depleted rat, normal responses to PTH were observed when the serum Mg concentration was 0.95 mg/dl (64); however, in another study rats with a mean serum Mg of 0.46 mg/dl were refractory to PTH (53). In addition, a longitudinal study of Mg deficiency in dogs demonstrated a progressive decline in responsiveness to PTH with increasing degrees of Mg depletion (56). Calcium release from the skeleton also appears to be dependent on physicochemical processes as well as cellular activity (65,66). Low Mg will result in a decrease in calcium release from bone (65,66) and may be another mechanism for hypocalcemia in Mg deficiency.

The renal response to PTH has also been assessed by determining urinary excretion of cAMP and/or phosphate (Figs. 5 and 6) in response to exogenous PTH. In some patients, a normal effect of PTH on urinary phosphate and cAMP excretion has been noted (42–44,50,62,63). In general these were the same subjects in whom a normal calcemic effect was also seen (42,62,63). In other studies, of more severely Mg-depleted patients, an impaired response to PTH has been observed (22,49,67). Figure 6 shows the effect of PTH on urinary cAMP in one hypocalcemic Mg-deficient patient prior to and following Mg therapy; prior to Mg treatment, PTH did not increase urinary cAMP excretion, but following Mg repletion the rise in cAMP was normal. A decrease in urinary cAMP excretion in re-

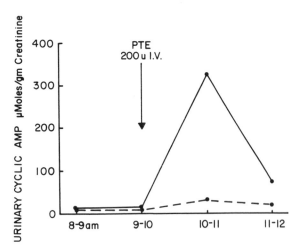

FIG. 6. Effect of an intravenous injection of 200 units of parathyroid extract on the excretion of urinary cAMP in a magnesium-deficient patient before (*dashed line*) and after (*solid line*) 4 days of magnesium therapy. Urine was collected for four consecutive 1 hr periods, two before and two after the PTE injection. While Mg deficient, the patient had a minimal rise in urinary cAMP in response to PTH, but, following Mg therapy, the response was normal. (Reprinted from ref. 22 with permission.)

sponse to PTH has also been described in the Mg-deficient dog and rat (56,57).

EFFECT OF MAGNESIUM DEFICIENCY ON VITAMIN D METABOLISM AND ACTION

Magnesium may also be important in vitamin D metabolism and/or action as suggested by a number of clinical observations. Patients with hypoparathyroidism who have been resistant to therapeutic doses of vitamin D have been reported to become more responsive to vitamin D after Mg therapy (68–70). The treatment of malabsorption syndromes with vitamin D may not be effective until Mg is simultaneously administered (71,72). Rickets, thought to be secondary to vitamin D resistance, have healed with Mg therapy (73). Patients with hypocalcemia and Mg deficiency have been reported to be resistant to pharmacological doses of vitamin D (71,74,75), 1α-hydroxyvitamin D (76,77), and $1,25(OH)_2D$ (78). Similarly, impaired calcemic response to vitamin D has been found in Mg-deficient rats (79–81), lambs (82), and calves (83).

Intestinal calcium transport in animal models of Mg deficiency has been found to be reduced in some (84,85) but not all (80,86) studies. Calcium malabsorption was associated with low serum levels of $25(OH)_2D_3$ in one study (79), but not in another (86), suggesting that Mg deficiency may impair intestinal calcium absorption by more than one mechanism.

The exact nature of altered vitamin D metabolism and/or action in Mg deficiency is unclear. Patients with Mg deficiency and hypocalcemia frequently have low serum concentrations of $25(OH)_2D_3$ (87–90), so nutritional vitamin D deficiency may be one factor. Therapy with vitamin D, however, results in high serum levels of $25(OH)_2D_3$ without correction of the hypocalcemia (71), suggesting that the vitamin D nutrition is not the prime reason. In addition, conversion of radiolabeled vitamin D to $25(OH)_2D_3$ was found to be normal in three Mg-deficient patients (91). Serum concentrations of $1,25(OH)_2D_3$ have also been found to be low or low-normal in most hypocalcemic Mg-deficient patients (87–90). Mg-deficient diabetic children, when given a low-calcium diet, did not exhibit a normal rise in serum $1,25(OH)_2D_3$ or PTH (92). The response returned to normal following Mg therapy, supporting the possibility of altered vitamin D metabolism in Mg deficiency. Since PTH is a major agonist for $1,25(OH)_2D_3$ formation, the low serum PTH concentrations could explain the low $1,25(OH)_2D_3$ levels. In support of this is the finding that some hypocalcemic Mg-deficient patients treated with Mg have a rise in serum $1,25(OH)_2D_3$ to high normal or to frankly elevated levels (see Fig. 7) (87). Most patients, however, do not have a signifi-

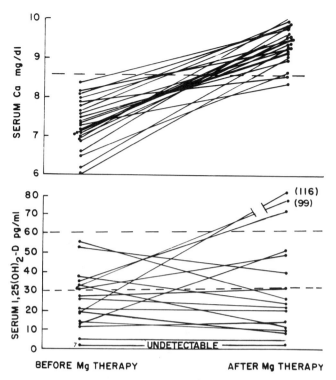

FIG. 7. Serum concentrations of calcium and 1,25(OH)₂D in hypocalcemic magnesium-deficient patients before and after 5–8 days of parenteral magnesium therapy. The *dashed lines* represent the upper and lower limits of normal for serum 1,25(OH)₂D and the lower limit of normal for the serum calcium. (Modified from ref. 87 with permission.)

cant rise within 1 week after institution of Mg therapy despite a rise in serum PTH and normalization of the serum calcium concentration, as is shown in Fig. 7 (87). These data suggest that Mg deficiency in man also impairs the ability of the kidney to synthesize $1,25(OH)_2D_3$. This is supported by the observation that the ability of exogenous administration of human PTH (1–34) to normal subjects after 3 weeks of experimental Mg depletion resulted in a significantly lower rise in serum $1,25(OH)_2D_3$ concentrations than before institution of the diet (39). It appears, therefore, that the renal synthesis of $1,25(OH)_2D_3$ is sensitive to Mg depletion. While Mg is known to support the 25-hydroxy-1α-hydroxylase in vitro (93,94), the exact Mg requirement for this enzymatic process is not known.

The association of Mg deficiency with impaired vitamin D metabolism and action therefore may be due to several factors. In some cases, vitamin D deficiency may contribute (87–90). The major reasons, however, appear to be due to a decrease in PTH secretion, with resultant decreased trophic effect on $1,25(OH)_2D_3$ synthesis as well as a direct effect of Mg depletion on the ability of the kidney to synthesize $1,25(OH)_2D_3$ (22,42–47,87–90). In addition, Mg deficiency may directly impair intestinal calcium absorption by resulting in low vitamin D metabolites (22,87–90) or by a direct mechanism (84,85). Skeletal resistance to vitamin D and its metabolites may also play an important role (76–83). It is clear, however, that restoration of normal serum $1,25(OH)_2D_3$ concentrations is not required for normal-

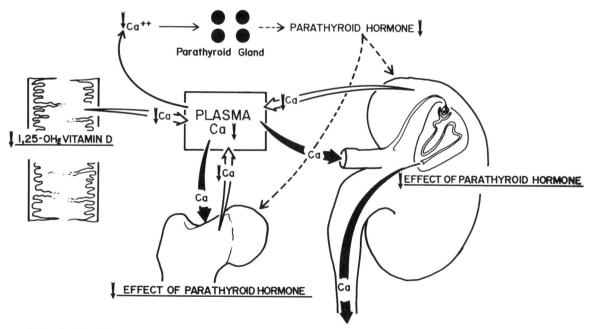

FIG. 8. Disturbance of calcium metabolism during magnesium deficiency. Hypocalcemia is caused by a decrease in PTH secretion as well as renal and skeletal resistance to the action of PTH. Low serum concentrations of 1,25(OH)₂D₃ may result in reduced intestinal calcium absorption. (Reprinted from ref. 2 with permission.)

ization of the serum calcium level. Most Mg-deficient patients who receive Mg therapy exhibit an immediate rise in PTH, followed by normalization of the serum calcium prior to any change in serum $1,25(OH)_2D_3$ concentrations (87–90). An overall view of the effect of Mg deficiency on calcium homeostasis is shown in Fig. 8.

MECHANISM OF IMPAIRED MINERAL HOMEOSTASIS IN MAGNESIUM DEFICIENCY

The mechanism for impaired PTH secretion and action in Mg deficiency remains unclear. It has been suggested that the presence of a high endogenous serum PTH concentration is more important in causing PTH resistance than the Mg deficiency; PTH administration has been demonstrated to result in diminishing peripheral effects of PTH (47). In the Mg-deficient patient, however, as Mg deficiency worsens, serum PTH concentrations fall (22,42–47). PTH resistance has been demonstrated in patients who had undetectably low PTH levels, suggesting that other mechanisms are operative (22,49–52). It has also been suggested that there may be a defect in the second messenger systems in Mg depletion. PTH secretion is thought to be mediated via cAMP (95), and PTH is also thought to exert is biologic effects through the intermediary action of cAMP (96). Adenylyl cyclase has been universally found to require Mg for cAMP generation both as a component of the substrate (Mg-ATP) and as an obligatory activator of enzyme activity (97). There appear to be two Mg^{++} binding sites within the adenylyl cyclase complex; one resides on the catalytic subunit and the other on the guanine nucleotide-regulatory protein Ns (98,99). The requisite role that Mg^{++} plays in adenylyl cyclase function suggests that factors that would limit the availability of Mg^{++} to this enzyme could have significant effects on the cyclic nucleotide metabolism of a cell and hence on overall cellular function. It is clear that some patients with severe Mg deficiency have a reduced urinary excretion of cAMP in response to exogenously administered PTH (22). In addition, PTH had a blunted effect in causing a rise in cAMP from isolated, perfused tibiae in Mg-deficient dogs (59). These observations correspond well with the impaired calcemic and phosphaturic effects of PTH in Mg-deficient patients and animals discussed above.

Adenylyl cyclase is regulated by both Mg^{++} and Ca^{++}. While Mg^{++} is stimulatory, Ca^{++} has been found to be inhibitory of enzyme activity in most tissues (100). In plasma membranes from parathyroid, renal cortex, and bone cells, Ca^{++} will competitively inhibit Mg^{++} activated adenylyl cyclase activity (100–103). In porcine parathyroid tissue, at an Mg^{++} con-

centration of 4 mM, Ca^{++} was found to inhibit adenylyl cyclase in a bimodal pattern described in terms of two calcium inhibition constants with K_i values of 1–2 μM and 200–400 μM (100). At a lower Mg^{++} concentration (0.5 mM), the only adenylyl cyclase activity expressed was that inhibitable by the high-affinity Ca^{++}-binding site. With increasing Mg concentrations, the fraction of total adenylyl cyclase activity subject to high-affinity calcium inhibition became progressively less. Thus, the ambient Mg^{++} concentrations can markedly affect the susceptibility of this enzyme to the inhibitory effects of Ca^{++}. Since total intracellular calcium has been observed to rise during Mg depletion (104,105), the combination of higher intracellular Ca^{++} and increased sensitivity to Ca^{++} inhibition due to Mg depletion could explain the defective PTH secretion in Mg deficiency. A similar relationship between Mg^{++} and Ca^{++} was described for adenylyl cyclase obtained from guinea pig bone (101). Ca^{++} caused a competitive inhibition of Mg^{++}-activated skeletal adenylyl cyclase, with a high-affinity Ca^{++}-binding site, with a K_iCa of 1–2 μM. Lowering the Mg^{++} concentration increased overall Ca^{++} inhibition. Thus, a fall in the intracellular Mg^{++} concentration would render adenylyl cyclase enzyme more susceptible to inhibition by the prevailing intracellular Ca^{++} concentrations and may be a mechanism by which both PTH secretion and PTH end-organ action are impaired in Mg deficiency.

Adenylyl cyclase is a widely distributed enzyme in the body and, if the above-mentioned hypothesis is true, the secretion and action of other hormones mediated by adenylyl cyclase might also exhibit impaired activity in Mg deficiency. The actions of adrenocorticotropic hormone (ACTH), TRH, GnRH, and glucagon have been demonstrated to be normal in hypocalcemic Mg-deficient patients (106). It was hypothesized that the adenylyl cyclase enzyme in these target tissues might have a lower Mg^{++} requirement or be less inhibitable by Ca^{++} than the parathyroid, kidney, and bone, which would afford selective protection from the effects of Mg depletion. Prior investigations have suggested that Mg affinity for adenylyl cyclase is higher (lower K_aMg) in liver (107), adrenal (108), and pituitary (109) than in parathyroid (100). In one study, investigation of K_aMg and K_iCa in tissues from one species (guinea pig) demonstrated that, under agonist stimulation, the K_aMg from liver is < thyroid < kidney = bone and the $KiCa^{++}$ for liver is > renal > kidney = bone (103). These data suggest that adenylyl cyclase regulation by divalent cations varies from tissue to tissue and may explain the greater propensity for disturbed mineral homeostasis in Mg deficiency.

While cAMP is an important mediator of PTH action, PTH has also been shown to activate the phospholipase C second messenger system (110). PTH activation of phospholipase C leads to hydrolysis of phosphatidylinositol 4,5-bisphosphate to inositol-1,4,5-triphosphate (IP_3) and diacylglycerol. IP_3 binds to specific receptors on intracellular organelles (endoplasmic reticulum, calciosomes), leading to an acute transient rise in cytosolic Ca^{++}, with subsequent activation of calmodulin-dependent protein kinases. Diacylglycerol activates protein kinase C. Mg depletion could perturb this system via several mechanisms. A Mg^{++}-dependent guanine nucleotide-regulating protein is also involved in activation of phospholipase C (111,112). Mg^{++} has also been shown to be a noncompetitive inhibitor of IP_3-induced Ca^{++} release (113). A reduction of Mg^{++} from 300 μM to 30 μM increased Ca^{++} release in response to IP_3 by two- to threefold in mitochondrial membranes obtained from canine cerebellum (113). In these same studies, Mg^{++} also was found to inhibit IP_3 binding to its receptor. Mg, at a concentration of 0.5 mM, decreased maximal IP_3 binding threefold (113). These Mg^{++} concentrations are within the estimated physiologic intracellular range (200–500 μM), so Mg^{++} may be an important physiological regulator of the phospholipase C second messenger system.

It is clear that the effect of Mg depletion on cellular function in terms of the second messenger systems is most complex, potentially involving substrate availability, G-protein activity, release and sensitivity to intracellular Ca^{++}, and phospholipid metabolism.

DIAGNOSIS OF MAGNESIUM DEFICIENCY

As was mentioned above, Mg is principally an intracellular cation. Less than 1% of the body Mg content is in the extracellular fluid compartments. The serum Mg concentration, therefore, may not reflect the intracellular Mg content. Nevertheless, measurement of the serum Mg concentration is the most available and commonly employed test to assess Mg status. The normal serum Mg concentration ranges from 1.7 to 2.2 mg/dl (0.71–0.91 mM); a value ≤1.7 mg/dl usually indicates Mg deficiency (2,3,12).

The total Mg content or concentration of a number of tissues, including red blood cells, skeletal muscle, bone, and peripheral lymphocytes, has been assessed as an index of Mg status. The Mg content of the peripheral lymphocyte has been under recent investigation, and it has been found to correlate with skeletal and cardiac muscle Mg content (2). This has been used in a number of research studies and, in general, seems to be a more accurate indicator of Mg status than the serum Mg concentration. A great deal of overlap with the normal range is seen, however, so lymphocyte Mg content is probably not a test sufficiently discriminatory to diagnose Mg deficiency in a given patient. The Mg tolerance test has been used for many years and appears to be an accurate means of assessing Mg status (2,12). Retention of a parenterally administered Mg load is greater than normal in both hypomagnesemic patients and normomagnesemic patients at risk for Mg deficiency. A suggested protocol for the Mg tolerance test is given in Table 5. Under this protocol, 23 normal controls retained 14% ± 4% (mean ± SEM) of the Mg load, while 15 hypomagnesemic patients retained 85% ± 3% (114). Twenty-four patients at risk for Mg deficiency (chronic alcoholics) also retained a significantly greater percentage of the Mg load than did the normal controls, 51% ± 5%. These data suggest that the Mg tolerance test is a more sensitive method to detect Mg deficiency than is the serum Mg concentration. While this test does appear to be quite discriminatory in patients with normal renal function, its usefulness may be limited if the patient has a renal Mg leak or is on a medication that induces renal Mg wasting.

TREATMENT OF MAGNESIUM DEFICIENCY

Patients who present with signs and symptoms of Mg deficiency should be treated with Mg. These patients will usually be hypomagnesemic and/or have an abnormal Mg tolerance test (2,3,12). These cir-

TABLE 5. *Suggested protocol for clinical use of magnesium tolerance test*

Collect baseline urine (spot or timed) for magnesium/creatinine ratio

Infuse 0.2 mEq (2.4 mg) elemental magnesium per kilogram lean body weight in 50 ml 5% dextrose over 4 hr

Collect urine (starting with infusion) for magnesium and creatinine for 24 hr

Percentage magnesium retained is given by the following formula:

$$1 - \frac{\text{Postinfusion 24 hr urine magnesium} - \text{Preinfusion urine magnesium/creatinine} \times \text{Postinfusion urine creatinine}}{\text{Total elemental magnesium infused}} \times 100$$

Criteria for Mg deficiency:
>50% retention at 24 hr = definite deficiency
>25% retention at 24 hr = probable deficiency

cumstances usually indicate treatment by parenteral administration. An effective treatment regimen is the administration of 2 g $MgSO_4 7H_2O$ (200 mg elemental Mg) as a 50% solution every 8 hr intramuscularly. These injections can be painful, and a continuous intravenous infusion of 600 mg elemental Mg over 24 hr therefore may be preferred and is better tolerated. Either regimen will usually result in a normal or slightly elevated serum Mg concentration. The restoration of a normal serum Mg concentration does not indicate repletion of body Mg stores, however, and therapy should be continued for ~3–7 days. By this time, symptoms should resolve and biochemical abnormalities such as hypocalcemia and hypokalemia should be corrected. Patients who are hypomagnesemic and have seizures or an acute arrhythmia may be given 100–200 mg Mg as an intravenous injection over 5–10 min, followed by 600 mg/day. Ongoing Mg losses should be monitored during therapy. If the patient continues to lose Mg from the intestine or kidney, therapy may have to be continued for a longer duration. Once repletion has been accomplished, patients usually can maintain a normal Mg status on a regular diet, provided the reason for the Mg deficiency has been corrected. If repletion is accomplished and the patient cannot eat, a parenteral maintenance dose of 100 mg of Mg should be given daily.

Patients who have chronic Mg loss from the intestine or kidney may require continued oral Mg supplementation. Magnesium salts in the form of sulphate, lactate, hydroxide, oxide, chloride, and glycerophosphate are available. An initial daily dose of 300 mg to as high as 600 mg elemental Mg may be used. The Mg is given in divided doses three or four times per day to avoid its cathartic effect.

Caution should be taken in Mg therapy in patients with any degree of renal failure. If a decrease in glomerular filtration rate exists, the dose of Mg should be halved, and the serum Mg concentration must be monitored daily. If hypermagnesemia ensues, therapy must be stopped.

REFERENCES

1. Aikawa JK. Biochemistry and physiology of magnesium. In: Prasad AS, Oberleas D, eds. *Trace elements in human health and disease.* New York: Academic Press, 1976;47–78.
2. Rude RK, Oldham SB. Disorders of magnesium metabolism. In: Cohen RD, Lewis B, Alberti KGMM, Denman AM, eds. *The metabolic and molecular basis of acquired disease.* London: Bailliere Tindall, 1990;1124–1148.
3. Wacker WEC, Parisi AF. Magnesium metabolism. *N Engl J Med* 1968;45:658, 663, 712–717, 772–776.
4. Quamme GA, Dirks JH. The physiology of renal magnesium handling. *Renal Physiol* 1986;9:257–269.
5. Quamme GA, Dirks JH. Renal magnesium transport. *Rev Physiol Biochem Pharmacol* 1983;97:69–110.
6. Rude RK, Ryzen E. TmMg and renal Mg threshold in normal man in certain pathophysiologic conditions. *Magnesium* 1986;5:273–281.
7. Brannan PG, Vergne-Marini P, Pak CYC, Hull AR, Fordtran JS. Magnesium absorption in the human small intestine: results in normal subjects, patients with chronic renal disease, and patients with absorptive hypercalciuria. *J Clin Invest* 1976;57:1412–1418.
8. Hodgkinson A, Marshall DH, Nordin BEC. Vitamin D and magnesium absorption in man. *Clin Sci* 1979;57:121–123.
9. Krejs GJ, Nicar MJ, Zerwekh HE, Normal DA, Kane MG, Pak CYC. Effect of 1,25-dihydroxyvitamin D_3 on calcium and magnesium absorption in the healthy human jejunum and ileum. *Am J Med* 1983;75:973–976.
10. Wong ET, Rude RK, Singer FR, Shaw ST. A high prevalence of hypomagnesemia and hypermagnesemia in hospitalized patients. *Am J Clin Pathol* 1983;79:348–352.
11. Ryzen E, Wagers PW, Singer FR, Rude RK. Magnesium deficiency in a medical ICU population. *Crit Care Med* 1985;13:19–21.
12. Rude RK, Oldham SB: Magnesium metabolism. In: Becker KL, ed. *Principles and practice of endocrinology and metabolism.* Philadelphia: J.B. Lippincott Co., 1990;531–536.
13. McNair P, Christensen MS, Christiansen C, Madsbad S, Transbol IB. Renal hypomagnesaemia in human diabetes mellitus: its relation to glucose homeostasis. *Eur J Clin Invest* 1982;12:81–85.
14. Zaloga GP, Charnow B, Pock A, Wood B, Zritsky A, Zucker A. Hypomagnesemia is a common complication of aminoglycoside therapy. *Surg Gynecol Obstet* 1984;158:561–565.
15. Shah GM, Alvarado P, Kirschenbaum MA. Symptomatic hypocalcemia and hypomagnesemia with renal magnesium wasting associated with pentamidine therapy in a patient with AIDS. *Am J Med* 1990;89:380–382.
16. Dominquez JH, Gray RW, Lemann J Jr. Dietary phosphate deprivation in women and men: effects on mineral and acid balances, parathyroid hormone and the metabolism of 24-OH-vitamin D. *J Clin Endocrinol Metab* 1976;43:1056–1068.
17. Wacker WEC, Moore FD, Ulmer DD, Vallee BL. Normocalcemic magnesium deficiency tetany. *J Am Med Assoc* 1962;180:161–163.
18. Iseri LT, Fairshter RD, Hardemann JL, Brodsky MA. Magnesium and potassium therapy in multifocal atrial tachycardia. *Am Heart J* 1985;110:789–794.
19. Dyckner T, Wester PO. Magnesium deficiency contributing to ventricular tachycardia. *Acta Med Scand* 1982;212:89–91.
20. Whang R, Oei TO, Aikawa JK, Watanabe A, Vannatta J, Fryer A, Markanich M. Predictors of clinical hypomagnesemia. *Arch Intern Med* 1984;144:1794–1796.
21. Shils ME. Experimental human magnesium depletion. *Medicine* 1969;48:61–82.
22. Rude RK, Oldham SB, Singer FR. Functional hypoparathyroidism and parathyroid hormone end-organ resistance in human magnesium deficiency. *Clin Endocrinol* 1976;5:209–224.
23. Buckle RM, Care AD, Cooper CW, Gitelman HJ. The influence of plasma magnesium concentration on parathyroid hormone secretion. *J Endocrinol* 1968;42:529–534.
24. Sherwood LM, Herrman I, Bassett CA. Parathyroid hormone secretion in vitro: regulation by calcium and magnesium ions. *Nature* 1970;225:1056–1057.
25. Oldham SB, Fischer JA, Capen C, Sizemore GW, Arnaud CD. Dynamics of parathyroid hormone secretion in vitro. *Am J Med* 1971;50:650–657.
26. Cholst IN, Steinberg SF, Troper PJ, Fox HE, Segre GV, Bilezikian JP. The influence of hypermagnesemia on serum calcium and parathyroid hormone levels in human subjects. *N Engl J Med* 1984;310:1221–1225.
27. Ferment O, Garnier PE, Touitou Y. Comparison of the feedback effect of magnesium and calcium on parathyroid hormone secretion in man. *J Endocrinol* 1987;113:117–122.
28. Toffaletti J, Cooper DL, Lobaugh B. The response of parathyroid hormone to specific changes in either ionized calcium, ionized magnesium, or protein-bound calcium in humans. *Metabolism* 1991;40:814–818.
29. Habener JF, Potts JT Jr. Relative effectiveness of magnesium and calcium on the secretion of biosynthesis of parathyroid hormone in vitro. *Endocrinology* 1976;98:197–202.

30. Mayer GP, Hurst JG. Comparison of the effects of calcium and magnesium on parathyroid hormone secretion rate in calves. *Endocrinology* 1978;102:1803–1807.

31. Wallace J, Scarpa A. Regulation of parathyroid hormone secretion in vitro by divalent cations and cellular metabolism. *J Biol Chem* 1982;257:10613–10616.

32. Brown EM, Thatcher JG, Watson EJ, Leombruno R. Extracellular calcium potentiates the inhibitory effects of magnesium on parathyroid function in dispersed bovine parathyroid cells. Metabolism 1984;33:171–176.

33. Hamilton JW, Spierto FW, MacGregor RR, Cohn DV. Studies on the biosynthesis in vitro of parathyroid hormone. *J Biol Chem* 1971;246:3224–3233.

34. Raisz LG. Effects of calcium on uptake and incorporation of amino acids in the parathyroid glands. *Biochim Biophys Acta* 1967:148;460–468.

35. Lee MJ, Roth SI. Effect of calcium and magnesium on deoxyribonucleic acid synthesis in rat parathyroid glands in vitro. *Lab Invest* 1975;33:72–79.

36. Shils ME. Magnesium, calcium and parathyroid hormone interactions. *Ann NY Acad Sci* 1980;355:165–180.

37. Gitelman HJ, Kukolj S, Welt LG. The influence of the parathyroid glands on the hypercalcemia of experimental magnesium depletion in the rat. *J Clin Invest* 1968;47:118–126.

38. Anast CS, Forte LF. Parathyroid function and magnesium depletion in the rat. *Endocrinology* 1983;113:184–189.

39. Fatemi S, Ryzen E, Flores J, Endres DB, Rude RK. Effect of experimental human magnesium depletion on parathyroid hormone secretion and 1,25-dihydroxyvitamin D metabolism. *J Clin Endocrinol Metab* 1991;73:1067–1072.

40. Targovnik JH, Rodman JS, Sherwood LM. Regulation of parathyroid hormone secretion in vitro: quantitative aspects of calcium and magnesium ion control. *Endocrinology* 1971; 88:1477–1482.

41. Mahaffee DD, Cooper CW, Ramp WK, Ontjes DA. Magnesium promotes both parathyroid hormone secretion and adenosine 3′,5′-monophosphate product in rat parathyroid tissues and reverses the inhibitory effects of calcium on adenylate cyclase. *Endocrinology* 1982;110:487–495.

42. Anast CS, Mohs JM, Kaplan SL, Burns TW. Evidence for parathyroid failure in magnesium deficiency. *Science* 1972; 177:606–608.

43. Suh SM, Tashjian AH Jr, Matsuo N, Parkinson DK, Fraser D. Pathogenesis of hypocalcemia in primary hypomagnesemia: normal end-organ responsiveness to parathyroid hormone, impaired parathyroid gland function. *J Clin Invest* 1973;52:153–160.

44. Chase LR, Slatopolsky E. Secretion and metabolic efficacy of parathyroid hormone in patients with severe hypomagnesemia. *J Clin Endocrinol Metab* 1974;38:363–371.

45. Wiegmann T, Kaye M. Hypomagnesemic hypocalcemia. *Arch Intern Med* 1977;137:953–955.

46. Rude RK, Oldham SB, Sharp CF Jr, Singer FR. Parathyroid hormone secretion in magnesium deficiency. *J Clin Endocrinol Metab* 1978;47:800–806.

47. Allgrove J, Adami S, Fraher L, Reuben A, O'Riordan JLH. Hypomagnesaemia: studies of parathyroid hormone secretion and function. *Clin Endocrinol* 1984;21:435–449.

48. Bethune JE, Turpin RA, Inoui H. Effect of parathyroid hormone extract on divalent ion excretion in man. *J Clin Endocrinol Metab* 1968;28:673–678.

49. Estep H, Shaw WA, Watlington C, Hobe R, Holland W, Tucker SG. Hypocalcemia due to hypomagnesemia and reversible parathyroid hormone unresponsiveness. *J Clin Endocrinol* 1969;29:842–848.

50. Muldowney FP, McKenna TJ, Kyle LH, Freaney R, Swan M. Parathormone-like effect of magnesium replenishment in steatorrhea. *N Engl J Med* 1970;281:61–68.

51. Connor TB, Toskes P, Mahaffey J, Martin LG, Williams JB, Walser M. Parathyroid function during chronic magnesium deficiency. *Hopkins Med J* 1972;131:100–117.

52. Woodard JC, Webster PD, Carr AA. Primary hypomagnesemia with secondary hypocalcemia, diarrhea and insensitivity to parathyroid hormone. *Dig Dis* 1972;17:612–618.

53. MacManus J, Heaton FW, Lucas PW. A decreased response to parathyroid hormone in magnesium deficiency. *J Endocrinol* 1971;49:253–258.

54. Reddy CR, Coburn JW, Hartenbower DL, et al. Studies on mechanisms of hypocalcemia of magnesium depletion. *J Clin Invest* 1973;52:3000–3010.

55. Brietenbach RP, Gonnerman WA, Erfling WL, Anast CS. Dietary magnesium, calcium homeostasis, and parathyroid gland activity of chickens. *Am J Physiol* 1973;225:12–17.

56. Levi J, Massry SG, Coburn JW, Llach F, Kleeman CR. Hypocalcemia in magnesium-depleted dogs: evidence for reduced responsiveness to parathyroid hormone and relative failure of parathyroid gland function. *Metabolism* 1974; 23:323–335.

57. Forbes RM, Parker HM. Effect of magnesium deficiency on rat bone and kidney sensitivity to parathyroid hormone. *J Nutr* 1980;110:1610–1617.

58. Raisz LG, Niemann I. Effect of phosphate, calcium and magnesium on bone resorption and hormonal responses in tissue culture. *Endocrinology* 1969;85:446–452.

59. Freitag JJ, Martin KJ, Conrades MB, et al. Evidence for skeletal resistance to parathyroid hormone in magnesium deficiency. *J Clin Invest* 1979;64:1238–1244.

60. Salet J, Polonovski CL, DeGouyon F, Pean G, Melekian B, Fournet JP. Tetanie hypocalcemique recidivante par hypomagnesemie congenitale. *Arch Fr Pediatr* 1966;23:749–767.

61. Stromme JH, Nesbakken R, Normann T, Skjorten F, Skyberg D, Johannessen B. Familial hypomagnesemia. *Acta Paediatr Scand* 1969;58:433–444.

62. Suh SM, Tashjian AH, Matsuo N, Parkinson DK, Fraser D. Pathogenesis of hypocalcemia in primary hypomagnesemia: normal end-organ responsiveness to parathyroid hormone, impaired parathyroid gland function. *J Clin Invest* 1973; 52:153–160.

63. Chase LR, Slatopolsky E. Secretion and metabolic efficacy of parathyroid hormone in patients with severe hypomagnesemia. *J Clin Endocrinol Metab* 1974;38:363–371.

64. Hahn TJ, Chase LR, Avioli LV. Effect of magnesium depletion on responsiveness to parathyroid hormone in parathyroidectomized rats. *J Clin Invest* 1972;51:886–891.

65. Pak CYC, Diller EC. Ionic interaction with bone mineral. *Calcif Tissue Res* 1969;4:69–77.

66. MacManus J, Heaton FW. The influence of magnesium on calcium release from bone in vitro. *Biochim Biophys Acta* 1970;215:360–367.

67. Medalle R, Waterhouse C. A magnesium-deficient patient presenting with hypocalcemia and hyperphosphatemia. *Ann Intern Med* 1973;79:76–79.

68. Homer L. Hypoparathyroidism requiring massive amounts of medication, with apparent response to magnesium sulfate. *J Clin Endocrinol Metab* 1961;21:219–223.

69. Jones KH, Fourman P. Effects of infusions of magnesium and of calcium in parathyroid insufficiency. *Clin Sci* 1966; 30:139–150.

70. Rossler A, Rabinowitz D. Magnesium induced reversal of vitamin D resistance in hypoparathyroidism. *Lancet* 1973;1: 803–806.

71. Medalle R, Waterhouse C, Hahn TJ. Vitamin D resistance in magnesium deficiency. *Am J Clin Nutr* 1976;29:854–858.

72. Heaton FW, Fourman P. Magnesium deficiency and hypocalcemia in intestinal malabsorption. *Lancet* 1965;2:50–52.

73. Reddy V, Sivakumar B. Magnesium-dependent vitamin D-resistant rickets. *Lancet* 1974;1:963–965.

74. Leicht E, Biro G, Keck E, Langer HJ. Die hypomagnesiaemie-bedingte hypocalciaemie: funktioneller hypoparathyroidismus, parathormon-und vitamin D resistenz. *Klin Wochenschr* 1990;68:678–684.

75. Coenegracht JM, Houben HGJ. Idiopathic hypomagnesemia with hypocalcemia in an adult. *Clin Chim Acta* 1974;50:349–357.

76. Selby PL, Peacock M, Bambach CP. Hypomagnesaemia after small bowel resection: treatment with 1α-hydroxylated vitamin D metabolites. *Br J Surg* 1984;71:334–337.

77. Ralston S, Boyle IT, Cowan RA, Crean GP, Jenkins A, Thomson WS. PTH and vitamin D responses during treat-

ment of hypomagnesaemic hypoparathyroidism. *Acta Endocrinol* 1983;103:535–538.

78. Graber ML, Schulman G: Hypomagnesemic hypocalcemia independent of parathyroid hormone. *Ann Intern Med* 1986; 104:804–806.

79. Lifshitz F, Harrison HC, Harrison HE. Response to vitamin D of magnesium deficient rats. *Proc Soc Exp Biol Med* 1967;125:472–476.

80. Rayssiguier Y, Carre M, Ayigbede O, Miravet L. Activite du 1-25 dihydroxycholecalciferol chez le rat carence en magnesium. *CR Acad Sc* 1975;281:731–734.

81. Miravet L, Ayigbede O, Carre M, Rayssiguier Y, Larvor P. Lack of vitamin D action on serum calcium in magnesium deficient rats. In: Cantin M, Seelig MS, eds. *Magnesium in health and disease.* New York: Spectrum, 1980;281–289.

82. McAleese DM, Forbes RM. Experimental production of magnesium deficiency in lambs on a diet containing roughage. *Nature* 1959;184:2025–2026.

83. Smith RH. Calcium and magnesium metabolism in calves. *Biochem J* 1958;70:201–205.

84. Winnacker JL, Anast CS. Vitamin D metabolism in magnesium and nutritional deficiency. Abstract, *Proceedings 56th Annual Meeting of the Endocrine Society,* Atlanta, 1974;A179.

85. Higuchi J, Lukert B. Effects of magnesium depletion on vitamin D metabolism and intestinal calcium transport. *Clin Res* 1974;22:617.

86. Coburn JW, Reddy CR, Brickman AS, Hartenbower DL, Friedler RM. Vitamin D metabolism in magnesium deficiency. *Clin Res* 1975;23:3933.

87. Rude RK, Adams JS, Ryzen E, et al. Low serum concentrations of 1,25-dihydroxyvitamin D in human magnesium deficiency. *J Clin Endocrinol Metab* 1985;61:933–940.

88. Fuss M, Cogan E, Gillet C, et al. Magnesium administration reverses the hypocalcaemia secondary to hypomagnesaemia despite low circulating levels of 25-hydroxyvitamin D and 1,25-dihydroxyvitamin D. *Endocrinology* 1985;22:807–815.

89. Fuss M, Bergmann P, Bergans A, et al. Correction of low circulating levels of 1,25-dihydroxyvitamin D by 25-hydroxyvitamin D during reversal of hypomagnesaemia. *Clin Endocrinol* 1989;31:31–38.

90. Leicht E, Schmidt-Gayk H, Langer HJ, Sniege N, Biro G. Hypomagnesaemia-induced hypocalcaemia: concentrations of parathyroid hormone, prolactin and 1,25-dihydroxyvitamin D during magnesium replenishment. *Magnesium Res* 1992;5:33–36.

91. Lukert BP. Effect of magnesium depletion of vitamin D metabolism in man. In: Cantin M, Seelig MS, eds. *Magnesium in health and disease.* New York: Spectrum, 1980;275–279.

92. Saggese G, Federico G, Bertelloni S, Baroncelli GI, Calisti L. Hypomagnesemia and the parathyroid hormone–vitamin D endocrine system in children with insulin-dependent diabetes mellitus: effects of magnesium administration. *J Pediatr* 1991;118:220–225.

93. Gray RW, Omdahy JL, Ghazarian JG, DeLuca HF. 25-Hydroxycholecalciferol-1-hydroxylase. *J Biol Chem* 1972;247:7528–7532.

94. Fisco F, Traba ML. Influence of magnesium on the in vitro synthesis of 24,25-dihydroxyvitamin D3 and 1α,25-dihydroxyvitamin D3. *Magnesium Res* 1992;5:5–14.

95. Abe M, Sherwood LM. Regulation of parathyroid hormone secretion by adenyl cyclase. *Biochem Biophys Res Commun* 1972;48:396–401.

96. Bitensky MW, Keirns JJ, Freeman J. Cyclic adenosine monophosphate and clinical medicine. *Am J Med Sci* 1973;266:320–347.

97. Northup JK, Smigel MD, Gilman AG. The guanine nucleotide activating site of the regulatory component of adenylate cyclase: identification by ligand binding. *J Biol Chem* 1982;257:11416–11423.

98. Maguire ME. Hormone-sensitive magnesium transport and magnesium regulation of adenylate cyclase. *Trends Pharmacol Sci* 1984;5:73–77.

99. Cech SY, Broaddus WC, Maguire ME. Adenylate cyclase: the role of magnesium and other divalent cations. *Mol Cell Biochem* 1980;33:67–92.

100. Oldham SB, Rude RK, Molloy CT, Lipson LG. The effects of magnesium on calcium inhibition of parathyroid adenylate cyclase. *Endocrinology* 1984;115:1883–1890.

101. Rude RK. Renal cortical adenylate cyclase: characterization of magnesium activation. *Endocrinology* 1983;113:1348–1355.

102. Rude RK. Skeletal adenylate cyclase: effect of Mg^{2+}, Ca^{2+}, and PTH. *Calcif Tissue Int* 1985;37:318–323.

103. Rude RK, Oldham SB. Hypocalcemia of Mg deficiency: altered modulation of adenylate cyclase by Mg^{++} and Ca^{++} may result in impaired PTH secretion and PTH end-organ resistance. In: Altura, Durlach, Seelig, eds: *Magnesium in cellular processes and medicine.* Basel: S. Karger, 1985;183–195.

104. George GA, Heaton FW. Changes in cellular composition during magnesium deficiency. *Biochem J* 1975;152:609–615.

105. Ryan MD, Ryan MF. Lymphocyte electrolyte alterations during magnesium deficiency in the rat. *Irish J Med Sci* 1979;148:108–109.

106. Cohan BW, Singer FR, Rude RK. End-organ response to adrenocorticotropin, thyrotropin, gonadotropin-releasing hormone, and glucagon in hypocalcemic magnesium deficient patients. *J Clin Endocrinol Metab* 1982;54:975–979.

107. Londos C, Preston MS. Activation of the hepatic adenylate cyclase system by divalent cations. *J Biol Chem* 1977;252:5957–5961.

108. Glynn P, Cooper DMF, Schulster D. Modulation of the response of bovine adrenocortical adenylate cyclase to corticotropin. *Biochemistry* 1977;168:277–282.

109. Porier G, DeLean A, Pelletier G, Lemay A, Labrie F. Purification of adenohypophyseal plasma membranes and properties of associated adenylate cyclase. *J Biol Chem* 1974;249:316–322.

110. Dunlay R, Hruska K. PTH receptor coupling to phospholipase C is an alternate pathway of signal transduction in bone and kidney. *Am J Physiol* 1990;258:F223–F231.

111. Babich M, King KL, Nissenson RA. G protein-dependent activation of a phosphoinositide-specific phospholipase C in UMR-106 osteosarcoma cell membranes. *J Bone Mineral Res* 1989;4:549–556.

112. Litosch I. G protein regulation of phospholipase C activity in a membrane-solubilized system occurs through a Mg^{2+}- and time-dependent mechanism. *J Biol Chem* 1991;266:4764–4771.

113. Volpe P, Alderson-Lang BH, Nickols GA. Regulation of inositol 1,4,5-trisphosphate-induced Ca^{2+} release. I. Effect of Mg^{2+}. *Am J Physiol* 1990;258:C1077–C1085.

114. Ryzen E, Elbaum N, Singer FR, Rude RK. Parenteral magnesium tolerance testing in the evaluation of magnesium deficiency. *Magnesium* 1985;4:137–147.

115. Rude RK. Parathyroid function in magnesium deficiency. In: Itokawa Y, Durlach J, eds. *Magnesium in health and disease.* London: John Libbey & Co., Ltd., 1989;317–321.

Subject Index